牛津神经外科教科书

Oxford Textbook of Neurological Surgery

原　著　Ramez W. Kirollos
Adel Helmy
Simon Thomson
Peter J.A. Hutchinson

主　译　孟凡刚　伊志强

副主译　倪石磊　卜　博　汤　劼
刘伟明　于　涛　魏俊吉

北京大学医学出版社

NIUJIN SHENJINGWAIKE JIAOKESHU

图书在版编目（CIP）数据

牛津神经外科教科书 / (英) 拉梅兹 · 基罗洛斯 (Ramez W. Kirollos) 等原著；孟凡刚，伊志强主译. — 北京：北京大学医学出版社，2024.9

书名原文：Oxford Textbook of Neurological Surgery

ISBN 978-7-5659-3070-6

Ⅰ.①牛… Ⅱ.①拉… ②孟… ③伊… Ⅲ.①神经外科学—教材 Ⅳ.①R651

中国国家版本馆CIP 数据核字(2024) 第038956 号

北京市版权局著作权合同登记号：图字：01-2020-6613

牛津神经外科教科书

主　　译：孟凡刚　伊志强
出版发行：北京大学医学出版社
地　　址：（100191）北京市海淀区学院路38 号　北京大学医学部院内
电　　话：发行部 010-82802230；图书邮购 010-82802495
网　　址：http：//www.pumpress.com.cn
E－mail：booksale@bjmu.edu.cn
印　　刷：北京信彩瑞禾印刷厂
经　　销：新华书店
策划编辑：冯智勇
责任编辑：阳耀林　**责任校对**：靳新强　**责任印制**：李　啸
开　　本：889 mm × 1194 mm　1/16　**印张**：61.5　**字数**：2000 千字
版　　次：2024 年 9 月第 1 版　2024 年 9 月第 1 次印刷
书　　号：ISBN 978-7-5659-3070-6
定　　价：450.00 元

译校者名单

主　译　孟凡刚　伊志强

副主译　倪石磊　卜　博　汤　劼　刘伟明　于　涛　魏俊吉

译校者（按姓氏汉语拼音排序）

安　旭　首都医科大学附属北京天坛医院
白金月　首都医科大学附属北京天坛医院
卞立松　北京市海淀医院
卜　博　中国人民解放军总医院第八医学中心
蔡国恩　福建医科大学附属协和医院
陈保东　北京大学深圳医院
陈国强　中国医科大学航空总医院
陈希恒　首都医科大学附属北京朝阳医院
程崇杰　重庆医科大学附属第一医院
崔志强　中国人民解放军总医院
戴　缤　北京世纪坛医院
范存刚　北京大学人民医院
范世莹　首都儿科研究所附属儿童医院
冯恩山　首都医科大学附属北京地坛医院
冯　涛　首都医科大学附属北京天坛医院
冯子超　山东大学齐鲁医院
高佳宁　北京市神经外科研究所
高献书　北京大学第一医院
高　源　北京市神经外科研究所
郭胜利　中国人民解放军总医院第八医学中心
郭旭飞　首都医科大学附属北京天坛医院
郭宇鹏　中国医科大学航空总医院
韩春雷　首都医科大学附属北京天坛医院
韩如泉　首都医科大学附属北京天坛医院
胡　威　美国佛罗里达大学
胡志强　北京世纪坛医院
黄亚波　苏州大学附属第一医院
季玉陈　郑州大学第一附属医院
贾　亮　河北医科大学第二医院
李春伟　北京大学第一医院
李　良　北京大学第一医院
李仁鹏　北京市神经外科研究所
李　晔　首都医科大学宣武医院
李志保　西安交通大学第一附属医院
梁　琨　首都医科大学附属北京地坛医院
刘　畅　北京大学第一医院
刘　冲　山东省立医院
刘二腾　首都医科大学附属北京地坛医院
刘方军　首都医科大学三博脑科医院
刘红杏　首都医科大学附属北京地坛医院
刘　江　中日友好医院
刘龙奇　北京积水潭医院
刘婷红　首都医科大学附属北京儿童医院
刘伟明　首都医科大学附属北京天坛医院
刘晓楠　首都医科大学附属北京天坛医院
刘亚欧　首都医科大学附属北京天坛医院
刘智明　首都医科大学附属北京天坛医院
鲁润春　北京大学第一医院
陆　军　北京医院
罗　芳　首都医科大学附属北京天坛医院
孟凡刚　北京市神经外科研究所
倪石磊　山东大学齐鲁医院

欧云尉 首都医科大学附属北京天坛医院
戚其超 山东大学齐鲁医院
亓 蕾 中国康复研究中心（北京博爱医院）
秦 涵 南京鼓楼医院
任连坤 首都医科大学宣武医院
任倩薇 北京市神经外科研究所
邵晓秋 首都医科大学附属北京天坛医院
沈胜利 北京大学第一医院
史 良 北京积水潭医院
司 雨 北京大学第三医院
苏亦兵 北京积水潭医院
孙玉晨 河北医科大学第二医院
汤 劼 首都医科大学宣武医院
汤 可 中国人民解放军总医院第八医学中心
汤韫钰 北京大学人民医院
田 艳 北京大学第一医院
田永吉 首都医科大学附属北京天坛医院
佟怀宇 中国人民解放军总医院第八医学中心
王安妮 北京市神经外科研究所
王 镔 吉林大学第一医院
王 虎 天津市环湖医院
王会志 北京市神经外科研究所
王开亮 首都医科大学宣武医院
王科大 北京积水潭医院
王 林 中国医科大学航空总医院
王 宁 中国医科大学航空总医院
王 乔 北京医院
王 群 首都医科大学附属北京天坛医院
王 拓 西安交通大学第一附属医院
王 伟 首都医科大学附属北京天坛医院
魏俊吉 北京协和医院
文俊贤 北京协和医院
文 龙 北京大学第一医院
吴 超 北京大学第三医院
吴嘉铭 北京协和医院
吴 量 首都医科大学附属北京天坛医院
吴世凯 北京大学第一医院
吴 涛 北京大学深圳医院
吴 越 重庆医科大学附属第一医院
肖以磊 聊城市人民医院
解自行 首都医科大学附属北京儿童医院
徐 丹 浙江大学医学院附属第四医院
许菲璠 北京大学第一医院
许海洋 吉林大学第一医院
薛 钦 首都医科大学附属北京天坛医院
薛 湛 首都医科大学附属北京天坛医院
阎 涛 北京积水潭医院
杨 程 首都医科大学附属北京天坛医院
杨鹏达 北京市神经外科研究所
杨希孟 北京医院
伊骏飞 北京大学第一医院
伊志强 北京大学第一医院
殷祥栋 北京大学第一医院
银 锐 北京协和医院
于 涛 北京大学第三医院
余晓帆 首都医科大学附属北京天坛医院
张超男 北京市神经外科研究所
张 衡 首都医科大学附属北京天坛医院
张建国 首都医科大学附属北京天坛医院
张 凯 首都医科大学附属北京天坛医院
张 敏 北京大学人民医院
张墨轩 北京市神经外科研究所
张庆九 河北医科大学第二医院
张晓炜 河北医科大学第二医院
张一博 中国人民解放军总医院第八医学中心
赵 博 中国人民解放军总医院第八医学中心
赵学敏 北京市神经外科研究所
钟 东 重庆医科大学附属第一医院
周思宇 北京市神经外科研究所
周文韬 首都医科大学附属北京天坛医院

原著者名单

Hadie Adams Cambridge University Hospitals NHS Foundation Trust, Cambridge, UK
43: Surgical management of head injury

Fardad T. Afshari Cambridge University Hospitals NHS Foundation Trust, Cambridge, UK
44: Complications of head injury

Wail Ahmed Consultant, Spinal Cord Injuries in Stoke Mandeville Hospital, Aylesbury, Buckinghamshire, UK
70: Spinal cord injury rehabilitation

Likhith Alakandy Consultant Neurosurgeon, Southern General Hospital, Glasgow, UK
68: Cervical spine injuries

Kieren Allinson Department of Pathology, Addenbrooke's Hospital, Cambridge, UK

Ossama Al-Mefty UAMS Medical Center, Little Rock, AK, USA; and Department of Neurosurgery, Brigham and Women's Hospital, Boston MA, USA
15: Chordomas and chondrosarcomas of the skull base

Rami O. Almefty Department of Neurosurgery, Temple University, Philadelphia, PA, USA
15: Chordomas and chondrosarcomas of the skull base

Nabeel Alshafai Assistant Professor, Neurosurgery, Antwerp, Belgium
40: Epidemiology of head injury and outcome after head injury

Fahim Anwar Consultant in Rehabilitation Medicine, Department of Rehabilitation Medicine, Cambridge University Hospital NHS, Foundation Trust, Cambridge, UK
70: Spinal cord injury rehabilitation

Vasileios Apostolopoulos University Hospital Southampton NHS Foundation Trust, Southampton, UK
32: Intraventricular tumours

Eric Arnaud Department of Pediatric Neurosurgery, Necker-Enfants Malades Hospital, Paris, France
86: Spinal development and spinal dysraphism

Keyoumars Ashkan Kings College Hospital, London, UK
76: Movement disorders

Tipu Aziz The Nuffield Department of Clinical Neurosciences, University of Oxford, Oxford, UK
75: Principles of deep brain stimulation

Matt Bailey Consultant Neurosurgeon, Salford Royal NHS Foundation Trust, Salford, UK
89: Paediatric hydrocephalus

Damiano G. Barone Department of Neurosurgery, Addenbrooke's Hospital, Cambridge, UK
70: Spinal cord injury rehabilitation

Chris Barrett Consultant Neurosurgeon, Southern General Hospital, Glasgow, UK
68: Cervical spine injuries

Janneke van Beijnum Salford Royal NHS Foundation Trust, Salford, UK
55: Cavernoma and angiographically occult lesions

Antonio Belli Reader in Neurotrauma, School of Clinical and Experimental Medicine, College of Medical and Dental Sciences, University of Birmingham, Birmingham, UK
44: Complications of head injury

Lorenzo Bello Associate Professor Neurosurgery, University of Milan, Italy
6: Low-grade glioma

Edward Benzel Chairman and Spinal Surgeon, Cleveland Clinic, OH, USA
67: Managing spinal cord trauma

Mitchel Berger Department of Neurological Surgery, University of California, San Francisco, CA, USA
13: Surgical techniques in the management of intrinsic tumours

René Bernays Department of Neurosurgery, Klinik Hirslanden, Zurich, Switzerland
37: Surgical management of pineal region lesions

Chris Bervoets Psychiatrist, UZ Leuven, Leuven, Belgium
80: Neurosurgical interventions for psychiatric disorders

Pierre-Aurelien Beuriat Hopital Chu de Lyon, Lyon, France
86: Spinal development and spinal dysraphism

Harjus Birk Department of Neurological Surgery, University of California, San Francisco, CA, USA
14: Meningiomas and haemangiopericytoma (HPC)—solitary fibrous tumour (SFT)

Peter Bodkin Aberdeen Royal Infirmary, Scotland, UK
2: Clinical assessment

Stana Bojanic Department of Neurosurgery, Oxford University Hospitals NHS Foundation Trust, Oxford, UK
96: Arachnoid cysts

Ciaran Bolger College of Surgeons, Dublin, Ireland
61: Thoracic spinal disease

Grainne Bourke Leeds General Infirmary, Clarendon Way, Leeds, UK
72: Entrapment syndromes

John Brecknell Queen's Hospital, Romford, London, UK
63: Spinal tumours

Andrew Brodbelt The Walton Centre NHS Foundation Trust, Liverpool, UK
8: Intracranial metastasis

Nicholas Brown University College Hospitals, London, UK
12: Chemotherapy for brain tumours

Karol P. Budohoski Neurosurgical Specialist Registrar, Cambridge University Hospital NHS Trust, Department of Neurosurgery, Addenbrooke's Hospital, Cambridge University Hospitals, Cambridge, UK
5: Perioperative care of the neurosurgical patient

Harry Bulstrode Clinical Lecturer in Neurosurgery, Neurosurgery Division, Department of Clinical Neurosciences, Cambridge Biomedical Campus, Cambridge, UK
7: High-grade gliomas and molecular biology of neurosurgical oncology

Diederik O. Bulters Department of Neurosurgery, Wessex Neurological Centre, Southampton General Hospital, Southampton, UK
46: Normal cerebrovascular physiology and vascular anatomy

John F. Burke Resident Physician, Department of Neurological Surgery, University of California, San Francisco, CA, USA
41: Pathophysiology of traumatic brain injury

Federico Cagnazzo Università di Pisa, Pisa, Italy
47: The pathophysiology of aneurysms

Joseph D. Chabot Department of Neurological Surgery, University of Pittsburgh, PA, USA
19: Surgical management of tumours of the orbit

Christopher Chandler Consultant Adult and Paediatric Neurosurgeon, King's College Hospital, London, UK
29: Ependymoma

Bedansh Roy Chaudhary Cambridge University Hospitals NHS Foundation Trust, Cambridge, UK
69: Thoracic and lumbar spine injuries

Randall M. Chesnut Professor, Neurological Surgery; Professor, Orthopedics and Adjunct Professor, Global Health, Harborview Medical Center, Department of Neurosurgery, Seattle, WA, USA
43: Surgical management of head injury

Omar Choudhri Assistant Professor, Department of Neurosurgery, University of Pennsylvania, PA, USA
53: Giant aneurysms and bypass surgery

Paul Chumas Consultant in Neurosurgery, Leeds Teaching Hospitals, Leeds, UK
33: Colloid cyst

Shlomi Constantini Director, Department of Pediatric Neurosurgery, Dana Children's Hospital, Tel Aviv Sourasky Medical Center, Sackler Faculty of Medicine, Tel Aviv University, Tel Aviv, Israel
34: Choroid plexus tumours; 88: Paediatric brain tumours

William T. Couldwell Professor, Neurosurgery, University of Utah, UT, USA
27: Surgical management of sellar and suprasellar tumours

Matt Crocker Consultant Neurosurgeon, St George's Hospital, London, UK
62: Lumbar spinal disease

Michael D. Cusimano Division of Neurosurgery, University of Toronto, ON, Canada; Keenan Research Centre for Biomedical Science, The Li Ka Shing Knowledge Institute, St. Michael's Hospital, Toronto, ON, Canada
21: Surgical management of anterolateral skull base lesions

Tilak Das Addenbrooke's Hospital, Cambridge University Hospitals, Cambridge, UK
3: Overview of neuroimaging

Hansen Deng Resident Physician, Department of Neurological Surgery, University of Pittsburgh Medical Center, Pittsburgh, PA, USA
41: Pathophysiology of traumatic brain injury

Chris Derham Consultant Neurosurgeon, Leeds General Infirmary, Leeds, UK
56: Surgical principles in spinal surgery

Federico Di Rocco The Hôpital Necker Enfants Malades, Paris, France
86: Spinal development and spinal dysraphism

Derek Duane Consultant in Neuroanaesthesia and Neurointensive Care, Cambridge University Hospital NHS Trust, Department of Anaesthesia, Addenbrooke's Hospital, Cambridge, UK
5: Perioperative care of the neurosurgical patient

Hugues Duffau Institute for Neurosciences of Montpellie, France
6: Low-grade glioma

Andrew Durnford Department of Neurosurgery, Wessex Neurological Centre, Southampton General Hospital, Southampton, UK
46: Normal cerebrovascular physiology and vascular anatomy

Rina Dvir Department of Pediatric Hemato-Oncology, Dana Children's Hospital, Tel-Aviv Medical Center, Tel-Aviv University, Tel-Aviv, Israel
34: Choroid plexus tumours

Frances Elmslie South West Thames Regional Genetics Service, St George's University Hospitals NHS Foundation Trust, London, UK
38: Neurophakomatoses

Rudolf Fahlbusch International Neuroscience Institute (INI), Hannover, Germany
26: Craniopharyngioma and Rathke's cleft cysts

Colin Ferrie Department of Paediatric Neurology, Leeds General Infirmary, Leeds, UK
84: Developmental disorders of the brain

Graham Flint Consultant Neurosurgeon, Queen Elizabeth Hospital, Birmingham, UK
65: Spinal cerebrospinal fluid dynamics

Petter Förander Karolinska Institute, Stockholm, Sweden
22: Schwannomas

Alan Forster Consultant Clinical Neurophysiologist, Aberdeen Royal Infirmary, Scotland, UK
71: Electrodiagnostics

Navin Furtado Queen Elizabeth Hospital, Birmingham, UK
60: Cervical spinal disease

Alexander Gamble Bedford, New Hampshire, USA
92: Hydrocephalus and normal CSF dynamics

Paul Gardner Department of Neurological Surgery, University of Pittsburgh, PA, USA
19: Surgical management of tumours of the orbit

H. Rao Gattamaneni Consultant in Clinical oncology, Christie Foundation Trust, Manchester, UK
25: Pituitary tumours

Fred Gentili Division of Neurosurgery, University of Toronto, ON, Canada
17: Esthesioneuroblastoma

George Georgoulis Department of Neurosurgery, General Hospital of Athens "Gennimatas", Athens, Greece
79: Cranial nerve vascular compression syndromes

V. Gerganov Consultant Neurosurgeon, Department of Neurosurgery, International Neuroscience Institute, Hannover; and Associate Professor, Hannover Medical School, Germany
26: Craniopharyngioma and Rathke's cleft cysts

Giorgio Gioffre Treviso, Italy
20: Skull lesions

Kanna Gnanalingham Salford Royal NHS Foundation Trust, UK
25: Pituitary tumours

Tony Goddard Consultant Interventional Neuroradiologist, Leeds General Infirmary, Leeds, UK
90: Paediatric neurovascular disorders

Lior Gonen Division of Neurosurgery, Department of Surgery, University of Toronto, Canada. Department of Neurosurgery, Aurora Neuroscience Innovation Institute, Aurora St. Luke's Medical Center, Milwaukee, Wisconsin
17: Esthesioneuroblastoma

John Goodden Consultant Neurosurgeon (Adult & Paediatric), Leeds General Infirmary, Leeds, UK
77: Spasticity

Alex Green The Nuffield Department of Clinical Neurosciences, University of Oxford, UK
75: Principles of deep brain stimulation

Fay Greenway Atkinson Morley Department of Neurosurgery, St George's University Hospitals NHS Foundation Trust, London, UK
38: Neurophakomatoses

Alexander Grote Department of Neurology, University of Bonn, Bonn, Germany
10: Glioneuronal and other epilepsy-associated tumours

Paul Grundy Department of Neurosurgery, Wessex Neurological Centre, University Hospital Southampton NHS Foundation trust, UK
32: Intraventricular tumours

Mathew Guilfoyle Department of Neurosurgery, Addenbrookes's NHS Trust, Cambridge, UK
52: Extracranial-intracranial bypass for cerebral ischaemia

Nigel Gummerson Consultant in Orthopaedic Trauma, Leeds General Infirmary, Leeds, UK
66: Scoliosis and spinal deformity

Nicholas Haden Plymouth Hospitals NHS Trust, Plymouth, UK
99: Spinal infection

Nicholas Hall Surgeon, Royal Melbourne Hospital Academic Centre, Parkville, VIC, Australia
24: Surgical management of cerebellopontine angle and petrous lesions

Richard M. Hall Professor of Spinal Biomechanics, School of Mechanical Engineering, University of Leeds, Leeds, UK
57: Spinal stability

Walter Hall Professor of Neurosurgery, Upstate Medical University, Syracuse, NY, USA
97: Microbiology

Seunggu J. Han Department of Neurological Surgery, University of California, San Francisco, CA, USA
14: Meningiomas and haemangiopericytoma (HPC)—solitary fibrous tumour (SFT)

Adel Helmy University Lecturer Neurosurgery, University of Cambridge, UK/Honorary Consultant Neurosurgeon, Addenbrooke's Hospital, Cambridge, UK
18: Malignant skull base tumours; 43: Surgical management of head injury

Catherine Hernon Consultant in Plastic & Reconstructive Surgery, Leeds General Infirmary, Leeds, UK
77: Spasticity

Shawn Hervey-Jumper Associate Professor, Neurosurgery, University of California San Francisco, USA
13: Surgical techniques in the management of intrinsic tumours

Nicholas Higgins Department of Radiology, Addenbrooke's Hospital, Cambridge, UK
95: Pseudotumour cerebri syndrome

Peter J.A. Hutchinson Professor of Neurosurgery, University of Cambridge, Cambridge, UK
43: Surgical management of head injury

Mohsen Javadpour Beaumont Hospital, Dublin, Ireland
51: Carotid artery disease and cerebral ischaemia

Michael D. Jenkinson Department of Neurosurgery, University of Liverpool, Liverpool, UK
36: Pineal tumours

Timothy Jones Department of Neurosurgery, St George's University Hospital Foundation Trust, London, UK
38: Neurophakomatoses

Sylvia Karcheva Consultant in Neuroanaesthesia, Cambridge University Hospital NHS Trust, Department of Anaesthesia, Addenbrooke's Hospital, Cambridge University Hospitals, Cambridge, UK
5: Perioperative care of the neurosurgical patient

Neal Kassell University of Virginia School of Medicine, Charlottesville, VA, USA
47: The pathophysiology of aneurysms

Andrew Kay Consultant Paediatric Neurosurgery, Queen Elizabeth Hospital, Birmingham, UK
87: Special considerations in paediatric head and spinal trauma

Andrew H. Kaye Surgeon, Royal Melbourne Hospital Academic Centre, Parkville, VIC, Australia
24: Surgical management of cerebellopontine angle and petrous lesions

Tara Kearney Salford Royal NHS Foundation Trust, UK
25: Pituitary tumours

Chris Kellett University College London Hospitals, London, UK
62: Lumbar spinal disease

Nicole C. Keong Consultant Neurosurgeon, National Neuroscience Institute and Duke-NUS Medical School, Singapore
94: Normal pressure hydrocephalus

Osaama H. Khan Department of Neurological Surgery, Northwestern University
31: Surgical approaches to posterior fossa tumours

Sadaquate Khan Department of Clinical Neurosciences, Western General Hospital, Edinburgh, Scotland, UK
58: Spinal physiology

Andrew King Manchester Skull Base Unit, Department of Neurosurgery, Manchester Centre for Clinical Neurosciences, Salford Royal Hospital, University of Manchester, Manchester, UK
23: Glomus tumours

Matthew A. Kirkman Specialty Registrar in Neurosurgery and Honorary Fellow in Neurocritical Care; and The National Hospital for Neurology and Neurosurgery, University College London Hospitals NHS Foundation Trust, Queen Square, London, UK
42: Intensive care management of head injury

Peter Kirkpatrick Department of Neurosurgery, Addenbrookes's NHS Trust, Cambridge, UK
52: Extracranial-intracranial bypass for cerebral ischaemia

Ramez W. Kirollos Consultant Neurosurgeon, Addenbrooke's Hospital, Cambridge Senior Consultant, National Neuroscience Institute, Singapore Associate Professor Duke's NUS Medical School
14: Meningiomas and haemangiopericytoma (HPC)—solitary fibrous tumour (SFT);
35: Surgical management of intraventricular lesions

Neil Kitchen National Hospital for Neurology and Neurosurgery, University College London Hospital NHS Foundation Trust, London, UK
4: The operating theatre environment

Georgios Klironomos Division of Neurosurgery, Department of Surgery, University of Toronto, Canada
17: Esthesioneuroblastoma

Angelos G. Kolias Clinical Lecturer Neurosurgery, Addenbrooke's Hospital, Cambridge, UK
43: Surgical management of head injury

Daniel Krell University College Hospitals, London, UK
12: Chemotherapy for brain tumours

Giuseppe Lanzino Mayo Clinic, Rochester, MN, USA
47: The pathophysiology of aneurysms

Michael Lawton Department of Neurosurgery, Barrow Neurological Institute, Phoenix, AZ, USA
49: Management of subarachnoid haemorrhage;
53: Giant aneurysms and bypass surgery

Bryan Lee Neurosurgeon, Barrow Neurological Institute, Phoenix, AZ
67: Managing spinal cord trauma

Boon Leong Quah Department of Neurosurgery, Queen's Hospital, Romford, London, UK and Division of Neurosurgery, Khoo Teck Puat Hospital, Singapore
9: Primary central nervous system lymphoma;
63: Spinal tumours

Shiong Wen Low Consultant Neurosurgeon, National University Hospital and Ng Teng Fong General Hospital, Singapore; and Associate Professor, Department of Surgery, National University of Singapore
69: Thoracic and lumbar spine injuries

Peter Loughenbury Leeds Teaching Hospital NHS Trust, Leeds, UK
57: Spinal stability

Ruichong Ma Department of Neurosurgery, Oxford University Hospitals NHS Foundation Trust, Oxford, UK
96: Arachnoid cysts

Andrew Maas University of Antwerp and Antwerp University Hospital, Department of Neurosurgery, Antwerp, Belgium
40: Epidemiology of head injury and outcome after head injury

Richard Mair Clinical Lecturer in Neurosurgery, Neurosurgery Division, Department of Clinical Neurosciences, Cambridge Biomedical Campus, Cambridge, UK
7: High-grade gliomas and molecular biology of neurosurgical oncology

Conor L. Mallucci Department of Paediatric Neurosurgery, Alder Hey Children's Hospital, Liverpool, UK
36: Pineal tumours; 89: Paediatric hydrocephalus

Geoffrey T. Manley Professor and Vice Chair, Department of Neurological Surgery, University of California San Francisco, San Francisco, CA, USA
41: Pathophysiology of traumatic brain injury

Richard Mannion Department of Neurosurgery, Addenbrooke's Hospital, Cambridge, UK
78: Pain pathophysiology and surgical management

Hani Marcus Faculty of Medicine, Department of Surgery and Cancer, Imperial College London, London, UK
39: Uncommon brain lesions

Henry Marsh Senior Consultant Neurosurgeon, St George's Hospital, London, UK
1: The History of Neurosurgery

Eleni Maratos Consultant Neurosurgeon, King's College Hospital, London, UK
1: The History of Neurosurgery

Tiit Mathiesen Department of Clinical Neuroscience, Karolinska Institutet, Stockholm, Sweden; and University of Copenhagen & Rigshospitalet, Copenhagen, Denmark
22: Schwannomas

Calan Mathieson Consultant Neurosurgeon, Southern General Hospital, Glasgow, UK
68: Cervical spine injuries

Tomasz Matys University Lecturer and Honorary Consultant Neuroradiologist, Department of Radiology, University of Cambridge, Cambridge, UK
3: Overview of neuroimaging

Donald McArthur Consultant Adult and Paediatric Neurosurgeon, Nottingham University Hospitals NHS Trust, Nottingham, UK
30: Haemangioblastoma

Helen McCullagh Leeds General Infirmary, Leeds, UK
90: Paediatric neurovascular disorders

Michael McDermott Department of Neurological Surgery, University of California, San Francisco, USA
14: Meningiomas and haemangiopericytoma (HPC)—solitary fibrous tumour (SFT)

Andrew McEvoy National Hospital for Neurology and Neurosurgery, University College London Hospitals NHS Foundation Trust, UK
16: Dermoid and epidermoid cysts;
82: Classification of seizures and epilepsy

Eavan McGovern University College Dublin and St. Vincent's University Hospital, Dublin, Ireland
59: Medical pathologies of the spinal cord

Chris McGuigan University College Dublin and St. Vincent's University Hospital, Dublin, Ireland
59: Medical pathologies of the spinal cord

Iain McGurgan University College Dublin and St. Vincent's University Hospital, Dublin, Ireland
59: Medical pathologies of the spinal cord

Jason McMillen Consultant Neurosurgeon, Royal Brisbane and Women's Hospital, Brisbane, Queensland, Australia
48: The pathophysiology of subarachnoid haemorrhage

Harry Mee Department of Rehabilitation Medicine, Cambridge University Hospital NHS Foundation Trust, Cambridge, UK
70: Spinal cord injury rehabilitation

Michael P. Meier Department of Surgery, Division of Neurosurgery, St. Michael's Hospital, University of Toronto, ON, Canada
21: Surgical management of anterolateral skull base lesions

H. Metwali International Neuroscience Institute (INI), Hannover, Germany
26: Craniopharyngioma and Rathke's cleft cysts

Samantha Mills Department of Neuroradiology, The Walton Centre NHS Foundation Trust, Liverpool, UK
36: Pineal tumours

Catherine Moran College of Surgeons, Dublin, Ireland
61: Thoracic spinal disease

Jacques J. Morcos Department of Neurological Surgery, University of Miami Miller School of Medicine, FL, USA
31: Surgical approaches to posterior fossa tumours

Michael Morgan Cerebrovascular Neurosurgeon, Macquarie University Hospital, Sydney, NSW, Australia
50: Cerebral arteriovenous malformation and dural arteriovenous fistulae

Robert Morris Consultant Neurosurgeon, Addenbrooke's Hospital, Cambridge, UK
71: Electrodiagnostics

Paul Mulholland University College Hospitals, London, UK
12: Chemotherapy for brain tumours

Thangaraj Munusamy Department of Neurosurgery, Addenbrooke's Hospital, Cambridge, UK; and Division of Neurosurgery, Khoo Teck Puat Hospital, Singapore
9: Primary central nervous system lymphoma; 98: Cranial infections

Ammar Natalwala Specialist Registrar in Neurosurgery, Queen's Medical Centre, Nottingham, UK
30: Haemangioblastoma

Lamia Nayeb South Thames Foundation Trust, London, UK
58: Spinal physiology

Jayson A. Neil Midwest Neurosurgery Associates, Kansas City, MO, USA
27: Surgical management of sellar and suprasellar tumours

Vincent Nga Consultant Neurosurgeon, National University Hospital Singapore, Singapore
74: Peripheral nerve tumours

Bart Nuttin Neurosurgeon, UZ Leuven, Leuven, Belgium
80: Neurosurgical interventions for psychiatric disorders

Karen O'Connell University College Dublin and St. Vincent's University Hospital, Dublin, Ireland
59: Medical pathologies of the spinal cord

A. O'Hare Beaumont Hospital, Dublin, Ireland
51: Carotid artery disease and cerebral ischaemia

Berk Orakcioglu Ethianum, Heidelberg, Germany; and Department of Neurosurgery, University of Heidelberg, Heidelberg, Germany
54: Spontaneous intracranial haematoma

Brian P. Walcott Department of Neurosurgery, University of Southern California, Los Angeles, USA
49: Management of subarachnoid haemorrhage

Benedict Panizza University of Queensland, Princess Alexandra Hospital, QLD, Australia
18: Malignant skull base tumours

Chris Parks Department of Paediatric Neurosurgery, Alder Hey Children's Hospital, Liverpool, UK
89: Paediatric hydrocephalus

Tufail Patankar Consultant Interventional Neuroradiologist, Leeds General Infirmary, Leeds, UK
90: Paediatric neurovascular disorders

Hiren Patel Salford Royal NHS Foundation Trust, Salford, UK
55: Cavernoma and angiographically occult lesions

Omar Pathmanaban Manchester Skull Base Unit, Department of Neurosurgery, Manchester Centre for Clinical Neurosciences, Salford Royal Hospital, University of Manchester, Manchester, UK
23: Glomus tumours

Erlick Pereira Senior Lecturer and Honorary Consultant at St George's, London, UK
75: Principles of deep brain stimulation

Jonathan R Perera Speciality Registrar, Royal National Orthopaedic Hospital, Stanmore, UK
73: Supraclavicular brachial plexus and peripheral nerve injuries

David Pettersson Karolinska Institute, Stockholm, Sweden
22: Schwannomas

John D. Pickard Division of Neurosurgery, Department of Clinical Neurosciences, University of Cambridge, Cambridge, UK
95: Pseudotumour cerebri syndrome

Ian K. Pople Department of Neurosurgery, Southmead Hospital, Bristol, UK
93: Shunt technology and endoscopic ventricular surgery

Stephen Price Addenbrooke's Hospital, Cambridge University Hospitals, Cambridge, UK
7: High-grade gliomas and molecular biology of neurosurgical oncology

Harold Rekate Hofstra University, Hempstead, NY, USA
92: Hydrocephalus and normal CSF dynamics

Eduardo C. Ribas Division of Neurosurgery, University of São Paulo Medical School, and Albert Einstein Hospital, São Paulo, Brazil
35: Surgical management of intraventricular lesions

Guilherme C. Ribas Professor of Surgery, Department of Surgery, University of São Paulo Medical School, Department of Surgery and Neurosurgeon, Albert Einstein Hospital, São Paulo, Brazil
35: Surgical management of intraventricular lesions

Desiderio Rodrigues Consultant Paediatric Neurosurgeon, Queen Elizabeth Hospital, Birmingham, UK
87: Special considerations in paediatric head and spinal trauma

Roberto Rodriguez Rubio Department of Neurological Surgery, University of California, San Francisco, USA
49: Management of subarachnoid haemorrhage

Federico Roncaroli Clinical Reader in Neuropathology, University of Manchester, Manchester, UK
25: Pituitary tumours

Jonathan Roth Department of Pediatric Neurosurgery, Dana Children's Hospital Tel-Aviv Sourasky Medical Center, Tel Aviv University, Israel
34: Choroid plexus tumours; 88: Paediatric brain tumours

James Rutka Neurosurgeon and Senior Scientist, The Hospital for Sick Children (SickKids), Toronto, ON, Canada
28: Medulloblastoma

Thomas Santarius Department of Neurosurgery, Addenbrooke's Hospital, Cambridge, Cambridge, UK
6: Low-grade glioma; 14: Meningiomas and haemangiopericytoma (HPC)—solitary fibrous tumour (SFT); 39: Uncommon brain lesions

Johannes Schramm Department of Neurosurgery, University of Bonn, Bonn, Germany
83: Surgical management of epilepsy

Daniel. J. Scoffings Addenbrooke's Hospital, Cambridge University Hospitals, Cambridge, UK
3: Overview of neuroimaging

Brian Scott Consultant Paediatric Orthopaedic Surgeon, Leeds General Infirmary, Leeds, UK
77: Spasticity

Alessandro Scudellari Consultant in Neuroanaesthesia, Addenbrooke's Hospital, Cambridge University Hospitals, Cambridge, UK
5: Perioperative care of the neurosurgical patient

Senthil Selvanathan Consultant Neurosurgeon, Leeds Teaching Hospital NHS Trust, Leeds, UK
56: Surgical principles in spinal surgery

Richard Selway King's College Hospital NHS Foundation Trust, London, UK
81: Diagnosis and assessment

Ashish H. Shah Department of Neurological Surgery, University of Miami Miller School of Medicine, FL, USA
31: Surgical approaches to posterior fossa tumours

Jonathan Shapey The National Institute of Neurology and Neurosurgery, London, UK
4: The operating theatre environment

Melanie Sharp Consultant Paediatric Neurosurgeon, Queen Elizabeth Hospital, Birmingham, UK
87: Special considerations in paediatric head and spinal trauma

Asim Sheikh Consultant Neurosurgeon, Leeds General Infirmary, Leeds, UK
33: Colloid cyst

Susan Short Professor of Clinical Oncology and Neuro-Oncology, Leeds Institute of Cancer and Pathology, Leeds, UK
11: Radiotherapy and radiosurgery for brain tumours

Adikarige Haritha Dulanka Silva Queen Elizabeth Hospital, Birmingham, UK
60: Cervical spinal disease

Matthias Simon Department of Neurology, University of Bonn, Bonn, Germany
10: Glioneuronal and other epilepsy-associated tumours

Marc Sindou Department of Neurosurgery, University of Lyon 1, Hôpital Neurologique P. Wertheimer, Groupement Hospitalier Lyon, Lyon, France
79: Cranial nerve vascular compression syndromes

William Singleton Department of Neurosurgery, Southmead Hospital, Bristol, UK
93: Shunt technology and endoscopic ventricular surgery

Marco Sinisi Consultant Neurosurgeon, Royal National Orthopaedic Hospital, Stanmore, UK
73: Supraclavicular brachial plexus and peripheral nerve injuries

Martin Smith Martin Consultant in Neuroanaesthesia and Neurocritical Care, National Hospital for Neurology and Neurosurgery, University College London Hospitals, UK
42: Intensive care management of head injury

Saksith Smithason Cleveland Clinic, OH, USA
67: Managing spinal cord trauma

Guirish Solanki Consultant Paediatric Neurosurgeon, Queen Elizabeth Hospital, Birmingham, UK
87: Special considerations in paediatric head and spinal trauma

S. Tonya Stefko Department of Ophthalmology, University of Pittsburgh, PA, USA
19: Surgical management of tumours of the orbit

Catherine Suen Department of Neurology, University of Utah School of Medicine, UT, USA
41: Pathophysiology of traumatic brain injury

Yuval Sufaro Skull Base Fellow, Royal Melbourne Hospital, Australia
24: Surgical management of cerebellopontine angle and petrous lesions

Kieron Sweeney Department of Paediatric Neurosurgery, Children's University Hospital, Dublin, Ireland
51: Carotid artery disease and cerebral ischaemia; 61: Thoracic spinal disease

Mobin Syed Consultant Plastic surgeon Guys and St Thomas Hospital, London
Mobinsyed@doctors.org.uk

Tamara Tajsic Department of Neurosurgery, Cambridge University Hospital NHS Foundation Trust, Cambridge UK
70: Spinal cord injury rehabilitation

Rokas Tamosauskas Consultant in Anaesthesia and Pain Medicine, Cambridge University Hospitals NHS Foundation Trust, Department of Pain Medicine, Addenbrooke's Hospital, Cambridge, UK
78: Pain pathophysiology and surgical management

Boon Hoe Tan Division of Neurosurgery, Khoo Teck Puat Hospital, Singapore
98: Cranial infections

Mario Teo Consultant Neurosurgeon, Bristol Institute of Clinical Neuroscience, UK
53: Giant aneurysms and bypass surgery

Dominic Thompson Consultant in Paediatric Neurosurgery, Great Ormond Street Hospital, London, UK
85: Spinal development and spinal dysraphism

Simon Thomson Leeds Teaching Hospital NHS Trust, Leeds, UK
56: Surgical principles in spinal surgery

Martin Tisdall Consultant Paediatric Neurosurgeon, Great Ormond Street Hospital, London, UK
91: Paediatric epilepsy

Ivan Tmofeev Department of Neurosurgery, Addenbrookes's NHS Trust, Cambridge, UK
20: Skull lesions

Nicolas de Tribolet Professor of Neurosurgery, University of Lausanne, Switzerland
37: Surgical management of pineal region lesions

Rikin Trivedi Department of Neurosurgery, Addenbrooke's Hospital, Cambridge, UK
74: Peripheral nerve tumours

Kevin Tsang Consultant Neurosurgeon, Imperial College NHS Trust, London, UK
58: Spinal physiology

Georgios Tsermoulas Queen Elizabeth Hospital, Birmingham, UK
60: Cervical spinal disease

Atul Tyagi Consultant Neurosurgeon (Adult & Paediatric), Leeds General Infirmary, Leeds, UK
84: Developmental disorders of the brain; 90: Paediatric neurovascular disorders

Ismail Ughratdar University Hospitals Birmingham NHS Foundation Trust, Birmingham, UK
76: Movement disorders

Andreas W. Unterberg Department of Neurosurgery, University of Heidelberg, Heidelberg, Germany
54: Spontaneous intracranial haematoma

Sophia Varadkar Consultant Paediatric Neurologist, Great Ormond Street Hospital, London, UK
91: Paediatric epilepsy

Elizabeth Visser Aberdeen Royal Infirmary, Scotland, UK
2: Clinical assessment

Daniel Walsh Consultant Neurosurgeon, Kings College Hospital, London, UK
64: Vascular lesions of the spinal cord

Yizhou Wan Resident Physician, Department of Neurosurgery, Oxford University Hospitals, Oxford, UK
39: Uncommon brain lesions

Mueez Waqar Department of Neurosurgery, The Walton Centre NHS Foundation Trust, Liverpool, UK
36: Pineal tumours

Daniel Warren Consultant Neuroradiologist, Leeds General Infirmary, Leeds, UK
84: Developmental disorders of the brain

Colin Watts Professor of Neurosurgery/Honorary Consultant Neurosurgeon, University of Birmingham
9: Primary central nervous system lymphoma

Tim Wehner Formerly Department of Clinical Neurophysiology, National Hospital for Neurology and Neurosurgery, Department of Clinical and Experimental Epilepsy, Institute of Neurology, University College London, London, UK
82: Classification of seizures and epilepsy

Edward White Consultant Neurosurgeon, University Hospitals Birmingham, UK
99: Spinal infection

Peter C. Whitfield University Hospitals Plymouth, Derriford Road, Plymouth, UK
44: Complications of head injury

Mark Wilson St Mary's Hospital, London, UK
45: Concussion and sports-related head injury

Ethan A. Winkler Resident Physician, Department of Neurological Surgery, University of California, San Francisco, CA, USA
41: Pathophysiology of traumatic brain injury

Christoph M. Woernle Department of Neurosurgery, Klinik Hirslanden, Zurich, Switzerland
37: Surgical management of pineal region lesions

Victoria Wykes Department of Neurosurgery, National Hospital for Neurology and Neurosurgery, University College London, London, UK
82: Classification of seizures and epilepsy

Eugene Yang Division of Neurosurgery, Khoo Teck Puat Hospital, Singapore
98: Cranial infections

John K. Yue Resident Physician, Department of Neurological Surgery, University of California, San Francisco, CA, USA
41: Pathophysiology of traumatic brain injury

Zsolt Zador NIHR Academic Clinical Lecturer and Specialty Registrar in Neurosurgery, Department of Neurosurgery, Salford Royal NHS Foundation Trust, University of Manchester, Manchester, United Kingdom
25: Pituitary tumours

Rashed Zakaria The Walton Centre NHS Foundation Trust, Liverpool, UK
8: Intracranial metastasis

中文版序一

北京市神经外科研究所孟凡刚教授和北京大学第一医院伊志强教授主译的《牛津神经外科教科书》（*Oxford Textbook of Neurological Surgery*）即将付梓，受邀作序，谨表祝贺。

《牛津神经外科教科书》是牛津外科教科书系列丛书之一，是世界通用的神经外科教材。原著编者200余位，主要来自欧洲和北美洲的大学医院，撰写内容充分反映了当前世界神经外科的发展水平。本书在国外神经外科学界备受推崇，影响很大。

北京大学医学出版社将《牛津神经外科教科书》的主译工作交予北京市神经外科研究所和北京大学第一医院共同完成。两位主译邀请全国各地从事神经外科工作的知名专家和卓有建树的中青年医师共同翻译，期望本书成为中国神经外科医师了解世界神经外科前沿领域的一个窗口，为我国神经外科医师开阔思路，充实临床经验发挥作用。

本书共99章，逾1000个图表，图文并茂，内容丰富，几乎涵盖了神经外科临床的各个方面，读者能从中获取所需内容，是对临床神经外科医师有重要参考价值的医学译著，对中青年医师更新观念和获取新知识多有裨益，同时对其他相关学科的医师也有所帮助。

感谢所有译者和编辑兢兢业业付出的辛勤劳动！

赵继宗

中国科学院院士

国家神经系统疾病临床医学研究中心主任

首都医科大学神经外科学院院长、教授、主任医师

中文版序二

医生是一个终身学习的职业。因为这是患者对我们的要求，要求我们以最好、最先进和最有效且安全的方法来诊治疾病，以求达到既治好病又获得最好的生存质量。据统计，现在全球生物医学类杂志有2万多种，每天有4000篇论文发表，医学“三新”（新理论、新设备、新技术）层出不穷。因此，医生要跟上医学专业的发展，必须每天学习，才能满足患者的需求。

近来，历史悠久、素以出版权威性学术专著享有盛誉的牛津大学出版社，推出了医学系列参考巨著，其中包括《牛津神经外科教科书》（*Oxford Textbook of Neurological Surgery*）。该书由英国著名神经外科教授Kirollos等主编，邀请欧洲、北美洲等地区200多位神经外科专家组成国际编委，系统介绍了脑肿瘤、颅底肿瘤、颅脑外伤、脑血管病变、脊髓病变、脊髓外伤、周围神经病变、功能神经外科、癫痫、小儿神经外科、脑脊液病变、颅内和椎管内感染等。本书将临床基础和“三新”紧密结合，内容翔实、图文并茂，可读性强，适用于神经外科实习医生、住院医生、研究生和各级神经外科专家以及相关学科的专家。

北京市神经外科研究所孟凡刚教授和北京大学第一医院伊志强教授联合主译，组织国内同仁，不辞辛劳，精心翻译本书，为大家献上一本值得学习和参考的神经外科专著，为我国神经外科事业进一步发展作出贡献，造福广大病患。

周良辅
中国工程院院士
国家神经疾病医学中心复旦大学神经外科研究所
复旦大学附属华山医院神经外科
上海神经外科临床医学中心

中文版序三

在神经外科蓬勃发展、日新月异的时代，终身学习是临床医生职业生涯的必备技能，与世界先进科技保持同步也是每一位临床医生的毕生追求。我国广大的神经外科医生更是肩负着更新知识、提高水平、保持与国际神经外科新技术进展同步的重任，这对我国广大的神经外科医生也提出了更高的要求，因此学习世界神经外科最新专业书籍的需求更加迫切。《牛津神经外科教科书》(*Oxford Textbook of Neurological Surgery*)中文版的问世，打开了一扇了解国外神经外科先进知识的窗口，为我国神经外科医生更新观念、获取新知识提供宝贵的途径，也必将促进我国神经外科事业的不断发展和进步。

英国作为现代神经外科学的发源地之一，见证了现代神经外科的兴起和蓬勃发展。《牛津神经外科教科书》原著由享有盛誉的牛津大学出版社出版，作为神经外科方面的权威教材，凝聚了欧洲和北美洲等地区200余位顶级神经外科专家的智慧，超过1000页的篇幅承载着深厚的历史和丰富的学术传统，涵盖了神经外科领域的各个方面，展现了世界神经外科发展的重要节点。这部巨著既包含神经外科基础知识，又展示了神经外科最新的技术和研究进展。这不仅是一部重要的参考书，更是一部可资神经外科医生参照的全面系统又细致入微的学科教科书。

北京市神经外科研究所孟凡刚教授和北京大学第一医院伊志强教授，以及来自国内各地所有参与翻译的神经外科医生们，勇于担当作为，敢于直面挑战，勤于研究破解，成功完成了这一艰巨但意义非凡的重任，在此谨表祝贺！奋楫笃行，筑梦医学，愿这部中文版的《牛津神经外科教科书》能够成为中国神经外科医学事业发展的推动力，为我国医学同仁提供更深入、更广阔的学术指导，助力我国神经外科高质量发展，为我国神经外科走上国际舞台做出更加卓越的贡献！

江 涛
中国工程院院士
北京市神经外科研究所所长
首都医科大学附属北京天坛医院神经外科中心主任

译者前言

《牛津神经外科教科书》是一部全面、系统的神经外科教科书，是传统的基础理论和新知识的结合，反映了神经外科领域发展的广阔性和复杂性。本书主编组织了来自全球各地的200多位神经外科专家，齐心协力编写了这部布局清晰、可读性强、插图精美的图书。

《牛津神经外科教科书》开篇主要阐述神经外科的发展历史和临床规范，掌握这些知识是科学合理地从事和开展神经外科工作所必需的。而在随后各个章节中，既有历史的回顾又有新的临床研究进展，既包括神经外科疾病的背景和一般特征，也包括实用的外科技术，使读者能够全面地获取知识。

本书的翻译出版是我国神经外科领域的一大喜事。近年来，随着医学新技术在临床的推广和普及，我国的神经外科事业得到了飞速的发展，取得了巨大的进步，整体的医疗水平也得到了很大的提升，但是与国外先进水平仍然存在差距。各位译者通过辛勤的工作，将国外神经外科的理念引介到国内，必将促进中国神经外科事业的进步，推动我国神经外科事业的发展，造福于广大患者。本书内容全面，既有传统的基本内容，又有科研临床的最新进展，相信不管是刚刚入门的神经外科医师，还是已经事业有成的专家，都会从本书中受到启发。在此我们也希望中国的神经外科医生能够利用本书，掌握更详细的知识、技能和经验，共同推动我国神经外科的发展。

最后，衷心感谢本书99章的每一位译者，大家的辛勤工作将助力我国神经外科的进步，也将被我国神经外科事业的发展历程所铭记。由于译者的能力所限，不当之处在所难免，敬请各位读者谅解和指正。

孟凡刚　伊志强

原著丛书序

外科学教科书的出版有了新的进展，新版《牛津外科教科书》将替代之前的两个版本，并由单本外科教科书改为包含各亚专业的系列教科书。出版系列教科书的原因在于：首先，对于单本外科教科书，如果需要囊括所有的专业知识，所需的篇幅将越来越大，例如《牛津外科教科书》(第2版)为3卷；其次，读者的需求也正在转变，新的专业教科书既要符合接受高等外科培训人员的需要，也要具有互联网的可及性。

因此，我们首先编写了一本涵盖外科学基础知识的大纲式书籍，包括解剖学、生理学、生物化学、循证医学等内容。随后我们还编写了涵盖各个亚专业的专科书籍，每一本都作为独立的教科书呈现，并可在牛津医学网(Oxford Medicine Online)上查阅。

尽管不同专业之间难免会有重叠，但按照编写计划，不同亚专业的教科书之间都将彼此独立。然而，《外科学基础知识》这本核心书籍将支撑起其他每个亚专业所需的理论与实践知识。

在接下来的几年中，我们将致力于实施这一雄心勃勃的计划，并充分运用在线平台定期更新上述诸多亚专业教科书。

各教科书都将满足外科专家委员会规定的培训和学习的要求，专家委员会由大不列颠及爱尔兰四家外科学院认证，并将继续适用于来自全球的读者。

这项工作完成后，“牛津外科系列教科书”将在未来很长一段时间内，对于外科学丛书的出版起到引领的作用。

Peter J. Morris
纳菲尔德外科名誉教授
外科系前主席
牛津大学移植中心主任
英国牛津大学和牛津大学拉德克利夫医院

原著序一

《牛津神经外科教科书》是“牛津外科系列教科书”所推出的一部新书。该书作为第一部由英国主导编写的综合性教科书，几乎涵盖了从《诺斯菲尔德中枢神经系统外科学》一书问世以来的所有神经外科内容。

尽管本书是由英国方面构思与编写的，但是它已然获得了深远的国际影响，对于世界上所有国家的医学专业人员而言，也都具有极其重要的价值。

本书填补了简明手册类型的教科书和大型百科全书之间的空缺，不仅适用于初级和中高级神经外科学员和医生，而且对其他学科的专业人员也有助益。此外，本书对那些参加英国大学神经外科考核、欧洲神经外科考核和其他国家的同等考核的人员也大有裨益。本书的写作架构突出了临床上严谨求实的科学精神。

本书共分为 20 篇，涵盖了 99 章，在这 1000 余页的鸿篇巨制中包含着超过 1000 个图片和表格，所有的章节都经过精心编排。本书的所有章节都采用统一的格式，图文并茂，以清晰的图表对各章节的主要内容进行阐述。

本书涵盖了最前沿的神经外科领域的新发现，例如其中所包含的最新临床试验结果，甚至在校稿阶段还保持着对内容上的更新。

最后，我想要向所有参与本书编写的来自世界各地不同神经外科亚专业的专家们表示祝贺！是大家共同努力成就了这样一部布局清晰、可读性强且插图精美的图书。我相信本书将会成为全世界所有神经外科医生书架上重要的参考书。

Franco Servadei

原著序二

过去的四十年时间见证了神经外科在发展规模和速度上的巨大进步，单以我从事的亚专业来看，神经外科的实践内容已焕然一新。20世纪70年代显微神经外科和断层成像技术的出现，伴随着术前和术中管理的进步，促进了神经外科的数次革新和蓬勃发展。为了充分利用新机遇来提升患者的治疗效果，专业化变得非常必要。神经外科医师应当积累专业且详尽的知识、技能和经验，以推动神经外科发展，并使之变得越来越精细和多样化。

《牛津神经外科教科书》的编委面临着巨大的挑战：需要把现代神经外科学的所有复杂的实践知识囊括在一本书里。因此，除了知识层面的深度之外，本书在编撰中还考虑到了两个重要层面：基础科学的严谨性和神经外科手术的精细性。

本书成功地填补了神经外科现有文献中的空白：无论是实习生还是经验丰富的医生们，本书都将提供全方位的神经外科知识。本书的研究方法具有前瞻性，着重强调基础和临床研究以及循证医学的重要性。神经外科手术的安全与成功需要越来越扎实的人体解剖学知识、精准的临床判断思维和更高水平的专业技能，同时还要具备将不断增长的复杂文献转化为临床实践的能力。

英国的神经外科有着悠久的历史。1879年现代神经外科手术在苏格兰（格拉斯哥）诞生。英国神经外科医师学会虽然是世界上最古老的国家级学会之一，但是它依旧保持着开放的发展理念，超越不断变化的国家政治边界的束缚，学会不停地吸引全球的神经外科学界的同事们加入其中，这一点也体现在本书的编撰中——虽然本书主要由英国的神经外科医生所编写，但也成功地邀请到了来自世界各地拥有着最熟练的技术和最丰富经验的神经外科医生以及最有见识的科学家们加入其中。因此对于神经外科医生而言，从早期接受入门培训到后来的亚专业经验与咨询实践的积累，《牛津神经外科教科书》是其在整个过程中的珍贵陪伴。毋庸置疑，对于世界范围内的神经外科医生们来说，本书将是最具有权威性的教科书。

Graham Teasdale 爵士

符号和缩写

Ω	omega	欧米伽
α	alpha	阿尔法
β	beta	贝塔
γ	gamma	伽马
μg	micrograms	微克
AAA	asleep-awake-asleep	睡眠 - 唤醒 - 睡眠（麻醉）
AAICH	anticoagulation-associated intracerebral haemorrhage	抗凝相关脑出血
AANS	acute and chronic settings	急性和慢性环境
ABC	aneurysmal bone cyst	动脉瘤性骨囊肿
ABI	auditory brainstem implants	听觉脑干植入物
ABR	auditory brainstem responses	听觉脑干反应
AC	anterior and posterior commissure	前连合和后连合
	arachnoid cyst	蛛网膜囊肿
ACA	anterior cerebral artery	大脑前动脉
ACD	anterior cervical discectomy	颈椎前路椎间盘切除术
ACPP	atypical choroid plexus papilloma	不典型脉络丛乳头瘤
ADC	apparent diffusion coeffecient	表观弥散系数
ADI	atlantodental interval	寰齿间距
ADL	activities of daily living	日常生活活动
ADNFLE	autosomal-dominant nocturnal frontal lobe epilepsy	常染色体显性夜间额叶癫痫
ADPKD	autosomal dominant polycystic kidney disease	常染色体显性多囊肾病
AED	antiepileptic drug	抗癫痫药物
AF	atrial fibrillation	心房颤动
AGNIR	Advisory Group on Non-ionising Radiation	非电离辐射咨询小组
AICA	anterior inferior cerebellar artery	小脑下前动脉
AIDS	acquired immunodeficiency syndrome	获得性免疫缺陷综合征
AIP	aryl hydrocarbon receptor-interacting protein	芳基烃受体相互作用蛋白
AIS	Abbreviation Injury Score	简略损伤评分
	ASIA Impairment Scale	美国脊柱损伤协会损伤评分
ALI	acute lung injury	急性肺损伤
ALIF	anterior lumbar interbody fusion	前路腰椎椎间融合
ALL	acute lymphatic leukaemia	急性淋巴白血病

ALL	anterior longitudinal ligament	前纵韧带
AP	anteroposterior	前后位
ASA	American Society of Anesthesiologists	美国麻醉医师协会
	anterior spinal artery	脊髓前动脉
ASIA	American Spinal Injuries Association	美国脊柱损伤协会
ASPECTS	Alberta Stroke Programme Early CT Score	艾伯塔脑卒中早期 CT 评分
AT	anaplastic transformation	间变性转化
ATA	anterior temporal artery	颞前动脉
AT Ⅲ	antithrombin Ⅲ	抗凝血酶Ⅲ
ATLS	advance trauma life support	高级创伤生命支持
ATRT	atypical teratoid rhabdoid tumour	非典型畸胎样横纹肌样肿瘤
AVF	arteriovenous fistula	动静脉瘘
AVM	arteriovenous malformation	动静脉畸形
AZ	annulus of Zinn	总腱环
BAEP	brainstem auditory evoked potentials	脑干听觉诱发电位
BBB	blood–brain barrier	血脑屏障
BECTS	benign epilepsy with centrotemporal spikes	良性癫痫伴中央颞叶棘波
BIS	bispectral index	双谱指数
BMD	bone mineral density	骨密度
BMI	body mass index	体重指数
BOLD	blood oxygen level dependent	血氧水平依赖
BP	blood pressure	血压
BRAT	Barrow Ruptured Aneurysm Trial	Barrow 破裂性动脉瘤试验
BTF	Brain Trauma Foundation	脑外伤基金会
CA	cerebral autoregulation	脑血流自身调节
CAA	cerebral amyloid angiopathy	脑淀粉样血管病
CAD	coronary artery disease	冠状动脉疾病
CAMS	cerebrofacial metameric arteriovenous syndromes	脑面体节性动静脉畸形综合征
CAPECTH	craniectomy-associated progressive extra-axial collections with treated hydrocephalus	颅骨切除术后进展性轴外脑积水
CAR	cerebral autoregulation	脑血流自身调节
CAS	carotid angioplasty and stenting	颈动脉血管成形术和支架置入术
CBF	cerebral blood flow	脑血流量
CBV	cerebral blood volume	脑血容量
CCA	common carotid artery	颈总动脉
CCM	cerebral cavernous malformations	脑海绵状畸形
CDC	Centers for Disease Control	疾病控制中心
CDK	cyclin dependent kinases	细胞周期素依赖性激酶
CFAM	cerebral function analysing monitor	脑功能分析监测
CHF	congestive heart failure	充血性心力衰竭
CHLA	Children's Hospital Los Angeles	洛杉矶儿童医院
CISS	Constructive Interference in Steady State	稳态干扰序列

CM	cavernous malformations	海绵状畸形
	central myelin	中央髓鞘
CMAP	compound motor action potential	复合运动动作电位
$CMRO_2$	cerebral metabolic rate of oxygen consumption	脑代谢耗氧率
CN	cranial nerve	脑神经
CNS	central nervous system	中枢神经系统
	Congress of Neurological Surgeons	神经外科医师协会
COPD	chronic obstructive pulmonary disease	慢性阻塞性肺疾病
COSS	Carotid Occlusion Surgery Study	颈动脉闭塞手术研究
CPA	cerebellopontine angle	桥小脑角
CPC	choroid plexus carcinoma	脉络丛癌
CPH	choroid plexus hyperplasia	脉络丛增生症
CPP	cerebral perfusion pressure	脑灌注压
	choroid plexus papilloma	脉络丛乳头状瘤
CPT	choroid plexus tumour	脉络丛肿瘤
CRF	corticotrophin-releasing factor	促肾上腺皮质激素释放因子
CRH	corticotrophin-releasing hormone	促肾上腺皮质激素释放激素
CRP	C-reactive protein	C 反应蛋白
CRPS	complex regional pain syndrome	复杂区域疼痛综合征
CRW	Cosman-Roberts-Wells	Cosman-Roberts-Wells 系统
CSF	cerebrospinal fluid	脑脊液
CSW	cerebral salt wasting	脑性盐耗
CSWS	cerebral salt wasting syndrome	脑性耗盐综合征
CT	computed tomographic	计算机断层扫描
CTA	computed tomography angiography	CT 血管造影
CTP	cerebellar tonsillar prolapse	小脑扁桃体脱垂
CTS	carpal tunnel syndrome	腕管综合征
CTV	clinical target volume	临床靶体积
CUSA	cavitron ultrasonic surgical aspirator	超声外科吸引装置
DBS	deep brain stimulation	脑深部（电）刺激术
DEBS	direct electrical brain stimulation	直接脑电刺激
DES	drug-eluting stents	药物洗脱支架
DESD	detrusor external sphincter dyssynergia	逼尿肌外括约肌协同失调
DEXA	dual-energy X-ray absorptiometry	双能 X 射线吸收法
DI	diabetes insipidus	尿崩症
DIND	delayed ischaemic neurological deficits	延迟缺血性神经功能缺陷
DISH	diffuse idiopathic skeletal hyperostosis	弥漫性特发性骨骼肥大症
DLGG	diffuse low-grade gliomas	弥漫性低级别胶质瘤
DNP	dynamic nuclear polarization	动态核极化
DNT	dysembryoplastic neuroepithelial tumours	胚胎发育不良性神经上皮肿瘤
DPG	diffuse pontine glioma	弥漫性脑胶质瘤
DRG	dorsal root ganglion	背根神经节

DRIFT	Drainage, Irrigation and Fibrinolytic Therapy	引流、冲洗和纤溶治疗
DSA	digital subtraction angiography	数字减影血管造影
DSB	double-strand break	双链断裂
DTI	diffusion tensor imaging	弥散张量成像
DVA	deep venous anomaly	深静脉异常
DVA	developmental venous anomaly	发育性静脉异常
DVT	deep vein thrombosis	深静脉血栓形成
DWI	diffusion-weighted imaging	弥散加权成像
DWMH	deep white matter hyperintensities	深部白质高信号
DXA	dual X-ray absorbitometery	双 X 射线吸收仪
ECA	external carotid artery	颈外动脉
ECG	electrocardiogram	心电图
ECoG	electrocorticography	皮层脑电图
EDF	elongation derotation flexion	伸长 - 反旋 - 屈曲
EDL	extensor digitorum longus	指长伸肌
EEA	endoscopic endonasal approach	内镜经鼻入路
EEG	electroencephalography	脑电图
EGFR	epidermal growth factor receptor	表皮生长因子受体
EIEE	early infantile onset epileptic encephalopathies	早期婴儿发作癫痫性脑病
ELISA	enzyme-linked immunosorbent assay	酶联免疫吸附试验
EMA	epithelial membrane antigen	上皮膜抗原
EMG	electromyography	肌电图
ENT	ear, nose, and throat	耳鼻喉
EOIS	early onset idiopathic scoliosis	早发性特发性脊柱侧凸
EOR	extent of resection	切除程度
EORTC	European Organization for Research and Treatment of Cancer	欧洲癌症研究和治疗组织
EP	evoked potential	诱发电位
EPC	epilepsia partialis continua	部分癫痫持续
ES	ethmoid sinus	筛窦
ERG	Electroretinogram	视网膜电图
ES	Ewing's sarcoma	尤因肉瘤
ESO	European Stroke Organisation	欧洲卒中组织
ESR	erythrocyte sedimentation rate	红细胞沉降率
ET	essential tremor	特发性震颤
ETT	endotracheal tube	气管内导管
ETV	endoscopic third ventriculostomy	内镜下第三脑室造瘘术
EVD	external ventricular drain	脑室外引流
EZ	epileptogenic zone	致痫区
FA	fractional anisotropy	分数各向异性
FCD	focal cortical dysplasias	局灶性皮质发育不良
FCU	flexor carpi ulnaris	尺侧腕屈肌
FD	fibrous dysplasia	纤维性结构不良

FDA	Food and Drug Administration	食品药品监督管理局
FEF	frontal eye field	额叶视区
FES	functional electric stimulation	功能性电刺激
FFP	fresh frozen plasma	新鲜冷冻血浆
FGN	French Glioma Network	法国神经胶质瘤网络
FIESTA	fast imaging in steady state	稳态快速成像
FIPA	familial isolated pituitary adenoma	家族性孤立性垂体腺瘤
FLAIR	fluid attenuated inversion recovery	液体抑制反转恢复
FLE	frontal lobe epilepsy	额叶癫痫
FM	Foramen of Monro	室间孔
FSH	follicle-stimulating hormone	促卵泡激素
FSU	functional spinal unit	功能性脊柱单位
FTT	failure to thrive	成长受阻
FV	flow velocities	流速
FZS	fronto-zygomatic suture	额颧缝
GABA	gamma aminobutyric acid	γ 氨基丁酸
GAF	Global Assessment of Function	功能大体评定量表
GCS	Glasgow Coma Scale	格拉斯哥昏迷量表
GCT	germ cell tumours	生殖细胞肿瘤
	granular cell tumour	颗粒细胞肿瘤
GFAP	glial fibrillary acid protein	胶质细胞原纤维酸性蛋白
GFR	glomerular filtration rate	肾小球滤过率
GH	growth hormone	生长激素
GHIH	growth hormone-inhibiting hormone	生长激素抑制激素
GHRH	growth hormone release hormone	生长激素释放激素
GI	gastrointestinal	胃肠道
GMFM	Gross Motor Function Measure	运动功能总指标
GSPN	greater superficial petrosal nerve	岩浅大神经
GTCS	generalized tonic-clonic seizures	全面性强直 - 阵挛性发作
GTR	gross total resection	全切除
GTV	gross tumour volume	肿瘤总体积
GW	gliadel wafers	卡莫司汀植入剂
H&E	haematoxylin and eosin	苏木精和伊红
HBO	hyperbaric oxygen	高压氧
HDDST	high-dose dexamethasone suppression tests	大剂量地塞米松抑制试验
HGG	high-grade glioma	高级别胶质瘤
HHT	hereditary haemorrhagic telangiectasia	遗传性出血性毛细血管扩张症
HIF	hypoxia inducible factor	低氧诱导因子
HIFU	high-intensity focused ultrasound	高强度聚集超声
HIV	human immunodeficiency virus	人类免疫缺陷病毒
HLA	human leukocyte antigen	人类白细胞抗原
HMSN	hereditary motor, and sensory neuropathy	遗传性运动感觉神经病

HO	heterotrophic ossification	异位骨化
HPA	hypothalamic-pituitary axis	下丘脑 - 垂体轴
HPC	haemangiopericytoma	血管外皮细胞瘤
HR	homologous recombination	同源重组
HRQOL	health-related quality of life	健康相关的生活质量
HS	hippocampal sclerosis	海马硬化症
HS	hypertonic saline	高渗盐水
HSV	herpes simplex virus	单纯疱疹病毒
HU	Hounsfield units	亨氏单位
IA	intra-arterial	动脉内
IAC	internal auditory canal	内听道
IAM	internal auditory meatus	内耳道
IBE	International Bureau for Epilepsy	国际癫痫局
ICA	inferior cerebellar artery	小脑下动脉
ICA	internal carotid arteries	颈内动脉
ICBP	infraclavicular brachial plexus	锁骨下臂丛神经
ICE	ifosfamide, carboplatin, and etoposide	异环磷酰胺、卡铂和依托泊苷
ICH	intracerebral haemorrhage	脑出血
ICP	intracranial pressure	颅内压
ICU	intensive care unit	重症监护病房
IFOF	inferior fronto-occipital fasciculus	下额枕束
IJV	internal jugular vein	颈内静脉
ILAE	International League Against Epilepsy	国际抗癫痫联盟
IO	inferior oblique	下斜肌
IOF	inferior orbital fissure	眶下裂
IOM	Intraoperative monitoring	术中监测
IPG	implantable pulse generator	植入式脉冲发生器
IPG	implanted battery-operated pulse generator	植入式电池驱动脉冲发生器
IPSS	inferior petrosal vein sampling	岩下静脉取样
IR	inferior rectus	下直肌
IR	iterative reconstruction	迭代重建
ISAT	International Subarachnoid Aneurysm Trial	国际蛛网膜下腔动脉瘤试验
ISCoS	International Spinal Cord Society	国际脊髓学会
ISNCSCI	International Standards for Neurological Classification of Spinal Cord Injury	脊髓损伤神经分类国际标准
ITB	intrathecal baclofen	鞘内注射巴氯芬
IVC	inferior vena cava	下腔静脉
IVP	intraventricular pressure	心室内压力
JET	Japanese EC-IC Bypass Trial	日本 EC-IC 旁路试验
KOLT	Kendrick object learning test	肯德里克对象学习测试
kPa	kilopascal	千帕
KPS	Karnofsky Performance Status	卡氏健康状况

LCH	Langerhans cell histiocytosis	朗格汉斯细胞组织细胞增生症
LDD	L'hermitte-Duclos disease	莱尔米特 - 杜克洛病
LDDST	low-dose dexamethasone suppression test	小剂量地塞米松抑制试验
LDL	low-density lipoprotein	低密度脂蛋白
LDM	limited dorsal myeloschisis	局限性背侧脊髓裂
LFS	Li-Fraumeni syndrome	利 - 弗劳梅尼综合征
LG	lacrimal gland	泪腺
LGG	low-grade glioma	低级别胶质瘤
LH	luteinizing hormone	黄体生成素
LINAC	linear accelerator	直线加速器
LMN	lower motor neuron	下运动神经元
LMWH	low molecular weight heparin	低分子量肝素
LOC	level of consciousness	意识水平
LOH	loss of heterozygosity	杂合性丢失
LOIS	late onset idiopathic scoliosis	迟发性特发性脊柱侧凸
LOR	line of response	反应线
LOVA	longstanding overt ventriculomegaly in adults	成人长期显著性脑室扩张症
LP	levator palpebrae	眼睑提肌
LP	lumbar puncture	腰椎穿刺
LR	lateral rectus	外直肌
LR	Lindegaard ratio	林德加比
LSO	lumbar sacral orthosis	腰骶矫形器
LSR	lateral spread responses	横向扩散反应
MAC	minimal alveolar concentration	最小肺泡浓度
MAP	mean arterial pressure	平均动脉压
MC	Meckel cave	Meckel 腔隙
MCA	middle cerebral artery	大脑中动脉
MCD	malformation of cortical development	皮质发育畸形
MDT	multidisciplinary team	多学科团队
MEG	magnetoencephalography	脑磁图
MEP	minimally endoscopic procedures	微创内镜手术
MEP	motor evoked potential	运动诱发电位
MHC	major histocompatibility complex	主要组织相容性复合体
MI	myocardial infarction	心肌梗死
MIP	maximum intensity projection	最大密度投影
MIT	minimally invasive techniques	微创技术
MLF	medial longitudinal fasciculus	内侧纵束
MM	multiple myeloma	多发性骨髓瘤
MMD	moya moya disease	烟雾病
MMS	moya moya syndrome	Moyamoya 综合征
MMSE	mini-mental state examination	简易精神状态检查
MND	motor neurone disease	运动神经元疾病

MOG	myelin oligodendrocyte glycoprotein	髓鞘少突胶质细胞糖蛋白
MPBT	malignant paediatric brain tumours	儿科恶性脑肿瘤
MPNST	malignant peripheral nerve sheath tumours	恶性周围神经鞘瘤
MR	magnetic resonance	磁共振
	medial rectus	内直肌
MRA	magnetic resonance angiography	磁共振血管成像
	MR-angio	磁共振血管成像
MRC	Medical Research Council	医学研究委员会
MRI	magnetic resonance imaging	磁共振成像
MRM	magnetic resonance myelography	磁共振脊髓成像
MRN	magnetic resonance neurography	磁共振神经成像
MRS	magnetic resonance spectroscopy	磁共振波谱
MRSA	methicillin-resistant Staphylococcus aureus	耐甲氧西林金黄色葡萄球菌
MRV	magnetic resonance venography	磁共振静脉成像
MS	multiple sclerosis	多发性硬化症
MSH	melanocyte-stimulating hormone	黑色素细胞刺激激素
MTG	middle temporal gyrus	颞中回
MTLE	mesial temporal lobe epilepsy	颞叶内侧癫痫
MTT	mean transit time	平均通过时间
MUAP	motor unit action potential	运动单位动作电位
MVA	motor vehicle accidents	机动车辆事故
MVC	motor vehicle collisions	机动车碰撞
MVD	microsurgical vascular decompression	显微血管减压术
Na+	sodium	钠
NAA	N-acetyl aspartate	N- 乙酰天冬氨酸
NASCIS	National Acute Spinal Cord Injury Studies	国家急性脊髓损伤研究
NCS	nerve conduction studies	神经传导研究
NeuN	neuronal nuclei	神经元核
NFPA	non-functioning pituitary adenomas	无功能垂体腺瘤
NHEJ	non-homologous end-joining	非同源末端连接
NHL	non-Hodgkin's lymphoma	非霍奇金淋巴瘤
NICE	National Institute of Clinical Excellence	国立临床规范研究所
NIRS	near infrared spectroscopy	近红外光谱
NLI	neurological level of injury	神经损伤程度
NMDA	N-methyl-D-aspartate	N- 甲基 -D- 天冬氨酸
NMS	non-motor symptoms	非运动症状
NOAC	new oral anticoagulants	新型口服抗凝剂
NOS	not otherwise specified	没有其他说明
NPH	normal pressure hydrocephalus	正常压力脑积水
NPSA	National Patient Safety Agency	国家患者安全局
NPUAP	National Pressure Ulcer Advisory Panel	国家压疮咨询小组
NSAID	non-steroidal anti-inflammatory drug	非甾体抗炎药

OC	optic canal	视神经管
OCR	optico-carotid recesses	视神经颈动脉隐窝
OCT	optical coherence tomography	光学相干层析成像
ODI	Oswestry Disability Index	Oswestry 残疾指数
OEF	oxygen extraction fraction	氧摄取分数
OLE	occipital lobe epilepsy	枕叶癫痫
OLF	ossification of the ligamentum favum	黄韧带骨化
ON	optic nerve	视神经
OPG	optic pathway glioma	视神经通路胶质瘤
OPLL	ossification of the posterior longitudinal ligament	后纵韧带骨化
OS	overall survival	总体生存率
OSA	obstructive sleep apnoea	阻塞性睡眠呼吸暂停
PA	pilocytic astrocytoma	毛细胞星形细胞瘤
PAR	protease-activated receptors	蛋白酶激活受体
PBI	penetrating brain injury	穿透性脑损伤
PBT	paediatric brain tumour	儿科脑肿瘤
PCA	posterior cerebral artery	大脑后动脉
PCC	prothrombin complex concentrate	凝血酶原复合物浓缩物
PCNSL	primary central nervous system lymphoma	原发性中枢神经系统淋巴瘤
PCR	polymerase chain reaction	聚合酶链反应
PCV	procarbazine, CCNU, vincristine	丙卡巴肼、洛莫司汀和长春新碱
PD	Parkinson's disease	帕金森病
	proton density	质子密度
PDGFR	platelet-derived growth factor receptor	血小板源性生长因子受体
PE	preoperative embolization	术前栓塞
PE	pulmonary embolism	肺栓塞
PEDI	Pediatric Evaluation of Disability Inventory	残疾儿童评估目录
PEEK	poly-ether-ether-ketone	聚醚醚酮
PEEP	positive end-expiratory pressure	呼气末正压
PEG	percutaneous endoscopic gastrostomy	经皮内镜下胃造瘘术
PET	positron emission tomography	正电子发射断层扫描
PFO	patent foramen ovale	卵圆孔未闭
PFS	progression-free survival	无进展生存期
PI	pelvic incidence	盆腔发病率
PICA	posterior inferior cerebellar artery	小脑后下动脉
PIH	prolactin-inhibiting hormone	催乳素抑制激素
PIOL	primary intraocular lymphoma	原发性眼内淋巴瘤
PLL	posterior longitudinal ligament	后纵韧带
PML	progressive multifocal leukoencephalopathy	进行性多灶性白质脑病
PNET	primitive neuroectodermal tumour	原始神经外胚层肿瘤
PONV	postoperative nausea and vomiting	术后恶心呕吐
PPTID	pineal parenchymal tumours of intermediate differentiation	中分化松果体实质肿瘤

PRH	prolactin-releasing hormone	催乳素释放激素
PSA	posterior spinal arteries	脊髓后动脉
PSO	pedicle subtraction osteotomy	经椎弓根椎体截骨术
PT	pelvic tilt	盆腔倾斜
	prothrombin time	凝血酶原时间
PTA	pure-tone audiogram	纯音听力图
PTH	post-traumatic hydrocephalus	创伤后脑积水
PTPR	papillary tumour of the pineal region	松果体乳头状瘤
PTS	post-traumatic seizures	创伤后癫痫发作
PTSD	post-traumatic stress disorder	创伤后应激障碍
PTT	partial thromboplastin time	部分凝血活酶时间
PTV	planning target volume	计划靶区
PVA	poly-vinyl-alcohol	聚乙烯醇
QoL	quality of life	生活质量
QOLIBRI	Quality of Life after Brain Injury	脑损伤后的生活质量
RA	rheumatoid arthritis	类风湿关节炎
RANKL	receptor activator of NF- κ B ligand	NF- κ B 配体受体激活剂
RANO	Response Assessment in Neuro-Oncology	神经肿瘤学研究的反应评估
RAPD	relative afferent pupil defect	相对性传入性瞳孔障碍
RCC	renal cell carcinoma	肾细胞癌
RCN	Rare Cancer Network	罕见癌症网
RCT	randomized clinical trials	随机临床试验
REM	rapid eye movement	快速眼动
REZ	root entry zone	神经根入髓区
RF	rheumatoid factor	类风湿因子
RNFL	retinal nerve fibre layer	视网膜神经纤维层
RT	radiation therapy	放射治疗
RT	resistance in the tube	管内阻力
RVAD	rib-vertebral-angle difference	肋椎角差
SAH	subarachnoid haemorrhage	蛛网膜下腔出血
SARS	sacral anterior nerve root stimulator	骶神经前根刺激器
SBP	supraclavicular brachial plexus	锁骨上臂丛神经
SCA	superior cerebellar artery	小脑上动脉
SCAVM	spinal cord arteriovenous malformations	脊髓动静脉畸形
SCI	spinal cord injury	脊髓损伤
SCID	severe-combined immunodeficiency disease	重症联合免疫缺陷病
SCM	strap muscles	束带肌
SCO	spindle cell oncocytoma	梭形细胞瘤
SCPP	spinal cord perfusion pressure	脊髓灌注压力
SDAVF	spinal dural arteriovenous fistula	脊髓硬脑膜动静脉瘘
SDR	selective dorsal rhizotomy	选择性背神经后根离断术
SDS	speech discrimination score	言语识别率

SEA	spinal epidural abscess	硬脊膜外脓肿
SEEG	stereoencephalography	立体脑电图
SEER	surveillance Epidemiology and End Results	监测流行病学和最终结果
SEGA	subependymal giant cell astrocytomas	室管膜下巨细胞星形细胞瘤
SEP	somatosensory evoked potential	体感诱发电位
SESH	spontaneous epidural spinal haemorrhage	自发性脊髓硬膜外出血
SFT	solitary fibrous tumour	孤立性纤维肿瘤
SGCT	subependymal giant cell tumour	室管膜下巨细胞肿瘤
SIADH	syndrome of inappropriate antidiuretic hormone	抗利尿激素异常分泌综合征
SIVMS	Scottish Intracranial Vascular Malformation Study	苏格兰颅内血管畸形研究
SLE	systemic lupus erythematous	系统性红斑狼疮
SLF	superior longitudinal fasciculus	上纵束
SMA	supplementary motor area	运动辅助区
SNAP	sensory nerve action potential	感觉神经动作电位
SNO	Society for Neuro-Oncology	神经肿瘤学会
SNUC	sinonasal undifferentiated carcinoma	鼻窦未分化癌
SO	superior oblique	上斜肌
SOF	superior orbital fissure	眶上裂
SOM	spheno-orbital meningiomas	蝶眶脑膜瘤
SOV	superior ophthalmic vein	眼上静脉
SPECT	single photon emission computed tomography	单光子发射计算机断层扫描
SPES	single pulse electrical stimulation	单脉冲电刺激
SPN	selective peripheral neurotomy	选择性外周神经切除术
SPV	superior petrosal venous	岩上静脉
SR	superior rectus	上直肌
SSFP	steady state free precession	稳态自由旋进
SSI	surgical site infection	手术部位感染
SSMA	supplementary sensorimotor area	感觉运动辅助区
SSS	superior sagittal sinus	上矢状窦
SST	Short Synacthen Test	短同步测试
STA	superficial temporal artery	颞上动脉
	superior thyroid artery	甲状腺上动脉
STASCIS	Surgical Treatment of Acute Spinal Cord Injury Study	急性脊髓损伤外科治疗研究
STG	superior temporal gyrus	颞上回
STIR	short tau inversion recovery	短时间反转恢复序列
STR	subtotal resection	次全切除术
SUDEP	sudden unexplained death in epilepsy	癫痫猝死症
SUNCT	short-lived, unilateral neuralgic headache with conjunctival injection and tearing	短暂单侧神经痛样头痛发作伴结膜充血和流泪
SVA	sagittal vertical axis	矢状轴
SVM	spinal vascular malformation	脊柱血管畸形
SWI	susceptibility weighted imaging	磁敏感加权成像

TBI	traumatic brain injury	创伤性脑损伤
TCD	transcranial Doppler	经颅多普勒
TCGA	The Cancer Genome Atlas	癌症基因组图谱
TF	tissue factor	组织因子
TFPI	tissue factor pathway inhibitor	组织因子途径抑制剂
TIVA	total intravenous anaesthesia	全静脉麻醉
TLE	temporal lobe epilepsy	颞叶癫痫
TLSO	thoracolumbar sacral orthosis	胸腰骶矫形器
TMG	transmural pressure gradient	跨壁压力梯度
TMS	tumefactive multiple sclerosis	肿瘤样多发性硬化
TN	trigeminal neuralgia	三叉神经痛
TOF	time of flight	时间飞跃法
TORCH	Toxoplasmosis, Other (syphilis, varicella-zoster, parvovirus B19), Rubella, Cytomegalovirus (CMV), and Herpes infections	弓形虫、其他(梅毒、水痘-带状疱疹、细小病毒B19)、风疹、巨细胞病毒和疱疹感染
TREZ	trigeminal root entry zone	三叉神经根入髓区
TRH	thyroid-releasing hormone (also thyrotropin-releasing hormone)	促甲状腺激素释放激素
TSC	tuberous sclerosis complex	结节性硬化症
TSH	thyroid-stimulating hormone	促甲状腺激素
TT	thrombin time	凝血酶时间
TTM	targeted temperature management	目标体温管理
TTP	time to peak	达峰时间
TZ	transitional zone	过渡区
UH	unfractionated heparin	普通肝素
UMN	upper motor neuron	上运动神经元
UMNL	upper motor neuron lesions	上运动神经元病变
VA	vertebral artery	椎动脉
VAD	ventricular access device	脑室通路装置
VAE	venous air embolism	静脉空气栓塞
VASO	vascular space occupancy	血管空间占用
VBA	vertebrobasilar artery	椎基底动脉
VDE	velocity of diametric expansion	直径扩张速度
VEGF	vascular endothelial growth factor	血管内皮生长因子
VEP	visual evoked potential	视觉诱发电位
VGAM	vein of Galen malformations	Galen 静脉畸形
VGPN	vago-glossopharyngeal neuralgia	迷走-舌咽神经痛
VHL	von Hippel-Lindau syndrome	希佩尔-林道综合征/VHL 综合征
VMAT	volumetric modulated arc therapy	容积弧形调强放射治疗
VNS	vagus nerve stimulation	迷走神经刺激
VP	vancomycin powder	万古霉素粉末
VP	ventriculoperitoneal	脑室腹腔
VRE	vancomycin-resistant enterococci	万古霉素耐药肠球菌

VS	vestibular schwannoma	前庭神经鞘瘤
	ventral striatum	腹侧纹状体
VTE	venous thromboembolism	静脉血栓栓塞
vWF	von Willebrand factor	血管性血友病因子
WBC	white blood cell	白细胞
WBRT	whole-brain radiation therapy	全脑放射治疗
WFNS	World Federation of Neurosurgical Societies	世界神经外科学会联合会
WFSBP	World Federation of Societies of Biological Psychiatry	世界生物精神病学会联合会
WHO	World Health Organization	世界卫生组织
YBOCS	Yale-Brown Obsessive-Compulsive Scale	耶鲁 - 布朗强迫症量表

目 录

第十一篇 血管神经外科

第十二篇 脊柱外科原则

第十三篇 脊柱外科

第十四篇 脊柱损伤

第十五篇 周围神经外科

第十六篇 功能性神经外科

第十七篇 癫痫

第十八篇 小儿神经外科

第十九篇 脑脊液循环障碍

第二十篇 感染性疾病

第一篇　神经外科原则

第1章　神经外科简史

Eleni Maratos・Henry Marsh 著
高源、徐丹、李志保 译，孟凡刚、胡威 审校

引言

神经外科的历史始于前现代时代，最初是对颅骨和头部外伤的外科手术史。而自19世纪以来，随着大脑定位理论、消毒和麻醉学的发展，神经外科逐渐成为对大脑本身的外科手术史。

已知的第一个神经外科手术是颅骨环形钻孔，可能在生者和逝者身上都进行过。目前还不清楚这些手术的目的是出于治疗还是某种仪式。来自世界各地的遗址中发现许多带穿孔的头骨，这些可以追溯到几千年前的新石器时代，甚至更早。

古埃及

最早的神经外科著作可以追溯到古埃及，保存在公元前1600年的《艾德温·史密斯纸草文稿》（Edwin Smith Papyrus）中。这是首次使用理性的科学方法处理头颅损伤而不是巫术。其风格能让人联想到现代的病例报告，前十个病例集中于头部创伤，同时也包含了已知最早的关于大脑本身（而非颅骨）的参考文献，它描述了"曲折的结构，就像熔炼铜时发生的涟漪"。这些病例生动地描述了一种有条不紊的治疗方法：首先确定受伤的深度，以及是否存在潜在的颅骨骨折或大脑外露，然后根据检查所见提出不同的治疗策略。《艾德温·史密斯纸草文稿》已由美国国立卫生研究院翻译和转载，可在线进行研究学习（https://ceb.nlm.nih.gov）。和已知最早的头部损伤管理建议一样，《艾德温·史密斯纸草文稿》也首次记录了为防止进一步损伤而进行的脊柱固定术。

古希腊和拜占庭

希波克拉底（Hippocrates，公元前460—370年）在《头外伤》一书（De capitis vulneribus/On Head Wounds）中对头部损伤做了大量的描述。他的治疗策略几乎完全建立在骨折分类的基础之上，而不是患者的临床症状。他描述了包括对冲伤在内的五种类型的颅骨骨折。关于头部损伤，他写到"nullum capitis vulnus contemnendum est"（任何头部损伤都不可轻视）。他的著作不仅局限于头部外伤，他还被认为是第一个描述蛛网膜下腔出血的人：

> 如果一个健康的人突然感到头痛，立即躺下，说不出话，喘不过气，除非开始发烧，否则7天内就会死亡。

他还描述了与脑损伤相关的对侧肢体抽搐。因此，他被认为可能是第一个描述脑功能定位的医生。

大约公元前300年，亚历山大（Alexander）学派引入了正式的解剖学。也是在这个时候，赫罗菲拉斯（Herophilus）开始发展我们今天使用的解剖学命名法（**图1.1**）。他发现神经和肌腱确实是不同的结构，这与古埃及人的想法相反。他也是第一个描述脑室和静脉窦解剖结构的人。鼻窦汇合处仍以他的名字"Torcula Herophili"命名。他还描述了位于第四脑室底部"αναγλυφη τηςχ αλαμης"和脉络丛（得名于它与胎盘血管相似）。

塞尔苏斯（Celsus）生活的时间大约在公元前25年到公元50年，是第一个描述炎症（红疹、疼痛和肿瘤）的人，他还撰写了有关硬膜外出血、脑积水、三叉神经痛和脊柱骨折的文章。他主张将开颅手术作为头部外伤最后的治疗手段，他描述了钻孔的技术，并将锤子和带有保护性刀片的凿子与这些技术联系起来。在另一项关于脑部定位的早期研究中，他建议在疼痛最严重的一侧进行手术。

Galen（129—200）

随着盖仑（Galen）提出了科学和医学的脑中心模型，大脑逐渐被认为是智力和自主运动的中枢。他识别出了软脑膜（与硬脑膜不同）、胼胝体、脑室（与Herophilus一起）、松果体和垂体腺。他还为神经

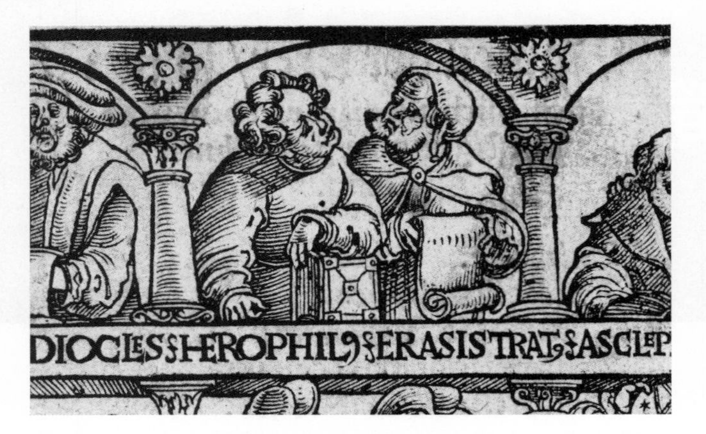

图 1.1 卡尔西登的赫罗菲拉斯（Herophilus）（约公元前 330—前 260 年），一位在亚历山大港行医的希腊医生。这里可以看到他正在与喀俄斯岛的埃拉西斯特拉图斯（Erasistratus）进行讨论

Wellcome 收藏

科学做出了其他的重要贡献：在现代解剖学家命名之前就描述了 Sylvius 导水管和 Monro 孔；确定横断脊髓会导致损伤水平以下的神经功能丧失；描述了我们现在所说的 Brown-Séquard 综合征。此外，他还指出，喉返神经反复受伤导致他的实验犬的声音嘶哑。他还主张修复颅骨凹陷性骨折并使用冲洗来减少因环钻术而产生的热量。在后来的 1500 年的时间里，他的学说一直被接受，基本上没有受到质疑。

在中世纪时期（750—1200 年），最具创新性的医学著作都来自阿拉伯伊斯兰世界，这也使赫罗菲拉斯和盖仑的学说得以延续。传统的床边教学就是在这个时期建立起来的。

科学时代的开始

16、17 世纪在科学和哲学的各个方面都取得了显著进步。在维萨里（Vesalius）之前的中世纪，欧洲就已经开始进行尸体解剖了，但维萨里的解剖更加广泛和系统，是第一个挑战盖仑和亚里士多德（Aristotle）学说的人。威廉·哈维（William Harvey，1578—1657）在 *de motu Cordis et Sanguinis in Animalibus*（1628）中发表了他关于心脏功能和血液循环的开创性著作。威尔斯（Willis，1621—1675）将这一知识应用到他对大脑解剖结构的理解中，并表明阻塞其同名环（Willis 环）的一部分并不会影响血流，从而证实了它们的吻合性。

这一时期，尽管神经外科仍局限于创伤，但其他领域的外科手术却在继续发展。在对传统的挑战中，Yonge（1646—1721）指出，一旦硬脑膜被破坏，死亡“并非不可避免”。Percival Pott 不仅研究了脊柱结核（最近在神经外科实践中又有了复兴），而且在我们对头部外伤的理解上做出了重大贡献。他断言，在头部受伤时，钻孔术可以缓解血液渗出产生的压力，从而为最古老的神经外科手术提供依据。与此同时，Jean Louis Petit（1674—1750）将与硬膜外血肿相关的经典“清醒期”描述为短暂的意识丧失，随后由于血液积聚压迫大脑而逐渐恶化。人们开始认识到脑损伤而不是头部受伤的重要性。Bell（爱丁堡，1749—1806）描述了瞳孔对光反应的丧失，并认为这是对硬膜外血肿进行“快速排出”手术的一个指标。Bell 还发现脑积水可能与脊柱裂有关。

虽然大多数手术仍然是与创伤有关的，但一个关键的例子是 Morand（1697—1773）成功清除了继发于中耳乳突炎的颞部脓肿。他描述了用手指对其探索并洗净腔体，然后放下一条可以缓慢抽出的银管——这种方法在今天仍有意义，银因其杀菌特性再次在医学上发挥作用。

Cotugno（1736—1822）进一步描述了脑脊液通路，并首次描述了坐骨神经痛的“神经起源”。他还认为代偿性脑积水是继发于脑萎缩的。

外科医生兼解剖学家 John Hunter（1728—1793）是 Pott 的学生，对普通外科和神经外科都做出了重大贡献。他的解剖学作品中收藏了这位爱尔兰巨人（Cushing 最初的肢端肥大患者），现在仍然可以在伦敦皇家外科医学院的亨特利（Hunterian）博物馆中看到。

然而，在这段时间里，神经外科手术仍然受到感染的困扰，而麻醉剂的缺乏意味着手术速度快但不精准。脑定位的临床技能尚未描述，因此手术仅限于具有外部表现的病变。

早期现代至 19 世纪

我们今天所知道的现代神经外科手术始于 19 世纪。麻醉和抗菌术的同步发展使死亡率降低到可接受的水平，仅凭临床检查就可以定位脑部病变的能力使外科医生能够应对隐匿性病变，从而大大拓宽了该专业的范畴。这些进步最终促成了神经外科作为一门专业的诞生。

并行发展

麻醉

在 19 世纪 40 年代，乙醚的引入使得外科手术能够以一种无痛的方式进行，而无须外科医生短时间内完成手术或使用约束装置。1846年，在马萨诸塞州总医院，牙医William Morton说服Warren医生使用乙醚切除了一个颌下肿瘤。此后不久，Marie Jean Pierre Flourens在1847年成功地使用了氯仿麻醉。这并非没有风险，但对外科医生和患者而言都有明显的好处。随着麻醉越来越安全，可以处理的病理范围也在扩大，复杂的手术方法也随之发展。

抗菌术

在抗菌术之前，由于感染，神经外科手术几乎是致命的。Louis Pasteur（1822—1895）发展了他的微生物理论，并从根本上改变了人们对感染起源的看法。他推测肉的腐败和发酵不是由于“自发”退化，而是由于活的微生物产生的。Joseph Lister（1827—1912）是格拉斯哥大学的外科教授，他将巴斯德的微生物理论应用于外科手术，特别是伤口感染。他开始使用石炭酸（苯酚），并评论说，他的伤口愈合过程中没有脓。因此，截肢的死亡率从45%大幅下降到15%。与此同时，美国的William Keen（1837—1932）在他的手术室中采用了Lister的原则，把它们应用到外科医生、患者和手术室环境中，这是今天仍在奉行的原则。他坚持要用石炭酸清理所有表面，并除去地毯和家具。外科医生用肥皂、酒精和升华物洗手，患者也开始接受剃发、肥皂水、乙醚、湿升华物敷料和氯化汞清洗等术前准备。

Holmes Semmelweiss还发现洗手可以从根本上减少产科和妇科的感染。Keen将他的手术器械在术前煮沸2小时以加热灭菌，这种方法是在1891年由Ernst von Bergman提出的。1883年，Neuber开始使用无菌工作服和无菌帽，但直到1890年William Stewart Halsted（1852—1922）委托Goodyear制作一些橡胶手套来保护护士的手免受氯化汞的伤害的时候，手套才被常规用于外科手术（图1.2）。Mikulicz随后在1897年推出了面罩。

Cushing自己在1915年说过，“感染当然不能归咎于魔鬼的干预，而必须归咎于外科医生的门上”。他发表了自己130例的系列病例，其中只有一例感染——感染率不到1%，这在今天仍然令人羡慕。疾病控制和预防中心（Centre for Disease Control and prevention，CDC）对1992—2003年开颅手术感染率的审计报告中显示，低风险病例的感染率为0.86%，高风险病例为2.32%。在同一系列中，Cushing也报告了高达8.4%的死亡率（Cushing，1915）。在20世纪40年代，开始采取抗生素预防措施以减少术后感染。

脑定位

19世纪60年代，神经症状和体征与脑损伤位置之间的关系开始改变神经外科手术的范围。神经系统检查在我们目前的实践中仍然十分重要，以至于很难想象脑定位之前的时代。在19世纪初，定位理论与不可信的颅相学伪科学联系在一起。随后，Paul Broca（1824—1880）证明了语言只局限于大脑的左半球，John Hughlings Jackson（1835—1911）描述

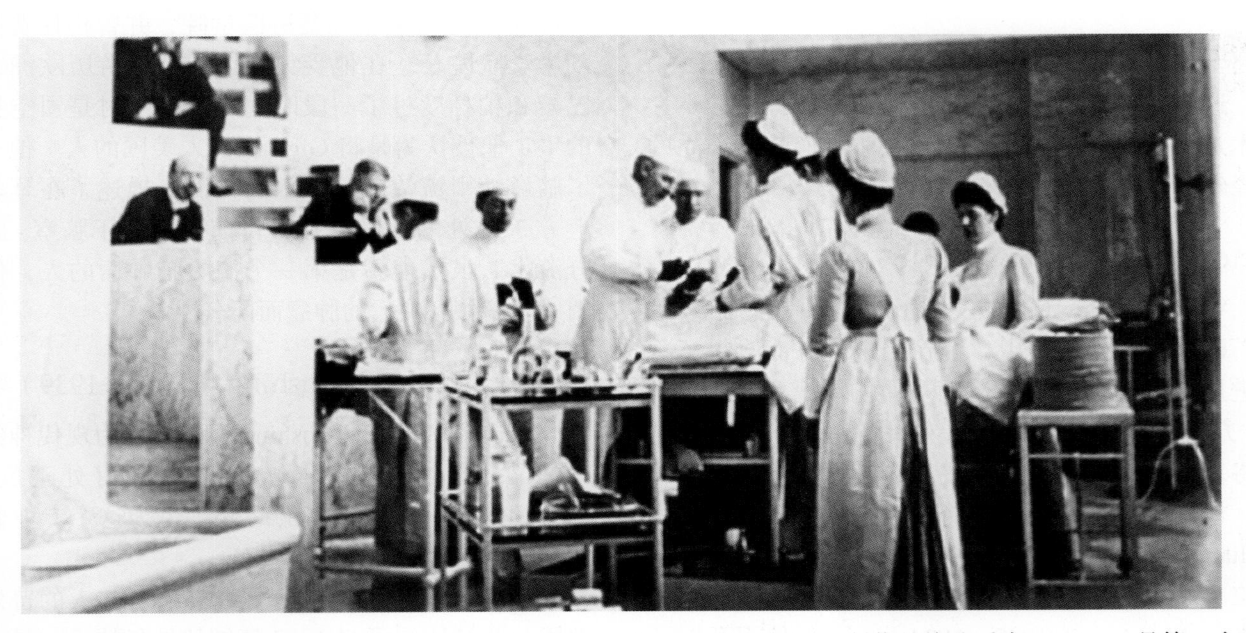

图1.2 Harvey Cushing和William Halsted在手术室的照片。注意一下Goodyear制作的橡胶手套，Halsted是第一个在外科手术中常规使用手套的人

了后来被称为“杰克逊癫痫”的局灶性运动活动，即“身体的各个部位接连受到影响”。他还正确地识别出第三脑神经麻痹使血肿偏向瞳孔固定和扩大的一侧。他指示 Jonathan Hutchinson（1828—1913）根据他判断的位置进行手术，同侧瞳孔扩大被称为“哈钦森瞳孔”。

就在同一时期，David Ferrier（1843—1928）在包括灵长类动物在内的动物身上使用电刺激创建了第一个皮质图谱，其中包括运动皮质的正确位置。他称赞 Hughlings Jackson 预测了他的动物研究结果。Fritz 和 Hitzig 在同一时期使用了类似的皮质刺激技术绘制了狗的脑皮质图谱。

Alexander Hughes Bennett 博士（1848—1901）被认为是第一个仅通过脑定位来指导切除肿瘤的神经病学家。1885 年，他指导 Rickman Godlee（1849—1925）从一位出现对侧局灶性运动癫痫并继发进行性偏瘫的患者身上切除运动区肿瘤。手术很成功，但患者后来死于感染，这种情况在当时经常发生（Bennett and Godlee，1965；Kerr et al.，2005）。

止血法

神经外科手术的发展需要新的方法来应对开颅手术中的大出血。William Bovie（1882—1958）发明了电灼止血的方法，并于 1926 年由 Cushing 首次使用。在 20 世纪初期，输血的发展也很重要。在此之前，开颅手术有时会分阶段进行，每次手术之间要间隔一定的时间，让患者自己的造血功能来补充打开头皮和颅骨时损失的血液。

早期的先驱

这些在麻醉、抗菌、脑定位和止血方面的重大技术进步，为神经外科的早期先驱者们建立独立的神经外科专业奠定了基础。

Victor Horsley（1857—1916）

Victor Horsley（1857—1916）是一名临床医生、研究员和外科医生，他在脑定位方面取得了重大进展。他发表了有关运动皮质的图谱和“内囊排列”方面的著作，并在“颅骨和大脑表面的位置关系”中将表面解剖学与潜在的皮质特征联系起来。1888 年，他是第一个成功切除脊髓肿瘤的人（神经学家 William Gowers 于 1845—1915 年对脊髓肿瘤进行了定位）。他并不是第一个摘除脑肿瘤的人——那是 William Macewen（1848—1924）——但他因开展了几项开创性手术而享有盛誉，其中包括因颅内压升高而施行的颅缝早闭手术和因神经痛而实施的三叉神经后根切断术。他也是第一个做垂体手术的人。他的技术进步包括开发用于治疗骨出血的抗菌骨蜡（至今仍在使用）和 Horsley-Clark 立体定向装置。他本人是一名普外科医生，但在发展神经外科专科领域方面一直走在前列。在皇后广场，他被任命为第一个专门的神经外科医生。遗憾的是，他在第一次世界大战中死于沙漠热。

William Macewen（1848—1924）

William Macewen（1848—1924）出生于苏格兰布特岛的班纳廷港。从 1892 年到 1924 年，他是格拉斯哥大学的外科讲座教授，1909 年被授以爵位，成为国王的外科医生。他对外科的主要贡献是在骨科，创立了植骨术，并为没有四肢的士兵和水手建立了路易斯公主苏格兰医院，他还在那里设计了 Erskine 假肢。1879 年，他成功地从一名 14 岁的女孩身上摘除了脑膜瘤，这被认为是首例脑瘤手术。他不需要当时新颖的脑定位新技术，指导他完成手术的是脑膜瘤外部覆盖着骨质增生。患者出现了外观畸形，随后在病灶对侧出现了难治性癫痫，这为 Macewen 提供了尝试切除的适应证。他坚信无菌外科手术技术，并且在死于其他原因之前，患者还存活了 8 年，且能够工作。他的脑脓肿手术死亡率低，可与现代技术媲美。

William W. Keen（1837—1924）

美国第一位神经外科医生是 William Williams Keen Jr.，他就读于杰斐逊医学院，并曾担任费城解剖学学院院长。在他受教育期间，他游历欧洲，在巴黎和柏林度过了一段时间，这在当时是司空见惯的事。他被认为是将 Gigli 锯引入美国的人。他开创了脑脊液引流治疗脑积水的先河，描述了在耳郭后上方 3cm 处的顶骨钻孔，目前仍常用于脑室 - 腹腔分流术。虽然他不是第一个摘除脑肿瘤的人，但他因成功摘除一些大的肿瘤而闻名。

Harvey Williams Cushing（1869—1939）

Harvey Williams Cushing 通常被视为现代神经外科之父（**图** 1.3 和**图** 1.4）。Cushing 正好处于抗菌、麻醉和脑定位开始发展的时候，也为这个专业做出他的贡献。

他接受了当时的外科教授 Halsted 本人的普外科训练，并被传授了 Halsted 精细的外科技术。另一个对 Cushing 产生重大影响的是 William Osler（1849—

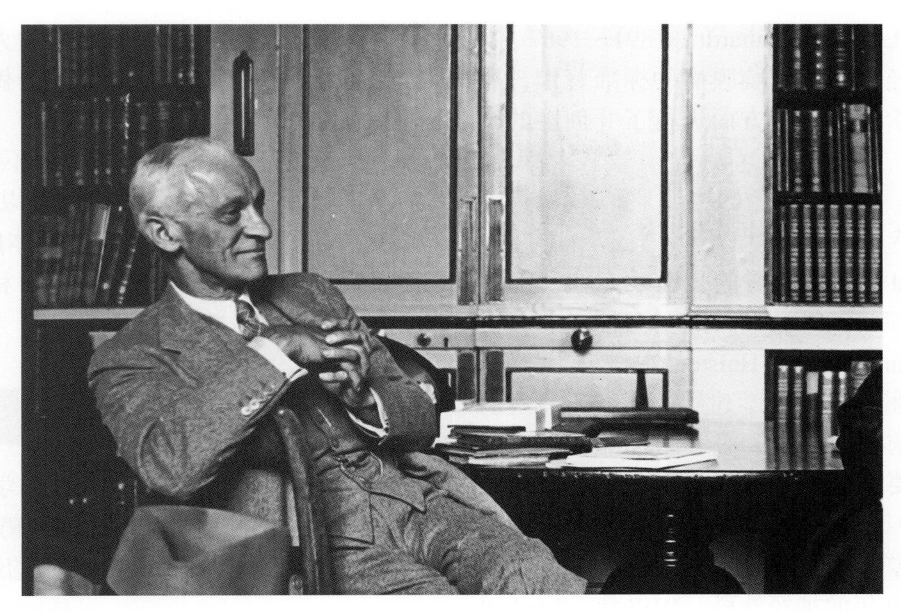

图 1.3　现代神经外科之父 Harvey Cushing

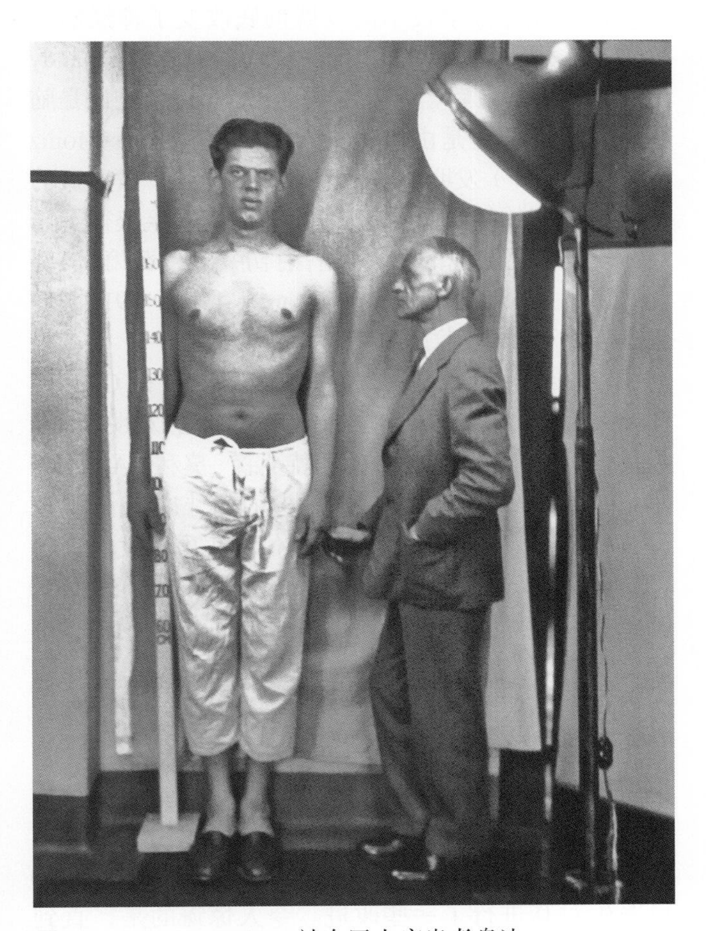

图 1.4　Harvey Cushing 站在巨人症患者身边

Reproduced from Shin P. Harvey Cushing's Ghosts: Death and Hauntings in Modern Medicine. Yale J Biol Med. 2011; 84(2): 91-101

1919），他鼓励 Cushing 在医学的哲学层面进行研究，包括医学史的研究。Cushing 是 Osler 的"锁门者"之一，即住在 Osler 隔壁的学生们，他们被给予了 Osler 拥有大量藏书的图书馆的"锁门钥匙"。

在那些日子里，美国医生花时间去拜访欧洲的同行是很常见的，Osler 鼓励 Cushing 也这样做。Cushing 在伦敦拜访了 Horsley，据他自己说，他对 Horsley"有些失望"。Cushing 本人是一名一丝不苟的外科医生，他形容 Horsley 的技术"是恶劣的"，并评论说 Horsley 身上一定有很多"脓毒性伤口"。事实上，Horsley 当时认为"脑真菌感染"（即感染）的死亡率为 30%~50%。

Cushing 随后前往法国和瑞士，在伯尔尼与 Kocher 一起工作。与他所写的关于 Horsley 的文章相反，他评论 Kocher 的技术是"详细的""烦琐的"和"绝对止血的"。Cushing 在颅内压方面的开创性工作就是当时在 Kronecker 实验室开始的。正是在这里，他发现了"当颅内张力升高时，血压会上升到略高于对髓质施加压力的水平"——现在被称为库欣反射。之后，他又去了意大利，在那里，他对 Scipione Riva-Rocci 设计的血压计印象深刻，于是他将其带回了美国。

1901—1910 年是神经外科的关键十年。Cushing 认识到颅内压升高和精细的手术技术的重要性。于是，他主导引入了术中血压监测，并根据他自己的患者在手术台上死亡的经验，还引入了麻醉图表来记录手术过程中的脉搏和呼吸。他与 Percival Bailey

（1892—1973）和 Louise Eisenhardt（1891—1967）共同撰写了有关神经胶质瘤和脑膜瘤的标准著作，并在脑垂体疾病的诊断和治疗方面进行了开创性的工作。

Walter Dandy（1886—1946）

Walter Edward Dandy 学习的是医学专业，随后在约翰·霍普金斯医院度过了他的整个职业生涯（**图 1.5**）。他和 Cushing 同属于 Halsted 外科时代，是 Cushing 在约翰·霍普金斯大学建立的亨特实验室的研究助理。他在脑脊液产生和吸收方面的工作证实了脉络膜丛的重要性，并使我们对婴儿脑积水的认识取得了进展。

他在"脑室充气造影术"（1918）方面的工作彻底改变了接下来 60 年的神经外科。1913 年，Luckett 描述了颅腔积气的放射学表现，但 Dandy 发明了一种技术，通过这种技术，脑室气体造影（也被称为气脑造影）可以让阅片者通过脑室中产生的扭曲来推断髓内肿块的位置。在 20 世纪 70 年代计算机断层扫描（computed tomography，CT）扫描仪问世之前，这一技术与 1927 年 Moniz 发现的脑血管造影技术一起成为影像诊断的基石。此前，Cushing 等曾使用 X 射线来识别髓外肿块，如鞍区病变，但在气脑造影技术被引入之前，髓内病变只能通过大脑定位的临床技能来诊断。1921 年，他是第一个做胶样囊肿手术的外科医生。

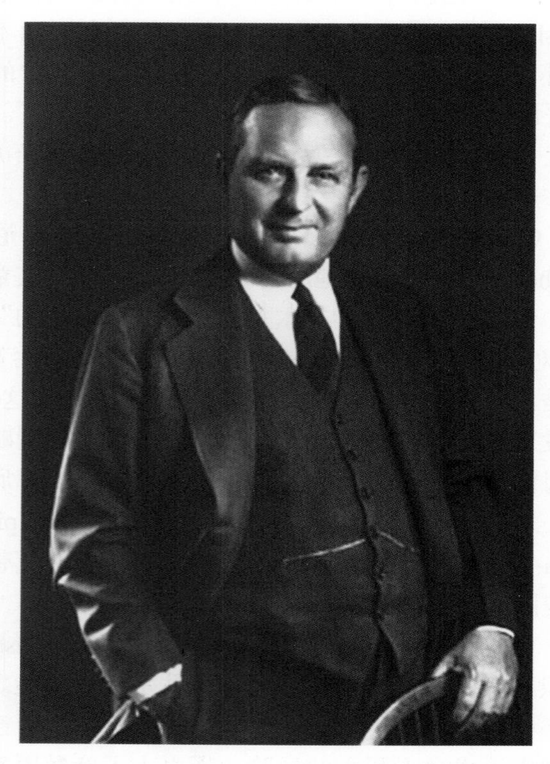

图 1.5 Walter Dandy 是 Cushing 的学生及后来的竞争对手，对神经外科做出了数个关键的贡献

他主张全切除听神经瘤，而不是 Cushing 更保守的不全切除，他切除第五脑神经以治疗三叉神经痛，并发展了经胼胝体入路到松果体的方法。1929 年，他发现椎间盘破裂是马尾综合征和双侧坐骨神经痛的病因。

从 20 世纪末至今

近几十年来，随着介入放射学治疗动脉瘤和立体定向放射外科治疗小前庭神经鞘瘤等技术的发展，技术的发展在很大程度源于科技的进步。

技术的进步

诊断性影像学

诊断性影像学技术的发展彻底改变了神经病学的诊断（并引入了偶然发现的现代问题）。继 Dandy 的气脑造影术之后，成像技术的下一个主要进展是脑血管造影术。这是由 Antonio Caetano de Egas Moniz（1874—1935）发明的，他后来因发明了广遭质疑的治疗精神病的脑叶白质切除术而在 1949 年获得了诺贝尔奖（他还被他的一个患者射伤并导致截瘫）。脊髓造影术是由 Jean Athanase Sicard（1872—1919）提出的，它可以识别脊柱的较大病变。

X 射线和计算机技术的并行发展使得 Godfrey Hounsfield（1919—2004）在 EMI 基础上发明了 CT 扫描仪。1971 年，在伦敦的阿特金森·莫利（Atkinson Morley）医院，第一次对患者进行 CT 扫描，证实他患有右额叶肿瘤。20 世纪 80 年代，正电子发射型计算机断层显像（positron emission tomography，PET）和磁共振成像（magnetic resonance imaging，MRI）迅速发展起来。

手术显微镜

1927 年斯德哥尔摩的 Gunnar Holmgren 是双目显微镜的先驱之一，它的第一次临床应用是由耳鼻喉科医生用于治疗中耳炎。并且，耳鼻喉（ENT）科医生对其进行了一些改进。令人惊讶的是，直到 1957 年显微镜才首次用于神经外科。Theodor Kurze 显然是受到耳鼻喉科医生 William House 使用手术显微镜的电影的启发，用它来切除一个 5 岁孩子的神经鞘瘤。

在神经外科领域还有无数其他的进步。例如，内镜的使用改变了颅底外科手术，脑室 - 腹腔分流术的引入从根本上改变了我们治疗脑积水的方法。相对而言，这些技术仍处于起步阶段，至少在本世纪内还会继续发展。

脊柱神经外科史

虽然本章主要关注颅脑神经外科的历史，但脊柱外科的发展也不应被忽视。《艾德温 · 史密斯纸草文稿》再一次向我们生动地描述了古埃及处理脊柱创伤的方式。古埃及人，尤其是 Imhotep（被认为是世界上第一个医生）将临床图景与管理计划和预后联系起来的能力是显著的。病例 31 清楚地描述了继发于颈椎脱位的完全性脊髓损伤——早于 1858 年 Brown-Séquard 关于脊髓定位的论文几十个世纪。

古希腊 Herophilus 学派描述了第一个牵引装置，主张矫正创伤后继发的脊柱后凸。Hippocrates 认为，移位的椎骨对“脊髓”的压迫是导致瘫痪的原因。与古埃及一样，如果患者是瘫痪的，则不建议进行治疗。Celsus 和 Galen 也不主张手术，他们认识到脊髓损伤的不良预后，特别是发生排尿功能障碍。Celsus 认识到高颈椎病变与四肢瘫痪和呼吸障碍有关，而胸腔病变导致截瘫。Galen（131—201）创造了脊柱后凸、脊柱前凸和脊柱侧凸等术语。值得注意的是，他也是在 Percival Pott（1713—1788）之前几百年第一个描述结核性脊髓疾病的人。在实验中，他证明了脊髓横断导致病变水平以下功能丧失，他还提出了自主行为的信号是沿着脊髓传递的新的脑概念。埃伊纳岛的 Paulus（624—690）是第一个提倡脊椎手术的人，他切除了瘫痪的受伤患者身上的骨片。有趣的是，在早期提及“知情同意”时，他形容自己的手术是“在告知危险之后”进行的。

在中世纪和欧洲的“黑暗时代”，脊柱外科进展甚微。医学的中心地位转移到了阿拉伯世界。以前从 Alexander 学派和 Herophilus 学派获得的知识通过将拉丁文献翻译成阿拉伯语得以保存，但并没有取得任何重大进展。一个值得注意的例外是土耳其医生 Sabunuoglu（公元前 1385 年），他为我们提供了治疗坐骨神经痛的第一个描述——也是第一个描述退行性而非创伤性的脊柱疾病。直到 1764 年，Cotugno 才推测神经压迫是坐骨神经痛的根源，后来法国神经学家 Lasegue、Dejerine 和 Sicard 才建立了这个模型。

在 18 世纪和 19 世纪，欧洲启蒙运动时期，现代脊柱外科的基础建立起来。Percival Pott（1713—1788）描述了他现在同名的结核性脊柱疾病，并成功冲洗了椎旁脓肿。John Bell（1763—1826）描述了与脊髓损伤有关的弛缓性痉挛性瘫痪和括约肌障碍。关于脊椎手术，他在 1799 年曾说过“切开脊椎是一场梦”。1814 年，伦敦圣托马斯医院的外科医生 Cline 先生为一名从阳台上摔下来后截瘫的男子手术，这被誉为脊椎第一次“钻孔术”。他进行了椎板切除术并摘除小关节以减少脱位，但患者死亡。有军史上的报道说 Villedon 上尉因胸部枪伤导致脊髓受伤，Louis 外科医生给 Villedon 上尉做过手术，据报道 Villedon 上尉术后恢复了一些远端功能。

手术仍因其高死亡率和发病率而备受争议，直到抗菌术（Lister 1882—1912 和 Semmelweiss 1818—1865）和安全的全身麻醉的出现。脊髓定位反映了大脑定位（Blesius 在 1666 年进行的早期工作，他描述了灰质 - 白质的分化）和前后脊髓神经根。Mistichelli 在 1709 年描述了锥体的交叉，Huber 在 1739 年描述了齿状韧带。Rolando 在 1809 年描述了胶质区，Brown-Séquard 在 1846 年发表了对感觉束交叉的描述。Brown-Séquard 是脊髓损伤手术的有力倡导者，他对脊髓定位的贡献和对脊髓束的描述跟与他的同名的脊髓半切综合征永记史册。19 世纪，Rauber、Weber 和 Messerer 在体内和体外对脊柱的生物力学做了进一步的研究。

在 19 世纪晚期，脊柱手术仍然主要局限于创伤和感染（trauma and infection，TB）。在 Cotugno 描述坐骨神经痛的神经压迫大约两个世纪后，Oppenheim 和 Kruse 描述了首个椎间盘突出手术（1909）。Mixter 和 Barr 在 1933 年充分描述了椎间盘突出的发病机制，并提出“经硬膜”入路治疗椎间盘突出。1977 年，Caspar 和 Yasargil 描述了现今使用的椎板内硬膜外入路显微手术。对这些发展至关重要的还是 1895 年 Roentgen 发现了 X 射线，这从根本上改善了脊柱骨折的诊断。以前认为脊柱骨折几乎总是与神经功能缺陷有关（90%）。Sudeck 对 X 射线进行了系统的解释，并确定大多数完整患者的骨折都被遗漏了，因此瘫痪的真实概率更接近 15%~20%。影像学技术的出现，如 CT（70 年代）和 MR（80 年代），对退行性脊柱疾病手术的发展同样产生了巨大的影响。

尽管一些关键的脊柱手术“第一次”是由 19 世纪的外科医生创造的，但直到 20 世纪，成像和材料科学的进步才使脊柱手术领域扩展到脊柱固定。脊柱所有部位的前、后、外侧入路均得到发展。由于颈椎的生物力学强度较差，且邻近重要的神经和血管结构，颈椎具有特殊的挑战。在过去的 50~100 年里，我们看到了从上世纪50年代Bailey和Badgley首次提出的不带任何植骨的前路椎间盘减压（anterior cervical discectomy，ACD）的颈椎前路手术到1958年Cloward与之后的Smith和Robinson提出的ACD和颈椎前路间盘切除减压融合术（anterior cervical discectomy fusion，ACDF）的发展。第一个颈椎前路钢板是由Orozco和Lovet设计的，需要双皮质螺钉，这在技术上是具有挑战性的地方。由于技术和生物力学的进步，笔者在2000年引入了单皮质锁定螺钉和可变角度螺钉的动态载荷共享板。在此期间，下位脊柱的后入路也受益于材料科学的进步，其中包括强低突型螺钉，并且颈椎后路固定已经从第一次在1891年的颈椎后路固定中银导线的使用，经过椎间导线（Rogers 1942）、椎板下导线（1970）和锥面导线，最终80年代发展到Roy-Camille侧块螺钉。脊柱固定的历史本身就值得用单独一章进行介绍。关键的进展是提出骨科医生用于长骨骨折的切开复位内固定的原则，并将其应用于脊柱。1953年，Holdsworth和Hardy描述了一种钢板和螺钉系统。经椎弓根螺钉内固定术于1944年由King提出，但直到1959年Boucher才应用。1958年，Harrington介绍了他的脊柱侧凸矫正系统——最初是用于脊髓灰质炎引起的脊柱侧凸，后来用于特发性病变。腹侧脊柱侧凸手术于1964年由Dwyer首次提出。椎间盘手术的早期重点是保持运动和避免僵硬，后来，当椎间盘突出的病理被发现是继发于不稳定和融合时，这个问题就受到了挑战。与此相反，其他人则专注于开发Fernstrom于1966年提出的能保持运动的椎间盘置换，并于1975年由Froning申请专利（尽管从未植入）。charité椎间盘是目前最常用的人工椎间盘。

硬膜内脊髓肿瘤手术的进展与颅脑手术相似，1887年Horsley首次成功切除了硬膜内肿瘤。1907年，Elsberg进行了首次成功的髓内肿瘤切除手术，并描述了脊髓切开术的两个阶段技术，然后在第二次时进行肿瘤切除。Dandy发明的气脑造影技术对脊柱也很有用，当然，手术显微镜的引入大大提高了硬膜内和髓内切除术的成功率。

脊柱外科的技术进步日新月异。在微创手术、图像引导螺钉置入和内镜入路方面的最新进展都是在过去30年里发展起来的。20世纪90年代的胸腔镜椎间盘切除术和融合术已经发展到使用最小通路治疗脊柱侧凸和椎体切除。腹腔镜椎间盘切除术也在同一时期发展起来。内镜之父Desormenaux在1853年也很难预见到它现在的无数应用。脊柱外科仍然是一个快速发展的领域，目前的人口结构意味着将不乏对脊柱创伤、感染，当然还有退行性脊柱疾病的治疗需求。

神经外科的未来

在过去的100年里，神经外科在实践中取得了巨大的进步。未来很可能会看到从开颅手术到微创、内镜和放射引导介入技术的进一步发展。

参考文献

扫描书末二维码获取。

第2章 临床评估

Peter Bodkin・Elizabeth Visser 著
秦涵、韩春雷、王会志 译，孟凡刚、蔡国恩、冯涛 审校

引言

现代神经外科的实际临床评估过程与传统模式略有不同。由 William Osler 和其他临床方法学先驱制订的病史采集和查体的基本规则，仍然是目前临床评估的核心，但我们也必须考虑到患者在神经外科医生首诊之前的病史情况。如今，无论是在病房还是门诊，我们已很少会去了解相关的病史资料——事实上，我们往往会看到能非常详尽描述患者的病理解剖学细节的高质量的影像资料。转诊医生很可能已提供了鉴别诊断列表。换句话说，在我们接诊患者之前，患者的病情资料通常已被整齐地准备好了。

然而，我们的工作不仅仅是为既定的问题提供手术治疗。我们不仅仅是手术技术人员。虽然必须认真考虑提供给我们的信息，但我们决不能粗浅地来看待这些信息。临床评估中各种失误和错误的结论可能一直存在。同样，虽然影像学非常有价值，但不应脱离临床背景。MRI 扫描能比顶尖的临床医生更准确地定位病变，但检查技术不能让我们从一个握手中拟诊出肢端肥大症，或从患者进入门诊的脚步声音诊断出是否存在腓总神经麻痹。

当我们收集并了解这些病史信息时，临床中有一项同样、甚至是更加重要的工作。通过将患者的症状置于其日常生活的背景下，我们开始与患者建立相互信任和理解的关系。这里建立的融洽的医患关系将是患者衡量我们干预措施成败的基础。

大多数教科书中描述的传统神经病学临床评估与神经外科医生所需的评估存在细微差异。本章旨在为神经外科执业医师和培训医生提供所需要的临床评估方法。

神经外科病史采集

神经外科病史采集的主要目的是获得充足的信息来定位病变的解剖位置，并在工作中获得对发病过程的印象。特别是症状的持续时间和严重程度，这将成为是否需要手术干预以及何时进行干预的重要指导。

与任何重要事件一样，充分的准备将提供良好的第一印象，并且从长远来看也会节约时间。应仔细查阅转诊记录、临床记录、影像学和其他检查。事先与相关团队成员进行讨论也是有益的。

在门诊，自己亲自从候诊室召唤患者是非常有价值的。可通过查看患者与谁在一起，以及他们的关系密切程度来获悉患者的社交情况。可以通过了解患者站立和进入诊室需要的时间，以及气喘程度来粗略评估其麻醉耐受性。这也是一个评估步态和是否需要辅助行走以及其他事项的合适时机。

会诊的环境也需要注意。患者和医生应尽可能处于同一水平面上。应该意识到，俯视或坐在桌子后面可能会产生会令人生畏的印象，会降低此次会诊的效果。若需要查看影像资料，软件平台需提前打开并下载完毕相关的图像。

自我介绍要清楚，介绍您的名字和职位。其他重要的人也可一并进行介绍，但应该明确患者才是谈论的核心。

如何开始问诊很重要。应该从开放性问题开始，“有什么不舒服吗”或“需要我提供什么帮助”。转诊记录或会诊记录倾向于强调症状，这会吸引您首先去看患者的症状。因此，明智的做法是避免说“你的医生是要让我看你的面部疼痛吗”。假设可能具有误导性，并可能会使患者告诉您预期想听到的内容。

一旦您让患者讲述他们的病史时，可能需要补充询问一些内容。患者可能只讲了大致情况，但可能遗漏很多内容或只有粗略的基本细节。当涉及可能影响您治疗决策的信息时，应继续进一步追问，直至您感觉有满意的细节可以得出结论。在此过程中，询问患者的职业和惯用手很重要。患者仅说“退休”是不够的。因退休的大学教授与退休的造船师对生活的期望值会有很大的不同。

病史采集需要包括时间进程、症状的解剖定位、不同的症状和特征。须详细询问来定位病变或获得关于潜在病理过程的线索。如果有患者未主动说出的症状，则必须考虑可能相关的症状，并直接询问这些症状。例如，在评估因右顶叶肿瘤导致空间定向障碍的患者时，需要记住询问其视野问题，如考虑是否累及视放射等，以此类推。

病史中最重要的部分通常是询问病情对患者生活方式的影响。看似不必要，其实大多数患者很高兴让您知道他们的问题，以及疾病对他们的家庭、工作和生活的一系列影响。当您不仅对处理患者特定的疾病本身感兴趣，而且希望帮助患者回到他们喜欢的事情上来，您已经将医学会诊转变为更有意义的对话。患者将明白您正在治疗他们，而不仅仅是治疗他们的肿瘤或突出的椎间盘。

收集线索，留心不协调的地方。如果你听到的信息没有意义，那就去继续深入问诊，不要忽略有用的信息。了解到截至目前的疾病诊疗过程也很有用：止痛药、理疗、注射、其他医生的诊断等。患者适合麻醉吗？手术前是否需要停用药物？不健康的生活方式会导致该病吗？

根据病史得出结论，患者应感觉其问题已得到充分解决。“您还有什么想了解的吗？”是允许表达任何附加信息的有用方式。到会诊的这一阶段，患者有望处于更放松和开放的心态，并可能揭示潜在的目的和担忧。最后，确定一个简短的病情摘要，并尽力理清任何不确定或不一致之处。

神经外科体格检查

意识障碍患者的检查

对意识水平改变的患者，所采用的检查方法会因患者无法听从指示并进行口头反馈而受到明显限制。因此，我们只能进行粗略的和基本的床旁检查［即检查瞳孔对光反应和格拉斯哥昏迷评分（Glasgow Coma Scale，GCS）］。通常高风险的决定是根据这些评估作出的，因此要极其谨慎地进行这些评估，同时注意可能的干扰因素（**表 2.1**）。

瞳孔反应障碍可能是由于传入和传出通路中多个位置受损所致。眼眶的直接创伤可引起瞳孔括约肌断裂，产生外伤性瞳孔散大。外伤性视神经病变可能是由于穿透伤所致的直接破坏，也可能是头部钝性创伤中剪切力间接破坏所致。顶盖前核或中脑头侧的Edinger-Westphal核的病变也会引起瞳孔散大。

表 2.1　GCS 评估中的干扰因素

格拉斯哥昏迷评分（GCS 评估）	干扰因素
睁眼 （4 = 自动睁眼，3 = 呼唤睁眼，2 = 刺痛睁眼，1 = 不睁眼）	眼眶损伤 眼睑淤血 畏光
言语反应 （5 = 定向正常，4 = 言语混乱，3 = 言语错误，2 = 言语难以理解，1 = 不语）	非母语者 颌面部损伤 气管插管 / 气管切开 失聪
运动反应 （6 = 遵嘱运动，5 = 刺痛定位，4 = 刺痛屈曲 / 退缩，3 = 刺痛异常屈曲，2 = 刺痛伸展，1 = 无运动）	脊髓损伤 上肢骨折、石膏和固定

包括同侧下丘脑在内的多种来源的复杂调节通路调节交感神经性瞳孔张力。皮质下行控制癫痫发作后瞳孔异常，表现为同侧或对侧瞳孔散大或瞳孔缩小，目前对此知之甚少（Plum and Posner, 2007）。因此，许多脑区的损伤可能导致瞳孔异常（**图 2.1**）。在神经外科临床实践中，颞叶钩回疝沿第Ⅲ对脑神经压迫副交感神经纤维是瞳孔异常的常见原因。

格拉斯哥昏迷评分（GCS）纳入了多种临床特征，为评估整体脑功能提供了指导。在三个部分（睁眼、言语反应和运动反应）中，运动反应最有可能区分损伤的严重程度。红核以上的病变产生去皮质强直（上肢屈曲和下肢伸展，红核脊髓束功能），红核以下的病变产生去大脑强直（上下肢伸展，前庭脊髓束功能）。正常屈曲（M4）为屈曲伴旋后；异常屈曲（M3）为屈曲伴旋前，类似于去皮质强直和如前所述的红核脊髓束功能的释放；伸展（M2）类似于去大脑强直和前庭脊髓束功能的释放。在脊髓损伤引起外周感觉麻木的情况下，最好的方法是对三叉神经区域施加疼痛刺激，如压迫眶上切迹。

血压升高、心率下降和呼吸模式改变（库欣三联征）是颅内压升高的典型反应，但通常是晚期的濒死特征。

语言和言语障碍检查

认识到任何言语和语言的异常非常重要，因为这可能影响病史采集、神经系统检查和高级功能评估，从而总体上影响接诊的结果。正确识别言语障碍有助于神经系统病变的定位。当我们通过语言进

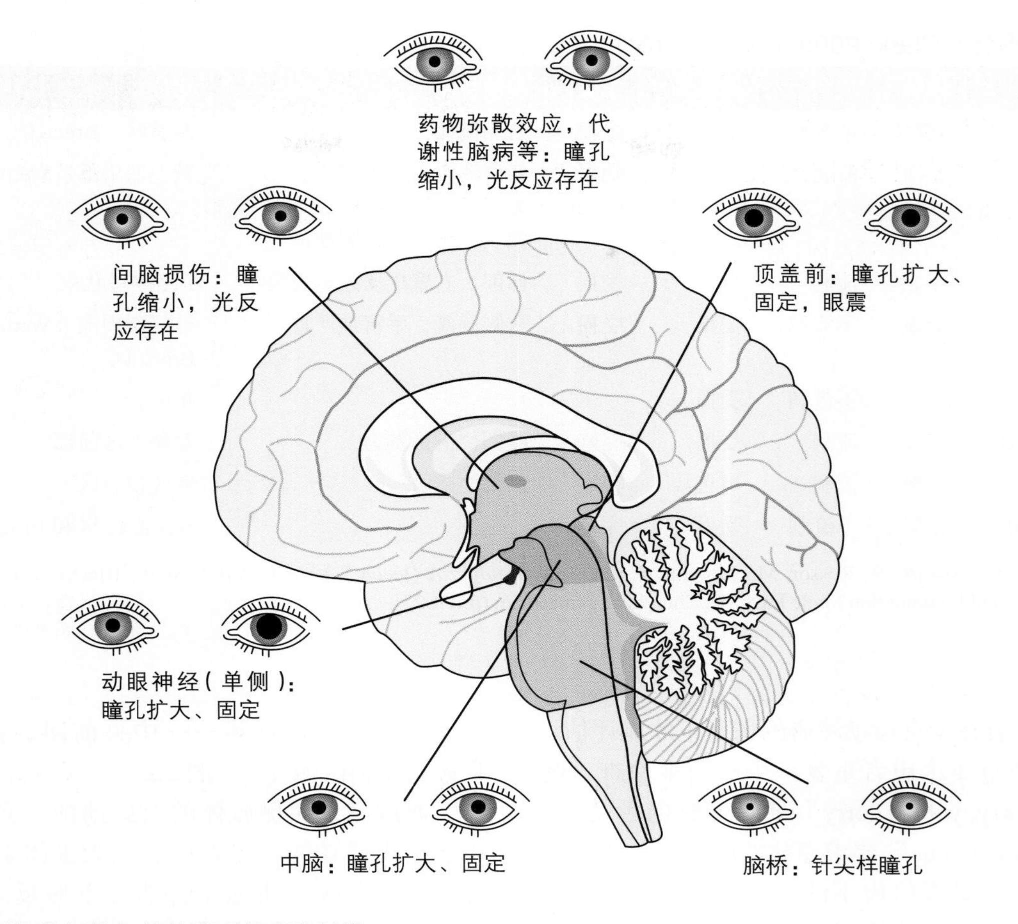

图 2.1　与解剖部位损伤相关的典型的瞳孔异常

行交流时，听力、理解、发声、发音、意识、思维和找词功能必须完好无损。语言是声音、写作和意义组合的复杂相互作用，通常与文化背景相关联。

通过让患者参与正常的对话并询问简单的问题，以评估患者的语言理解情况：您的名字是什么？您的职业是什么？您今天是怎么来的？确保患者能清楚地听到您的声音，并询问他们的母语是什么。确定患者是左利手还是右利手。根据经验，99% 的右利手患者的优势半球在左脑；左利手患者中，60% 的人为左半球优势，20% 为双侧优势，20% 为右半球优势。

以下为不同类型的语言障碍：

1. 失语症——定义为一种口语障碍。分为以下几个亚类：
   1.1 非流畅性失语（前头部、运动性或 Broca 失语）；
   1.2 流畅性失语（后头部、感觉性或 Wernicke 失语）；
   1.3 传导性失语症；
   1.4 经皮质性失语（感觉性和运动性）。
2. 失读症或阅读障碍是一种获得性阅读能力障碍。
3. 失写症或书写不能，定义为书面语言障碍。
4. 构音障碍是一种发音或言语障碍。
5. 发声困难是指呼气在振动的声带上产生声音的异常。

对这些异常的进一步检查包括评估自发言语、流畅性、命名、重复、发音、言语量、阅读和书写，并将有助于病理定位。

1. 失语症评估

   评估自发言语、流畅性以及患者是否使用了错误的单词（失语症）。要求患者在 1min 内说出以“F”开头的动物名称或单词。这测试了找词能力。还要求他们说出熟悉的物体的名称：一支钢笔、一只手表、一条领带等。然后要求患者重复短语。**表** 2.2 总结了检查和病理定位的结果。
2. 评估失读症或阅读障碍，要求患者阅读句子或执行书面命令。
3. 失写症或书写不能，可以通过要求患者写出句子

表 2.2 失语评估（Clark, 2009; Fuller, 2013）

	理解	流利	命名	重复	其他特点	定位
非流畅性失语	完好	不流利	受损	受损	右侧偏瘫，抑郁	左额叶、Broca 区
流畅性失语	受损	流利	可正常	受损	新词的使用 无意义言语 偏执，可能有视野缺损	颞上回后部、Wernicke 区
传导性失语	完好	流利	受损	受损	抑郁，右臂皮质感觉丧失	顶盖 / 弓状束
完全性失语	受损	不流利	受损	受损	右侧偏瘫，手臂最严重	外侧裂周围、Wernicke 区和 Broca 区
命名性失语症		不流利	受损			角回
皮质运动性失语	完好	流利	受损	完好	停顿，讲话费力	左额上区前部
皮质感觉性失语	受损	流利	可正常	完好	语义性错语	颞枕顶后区
皮质混合性失语	受损	不流利	受损	完好		Wernicke 区和 Broca 区同时受损

Data from Clarke, C; Howard, R; Rossor, M; Shorvon, S. (2009) *Neurology: A Queen Square Textbook*. Wiley-Blackwell (p. 252–4), Fuller, G. (2004) Neurological Examination Made Easy, 3e. Churchill Livingstone. (p. 17–25).

来检查。只有在没有运动障碍的情况下才能评估。

4. 构音障碍通过要求患者重复一个短语来检查。例如，“red lorry, yellow lorry”要求完整的舌功能，“baby hippopotamus”要求完整的唇功能。注意说话的节奏以及是否口齿不清。构音障碍可以描述为痉挛性（由假性延髓麻痹引起，如运动神经元病）、锥体外系（与帕金森综合征相关，通常与发声困难相关）、小脑性构音障碍（与多发性硬化、酒精中毒或遗传性共济失调相关）和下运动神经元性构音障碍（累及腭部运动的病变引起的鼻音，累及舌运动的病变引起字母“T”和“S”费力，以及累及面部运动的病变导致字母“B”“P”“M”和“W”发音困难，常累及后组脑神经）。
5. 最后听讲话的音量，如果下降，则描述为语音发音困难。

脑叶检查

对每个脑叶功能的检查应是神经外科医师评估中熟知的部分。然而，我们应该了解脑叶之间的大致分界，而且，如果病变在分界脑沟上或附近时，我们应检查多个脑叶。在解剖学上，Yasargil 的 7 脑叶系统广为人知（额叶、中央叶、顶叶、枕叶、颞叶、岛叶和边缘系统；参见 Ribas，2010），但在这里我们将使用额叶、顶叶、颞叶、枕叶和小脑。

额叶

由于额叶体积最大，因此，额叶检查的部位也最多，复杂性也最大（**专栏 2.1**）。在解剖学上，需考虑四个不同的区域——中央前回、背外侧皮质、眶额皮质和内侧皮质（**图 2.2**）。

通过测试对侧肢体的上运动神经元体征评估初级运动皮质功能。患者可表现为锥体束无力的典型姿势（即上肢屈肌强于伸肌，下肢反之）。手旋前试验是典型的神经外科测试方法，有助于检出细微的肌力下降。初级运动皮质前方的外侧区域为前运动皮质，内侧为辅助运动区（supplementary motor area，SMA）。这些区域的功能复杂，但与初级运动皮质有共同作用。紧邻初级运动皮质前方的皮质区（Brodmann 区 6）包括外侧的运动前区和内侧半球间的 SMA 区。外侧的运动前区与小脑有相互联系，并与外部感觉信息的运动细化有关。SMA 与基底神经节具有相互联系，并参与内部感觉信息的运动启动。与初级运动皮质的“小矮人图（homunculus）”（腿内侧、上肢、面部和舌外侧）相反，SMA 的“小矮人

专栏 2.1 额叶评估方案

- 询问左右利手情况并评估言语
- 观察行为——不语、衣着不当、言语障碍
- 姿势 / 步态——去皮质，“磁性步态”（magnetic）
- 锥体束性无力
- 眼球扫视运动
- 原始反射
- 需要导尿
- 嗅觉丧失和 Foster Kennedy 综合征
- 神经心理学测试——模仿动作、持续动作、概念化、工作记忆

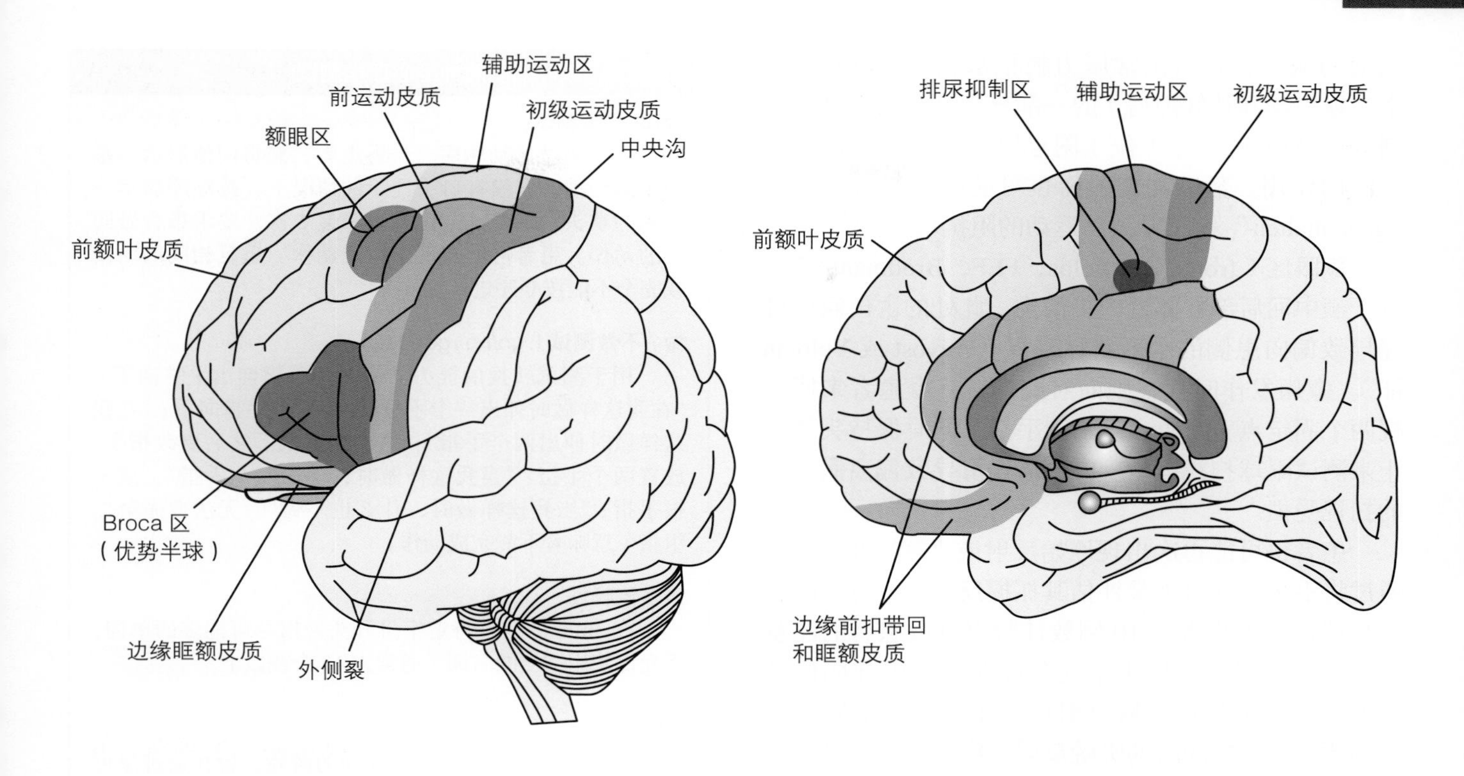

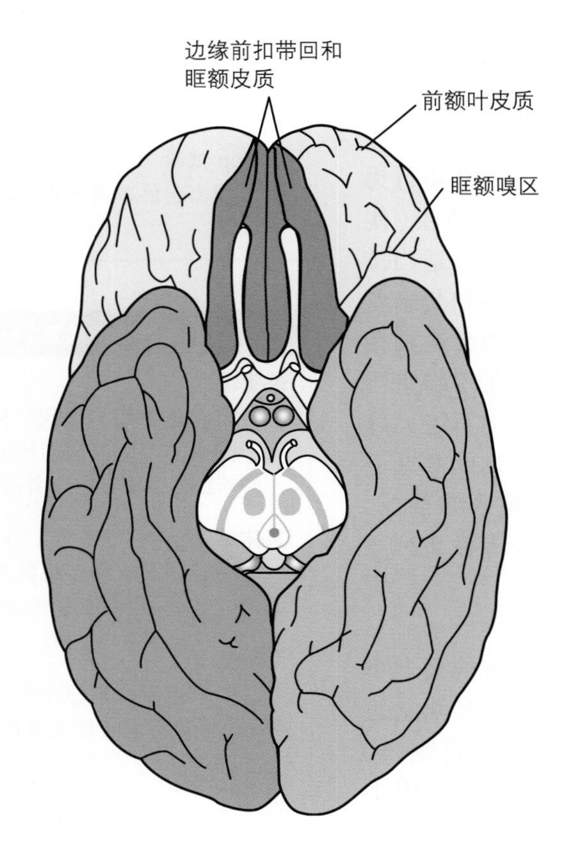

图 2.2 额叶

Neuroanatomy through Clinical Cases, 1st Edition by Blumenfeld (2002) Fig.19.11 p. 848. By permission of Oxford University Press, USA.

图”呈水平排列（腿后部邻近旁中央小叶，腿部、上肢为初级运动区，然后面部和舌更靠前）。SMA 在行走启动、序列化运动中的保持姿势稳定性以及身体两侧的协调中发挥作用。额叶共济失调引起特征性的磁性步态，患者走路时脚好像粘在地板上（Brun 失用症）。这与帕金森步态有相似之处，但没有手臂摆动的减少。它是正常压力脑积水临床三联征（步态、尿失禁和认知障碍）的一部分。这反映了排尿抑制区（SMA 正下方）位于附近以及额叶在认知中更广泛的作用。额叶功能障碍也可能引起非自主抗拒“gegenhalten”——对被动运动的阻抗增加。

额眼区（frontal eye fields，FEF，Brodmann8 区）位于额中回后部并邻近中央前沟。此处的占位病变可能导致偏向患侧的水平共轭凝视（Prévost 或 Vulpian 征）。癫痫发作时视线则向对侧偏转。令患者来回注视两个固定点（例如，拳头和手指）同时保持头部静止来测试眼球扫视运动。FEF 损伤可导致偏离病变侧的扫视受损。

患者也可能再次出现原始反射或“额叶释放征”。通过将手指轻穿过手掌评估其抓握反射。最可靠的方法是通过要求患者从 10 倒数计数以分散患者的注意力。掌颏反射是抚摸手掌大鱼际肌时，引起同侧颏肌的短暂收缩反应。唇反射可见于在敲击上唇时或当物体压在两唇间时的吸吮反射。眉间敲击也可能引起持续眨眼，在正常个体中此反射减弱。应该记住，这些反射很可能见于正常个体，尤其是老年人（25% 的正常成人有掌反射；见 Brazis et al.，2011）。

前额叶区域包含大量在行为控制中具有复杂作用的脑区。这些行为控制作用可分为克制性（将行为限制在社会和文化上可以接受的行为）、主动性（使想法付诸行动的动机）和秩序性（对任务进行适当排序；参阅 Blumenfeld，2002）。简单地观察和与患者交谈就可以深入了解这一点。显然，可能会遇到相当矛盾的行为，一些患者缺乏任何类型的“起立行走”（get up and go），而另一些患者则滔滔不绝、过度自来熟或不老练。一般而言，意志缺失更常见于背外侧凸面的病变，去抑制通常是眶额区的特征。有许多反应额叶功能的神经心理学测试（**专栏 2.2**）。

顶叶

顶叶（**图 2.3**）可分为中央后回、后方的顶上小叶和顶下小叶（角回和缘上回）。躯体感觉和知觉的处理位于中央后回（单模态）；后部接收来自躯体、视觉和其他感觉模式的多模态同化输入，主要用于控制运动，尤其是手和上肢（Kolb and Whishaw，2009）。左顶下小叶在语言中起作用，这将在语言部分进行讨论。顶叶疾病可致感觉受损。然而，由于许多躯体感觉是在丘脑处理的，因此不会有完全的麻木，而是更细微的损伤。这些可以通过感觉消退、姿势失认症、感觉障碍和两点辨别觉来测试（**专栏 2.3**）。

专栏 2.2 额叶功能的神经心理学测试

Luria 三步测试

用于测试运动顺序。告诉患者，您将向他展示一系列手部运动。在没有口头提示的情况下，按顺序演示一系列的拳头、掌缘、掌面，并重复 5 次。要求患者做同样的动作。患者可能表现出持续动作、重复相同的动作或完全不能按顺序进行。

做 / 不做测试（go/no-go test）

用于测试转换的能力。将两个手指伸出手掌向下：“在我这样做时伸出一个手指”，将一个手指向下；“在我这样做时伸出两个手指”。这样做几次。然后更改指令。放置两个手指：“当我这样做时，伸出一个手指”，放一根手指；“当我这样做时，什么也不做”。无法遵循第二组指令意味着不能完成动作。

语言流畅性

在 1min 内，以特定字母开头说出尽可能多的单词，不允许使用适当的名词。通常为 12 个或以上。

汉诺塔游戏

将堆栈的碟子在立柱间移动的游戏，旨在通过尽可能少的移动来实现目标。

Wisconsin 卡片分类测验

这是一个测试执行功能卡片匹配试验。

Stroop 试验

读出彩色单词列表（即黄色文本中的绿色单词）。约束试验。

专栏 2.3 顶叶功能检查（任意半球）

感觉减退

要求患者闭上眼睛、伸出手臂。触摸身体相应部位的一侧或双侧，并询问他被触摸的部位。当患者说只有一侧被触碰而实际上两者都被触碰时，即为感觉减退。

实体觉

患者闭上眼睛，将熟悉的物体放在手中，要求他们识别。可使用不同面值的硬币。

图形觉

要求患者识别您在其手掌上描出的数字或字母。在测试开始之前，应该就采用哪种测试方式达成一致。

两点分辨觉

使用卡尺或弯曲的纸夹，询问患者是否能感觉到一个点或两个点。在指尖上应该能够识别两个相距约 2~4 mm 的点，手掌上为 8~15 mm。

视野

检查同侧下象限盲。

结构性失用

要求患者临摹 3D 绘图。

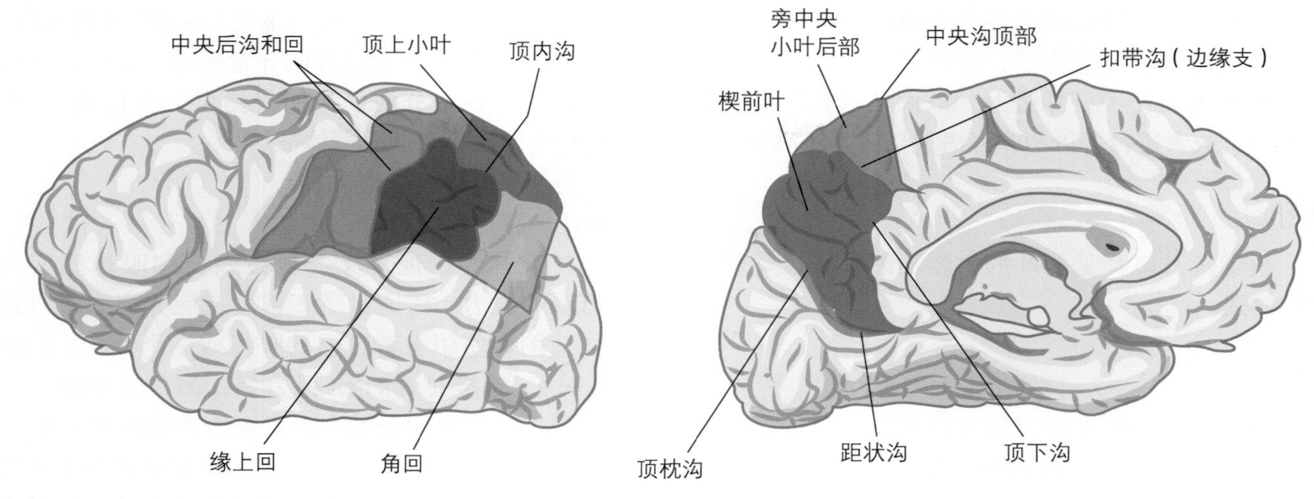

图 2.3 顶叶

优势侧顶叶病变与一系列被称为 Gerstmann 综合征的体征相关。尽管很少会都出现，但为了检查的完整性，牢记这四个体征仍然是有用的（**专栏 2.4**）。对于非优势侧顶叶（**专栏 2.5**），对侧忽略占优势。根据患者外观（身体一侧缺乏打理），可能会观察到这种情况。其他症状可能变得明显，如地理定向丧失（在熟悉的地方迷路）、穿衣失用症和疾病感缺失（缺乏疾病意识）。

专栏 2.4 顶叶检查—优势半球（Gerstmann 综合征）

计算困难

要求患者计算从 100 减去 7，继续按顺序减去 7。

书写困难

要求患者写一个简单的句子。

手指异常和左右定向障碍

可以通过交叉患者双手后询问患者，"我在摆动您的哪个手指？"来检查（图 2.4）。也可要求患者用左手无名指触摸右耳。还需记住评估语言功能（见前文）。

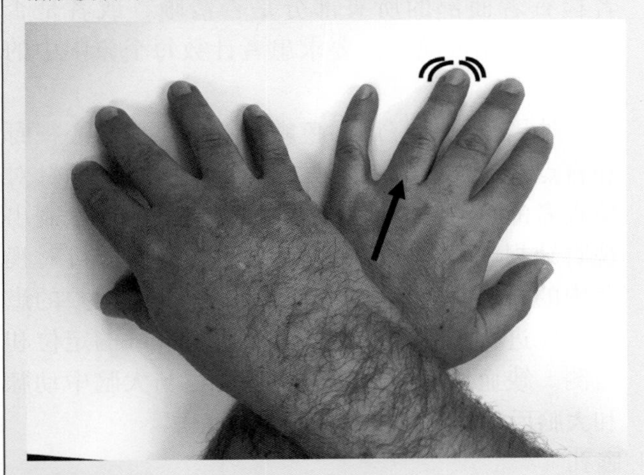

图 2.4 测试手指异常和左右定向障碍："我在摆动哪个手指？"正确答案为"左手无名指。"

专栏 2.5 顶叶检查—非优势半球

单侧空间忽略

要求患者标记水平线的中间位置。中心向脑损伤侧（通常为右半球）的位移表明存在单侧忽略。也可以使用目标消除测试。这是要求患者在页面或类似内容上圈出每个"a"的地方。单侧忽略时只有一侧页面会被注意到。

交叉反应试验

要求患者移动被触摸肢体对侧的肢体（运动忽略）。

穿衣失用症

要求患者脱掉针织套衫或其他衣物。将其由内翻出，并要求患者以正确方式传回。

剪纸

要求患者使用一把剪刀从一张纸上剪下一个形状。

颞叶

颞叶在处理听觉信息（Heschl 回）、视觉信息（颞下皮层）、情绪（杏仁核）以及记忆和空间定位（海马）中发挥作用。它在语言中的作用尤其是在语言（情绪韵律）中的发声（主导）和感知（非主导）情绪方面很重要。需要记住的是，Meyer 袢越过颞角顶部，因此，病变可能导致一个"难以实现的幻象（pie in the sky）"的四分象限盲。除了简单的记忆、言语和视野检查外，颞叶的床旁检查有限。神经心理学家可以进行双耳分听测试，将不同的录音内容呈现在一对耳机的任一只耳朵上，以评估选择性的听觉注意力，或者进行言语和非言语记忆的高级测试。

枕叶

视觉及其解释是枕叶的主要功能，在视觉部分进行阐述。

小脑

小脑通过分析来自大脑和脊髓的广泛的感觉输入，协调平稳的、有计划的运动行为。中线结构（蚓部和绒球小结叶）控制躯干和眼球运动的协调。小脑半球维持对肢体运动的控制，并帮助运动计划。由于小脑保持同侧或交叉两次输出，小脑半球的病变将引起同侧缺陷。共济失调是小脑功能障碍的特征性体征。当主动肌和拮抗肌之间的协调较差时，动作会显得笨拙。通过空间的轨迹不精确，运动的时机也不精确。躯干共济失调甚至可能使患者在床上坐起也非常困难。可能有宽基底步态和蹒跚步态。检测其他肢体共济失调的方法是要求患者重复快速的肢体轮替运动（例如一只手内旋/外旋）。出现异常时为轮替动作障碍。也可以要求患者伸出手臂，然后触摸他们的鼻子，或者触摸检查人员的手指，再触摸患者自己的鼻子，可能引起意向性震颤。Holmes 反跳试验揭示运动过度。例如，在手臂伸展和闭上眼睛的情况下，检查者将患者的一只手臂向下推。松开后，患者的手臂高于最初的位置。可有同侧肌张力减退和摆动性膝跳。小脑在发音中起作用，当受损时将引起说话费力、发音不清的构音障碍。缄默症是中线手术切除后公认的问题，常见于髓母细胞瘤切除后的儿童。解剖学基础是由于齿状核-丘脑-皮质通路的破坏，使双侧齿状核损伤引起缄默。这解释了为什么优势半球 SMA 损伤、双侧丘脑切开术和中脑卒中（红核）可导致相同的综合征。由于齿状核与中线非常接近，小脑缄默症最初被错误地认为是分开蚓部所致。快速朝向异常侧也可出现眼球震颤。垂直眼震（如 Chiari 畸形可见下视眼震）。颅后窝病变患儿可出现头部倾斜。认知-情感症状在小脑疾病中也越来越多地被认识到。

视觉系统检查

本节将详细介绍眼睛和第Ⅱ、Ⅲ、Ⅳ和Ⅵ脑神经的检查。有必要进行全面的病史询问，以了解患者的视觉症状范围。这些可包括上睑下垂、视力模糊、复视、“异常光影”、视力丧失（一过性或持续性、部分或完全）、可视化世界的异常运动、眼痛、头痛或眼眶痛。在本节中，我们将提供一个检查示例，以避免遗漏最重要的眼部体征。

神经眼科检查应包括：

1. 视力

视神经、视交叉、视束病变和眼球病变均可影响视力。需通过矫正视力或屈光视力进行评估，例如使用患者自己的眼镜或一个针孔（a pin hole）。标准是 Snellen 视力表，测量 6 米距离处的视力。结果用分数[距离视力表的距离（米）/应看到字母的距离（米）]表示。如果视力下降但可通过验光矫正，是由于眼部缺陷所致。如果视力无法矫正，则表示视觉通路存在问题。如果患者无法看到最大的标志，则可以通过靠近图表，或手指计数、手部运动感知、光感知来评估视力。

2. 色觉

这对于评估视神经功能最有用。使用 Ishihara 盘进行评估，并通过正确识别的色板数对每只眼睛进行单独评分。在对眼睛进行比较时，还应考虑识别色板的速度。请记住，8% 的男性和 0.5% 的女性可能患有 X 连锁隐性先天性色觉缺失或色盲症。在这些患者中，色觉丧失为双侧性，视力和视野正常。评估色觉的一种更粗略的方法是要求患者注视一个有色目标，如红帽，在眼睛有病变时，有色目标看起来会褪色或“颜色被洗脱”。

3. 视野检查

可以直接面对面进行视野测试，并对每只眼睛进行单独评估。患者应注视检查者的鼻子，依次遮盖每只眼睛。该试验可检测偏盲、象限盲、垂直视野和中心视野缺损。遮住眼睛后，询问患者检查者面部的所有部分是否清晰，或者是否有部分模糊或缺失。要求患者计数每个象限中的手指。

外周视野最好用白色帽针评估，而中心视野和盲点应用红色帽针测试。后者通过移动帽针对检查者的盲点进行评估。根据患者的描述绘制出视野缺损。异常图示如下（见**图** 2.5），并可对视路中的缺损进行定位。所有怀疑有视野缺损的患者均应进行正式的视野检查，进行准确的定位和监测。缺血性枕叶病变的黄斑保留与大脑中动脉和大脑后动脉对枕极的双重供血有关。

4. 瞳孔

瞳孔光反应通路包括视神经（传入）和第Ⅲ脑神经的副交感神经部分（传出）。调节反射来自

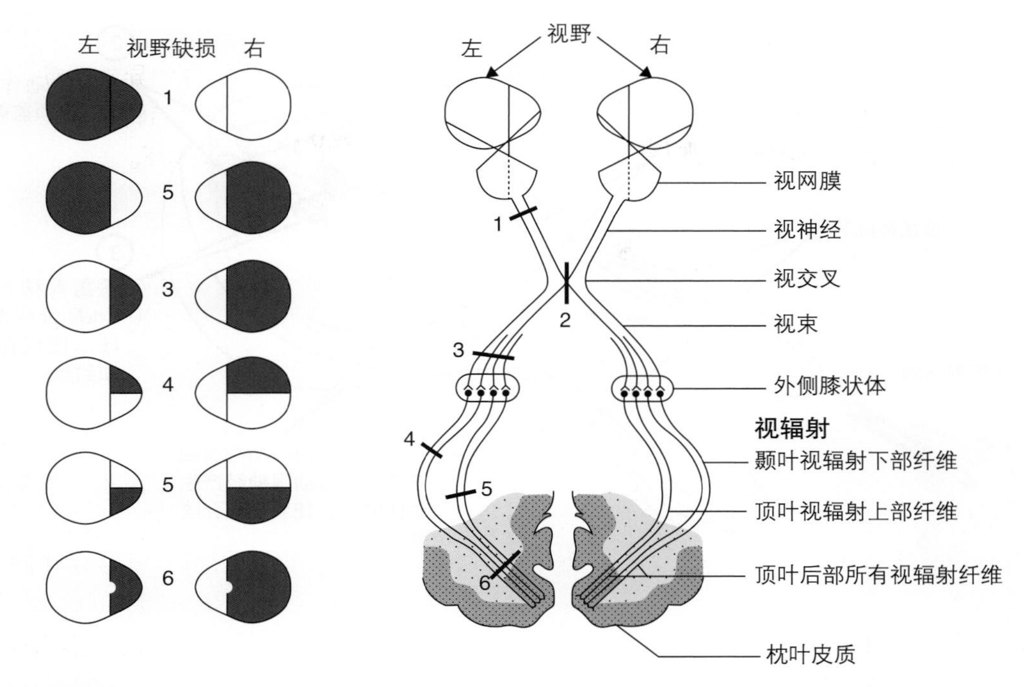

图 2.5　视野的评估和缺损的定位

From: *Macleod's Clinical Examination*, Ninth edition figure 7.8 page 211, J. Munro and C.R.W. Edwards.

额叶（传入）和第Ⅲ脑神经的副交感神经部分（传出）。

检查有无瞳孔不等大，然后让患者注视远处的目标，测试直接和间接对光反射、瞳孔调节反射，最后进行摆动光试验。

4.1 大小

瞳孔的检查首先要在室内光线下进行，如果瞳孔不等大且在光照下比在黑暗下明显，则副交感神经系统异常，瞳孔较大侧异常。第Ⅲ脑神经麻痹、Adie 瞳孔或虹膜括约肌受损是属于副交感神经通路。然后在暗光下检查瞳孔不等大，如果在暗光下瞳孔不等大且较在光照下明显，则存在交感神经功能障碍，瞳孔变小侧异常。Horner 综合征是交感神经疾病的一种表现。如果在两种情况下瞳孔不等大程度相同，则不表明存在神经系统问题。

对光反应受损但调节反射正常（light-near dissociation）的疾病包括 Parinaud 综合征（**专栏 2.6**）、神经梅毒、糖尿病、Adie 瞳孔、双侧视神经病变和第Ⅲ脑神经的异常刺激。

4.2 光反应（直接和间接）

用亮光照射每只眼睛，观察瞳孔收缩的速度和幅度（见**图 2.6**）。如果瞳孔对光线没有正常反应，通过观察近物来检查反应。再次，检查瞳孔对观察近物的收缩速度和幅度，以及观察远目标时的扩张速度。

专栏 2.6　Parinaud 综合征

- 眼球上视不能
- 瞳孔变大不规则，光反应消失，调节反射存在（光 - 近分离）
- 眼睑异常——眼睑内陷或下垂
- 辐辏受损
- 退缩性眼球震颤

4.3 光摆动试验（swinging light test）

患者注视远处的目标时，灯光变暗。将光线从一只眼睛移动到另一只眼睛，一次大约 1 秒。观察每个瞳孔的初始运动（通常是收缩）。为了诊断相对传入性瞳孔缺损（relative afferent pupil defect，RAPD），一个瞳孔应持续扩大而不是收缩。RAPD 的存在提示视神经病变（**表** 2.3）。

5. 眼底镜检查

建议对所有患者进行眼底镜检查，检查有无苍白的视盘水肿，因其可能提示颅内压升高和视神经萎缩。系统性地检查视盘、血管和视网膜。**表** 2.4 总结了通过目前的技术检查出的有助于病变定位的视觉症状。

6. 眼球运动

6.1 固定、眼球震颤和扫视

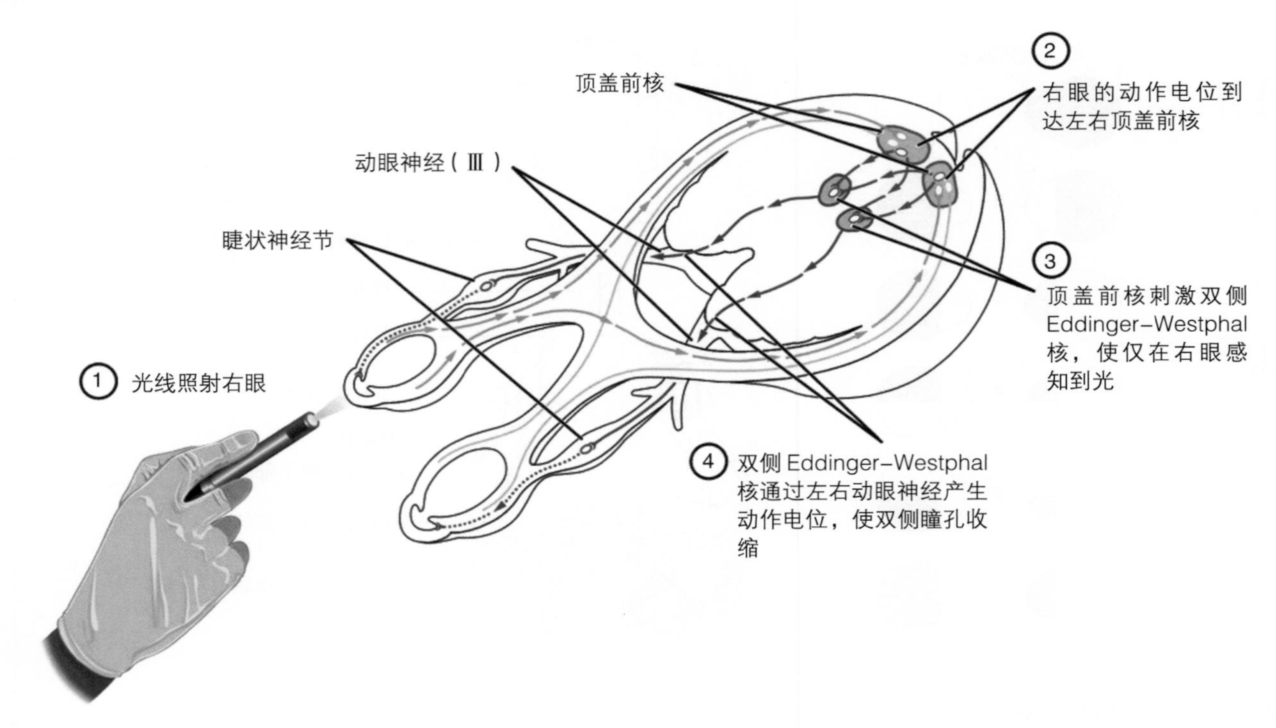

图 2.6 对光反射

Authored by: OpenStax College. Provided by: Rice University. Project: Anatomy & Physiology. http://cnx.org/content/col11496/latest/

表 2.3 相对传入性瞳孔缺陷（Pane, 2007）

正常瞳孔		
光刺激	右侧瞳孔	左侧瞳孔
无	●	●
左侧	•	•
右侧	•	•
左侧相对传入性瞳孔缺损		
光刺激	右侧瞳孔	左侧瞳孔
无	●	●
左侧	●	●
右侧	•	•

This article was published in *The Neuro-ophthalmology Survival Guide*, A Pane, p 379, Copyright Elsevier (2007).

注视障碍包括眼球震颤和眼球跳动性病变。检查眼部不自主运动或眼球振荡病史。先天性固定障碍通常无症状，多偶然被注意到。

眼球震颤是眼球的节律性振荡。首先检查眼睛处于平视位，然后处于不同的凝视位时的眼震情况。检查开始时，注意眼球震颤的快相和方向或是否呈摆动性。还应注意双眼的眼球震颤是否相似，以及是否有潜伏成分或覆盖一只眼睛时眼球震颤是否增加。不同类型的眼球震颤有助于病理定位，总结见**表** 2.5。

通过扫视测试，评估患者注视偏侧目标的速度和准确性，可以暴露细微的核间性眼肌麻痹或第Ⅵ脑神经麻痹。具体通过让患者注视其头部两侧的两个

表 2.4 视觉系统中病变的定位（Beck and Smith, 1988）

	视神经	视交叉	视束	颞叶	顶叶	枕叶
视力	正常或降低	正常或降低	正常或降低	正常	正常	正常
色觉	正常或降低	正常或降低	正常或降低	正常	正常	正常
视野	中心盲点	双眼颞侧偏盲	同向性偏盲	同向性上象限盲	同向性下象限盲或偏盲	同向性偏盲，黄斑回避
相对性传入性瞳孔缺损	有	有或无	有或无	无	无	无
视盘苍白	有或无	有或无	有或无	无	无	无

Beck & Smith, *Neuro-Ophthalmology: A Problem-Oriented Approach*, 1e, Little Brown & Co, USA, Copyright © 1987.

表 2.5 眼球震颤类型和神经系统定位

眼球震颤类型	定位
向下	颅颈交界区
周期交替	颅颈交界区
凝视诱发	前庭、小脑
向上	小脑、延髓
垂直向	间脑、中脑
扭转	中央前庭的
会聚 - 回缩	背侧中脑
反跳	小脑

Beck & Smith, *Neuro-Ophthalmology: A Problem-Oriented Approach*, 1e, Little Brown & Co, USA, Copyright © 1987.

不同物体来进行测试。要求患者交替注视物体。注意扫视起始、速度和准确性，这可能太小（低于度量）或太大（超过度量）。

6.2 眼球运动及第Ⅲ、Ⅳ、Ⅵ脑神经

眼球运动包括由额叶控制的扫视运动、由枕叶控制的追逐运动（促进注视运动物体的缓慢运动）、由小脑前庭核控制的前庭眼反射（允许身体或头部运动的眼位补偿）和由中脑控制的调节反射（注视靠近面部的物体）。来自不同控制中枢的输入活动通过整合以同步眼球运动。中脑内侧纵束（medial longitudinal fasciculus，MLF）走行于中脑第Ⅲ、Ⅳ脑神经核和脑桥的第Ⅵ脑神经核之间。眼肌中的外直肌由第Ⅵ脑神经控制，上斜肌由第Ⅳ脑神经控制，其余均为第Ⅲ脑神经控制。

6.2.1 第Ⅲ脑神经麻痹（动眼神经）

完全性动眼神经麻痹表现为上睑下垂、瞳孔散大和光反应消失三联征，眼球位于“下外”方（图 2.7）。瞳孔受累可能是由于缺血影响了动眼神经内部的神经纤维所致。副交感神经纤维位于动眼神经的外围，更常受到压迫性病变的影响，通常是后交通动脉瘤。

核间性眼肌麻痹是由MLF病变引起。患者有眼球共轭运动障碍；侧视检查时，一只眼睛内收不完全，另一只外展性眼球震颤。向右注视时左眼内收障碍时描述为左侧核间性眼肌麻痹（图 2.8）。水平共轭凝视中心位于第Ⅴ脑神经核水平的脑桥旁正中网状结构中。眼球沿水平方向转动时，外展正常（Ⅵ），但传递至动眼神经的信号无法通过MLF传递给第Ⅲ脑神经核，导致内收受限。为克服由此产生的复视，可引起外展眼球的震颤。垂直凝视中心位于第Ⅲ脑神经 / 上丘水平的内侧纵束喙侧间质核（the rostral interstitial nucleus of the MLF, riMLF）。

6.2.2 第Ⅳ脑神经麻痹（滑车神经）

表现为向下看时复视，头部倾斜远离患侧，无明显斜视（图 2.9）。患眼瞳孔可略高于健侧，但不明显。

当怀疑有第Ⅳ脑神经麻痹时，让患者观察水平物体（例如，每只眼睛交替

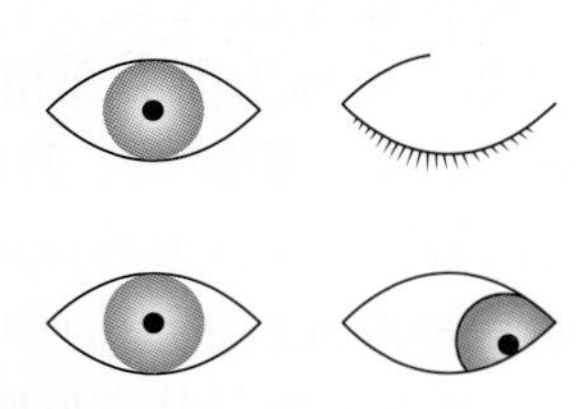

图 2.7 左侧第Ⅲ脑神经麻痹

From Fuller, G. (2004) *Neurological Examination Made Easy*, 3e, Churchill Livingstone, p. 88, Fig 9.4.

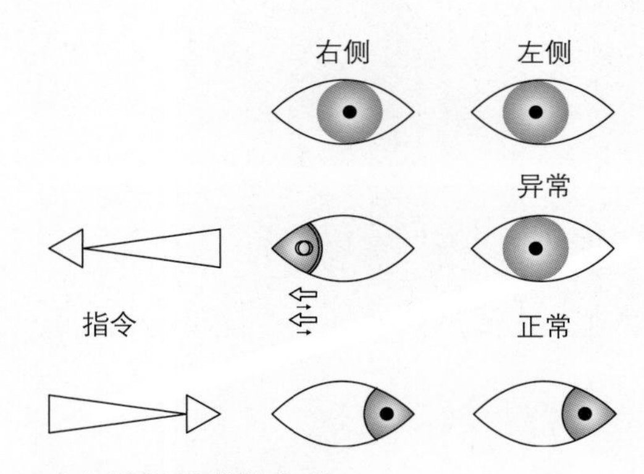

图 2.8 左侧核间性眼肌麻痹

From Fuller, G. (2004) *Neurological Examination Made Easy*, 3e. Churchill Livingstone, p. 88, Fig 9.6.

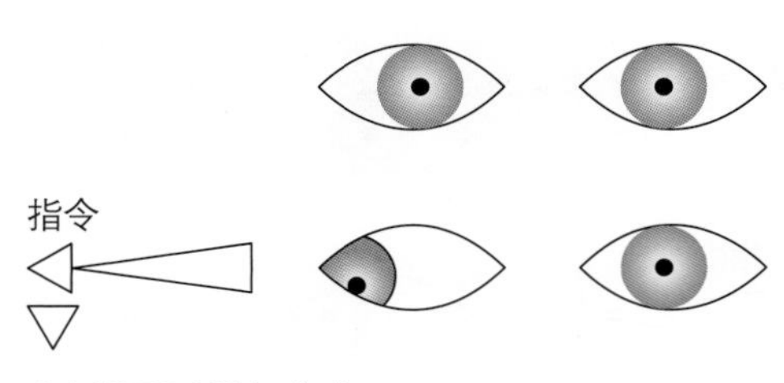

图 2.9 左侧第Ⅳ脑神经麻痹

From Fuller, G. (2004) *Neurological Examination Made Easy*, 3e. Churchill Livingstone, p. 88, Fig 9.4.

看门框顶部）很有帮助。滑车神经麻痹会产生两个向患侧成角的图像（**图** 2.10）。

6.2.3 第Ⅵ脑神经麻痹（展神经）

表现为复视，出现水平分离的两个图像（**图** 2.11）。因麻痹的眼肌出现斜视、复视。患者瞳孔正常。

7. 眼睑位置

检查眼睑位置、轮廓，并测量眼睛处于正常位置时的睑裂。上眼睑通常覆盖角膜 1 mm，超过该值表明上睑下垂。还需检查眼球向不同方向注视时不同的上睑下垂，如先天性上睑下垂和 Duane 综合征。向上凝视时出现的疲劳性上睑下垂（2 min 后 > 2 mm）提示神经肌肉无力，如重症肌无力。

8. 眼眶

最后，在检查眼眶时，应注意是否存在眼球突出、眼球内陷或眼球充血。须站在患者身后，从前额向下看，以评估眼球突出情况。Hertel 眼球突出计可进行更准确的测量。在闭合的眼睑上听诊到杂音提示颈动脉 - 海绵窦瘘的可能。

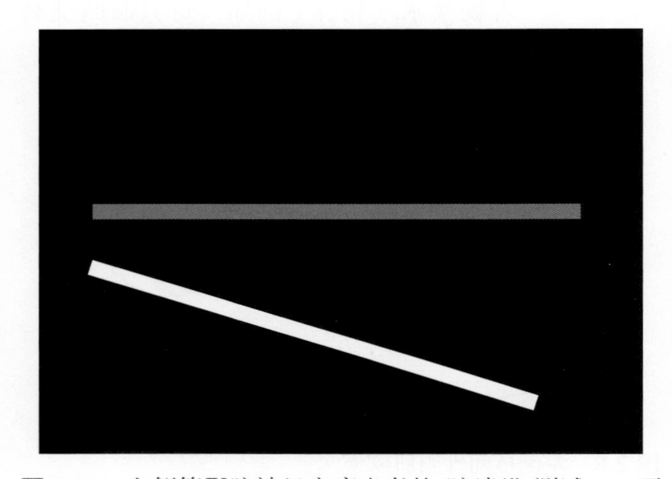

图 2.10 左侧第Ⅳ脑神经麻痹患者的“门框”测试——两幅图像指向患侧

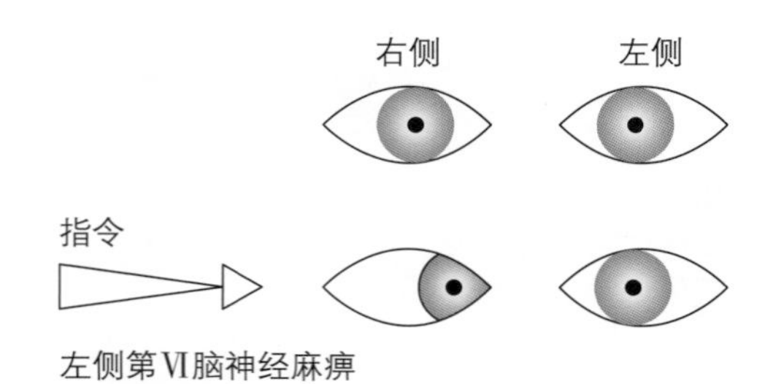

图 2.11 左侧第Ⅵ脑神经麻痹

From Fuller, G. (2004) *Neurological Examination Made Easy*, 3e. Churchill Livingstone, p. 88, Fig 9.4.

脑神经检查

本节将包括眼部检查章节中未讨论到的脑神经检查。

1. 第Ⅰ脑神经（嗅觉）。询问患者是否注意到嗅觉的任何变化。使用两种不同的气味（例如咖啡或橙子）进行检查。可用嗅觉检查试剂盒。
2. 第Ⅱ脑神经（主要为视力、视野和瞳孔功能）。完整的检查还应包括眼底镜检查、盲点检查和色觉检查。
3. 第Ⅲ、Ⅳ、Ⅵ脑神经（眼球运动）。
4. 第Ⅴ脑神经（面部感觉和咀嚼肌）。三叉神经具有运动和感觉成分：上颌支是颧弓处分出的第一支神经。通过咬牙时触诊咀嚼肌或要求患者对抗阻力张口观察其下颌运动来检查运动功能。通过轻触三叉神经的三个分支（眼支、上颌支和下颌支）进行感觉检查。最后，用一小块棉絮轻触角膜，进行角膜反射（传入支Ⅴa，传出支Ⅶ）检查，应该从视野外侧轻触角膜。另一种方法是轻吹眼睛并检测反应情况。还应注意正常结膜反应，如流泪和充血。
5. 第Ⅶ脑神经（面部表情、舌前 2/3 味觉）。面神经支配面部表情肌，茎突舌骨肌、镫骨肌和二腹肌后腹的肌肉受第二颧支支配（**图** 2.12）。当面部肌肉力弱时，首先要确定是上运动神经元（upper motor neuron，UMN）性质的还是下运动神经元（lower motor neuron，LMN）性质。面肌上部由双侧面神经核团支配，由此解释不同的临床特征。首先，寻找面部运动的不对称性，这可能是非常微妙的：仅仅是眼睛闭合不完全、眨眼缓慢或笑容延迟的暗示。然后，嘱患者皱眉（额、颞支），闭眼（眼轮匝肌、颧支），鼓腮（颊肌）或吹哨（口轮匝肌、双颊支），示齿（颧大肌、颊或下颌缘支），皱下巴（颏肌、下颌缘支），并耸肩（颈阔肌、颈支）。可使用 House–Brackmann 量表对面瘫的严重程度进行分类（见**第 24 章**）。

在上运动神经元性肌无力中，可见额部肌肉力量强于下面部，也称为前额保留。单侧面肌无力可能是由于血管病变、脱髓鞘、肿瘤或脑干病变所致。双侧无力可因假性延髓性麻痹或运动神经元病所致。

在下运动神经元性肌无力中，可见下面部与前额一样瘫痪。Bell 麻痹是其常见原因，通常在发病后 12 小时内最严重，可伴有乳突周围疼痛、味觉丧失和听觉过敏。下运动神经元性面瘫的其他原因为脑桥病变、桥小脑角病变和腮腺肿瘤。双侧下运动神

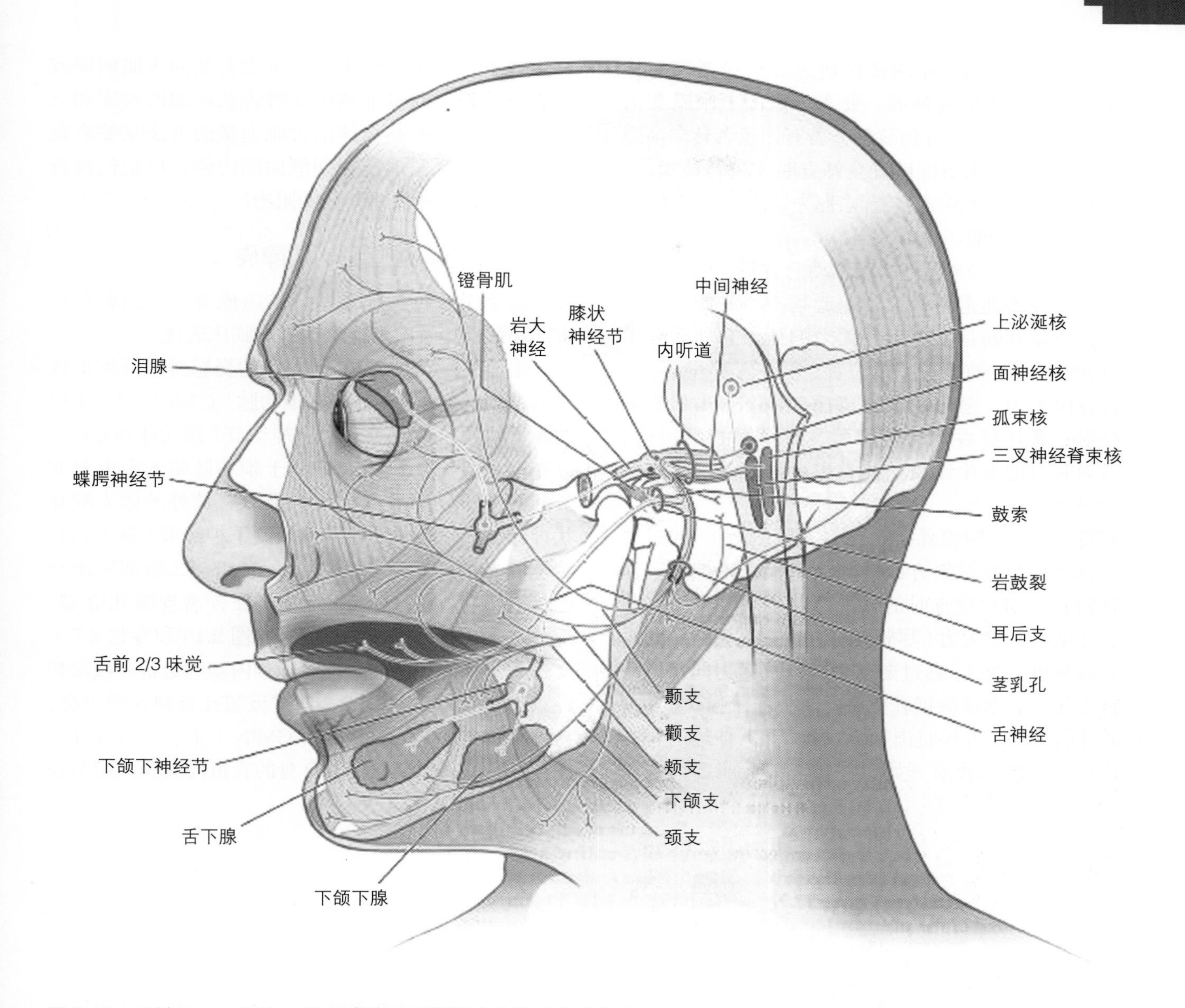

图 2.12 面神经——运动、副交感神经和特殊感觉神经支配分布

Blumenfeld, Hal. (2002) *Neuroanatomy through Clinical Cases*. Sunderland, Massachusetts: Sinauer. Fig 12.10, chapter 12 p. 480.

经元性面肌无力的原因是神经肌肉接头疾病，如重症肌无力、运动神经元疾病、肌病、神经结节病或吉兰 - 巴雷综合征。

6. 第Ⅷ脑神经（蜗神经和前庭神经）。通过分别测试双耳进行听力测试。遮盖另一侧耳朵，摩擦手指或耳语来测试听力。若听力下降，则进行 Rinne 和 Weber 测试。测试时需要一个 512 Hz 音叉。通过 Rinne 测试比较骨传导与气传导。敲击音叉，将基部置于乳突上（骨传导，简写为 BC）。当音调消失时，音叉置于外耳道（气导，简写为 AC）上方。正常反应是音叉在外耳道前方移动时再次出现音调（即气导优于骨导，AC>BC）。这反映了鼓室和中耳听小骨提供的放大作用。Weber 试验为敲击音叉，将基部置于前额中线上。双耳应同样听到音调的声音。如果它偏向一侧，说明对侧感觉神经性听力缺陷，或者同侧的感觉神经性耳聋增加了该耳的敏感性。这些测试有时可能难以解释，标准检查是纯音测听和内耳道听觉障碍成像。

前庭功能检查包括步态和眼震。其他有价值的检验还有 Hallpike 检验，用于体位性眩晕患者。患者坐位，头偏向一侧，快速仰卧，头部伸展，检查者应支撑患者的头部。观察眼球震颤、相关延迟以及是否疲劳。询问患者是否出现眩晕。对侧重复该步骤。如果眼球震颤疲劳和延迟，提示外周前庭障碍，如良性阵发性位置性眩晕。如果不疲劳，则由中枢异常所致。Unterberger 测试是通过要求患者面对检查者站立，手臂向前伸展。要求患者闭上眼睛并向前行走。观察是否有任何旋转。若有则患者转向前庭病变侧。只有在患者能够安全站立时才进行该操作。Romberg 试验是评估本体感觉丧失，而不是专门评估平衡或前庭功能。

7. 第Ⅸ、Ⅹ脑神经（腭部肌肉运动、吞咽、咽反射）。舌咽神经和迷走神经通常一起检查。先倾听患者声音质量判断是否有延髓无力的征象，然后要求患者咳嗽。检查悬雍垂的位置，嘱患者发“啊”声。若肌肉无力，悬雍垂会偏离病变侧。很少检查咽反射；若怀疑吞咽功能障碍，不应检查咽反射，因为有可能发生误吸。此类患者采用透视检查更为安全。
8. 第Ⅺ脑神经（胸锁乳突肌、斜方肌肌力）。通过要求患者耸肩测试斜方肌的力量来检查副神经，注意初始运动和检查时的任何两侧不对称性。翼状肩可见斜方肌无力（尽管胸长神经损伤引起的前锯肌麻痹更常见）。通过要求患者抵抗阻力向对侧旋转头部，来测试胸锁乳突肌的肌力和肌容积。
9. 第Ⅻ脑神经（舌部肌肉和运动）。舌下神经的检查从位于口底的舌肌开始。注意任何舌肌萎缩或肌束震颤。当患者伸舌时，舌尖会朝向舌肌弱侧或患侧偏斜。双侧锥体病变时舌肌运动的速度和流畅性会受到影响。评估舌肌力量的方法是要求患者用舌头紧紧地压在同侧面颊内侧，以抵抗检查人员手指压在面颊外侧的阻力。

自主神经功能检查及功能障碍

需要了解自主神经系统的组成方式，以解释在头部和颈部检查时可能会遇到的临床表现。

来自 T1-4 侧柱的节前胞体的交感神经纤维形成交感神经链，并通过颈下（椎动脉，C7-8）、颈中（甲状腺下动脉和 C5-6）和颈上神经节（颈动脉和 C1-4）分布节后纤维。该神经链位于颈动脉鞘的后内侧和长肌的前方。然后，节后纤维沿着颈外动脉支配睫状神经节和瞳孔开大肌，以及颌下神经节（颌下腺和舌下腺）和耳神经节（腮腺）。一级、二级或三级交感神经病变可引起 Horner 综合征，出现瞳孔收缩、部分上睑下垂和半侧面部无汗（**图** 2.13 和**专栏** 2.7）。支配头颈部的其余交感神经随颈内动脉走行：颈深神经颈动脉岩骨段上形成，通过破裂孔延伸到颅中窝，与副交感神经岩大浅神经（GSPN）汇合形成 Vidian 神经。Vidian 神经通过其自身的管道向翼腭神经节提

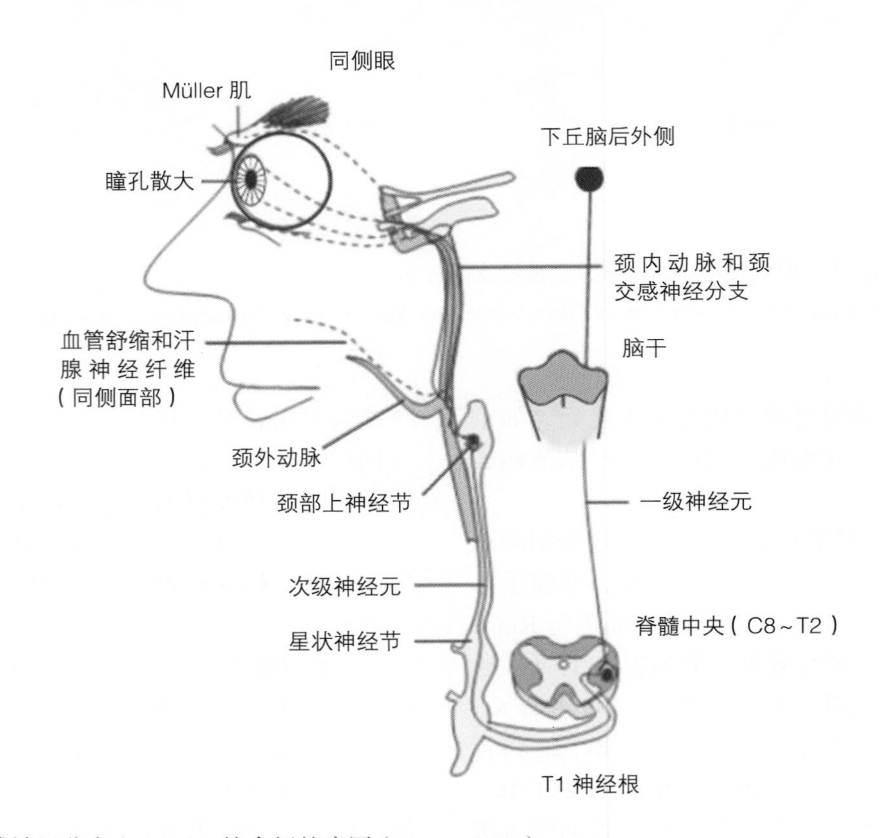

图 2.13 瞳孔的交感神经分布和 Horner 综合征的病因（Kong, 2007）

专栏 2.7 Horner 综合征鉴别诊断

一级神经元病变
Arnold–Chairi 畸形
颅底脑膜炎（如梅毒）
颅底肿瘤
脑血管意外 / 延髓外侧综合征
脱髓鞘疾病（如多发性硬化）
脑桥出血
颈部创伤
垂体瘤
脊髓空洞症

二级神经元病变
肺上沟瘤（Pancoast 瘤）
产伤伴臂丛下段损伤
颈肋
主动脉、锁骨下动脉或颈总动脉动脉瘤 / 夹层
中心静脉置管
创伤 / 手术损伤（根治性颈部清扫术、甲状腺切除术、颈动脉血管造影术、冠状动脉旁路移植术、上脊椎整脊手法）
胸管引流放置
淋巴结病（如霍奇金病、白血病、结核病、纵隔肿瘤）
下颌牙脓肿
中耳病变（如急性中耳炎）
神经母细胞瘤
腰椎硬膜外麻醉

三级神经元病变
颈内动脉夹层
丛集性 / 偏头痛
颈动脉血栓形成
颈动脉海绵窦瘘
带状疱疹
眶尖肿瘤
原发性

供自主神经纤维，副交感神经分布于三叉神经的上颌支。

副交感神经含四个脑神经内：第Ⅲ、Ⅶ、Ⅸ和Ⅹ脑神经。有 4 个同样重要的脑干副交感神经核：Edinger Westphal 核（Ⅲ）、上泌涎核（Ⅶ）、下泌涎核（Ⅸ）、迷走神经背核（Ⅹ）。迷走神经不参与颅神经中副交感神经部分，但分布于胸腔和腹部所有脏器，直至中肠（占横结肠的 2/3）。其余三个脑神经的节前副交感神经纤维终止于四个神经节：睫状神经节（Ⅲ经神经至下斜肌）、翼腭神经节（Ⅶ经 GSPN）、下颌下神经节（Ⅶ经鼓索）以及耳神经节（Ⅸ经岩浅小神经）。因此，面神经有两个副交感神经分支，起源于脑干水平的中间神经（**图 2.12**）。鳄鱼泪综合征是一种罕见的面神经损伤症状，面神经损伤导致支配唾液分泌的神经错生长进入支配泪腺的神经，出现进食时流泪症状。

节后副交感神经纤维通过三叉神经的一个分支传递到靶腺体。睫状神经节的纤维沿着短睫状神经（鼻睫状神经分支，Va）传递，控制瞳孔收缩和调节。翼腭神经节的纤维通过颧颞神经（Vb）和泪腺神经（Va）进入泪腺。其余的纤维来自翼腭神经节，通过三叉神经的上颌分支分布于鼻子、上颚和鼻咽窦。下颌下神经节的神经纤维经舌神经（Vc）分布于下颌下腺和舌下腺。

周围神经系统检查：上肢和下肢

四肢的神经系统检查基于一般检查、肌张力、肌力、反射、共济和感觉的评估。依据病史，进一步定位将依赖于关键检查结果（例如，对疑似脊髓病的患者，确认是否有长束体征；对于神经根病，将相应的肌病和皮节的缺陷进行关联；对于脊髓空洞症，测试脊髓丘脑与后索功能；臂神经痛和坐骨神经痛，需注意区分是周围神经病变或神经根病变）。了解上下运动神经元体征之间的差异当然是至关重要的。考虑到这一点，应该有一个合乎逻辑的排除过程，其顺序取决于个人的选择和情况。

一般检查

首先进行一般检查，注意有无姿态异常或惯用一侧肢体。类风湿性关节炎等全身性疾病的皮肤红斑可能非常明显，此时可进行步态评估。特征性的病理性步态指向特定的神经解剖学疾病（**专栏 2.8**）。

专栏 2.8 步态异常

- 偏瘫——由于固定跖屈和膝关节伸展姿势，痉挛的下肢呈划圈动作
- 双侧瘫痪——通常由于脑瘫引起的内收的剪切步态
- 脊髓病——宽基底笨拙步态
- 跨阈步态——L5 神经根病或腓总麻痹导致足下垂的患者
- 肌病步态——交替侧骨盆下落的摇摆步态
- 帕金森步态——小碎步前冲步态
- 小脑步态——转向不受控步态
- 磁性步态——脚似乎粘在地板上，见于正常压力脑积水

足跟-趾（串联）步行和 Romberg 试验是有价值的辅助手段。通常，Romberg 试验仅在本体感觉障碍时呈阳性。值得注意的是，这不是对小脑功能的测试，因为在闭眼的情况下，有或无小脑疾病均会出现共济失调。应继续检查肌群萎缩、肌束震颤、震颤和皮肤瘢痕，如曾行腕管减压术。

肌张力和反射

关节周围肌群的阻力是一个复杂系统的结果，涉及肌梭和高尔基体肌腱器官的反馈、激动剂和拮抗剂 α 运动纤维的单突触反射、抑制性脊髓上控制和小脑的处理。肌张力可以降低（肌张力减退）或升高（痉挛或强直）。痉挛是对被动牵张反应的肌张力的速度依赖性增加，伴有过度的肌腱抽搐，与上运动神经元综合征的其他特征相关（Lance，1980）。在被动运动结束时，通常有一个特征“阻力减小”（折刀样）。肌强直不依赖于速度或阻力，缺乏任何“阻力变化”。痉挛更常与皮质脊髓损伤相关，而强直通常起源于锥体外系。可通过轻轻内旋和外旋腿部、快速抬高膝盖或腕部旋前/旋后进行评估。

腱反射是单突触反射。高尔基体腱器官的活动刺激传入神经元，传出神经为 α 运动神经元。最常测试的反射是肱二头肌（C5）、旋后肌（C6）、肱三头肌（C7）、膝关节（L3/4）和踝关节（S1）反射。患者应保持放松姿势，使用叩诊锤轻敲肌腱。如果反射未引出，可以通过要求患者咬紧牙或将手指交锁对抗阻力来做加强试验。

上运动神经元功能障碍的特异性检查包括 Hoffmann 征、跖反射和阵挛。Hoffmann 征阳性是当迅速向下轻弹中指末节指骨时引起拇指屈曲。应在屈膝的情况下测试阵挛，任何超过 5 次的踝关节跳动都是病理性的。

肌力

肌肉群可以通过几种方式进行测试。可以要求患者最大限度地收缩肌肉，然后尝试抵抗肌肉（等长收缩）。或者，可以尝试通过一系列运动抵抗肌肉群（等张收缩）。医学研究委员会（Medical Research Council，MRC）量表提供了可重复的肌力分级系统（**表** 2.6）。重点检查不同的肌肉群将取决于是否寻找锥体束瘫痪、长束症疾病、神经根性疾病或周围神经相关的问题。在测试神经根或脊髓功能障碍节段时，美国脊柱损伤协会工作手册（ASIA，2015）提供了一个极好的、合乎逻辑的模式（**图** 2.14）。对于每个脊髓节段，指定特定的动作来测试单个神经根。

表 2.6 MRC 肌力分级

级别	描述
5 级	正常肌力
4 级	运动可对抗阻力，但不完全
3 级	运动可抵抗重力，但不能对抗阻力
2 级	运动不能抵抗重力
1 级	运动微弱
0 级	无运动

感觉

对于感觉系统检查，应以神经根范围或根据周围神经分布进行检查（**图** 2.15）。除外周定位外，还需要考虑不同的模式。需注意，辨别性的轻触觉、本体感觉、振动觉和两点辨别觉是通过后索中的大的快速传导纤维进行的。针刺（浅表疼痛）和温度觉是通过脊髓丘脑束中较小、较慢的纤维传导。同样，ASIA 图表是测试感觉最佳点的一个非常有价值的指南。应测试轻触和针刺部位的皮肤上的精确点。在进行检查时，两侧对比至关重要。应仔细绘制感觉减退或感觉过敏的区域。要求患者闭上眼睛可能会提供更多客观信息。

在测试关节位置感觉时，重要的是要记住，患者可通过对手指施加的压力来判断运动方向。因此，应捏住患者拇指或大脚趾两侧而不是上下侧。如果本体感觉丧失，应检查下一个近端关节。

一些常见的周围神经病变的检查方法详见**专栏** 2.9、**专栏** 2.10 和**表** 2.7。

信息整合

随着病史采集和体格检查的进行，病史信息不断被提炼，因此应精炼询问方式，定位查体重点。最终，必须将这些不同的病史信息汇集在一起，理解它们，并试图确定患者主诉最可能的解剖来源和可能导致主诉的潜在病理过程。一旦达到这一点，就有必要决定是否需要进一步检查，以及可能的检查结果。

在决策过程中，必须严格确保客观。

相对于无法治疗的患者，医生对他们能够帮助的患者和能够治愈的疾病更感兴趣。因此，医生倾向于使诊断适合他们的专业技能，甚至是他们可以治愈的疾病（Handy，1990）。

在考虑是否给患者做手术时，始终要找到一个

INTERNATIONAL STANDARDS FOR NEUROLOGICAL CLASSIFICATION OF SPINAL CORD INJURY (ISNCSCI)

ASIA — AMERICAN SPINAL INJURY ASSOCIATION | ISCOS — INTERNATIONAL SPINAL CORD SOCIETY

Patient Name ______ Date/Time of Exam ______

Examiner Name ______ Signature ______

RIGHT

	MOTOR KEY MUSCLES		SENSORY KEY SENSORY POINTS Light Touch (LTR)	Pin Prick (PPR)
		C2		
		C3		
		C4		
UER (Upper Extremity Right)	Elbow flexors C5			
	Wrist extensors C6			
	Elbow extensors C7			
	Finger flexors C8			
	Finger abductors (little finger) T1			
		T2		
		T3		
		T4		
		T5		
		T6		
		T7		
		T8		
		T9		
		T10		
		T11		
		T12		
		L1		
LER (Lower Extremity Right)	Hip flexors L2			
	Knee extensors L3			
	Ankle dorsiflexors L4			
	Long toe extensors L5			
	Ankle plantar flexors S1			
		S2		
		S3		
(VAC) Voluntary Anal Contraction (Yes/No)		S4–5		
RIGHT TOTALS (MAXIMUM)	(50)		(56)	(56)

Comments (Non-key Muscle? Reason for NT? Pain?):

LEFT

SENSORY KEY SENSORY POINTS Light Touch (LTL)	Pin Prick (PPL)		MOTOR KEY MUSCLES	
		C2		
		C3		
		C4		
			C5 Elbow flexors	UEL (Upper Extremity Left)
			C6 Wrist extensors	
			C7 Elbow extensors	
			C8 Finger flexors	
			T1 Finger abductors (little finger)	
		T2		
		T3		
		T4		
		T5		
		T6		
		T7		
		T8		
		T9		
		T10		
		T11		
		T12		
		L1		
			L2 Hip flexors	LEL (Lower Extremity Left)
			L3 Knee extensors	
			L4 Ankle dorsiflexors	
			L5 Long toe extensors	
			S1 Ankle plantar flexors	
		S2		
		S3		
		S4–5	(DAP) Deep Anal Pressure (Yes/No)	
(56)	(56)		(50) LEFT TOTALS (MAXIMUM)	

MOTOR (SCORING ON REVERSE SIDE)

0 = total paralysis
1 = palpable or visible contraction
2 = active movement, gravity eliminated
3 = active movement, against gravity
4 = active movement, against some resistance
5 = active movement, against full resistance
5* = normal corrected for pain/disuse
NT = not testable

SENSORY (SCORING ON REVERSE SIDE)

0 = absent
1 = altered
2 = normal
NT = not testable

MOTOR SUBSCORES

UER ___ + UEL ___ = UEMS TOTAL ___ ; LER ___ + LEL ___ = LEMS TOTAL ___

MAX (25) (25) (50) ; MAX (25) (25) (50)

SENSORY SUBSCORES

LTR ___ + LTL ___ = LT TOTAL ___ ; PPR ___ + PPL ___ = PP TOTAL ___

MAX (56) (56) (112) ; MAX (56) (56) (112)

NEUROLOGICAL LEVELS
Steps 1–5 for classification as on reverse

	R	L
1. SENSORY		
2. MOTOR		

3. NEUROLOGICAL LEVEL OF INJURY (NLI) ___

4. COMPLETE OR INCOMPLETE? ___
Incomplete = Any sensory or motor function in S4–5

5. ASIA IMPAIRMENT SCALE (AIS) ___

(In complete injuries only)
ZONE OF PARTIAL PRESERVATION
Most caudal level with any innervation

	R	L
SENSORY		
MOTOR		

REV 11/15

图 2.14 国际脊髓损伤神经分型标准品工作手册

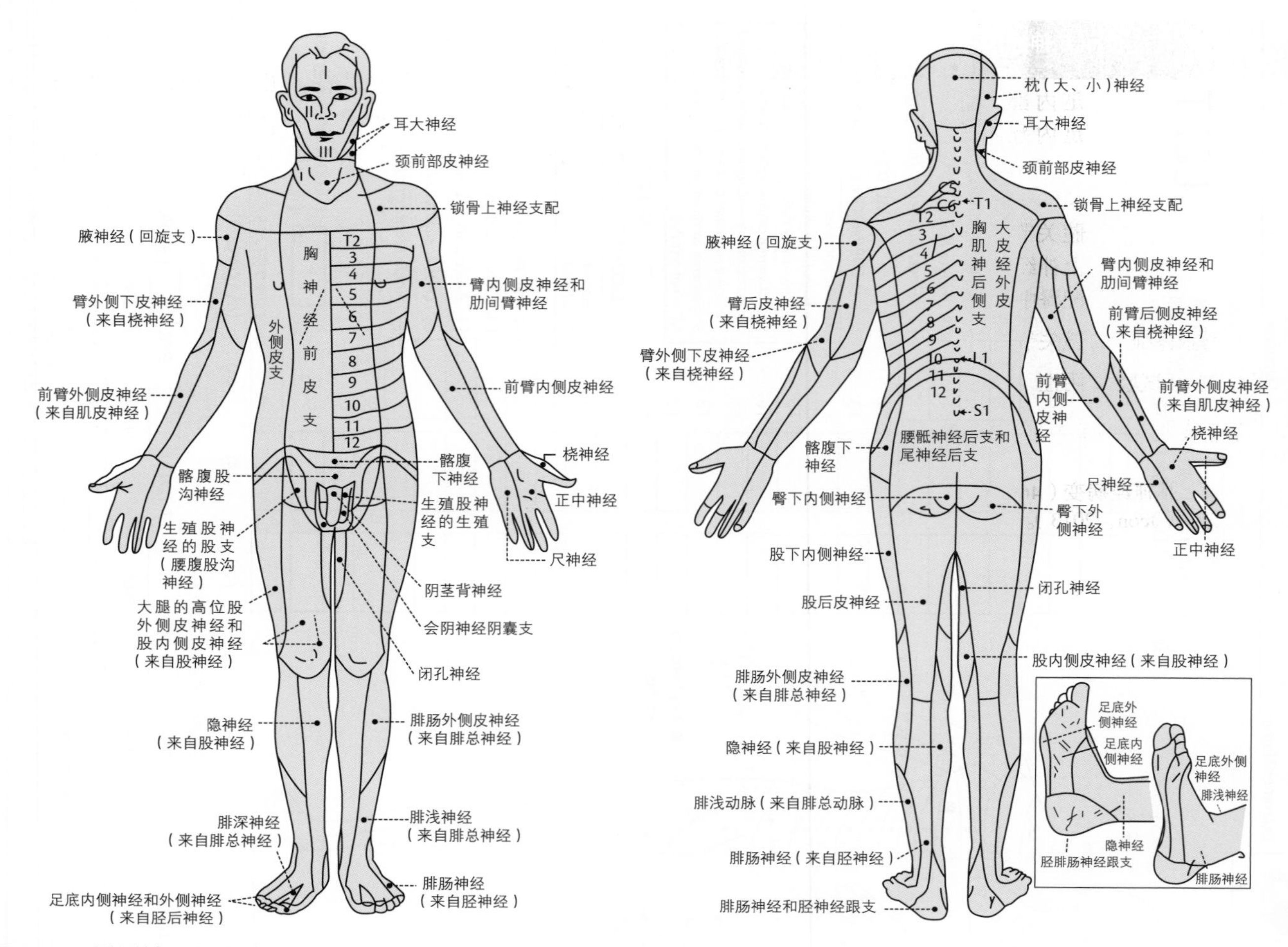

图 2.15 周围神经的皮肤分布

专栏 2.9 腕管综合征的检查

- 大鱼际隆起萎缩
- 用拇指做 O 形来测试对掌功能
- 测试拇指外展，手背朝下，拇指朝上
- 无名指感觉分裂，尺侧感觉更敏感
- 因手掌皮支走行于屈肌支持韧带上方，中央手掌区无感觉丧失
- Phalen 征（预测价值高）
- Tinel 征（预测价值低）
- 无 benediction 征（尝试握拳，但拇指和示指保持伸展），病因为正中神经的近端受到压迫

专栏 2.10 肘部尺神经病变检查

- 第一背侧骨间肌和小鱼际隆起萎缩
- Wartenberg 征—小指处于外展状态，容易卡住口袋
- 测试指外展
- 尺侧异常—尺侧爪形手见于腕部尺神经损伤，肘部近端无病变
- Froment 试验—为拇内收肌试验，其中大鱼际隆起为尺神经支配的唯一肌肉。嘱患者用拇指与示指夹住一张纸。抽纸时拇指屈曲提示试验阳性
- 尺神经沟内尺神经触痛和肿大，Tinel 试验阳性
- 无名指感觉分裂，桡侧感觉增强
- 需排除 C8 神经根病、肺上沟瘤和胸廓出口综合征（据 Horner 综合征鉴别诊断）

表 2.7　区分 L5 神经根病和腓总神经麻痹的临床特征[a,b]

	L5 神经根病	腓总神经麻痹
无力模式	足内翻（胫骨后肌、足内翻肌，由 L4 和 L5 经由胫神经而非腓神经支配） 髋关节外展（通过臀上神经经由 L4/L5/S1 支配臀中肌和臀小肌）	足外翻
神经根紧张体征	髋关节屈曲	踝关节内翻
腓骨颈 Tinel 试验	阴性	阳性

[a] 始终牢记足下垂的中枢原因，尤其是压迫运动皮质的大脑镰旁脑膜瘤。

[b] 外周原因：腓神经病变（46%）、腰神经根病（15%）、坐骨神经疾病（5%）（Jeon，2013）。

平衡点。做手术和不做手术的风险有什么区别？清楚地了解疾病的自然史是必要的，就像详细了解特定手术的潜在并发症一样。

病史和体格检查是管理患者的基础。必须以我们对神经外科疾病的了解为指导，针对患者病史和查体信息进行处理，相关内容将在后续章节中进一步介绍。

延伸阅读、参考文献、EBRAIN 的相关链接

扫描书末二维码获取。

第 3 章　神经影像概述

Tomasz Matys · Daniel. J. Scoffings · Tilak Das 著
刘婷红、王乔、李俊杰 译，孟凡刚、肖以磊、刘亚欧 审校

引言

过去四十年中，电子计算机断层扫描（computed tomography，CT）（Hounsfield，1995）和磁共振成像（magnetic resonance imaging，MRI）（Mansfield and Maudsley，1977；Lauterbur，1989）快速发展使神经影像发生了革命性变化，克服了以往间接显示颅内血管或脑室位移等方法的局限性，可直接显示颅内病灶（Hoeffner et al.，2012）。CT 首次临床应用于一名脑肿瘤患者，毫无疑问，断层成像技术的发展带给神经科学带来的益处，远超其他医学领域。MRI 和核医学方法在不断发展，特别是正电子发射计算机断层显像（positron emission tomography，PET），该设备可实现对中枢神经系统特定功能的成像，如血流、组织微环境和代谢。未来的发展方向将注重提高解剖成像的空间分辨率和软组织分辨率，同时进一步拓展功能成像的应用。分子成像也有望得到全面充分的临床转化，除了对疾病的病理和功能成像外，还可对特定的细胞和分子进行成像（Hoffman and Gambhir，2007；Massoud and Gambhir，2007）。

在本章中，我们讨论了目前对神经外科有帮助的神经放射学成像技术。由于篇幅有限，仅简单介绍部分物理原理的基础知识，需要更全面了解可查阅相关文献（Allisy-Roberts and Williams，2007）。我们将介绍神经放射学方法的适用性及局限性，关于具体疾病的发生发展和影像学表现可参考本书其他章节。感兴趣的读者可在神经放射学专著中找到更多相关资料（Nadgir and Yousem，2016）。

成像原理

射线照相和透视

射线照相（“普通 X 线”）原理是将准直 X 射线束透过患者投射至影像接收器上，传统的影像接收器是包含荧光屏和胶片的片匣，而现在临床中常用的是数字影像探测器。X 线通过人体不同组织衰减程度不同，到达探测器表面的强度不同，故 X 线图像可区分空气（黑色）、脂肪（深灰）、软组织、水（浅灰）和骨骼（白色）。X 线图像是三维立体结构的二维表示，通过获取不同位置（通常是正位）的投影图像，以判断病灶在患者体内的位置。

随着 CT 和 MRI 的日益普及，除了某些特殊情况，传统 X 线在神经外科患者中的使用已经减少。X 线的优点包括易获取、成本低、用途广、可在床旁拍摄以及可根据患者处于不同位置（如站立、屈曲和脊柱伸展）时的 X 线片来获取患者的动态信息。虽然 X 线片具有很高的空间分辨率，但其主要缺点是软组织分辨率有限。X 线可评估脑室分流术颅外部分的连续性，脊柱植入物和假体的位置及完整性，并且还可随访脊柱骨折患者椎体的形态和压缩程度。在诊断脊柱骨折和疑似脊柱损伤的初步评估中，X 线不如 CT 敏感，提供的价值有限。屈伸位 X 线常用于评估患者腰椎退行性变或腰椎滑脱的不稳定性。

透视通过将连续或脉冲 X 线束穿过患者传递到影像增强器上，提供感兴趣区的实时图像，最常见的方法是 C 臂，该设备可在患者周围旋转和定位，以提供所需角度的视野。透视的主要用途包括确定脊柱手术时正确椎体水平，监测脊柱固定装置或假体的位置，以及对因肥胖或退行性变而导致床边腰椎穿刺（lumbar puncture，LP）失败的患者进行腰穿引导。

CT

CT 的基础知识及技术

1973 年，CT 作为首个直接对大脑进行成像的设备进入临床应用（Wolpert，2000）。与 X 线成像类似，CT 成像基于不同组织对 X 线的衰减程度不同，使用不同的准直射线束以圆形方式扫过患者，投射至大量单排探测器上，然后使用数学算法重建图像。简而言之，当 X 线光子沿特定路线穿过患者的身体时，

其能量的损失取决于路线上穿过组织的衰减系数。通过测量物体多个方向X线光子的能量，可计算出检查范围内每个体素的衰减系数。然后，基于水和空气，将衰减系数值转换更常用的射线密度值（“CT值”），并以单位Hounsfield（HU）表示。CT值的范围从−1000 HU（空气）到3000 HU以上（骨皮质），其中0 HU是蒸馏水的衰减系数。**表**3.1给出了中枢神经系统不同组织的常见HU值。

随着技术的进步，获取多方位信息的方式和速度已经发生了巨大的变化，原始的机器是“铅笔状”X线束，现在是扇形的X线束，并且探测器的数量随着机架的长度和行数增加（Ginat and Gupta，2014）。螺旋CT是CT扫描技术的一个重要发明，在螺旋CT中，数据是以连续的方式获得的，患者在机器内平稳地移动，而X线球管在患者周围连续螺旋样旋转。这种数据采集方式显著改善了人体CT扫描，但会引起“风车伪影”（Barrett and Keat，2004），然而对于颅脑成像，连续CT扫描可能更具优势。在神经放射学应用中，螺旋CT评估颈部和颅内血管图像质量较好，并且可以提供任一平面上同向高分辨率的容积重建图像。

将放射密度矩阵显示为灰度影像可使原始CT数据转换成可用的医学图像。从Hounsfield所示的范围来看，CT值可能超过了4000多个放射密度等级，理论上人类在最佳条件下可以看到大约720个灰度级（Kimpe and Tuytschaever，2007），然而在实际中更低。因此，不可能同时将CT数值的整个动态范围映射到灰度，这就需要使用以特定水平和特定宽度为中心的“窗口”来显示该范围。窗口内的射线密度值显示为灰色，而窗口边界值以下和以上的值分别显示为黑色和白色。由于大脑中大多数感兴趣的组织位于0~100 HU的范围，因此使用40 HU左右的窗位和80 HU的窗宽可较好的显示这些组织（**图**3.1A）。由于急性出血的密度接近标准窗的上限，故出血为很明显的高密度；但是紧邻骨骼的出血则难以被发现。使用窗位略高、窗宽略大的“硬膜下窗口”（如L/W 70/200），可以更好地鉴别急性出血和邻近骨骼（**图**3.1B）。将窗位设置为负值可以区分脂肪和空气。要查看骨骼细节，需要将窗口设置为更高的窗位和窗宽（例如，L/W 500/3000，**图**3.2）

影响图像质量的最重要因素之一是数学重建算法，也称为重建滤波核或重建滤波器。应用不同核函数平衡图像的空间分辨率和噪声。核平滑生成的图像噪声低，且检测低对比度能力更好，更适合于颅脑检查，但其空间分辨率降低。核锐化算法的图像空间分辨率高，更适合于评估骨性结构。骨核算法的使用对于骨折的检测是必不可少的（**图**3.2），可应

表3.1 神经影像主要组织的CT值

组织	HU值
急性出血	56 ~76
空气	−1000
骨	1000~3000
钙化	140~200
脑脊液	0
脂肪	−30~−100
灰质	32~41
白质（半卵圆中心）	23~34

This table was adapted from *Neuroradiology: The Requisites*, David Yousem, Robert Zimmerman, Robert Grossman, Copyright Elsevier (2010).

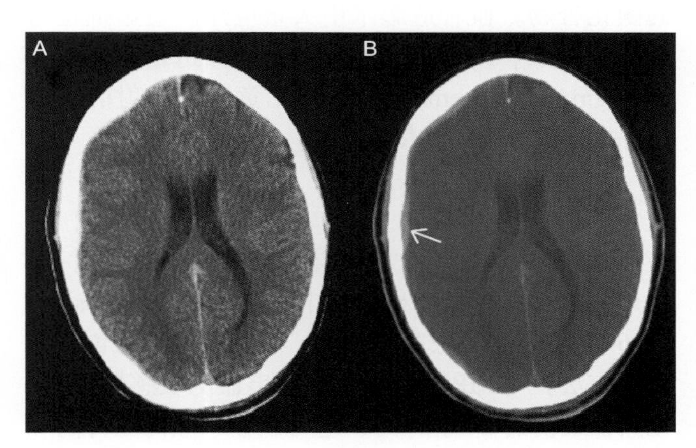

图3.1 标准窗（A，窗位/窗宽为40：80）能很好地区分灰质和白质，但颅骨附近的高密度出血很难鉴别。扩大窗（B，“硬膜下窗”70：200）使右侧少量硬膜下出血（箭头）更加明显

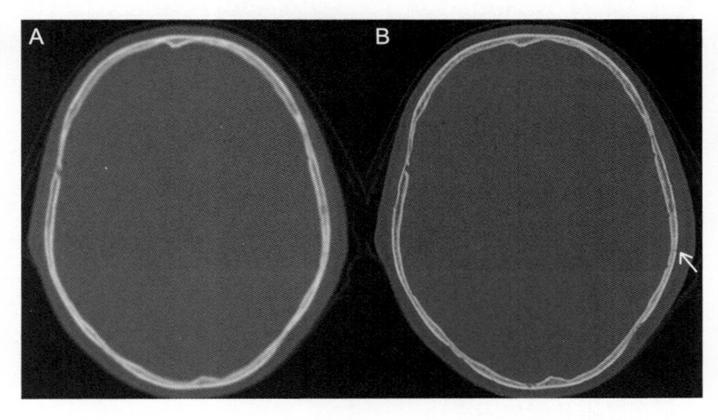

图3.2 使用标准（A）和骨核（B）重建的颅骨图像，骨窗（窗位/窗宽为500：3000）。使用骨核重建（箭头）可明显地看到左侧颞骨鳞部的线状骨折

用于外伤时的任一部位，也可用于鼻窦和颞骨检查。

CT 造影剂和风险

由于碘化合物具有高原子序数和高衰减性，因此碘造影剂历来是X线和CT的首选造影剂（Lusic and Grinstaff，2013）。在CT颅脑成像中，造影剂用于检测血脑屏障破裂的区域（即造影剂漏入脑实质）；或使血管密度升高，用于CT血管成像（包括静脉成像）。

碘造影剂的风险包括过敏反应和其引起的急性肾损伤。为了尽量避免发生不良反应，要尽早识别危险人群（**专栏 3.1**）并采取适当的预防措施（Iodinated Contrast Media Guideline，Royal Australian and New Zealand College of Radiologists）。

当前的标准是使用非离子型、低渗透压的化合物。此类物质严重反应的发生率为0.04%，非常严重反应的发生率为0.004%（Hunt et al.，2009）。成人颅脑CT静脉造影常用剂量为50 ml，含300 mg/ml的碘化合物。血管造影术中大量应用。造影剂也可以通过腰椎、颈椎、脑池或脑室入路进行鞘内注射（Nadgir and Yousem，2016）；儿童鞘内注射的实现有待批准更低浓度的化合物。

CT 的优点及缺点

CT在神经影像中发挥着极其重要的作用，尤其是在急诊和神经外科手术中（Nadgir and Yousem，2016）。它是一种快速、方便、有效筛查严重创伤患者的方法。与MRI相比，CT对出血的敏感性较高，尤其在最初的24小时内，它可以显示颅内压升高和脑疝，从而在创伤早期迅速做出治疗决策。对可疑的蛛网膜下腔出血（subarachnoid haemorrhage，SAH），CT是首选的影像学检查，一旦确诊SAH，可迅速进行CT血管造影。同时，CT是评估脑梗死的有效手段，结合CT血管造影和CT灌注，指导疑似缺血性卒中患者的溶栓治疗（Kidwell and Wintermark，2010）。

CT有助于评估脑部和脊柱术后并发症（如出血、梗死或脑积水）以及定位脑室引流管或其他植入物。便携式头部CT扫描仪可以在神经重症监护病床床旁进行检查，无须运送体征不稳定的患者。

CT静脉造影通常可以作为MR静脉造影的替代方法或当MRI出现伪影时，帮助进行辅助诊断。

CT是评估骨病变的最佳方式，对于评估颅骨、颅底、面部和脊柱骨折至关重要。CT也是评估颞骨和鼻窦的首选手段。

CT对钙化的敏感性有助于诊断含钙的CNS肿瘤（如脑膜瘤、少突胶质细胞瘤、颅咽管瘤）、代谢紊乱（如甲状旁腺功能亢进）和先天性病变（如TORCH感染、结节性硬化）。最后，对于MR绝对禁忌证的患者，CT脊髓造影是一种可替代MR脊柱成像的方法。

辐射是CT的缺点之一。颅脑CT平均有效剂量约为2毫希弗（mSv），而每人每年辐射量为2~5 mSv。其他神经放射学检查需要更高的剂量（**表 3.2**）。辐效应可分为确定性（可预测并取决于辐射累积量，例如照射晶状体引起的白内障）和随机性（偶然的，例如诱发恶性肿瘤）（Allisy-Roberts and Williams，2007）。尤其是儿童应用时需要考虑白内障的风险（Michel et al.，2012）。

在怀孕期间，头颈部CT对胎儿的暴露剂量较低，诱发儿童癌症的风险被认为小于1/1000000。直接暴露胎儿位置的CT检查（如脊柱CT）风险较高（1/1000~1/10000），应尽量避免（The Royal College of Radiologists，2009）。理论上，使用碘造影剂会抑制胎儿甲状腺，应在胎儿出生后第一周检查甲状腺功能。

CT技术的进步包括保证图像质量的同时，减少必要的辐射剂量，这对小儿成像尤为重要。减少辐射剂量的主要方法是根据患者的体型、体重和特定的成像方式改变管电压和管电流（从而改变X线光子能量和X线束强度）调整剂量。与传统重建技术“滤波反投影”不同，迭代重建（iterative reconstruction，IR）在保持图像质量的同时剂量也较低，迭代重建需要较长的计算时间，其生成的图像噪声低和空间分辨率高，同时射线硬化伪影和金属伪影少。尽管

专栏 3.1 造影剂引起的急性肾损伤（CI-AKI）和过敏反应危险因素

CI-AKI 危险因素

肾病（包括肾移植）
糖尿病
二甲双胍（乳酸酸中毒）

过敏反应危险因素

既往有碘造影剂过敏史
既往药物过敏史或湿疹史
哮喘病史
正在服用β受体阻滞药

The Royal Australian and New Zealand College of Radiologists. Iodinated Contrast Media Guideline. Sydney: RANZCR；2018.

表 3.2 CT 神经放射检查中的常见辐射剂量（Cohnen et al., 2006; Mettler et al., 2008）

检查项目	平均剂量（范围）
头颅 CT	1.75 mSV
头部血管造影	1.9 mSv
颈部血管造影	2.8 mSv
CT 脑灌注	1.1~5.0 mSv
脑卒中综合防治方案	高达 9.5 mSV
脊柱 CT	6 mSV

Data from Cohnen, M et al., Radiation exposure of patients in comprehensive computed tomography of the head in acute stroke, *AJNR. American Journal of Neuroradiology*, volume 27, issue 8, pp. 1741–5. 2006, and Mettler, F.A et al., Effective doses in radiology and diagnostic nuclear medicine: a catalog, *Radiology*, volume 248, issue 1, pp. 254–63. 2008.

在体部成像中效果更为明显，但在脑部成像也已证明剂量降低（Kilic et al., 2011; Mirro et al., 2016）。两种重建技术的图像在主观上似有所不同，因此 IR 仍在临床评估中。

磁共振（MRI）

MRI 基础知识及技术

MRI 利用了原子核的磁共振现象，这种现象是由于原子核的质子或中子数量不等而产生，主要是包含单质子的氢原子核（^{1}H）。MRI 基于射频信号的发生，当与强磁场对准的质子被外部施加的射频脉冲打乱时，返回到平衡状态发出的射频信号（**图 3.3**），以空间有序的方式识别出所发射的信号，并重建图像，反映了给定体素的信号强度。激发脉冲的类型、信号、被识别的时间以及激励间隔的不同可在图像中产生不同的对比度（Allisy-Roberts and Williams, 2007）。两种主要的 MRI 序列根据组织的 T1 或 T2 弛豫时间提供了图像加权（**表** 3.3）；颅脑成像最常用序列如**图** 3.4 所示。质子密度（proton density, PD）加权图像可以与 T2 加权图像一起获得，无需额外的扫描时间；它们在灰质和白质之间具有良好的对比度，在特定情况下有价值，但在神经放射学中应用并不普遍。水在 T2 加权序列上表现为高信号，因为大多数病理过程与水含量增加有关（水肿），故在 T2 加权像上表现为高信号。脂肪在 T2 加权像上呈高信号，与水不同，它在 T1 上也呈高信号。除了脂肪，T1 高信号也可能是由于黑色素、富含蛋白质的液体、钙化和钆螯合造影剂（见下文）。出血在 MRI 上表现复杂，其信号强度取决于出血的时期（**表** 3.4）。

MRI 的信号可以通过自旋回波或梯度回波序列产生（Bitar et al., 2006; Allisy-Roberts and Williams, 2007）。自旋回波更常用，可提供更好的信噪比，但比梯度回波慢。因此，使用梯度回波序列来采集神经外科导航所需的大容量数据。梯度回波序列的一个重要特征是缺乏对磁场不均匀性的补偿，导致其对局部磁场的不均匀性敏感。梯度回波序列在临床中常用于检测出血，因为含铁血黄素中铁的局部磁敏感性效应所致信号非常低，即“晕染效应”。磁敏感加权成像（susceptibility weighted imaging，SWI）利用高分辨率完全速度补偿的 3D 梯度回波序列（DiIeva et al., 2015）可以更好地显示含铁血黄素，例如，创伤脑损伤时的微出血。梯度回波序列图像对比度取决于磁敏感效应，如动态磁敏感对比灌注成像和血氧水平依赖等。

MRI 图像对比度可通过抑制技术来改变，抑制技术将特定组织的信号设为零。在脑成像中用液体衰减反转恢复序列（fluid-attenuated inversion recovery, FLAIR），即抑制脑脊液信号；通常与 T2 加权一起使用，以使脑实质的 T2 高信号更明显（T2-FLAIR，通常简称为 FLAIR）。勿与不常用的 T1-FLAIR 序列相混淆，例如，T1-FLAIR 序列用于改善灰白质对比度，否则在较高磁场强度下对比度会降低。

脂肪抑制技术可以提高 T2 加权图像上液体的信号或者在脂肪存在的情况下提高 T1 增强加权图像上的对比度（例如，检测到脊柱或脊柱旁软组织中的水肿，或颅底的对比度增强）。脂肪抑制可以通过短反转时间恢复序列（short tau inversion recovery, STIR）或频率饱和技术来实现。STIR 在含骨结构周围（眼眶、颅底、鼻窦）、金属异物和大视野（例如在脊柱成像中）非常有用。然而，当 STIR 序列与造影剂一起使用时存在不足，可用频率饱和脂肪抑制技术。

平衡稳态自由进动（steady state free precession, SSFP）序列混合 T2/T1 加权，具有高分辨率和良好的信噪比等优势。在神经影像学中，SSFP 通常用重 T2 加权进行，为脑脊液和脑脊液包含的结构（如脑神经脑池段和邻近血管）提供高对比度分辨率。因此，平衡 SSFP 技术如稳态进动快速成像（fast imaging in steady state, FIESTA）或稳态进动结构相干成像，可用于研究血管袢导致的三叉神经痛或面肌痉挛、筛查桥小脑角区肿瘤。其他用途包括评估内耳结构和脑脊液漏（Saindane, 2015）。

弥散加权成像（diffusion-weighted imaging, DWI）对水分子的运动敏感。DWI 加权通常是沿三个主要空间方向编码的特殊扩散梯度序列，并将信号合并

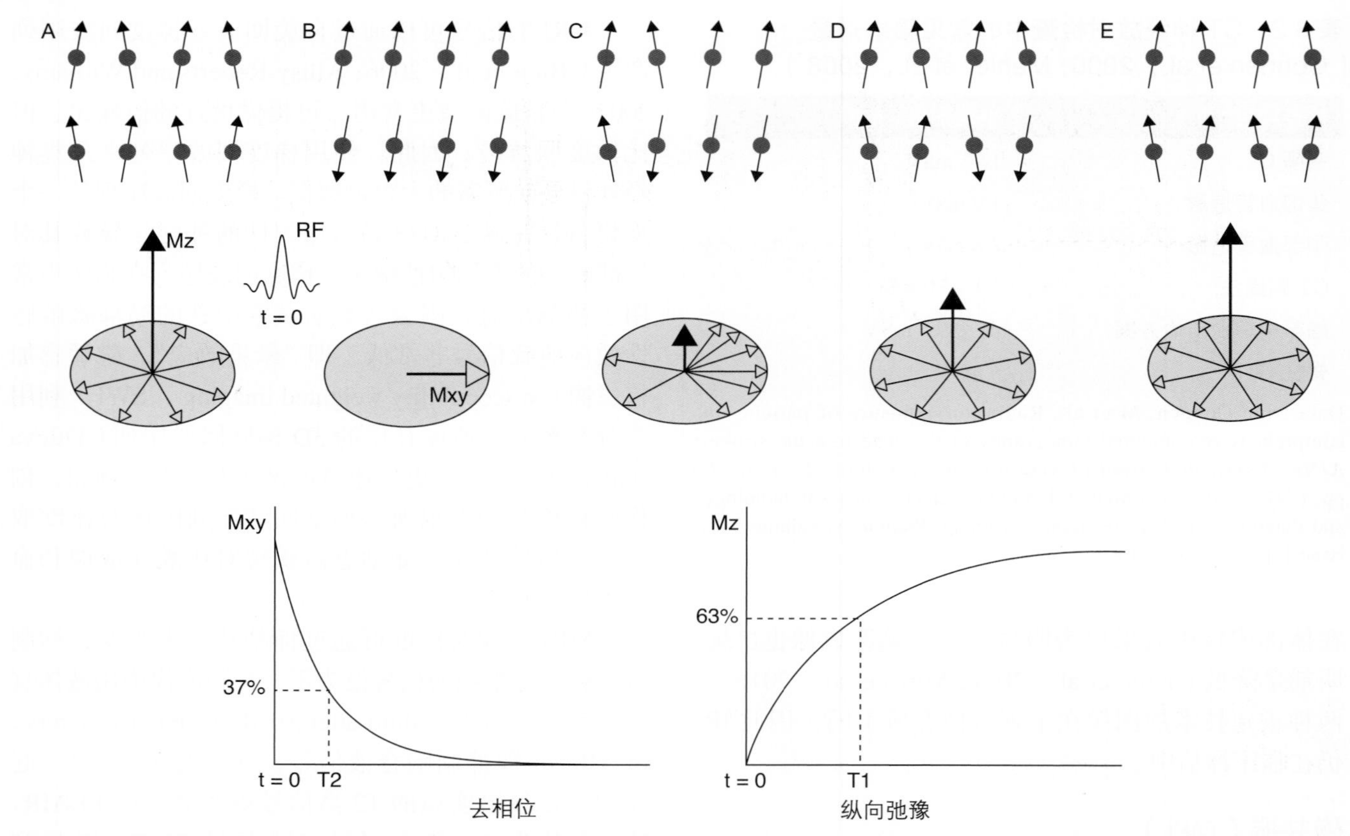

图 3.3 由于有电荷和自旋，质子具有磁性，表现出磁偶极子的特性。磁场外的偶极子是随机分布的，净磁化强度在任何方向都为零。当置于磁场中时，磁偶极子与磁场平行（“自旋向上”）或反平行（“自旋向下”）时并开始进动（绕轴摆动），其频率取决于磁场强度（拉莫尔频率）。（A）因为有少量多余的偶极子（大约 3%）“自旋向上”，它们的纵向磁化矢量加起来形成净纵向磁化 Mz。由于进动，每个偶极子也会产生横向磁化矢量。然而，由于偶极子在不同的相位进动，它们的横向磁化矢量相互抵消，净横向磁化保持为零。（B）外部射频（radiofrequency，RF）脉冲使一些偶极子自旋向下；90°RF 脉冲正好使一半多余的偶极子自旋向下，因此任一方向偶极子数量相等，净 Mz 矢量为零。射频脉冲还引起进动相位的同步，因此所有偶极子进动一致（达到相位一致），且它们的横向磁化加起来产生净横向磁化矢量 Mxy，在横向平面上旋转。（C~E）在射频脉冲停止后，质子在短时间内因失相位（失相位，导致横向磁化 Mxy 的损失）返回到自旋向上状态（纵向弛豫，导致纵向磁化矢量 Mz 的“再出现”），最后返回到其初始状态。上述过程取决于时间常数 T2 和 T1 呈指数相关，T2 表示去相位完成 63% 的时间（37% 的相位保留），T1 是纵向磁化恢复到 63% 的时间（底部图）。T2 时间相对较短，在纵向弛豫（E）之前完全去相位（D）。T1 和 T2 时间长短取决于组织类型，可确定 T1 和 T2 加权序列上的组织对比度。短 T1 的组织在 T1 加权序列上亮度高，而长 T2 的组织在 T2 加权序列上表现为低信号（例如，由于脂肪组织 T1 短、T2 长，故在 T1 和 T2 加权序列上表现为高信号）

表 3.3 在 T1 和 T2 加权 MRI 序列上不同物质和组织的信号强度

物质	T1- 加权序列	T2- 加权序列
水 / 脑脊液	↓	↑
脂肪	↑	↑
空气	↓	↓
骨皮质	↓	↓
红骨髓	=/ ↑	↑
黄骨髓	↑	↑

到弥散加权图像中。由于 DWI 弥散加权图像既有弥散加权，又有 T2 加权，明显的高信号可能是由于弥散受限所致，也可能是 T2 高信号的“穿透”效应。因此，有必要观察表观弥散系数（apparent diffusion coefficient，ADC）图。它消除了 T2 加权的影响，并使弥散受限表现为低信号。弥散受限可能提示细胞外空间的缩小，可能由细胞肿胀（例如缺血性卒中）或高细胞密度（例如淋巴瘤或髓母细胞瘤）及胆脂瘤或表皮样囊肿等病变造成。在神经外科中，DWI 最重要的应用是鉴别脓肿与其他环状强化病变，脓肿内容物表现出明显的弥散受限。

弥散张量成像（diffusion tensor imaging，DTI），

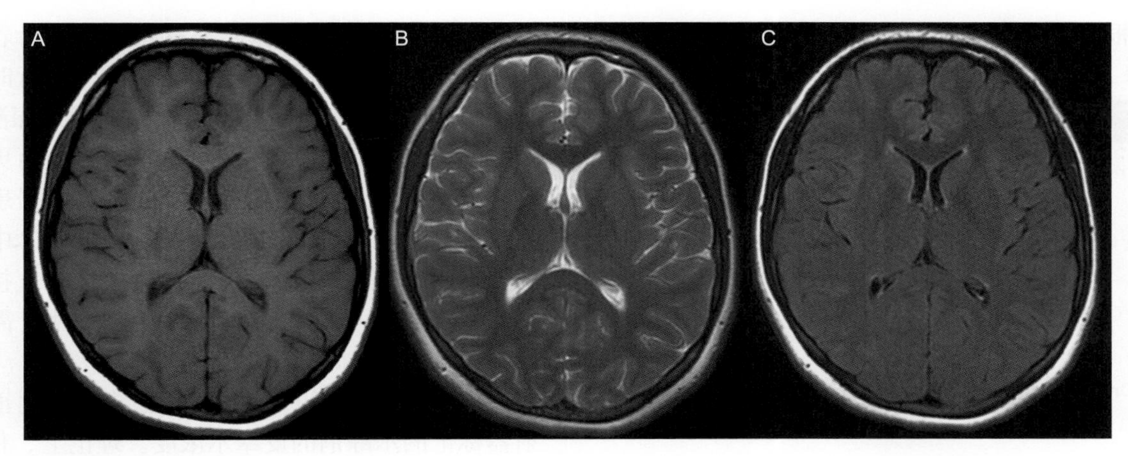

图 3.4　颅脑常规磁共振成像。（A）在 T1 加权图像上，灰质比白质暗（"更灰"）。（B）在 T2 加权像上，白质比灰质暗，液体呈高信号。（C）T2-FLAIR 显示灰质和白质的对比度与 T2 加权像相似，但脑脊液无信号

表 3.4　T1 和 T2 加权 MRI 序列上出血不同阶段的信号强度

出血阶段	血红蛋白产物	T1- 加权序列	T2- 加权序列
超急性期（<24 小时）	氧合血红蛋白	=	↑
急性期（1~3 天）	脱氧血红蛋白	=	↓
亚急性期早期（3~7 天）	胞内正铁血红蛋白	↑	↓
亚急性期晚期（1~4 周）	胞外正铁血红蛋白	↑	↑
慢性期（>1 月）	血铁黄素	↓	↓↓

至少在六个不同的方向采用扩散梯度扫描，可以计算给定体素中的主要扩散方向。由于水在白质束上的运动相对不受限制，DTI 可计算神经纤维的方向并重建白质束（DTI 纤维束成像），在神经外科手术计划中有较高价值（Waldman et al.，2009；Saindane，2015）。DTI 还可以评估多种扩散各向异性，在创伤性脑损伤（Hulkower et al.，2013）和高级别胶质瘤（Price et al.，2007；Yan et al.，2016）的成像和预测方面具有很好的价值。

功能磁共振成像（functional MRI，fMRI）是基于氧合血红蛋白（逆磁性）和脱氧血红蛋白（顺磁性）的不同磁性引起的血氧水平依赖（blood oxygen level dependent，BOLD）效应。大脑皮质神经元活动增强的区域表现出较高的耗氧量，但因神经血管耦合也导致灌注增加；灌注增加占主导的结果是 MRI 信号增加。不同的激活模式有助于重要皮层功能的定位，如定位感觉运动皮质和语言皮质（Stippich and Blatow，2007）。

MRI 造影剂

MRI 常用的造影剂主要是基于钆化合物的顺磁性造影剂。这类造影剂的药代动力学与碘造影剂相似，能快速从血管腔内到组织间，但钆磷维塞除外，它是一种与白蛋白结合并留在血管腔内的药物。钆化合物不能通过完好的血脑屏障，因此出现对比度增强反映了血脑屏障的破坏。而脑室周围结构血脑屏障不完整，会出现生理性增强，勿认为异常病变（Horsburgh and Massoud，2013）。造影剂对比度增强在 MRI 上比 CT 上更明显，在评估脑和脊柱的肿瘤、血管疾病、炎症和感染中具有重要价值。

钆化合物通常是安全的，但其螯合物和积累在组织中释放的游离钆可能存在副作用。肾源性系统性纤维化是一种罕见但致残的皮肤病，类似硬皮病和嗜酸性筋膜炎，首次在接受钆造影增强 MRI 的透析患者中观察到。大多数病例与使用不稳定的线性造影剂有关，这些药物现在被归类为高风险药物（**表 3.5**）。这类化合物使用需要肾功能监测，在肾小球滤过率（GFR）低于 30 ml/（min · 1.73 m^2）的患者、新生儿和肝移植围术期禁用；母乳喂养应在注射造影剂 24 小时后进行。对中、低风险造影剂的预防措施建议类似，但不是强制性的。

最近人们认识到，多次使用钆造影剂会导致脑内钆积聚，以齿状核和苍白球中浓度最高（Kanda et al.，2015b；McDonald et al.，2015）。不稳定的线性化合物比非大环类化合物在患者中发生钆蓄积更为常见（Kanda et al.，2015b），甚至在肾功能正常的情

表 3.5 根据肾源性系统性纤维化的风险对 MRI 造影剂的分类

高风险	中风险	低风险
钆双胺（欧乃影）	钆塞酸（卜迈维斯）	钆特酸（多它灵）
钆弗塞胺（安力磁）	钆贝酸（莫迪司）	钆特醇（普海司）
钆喷酸（马根维显）	钆膦维塞（三钠钆膦维司）	钆布醇（加乐显）

Data from Drug Safety Update Jan 2010, vol 3 issue 6: 3. https://www.gov.uk

况下也会出现蓄积（Kanda et al., 2015a；McDonald et al., 2015）。然而，这些发现的临床意义尚不清楚。

MRI 在神经外科手术中的常见应用

MRI 结构成像与 CT 相比有许多优点，除少数特殊情况下，MRI 是评价颅内和脊柱病变的首选方法。在结构成像中，MRI 提供了良好的组织对比度，对实质和增强病变更敏感，更好地显示解剖结构，并且可任一平面成像而不用接受电离辐射，且通过功能序列可以获得更多信息。MRI 的缺点是扫描时间长，在临床情况不稳定的患者中应用存在困难，且更容易出现运动伪影；因此，CT 在显示颅内出血和骨折方面具有较高的价值，在紧急情况下，特别是创伤时首选的检查方法。CT 对骨皮质和钙化的显示更好，而且更易获取图像，费用更低。MRI 的应用受到静磁场、射频脉冲和梯度场等有关的安全问题限制。装有起搏器、铁磁性动脉瘤夹、植入物或异物的患者一般不适合 MRI 检查。在对装有分流阀、人工耳蜗和心脏瓣膜患者以及孕妇扫描时，需谨慎小心；各情况扫描方法各不相同。最后，幽闭恐惧症可能导致许多患者无法接受 MRI 检查或长时间扫描。

正电子发射断层扫描（PET）

PET 是一种核医学技术，使用标记有正电子发射同位素的示踪剂。最常用的放射性核素是氟 -18（^{18}F），因为它的半衰期相对较长，接近 2 小时，足够从外部回旋加速器设备中运输到影像中心。半衰期短的放射性核素（^{11}C、^{13}N、^{15}O）需要当时使用回旋加速器或在放射性核素发生器（^{68}Ga、^{82}Rb）中生产。在靶器官中，放射性核素发射的正电子短距离传播后与邻近原子中的电子相互作用发生湮灭，并发射两个方向相反的高能光子，这两个光子可被环形排列的固态闪烁探测器探测到。通过配准两个相对的探测器对之间的脉冲来重建图像，沿着特定的路线确定湮灭发生的位置（**图** 3.5）。飞行时间 PET（time of flight PET，TOF-PET）技术通过探测两个光子到达相对探测器时间的微小差异，从而更精准地确定湮灭发生的具体位置。数据需要根据患者体内光子衰减进行校正；衰减信息在单独 PET 中使用旋转放射源或在 PET-CT 扫描仪中使用 CT 直接扫描获得。MRI-PET 中的数据校正更具挑战性，需要从解剖 MRI 图像中计算衰减值。

PET 具有极高的灵敏度，能够检测到正电子发射器标记的示踪剂的皮摩尔浓度。理论上，任何生理上存在的物质、药物或受体配体都可以被标记，故 PET 成为功能和分子成像最有前景的技术。应用最广泛的示踪剂是 ^{18}F- 氟脱氧葡萄糖（^{18}F-FDG），其摄取量反映了葡萄糖代谢的速率。由于脑内生理葡萄糖代谢率高，故其在大脑中的使用存在不足；其潜在应用包括高级别脑肿瘤的成像，低级别胶质瘤的间变性转化，放射性坏死与肿瘤进展的鉴别，免疫缺陷患者淋巴瘤与弓形虫病的鉴别，以及检测癫痫中局灶性皮质发育不良。PET 示踪剂的设备和在脑成像中的潜在应用在不断发展，详见**表** 3.6 中的总结。

目前临床上使用的大多数 PET 扫描仪是独立的机器或 PET-CT 组合。PET-MRI 的使用也越来越多。鉴于 MRI 在脑组织中优越的组织对比度和分辨率，PET-MRI 在神经成像方面具有优势。目前在单独的扫描仪上融合连续的 PET 和 MRI 图像是可实现的，PET-MRI 组合成像极大地促进了图像融合，无需后续配准。更重要的是，同时获取 PET 和 MRI 图像，在扫描参数发生突变时（如脑灌注或缺氧）有重要价值（Catana et al., 2012）。这些方法目前主要局限于神经影像学研究，临床实用性尚待明确。

其他核医学技术

大多数核医学技术使用放射标记的示踪剂发射伽马射线。最常用的放射性核素是 ^{99m}Tc（锝），因为它具有最佳半衰期、易于生产和易于融入其他放射性药物的特点。其他用于神经成像的同位素包括 ^{111}In（铟）和 ^{133}Xe（氙）。在单光子发射计算机断层扫描（single-photon emission computed tomography，SPECT）中，可以使用平面伽马相机或旋转伽马相机来探测发射的伽马射线。SPECT 在神经放射学中的应用包括使用 ^{99m}Tc-HMPAO、^{99m}Tc-ECD 和 ^{133}Xe 的脑灌注测量、痴呆的诊断、癫痫致痫灶的识别、帕金森综合征多巴胺转运体的成像和脑肿瘤评估（McArthur et al., 2011）。平面伽玛照相机图像是从放射性核素脑池造

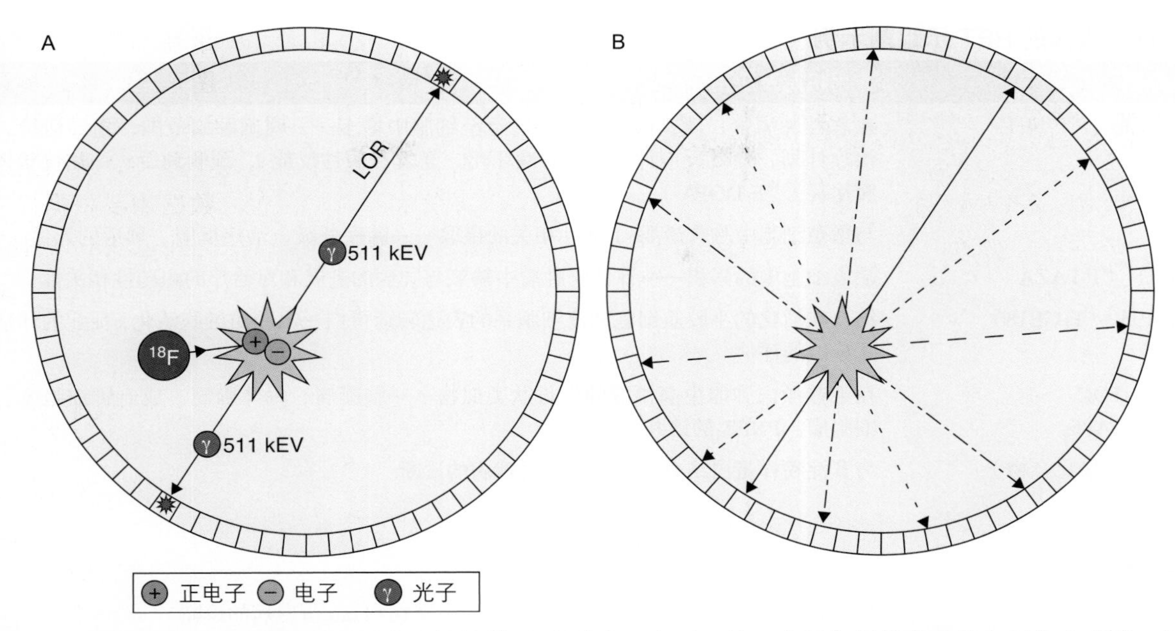

图 3.5 （A）发射正电子的放射性核（最常见的是 ^{18}F）释放出正电子，该正电子与靶器官中的电子发生碰撞，从而导致一系列湮灭。每次湮灭都会导致两个高能（511 keV）光子以光速沿相反方向（彼此成 180°）直线传播。这两个光子同时（湮灭发生在机架中心时）或在很短的时间窗前后（湮灭发生在机架偏中心位置时）到达机架周围的环状检测器。监测这类事件可沿着响应线（line of response，LOR）定位光子位置，该响应线与记录光子的一对探测器相连。在飞行时间（time of flight，TOF）PET 中，即使偏离机架中心时，每个光子到达探测器所需时间的微小差异也被考虑在内，这使得湮灭沿着 LOR 定位更精准。（B）当一系列湮灭产生的光子沿着不同的响应线传播时，结合多个探测到的信息可以定位辐射源

影中获得的，通常使用 ^{111}In-DTPA，用于检查脑积水或脑脊液漏。

脊髓造影术

尽管 MRI 是大多数脊柱病变首选的检查方法，但脊髓造影术适用于不能接受 MRI 检查的患者（例如，起搏器植入后），也可用于检测自发性低颅压患者的脑脊液漏出部位（Kranz et al.，2016）。将碘造影剂经腰椎穿刺注入脊髓蛛网膜下腔，如果不能进行腰椎穿刺，则可在 C1-2 侧位穿刺注射。穿刺常在透视下引导，造影剂的注射需要通过间歇荧光屏监测，以确保不会注射至硬膜外或硬膜下。然后通过倾斜检查台将对比剂沿着椎管流动到适当的位置，并在患者仰卧位、俯卧位和斜卧位拍摄 X 线片。脊髓造影术后常会进行脊柱 CT 检查，后者比 X 线片提供了更多的解剖学信息，并且在同一图像上对骨骼和脊神经根解剖显示得更好。

脊髓造影的禁忌证包括对碘化造影剂过敏、癫痫发作、出血性疾病、服用抗凝剂或抗血小板药物的患者、怀疑颅内压升高的患者和不合作的患者。现代水溶性碘造影剂的并发症少见，具体包括穿刺硬膜后头痛、癫痫发作、穿刺部位出血、神经根损伤和蛛网膜炎（Sandow and Donnal，2005）

超声（ultrasound，US）

超声是一种约 20 kHz 的声波，高于人类听觉上限的频率。用于医学成像的超声通常频率在 2~18 MHz。当超声束从探头传输到人体时，随着通过组织的密度和组织的压迫发生反射和折射。US 探头可以检测反射的回声，并根据回声在组织中的传播时间和速度来确定其在患者体内的距离。回声的强度受组织的反射率及其衰减程度影响。因此，可以重建二维灰度图像，其中每个像素的位置和亮度与患者体内产生回声的位置和强度相对应，即 B 型超声（Allisy-Roberts and Williams，2007）。

骨骼和钙化都具有高反射性和衰减性，阻止了声波的穿透传播，因此呈现明亮的白色，在该区域之后有一个“声影”，无法获得影内任何信息。相反，液体的反射性很低，对声束的衰减较弱，表现为无回声区，在回声区之外与邻近组织的声音传播增强，其后部回声增强。

骨骼对声束的衰减限制了 B 型超声在成人和儿童大脑评估中的应用。新生儿和婴儿的经囟门超声检查可评估脑室大小，检测早产儿的脑室内和实质出血，以及评估缺氧缺血性脑病的脑实质情况。新生儿也可进行脊柱超声检查，以评估可疑脊柱闭合

表 3.6 神经成像的 PET 示踪剂示例

PET 示踪剂	作用机制及应用
^{11}C- 甲硫氨酸、^{18}F-FET	在恶性肿瘤中，氨基酸转运蛋白转运至细胞中增多——明确肿瘤范围，指导活检，制订治疗计划，疗效反应评估（放射性坏死、复发、假性反应），预测预后；评估纹状体多巴胺途径（^{18}F-DOPA）
^{18}F-FLT	与增殖细胞中胸苷激酶 -1 活性相关的摄取——肿瘤分级、治疗反应、预后的评估
^{18}F-FMISO、^{18}F-FAZA	缺氧细胞中的累积——评估脑肿瘤中缺氧与肿瘤的进展和对治疗的耐药性相关性
^{11}C-PK11195、^{18}F-GE180	结合在活化的小胶质细胞和癌细胞系的表达转运蛋白—小胶质细胞活化 / 炎症的评估，肿瘤分级的评估
^{68}Ga-DOTA-TOC ^{68}Ga-DOTA-TATE	在某些颅内肿瘤中高摄取的生长肽类似物——脑膜瘤、垂体腺瘤、成血管细胞瘤、髓母细胞瘤、PNET 的诊断
^{11}C-PiB（匹兹堡化合物） ^{18}F- 氟比他班 ^{18}F- 氟贝他吡 ^{18}F- 氟美他酚	与 β 淀粉样蛋白结合——阿尔茨海默病的诊断
^{11}C-PBB3 ^{18}F-FDDNP	与 tau 蛋白 / 神经原纤维结合——阿尔茨海默病和 tau 蛋白病的诊断
^{11}C- 氟马西尼 ^{11}C- 二丙诺啡 ^{11}C-SCH23390 ^{11}C- 雷氯必利	苯二氮䓬受体配体——受体结合研究 阿片受体配体——受体结合研究 多巴胺 D 1 受体配体——受体结合研究 多巴胺 D 2 受体配体——受体结合研究
$^{15}O_2$ 和 $[^{15}O]H_2O$ ^{11}C- 亮氨酸、^{11}C- 酪氨酸 ^{11}C- 白蛋白 $^{11}CO_2$、^{11}C-DMO	脑血流量、氧代谢 蛋白合成率 血浆容量 pH

不全其脊髓圆锥的位置、是否存在脊髓纵裂或椎管内占位。

当超声被一个移动的界面反射，其频率因多普勒效应改变，界面向传感器移动则频率增加；反之则频率降低。频率的变化量受反射物运动速度的影响。脉冲多普勒超声利用这种效应获得血管的波形，显示血流速度和方向。在彩色多普勒成像技术中，将血流方向和速度信息以彩色编码图叠加在 B 型超声灰度图像上。

多普勒超声可用于检测颈动脉杂音、短暂性缺血发作或缺血性中风患者的颈动脉狭窄。颈动脉狭窄的程度通常是根据狭窄区血流速度的增加而确定一个百分比范围。经颅多普勒（transcranial Dopple，TCD）也可以评价颅内主要动脉的血流。TCD 需要使用低频（2~3 MHz）换能器，从而可穿透相对较薄的翼骨或经枕骨大孔扫描。TCD 可对动脉瘤性蛛网膜下腔出血患者进行床旁监测，以寻找血流速度增加导致的痉挛血管（Marshall et al.，2010）。一些机构使用术中彩色多普勒超声评估 Chiari I 型畸形患者枕大孔的脑脊液流量。

血管成像

数字减影血管造影

尽管随着 CT 血管造影和 MR 血管造影的发展，数字减影血管造影（digital subtraction angiography，DSA）（Wolpert，1999）作为一线检查的适应证有所减少，但仍然是脑和脊柱血管疾病成像的金标准。DSA 通常在局麻下进行，但对于不合作的患者、介入性神经放射手术和诊断性脊髓血管造影（根据操作者需求），可能需要镇静或全身麻醉。DSA 常见入路是股总动脉；如操作困难，则可采用经桡动脉或经肱动脉入路。用针穿刺后，软头导丝穿过针头进入动脉，然后取下针头并更换聚乙烯导管。有多种形状导管可供选择，取决于术者的习惯和动脉迂曲的程度。在透视引导下，根据 DSA 的适应证，导管可以放置在颈内动脉、颈外动脉和椎动脉中。神经血管造影通常使用双平面血管造影设备进行，双平面血管造影装置有两个 X 射线管和图像增强器，或者增加平板数字探测器。这样可以同时从两个不同的投影中获取图像，减少检查的时长和注射的对比剂剂量。获取在对比剂注入动脉之前（即“掩模图像”）图像和注射对比剂过程的图像。注射对比剂期间获得的图像减去掩模图像，生成的图像消除了骨骼和软组织，仅显示血管。如果患者在图像采集过程中移动，掩模图像将无法与之后的对比图像正确配准，可能需要手动配准。在注射对比剂期间，也可以旋转C形臂围绕患者头部来获得三维图像（3D DSA）。

脑DSA可能的并发症包括所有侵入性血管造影常见的并发症，如穿刺部位血肿（约5%）、动脉夹层和造影剂反应。主动脉弓和颈动脉导管的操作会有小概率致神经功能缺损，通常是暂时性的（约2.5%），少数是永久性的（约0.2%）。神经系统并发症取决于术者的经验，老年患者和手术时间长会增加风险。

CT动脉造影和CT静脉造影

CT动脉造影（CT angiography，CTA）是在第一次团注碘造影剂期间快速获取感兴趣区域的薄扫数据。动脉期图像采集可以通过团注追踪法或测试团注追踪法。团注追踪是在造影剂注射后所选血管（通常是颈内动脉）的衰减达到预定水平时触发扫描。测试团注追踪法通过单独注射少量造影剂来确定开始扫描的最佳时间。尽管图像判读需要回顾轴向采集的源图像，但使用多平面重建、最大密度投影（maximum intensity projection，MIP）和容积再现重建三维图像有助于识别异常并帮助鉴别与周围血管的关系。

与DSA相比，CTA的优点包括无创性、更广泛的可用性以及简单和快速。传统CTA的缺点包括其时间分辨率较差，图像本质上是“独立照片”，不能提供动态信息，而DSA空间分辨率低，可能掩盖邻近骨骼的小血管异常。骨减影CTA图像可以在注入对比剂之前获取CT掩模图像，类似于DSA的方式从注射对比剂后的图像中减去，或者通过双能X线采集（需专用的双能CT扫描仪）。

CT静脉造影在原理上与CTA相似，不同之处在于图像采集时间是注射对比剂后处于静脉期时。图像采集时机不太关键，通常在对比剂注射后40秒进行延迟扫描。

磁共振血管成像和静脉成像

MRI进行血管成像有以下几种方法。无对比剂血管成像技术依赖于流动血液和周围静止组织之间的信号差异（Lim and Koktzoglou，2015）。时间飞跃法磁共振血管成像（time-of-flight magnetic resonance angiography，TOF-MRA）依赖于流入增强效应，其中射频脉冲反复作用于静止组织，使层面内静质子达到饱和，显示低信号，而流动质子刚进入层面，非饱和的血液呈现高信号。相位对比血管造影（phase-contrast angiography，PC-MRA）使用双梯度引导血液沿梯度方向流动，与流速成正比。通过改变梯度强度，调整速度编码值（Venc）显示动脉或静脉血流。TOF-MRA和PC-MRA都可以在二维（2D）或三维（3D）上进行采集。对比增强MRA（contrast-enhanced MRA，CE-MRA）原则上与CTA相似，通过静脉注射造影剂显示血管。在实际应用中，3D TOF-MRA是目前颅内血管成像的主要手段，与CTA相似，在3.0 T扫描中对动脉瘤具有灵敏度高、特异性高等优点（Lim and Koktzoglou，2015）。CE-MRA可以更好地显示大动脉瘤或血流缓慢的动脉瘤，也可以作为时间分辨检查手段（Saindane，2015）来评估动静脉畸形或硬脑膜瘘。检测颈动脉狭窄时，TOF-MRA不如CE-MRA敏感和特异（Gough，2011），并且可能高估狭窄程度。MRV常用相位对比法，因为时间飞跃可能被亚急性血栓的高信号混淆，它可模仿正常的流入增强效应（Nadgir and Yousem，2016）。MRV也可用于增强检查（Sadigh et al.，2016）。

其他血管技术

如前文所述，SWI对少量血代谢产物的高度敏感性使其在检查颅内出血方面非常有用，例如脑淀粉样血管病或创伤性脑损伤中的微出血。此外，SWI对脱氧血红蛋白的顺磁性敏感，可以很好地显示静脉结构（Di Ieva et al.，2015）。SWI可显示动静脉畸形（arteriovenous malformations，AVM）的静脉引流，并评估其神经外科切除范围以及显示微动静脉畸形（Mossa Basha et al.，2012；Saindane，2015）。

除了评估血管腔，血管壁的评估也越来越受到重视。在颈动脉成像中，重点评估动脉粥样硬化斑块，特别是其的稳定性和破裂倾向（Young et al.，2011）。颅内血管壁成像可用于评估颅内动脉粥样硬化、烟雾病、血管炎、可逆性脑血管收缩综合征和颅内动脉夹层（Mandel et al.，2017）。

脑血流和代谢的成像方法

脑灌注和代谢成像具有重要的研究意义和广泛的临床应用，临床应用包括评估急性卒中、缺氧性脑损伤、血管痉挛、脑血流量储备和创伤性脑损伤（Coles，2006；Dani and Warach，2014）。主要应用在神经肿瘤学中，结合多种方法评估肿瘤类型和分级、鉴别非肿瘤性病变、指导活检、反应评估以及鉴别放化疗反应与肿瘤进展（Herholz et al.，2007；Waldman et al.，2009；Kim et al.，2016）。脑局部血流和代谢的差异也为痴呆和神经退行性疾病的诊断提供了更多的信息（Schuff，2013；Ishii，2014）。由于篇幅有限，本章仅对可用方法做简要描述，更全面的介绍可查看相关参考文献以及专著（Gillard et al.，2010；Barker et al.，2013）。

脑血流检测

脑灌注的成像方法可以使用惰性扩散示踪剂或非扩散血管内示踪剂（Coles，2006）。前者依据的是Fick原则，即靶器官对任何物质的摄取取决于其动静脉浓度差异和器官灌注。应用扩散示踪剂的技术包括非放射性 ^{131}Xe 增强 CT 以及应用 SPECT 和 ^{99m}Tc-HMPAO、^{99m}Tc-ECD 或放射性核素 ^{133}Xe 等核医学方法，还有应用 $^{15}O_2$ 的 PET。定量 $^{15}O_2$ PET 和氙气 CT 被认为是测量脑灌注的金标准，但在临床中并未常规应用（Thompson et al.，2010）。在磁共振灌注中动脉自旋标记水分子作为示踪剂，这种方法可能会越来越多地应用于临床（Grade et al.，2015）。

血管内注射非扩散示踪剂的技术应用越来越广泛，并且在卒中和神经肿瘤成像中逐渐成为临床常规检查的一部分。与 CT 或 MRI 测量灌注情况的基本原理相似，关键在于第一次扫描注射对比剂时快速成像（Konstas et al.，2009a）。简而言之，如果造影剂在血管内，颅内组织的衰减（CT）和信号强度（MRI）的变化取决于组织固有的灌注特点和感兴趣区动脉（动脉输入功能）的造影剂流量。对比剂浓度曲线下面积和对比剂的容量可评价脑血容量（cerebral blood volume，CBV）和平均通过时间（mean transit time，MTT），脑血流量（cerebral blood flow，CBF）可根据中心容积定理（CBF=CBV/MTT）计算。CT 灌注成像（CT perfusion，CTP）目前广泛用于评估急性卒中（Konstas et al.，2009a；Konstas et al.，2009b）梗死核心和缺血半暗带的程度以及蛛网膜下腔出血后血管痉挛的诊断和治疗（Mir et al.，2014）。CTP 最大的优点是碘浓度与组织衰减值呈线性关系，可以直接测量动脉输入和静脉输出功能，从而可以直接计算血管参数。与 MRI 相比，灌注 CT 的缺点是有电离辐射，覆盖范围有限，现在多排 CT 扫描仪和移动床技术可克服部分缺点。

磁共振成像灌注技术的基础是钆造影剂的磁敏感效应导致 T2* 信号的降低 [动态敏感性对比增强（dynamic susceptibility contrast，DSC）]，或通过增加 T1 信号反映的弛豫效应 [动态对比增强（dynamic contrast enhancement，DCE）]。绝对灌注参数的量化比 CTP 更为困难，需要对造影剂进行数学和药代动力学建模，并校正漏入血管外的造影剂（Jackson，2004）。为了便于比较，DSC 得出的灌注参数可以表示为相对值，通常与对侧脑白质进行标准化。DCE 可表征包括渗透性在内的多个微血管环境的参数。最常用的指标包括血流量（F）、单位组织的渗透面积（PS）、容量转移常数（K_{trans}）、血管外细胞外间隙（Ve）和血浆（Vb），以及根据增强曲线形状得出的半定量指数（Thompson et al.，2010；Griffith and Jain，2015）

血流容积成像（vascular space occupancy imaging，VASO）在 T1 上利用血液和组织之间的差异来分离二者，是定量脑血流量的一种新兴技术。VASO MRI 不用注射对比剂，可高时间分辨率的监测脑 CBV 的变化，注射造影剂后能测量 CBV 绝对值的变化（Lu and Uh，2013）。

磁共振弥散加权成像中的信号不仅取决于弥散本身，而且依赖于毛细血管内的血流（伪弥散），近年来，利用脑体素内不相干运动成像（intravoxel incoherent motion imaging，IVIM）来测量脑灌注重新引起了学者们的兴趣。通过应用弥散梯度强度和双指数拟合或峰度模型，可以鉴别毛细血管血流和真正的弥散，从而评估脑灌注（Federau et al.，2014）。

还有使用于基于灌注和氧气代谢的评估脑含氧量的方法。金标准方法是 $^{15}O_2$ PET，可作为 $[^{15}O]H_2O$ 和 $[^{15}O]CO$ 的补充（三重态氧 PET），除了评估脑灌注指数外，还可评估脑氧代谢率（cerebral metabolic rate of oxygen，CRMO2）和氧摄取分数的绝对值。新兴的基于 MRI 的方法包括定量 BOLD、基于相位和磁敏感成像以及基于 T2 的血管内成像等方法（Christen et al.，2013）。

脑代谢评估

目前用于评估脑代谢的两种主要成像方式是 PET 和磁共振波谱（magnetic resonance spectroscopy，MRS）。如上文所述，不同示踪剂 PET 评估局部或区域葡萄糖代谢（^{18}FDG-PET）和氧代谢（$^{15}O_2$，三重态氧）。在脑肿瘤中，PET 可以评估氨基酸转运（^{11}C- 蛋氨酸，^{18}F-FET）、蛋白质合成（^{11}C- 蛋氨酸和 ^{11}C- 亮氨酸）、DNA 合成（^{18}F-FLT）、组织的缺氧水平（^{18}F-FMISO 和 ^{18}F-FAZA）。

MRS 基于化学位移，化学位移是由于感兴趣原子与化合物结合时，电子所受屏蔽引起的共振频率的特定变化。MRS 允许在既定的感兴趣体素（单体素光谱）中评估生化环境，或从 2D 或 3D 磁光谱成像（CSI）绘制出整个大脑中既定化合物的浓度。MRS 由于灵敏度低、信噪比低，对磁场强度和匀场精度要求较高，是一项具有挑战性的技术。由于靶核充裕，MRS 最常用的是氢质子波谱（^{1}H-MRS）。在大脑中，^{1}H-MRS 可检测到被认为是几种特定代谢标志物的波谱，如 N- 乙酰天冬氨酸（NAA，神经元完整性的标志物）、胆碱（Cho，细胞膜代谢的标志物）、肌酸和肌醇（细胞能量代谢的标志物）。病理状况会导致波谱模式改变，或出现异常代谢物峰，如乳酸（Lac，代谢性酸中毒和细胞死亡的标志物）或脂质（组织分解的标志物）；例如，高级别脑胶质瘤表现出 NAA 减少和 Cho 升高，伴有脂质和乳酸峰（Herholz et al.，2007）。更具技术难度的 ^{31}P-MRS 可以通过检测含磷的 ATP 分子、磷酸肌酸和无机磷酸盐的波谱评估能量代谢以及通过检测磷酸单酯和磷酸二酯来评估神经元细胞膜代谢（Herholz et al.，2007）。

近年来，动态核极化（dynamic nuclear polarization，DNP）或超极化技术引起了人们的广泛关注，DNP 是通过增加产生磁共振信号的原子核的比例来解决 MRS 低灵敏度问题。通常在磁场中极化的原子核的磁矩或与磁场平行（自旋向上）或反平行（自旋向下）；净磁共振信号由指向每个方向的原子核数之间的微小差异导致（每百万个核中只有几个原子核指向自旋向上）。DNP 将含有固态未配对电子的感兴趣原子核和自由基进行极端冷却，然后将其置于强磁场中。在上述条件下，电子自旋变得高度极化，通过微波辐射使部分极化转变成核自旋，可使信噪比增加 10000 倍以上（Ardenkjaer-Larsen et al.，2003）。DNP 目前不能在人体内进行，但可超极化含有 MRS 可检测的原子核，使其活跃，注射到患者体内，从而增加图像的信噪比。现已有可系统性应用于人体的 DNP，且已有大量相关研究。目前 DNP 中最常用的代谢物是 [1-^{13}C] 丙酮酸，注射后通过乳酸脱氢酶（LDH）转化为 [1-^{13}C] 乳酸，经丙氨酸转氨酶转化为 [1-^{13}C] 丙氨酸，经丙酮酸脱氢酶（PDH）转化为 $^{13}CO_2$，后者进一步转化为 [^{13}C] 碳酸氢盐。在恶性肿瘤中，即使存在足够的氧气（Warburg 效应），丙酮酸转化为乳酸的过程会增加，有助于癌症诊断和治疗反应评估（Kim et al.，2016）。其他在动物模型中表现出潜力的标志物包括用于检测细胞坏死的 [1，4-^{13}C] 富马酸盐，[^{13}C] 碳酸氢盐用于体内 pH 测量，[5-^{13}C] 谷氨酰胺用于评估肿瘤代谢，而 [1-^{13}C] 尿素可以用作灌注标志物。只要化学位移足以在波谱上鉴别，也可以同时注入和检测多种超极化底物（Brindle et al.，2011）。

未来研究方向

目前的常规放射学方法能够以高灵敏度和高分辨率显示疾病的解剖和宏观病理特征。如前文所述，功能成像方法是从解剖学成像朝着更精确地描述疾病过程迈出的重要的第一步，因为它使人们更加了解各种疾病的生理病理变化。然而这些方法仍然是非特异性的，提示许多病理途径中可能存在最终的转化。获得更具体信息的方法之一是放射组学，将放射学图像转换为高维数据，然后以类似于基因组学、蛋白质组学或代谢组学方法的方式进行特征提取和数据挖掘，以获得与疾病特定特征相对应的影像组学特征（Gillies et al.，2016）。放射组学特征包括语义学特征（例如形状、大小或血管）和数学特征（例如直方图偏斜或峰度，分形和纹理分析）。放射组学为诊断、治疗选择和预后提供了有价值的信息，但其缺点是原始图像获取的方式相同。最终目标是通过使用特定分子靶点或生物化学的探针，获得在观察到的解剖和功能并发症之前和之后的细胞和分子事件的信息。这将更好地了解生物学的异常，实现早期检测，提供准确的诊断和疾病分期。分子成像还可以在药物开发过程中提供可靠的生物标志物，在出现反应表型之前，就可在分子水平上快速评估治疗效果（Massoud and Gambir，2007）。故此方法最重要的应用将是在神经肿瘤学中，已经有一些检测特定受体或特定酶亚型的蛋白质产物的临床应用（Kim et al.，2016）。由于光学，光声或超声技术在颅内成像方面的局限性（部分技术可用于术中或内镜检查期间），PET 和 MRI 很可能用于成像探针。纳米颗粒正在成为一种理想的显像剂（Thakor and Gambir，2013），它可以通过既定的方法或多种途径靶向标记特定组织，例如通过 MRI 进行术前成像以及使用光声和光学成像进行术中定位（Kircher et al.，2012）。纳米颗粒与治疗药物的结合，可同时实现诊断和治疗——诊断治疗学（Kelkar and Reineke，2011；Thakor and Gambir，2013），例如将成像与靶向化疗、基因沉默剂、放射性同位素、辐射增敏药物、光动力或光热干涉结合起来。未来，成像无疑将成为精准医疗的关键环节，为患者或病变靶向治疗制订精确诊断、个性化治疗方案（Kim et al.，2016）。

参考文献、EBRAIN 的相关链接

扫描书末二维码获取。

第 4 章　手术室环境

Neil Kitchen · Jonathan Shapey 著
梁琨、任倩薇 译，刘晓楠、王伟、孟凡刚 审校

神经外科手术室

20 世纪，神经外科手术室在照明、设备、气流和无菌性方面有了显著的进步。术中成像和集成导航系统也开始出现（**图 4.1**）。

现代化标准手术室被划分成不同的区域，以尽量减少细菌污染。手术室为无菌区，麻醉室为洁净区，其他区域为污染区。标准手术室设有单向气流系统，以每小时至少进行 20 次换气的方式降低空气传播污染的风险。空气在进入手术室之前会经过过滤，然后从最干净的区域传播到较为污染的区域，但是如果手术室的门保持打开状态，则会阻碍空气流通。烟雾测试可用于评估空气如何流过手术室。现在带层流罩的超净手术室已被用于骨科植入手术，但由于定位设备，尤其是手术显微镜的问题，使得超净手术室在神经外科中的应用存在困难。

手术室的温度和湿度也有规定。20~22 ℃的平均温度对大多数手术团队来说是舒适的，但必须使用保暖毯和加温静脉输液来防止患者体温过低。

在脊柱内固定和植入手术中，需要特别重视无菌原则。包括尽量减少手术室人员的数量和人员的进出次数，使用“非接触技术”进行皮肤准备，设备灭菌和术中抗生素预防等措施以最大限度地降低感染风险，这将在**第 94 章**中进行详细讨论。

2009 年，世界卫生组织（WHO）发表了一项具有里程碑意义的研究。该研究发现，实施系统的检查可以减少多达 1/3 的安全事故（Haynes et al., 2009）。国家患者安全局（National Patient Safety Agency，NPSA）在 2010 年启动了“手术安全步骤”倡议，所有 NHS 医疗保健机构现在都有义务使用世卫组织的外科手术安全检查表（**图 4.2**）。该计划的目的是减少围术期护理不当带来的危害，并支持手术室环境内文化的改变，从而更好地促进整个团队的沟通。这五个步骤是：①术前团队概要；②术前登记；③手术时间；④术后登记；⑤术后团队小结。

手术患者定位

手术室中的核心设备是手术台。现代的神经外科手术台具有射线透过性，头部和腿部可互换，安装在偏置的柱基上，实现手术台面向颅骨或尾部移动并在所有平面上倾斜。抬头位可用于大多数神经外科手术，因为它可以降低颅内压和静脉出血风险。但是，因为存在空气栓塞、术后硬膜下积气和分水岭梗死的风险，通常应避免过分抬头。在大多数显微外科手术中都需要进行颅骨固定，以确保将头部固定在最佳位置，同时要考虑到颅骨基部的最终角度、所需的手术路径以及最小化脑部回缩的需要。使用术中图像引导系统时，颅骨固定尤其重要，许多颈椎手术也需要颅骨固定。

通过使用销钉固定装置，例如三点固定的 Mayfield 头架，可实现颅骨固定。在摇杆销上标出 20、40、60 和 80 磅的拉力环，拉力为 60 磅，可在成人中安全固定。在放置销钉时，重要的是要避开颞骨鳞部、眶上、植入的分流装置和大额窦。儿科患者应谨慎使用或避免使用颅骨固定装置，因为这可能导致颅骨穿孔和硬膜外出血。

神经外科中有多种手术体位，外科医生会根据具体情况确定首选体位。常见的手术位置包括仰卧位、俯卧位、公园长椅位和坐位（**图 4.3**）。与麻醉师的密切合作对于确保患者处于最佳手术位置至关重要，但是手术团队的每个成员都必须注意，以防不当定位的潜在并发症。骨突出在手术过程中有造成压力性损伤的危险，必须加以很好的衬垫，同时还必须遮盖患者的眼睛以保护其免受挤压与酒精清洁溶液伤害。因受压或牵拉性麻痹会造成周围神经损伤，以尺神经和腓总神经最易受损，特别是在侧卧（长椅）位手术时。坐位手术增加了发生空气栓塞的风险（大多数是潮气末 CO_2 快速上升）。俯卧位时由于眼压升高和视神经灌注压降低，患者有一定的失明风险。颅骨固定不当也会导致头皮坏死或局部

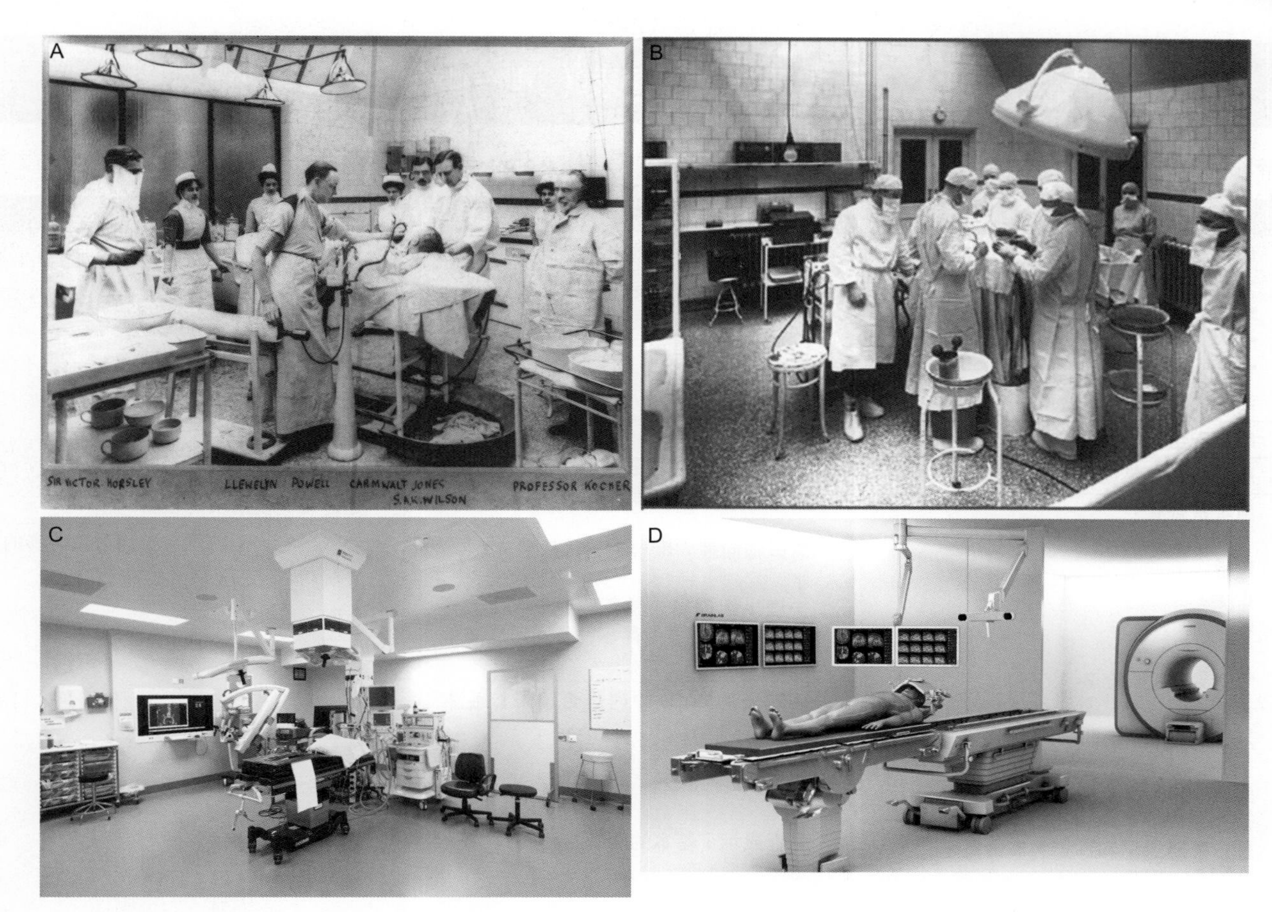

图 4.1 神经外科手术室。(A)Victor Horsley 在皇后广场医院的手术室(1906 年);(B)20 世纪 30 年代手术室;(C)现代神经外科手术室;(D)术中 MRI 室

血肿。

手术室内的设备位置可优化手术操作

外科医生在手术过程中需要考虑手术室人员的位置。手术助手不应位于外科医生和清洁护士之间，手术室不应该放置多余的未使用设备。钻头、超声吸引器和双极器的位置必须明确，导线不应穿过手术野，这样外科医生就可以用他们的惯用手进行操作。图像引导摄像机的位置应确保显微镜和手术室工作人员不会妨碍到患者所在的位置。手术室的声音不应该影响外科医生、麻醉师和其他手术室工作人员的有效沟通。

低血糖、咖啡和膀胱充盈等情况都可能对外科医生的手术造成影响。给予外科医生舒适的环境并不是过分的要求，而是安全手术所必需的。手术牵开器系统和座椅可以让外科医生的手肘和手腕在坚实的表面上休息，这对减少疲劳非常有用。一些手术体位，尤其是坐姿，要求医生在手术时抬高手臂，这样会造成疲劳。长时间的手术最好由手术小组进行，这样就可以根据需要进行休息。

手术室设备

神经外科医生需要熟悉许多类型的手术设备。虽然该内容超出了本章的范围，但是以下设备值得特别考虑。

手术显微镜

关于第一台真正的显微镜的发明者仍有很多争议，一般认为它是在 16 世纪后期发展起来的。与物理学家恩斯特·阿贝(Ernst Abbé)合作的德国机械师卡尔·蔡司(Carl Zeiss)革新了透镜制造和显微镜制造技术。20 世纪初，显微镜已是实验室医学研究中不可或缺的一部分，但直到 1921 年，瑞典耳鼻喉科医生 Carl Nylén 使用显微镜对患有慢性中耳炎的患者进行手术后，显微镜才在手术室中使用。 蔡司于 1953 年推出了他们的第一台系列手术显微镜。1957

World Health Organization

手术安全核查表（第一版）

麻醉诱导前 ▶▶▶▶▶▶▶▶▶▶▶▶▶▶▶▶▶	皮肤切开前 ▶▶▶▶▶▶▶▶▶▶▶▶▶▶▶▶▶	患者离开手术室之前
术前登记	**手术时间**	**术后登记**
☐ 患者已确认 • 身份 • 部位 • 步骤 • 同意 ☐ 治疗中心标记 / 不适用 ☐ 麻醉安全检查完成 ☐ 患者脉搏血氧仪和功能 患者是否有： 过敏 ☐ 否 ☐ 是 气道 / 吸入风险？ ☐ 否 ☐ 是，且设备 / 辅助装置可用 失血 >500 ml（儿童 7 ml/kg）？ ☐ 否 ☐ 是，静脉通路和计划的液体充足	☐ 确认所有团队成员的名字和职责 ☐ 外科医生、麻醉专家和护士确认 • 患者 • 手术部位 • 手术流程 预期的关键事件 ☐ 外科医生：哪些是关键的或意外的步骤，手术时间，预期的出血量？ ☐ 麻醉师回顾：患者有无特殊情况？ ☐ 护理小组回顾：是否确认无菌（包括指标结果）? 是否存在设备问题或其他问题？ 在过去的 60 分钟内是否给予抗生素预防治疗？ ☐ 是 ☐ 不适用 是否显示了基本的图像？ ☐ 是 ☐ 不适用	护士与团队确认： ☐ 记录的过程名称 ☐ 仪器、海绵和针数是否正确（或不适用） ☐ 标本的标签（包括患者姓名） ☐ 是否有需要解决的设备问题 ☐ 外科医生、麻醉师和护士对该患者的康复和管理的关键问题进行评估

本清单并不全面。建议适当增加和修改相关内容以适应当地的实际情况。

图 4.2 世界卫生组织手术安全检查表

Reproduced with permission from the World Health Organization.

年，Theodore Kurze 成为第一位对患者使用显微镜的神经外科医生，切除了一位 5 岁儿童的面神经瘤。1960 年 Raymond Donaghy 进行了第一例显微神经血管手术。他还在佛蒙特州建立了一个显微外科培训实验室，年轻 Gazi Yasgaril 被派去学习这项新兴技术。Yasgaril 宣传了显微神经外科的优势，并使手术显微镜成为现代神经外科的组成部分（Kriss and Kriss，1998）。

手术医生能够可以借助现代显微镜以高放大倍率看到术区的三维图像。现代显微镜的主要组件是物镜、双目镜筒、光源、电动变焦系统和悬架系统。手术显微镜的设计可确保高质量的照明完全平行且非常接近光路。两个视场也彼此靠近，可以在深而狭窄的伤口底部实现双眼视觉。显微镜放大的倍数越大，外科医生的视野就越小，因此外科医生应尝试使显微镜尽可能地靠近患者。但是，在显微镜和伤口之间需要有一个良好的工作距离，以允许手术器械在使用过程中不会彼此碰撞或与显微镜发生摩擦。现代显微镜具有从 200~500 mm 的电动可变焦距的物镜，焦距实际上与工作距离相同。目镜用于将中间图像放大 10 倍，并且补偿屈光不正。为了允许显微镜自由移动，术前调试是必不可少的，并且要求洞巾不能限制显微镜的移动。

现代显微镜通常还装有两个附加光源。红外 800 nm 灯可通过术中荧光观察血流，蓝色 400 nm 灯用于荧光引导的肿瘤手术。

神经内镜

神经内镜首次应用于 1910 年，当时泌尿科医师 Victor Lespinasse 使用小儿膀胱镜尝试通过内镜下凝固脉络膜丛来治疗小儿脑积水（Abd-El-Barr and Cohen，2013）。之后，Dandy 和 Mixter 在 20 世纪 20 年代尝试对第三脑室进行内镜开窗术以治疗脑积水，但随着光学和电子技术的发展，神经内镜的真

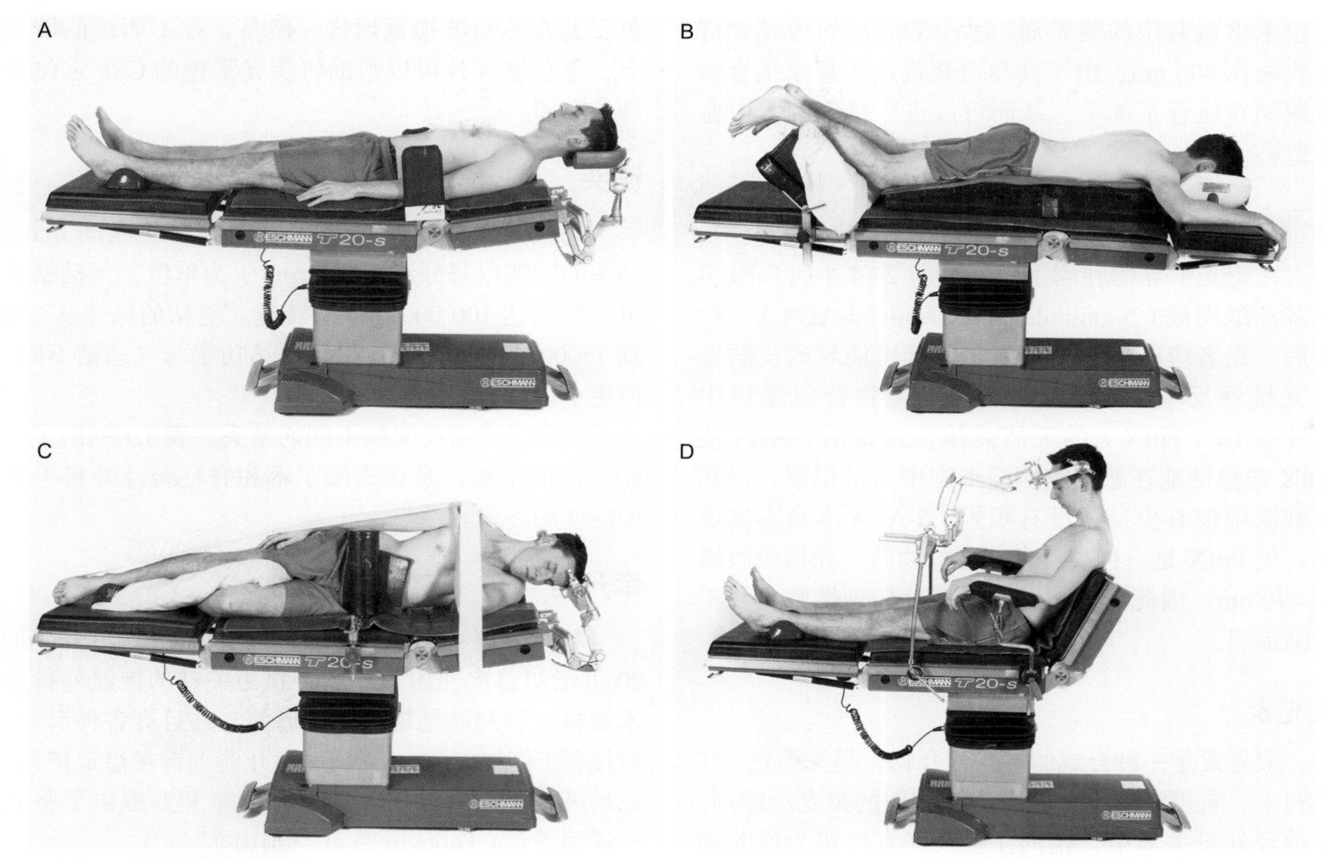

图 4.3　神经外科常用的患者体位。（A）仰卧位：翼点开颅，额 / 额下 / 眶上开颅，顶开颅，颞开颅（肩滚置于同侧肩下），经蝶窦手术。（B）俯卧位：中线枕下颅骨切除术，脊柱手术。（C）外侧 / 公园 - 长凳 /3/4 俯卧位：乙状窦后 / 外侧枕下颅骨切除术，脊柱手术。（D）坐位：枕下颅骨切除术，颈椎手术

正进步出现在 20 世纪 70 年代（Liu et al.，2004）。

显微镜下的术中照明和视野量由手术方法决定，在手术通道又长又窄的情况下可能会受到很大限制。现代内镜能够将更强的光带入手术视野，并在近距离位置提供更广阔的视角和更好的放大倍率。内镜手术的其他潜在优势包括降低组织破坏和脑组织牵拉，有利于切口美观，缩短住院时间并降低手术并发症的发病率。

内镜有两种主要类型：即柔性光纤和刚性杆状透镜系统。两种类型的内镜都使用氙气光源，该氙气光源通过光纤传输到内镜。光纤柔性内镜通过一组紧密堆积的光纤线传输图像，并且比刚性透镜内镜更小且更具延展性。刚性内镜比光纤内镜更昂贵，但它通过一系列透镜提供了卓越的图像分辨率和透射光。一些内镜具有工作通道，允许插入兼容的仪器，例如微型镊子、内镜剪刀、单极手术电极或 Fogarty 球囊导管。冲洗通道可以清除透镜上的碎屑和手术区域的出血。内镜具有各种角度（0°、30°、70° 和 120°），以便可视化手术视野的隐藏部分，但通常手术者仅在 0°～30° 进行操作。

最初，神经内镜手术仅限于脑室，但现在内镜已用于治疗多种神经外科疾病。H.D. Jho 开创了经鼻内镜下垂体手术的方法（Jho and Alfieri，2001）。内镜在其他颅底病变中的应用也在不断扩展（Paluzzi et al.，2012）。内镜还用于脊柱外科，特别是用于胸腔手术。内镜手术中重要的是要为手术选择合适的内镜。例如，无通道的纤维内镜可能适用于诊断性脑室造口术，但在进行经鼻内镜手术时，最好使用坚固的多通道透镜内镜。尽管内镜是一个迅速发展的领域，但并不是所有的神经外科医师都在常规进行内镜手术，其存在陡峭的学习曲线。适当的培训是必不可少的，通过与其他专业专家合作，比如内镜方面经验丰富的耳鼻喉专家，可以减少学习的困难，并减少手术时间和手术并发症的发病率。

荧光剂

吲哚菁绿

吲哚菁绿（indocyanine green，ICG）是术中血管

造影术中最常用的荧光剂。术中静脉注射后其光谱吸收峰在 800 nm，由于其与血浆蛋白的紧密结合而被限制在血管系统中，从而可以进行良好的术中血管造影。

5- 氨基乙酰丙酸

在荧光引导的肿瘤手术麻醉前 2~4 小时口服 5-氨基乙酰丙酸（5-aminolevulinic acid，5-ALA）。给药后，患者应避免阳光直射，因其可能导致皮肤发生光敏性反应。5-ALA 是血红素生物合成途径中原卟啉 IX（PpIX）的天然前体，过量的 5-ALA 使 PpIX 选择性地在恶性胶质瘤细胞中大量积累，但在正常脑中仅有少量或没有积累。5-ALA 本身不发荧光，但 PpIX 是一种高度发荧光的物质，光谱吸收峰在 440 nm，因此可以帮助术者区分病理性肿瘤和正常脑组织。

荧光素

荧光素是一种合成的有机化合物，呈深橙色 / 红色粉末。它可溶于水，是被广泛应用的荧光示踪剂。在神经外科手术中，鞘内注射荧光素已成为诊断和定位脑脊液（cerebrospinal fluid，CSF）渗漏的重要工具，并且在术中用于协助定位颅底缺陷的部位。目前建议除去 10 ml 的患者 CSF，并用等量的荧光素稀释溶液注入鞘内腔来代替。稀溶液的颜色为鲜绿色，通常不需要视觉增强。但是，在不明确的情况下，蓝色滤光片可以帮助将荧光素色的 CSF 定位在颅骨底部。

钻头

现代高速外科骨钻可以采用气动或电动方式。钻头的转速以每分钟转数（rpm）为单位，气动钻头可产生高达 100 000 rpm 的转速。电钻的钻速从 200 到 75000 rpm 可调节，尽管电钻功率与气动钻不同，但更小、更轻，更易于操纵。

根据手术需要安装不同的钻头。**表 4.1** 列出了一些常用的钻头以及在头颅手术和脊柱神经外科手术中的使用方式。

牵开器

脑牵开器由 Harvey Cushing 和 Victor Horsley 于 20 世纪初首次使用，此后一直是关键的神经外科手术器械。脑刮匙是矩形或锥形的，并且有各种尺寸。铰接臂（例如 Yasargil Leyla 牵开器）旨在稳定铲刀，此后开发的各种牵开器系统，为牵开器提供了坚实的锚固平台（Dujovny et al.，2010）。

牵开器的不当使用或者牵开时间过长可能会引起皮质挫伤、血管损伤、脑肿胀和神经功能缺损。因牵开器使用不当造成的损伤发生率高达 10%（Spetzler et al.，1992）。有的外科医生主张完全避免

表 4.1　颅、脊柱神经外科用普通钻头及附件

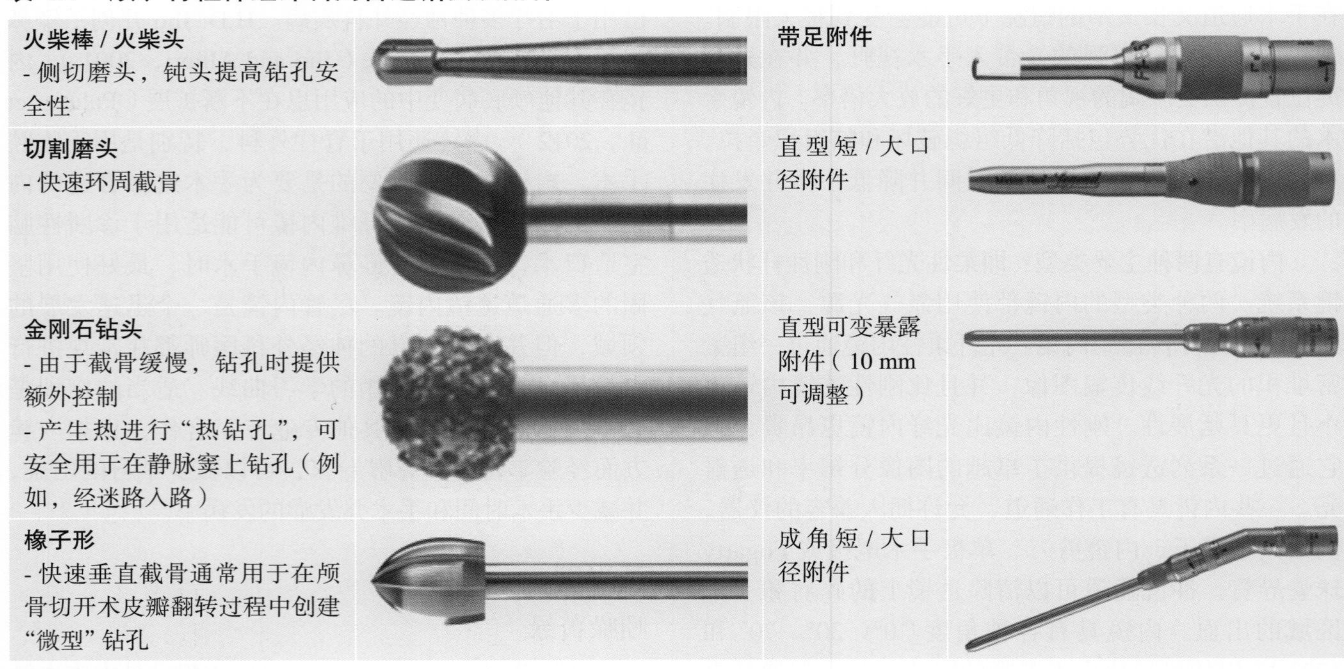

钻头	附件
火柴棒 / 火柴头 - 侧切磨头，钝头提高钻孔安全性	**带足附件**
切割磨头 - 快速环周截骨	直型短 / 大口径附件
金刚石钻头 - 由于截骨缓慢，钻孔时提供额外控制 - 产生热进行“热钻孔”，可安全用于在静脉窦上钻孔（例如，经迷路入路）	直型可变暴露附件（10 mm 可调整）
橡子形 - 快速垂直截骨通常用于在颅骨切开术皮瓣翻转过程中创建“微型”钻孔	成角短 / 大口径附件

Medtronic, Midas Rex.

使用牵开器，认为选择好的手术体位可以使重力作为辅助而不会妨碍外科医生，适量排出脑脊液、输注甘露醇、熟练的麻醉师以及对手术的耐心等因素都可以避免不必要的过度牵开。明智而谨慎地使用牵开器可以最大限度地减少与牵开器使用相关的并发症，此类技术包括将手术纱布放置在牵开器下方，避免牢固的牵开以及使用硅涂层的牵开器。

电凝疗法

电凝疗法用于切割组织和止血。高频交流电通过人体组织时会产生热量。在 400 kHz~10 MHz 的频率下，高达 500 mA 的电流是安全的，局部的高密度电流产生的温度可以高达 1000 ℃。在高于 50 kHz 的频率下不会刺激神经肌肉组织。

有两种不同类型的电凝疗法：

单极电凝疗法

单极透热疗法使用高功率装置（400 W）产生从头端电极（高电流密度）经接地板（低电流密度）返回发生器的高频交流电。不同的电压会影响热凝的模式。切割电凝使用连续低电压输出（500~1000 V）产生局部高温，造成浅表组织破坏和水的气化，同时凝固血管和止血作用弱。替代凝固在短时间间隔内产生高频电流的脉冲高压输出（高达 6000 V），导致组织水汽化和血管凝固。许多电凝设备可以同时切割和凝固组织。

单极热凝在潮湿环境中不起作用，可引起热量扩散，损伤周围（1~2 cm）组织。患者电极板放置不正确是电凝灼伤的最常见原因。为最大限度地降低并发症风险，患者电极板的表面积应至少为 70 cm^2，并且保证其接触良好，同时要远离骨突起、金属假体（如髋关节置换）和瘢痕组织，一般是粘贴在备皮后的干燥的皮肤处。

有心律失常病史的患者应慎用单极热凝，单极热凝也不能用于植入心脏起搏器的患者，会引起心脏停搏。有病例报告称，在使用单极热凝之前，如果皮肤上的酒精没有挥发，有燃烧风险。

双极电凝疗法

双极电凝使用较低的功率（50 W）在两个头端之间产生高频交流电。它使用 1 MHz 波形进行切割和凝固，并且由于其仅使用 140 V，因此可用于植入起搏器和除颤器的患者。不需要使用患者电极板，双极电凝可以在潮湿的环境中有效使用。

双极镊的长度和尖端锋利度各不相同。凝固、炭化的组织会粘在活检钳上，必须保持干净。可用改良包括灌注双极镊和冷头镊，使该风险的可能性降低。

超声吸引器

超声吸引器是一种振动外科器械，它利用超声作为一种物理能量来破碎（空化）、乳化并去除不需要的组织。用于神经外科的超声吸引器的例子包括 Cavitron 超声外科吸引器（CUSA）（Integra）和 Sonopet（Stryker）。空心钛尖端沿其纵轴振动，产生 20~60 kHz 的超声，所有模型均允许外科医生指定振动、冲洗和抽吸的水平，以便在组织解剖期间实现最大程度的控制。CUSA 包含辅助组织选择功能，可进一步调节相对组织碎裂率，一些抽吸器（例如 Sonopet）可通过将纵向振动与扭转振动耦合来进行精细的解剖。

超声外科吸引器可在单个手持式设备中提供超声空化、冲洗和抽吸，可减少手术区域内的器械更换并改善医生视野。目标神经组织的选择性破碎也降低了血管损伤的风险，但是必须谨记由热损伤引起的附带损害以及出现模糊的“假”组织平面的风险。

止血材料

在神经外科手术中实现和维持止血对手术结局至关重要。针对凝血级联反应中的不同靶点已经开发了各种止血材料（**图 4.4** 和**表 4.2**）（Grant，2007）。其中一些在术后可能会引起肿胀，应注意避免止血药残留，其在肿胀后会引起神经压迫。这在脊椎中尤其重要。某些止血剂可能会导致 MR 伪影，使残留肿瘤的术后评估变得困难。

出血问题也可以通过更改患者体位、氨甲环酸、止血钳或肌肉贴片来控制。Victor Horsley 首先将骨蜡用于神经外科手术，现已广泛用于骨边缘出血的止血。

神经导航

影像技术彻底改变了神经外科的临床实践，并已成为指导诊断、术前计划和术中导航的关键。尤其是图像引导手术已成为现代神经外科必不可少的技术，并且适用于许多神经外科手术，包括神经肿瘤、血管和功能神经外科。

立体定向外科手术的目的，是通过解剖或影像注册，定位患者所在的手术空间。图像引导可实现更小、更精确定位的切口以及对病变的精确定位。

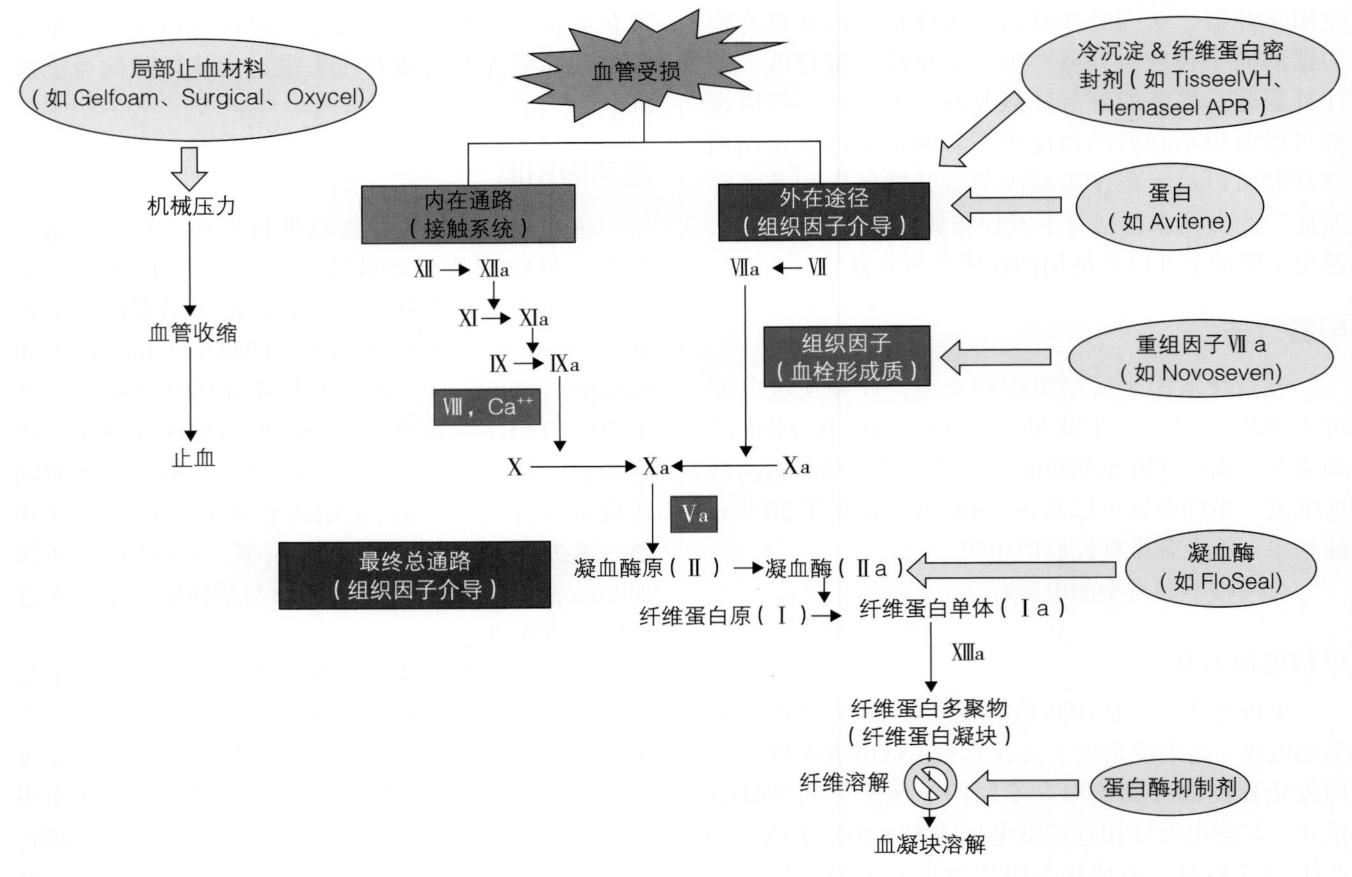

图 4.4 止血材料及其作用机制

Adapted from *Surgery*, Volume 142, issue 4, Gerald A. Grant, Update on hemostasis: neurosurgery, pp. S55–S60, Copyright (2007), with permission from Elsevier.

表 4.2 止血材料及其作用机制

止血辅助	品名	活性组分
局部止血剂	Gelfoam	海绵胶
	Surgical	氧化再生纤维素
	Oxycel	氧化纤维素
蛋白	Avitene	微晶胶原（与血小板反应）
血纤蛋白黏合剂	Tisseel Haemaseel APR	纤维蛋白原 / 因子ⅩⅢ浓缩物（冷沉淀）和凝血酶混合物
凝血酶	FloSeal	明胶基质和凝血酶混合物
蛋白酶抑制剂		纤溶酶抑制剂（抑制纤溶）

Adapted from *Surgery*, Volume 142, issue 4, Gerald A. Grant, Update on hemostasis: neurosurgery, pp. S55–S60, Copyright (2007), with permission from Elsevier.

立体定向神经外科手术可以是基于框架的或无框架的。

基于框架的立体定向神经外科

立体定向定位的概念最早是在 1908 年由 Victor Horsley 和 Robert Clark 提出的，当时这种装置仅适用于中小型实验动物（**图 4.5A**）。Ernest Speigel 和 Henry Wycis 于 1947 年首次将立体定向手术成功应用于人类，1949 年瑞典神经外科医师 Lars Leksell 在参观了费城的 Wycis 后开发了以弧弓为中心的立体定向框架系统。Leksell 的框架由一个矩形的基环组成，该基环通过四个销钉固定在头骨上，并使用了三个极坐标（角度、深度和前后位置）。这三个坐标始终表示圆弧的中心，代表靶点，并且圆弧中心的装置使选择探针入口和轨迹时具有最大的灵活性。该框架在随后的几年中进行了修改，但在功能和外观上仍与原始 1949 年的设备非常相似（**图 4.5B**）。

另一个常用的框架系统是 Cosman-Roberts-Wells（CRW）Precision™ Arc 系统（**图 4.5C**）。它具有 N

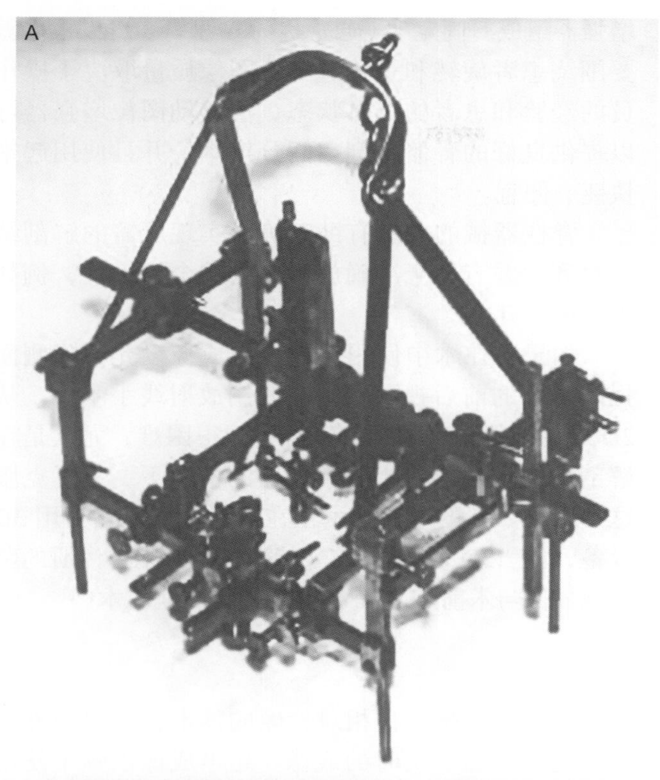

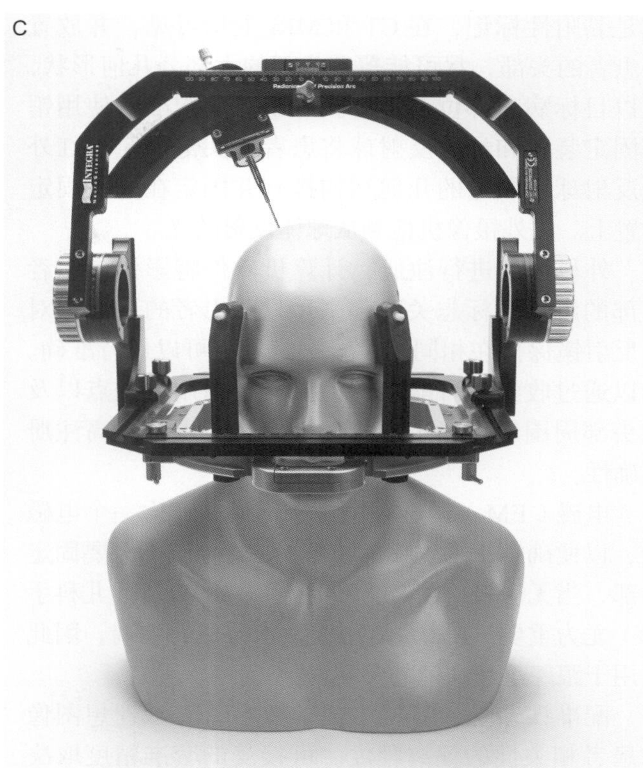

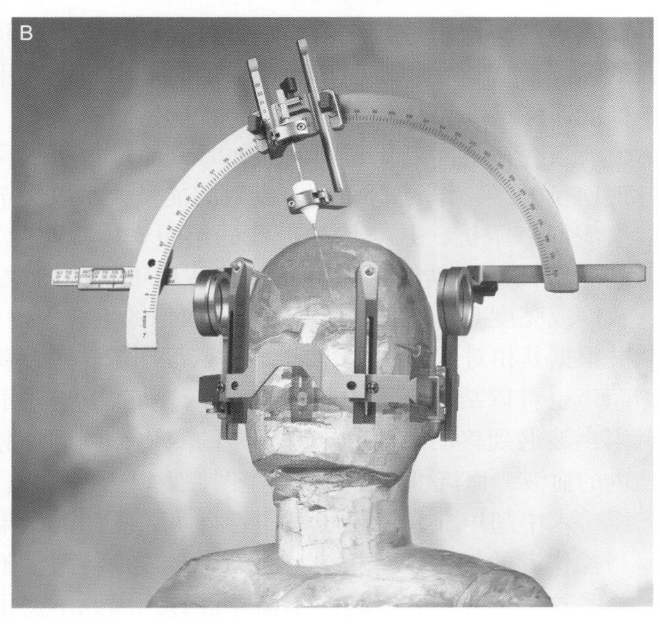

图 4.5　立体定向框架：（A）Horsley-Clarke 立体定向框架（1908）；（B）Leksell 立体定向框架；（C）CRW Precision™ 弧弓系统

形的“小围栏”定位环，病变位于具有固定半径的立体定向球体的中心，可以自由选择无限数量的入颅点。CRW Precision™ Arc 系统还具有幻象底座，可用于在将设置应用于患者之前确认靶点。Leksell 和 CRW Precision™ 系统的 CT 和 MRI 兼容模型均已推出。

高分辨率 MR 成像的出现改变了立体定向手术计划。立体定位不再依赖于解剖图谱，通常在计算机工作站上实现，该工作站可以在计算机生成的 3D 模型上制定靶点和手术路径。基于框架的立体定位具有较高的精确度，尽管在颅内实践中已被无框架立体定位技术所取代，但仍继续用于重要的靶点定位，例如功能性病变和电极或导管定位，小或深部病变的活检以及伽玛刀立体定向放射外科。

无框架立体定向神经外科

无框立体定位使用骨性标志、面部特征或基准标记与手术前获得 3D 立体图像进行共配准。基准点是黏附性标记，在CT和MRI上均可见，并放置在患者的头部，尽可能覆盖头部的大部分几何形状，但以目标病变部位为中心。对于光学配准，使用销钉固定装置和红外反射球将患者的头部固定，红外线反射球以预定的几何结构排列并固定在同一固定装置上。红外摄像机检测从球体反射的光。

外科医生进行注册，计算机软件将影像与患者头部的解剖学标志关联起来。只要患者的头部相对于反射镜保持在相同的位置，定位就可以保持准确。可以通过收集尽可能多的注册点，使用基准点以及在头部周围尽可能多地分布模拟注册点来提高注册准确性。

电磁（EM）配准在患者头部周围产生一个电磁场，以便确定手术器械的位置。EM导航不需要固定头部，当无法轻松固定头部时（例如，分流或儿科手术）尤为重要。EM系统跟踪手术器械的尖端，因此可用于跟踪柔性内镜的尖端。

配准误差是计算机生成的数字，表示理想图像与患者相关性的偏离程度。可接受的套准精度取决于目标病变的大小。体积配准使外科医生可以在三个正交平面上查看图像，配准后，外科医生可以使用装有反射球的仪器将仪器的位置与图像实时关联。还可以将其他图像序列（例如功能成像和纤维束示踪成像）与体积数据合并，使外科医生可以在术中查看这些图像。图像引导系统还适用于脊柱内固定手术，并且可以与手术显微镜连接，以便将显微镜的焦点用作图像引导指针，并可以将图像引导数据覆盖在操作员在显微镜下的视野上。

无框架图像导航系统是一项重要的技术进步，是现代神经外科设备的重要组成部分，但是我们必须意识到它们的局限性。由于患者、参考镜架或基准的移动，以及由于照相机和红外线反光镜之间视线的损失，脑脊液丢失或切除后因术中脑漂移而导致配准不准确。在要求亚毫米精度并且可接受固定轨迹的情况下，优先选择框架系统。

术中实时影像

X射线

移动式X射线图像增强器在神经外科手术室广泛应用，包括脊柱外科手术时进行解剖结构定位，在脊柱内固定中进行成像以及在其他骨骼解剖结构定位（如第四脑室或垂体窝）。

移动式图像增强器通常由一个具有低强度X射线源的部件和一个在安装座上彼此相对放置的图像增强器组成。固定架（通常称为C型臂）可以根据需要围绕患者旋转和平移。尽管图像质量取决于操作员的经验和患者的身体状态，但移动图像增强器可以提供良好的骨骼解剖空间分辨率，并且使用起来快捷、便宜。

脊柱器械的成像有助于确保实现所需的解剖结构对齐，并有助于准确放置植入的金属工件，例如椎弓根螺钉。

如果要在术中使用荧光透视成像以允许除侧面视图之外的前后视图，则应使用放射线手术台。从2D成像确保精确的螺钉定位可能很困难，尤其是在解剖结构异常或使用复杂仪器的情况下。为了克服这一困难，新的成像技术正在被引入，包括专用3D设备，如“3D C臂”或“O臂”，以及结合注册的荧光镜显像与术前3D CT扫描的神经导航技术。

超声

术中超声是一种相对价廉的技术，可以为外科医生提供快速、实时的成像。超声成像依赖于使用高频声波对组织进行成像。声音被设定为疏密相间的纵波形式，在物质间传递机械能。术中超声利用换能器将5~10 MHz的超声波传入组织。

当存在不同组织密度的界面时，能量被组织反射回换能器，作为“回声”。反射的能量大小取决于组织的声阻抗，其与传播声波的组织密度成正比。然后将回波振动转换为电脉冲，并用于生成图像。灰度或亮度（B模式）是解剖超声成像的主要手段，并根据其相对回声提供组织的2D灰度图像。多普勒超声也可以结合到术中超声中。多普勒效应描述了当声波遇到移动界面时声音频率的变化，例如动脉内的血液，血流可以在实时超声图像上以彩色映射。

术中超声非常依赖于操作者自身，图像的结果与操作者的知识储备相关，因为大多数外科医生不熟悉这种成像模式。超声不能穿透骨，因此不能用于计划颅骨切开术，并且穿透更深的结构有限，这意味着需要仔细选择病例。术中超声已被用于治疗各种疾病，最常用于胶质瘤手术。一些导航设备现在也能够将超声图像与术前MR扫描的重建平面配准。术中多普勒超声在神经血管手术中发挥作用，一些外科医生在枕骨大孔减压术使用超声证实CSF流动充分。

术中MRI（iMRI）

神经外科医师越来越依赖影像引导来进行理想、安全和高效的手术。常规神经导航系统不允许神经外科医师对术中产生的脑漂移进行调整，这促使了术中 MRI 系统的开发（**图 4.1D**）（Hall and Truwit，2008）。iMRI 系统的主要特征是能够在手术过程中获得同步成像，以告知外科医生所实现的切除范围，从而指导进一步的手术决策，大多数 iMRI 系统还允许将新图像配准到神经导航系统上。

iMRI 系统可以垂直或水平打开。在垂直开放系统中，患者保持在固定位置，外科医生在扫描仪范围内工作。所有手术工具必须与 MR 兼容，并且必须保持其他设备的不同屏蔽水平。图像可以在手术过程中的任何时间点轻松、快速地采集，而不移动患者或磁体，但是垂直开放系统通常是低场强的（0.3~0.5 T），因此图像的质量与标准诊断成像技术产生的图像质量不同。

水平开放的 iMRI 系统包括一个位于集成手术室内的高场磁体（1.5~3.0 T）（**图 14.1D**）。扫描床可以从标记的磁场线（5 高斯线）滑动或旋转，允许在进行扫描之前使用标准仪器以常规方式进行手术。新的高场强开放 iMRI 扫描仪可以提供更高质量的图像，允许功能 MRI、MR 血管造影、MR 静脉造影、MR 波谱和纤维束成像等功能。该系统的缺点包括构建术中 MRI 手术室高昂的成本以及患者进出扫描仪导致手术时间的增加。

术中神经电生理监测

术中神经生理学监测提供了对神经系统完整性的实时、连续评估，对于各种类型的神经外科手术都至关重要（Gonzalez et al.，2009）。术前咨询神经生理学家以确保选择最恰当的模式，结果必须始终在进行外科手术的背景下进行解释。因此，术中在手术室配备神经生理学家是有帮助的。术中监测可能受到麻醉剂的显著影响，因此与麻醉师密切合作也至关重要。

感觉诱发电位

可以通过刺激视觉、听觉和躯体感觉系统，产生诱发电位，记录神经系统对这些外界刺激的生物反馈反应。这些记录提供了从周围神经到皮质水平的感觉通路信息。

体感诱发电位（SSEP）

体感诱发电位（somatosensory evoked potentials，SSEP）由周围神经的短时（0.1~1.0 ms）电刺激（1~5 Hz）产生，在神经的近端部分或感觉通路记录产生的反应。将记录电极放置在指定的可重现位置。每个位置用字母标示；N（负偏转）或 P（正偏转）和对应于波潜伏期的数字。通常刺激正中神经或胫神经，并监测 SSEP 的潜伏期和振幅。

SSEP 波形通常变化很大，因此应在手术开始前和整个手术过程中进行监测。为了将 SSEP 信号与背景噪声分开，采用了一种称为信号平均的技术来结合大量的 SSEP 信号。进行信号平均需要时间，这意味着在神经损伤发生后几分钟内可能不会观察到 SSEP 变化。SSEP 波形的振幅降低约 50% 或潜伏期延长 10% 被认为是有意义的。吸入麻醉剂、血压波动、低体温和氧合均可不同程度地影响 SSEP，因此需要事先与麻醉师密切协商，以确保实现稳定的麻醉。在胸椎手术中，上肢 SSEP 信号可作为对照。脊柱 SSEP 持续监测通常用于脊髓和复杂脊柱手术，在脊柱侧凸手术中也是必不可少的（Thirumala et al.，2014）。SSEP 的皮质标测也可用于癫痫手术或感觉运动和岛叶皮质肿瘤手术。

视觉诱发电位（VEP）和脑干听觉诱发电位（BAEP）

术中视觉诱发电位（visual evoked potentials，VEP）和脑干听觉诱发电位（brainstem auditory evoked potentials，BAEP）不太常用。VEP 可由固定模式或非固定模式的刺激诱发，可在手术期间在视交叉或视束周围使用，但麻醉下的结果并不可靠。BAEP 记录听觉刺激递送至外耳道后由 7 个离散波组成的波形。每个波对应于从 Corti 器到听觉皮质的听觉系统特定位点。BAEP 可用于保留听力的前庭神经鞘瘤手术或面肌痉挛的微血管减压术。

运动诱发电位

运动诱发电位（motor evoked potentials，MEP）是通过电或磁刺激运动皮质、脊髓或周围神经产生的。在术前标测中首选经颅磁刺激，因为其创伤较小，但通常在术中使用螺旋或针电极进行经颅电刺激。神经源性 MEP 直接从脊髓或周围神经记录。神经源性 MEP 产生两种类型的波：刺激沿皮质脊髓束的直接传播产生直接波（D 波），而间接波（I 波）由相邻皮质的激活产生。肌源性 MEP 使用肌电图（EMG）记录特定的肌肉反应（M 反应）。M 反应反映了运动单位动作电位（motor unit action potential，MUAP），并反映了一个运动单位肌纤维的总和动作电位。

吸入麻醉剂对 MEP，特别是 I 波反应有显著影响。D 波不受吸入麻醉剂的影响，但 α 运动神经元在较高剂量下被阻断，即使是在经颅电刺激下也是如此。静脉麻醉药仅对 MEP 有轻度影响，当使用 MEP 时，通常首选使用丙泊酚和依托咪酯的全静脉麻醉，因为它们的抑制作用低于相似麻醉深度下的气体。然而，过高剂量的丙泊酚可能与吸入剂具有相似的抑制作用。通常避免使用苯二氮䓬类药物，因为它们可消除 MEP 反应。神经肌肉阻滞剂不影响神经生理学监测，实际上可以增强 I 波记录，但当乙酰胆碱的神经肌肉传递被完全阻断时，不能记录 MUAP。麻醉师观察 M 反应，以评价神经肌肉阻滞的程度。

MEP 可在脊髓和复杂脊柱手术期间监测脊髓背外侧和腹侧束，是背柱 SSEP 监测的补充（Schwartz et al.，2007）。在进行选择性背根切断术治疗痉挛时，会阴部 MEP 监测和肛门括约肌的骶骨 EMG 记录有助于识别可以选择性切断的神经根。

与 SSEP 不同，MEP 通常不连续监测，因为患者可能在刺激后移动。外科医生和神经生理学家还需要合作，以确保在不中断手术的情况下获得充足的 MEP。

肌电图

将记录电极置于针头内，插入肌肉，记录该肌肉的 MUAP。然后将信号转换成声音，以证明肌肉活动。诱发 EMG 使用电刺激识别特定神经，而自由运行 EMG 用于识别神经正常放电的任何中断。自发性良性放电产生短暂的非持续性放电（类似于“爆米花”的声音），表明刺激接近神经，而神经紧张性放电延长，表明持续的神经损伤。

面神经监测是脑神经外科手术中最常用的术中 EMG 类型，记录电极放置于口轮匝肌和眼轮匝肌中。在外科医生故意刺激神经或操作过程中的机械或热损伤意外刺激神经时记录肌肉活动。当避免神经肌肉阻滞但面部肌肉对肌肉松弛剂的作用相对抵抗时，获得最佳的面神经 EMG 记录。应使用哈特曼氏（Hartman）溶液冲洗代替生理盐水冲洗，以避免刺激面神经。EMG 还用于监测选择性背根切断术期间的肌群活动，以治疗痉挛，脊髓神经根监测被认为是脊柱内固定期间使用的多模态脊柱监测的关键组成部分。

术中皮质刺激定位（脑定位）

术中脑映射通常用于在癫痫或肿瘤手术期间定位功能区及其周围的运动、感觉或语言皮质。相位反转 SSEP 可用于麻醉患者，以定位初级感觉或运动皮层，由此将条形栅放置在与中央沟预期方向垂直的大脑表面。N20/P20 峰值的相位反转表明这些电极跨越中央沟。在清醒患者中，可使用直接皮质刺激绘制运动皮质图。

对于颞叶的语言定位，将记录电极条置于脑表面，然后使用双极皮质刺激器刺激皮质。刺激电流以 2 mA 的低电压缓慢增加，最大可达 10 mA，同时观察后放电（类似于局灶性发作）。确定患者后放电的阈值后，要求患者说出图片卡上显示的物体，同时继续刺激皮质，并记录任何失语错误或言语骤停。然后重复上述步骤，使患者的语言区可以映射到大脑表面。脑皮质图谱的描绘常需要开颅手术中保持患者意识清醒，尤其是语言区的开颅手术。

患者的术前准备是清醒手术的关键。因为手术中需要患者的良好配合，所以应仔细筛选患者，以确保患者完全理解手术过程中会发生什么。清醒开颅手术的文章中已经介绍了各种麻醉和手术技术，但是成功的手术还需要对特定临床问题的预案（Erickson and Cole，2012）。完全清醒手术是在局麻药物浸润头皮后或头皮局部神经阻滞后进行的。睡眠 - 觉醒 - 睡眠（asleep- awake- asleep，AAA）技术在开关颅期间使用全身麻醉，术中让患者从麻醉中苏醒。然而，开关颅过程中更常应用的麻醉技术被称为监测麻醉管理（也称为清醒镇静），在 AAA 技术中使用药物（丙泊酚和芬太尼），但以脉冲和较低剂量的方式给药，目标是使患者平稳过渡到清醒状态，并避免气道干预的问题（Erickson and Cole，2012）。

延伸阅读、参考文献、EBRAIN 的相关链接

扫描书末二维码获取。

第5章 神经外科患者的围术期管理

Karol P. Budohoski · Alessandro Scudellari · Sylvia Karcheva · Derek Duane 著
徐丹、任倩薇、王开亮 译，孟凡刚、韩如泉 审校

引言

时至今日，减少神经外科手术患者的围术期并发症并取得良好的预后需要多学科共同参与。在围术期，临床管理的失败可导致严重的残疾或死亡（Wacker and Staender，2014）。在积极防治围术期并发症的同时，为患者做好手术和康复阶段的临床和心理准备是神经外科医师和麻醉医师的共同目标。这需要遵循既定的围术期流程，包括术前评估、术前访视、医患沟通、尊重患者意愿、加强团队合作以及制订围术期的管理策略。这些流程将在下面的章节中进行详细讨论，以强调它们在围术期神经保护功能方面发挥的重要作用。

术前麻醉评估

术前评估的目的是评估患者的并发症并制订围术期麻醉管理计划。评估应遵循临床规则，即病史记录、体格检查、必要的化验及辅助检查、风险评估和获取患者的知情同意。术前评估使用美国麻醉医师协会（American Society of Anesthesiologists，ASA）分级标准，根据患者体质状况和对手术危险性进行分类（**表5.1**）。

表5.1 ASA 麻醉病情评估分级

ASA 分级	标准
Ⅰ	无器质性疾病，发育、营养良好，能耐受麻醉和手术
Ⅱ	除外科疾病外，有轻度病变，但功能代偿健全
Ⅲ	并存病变严重，体力活动受限，但尚能应付日常活动
Ⅳ	并存病变严重，丧失日常活动能力，威胁着生命安全
Ⅴ	病情危重，随时有死亡的威胁
Ⅵ	脑死亡，其器官将被摘除用作器官移植手术
	注：如系急症，在每级数字前标注“急”或“E（emergency）”字

ASA Physical Status Classification System is reprinted with permission of the American Society of Anesthesiologists, 1061 American Lane, Schaumburg, Illinois 60173–4973.

气道

困难气道可导致缺氧和高碳酸血症，是麻醉相关并发症和死亡的最重要的独立危险因素。因此，术前对气道进行全面评估至关重要。目前已有许多预测困难气道的评估方法，如张口度、马氏评分、颈部活动度和口咽解剖径线测量等，但均不具备良好的特异性和灵敏度。在神经外科，颈椎疾病导致颈部活动受限、颈椎不稳需佩戴颈托或颈椎牵引的患者以及肢端肥大症的患者，都存在插管困难的可能。为了更好地保障术前容量补充和避免插管时胃内容物反流误吸，最新的指南支持麻醉医师允许成人和儿童在择期手术前2小时饮用清水、6小时内禁止食用固体食物（Smith et al.，2011）。

呼吸系统

术前改善肺功能是十分重要的，以确保患者术中得到充分的氧合和通气，满足脑组织氧气供应。神经系统疾病患者发生吸入性肺炎和神经源性肺水肿的风险较高，这对神经功能和生存率均会产生不利影响。

吸烟患者应在术前至少6~8周停止吸烟，改善肺功能，以达到更好的手术预后。感染性或炎症性呼吸道疾病的急性加重期需要进行治疗干预，并将手术推迟6周，以改善气道敏感性。慢性肺部疾病应进行临床评估，如果有证据表明疾病进展恶化，还需要进一步的影像学和肺功能检查，以明确相关并发症（包括术后辅助通气）的风险。患有阻塞性睡眠呼吸暂停的患者，特别是肢端肥大症或库欣病的

患者，往往对阿片类镇痛药和镇静剂非常敏感，如果术前没有常规采取持续气道正压治疗，这些患者可能会出现通气障碍、肺不张和肺部感染。

心血管系统

心脏疾病在神经外科患者中很常见，仔细评估心血管系统的功能状态对于预测围术期和远期的心血管并发症十分必要（Fleisher et al., 2014）。伴有常见危险因素的患者，以及在进行日常活动时有呼吸短促、疲劳或胸痛史的患者，通常提示心功能不全，需要进一步评估。修订的心脏风险指数（**表 5.2**）使用六个独立变量，有助于评估神经外科患者心脏并发症和死亡的风险（Ford et al., 2010）。

高血压控制不佳［收缩压＞180 mmHg，平均动脉压（mean arterial pressure，MAP）>110 mmHg］会增加脑血管阻力，并导致脑血流自动调节曲线右移以及对急性低血压的耐受性差。若手术可以推迟，则需要数周或数月来调整血压。此外，急诊手术可以采用静脉给药方式进行诱导及维持，但会增加并发症的风险。

近期有过心肌梗死或冠状动脉支架介入治疗的患者，如果在 6 个月内接受手术，心肌发生进一步损伤的风险更高。心力衰竭是围术期死亡的重要危险因素，术前需要根据国际指南和当地心脏病学协会建议进行最佳治疗，以确保良好的预后（Yancy et al., 2013）。

怀疑有新发心脏瓣膜病变的患者需要超声心动图评估其严重程度。一些患者在进行择期神经外科手术前，可能需要进行瓣膜介入治疗，以降低围术期心脏风险。一般来说，评估心脏瓣膜疾病的严重程度有助于选择适当的麻醉方式，以提供最佳的术中监测和术后护理。

表 5.2 心脏风险指数（修订版）

	评估项目
1	高危风险型手术
2	缺血性心脏病（包括以下任何一种：心肌梗死史、运动试验阳性、当前认为继发于缺血性心脏病的胸痛、使用硝酸盐治疗或具有病理性 Q 波的心电图）
3	充血性心力衰竭
4	脑血管病史
5	术前胰岛素治疗
6	术前血清肌酐 >2.0 mg/dl

Reproduced with permission from Thomas H. Lee et al., Derivation and Prospective Validation of a Simple Index for Prediction of Cardiac Risk of Major Noncardiac

随着年龄的增长，心律失常的发生率越来越高，因此所有 55 岁以上的患者都建议在术前常规进行心电图检查。术前出现心律失常应立即寻找其潜在的原因。房颤（atrial fibrillation，AF）是最常见的快速性心律失常。对于临床心率控制稳定的房颤患者，除了调整抗凝药物外，一般不需要在围术期进行特殊评估。出现传导型心律失常，或发生室上性或室性心动过速的患者需要转诊到心内科进行进一步评估，并尽可能转复为窦性心律或经静脉植入永久性起搏器。对于那些在神经外科手术前植入心脏起搏器或除颤器的患者，如果术中使用了电凝，术后需要检查他们的设备是否出现故障。

神经系统

术前应使用格拉斯哥昏迷量表（Glasgow Coma Scale，GCS）评估患者的神经功能状态，明确已存在的神经功能缺失。评估瞳孔大小和对光反应。评估脑神经的完整性对于确定延髓功能以及呕吐和呛咳反射十分重要。评估感觉和运动功能检查是否正常，对比患者术前及术后神经功能状态，可以发现任何可能的神经功能缺失。

其他系统疾病

在神经外科手术之前，需要改善影响内分泌、肾、肝、神经肌肉和代谢系统的其他疾病。由脑盐耗（cerebral salt wasting，CSW）综合征、抗利尿激素分泌异常（inappropriate antidiuretic hormone secretion，SIADH）或尿崩症（diabetes insipidus，DI）等引起的电解质（尤其是钠和钾）和水紊乱，在术前需要适当治疗，以确保麻醉安全实施。高血糖是神经外科患者常见的问题，主要是由于皮质醇的使用引起，已有充分的证据证明它对颅脑损伤有不良影响（Kramer et al., 2012）。术前必须按照治疗指南使用胰岛素来改善血糖水平。

院前用药及过敏状态

患者的院前药物治疗通常持续到手术当天。然而，神经外科通常会改变糖皮质激素和抗惊厥药物的使用。大多数降压药和治疗慢性疼痛的镇痛药应继续使用至术前。糖尿病患者有时可暂停使用口服降糖药，但为了控制血糖水平，可能需要在术前静脉注射胰岛素治疗。术前请血液科或心血管科会诊，在适当的时间停用抗凝和抗血小板药物，使凝血和血小板功能恢复正常，并综合考虑手术的紧迫性以及与出血和血栓形成的潜在风险。

麻醉前应记录患者的药物过敏史。任何与特定药物相关的过敏反应、面部肿胀、支气管痉挛、低血压或严重的皮肤红斑的记录都非常重要，避免遗漏。详细记录对抗生素、静脉注射造影剂和麻醉药物过敏，以及对手术过程中使用的乳胶、碘、氯己定、胶带和其他物质相关的过敏反应。

术前检查

美国ASA和美国国家健康和护理优化研究所（National Institute for Health and Care Excellence，NICE）的指南并不提倡模板化的术前检查，而是提倡基于手术类型（从简单到复杂）和并发症所导致的功能障碍进行检查。通过血生化、血液学和电生理测试以及影像学评估特定器官的病理损害程度和功能障碍，从而提供患者的生理状况和麻醉药物相关的潜在风险的信息。基于病史和检查结果，术前评估血红蛋白水平。当预计手术有大量出血风险时，需要血型检测和交叉配血试验。对有家族性出血性疾病病史或有其他凝血障碍危险因素的患者需要常规进行术前凝血功能检查。然而，没有证据能表明这些凝血异常值可以预测围术期出血情况（Seicean et al.，2012）。

伴有直接或间接影响肝肾功能的并发症，则需要检查钠、钾、肌酐、尿素、估计肾小球滤过率和肝酶水平。对于惊厥性疾病的患者应评估镁、钙和抗惊厥药物浓度水平。当怀疑内分泌系统异常时，应按照下丘脑 - 垂体 - 靶器官轴进行检查。其他血液检查应根据并发症的严重程度和相关功能损伤来制订。

对伴有缺血性心脏病体征和症状的患者应进行心电图检查，以筛查高血压心脏病、心律失常或隐匿性心肌缺血。术前存在劳力性呼吸困难或胸痛的患者需结合运动负荷测试、超声心动图、MRI和冠状动脉造影对心血管状况进一步评估。对于患有心脏疾病和潜在肺部疾病进展期的患者有必要进行术前胸片和肺功能检查。

术中麻醉管理

麻醉诱导与维持

神经外科麻醉有两个基本原则：①松弛大脑使之具有良好的手术条件；②维持脑灌注压（cerebral perfusion pressure，CPP）和脑氧合。关于最佳麻醉的管理方式仍存在争议，因此这些干预措施往往是经验性的，而非以临床研究证据为基础的。

静脉通路

适宜手术的患者从麻醉诱导到苏醒的过程需经过特定的麻醉管理。常见的是在建立静脉通路后使用静脉诱导，除外儿童和不合作或怕针的成人患者使用吸入诱导。一般来说，全身麻醉下需建立动脉和静脉通路。根据手术类型和并发症的严重程度，有时需要使用中心静脉导管。

麻醉诱导类型及用药

静脉麻醉诱导通常使用短效药物，如异丙酚、硫喷妥钠、依托咪酯或氯胺酮（见**表**5.3和**图**5.1）。每种诱导药物都有各自的优缺点，但是可选择药物种类较少。一般来说，异丙酚和硫喷妥钠起效快，但可能导致严重的低血压。依托咪酯和氯胺酮对血流动力学的影响较小，但前者可抑制肾上腺皮质活动数小时，后者可引起术后幻觉和噩梦。如果起初不能建立静脉通路，或者患者为儿童，则要考虑气道控制问题，可使用挥发性药物和空氧混合物进行吸入诱导（见**表**5.4）。但这种诱导方式通常需要较长时间，与兴奋性现象有关，并且如果出现气道问题，不能立即通过静脉通路给予肌肉松弛剂处理。

气道管理

麻醉诱导后，使用非去极化肌松药（如阿曲库铵或罗库溴铵）有助于插管或置入声门上气道装置。根据剂量不同，药效可在1~3分钟内达峰，它们常引起组胺释放但却很少引起过敏反应。在大多数神经外科手术中，普通型或加强型气管导管（endotracheal tube，ETT）常用于气道管理。术中应妥善固定好ETT，避免脱出，特别是俯卧位患者。如果术前评估预测为困难气道，且患者存在颈椎病变，则可能需要纤支镜辅助下清醒或镇静插管。相比于普通外科患者，神经外科患者中未预测的困难气道并不常见，实践中应遵循标准管理办法处理。插管后，患者应使用空 / 氧混合气体进行通气，必要时吸入挥发性麻醉剂。

紧急情况下，通常采用快速序贯诱导。具体包括使用100%氧气给患者预充氧5分钟，给予短效静脉镇静剂（如异丙酚或硫喷妥钠），同时应按压环状软骨以避免误吸，一旦患者失去意识，立即注射去极化肌松剂（如琥珀胆碱）或较高剂量的非去极化肌松剂。按照该方案，达到适宜插管条件的时间通常

表 5.3 静脉麻醉药对脑血管、呼吸和心血管参数的影响

	靶向受体	颅内压	脑血流	$CMRO_2$	CO_2 反应性	自动调节	呼吸抑制	心血管抑制	适应证
丙泊酚	GABA	↓↓	↓	↓↓	→	→	++	++	麻醉诱导与维持
硫喷妥钠	GABA	↓↓	↓	↓↓	→	→	++	+	麻醉诱导，巴比妥深度昏迷
依托咪酯	GABA	↓↓	↓	↓↓	→	→	++	-/+	麻醉诱导（心血管不稳定患者）
氯胺酮	NMDA	↑/↓	↑	↑	→	→	-	-	低血容量创伤患者
右旋美托咪啶	α_2 肾上腺素受体	↓	↓	↓	→	→	-	浓度依赖性	功能神经外科手术
苯二氮䓬类药物	GABA	↓	↓	↓	→	→	+	+	镇静前用药，ICU 镇静

↓，减少；↑，增加；→，不变

a) Reproduced with permission from Srejic, U., 'Volatile Anesthetic Agents', pp. 62-6, in R. Adapa, D. Duane, A. Gelb, & A. Gupta (Eds.), *Gupta and Gelb's Essentials of Neuroanesthesia and Neurointensive Care*, 2018 © Cambridge University Press.

b) This article was adapted from *Cottrell and Young's Neuroanesthesia*, James Cottrell William Young, Effects of Anesthetic Agents and other Drugs on Cerebral Blood Flow, Metabolism and Intracranial Pressure, pp. 78-95, Copyright Elsevier (2010).

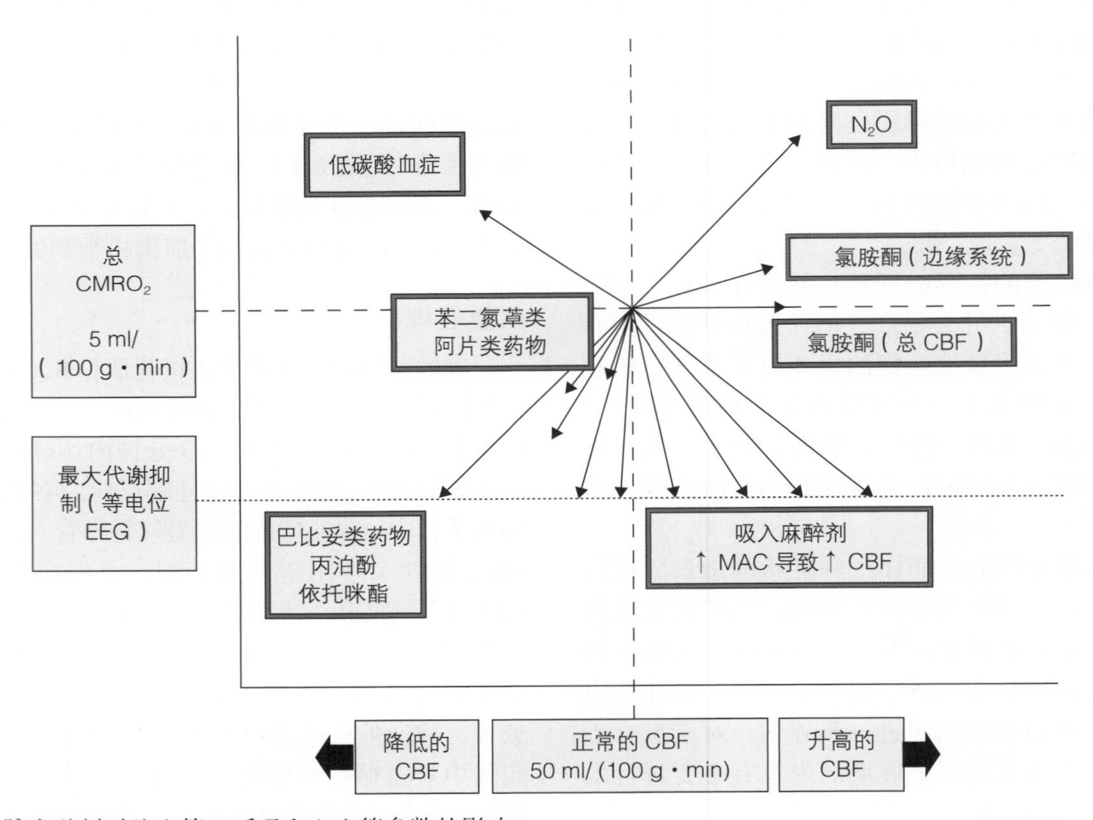

图 5.1 静脉麻醉剂对脑血管、呼吸和心血管参数的影响

是 90 秒。

麻醉监测

神经外科麻醉需要进行标准的生理监测。包括：心率、三导联或五导联心电监护、脉搏氧饱和度、无创或有创血压、呼吸频率、呼气末二氧化碳分压、鼻咽温度以及氧气和吸入麻醉剂的浓度。调节通气参数［（潮气量、吸气峰压、呼气末正压（positive end-expiratory pressure，PEEP）］，使动脉血氧分压大于 13 kpa，血二氧化碳水平在 4.5~5 kpa。若手术时间

表 5.4 吸入麻醉药对脑血管参数的影响

	颅内压	脑血流	脑耗氧代谢率	CO_2 反应性	自动调节	心血管抑制
七氟烷	→或↑	↑或→	↓↓	剂量相关↓	剂量相关↓	+
地氟烷	↑或→	↑或↓	↓↓	剂量相关↓	剂量相关↓	+
异氟烷	→或↑	↑或→	↓↓	剂量相关↓	剂量相关↓	+

较长，预计有大量失血或需要高渗治疗时，应插入导尿管监测尿量。麻醉过程通常需要保持肌松状态，因此肌松监测非常重要。

在某些情况下，脑电图（EEG）、神经电生理监测、运动或体感诱发电位监测有助于减少术后神经功能损伤。对于采用全凭静脉麻醉（total intravenous anaesthesia，TIVA），或不使用肌松药的深度麻醉以及术中知晓风险较高的患者，推荐使用脑电双频谱指数或谱熵进行基于脑电分析的麻醉深度监测（Escalier et al.，2014）。

体位

麻醉诱导后，置入喉镜、导尿、留置中心静脉导管、上头架和摆体位等强烈刺激可能引起血压增高，必须加以控制，以避免颅内压意外升高。颅内压升高还可能由以下情况导致，如：头位没有抬高15°~30°，颈部扭转引起静脉回流受阻，PEEP大于10 cmH_2O，以及俯卧位手术通气受阻。颈部过度扭曲还可能导致舌头和气道水肿，妨碍术毕安全拔管，应尽量避免。

众所周知，坐位手术有其特殊的并发症，如低血压、静脉空气栓塞（venous air embolism，VAE）、巨舌症、气颅和神经损伤。尽管如此，如果遵循严格的团队合作，该体位仍是可以接受的，并能提供良好的手术条件。在俯卧位中，手术和麻醉团队都有责任采取措施，最大限度地降低器官压力性损伤、皮肤坏死、周围神经病变和眼部并发症（DePasse et al.，2015）。

麻醉维持

全身麻醉包括镇静、镇痛和肌松三部分。一般情况下，静脉麻醉药可以降低脑氧代谢率（$CMRO_2$）和脑血流（CBF），在抑制兴奋性毒性和自由基介导的脂质过氧化的同时，保持脑血管自动调节能力（CAR）和二氧化碳反应性。但是，它们可以降低MAP和CPP，从而对脑氧合和颅内压（ICP）产生潜在的有害影响。相比之下，吸入麻醉剂呈剂量依赖性抑制 $CMRO_2$，但可引起脑血管舒张（地氟醚＞异氟醚＞七氟醚），增加CBF，进而升高ICP，除非被低碳酸血症引起的血管收缩所代偿。这些药物还会剂量依赖地引起CPP、CAR和二氧化碳反应降低。

静脉麻醉剂和吸入麻醉剂对脑血流动力学的影响存在差异，最佳的麻醉方式尚未达成共识（Chui et al.，2014）。然而，对于已经存在颅内压升高的患者，静脉麻醉似乎具有理论上的优势，而吸入麻醉剂则应由经验更丰富的麻醉医师使用。对于需要电生理监测的颅脑和脊髓手术，和吸入麻醉剂相比，TIVA对测量电位的影响更小。脊髓脊柱手术中需要考虑的麻醉因素与颅脑手术相同。

术中事件及麻醉事件

呼吸系统及心血管系统

通过调节通气量来控制动脉血氧和二氧化碳水平在颅内高压患者的管理中至关重要。通气不足和需要立即纠正的情况主要包括：①气管插管误入支气管；②导管打折或痰液阻塞；③支气管痉挛；④错误的俯卧位姿势；⑤中心静脉置管或脑脊液分流术开通皮下隧道后未及时识别的气胸。

术中低血压（收缩压<90 mmHg）与创伤性脑损伤（traumatic brain injury，TBI）患者预后不良有关，通常需要减少麻醉剂量，增加液体和正性肌力支持。ICP介导的迷走神经刺激，三叉神经心脏反射激活，脑干操作和利多卡因毒性可诱发心律失常。停止刺激通常可以终止外部干扰或在药物辅助下恢复至窦性节律。如果术中发生心脏停搏，应遵循常规的高级生命支持方案，应考虑尽早将患者的头部固定器去除并采用仰卧位[Resuscitation Council（UK），2014]。

术中液体管理

一般来说，除非有明显的出血或血流动力学不稳定，否则应尽量减少术中输液量。最常用的是无葡萄糖等渗晶体溶液。高渗剂和其他利尿剂会显著影响体液和电解质平衡，有时需要积极的补充以避免代谢紊乱。

神经外科手术期间的失血量是不可预知且严重的，可导致低血压、脑氧合降低、凝血障碍和贫血。必须快速使用晶体液和血液制品恢复血容量。凝血试验和血液学建议可用于指导凝血因子的使用。输血的最佳血红蛋白标准是有争议的。几项研究的报告显示，贫血和红细胞输注均与患者预后不良相关（Alan et al.，2014；Gruenbaum and Ruskin，2014）。

其他意外事件

在神经外科手术过程中，可能会发生灾难性的意外事件，需要外科医师和麻醉医师共同采取措施。这些事件包括：过敏反应、癫痫发作、急性脑肿胀、动脉瘤破裂和 VAE。处理这些突发事件的基本原则包括识别和消除病因，然后进行治疗，以防止或减少任何对患者不利的结果。总之，努力的方向是：①使用液体和正性肌力药物恢复 CPP 来改善大脑氧合；②尝试使用麻醉药、抗惊厥药和低体温降低 $CMRO_2$ 来保护神经功能；③用高渗药物和短期过度通气降低颅内压。

在神经外科，特别是神经肿瘤手术，一直推荐预防性使用抗癫痫药物。有研究显示，术后第一周癫痫发作的发生率降低了 40%～50%，但对晚期癫痫发作影响很小甚至没有影响（Temkin，2002）。

麻醉苏醒期

手术结束后的麻醉苏醒期应谨慎管理。其目的是保持血流动力学稳定，避免过度呛咳和 ETT 抵抗的同时，快速、平稳地过渡到正常的认知功能。这样可以迅速进行神经系统功能评估，尽早发现需要紧急干预的功能障碍。在神经外科，无论静脉麻醉还是吸入麻醉，在恢复正常认知的时间方面没有显著差异（Chui et al.，2014）。

对苏醒期的不当管理可能会导致血流动力学不稳定，以及颅内出血、脑高灌注综合征或缺血性心肌功能障碍。通常需要使用降压药将收缩压控制在 160 mmHg 以下。一般来说，大多数患者应该在不需要气道支持、呼吸自主、血流动力学稳定、意识清醒、反应机敏、体温正常和舒适的情况下送至麻醉后恢复室。

术后麻醉管理及相关并发症

呼吸系统

手术结束后，患者通常在手术室或加强监护区拔除气管导管。颅脑术后早期呼吸系统并发症的发生率高达 20%（Ali，2015），表现为气胸继发的低氧及高碳酸血症、肺不张、痰潴留、吸入性肺炎、支气管痉挛或神经源性肺水肿。可选择辅助氧疗、物理治疗、抗生素、支气管扩张剂、利尿剂、无创通气和影像学检查后胸腔穿刺术等治疗方式。如果动脉血氧和二氧化碳水平继续恶化，应尽早进行二次插管和机械通气，从而避免继发性脑损伤。

心血管系统

拔管时出现的一过性高血压并不少见，但也可能延续为术后持续高血压。治疗术后疼痛可能使患者血压降至正常范围。然而，持续的收缩期高血压可导致颅内出血或脑高灌注综合征，需要立即使用短效降压药物治疗。但应避免过度的降压治疗，这会增加脑缺血的风险。术后低血压通常可使用液体治疗，但有时需要进一步排除心肌功能障碍。

苏醒延迟

苏醒延迟可能与麻醉药物的残留抑制作用、肌肉松弛剂拮抗不充分、低血糖或低体温有关。在停止麻醉后的合理期限内，如果患者的意识水平降低或有神经病学异常体征，则需要进行计算机断层扫描（CT）。病因可能是颅内积气，高氧治疗 12 小时后病情通常好转。在 CT 扫描没有任何异常又难以解释苏醒延迟时，常通过排除法来诊断亚临床癫痫发作，应静脉注射抗惊厥药物，并进行脑电图检查。在所有患者中，尤其是癫痫发作导致意识状态改变的患者，可能需要为患者提供呼吸支持并将其转至神经重症监护室。

术后恶心呕吐

术后恶心呕吐（postoperative nausea and vomiting，PONV）发生率为 30%～50%，高危患者超过 70%。神经外科手术后持续性 PONV 可能导致颅内出血和脑肿胀。其危险因素包括女性、年轻、既往恶心呕吐史、颅内病理类型、幕下手术、使用一氧化氮、对阿片类药物敏感和术后低血压。在对包括抗胆碱能药、抗组胺药、多巴胺受体拮抗剂、5-HT3 拮抗剂、类固醇和神经激肽 -1 受体拮抗剂在内的各种止吐药的研究中，没有发现哪一种药物优于其他类别。在预防或治疗 PONV 时，大多数麻醉医师会采用 2~3 种药物结合的多模式方法（Kranke，2015）。

疼痛管理

在神经外科手术后的最初 24~48 小时，2/3 的患者会经历中度至重度疼痛。由于可能涉及多种假设的疼痛机制，目前还没有大规模的研究为某种特定术后镇痛方案提供一级证据。多模式的疼痛管理方法是必要的，目标是针对几种疼痛信号通路。阿片类药物是治疗颅脑或脊柱手术后中度至重度疼痛的主要药物。顾虑到其使用会增加 PONV、尿潴留、瞳孔变化、镇静和呼吸抑制等副作用的发生，因此必须与患者疼痛评分、躁动、脑血流动力学改变和因镇痛不足而引起的颅内压升高相结合使用。

以可待因为基础的药物、对乙酰氨基酚（扑热息痛）、非甾体抗炎药（NSAIDs）、加巴喷丁类、中枢 α_2 激动剂、氯胺酮、利多卡因溶液和镁作为单药治疗效果较差，但在多模式治疗方案中使用时，在减少阿片类药物使用和缓解疼痛方面更有效（Devin and McGirt，2015）。在使用非甾体抗炎药时，必须考虑出血、胃溃疡、肾毒性、骨融合受损和冠状动脉血栓形成的风险。氯胺酮可引起幻觉、镇静和复视，而加巴喷丁则与镇静、头晕、头痛和视觉障碍有关。一些研究表明，幕下手术往往疼痛更强，也有一些报道表明了患者自控镇痛的效果。

在所有接受开颅手术的患者中，都应考虑使用局部麻醉药以头皮阻滞的形式进行头皮浸润麻醉。有证据表明，这会使术后 24 小时内阿片类药物需求减少，疼痛评分降低（Guilfoyle et al.，2013）。硬膜外和神经鞘内镇痛药物联合使用已被提倡用于缓解脊柱手术后的术后疼痛。然而，很少有证据表明与手术类型相关的最佳方法或药物使用剂量（Sharma et al.，2012）。

液体及电解质管理

大多数患者在平稳的神经外科手术后不需要常规静脉输液。可能需要术后输液来维持血容量的临床情况包括：意识恢复延迟，脑血管痉挛、延髓功能紊乱、持续性 PONV、术中大量失血、高渗治疗导致大量利尿、血流动力学不稳定以及如糖尿病、DI 和 CSW 综合征等内分泌问题。一般用等渗晶体溶液，有时需要添加氯化钾。含葡萄糖的液体可能加重神经损伤并增加大脑游离水含量。

蛛网膜下腔出血、颅脑外伤、颅内肿瘤和垂体手术后常出现水平衡失调导致低钠血症或高钠血症（<136 mmol/L或>150 mmol/L）比较常见。这些患者可以通过在术后 24~48 小时测量尿量和血清钠来获得改善。低渗性多尿时，血浆钠浓度的升高是急性 DI 的有力证据，需要果断采取干预，通常在内分泌学检查的指导下给予去氨加压素和液体复苏。

由 SIADH 或脑盐消耗综合征（cerebral salt wasting syndrome，CSWS）引起的低钠血症在神经外科患者中比较常见。排除肾上腺和甲状腺功能减退后，如果血容量正常的患者尿量降低同时伴血浆钠和尿素下降，则可以考虑诊断为 SIADH。如果存在低钠血症、尿量增加、低容量血症、血压下降和血尿素升高（在没有利尿治疗的情况下），则应考虑诊断 CSWS。24 小时尿钠排出量有助于区分 SIADH 和 CSWS。

CSWS 的治疗包括静脉注射足够的氯化钠，以补充尿钠丢失量，在难治性病例可使用氟氢化可的松。然而，神经外科背景下的 SIADH 应在限制液体输注和使用高渗盐水、地环素和选择性加压素 -2 受体拮抗剂的方面采纳专家建议。必须仔细监测低钠血症的纠正速度，以避免脑桥中央脱髓鞘等神经系统并发症。一般认为纠正速度不超过 12 mmol/（L · d）是安全的。

神经外科患者常因围术期渗透性治疗、相关肾衰竭或外伤而出现钾离子紊乱。低钾血症（K^+ <3.5 mmol/L）和高钾血症（K^+>5.5 mmol/L）应及时治疗，以避免危及生命的心律失常和血流动力学波动。

术后护理设施

至关重要的是，所有神经外科患者都应在一个专门监测、评估和识别神经外科并发症的区域接受术后护理。这需要专业的知识，包括：持续的神经功能评估，血流动力学指标的维持，气体交换参数的解读，伤口出血的观察，脑室外引流的管理，及时给予锥体外系疾病药物治疗和在神经放射介入手术后给予抗血栓药物。有证据表明，除神经重症监护病房外，行择期手术的神经外科患者在这些术后护理区域进行护理也是安全的且具有成本效益的（Smith，2015）。

特殊神经外科手术的麻醉

创伤性脑损伤

在创伤性脑损伤手术中，麻醉医师的主要任务是保护大脑免受进一步的继发性损伤。术中处理包括维持足够的脑灌注压，同时保持氧气和二氧化碳水平，以及体温和血糖水平在正常范围内。

许多患者是事故导致多发伤的受害者，在进入手术室之前可能已经进行了气管插管和辅助通气。为了稳定心肺功能，在神经外科干预前，要优先处理危及生命的损伤。应尽力评估和记录 GCS 评分、瞳孔大小、反应性、已存在的神经功能缺失、脊柱轴向稳定性以及任何其他可得到的相关医疗 - 社会史。除了常规生化和血液学检查外，在采取任何干预措施之前，必须确认凝血功能和血液制品可获取。

麻醉诱导通常使用异丙酚或硫喷妥钠，两者均可显著降低 $CMRO_2$，从而降低 ICP。然而，除了氯胺酮和依托咪酯外，大多数麻醉剂都会引起一定程度的低血压，而这种低血压可以用血管升压药来改善。琥珀胆碱是一种去极化的神经肌肉阻滞剂，常作为快速诱导剂以便于气道管理。去极化剂和非去极化制剂对 ICP 均无显著影响。对于神经创伤患者来说，插管可能很困难，因为他们需要颈托和手动线性固定，以应对可能出现的颈椎损伤。为避免缺氧和高碳酸血症导致的颅内压升高，为气管插管失败制订后备计划是至关重要的。

在手术过程中，通过测量体温、尿量和神经肌肉功能来加强标准监测。有创动脉血压监测必不可少，它可以定期测量血气。在大多数病例中，大口径外周静脉通路是足够的，除非必要，中心静脉通路的建立不应延误手术。

使用异丙酚和瑞芬太尼的全静脉麻醉是一种广泛应用于脑损伤患者的麻醉维持技术。也可以使用吸入麻醉药，但应该使用低浓度（<1 MAC），并且要避免使用一氧化二氮。使用小于 8 cmH_2O 的 PEEP 以达到 PaO_2 在 11 kpa 以上和 $PaCO_2$ 在 4~4.5 kPa。应避免长期低碳酸血症可能引起的脑缺血。在成人中，根据需要使用液体（血液制品或无葡萄糖晶体液）和血管升压药将 CPP 维持在 60 mmHg 以上。甘露醇（0.25~1 g/kg）和（或）高渗盐水（5%，2~3 ml/kg）的高渗疗法可用于减轻脑肿胀。另一方面，应维持血糖、体温及电解质水平在正常范围内，并维持代谢稳定。

损伤严重的患者需要进行术后颅内压监护，并需要在神经重症监护室进行一段时间的镇静和辅助通气。一些患者可能适合拔管，但需要加强Ⅱ级护理，包括神经系统监测、镇痛以及液体和电解质管理。应依据神经外科团队的建议给予抗惊厥药物治疗和血栓预防。

脑肿胀及神经保护

术中严重脑肿胀的病因是多因素的，是脑外伤手术中公认的并发症。在许多病例中，临床治疗并不令人满意，而且没有立竿见影的效果，因此不能还纳骨瓣，而需紧急头皮缝合以覆盖疝出的脑组织。调节基本神经生理参数会带来一些好处。可采用液体或血管升压药物，纠正低氧血症和轻度一过性高碳酸血症（$PaCO_2$ 4~4.5 kPa）等方法来改善 CPP。患者应该取仰卧位，头部抬高 30°，追加异丙酚、硫喷妥钠或阿片类药物来增加麻醉深度，使用神经肌肉阻滞剂，并开始高渗或利尿治疗。通过降低环境温度和静脉输注冷晶体溶液积极治疗高热，并应考虑实施亚低温（35~36 ℃）治疗。高血糖需要静脉注射胰岛素，如果癫痫发作是诱因，可用抗惊厥药物治疗。输注硫喷妥钠造成脑电图爆发抑制以及采取脑脊液引流术可能会给治疗带来一定好处。

颅内动脉瘤手术

围术期，对颅内血管手术患者的麻醉管理旨在减少与神经系统、全身系统、麻醉和神经外科并发症相关的风险来改善预后。

紧急颅内血管手术的患者通常难以进行全面的术前评估。然而，建立基线神经功能评估和改善患者的一般状况是减少脑积水、心肺功能障碍和电解质异常相关并发症的重要措施。这可能涉及治疗心律失常、低血容量、低血压、神经源性肺水肿引起的缺氧，以及由抗利尿激素分泌异常综合征或脑性盐耗综合征引起的钠代谢紊乱。术前基础检查应包括血常规、电解质检查、心肌肌钙蛋白、凝血功能、血型、12 导联心电图、超声心动图（必要时）和胸片。继续治疗基础疾病的同时配合尼莫地平和抗惊厥药物治疗。对于择期颅内血管手术患者，要进行全面的术前评估，重点放在相关的并发症上。手术前，对抗凝和抗血小板药物进行药效评估，并与血液科专家共同制订围术期管理计划。

在麻醉过程中，除了常规的心脏、呼吸、尿量和体温监测外，可能还需要对心输出量进行更专业的血流动力学评估，以了解血管充盈程度，特别是怀疑有心肌功能障碍时。中心静脉通路是输送血管活性药物的必要途径。静脉麻醉诱导应避免平均动脉压和颅内压的大幅波动，因为这可能改变动脉瘤的跨壁压力梯度（TPG = MAP-ICP），并导致动脉瘤破裂。喉镜检查、插管和应用头颅骨钉的刺激都可造成血压升高，应加以预防和预见。平均动脉压应维持在患者术前正常水平的正负20%以内，以达到足够的脑灌注压。

脑动脉瘤手术可以在吸入麻醉或全凭静脉麻醉下进行。通常使用短效静脉药物，如丙泊酚、芬太尼、瑞芬太尼或舒芬太尼。吸入麻醉药物可能引起脑血管扩张，从而增加脑血容量，导致颅内压增高，在使用时不应超过最低肺泡浓度（MAC<1）。短效神经肌肉阻滞剂有助于促进充分的通气。应避免高碳酸血症，$PaCO_2$需保持在4.5~5 kpa。在维持正常体温和血糖的同时，PaO_2应保持在11 kpa以上。应推迟应用高渗溶剂，如甘露醇（0.5~1 g/kg）或高渗盐水（2 ml/kg 5% NaCl），最好推迟至硬脑膜打开。

在手术中，临时阻断动脉超过15~20分钟有致缺血的风险，因此，通常需要升高平均动脉压以改善侧支循环。但是，目前缺乏使用吸入麻醉剂、低温、巴比妥、丙泊酚和额外剂量的甘露醇来延长安全阻断时间的证据。动脉瘤夹闭后，可以使用甲硝胺、去甲肾上腺素或去氧肾上腺素轻度至中度升高血压来改善脑灌注。在动脉瘤手术顺利结束后，应在患者咳嗽和血流动力学波动最小的情况下拔出气管插管，并使患者迅速恢复意识，以便进行早期神经学评估。颅内血管疾病患者应在神经外科加强监护病房或重症监护室接受治疗，以确保适当的镇痛、持续的血流动力学监测、充足的氧合、最佳的液体和电解质管理以及能够及时发现并发症。

术中动脉瘤破裂的处理

急诊患者术中动脉瘤破裂的发生率在5%~10%。良好的预后依赖于迅速控制出血，同时维持足够的脑灌注。麻醉医师与神经外科团队的有效沟通至关重要。动脉瘤破裂患者应使用100%的氧气进行通气。腺苷诱导的短暂性心脏停搏，麻醉药或血管活性药物导致的短期低血压有助于控制术中出血。用血液、凝血药物和晶体溶液恢复血容量以维持最低安全脑灌注压。进一步注射丙泊酚、硫喷妥钠或依托咪酯可用于抑制脑电图爆发，从而将脑代谢率降至最低。可通过高渗药物或轻度升高体温（34~35℃）治疗，但目前缺乏良好的证据证明其疗效。动脉瘤夹闭后，脑灌注压应维持在正常水平。

颅后窝手术

在颅后窝手术患者围术期管理中，需注意心律失常的风险、体位相关的并发症和静脉空气栓塞的风险。

除了常规的术前评估外，详细的神经系统检查对于制订围术期管理是至关重要的。特别是寻找与脑干、脑神经和小脑病理相关的颅内压升高和功能障碍的征象。应与神经外科医师讨论相关影像资料，并制订体位、脑脊液引流、神经生理监测和任何潜在的重大并发症的管理计划。

除了标准的监测外，建议留置动脉内导管。置入中心静脉导管可治疗静脉空气栓塞。电生理监测应根据手术部位和病变部位进行调整。过度屈颈会增加血流动力学不稳定、静脉空气栓塞和脊髓受压的风险，因此颅后窝手术的坐位使用率有所下降。现在手术通常采用俯卧位或半俯卧位，需要注意的是，应避免气管水肿、皮肤、周围神经和腹部器官损伤等相关并发症。

没有证据表明特定的麻醉技术能改善颅后窝手术的预后。颅后窝手术的总体麻醉目标是充分镇痛，维持脑灌注压、血流动力学稳定和避免咳嗽。脑干操作可引起心律失常，特别是心动过缓以及室性和室上性心动过速。但大多数心律失常会随手术停止而终止，很少需要药物干预或更罕见的情况下需要心外按压。三叉神经心脏反射也可引起术中明显的高血压，可通过加深麻醉来治疗。

与所有神经外科手术一样，术后早期对患者进行神经系统评估至关重要。然而，在长时间的俯卧位手术后，一些麻醉医师会在拔管前进行“漏气试验”，检查是否存在气管水肿、是否需保留气管插管。如果出现上述情况，或者气道反射恢复缓慢，可以保留气管插管，并在重症监护室进行辅助通气，直到安全完成拔管。术后早期要避免高血压，以降低脑水肿和颅内出血的风险。

静脉空气栓塞

在颅后窝手术中，血流动力学明显改变的静脉空气栓塞（venous air embolism，VAE）的发生率在坐位手术中为8%~15%，俯卧位或公园长椅位为3%~5%。危险因素包括心脏水平以上的手术部位和存在不可塌陷的静脉（静脉窦）。近25%的成人有卵圆孔未闭，这增加了空气栓塞的风险，从而导致心肌和脑缺血。VAE的术中临床表现多种多样，从最少量空气夹带所致轻微症状到心脏停搏，再到大量气体栓塞所致死亡。

VAE的病理生理包括：右心室流出功能受损、肺毛细血管机械性阻塞、肺内分流增加导致缺氧和高碳酸血症、肺动脉压力升高、支气管收缩、心输出量减少、低血压、心律失常、心肌衰竭和心脏停搏。心前区多普勒超声和呼气末二氧化碳是颅后窝手术期间 VAE 的推荐监测手段，可以在临床症状出现之前发现。在出现 VAE 时，通知外科医师用生理盐水浸泡伤口以防止进一步的空气进入。压迫颈静脉可暂时增加静脉压力，使破损部位得以定位和修复。也可采取降低心脏和手术部位之间的梯度，吸入 100% 氧气，停止吸入一氧化二氮的方式。如果需要，尝试通过中心静脉导管吸出空气并提供血流动力学支持。如果患者血流动力学仍不稳定，可能需要放弃手术，并取仰卧位，必要时采取进一步复苏措施。

神经肿瘤

原发性或转移性脑肿瘤患者的术前评估包括症状评估、癫痫发作史、发病前状况评估和入院前药物治疗史。除语言功能异常外，还应检查患者的意识水平、周围神经功能。实验室检查应排除严重的生化、血液和凝血功能障碍。原发性脑部病变的影像学检查需要了解病灶的位置、大小、颅内压升高的征象和血管分布，而继发性肿瘤则需仔细评估原发病灶的转移情况。在麻醉诱导前 4 小时，有时可能会使用 5- 氨基乙酰丙酸（5-ALA）荧光来提高肿瘤完全切除的可能性。如果需要，应考虑在神经外科病房或重症监护病房进行患者的术后管理。

全身麻醉的诱导通常使用静脉注射药物、阿片类药物和非去极化肌肉松弛剂。减轻喉镜检查和头钉植入时的血流动力学反应有助于维持稳定的 CPP，避免 ICP 过度升高。除了标准的监测外，长时间的复杂手术或根据并发症需求可能还需要动脉导管、中心静脉通路、体温和尿量测量，以及更先进的血流动力学监测。在特殊的情况下，需要进行电生理监测。在开颅过程中可能需要高渗药物治疗，随后需进行血气分析以监测电解质变化。在摆体位时，适当的头部抬高和避免静脉阻塞可以限制 ICP 的升高，同时尽量减少颈部屈曲以避免术后气管水肿。

麻醉通常由全凭静脉麻醉或吸入麻醉剂辅以阿片类药物来维持，有时需要使用非去极化肌肉松弛剂。丙泊酚可降低脑血容量（CBV），保持自动调节和 CO_2 反应性，而挥发性药物因会引起脑血管舒张而增加 ICP。在进行电生理监测时，静脉麻醉对信号特征的干扰较小。手术期间应使用无糖等渗晶体溶液进行补液。大量失血的情况下需要输血来维持血流动力学稳定和保障充分的脑氧合。一般来说，开颅手术麻醉的主要任务是避免缺氧、高碳酸血症、低体温、低血糖、ICP 升高，并在提高脑顺应性的同时维持稳定的 CPP。与神经外科肿瘤相关的并发症处理可能涉及急性出血的血液制品和凝血因子，静脉麻醉药物，控制癫痫的抗惊厥药物，以及术后血肿的影像学检查。VAE 和急性脑水肿的治疗已在其他章节中提到。

麻醉恢复期尽量减少咳嗽和用力，避免颅内压增加。在恰当的时间停止麻醉维持药物，以便于迅速恢复意识并进行早期的神经功能评估。如果气颅严重，可能会延迟苏醒。及时发现气颅有利于患者预后，气颅患者可进行高浓度氧疗。术后高血压通常用短效 β 受体阻滞剂来治疗，使 MAP 小于 160 mmHg。强阿片类药物的镇痛作用需要与其镇静性能相权衡，但如果在患者苏醒之前行头皮神经阻滞，则可能需要减少这些药物的使用。

术中唤醒

神经外科的发展使人们更加关注术中唤醒，目前这种手术常用于癫痫手术和切除涉及重要功能区病变的手术。手术可以在局部麻醉加或不加镇静的情况下进行，也可以最初为全麻（使用气管插管或声门上气管装置），然后使患者苏醒（睡眠 - 觉醒），或再次麻醉（睡眠 - 觉醒 - 睡眠）下进行。为了确保这些手术的成功，需要对患者进行仔细的选择、咨询并获得同意。麻醉医师的工作至关重要，需确保：①维持气管通畅和通气良好；②维持血流动力学稳定；③根据手术需要给予足够的镇痛和镇静；④确保患者配合进行持续的神经功能评估；⑤及时处理任何癫痫发作。持续的麻醉和清醒状态对于避免潜在的颅脑损害和危及生命的并发症有至关重要的作用。

脊柱脊髓外科

为确保良好的预后，脊柱脊髓手术的麻醉需要综合考虑各种问题。具体包括：处理由创伤性或退行性颈椎疾病引起的潜在困难气道；处理俯卧位的病理生理改变；采用恰当的麻醉技术以便于准确的神经电生理监测，处理失血和凝血问题；提供有效的多模式术后镇痛，以实现术后早期活动和出院（Bajwa and Halder，2015）。

由于脊柱脊髓手术患者的年龄范围，只有采用系统的术前评估方法，才能确保识别出任何已有的因近期创伤或慢性病导致的局灶性神经学症状或已改变的生理状态。在颈椎或上胸部手术的患者中，需要处理困难气道的情况并不少见。既往颈椎内固定手术史或关节炎病史可导致颈部活动受限、颈椎不稳和脊髓受压，通常需要在清醒或镇静状态下使用纤维支气管镜或其他视频喉镜设备进行插管，以避免对脊髓造成进一步损伤。需要手术治疗的脊柱侧凸或其他神经肌肉疾病的患者，其呼吸功能（如肺容量和肺顺应性）可能会受到影响。胸部创伤可导致多处肋骨骨折、连枷胸、气胸和肺挫伤，导致术中充分供氧和通气困难，特别是对于俯卧位的患者，术后可能需要进一步的重症监护。

接受脊柱手术以稳定脊髓损伤的患者可能会由于脊髓休克或自主神经反射障碍而出现血流动力学不稳定，需要血管活性药物来维持心率和平均动脉压平稳。合并心脏病但因脊柱退行性疾病导致活动受限的患者通常需要在手术前进行负荷超声心动图检查。由于药物或外伤引起的获得性凝血异常需要恢复至正常后进行手术，以避免血肿形成导致脊髓受压。大型脊柱脊髓手术有大量出血的风险，需确保可以随时获得血液和凝血因子，使用自体血液回收和氨甲环酸有助于减少异体输血需求（Cheriyan et al.，2015）。

在脊柱手术中，主要的麻醉目的是始终保持足够的脊髓灌注。麻醉的措施通常包括：①大口径静脉通路；②标准监控；③测量有创动脉和（或）中心静脉压力、温度和尿量；④静脉诱导；⑤如果计划进行经胸手术，使用双腔气管导管进行合理的气道管理；⑥如果使用神经生理监测应避免诱发电位信号的幅度降低，可使用吸入麻醉剂或全静脉麻醉维持；⑦采用强制热通风装置；⑧在预计会发生大量失血时，可使用术中血液回收。

应有计划地从麻醉中苏醒，并注意识别长时间俯卧位后的气道水肿。患者应小心仰卧，头部抬高 30° 以上，应在能对指令做出反应时拔管，并尽量减少咳嗽。使用 β 受体阻滞剂或其他血管活性药物对血压进行预先控制，避免收缩期高血压超过 160 mmHg。出现任何新的运动障碍症状都需要立即进行神经外科体格检查、影像学检查，可能还需要进行手术探查。术后疼痛管理应该是多模式的，包括使用硬膜外麻醉、患者自控镇痛、间歇性静脉或口服阿片类镇痛药、非甾体抗炎药、加巴喷丁、α_2 激动剂（如可乐定）和氯胺酮。

俯卧位的注意事项

俯卧位需要正确的装置和足够的人员来移动、搬运患者。至少需要六个人进行滚木手法搬运以保持脊柱对齐。患者可以被放置在不同的框架（如 Wilson、Allen）、桌子（如 Jackson）和床垫（如 Montreal）上。不应收缩腹部，从而可以使横膈膜自由移动，并以尽可能低的胸内压进行通气，避免可能导致术野出血的静脉充血。腹部器官缺血与不明原因的代谢性酸中毒可能是体位不佳造成的。由于前负荷减少，心排血量通常在转为俯卧时下降，这需要补液和血管升压药物来恢复血流动力学的稳定。无论是使用 Mayfield 头架还是泡沫垫，头部和颈部应处于中立位置。用胶带和填充物包裹的眼睛不应该有压力。手臂应该放在患者身边，或者外展角度不超过 90°。四肢及受压点均需填塞支撑，以避免损伤臂丛、尺神经、正中神经、外侧皮神经、腓总神经和坐骨神经。脊柱手术后视力丧失的发生率为 1/30000，可能是由于缺血性视神经萎缩、皮质缺血或视网膜中央动脉闭塞所致。导致该并发症的病因包括：手术时间超过 6 小时、术中大量失血量和低血压、头部位置不中立、头架使用不当以及其他可能的患者相关因素（Shmygalev and Heller，2011）。

垂体手术

这些患者围术期评估的重点是处理垂体病变引起的 ICP 升高、占位效应和激素分泌紊乱所导致的一系列生理改变。术前，影像学检查确定病变的范围，同时其他的检查可确定患者是否出现电解质紊乱、激素分泌异常综合征、心肺储备减少和上气道结构功能障碍。

肢端肥大症，由功能性垂体大腺瘤分泌过多生长激素所引起，可导致与上气道改变有关的麻醉问题，包括下颌前突、巨舌、组织肥大导致声门开口变小和喉返神经损伤引起的声音嘶哑。该疾病还与阻塞性睡眠呼吸暂停（obstructive sleep apnoea，OSA）、高血压、心肌传导异常、糖尿病、脊柱后凸畸形和近端肌病有关。患者可能需要术前经胸超声心动图来评估左心室功能，检查肺功能，并考虑对潜在的困难气管进行清醒纤支镜引导插管。

由垂体腺瘤分泌的促肾上腺皮质激素过多而导致的糖皮质激素过多被称为库欣病。患者常伴有躯干肥胖、满月脸、四肢消瘦、OSA、心功能障碍、凝血功能异常、骨质疏松、皮肤薄、糖尿病等。在这些患者中，麻醉医师要考虑困难气道和术中心肺不稳定的问题。

由促甲状腺激素分泌腺瘤引起的甲状腺功能亢进术前需要应用生长抑素类似物、抗甲状腺药物和 β 受体阻滞剂进行治疗。某些患者在麻醉诱导时需要补充糖皮质激素，以缓解麻醉和手术时的代谢紊乱。

垂体手术患者最重要的麻醉问题与气道管理和血流动力学不稳定有关。应具备各种插管技术的专业知识，包括可视喉镜和清醒纤支镜插管。加强型经口气管插管常用于经鼻垂体手术。口咽部通常用纱布填塞以防止血液进入呼吸道，在拔管前必须将其取出。心血管疾病在激素分泌型肿瘤的患者中很常见。术中由于高血压、心律失常、心肌缺血和心室功能障碍引起的血流动力学不稳定可能需要有创动脉压监测和血管活性药物来维持足够的脑灌注压。

垂体瘤手术的麻醉方法可以选择静脉或吸入麻醉。除常规监测之外还要辅以有创动脉压、体温和尿量的监测。疼痛刺激导致的高血压，在鼻腔蝶窦分离时很常见，但在手术操作鞍区病变本身时很少发生。在鼻腔黏膜应用含肾上腺素的局麻药可进一步对血流动力学造成不利影响。可使用瑞芬太尼、短效β受体阻滞剂和血管扩张剂来保持心血管功能稳定。适度过度通气产生的高碳酸血症和腰椎鞘内置管可以暂时性升高ICP，将肿瘤推入手术区域。血容量不足可用无葡萄糖晶体溶液补充，以保持渗透压平衡，同时应避免电解质紊乱。垂体瘤手术出血量一般很少，但若损伤海绵窦，则需要输血治疗。鞍区脑脊液漏，有时可通过Valsalva捏鼻鼓气法来识别，通常用自体腹部或大腿脂肪及筋膜封堵术腔。

从麻醉中苏醒之前，先抽吸口咽内容物并取出纱布包。平稳轻柔的拔管可防止手术放置的鼻腔止血材料移位。已知有困难气道的患者应在头向上倾斜的位置拔管最为安全。肌源性疾病患者可因为肌肉无力而不能拔管，需要在重症监护室进行一段时间的术后机械通气。所有患者在麻醉恢复室都应该给予适当的镇痛药和止吐药。出院后，要与内分泌科医师进行联合管理，除了协助早期识别和治疗其他神经内分泌并发症外，还可指导进一步的类固醇和激素替代治疗。

凝血功能障碍及静脉血栓栓塞性疾病

凝血的病理生理学机制

级联模型

凝血是一种蛋白水解酶级联反应，这个概念在1964年被两个团队首次提出（Davie and Ratnoff，1964；Macfarlane，1964）。从示意图上看，凝血途径可以分为外源性途径和内源性途径（**图5.2**）。当血液与血管外细胞（如血管壁内的成纤维细胞）表面的组织因子（tissue factor，TF）接触时，外源性凝血途径被激活。内源性凝血途径在体内的作用机制尚不清楚。当血管壁内部受损或机械装置接触到血液时，它就会被激活。然而，无论是外源性途径还是内源性途径，都有助于理解常规凝血试验的生化反应，如凝血酶原时间（prothrombin time，PT）和部分凝血酶时间（**表5.5**）。

外源性和内源性途径最终导致因子X转化为Xa

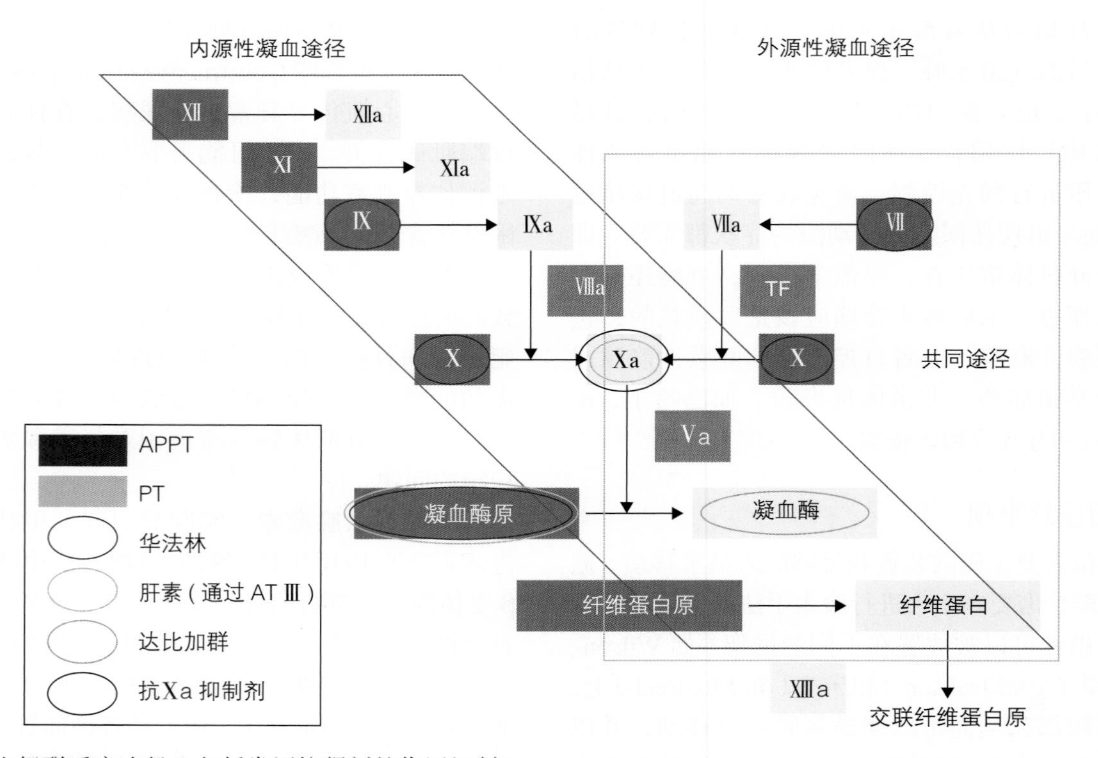

图5.2 凝血级联反应途径，包括常用抗凝剂的作用机制

表 5.5　凝血试验、相关凝血因子及临床应用

化验	遗传性	获得性	作用途径	临床应用
aPTT	vWF、Ⅷ、Ⅸ、Ⅺ、Ⅻ因子缺乏症（血友病）	肝素；抗磷脂抗体	内源性、共同的途径	出现异常前因子缺乏 20%~40%；监测肝素治疗
PT	Ⅶ缺乏症	华法林；凝血因子Ⅶ抑制剂；维生素 K 缺乏；肝病	外源性、共同的途径	筛查因子Ⅶ缺乏症；筛查因子Ⅹ、Ⅶ、Ⅰ（联合 aPTT）；监测华法林使用（INR）；INR 不适用于肝病
TEG			包括血小板功能在内的凝血全过程	区分手术出血和凝血障碍

（因子Ⅹ是共同途径的第一个因子），Ⅹa 是凝血酶原复合物的重要组成部分。凝血酶原复合物由Ⅹa 和Ⅴa 因子通过钙离子结合在磷脂膜上组成。凝血酶原复合物将凝血酶原（因子Ⅱ）转化为凝血酶（因子Ⅱa），进而激活因子ⅩⅢ。通过在纤维蛋白分子之间形成共价交联可以用来稳定血栓。

细胞依赖模型

虽然经典模型解释了实验室凝血试验的功能和特定凝血因子之间的相互作用，但这并不足以让我们充分了解体内的凝血机制。以细胞为基础的模型更能反映人体中的凝血过程，并可以更好地描述一些临床遇到的凝血障碍，如血友病中所观察到的外源性途径无法弥补内源性途径的因子缺陷（Hoffman and Monroe，2001；Hoffman，2003）。

细胞模型将重点放在凝血过程中的特定细胞及其细胞表面受体上，该过程发生在起始、扩增和增殖的三个重叠阶段。起始反应发生于含 TF 的细胞（如基质成纤维细胞，通常位于血管系统外）、血液单核细胞或炎症状态的内皮细胞。血管壁的破裂使含 TF 的细胞暴露于血浆中。因子Ⅶ与细胞表面的 TF 结合，然后被激活为因子Ⅶa。Ⅶa/TF 复合物激活因子Ⅹ和因子Ⅸ。当局限于细胞表面时，因子Ⅹa 与因子Ⅴa 结合，导致凝血酶原产生凝血酶，开始扩增过程。重要的是，当组织因子途径抑制剂和抗凝血酶Ⅲ（ATⅢ）从细胞表面分离时，因子Ⅹa 被迅速抑制。

凝血酶在含 TF 的细胞上产生，通过蛋白酶激活受体发挥作用，导致血小板激活，在组织损伤状态下血小板已经黏附在血管外基质上。这些活化的血小板，导致活化因子Ⅴ和Ⅷ的产生。血小板 α 颗粒释放因子 Va，而血管性血友病因子（vWF）释放因子Ⅷa。这些因素共同导致凝血酶的大规模产生，凝血酶在活化血小板表面的酶复合物的帮助下形成稳定的纤维蛋白凝块。Ⅷa/ Ⅸa 复合物可以激活Ⅹa 因子。在以细胞为基础的凝血模型中，血小板细胞表面在各个阶段都是必不可少的。血小板的特殊功能与其通过多种受体和途径黏附损伤表面的能力有关。血小板表达糖蛋白Ⅰb/Ⅸ和 vWF，有助于将血小板定位到损伤部位。重要的是，抗凝的启动通常被局限在不同的细胞表面，以限制不必要的凝血激活。**表** 5.5 显示了常用抗凝剂的作用机制。

神经外科术前凝血功能紊乱的患者处理

神经外科的凝血功能紊乱通常与术前使用抗血小板或抗凝药物预防原发性或继发性心血管疾病有关。此外，使用纤溶药物治疗脑血管和心血管急症增加了需要干预的颅内出血发生率。

择期手术

在择期手术的患者中，可疑的或已知的凝血功能障碍应得到充分的诊断和适当的因子替代治疗。术前使用抗血小板药物或抗凝药物引起的凝血功能障碍，应在术前停止使用这些药物以使凝血系统恢复正常（**表** 5.6）。在处理围术期抗凝治疗时，必须在手术出血风险、术前和术后发生静脉血栓栓塞（venous thromboembolism，VTE）事件的可能性以及停用和重新使用抗凝药物的最短和最安全的时间间隔之间取得平衡。

口服或静脉注射抗血小板药物以预防脑、冠状动脉或颈动脉血栓栓塞性疾病，并可逆或不可逆地抑制环氧化酶 -1（COX-1）和血栓素 A2 的合成和 P2Y12 受体以及影响血小板功能长达 10 天。为了在术前获得血小板再生，应停止抗血小板药物治疗，直到可以产生新的血小板（通常每天产生 2 万个血小板，即需要 5 天产生 10 万个新血小板）。某些神经外科手术通常在不停用抗血小板药物的情况下进行（例如颈动脉内膜剥脱术或脑血管搭桥术），以最大限度地减少围术期卒中和（或）血管闭塞的风险。

表 5.6 择期手术前停用抗血小板和抗凝药的用药时间

药物	时间	检验	半衰期
阿司匹林	5 天		每天产生 20 K 血小板（5 天 =100 K）
氯吡格雷	5~7 天		每天产生 20 K 血小板（5 天 =100 K）
华法林	3~5 天	INR（手术当天）	36~42 小时
LMWH	12 小时	抗 Xa 化验	4 小时
UH	4 小时	检查 APTT 比率	1 小时
NOAC	2 天		9~17 小时（约 12 小时）

LMWH，低分子肝素；NOAC，新型口服抗凝剂；UH，普通肝素

关于心血管疾病，大多数指南一致认为，血栓形成的风险在裸露金属心脏支架置入后长达 6 周、药物洗脱支架置入后 6 个月和心肌梗死、卒中或深静脉血栓形成（deep venous thrombosis，DVT）后 3 个月处于最高水平（Rabbitts et al.，2008）。12 个月后，这种风险会大大降低。在这些患者中，即使短时间不进行双重抗血小板治疗就会增加支架内血栓形成和心血管事件的风险。因此，在这些患者中，任何择期手术都应该推迟。血栓形成风险高的患者，如心脏机械瓣膜患者，需要在手术前 3 天停用华法林，但通常需要在手术前 12~24 小时使用治疗量低分子肝素（low molecular weight heparin，LMWH）进行桥接治疗。通常应在术后 24~48 小时内重新开始抗凝药物治疗。

急诊手术

对于接受急诊神经外科手术的患者，无论是医源性还是与疾病相关的凝血障碍的处理都几乎没有好的证据来支持最佳治疗方案。极少会发生有凝血障碍但仍然需要进行紧急手术的情况。一般来说，通常有时间对患者进行评估、实验室检测和制订适当的治疗方案。

抗凝相关性颅内出血

有时需要神经外科干预的情况是先前使用抗凝和抗血小板药物所导致的。最常见的问题是抗凝相关的脑出血（anticoagulation- associated intracerebral haemorrhage，AAICH）。口服抗凝剂如维生素 K 抑制剂，使 AAICH 的发生率增加到所有脑出血的 15%，而这些患者发生脑出血的风险增加了 11 倍（Wintzen et al.，1984；Flaherty et al.，2007）。此外，口服抗凝药物的患者出现血肿扩大的风险明显升高，预后更差（Flibotte et al.，2004）。AAICH 的管理基于四个原则：稳定出血（即防止血肿扩大），解决实施任何干预的安全问题，紧急抗凝逆转，监测血栓栓塞并发症的影响及预防栓塞。

严格的收缩压管理可用于防止血肿扩大。最近的一项对 4 个大型随机试验的 meta 分析评估了 ICH 管理中血压目标（急性脑出血快速降压；INTERACT；ICH ADAPT；INTERACT2），表明了将收缩压降低到 140 mmHg 以下与减少 24 小时内血肿扩大和改善 3 个月后的预后相关（Tsivgoulis et al.，2014）。因此，目前的指南建议收缩压目标降低至 140 mmHg 以下（Hemphill et al.，2015）。

逆转抗凝和抗血小板药物

紧急逆转抗凝通常难以实现，需要一定的时间及输注特定的血液制品。关于特定干预措施的有效性，目前证据是不足的，但是一些原则已被广泛接受。**表** 5.7 总结了常用抗凝血药物和抗血小板药物的逆转策略。

华法林

华法林是 AAICH 中最常见的药物。对于国际标准化比值（international normalized ratio，INR）大于 1.4 的患者，应给予维生素 K。但要注意的是，维生素 K 可能需要 24 小时才能充分发挥作用，因此，应采取其他治疗方案。目前的建议包括：输血新鲜冷冻血浆（fresh frozen plasma，FFP）或凝血酶原复合物浓缩物（prothrombin complex concentrate，PCC）。FFP 包含所有凝血因子，但交叉配血需要时间，大量输血也可能导致肺损伤、容量超载和过敏反应。包含 3 个因子（Ⅱ、Ⅸ和Ⅹ）和 4 个因子（Ⅱ、Ⅸ、Ⅹ和Ⅶ）的 PCC 也是可以使用的。在一项涉及 202 名华法林相关出血患者的研究中，约 60% 的病例中 PCC 能在 30 分钟内使 INR 恢复正常，而接受 FFP 的患者只有 10%（Sarode et al.，2013），这使得 PCC 成为大多数医疗中心的首选治疗方法。

新型抗凝药物

非维生素 K 口服抗凝剂（non-vitamin K oral anti-coagulants，NOACs）——也被称为 DOACs（直接口服抗凝剂），是一组不同的药物，包括Ⅹa 因子抑制

表 5.7　神经外科紧急逆转抗凝

药物	试验	治疗
阿司匹林	PFA-100	1~2 U 血小板；DDAVP 0.4 mcg/kg（至少 30 分钟）
氯吡格雷	血小板聚集试验	1~2 U 血小板；DDAVP 0.4 mcg/kg（至少 30 分钟）
替格瑞洛		1~2 U 血小板；DDAVP 0.4 mcg/kg（至少 30 分钟）
UH	APTT 比率	若服用 UH 时间在 2~3 小时内，每 100 U UH 给予鱼精蛋白 1 mg（如果 APTT 持续升高，重复剂量为每 100 U UH 给予 0.5 mg）
LMWH	抗Xa 试验	1 mg（依诺肝素）/100 U（达肝素）给予鱼精蛋白 1 mg。若服用 LMWH 超 8 小时则半量给药
戊多糖	抗Xa 试验	4 因子 PCC 20 U/kg；rfVIIa 90 mcg/ kg
华法林	INR	维生素 K 5~10 mg；FFP 15 ml/kg；4 因子 PCC 20 U/kg；rfVIIa
直接凝血酶抑制剂	APTT/TT	达比加群 - 依达赛珠单抗 5 mg，每 15 分钟 2 次；血液透析；若服用时间在 2 小时内给予 TXA，4 因子 PCC，活性炭 50 g
凝血因子 Xa 抑制剂	抗Xa 试验	4 因子 PCC 50 U/kg；若服用时间在 2 小时内给予活性炭 50 g

LMWH，低分子肝素；NOAC，新型口服抗凝剂；PCC，凝血酶原复合物浓缩物；TXA，氨甲环酸；UH，普通肝素

剂（利伐沙班、阿哌沙班、伊多沙班）和直接凝血酶（Ⅱa）抑制剂（达比加群）。这些药物起效快，剂量依赖性强，半衰期短（平均 5~15 小时），经肾和肝代谢，其药代动力学特征更具有可预测性。因此，其主要优点是对常规药物监测的要求低得多。如果患者正在使用 NOAC 药物，肾功能和肝功能正常，且手术出血风险较 VTE 低，则停药 2~3 个半衰期即可。如果出血风险高，则停药 4~5 个半衰期即可。NOACs 的平均半衰期为 12 小时，因此人们认为停用 48 小时可以保证手术的安全。一旦术后认为止血稳定，应尽快重启 NOACs。

然而，除了达比加群，这些药物并没有特定的逆转剂。idarucizumab 是一种抗达比加群的单克隆抗体，目前已获准用于快速逆转与其使用相关的出血。在紧急情况下或没有逆转剂时，专家意见建议使用活化四因子凝血酶原复合浓缩液、活化重组因子Ⅶ、可能使用口服活性炭（患者在摄入 NOAC 2 小时内发生出血）和血液透析。必须承认，通常检测的止血化验评估不是延长就是不受 NOACs 的影响，正常值可能不排除临床相关的药物浓度。抗Xa 试验、稀释凝血酶时间（thrombin time，TT）试验、蛇静脉酶凝血时间和 NOAC 逆转剂目前正在临床试验中进行评估，以便制定 NOAC 逆转的循证指南（Gehrie and Tormey，2015）。

肝素

与普通肝素（unfractionated heparin，UH）治疗相关的脑出血患者只占 0.1%。紧急逆转措施包括停止输注和注射鱼精蛋白。监测 APTT 是必需的，因为可能需要反复注射鱼精蛋白。低分子肝素通过抗凝血酶抑制Xa 因子，但对凝血酶的作用有限。鱼精蛋白（1 mg/1 mg 依诺肝素或 100 U 达肝素）仅能部分逆转低分子肝素，抗Xa 因子试验可监测残留效应。

抗血小板药物

在最新的文献报道中，抗血小板药物与脑出血的关系存在争议且未得到证实（Sansing et al.，2009）。一般来说，当发现脑出血时，应停止使用抗血小板药物。PATCH 研究（Baharoglu et al.，2016）是首个血小板输注与抗血小板药物治疗脑出血的随机对照试验，该研究显示输注血小板出现了向不良预后的转变。尽管证据不是决定性的，除非计划进行手术治疗，否则不推荐血小板输注（Frontera et al.，2016）。一项小型研究表明，DDAVP 可改善血小板功能，可考虑用于治疗阿司匹林、ADP 受体抑制剂或 COX-1 抑制剂相关 ICH 的患者（Kapapa et al.，2014；Naidech et al.，2014；Frontera et al.，2016）。

神经外科手术相关静脉血栓疾病

发生率

目前认为高达 90% 的肺栓子来源于下肢或上肢 DVT。静脉血栓栓塞一词通常是指这两种现象。静脉血栓是发生肺栓塞的常见因素，50%~60% 的死亡与肺栓塞有关，预防肺栓塞对患者预后至关重要。在神经外科患者中，静脉血栓栓塞的主要危险因素包括：神经系统恶性肿瘤、外伤性脑损伤、脊髓损伤、脑血管疾病、手术时间长、使用激素、脓毒血症症和长期卧床不活动。仅使用机械性预防设备，神经外科手术后发生 DVT 的风险约为 16%。如果在术后 24 小时内使用低分子肝素进行预防，风险可降至 9%。一般认为肺栓塞的风险为 1.5%~5%。最近的研究证实，相比于出血问题，早期使用低分子肝素更能够降低症状性静脉血栓栓塞的发生（Rolston et al.，2014）。

预防性治疗

开颅脑肿瘤切除术

Kimmell 和 Jahromi（2015）在 4000 多名接受开颅手术的患者中发现，VTE 的发生率高于其他神经外科手术患者。进一步分析表明，神经外科肿瘤手术、并存内科并发症、年龄大于 60 岁、使用激素、手术时间大于 4 小时以及发生术后并发症等因素均显著增加了静脉血栓栓塞的风险。Salmaggi 等（2013）在一项系统综述得出结论，所有接受神经外科肿瘤手术的患者都应该在手术前开始对 VTE 进行机械性预防，并一直持续到出院，而那些被认为大出血风险较低的患者应在术后 24 小时进行低分子肝素预防治疗。然而，在实际临床工作中，所有接受肿瘤开颅术的患者，除非有相关禁忌证，否则应从术后第 1 天进行低分子肝素治疗来预防 DVT。

脊髓脊柱外科

在脊柱手术患者中，VTE 的发生率根据手术的脊柱水平、手术范围和围术期活动度的不同而不同。胸腰椎内固定手术和融合术的患者发生静脉血栓栓塞的风险较高。一些术中机械性预防手段被认为收益很小，但对于接受长时间、前后入路的复杂脊柱手术的患者，以及那些具有已知血栓栓塞危险因素（如脊髓损伤、恶性肿瘤和高凝状态）的患者，应该考虑术后药物预防。考虑到硬膜外血肿形成以及出血、输血和伤口并发症等明确导致的神经功能恶化风险因素，需要对所有接受脊柱手术的患者进行药物预防的个体化风险 - 收益分析。

创伤性颅脑损伤

在无预防措施的创伤性颅脑损伤患者中，DVT 发生率可高达 54%（Foreman et al.，2014）。研究表明，通过机械预防 DVT 和肺栓塞的发病率分别下降到 30% 和 3%。考虑到可能出现颅内出血扩大，药物预防在这种情况下是存在争议的。几项研究已经显示稳定的颅内损伤（低风险的创伤性脑损伤）的进展率为 3% 左右，从而制订了相关的治疗方案（例如 Parkland 方案），建议在 TBI 后 24 小时内反复行颅脑 CT 检查，以便于可以安全使用 LMWH（Phelan，2012）。如果患者有多处挫伤或是硬膜外、硬膜下、蛛网膜下腔或脑室内出血，则认为他们是中度风险的 TBI，只有在 72 小时后 CT 扫描显示出血稳定时才能使用低分子肝素。需要开颅血肿清除术或脑室外引流的高风险 TBI 患者应考虑植入下腔静脉滤器，这已被证明可以减少肺栓塞，但可能增加 DVT 的复发。

延伸阅读、参考文献

扫描书末二维码获取。

第二篇　肿瘤和颅底——脑内肿瘤

第 6 章　低级别胶质瘤

Thomas Santarius · Lorenzo Bello · Hugues Duffau 著
王虎 译，伊志强 审校

引言

根据 2016 年最新修订的世界卫生组织（WHO）中枢神经系统肿瘤分类（Louis et al.，2016），低级别胶质瘤通常指低于间变期的胶质瘤。在本章中，我们将重点关注幕上 2 级弥漫性低级别胶质瘤（diffuse low-grade gliomas，DLGG）的成年患者的治疗，即星形细胞瘤和少突胶质细胞瘤。近年来，组织学诊断并不只单纯描述肿瘤实体，而是描述具有不同生物学和临床行为的异质性肿瘤疾病；与此同时，一些放射学分子标志物正在被逐步发现识别，逐渐提高了预后判断的准确性。

人们曾经普遍认为，低级别胶质瘤在生物学上是稳定的，但现在我们知道低级别胶质瘤像大多数其他肿瘤一样经历了变化，从而成为生物学上更具侵袭性的实体，最终达到 WHO 3 级或 4 级的组织学标准。这通常被称为恶化或间变化（anaplastic transformation，AT），即从非恶性变为恶性实体的变化。虽然这种变化在某些病例中可能是突然和巨大的，特别是从临床的角度来看，但大多数患者在生物学水平上可能是渐进的。换言之，DLGGs 并不是一种疾病，而是一种疾病进化过程中的一个阶段。

过去几十年间，认知神经科学、影像和遗传学方面有了重大的技术和概念进步，DLGG 作为一种脑部疾病和个体化治疗的开创性概念被提出。将 DLGG 作为是脑内的一类肿瘤是错误的。相反，它应该被看做是一种进行性的、侵袭性的中枢神经系统慢性疾病。它对大脑的影响以及对患者的影响是一种动态的变化，且特定于个别患者。脑功能对定义一个人非常重要，因为他 / 她在家庭和更广泛的社会中的承担不同的角色，即使是最细微的损伤和改变都可能对患者的生活质量和社会功能产生深远的影响。因此，DLGG 患者的治疗已经脱离了经典的、严格的治疗方式顺序（不全切除的情况下，手术后放疗，复发时再进行化疗），此种治疗方式没有考虑到任何针对不同患者的个性化治疗顺序。这里我们提出一个现代化的多通道、个性化、针对患者长期的动态管理方式，这种方式可以灵活地对所提供的临床、放射和组织分子数据做出反馈，从而最大化延长每个患者的生存时间并提高生活质量。

发病率

根据来自欧洲和美国的数据，DLGG 的发病率为 1~1.5/（100000 患者 · 年）[星形细胞低级别胶质瘤，0.6~1.2/（100000 患者 · 年）；少突胶质细胞低级别胶质瘤，0.3/（100000 患者 · 年）]，占所有原发性脑肿瘤的 10%~15%（Crocetti et al.，2012；Ostrom et al.，2014）。在诊断时，DLGG 患者的年龄通常在 30~45 岁（Capelle et al.，2013）。在法国对 1295 例 DLGG 的研究中，47 例是偶然发现。影像学诊断偶然发现的 DLGG 患者的年龄比症状性 DLGG 患者年龄稍低（中位数为 35.5 岁 *vs*. 37.0 岁；Pallud et al.，2010b）。随着全球颅脑影像技术的普及，DLGG 的发病率可能会增加。

DLGG 好发于功能区，如岛叶或辅助运动区（Duffau and Capelle，2004）。这一位置的多发可能是由于发生症状的阈值在大脑的这些区域较低（Pallud et al.，2010b）。这与偶发患者在功能区出现 DLGGs 的可能性较小的观察结果是一致的（Pallud et al.，2010b；Potts et al.，2012；Zhang et al.，2014）。

男性约占 DLGG 患者的 60%（McGirt et al.，2008；Schomas et al.，2009；Pallud et al.，2010a）。但 Pallud 等分析发现，在偶发 DLGG 患者（女性 58%）中，这种轻微的男性优势被逆转，随后 Potts 等证实了这一点（Pallud et al.，2010b；Potts et al.，2012）。症状性和偶发性 DLGG 的性别分布原因尚不清楚。基于头痛被列为最常见的行 MRI 检查的原因，作者推测，性别在有症状和无症状人群中的区别（$P<0.001$）可能与女性头痛的发生率较高（Pallud et al.，2010b）或女性通常比男性更有可能求医有关（Potts et al.，2012）

临床表现

80% 以上的 DLGG 患者会伴有癫痫发作。其他患者表现为局灶性功能障碍、精神状态改变或颅内压增高（Pallud et al.，2010b; Pallud et al.，2014）。癫痫发作通常与皮质肿瘤相关，特别是位于额叶、颞叶、岛叶和中心部位的少突胶质肿瘤（Pallud et al.，2014）。

近年来表现为神经功能障碍的患者越来越少见。在一项对 852 名成年患者的回顾性研究中，Youland 等人比较了 1960 年至 1989 年和 1990 年至 2011 年两个历史队列患者的临床表现（Youland et al.，2013）。研究发现，与近期队列相比，早期队列中的患者在诊断时出现多种症状的人数更多（51% *vs*. 24%；*P*<0.0001）参见**表** 6.1。

DLGG 患者临床表现为神经功能障碍的比例相对较少，癫痫发作可出现几月甚至几年的滞后，这都有些令人惊奇，特别是这些肿瘤常位于大脑功能区（Duffau and Capelle，2004）。这与高级别胶质瘤，特别是多形性胶质母细胞瘤的表现形成了鲜明对比。这与以下几个因素相关，包括 DLGG 缺乏或仅有轻微的脑水肿、生长缓慢以及 DLGG 允许受累的大脑功能回路重新定位，即大脑功能的重新映射，这一现象被称为大脑可塑性（Duffau，2005）。越来越多 DLGG 是由于越来越精细的影像学诊断，而不是怀疑胶质瘤而进行的影像扫描。在上述的 1960 年至 1989 年的 Youland 等人的队列中没有偶发的 DLGGs，而在 1990 年至 2011 年的队列中有 11 例（Youland et al.，2013）。

虽然严重的神经功能障碍如言语障碍和偏瘫在 DLGG 的临床表现中很少见，但在诊断时进行客观的神经心理学评估时，往往会观察到更多细微的认知功能障碍。执行能力、注意力、集中力、工作记忆或情绪障碍经常被检测到（Klein et al.，2012; Duffau，2013; van Loon et al.，2015; Racine et al.，2015）。这些缺陷可归因于肿瘤本身、癫痫发作和抗癫痫药物。现在建议在肿瘤治疗前对高级心理功能和健康相关生活质量进行系统评估。这有几个重要的目的：①检测细微的神经心理缺陷；②针对特定个体调整治疗策略（例如，对于弥漫性认知障碍的 DLGG 患者，选择新辅助化疗而不是先手术）；③根据所检测到的功能障碍和肿瘤的位置设计手术策略（即选择在清醒手术中应进行的最合适的神经学评估）；④建立预处理基线，以检测治疗后的功能障碍，并促进术后个性功能康复计划。

影像学诊断

MRI 是诊断和评估 DLGG 的主要工具。T1 呈低信号，T2 呈高信号。肿瘤的范围与 FLAIR 序列高信号一致（Price，2010）。然而，需要特别注意的是，DLGG 是一种弥漫性肿瘤疾病，胶质瘤细胞已被证明存在于 FLAIR 信号异常之外，最远达 2cm（Pallud et al.，2010c）。

通常，DLGGs 缺乏强化导致影像学诊断为低级别胶质瘤，而强化的肿瘤，更有可能怀疑为 3 级或 4 级。虽然这对大多数人来说是正确的，但超过 30% 的无增强的病例将被重新划分为 3 级或 4 级，15%~30% 的 DLGG 会显示增强（Cavaliere et al.，2005）。非强化胶质瘤的组织学分级高于 2 级的可能性随着年龄的增长而增加（Barker et al.，1997）。

在 DLGG 中，增强在少突胶质细胞瘤中更常见（20%~50%），使得增强在少突胶质细胞瘤中成为一个级别特异性相对较低的特征，62%~72% 的间变性少突胶质细胞瘤会出现增强（White et al.，2005）。

表 6.1 两个历史队列（1960—1989 年和 1990—2011 年）中 DLGG 患者的表现

症状	总数 *n*=852(%)	1960—1981 年 *n*=281(%)	1990—2011 年 *n*=571(%)	*P* 值
癫痫	610(72)	218(78)	392(69)	0.008
头痛	258(30)	130(46)	128(23)	<0.0001
语言	61(7)	26(9)	35(6)	0.12
感觉 / 运动症状	271(32)	113(40)	158(28)	0.003

出血和钙化在少突胶质细胞瘤中也很常见。大约1/4的少突胶质细胞瘤出现钙化，CT扫描可清晰显示（Khalid et al.，2012）。间变性少突胶质细胞瘤钙化是低级别少突胶质细胞瘤的两倍，钙化与肿瘤随时间由低级别到高级别的进展一致（Khalid et al.，2012）。

弥漫性低级别胶质瘤具有特征性的形状、位置以及沿白质纤维束扩散的特点。MRI表现或DLGG不均匀，表现为一端界限明显，另一端胶质增生（**图6.1**）。在影像学上诊断DLGG通常是可能的，根据临床表现和重复扫描，通常是在3个月或更早的时间，这取决于对DLGG以外的病理学的怀疑程度和延迟诊断的有害后果的可能性。影像学鉴别诊断包括：脑炎、脑缺血/梗死和其他低分级肿瘤（如DNET，神经节胶质瘤）或更高分级的胶质瘤。然而，在准确的临床病史背景下，神经胶质瘤的诊断很少有疑问。活检以区别于其他诊断（如Rasmussen脑炎）很少有必要。只有当另一种诊断更有可能且需要组织学证实时，才进行穿刺活检（**图6.2**）。在适当的时候，间隔MRI扫描不仅有助于鉴别诊断，而且对患者的后续治疗也很重要，因为生长速度是DLGG预后因素（详见后面的详细信息；参见Pallud et al.，2013）。磁共振波谱也可以用于区分肿瘤和非肿瘤病变（Oz et al.，2014）

间变性恶化是这些患者的主要致死因素，Capelle等人的一系列与间变性肿瘤平行的生存曲线证明了这一点（Capelle et al.，2013）。因此，监测肿瘤的变化是很重要的。在放射治疗的胶质瘤的背景下，正电子发射断层扫描（positron emission tomography，PET）不仅有助于细化鉴别诊断，还有助于识别潜在的间变性位点（Ewelt et al.，2011；la Fougère et al.，2011；Thon et al.，2015）。然而，对于常规监测和检测AT，特别是当需要频繁（例如三个月）监测时，灌注MRI测量相对脑血容量（rCBV）更实用（Danchaivijitr et al.，2008；Hu et al.，2012）。

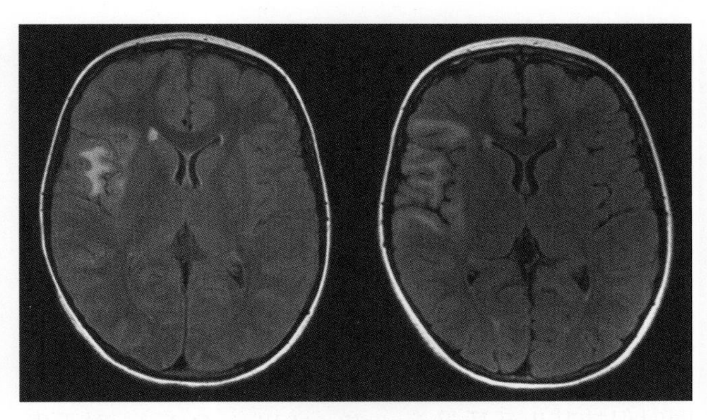

图6.2 DLGG的鉴别诊断包括自身免疫性脑炎。图示患者14岁，表现为进行性的顽固性癫痫发作。扫描间隔一个月进行

影像诊断后的治疗

DLGG的影像学诊断意味着一个行程的开始，行程的进程取决于癌症、大脑，以及患者与治疗团

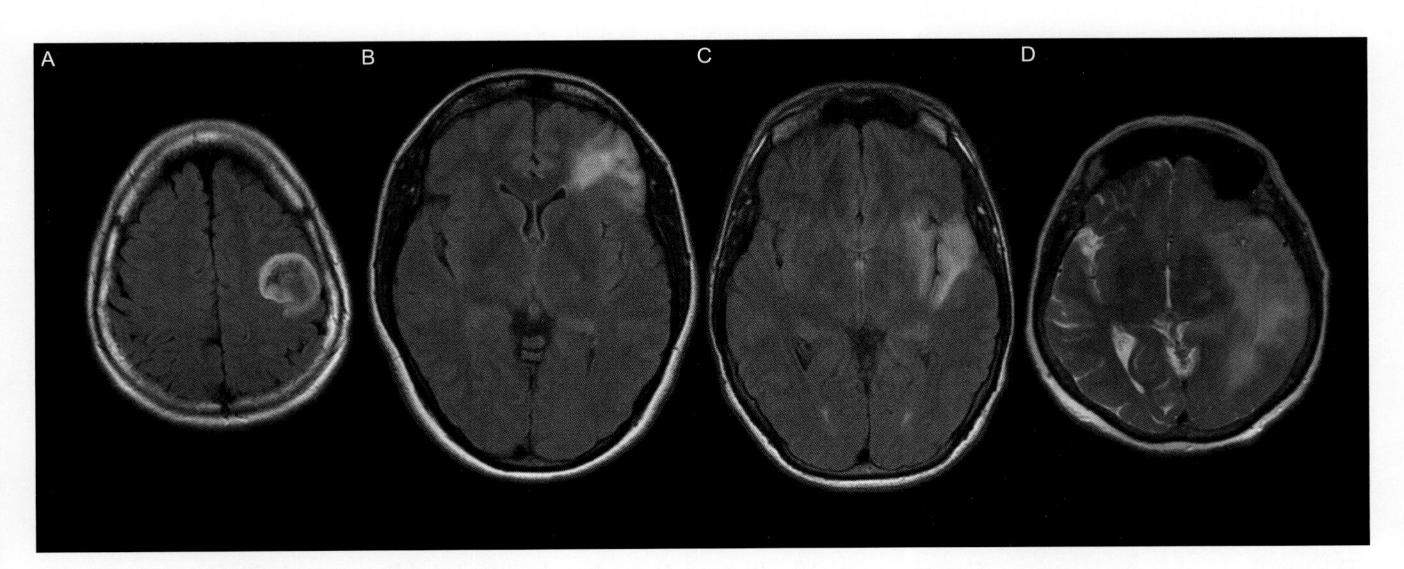

图6.1 DLGG的弥漫性光谱，从相对局限（A）到弥漫性更强，但包含在一个叶内（B），扩散到相邻叶（C）到大脑胶质瘤病（D）

Courtesy of Dr Kieren Allinson，Department of Pathology，Addenbrooke's Hospital，Cambridge

队的合作所做出的选择。然而，长期的OS以及我们对DLGG的本质、治疗以及对其影响的理解的不断发展，增加了另一个层次的复杂性。目前，DLGG仍然是不可治愈的，经过几年的时间，它们通过一系列间变性转变不断地向明确的终点死亡发展。在这一过程中，肿瘤体积会增加，侵犯挤压周围的大脑，并逐渐对大脑的正常功能产生越来越大的干扰。患者的行程是复杂的，治疗团队需要和患者一起制订一种策略，在最大限度地提高患者的生存长度的同时保持其生活质量（quality of life，QoL）。对于患者，因为每个肿瘤都是个体化的，所以都需要个体化的治疗方法（即个体化治疗）。

表6.2列出了与DLGG患者结局（总生存期和间变性进展时间）相关的最重要变量（预后因素）。这些变量单独和综合对疾病自然史和生活质量的影响都需要考虑。重要的是，患者要尽可能多地了解这些变量，包括每个变量相关的不确定性。本质上，一些变量是确定的（临床、放射学、组织学和分子预后因素），其他变量是可以改变的（肿瘤体积）或选择的（治疗：手术、化疗和放疗）。以下将分为五个部分讨论这些问题。在最后一节中，将描述我们机构使用的典型治疗方式。

临床预后参数

患者年龄被长期确定为DLGGs的预后因素（Bauman et al.，1999；Pignatti et al.，2002；Capelle et al.，2013；Jakola et al.，2013）。有趣的是，年龄也与非强化胶质瘤间变率较高有关（Barker et al.，1997）。

年龄、出现神经功能障碍或在发病时没有癫痫发作以及较差的身体状态（KPS<70%）与较差的预后相关（Leighton et al.，1997；Pignatti et al.，2002；Jakola et al.，2012；Capelle et al.，2013）。

影像学预后参数

在许多研究中，肿瘤体积与OS呈负相关（Berger et al.，1994；Lote et al.，1997；Pignatti et al.，2002；Shaw et al.，2002；Chang et al.，2008）。

肿块效应、局灶性功能障碍和（或）导致功能状态较差的颅内高压在单因素分析中是重要因素，而在多因素分析中则不是，可能是因为它们与肿瘤体积有关。较大的肿瘤体积限制了治疗的可能性，并增加了治疗相关并发症的风险（Shaw et al.，2002；Smith et al.，2008）。同样，延伸到功能区或位于功

表6.2 DLGG患者预后相关因素

相关因素	OS	TAT	参考文献
年龄	√		(Leighton et al., 1997; Bauman et al., 1999; Pignatti et al., 2002; Capelle et al., 2013; Jakola et al., 2013)
KPS	√		(Leighton et al., 1997; Capelle et al., 2013; Jakola et al., 2013)
存在神经功能障碍	√		(Pignatti et al., 2002)
有癫痫发作	√		(Leighton et al, 1997; Pignatti et al., 2002)
肿瘤体积	√		(Berger et al, 1994; Lote et al., 1997; Pignatti et al., 2002; Shaw et al., 2002; Chang et al., 2008; Capelle et al., 2013; smith et al., 2008; Jakola et al., 2013)
肿瘤过中线	√		(Pignatti et al., 2002; van den Bent et al., 2005)
肿瘤位于额叶	√		(Capelle et al., 2013)
生长速度	√	√	(Pallud et al., 2013)
rCBV	√		(Bisdas et al,2009; Caseiras et al 2010)
组织学：星形细胞瘤而非少突胶质细胞瘤	√		(Leighton et al., 1997; Pignatti et al., 2002; Mehta et al., 2014)
1p19q共缺失	√	√	(Kaloshi et al., 2007; Cancer Genome Atlas Research Network et al., 2015; Eckel-Passow et al., 2015)
IDH突变	√	√	(Cancer Genome Atlas Research Network et al., 2015; Eckel-Passow et al., 2015)
TERT突变	√	√	(Cancer Genome Atlas Research Network et al.. 2015; Eckel-Passow et al., 2015)
切除程度	√	√	(Leighton et al., 1997; Smith et al., 2008; Jakola et al., 2012; Capelle et al., 2013)

OS，总生存率；TAT，间变性进展时间

能区与较短的 OS 相关，这可能是因为切除范围的限制，也可能是因为神经功能障碍的早期进展（Chang et al.，2008）。

肿瘤生长的速度，表示为直径的扩张速度（velocity of diametric expansion，VDE），即最初的肿瘤体积和增加的体积（Pallud et al.，2012），被发现是一个与 OS 和恶性 PFS 的相关的独立预后因素，无论组织病理学与分子结果（Pallud et al.，2013）。VDE 作为预测和监测工具的优势之一是它相对较好的抽样偏差，因为它将肿瘤作为一个整体来考虑。此外，该方法具有无创、简单、重现性好、成本低廉等优点。

PET、MR 波谱和 MRI 测量的高脑血容量（rCBV）可以检测恶性转化的迹象，并与较短的 OS 相关（Bisdas et al.，2009；Caseiras et al.，2010），而磁共振波谱上乳酸盐和脂类的存在与更具侵袭性有关（Guillevin et al.，2012）。胆碱肌酸比（Cho/Cr）与肿瘤细胞增殖相关（Herminghaus et al.，2002）。Cho/ Cr 和 NAA（N- 乙酰天冬氨酸）/Cr 比值有助于区分低级别和高级别胶质瘤，其敏感性和特异性约为 80%~85%（Server et al.，2011；Zou et al.，2011；Collet et al.，2015），包括 2 级和 3 级的区分（Collet et al.，2015）。在 27 例脑胶质瘤患者中，磁共振波谱检测到 IDH1 突变的脑胶质瘤患者中 2- 羟基戊二酸（2HG）比 IDH1 野生型水平升高（P=0.003；Pope et al.，2012）。

Floeth 等人前瞻性地随访了 21 例小的非增强 T2 高信号偶发肿瘤的患者，采用系列 MRI 扫描和 18F-FET PET 作为随访指标（Floeth et al.，2008）。两名患者的病变显示生长缓慢和阴性的 18F-FET PET，随后的组织诊断为 WHO 2 级星形细胞瘤。第二组患者生长迅速，18F-FET PET 阳性，被发现为高级别胶质瘤。然而，对于间变性转化的常规监测和检测，灌注 MRI 测量 rCBV 更实用，特别是当需要频繁（如 3 个月）监测时（Danchaivijitr et al.，2008；Hu et al.，2012）。

功能性 MR、DTI 神经束显影和脑磁图（MEG）对术前规划有帮助，但讨论它们在治疗 DLGG 中的作用超出了本章的范围（Ottenhausen et al.，2015）。

组织学和分子预后参数

基于组织学检查，根据 2016 年世界卫生组织中枢神经系统肿瘤分类（Louis et al.，2016）将胶质瘤分为四个等级；分级越高，预后越差（**表 6.3**）。1 级星形细胞瘤，如毛细胞星形细胞瘤和巨细胞星形细胞瘤，构成了完全不同的一类疾病，这里不作讨论。虽然 2 级弥漫性幕上胶质瘤（星形细胞瘤和少突胶质细胞瘤；**图 6.3**）是本章的主题，这些不能在没有参考 3 级和 4 级胶质瘤的情况下讨论，尤其是因为 2~4 级是一个连续的分类，而不是独立的分类，更重要的是，2 级肿瘤总是进展到更高级别。因此，2 级胶质瘤是疾病的一个阶段，而不是疾病本身。

表 6.3 2~4 级弥漫性胶质瘤 5 年和 10 年生存率

弥漫性胶质瘤（WHO 分级）	5 年相对生存率（%）	10 年相对生存率（%）
少突神经胶质瘤（2）	78.5	62.8
间变少突神经胶质瘤（3）	52.2	39.3
星形细胞瘤（2）	47.4	37.0
间变性星形细胞瘤（3）	27.3	19.0
胶质母细胞瘤（4）	5.0	2.6

Reproduced with permission from Ostrom, Quinn T.; Gittleman, Haley, CBTRUS Statistical Report: Primary Brain and Central Nervous System Tumors Diagnosed in the United States in 2007–2011, *Neuro-Oncology*, Volume 16, suppl 4, pp. 1–63. Copyright © 2014 Oxford University Press and the Society for NeuroOncology (SNO).

尽管总生存率与每种组织学诊断有广泛的相关性（**表 6.3**），但有大量证据表明，具有相同组织学诊断的个体患者的肿瘤不一定具有相同的生物学特性，其结果可能存在很大差异（Gravendeel et al.，2009；Gorovets et al.，2012）。这会有许多原因，但最重要的两个可能是错误的分级和肿瘤的内在因素。

诊断误差的两个主要来源是抽样和观察者间的可变性。后者与一些分类标准的描述性和模糊性有关，特别是区分 2 级和 3 级肿瘤的标准（Louis et al.，2007）。例如，星形细胞瘤的 3 级判定标准（有丝分裂活性）没有明确规定任何有丝分裂分界点，因此是主观的，通常基于病理学家的个人经验和偏见。在一项调查神经病理学专家诊断不一致率的大型研究中，约 40% 的病例回顾与最初的诊断存在某种类型的不一致，其中约 9% 对即时的治疗效果产生严重影响（Bruner et al.，1997）。同样，2007 年版的混合少突星形细胞瘤类别的标准（识别肿瘤和令人信服的星形胶质细胞少突胶质表型）分类，现在被认为也是非常主观的，这种诊断分类在 2016 修订中被剔除（Louis et al.，2016）。

组织学分级肿瘤内的异质性和随之而来的取样误差可能是误诊的另一个重要来源。Kunz 等发现间变灶体积在 0.6~8.7 ml，覆盖整个可见肿瘤体积的 44%（Kunz et al.，2011）。取样不充分（特别是穿

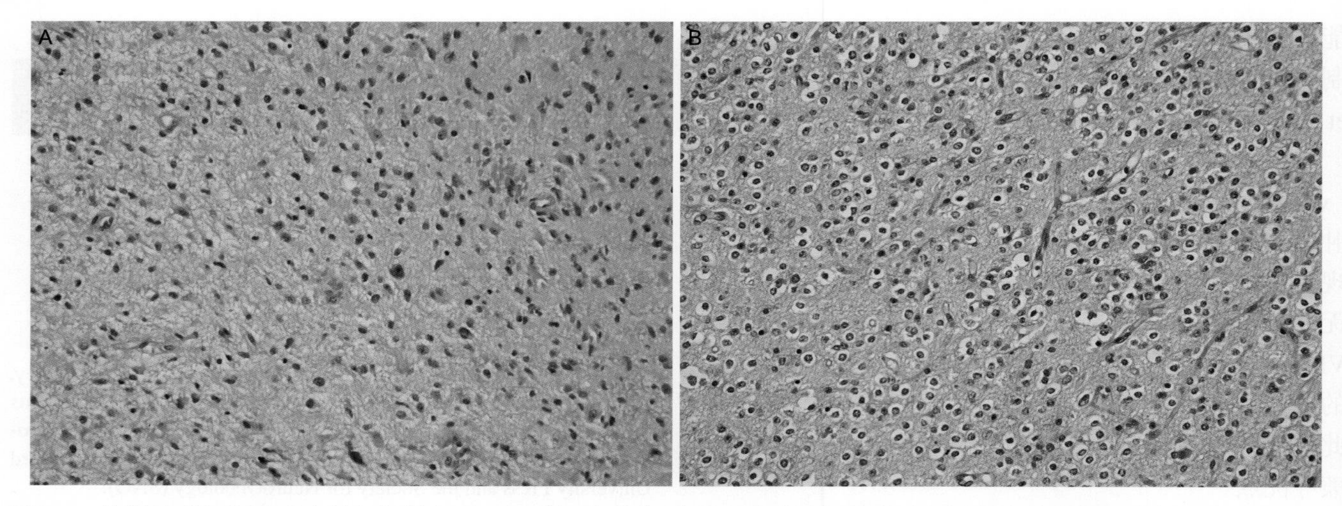

图 6.3　弥漫性低级别胶质瘤的组织学表现：星形细胞瘤（A）和少突胶质细胞瘤（B）（苏木精和伊红染色，20 倍放大）

（A）与正常白质相比，星形细胞瘤是多细胞区域。核多形性和小微囊。未见血管增生和坏死。（B）少突胶质细胞瘤由单核细胞组成，细胞核均匀圆形，核周晕（煎蛋状或蜂窝状外观）。由于固定，核周晕是人工形成的，在冷冻切片中不存在。在这张幻灯片上看到的另一个典型特征是树枝状细毛细血管，通常被描述为铁丝网状

Courtesy Dr Kieren Allinson, Consultant Neuropathologist, Addenbrooke's Hospital, Cambridge.

刺活检和次全切除），未能处理和组织学检查整个标本，可能导致忽视间变灶，从而导致错误诊断，通常是对疾病的低估。无论是穿刺活检还是切除，PET 引导下的取样准确性都可以得到提高（Kunz et al.，2011；Thon et al.，2015）。5-ALA 的使用也有助于术中识别术前 PET 显示的热点（Ewelt et al.，2011）。当诊断是建立在穿刺活检和旧的研究标准上时，应该更需要考虑。

组织学诊断具有，因而局限性是需要不断寻找更准确、客观和临床相关的 DLGG 患者分级标志物。由于癌症本质上是一种遗传疾病（Vogelstein and Kinzler，2004），毫无疑问，分子生物学将提供许多这样的标志物。事实上，已经发现了许多与胶质瘤相关的分子标志物，它们在预测预后方面似乎优于组织学（Gorovets et al.，2012）。这些包括突变或 IDH1 或 IDH2、ATRX 和 TERT 基因，以及 1p/19q 染色体臂的缺失，并首次被纳入世界卫生组织最新的分类中（Louis et al.，2016）。事实上，即使组织学上看起来像星形细胞瘤，则诊断为少突胶质细胞瘤，如果肿瘤具有少突胶质细胞瘤的分子特征（IDH-突变和 1p/19q- 共缺失）。同样，如果肿瘤在显微镜下看起来像少突胶质细胞瘤，但发现有 IDH、ATRX 和 TP53 突变，但 1p/19q 完整，则诊断为弥漫性星形细胞瘤（另见**图** 6.4）。这将留下一个相当模糊的少突胶质细胞瘤的分类，仅适用于分别表现出少突胶质细胞和星形胶质细胞分子特征的细胞群，或在组织学上（表型上）同时表现出少突胶质细胞和星形胶质细胞肿瘤细胞的情况。后者仅适用于无法进行分子诊断试验的情况。

编码异柠檬酸脱氢酶 1 或 2（IDH-1 和 2）的基因失活突变约发生在 75% 的 2 级和 3 级弥漫性胶质瘤和 80% 的继发性胶质母细胞瘤中，而这些基因本身仅占胶质母细胞瘤的少数（~10%）。IDH 突变在继发性胶质母细胞瘤中非常罕见（<5%）。这些情况与 IDH 突变是胶质瘤进展的早期变化的概念是一致的。IDH 突变的 DLGG 似乎是一种独立的、相互排斥的 DLGG 谱系，以 ATRX 和 p53 或 TERT 突变为特征（Eckel-Passow et al.，2015）。这些谱系与星形细胞表型有关，1p19q 共缺失则与少突胶质表型相关。

最近，两项主要的分子研究由癌症基因组图谱（TCGA） 小组（Cancer Genome Atlas Research Network et al.，2015）和梅奥诊所 - 加州大学旧金山分校（Mayo-UCSF；Eckel-Passow et al.，2015）合作发表。在 TCGA 研究中，显示 IDH 突变和 1p/19q 共缺失（1p/19q-del）的弥漫 2 级和 3 级肿瘤预后最好，其次是 IDH 突变和没有 1p/19q 共缺失的肿瘤。IDH 野生型肿瘤与胶质母细胞瘤生存率相同（Cancer Genome Atlas Research Network et al.，2015）。 在 Mayo-UCSF 的研究中，2 级和 3 级弥散肿瘤通过三种变形被分为 5 个胶质瘤分子群：TERT 启动子和 IDH 突变，1p/ 19q 共缺失（Eckel-Passow et al.，2015）。只有 IDH 突变的肿瘤是最常见的（45%），预后中等。它们占所有具有少突胶质细胞成分的胶

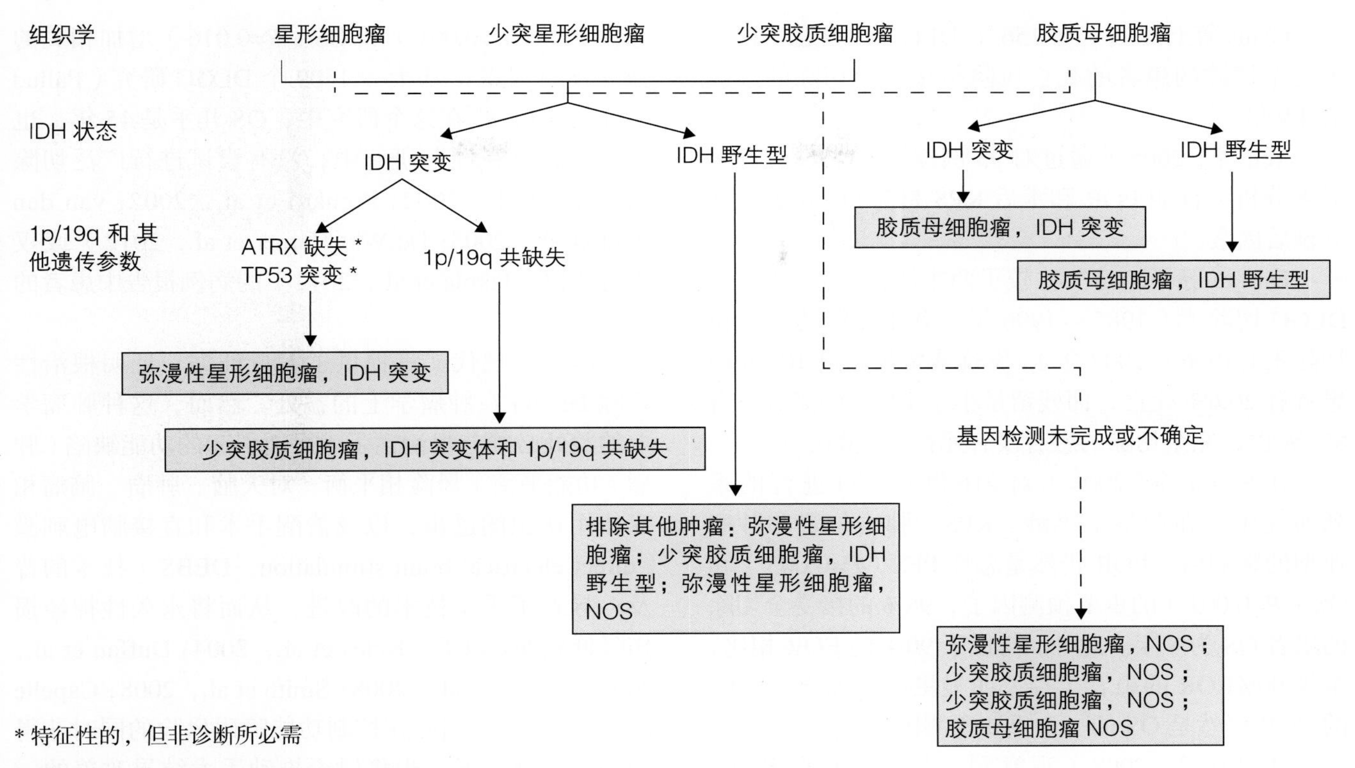

图 6.4　基于组织学和遗传特征的弥漫性胶质瘤分类简图

Data from Louis, D.N. et al., *WHO classification of tumours of the central nervous system*, IARC Press. 2016.

质瘤患者的一半，占Ⅱ级或Ⅲ级星形细胞瘤患者的2/3。这些肿瘤几乎总是获得 TP53 和 ATRX 突变。三联阳性（IDH- 和 TERT- 突变，1p/19q 共缺失）肿瘤是第二常见的（29%），预后良好。它们几乎没有额外的获得性改变，并与少突胶质组织类型密切相关。IDH- 和 TERT- 突变而无 1p/19q 共缺失的预后相似，但罕见（5%）。三阴性肿瘤的发生率与其相似（7%），且预后差，EGFR、PTEN 和 NF1 基因突变。预后最差的是仅 TERT 突变（野生型 IDH，无 1p/19q 共缺失）。这些肿瘤占 2 级和 3 级人群的 10%。与三阴性组相似，他们有许多其他基因突变，包括 EGFR、EGFRv Ⅲ、PTEN、NF1、RB1 和 PIK3CA 或 PIK3R1。

肿瘤的分类是一个不断发展的过程。分子标志物的发现和对胶质瘤生物学的更好理解无疑将加速并进一步改变当今胶质瘤的分类方式。

手术

手术治疗 DLGG 的价值一直存在争议。然而，在过去的 20 年里，越来越清楚的是，手术切除可能是影响 DLGG 患者自然史的主要积极因素。更好的信息收集，基于理解大脑和肿瘤 / 大脑相互作用的完善的外科技术，都促进了这些发展。

经典的低级别胶质瘤文献在数据收集方面存在一些不足，包括缺乏组织学诊断、长期高质量的随访和切除范围的准确报告，切除范围主要是基于外科医生的术中印象（Sanai and Berger，2008）。系统的运用术后影像进行预后等判定并没有被完全、客观地使用（Sanai and Berger，2008）。由于 DLGG 的侵袭性，许多研究低估了残余肿瘤的程度，从而得出了有关手术获益的错误结论。目前，FLAIR MRI 是客观计算术后残余体积的金标准。

在最近所有基于 FLAIR MRI 容量评估的客观术后切除范围（extent of resection，EOR）评估系列中（稍后回顾），切除程度预测了 OS 的显著改善。当术后 MRI（完全切除）未见信号异常时，患者的 OS 明显长于有残留异常的患者。此外，即使是不完全切除，更大程度切除的患者的 OS 也明显更长。这是由于手术延迟了组织学升级，残余肿瘤的体积可以作为 AT 的预测因子（Berger et al.，1994）。这种影响可能的潜在机制是移除所有或许多间变性病灶，这些病灶可能导致组织学快速升级，并将该病例排除低级别队列，手术可以降低肿瘤生物学分级，事实上，这种降级不是一个二元事件，而是残余肿瘤间变性潜能的分级减少，这体现在 OS 与残留肿瘤体积呈反比关系的连续性特征上。

Claus 等（2005）在 156 个 DLGG 中报道，接受不完全切除的患者的死亡风险是接受全切除的患者的 4.9 倍。

Yeh 等（2005）通过对 93 例连续 DLGG 进行多因素分析，证明 EOR 和术后 KPS 是与 OS 相关的独立预后因素。

Duffau 等（2005）比较了两个历史队列：100 例 DLGG 切除术（1985 — 1996 年）和 122 例功能定位切除术（1996 — 2003 年），发现残留量超过 10 ml 的患者有 20.6% 死亡，而残留量小于 10 ml 的患者只有 8% 死亡，完全切除的患者没有死亡（P=0.02）。

在 Smith 等（2008）对 216 例 DLGG 进行的系列研究中，在调整了年龄、KPS、肿瘤位置和肿瘤亚型的影响后，EOR 仍然是恶性 PFS（P=0.005）和 OS（P=0.001）的重要预测因子，98% 的接受全切除的患者 OS 为 8 年。此外，与低于 90% 的 EOR 相比，至少 90%EOR 的患者生存率明显更好，而至少 80% 的 EOR 仍然是 OS 的一个重要预测因子。

McGirt 等（2008）观察到，与次全切除相比，全切除（术前 FLAIR 信号异常完全切除）与 OS 增加独立相关（P=0.017）。在 191 例连续的 DLGG 中，同样的研究小组也表明，全切除是间变性的独立因素（P= 0.05；Chaichana et al.，2010）。

Ahmadi 等（2009）对 130 例 DLGG 进行了研究，通过多变量分析，作者发现 90% 以上的切除与 OS 相关。

Schomas 等（2009）对 314 名随访 13.6 年的 DLGG 患者进行多因素分析，发现小于次全切除是 OS 的不良预后因素。该团队最近还证实，在一 852 DLGG 研究中，全切除和次全切除是与 OS 改善相关的因素（Youland et al.，2013）。

基于对 190 例 DLGG 的回顾，Ius 等（2012）证明，EOR 等于或大于 90% 的患者 5 年生存率估计为 93%，EOR 在 70%~89% 的患者 5 年生存率为 84%，EOR 小于 70% 的患者 5 年生存率为 41%（P=0.001）。

Jakola 等（2012）调查了两所医院采用不同手术策略的 DLGG 人群平行队列的生存率。倾向于早期手术切除的中心的治疗比倾向于活检和观察等待（中位生存期 5.9 年）的中心的治疗具有更好的 OS（未达到中位生存期）。

最近，法国胶质瘤网络（French Glioma Network，FGN）公布了迄今为止报道的最大的 DLGG 手术研究（1097 例患者），显示 EOR 和术后残余体积是与较长 OS 显著相关的独立预后因素（Capelle et al.，2013）。同一组还发现手术切除是与恶性 PFS（P=0.001）和 OS（P=0.016）增加相关的独立预后因素，基于一 1509 个 DLGG 研究（Pallud et al.，2014），在这个研究中，OS 几乎是 15 年，也就是说，是在经典研究中，没有尝试进行广泛切除（Karim et al.，2002；Pignatti et al.，2002；van den Bent et al.，2005；De Witt-Hamer et al.，2012）或仅进行活检（Jakola et al.，2012）的病例报告中患者的两倍。

因此，现代文献提供了大量证据，证明根治性切除 DLGG 在肿瘤学上的益处。然而，这种肿瘤学上的益处必须与根治性手术可能引起的功能缺陷（肿瘤 - 功能平衡）风险相平衡。对大脑、肿瘤、脑瘤相互作用认识的进步，以及清醒手术和直接脑电刺激（direct electrical brain stimulation，DEBS）技术的普及，导致了手术技术的改进，从而将永久性神经损伤降低到 5% 以下（Keles et al.，2004；Duffau et al.，2008；McGirt et al.，2008；Smith et al.，2008；Capelle et al.，2013）。因此在控制功能障碍风险的同时获得肿瘤学益处。下一步将讨论推动手术结果改善的一些因素，包括技术和概念上的。

近年来，人们对大脑功能的认识取得了很大的进展，在理解大脑功能方面已经取得了很大的进展，从具有特定功能的"皮质区域"的概念转移到功能网络的概念，也被称为 hodotopical 模型（hodos- 通路，topos- 区域；见 Duffau，2015）。由于脑回和脑沟在手术中很容易辨认，外科医生传统上把重点放在识别和保存已知与某些功能相关的皮质上，例如中央前回，它容纳皮质脊髓束的神经元。另一方面，白质则是无定形的，因此在很大程度上被忽视了，其后果要么是切除程度非常保守，要么是神经功能缺损风险失控，要么两者兼而有之。

另一个重要的概念是大脑可塑性，即大脑功能从一个解剖位置重新定位到另一个位置的能力（"大脑重组"）。脑可塑性是 DLGG 患者神经功能缺损罕见的根本原因，即使这些肿瘤经常位于功能区（Duffau and Capelle，2004）。这些肿瘤生长缓慢的特点允许大脑进行功能性重新映射，从而允许对传统上认为无法手术的大脑区域进行广泛的外科切除（Desmurget et al.，2007；Duffau，2014）。例如，在没有造成永久性神经功能缺损的情况下，广泛切除侵犯左侧半球经典"Broca 区"的弥漫性侵袭肿瘤（Benzagmout et al.，2007；Lubrano et al.，2010）。此外，切除左额下回的盖部和（或）三角部同时不会有失语症的危险是可能的，原因有二。第一，在基于 771 个刺激位点构建的关键区域概率图的人脑网络模型中，最近已经证明Broca区不是语言输出区（Tate et al.，2014；Tate et al.，2015）。第二，这个区域的组织损失可以通过邻近区域的补充来代偿，主要是腹侧运动前皮质（语音发音的关键区域）、额下回的眶部、背外侧前额叶皮质或脑岛以及偏远区域，例如对侧同源区（Benzagmout et al.，2007；Duffau，2012a）。

即使有些DLGG看起来“界限清楚”，但它们都沿着白质束深入大脑，肿瘤和组织混合在一起。以“切除肿瘤”为主要目标，要么会导致神经功能缺损的不可控风险，要么会导致切除程度低于可能的程度。相反，将DLGG手术视为大脑手术而不是肿瘤手术是有帮助的。切除范围不应局限于肿瘤边界，而应局限于脑功能边界。因此，图像导航是有用的，但它是通过组合DEBS和合适的神经生理学和临床反馈工具来识别关键大脑“hodos”和“topos”（Coello et al.，2013；Bello et al.，2014）。因此，与没有DEBS的手术相比，术中使用DEBS更大程度的切除（总切除率为75% *vs*. 58%）和更低的永久性神经功能缺损率并不奇怪（3.4% *vs*. 8.2%；De Witt-Hamer et al.，2012）。清醒手术是DLGG手术器械中的另一个重要工具，对于浸润或邻近大脑语言有关区域的病例获得功能性反馈是绝对必要的。一项由欧洲低级别胶质瘤网络进行的前瞻性研究发现，清醒手术耐受性好，安全性高（Beez et al.，2013）。切除概率图是一种胶质瘤切除手术的质量评估工具，由De Witt-Hamer等（2013）开发。DLGG手术的技术细节超出了本章的范围，在本教科书的其他地方有介绍。

功能边界的概念是切除的界限，在某些情况下，可以进行扩大切除（即切除范围超出MRI信号异常范围）。最近的一项研究表明，在非功能区的DLGG患者中，行扩大切除术可以阻碍AT的发生，平均随访35.7个月，最大随访135个月（Yordanova et al.，2011）。这一研究与对照组（仅行完全切除术的DLGG）进行比较。对照组中有7例患者出现AT，但所有接受扩大全切除术的患者均未出现AT（P=0.037）。此外，对照组10例患者接受辅助治疗，而扩大全切除组仅1例（P=0.043）。

除了肿瘤学上的益处外，手术切除通常可以改善症状（Teixidor et al.，2007；Duffau et al.，2009）。对于癫痫患者尤其如此，癫痫是DLGGs患者最常见和使人衰弱的症状。两项机构研究发现，完全切除可控制癫痫的发作（Englot et al.，2011；You et al.，2012）。在FGN的一个大型研究（n=1509）中，发现不仅全切，而且次全切都可以控制术后癫痫发作（Pallud et al.，2014）。

对于DLGG患者，再手术不仅应在复发时考虑，而且应作为长期、多模式治疗计划的一部分。在使用多变量分析的FGN研究中，后续的手术切除是与较长OS显著相关的独立预后因素（Capelle et al.，2013）。与初次手术一样，切除程度影响OS（Ramakrishna et al.，2015）。所有复发性肿瘤，包括位于功能区的肿瘤，都应考虑再次手术，因为可以达到更大程度的切除。在Martino等的研究中，尽管涉及功能区，73.7%的患者在再次手术期间实现了全切除或次全切除（Martino et al.，2009）。在这个研究中，手术间隔的中位时间是4.1年。由于再次手术时发现的间变性转化率很高（42%~58%；Schmidt et al.，2003；Martino et al.，2009；Ramakrishna et al.，2015），并且由于恶化肿瘤到第二次手术的时间更长（49个月 *vs*. 22.5个月；Schmidt et al.，2003），有人建议在AT已经发生后，进行早期再干预，而不是进行晚期手术（Martino et al.，2010）。

这种多阶段手术方式从最初的功能导航下切除开始，然后持续数年，然后在保持生活质量的同时，可以行第二次手术适当切除肿瘤，这要归功于大脑的可塑性（Duffau，2005；Duffau，2014）。第一次手术本身、术后功能康复和DLGG的缓慢生长特性可以诱发大脑重塑（Duffau，2011）。定期的神经认知评估和连续的功能神经成像可以为预测第二次甚至第三次或第四次手术提高切除率提供有用的数据。（Duffau，2013；Duffau，2014）。因此，只有考虑到DLGG的生长与脑重塑的关系，才能为每位患者找到多次手术的最佳肿瘤-功能平衡（Duffau，2012c）。

然而，只有当切除至少是次全切除时，手术才显示出显著的肿瘤学益处。因此，当胶质瘤非常弥漫，特别是皮质-皮质下结构广泛浸润，或双半球浸润，大脑的重塑性可能被限制（Duffau and Taillandier，2015），手术预计只能部分切除。（Duffau，2011；De Witt-Hamer et al.，2013）。在这些病例中，因为即使部分切除也可能缓解癫痫的发作，所以除了难治性癫痫患者外，其余没有进行（再）手术的指征，对于位于岛叶或近颞叶结构内的肿瘤尤其如此。非常少见的情况下，次全切除术治疗的放射治疗引起的局灶性增生或颅内压升高。对于难治性癫痫，还应考虑化疗（ChT）和（或）放疗（RT）。

虽然绝大多数GLGG都伴有癫痫发作，但越来越多的DLGG是在头颅影像学检查中发现的，而不是因为怀疑是胶质瘤，最常见的原因是头痛和创伤（另见发病率部分；Pallud et al.，2010b；Potts et al.，2012；Zhang et al.，2014）。与症状性DLGG相比，偶发性DLGG不太可能位于大脑的功能区，且术前体积较小，全切除的可能性较大，OS较长（Pallud et al.，2010b；Potts et al.，2012；Zhang et al.，2014）。偶发性与生存益处显著相关（P=0.04）（Pallud et al.，2010b）。由于EOR是OS、PFS和AT的一个主要预测因素，并且由于在偶发性DLGG中更可能实现全切和超全切，因此提出了早期和根治性手术切除（Duffau，2012b），目前正在讨论DLGG的筛查（Mandonnet et al.，2014）。

化疗

化疗（ChT）和放疗对于手术后进展患者的有效性已经得到证实（Soffietti et al.，2010）。PCV［丙卡巴嗪、洛莫司汀（也称为CCNU）、长春新碱］和替莫唑胺（TMZ）在MRI上的缓解率（45%~62%）和缓解持续时间（10~24月）相似。然而，由于具有更好的耐受性（特别是减少了骨髓毒性）和更好的生活质量，更倾向于选择TMZ（Soffietti et al.，1998；van den Bent et al.，1998；Quinn et al.，2003；van den Bent et al.，2003；van den Bent et al.，2012；Fisher et al.，2015）。ChT可以改善患者的生活质量，特别是对影像学稳定和一些癫痫发作和神经功能障碍较少的疾病稳定的患者（Quinn et al.，2003；Koekkoek et al.，2015）。

有人研究ChT作为手术后的初始治疗在不完全切除、持续癫痫发作或MRI随访进展迅速的DLGG患者中效果（Hoang-Xuan et al.，2004）。通过客观地计算重复MRI上肿瘤生长速率，在大多数情况下，可以观察到对生长速率的影响，至少轻微，甚至部分肿瘤缩小（Ricard et al.，2007）。少部分患者肿瘤体积的减少可持续24~30个月，甚至可能在终止ChT后继续减少。大多数癫痫发作的患者即使影像学上没有改变，但临床上可能得到改善（Koekkoek et al.，2015）。少突胶质细胞肿瘤的患者可能更有敏感，但混合或星形细胞肿瘤患者也可能有效果（Koekkoek et al.，2015）。尽管绝大多数DLGGs对TMZ治疗表现出一定的效果，但与1p/ 19q完整的患者相比，1p/19q缺失患者的效果更显著，效果持续时间更长，导致PFS和OS更长（Kaloshi et al.，2007；Kesari et al.，2009）。虽然甲基化的MGMT启动子患者在使用TMZ治疗时OS更长，但与标准TMZ方案相比，长时间低剂量的TMZ即使在未甲基化的MGMT启动子患者中也会导致OS和PFS延长（Kesari et al.，2009）。这应该与TMZ相关毒性的增加有关。

Johnson等（2014）描述了TMZ治疗的DLGG患者中发生的多重突变。10个接受TMZ治疗的患者中有6个复发为高级别胶质瘤。然而，研究队列（n=23）不能代表整个DLGG，因为只有一例是少突胶质细胞瘤，所有样本都有ATRX或p53或两种基因突变，近3/4的肿瘤复发为高级别胶质瘤。目前尚不清楚本研究中发现的TMZ诱导的高突变基因型是否是一种普遍存在于DLGG中的现象，更不清楚高突变基因型是否影响DLGG的结局。因此，这些发现只能被视为实验室发现（van den Bent，2014）。

放疗

两项Ⅲ期随机试验表明，高剂量与低剂量辐射相比没有优势，并且高剂量辐射的毒性增加（Karim et al.，1996；Shaw et al.，2002）。关于放射治疗（RT）的时机，欧洲癌症研究与治疗组织（EORTC）22845 Ⅲ期随机试验表明，尽管PFS增加，但早期放射治疗对OS没有影响（Karim et al.，2002；van den Bent et al.，2005）。虽然放疗（RT）可能有助于控制癫痫发作，但平均随访12年且无肿瘤进展的患者如果不接受放疗，仍能保持其认知状态，而接受RT的患者则经历了注意力和执行功能以及信息处理速度的恶化（Douw et al.，2009）。不过，必须承认这项研究有一定的局限性，如缺乏基线、选择偏倚、接受放射治疗的患者有更严重疾病，以及使用过时的技术，如全脑放射治疗。

2014年美国临床肿瘤学会会议上公布的RTOG 9802试验结果（18~39岁年龄段次全切除或活检，或40岁及以上年龄段进行任何程度的切除）显示，与单纯RT相比，接受早期RT和PCV治疗后OS有所改善（13.3年 *vs*. 7.8年，P=0.03；Mehta et al.，2014）。对PFS，早期联合RT和PCV也比单纯RT具有优势（10.4年 *vs*. 4.0年，P=0.002）。这项研究经常被误解为证明早期联合使用放化疗的好处。相反，它显示了早期使用化疗的好处。由于化疗潜在的迟发性神经毒性和在无论治疗时间（早期或晚期）在OS方面的等效结果，RT正越来越多应用于因为风险较高不能手术或不能手术切除肿瘤，以及ChT后进展的患者，而不是作为首选治疗（Youland et al.，2013）。

我们机构使用的多模式和多阶段治疗策略

在本节中，我们简要总结了目前治疗 DLGG 患者的方法（**图** 6.5）。这是一个不断演变的过程，取决于我们对疾病的理解，而这种理解反过来又取决于公布的数据，无意中也取决于我们的个人经验。

首先，必须对患者和疾病进行适当的评估。这包括计算肿瘤体积和生长情况（至少需要两次扫描，间隔至少两个月）和广泛的神经心理学评估。影像和临床信息用于讨论手术的具体方式和风险，以及选择特定的工具进行术中计划，这将有助于最小化永久性神经功能缺陷的风险，最大化切除范围（Coello et al.，2013）。

如前所述，治疗计划应与患者共同制订。他或她应适当地了解这种疾病的慢性和不可治愈性，以及在今后几年内需要多种治疗措施，其类型和时间将视每一种疾病的演变而定。重要的是，讨论当前、中期和长期的获益和可用干预措施的风险，为了相对较长的生存期，新疗法的可能性也需考虑在内。

根据 2010 年发表的欧洲指南（Soffietti et al.，2010），早期最大限度的手术切除是治疗 DLGG 的首选。穿刺活检仅用于那些不愿意或由于医学原因不能进行切除的患者。当一些弥漫性病变，如胶质增生病，不能次全切除时，可以考虑活检。

一旦确定了组织学诊断，就需要考虑某些临床参数来决定是否应该进行辅助治疗。以下临床特征更可能建议辅助治疗：年龄超过 40 岁，部分切除 / 残

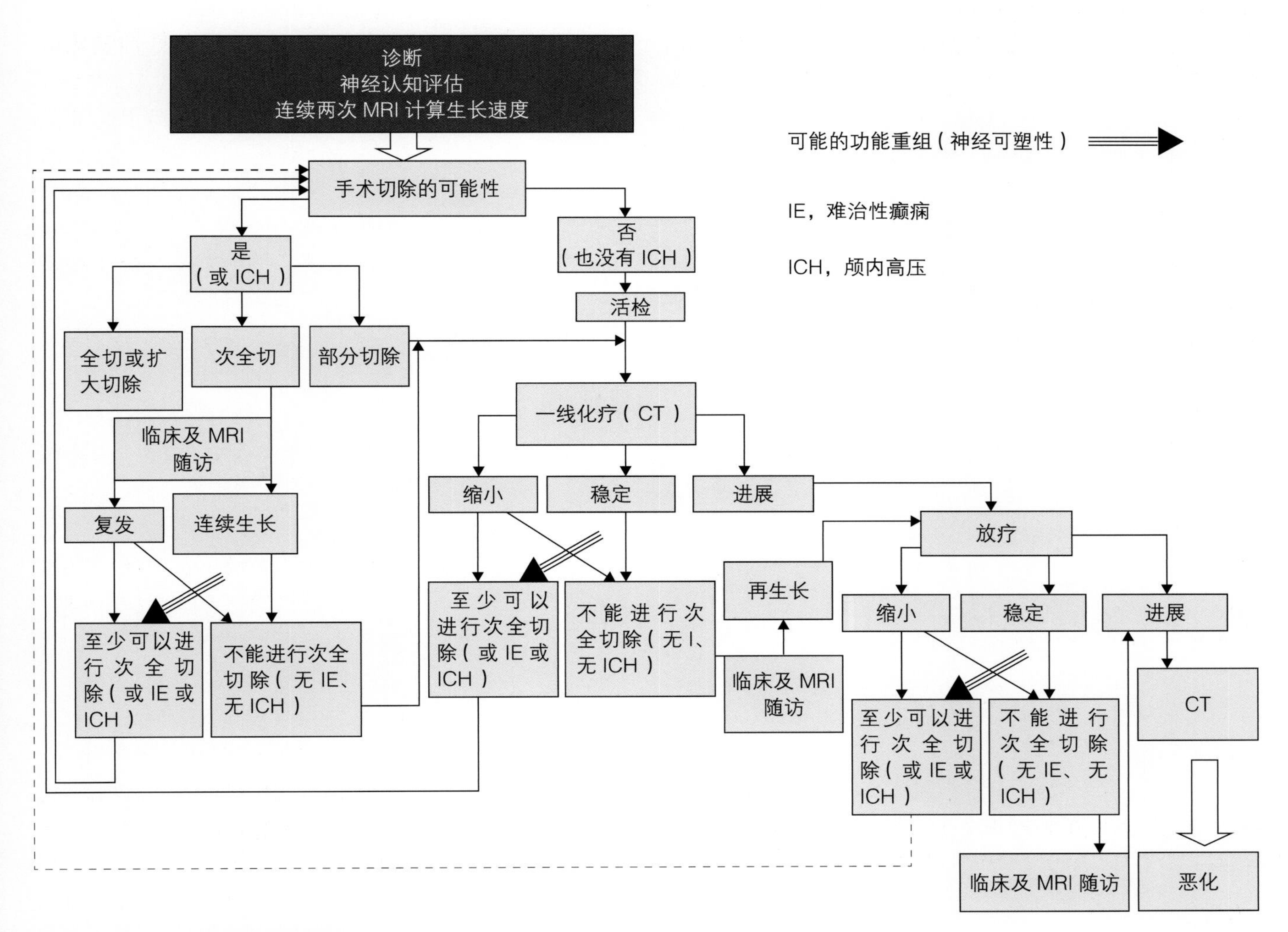

图 6.5　我们机构使用的治疗策略示意图

留超过 10 ml，星形细胞瘤，三重阴性，或 TERT 突变，生长迅速，癫痫难以控制。考虑到星形细胞瘤、TERT 和三阴性肿瘤的 OS 较差和对 ChT 反应较差，放疗的阈值可能较低。然而，分子标志物的重要性应该谨慎考虑，特别是因为它们有待更广泛的验证。

参考文献、EBRAIN 的相关链接

扫描书末二维码获取。

第7章 高级别胶质瘤与神经外科肿瘤的分子生物学

Stephen J. Price · Harry Bulstrode · Richard Mair 著
王虎 译，伊志强 审校

神经外科肿瘤学的分子基础

正常的人类细胞通过基因组和表观基因组逐步改变发展成癌细胞。在一个相对宽松的组织微环境的背景下，这些变化共同降低对细胞的生长、增殖和生存的控制，导致肿瘤的发展。最近的概念认为肿瘤不是不受控制地增殖的细胞球，而是有自身规律的复杂组织：肿瘤的起始、维持和发展代表了组织维持和更新机制解除管制后的复杂突发性产物。

癌症基因组学基础

体细胞突变

在过去的十年里，了解癌症基因组的情况在技术上是可行的。这在很大程度上得益于下一代测序技术的发展和完善（Goodwin et al.，2016）。肿瘤平均包含33~66个影响蛋白质产生的突变，但这也因癌症病因和癌症发病患者年龄而异（Vogelstein et al.，2013）。与增殖组织对诱变剂的反应相比，脑肿瘤含有相对较少的突变。例如，胶质母细胞瘤（glioblastomas，GBM）平均每个肿瘤有35个非同义突变（即导致氨基酸序列改变的突变），相比之下，紫外线辐射引起的黑色素瘤平均有135个突变，吸烟引起的小细胞肺癌平均有163个突变（Meyerson et al.，2010）。具有选择性生长优势并在特定肿瘤类型中反复遇到的突变被称为“驱动”突变。驱动突变可细分为癌基因（其突变产物驱动肿瘤生成）和肿瘤抑制基因（其功能丧失导致肿瘤进展）（如NF2）。一个典型的GBM细胞会有2~5个驱动突变。癌基因和肿瘤抑制基因在胶质瘤中表现出明显不同的突变模式（Vogelstein et al.，2013）。癌基因通常在关键部位表现出错义点突变：这些DNA编码中的单碱基替换引起了氨基酸序列的特殊功能改变，导致癌基因活性的启动。特定位置的特定突变是达到这种效果的必要条件，但单个等位基因的突变就足以促使癌症的形成。另外，染色体重排可导致具有致癌活性的融合蛋白的表达。相反，肿瘤抑制基因会因任何突变而失活，导致阅读框内终止密码子的发生，包括插入、缺失，或者在整个编码序列中任意位置发生单碱基替换。通常情况下，两种肿瘤抑制等位基因的缺失会使癌症发展，或者是两种等位基因的体细胞突变，或者是在一种等位基因的种系突变的情况下单个等位基因的体细胞突变——例如，在一些错构瘤疾病中如神经纤维瘤病和视网膜血管瘤病。

尽管单个肿瘤细胞克隆通常仅表现出少数驱动突变，但遗传不稳定性意味着在肿瘤体积中少数细胞的亚克隆中以低频率存在大量额外的驱动突变。因此，针对特定突变的靶向治疗往往表现出显著的初始反应，随后治疗失败，因为一个预先存在的耐药亚克隆生长起来以取代失去的细胞。肿瘤也有许多不利于生长的突变。这些“乘客”突变代表了一个偶然的有效位点，在肿瘤之间和肿瘤内部是不同的，可以用来绘制肿瘤的进化图。

染色体改变

癌症细胞中的染色体非整倍性变化是常见的，在各种来源的癌症中均可观察到。拷贝数变异在癌细胞中普遍存在，通过增加每个细胞的基因拷贝数量来扩增基因表达。例如，表皮生长因子受体（epidermal growth factor receptor，EGFR），伴随着肿瘤抑制基因缺失而缺失［例如，磷酸酶和紧张素同源物（phosphatase and tensin homolog，PTEN），导致其表达减少或缺失（Cancer Genome Atlas Research，2008）］。染色体臂1p和19q发生不平衡易位，随后丢失一条衍生染色体，是少突胶质细胞瘤具有预测意义的分子标志（Cairncross et al.，1998）。稍后将对此进行更详细的描述。

染色体也可以发生融合，DNA断裂和随后的异常重组导致致癌靶点的产生，例如，幕上室管膜瘤中的C11orf95-RELA（Parker et al.，2014）。这些重排可以是染色体间的、染色体内的或基因内的，它们会使基因组的不同区域错误地排列。

癌症的功能

突变对12条细胞内信号通路有下游效应，使癌细胞产生肿瘤表型。这是通过发展8种“标志性”能力实现的，这8种能力由Hanahan和Weinberg（Hanahan and Weinberg，2011）描述，并与细胞命运、细胞存活和基因组维持的三个基本细胞过程相关。

信号通路

细胞通过信号通路的发展对外部环境作出反应。癌症通过多种机制破坏了这些通路，如受体蛋白、自分泌增殖信号、组成性受体激活的上调（即使没有配体也会激活，如GBM中的EGFRvⅢ扩增）和细胞内负反馈回路的破坏（PTEN丢失）。

逃避抑生长因子

正常细胞周期调节蛋白在癌症中常发生突变。TP53主要检测细胞内压力，诱导细胞凋亡，视网膜母细胞瘤（retinoblastoma，Rb）TP53突变后，细胞内抑制信号转导缺失，从而导致细胞周期不受控制。

逃避接触抑制

细胞接触抑制在癌症中经常被忽略。NF2的突变影响merlin（神经鞘蛋白）的产生，这是一种细胞骨架蛋白，通过细胞内酪氨酸激酶结合限制有丝分裂信号的产生。因此，在接触抑制通常被抑制的情况下，会导致细胞增殖（Okada et al.，2005）。超过一半的脑膜瘤含有NF2肿瘤抑制基因突变。NF2突变和染色体22缺失与半球脑膜瘤发生相关（Arnold et al.，2013）。

基因组不稳定、突变和逃避细胞死亡

TP53诱导DNA链断裂和染色体损伤后的细胞凋亡（如细胞应激或细胞分裂时）。因此，p53蛋白的丢失使细胞能够逃避程序性细胞死亡并继续增殖。TP53突变的细胞由于丢失了这个检查位点，其突变率持续增加。替莫唑胺治疗LGG后发生的错配修复基因突变也被证明会导致高突变表型的发展（Turcan et al.，2012）。有趣的是，细胞内凋亡的缺失并不总是导致细胞的持续增殖，一些细胞往往无法存活，虽然不能发生凋亡，但会发生坏死。这是潜在的致瘤原因子，因为它诱导了促炎症微环境，刺激细胞因子分泌，诱导血管生成，促进肿瘤细胞侵袭和增殖（Grivennikov et al.，2010）。

无休止的复制

正常细胞只能进行有限次数的细胞分裂：分裂过程中固有的染色体末端遗传物质的丧失导致只能进行大约50次的分裂，即Hayflick极限。神经肿瘤学中存在各种与端粒DNA的延伸和维持相关的突变。胶质瘤中常见的影响这一过程的两种突变是ATRX和TERT。后来都被描述为分子生物标志物。

促进新生血管生成

血管生成是引发、维持和发展各种肿瘤过程的关键因素，无论是局部的原发灶还是远处的肿瘤，血管生成已被证明是GBM不良预后的独立预测因子（Jain et al.，2007）。在所有实体肿瘤中，GBM表现出最高程度的血管增生和内皮细胞增生（Folkman，1972）。

神经胶质瘤需要血液供应来促进肿瘤生长。初始阶段包括血管协同选择，此时肿瘤取代正常的脑血管。下一个阶段是血管生成，这时新的血管开始生长。血管内皮生长因子（vascular endothelial growth factor，VEGF）是肿瘤血管生成的关键驱动因素，VEGF受体抑制剂贝伐珠单抗对肿瘤生长具有有效但短暂的作用，但也可能促进肿瘤侵袭。

异常细胞代谢

异常细胞代谢在肿瘤的发展中起着基础性的作用，因为它可以为过多的细胞增殖提供能量需求，并产生细胞快速周转所需的生物合成前体（Vander Heiden et al.，2009）。异柠檬酸脱氢酶是一种细胞内酶，催化异柠檬酸氧化脱羧，形成α-酮戊二酸和CO_2。它有三种亚型：胞质的IDH1，以及位于线粒体内的IDH2和IDH3。IDH1或IDH2的突变通过改变底物特异性改变酶的功能，从而导致2-羟基戊二酸的错误生成（Dang et al.，2009）。这种共生代谢物影响细胞内双加氧酶的活性。在低级别胶质瘤（胶质瘤CpG岛甲基化表型或G-CIMP）中，10-11易位（ten-eleven translocation，TET）酶（以及其他酶）受到抑制，导致高甲基化表型，并导致肿瘤形成（Turcan et al.，2012）。最后，癌细胞到基质细胞的代谢共生已经被证明，基质细胞以类似中枢神经系统内神经胶质和神经元关系的方式喂养癌细胞（Feron，2009）。

肿瘤促炎反应

如前所述，单独的基因组不稳定性不足以维持肿瘤进展。合适的微环境也会驱动肿瘤的进展。肿瘤和免疫系统之间的复杂相互作用导致抑制性细胞因子和趋化因子的表达（Qian and Pollard，2010）。GBM 内的研究表明，GBM 亚型和免疫特征之间存在相关性。免疫细胞浸润和不同的潜在突变环境之间的相关性，以及特殊细胞因子（如 TGF-b）调节间叶细胞性胶质母细胞瘤的增殖、迁移和致瘤性的能力，进一步定义了免疫微环境在胶质母细胞瘤中的作用。

表观基因组学

表观基因组学是指 DNA 修饰导致基因表达的改变，而不改变碱基对序列。例如，MGMT 启动子的甲基化是一种表观基因组修饰，导致该 DNA 修复基因的表达降低，从而使 GBM 对烷基化化疗的敏感性增加。在实际中，肿瘤发生涉及基因组和表观基因组进化的一个过程，融合到具有选择性优势和恶性的特征上，例如不受限制的细胞分裂。基因组突变也可以驱动表观基因组进展：基于无偏基因组测序的方法已经反复和意外地发现了与基因表达的细胞调节有关的基因中的驱动突变的例子，包括负责儿童 GBM 中 DNA 包装的组蛋白（H3K27M 和 H3G34R/V 突变）（Wu et al.，2012）和 IDH 突变驱动肿瘤代谢物 2- 羟基戊二酸的产生，后者抑制弥漫性胶质瘤中的 DNA 甲基化转换（Dang et al.，2009）。

胶质瘤干细胞

干细胞的特征是它们具有自我更新能力（无限分裂产生更多同种类型细胞的能力）、多能性（分化为多种谱系的能力，例如胶质细胞和神经元），以及它们在体内产生肿瘤的能力。

胶质母细胞瘤和髓母细胞瘤是两种典型的肿瘤，它们的干细胞部分可以被分离并高效地移植到小鼠体内形成肿瘤，而大多数肿瘤细胞群没有这种特性。肿瘤干细胞和大量肿瘤子代具有相同的突变，因此子代细胞突变是明确的，但不足以确定干细胞的特性，基因表达和基因组结构（表观基因组学）以及微环境也起着关键作用。在实际中，在 GBM 中发现的癌干细胞始终显示出与胚胎大脑中的神经干细胞和祖细胞群相关的基因表达模式，而这也是可预期的，因为这些细胞程序已经进化到支持特定中枢神经系统（central nervous system，CNS）生态位的快速增殖，并且这些干细胞的起源细胞可能是中枢神经系统的祖细胞或其衍生细胞。初步实验表明，包括 CD133 和 CD15/SSEA-1 在内的神经干细胞表面标志物也可用于脑肿瘤干细胞（Singh et al.，2004）。这些脑瘤干细胞可能对放疗和化疗有选择性的抵抗（Bao et al.，2006）。

髓母细胞瘤中的干细胞

髓母细胞瘤提供了一个很好的例子，说明共同选择神经干细胞途径如何推动脑肿瘤干细胞增殖。不同的髓母细胞瘤亚群表现出 sonic hedgehog 通路或 Wnt/B-catenin 通路的不同基因突变。这些通路显示出一定程度的功能冗余，聚合在一起驱动肿瘤干细胞自我更新增殖以及髓母细胞瘤组织学。世界卫生组织（WHO）2016 年 CNS 分类中纳入的分子亚型反映了生物学和预后的主要差异（Louis et al.，2016）。WNT 激活髓母细胞瘤（通常表现为 CTNNB1 突变）和 Shh 激活髓母细胞瘤（通常为 PTCH1、SMO、SUFU 突变）与第 3 组和第 4 组髓母细胞瘤一起被发现，特征不太明确，预后通常较差。髓母细胞瘤分类是新一代分子肿瘤分类系统的典型代表，其希望在理解机制的基础上，获得突变和基因表达谱的关联性。虽然这里描述的分类是基于基因表达，但亚组中同时发生的基因组突变的鉴定进一步确定了预后组（例如 SHH 组中的 TP53 突变预测预后较差）。同样，在脑膜瘤中，SMO 突变导致 sonic hedgehog 通路的激活与发生于前颅底的肿瘤有关。脑膜瘤内的突变也与组织学亚型相关。对于其他肿瘤，包括 GBM，存在基于表达的分类系统。癌症基因组图谱分类（总结在**表 7.1** 中）可能是迄今为止最为人所知的胶质母细胞瘤分子分类系统，但绝不是全确定的（Verhaak et al.，2010）。前神经元型组显示生存率提高，但有趣的是，与单纯放疗相比，放化疗组无生存优势。进一步的工作正在进行中，以了解这种分类对个别患者的意义。抗血管生成药物试验的分析

表 7.1　肿瘤基因组图谱 GBM 亚型的分类

亚型	突变特征	表达信号
前神经元型	*TP53, PDGFRA, PI3K, IDH1*	*OLIG2, NKX2-2*
神经元型	*TP53, EGFR*	*MBP, SYT1*
经典型	*EGFR, Chr10, PDGFRA*	*EGFR, AKT2*
间质型	*NFkB, NF1*	*CD44, YKL40*

表明，这一前神经元型组可能从抗血管生成治疗中获益（Sandmann et al.，2015）。

高级别胶质瘤的概述

高级别胶质瘤（high- grade glioma，HGG）包括一些被 WHO 分类为 WHO Ⅲ级和Ⅳ级肿瘤的组织学实体。传统意义上，人们认为它们有类似的特性，并以类似的方式进行治疗。然而，我们在肿瘤生物学的理解上的最新进展，使我们识别了分子标志物，这些分子标志物现在是这些肿瘤分类的核心。我们认为这些肿瘤是分子上不同的亚型，它们的特性不同，应该用特定的方式来治疗。

高级别胶质瘤的分类

高级别胶质瘤产生于大脑中的支持神经胶质细胞，主要的细胞类型决定病理分类。肿瘤根据 WHO 分级系统（Ⅰ~Ⅳ级）在光镜下的表现进行分级。HGG 包括 WHO 分级Ⅲ级肿瘤（间变性星形细胞瘤和间变性少突星形细胞瘤）和Ⅳ级肿瘤（胶质母细胞瘤、含少突胶质细胞成分的胶质母细胞瘤和胶质肉瘤）。2016 年版的 WHO 分级系统删除了混合胶质瘤（即少突星形细胞瘤），现在根据其分子分类对其进行分类。

组织学上，Ⅲ级肿瘤为弥漫浸润性胶质瘤，伴有局灶性或分散性间变，具有明显的增殖潜能，细胞增多，明显的核非典型性和高有丝分裂活性。Ⅳ级肿瘤表现为细胞多形性、核非典型性、活跃的有丝分裂活性、血管血栓形成、微血管增生和坏死。示例如**图 7.1** 所示。

肿瘤按肿瘤最恶性的部分进行分级。因此，充分的取样来确定适当的分级是必要的，尤其是在活检过程中。

流行病学

高级别胶质瘤是最常见的原发性内源性脑瘤，占所有新诊断的原发性恶性脑肿瘤的 85%。据报道，在欧洲和北美，这些肿瘤的发病率约为

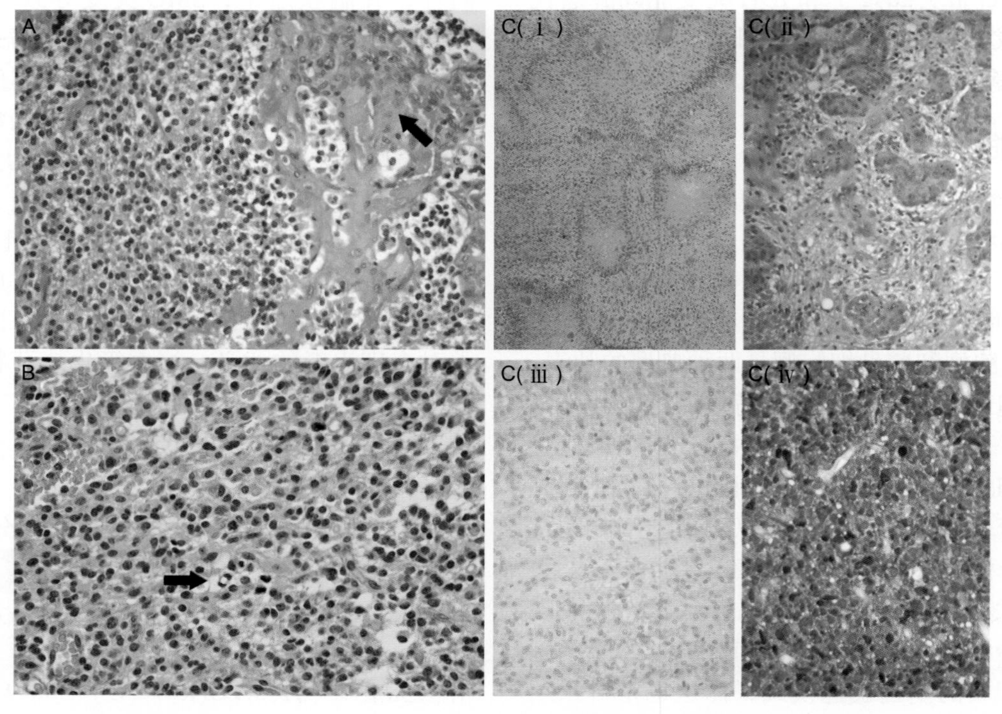

图 7.1 （A）间变性少突胶质细胞瘤（Ⅲ级）：圆形核伴核周晕，表明少突胶质细胞谱系；微血管增生（箭头）、坏死和活跃的有丝分裂活性是高级别特征。这种组织学诊断与 IDH 突变和 1p/19q 共缺失密切相关。（B）间变性星形细胞瘤（Ⅲ级）：高细胞密度，核多形性，有丝分裂象（箭头所示）是高级别特征。没有Ⅳ级胶质母细胞瘤中的坏死和微血管增生。（C）胶质母细胞瘤（Ⅳ级）：（i）肿瘤细胞的多细胞带突出了坏死肿瘤的边界，称为栅栏状（或假栅栏状）坏死。胶质母细胞瘤的典型组织学特征。（ii）形成这些肾小球样结构的微血管增生是胶质母细胞瘤的另一个典型组织学特征。对 IDH1 R132H 突变的免疫染色可区分 IDH 野生型（iii）和 IDH 突变型（iv）肿瘤

Courtesy of Dr Kieren Allinson, Department of Pathology, Addenbrooke's Hospital, Cambridge.

5/（10 万人·年）。英国肿瘤登记处关于胶质母细胞瘤的最新数据发现，总体全国年标准化发病率为 4.64/（10 万人·年），平均每年超过 2100 例（Brodbelt et al.，2015）。这可能低估了真实数据，因为有 1/5 的人没有住院（Pobereskin and Chadduck，2000）。

在所有高级别胶质瘤中，胶质母细胞瘤占 60%~70%，间变性星形细胞瘤占 10%~15%，间变性少突胶质细胞瘤约占 10%，其余为间变性室管膜瘤和间变性神经节胶质瘤。

最近在西方，HGG 的发病率有所增加，尤其是在老年人中。这可能反映了改进后的影像诊断的增多（Wen and Kesari，2008）。胶质母细胞瘤的发病率随着年龄的增长而增加，在 65~75 岁达到高峰（Brodbelt et al.，2015）。男性的发病率是女性的 1.66 倍（Brodbelt et al.，2015）。

高级别胶质瘤的病因学

在大多数情况下，不能确定是什么原因造成的。然而，暴露于电离辐射，如既往癌症治疗是一个确定的危险因素（Walter et al.，1998）。许多其他因素也被研究过，包括头部损伤、含有 N- 亚硝基化合物的食物、电磁场、吸烟以及最近使用手机，但这些都没有被证明是 HGG 发展的危险因素（Inskip et al.，2001；Kleinerman et al.，2005；Holick et al.，2007）。

胶质瘤的发生确实有一定的遗传风险。有胶质母细胞瘤家族成员的个体发生 GBM 的风险似乎是无家族史者的 2 倍（Schwartzbaum et al.，2006）。大约 5% 的 HGG 患者有胶质瘤家族史（Bondy et al.，1994）。其中一些是家族性的，与遗传综合征有关，如 1 型和 2 型神经纤维瘤病、Li-Fraumeni 综合征和 Turcot 综合征。研究还显示了 DNA 修复基因与肿瘤侵袭性之间的联系（Bhowmick et al.，2004；Okcu et al.，2004；Simon et al.，2006）。端粒 - 保护蛋白基因复合物的突变，特别是 POT1，最近证明与这些家族性胶质瘤综合征相关（Bainbridge et al.，2015）。目前尚无明确的家族性胶质瘤筛查指南。

巨细胞病毒在胶质母细胞瘤病因学中的作用

人们对病毒感染参与神经胶质瘤多步骤发展的可能性非常感兴趣。当一项研究在 100% 的胶质母细胞瘤样本中发现巨细胞病毒（cytomegalovirus，CMV）基因产物，但未能在正常组织中发现它时（Cobbs et al.，2002），人们对这可能是胶质瘤发生的一个重要原因产生了极大的兴趣。但其他研究未能复制这些结果（Dey et al.，2015）。一项随机、双盲的关于缬更昔洛韦的试验，一种抗巨细胞病毒疗法，用于放化疗（VIGAS 研究），未能显示任何生存获益（Stragliotto et al.，2013）。然而，该组织随后给《新英格兰医学杂志》（*the New England Journal of Medicine*）写的一封信引起了广泛的关注（Stragliotto et al.，2013）。他们报道说，在一项回顾性分析中，与同时代的对照组相比，接受缬更昔洛韦治疗的患者（作为试验的一部分和出于同情的理由）的生存率有所提高。这项研究存在几个缺陷，目前的共识结论是，文献支持巨细胞病毒在恶性胶质瘤中的肿瘤调节作用，但未来的研究需要重点确定巨细胞病毒作为胶质瘤启动因素的作用（Dziurzynski et al.，2012）。

特应性疾病可能有保护作用

一个不寻常的发现是，特应性疾病（如哮喘、湿疹或过敏）是神经胶质瘤发生的保护性因素。与对照组相比，胶质瘤患者的特应性症状更少。由于特异反应可能是免疫功能障碍的标志，它可能表明免疫因素在胶质瘤病因中的作用。

高级别胶质瘤的病理学及发病机制

高级别胶质瘤的分子生物学

世界卫生组织（WHO）中枢神经系统肿瘤分类的引入导致了高级别胶质瘤分类的广泛变化（Louis et al.，2016）。分子亚群的定义将神经胶质源性肿瘤大致划分为 IDH 野生型、IDH 突变型和未指定的 IDH（即未寻找 IDH 突变；Louis et al.，2016）。在这种分类中（包括少突胶质细胞瘤的 1p19q 染色体共缺失），弥漫性胶质瘤、少突胶质细胞瘤、间变性星形细胞瘤、间变性少突胶质细胞瘤和胶质母细胞瘤现在都已被定义。

胶质母细胞瘤的突变和瘤内异质性

确定发生的突变倾向集中于三种细胞内信号通路：具体来说，PI3K、TP53 和 Rb（Cancer Genome Atlas Research，2008）。经典的“刺激”包括激活生长信号受体 EGFR、PDGFR 和 MET 的突变，以及它们的下游靶点 PI3K、AKT、mTOR 和 RAS。同样，负责调节这些级联的肿瘤抑制因子也会在 GBM 中发生功能缺失突变，包括 PTEN、NF-1、RB1 和 TP53。**图 7.2** 总结了这些途径。

尽管存在这种趋同，但 GBM 的肿瘤间和肿瘤内

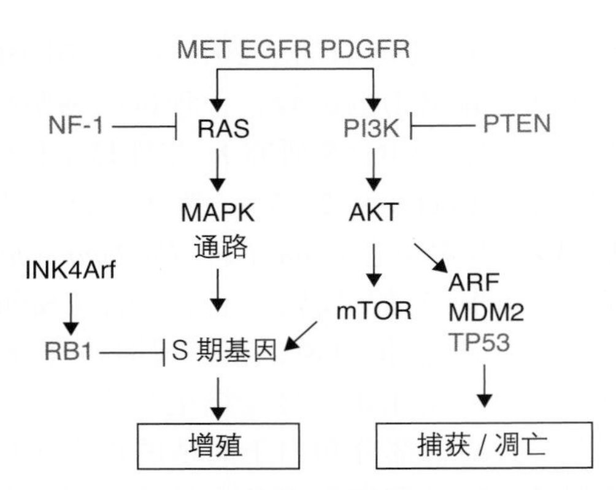

图 7.2 参与胶质瘤形成的代谢途径。这些途径的常见突变成分在图中用红色突出显示

异质性仍被认为是治疗失败和疾病复发的主要原因。GBM 存在基于基因表达的分类系统，但迄今为止证明不太可靠（Verhaak et al.，2010），并且已确定单个肿瘤中不同组的广泛共存（Sottoriva et al.，2013）。

高级别胶质瘤的发展与进展

胶质母细胞瘤可以为原发性肿瘤，也可以起源于先前存在的低级别胶质瘤。这些原发性和继发性胶质母细胞瘤构成独立的和不同的疾病实体。它们影响不同的流行病学群体，具有不同的预后。

原发性胶质瘤通常是新发的表现，患者主要为年龄较大且临床病史较短者。继发性胶质瘤通常是由低级别恶性发展到高级别恶性的肿瘤，患者主要为年轻人，发病间隔在 1~10 年。

高级别胶质瘤的转移和进展

肿瘤侵袭

局部白质侵袭是胶质瘤的主要病理特征，也是治疗失败的主要原因。这种入侵程度因人而异。针对侵袭边界的组织学研究表明，20%~27% 的 GBM 具有有限的侵袭，定义为小于 1 cm 的扩散（Scherer，1940；Burger et al.，1988），而约 20% 的患者有弥漫性浸润，定义为大于 3 cm 的扩散（Burger et al.，1988）。

侵袭细胞的基因表达发生变化，促进迁移的基因表达上调，促凋亡基因表达降低（Hoelzinger et al.，2005）。胶质瘤的侵袭过程有三个阶段，首先是细胞黏附分子的表达，使胶质瘤细胞黏附于细胞外基质的成分（特别是肌糖蛋白 -C）。其次是蛋白酶（如金属蛋白酶）的产生，降解基质，消除细胞运动的障碍。在胶质瘤中，金属蛋白酶（metalloproteinases，MMP）的产生，特别是分泌的 MMP-2、MMP-9 和组织结合的 MT1-MMP 对侵袭是至关重要的（Lampert et al.，1998；Beliveau et al.，1999）。分泌的 MMP 受到其组织抑制剂 TIMP-1 和 TIMP-2 的调控，而 TIMP-1 和 TIMP- 2 在胶质瘤中被下调（Beliveau et al.，1999）。最后，细胞迁移到蛋白酶活性降解的基质区域。这是由趋化因子 CXCL12 的增加分泌而促进的（Zhang et al.，2005），该趋化因子与 CXCR4 受体结合，而 CXCR4 受体在侵袭性胶质瘤细胞中上调。

最近，胶质母细胞瘤已被证明含有少量具有自我更新和肿瘤形成能力的细胞。这些细胞在分子遗传学水平上已被证明是母体肿瘤的代表。它们在体外高度活跃，在体内表现出广泛的宿主侵袭。初步基因表达分析表明，它们表达多种与侵袭和迁移相关的标志物，包括膜结合蛋白如 MT1- MMP、NG2 和 B1- 整合素，以及可溶性因子如纤溶酶原、MMP-2 和 MMP-9。

神经胶质瘤播散及转移

如前一节所述，高级别胶质瘤主要通过侵犯白质束而进展。Scherer 描述了肿瘤生长的其他机制（Scherer，1938），包括沿软脑膜表面的软脑膜下生长和沿脑室表面的室管膜下生长。这可能导致偶尔播散到脊柱。

HGG 的转移是非常罕见的，但已被描述。它主要沿脑室 - 腹腔分流器扩散至腹腔或头皮，特别是在骨瓣缺失的部位。有病例表明，移植了 HGG 患者器官的患者发生了 HGG 转移，这表明免疫系统的抑制是这些细胞生长所必需的。

胶质瘤进展中的“缺氧开关”

在白质束中生长的侵袭性细胞与中枢肿瘤细胞有不同的生物学和行为。这些细胞更活跃，但不分裂（Giese et al.，1996）。随着它们数量的增加，可用的代谢产物受到挑战。在高级别胶质瘤的快速分裂区域，这种竞争将导致缺氧的发展。“缺氧开关”在这些肿瘤中导致三种主要的特性改变（Bjerkvig et al.，2009），缺氧促进癌症干细胞分裂，由于 VEGF 等因子的产生促进血管生成，最后通过上调侵袭因子促进侵袭。

随着恶性程度的增加，缺氧将导致最终的坏死和微血管增生，这两者都是胶质母细胞瘤的组织学特征。

缺氧是胶质瘤干细胞“迁移或生长”的趋势中心（Giese et al.，1996）。在缺氧条件下，这种趋势是迁移和侵入，而在较高的氧分压下，倾向于增殖：两种表型在临床上都不可取。

高级别胶质瘤的分子生物标志物

我们已经可以识别几种肿瘤发生的分子生物标志物。生物标志物是一种客观测量和评估的因素，作为正常生物或致病过程或药物对治疗干预反应的指标。这些生物标志物可以是诊断、预后或对治疗反应的预测因素。在高级别胶质瘤中，已经发现了许多这样的标志物，现在正被用来更好地对这些肿瘤进行分类。

异柠檬酸脱氢酶突变

异柠檬酸脱氢酶（isocitrate dehydrogenase，IDH）基因编码一种细胞质酶，将异柠檬酸转化为α-酮戊二酸。该基因的突变导致2-羟基戊二酸的产量增加了10倍，而不是α-酮戊二酸（Dang et al.，2009）。在5.6%~12%的GBM患者中发现了IDH1基因突变，并且似乎无进展生存期和中位生存期更好（3.7年 *vs*. 1.1年）（Parsons et al.，2008；Weller et al.，2009），表明IDH突变是预后性的，而不仅仅是预测性的（van den Bent et al.，2010）。大多数突变是点突变，涉及精氨酸132（R132H）突变。这允许对石蜡包埋组织进行免疫组化检测，已证明与DNA测序有88%~99%的一致性（Zou et al.，2015）。免疫组化IDH R132H突变的例子如**图7.1C**所示。其他突变可能包括IDH1的其他点突变或线粒体IDH2的突变。

越来越清楚的是，无突变的低级别胶质瘤预后非常差（Eckel-Passow et al.，2015）。这表明高级别和低级别胶质瘤的划分现在应该基于IDH突变状态而不是组织学（Brandner and von Deimling，2015）。

染色体1p/19q缺失

在WHO 2016年分类中，IDH突变肿瘤中1p19q异质性缺失可诊断为少突胶质细胞瘤或间变性少突胶质细胞瘤。这种突变在化疗中提高了生存率，最初被认为是对化疗敏感性的预测。放疗与放化疗对比试验的结果显示，1p19q缺失的单纯放疗组优于1p19q未缺失的放化疗组，再次表明这些分子标志物的预后性质（van den Bent et al.，2006）。然而，两项类似研究的长期随访现在已经清楚地显示，放疗和化疗治疗1p19q缺失肿瘤具有生存优势，这表明这应该是我们对这些肿瘤标准治疗的一部分（van den Bent et al.，2013；Cairncross et al.，2013）。

O-6-甲基鸟嘌呤-DNA甲基转移酶（MGMT）的甲基化

MGMT基因编码O-6-甲基鸟嘌呤-DNA甲基转移酶，这是一种DNA修复酶，可以去除鸟嘌呤O-6位点上的烷基，这是DNA烷基化的重要位点。MGMT甲基化状态已被用于预测对烷基化化疗药物如替莫唑胺的反应。在甲基化形式下，它是非功能性的（即不产生酶，从而限制了DNA修复）。MGMT甲基化发生在高达45%的GBM病例中（Hegi et al.，2005；Stupp et al.，2005），并且与中位生存期的改善相关，在与替莫唑胺联合放疗后，中位生存期明显长于单独放疗的患者（Hegi et al.，2005；Weller et al.，2009）。相比之下，未甲基化组的生存率差异不显著，但放化疗组存在生存差异（Stupp et al.，2005）。单独进行放疗的甲基化组比未甲基化组有更好的生存率，这表明MGMT甲基化是一种预后标志而不是预测标志。

MGMT甲基化状态的评估并非没有技术问题。已经确定了多个突变位点，使得这种标志难以评估。此外，结果是半定量的，没有明确的界限来定义阳性或阴性状态，导致没有明确的临床标准试验来解释结果。

TERT启动子突变

TERT（一种编码端粒酶的基因）的突变已经在一些脑肿瘤中被发现。有趣的是，在胶质母细胞瘤和低级别胶质瘤中都发现了突变。这表明端粒的维持可能对胶质瘤的形成很重要（Killela et al.，2013；Vinagre et al.，2014）。

组蛋白H3突变

组蛋白H3家族3A（H3F3A）的突变已在儿童脑干和中线胶质母细胞瘤中被发现（Wu et al.，2014）。这些是H3F3A内甘氨酸-精氨酸/缬氨酸密码子34（G34R/V）改变之间的点突变。在成人中，它们的发生率占所有胶质母细胞瘤的3.4%（Yoshimoto et al.，2017）。对于年轻人，往往是中线肿瘤。

争议：我们应该用组织学标准还是分子标志物来对高级别胶质瘤进行分类

现在很清楚的是，基于组织学标准的肿瘤诊断包括几个不同的肿瘤亚类，分子标志物在我们的

HGG 亚类中是非常重要的。目前的问题是这些分子标志物在我们对这些肿瘤的分类中应该发挥多大的作用?

结合三种标志物(即 IDH 突变、1p19q 编码缺失和 TERT 突变)的研究已经能够确定胶质瘤的五个分子亚类(Eckel-Passow et al., 2015;**表** 7.2)。在 WHO Ⅱ/Ⅲ级肿瘤中,大多数具有所有标志物突变(三阳型)、TERT 和 IDH 突变,或仅 IDH 突变。这些突变具有良好的预后。然而,约 17% 的肿瘤仅有 TERT 突变或无突变,这些预后与胶质母细胞瘤相似。最近,国际神经病理学协会(International Society of Neuropology Consenses of Haarlem)强调了将这些分子标志物纳入诊断的重要性(Louis et al., 2014)。

WHO 2016 年最新分类系统现已纳入分子诊断,以提供分层诊断。这种分层诊断方法确保了这种分类方法可以应用于资源有限的国家,因为这些国家没有分子诊断方法。综合诊断允许结合分子信息和基于组织学的诊断,以提供特定的诊断。在分子诊断不可用的情况下,肿瘤被归类为未分类(NOS)。这些分层诊断为:

第 1 层:综合诊断(整合所有组织信息)
第 2 层:组织学诊断
第 3 层:WHO 分级(自然史)
第 4 层:分子信息
如**表** 7.3 所示。

临床表现

许多 HGG 患者表现为占位效应、水肿或出血引起的颅内压升高的体征和症状。这些症状通常表现为头痛、恶心、呕吐、视力下降、复视、嗜睡和精神错乱。其他表现包括局灶性神经功能障碍、与肿瘤位置相关的症状(如失语症、肢体无力、感觉改变)和神经认知缺陷(包括去抑制和人格改变)(Tucha et al., 2000)。大约 50% 的Ⅲ级和 25% 的Ⅳ级肿瘤表

表 7.2 基于三种分子标志物的胶质瘤分子亚分类

	三阳型	TERT 和 IDH	单 IDH	三阴型	单 TERT
分组改变	IDH-1、1p/19q 和 TERT 突变	TERT 和 IDH 突变	IDH 突变	-	TERT 突变
共同突变	CIC、FUBP1、NOTCH1、PIK3CA 或 PIK3R1	TP53 和 ATRX	TP53 和 ATRX	EGFR、PTEN 和 NF1	EGFR、EGFRv Ⅲ、PTEN、NF1、RB1、PIK3CA、PIK3R1
平均年龄	44 岁	46 岁	37 岁	50 岁	59 岁
TGCA 亚型	前神经元型	间质型、神经元型、前神经元型	前神经元型	经典型、间质型、神经元型和前神经元型	经典型和间质型
常见组织学	少突胶质细胞瘤	星形细胞瘤,WHO Ⅱ级或Ⅲ级	星形细胞瘤,WHO Ⅱ级或Ⅲ级	67% GBM	90% GBM 10% Ⅱ级或Ⅲ级

Source data from Eckel-Passow, J., Lachance, D., Molinaro, A., et al., Glioma groups based on 1p/19q, IDH, and TERT Promoter Mutations in Tumors, *N Engl J Med* 2015; 372: 2499–508. DOI:10.1056/NEJMoa1407279.

表 7.3 分层诊断示例(WHO 2016 年分类)

	胶质母细胞瘤	间变性星形细胞瘤	间变性少突胶质细胞瘤
第 1 层:综合诊断	胶质母细胞瘤 - IDH 野生型	间变性星形细胞瘤 -IDH 突变,1p/19q 非共缺失	间变性少突胶质细胞瘤 - IDH 突变,1p/19q 共缺失
第 2 层:组织学诊断	胶质母细胞瘤	间变性星形细胞瘤	间变性少突胶质细胞瘤
第 3 层:分级	Ⅳ级	Ⅲ级	Ⅲ级
第 4 层:分子信息	IDH 野生型 TERT 突变 MGMT 甲基化	IDH 突变,1p/19q 非共缺失	IDH 突变,1p/19q 共缺失
无分子信息诊断	胶质母细胞瘤,未分类	间变性星形细胞瘤,未分类	间变性少突胶质细胞瘤,未分类

现为癫痫发作，而 80% 的低级别胶质瘤表现为癫痫发作。

高级别胶质瘤的影像

最初的成像方式通常是增强计算机断层扫描（CT），然而，磁共振成像（MRI）更加敏感，现在是所有脑肿瘤患者的首选成像方式。

在 CT 和 MRI 上，HGG 通常表现为不规则、界限不清的肿块并伴有血管源性水肿。通常肿块边缘强化，中心区域为非强化。增强本身不能作为诊断特征，因为 30%~50% 间变性肿瘤在 CT 上没有增强（Chamberlain et al.，1988），16% 在 MRI 上没有增强（Al Okaili et al.，2007）。此外，20% 的低级别胶质瘤（特别是少突胶质细胞瘤）CT 上有强化（Chamberlain et al.，1988），35% 的低级别胶质瘤 MRI 上有强化（Al Okaili et al.，2007）。

肿瘤的位置主要在幕上。额叶是最常见的部位（24.9%），其后依次是颞叶（21.8%）、顶叶（16.7%）、枕叶（4.8%）、小脑（0.5%）、脑干（0.4%）或未分类 / 其他（30.9%）（Brodbelt et al.，2015）。

使用影像学制订治疗计划的主要问题之一是影像学解剖无法确定肿瘤边缘。尸检和活检研究均显示肿瘤实际边界超出 CT（Lilja et al.，1981；Selker et al.，1982；Burger et al.，1983；Kelly et al.，1987）、增强 T1 加权 MRI（Lunsford et al.，1986；Kelly et al.，1987；Price et al.，2006）和 T2 加权 MRI 上的边界（Lunsford et al.，1986；Kelly et al.，1987；Johnson et al.，1989；Watanabe et al.，1992；Price et al.，2006）。这些影像技术不能确定肿瘤的边缘或侵袭性。高级的影像学方法已被开发用于评估这些肿瘤。这些正在临床实践中使用，并在其他地方进行了总结（Price，2007）。

术后 MRI 是唯一客观评估切除范围的方法。研究表明，与外科医生的判断相比，它能识别更多的不完全切除病例（Albert et al.，1994）。72 小时内进行影像学检查可以避免术后发生改变的影响。

HGG 的高级 MRI 检查

一些高级的 MRI 方法现在在常规实践中评估肿瘤，提供肿瘤生理学和病理学信息，并在下文和其他地方进行总结（Price et al.，2007；**图 7.3**）。

弥散成像是一种对图像中质子的扩散非常敏感的成像方法。有质子运动受限的区域，如缺血细胞毒性水肿、表皮样囊肿或脓肿，弥散加权成像（diffusion- weighted imaging，DWI）显示明亮。由于 DWI 具有 T2 加权信号的分量，因此不能作为定量

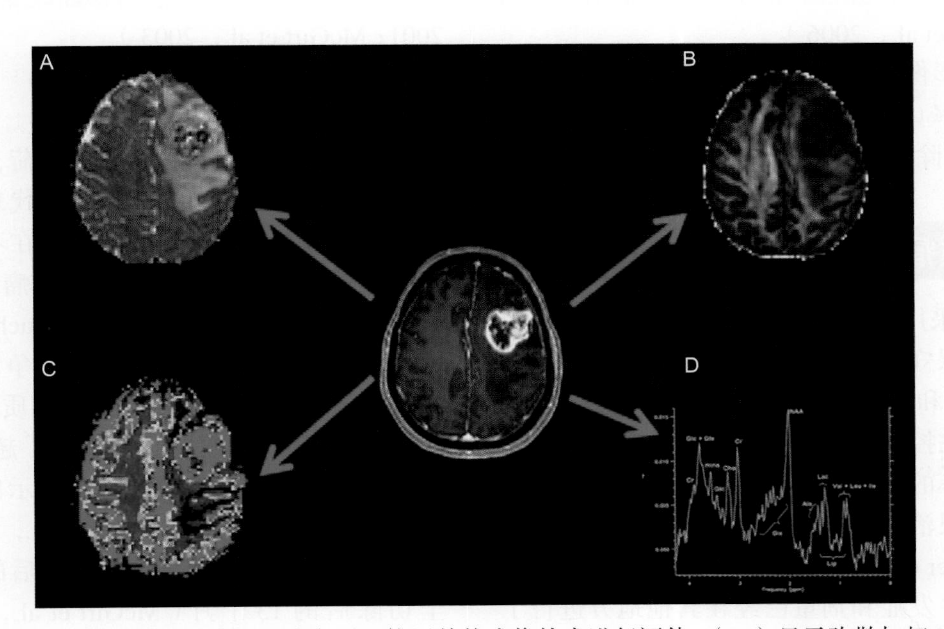

图 7.3 高级肿瘤影像。这种增强胶质母细胞瘤可以使用其他成像技术进行评估。（A）显示弥散加权 MRI 的表观弥散系数（ADC）图像。ADC 降低可能是由于肿瘤细胞增多。由于肿瘤细胞增多，肿瘤内 ADC 普遍减少。（B）显示来自 MRI 弥散张量成像（DTI）的分数各向异性（FA）图像，显示白质束的破坏，可用于引导白质束并观察它们与肿瘤的关系。（C）是灌注成像，显示相对脑血容量（rCBV），衡量血管分布和血管生成。（D）磁共振波谱可用于寻找高级别胶质瘤的代谢谱。在这个例子中显示的光谱是正常的大脑

测量。表观弥散系数（apparent diffusion coefficient，ADC）是一种定量的测量方法，它与质子扩散的距离有关。在自由弥散区域（如脑脊液间隙）ADC很大。当弥散受限时，ADC较低。在HGG中，由于水肿引起的水分增加，ADC比正常大脑大，但随着细胞数量的增加，ADC减少。因此，低级别胶质瘤的ADC低于高级别胶质瘤（Sugahara et al.，1999）。

弥散张量成像是DWI成像技术的延伸，它对水分子的定向扩散非常敏感。它被用来评估白质束的破坏和靠近肿瘤的白质束位置。

灌注MRI评估血流。分级较高的肿瘤往往具有较高的灌注，有证据表明，灌注可以在低分级胶质瘤中识别间变灶（Danchaivijitr et al.，2008）。

磁共振波谱可以识别出大量感兴趣的肿瘤代谢产物。高级别胶质瘤的光谱表现为N-乙酰天冬氨酸（白质完整性的标志）减少，总胆碱（膜转换的标志）增加，脂质和乳酸（坏死）信号增强。

HGG的正电子发射断层扫描成像

在正电子发射断层扫描（positron-emission tomography，PET）成像上，与正常皮质相比，高级别胶质瘤倾向于高代谢。在FDG PET中，肿瘤可能很难与功能性皮质区分开。此外，FDG摄取增加并非肿瘤特异性，可在炎症区域看到。使用[^{11}C]-蛋氨酸（MET PET）或[^{18}F]-乙基酪氨酸（FET PET）的氨基酸PET对肿瘤更有特异性，似乎能更好地描绘肿瘤的范围（Pirotte et al.，2006）。

使用PET影像引导活检的研究表明，它提高了活检的诊断效率（Levivier et al.，1995），并有助于确定需要手术切除的区域（Pirotte et al.，2009）。

高级别胶质瘤的治疗

HGG最好采用多学科团队方法进行管理。治疗的选择范围从保守治疗到手术和辅助治疗。治疗的主要目的是诊断和延长无进展生存期。

地塞米松在控制与肿瘤相关的脑水肿方面至关重要。对类固醇的反应可能非常快。类固醇治疗未能改善，提示根治性手术切除可能导致神经功能障碍恶化（Stummer et al.，2011a）。类固醇在神经肿瘤学中的作用、并发症和剂量已经在其他地方进行了综述（Ryan et al.，2012）。

保守治疗是一种有效的选择，对于预后差的患者，如年龄和不良的表现状态，特别是肿瘤被认为是不可切除的情形。在这种情况下，良好的姑息性和支持性护理是很重要的。

由于肿瘤的位置和治疗的效果，脑瘤患者的行为和性格变化非常常见。对心理社会功能的支持很重要，神经心理学家应该参与进来。HGG患者的重度抑郁比正常人群更常见，且影响生活质量。

HGG手术

手术的目的是获得肿瘤的代表性组织样本，用于组织学和分子标志物评估，安全地切除肿瘤，以改善压力症状，提高辅助治疗的疗效，延缓恶化，提高生存率，最后，还有通过手术进行治疗的潜力。

影像引导肿瘤活检

活检具有微创性，耐受性好，适用于任何部位或任何大小的病变，但通常只在切除的风险大于益处时才考虑。当最初的诊断可能影响后续治疗时，最好使用活检。然而，它也有不足，取样存在误差，特别是在小的或异质性的样本，以及出血并发症。影像引导现在通常用于降低非诊断性活检的风险。

HGG活检时，取样误差是一个问题，当比较一系列接受活检和切除的患者的诊断时，存在差异。在接受切除术的患者中，82%患有胶质母细胞瘤，18%患有间变性星形细胞瘤，而在接受活检的患者中，49%患有胶质母细胞瘤，51%患有间变性星形细胞瘤（Glantz et al.，1991）。在切除前进行活检的患者中，39%~49%的患者诊断改变（Jackson et al.，2001；McGirt et al.，2003）。

肿瘤切除

减瘤手术有利于减少肿瘤负荷，从而降低颅内压升高的不良反应，并提供更有代表性的组织学样本。胶质母细胞瘤手术的目的是在不损伤周围正常大脑的情况下尽可能多地切除肿瘤。据估计，50%的患者适合进行根治性切除（Schucht et al.，2012）。手术是否能提高生存率一直存在争议。Cochrane的文献综述强调了这一领域缺乏高质量的研究（Hart et al.，2000）。回顾性研究表明，超过98%的肿瘤切除术后MRI表现为全切除，显示出更好的生活质量和无进展生存期（Lacroix et al.，2001）。根据一项研究，中位生存期从次全切除后的8个月改善到全切除后的13个月（McGirt et al.，2009b）。一项涉及RPA分析的研究再次证实了这一点，该研究显示，年龄、表现状态、神经病学和精神状态的较严重基线疾病患者的生存获益最大（Pichlmeier et al.，2008）。当联合化疗和放疗时，强化影像上完全切除与延长生存期相关（Stummer et al.，2012）。三项主要随机对照研究的结果也证实了根治性切除的生存期改善（Stummer et al.，2011b）。

这些队列研究的困难在于存在肿瘤可切除性偏倚。具有良好预后特征的患者（即年轻、表现良好、非功能区肿瘤较小的患者）比表现较差、功能区肿瘤较大的老年患者更有可能进行全切除（Stummer et al.，2008）。此外，现在大多数外科医生都认为随机让患者进行部分切除是不道德的。

对这些肿瘤实施全切除的困难（即在术后早期成像上完全切除肿瘤的增强部分）（Vogelbaum et al.，2012）在于确定这些肿瘤的边界。由于肿瘤和正常大脑之间的边界较差，大多数研究表明，进行了全切除的患者少于30%（Wood et al.，1988；Vecht et al.，1990；Albert et al.，1994；Barker，1996；Kowalczuk et al.，1997）。为了提高切除率，人们开发了各种工具。

影像指导对于计划开颅手术至关重要，但不可预测的脑转移限制了其在识别肿瘤界限方面的应用。

术中超声检查是一种有用的方法，但取决于使用者经验。通过活组织检查评估肿瘤边界，切除前显示了95%的高特异性和敏感性，但在切除过程中降低（敏感性87%，特异性42%）（Rygh et al.，2008）。

术中磁共振成像提供了最精确的方法，但非常昂贵，而且确实增加了肿瘤切除的时间。队列研究表明，术中MRI最大化切除可提高生存率（Mehdorn et al.，2011）。

5-氨基酮戊酸（5-ALA）荧光引导提供了一种可用于所有神经外科中心并有助于识别肿瘤的方法（**图7.4**）。5-ALA是一种新的用于在蓝光（400 nm）下识别胶质瘤组织的外科辅助剂。5-ALA在正常的血红素生物合成途径中被吸收和转化。肿瘤中缺乏铁螯合酶，导致荧光团原卟啉Ⅸ在蓝光下发出荧光。使用5-ALA可以更完整地切除对比增强的肿瘤，从而改善恶性胶质瘤患者的无进展生存期。Stummer等人表明，与白光组相比，5-ALA组的完全切除率增加了29%。5-ALA组也比白光组有更高的6个月无进展生存率（41% *vs.* 21.1%）（Stummer et al.，2006）。

对于外科神经肿瘤学家来说，关键是尽量扩大切除范围，同时避免引起神经损害。很明显，运动和语言障碍不仅影响生活质量，而且与更差的生存率相关（McGirt et al.，2009a）。术中使用皮质和皮质下的功能绘图（De Witt Hamer et al.，2012）可以使术后神经功能缺损的发生率降低一半。

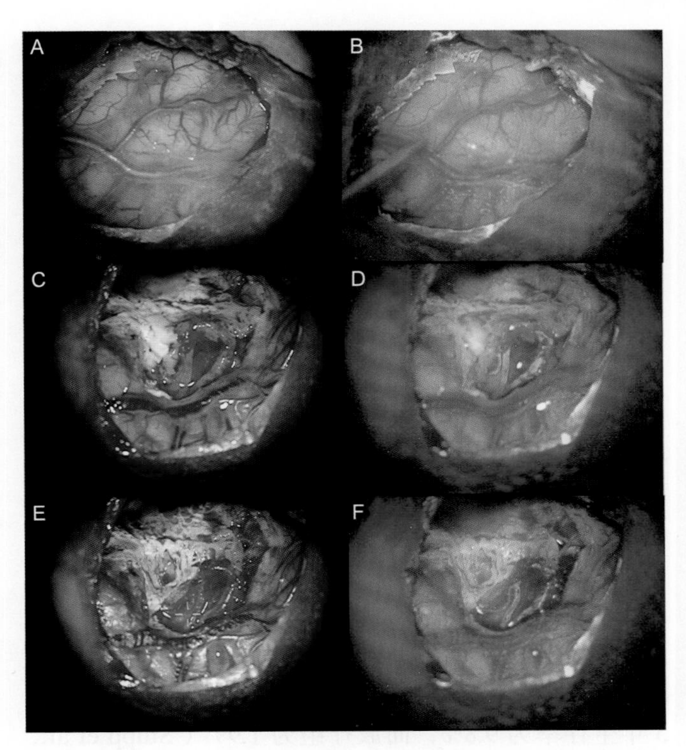

图7.4　切除术野和5-ALA。白光（A）和5-ALA荧光（B）下皮质前切开大脑皮质。可见肿瘤后部的荧光肿瘤。中间一排为白光（C）和5-ALA（D）下的术中视图。荧光区域在白光下表现正常。在切除结束时，可以完全切除荧光肿瘤（E，白光；F，5-ALA），为切除提供了一个合适的终点

HGG放疗

放射治疗已成为高级别胶质瘤辅助治疗的主要手段。20世纪70年代的多项研究显示了生存获益（Walker et al.，1978）。试图通过增加辐射剂量来改善初始的获益已经失败。不幸的是，脑放射治疗的治疗窗口很窄，随着放射剂量的增加，放射性坏死的发生率也在增加。部分原因是常规影像学无法识别浸润性肿瘤。因此，放疗计划将明显的肿瘤概括为肿瘤总体积（gross tumour volume，GTV）。然后应用2.5 cm的边缘形成临床靶体积（clinical target volume，CTV）。增加0.5 cm的边距，以考虑设置误差和患者移动，形成计划目标体积（planning target volume，PTV）。换言之，在包含正常大脑的肿瘤周围应用3cm的边缘。同时，为了降低放射性坏死的风险，放射剂量被限制。

HGG通常采用两种放疗方案。根治性放疗在30天内给予60 Gy剂量，而短程或姑息性放疗在2周内给予6次30 Gy剂量。姑息性放射治疗要求较少，因此患者可以很快开始治疗，并且耐受性良好。在患者病情严重恶化的情况下，它很有用。

HGG 化疗

在替莫唑胺出现之前，丙卡巴肼、洛莫司汀和长春新碱（PCV）是标准的辅助化疗方案。这种以亚硝基脲为基础的化疗提供了很小的生存获益；2 年生存率增加了 5%（Stewart，2002）。治疗包括 10 天的口服丙卡巴肼，单次口服 CCNU（洛莫司汀），单次静脉滴注长春新碱，每 6 周一次。

替莫唑胺的使用提高了患者的生存率。每 28 天一个周期口服 5 天。白细胞减少和血小板减少通常是这种治疗的副作用。根治性放疗加每日联合替莫唑胺治疗，再加上 6 个疗程的替莫唑胺辅助治疗，可显著改变 GBM 的预后。Stupp 等人在一项多中心试验中显示，中位随访期为 28 个月，放疗加替莫唑胺组的中位生存期为 14.6 个月，而单纯放疗组为 12.1 个月。2 年生存率分别为 26.5% 和 10.4%（Stupp et al.，2005），而对同一人群的 5 年回顾显示，替莫唑胺组 5 年生存率为 9.8%，而放疗组为 1.9%（Stupp et al.，2009）。这比以往高级别胶质瘤的生存率统计有了显著的进步。MGMT 状态被认为是一个有利结果的最重要的预测因素。

目前公认，放化疗后立即出现的 MRI 表现可以显示疾病的明显进展，Stupp 等（2009）报告的研究中，22% 的患者由于假定的肿瘤进展而没有接受辅助化疗，随后的成像显示这种情况稳定或改善。这种假性进展在甲基化 MGMT 患者中更常见，被认为是治疗反应的良好预后标志。

局部化疗

另一种辅助手术是用含有卡莫司汀（BCNU）的晶片进行局部治疗。这些晶片可以绕过血脑屏障局部输送高浓度化疗药物。一项针对进展期患者的安慰剂对照研究显示，与安慰剂相比，进展期患者的中位生存期（31 周 vs. 23 周）和 6 个月生存率（6 个月时 44% 死亡 *vs.* 64%）均有显著改善（Brem et al.，1995）。一项对新诊断 HGG 的进一步研究也显示了生存优势。

然而，这些药物的使用仍然存在争议，人们对其疗效和不良反应提出了质疑，包括高达 28% 的中枢神经系统和伤口感染率（Engelhard，2000；McGovern et al.，2003）。然而，有大量证据表明 BCNU 晶片可用于辅助治疗。一项关于 BCNU 晶片植入联合替莫唑胺和放疗，治疗新诊断 GBM 的回顾性研究显示，中位生存期为 20.7 个月，2 年生存率为 36%（McGirt et al.，2009b）。显然，需要更广泛的切除（>90%）才能获益（Stummer et al.，2012）。

靶向分子治疗

靶向分子治疗是一种令人兴奋的新的治疗选择，目前正处于不同的研究和发展阶段。这些药物通过与受体相互作用或影响下游靶点来靶向神经胶质瘤的致瘤途径。目前为止，阻断 EGFR、血小板源性生长因子受体、磷脂酰肌醇 3- 激酶（PI3K）以及相关通路和 SRC 相关通路的药物临床试验都令人失望。Wick 等（2011）总结说，很明显，单药治疗效果甚微，目前正在进行联合治疗的试验。这种不良反应的原因被认为是神经胶质瘤的发展过程中激活了多个受体酪氨酸激酶，所以阻断一个受体对整个通路的影响很小（Stommel et al.，2007）。靶向治疗的组合可能是前进的方向

抗血管生成治疗

一种靶向治疗阻断了血管内皮生长因子参与肿瘤血管生成的途径。一项关于贝伐珠单抗治疗肿瘤复发的小型非随机Ⅱ期研究显示，有较高的缓解率（6 个月时 PFS 为 46%；6 个月时 OS 为 77%）（Vredenburgh et al.，2007）。这项试验为 FDA 的批准铺平了道路。但这项研究的非随机性和非标准终点使得欧洲药品管理局（EMEA）拒绝在欧洲使用它。使用抗血管生成药物研究的一个问题是，由于血脑屏障的关闭，增强效果明显降低。这种所谓的假反应并不能预测对这些药物的反应，随后的进展可能在没有明显增强的情况下发生（Norden et al.，2008）。

两项大型Ⅲ期研究——欧洲 AVAGlio 研究（Chinot et al.，2014）和北美 RTOG 0825 研究（Gilbert et al.，2014）均未显示在标准治疗中加入贝伐珠单抗有任何生存优势。RTOG 0825 发现患者在接受贝伐珠单抗治疗后病情恶化，而 AVAGlio 研究显示患者在肿瘤进展前生活质量稳定（Taphoorn et al.，2015）。

免疫疗法

大脑通常被认为是免疫特权器官，由于其缺乏淋巴管，血脑屏障阻断细胞因子和细胞进入大脑的通道，主要组织相容性复合体（major histocompatibility complex，MHC）低基线的表达和高水平的蛋白质免疫调节细胞减少基线功能。近年来这些假设被人反驳。然而，脑肿瘤通过极低表达 MHC 蛋白、降低单核细胞吞噬功能和抗原呈递、降低 T 细胞激活和表

达促进免疫细胞凋亡的标志物进一步逃避和抑制免疫应答。克服这些机制将允许特异性识别和破坏肿瘤细胞，而不会损伤正常的大脑。免疫疗法似乎是对付分布在正常大脑中的侵入性细胞的理想疗法。免疫疗法是一种令人兴奋的方法，它可以靶向单个肿瘤细胞而不损伤正常组织，并且与细胞是否处于周期无关（细胞毒性疗法的问题也是如此）。

有三种方法可以克服肿瘤诱导的免疫抑制。

细胞因子疗法：这是基于这些强大的免疫调节因子激活免疫系统。困难在于通过血脑屏障的传递，人们尝试通过注射和输注细胞因子或基因疗法来促进细胞因子的表达。某些早期研究已经表明，这是安全的，具有不同的疗效，这些方法可能对其他疗法提供一个有用的辅助。

被动免疫疗法。包括血清疗法，其中单克隆抗体指向肿瘤特异性抗原，传递毒素或放射性物质，选择性地杀死细胞。神经胶质瘤中发现的肌糖蛋白或突变的EGFRvⅢ等靶点已被使用，但早期研究结果令人失望。过继免疫疗法的主要目的是通过使用IL-2刺激收获的淋巴细胞产生淋巴因子激活的杀伤细胞来增强肿瘤反应。早期的研究结果显示，这种方法有少量的益处，但由于IL-2的毒性诱导脑水肿而受到限制。

主动免疫疗法：这些方法包括通过接种抗肿瘤特异性抗原的疫苗来启动免疫应答。这种方法的困难在于大脑内抗原呈递能力较差。最近人们的兴趣集中在树突状细胞上，树突状细胞在受到抗原刺激时，可以激活T淋巴细胞增殖并破坏这些细胞。方法包括从血液或骨髓中提取自体树突状细胞，用抗原刺激它们，然后通过皮下注射将它们输送回患者体内。所使用的抗原要么是肿瘤内常见的抗原，要么是患者肿瘤的个体化抗原。早期研究显示出了希望和很小的毒性，因此允许其中一些方法进入Ⅲ期研究（Hdeib and Sloan，2015）。

饮食疗法

饮食在控制神经系统疾病中的作用已经得到很好的证实。生酮饮食用于控制医学上难治性癫痫已有多年。由于神经胶质瘤优先代谢葡萄糖，而酮体代谢不好，因此使用高脂肪、低碳水化合物饮食导致酮症状态。临床前研究表明，在包括胶质瘤在内的癌细胞系中，阻断这些糖酵解途径具有抗肿瘤、促凋亡和抗血管生成的作用。很明显，生酮饮食对大多数患者来说是不能容忍的，因此建议采用改良的Atkin饮食法。迄今为止，各种质量的研究都未能显示出明确的疗效。

肿瘤电场治疗

肿瘤电场治疗是一种新的治疗脑肿瘤的方法。临床前研究表明，使用低强度和中频电场可以在不引起加热或去极化神经元的情况下破坏有丝分裂。最近一项Ⅲ期研究报告显示，在辅助化疗阶段使用该方法具有显著的生存优势（Stupp et al.，2015）。现在有一项提议认为这应该被视为一种标准的治疗（Mehta et al.，2017），但其成本目前可能禁止常规使用。

老年HGG治疗

随着人口老龄化的加剧，老年人的神经胶质瘤越来越成为一个常见的问题。老年人往往具有更强的表现型，通常由于虚弱和其他共病，对治疗的反应较差。他们往往被排除在临床试验之外。因此，60岁以上的患者不太可能接受最彻底的治疗（Brodbelt et al.，2015）。

根治性手术治疗这些肿瘤似乎是一种有效的治疗方法，可以改善预后（Ewelt et al.，2011）。两项大型研究表明，在MGMT甲基化胶质母细胞瘤的老年患者中，单独使用替莫唑胺比放疗有更好的生存率（Malmström et al.，2012；Wick et al.，2012）。

进展期肿瘤的治疗

尽管采取了最好的治疗方法，但几乎所有HGG患者的肿瘤都会在某一时刻复发。根据患者的临床情况，可以考虑挽救性治疗。

手术：再手术比原手术的发病率和死亡率更高。然而，对于长期无进展生存期且肿瘤可最大限度切除的患者，这是一种选择。在这个阶段插入卡莫司汀晶片已被证明可以提高生存期（Brem et al.，1995）。

放疗：有些人认为重复照射的毒性被高估了。重复照射是一个越来越多的选择，精确分割放射治疗是最理想的技术。也有人建议，为了对复发性肿瘤进行精确的局部放疗，可以考虑进行放射外科治疗。到继发进展的平均时间是几个月。

细胞毒性化疗：传统的化疗方案也能延长继发进展的时间，但疗效有限，且骨髓抑制等与治疗相关的毒性发生率很高（Niyazi et al.，2011）。最近的Ⅲ期试验未能显示替莫唑胺比PCV疗法有生存期优势（Brada et al.，2010）。最近的数据表明，MGMT

甲基化是否是高剂量替莫唑胺预后分子标志物受到挑战（Weller et al.，2015）。

目前几乎没有数据支持靶向治疗的常规使用。因此，这些只是临床试验的一部分。

预后

尽管在治疗上取得了许多进步，但诊断为 HGG 仍然有一个令人沮丧的预后。无任何治疗的中位生存期少于 6 个月，治疗后增加到 18 个月。较差的生存率与年龄增加、较差的初始神经病学、较差的一般状况有关，这一点由 Karnofsky 表现评分（KPS）和 MGMT 甲基化缺失得到证实。接受手术和放化疗的患者显示出更好的长期疗效。为什么某些患者比其他患者活得更长还不清楚。死亡通常是由于脑水肿和颅内压升高。

延伸阅读、参考文献、EBRAIN 的相关链接

扫描书末二维码获取。

第 8 章　颅内转移瘤

Andrew Brodbelt・Rasheed Zakaria 著
文龙 译，伊志强 审校

引言

颅内转移患者的治疗原则详见**专栏 8.1**。

流行病学

颅内转移瘤是最常见的颅内肿瘤。基于西方人群的研究表明，颅内转移瘤年龄调整后的年发病率为 7~14 人/10 万人（Fox et al.，2011），而胶质母细胞瘤为 4.6 人/10 万人，脑膜瘤为 7.6 人/10 万人（Ostrom et al.，2014；Brodbelt et al.，2015）。尸检研究表明，高达 24%的实体肿瘤患者可能会有脑转移，尽管只有 6%的患者会在其病程中出现颅内转移的症状（Posner and Chernik，1978）。脑转移瘤发病率的增加，部分原因是由于更好的系统性肿瘤治疗和更灵敏的检测方法提高了生存率（Fox et al.，2011）。年龄和性别对脑转移发病率的影响取决于原发肿瘤。罹患肺癌和乳腺癌的女性患者比男性患者更容易发生脑转移，而黑色素瘤、肾癌和结直肠癌则恰恰相反（Davis et al.，2012）。虽然年轻乳腺癌和肺癌患者（<40 岁）的脑转移发生率大约是 70 岁以上患者的两倍，但老年患者癌症患病率的增加意味着老年患者总体上仍可见更多的脑转移。因此，对于任何伴发可疑症状的患者，临床医生不应认为其“太年轻”就不会发生脑转移。

专栏 8.1　颅内转移瘤患者的治疗原则

- 治疗是非治愈性的，其目的在于改善生活质量。
- 患者的表现评分对预后至关重要。
- 年龄越大，预后越差。
- 最基本的分期包括颅脑 MRI 及胸部、腹盆腔的 CT 或 PET-CT。
- 不仅要评估颅脑转移情况，也要评估患者整体状态和肿瘤负荷。
- 对于有肿瘤病史的患者，新的颅内病变可能是不同肿瘤或者脓肿。

约有 1/3 的患者出现单发病灶，1/3 为寡转移灶（2~3 个病灶），1/3 为多发转移灶（>4 个病灶；Norden et al.，2005）。转移发生率因肿瘤类型而异，高达 20%的肺癌患者可发生脑转移，而甲状腺癌、前列腺癌、胃癌和卵巢癌患者的转移率则不到 1%（National Cancer Institute，2015）。30%~60% 的脑转移患有肺癌（Fox et al.，2011），其中非小细胞癌最为常见（Delattre et al.，1988）。其他常见的原发肿瘤包括乳腺癌、黑色素瘤、肾癌和结直肠癌（Delattre et al.，1988）。从原发病确诊到出现脑转移的中位时间约为 12 个月，但从 3 个月（非小细胞癌）至 46 个月（卵巢癌）不等（Nussbaum et al.，1996；Kolomainen et al.，2002）。某些遗传亚型也可以促进脑转移，例如在乳腺癌中，三阴型（雌激素受体、孕激素受体、HER2 受体均阴性）和 HER2 受体阳性的亚型，都与脑转移的高风险有关（Pestalozzi et al.，2006）。

肿瘤患者出现颅内占位并不一定是脑转移。一项小样本量的研究结果显示，在 21 例有恶性肿瘤病史的患者中，有 4 名患者被误诊为脑转移瘤并接受了全脑放疗，而实际上，他们罹患的是原发性恶性脑肿瘤（Maluf et al.，2002）。当出现以下情况时应考虑可能患第二种恶性肿瘤，而非转移瘤：缺乏活动性全身病变（尤其是肺癌），无病间隔时间较长，很少转移至脑部的原发性肿瘤类型（例如前列腺癌），以及颅脑放疗暴露史。1/3 罹患新发脑转移瘤的患者没有肿瘤病史。在这些病例中，原发肿瘤通常在 2 个月内被发现（同期症状），而 5%~10% 则无法发现。原发灶不明的肿瘤患者预后很差，并且可能无法从传统的化疗和放疗策略中获益（Norden et al.，2005；NICE，2010）。

病理学

与原发性脑肿瘤不同的是，脑转移瘤来自肿瘤细胞的血行播散，因此多发于脑灌注相对较高的区域。80% 的转移灶位于大脑半球，15% 位于小脑，5% 位于脑干（Delattre et al.，1998）。在大脑半球中，转移细胞优先黏附在灰白质交界处狭窄的血管分支点（Louis et al.，2007）。脑转移瘤周围毛细血管具有异常的微结构和缝隙连接，外加局部细胞因子的释放，使其可被大分子物质和水渗透，进而发生渗透作用。这种严重的血管源性水肿中包含少量肿瘤细胞，可使用类固醇或转移灶切除术减轻水肿。

转移级联反应描述了癌细胞从原发部位到脑部的运动，是一个复杂而低效的过程（**图 8.1**）。每一阶段都是潜在的药物或其他治疗的靶点。例如，在常规对比增强磁共振成像（MRI）之前，用附着在细胞黏附分子 VCAM-1 上的标记铁颗粒检测早期转移，可为未来的治疗提供机会（Serres et al.，2012）。

转移灶的外观可能是实心或橡胶状的，伴有中心区域的坏死。通常是黄色或者棕褐色，但黑色素

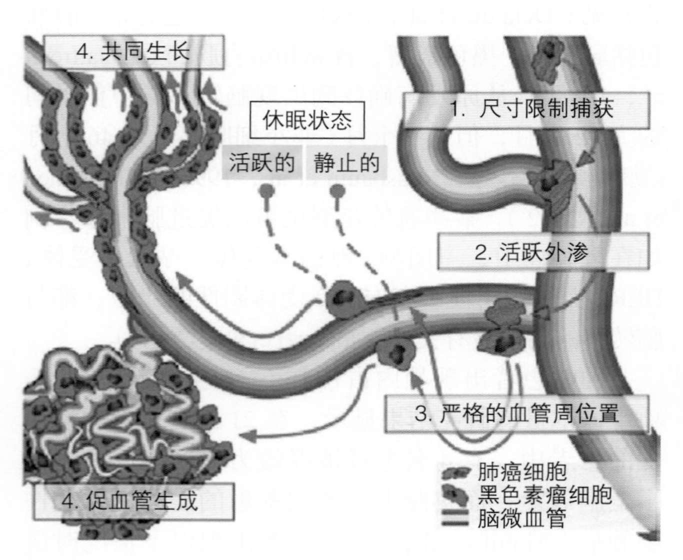

图 8.1 转移级联：由 TGF-β、IGF 和 EGF 等生长因子驱动的实体器官肿瘤细胞从静态的“上皮型”转变为更具流动性的“间质型”细胞表型，脱离其邻近结构，并侵入局部细胞外基质（这需要钙黏着蛋白破坏和蛋白水解酶，例如基质金属蛋白酶）。侵袭性伪足、富含肌动蛋白的胞膜突出物（引导细胞通过其微环境）的形成以及组织纤溶酶原激活剂的释放，促进了血管内浸润（进入血流）。1. 一旦进入循环系统，这些细胞必须在强大的剪应力和免疫攻击中生存下来，这涉及增强的细胞骨架。细胞在血管分叉和狭窄处附着于内皮。2. 透过血脑屏障需要整合素和细胞黏附分子介导。3. 转移的肿瘤细胞黏附于在血管周围。4. 脑部侵袭是肿瘤特异性的，黑素瘤细胞沿血管生长（共同生长），而肺癌细胞产生新血管（新生血管生成）。

瘤转移灶通常因富含黑色素而呈现黑色。出血最常出现在肾癌、黑色素瘤、绒毛膜癌、甲状腺癌和肝细胞癌的转移瘤中。转移瘤常常边界清晰，压迫邻近的胶质组织，形成假包膜（**图 8.2**）。

尽管有明显的宏观平面，但越来越多的证据表明脑转移瘤存在局部侵袭，这对治疗和预后都有影响（**图 8.2**）。浸润越强，预后越差（Siam et al.，2015）。肿瘤与脑组织交界处的弥散 MRI 征象改变可预测局部复发，也可用于辅助治疗策略，包括扩大切缘或立体定向放疗（stereotactic radiosurgery，SRS）（Zakaria et al.，2014）。

症状和体征

脑转移瘤患者的症状和体征包括颅内压增高、脑脊液循环受阻、神经肿瘤占位效应，以及在未经治疗的情况下，会出现疾病进展和死亡。皮质刺激可导致 15%~20% 的患者出现局灶性或全身性癫痫发作，但在黑色素瘤患者中比例更高（50%）（Taillibert and Delattre，2005）。单发或寡转移表现为头痛（80%）、局灶性神经功能障碍（30%~40%）和视觉障碍（6%），而多发转移可表现为脑病或急性意识障碍（Gaspar et al.，1997）。尽管有一项研究发现 40% 的肺癌脑转移患者无症状，但明确的癌症患者出现任何上述特征均应考虑颅内转移（Ohana et al.，2014）。

检查

第一步是记录病史并进行临床检查，应包括询问肿瘤指标（体重减轻、大便习惯改变、吸烟）、既往肿瘤病史和其他医疗问题，进行乳房或直肠查体，应计算并记录评分值。使用 WHO 及 EORTC 体力状态评分和 Karnofsky 功能状态评分标准，但结果的主要决定因素与患者在日常活动方面是否需要帮助有关。WHO 和 EORTC 体力状态评分 2 分或 2 分以上，或 Karnofsky 评分低于 70 分，说明患者日常生活需要帮助。

初次的放射学检查包括头部的 CT 扫描，这通常足以提示诊断。MRI 对诊断和治疗计划至关重要（**图 8.3**）。MRI 可比 CT 检测到更小的肿瘤，但确切的大小取决于扫描层厚。双倍和三倍的造影剂剂量可提高检出率，但增加肾毒性风险和假阳性。

影像学检查应该有助于解答这些问题，包括是否为脑转移；是否可以排除感染、高级别胶质瘤、

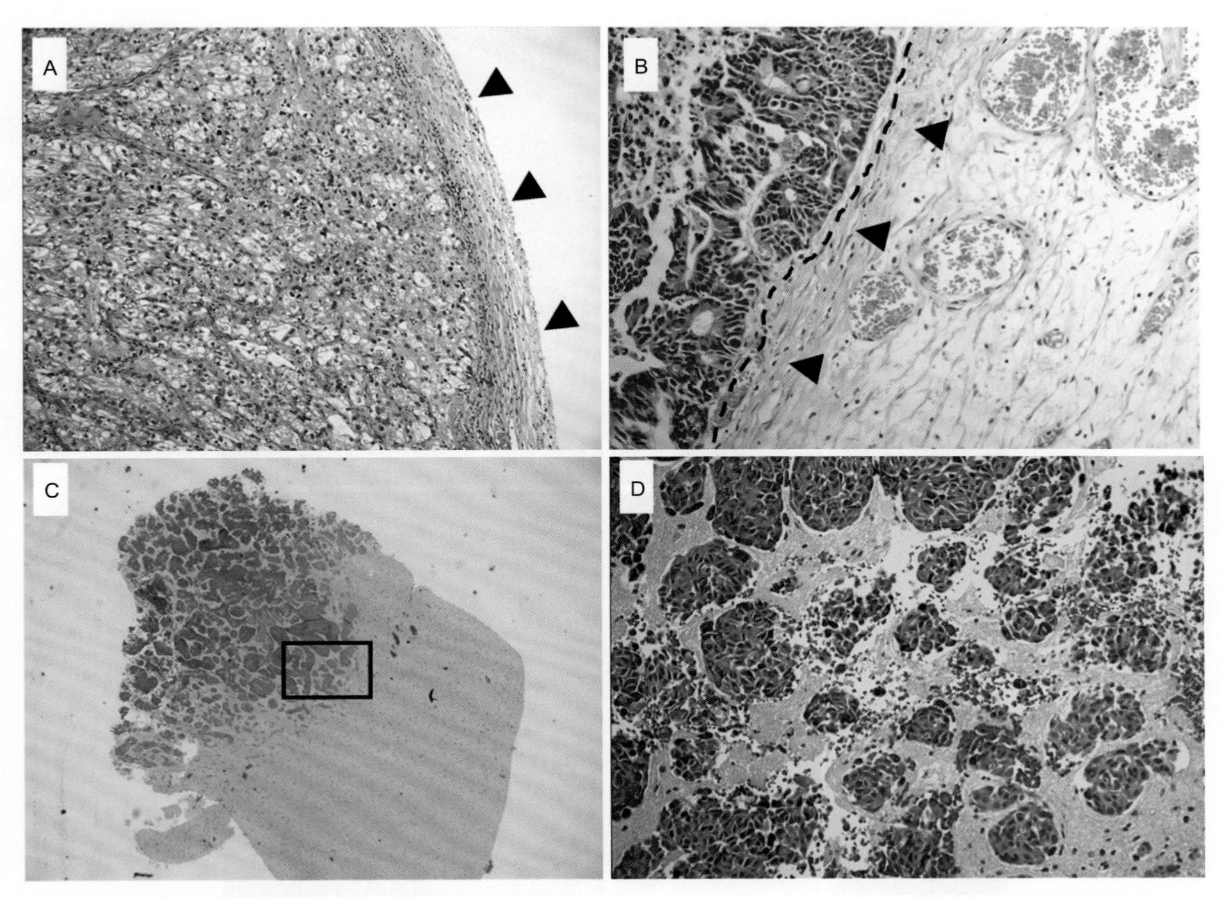

图 8.2 （A）和（B）脑转移灶与周围脑组织有清晰的分界平面。肾（A，×100）和肺腺癌（B，×200）转移灶显示了挤压白质的假包膜（箭头），在脑组织与肿瘤之间有清晰的边界（虚线）。（C）和（D）在多达 1/3 的转移灶中发现了弥漫性浸润边缘（Neves et al.，2001；Berghoff et al.，2013）。C（×50），D（×200）黑色素瘤转移灶内显示了周围脑实质中的微观瘤巢

淋巴瘤以及包括多发性硬化或弓形虫病在内的其他病变；转移灶的数量、大小和体积是多少；原发部位在哪；颅外病变累及范围多大；手术安全性如何。

多模式 MRI 有助于鉴别转移灶和影像学上的其他异常病变。与浸润性胶质瘤相比，转移瘤可能表现出更低的瘤周灌注和更高的弥散性，而磁共振波谱特征有助于鉴别脑膜瘤或淋巴瘤。在临床实践中，最好的特征仍然是存在周围血管源性水肿，以及在标准 T1、T2 和钆增强 T1 加权 MRI 序列上出现的病灶。弥散加权成像（diffusion-weighted imaging，DWI）和表观弥散系数（apparent diffusion coefficient，ADC）的 MRI 可以被快速获取，并显示由于液体运动受限而形成的脓肿，但在黏液转移灶中弥散受限也可以发生（**图 8.4**；见 Ebisu et al.，1996）。[18F]FDG-PETCT 是检测已确诊或疑诊实性肿瘤患者颅内转移的敏感方式，可能鉴别脑转移瘤和淋巴瘤，但不能除外高级别胶质瘤，因其空间分辨率差，所以需要临床评价和 MRI 来完成评估。

治疗后的生活质量影响生存率，诸如功能磁共振成像和纤维束造影等先进技术越来越多地应用于转移瘤手术（**图 8.5**）。

肿瘤分期决定治疗方案，全血细胞计数、肌酐、电解质、凝血功能和肝功能化验都有助于评估全身性肿瘤。特定的肿瘤分期需要全身PET-CT扫描或胸、腹、盆腔增强 CT 扫描。同步发现或未知原发灶的患者，可以考虑监测肿瘤标志物，包括用于生殖细胞肿瘤的人绒毛膜促性腺激素（ß-HCG），用于肝细胞癌的 α 胎蛋白（αFP），用于胃肠道、肺癌和乳腺癌的癌胚抗原，以及用于卵巢肿瘤的 CA125。进一步的影像学评估包括骨扫描、乳腺钼靶、超声检查和 MRI 检查。在 2~7 天内快速、恰当的分期有助于有效决策的制订，避免临床相关的肿瘤进展（这可能会减少治疗选择）。

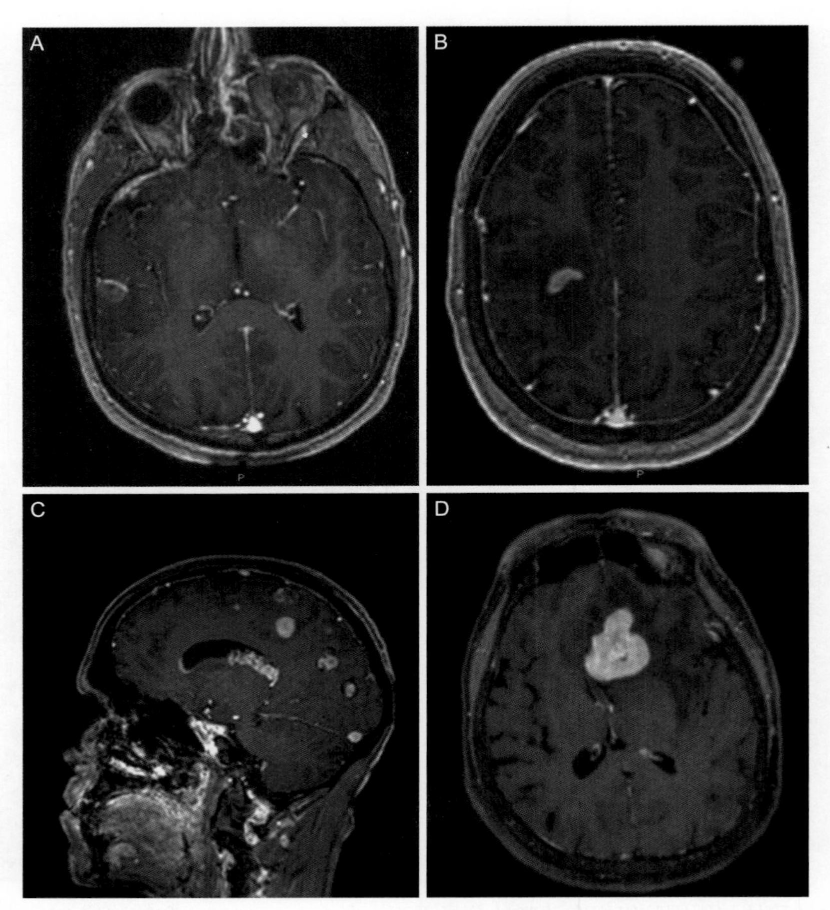

图 8.3 T1 MRI 增强像上强化肿块的鉴别诊断。（A）现年 55 岁，分期检查阴性，无原发肿瘤史，切除后提示高级别神经胶质瘤。（B）22 岁，左侧麻木、无力的短期病史，全身 CT 正常，腰穿提示炎性征象，诊断为多发性硬化斑块。（C）42 岁，黑色素瘤病史的 HIV 阳性男性，活检病理证实为弓形虫病。（D）70 岁，吸烟史，表现为意识障碍和胸部 CT 上的肺门肿块，胸外科医生无法取病理。活检提示淋巴瘤

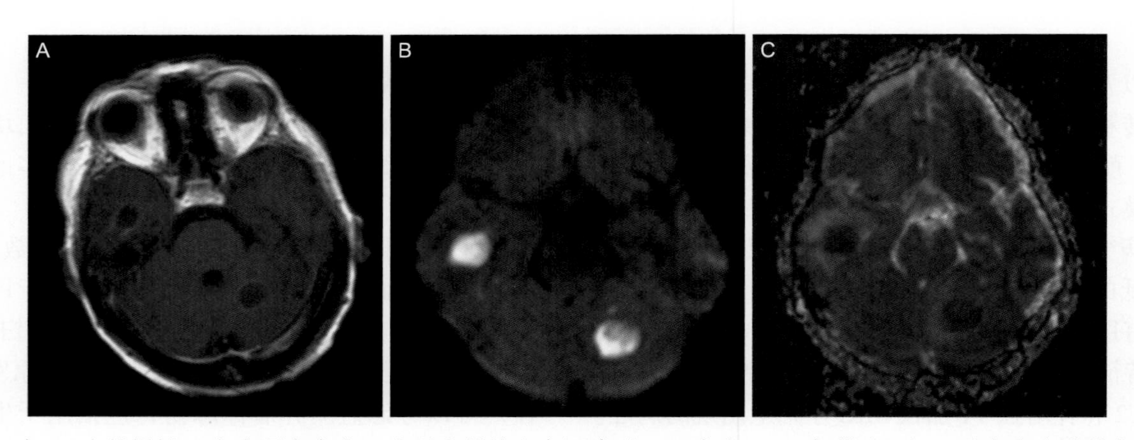

图 8.4 一名 53 岁的男性，有头颈癌病史，表现为低热和意识障碍。T1 加权 MRI 扫描（A）显示有多个增强病变。弥散加权 MRI（B）和表观弥散系数图（C）显示扩散受限。抽吸显示脓液（链球菌），调查发现心内膜炎。经过长期静脉使用抗生素治疗后，病情完全缓解

治疗

口服或静脉注射皮质类固醇治疗（地塞米松）可以显著减轻由肿瘤血管源性水肿引起的症状。地塞米松的起始剂量为每天 16 mg，分 2 次或 4 次服用，但应根据耐受性尽快逐渐减少。地塞米松的副作用包括但不限于消化性溃疡、失眠、肌病、体重增加、精神障碍、皮肤菲薄、库欣综合征、肾上腺抑制和

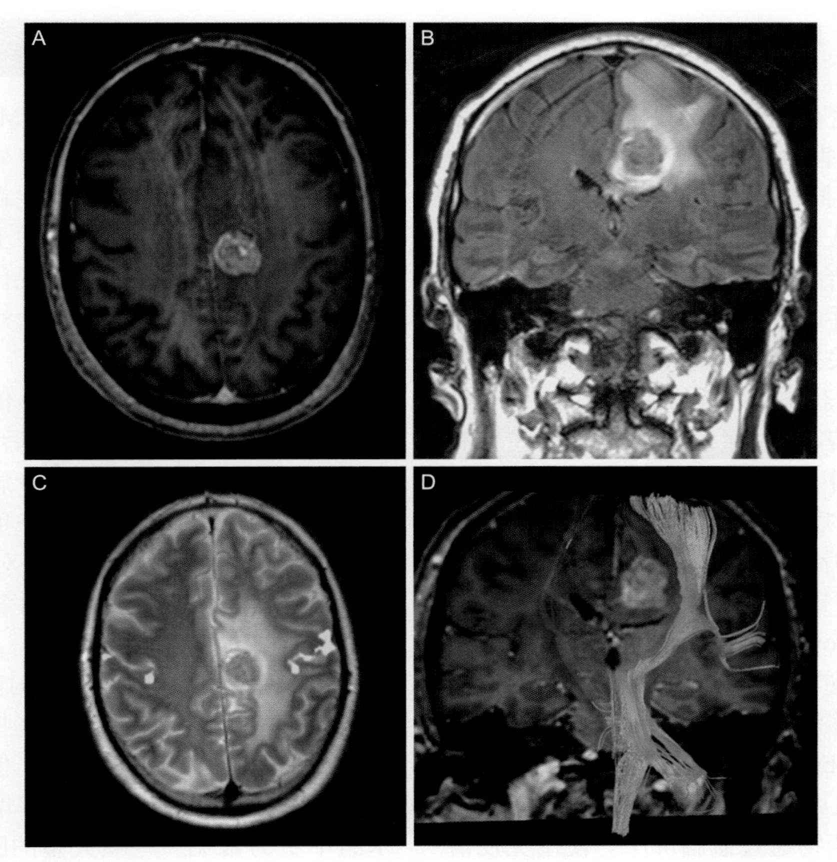

图 8.5 一名 58 岁男性，出现右侧偏瘫，应用类固醇后改善，并怀疑有脑转移。（A）对比后 T1 加权 MRI 显示强化肿块。（B）矢状位 FLAIR 确认肿块位于扣带回，伴水肿。该患者是重度吸烟者，CT 发现了一个小的肺门肿块。肺门活检和支气管灌洗未成功。（C）使用手指敲打试验的功能性 MRI 定位了初级运动皮质。（D）带有弥散张量成像（DTI）的种子束摄影图显示皮质脊髓束侧方移位。经半球间切除病灶，病理提示腺癌，无新发神经系统并发症，在治疗后生存了近一年，直至死于原发肿瘤

感染风险增加，应常规、同步应用质子泵抑制剂保护胃黏膜，应尽可能短时间、低剂量使用地塞米松。

个性化治疗选择可分为局部治疗（手术、SRS、激光治疗、聚焦超声治疗）和全脑或全身治疗（全脑放疗（whole- brain radiotherapy，WBRT）、化疗、靶向或免疫治疗。最终的治疗目标是通过单独或联合的治疗方案，加强局部控制，延长生命，预防进一步的神经系统并发症。

手术治疗颅内转移瘤可提供诊断组织标本、减轻肿瘤占位效应，孤立性或寡转移性疾病可考虑手术。随机对照试验的 meta 分析表明，与单纯 WBRT 相比，手术可改善生存率和功能状态（Hart et al.，2005）。但是，即便应用了包括术中唤醒、综合多模态 MRI 和影像导航（**图 8.4**）的现代显微神经外科技术，手术治疗仍存在危及生命、感染和神经功能障碍的风险。最初用于其他系统肿瘤切除的外科技术，包括整块切除和扩大切缘，现在已用于脑转移瘤切除术，以降低局部复发率和软脑膜扩散（Yoo et al.，2009；Patel et al.，2010）。如果需要病理诊断标本，并且 SRS 不可行，手术仍然是有占位效应的大肿瘤、囊性肿瘤或放疗抵抗性肿瘤的首选方式。

立体定向放疗是一种将大功率能量集中在单一或者少量目标的电离辐射治疗方法。其优点是可以为日间病例使用，可以使用热塑性面罩而不是框架，可以避免外科手术，可以针对深部或语言皮质的多个病变，效果可以与手术相媲美。其缺点在于并非适用于所有肿瘤，病变大小需≤4 cm 或 20 ml，邻近视神经或者脑干的肿瘤有发生局部放射性坏死的风险，而囊性和放疗抵抗的肿瘤（通常是肾和黑色素瘤）反应欠佳。治疗后肿瘤会肿胀，导致类固醇治疗延长，并伴有副作用，这使 SRS 不适用于某些颅后窝转移。SRS 无法取得标本进行病理诊断。在可用的不同平台（伽马刀、射波刀和直线加速器）之间没有确切的功效或安全性差异。放疗坏死率随肿瘤体

积的增大而增加，对于大于 20 ml 的病变，可采用大分割放疗。

WBRT 改善了生存率和颅内肿瘤的控制，但目前的担忧涉及认知损害。90%的脑转移患者在诊断时已有神经认知功能受损，多达 2/3 的患者会在 WBRT 后的 2~6 个月出现认知功能的进一步下降（Pinkham et al.，2015）。局部治疗后不做全脑放疗会延缓认知功能下降的时间，并改善言语记忆，但有不同观点认为肿瘤进展和相关挽救治疗带来的损害会超过免除放疗副反应带来的获益。最近的证据表明，WBRT 并不能改善所有患者的生存，特别是在那些患有 NSCLC 的老年患者中，表现评分差，简单的类固醇治疗和良好的姑息治疗可能更合适（Mulvenna et al.，2016）。新的分级放疗策略可通过保护海马，针对瘤床以减少全脑区域，或使用神经保护剂（如美金刚）来减少认知损害（Brown et al.，2013）。

最近的发展挑战了以下观点，即全身药物治疗不能有效治疗脑转移瘤。正在研究的领域包括确定跨血脑屏障（blood– brain barrier，BBB）的药物之间的抗转移作用，开发可全身作用的预防脑转移药物，以及促进传统化疗药物通过血脑屏障。使用免疫治疗剂伊匹单抗（ipilimumab）进行黑色素瘤预处理可改善手术效果（Jones et al.，2015），一半的患者伴有 B-Raf 原癌基因（BRAF）突变，抑制该通路可以延长未经治疗的脑转移患者的总体生存期（>7 个月）（Goyal et al.，2015）。一项针对酪氨酸激酶抑制剂的英国新近研究（CAMBT1）正在测试，对准备接受肺或乳腺癌转移灶切除的患者进行术前低剂量、针对转移灶的靶向放疗是否能够提高药物的通过率。

新的治疗方法包括间质激光热疗法，该疗法通过几乎实时的 MR 热像仪控制激光穿过颅孔以加热肿瘤（Hawasli et al.，2013）。MR 引导聚焦超声（MRgFUS）使用受 MR 热像仪控制的超声瞄准深部病变。最初用于纤维瘤，MRgFUS 已开始用于颅内病变（Coluccia et al.，2014）。据报道，术中植入腔内的卡莫司汀晶片（Gliadel）可减少局部复发（Abel et al.，2013），但很少使用。

由于脑转移不太可能被治愈，因此，无论制订何种治疗计划，患者及家属都需要持续的支持和对症治疗。具体问题包括认知能力下降、活动障碍、血栓栓塞、疼痛、自理能力下降、焦虑、抑郁和癫痫（Taillibert and Delattre，2005）。姑息治疗团队的早期参与对于最大限度提高患者的生活质量至关重要。

治疗选择

成立定期的多学科团队（MDT 或肿瘤委员会），以便完善患者计划内治疗的有效评估。由经验丰富的神经放射医生回顾阅片，并在肿瘤科医生、神经外科医生、病理医生、专科护士和姑息治疗团队之间进行充分讨论，确保遵循现代治疗方法，并提高临床试验的招募率。最终的治疗选择仍然是主诊医生和患者共同决定。

有许多可能的治疗组合。传统上，手术治疗之后进行 WBRT。在局部治疗后使用 WBRT 可降低局部复发率，并控制颅内其余病灶，但相关的认知能力下降仍然令人担忧。在一项将手术联合 WBRT（*n*=49）与单纯手术（*n*=46）对比的随机对照试验中，联合 WBRT 可将颅内控制率从 30%提高到 82%（Patchell et al.，1998）。然而，总体生存率和生活质量（以表现良好状态所花费的时间形式）仅是次要观察指标，两者均未见改善。这些结果已被用来证明手术后不做 WBRT 的合理性。但是，本研究中的局部复发与神经系统相关死亡率增加有关，这在仅手术组中更为常见。一项大型的欧洲研究（Kocher et al.，2011）将接受手术治疗的患者随机分为观察组或 WBRT 组。WBRT 将瘤床的复发率从 60%降至低于 30%，但无进展生存率仅轻度增加，总体生存率没有变化。该研究的生活质量数据显示，WBRT 在 8 周时导致身体机能下降和疲劳，在 9 个月时全身健康状况恶化，并使认知功能下降。

如果应用 SRS，则可在 WBRT 之后。一项大型研究（Kocher et al.，2011）将接受 SRS 的患有 1~3 个脑转移灶的患者随机分为观察组或 WBRT 组。联用 WBRT 不会使总生存期有所差异，但是致死性的颅内进展从 44%降至 28%，并且挽救疗法也更少。一项 meta 分析得出的结论是，在 SRS 联合 WBRT 可改善局部控制，但不改善整体生存率，但由于对认知功能的不利影响，因此建议不做 WBRT（Tsao et al.，2012）。

术后进行 SRS 是改善局部控制、减少认知不良反应的一种方法。一项随机对照研究表明，针对术腔内的 SRS 与 WBRT 相比，具有与手术相当的生存率，但认知结果有所改善（Brown et al.，2017），这种范例越来越受欢迎。先进的 MRI（例如 DWI 序列）可预测微观浸润和肿瘤残留，在未来可用于改进 SRS 方案和治疗选择。

尽管 WBRT 仍然是多发脑转移患者的标准治疗方法，但改进的算法已使这些患者适用 SRS。一项前瞻观察性研究纳入了1194例接受单独SRS的患者，这些患者可多达10处转移（总体积<15 ml）并且表现得分在70或以上，结果显示，伴有2~4个和5~10个转移灶的患者在总体生存率、并发症率和局部复发率之间没有差异（Yamamoto et al.，2014）。目前在多发转移的疾病中，尚无将SRS与WBRT进行比较的随机对照研究。SRS对正常脑组织提供较低的剂量，可作为日间病例，有望为该组患者提供有希望的结果。

选择治疗的原则至关重要（**专栏**8.2）。在孤立性或寡转移的疾病中，仍可自我照顾（KPS>70，WHO≤2）且全身疾病负荷预期生存3~6个月的患者，应考虑进行积极治疗。适当的手术或SRS可提供局部控制，可能改善神经功能，并可以延长生命。联用WBRT可减少局部和远处复发，从而减少神经系统恶化和死亡。术后针对术腔的SRS有助于局部控制。避免WBRT可降低认知能力下降的风险，但需持续随访和进一步的挽救治疗。在多发转移性疾病中，WBRT仍是可行的治疗方法，但SRS变得越来越重要。随着个性化全身性化学疗法和免疫疗法的发展，可能会出现新的手术或放疗替代方案以及新的联合治疗方法。患者、神经外科医生和肿瘤治疗医师间应进行密切讨论，以平衡可选治疗方案的风险和获益（见**专栏**8.2）。

恶性脑膜炎

5%的脑转移患者将进展为恶性脑膜炎（癌性脑膜炎，软脑膜转移），并可能出现脑神经病变，原因不明的脑积水或意识障碍（Le Rhun et al.，2013）。对比增强的T1和FLAIR MRI序列或腰穿（lumbar puncture，LP）可以检测到蛛网膜下腔内沿神经分布的肿瘤细胞。反复、大剂量腰穿的即刻检出率为80%（Le Rhun et al.，2013）。对较大沉积物进行开放式活检是存在质疑的，脑脊液分流的手术具有肿瘤播散至腹腔的风险，尽管两者都有可能起作用。虽然预后很差（未经治疗为6周），但通过CSF池中的脑脊髓放疗和鞘内化疗仍然是治疗的主要手段。

专栏8.2　治疗决策制订原则

- 治疗是非治愈性的；其目的是延长生命、提高质量。
- 患者的心理和支持治疗与转移治疗一样重要。
- 如果患者无法生活自理，则不太可能从治疗中受益。
- WBRT是改善术后颅内控制的标准方案，但应考虑到神经认知功能下降的风险。
- 局部治疗（手术和SRS）可提高预期生存并改善局部控制。
- 单独进行局部治疗比WBRT的认知功能副作用小，但需要持续监测以控制远期神经系统疾病。
- 全身性肿瘤治疗方法正在不断发展。与肿瘤科医生进行讨论可能会为放疗和外科手术提供替代方案。

预后

现已存在多种预后评分系统（**表**8.1）。这些系统强调了患者评分在治疗决策中的重要性。低评分患者的唯一例外是通过手术减小占位效应或治疗脑积水进而改善功能。最新的评分系统结合了肿瘤亚型、生化参数和影像数据（Sperduto，2010）。目前，对无症状患者进行筛查似乎并未提高生存率。

里程碑式文章

Patchell及其同事在20世纪90年代进行了两项里程碑式的研究，确定了颅内转移的现代治疗方法。他们提出了两个问题?

我们应该切除颅内转移瘤吗？

在第一项研究中，他们将48例患有孤立性脑转移的患者随机分为肿瘤切除组或活检后WBRT组（Patchell et al.，1990）。与放疗组相比，手术组的原转移部位复发率更低（25例中有5例[20%] *vs*. 23例中有12例[52%]；$P<0.02$）。手术组的生存期显著延长（中位时间，40周 *vs*. 15周；$P<0.01$），手术组患者的功能独立保持时间更久（中位时间，38周 *vs*. 8周；$P<0.005$）。

如果我们完全切除了转移，我们是否应该进行术后放疗？

95名患者在肿瘤切除后被随机分配至接受WBRT或不再接受进一步治疗。接受术后脑部MRI以确认肿瘤完整切除（Patchell et al.，1998）。接受放疗的患者脑内复发或死于神经系统疾病的可能性更小。

争议：SRS还是神经外科手术？

关于SRS和手术是否能提供更好的局部治疗的争论还在持续，但是尚未有一个直接的对照研究比较手术和SRS。一项回顾性的病例研究发现，当同时进行WBRT时，SRS或手术之间没有区别（Schöggl et al.，2000）。在另一项研究中，仅将SRS

表 8.1 脑转移患者的预后可通过复杂性增加的评分系统进行评估。递归分区分析（RPA）文章对一系列接受放疗的患者进行了统计，描述了三级系统，并发现表现评分较差的患者没有任何获益。预后分级评估（GPA）纳入来自了采用不同治疗策略的各类试验的患者，将每个特征分开，并涵盖了转移灶数目，而 DS-GPA 则包括不同的原发肿瘤类型。对于每种评分系统和疾病而言，一个共同的因素是 Karnofsky 评分

评分系统	分类	因素				结局（中位总体生存时间）						
RPA	分类Ⅰ	年龄 <65，KPS ≥ 70，原发肿瘤可控，无颅外转移				7.1 个月						
	分类Ⅱ	所有不属于分类Ⅰ和分类Ⅲ的患者				4.2 个月						
	分类Ⅲ	KPS <70				2.3 个月						
GPA	0 分	年龄 >60	KPS <70	>3 个转移灶	颅外转移	GPA 0~1		2.6 个月				
	0.5 分	年龄 50~59	KPS 70~80	2~3 个转移灶		GPA 1.5~2.5		3.8 个月				
	1 分	年龄 <50	KPS 90~100	1 个转移灶	无颅外转移	GPA 3		6.9 个月				
						GPA 3.5~4.0		11.0 个月				
DS-GPA	原发肿瘤	评分	0	0.5	1	–	–	DS–GPA	0~1	1.5~2.5	3	3.5~4
	非小细胞肺癌 / 小细胞肺癌	年龄	>60	50~60	<50	–	–	非小细胞肺癌	3.0	6.5	11.3	14.8
		KPS	<70	70~80	90~100	–	–					
		颅外转移	有	–	无	–	–	小细胞肺癌	2.8	5.3	9.6	17.0
		转移灶数目	>3	2~3	1	–	–					
	黑色素瘤 / 肾细胞癌	评分	0	1	2	–	–	黑色素瘤	3.4	4.7	8.8	13.2
		KPS	<70	70~80	90~100	–	–	肾细胞癌	3.3	7.4	11.3	14.8
		转移灶数目	>3	2~3	1							
	乳腺癌	评分	0	0.5	1	1.5	2	乳腺癌	3.4	7.7	15.1	25.3
		KPS	≤50	60	70~80	90~100	–					
		亚型	基底型	–	LumA	HER2	LumB					
		年龄	≥60	<60	–	–	–					
	消化道肿瘤	评分	0	1	2	3	4	消化道肿瘤	3.1	4.4	6.9	13.5
		KPS	<70	70	80	90	100					

RPA，递归分区分析；GPA，预后分级评估；DS，疾病特异；KPS，卡诺夫斯基（Karnofsky）功能状态评分。

Data from Gaspar et al., Recursive partitioning analysis (RPA) of prognostic factors in three Radiation Therapy Oncology Group (RTOG) brain metastases trials, *International Journal of Radiation Oncology, Biology, Physics*, Volume 37, pp. 745–51, 1997; Sperduto PW, Berkey B, Gaspar LE, Mehta M, Curran WJ, A new prognostic index and comparison to three other indices for patients with brain metastases: An analysis of 1960 patients in the RTOG database, *International Journal of Radiation Oncology, Biology, Physics*, Volume 70, pp. 510–14, 2008; Sperduto PW, Chao ST, Sneed P, et al., Diagnosis-specific prognostic factors, indices and treatment outcomes for patients with newly diagnosed brain metastases: a multi-institutional analysis of 4259 patients, *International Journal of Radiation Oncology, Biology, Physics*, Volume 77, Issue 3, pp. 655–61, 2010.

与手术和 WBRT 进行了比较，结果显示在 6 个月时无差异（Muacevic et al.，2008）。在英国的临床实践中，SRS 被用于治疗 1~3 个较小的转移瘤（上限为体积 20 ml 或直径 30 mm），这些肿瘤几乎没有水肿或肿块占位效应，并且预计患者可以存活 6 个月。SRS 无疑比神经外科手术更快、侵入性更小，但是某些亚型的肿瘤已知具有一定的耐放射性（例如，黑色素瘤和肾细胞癌）。对于适合麻醉的患者，神经外科手术具有消除占位效应和减轻水肿的优势，从而潜在地增加 CSF 流量和神经损伤，特别是对颅后窝或较大、非功能区的幕上病变。至关重要的是，手术能为未知原发肿瘤的患者提供诊断标本。已证实，对于患者有囊性转移灶的患者，手术行囊肿引流和SRS的联合治疗是有效的（Franzin et al.，2008）。未来，针对较大的肿瘤，联合SRS、间质性激光热疗法或MRgFUS与手术相联合的杂交方法，对于较小的难以接近的病变可能会成为标准方法，除非化疗和免疫治疗上取得显著成果。

结论

颅内转移瘤变得越来越普遍，这些患者的治疗具有挑战性，并涉及多个亚专业。尽管外科手术、SRS和WBRT仍是核心选择，但治疗方法正在进步。患者表现评分是治疗结果的关键，必须注意使生活质量最大化。肿瘤管理方面的进展已开始为该患者群体带来更好的预后。

延伸阅读、参考文献、EBRAIN的相关链接

扫描书末二维码获取。

第 9 章 原发性中枢神经系统淋巴瘤

Boon Leong Quah・Thangaraj Munusamy・Colin Watts 著
刘畅 译，伊志强 审校

引言

原发性中枢神经系统淋巴瘤（primary central nervous system lymphoma，PCNSL）是一种罕见的非霍奇金淋巴瘤（non-Hodgkin's lymphoma，NHL），治疗上由于其恶性的特点而具有挑战性。其背后的原因在于对于这种全身性疾病，治愈率约 70%，而在免疫方面，PCNSL 的治愈率较差，尤其是 HIV 相关的 PCNSL 更差。幸运的是，自从 20 世纪 70 年代以来，该病的中位生存期有了近两倍的提升，这也反映了该病的治疗手段更具有效性。本章中，我们将会阐述生存率上升的相关原因，并从神经外科的角度说明该病治疗方案的选择。

流行病学

PCNSL 是一种罕见的肿瘤，发病率为十万分之 0.48，占原发性中枢神经系统肿瘤的 2%~3%，且该肿瘤级别较高，具有侵袭性。PCNSLs 是一种非霍奇金淋巴瘤，大约占所有 NHL 的 2%。大部分的 PCNSL 由弥漫性大 B 细胞组成。有关免疫学方面，该病的发病率高峰在 60 岁及以上，如果是 HIV 相关的 PCNSL，其中位发病年龄在 37 岁（Norden et al., 2011）。HIV 相关的 PCNSL 常与 EB 病毒相关，而 AIDS 相关的淋巴瘤只有 20%（Wang et al., 2014）。相比免疫功能缺陷组中男性比例显著占优，免疫功能正常组的男女患病比例为 1.2~1.7：1（**表** 9.1）。

流行病学数据显示，从 20 世纪 90 年代开始，免疫病因相关的 PCNSL 的发病率逐年提升，尤其是在 65 岁以上的患者。与之相反，由于高效的抗病毒治疗的广泛应用，HIV 相关的 PCNSL 的发病率逐步下降。

临床表现

PCNSL 的累及范围包括脑组织、软脑膜、脑神经、脊髓、脑脊液或眼睛，且没有全身系统感染的相关证据。患者经常表现为神经系统相关症状，该症状与病灶所在的神经解剖位置相关。大部分患者有躯体性的、认知相关的、神经精神相关的或运动相关的症状，约 20% 的患者有癫痫发作。侵袭软脑膜的患者占 15%~20%，可能伴有多个脑神经麻痹的相关症状。20%~30% 的患者在确诊时伴有眼部受累，常累及双眼，引起非特异性症状，包括疼痛、红肿、畏光、视力模糊和视力下降。HIV 相关的 PCNSL 是 AIDS 患者以 CD4 计数偏低和 EB 病毒感染为特征的一类疾病，该类患者更容易出现脑病和相关的感染病史。不同的患者疾病进展的情况不同。有些在确诊的前几年即表现出慢性症状，有些则进展迅速，且极具侵袭性。

诊断

影像学

PCNSL 侵袭的常见部位包括脑室旁区域、基底节、胼胝体和深部白质。额叶最常受累，其余部位包括顶叶、颞叶和枕叶。MRI 的影像特点包括病灶出现均一的明显强化（**表** 9.1）。

然而，10% 的与免疫相关的患者病灶无明显强化，特别是那些反复复发的病例。与 AIDS 相关的 PCNSL 患者中，约 70% 可见多重性，即病灶出现不均一的环形强化。PCNSL 的特征是沿着 Virchow-Robinson 血管周围间隙扩散。钙化、出血、坏死等情况相对少见，但在后续的治疗过程中越来越常见。磁共振波谱成像常常证实相对于胶质瘤，PCNSL 的

表 9.1　免疫功能正常和免疫功能缺陷的 PCNSL 患者的比较

PCNSL		免疫功能正常	免疫功能缺陷
	年龄（年）	60 余岁（中位年龄 56 岁）	30 余岁（中位年龄 35 岁）
	诊断时间	3 个月	2 个月
症状		神经功能缺失（与肿瘤的部位相关） 癫痫和脑神经麻痹症状少见	神经功能缺失（与肿瘤的部位相关） 癫痫、脑病和脑神经麻痹症状常见
中枢神经系统部位	成人	孤立性（70%）、幕上（85%）、脑室旁（60%）、胼胝体（12%）	多发性（50%），幕上
	儿童	孤立性 顶叶和额叶、小脑、垂体柄、下丘脑 软脑膜扩散更常见（18%）	
鉴别诊断		高级别胶质瘤 多发性硬化 转移瘤 神经结节病	弓形虫病 脓肿 进行性多病灶脑白质病
影像学特点	CT	灰质高密度 增强扫描出现均一强化	增强扫描不均一环形强化
	MRI	T1 低信号，T2 高信号，增强扫描均一强化	不均一环形强化（儿童患者中也常见）
亚分类		低级别到高级别 95% 为 DLBCL 与 EB 病毒的相关性：罕见	常与 EB 病毒有关 通常为高级别、DLBCL、免疫母细胞亚型 （类似于 AIDS 和移植的患者）

缩写：AIDS，获得性免疫缺陷病；BCL-6，B 细胞淋巴瘤 6 蛋白；CNS，中枢神经系统；CT，电子计算机断层扫描；DLBCL，弥漫大 B 细胞淋巴瘤；DWI/ADC，弥散加权成像 / 表观扩散系数；EBV，EB 病毒；MRI，磁共振成像；MRS，磁共振波谱成像；PCNSL，原发性中枢神经系统淋巴瘤；T1WI，T1 加权像；T2WI，T2 加权像

胆碱 / 肌酸比值更高。并且单体素质子的大脂质峰是其特点（Yamasaki et al.，2015）。

PET 和 SPECT 显示，PCNSL 的病灶为高代谢的。这有助于鉴别 AIDS 引起的弓形虫病，该病往往是低代谢的。**图** 9.1 和**图** 9.2 展示了 PCNSL 诊断和鉴别诊断的影像学相关病例。

眼科检查（裂隙灯检查和玻璃体切割术）

所有怀疑 PCNSL 的患者需行完整的眼科学检查和脑脊液检查，排除有无相关禁忌。大约 25% 的 PCNSL 患者可进展为眼部受累。与之相反，约 90% 的原发性眼内肌淋巴瘤（primary intraocular

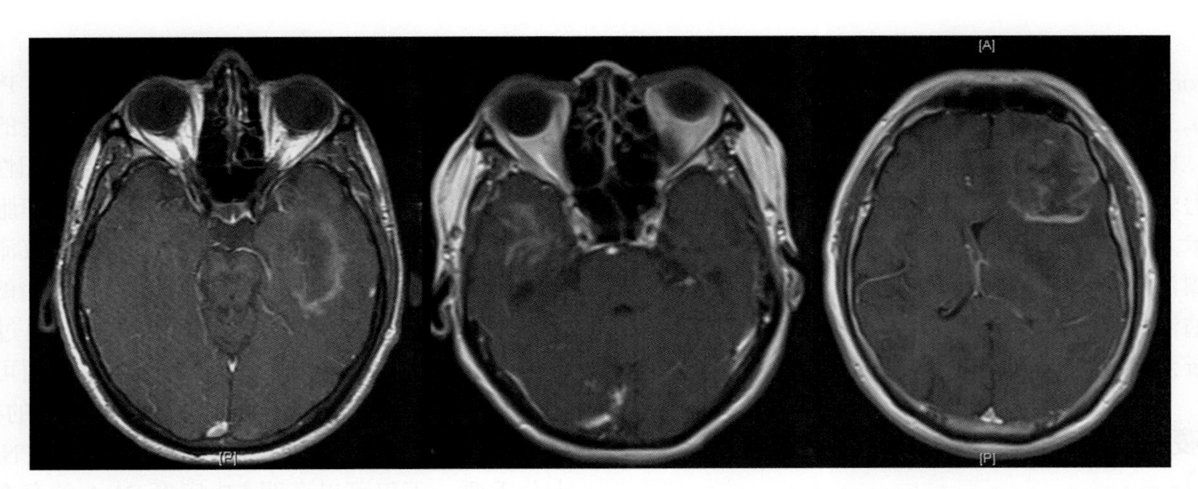

图 9.1　与 PCNSL 病理表现类似的其他疾病的增强 MR 表现。左侧：左颞肿胀的多发性硬化。中间：右颞弥漫大 B 细胞淋巴瘤。右侧：左额胶质母细胞瘤 WHO Ⅳ级

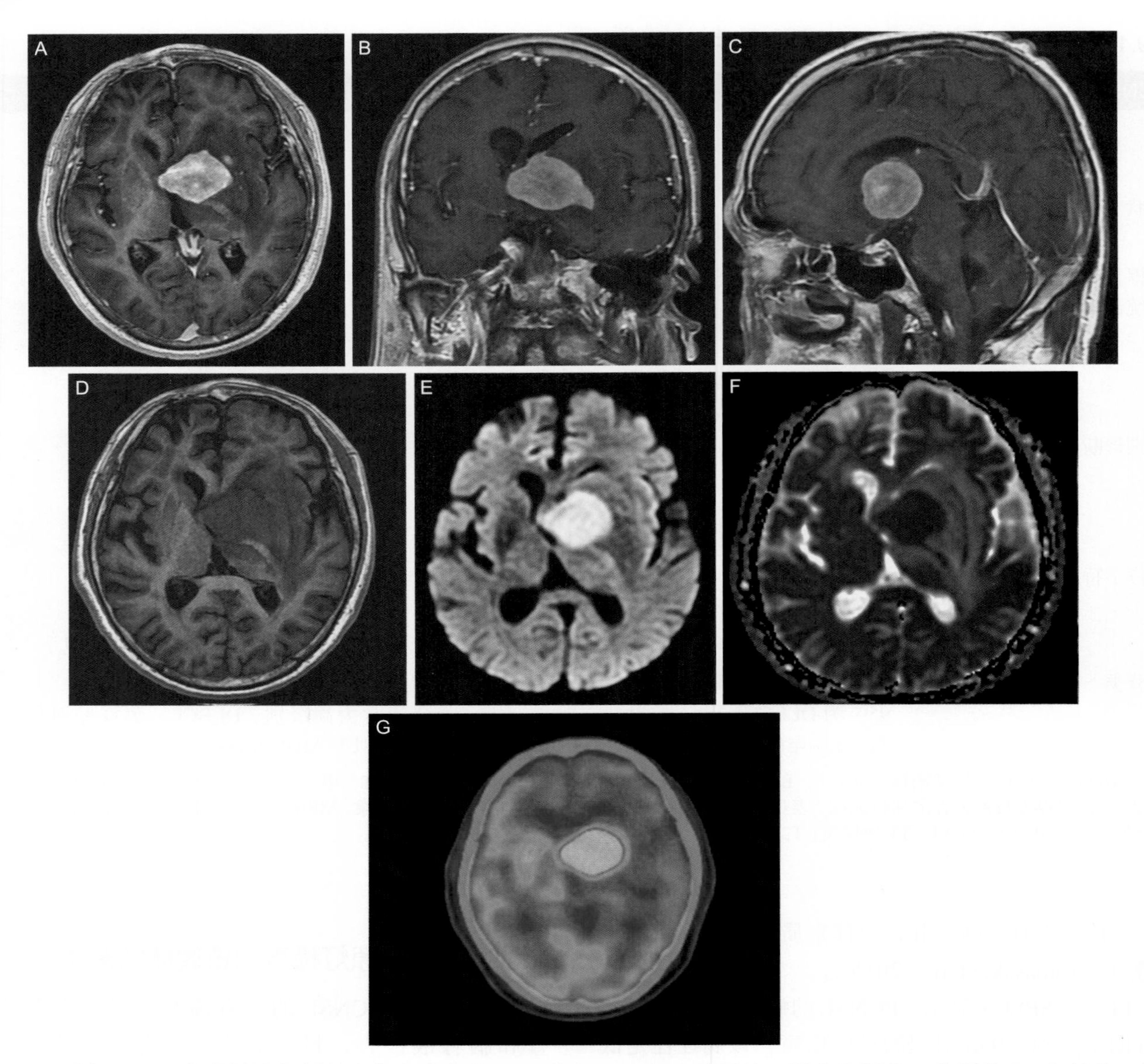

图 9.2　一例 PCNSL 患者累及左侧基底节和内囊的 MRI 表现。T1 相上显示均一强化的图像，分别为（A）轴位、（B）冠状位、（C）矢状位。（D）T1 平扫可见低信号病灶。（E）和（F）分别为 DWI 和 ADC 图像。（G）PET 可见高代谢 PCNSL 病灶

lymphoma，PIOL）可进展为 PCNSL（Gündüz et al., 2003）。如果裂隙灯检查中发现与 PCNSL 的表现相一致，则建议对玻璃体标本进行细针穿刺活检，或对视力较差或患病较重一侧的眼睛行诊断性玻璃体切割术。玻璃体切割术还可以通过清除造成视力模糊和漂浮物的细胞碎片来改善视力。该方法的侵入性比脑活检低，并且有可能在大约 25% 的患者中做出诊断，而不必使他们遭受立体定向脑活检的危害。

脑脊液检查（细胞学、流式细胞术和聚合酶链反应）

多模态的脑脊液分析包括细胞学、流式细胞术和聚合酶链反应（polymerase chain reaction，PCR），是相辅相成的重要附加检查工具，存在可疑的放射学发现时，有助于 PCNSL 的诊断。脑脊液阳性的细胞学检查几乎总是代表软脑膜受累，但在细胞密度低的标本中灵敏度有限。另一方面，脑脊液流式细胞术不受限于上述限制，展现出 PCNSL 诊断的良好的灵敏性和特异性（Craig et al., 2011）。通过 PCR 可证明脑脊液中淋巴细胞的单克隆性，从而可明确诊断，并且该技术也可以用于玻璃体切割术的标本，以诊断 PIOL。脑脊液检查在 AIDS 相关的 PCNSL 中十分重要，不仅可以证明 EB 病毒 DNA 的存在，而且可以免除立体定向活检的手术操作。

组织学检查

诊断PCNSL的金标准是阳性的组织活检和组织病理结果。对比2007年中枢神经系统恶性肿瘤的分类，2016年修订版的WHO分级明确并扩展了中枢神经系统恶性肿瘤的范围，使其与2008版WHO分类的造血和淋巴组织保持一致（Louis et al.，2016）。中枢神经系统弥漫大B细胞淋巴瘤或PCNSL严格定义为局限在中枢神经系统的大B细胞淋巴瘤。PCNSL是一种独特的成熟B细胞淋巴瘤，这种淋巴细胞属于晚期生发中心B细胞，其终末B细胞分化受阻。免疫组化显示CD20阳性（也包括CD79A，PAX5），大部分BCL6阳性（60%~80%），MUM1/RF4阳性（90%），少量的CD10表达（<10%）。它们携带重新排列并发生体细胞突变的免疫球蛋白（IG）基因，并且有体细胞过度突变的证据。

PCNSL不同于其他的淋巴瘤，也可能原发于中枢神经系统，包括起源于硬膜、血管内的大B细胞淋巴瘤、T细胞淋巴瘤或NK细胞淋巴瘤。PCNSL还需要和免疫缺陷相关的原发性中枢神经系统淋巴瘤相鉴别，包括免疫缺陷相关的原发性中枢神经系统淋巴瘤（遗传性或获得性）、AIDS相关的弥漫性大B细胞淋巴瘤、EB病毒阳性的弥漫性大B细胞淋巴瘤、淋巴瘤样肉芽肿。

从组织学上讲，PCNSL类似于其系统性对应物，具有弥漫性实质浸润和血管中心生长模式的细胞构筑特征（Mrugala et al.，2009）。中小型血管周围环绕着一圈恶性淋巴细胞，有些可能侵入血管壁，从而导致血脑屏障破裂。这些淋巴瘤细胞缺乏细胞间凝聚力，不会形成腺体或其他结构（**图**9.3和**图**9.4）。它们具有突出的核仁，周围是嗜碱性细胞质的边缘。汇合区域可见凋亡细胞或坏死。此外，还有各种反应性T细胞和星形胶质细胞，类似于脑炎的表现。

免疫功能低下

免疫功能低下可导致患PCNSL的风险增加，根据其免疫相关表型可分为三组：获得性（HIV相关）、医源性（移植受体相关）和先天性免疫缺陷状态（**表**

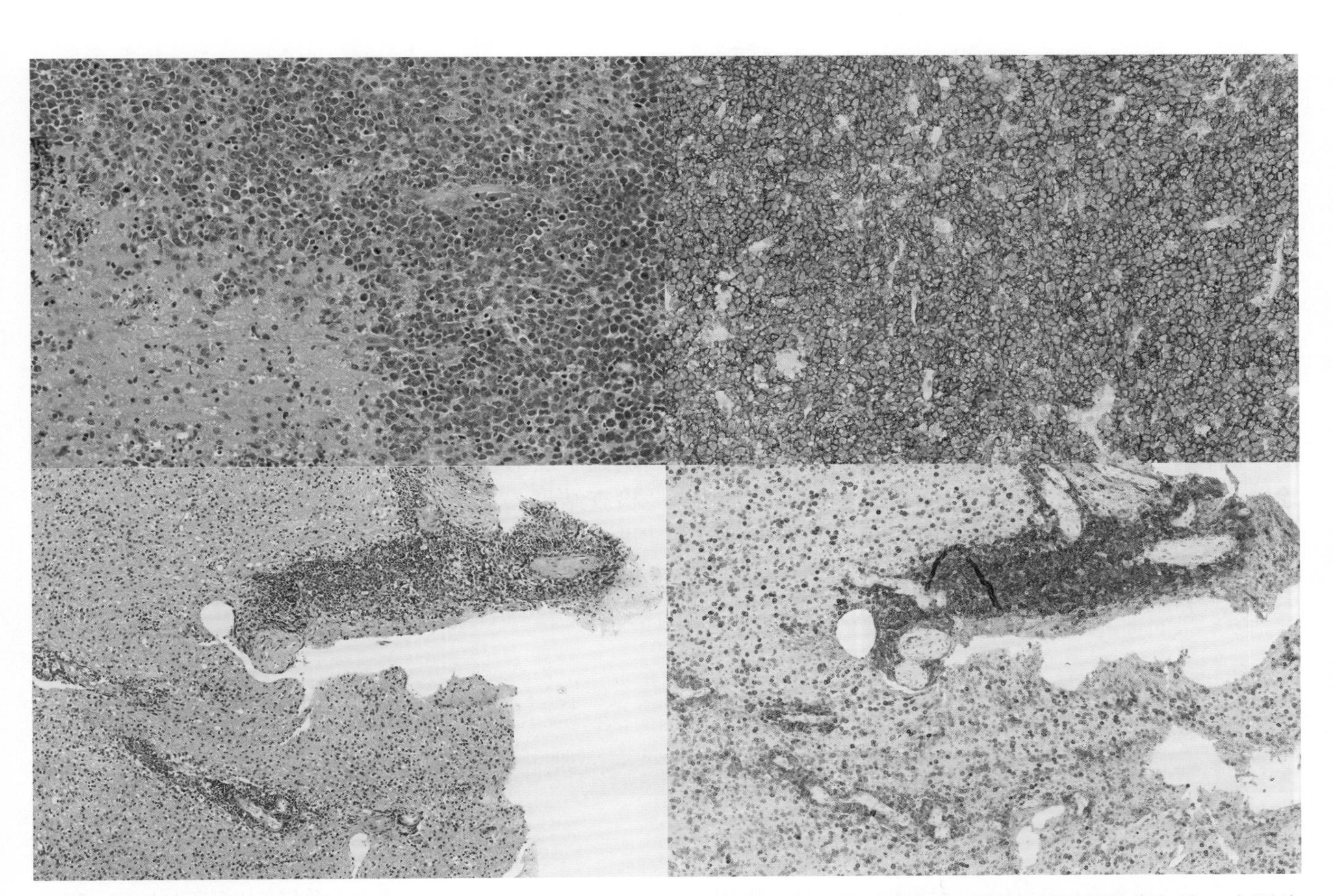

图9.3 两例弥漫大B细胞淋巴瘤。左上：脑活检示弥漫大B细胞淋巴瘤，在图片右上区域有活跃的肿瘤细胞，在图片的左下区域有坏死（H&E染色，放大倍数20倍）。右上：CD20免疫组化染色。左下：脑活检示不同的淋巴瘤，沿血管周围间隙生长排列（H&E染色，放大倍数10倍）。右下：CD79A免疫组化染色

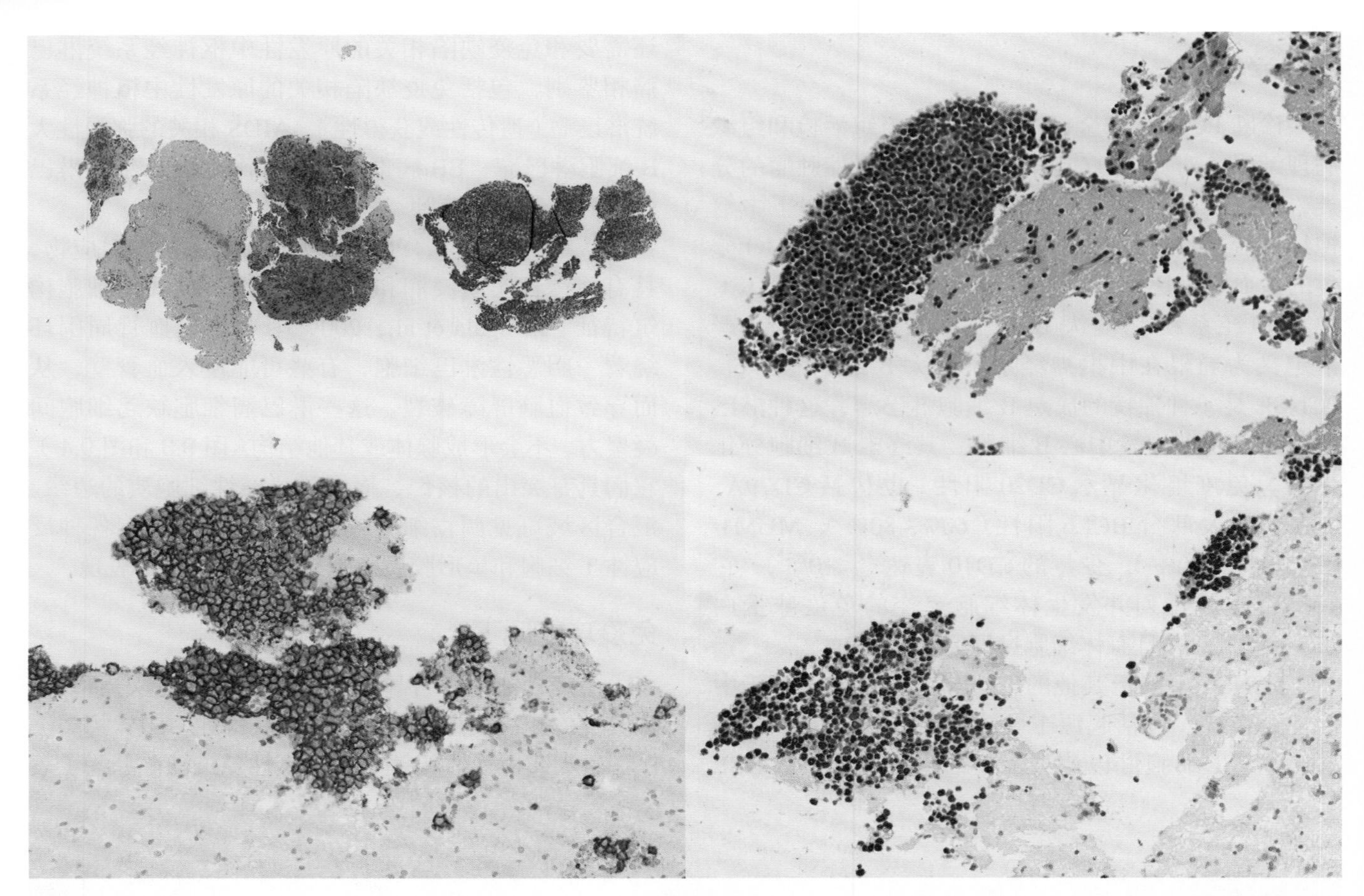

图 9.4　弥漫大 B 细胞淋巴瘤，EB 病毒阳性。左上：三块肿瘤组织显示，从左到右依次为坏死、出血和活跃的肿瘤细胞（H&E 染色，放大倍数 4 倍）。右上：活跃的肿瘤细胞临近正常脑组织周围（H&E 染色，放大倍数 20 倍）。左下：CD20 免疫组化染色。右下：EBER 原位杂交

9.2）。三组间的发病率和预后也有显著的不同。但其总体的治疗原则是基本相同的，目标是恢复免疫功能。

在免疫功能低下方面，PCNSL 的诊断没有明显的不同，从针对当前的免疫功能推荐中，组织学的诊断仍为金标准（**图** 9.3）。然而，患者面临的潜在发病率和医护人员面临的潜在风险提示，对这类疾病的患者进行侵入性较小的检查是合理的。若患者 MRI 检查具有典型的 PCNSL 特点，PET 病灶为高代谢的，且脑脊液 PCR 可发现 EB 病毒阳性，那么极有可能诊断为 PCNSL。另外，抗弓形虫病治疗试验的阴性反应提示 PCNSL，但由于一些原因，该方法遭到了反对，原因有三。首先，未获取组织学病理检查结果。其次，正确的诊断会被延误，从而导致进一步的神经功能退化。最后，有可能弓形虫病和 PCNSL 共存。

表 9.2　免疫正常和免疫缺陷状态的 PCNSL 风险

免疫状态	组别	疾病 / 综合征	PCNSL 的风险
免疫正常			小于十万分之 0.5
免疫缺陷	获得性	HIV 相关的（AIDS）	HIV 感染患者中占 2%~6%
	医源性（PTLD）	肾源性、心源性、肺源性、肝移植	移植受体患者中占 1%~7%
	先天性	SCID、Wiskott-Aldrich 综合征、共济失调 - 毛细血管扩张症	4% 的风险

AIDS，获得性免疫缺陷病；HIV，人类免疫缺陷病毒；PTLD，移植后淋巴组织增生性疾病；SCID，重症联合免疫缺陷症

分子肿瘤细胞生物学

正常的 B 细胞来自造血干细胞，从骨髓中出现，为成熟但幼稚的 B 细胞。随后，它们在外周淋巴组织中遇到抗原后经历体细胞过度突变和亲和力成熟，并最终分化为浆细胞或记忆 B 细胞（**图** 9.5）。

目前学术假说认为 B 细胞淋巴瘤的分子发病机制与正常 B 细胞生长通路的扰动有关，例如与 B 细胞生长或生理至关重要的基因突变有关。这些改变可能发生于细胞分化进程的任一阶段。一些 PCNSL 相关的重要基因和介质以及它们的作用总结在**表** 9.3 中。其中 10% 的肿瘤表达 CD10，50%~90% 表达 BCL2 和 BCL6（Braaten et al.，2003）。超过 95% 的 MUM1 染色为阳性（Camilleri-Broët et al.，2006），这意味着这些 B 细胞即将离开生发中心。但是，由于大脑没有生发中心，因此尚不知道 PCNSL 中 B 细胞的恶性转化是否发生在迁移到中枢神经系统之前。

微环境在 PCNSL 的发病机制中起着基本作用，其中包含的趋化因子可作为神经营养因子或生存因子。在脑脊液中检测这些因素可以将其用作 PCNSL 的生物标志物，有助于诊断和监测治疗反应。发现脑脊液中 CXCL13 和 IL-10 的水平升高，对 PCNSL 的诊断有 99.3％的特异性，并具有良好的敏感性（Rubenstein et al.，2013）。对于高危患者以及预计活检检出率较低的患者，测试这些生物标志物的好处可能更为明显。

在 Knowles（2003）的一项研究中，在几乎 100％的 HIV 阳性 PCNSL 患者的脑脊液中检测到高水平的 EB 病毒 DNA。AIDS 相关的 PCNSL 的发病机制为 CD4＋淋巴细胞计数低于每微升 100 个细胞，且可能与其有免疫活性的对应物不同。这可能与受损的 T 细胞反应和激活的 B 细胞恶性转化有关。

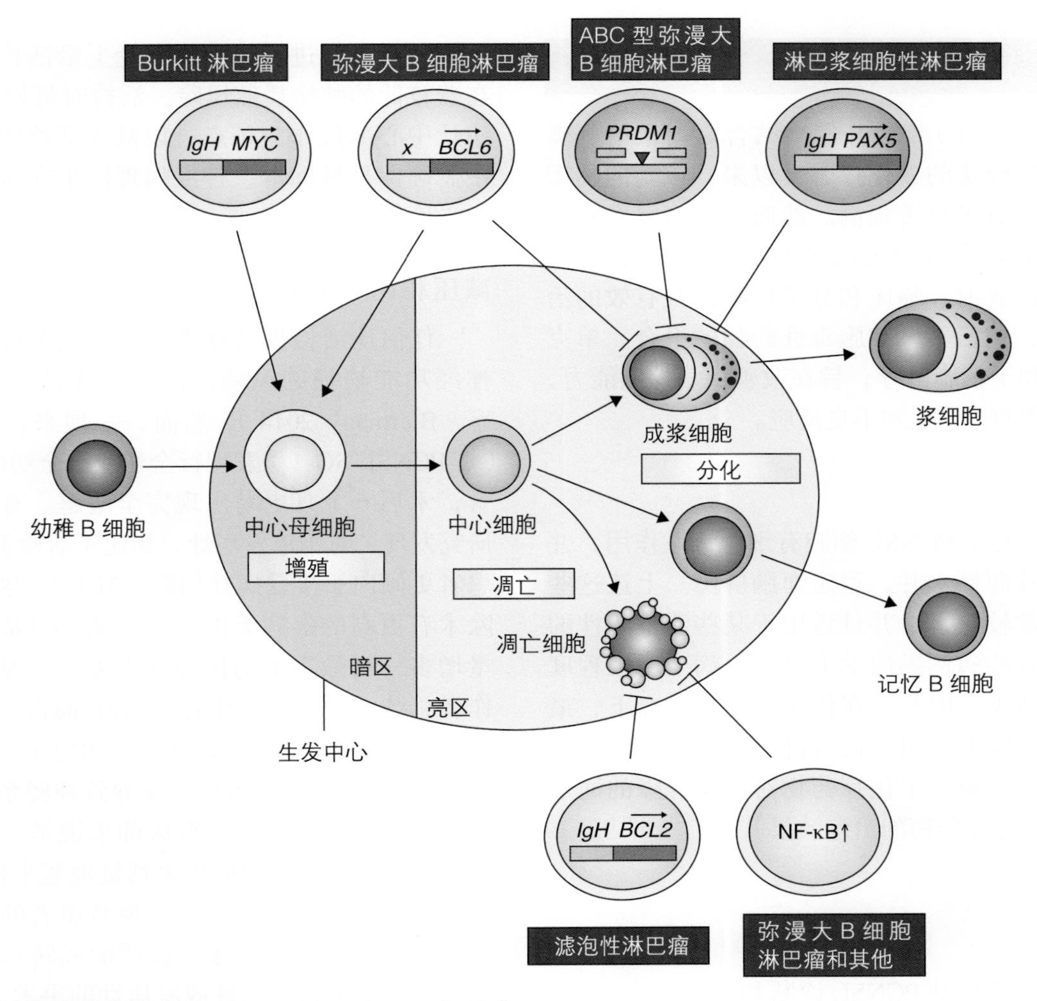

图 9.5　正常 B 细胞发育史（Klein and Dalla-Favera，2008）

表 9.3 PCNSL 基因和调节因子的作用

基因 / 调节因子	作用	作者
HLA（6p21）	抗原处理，信号通路	Cady et al.，2008
PRDM1（6q21）	调节 B 细胞分化为浆细胞	Courts et al.，2008
PTPRK	细胞黏附	Cady et al.，2008
TNFAIP3	调节核因子 NF-κB 信号通路	Paik et al.，2013
MALT1	NF-κB 信号通路的激活	Schwindt et al.，2009
TBL1XR1	NF-κB 信号通路的转录调控	Nakamura et al.，2004
MYD88	NF-κB 和 JAK/STATb 信号通路的激活	Nakamura et al.，2016
CD79B	B 细胞受体信号通路	Nakamura et al.，2016
CDKN2A	细胞周期的调节	Schwindt et al.，2009
MYC	转录调控	Rubenstein et al.，2006；Cady et al.，2008
IL4	JAK/STAT 通路的上调促进因子	Rubenstein et al.，2006

CD，白细胞分化抗原；CDKN，细胞周期素依赖性激酶抑制物；HLA，人类白细胞抗原；IL，白细胞介素；JAK，酪氨酸激酶；PRDM，正向调节区；PTPRK，酪氨酸磷酸酶受体蛋白 K；MALT，黏膜相关的淋巴组织淋巴瘤异位；MYC，骨髓细胞组织增生；MYD，髓样分化；NF-κB，核因子 KB；STAT，转录信号诱导与激活因子；TBL1XR1，转导素 β 样 X 连锁受体 1；TNFAIP3，肿瘤坏死因子 α 诱导蛋白 3

治疗

自从 20 世纪 80 年代开发出结合高剂量甲氨蝶呤和全脑放射疗法的放化疗方案以来，该病的临床预后和生存率有了显著提高。然而，疾病复发和药物的神经毒性成了治疗上的主要挑战。当前的治疗模式逐步向精准放射、临床和分子诊断以及有效的治疗方案转变，包括新型细胞毒性药物的组合、单克隆抗体治疗和干细胞治疗，旨在改善疾病控制能力，同时减少药物的神经认知不良反应。

类固醇类药物

地塞米松对于 PCNSL 细胞有细胞毒性作用，并可以减少血管源性水肿，稳定血脑屏障。上述这些作用效果常常较短暂，并且适用于某些活检阴性的病例，其中有些病例影像学上可显示病变增强程度及范围显著减少。因此，在任何可能的情况下，最好先确诊或排除 PCNSL 后，再使用类固醇类药物。此外，地塞米松减少了化疗药物对血脑屏障的通透性，从而降低化疗药物的治疗效果。

手术治疗

活检

立体定向活检是 PCNSL 诊断和分类的金标准。活检的优点在于患者耐受性好，且只需承受较小的风险即可获得较迅速的诊断。整个手术可以选择局部麻醉的方式进行，而且理论上沿活检路径可能存在着较低的肿瘤播散风险。活检时最好选取 PCNSL 病灶中心部位作为靶点，以减少活检阴性可能。术中需确保足量标本，神经病理医生在术中即可得出初步诊断。

减压和切除手术

任何比活检更具侵袭性的方法都被认为会冒着神经功能缺损的风险，同时又无法改善整体生存率（Bierman，2014）。然而，一项来自德国的研究（G-PCNSL-SG-1）发现行全切或次全切的 PCNSL 患者，术后 6 个月更易出现完全缓解。有趣的是，有研究发现，对于单发病灶，相比于活检手术（19%），患者更倾向于接受病灶切除（31%）。尽管单病灶切除术有更高的疾病无进展生存期，但是一旦病灶数量增多，切除手术的优势就丧失了。因此该研究的作者总结，对于单病灶的 PCNSL 而言，应该重新考虑病灶切除手术（Weller et al.，2012）。

继发于 PCNSL 占位效应导致神经系统症状迅速恶化的情况，对神经外科医师来说是一项独特的挑战。通常起始治疗即应用大剂量地塞米松和甘露醇，迅速决定外科手术治疗可以挽救患者的生命。最初的影像学检查往往更像是胶质瘤或转移瘤，因此在紧急情况下可行切除性或减压性的手术。有趣的是，Lee 等的一项研究（2014）描述了一例患者，出现了快速的神经功能恶化，由于应用了高渗疗法、地塞米松和化疗而免于外科手术治疗。上述治疗可使得瘤周水肿、肿瘤大小以及占位效应显著减小。

化疗和放疗

目前的证据支持将PCNSL的治疗策略从全脑放射治疗或高剂量甲氨蝶呤单一治疗转向基于高剂量甲氨蝶呤的联合化疗方案。与单独使用全脑放射治疗或单药高剂量甲氨蝶呤化疗所获得的治疗效果相比，联合化疗方案可提高患者的总体生存率（**表** 9.4）。

治疗分两期：诱导期和巩固期。诱导期为基于高剂量甲氨蝶呤的化疗方案，其目的是控制疾病，并诱导缓解。目前正在进行的临床试验所应用的免疫治疗包括利妥昔单抗，一种抗CD20的单克隆抗体（IELSG-32 和 HOVON105 PCNSL/ALLG NHL24 试验）。鞘内注射甲氨蝶呤曾经作为PCNSL的一种治疗方式，但有证据表明出现弥漫性脑膜以及脊髓受累的情况。但是，鞘内注射化疗的好处尚不清楚，因为甲氨蝶呤的治疗浓度很容易通过静脉途径达到。血脑屏障破坏后进行化疗是一种新的方法，旨在改善化疗效果，但仅限于具备适当设施和技术能力的研究中心（参考国际血脑屏障破坏联盟）。应用上述方法，McAllister等（2000）显示了其他应用高剂量甲氨蝶呤的治疗方案，但是报告了4例患者死亡，癫痫、短暂性脑缺血发作、卒中等概率增加。尽管这种治疗方法有望通过增强化疗的有效性和减少化疗药物的剂量而大有希望，但仍需要进一步评估研究。

巩固期的目的是消除化疗诱导期后的残留病灶。此期的方案为全脑放射治疗和（或）化疗。在相对年轻和健康的患者中，高剂量化学疗法和自体干细胞移植可被视为替代疗法（Schorb et al.，2013）。

当前的治疗选择尚未被证实可以产生持续完全缓解或治愈的结果。由于没有标准的治疗方法，疾病复发几乎是不可避免的，因此这是一个特别具有挑战性的领域。目前可选择的治疗方案包括放疗和二线的化疗方案。

预后

文献中很少有关于未接受过PCNSL治疗的患者预后的数据，因为获得的大多数数据都反映了接受治疗患者的总体生存期和无进展生存期。对于这种罕

表 9.4　联合治疗方案及生存率

年份	文献	方案	患者数量	中位随访（月）	OS（%）	中位OS（月）	2年PFS（%）	中位PFS(月)
2002	DeAngelis et al.（2002）	MTX、PCB、长春新碱，IT-MTX、全脑放疗	98	56	NA	37	NA	24
2006	Illerhaus et al.（2006）	MTX、ASCT、全脑放疗	30	63	（3年OS）68.5	NA	NA	NA
2007	Montemurro et al.（2007）	MTX、塞替派、ASCT、全脑放疗	28	15	（2年OS）48	48	45	45
2009	Ferreri et al.（2009）	MTX、ARA-C、全脑放疗	79	30	（3年OS）46	NA	NA	NA
2012	Wieduwilt et al.（2012）	MTX、TMZ、利妥昔单抗、依托泊苷、ARA-C	31	79	NA	66	79	24
2013	Morris et al.（2013）	MTX、利妥昔单抗、长春新碱、PCB、ARA-C、减量全脑放疗	52	70	（5年OS）80	79	77	39
2015	Omuro et al.（2015）	MTX、利妥昔单抗、长春新碱、PCB、ASCT	33	45	（2年OS）81	NR	79	NR

ARA-C，阿糖胞苷；ASCT，自体干细胞移植；IT，鞘内的；NA，未予以提供；NR，未达到；OS，总生存期；MTX，甲氨蝶呤；PCB，甲基苄肼；PFS，无进展生存期；TMZ，替莫唑胺

见的肿瘤，未经治疗的预后是令人遗憾的，生存期可能仅持续数周到数月。Henry 等（1974）报告如果仅提供支持治疗，生存期仅有 3.3 个月。Norden 等（2011）分析了 SEER 数据库并发现从 20 世纪 70 年代以来，PCNSL 的中位生存期仅有 7.5 个月。上述数据表明，有免疫能力的患者接受治疗后的中位生存期约为 14 个月，而与 HIV 相关的 PCNSL 的生存期约为 2 个月。韩国的另一项基于人群的研究分析了 1999 年至 2007 年间 688 例患者的数据，中位生存期为 21 个月（Shin S-H et al.，2015），但未说明患者的免疫状况。尽管如此，这个数据提供了有关 PCNSL 患者真实的生存期情况。

另一方面，试验数据报告的数字明显好于流行病学数据（**表** 9.4）。这主要与患者准入标准相关。所有有关 PCNSL 治疗的试验均需排除免疫功能缺陷的患者，以及弥漫性病变的患者，而剩下的患者均是相对局灶性病变的患者。虽然选择标准对于确保研究人群的统一并获得有意义的结果是必不可少的，但研究的人群并不总是 PCNSL 患者整体的真实代表。尽管如此，现有的数据表明，经过正规的治疗后，生存期可以得到提高。

免疫功能缺陷的患者

总体而言，与 HIV 相关的 PCNSL 均为致命性疾病，中位生存期约为 3 个月。在未接受过治疗的患者中开始使用 HAART（高效抗逆转录病毒疗法），或改变药物组合，目前被认为与提升疾病控制和总体生存率相关。我们对获得性和先天性免疫抑制的相关 PCNSL 的治疗遵循相同的原理，即改善或消除免疫抑制状态。这就需要仔细考虑移植排斥和疾病进展的风险。类固醇类药物和全脑放射治疗是主流的治疗方案。其他治疗方案包括化疗、减少剂量的全脑放射治疗，尽管上述治疗前景广阔，但应仅限于合适的研究中心作为试验研究来使用。Jacomet 等（1997）研究了高剂量甲氨蝶呤作为单独治疗方案应用于 HIV 相关的 PCNSL 之中，并证明可以提升 9.7 个月的生存期。这类治疗的理想患者是神经系统状况良好且无活动性机会感染的患者。脑脊液 EB 病毒 DNA 水平可作为衡量肿瘤对化疗反应的替代肿瘤标志物。

争议：放疗治疗 PCNSL 的作用

反对放疗的观点

全脑放射治疗一直以来被当做治疗 PCNSL 的主要治疗方式，尽管治疗初始的效果显著，但 Nelson 等（1992）发现超过 60% 的接受全脑放疗作为唯一治疗方案的患者，在放疗区域内有病灶进展的情况。同组中位生存期仅有 11.6 个月。随着高剂量甲氨蝶呤的应用，越来越多结果证实全脑放疗联合高剂量甲氨蝶呤的预后更佳。然而，来自 G-PCNSL-SG-1（Thiel et al.，2010）的数据表明，不增加全脑放疗的一线化疗方案并不会降低总生存率。此外，对治疗有持续完全反应的患者，往往需遭受延迟的神经毒性反应，且增加了发病率和死亡率（Doolittle et al.，2013）。且超过 60 岁以上的患者极易受到影响，幸存者也往往需要监护。为了减少这种并发症，减量的全脑放疗作为巩固期的一种治疗方案，但结果却喜忧参半。Bessell 等（2002）报道了联合化疗后减量的全脑放疗（30.6 Gy）的结果不佳。Morris 等（2013）报道了联合化疗后再行 23.4 Gy 放射治疗，显示出令人鼓舞的结果，但 60 岁以上的组别中，预后明显较差。Wang 等（2014）总结的一篇综述提出，限制全脑放疗应用的三点不足：对病灶的局部控制不足，放疗照射视野外的放射隐匿性淋巴瘤细胞的扩散，以及放射线对脑功能的有害影响。

支持放疗的观点

联合化疗方案后巩固放疗的基本原理在于，PCNSL 是一种弥漫性疾病，巩固期的全脑放疗与无进展生存期和总生存期升高相关。G-PCNSL-SG-1 试验提供了包括全脑放疗在内的无进展生存期适度改善的证据，但未能显示总生存期有任何显著改善。这项研究由于执行过程中的一些缺陷而受到批评：未能达到其主要终点、违背方案以及存在高风险的偏倚。Cochrane 合作组织发表了一篇有关附加放射疗法在治疗 PCNSL 作用的综述。作者发现，没有充分的数据表明，联合放化疗方案与单纯化疗方案相比，两组患者的总生存期相似。该综述还表明，无进展生存期的证据不足（Zacher et al.，2014）。Ferreri 等（2009）比较了两种化疗（高剂量甲氨蝶呤组对比高剂量甲氨蝶呤加阿糖胞苷组）加全脑放疗方案。尽管研究中未将全脑放疗作为主要结果，全脑放疗无论衔接哪种化疗方案，完全缓解率分别为 64% 和 30%。Prica 等（2012）发表的一项有关决策分析研究的结果表明，接受化疗后联合全脑放疗的 60 岁以下患者的生存期和生活质量都有所改善。

深层的研究和思考

在写本章的同时，有三项正在进行的有关全脑放疗治疗 PCNSL 的研究。PRECIS 是在法国正在进行的一项前瞻性随机Ⅱ期研究，旨在比较高剂量甲氨蝶呤加全脑放疗与高剂量甲氨蝶呤对于造血干细胞的影响。英国发起的 IELSG32 是一项随机的Ⅱ期临床试验，评估了三种不同的化疗方案，其中达到完全缓解的患者将接受后续的全脑放疗或自体干细胞移植。RTOG-1114 是一项在美国进行的随机的Ⅱ期临床试验，评估采用 R-MVP 化疗方案治疗，然后单独使用阿糖胞苷或阿糖胞苷加全脑放疗进行治疗。

在寻找更有效的治疗 PCNSL 的方法以达到与全身性非霍奇金淋巴瘤有相似效果的同时，可以预见放疗将继续发挥重要作用。从 G-PCNSL-SG-1 试验获得的数据尚不清楚有效化疗方案后应用放疗方案的作用。但是，在获得更高级别的证据之前，对“赞成”和“反对”全脑放疗的论点需要仔细考虑。

对于 60 岁以下的患者，全脑放疗与有效的化疗方案相结合，具有改善缓解率、延长无进展生存期和总生存期的潜力。但是，需要仔细权衡其益处与延迟性神经毒性可能造成的破坏性影响，尤其是对于 60 岁以上的患者。此外，挽救性全脑放疗是治疗全脑放疗后初次复发患者的潜在选择。治疗前，必须考虑患者的期望以及任何形式的治疗对患者生活质量的潜在影响。

致谢

本章“组织学”部分的内容由来自荷兰奈梅亨大学（Radboud University Nijmegen）神经病理科 Pieter Wesseling 医生完成。

病理图片（**图 9.3 和图 9.4**）由来自新加坡国立大学医学院病理科的 Seet Ju Ee 医生提供。这些病例均来自该科室。

参考文献、EBRAIN 的相关链接

扫描书末二维码获取。

第 10 章　胶质神经元和其他癫痫相关性肿瘤

Matthias Simon · Alexander Grote 著
刘畅 译，伊志强 审校

引言

神经元和神经胶质细胞肿瘤占颅内肿瘤不足5%，其中节细胞胶质瘤和胚胎发育不良性神经上皮瘤（dysembryplastic neuroepithelial tumours，DNTs）最常见，这两种类型常见于药物难治性癫痫的外科手术中。虽然任何一种颅内肿瘤都可能会引起癫痫发作，但是某些特定类型的肿瘤与慢性或药物难治性癫痫密切相关。除了上述提到的节细胞胶质瘤和DNTs，与癫痫相关的有毛细胞和多形性星形细胞瘤，又称为血管中心型胶质瘤（angiocentric glioma，ANET），还有一些 WHO Ⅱ级和Ⅲ级的弥漫性胶质瘤。上述提到的这些与癫痫相关的肿瘤统称为长期癫痫相关性肿瘤（longstanding or long-term epilepsy-associated tumours，LEATs）。由于大多数病例在癫痫发病后的 2 年内已行外科手术治疗，LEATs 又常被称为“低级别癫痫相关性神经上皮细胞肿瘤”（Blumcke et al.，2016）。

慢性或难治性癫痫的刻板的临床表现，通常是一个非常良性的临床过程，与混合性（神经胶质及神经元）肿瘤的性质表明不同组织学 LEAT 的生物联系（Blumcke et al.，2014）。然而，目前大多数分子遗传学和免疫组化研究显示出另一种情况。值得注意的是，有 LEAT 组织学接受过癫痫手术治疗的患者预后更差。这有重要的临床意义。笔者认为，LEAT 患者通过影像学检查，或者因单次癫痫发作偶然发现病变，应早期行外科手术治疗，而不应该简单地进行定期影像学复查。目前尚不清楚这类病例的转归，是良性过程进展为长期的癫痫发作，还是会向肿瘤疾病进展。

本章内容将回顾分析神经元和神经胶质细胞肿瘤，包括非神经胶质细胞 LEAT 变异型肿瘤的临床、病理和影像的相关特点。我们描述了相对常见的节细胞胶质瘤、DNTs 和中枢神经系统特异相关的罕见的家族性错构瘤综合征（发育异常的小脑性神经节细胞瘤，Lhermitte-Duclos 病）。本章还介绍了目前 WHO 分级中更为罕见的一些胶质神经元肿瘤（乳头状胶质神经元肿瘤、第四脑室伴菊心团形成的胶质神经元肿瘤、婴儿促纤维生成型节细胞胶质瘤 / 星形细胞瘤、脑室外神经细胞瘤、小脑脂肪神经细胞瘤）和非胶质神经元相关的 LEAT。最后，针对颞叶癫痫相关性肿瘤的海马切除手术治疗，我们简要总结了该手术方式的利弊。

节细胞胶质瘤

节细胞胶质瘤最常见于儿童和青壮年阶段。成人的发病率为 0.3%~5.2%，儿童则可达 14%。最常见的发病位置位于颞叶，其次位于额叶，也可位于幕上中线、基底节和丘脑、小脑、脑干以及脊髓，但相对罕见。

组织学上，节细胞胶质瘤由混合型神经节细胞和新生胶质细胞成分组成（**图 10.1**）。而两者组成成分的比例有较大变化，从而导致肿瘤形态学上以神经元细胞群（神经节细胞瘤）为主，或者以胶质成分为主。绝大多数节细胞胶质瘤为 WHO Ⅰ级。间变性的肿瘤一般为 WHO Ⅲ级，只占节细胞胶质瘤的 1%~2.6%。目前，WHO 分级不再承认介于中间型的“非典型”WHO Ⅱ级的节细胞胶质瘤（即，非良性非间变型），有一些临床证据显示三分类而非二分类系统。节细胞胶质瘤有一定的概率转变为胶质母细胞瘤。有文献报道，11 例已行继发性胶质母细胞瘤的手术患者中，有 5 例第一次手术的病理为节细胞胶质瘤（Luyken et al.，2004；Majores et al.，2008）。有超过 50% 的节细胞胶质瘤患者发现特异性的 BRAF 肿瘤基因突变（BRAF *c*.1799T>A/BRAF V600E）（Koelsche et al.，2013）。BRAF V600E 突变可能提示预后不佳（Dahiya et al.，2013）。节细胞胶质瘤极少出现 IDH1 突变。

典型的节细胞胶质瘤患者伴随症状性癫痫，而

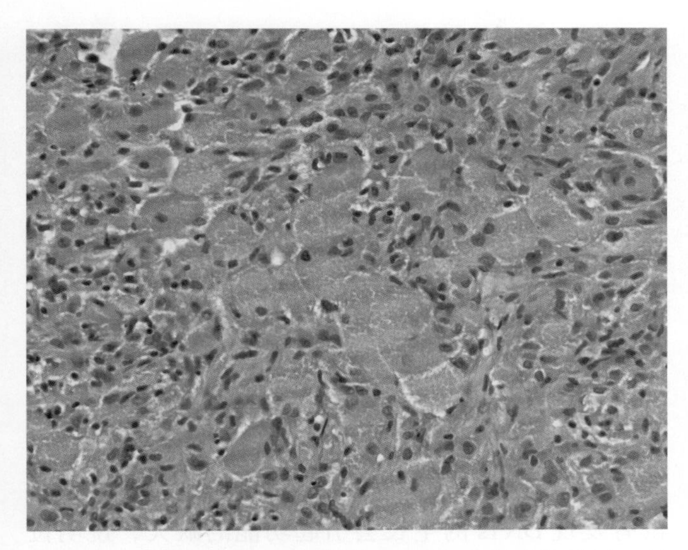

图 10.1 异常神经节细胞巢是神经节细胞肿瘤的特征，其可能包括新生性神经胶质成分。嗜酸性粒状体和血管周围淋巴细胞为一般特异性特点

Courtesy of Dr Kieren Allinson, Department of Pathology, Addenbrooke's Hospital, Cambridge.

不伴有癫痫发作的节细胞胶质瘤患者需警惕非良性临床病程的可能性。位于脑组织深部、小脑、脑干、脊髓等部位的节细胞胶质瘤会表现出与解剖位置相对应的临床症状和体征（**图** 10.2）。节细胞胶质瘤在MRI 的 T2 和 FLAIR 相上为高信号，在 T1 相为低或等信号。肿瘤囊变和斑片或结节状增强是 MRI 的常见特点，而钙化并不罕见。间变性肿瘤的 MRI 表现并不具有特异性，但通常都表现为类似于良性的节细胞胶质瘤。

节细胞胶质瘤的治疗可选择外科手术。手术并发症出现概率较低，这也反映出大多数节细胞胶质瘤患者具有良好的病灶位置、年轻以及较好的身体状况。术后患者癫痫发作控制良好。本中心的手术随访结果表明，伴有 2 年以上癫痫发作的 LEAT 患者共 207 例，行外科手术治疗并随访 10 年，其中节细胞胶质瘤 86 例，Engel Ⅰ级（无癫痫发作或偶尔有非致残性的癫痫发作）近 80%（Luyken et al.，2003）。据我们的经验，WHO Ⅰ级的节细胞胶质瘤患者行肿瘤全切后，绝大部分均可治愈，只有极少的患者预后不佳（Luyken et al.，2004）。相反，非典型和间变性节细胞胶质瘤的 5 年无进展生存期仅分别接近 70% 和 30%。临床表现为长期或难治性癫痫是临床预后

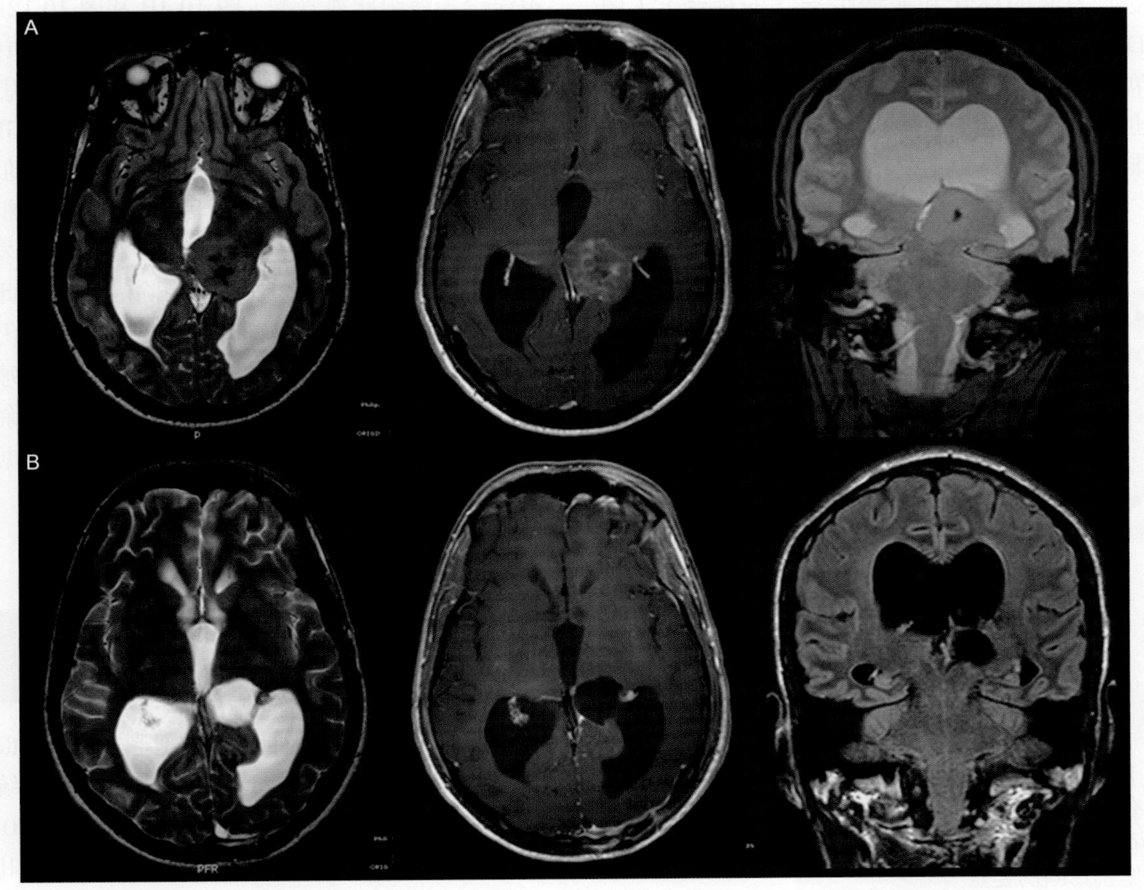

图 10.2 一例 26 岁的男性患者，节细胞胶质瘤位于左侧丘脑，出现了梗阻性脑积水的症状和体征。该患者经顶叶皮质 - 侧脑室入路成功切除了肿瘤，不伴有继发的神经功能缺损。（A）术前 MRI ；（B）术后 MRI

的重要指标（Majores et al.，2008）。在除慢性癫痫和癫痫手术外的病例占比高的中心，肿瘤预后更差。最近的一篇文献表明 88 例患者 5 年无进展生存期只有 58%（Compton et al.，2012）。

考虑到 WHO Ⅲ级的间变性节细胞胶质瘤患者预后相对不佳，与其他间变性胶质瘤类似，放射治疗应该被推荐为常规治疗方式，即使该方案不是基于非常实质性的证据。放射治疗可作为复发性、不可切除性或不完全切除性肿瘤的一种治疗选择，该类肿瘤的组织学表现为非典型特征，但并未完全满足 WHO Ⅲ级的标准。化疗的证据尚不充足。

胚胎发育不良性神经上皮瘤

DNTs 是第二常见的神经胶质肿瘤，男性患者的发病率略高，且更常见于 20~40 岁。儿童患者可占到一定比例。DNTs 最常见于颞叶，也可出现在幕上脑组织的任何部位。幕上深部脑组织（尾状核、透明隔）和颅后窝（脑干、小脑）的病灶也有报道。

DNTs 的组织学特点表现为多结节外观和特殊的神经胶质成分，混合有少突胶质细胞样细胞排列成垂直于皮质表面的柱状和非增生异常的神经元（**图 10.3**）。DNTs 大多数属于 WHO Ⅰ级。WHO 分级可分为简单型和复杂型两个亚型。弥漫型变异存在争议，这也反映出 DNTs 与弥漫型低级别胶质瘤鉴别诊断的难度。混合型 DNTs/ 节细胞胶质瘤也有报道

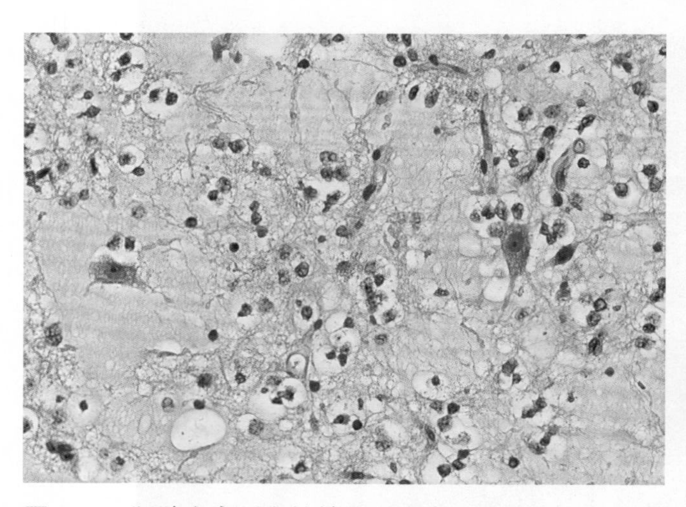

图 10.3 胚胎发育不良性神经上皮瘤（H&E 染色，放大倍数 400 倍）。这些肿瘤通常以混在黏液池中的大锥体神经元为特征。该特征在少突胶质细胞瘤中比较少见，可作为组织学鉴别诊断的要点

Courtesy of Dr Kieren Allinson, Department of Pathology, Addenbrooke's Hospital, Cambridge.

（Thom et al.，2011）。既往文献报道，32 例 DNTs 的患者，既无 BRAF V600E 突变，又无 IDH1 突变（Grote and Simon，2015）。有些文献报道 DNTs 患者中，有 LOH 1p/19q 或者 IDH1 突变（Thom et al.，2011）。部分 DNTs 的病例报道中，发现 70%~80% 的病例伴有局灶性皮质发育不良（focal cortical dysplasias，FCDs）。FCDs 与肿瘤相关的致病关系目前尚未阐明。一种假设认为这些变化为之前瘤床的遗迹，已经部分转化为实际的 LEAT。更可能的是，FCDs 与 LEATs 同时生长或继发于肿瘤的生长（Thom et al.，2012）。

DNTs 最常表现为药物难治性癫痫，我们目前还没有发现 DNTs 的生长会引起功能的缺失，说明位于重要功能区的 DNT 的生长会引起功能重塑，切除功能区的 DNT 并不引起功能缺失。我们的经验是伴随的 DNTs 并不少见。典型的 MRI 表现为肿瘤呈多囊性，伴有小块占位或水肿，T2 相和 FLAIR 相为高信号，T1 相为低信号。对比增强和钙化并不少见（15%~20%）。DNTs 对周围颅骨有一定概率的侵蚀（20%~70%）。鉴别诊断包括与节细胞胶质瘤或其他的 LEAT 伴随弥漫性胶质瘤。有些 DNTs 在术前容易被误诊为海绵状血管瘤（**图 10.4B** 和**图 10.12B**）。

DNTs应行外科手术治疗。与节细胞胶质瘤一样，其手术并发症发生概率较低。难治性癫痫患者中有将近 80% 的 DNTs 术后多年随访可达 ENGEL Ⅰ级（Luyken et al.，2003）。不完全的切除或伴随 FCD 是癫痫发作或复发的主要预后因素。DNTs 的组织病理学上主要为良性。我们仅观察到 1 例个案，发现肿瘤复发的原因是 DNT 未被完全切除。尽管如此，即使手术完全切除肿瘤，或有恶变转化现象，仍然有一小部分且数量在持续增加的复发肿瘤的病例（Thom et al.，2011）。因此对于残存肿瘤和部分切除的 DNT 患者，建议进行影像学随访。目前没有证据支持对 DNTs 患者进行放化疗。特别引起注意的是，辅助治疗可能对恶变转化的病例有效。

发育不良性小脑神经节细胞瘤（Lhermitte-Duclos 病）

发育不良性小脑神经节细胞瘤（Lhermitte-Duclos disease，LDD）是 Cowden 病的中枢神经系统主要临床表现。Cowden 病（OMIM 数据库 158350）是常染色体显性遗传病，最常见为 PTEN 生殖细胞突变。Cowden 综合征中的 LDD 也可能为 PIK3CA 突变引起。该病的临床表现为多发性错构瘤，其起源于三

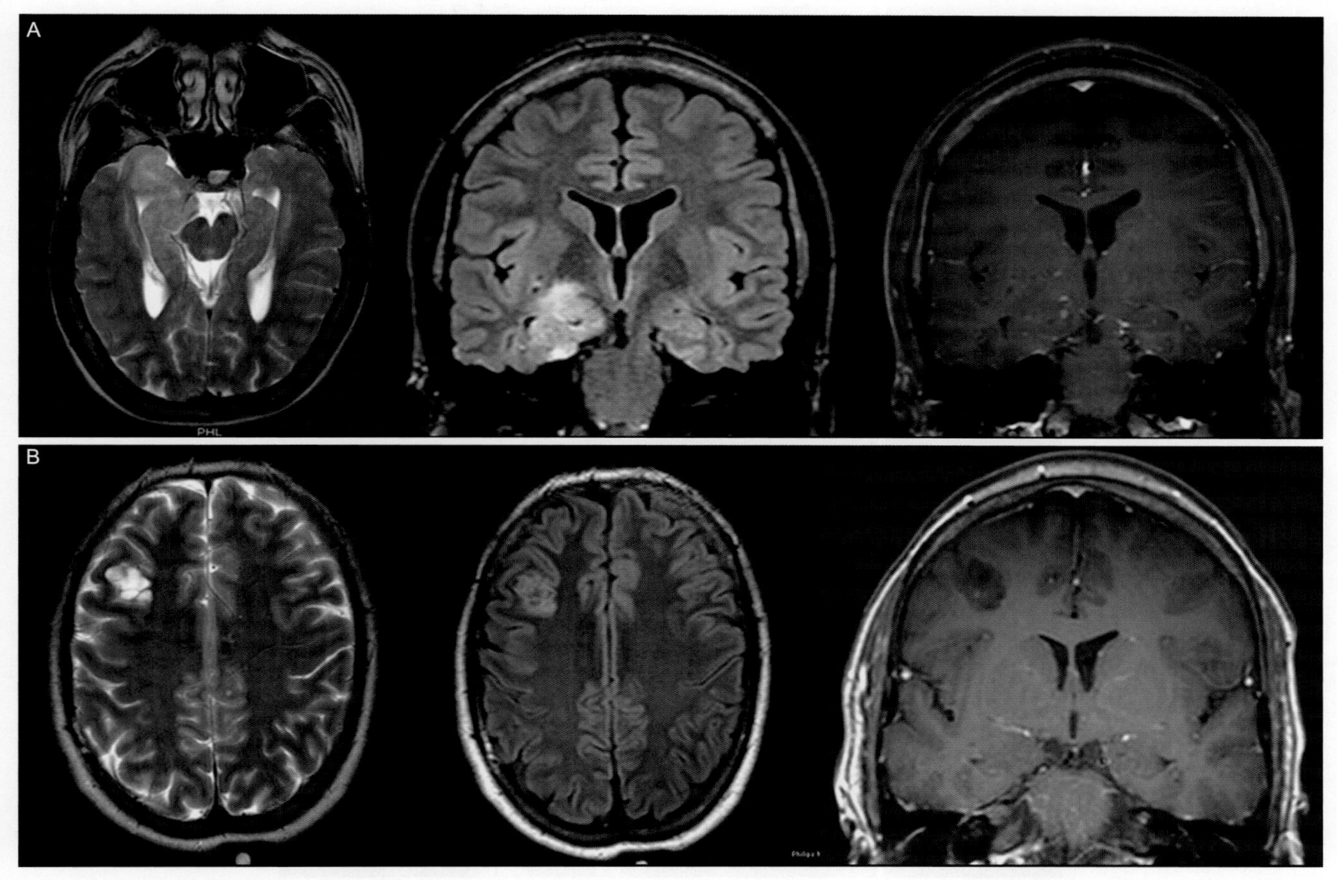

图 10.4　长期癫痫相关的节细胞胶质瘤和胚胎发育不良性神经上皮瘤。（A）一例 19 岁药物难治性癫痫患者，1 岁起病，发现颞叶内侧的节细胞胶质瘤，为 WHO I 型。肿瘤累及颞极内侧、钩回、杏仁核、海马、海马旁回以及向后延伸超过背侧中脑的水平。（B）一例 22 岁药物难治性癫痫男性患者，病史 6 年，发现位于右额的胚胎发育不良性神经上皮瘤

个生殖细胞层，乳腺癌、非髓样甲状腺癌和内膜癌的风险也随之增加。PTEN 突变携带者患乳腺癌、甲状腺癌、内膜癌的生存风险分别达 85%、38% 和 28%。孤立性和散发性的 LDD 也可以出现，并归因于体细胞的 PTEN 突变。儿童 LDD 患者中，也有罕见的非 PTEN 突变的报道（Pilarski et al.，2013）。

LDD 可引起小脑分子层和内颗粒细胞层的增大，并充满了发育不良的神经节细胞（图 10.5）。这在大体标本上显示出增厚且多形的小脑脑叶。MRI 上 T2 相显示了“虎纹样”的特点，增强扫描可见片状强化。由于 MRI 的特点非常具有特异性，往往不需要组织病理学即可诊断该病（图 10.6）。LDD 可伴有脑积水、巨脑畸形、脊髓空洞、脑膜瘤、海绵状血管瘤和静脉血管瘤。目前为止还不清楚 LDD 属于错构瘤还是真正的肿瘤。有些既往被认为是 LDD 的患者，最终被诊断为真正的神经胶质细胞肿瘤。LDD 的临床表现可能为偶然间发现或小脑肿物的逐渐增大。减压手术是首选的治疗方法，病灶边界不清是外科手术的主要技术难点，这也与远期生存相关。放射治疗可使患者症状稳定，但会加重神经功能的退化（Prestor et al.，2006）。

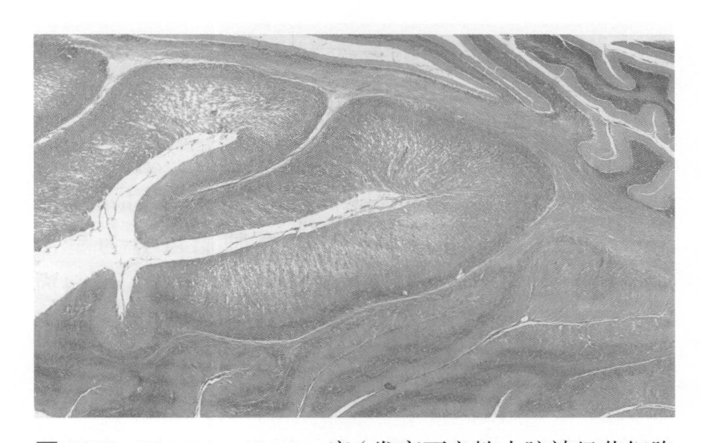

图 10.5　Lhermitte-Duclos 病（发育不良性小脑神经节细胞瘤），最好于显微镜低倍视野下观察，最显著的特点为受累的小脑皮质增厚，并且缺少深染的颗粒细胞层。可与图中右上角的正常皮质做比较

Courtesy of Dr Kieren Allinson, Department of Pathology, Addenbrooke's Hospital, Cambridge.

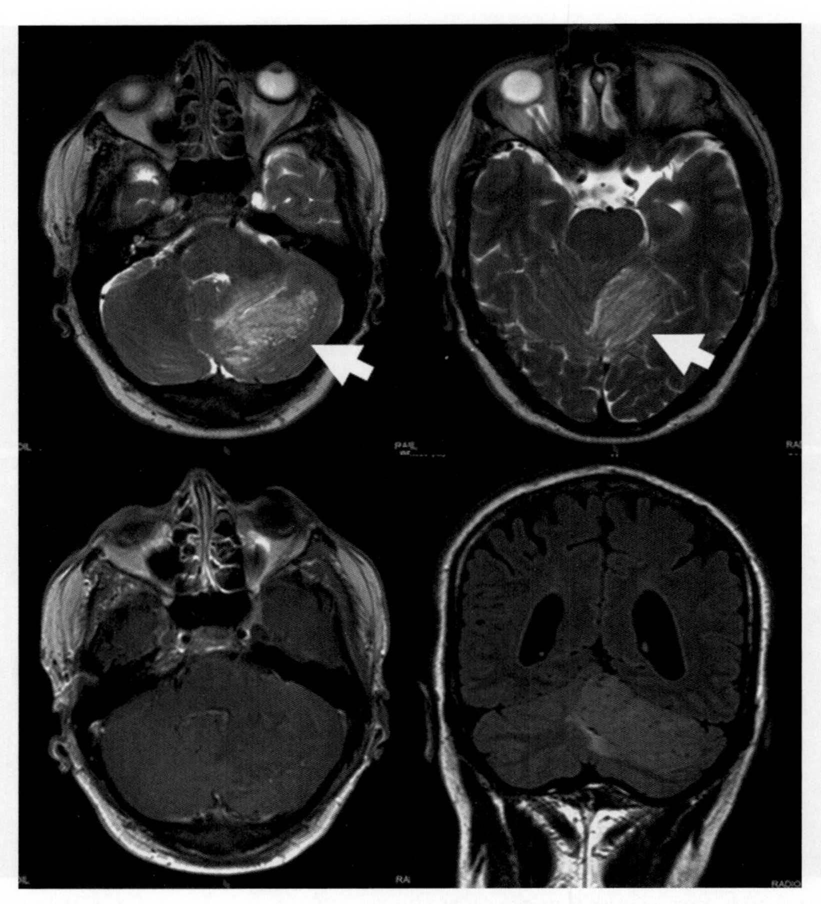

图 10.6 一例有 PTEN 基因突变的 50 岁男性，患有发育不良性小脑神经节细胞瘤（Lhermitte-Duclos 病），伴 Cowden 综合征。影像上可观察到条纹状增厚的小脑叶（箭头处）

非胶质神经元的 LEATs

弥漫性星形细胞肿瘤和少突胶质细胞肿瘤在癫痫外科手术中并不少见。近期本中心的一组研究中，26/158 例（16.5%）的病例可归为此类（Grote and Simon，2015）。组织学上，这类肿瘤可分为星形细胞瘤、混合型胶质瘤和少突胶质细胞瘤，可归为 WHO Ⅱ级和Ⅲ级。各类肿瘤常发生 IDH1 突变（本组病例占 39%），然而，这个数据明显低于弥漫性胶质瘤的 IDH1 突变率，60%~90%。这也是 LEAT 生物学的特点。肿瘤主要分布于颞叶和额叶，也可分布于旁边缘系统（比如岛叶）。影像学表现上，LEAT 和非 LEAT 的弥漫性胶质瘤无明显不同。无论是肿瘤还是癫痫相关的预后均较好，在本中心的一组数据中，35 例 WHO Ⅱ级和 3 例 WHO Ⅲ级星形胶质细胞瘤的患者因肿瘤及难治性癫痫行肿瘤切除手术，10 年无进展生存期和总生存期分别为 75% 和 90%（Luyken et al.，2003），术后 1 年癫痫无发作率约 70%。同构星形细胞瘤是一种非常罕见的弥漫性星形细胞瘤变型，其临床病程非常良好（Schramm et al.，2004）。

毛细胞型星形细胞瘤占癫痫外科手术的 2.5%~10% 以上。特征是由双极性星形细胞和 Rosenthal 纤维组成的双相生长模式。毛细胞型星形细胞瘤和节细胞胶质瘤鉴别诊断困难，这可能也在一定程度上解释了已发表的临床队列研究中发病率有相对变化的原因。毛细胞型星形细胞瘤与丝裂原活化蛋白激酶（mitogen-activated protein kinase，MAPK）通路的改变相关。小脑外的毛细胞型星形细胞瘤包含的变异包括：BRAF：KIAA1549 的融合和复制（大约 60% 的病例），BRAF V600E、FGFR1、KRAS，NF1 和 PTPN11 突变，NTRK2 的融合（Jones et al.，2013）。致痫性的毛细胞型星形细胞瘤常见于颞叶。MRI 常见囊性改变并伴有近期出血。最典型的影像表现为大的囊性改变，囊壁和瘤结节强化明显。增强扫描可为明显强化或无强化（**图 10.7**）。肿瘤学和癫痫相关的预后较好，与节细胞胶质瘤相似。并非所有患者均如此。我们发现在一组 44 例毛细胞

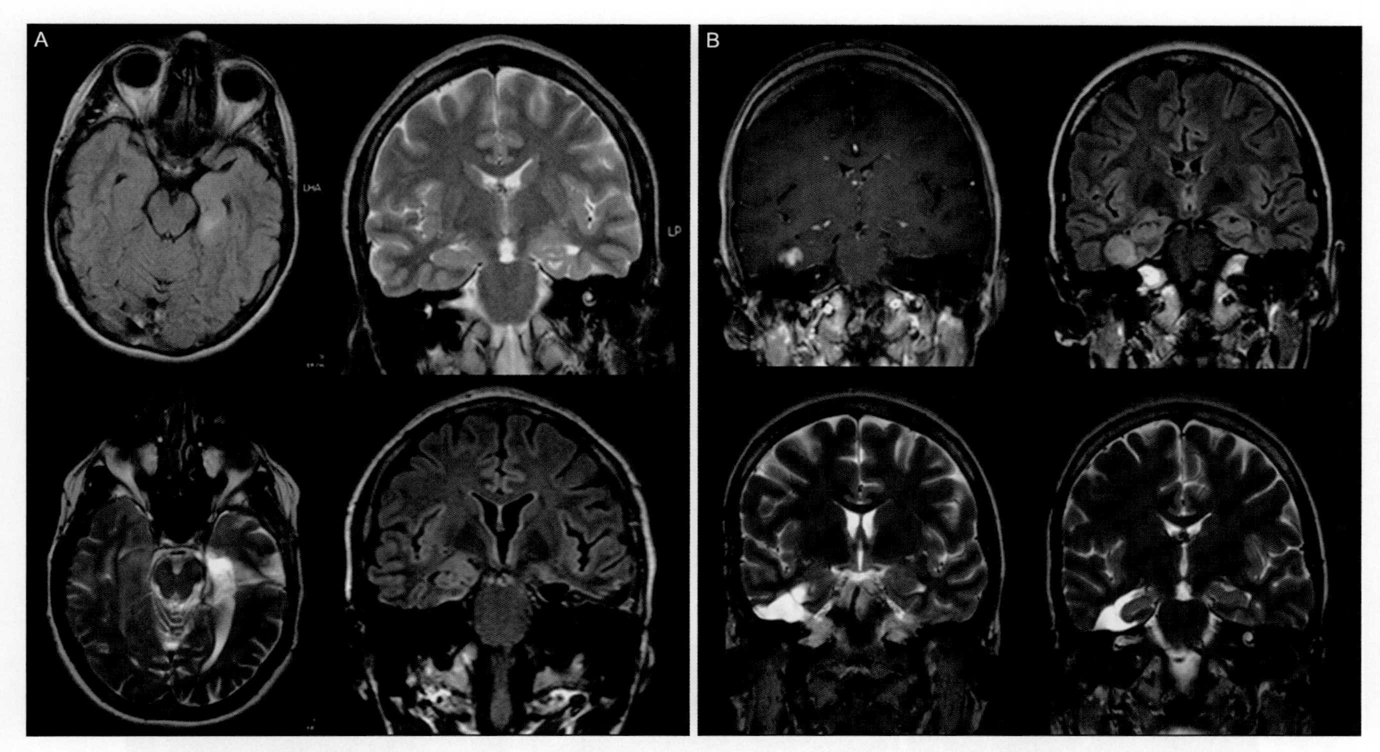

图 10.7 外科手术治疗颞叶内侧基底节相关的长期癫痫相关性肿瘤：切除或保留海马。（A）上排：一例 36 岁女性患者，有 32 年癫痫病史，在左侧海马旁回发现节细胞胶质瘤（WHO Ⅰ级）。肿瘤累及部分海马结构，伴海马硬化。下排：手术为扩大病灶切除术，包括切除杏仁核和海马。患者术后 3 年无癫痫发作，术后一直在幼儿园做一名全职老师。海马切除不仅控制了癫痫，且未造成神经心理功能损伤。（B）上排：一例 34 岁女性，5 年癫痫病史，在颞枕脑回的外侧发现胚胎发育不良性上皮细胞瘤（DNT）。下排：手术为扩大病灶切除，由于影像学、症状学、脑电图均未提示癫痫为海马起源，故手术保留了海马和杏仁核结构。患者术后 3 年无癫痫发作

型星形细胞瘤的成人病例中，5 年无进展生存率和总生存期分别为 72% 和 87%。组织学上，14% 的病例为不典型，而 6% 的病例为间变性特点。该类患者可受益于肿瘤全切和部分切除或活检等治疗，目前没有证据表明放疗或化疗可阻止肿瘤的进展（Stuer et al.，2007）。

多形性黄色星形细胞瘤（pleomorphic xanthoastrocytomas，PXAs）常见于儿童和青年。组织学表型十分多变，单核与多核的巨型星形细胞和黄色瘤细胞相混合（图 10.8）。MRI 常见一囊性团块，伴有局灶性增强和浅表脑皮层软膜生长（图 10.9）。大多数肿瘤分布在幕上，尤其是颞叶。大部分 PXAs 属于 WHO Ⅱ级。病灶间变性特点和有丝分裂增强（核分裂象大于每 10 个高倍视野下 5 个有丝分裂）达到近 1/3 的病例。PXAs 常可监测到 BRAF V600E 的基因突变（65%~80%），但无 IDH1 突变。与间变性肿瘤相比，BRAF V600E 突变更常见于 WHO Ⅱ级的肿瘤，并且可能与位于颞叶以及患者年龄较小相关。大多数患者症状表现为癫痫（大于 60%~80%），且所有肿瘤癫痫手术的患者超过 5% 为 PXA（Luyken et al.，

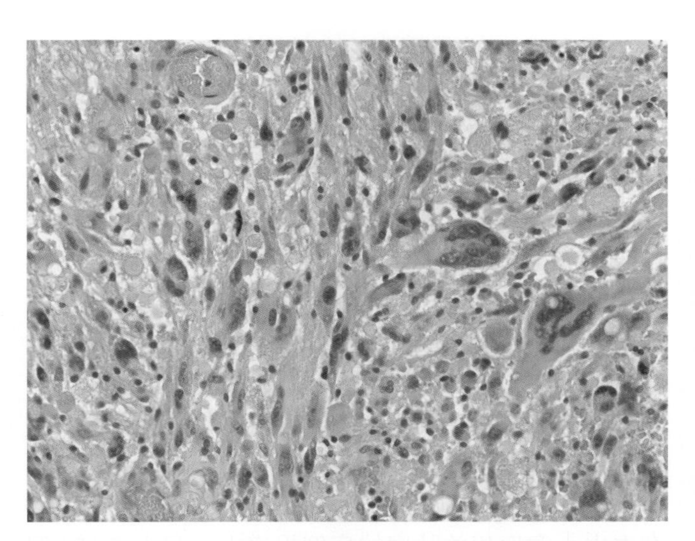

图 10.8 多形性黄色星形细胞瘤（WHO Ⅱ级）可见纺锤形的星形细胞，并伴有较大的多核多形性细胞。脂质液泡、嗜酸性颗粒体和血管旁淋巴细胞也是其共同特点

Courtesy of Dr Kieren Allinson, Department of Pathology, Addenbrooke's Hospital, Cambridge.

2003；Ida et al.，2014；Grote and Simon，2015）。针对 PXA 及相关癫痫的治疗手段，外科手术是选择之

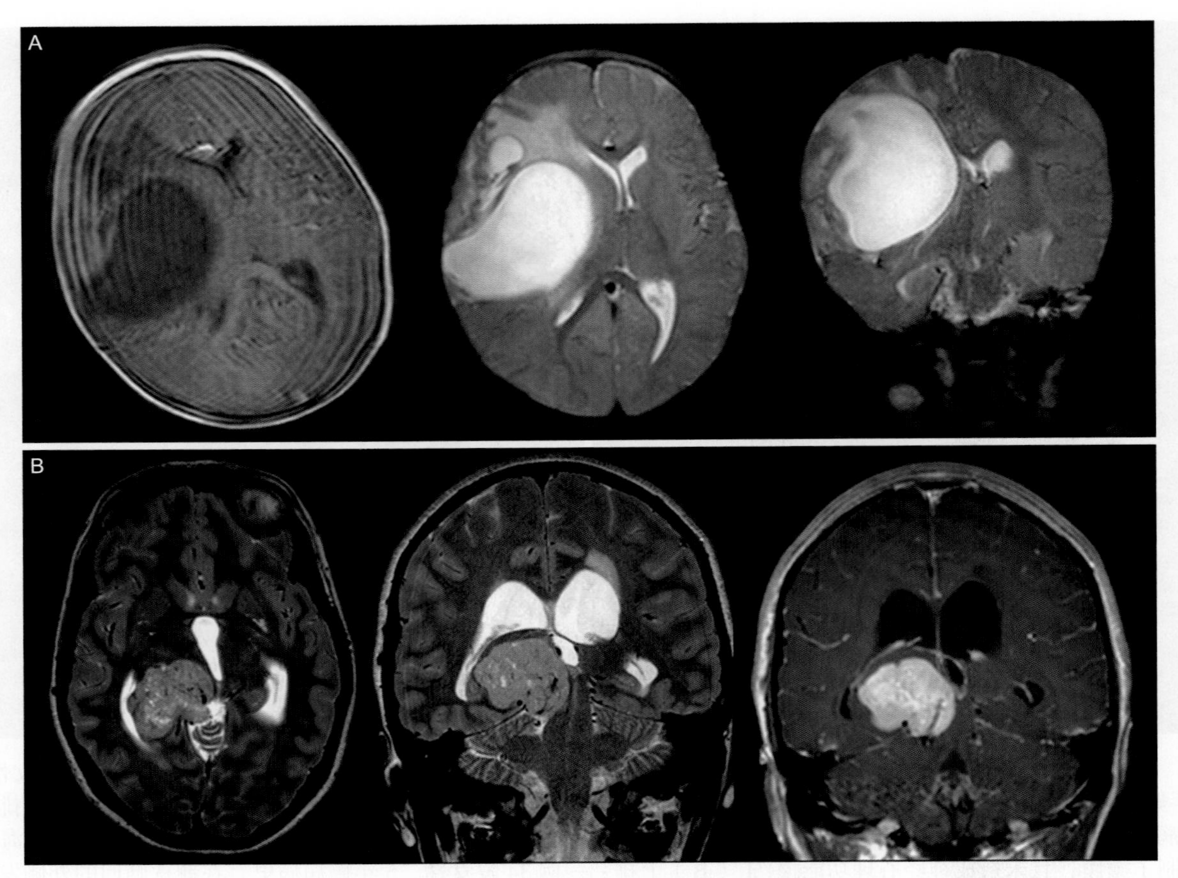

图 10.9 （A）一例 8 个月大的女婴，右侧额顶区可见婴儿发育不良性节细胞胶质瘤。（B）一例 25 岁女性，有脑积水的症状，影像学发现背侧丘脑和颞枕脑回的中部可见不典型的脑室外神经细胞瘤（WHO Ⅱ级）

一。在 Luyken 的研究中，一项平均随访了 8 年的队列研究，5 例与癫痫相关的 PXA 无一例复发（Luyken et al.，2003）。而如果包含无长期癫痫的 PXA 患者，结果显示不佳：PXAs WHO Ⅱ级的术后患者，5 年无进展生存率和总生存率分别为 71% 和 90%。而间变性 PXA 患者，5 年无进展生存率和总生存率分别仅有 49% 和 57%。与次全切除或活检的患者相比，肿瘤全切可显著提高生存期（Ida et al.，2014）。针对间变性 PXA，一些研究支持放射治疗和烷化剂化疗的有效性。BRAF 的抑制剂维罗非尼对有些病例有效，而有些则无效。

血管中心型胶质瘤（angiocentric gliomas，ANETs）在本中心癫痫相关肿瘤的病例报道中，只占 5/158 例（3.1%）（Grote and Simon，2015）。ANETs 好发于儿童和青年患者中，最主要的临床表现为癫痫发作。组织学上，ANETs 的特点是双极细胞组成的血管中心生长模式，和室管膜瘤样的特征，比如像假玫瑰花结一样，属于 WHO Ⅰ级。肿瘤好发于额叶和颞叶（Chen et al.，2014）。本中心报道的 5 例患者中，无 BRAF V600E 或者 IDH1 突变。在某些 ANETs 中，可见 MYB 或 MYB11 异常（Zhang et al.，2013b）。在这些肿瘤中，也未见染色体 1p/19q 杂合性缺失。影像学通常提示累及白质的病灶不强化（**图 10.10**）。该类肿瘤的预后通常较好，但个别间变性肿瘤的病例会出现肿瘤复发。

其他胶质神经元性的肿瘤

乳头状胶质神经元肿瘤（papillary glioneuronal tumour，PGNT）被认为是非常罕见的肿瘤类型。组织学上，这些肿瘤的特点是假乳头状生长和乳头间片状或局灶性的神经元细胞聚集。MRI 和 CT 的特点类似于节细胞胶质瘤，然而，与节细胞胶质瘤相比，PGNT 的环形强化并不少见，且位置并不常好发于颞叶，脑室旁生长相对常见。有报道发现 1 例 FGFR1 突变的患者（Gessi et al.，2014a）。肿瘤全切往往提示预后良好。然而，尽管 PGNT 属于 WHOI 级，肿瘤复发并不少见。最近的一篇综述分析了 71 例病例后发现该肿瘤 2 年无进展生存率为 82%。甚至还有一例原发性转移性播散的病例报道。少数病例（其中

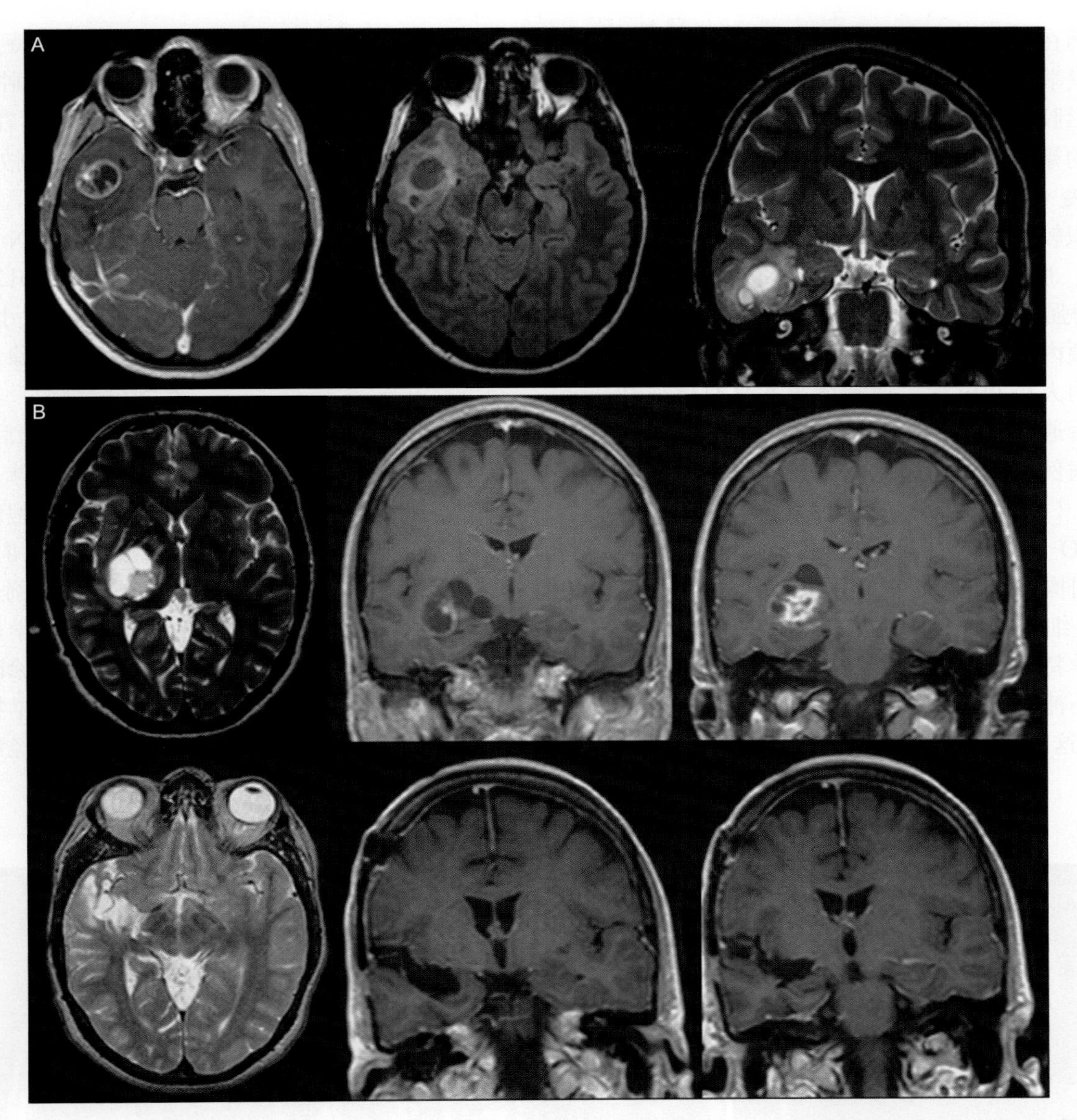

图 10.10 （A）一例 17 岁女性患者，病灶位于右侧颞叶，出现全面性癫痫发作，诊断为毛细胞型星形细胞瘤，WHO Ⅰ级，已手术治疗。（B）上排：位于杏仁核背侧和基底节的毛细胞型星形细胞瘤，WHO Ⅰ级。一例 50 岁的女性，主诉头痛，伴有其他非特异性的症状。（B）下排：术后 MRI 示无肿瘤残留。术后未出现新发神经功能缺陷

多数病例为残余肿瘤）需行放射治疗（Schlamann et al.，2014）。

第四脑室伴菊形团形成的胶质神经元肿瘤（rosette- forming glioneuronal tumour of the fourth ventricle，RGNT）起初被认为是位于小脑的 DNT，但是目前被认为 WHO 分类的一类特殊疾病，被归为 WHO Ⅰ级。大约 20% 的病例位于颅后窝的外侧，常临近三脑室，甚至位于脊髓。病理表型上，一方面这种双相的肿瘤伴有均一的神经细胞，形成菊形团和血管周假菊形团，另一方面，有类似于毛细胞星形细胞瘤的星形胶质细胞成分。8 例患者中可出现 2 例 FGFR1 突变（Gessi et al.，2014b）。MRI 通常显示囊性和实性混合，并且占位通常不强化。治疗上，通常选择手术治疗，目标是完全切除肿瘤。然而，也有其他观点，最近有 41 例患者的文献报道显示，全切并不比次全切更具优越性（Zhang et al.，2013a）。由于肿瘤的位置以及与周围组织结构的粘连或浸润，外科手术较为困难，且很容易出现术后新发的功能缺失。2014 年的一篇综述指出，转移性播散的比例大约 7%，死亡患者约 6%（Schlamann et al.，2014）。

婴儿发育不良性节细胞胶质瘤（desmoplastic infantile gangliogliomas，DIG）和婴儿发育不良性星形细胞瘤（desmoplastic infantile astrocytomas，DIA）是非常罕见的位于额顶脑膜的 WHO Ⅰ级的肿瘤。大

多数病例在 1 岁以内即被诊断，且男性的发病率略高。组织学上，典型表现为增生性间质具有混合的新生星形胶质细胞，成分可变的神经元细胞和未分化细胞的聚集体。DIG/DIA 可出现 BRAF V600E 的基因突变（Koelsche et al.，2014）。影像学通常表现为体积较大位于硬膜基底的囊性分隔的占位（**图 10.11A**）。肿瘤的实性部分通常附着于脑组织皮层和硬膜。增强可见肿瘤的实性部分强化明显。患者通常表现为颅内压增高。治疗上，可考虑外科治疗，基于肿瘤的大小和位置，通常该手术具有挑战性。全切的预后通常较好。然而，在大龄儿童中，通常约 40% 的病例需术后辅助化疗和放疗。播散性的病例并不少见（Hummel et al.，2012）。

WHO 分类列举了几种肿瘤变异，组织学上通常以小的同构神经元为特征，因此被称为神经细胞瘤。中枢神经细胞瘤会在本书的其他章节描述。具有相似的组织学特性，但不伴有脑室内生长的类似肿瘤称为脑室外神经细胞瘤（extraventricular neurocytomas，EVN）。这种肿瘤可在脑内生长，也可在颅顶外生长。EVN 通常属于 WHO Ⅱ级。影像学特点包括囊性占位，异质性增强，占位效应和周围水肿反应（**图 10.11B**）。非典型的组织病理学特点包括在大约 1/4 的患者中，观察到有丝分裂活动增加（例如：MIB-1 指数＞3%）。不典型的EVN通常预后较典型EVN差。近期的文献回顾报道，非典型和典型 EVN 的 5 年缓解率分别为 36% 和 68%（Kane et al.，2012）。全切对控制 EVN 效果显著，但基于肿瘤的大小和位置，全切的难度较大。放疗可作为不完全切除术后的补充治疗方案。

许多小脑脂肪神经细胞瘤是典型的颅后窝肿瘤。该类肿瘤通常起源于小脑蚓部和小脑半球，生长可延伸至脑池。肿瘤细胞由同形神经元细胞组成，伴有局部的脂肪瘤分化，通常被归为 WHO Ⅱ级。MRI 影像特点反映了脂质化结构的分布和比例。增强扫描可见肿瘤不均匀强化。对于神经影像学医师和神经病理学医师而言，该病最主要的鉴别诊断是髓母细胞瘤和室管膜瘤。实际上，这些肿瘤早期也被称之为脂质化的髓母细胞瘤。小脑脂肪神经细胞瘤有

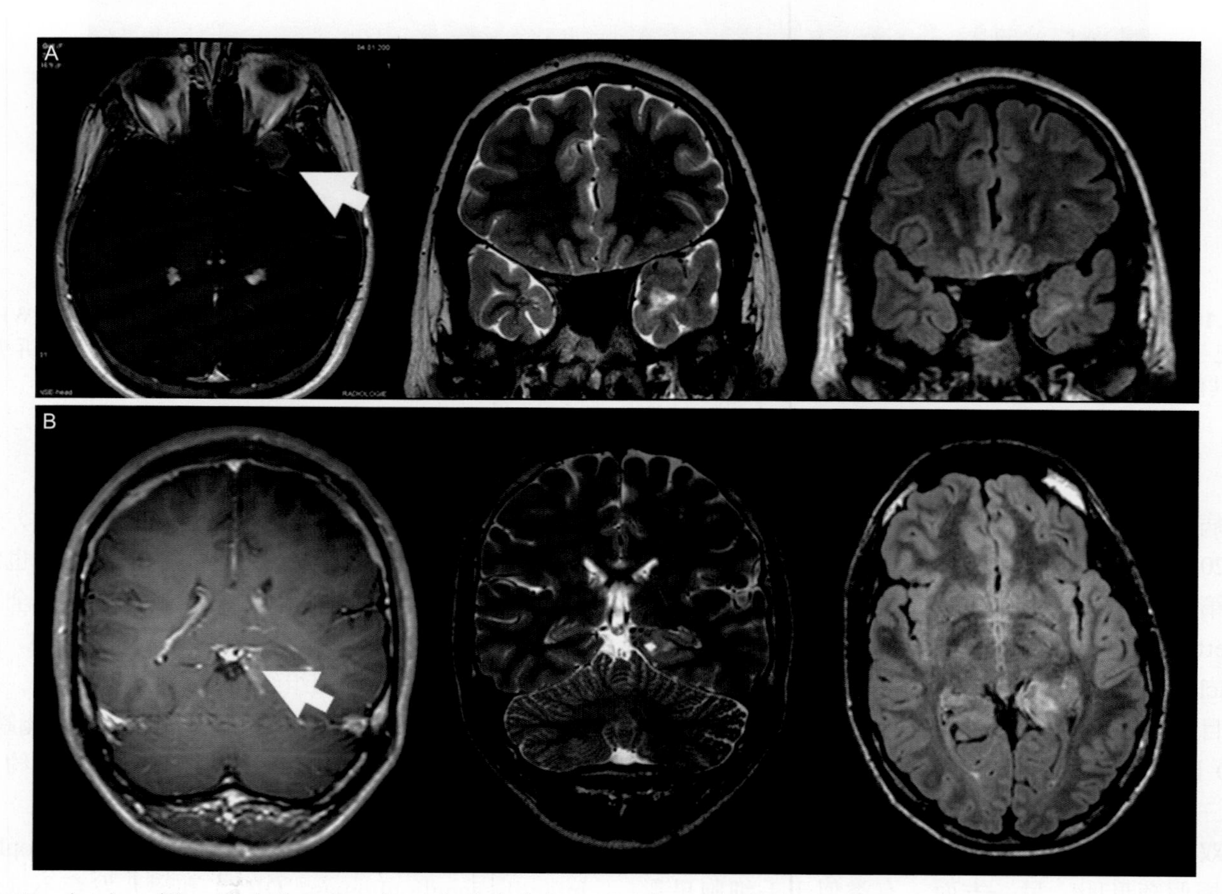

图 10.11 （A）一例 20 岁女性患者，有 18 年癫痫病史，可见位于颞极的多形性黄色星形细胞瘤，WHO Ⅱ级。（B）一例 19 岁男性患者，因一次复杂部分性癫痫发作被诊断为多形性黄色星形细胞瘤（WHO Ⅱ级），肿瘤位于颞枕脑回的中间偏背侧。可以观察到软脑膜的明显生长（箭头处）

较高复发率，并降低了总体生存期。一篇 19 例病例报道的综述显示，该病 5 年生存期仅 48%，并且个案报道描述了肿瘤的临床进展性和组织学的间变性。小脑外幕上的脂肪神经细胞瘤也有相关报道。手术可作为该病的治疗方式（Chakraborti et al.，2011）。放疗的作用仍有争议。

争议

针对手术治疗颞叶相关的 LEATs，是否需行海马切除？

相比于肿瘤的生长，手术治疗 LEATs 的目的更偏重于控制肿瘤相关的癫痫发作。为了达到这个目的，外科医生采取了各种手术策略，从单纯的肿瘤切除或“病灶切除术”，到肿瘤加周围皮质的切除（病灶扩大切除术）。该种切除包括了额外的皮层切除，或颞叶内侧结构的切除，以达到完整切除致痫灶的目的（Zaghloul and Schramm，2011）。后一种手术策略有时需要在术前做侵袭性的癫痫相关检查，或需要术中行皮层脑电图监测。

针对是否切除，以及何时切除肿瘤及周围皮质，仍然是一个有争议的问题。支持单纯病灶切除的第一个观点是行这种术式的患儿常常有良好的预后。根据近期的文献回顾报道，约 80% 的颞叶低级别肿瘤的患者行肿瘤全切后，均可达到癫痫无发作的水平（Englot et al.，2012）。第二个观点是有关神经功能的保护。即使经验丰富的术者行颞叶内侧切除，也会有较低的概率出现偏瘫、失语和显著的视野缺损。与整个颞叶切除相比，行局限性颞叶病灶切除术的患者，其神经心理学结果可能更好（Schramm，2008）。切除了 MRI 阴性并且组织病理学阴性的海马结构，会明显增加记忆受损的风险（特别是累及优势半球侧的手术）。而对于术前海马已有病变的手术来说，切除病变的海马后，记忆倒退的情况相对少见（Helmstaedter et al.，2011）。有趣的是，在一项 207 例颞叶内侧癫痫患者的随机对照组中（>95% 的患者均为颞叶内侧海马硬化），范围更广的海马切除并不意味着更好的癫痫预后（Schramm et al.，2011）。

然而，另一种情况是颞叶 LEAT 的手术可以进行颞叶内侧结构的切除。首先，相比于只切除肿瘤，如果手术切除全部海马和周围的颞叶皮层，更多的患者会有良好的预后（最近的文献报道两者的癫痫无发作率分别为 79% 和 86%~87%）（Englot et al.，2012）。值得注意的是，这些数字可能低估了扩大切除术对癫痫预后的影响，因为难治性的癫痫可能常常接受更为广泛的切除性手术。其次，合适的手术策略需要考虑到癫痫的病理生理特点。同时伴有药物难治性癫痫和神经胶质 LEATs 的患者，可能具有其他病理结果的情况并不少见。至少有 1/4 的节细胞胶质瘤的患者伴有皮质发育不良，这种病理类型在 DNTs 的患者中可能更常见（Thom et al.，2012）。在 LEAT 的病例中，也可能伴有海马硬化（**图 10.12A**）。此外，肿瘤不仅可能通过对周围脑部施加压力和刺激而引起癫痫发作（单纯病灶切除术的基本原理）。肿瘤相关的癫痫常常起源于肿瘤边界，即在肿瘤和周围正常脑组织之间，也有可能出现在肿瘤远隔的脑组织（需术中皮层脑电图证实）（Zaghloul and Schramm，2011）。

我们的手术策略是对于那些由于颞叶外或颞叶新皮层的 LEATs 导致的颞叶新皮层癫痫，采取扩大病灶切除的手术方法（例如：肿瘤全切加切除 0.5 cm~1 cm 的肿瘤外侧边界）。如果病灶位于重要功能区边界或功能区上，我们采取单纯病灶切除的手术方式。术前的影像学检查非常重要，目的是为了判断有无其余的致痫病灶（例如：通过影像学辨认致痫病灶和肿瘤病灶的边界）。若肿瘤累及颞叶内侧结构，手术范围应涉及颞叶内侧结构，包括海马、海马旁回和临近的颞叶内侧组织边界（**图 10.12**）。如

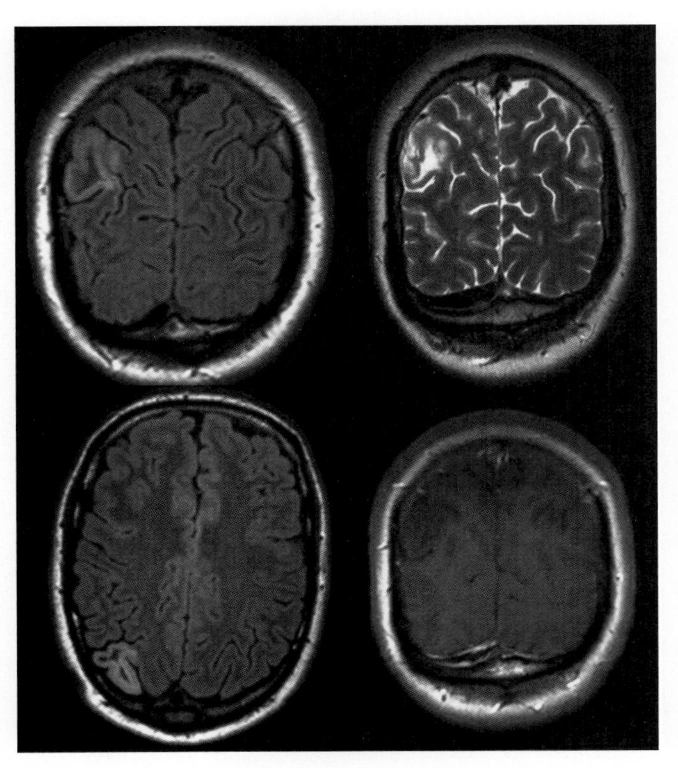

图 10.12 一例 20 岁男性患者，有 3 年癫痫病史，可见位于右侧顶叶的血管中心型胶质瘤（ANET）

果认为癫痫方面的获益超过潜在的不良神经心理后遗症，那么术前的深部电极脑电图结果或术中皮层脑电图结果可为切除范围提供相关的临床证据。经验证实优势半球侧的海马切除手术有更高的神经认知倒退的相关风险（例如记忆丧失）。

延伸阅读、参考文献

扫描书末二维码获取。

第 11 章　脑肿瘤放射治疗与放射外科

Susan Short 著
张敏 译，高献书 审校

病史：恶性脑肿瘤患者的管理和治疗

所有疑似脑瘤的患者都应通过一个包含所有相关临床和医疗专家组成的多学科综合治疗团队（multidisciplinary team，MDT）来进行检查和治疗。在多学科讨论之前，需要提供临床病史和相关的影像学资料（一般为颅脑增强 MRI 扫描）。

大多数情况下首选手术，既可以切除肿瘤、缓解占位效应等症状，又可为组织学诊断提供材料。但肿瘤往往具有高度侵袭性，手术不能切除显微镜下的亚临床病灶，单独手术很难治愈。因为伦理原因，不可能开展随机研究来比较不同手术切除范围的疗效，但在大多数恶性肿瘤中，手术切除范围与总体疗效呈正相关。

最近的研究通过采用 5- 氨基乙酰丙酸（5-aminolevulinic acid，5-ALA）荧光引导或术中 MRI 图像引导手术切除的技术，可以实现最大范围安全切除（Schatlo et al.，2015）。手术后，汇总临床病史、影像资料和组织病理学等数据，进行多学科讨论，制订后续治疗策略，尽快转诊。大多数情况下，根据肿瘤组织学以及临床因素（包括患者的年龄和一般情况）等，患者需要进行辅助放疗和（或）化疗。同时，多学科讨论也是一个重要的机会，可以判定患者是否应加入临床研究，以测试新疗法的效果。

放疗仍然是原发性脑肿瘤术后最有效的治疗手段，meta 分析结果已经证实了其对Ⅲ、Ⅳ级胶质瘤的疗效。关于最常见的成人胶质瘤 GBM（胶质母细胞瘤），2005 年 EORTC 发表了一项具有里程碑意义的研究，确立了其标准治疗模式，即术后放疗 6 周（60 Gy/30 次，周一至周五），同步使用替莫唑胺（temozolomide）化疗，其疗效优于单独放疗（Stupp et al.，2005）。联合治疗后中位生存期达 14 个月。

在间变性星形细胞瘤（WHO Ⅲ级星形细胞瘤）中，最大限度安全切除后采用类似剂量的外照射仍然是标准的治疗方法。但联合模式治疗是否会像 GBM 那样进一步改善疗效，尚有待观察，目前正在进行相关研究（EORTC 26053-22054）。对Ⅲ级少突胶质细胞瘤，放射治疗也是重要治疗方法。EORTC 26951 和 RTOG 9402 两项研究均比较了放疗伴或不伴辅助化疗 [甲卞肼、CCNU、长春新碱（PCV 方案）] 的疗效，长期随访数据显示术后联合治疗有明显的生存获益（大于 10 年）。

在低级别胶质瘤中，放射治疗的作用仍有待商榷。对存在临床高危因素而不适合行根治性手术等有适应证的患者，放射治疗仍然是标准治疗。最近一项欧洲Ⅲ期临床研究（EORTC 22033-26033）比较了替莫唑胺化疗作为一线治疗与放射治疗疗效，二者无进展生存相当，目前正在等待分子病理学定义的亚组分析结果（Baumert et al.，2016）。低级别胶质瘤往往是广泛性生长的，也就意味着对相对年轻的患者要进行大范围的脑组织照射，限制了放射治疗的应用。目前还不能确定是否需要和高级别肿瘤一样高的放疗剂量，尚无比较照射 45 Gy 和 60 Gy 疗效的大型研究。低级别少突胶质细胞瘤，根据 WHO 2016（Louis et al.，2016）报告的分子病理分型，如果存在 1p19q 染色体缺失，其对放疗联合 PCV 化疗的反应特别好，与高级别胶质瘤类似。

放射治疗基础科学

放射生物学原理

放射是一种有效的治疗肿瘤的方法。当射线作用于细胞时，会造成细胞损伤；而癌细胞对射线的耐受性比正常细胞差，因此射线可以选择性地杀灭肿瘤细胞。真核细胞受照后，主要毒性损伤是 DNA 双螺旋的双链断裂（double- strand break，DSB），所有细胞都有一系列复杂的机制来识别和修复这些损伤。哺乳动物细胞中有两种主要的 DNA DSB 修复通路，包括非同源末端连接（non-homologous end-joining，NHEJ）和同源重组（homologous recombination，

HR)。非同源末端连接在整个细胞周期中都是活跃的，而同源重组只有当姐妹染色单体作为修复受损链的模板时，可在细胞周期 S 和 G2 期起作用。两个通路的修复平衡均受初始修复的动力学和其他一些可影响染色质结构的蛋白质影响。两者之间一个重要区别是：同源重组采用正常的模板来再生受损的 DNA，通常不出错；而 DNA 序列可能在重新连接的链端之间丢失，因此非同源末端连接容易出错。也是因为这个原因，非同源末端连接的修复可能致突变并导致辐射诱发恶性肿瘤。**图 11.1A** 总结了每个通路中的信号事件和主要效应蛋白。

原则上，通过靶向癌细胞中独特的修复通路或与正常细胞相比表现出过度依赖的通路，可以有效地增强辐射的细胞毒性效应。比如合成致死性，其修复抑制剂靶向特定的、在修复能力异常的肿瘤细胞中活跃的修复路径。在胶质瘤中，虽然放疗联合替莫唑胺化疗已被证明能显著改善 GBM 患者的预后（Stupp et al.，2005；Stupp et al.，2009），但几乎没有证据将其直接归功于放射增敏。放射增敏指的是，临床前研究中，两种治疗方式联合起来产生的一种附加效应。目前关于详细的 DNA 修复分子生物学研究仍在持续，以寻找到新的放化疗增敏靶点。

多种方法可用于评估辐射对细胞的影响，包括使用免疫荧光（immunofluorescent，IF）染色技术显示蛋白质在受损 DNA 位点的再定位。目前已经证明对磷酸化的组蛋白 H2AX 的免疫荧光染色非常有效，这种蛋白在 DNA DSB 的位点被快速磷酸化，而 DSB 修复时又被快速去磷酸化。细胞核中可以看见磷酸化蛋白的单个斑点，其数量与诱导的 DNA DSB 呈线性关系，从而可以量化损伤和分析修复动力学。辐射后早期显示的斑点数也可用于间接测量辐射剂量。**图 11.1B** 为这种方法的示例。

受照射后细胞存活和剂量的关系更复杂，反映出细胞修复损伤的能力存在差异。对于大多数暴露于 X 射线下的细胞，例如，用细胞克隆形成试验测定的存活剂量 - 反应关系是线性二次曲线，其存活曲线存在一个拐点，当辐射剂量超过该剂量时，细胞对每单位剂量敏感性更高。不同类型细胞的拐点不同，但正常组织的拐点往往低于肿瘤细胞。因此一个重要的和长期确立的放射生物学原则是，将大的总辐射剂量分割成小剂量每周五次进行放疗，耐受性更高。分次放疗允许对单次大剂量耐受性差的正常组织在治疗后修复和再生，因此标准的放射治疗模式是每日剂量（分次）约 2Gy，根治性剂量（约 60 Gy），6 周内完成。将正常组织排除在治疗范围之外，每天更大的剂量或单次大剂量，即放射外科手术，是可以耐受的。

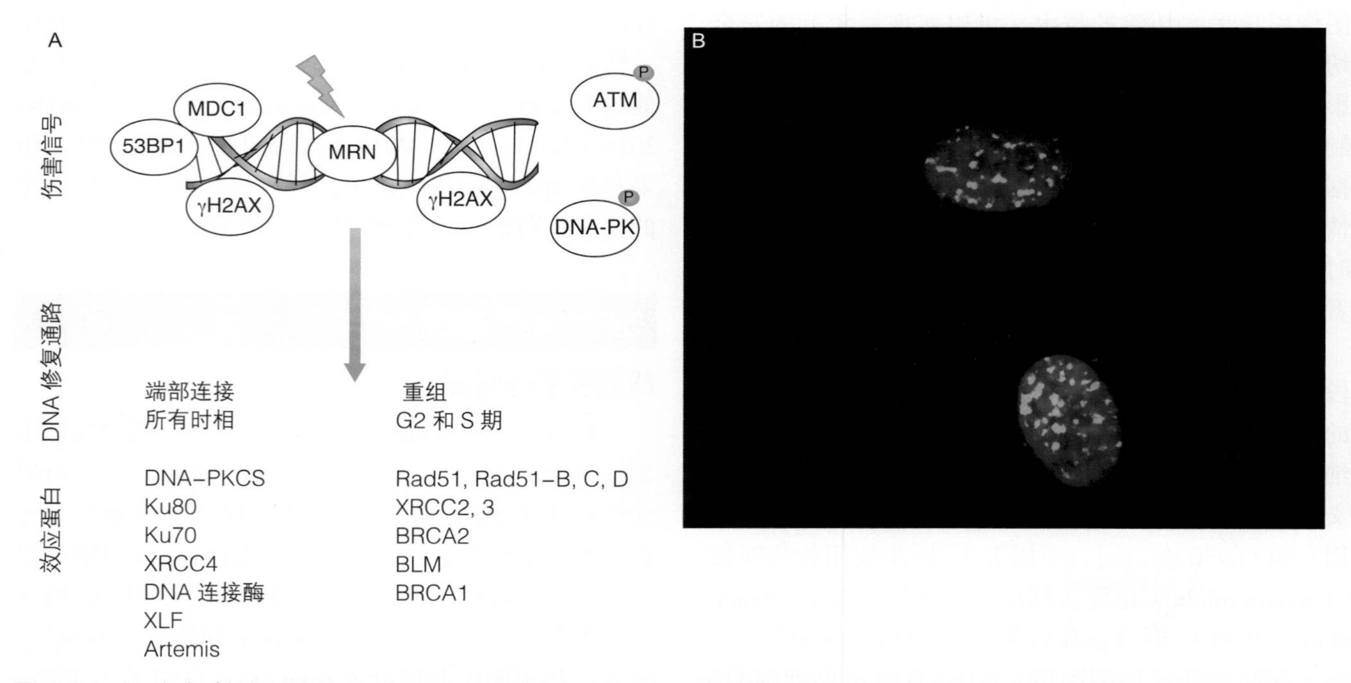

图 11.1 （A）辐射致 DNA 双链断裂后激活的、哺乳动物细胞中存在的两种主要 DNA 损伤修复途径以及涉及的主要信号和效应蛋白。（B）受辐射后，胶质瘤细胞修复蛋白 γH2AX 染色的范例。细胞核用 4'，6- 二氨基 -2- 苯基吲哚（4'，6-diamidino-2-phenylindole，DAPI）染色（蓝色），磷酸化蛋白染色为绿色

放射物理

现代放射治疗通过有效传送高能（兆伏级）X射线进行治疗。临床所用射线最常由直线加速器产生，其采用微波电场将电子加速到高能，通过撞击金属靶产生次级X射线，其后通过两级准直器的滤过和均整，产生满足一定平坦度和对称性要求的具备特定能量范围和形状的治用射野。射线能量决定了大部分能量沉积及后续发生细胞损伤的组织深度。对于高能射线，这个组织深度在几厘米范围内。为了在组织深部产生剂量的高能沉积区，可将不同方向的多个光束聚焦在肿瘤靶区上，使得射线交叉处产生剂量累积，同时减少入射通路上正常组织的剂量。在三维空间中设计治疗计划时，将靶区置于射线交叉处，以达到高剂量射线沉积于肿瘤以及保护周围正常组织的目的。增加照射野数量或采用动态野照射，使得更小体积正常组织受到给定肿瘤剂量的照射，以实现对正常组织的进一步保护。

放射治疗技术

外照射适形放疗

常规适形放射治疗通常采用由MRI和计算机断层扫描（CT）相结合的三维诊断成像。其中一个数据集（通常是CT）是在患者处于预定治疗位置时（模拟定位）得到的，这样解剖结构就可以与治疗情况交叉参考。然后二次成像数据集[通常是MRI，有时是正电子发射断层扫描（positron emission tomography，PET）]可以以数字方式叠加在CT图像上。患者被固定在个体化的热塑膜中，用于CT成像和后续治疗，确保不同类型肿瘤治疗的准确、适形和可重复性。随后进行如前所述照射野的计划设计，通常采用3~4个静态光束，剂量按比例从不同光束方向依次给予，使肿瘤获得高剂量照射，同时减少正常组织剂量。当三维靶区非常复杂，或辐射敏感的危及器官邻近肿瘤靶区的凹陷处时，这种方法的局限性也很明显，三维适形放疗无法实现在保护正常组织的同时给予肿瘤高剂量放疗。在中枢神经系统中，靠近眼眶后部和颅底的区域尤为相关。

调强放疗

调强放射治疗（intensity-modulated radiotherapy，IMRT）通过动态调节辐射束来进行治疗。它是通过使用多叶准直器来实现的，当光束离开机头时，多叶准直器在光束路径内移动，以便对光束在到达患者之前进行3D调制。从而可以实现对更复杂形状靶区，尤其是凹陷形肿瘤靶区的高度适形治疗。

在临床和剂量学研究中已经评估了调强放射治疗颅脑肿瘤的适用性，它可以有效地靶向治疗这些肿瘤（Khoo et al.，1999；Narayana et al.，2006）。随着技术的进一步发展，出现了可以更快速进行放射治疗的Arc（弧）模式，其通过减少放射束的“准备时间”来优化调强放射治疗，减少患者需要在治疗床上的时间。由于使用多个照射野时内部散射高，该方法还降低了人体总剂量。图11.2比较了胶质瘤患者的三维适形与调强放疗方案。

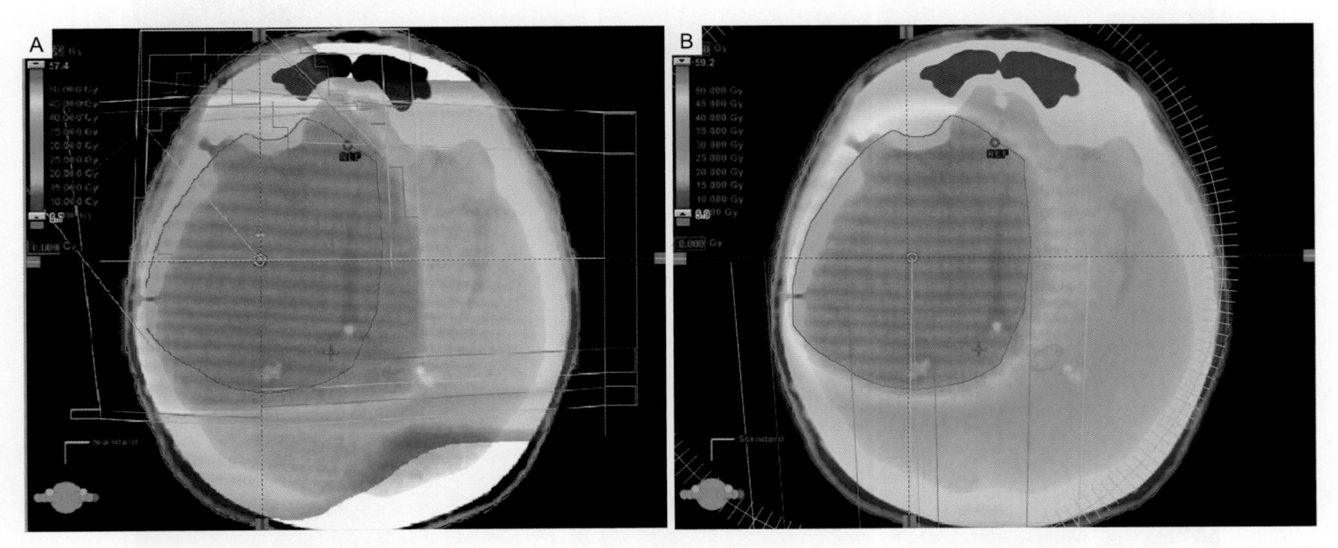

图11.2　一例胶质瘤患者的CT轴位图，分别为相同靶区下的三维适形放疗计划（A）和IMRT放疗计划（B）的等剂量曲线。红线内为靶区。红色区域为高剂量区，蓝色区域代表靶区外的低剂量区（<30%）。海马作为危险器官单独勾画（左，橙色线；右，蓝色线）

立体定向放射外科

放射外科指以产生局部肿瘤消融为目的的单剂量高聚焦放射治疗。如前所述，正常组织从大的单次辐射剂量中修复的能力有限，这意味着这种方法的应用通常限于小的、特定的可以将局部正常组织排除在照射野之外的靶区。历史上，放射手术最常用的是基于钴的技术（伽玛刀），它将多个源瞄准在一个点上，在辐射束的交叉点（等中心）产生非常高的剂量，且光束前方具备陡峭的剂量跌落。在这种方法中，患者被固定在头部框架中，以确保在三维空间中的准确照射。同样的治疗也可以使用其他技术来实现，例如赛博刀，它在图像引导下通过机器人手臂传送辐射剂量，而不需要固定框架。

因为肿瘤体积很大，呈浸润性生长，无法精确勾画靶区，因而大多数恶性脑肿瘤不适于放射外科。利用放射外科手术为高级别胶质瘤靶区内部推量提高放疗总剂量的临床研究，并没有获益（Baumert et al.，2003；Baumert et al.，2008）。但放射外科是目前治疗脑转移的标准方法，因为脑转移灶往往比较小，易于勾画（**图 11.3**）。

近距离放疗

近距离放疗是将放射源直接放置在肿瘤内或肿瘤术床的放射治疗。尽管既往曾有大量研究使用多种近距离治疗技术，试图给预后不良的肿瘤采取局部推量放疗，但目前近距离放疗在颅内肿瘤的应用并不常见。总的来说，近距离放疗对脑瘤疗效欠佳，几乎没有局部肿瘤控制良好的报道，但大多数研究表明放射性坏死的风险增加。最近，有些研究开始探索将近距离放疗作为有争议部位肿瘤手术的替代方法，然而，这种方法的有效性有待于随机研究的评估（Ruge et al.，2013）。

硼中子俘获治疗

硼中子俘获疗法是基于辐射剂量局部增强的原理。将含硼化合物（通常是硼化氨基酸，如苯丙氨酸）输注入肿瘤内，然后用局部低剂量中子束照射，激活硼发射 α 粒子来实施放疗。肿瘤细胞氨基酸膜转运系统增强，可选择性地摄取硼 - 氨基酸化合物，从而可以选择性地使肿瘤细胞对中子照射敏感。原则上，这也适用于照射范围内任何部位的侵袭性肿瘤细胞，使这一方法更具吸引力。这一治疗方式所面临的挑战包括提供放疗时所需的足量硼化合物，以及产生和靶向低能中子束所需的专业设备。世界上有几个研究团体正在研究这项技术，但尚未广泛应用，也尚未在临床研究中正式与常规放射治疗进行比较（Miyatake et al.，2009）。

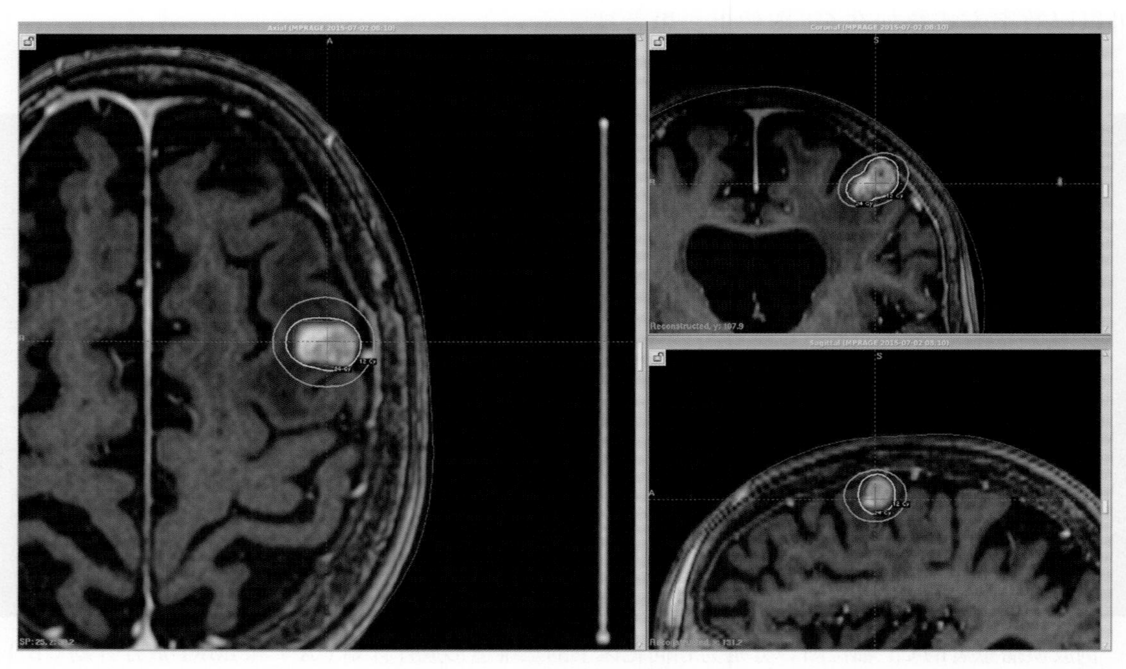

图 11.3 脑转移患者放射外科治疗计划图（轴向、冠状、矢状）。黄线所示区域为高剂量靶区，绿线所包为高剂量区域，显示各个方向上肿瘤外的剂量跌落

质子治疗

质子放疗利用带电质子代替 X 射线进行放射治疗。其优点来自组织中带电粒子的特殊剂量分布。质子能量大量沉积在一个小范围内，称为布拉格峰，它的位置取决于射线的能量和射线穿过的组织。可以利用特定光束对特定点进行高剂量照射，而其深部组织几乎不受到照射。正常组织紧邻肿瘤靶区或大体积的放射敏感组织位于照射野出射路径中的情况下，优势特别明显。因此，质子束放射治疗可用于常规 X 射线束治疗可能会导致正常组织毒性风险极高的情况，例如临近视路和脑干或脊髓的颅底病变。这对许多儿科肿瘤来说也是一个优势，发育中的正常组织对辐射暴露特别敏感，因此去除照射路径中的放射剂量可以显著降低远期毒性的风险。**图 11.4** 所示为质子束在组织中的剂量沉积示意图（A）和颅底肿瘤患者的质子束治疗计划（B）。

放疗的局限性和副作用

尽管优化了复杂的放疗方法，治疗期间非肿瘤组织也不可能被完全排除在照射野外。在中枢神经系统中，相关正常组织包括头皮的皮肤和头发、未受侵的脑功能区（non-involved eloquent brain）、试听器官、垂体和脑血管。这些组织都表现出剂量依赖性毒性，根据所涉及的组织在不同的时段出现。通常按出现的时间早晚将副作用分成早期反应和晚期反应，早期反应在数周内出现，晚期反应在数月至数年内出现。还有一种副作用可发生在中间时间，表现为嗜睡综合征（Powell et al.，2011）。常见的早期反应包括脱发和皮肤红斑，在开始治疗后 3~4 周内出现。晚期反应包括垂体功能衰竭、视听通路受损以及认知缺陷。**图** 11.5 显示了一组描述放射治疗急性副作用发生时间的数据。

正常脑组织的一种重要辐射诱发病变表现为正常组织坏死，可发生在治疗后 6 个月至数年之间。这种并发症的发生率与总剂量、分次剂量和正常脑组织受照体积相关。放射性坏死可能无症状，也可引起颅内压升高或产生局灶性神经症状。最佳预估放射性坏死发病率在接受常规分割放疗的患者中不到 5%；但当提高分次剂量或者正常脑组织受照体积增大，其发病率升高，放射外科术后出现脑组织放射性坏死发生率高达 25%。MRI 扫描上很难鉴别放射性坏死和高级别肿瘤进展。放射性坏死典型的表现是区域局部强化，因为血脑屏障被破坏导致，无法与有活性的肿瘤组织鉴别，且发生时间与肿瘤复发高发时段重合。开发能够可靠地区分辐射坏死和肿瘤复发的成像技术，包括使用 PET、SPECT 或改进 MRI 技术，是一个活跃的研究领域。如果后续治疗选择依赖于是否有活性肿瘤成分的存在这一判断，那么活检仍然是区分这两种情况的决定性方法。

在大多数情况下，疑似放射性坏死时采用支持治疗，可使用类固醇药物来减少水肿，必要时可在

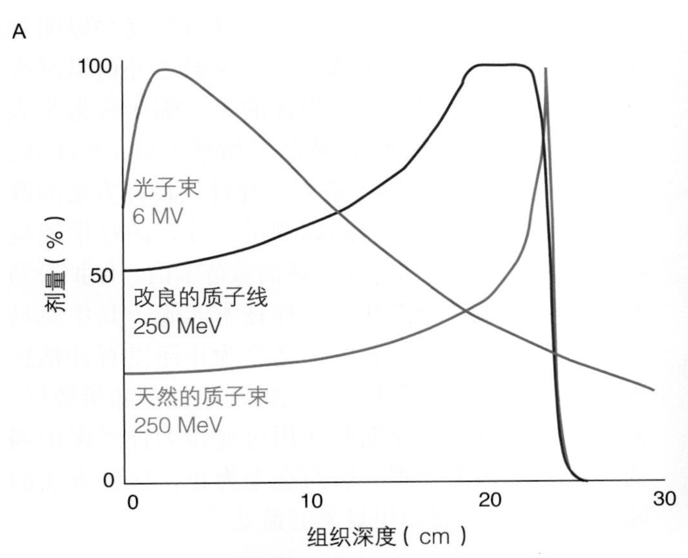

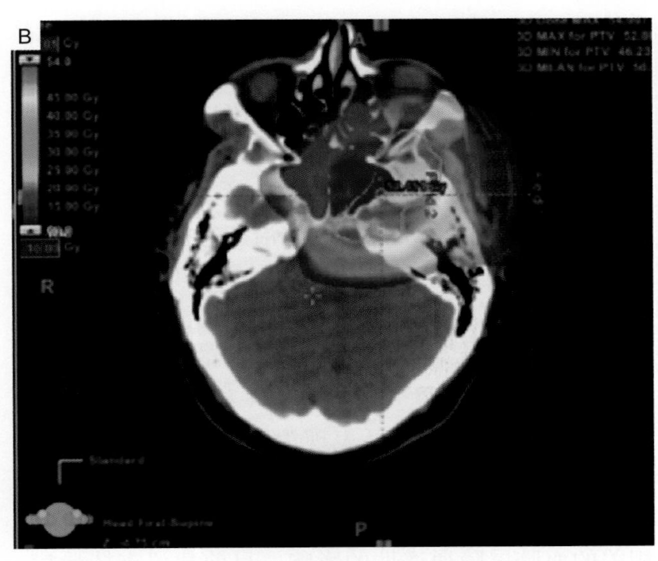

图 11.4 （A）光子束在组织中的能量沉积不同，最大剂量邻近表面，显著剂量超出组织最大范围（粉线）。相比之下，质子束的能量沉积在布拉格峰这一较窄的深度范围内，布拉格峰外其剂量呈陡峭下降（天然质子束，红线）。可以加宽组织中布拉格峰的范围（改良的质子束，蓝线），代价是接近表面剂量增加。（B）颅底肿瘤患者的质子束计划剂量分布图。蓝色等剂量线代表低剂量区域，在肿瘤靶区外急剧跌落

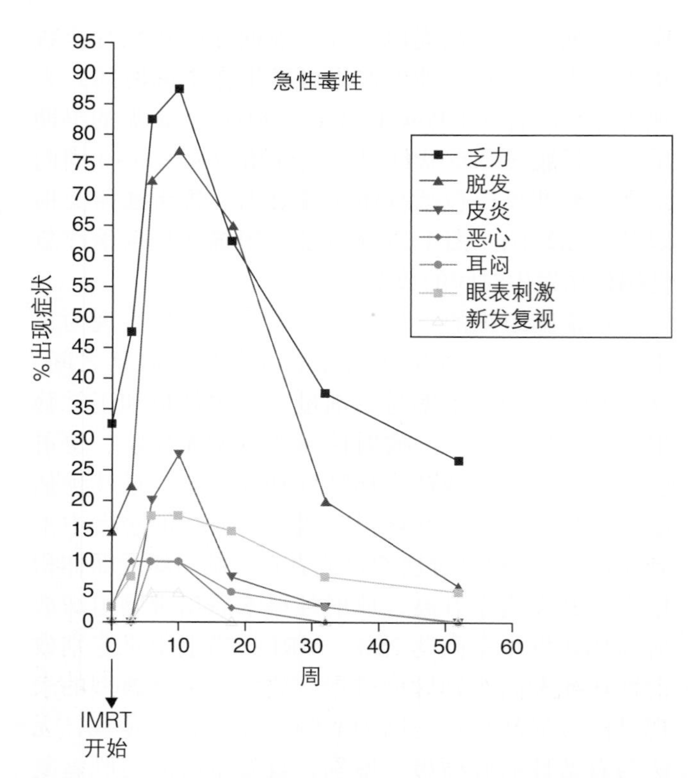

图 11.5 50 例接受颅底调强放疗的患者放疗急性期毒副作用的发生发展过程

Reproduced by agreement with Dr J. Maclean.

严密的临床和放射监测下使用脱水药物。这种情况下应用血管内皮生长因子（vascular endothelial growth factor，VEGF）抑制剂的文献越来越多，一些小型研究报道了贝伐珠单抗（一种人源化抗 VEGF 单克隆抗体）在对类固醇无反应的症状性放射性坏死患者中的良好疗效。一系列小型研究还报道了高压氧治疗（hyperbaric oxygen therapy，HBO）有效，其原理是通过增加血浆载氧量来增加对受损组织内输送氧的能力，从而促进恢复。HBO 一个疗程至少 20 次。HBO 应用不广，一般用于其他治疗选择受限的患者。如果病变占位效应明显且对类固醇或其他药物治疗没有反应，应考虑手术切除。

在接受手术和辅助放（化）疗的患者中，存在"假性进展"的问题。早期随访（放疗后 1~2 个月）时磁共振成像图像上可表现为肿瘤体积增大强化；通常无症状，无需特殊干预即可消退。这表明其发生的潜在原因是治疗引起的与神经或血管组织损伤相关的血脑屏障通透性的影响。目前建议支持治疗，4~6 周后重新评估，此时假性进展可开始逐渐消失。

最常见的辐射诱发肿瘤是脑膜瘤，辐射诱发恶性肿瘤很少，包括胶质瘤和肉瘤（Brada et al.，1992；Minniti et al.，2005）。真正的辐射诱发恶性肿瘤的发病率很难确定，特别是在中位生存期很短的人群中。来自儿科人群的数据表明，尽管暴露时低龄也被认为是导致规定剂量风险增加的一个重要因素，脑照射后的风险很高，可能比未照射人群高 5~10 倍。流行病学数据，例如原子弹存活数据证实了与剂量成正比的恶性肿瘤的风险，但这些全身剂量很难转化为仅部分器官体积暴露于高剂量治疗的患者的风险估计，而且这些患者的风险可能较低。然而，目前已确定的辐射致突变潜力和现有数据，特别是儿童癌症幸存者的数据，表明：随着治疗效果的提高，降低辐射诱发恶性肿瘤的风险非常重要。现代放射治疗技术可以更精准地照射肿瘤并减少暴露于高剂量的周围正常组织，有助于降低辐射诱发恶性肿瘤的风险。然而，其中一些技术，包括调强放射治疗，也可能增加暴露于极低剂量辐射的正常组织的体积，目前尚不清楚低剂量照射对总体长期风险的影响。迄今为止，还没有关于使用调强放射治疗或质子束治疗的脑部后的第二种癌症风险的研究。

晚期毒性发生机制与中枢神经系统内皮和胶质细胞受损有关（Benczik et al.，2002；Otsuka et al.，2006）。中枢神经系统内的大多数细胞是有丝分裂后的细胞，因此对辐射不敏感。中枢神经系统中最敏感的分化细胞类型是少突胶质细胞群体，较低剂量照射后即可发生脱髓鞘（Panagiotakos et al.，2007）。目前的脑放疗后迟发毒性模型包括位于特定解剖和生物部位（包括脑室下区和海马）的干细胞样细胞群丢失的影响。在啮齿类动物模型中，这些细胞的丢失与认知缺陷有关，目前正在进行研究，以明确是否将富含干细胞的区域排除在辐射之外可以减少这些长期的副作用。令人担忧的是，临床数据集表明干细胞群体对极低辐射剂量敏感（Marsh et al.，2010）。这些数据引发了放射治疗计划设计方法的改变，如果不影响对肿瘤的高剂量放疗，治疗期间应将这些大脑区域特别排除在高剂量范围内。保护海马的技术可以通过调强放射治疗技术实施，其中海马被定义为一个危险器官，但迄今为止还没有评估这种方法对神经认知结果的影响的前瞻性的随机数据。另一种方法是在放疗期间使用可能作为神经保护剂的药物，例如美金刚。然而迄今为止，这种方法的随机研究还没有显示出显著的益处。

个案介绍

患者 70 岁，因驾驶时的实发反应迟钝就诊。体检发现患者的左侧肢体运动障碍，注意力不集中。完善检查，脑 MRI 代表性图像如图 11.6 所示。患者右额叶病变经活检证实为Ⅲ级少突胶质细胞瘤，伴 1p19q 杂合性缺失（loss of heterozygosity，LOH）。

伴有 1p19q LOH Ⅲ级胶质瘤的标准治疗是外照射联合化疗。但对年龄大于 70 岁的老年人，尚无随机对照研究进行疗效评估。对类似此患者的多灶性病变，因肿瘤总体积很大，可能临近多个危险器官，放射治疗难度极高。在这种情况下，病灶累及多叶，且临近视交叉，关注点在于照射野如何包括整个肿瘤。另一种方法是先化疗来减少肿瘤体积，以减少放疗范围，降低放疗的毒副作用。并非所有肿瘤都对化疗有效，但大多数 1p19q 杂合性缺失的患者对化疗敏感。

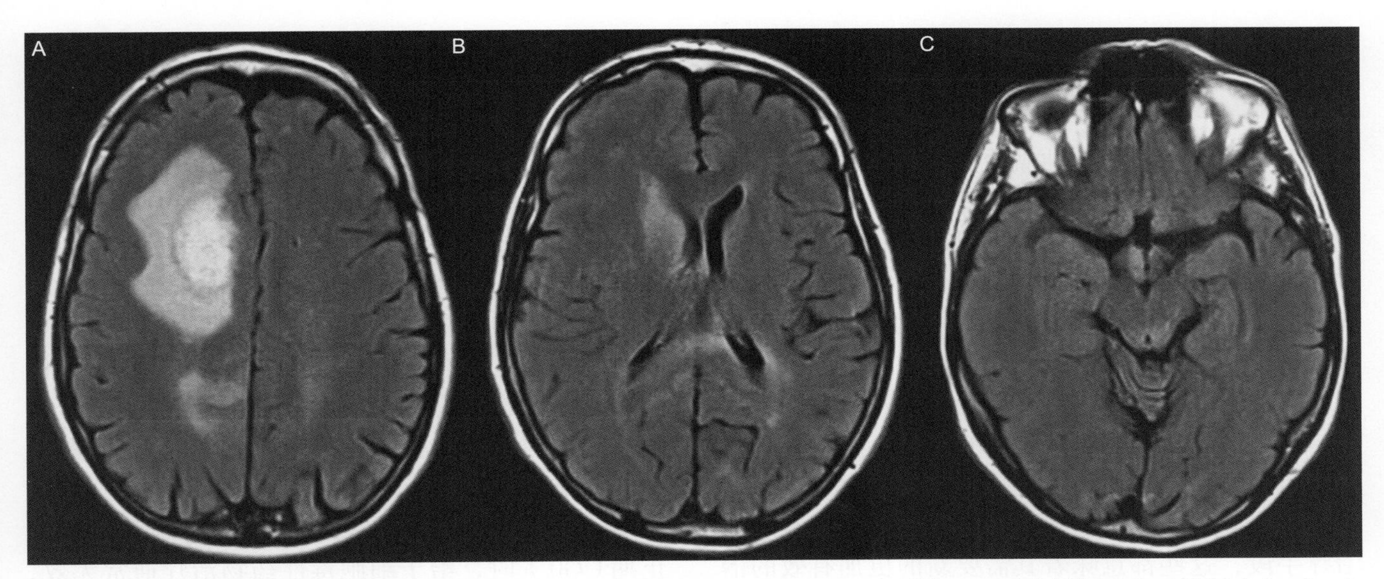

图 11.6 MRI 液体衰减反转恢复（fluid-attenuated inversion recovery，FLAIR）图像，显示右侧额叶和双侧顶叶（A）、右侧尾状核头和胼胝体（B）和右侧穹隆和右侧乳头体（C）的多灶高信号区

延伸阅读、参考文献、EBRAIN 的相关链接

扫描书末二维码获取。

第 12 章　脑肿瘤的化疗

Nicholas F. Brown • Daniel Krell • Paul Mulholland 著
田艳 译，吴世凯 审校

引言

手术切除虽然是脑肿瘤治疗的主要选择，但由于恶性脑肿瘤膨胀性生长和侵袭性特点，往往无法达到完全切除。扩大切除范围可以改善患者预后，但往往带来致残神经功能缺陷（Lacroix et al.，2001）。脑肿瘤一旦复发往往侵袭入正常脑组织当中，放疗等局部治疗应用也有一定局限性，这种情况下化疗通常会成为一种重要选择，因为化疗不仅延长生存期，还可以维持脑肿瘤患者的功能状态。

但与脑外肿瘤相比，化疗在脑肿瘤中的作用目前仍然有限。高级别脑肿瘤的预后差、缺乏有效的治疗手段，这些都意味着其需要新的更加有效的治疗方法。目前一些新的化疗药物正在临床试验阶段，可能为未来的脑肿瘤治疗提供选择。

在这一章中，我们将概述化疗的基本概念、分子标志物的应用、治疗反应的监测、化疗药物在神经胶质瘤中应用的药理学基础，以及未来的研究方向，但不包括其他原发性脑肿瘤（非胶质瘤）和脑转移性疾病的化疗。

化疗的基本概念

目的

化疗治疗癌症的基本原理是基于对单个转化细胞如何通过遗传不稳定和突变的累积最终发展成恶性肿瘤的理解。癌症的获得性标志性特征包括：发展出持续的增殖信号、逃避生长抑制因子、免疫抑制、避免细胞死亡、永不停止的复制，并诱导血管生成、侵袭和转移（Hanahan and Weinberg，2011）。这些标志性特征每一个都是现在和未来治疗的靶点。

脑肿瘤化疗的目的是延长患者生存期或缓解患者临床症状（姑息性），也可辅助其他治疗，提高其他治疗的有效性（辅助治疗）。尽管化疗在其他肿瘤中存在术前应用（新辅助治疗），但目前还没有证据表明脑肿瘤新辅助化疗可以提高患者的治愈率。

作用机制

细胞毒性药物作用于细胞分裂阶段，通过阻断DNA或其核苷酸前体合成的关键步骤来杀死细胞，也可通过破坏DNA结构的完整性来杀死细胞。这类药物应用于癌症的基本原理是癌细胞更加容易复制。然而，正常组织中也含有分裂细胞，因此细胞毒性药物的作用通常是非选择性的，这就解释了为什么化疗存在广泛的、常见的相关毒性，特别是骨髓抑制、胃肠道症状、疲劳、神经病变、不孕症、致畸、认知障碍和脱发。同理，当癌细胞处于细胞周期静止期（G0）时，给予细胞毒性药物治疗通常无效，当这些癌细胞再次进入细胞周期时，肿瘤将再次生长（Chabner and Loeffler，2015）。

应用原则

在一定时期内，一定剂量的化疗能够杀死一定比例的肿瘤细胞，而与肿瘤大小无关，即所谓的“部分杀伤”（Berenbaum，1972）。由于药物在肿瘤中浸润不良可降低肿瘤的杀伤作用，全身毒性也限制给药的剂量，因此，目前化疗主要采取反复多周期给药方案，其目的是通过连续杀死癌细胞来消除癌细胞群。化疗时的给药剂量通常是最大的耐受剂量，化疗间隔则需要足以使毒性恢复。这些参数在早期试验中已经被确定。化疗时通常采取联合给药方式，从而可以通过不同的作用机制增加疗效（相加或协同），又使毒性交叉重叠最小化。实际上，大多数化疗药物的剂量限制性毒性都是骨髓抑制，这也是联合给药时最常见的限制因素。

局限性

化疗存在多个缺陷。原发性耐药或获得性耐药会影响化疗的效果。耐药机制包括癌细胞表面转运泵的形成、基因扩增或化疗靶点的修饰、凋亡通路的缺陷和DNA修复基因的上调等。肿瘤内的遗传异质性降低了化疗杀死肿瘤内所有癌细胞的可能性，而随着时间的推移，不同位置肿瘤之间的“空间”遗传异质性和“时间”异质性进一步加剧了这一点。通常正常血管结构的破坏会限制药物进入肿瘤。对于脑肿瘤，尽管血脑屏障已经被破坏，但它对化疗来说仍然是一个独特的屏障。血脑屏障毛细血管之间的紧密连接可以阻止大分子和亲水性分子的运输，转运泵可以将药物从脑组织转移到脑脊髓液中，这些都限制了潜在有效化疗药物的浸润。虽然大多数化疗药物是通过静脉或口服给予的，但由于血脑屏障的存在，脑肿瘤治疗中出现了很多替代给药方法，包括外科局部给药和对流增强给药技术等。

其他疗法

非细胞毒性药物治疗包括靶向治疗和免疫治疗。靶向治疗是使用小分子或单克隆抗体对抗肿瘤细胞中突变或过表达的细胞内蛋白或细胞表面受体，目的是增加癌细胞杀伤，减少全身毒性。免疫疗法的目的是利用先天性和适应性免疫系统来靶向癌细胞，这将在本章后面详细讨论。

临床试验

临床试验是引进新疗法的基础，而新的化疗药物和联合方式也正在不断发展中。良好的临床实践（Good Clinical Practice，GCP）是一项国际质量标准，它提供了一个框架，以确保人体试验以规范、符合伦理和科学的方式进行。

- Ⅰ期临床试验主要目标是评估一种新化合物的安全性和毒性，是通过剂量递增设计来确定最大耐受剂量；次要目标是确定这种化合物药代动力学数据、药物活性和临床疗效。
- Ⅱ期临床试验是评估该化合物的活性，并继续评估其安全性和耐受性，试验过程通常被设计为随机的，并以安慰剂作为对照。
- Ⅲ期临床试验通常是以标准治疗方法作为对照，确立新疗法的疗效。它是药品监管机构（英国药品和健康管理局、美国食品和药品管理局以及欧盟的欧洲药品管理局）颁发药品许可证的基础。

胶质母细胞瘤是最常见的内在脑肿瘤，也是临床试验中最常被研究的肿瘤。其较短的预期寿命意味着以生存作为主要研究终点比其他肿瘤更容易获得。而胶质母细胞瘤的试验数据通常也被推荐用于其他脑肿瘤的临床试验。而使用分子标志物对患者进行分层，可以确定哪些患者可以从治疗中获益。

化疗药物

化疗通常是在肿瘤医生与患者讨论了化疗的目的、原理、常见和严重的不良反应，获得患者书面同意后开始的。化疗药物的剂量是根据患者的体重或体表面积（body surface area，BSA）、身体状态、器官功能（特别是骨髓、肾、肝）、并发症情况和既往化疗期间毒性反应来计算和调整的。在治疗期间需要对以上不良反应进行监测，并根据需要推迟化疗或减少化疗药物剂量。对于常见的不良反应，可以通过提前使用支持药物进行预防。受过专门培训的医生和护士需要密切监测患者，并积极处理化疗不良反应，以避免化疗延迟、遗漏或药物剂量的减少。在每周期化疗前和化疗期间需要定期进行血液学检查。患者也需要24小时开机，时刻与护士保持联系，随时讨论化疗毒性的管理，并注意观察自己的感染征象，必要时应紧急住院并静脉注射抗生素。患者还需要定期进行影像学检查评估化疗效果。

表12.1概述了被批准用于胶质瘤最常用的化疗药物的作用机制和常见的不良反应。这些药物的详细介绍可以在欧洲药品管理局（EMA）或美国食品和药品管理局（FDA）提供的药品管理网上找到。使用它们的证据将在本章后面讨论。

化疗的分子标志物

分子标志物在肿瘤学中常常被用作协助诊断和判断预后的指标。由于局部病变与中枢神经病理之间的一致性不足50%（Stupp et al.，2014），而分子标志物能够预测化疗疗效，因此分子标记有助于准确判断病情变化。此外，分子标志物可以作为化疗反应的独立预测因子，因此可以用来判断某些患者的化疗是否有效。确定辅助化疗方案的标志物将在后文讨论。其他协助诊断的标志物（如ATRX、TERT），但与化疗反应没有明确相关性的在此不做讨论。2016版WHO中枢神经系统肿瘤分类已经将分子标志物纳入了神经胶质瘤的诊断标准（Louis et al.，2016）。目前所有的神经胶质瘤都需要根据其IDH状态来确定。以前组织学特征相似的少突胶质细胞瘤，现在根据1p19q共缺失的存在与否被分为少突胶质细胞瘤和星形细胞瘤。然而，肿瘤的异质性使分子标志物对临床结果的解读存在很多不确定性（Forshew et al.，2013）。如果分子标志物只存在于肿瘤区域而不在其他部位，其对临床结果的判断力度就会下降，同样也可能导致假阴性结果的出现。

表 12.1 胶质瘤常用化疗药物

作用机制	特点	使用方法	不良反应
替莫唑胺			
一种达卡巴嗪口服衍生物。二者都是烷化剂 3- 甲基 -(三氮烯 -1- 基)咪唑 -4- 甲酰胺(MTIC)的前体药物。烷化剂能够不可逆地将一个烷基附着在 DNA 的鸟嘌呤上，干扰 DNA 复制，阻滞细胞复制和诱导细胞凋亡	一种相对较小的亲脂分子(194 Da)，具有很高的生物利用度。可以通过血脑屏障，自发水解成有活性的代谢产物。一般耐受性良好	联合放疗治疗胶质母细胞瘤时，75 mg/m² 口服，第 1~42 天，之后 150~200 mg/m² 口服第 1~5 天，每 28 天为一周期，共维持治疗 6 周期。治疗期间需使用抗生素预防肺孢子菌肺炎	非常常见(>10%)：厌食、便秘、恶心、呕吐、皮疹、皮肤干燥、不孕症、脱发、乏力。常见(1%~10%)：贫血、白细胞减少、血小板减少、肝功能异常、口腔念珠菌病、吞咽困难、口腔黏膜炎、高血糖、味觉减低、咳嗽、呼吸困难、肌肉骨骼疼痛、肌无力、疲劳、尿失禁、水肿、深静脉血栓、视物模糊、听力下降、耳鸣、焦虑、抑郁、失眠、头痛、抽搐。也有精子减少报道
洛莫司汀[CCNU，1-(2- 氯乙基)-3- 环己基 -1- 亚硝基脲]			
一种烷基化亚硝基脲。亚硝基脲是一种既含有亚硝基(R-NO)又含有尿素的化合物。亚硝基脲的非酶降解可以产生具有烷基化和氨基甲酰化活性的产物，导致 DNA 内或链间交联和有丝分裂停止	亲脂性，因此能透过血脑屏障	治疗胶质瘤时，可单药使用，或与丙卡巴肼和长春新碱联合(PCV 方案)使用。用法：每周期第一天口服，6~8 周为一个周期，共 6 个周期	非常常见(>10%)：皮疹、皮肤干燥、腹泻、肝功能异常、血小板减少(用药后 4 周达到最低水平)、白细胞减少(5~6 周达到最低水平)。常见症状(1%~10%)：疲劳、恶心、呕吐、厌食、不孕和贫血。其他明显副作用包括肝和肾损害、肺毒性，协调困难和意识混乱
卡莫司汀(BiCNU，双氯乙基亚硝脲类)			
一种与芥子气有关的亚硝基脲烷基化剂(参见洛莫司汀)	可静脉给予，也可作为凝胶片(Gliadel®)(阿伯制药，2014)植入，已在英国被批注用于胶质瘤	肿瘤切除术后，将 8 片晶片植入腔底，在 5 天内释放完卡莫司汀，以避免全身毒性	Gliadel 硅片：新发或加剧癫痫(54%)、脑水肿(23%)、伤口延迟愈合(16%)、脑膜炎(4%)。扁桃体突出和晶片移位引起阻塞性脑积水也有报道
PCV			
丙卡巴肼、洛莫司汀(CCNU)和长春新碱联合化疗方案		长春新碱静脉注射第 1 天，洛莫司汀口服第 1 天，丙卡巴肼第 1 或第 2 天开始口服，共 10 天，42 天为一周期，共 6 周期	
丙卡巴肼			
一种烷化剂(见替莫唑胺)，具体作用机制仍不清楚	细胞色素 P450 抑制剂，可与多种药物产生相互作用；单胺氧化酶抑制剂，能与酒精产生类似双硫的反应		非常常见(>10%)：恶心、呕吐、厌食。常见(1%~10%)：白细胞减少、贫血、血小板减少、疲劳、流感样症状、抑郁、失眠、神经病变、闭经和不孕不育。可发生过敏和酪胺反应，因此应避免摄入含有酪胺的食物，并应向患者提供避免的食物清单
长春新碱			
从马达加斯加长春花中提取的一种长春花生物碱。与微管蛋白结合成二聚体，抑制微管结构，从而在中期阻止有丝分裂	只能静脉使用，鞘内注射可产生致死性神经毒性，既往由于疏忽已发生多起死亡		非常常见(>10%)：神经病变、疲劳、严重便秘、腹痛、恶心、呕吐、脱发。常见(1%~10%)：白细胞减少、感染、肌无力、注射部位反应、尿潴留、过敏反应、口腔溃疡、下巴疼痛、麻痹性肠梗阻、皮疹

（续表）

作用机制	特点	使用方法	不良反应
贝伐珠单抗			
重组人源化血管内皮生长因子A（VEGF-A）单克隆抗体。血管生成在胶质母细胞瘤中很常见。缺氧是其主要的驱动因素，可导致肿瘤表达促血管生成因子（VEGF），促进内皮细胞增殖、迁移和侵袭。抗血管生成药物可以使血管正常化，降低血脑屏障的通透性（Friedman et al.，2009）		每2~3周静脉输注一次	非常常见（>10%）：高血压、恶心、呕吐、疲劳、白细胞减少、神经病变、厌食、便秘和头痛。常见（1%~10%）：蛋白尿、深静脉血栓形成、肠穿孔、出血、瘘管、伤口愈合障碍、后脑白质病、心力衰竭和心律失常

染色体1p/19q共缺失

1p和19q染色体的不平衡易位，可以导致染色体1p和19q染色体的遗传缺失，可以是共缺失或杂合性缺失（Cairncross et al.，2013）。这是一种特殊的实体肿瘤类型，其病理尚不完全明晰，但可以由此确诊少突胶质细胞瘤，而其在恶性胶质瘤中并不常见（<5%）（存在于15%的Ⅱ级弥漫型星形细胞瘤，30%~60%的Ⅱ级少突胶质细胞瘤/少突星形细胞瘤，15%的Ⅲ间变型星形细胞瘤，50%~80%的间变少突胶质细胞瘤/少突星形细胞瘤）（Stupp et al.，2014）。它与化疗敏感性和生存率的增加有关（Cairncross et al.，2013）。

6-甲基鸟嘌呤-DNA甲基转移酶（MGMT）启动子甲基化

替莫唑胺的细胞毒性作用体现在其对鸟嘌呤O6位点DNA的甲基化。MGMT是一种普遍存在的DNA修复酶，它可以去除鸟嘌呤O6位置的甲基，从而逆转甲基化，抑制替莫唑胺的细胞毒性作用。触发转录的启动子甲基化可以导致MGMT的表观遗传沉默，从而增加肿瘤对烷化剂（如替莫唑胺）的敏感性（Weller et al.，2010）。由于免疫组化缺乏标准，因此MGMT启动子的甲基化通常用甲基化特异性聚合酶链反应（methylation specific polymerase chain reaction，MSP）来检测。在40%~50% Ⅱ级弥漫型星形细胞瘤、60%~80% Ⅱ级少突胶质细胞瘤/少突星形细胞瘤、50% Ⅲ级间变型星形细胞瘤、70%间变型少突胶质细胞瘤和35%的胶质母细胞瘤中均存在MGMT启动子甲基化（Stupp et al.，2014）。它是间变型胶质瘤和胶质母细胞瘤的良好预后标志物，并且与烷化剂治疗间变型胶质瘤的有效性相关。MGMT启动子甲基化增加了化疗有效的可能性，这将在下文进行详述。

异柠檬酸脱氢酶（IDH）1和2突变

IDH 1或2的突变可以产生异常代谢物，即2-羟基戊二酸，其通过高甲基化可以产生表观遗传学变化。IDH 1和2突变是低级别胶质瘤的特征，如果在高级别肿瘤中被发现，提示肿瘤是从低级别胶质瘤转化而来。在70%~80%的Ⅱ级弥漫型星形细胞瘤和少突胶质细胞瘤、50%~80%的星形细胞瘤和间变型少突胶质细胞瘤中均可发现IDH突变，但胶质母细胞瘤只有5%~10%存在该突变。约90%的突变为IDH 1上的R132H突变，由免疫组化就可确定。基因测序可以帮助排除IDH 1其他位点和IDH 2的突变，这些均为阴性突变（Stupp et al.，2014）。IDH突变是良好预后的指标，并且已被证明可以预测间变型少突胶质细胞瘤对替莫唑胺的反应（van den Bent et al.，2013）。此外，以IDH为靶点的抑制剂（AG-221）的也正在被研究中。在免疫治疗中，2-羟基戊二酸可以通过磁共振检测，提供潜在的成像分子标志（Kang and Adamson，2015）。

表皮生长因子受体

表皮生长因子受体（epidermal growth factor receptor，EFGR）扩增或突变已在多种肿瘤中被发现，以EGFR为靶点的治疗已成为结直肠癌、肺癌和头颈部肿瘤的标准疗法。有一半的胶质母细胞瘤也存在EGFR扩增或突变，其中一半为EGFRvⅢ突变，是预后不良的指标。9% 的间变型星形细胞瘤也存在 EFGR 扩增或突变，而在其他胶质瘤中并不常见（Kang and Adamson，2015）。EGFR 是一个很有前景的治疗靶点，虽然目前还没有Ⅲ期临床试验证实 EGFR 靶向治疗的生存获益，但一些新的 EGFR 靶向药物仍在研发中，并正在进行相关临床试验。

BRAFV600

BRAF 突变是多种癌症发生的关键驱动因素，95% 以上为错义突变，是在第 600 个氨基酸位置上由缬氨酸取代谷氨酸（BRAFV600E）。虽然 BRAF 突变在整体胶质瘤中并不常见，但在 9% 的多形性黄色星形细胞瘤和毛细胞星形细胞瘤中可见（Schindler et al.，2011）。2016 版 WHO 中枢神经系统肿瘤分类已经将 IDH 野生型胶质母细胞瘤作为新类型进行收录，同时还收录了上皮样胶质母细胞瘤，这两种肿瘤常伴有 BRAF 突变（Louis et al.，2016）。BRAFV600 突变的肿瘤患者可以使用 BRAFV600E 小分子抑制剂来进行治疗。

疗效监测

临床上常用的反映疗效的观察指标包括中位总生存期（overall survival，OS）、无进展生存期（progression free survival，PFS）和客观缓解（objective response，OR）。在治疗开始后的各个时间点（如 6 个月或 12 个月）的 OS 和 PFS 也常被采用。认知功能、生活质量、症状、功能独立性和是否需要类固醇治疗也常作为临床疗效的次要观察指标（Lin et al.，2013）。

放疗疗效分为完全缓解（complete response，CR）、部分缓解（partial response，PR，30% 的单维收缩或 50% 的二维收缩）、疾病稳定（stable disease，SD，在 PR 和 PD 之间）和疾病进展（progressive disease，PD，增大 20%~25% 以上）。

实体瘤疗效评价标准（RECIST）适用于中枢神经系统以外的肿瘤，是根据靶病灶大小的变化对治疗疗效进行分类（Eisenhauer et al.，2009）。Macdonald 标准（Macdonald et al.，1990）是针对幕上恶性胶质瘤的，可以对肿瘤治疗反应进行客观的放射学评估，并根据胶质瘤的特异性进行分类，如类固醇使用和临床症状的改善。虽然它是为 CT 设计的，但也被外推用于磁共振成像。神经肿瘤学工作组（RANO）评价标准（**表** 12.2）是为了解决 Macdonald 标准的局限性而开发出来的，包括了缺乏评估非增强成分和使用增强对比剂作为肿瘤生长的替代方法。

注射造影剂后组织强化反映了造影剂穿过血肿瘤屏障的过程。一些非肿瘤性因素也可导致强化，如炎症、放射性坏死、癫痫发作、使用类固醇和抗血管生成药物。“假性进展”是病变在影像学上的非肿瘤性增加，这可能反映了治疗实际上是有效的，在接受替莫唑胺放化疗的患者中有 20%~30% 的患者出现了假性进展（Wen et al.，2010）。“假性反应”是病变的非肿瘤性减少，这可能反映了血肿瘤屏障通透性的降低，例如使用了抗血管生成药物治疗。为了解释这些情况，RANO 标准要求在治疗结束后的 12 周内对疗效进行重新评估，除非进展超出了放射治疗范围或病理证实。对于有潜在假性进展的患者，应继续给予治疗，直到后续影像学证实进展。

免疫治疗在神经胶质瘤中的应用目前仍处于临床试验阶段，同时免疫治疗也为确定治疗反应提出了新的挑战。免疫反应的产生需要一定时间，而肿瘤进展可能早已经发生，但却被炎性变化所掩盖。免疫治疗 iRANO 标准（**表** 12.2）已经解决了这些问题（Okada et al.，2015）。

胶质母细胞瘤（WHO Ⅳ级）

继 1980 年 RTOG-8302 试验之后，卡莫司汀成为第一个在手术和放疗之外的用于脑肿瘤的标准化疗药物。这项针对恶性胶质瘤的随机试验表明，卡莫司汀联合放疗对比单纯放疗或化疗提高了患者的生存率（Walker et al.，1980）。一项包括 12 项随机试验 3004 名高级别胶质瘤（Ⅲ级和Ⅳ级）患者的系统性回顾性分析表明，与单纯放疗相比，放疗联合卡莫司汀化疗使患者 OS 略有增加（HR，0.85；95%CI，0.78~0.91；$P<0.0001$），1 年 OS 从 40% 增加到 46%，2 年 OS 从 15% 增加到 20%，进展或死亡风险降低 17%（HR，0.83；95%CI，0.75~0.91；$P<0.0001$）（Stewart，2002）。

2005 年 EORTC-NCIC Ⅲ期临床试验结果公布。573 名胶质母细胞瘤患者随机接受替莫唑胺放化疗或单纯放疗，结果放化疗组患者的中位 OS 显著优于对照组（14.6 个月 *vs*. 12.1 个月）（HR，0.63；95%CI，0.52~0.75；$P<0.001$），2 年 OS 从 10.4% 提高到 26.5%（**图** 12.1）。根据此结果，同步放化疗成为目前胶质母细胞瘤术后的标准治疗：放疗剂量为 60Gy 分割 30 次，替莫唑胺每日口服，连续服用 6 周，之后休息 4 周，最后再口服 6 个周期辅助治疗。MGMT- 启动子甲基化是独立的生存预后良好指

表 12.2　RANO 和 iRANO 标准。iRANO 建议，如果在开始免疫治疗 6 个月，没有新的或严重恶化的神经功能障碍，并且这些障碍不是由于并发症或合并用药引起的，则在初次影像学进展三个月后重复进行影像学检查来确认疾病进展

	恶性胶质瘤	低级别胶质瘤
完全缓解	所有增强性病灶消失≥4 周；没有新发病变；非增强病灶（T2/FLAIR）稳定或改善；类固醇使用剂量不超过生理需求量；临床症状稳定或改善	所有增强和非增强病灶（T2/FLAIR）病变消失，持续时间≥4 周；没有新发病变；类固醇使用剂量不超过生理需求量；临床症状稳定或改善
部分缓解	增强性病灶的两垂直直径乘积总和减少≥50%，持续时间≥4 周；没有新发病变；非增强病灶（T2/FLAIR）稳定或改善；类固醇使用剂量稳定或减少；临床症状稳定或改善	非增强病灶（T2/FLAIR）两垂直直径乘积总和下降≥50%，持续时间≥4 周；没有新发病变；类固醇使用剂量稳定或减少；临床症状稳定或改善
微小有效	不适用	非增强病灶（T2/FLAIR）两垂直直径乘积总和下降25%~49%，持续时间≥4 周；没有新发病变；临床症状稳定或改善
疾病稳定	不符合完全缓解、部分缓解或疾病进展的条件；没有新发病变；非增强病灶（T2/FLAIR）稳定或改善；类固醇使用剂量稳定或减少；临床症状稳定或改善	不符合完全缓解、部分缓解或疾病进展的条件；没有新发病变；非增强病灶（T2/FLAIR）稳定或改善；类固醇使用剂量稳定或减少；临床症状稳定或改善
疾病进展	增强性病变的两垂直直径乘积总和增加≥25%；出现新发病变；非增强病灶（T2/FLAIR）明显恶化；显著的临床症状加重	非增强病灶（T2/FLAIR）的两垂直直径乘积总和增加≥25%；出现新发病变；显著的临床症状加重

Reprinted from *The Lancet Oncology*, Volume 16, issue 15, Okada et al., Immunotherapy response assessment in neuro-oncology: a report of the RANO working group, pp. e534–42, Copyright (2015), with permission from Elsevier.

Data from Wen PY, Macdonald DR, Reardon DA, et al. Updated response assessment criteria for high-grade gliomas: response assessment in neuro-oncology working group, *Journal of Clinical Oncology*, Volume 28, issue 11, pp. 1963–72, 2010.

Data from van den Bent M, Wefel J, Schiff D, et al. Response assessment in neuro-oncology (a report of the RANO group): assessment of outcome in trials of diff use low-grade gliomas. *Lancet Oncology*, volume 12, issue 6, pp. 583–93, 2011.

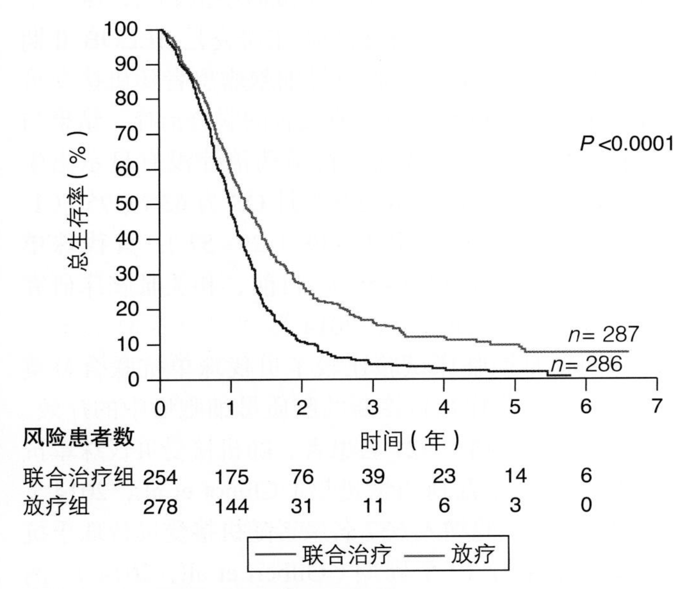

图 12.1　放疗联合替莫唑胺同步和辅助化疗对比单纯放疗对胶质母细胞瘤患者生存的影响

Reprinted from *The Lancet Oncology*, Volume 10, issue 5, Stupp et al., Effects of radiotherapy with concomitant and adjuvant temozolomide versus radiotherapy alone on survival in glioblastoma in a randomised phase III study: 5-year analysis of the EORTC-NCIC trial, pp. 459–66, Copyright (2009), with permission from Elsevier.

标（HR，0.45；95%CI，0.32~0.61；P<0.001），同时也是化疗有效的预测指标。在非甲基化患者中，给予甲基化催化剂，患者发生甲基化后，中位 OS 从 15.3 个月（95%CI，13~20 个月）增加到 21.7 个月（95%CI，17.4~30.4 月）（P=0.007），而在没有发生甲基化的患者中，两组患者的生存没有明显的统计学差异（Stupp et al.，2005）。

剂量密集型替莫唑胺化疗（口服第 1~21 天，28 天为一周期）会导致 MGMT 清除时间延长，从而提高临床疗效。然而，在一项纳入 833 例 GBM 患者的Ⅲ期随机试验中，无论 MGMT 状态如何，剂量密集型替莫唑胺治疗并不优于标准辅助治疗（第 1~5 天），中位 PFS 为 6.7 个月和 5.5 个月（HR，0.87；P=0.06），中位 OS 为 14.9 个月和 16.6 个月（HR，1.03；P=0.63），并且严重的不良反应明显增加（34% *vs*. 53%，P<0.01）（Gilbert et al.，2013）。

既往具有里程碑意义的放化疗试验均排除了 70 岁以上的患者，还有报道称患者超过 60 岁化疗获益就会降低（Stupp R. et al.，2009）。然而，虽然老年人体力状态不佳，化疗更容易产生毒副反应，但对老年患者的临床试验已经证明化疗仍然存在生存获益。Ⅲ期临床试验NOA-08将373名年龄大于65岁、患有高级别胶质瘤（89%胶质母细胞瘤）的患者随机分为替莫唑胺组和放疗组，并允许进展后交叉到另一组接受解救治疗（Wick et al.，2012）。结果替莫唑胺疗效不劣于放射治疗，中位OS分别为8.6个月和9.6个月（HR，1.09；95%CI，0.84~1.42；*P*=0.0330）。在有MGMT启动子甲基化患者中，化疗组较放疗组无复发生存时间更长，分别为8.4个月（95%CI，5.5~11.7）和4.6个月（4.2~5.0），相反，在没有MGMT启动子甲基化患者中，化疗组较放疗组无复发生存时间则缩短，分别为3.3个月（3.0~3.5）和4.6个月（3.7~6.3）。另一项北欧的Ⅲ期临床试验将291名年龄大于60岁的胶质母细胞瘤患者随机分为替莫唑胺化疗组和放疗组（低分割或标准分割）（Malmström et al.，2012），结果替莫唑胺组的中位OS明显优于标准放疗组（8.3个月 *vs*. 6.0个月，HR，0.7；95%CI，0.52~0.93；*P*=0.01），而低分割放疗组和替莫唑胺组的OS相似。在替莫唑胺治疗组，发生MGMT甲基化患者的生存期明显优于未发生甲基化的患者（9.7个月 *vs*. 6.8个月，HR，0.56；95%CI，0.34~0.93；*P*=0.02）；但在放疗组，MGMT甲基化与未甲基化患者的OS没有明显统计学差异（HR，0.97；95%CI，0.69~1.38；*P*=0.81）。因此，虽然这些试验支持替莫唑胺用于老年MGMT启动子甲基化的患者，但在未发生甲基化肿瘤患者中的疗效尚不清楚，尽管也有一些证据支持这一疗法。ORTC 26062-22061这项Ⅲ期临床试验将562名新诊断的年龄大于65岁的胶质母细胞瘤的老年患者随机分为两组，一组接受短期放疗（40 Gy分割15次），另一组接受替莫唑胺同步化放疗（Perry et al.，2016），结果接受替莫唑胺同步化放疗的患者耐受性良好，且中位OS从7.6个月增加到9.3个月（HR，0.67；95%CI，0.56~0.8；*P*<0.0001），发生MGMT甲基化患者的中位OS几乎翻倍（13.5个月 *vs*. 7个月；HR，0.53（0.38~0.73）；*P*=0.0001），但未发生MGMT甲基化的两组患者的OS则没有统计学差异（10个月对比7.9个月，HR 0.75（0.56~1.01，*P*=0.055）。

因此，对于可能不能耐受放化疗的患者，如老年人，可以考虑在甲基化肿瘤患者中使用替莫唑胺，而在无甲基化的肿瘤患者中使用放疗。

复发

目前复发性疾病还没有标准的治疗方法，尽管洛莫司汀或PCV（**表12.1**）方案常用，但临床试验并未发现其有显著的临床获益。如果患者已经接受过化疗，则推荐接受临床试验。

在几项试验中，洛莫司汀单药作为对照组使用后，证实其有适当的临床疗效。例如，REGAL Ⅲ期临床试验比较了西地尼布（一种VEGF抑制剂）单药、西地尼布联合洛莫司汀与洛莫司汀单药的临床疗效，结果洛莫司汀单药组中位OS为9.8个月，PFS为82天，西地尼布的增加没有提高患者的生存（Batchelor et al.，2013）。

争议

贝伐珠单抗

贝伐珠单抗是否应用目前仍存在争议，其在美国被批准用于复发疾病的治疗，但在欧洲并没有获得批准。一项非随机对照Ⅱ期临床试验纳入了167名复发胶质母细胞瘤的患者，比较了贝伐珠单抗单药与贝伐珠单抗联合伊利替康的临床疗效，结果贝伐珠单抗组6个月的PFS为42.6%，联合组为50.3%，历史对照为15%。该研究主要研究终点为OR，贝伐珠单抗组为28.2%，联合组为37.8%，历史对照为5%~10%，但三组之间的OS没有明显差异。由于潜在的假性反应，很难确定这些基于影像学的终点的临床意义。然而，随着时间的推移，那些服用糖皮质激素患者的激素使用量有稳定或减少的趋势。唯一一项对照组不含贝伐珠单抗的临床研究是BELOB Ⅱ期临床试验：153名复发胶质母细胞瘤患者随机接受贝伐珠单抗或洛莫司汀单药或二者的联合治疗，结果与洛莫司汀相比，贝伐珠单抗单药治疗没有显示出生存获益，而联合治疗组的9个月OS为63%（95%CI，49~75），洛莫司汀组为43%（29~57），贝伐珠单抗治疗组为38%（25~51）。目前，相关Ⅲ临床研究正在进行中（Taal et al.，2014）。

两项Ⅲ期临床试验比较了贝伐珠单抗联合替莫唑胺同步放化疗在新诊断的胶质母细胞瘤中的疗效。AVAGlio研究纳入921名患者，随机接受贝伐珠单抗或安慰剂治疗直到病情进展（Chinot et al.，2014）。RTOG0825试验纳入637名患者随机接受贝伐珠单抗或安慰剂治疗12个周期（Gilbert et al.，2014）。两项试验均显示贝伐珠单抗组的OS无明显获益，但PFS显著增加（AVAGlio试验为10.5个月 *vs*. 6.2个月（HR，0.64；95%CI，0.55~0.74；*P*<0.001）；RTOG0825试验为10.7 *vs*. 7.3个月（HR，0.79；95%CI，0.66~0.94；*P*=0.007）。考虑到假性反应的不确定性，两项试验均将生活质量评估作为次要终

点，结果却相互矛盾。虽然 AVAGlio 研究报告了应用贝伐珠单抗可以使患者基础健康相关生活质量维持时间更长、体力状态更好、糖皮质激素应用减少；但 RTOG0825 研究发现，贝伐珠单抗加重了患者的症状，恶化了患者的生活质量。因此，贝伐珠单抗在新诊断的胶质母细胞瘤中的疗效尚不确定。

卡莫司汀晶片植入物（卡氮芥®）

目前还没有任何前瞻性试验将卡莫司汀晶片植入物（卡氮芥®）与标准的替莫唑胺同步放化疗进行比较。一项包含 65 名高级别神经胶质瘤患者的回顾性研究比较了替莫唑胺同步放化疗后接受手术联合卡氮芥或单纯手术后患者的生存差异，结果两组的无复发生存期无显著性差异（12.9 个月 *vs*. 14 个月，*P*=0.89）（Noël et al.，2012）。另一项系统性分析则比较了卡氮芥或安慰剂联合放疗辅助治疗高级别胶质瘤的临床疗效（Hart et al.，2011）。两项随机对照试验的入组标准类似（*n*=32 和 240），在这项研究中，总体来讲，卡氮芥增加了患者的 OS（14 个月 *vs*. 11.5 个 月；HR，0.65；95%CI，0.48~0.86；*P*=0.003），而副作用除了颅内压升高外，其他没有显著增加（*P*=0.019）。尽管 OS 的改善与替莫唑胺同步放疗类似，但仍需谨慎解释。卡氮芥的优效性在纳入Ⅲ级肿瘤的更大的临床试验（与生存期和反应性增加相关）中更常见（16% *vs*. 12%）。在对胶质母细胞瘤患者的亚组分析中，卡氮芥的优效性没有达到统计学差异（*P*=0.1），尽管在调整了基线预后因素（年龄、体力状态）后变得有意义（*P*=0.04）。

一项单中心的回顾性研究并没有发现卡氮芥的生存获益。在这项研究中，222 名复发高级别神经胶质瘤患者手术后接受放疗联合卡氮芥或安慰剂的治疗，结果两组的中位 OS 分别为 31 周和 23 周（HR，0.83；95%CI，0.62~1.10；*P*=0.19），但如果考虑预后因素，则卡氮芥获得了显著的临床获益（Brem et al.，1995）。

因此，卡氮芥的确切疗效仍不清楚，不同的中心选择也不同。参见**专栏** 12.1。

WHO Ⅲ级胶质瘤

间变少突胶质细胞瘤（IDH 突变型，1p19q 共缺失）、间变星形细胞瘤（IDH 突变型）和间变星形细胞瘤（IDH 野生型）是 2016 年世界卫生组织中枢神经肿瘤分类中最常见的Ⅲ级胶质瘤（Louis et al.，2016）。传统上，Ⅲ级胶质瘤的治疗通常采用手术、术后辅助放疗的方式，一旦复发，则应选择化疗。然而，越来越多的证据表明，化疗联合放疗可以提高患者生存率，特别是对那些存在有利分子标志物的亚组人群。

EORTC-26951 试验比较了 368 例间变少突胶质细胞瘤患者在接受放疗联合或不联合 PCV 方案化疗后的生存差异（van den Bent et al.，2013），结果化疗增加了患者的 OS（42.3 个月 *vs*. 30.6 个月；HR，0.75；95%CI，0.6~0.95）。在这项研究中，有 80 名患者检测到了 1p19q 共缺失，结果亚组分析显示，在 1p19q 共缺失患者中，同步化疗的获益更加明显［中位 OS，未达到 *vs*. 112 个月；HR 0.56（0.31~1.03）］，而在无 1p19q 共缺失患者中则没有统计学差异［中位 OS，25 个月 *vs*. 21 个月；HR，0.83（0.6~1.10）］。RTOG9402 Ⅲ期临床试验进一步比较了 289 例间变型少突胶质细胞瘤患者放疗联合或不联合 PCV 方案化疗的生存差异（Cairncross et al.，2013）。虽然 PCV 化疗对总体人群的 OS 增加没有达到统计学差异（4.6 年 *vs*. 4.7 年；HR，0.79；95% CI，0.61~1.04；*P*=0.1），但在 1p/19q 共缺失的亚组患者中，接受 PCV 联合放疗患者的中位 OS 是单纯放疗组的 2 倍（14.7 年 *vs*. 7.3 年；HR，0.59；95%CI，0.37~0.95；*P*=0.03），而在无 1p/19q 共缺失的患者中则没有差异。进一步的分析发现，存在 IDH 突变的患者也能从 PCV 化疗中获益（中位 OS，9.4 年 *vs*. 5.7 年；HR 0.59；95%CI，0.40~0.86；*P*=0.006）（Cairncross et al.，2013）。值得注意的是，OS 的提高是在长期随访后才变得明显，两项试验的最初报告都没有显示化疗的生存获益。

CATNON 试验共纳入 748 名间变型胶质细胞瘤患者，其中期分析表明，替莫唑胺联合放疗改善了无 1p19q 共缺失患者的总生存（HR，0.645；95%CI 0.45~0.926；*P*=0.0014）（van den Bent et al.，2016）。

目前Ⅲ级胶质瘤的标准治疗方法仍然是手术加术后放疗。对于存在 1p/19q 共缺失的患者可以采取术后放疗联合 PCV 方案辅助化疗。而对于不存在 1p/19q 共缺失的患者，术后则接受放疗联合替莫唑胺的联合治疗，CATNON 试验的最终结果尚待公布。IDH 野生型间变星形细胞瘤患者的临床特征与胶质母细胞瘤患者相似，因此许多临床医生认为，使用与胶质母细胞瘤相同的方案治疗 IDH 野生型间变星形细胞瘤患者是合适的。这种方法正在 CATNON 试验中进行验证。CATNON 试验共分为三个化疗亚组：替莫唑胺同步放疗、放疗后序贯替莫唑胺、替莫唑胺同步并序贯放疗，参见**专栏** 12.2。

专栏 12.1 病例 1

图 12.2 患者，男，出现语言障碍后被诊断为多形性胶质母细胞瘤（图 A）。2011 年 10 月患者进行了脑肿瘤的手术切除，随后进行了辅助放化疗和 6 个周期的替莫唑胺的维持治疗，于 2012 年 8 月完成全部治疗（B）。2014 年 2 月患者肿瘤进展后（C）进行二次手术，之后应用替莫唑胺辅助化疗 3 个周期。2014 年 5 月肿瘤再次复发（D），患者在使用洛莫司汀、贝伐珠单抗和缬更昔洛韦的联合治疗后，应用伊匹木单抗继续治疗，肿瘤明显缩小（E）。但 2015 年 2 月患者肿瘤再次复发，进一步的治疗无效，于 2015 年 9 月去世。

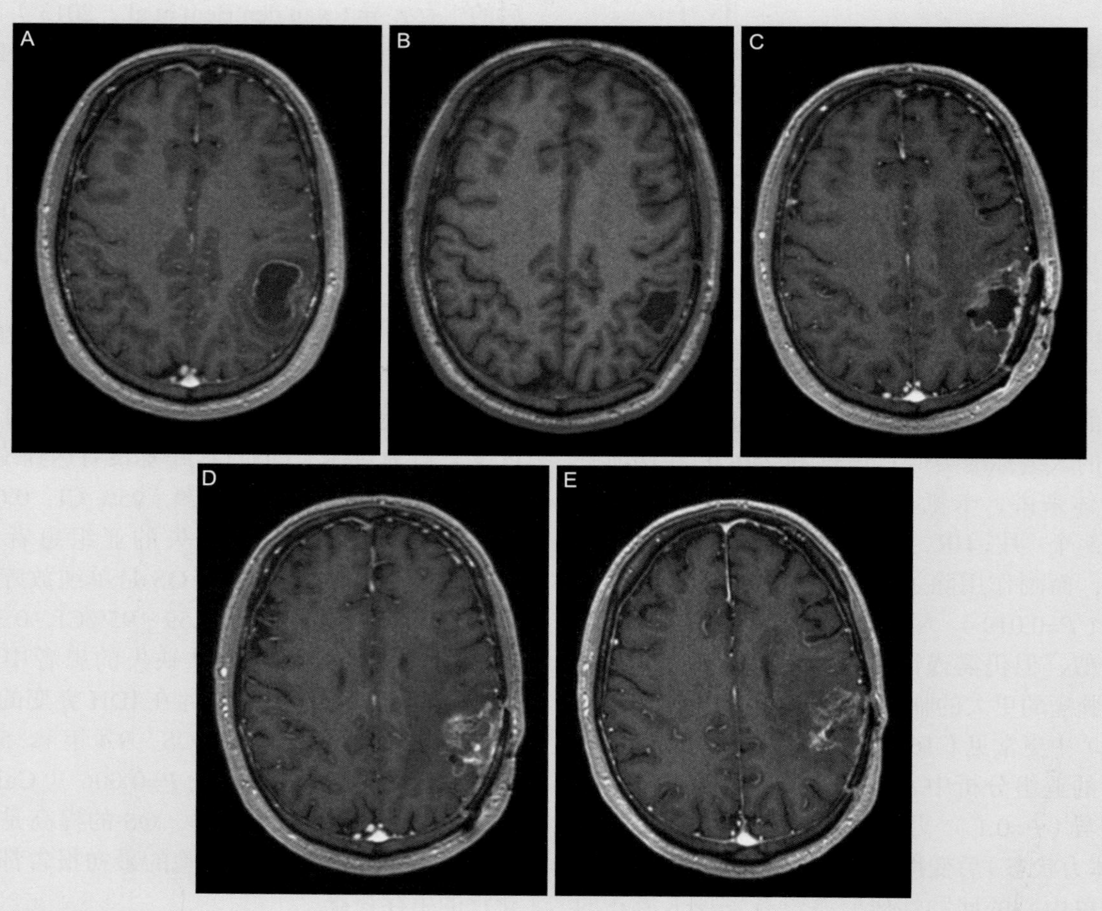

图 12.2 脑 MRI（T1+ 钆）

低级别胶质瘤（WHO Ⅰ、Ⅱ级）

Ⅰ级胶质瘤被认为是良性的，不需要化疗。传统上Ⅱ级胶质瘤在复发前也不需要化疗，但越来越多的证据表明早期化疗可以提高Ⅱ级胶质瘤患者的生存率。

RTOG-9802 3 期临床随机试验纳入了 256 名高风险Ⅱ级神经胶质瘤的患者，给予放疗后序贯 PCV 方案化疗，结果发现患者预后显著改善：中位 OS 从 7.8 年延长到 13.3 年（HR，0.59；*P*=0.03）；中位 PFS 从 4 年延长至 10.4 年（HR，0.5；*P*=0.002）；10 年生存率从 40% 提高至 60%（Buckner et al.，2016）。少突胶质细胞瘤对化疗最敏感，星形细胞瘤则对化疗不敏感。对于 IDH 突变的肿瘤患者加入 PCV 方案有显著的生存获益［HR，0.42（0.2~0.86）；*P*=0.02］，但对 IDH 野生型或存在 1p19q 共缺失的患者则无法得到此结论。

EORTC-22033 Ⅲ期试验比较了 477 名进展期、有症状或高风险低级别胶质瘤患者随机接受替莫唑胺单药化疗或单纯放疗的疗效差异。初步分析显示，两组间的 PFS 无明显统计学差异，对于无 1p 缺失的患者，替莫唑胺有降低 PFS 的趋势，而在有 1p 有缺失的患者中，替莫唑胺则可能能够增加 OS（Baumert et al.，2013）。

专栏 12.2 病例 2

图 12.3 患者，女，间变型少突胶质细胞瘤（WHO Ⅲ级，1p/19q 缺失）。2006 年 2 月行左侧开颅肿块切除手术，之后行辅助放化疗和替莫唑胺维持化疗。尽管多次复查提示肿瘤有轻微增长，但患者临床情况稳定，直到 2014 年 9 月，出现局灶性癫痫和右臂无力症状（MRI，A），之后患者接受了 6 个周期的 PCV 方案化疗，肿瘤几乎完全消失（B）。

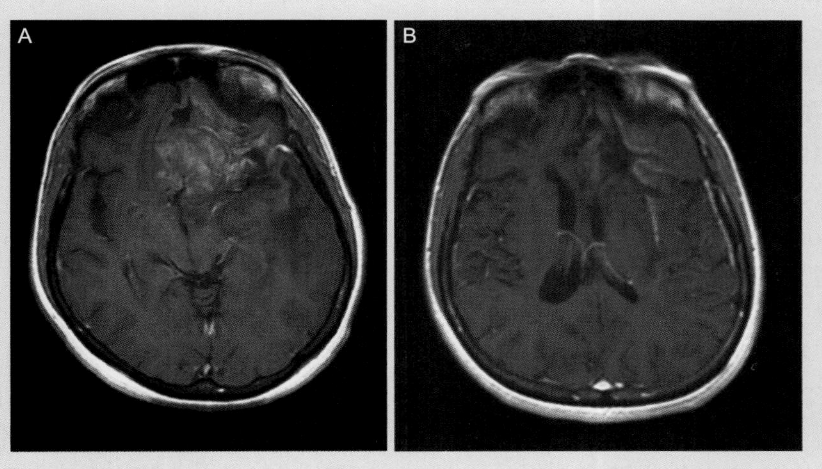

图 12.3 脑 MRI（T1+ 钆）PCV 治疗之前（A），PCV 治疗之后中线肿瘤几乎完全消失（B）

在复发性疾病中，EORTC-26972 前瞻性Ⅱ期临床试验在既往 PCV 方案治疗后复发的 28 例少突胶质细胞瘤患者中证实替莫唑胺有一定临床疗效（van den Bent et al.，2003），客观缓解率约为25%（95%CI，11%~45%），6 个月和 12 个月的 PFS 率分别为 19% 和 11%，中位进展时间为 8 个月。

低级别胶质瘤通常被认为是复发低风险的，因此患者术后通常采用观察等待的方法，一般不接受辅助化疗或放疗。然而，并没有明确的标准来确定复发风险。患者肿瘤次全切除、年龄超过 40 岁、症状加重或出现新症状一般被归为高风险。肿瘤的分子筛查可以帮助识别那些有不良预后的高风险患者，以及那些对化疗更有反应的患者。

新的化疗方法

高级别胶质瘤预后差，特别是复发性胶质瘤的患者，目前治疗效果有限，因此需要研发出新的治疗方法。深入分析患者分子标志物、基因表达和表观遗传学特点可以找到新的治疗靶点，并准确判断哪些患者可能从新疗法中受益。

替代输送疗法是一种新的治疗方法，目前正在研发中，可以使肿瘤暴露于无法穿透血脑屏障的疗法中。例如，纳米颗粒通过减少黏附相互作用可以增加血脑屏障的穿透性，医生通过手术在脑实质中植入导管可以将化疗药物直接输送至手术空腔。

靶向治疗

尽管在其他类型的肿瘤中找到了合适的分子靶点，但是在脑肿瘤中靶向治疗的临床试验结果却令人失望。

例如，EGFR 靶向治疗已广泛应用于肺癌、头颈部肿瘤和结直肠癌的治疗。在胶质母细胞瘤中，约 40% 的患者存在 EGFR 过表达。EGFR 单克隆抗体尼妥珠单抗和 EGFRvⅢ靶向疫苗 rindopepimut 尽管在早期试验中有良好的活性，但二者的Ⅲ期试验均未能显示出任何生存益处。虽然第一代酪氨酸激酶抑制剂（如厄洛替尼、吉非替尼、拉帕替尼）对胶质母细胞瘤无效，但第二代抑制剂目前正在临床试验中（Kang and Adamson，2015）。

如前所述，抗血管生成药物贝伐珠单抗是目前唯一在临床试验中显示出有限疗效的靶向药物，而其他靶向血管生成和侵袭的药物，如西伦吉肽（一种整合素抑制剂），其临床试验则以失败告终（CENTRIC，Stupp et al.，2014），还有一些其他靶向该途径的疗法正在早期临床试验进行中（例如 FAK 抑制剂 GSK2256098）。

BRAF 抑制剂达拉菲尼或维莫非尼与 MEK 抑制剂曲美替尼联合可增强抗肿瘤疗效，克服 BRAF 耐药，已经彻底改变了 BRAF V600 突变肿瘤患者的预后（Robert et al.，2015）。在进展期 BRAFV600 突变胶质瘤患者中，有个案报道和篮式临床试验表明在放化疗后序贯使用 BRAF 抑制剂有效（Hyman et al.，2015; Brown et al.，2016），然而，尚不清楚患者是否会从早期使用 BRAF 抑制剂中获得更多的益处。

治疗有效的靶点，理论上应存在于所有恶性细胞中，并且必须对肿瘤的生长或侵袭至关重要。靶向治疗虽然有良好的临床前活性，但在临床试验中却屡次失败有多种原因。我们尽管对神经胶质瘤分子特性的了解有所增加，但尚未建立起分子驱动机制（Kang and Adamson，2015）。另外脑肿瘤巨大的突变负荷产生的肿瘤异质性致使没有单一的驱动基因突变可以作为靶点，或者我们只是还没有确定一个潜在的治疗靶点，那么靶向治疗的失败就一定是不可避免的吗？由于潜在的有益药物被用于过度异质的患者中导致试验失败，是否隐藏了一组可能受益的患者，如果选择一个适当的分子标志物，这些患者是否就会被识别出来（**专栏 12.3**）？

免疫治疗

免疫系统可以潜在地识别和选择靶向特定的肿瘤抗原，并通过免疫记忆引起持久的应答。因此，免疫治疗是一种极具吸引力的抗肿瘤策略。目前免疫治疗已在黑色素瘤和肺癌中取得突破性进展，在其他肿瘤包括脑肿瘤中也成为一个令人期待的研究方向。尽管患者体内有针对肿瘤抗原的活化性 T 细胞，但大多数患者并没有产生足够的免疫反应来破坏肿瘤细胞，是因为癌细胞可以通过下调 MHC，产生抑制性细胞因子，调节 T 细胞浸润，增加免疫检查点受体的表达，诱导形成免疫抑制性微环境。这导致了肿瘤对能够诱导有效免疫反应的细胞（如树突状细胞、自然杀伤细胞和效应 T 细胞）产生耐受和逃逸。不同于全身免疫系统，因为白细胞无法穿透血脑屏障，中枢神经系统内缺乏天然 T 细胞且又没有明显的淋巴引流，因此中枢神经系统既往一直被认为是一个免疫豁免器官。然而在胶质瘤中，由于血脑屏障已被破坏，现在人们认为中枢神经系统完全可以与系统免疫相互作用，并且目前已经有研究发现从中枢神经系统到颈深部淋巴结的淋巴引流（Reardon et al.，2014）。免疫治疗的目的是调节免疫抑制肿瘤微环境（被动）或刺激肿瘤特异性免疫（主动）。下面将举例说明。

被动免疫

程序性死亡 -1（programmed-death 1，PD-1）是一种表达于 T 细胞和前 B 细胞表面的蛋白受体，当与其配体（PD-L1/PD-L2）结合时，可以通过促进抗原特异性 T 细胞的凋亡和减少调节性 T 细胞的凋

专栏 12.3 病例 3

图 12.4 患者，女，右侧顶叶多形性胶质母细胞瘤，2008 年 10 月手术切除，之后行辅助放化疗和替莫唑胺维持治疗。2009 年 6 月复发再次手术切除，但很快肿瘤再次复发（MRI，A），之后开始西仑吉肽治疗。之后的 3 年多时间里，患者临床症状保持稳定，强化病灶显著减少（MRI，B）。2012 年 12 月患者肿瘤进展，停用西伦吉肽。2013 年 2 月患者开始卡铂化疗，无效，3 个月后死亡。

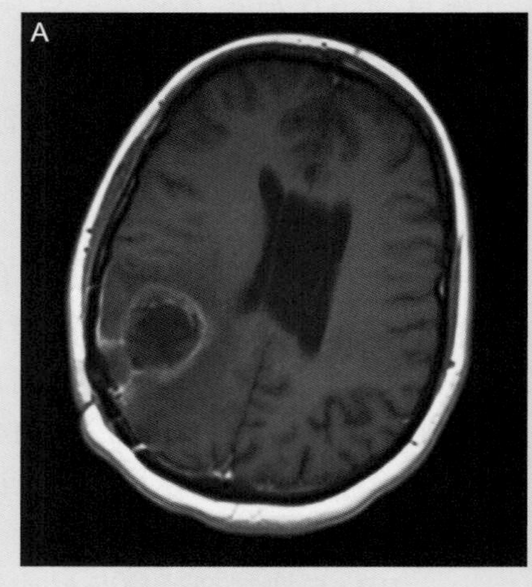

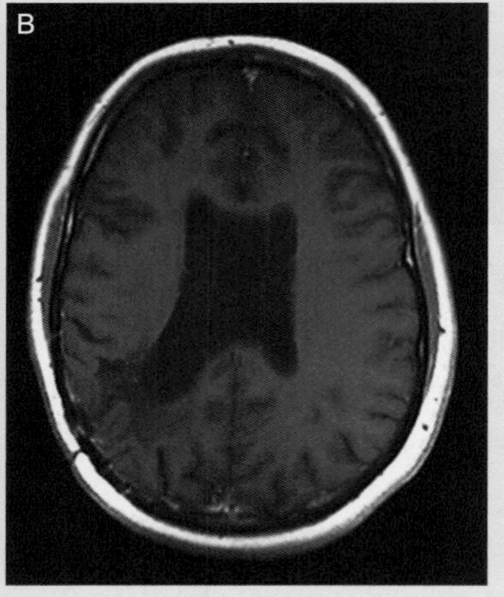

图 12.4 脑 MRI（T1+ 钆）西伦吉肽治疗前（2009 年 6 月，A），西伦吉肽治疗治疗期间肿瘤强化显著降低（2011 年 3 月，B）

亡来抑制免疫应答。PD-1 作为免疫检查点具有促进自我耐受和预防自身免疫的功能。细胞毒性 T 淋巴细胞相关蛋白 4（cytotoxic T lymphocyte-associated protein 4，CTLA-4）是另一个免疫检查点，当与抗原呈递细胞上的 CD80 或 CD86 结合时，可以下调免疫应答。增加免疫检查点受体的肿瘤表达有助于免疫系统对肿瘤产生耐受性。纳武利尤单抗和伊匹木单抗分别是抗 PD-1 和 CTLA-4 的单克隆抗体，已被批准用于治疗黑色素瘤和肺鳞癌，在脑肿瘤方面的临床试验也正在进行中。这些药物会使患者的非特异性 T 细胞增殖，并引起相应的不良反应，包括结肠炎、肝炎、弥漫性皮疹、眼部变化和内分泌失调（Reardon et al.，2014）。Checkmate-143 试验正在评估纳武利尤单抗联合或不联合伊匹木单抗治疗复发性胶质母细胞瘤的临床疗效，初步数据分析显示，在 20 例患者中，6 个月的 OS 为 75%（Sampson et al.，2015）。

其他正在研究的潜在免疫调节剂包括使用细胞因子（如干扰素、白介素 -1）促进炎症状态，以及通过抑制剂（如抗 CD25 和 IL-2 的巴利昔单抗）来抑制调节性 T 细胞（Kang and Adamson，2015）。

主动免疫

多肽治疗包括使用针对肿瘤特异性或肿瘤相关性抗原的疫苗。IMA-950 是一种含有 11 个人白细胞抗原（human leukocyte antigen，HLA）结合肿瘤相关肽的疫苗，可以在人胶质母细胞瘤组织中的 HLA 表面受体上被识别。其在一项纳入 45 名患者的 1 期临床试验显示出良好的疗效，6 个月的 PFS 为 74%（Halford et al.，2014）。

过继疗法需要在体外激活免疫细胞。树突状细胞（dendritic cells，DCs）是最有效的抗原呈递细胞，能够介导持久免疫，但由于肿瘤免疫抑制性微环境，通常处于失活状态。几种 DC 疫苗目前正在开发中，用以克服这种局部免疫抑制状态。DCVax-L 是一种通过白细胞分离技术从患者体内分离出的树突状细胞，将其与从患者手术中提取的裂解后的肿瘤抗原共培养后，再回输给患者的 3 期临床试验正在进行中（Northwest Biotherapeutics，2014）。

嵌合抗原受体是将肿瘤相关抗原的受体插入到效应 T 细胞。目前在胶质母细胞瘤中，针对一些靶点的嵌合抗原受体的临床试验正在进行中，包括 HER-2（80% 的胶质母细胞瘤过表达）（NCT01109095）和 EGFRvⅢ（NCT01454596）。

关键知识点

- 化疗可以延长脑肿瘤患者的总生存。
- 初诊的胶质母细胞瘤术后接受替莫唑胺同步放化疗是目前的标准疗法。对于不能耐受同步放化疗的老年患者，如果存在 MGMT 启动子甲基化，接受化疗比放疗更加获益。
- 卡氮芥对比替莫唑胺进行同步放化疗尚未进行前瞻性研究。
- 当胶质母细胞瘤复发时，洛莫司汀或替莫唑胺再挑战仍有一定的益处。贝伐珠单抗可能能够延长胶质母细胞瘤患者的 PFS 并减少糖皮质激素的使用。
- 发生 1p/19q 共缺失的间变型少突胶质细胞瘤（WHO Ⅲ级），应接受放疗序贯 PCV 方案化疗。“复发高风险”的低级别胶质瘤，特别是发生 1p/19q 共缺失的患者应接受化疗。
- 靶向治疗和免疫治疗可能成为未来治疗方案的基础。

里程碑式文献、延伸阅读、参考文献、EBRAIN 的相关链接

扫描书末二维码获取。

第 13 章　脑内肿瘤治疗的外科技术

Shawn Hervey-Jumper · Mitchel Berger
吴涛 译，陈保东 审校

引言

手术切除在内源性脑肿瘤的治疗中起着核心作用，越来越多的证据表明，手术的切除范围对改善患者的治疗效果和提升生活质量具有价值。由于肿瘤接近功能区结构和肿瘤边缘的不确定性，肿瘤的最大切除可能难以实现。皮质刺激定位、功能神经导航、术中 MRI 和荧光引导手术都是改善肿瘤切除范围的有用工具，同时将发病率降至最低。目前的证据表明，更广泛的手术切除与低级别或高级别胶质瘤患者生存期的延长和生活质量的改善密切相关。本章强调支持内源脑肿瘤手术作用的证据，包括神经外科解剖学，以及最大限度地扩大切除范围同时将发病率降至最低的技术。

神经外科解剖学

大脑半球与颅脑关系

见第 2 章图 2.2。

成人的大脑分为两个半球，包括额叶、顶叶、中央、颞叶、枕叶和岛叶。有六个主要连续的沟：外侧裂、胼胝体沟、顶枕沟、侧副沟、中央沟和距状沟。有两个间断的沟：中央前沟和颞下沟。

额叶被两个主要的沟分开：额上沟和额下沟，它们将额叶的侧表面分为额上回、额中回及额下回。这些从中央前沟延伸出来，并朝向前后方向。与中央沟平行的是中央前沟，它位于额叶的后端。额下回进一步被外侧裂的前支、升支及后支分为眶部、三角部和岛盖部。在额上沟和中央前沟之间的交叉点很容易辨识的标志是手区的运动皮质，形似希腊字母“Ω”（omega）。

顶叶的边界包括内侧的半球间裂，外侧裂和颞枕线，前部的中央沟和后部的颞顶线。顶叶主要有两个沟：中央后沟和顶间沟。顶间沟将顶叶表面分为顶上小叶和顶下小叶。顶上小叶位于内侧，体积较小，并继续作为楔前体的内侧，而顶下小叶由缘上回和角回组成。缘上回是颞上回的后延，角回是颞中回的后延。

颞叶的上界为外侧裂。颞叶有颞上沟和颞下沟，将颞叶分为颞上回、颞中回和颞下回。这三个颞叶脑回在前部汇聚，形成颞极。枕叶的边界包括内侧的距状沟和外侧的颞顶线。枕叶由几个短的水平沟组成，将枕叶外侧分为枕上回和枕下回。

分开额叶、顶叶和颞叶的是外侧裂，它由深层和浅层部分组成。岛叶位于外侧裂的深部。外侧裂的浅表部分包含一个干和三个支。外侧裂主干由内侧的钩回向外侧延伸至蝶翼外侧端，分为前水平支、前升支和后支。外侧裂的深部分为蝶部和岛盖部（Ribas et al.，2015）。蝶部位于岛阈处，自前向外侧延伸至前穿质。岛盖部是由外侧裂深部（在额顶盖和颞盖相对的唇之间）和外侧裂中部（上肢位于岛叶和额顶盖之间，下肢位于岛叶和颞顶盖之间）形成（Ribas et al.，2015）。介于颈动脉池内侧和外侧裂之间的是岛阈。岛的中央沟将岛的外侧表面分为前区和后区，前区分为三个短回，后区分为前、后长回（Ribas et al.，2015）。环绕岛叶的是环状沟，它将岛叶与上覆的岛盖分开。

白质束

见第 35 章图 35.5。

当代对人脑功能的看法已经从僵化的组织转变为更动态的大脑处理观点。大规模的皮质下白质网络促进了语言、运动和认知等复杂功能。关联纤维连接同一半球中不同叶的皮质区域，可分为短联络纤维和长联络纤维。短联络纤维连接相邻脑回，而长联络纤维（也称为纤维束）则连接远处的脑回，并形成明显的紧密束。临床上重要的主要分束是：①上纵束、②钩束、③枕额下束和④扣带回。上纵束绕着岛叶弯曲，连接额叶、顶叶和颞叶。钩束沿着岛阈位于岛叶前部，连接额叶基底和颞叶。扣带回位于海马旁回的胼胝体喙部下方。连接额叶和枕叶，以及颞叶和顶叶的后部的是额枕下束（inferior fronto- occipital fasciculus，IFOF）。IFOF 从额叶汇聚到基底神经节的外侧，然后沿着钩束之前走行。

从神经外科的角度来看，也许最重要白质区是那些与语言功能相关的白质区。早期的语言组织模型来自于皮质病变后的语言障碍。1861 年，Jean-Baptiste Bouillaud 发表了一系列额叶病变后长期言语丧失的患者。这些发现之后，Broca 观察到言语抑制与运动语言激活是分离的，但表达语言能力缺失（Chang et al.，2015）。几年后，Karl Wernicke 描述了颞上后叶的病变，导致重复、命名和理解能力受损，但流畅性完好。失语症以及影响言语产生或理解的语言障碍，可分为全面性失语症、Broca 失语症、Wernicke 失语症、混合性非流利性失语症或命名性失语症。

全面性失语症是失语症中最严重的一种，描述的是患者只能说出很少可辨认的单词，并且只能偶尔理解口头语言。因此，全面性失语症患者既不能读也不能写。Broca 失语症患者的语言输出减少，费力而笨拙，其特点是句子较短，少于四个字。Broca 失语症的患者通常能够理解语言，并保持阅读能力，但无法书写。

Wernicke 失语症的特点是理解能力受损，而言语的流畅性却得以保留，Wernicke 失语症患者的阅读和书写能力通常受到损害。混合性失语症是指言语少、费力，类似于严重的 Broca 失语症，但患者的理解能力有限，导致阅读和书写困难。命名性失语症患者无法说出名词和动词的名称，这就导致患者的流利程度相对正常，但由于患者找词困难，所以说话内容模糊不清。

目前的语言组织模型是基于背侧流和腹侧流处理的（Chang et al.，2015）。背侧流主要位于优势半球内，对感觉运动整合至关重要；而腹侧流是双侧的，对语言理解至关重要。通过皮质下电刺激图谱，现在我们对语言处理所必需的功能网络有了不断发展但更完整的理解。上纵束（superior longitudinal fasciculus，SLF）由四个主要部分组成（SLF Ⅰ、Ⅱ、Ⅲ和 SLF-tp）（Chang et al.，2015）。SLF Ⅰ不参与语言处理，SLF Ⅱ连接前运动皮质与角回，SLF Ⅲ连接前额叶腹侧皮质与缘上回，SLF-tp 连接顶下小叶与颞上后叶。刺激 SLF Ⅱ和Ⅲ引起构音障碍，而刺激 SLF Ⅲ和 SLF-tp 均引起错误或语言重复。弓状束通常被认为是连接 Broca 和 Wernicke 区域。现在我们了解到，弓状束连接额 - 盖和后颞皮质部位的方式更加多样化。刺激弓状束会导致失语和音位性言语错乱，而这条皮质下通路的损伤则会导致传导性失语（完整的理解、流畅的言语产生但重复性差；见 Chang et al.，2015）。

神经功能缺失

由于肿瘤的位置和疾病的程度不同，内源性脑肿瘤的神经功能缺失存在很大变化。颅内压升高时可出现非特异性的体征，包括视盘水肿（视盘水肿伴视网膜静脉充盈）和动眼神经麻痹（由于钩回疝）。额叶肿瘤可导致步态障碍、意志缺失、性格改变和偏瘫。失语症提示优势半球额叶或颞叶的皮质语言中枢受累。颞叶肿瘤也可能导致记忆力减退、听觉辨别力受损、癫痫发作及对侧上象限盲。顶叶肿瘤可导致感觉功能受损、注意力分散、对侧下象限盲、失语症或失认症。枕叶肿瘤会导致视觉障碍，而脑干肿瘤可能会损伤脑神经，导致长束征。松果体肿瘤影响中脑顶盖可导致 Parinaund 综合征，包括上视麻痹、眼睑回缩（Collier 征）或上睑下垂、瞳孔对光反射消失（对光反射无反应，但辐辏反射存在）和会聚 - 回缩性眼球震颤。

头痛是脑瘤患者最常见的症状，至少有 50% 的患者在某些时候会出现头痛。通常情况下，脑瘤患者的头痛在早晨醒来时加重，而且往往严重到足以将患者从睡眠中唤醒。

头痛的发生被认为是由睡眠期间卧床和二氧化碳分压（PCO_2）升高引起的颅内压暂时升高所致。肿瘤的占位效应加上 PCO_2 升高导致的脑血管扩张，最终导致头痛发生。

术前外科处理

术前计划

术前临床评估应包括手术前 24~48 小时进行的基线感觉运动和语言评估（Hervey-Jumper et al.，2015）。

术前成像包括增强和平扫脑 MRI，白质通路（包括皮质脊髓束、上纵束、弓状束、钩状束和眶前内束）的 DTI 成像，基于任务的功能性脑 MRI（fMRI）（Deng et al.，2015；Ille et al.，2015）（图 13.1）和灌注 MRI。

术前解剖影像可提供有关肿瘤位置、血管分布、占位效应、瘤周水肿以及是否接近潜在重要功能区域的信息。此外，这些解剖学研究可以重建，以创建可在手术（神经导航）中使用的三维模型。DTI 定义了肿瘤周围白质束的完整性，通常用于外科和放射治疗的计划（Alexander et al.，2007；Berman et al.，2007；Bello et al.，2008）。基于任务的功能磁

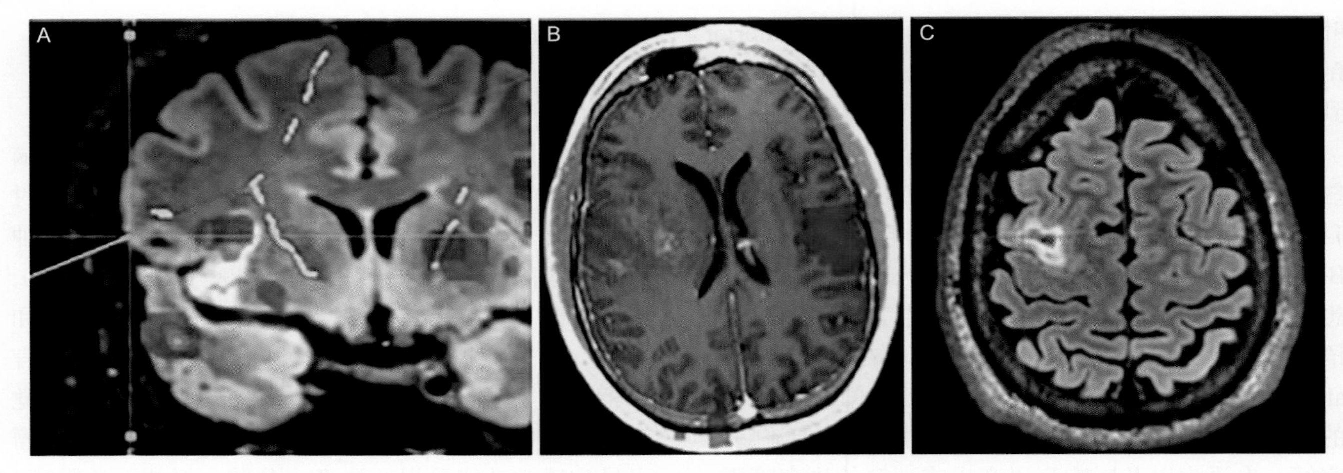

图 13.1 功能磁共振成像（fMRI）、脑磁图（MEG）和弥散张量成像（DTI）等成像手段为术前和术中应用提供了有价值的信息。（A）功能磁共振成像显示紫色区域为语言激活位点。（B）脑磁图蓝色标识区域为语言产生区。（C）DTI 显示皮质脊髓束位于胶质瘤外侧的纵束纤维的后方和上方

共振成像使用血氧水平依赖（blood oxygenation level dependent，BOLD）信号来识别皮质和皮质下的激活区域，以创建手术通道或切除计划，从而最大限度地减少对功能区周围结构的风险（Bogomolny et al.，2004；Nimsky et al.，2004）。最后，灌注 MRI 对评估肿瘤血管生成、内皮通透性和治疗反应是有用的。

结合解剖 MRI、功能 MRI、DTI 纤维束成像和灌注 MRI，临床医生可以做出更准确的术前诊断，并提供有关肿瘤组织与邻近功能皮质和皮质下通路的界面信息。

药物治疗

脑内肿瘤的治疗首选手术，目的是确定病理诊断并最大限度地安全切除肿瘤。术前药物治疗和手术计划是确保手术干预成功的关键。术前通常使用皮质类固醇来减轻占位效应和瘤周血管源性水肿的症状。虽然皮质类固醇的使用时间和剂量因外科医生的偏好而异，但成人常用的方案是每六小时静脉或口服地塞米松 4~6 mg。

出现癫痫症状的患者应开始服用抗惊厥药物。然而，除了极少数例外，没有数据表明预防性使用抗惊厥药物可以降低脑内肿瘤患者新发癫痫的风险（Chang et al.，2005；Chang et al.，2008；De Oliveira Lima，2015）。即便如此，在肿瘤累及高致痫区域（如运动皮质）的情况下，低级别胶质瘤、伴有大量血管源性水肿的多发性转移瘤或软脑膜疾病的患者通常会接受预防性癫痫药物治疗。苯妥英钠历来是一线抗癫痫药；然而，必须监测苯妥英钠的水平，以确保治疗性的血清药物浓度。左乙拉西坦现在被广泛使用，因为它的毒性很低，副作用最小，而且不需要监测血清浓度。

术中外科处理

活检和切除范围

近年来，一些研究加深了我们对肿瘤切除对脑内肿瘤患者无进展总生存率影响的理解（Hervey-Jumper and Berger，2014）。然而，外科手术的最初目标是建立明确的组织学诊断。决定手术切除还是活检取决于肿瘤的位置和大小、患者的年龄和一般状况。必须平衡肿瘤的自然病史及其随时间转化和生长的倾向。最近的数据将最大范围安全切除与患者年龄、肿瘤组织学、肿瘤表现状态和分子标志物一起作为长期结果的预测因素（Hervey-Jumper and Berger，2014）。因此，最大范围安全切除优先于活检。

手术切除治疗脑内肿瘤（尤其是低级别胶质瘤）的价值已被大量研究证实，该研究表明，肿瘤切除 90% 以上的患者可获得 60~90 个月的生存益处（Smith et al.，2008）。在一个基于大型人群的挪威患者研究显示，早期最大切除优于活检和观察等待，其 5 年生存率分别为 74% 和 60%，说明了切除优于观察等待（Jakola et al.，2012）。此外，低级别胶质瘤切除 90% 以上可以延缓和减少恶变可能，提高生存率。在大体完全切除脑内肿瘤后，也更有利于控制癫痫发作（Chang et al.，2008）。

影像引导

对于脑肿瘤外科医生来说，功能性和解剖学影

像引导是确定手术相关风险和解答患者术后潜在神经功能障碍相关咨询的重要部分。影像引导还可以提供一个概括性的术前印象，即功能通路可能被占位性病变移位。神经导航广泛应用于脑肿瘤手术，并可与DTI跟踪成像、脑磁图（MEG）或功能磁共振成像（fMRI）（通常称为“功能性神经导航”）相结合，以识别皮质和皮质下潜在感觉、运动、语言和视觉区域（Trin et al.，2014）（**图 13.1**）。因此，神经导航可以生成个性化的功能区地图，以及它们与大脑内肿瘤病变的关系。个体神经解剖学的变异性、占位效应造成的扭曲以及可塑性导致的功能重组使得经典的功能区域解剖学识别不足（Thiel et al.，2001；Duffau，2006）。与直接皮质刺激相比，fMRI对Broca区识别的敏感性和特异性分别为91%和64%，对Wernicke区的敏感性和特异性分别为93%和18%，对运动区的敏感性和特异性分别为100%和100%（Bizzi et al.，2008）。

用脑磁图或磁共振成像测量的静息状态连通性能够描绘大脑的功能连通性。静息状态连通性降低的脑内肿瘤术后神经功能缺陷的风险相对较低，而静息状态连通性增强的脑内肿瘤术后神经功能缺陷的风险较高（Guggisberg et al.，2008）。这些研究有助于确定与手术相关的风险、最佳手术入路，并告知患者有关潜在的术后神经障碍。皮质下通路的识别对于防止白质通路的损伤和保护功能至关重要（Sarubbo et al.，2015）。虽然目前评估皮质和皮质下功能组织的金标准是术中刺激试验，但术前和术中“可视化”白质束及其与脑肿瘤的空间关系是有利的。

清醒开颅手术与神经生理监测

直接皮质刺激描记最先由Wilder Penfield使用，可以在切除脑肿瘤的手术中识别语言、运动和感觉功能（Hervey-Jumper et al.，2015）。来自脑肿瘤的个体变异性和路径扭曲使得神经导航的可靠性降低。言语障碍、命名性失语和失读症通常位于Broca区解剖边界之外较远的地方（Sanai et al.，2008）。直接皮质刺激描记是识别和保护功能区的金标准。

皮质刺激使大脑的一个局部区域去极化，通过顺向和逆行传播电流的扩散来兴奋局部神经元。使用尖端2 mm和间隔5 mm的双极刺激允许局部扩散和更精确描记（Nathan et al.，1993）。早期的描记技术利用大范围开颅手术，目的是确定阳性功能部位；然而，也可以使用较小的开颅显露，依赖于阴性描记（Sanai et al.，2008）。阴性描记策略代表了描记技术的转变，避免显露和接触功能区。肿瘤外科医生必须在最大限度切除与保留运动和语言功能部位之间取得平衡。

专门的神经麻醉是完成安全清醒开颅手术的关键（Taylor and Bernstein，1999）。神经外科医生、麻醉师、言语病理学家和描记团队其他成员之间的清晰沟通确保了手术的准确性和患者安全。手术开始于应用患者监护仪（腋窝温度探头、血压袖带、动脉导管），并在定位前使用咪达唑仑、芬太尼或右美托咪啶（Hervey-Jumper et al.，2015）。镇静是使用异丙酚［高达100 μg/（kg · min）］或右美托咪啶［高达1 μg/（kg · min）和瑞芬太尼［0.07~2.0 μg/（kg · h）］实现的（Herrick et al.，1997；Bekker et al.，2001；Olsen，2008）。在插入Foley导尿管和安置Mayfield头架时也需要给予镇静。神经外科医生使用1%利多卡因和1∶100 000肾上腺素、0.5%丁哌卡因和8.4%碳酸氢钠混合物进行头皮阻滞。神经外科医师和麻醉师必须讨论好患者头部摆放的最佳位置，以便于操作、患者舒适度高和潜在的喉罩气道插入。在皮肤切开并取下骨瓣后，会停用所有镇静剂，然后要求患者在硬膜开窗前进行多次深呼吸以减少高碳酸血症。如需抑制术中癫痫大发作，可在专用静脉输液中注入异丙酚（1 mg/kg液体）。冰冻乳酸林格液可随时用于抑制术中癫痫发作。

术中刺激从1.5~2 mA的刺激电流开始，必要时增加到最大6 mA。恒流发生器以60 Hz的频率在4 s内发送1.25 ms的双相方波。数字标记被放置在手术区域上，间隔1 cm摆放（**图 13.2**）。连续皮质脑电图用于提高描记精度、监测亚临床发作活动和后放电电位。所有的语言测试在每个皮质部位至少重复三次，阳性部位被定义为刺激过程中至少三次中有两次无法计数、命名物体或阅读单词。语言描记试图通过刺激测试找出导致失语、命名不能和失读症的部位。言语抑制被定义为在没有同步运动反应的情况下停止计数。构音障碍与言语障碍的区别在于前者没有影响言语的不随意肌收缩（Sanai et al.，2008）。

5-氨基乙酰丙酸（5-ALA）

脑内肿瘤的大体全切除可能是具有挑战性的，而且大多数肿瘤复发都发生在先前切除腔的一厘米内，这一点已经得到了充分证实。大多数神经外科医生会高估切除程度。5-ALA是一种非荧光氨基酸前体，可在高级别胶质瘤中产生荧光卟啉（主要是原卟啉IX）的积聚（Stummer et al.，2006）。外源性5-ALA导致恶性胶质瘤细胞内荧光原卟啉的积累，在给药后6小时达到高峰，并持续升高12小时（Stummer

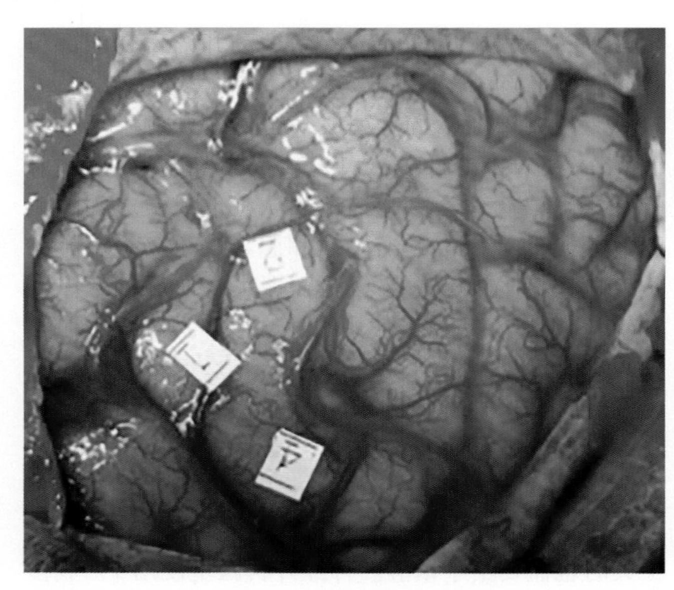

图 13.2 直接皮质和皮质下刺激描记是识别功能性语言和感觉运动区的金标准。皮质描记使用每隔 1 cm 放置的编号标志物来测试覆盖在肿瘤上并与肿瘤直接相邻的区域

et al.，2003）。原卟啉 IX 在 380+/-420 nm 光谱中有一个最强的吸收带，在 635 nm 和 704 nm 处发出红色荧光。最常见的既定方案是在手术前 3 小时口服 5-ALA，目标是在应用 5-ALA 后 4~5 小时切除肿瘤。当操作者在白光和紫光之间切换时，安装在手术显微镜上的长波通滤光片可以实现肿瘤的可视化（**图 13.3**）。

几项研究已经检验了 5-ALA 在提高恶性胶质瘤患者的切除范围和延长生存期方面的效果。完全去除所有荧光物质（5-ALA 完全切除）可以在不增加术后神经功能缺陷的情况下提高恶性胶质瘤的 6 个月和总体生存率（Stummer et al.，2006）。对接受常规白光显微手术或荧光引导手术并辅以 5-ALA 的疑似恶性胶质瘤患者进行的Ⅲ期临床试验发现，65% 的 5-ALA 患者接受了大体全切除，而接受传统白光显微手术的患者中这一比例为 36%。因此，研究组患者的 6 个月无进展生存率提高了 50%（41.0% *vs.* 21.1%）（Stummer et al.，2006）。

Gliadel 片

卡莫司汀片，也被称为 Gliadel wafers（GW）（Arbor Pharmaceuticals，LLC，Atlanta，GA），被批准用于治疗新诊断和复发的高级别胶质瘤（WHO Ⅲ级和Ⅳ级）。卡莫司汀是一种烷化剂，会干扰 DNA 的合成和修复。GW 是一种可生物降解的聚合物，含有 3.85% 的卡莫司汀。这些聚合物在肿瘤切除手术后被植入术腔，大约 5 天内释放 7.7 mg 的药物。由于几个原因，其广泛使用受到了限制。GW 的安全性和有效性一直是一个有争议的问题，一些发表的研究显示了极好的患者耐受性和提高了生存率，而另一些研究则没有发现通过在标准疗法中添加卡莫司汀片来改善生存率（Xing et al.，2015）。目前，卡莫司汀片的使用在大多数情况下都是有限的，因为担心伤口愈合问题，而且可能会影响后续临床试验入组。

深部肿瘤

深部肿瘤由于靠近重要的血管结构和位于功能区周围，治疗起来仍然具有挑战性。由于围术期并发症的高风险，位于脑岛、扣带回和丘脑的病变以前被认为是不能手术的。随着神经麻醉、先进的结

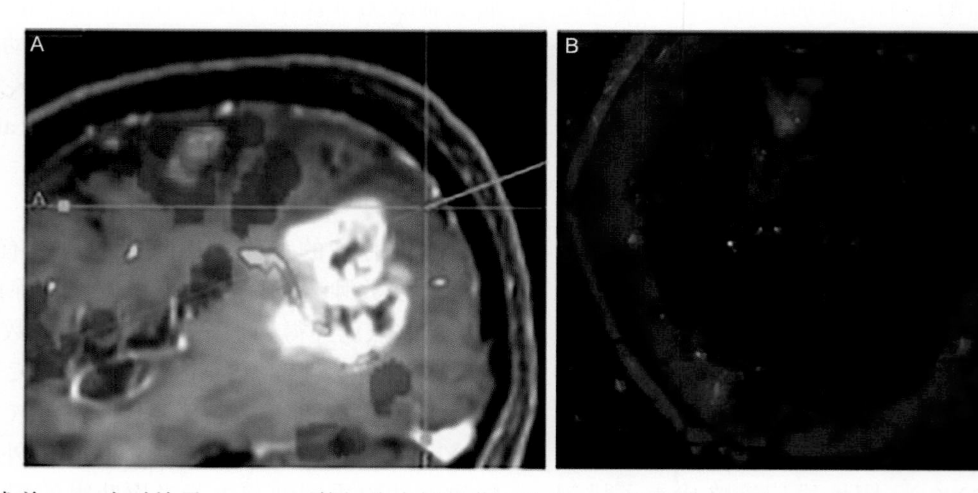

图 13.3 手术前 2~5 小时给予 5-ALA 可使细胞内摄取荧光卟啉。功能性神经导航显示肿瘤的皮质途径（A），在紫蓝色光下确认为粉红色（B）

构和功能成像，以及显微外科技术相结合，使得我们更容易治疗许多深部肿瘤。下一步将更详细地讨论岛叶、扣带回和丘脑深部肿瘤的手术入路和技术考虑。

岛叶病变

岛叶肿瘤是最具挑战性的神经外科病变之一。肿瘤的位置和语言优势半球决定了是否考虑经皮质入路或经侧翼入路（Benet et al.，2015）。患者半侧卧位，头部与地面平行（Sanai et al.，2010）。对于主要位于侧裂上方或下方的肿瘤，头顶分别朝向天花板或地板 15°。开颅手术是根据肿瘤的位置和覆盖的额叶或颞盖的受累情况量身定做的。可以利用皮质和皮质下感觉运动和语言描记技术。一旦确定了功能区，就通过岛动脉之间的非功能区（“皮质窗”）创建侧裂上方和下方的经皮质窗。将侧裂血管轮廓化后，可继行手术切除。沿着钩状束在侧裂下方进行手术。须识别和保存侧裂上豆纹动脉。皮质脊髓束的皮质下运动描记区标志着切除的内侧边界。早期识别走向内囊和放射冠的长豆纹动脉穿支，避免可能导致血管痉挛的过度操作，可最大限度地减少缺血性并发症。上纵束的水平纤维与上岛周沟相邻，钩状束与下岛周沟相邻。外囊水平的 IFOF 是通过皮质下刺激诱发语义性失语来识别的。

扣带回病变

扣带回覆盖胼胝体，位于大脑镰正下方。扣带回分为前部和后部，由沿其内侧表面的胼缘动脉覆盖。由于位于大脑半球间裂隙深处，前扣带回和后扣带回内的肿瘤手术困难。一般根据肿瘤的位置、大小、血供情况和病理，选择仰卧位或坐位，行单侧或双侧开颅手术。术前应仔细检查是否有桥静脉，这可能会影响手术入路。切开硬脑膜应慎重，避免损伤上矢状窦或近端引流静脉。手术时需要首先建立手术通路，然后行肿瘤血运阻断，并确定胼缘动脉和胼周动脉。依据肿瘤周围功能区、血运、大小和位置，确定大脑纵裂入路、额上回造瘘或顶上小叶造瘘入路（Talacchi et al.，2010）。

丘脑病变

丘脑肿瘤相对罕见，占所有脑肿瘤的 1%~5%（Sai Kiran et al.，2013）。虽然该部位的病变历来仅用立体定向活检和放射治疗，但先进的结构成像和显微外科技术使手术切除的术后发病率显著降低。术前增强影像显示边缘清晰的肿瘤可考虑手术切除，边缘模糊的非强化肿瘤应该通过活检进行治疗。手术入路的选择是基于肿瘤的位置（丘脑内的前部或后部）和是否接近内囊后肢。大多数深部肿瘤导致内囊后肢向前外侧移位，常用经颞中回入路。颞叶皮质切除后，经侧脑室沿肿瘤后外侧缘进入到达肿瘤。打开侧脑室颞角后，通过脉络膜裂到达肿瘤。这一入路确保了在岛叶下方和内囊后方进入手术区域。

如果肿瘤位于前方并进入侧脑室，特别是当脑室扩大时，适合经胼胝体入路，但对于向侧方延伸的较大病灶显露有限。若肿瘤向内突入第三脑室，需要注意避免损伤位于丘脑或脉络膜裂上方的穹隆脚。后侧半球间或幕下小脑上入路可用于探查那些位于丘脑枕后方的病变。因许多视束纤维与毗邻外侧膝状体的丘脑枕密切相关，故该入路有损伤视束纤维的危险。

术后外科处理

术后即刻，患者在重症监护病房中密切观察，做一系列的神经评估（Chang et al.，2005）。根据肿瘤的位置和切除程度，皮质类固醇可能会在术后几天逐渐减少。对于有癫痫病史的患者和已知有癫痫倾向区域的肿瘤，继续使用抗惊厥药物。长期使用抗癫痫药物进行预防仍然存在争议。考虑到手术切除范围对胶质瘤患者预后的重要意义，以及术中发现残留肿瘤的困难，术后 24 小时内做增强 MRI 以发现残留肿瘤已成为标准做法。

并发症

脑内肿瘤的手术有发生术后内科和外科并发症的风险。神经系统并发症可能导致视野、运动、感觉、认知或语言缺陷（Chang et al.，2005）。这些并发症的发生是由功能皮质和皮质下通路的破坏、脑水肿、血肿或血管损伤引起的。在大多数报道中，开颅手术切除脑内肿瘤后出现新的神经功能缺损的风险从 10% 到 25% 不等。手术风险增高与高龄、肿瘤位置深、肿瘤靠近功能区，以及较低的 Kanofsky 评分相关。依靠解剖和功能成像、皮质描记技术、最大限度地减少过度脑回缩、细致止血和早期识别主要血管结构，个体化设计手术入路，可以最大限度地减少神经系统并发症。

其他并发症与手术伤口和周围脑实质有关。这些疾病包括手术伤口感染、气脑、脑脊液（CSF）漏、脑积水、癫痫、脑脓肿、脑炎、脑膜炎和假性脑膜膨出。这些并发症在接受开颅手术切除脑内肿瘤的患者发生率为1%~5%，并且更容易发生在老年患者和接受再次手术的患者中。颅后窝手术和再手术与假性脊膜膨出、脑脊液漏、脑积水和伤口感染的发生率较高相关。幕上开颅术后伤口感染和蜂窝组织炎的发生率为1%~2%。通常是由金黄色葡萄球菌或表皮葡萄球菌引起的皮肤炎症导致的。幕上开颅术后癫痫发作的风险为0.5%~5%。预防性抗癫痫药物可以在术后常规使用，但其剂量和持续时间仍存在争议。

全身并发症包括不良事件，如深静脉血栓形成（deep vein thrombosis，DVT）、肺栓塞、肺炎、尿路感染、心肌梗死和脓毒症。这些医疗并发症发生在5%~10%的接受开颅手术切除脑内肿瘤的患者中，并且在老年患者和一般状态差的神经受损患者中更为常见。DVT是最常见的并发症，1%~10%的患者在开颅手术后的第一个月内发生。系统性癌症、多形性胶质母细胞瘤、偏瘫、长时间卧床和长时间手术的患者发生DVT或肺栓塞的风险尤其高。术后早期活动、应用间歇性加压装置、术后低分子肝素抗凝可降低术后DVT的发生率。

开颅手术切除脑内肿瘤是安全的，只要有周密的术前计划、细致的手术技巧和细心的术后护理，大多数并发症是可以预防的。

争论

清醒开颅与术中MRI（iMRI）比较

MRI引导下的脑肿瘤手术已被证明可以提高胶质瘤切除的范围和患者的生存率。许多研究试图量化iMRI对肿瘤切除范围的影响（Knauth et al.，1999；Wirtz et al.，2000）。iMRI和清醒开颅手术都是在降低神经功能缺失的同时最大限度地扩大切除范围的工具。使用iMRI结合传统的神经导航切除的主要原理是避免因脑脊液丢失和组织水肿而引起的脑移位（Nimsky et al.，2002）。随着手术的进展，神经导航变得越来越不可靠。术中MRI已被证明可以增加低或高级别胶质瘤患者的切除范围和生存率（Black et al.，1999）。在手术后神经功能缺损无差异的情况下，iMRI显著改善了肿瘤切除范围。在一系列涉及高级别胶质瘤患者的研究中发现，扩大切除范围能提高生存率（Schneider et al.，2005）。

关于清醒描记技术和iMRI引导的使用存在争议。唤醒技术允许实时语言和感觉运动描记和监测，这可能与功能和结构成像（功能神经导航）相结合。虽然这是确定功能区的最佳方法，但功能区和非功能区的切除范围可能是有限的。iMRI的主要优势是能够在整个过程中获得最新成像。许多患者因体重和身体习惯（清醒开颅手术）或心脏并发症等原因，都不是理想的选择。在iMRI中使用清醒描记和MRI引导手术是越来越被接受的，对于选择得当的患者，其优化了切除范围和患者的安全性。

延伸阅读、参考文献、EBRAIN的相关链接

扫描书末二维码获取。

第三篇 肿瘤和颅底——轴外肿瘤和颅骨病变

第14章 脑膜瘤和血管外皮细胞瘤 - 孤立性纤维瘤

Harjus S. Birk • Seunggu J. Han • Ramez W. Kirollos • Thomas Santarius • Michael W. McDermott 著
吴涛 译，陈保东 审校

引言

1922 年 Harvey Cushing 首次描述了脑膜瘤，此后被认为是最常见的颅内非神经胶质肿瘤（Ostrom et al.，2016）。这些生长缓慢的肿瘤连续发生于脑膜，起源于软脑膜的蛛网膜帽状细胞。它们有可能压迫脑组织，或较少见地侵入大脑、脊髓以及脑神经和周围神经，导致神经功能缺损。

根据部位的不同，脑膜瘤可产生广泛的症状。症状和体征可与邻近神经结构的压迫直接相关，也可继发于颅内压升高的影响。例如，如果肿瘤位于蝶骨嵴的内侧部分，视力下降和眼球活动麻痹可能是常见的；而位于颅后窝的肿瘤可能导致不同的症状群，包括脑积水和发声困难。

流行病学

脑膜瘤占所有原发性颅内肿瘤的 36.7%（Ostrom et al.，2016）。考虑到美国的人口增加，目前有 15 万人可能被诊断为脑膜瘤，发病率为 3/10 万 ~3.5/10 万（Claus et al.，2005）。据报道，脑膜瘤发病率越来越高，老年人的发病率上升更明显（Klaeboe et al.，2005）。这种增加可以通过引入先进的成像技术来解释，这些技术已被用于全面的患者检查，在这些技术上，偶发的脑膜瘤现在被普遍检测到。脑部 MRI 偶然发现脑膜瘤很常见，患病率随年龄增长而大幅增加（Morris et al.，2009）。这种趋势在未来很可能会持续。

发生脑膜瘤的风险随年龄增长而增加，受影响最大的年龄范围为 40~70 岁。好发于女性，所有脑膜瘤的女性与男性比例为 1.8∶1，症状性脑膜瘤的比例略高，为 2.3∶1（Radhakrishnan et al.，1995）。WHO 1 级与 2 级和 3 级脑膜瘤的女性 - 男性比率不同：分别为 2.3、1.2 和 1.1（Ostrom et al.，2016）。脑膜瘤在儿童中相当少见，仅占总数的 1.5%，在婴儿中极为罕见（Kotecha et al.，2011）。有趣的是，儿童期脑膜瘤在男性中的发生率略高于女性，比例为 1.3∶1（Kotecha et al.，2011）。高达 15%~25% 的儿童脑膜瘤病例与神经纤维瘤 1 型（NF2）或 2 型（NF2）相关（Baumgartner and Sorenson，1996；Kotecha et al.，2011）。这些病例倾向于发生在年轻个体中，男女比例相当。

放射性脑膜瘤

放射性脑膜瘤的风险取决于辐射剂量和照射野、可能的遗传易感性，最重要的是随访，因为有潜伏期的问题。这些脑膜瘤包括不同分级的脑膜瘤，其中超过 10% 为多发性脑膜瘤。平均潜伏期为 22.9±11.4 年，较高等级脑膜瘤的潜伏期较短（Yamanaka et al.，2017）。在一项接受头颅放射治疗的儿童癌症生存者的研究中，到 40 岁时，后续脑膜瘤的累积发生率为 5.6%，从原发性癌症到脑膜瘤诊断的中位间隔时间为 22 年，并且风险增加与辐射剂量增加相关（Bowers et al.，2017）。

病理

脑膜瘤被认为起源于脑膜上皮细胞（也称为蛛网膜帽状细胞）。脑膜上皮细胞在蛛网膜绒毛表面最丰富，分布于大静脉窦、大静脉、基底静脉丛、鸡冠等周围，但也见于中枢神经系统所有位置和其他部位的蛛网膜（Haines and Frederickson，1991）。然而，尽管经常重复，但这仅是基于观察到脑膜上皮和脑膜瘤细胞之间显著的相似性，以及高浓度脑膜上皮细胞与脑膜瘤常见位置之间的再定位的假设（Riemenschneider et al.，2006）。非常罕见的硬脑膜外脑膜瘤被认为是由脑膜上皮细胞包埋或其他一些“干细胞样”细胞引起的（Lang et al.，2000）。

与其他脑肿瘤一样，WHO 中枢神经系统肿瘤分类（WHO 分类）根据其组织学外观对脑膜瘤进行分级，其最后一次修订发表于 2016 年（Louis et al.，2016）。提示恶性程度更高的攻击行为和增加的组织学标准包括频繁有丝分裂、细胞过多区域、片状生长、高核质比、显著核仁和自发性坏死。

脑膜瘤扩大和移位，但一般不浸润邻近的脑或脊髓。硬脑膜和颅骨的侵袭确有发生，但对恶性肿瘤分级无意义。侵入颅骨可引起成骨细胞反应。所有恶性肿瘤级别的脑膜瘤均可发生脑浸润，表明复发的可能性更大，但在 2016 版 WHO 分类之前，仅认为不足以增加恶性肿瘤级别（Louis et al.，2016；Jenkinson et al.，2017）。然而，根据 2007 年版 WHO 分类，许多病理学家将伴有脑侵袭的脑膜瘤归类为非典型性。

在 2000 年分类之前，1 级脑膜瘤约占所有脑膜瘤的 90%，而非典型性（2 级）约 5%，间变性（3 级）1%~2%。在采用 2000 年 WHO 分类后，2 级脑膜瘤的比例增加至诊断为脑膜瘤的 15%~35%（Claus et al.，2005；Riemenschneider et al.，2006；Pearson et al.，2008）。在 2007 年分类中，具有其他 1 级组织学特征但显微镜下脑浸润的脑膜瘤可归类为非典型性，这导致非典型性脑膜瘤的比例进一步增加（Backer-Grøndahl et al.，2012）。在 Kshettry 等开展的基于人群的研究中，非典型性脑膜瘤的年发生率（每 100000 人）从 26%~28%（2004—2006）增加至 30%~32%（2008—2010）（Kshettry et al.，2015）。有趣的是，非典型性脑膜瘤在非颅底位置更常见（Backer-Grøndahl et al.，2012）。

WHO 3 级脑膜瘤，有时也称为恶性脑膜瘤，定义为高有丝分裂指数（每 10 个高倍视野超过 20 个有丝分裂）或其组织学外观类似于癌、肉瘤或黑色素瘤。它们是脑膜瘤最罕见的级别，仅包含 1%~2% 的新诊断脑膜瘤（Kshettry et al.，2015）。这些肿瘤患者的中位总生存期平均为 2~3 年（Sughrue et al. 2010；Perry，2013；Champeaux et al.，2015）。即使采用可能包括手术和放疗的积极治疗，局部控制通常无法实现，可能发生颅外转移。

Backer-Grøndahl 等（2012）报告的良性脑膜瘤亚型的相对频率（**图** 14.1）列于**表** 14.1。这些与其他报道的系列相似（Perry et al.，1999；Willis et al，2005）。区分脑膜瘤的良性亚型几乎没有预后意义，然而，它有助于区分脑膜瘤与其他肿瘤。分泌亚型通常可根据成像预测，因为这些脑膜瘤与大量水肿相关，可能危及生命（Regelsberger et al.，2009）。尤其是腹膜脑膜瘤可能进展为更高组织学分级（约 50% 的间变性脑膜由低级别脑膜瘤进展而来（Champeaux et al，2015）。因此应彻底采样，避免遗漏组织学更具侵袭性的潜在区域。

非典型性（**图** 14.2）和间变性脑膜瘤的诊断主要基于有丝分裂计数和**表** 14.2 中列出的其他“较软”标准。然而，一些以特定肿瘤细胞表型为特征的罕见脑膜瘤亚型与更频繁的复发相关，并自动（无论是否存在上述组织学“恶性肿瘤特征”）分级为 WHO 2 级（脊索样和透明细胞）或 WHO 3 级（乳头状和杆状）细胞脑膜瘤。然而，横纹肌样脑膜瘤不再自动归类为 3 级，而是应将缺乏恶性组织学特征的脑膜瘤归类为任何其他脑膜瘤，因为它们似乎与正常脑膜瘤分级相似（Louis et al.，2016）。

分子肿瘤细胞生物学

脑膜瘤是人类首个显示一致染色体异常的实体瘤之一，早在 1972 年就发现了 22 号染色体一个拷贝的丢失（Mark et al.，1972）。事实上，神经纤维瘤病 2 型（NF2）患者中第二常见的肿瘤是脑膜瘤，指出 NF2 基因是 22 号染色体上的靶标（Rouleau et al.，1993；Trofatter et al.，1993）。NF2 是 Knudson 二次打击假说后肿瘤抑制基因的教科书示例，其中第一次打击（一个等位基因的丢失）通常是杂合性缺失，第二次打击是丢失（缺失）或失活（通常是错义）点突变。随后在 40%~ 60% 的散发性脑膜瘤中发现 NF2 基因突变（Ruttledge et al.，1994；Riemenschneider et al.，2006）。NF2 基因编码 merlin，也称为神经纤维素 2，一种膜细胞骨架蛋白。该蛋白已被证明参与培养物中细胞生长和运动的控制（Shaw，2001；Lallemand，2003）。仅有一个野生型等位基因的基因工程小鼠显示发生许多肿瘤形式（McClatchey et al.，1998），而施万细胞或软脑膜细胞中的组织特异性失活分别导致神经鞘瘤或脑膜瘤的形成（Giovannini et al.，2000；Kalamarides et al.，2002）。

大量报道证实了 NF2 突变在脑膜瘤中的重要作用。利用新一代测序技术，2013 年 1 月发表的三篇论文发现了其他几个可能在脑膜瘤中很重要的基因，尤其是野生型 NF2（Brastianos et al.，2013；Clark et al.，2013；Reuss et al.，2013）。Clark 等（2013）和 Brastianos 等（2013）的研究已经确定了两个众所周知的癌症基因（SMO 和 AKT1）的突变，这两个基因都相互排斥，并且与 NF2 突变相互排斥。SMO 和 AKT1 突变频率分别为 5% 和 10%~15%。Clark 等还报道了 TRAF7（之前未与癌症相关（占所有肿瘤的

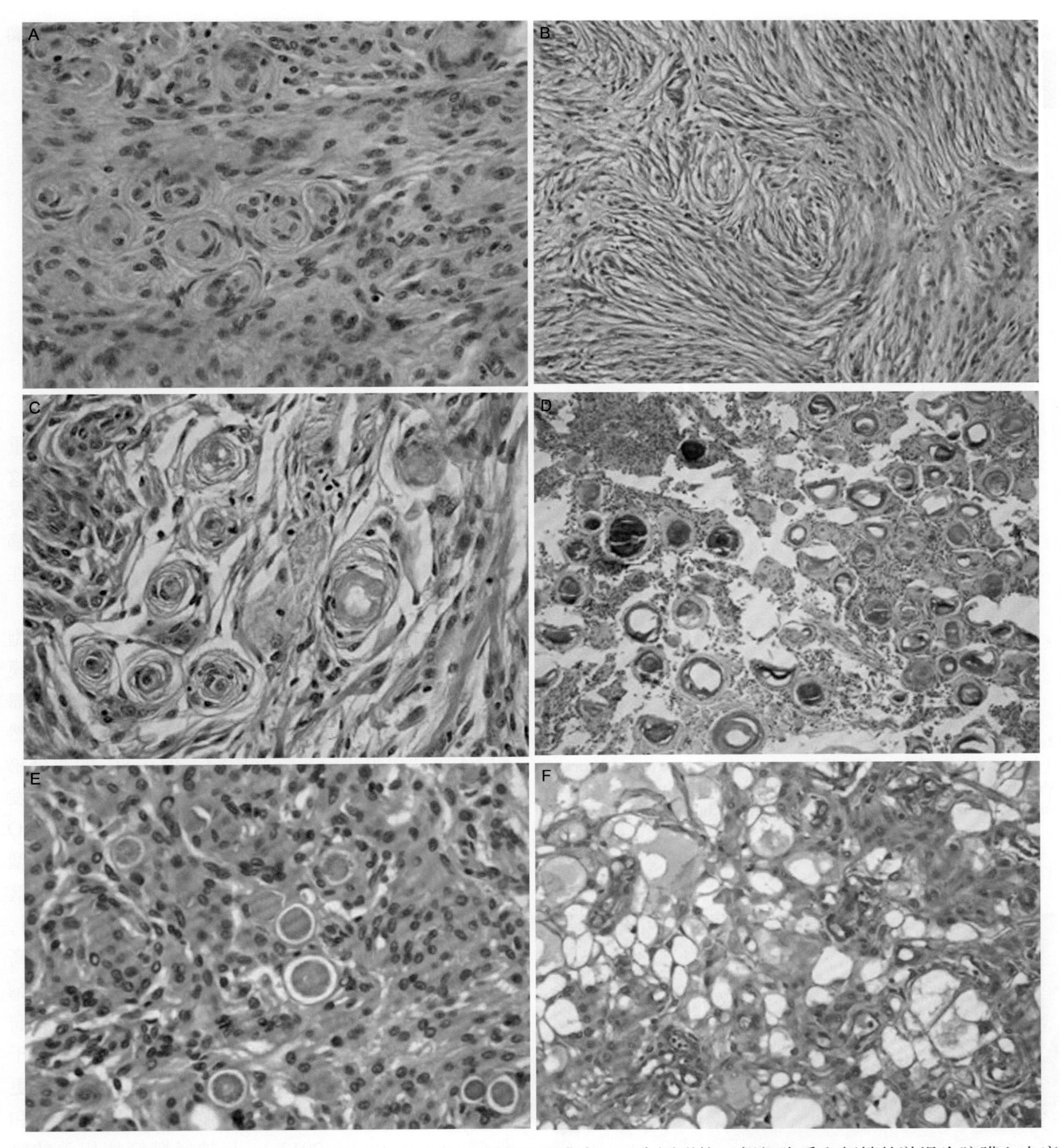

图 14.1　1 级脑膜瘤，组织学亚型示例。（A）脑膜上皮瘤型脑膜瘤——卵圆形核、假细胞质和频繁的漩涡为脑膜上皮瘤型脑膜瘤的特征。（B）成纤维细胞性脑膜瘤——呈束状排列的梭形细胞，常有中间的胶原，是成纤维细胞性脑膜瘤的特征。（C）移行性脑膜瘤——可能大多数脑膜瘤表现为脑膜上皮和成纤维细胞模式的混合物，即所谓的移行性脑膜瘤。（D）砂粒体脑膜瘤——虽然存在于绝大多数脑膜瘤中，但球形层状钙化结块，称为砂粒体，在胸髓区域经常遇到，这种亚型在组织学上占主导地位。（E）分泌性脑膜瘤——大量圆形、嗜酸性"分泌小体"是该 1 级亚型的特征，通常与 MRI 上的大量脑水肿相关。（F）微囊性脑膜瘤——一种蛛网样、微囊性结构例证了这种 I 级亚型，与分泌亚型一样，可伴有不成比例的脑水肿。这种亚型的光滑切面给实体提供了"湿性脑膜瘤"的旧称

Courtesy of Dr Kieren Allinson, Department of Pathology, Addenbrooke's Hospital, Cambridge.

表 14.1 脑膜瘤亚型的相对频率

WHO 分级	组织学亚型	近似比例（%）
良性（70%~80%）		
	• 脑膜上皮	17
	• 纤维（成纤维细胞）	7
	• 过渡型（混合型）	40
	• 砂粒状	1
	• 血管瘤性	1
	• 微囊	1
	• 分泌	1
	• 富含淋巴浆细胞	1
	• 化生	1
非典型性（20%~30%）	20~30	
	• 非典型	29
	• 脊索	
	• 透明细胞	1
恶性（1%~2%）	1~2	
	• 间变性	1
	• 乳头状	
	• 横纹肌样	

Reproduced with permission from Thomas Backer-Grondahl, Bjornar H Moen, Sverre H Torp, The Histopathological Spectrum of Human Meningiomas. *International Journal of Clinical and Experimental Pathology*, Volume 5, Issue 3, pp. 231–42. Copyright © 2012.

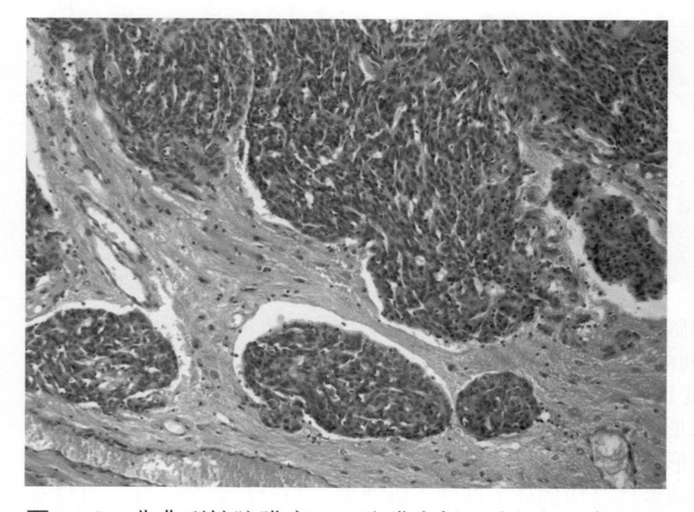

图 14.2 非典型性脑膜瘤——脑膜瘤侵入脑组织，如图所示，将该脑膜瘤定性为非典型性脑膜瘤，因此 WHO 分级为 2 级。与 2 级脑膜瘤相关的其他特征包括坏死和有丝分裂活性增加

Courtesy of Dr Kieren Allinson, Department of Pathology, Addenbrooke's Hospital, Cambridge.

表 14.2 世界卫生组织（WHO）2 级和 3 级脑膜瘤标准的比较

2 级	非典型性	4~19 个核分裂象 /10 HPF	**脑侵犯或以下组织学特征中的 3 种特征：** - 细胞增多 - 小细胞 N/C 比率高 - 大而突出的核仁 - 无模式，片状生长 - 局部坏死灶
3 级	间变性	20 个或以上核分裂象 /10 HPF	- 肉瘤或癌性组织

24%）和 KLF4（促进微分化体细胞多能性干细胞重编程的基因）的 10% 突变（Clark et al.，2013）。这些研究者也报道了 AKT1 突变可以与 TRAF7 共同发生，但不能与 KLF4 共同发生。发现 NF2 突变的脑膜瘤比 NF2 野生型具有更多的基因组重排，表明在 NF2 突变的肿瘤中存在更大的基因组不稳定性。

所有这些基因的突变似乎与不同的组织学亚型和肿瘤位置分离。Reuss 等人在 30/30 例分泌性脑膜瘤中观察到 KLF4 突变，在 29/30 例分泌性脑膜瘤中观察到 TRAF7 突变（Reuss et al.，2013）。虽然 KLF4 突变仅见于分泌性脑膜瘤，但在 8% 的非分泌性脑膜瘤中也观察到 TRAF7 突变。由于 NF2 突变发生的脑膜瘤倾向于横断性或成纤维细胞性，而 SMO 和 AKT1 突变的脑膜瘤倾向于主要为脑膜上皮亚型（Brastianos et al.，2013；Sahm et al.，2013）。对脑膜瘤进展为更恶性级别的遗传基础知之甚少。然而，高级别脑膜瘤的突变数量似乎更多，可能源于较高的基因组不稳定性（Weber et al.，1997；Brastianos et al.，2013；Clark et al.，2013）。当考虑颅底脑膜瘤时，发现 SMO 和 AKT1/TRAF7 突变的脑膜瘤位于中线；而 KLF/TRAF7 脑膜瘤，除中线外，还占据更多的外侧中颅窝。NF2 突变的脑膜瘤通常更靠后和外侧（Clark et al.，2013）。与神经鞘瘤病相关的脑膜瘤（由生殖系 SMARCB1 突变引起）主要见于大脑镰（van den Munckhof et al.，2012）。

具有一个以上脑膜瘤，但无 NF2 或神经鞘瘤病其他临床特征的病例可能由于独立的散发性肿瘤（Butti et al.，1989）、血液中未发现突变的镶嵌 NF2（Evans et al.，2005）或单个散发性肿瘤的克隆扩散（Larson et al.，1995；Stangl et al.，1997）而引起的。每个肿瘤中不同 NF2 突变的识别表明肿瘤是独立产生的。每个肿瘤中相同的双等位基因 NF2 突变表明镶嵌 NF2 或克隆扩散。其他基因的相同体细胞突变或相同 X 染色体的 X 失活（Evans et al.，2005）表明单个肿瘤的克隆扩散。在 NF2 疾病背景之外，还存在罕见家族，有脑膜瘤病史，以常染色体显性方式遗传（Aavikko et al.，2012；Smith et al.，2013）。

脑膜瘤受体

众所周知，脑膜瘤生长速率受性激素水平（如妊娠期间）和外源性药物（如抗雄激素醋酸环丙孕酮）的影响。尽管孕酮受体在高达 70% 的脑膜瘤中表达，但迄今为止尚未证实通过抗孕酮药物（如米非司酮（RU 486））控制这些受体对临床实践有效（Cossu et al.，2015；Ji et al.，2015）。目前正在研究其他药物，如生长抑素类似物和抗血管生成因子，以确定其治疗作用。奥曲肽是一种生长抑素类似物，靶向生长抑素受体亚型 2（SST2）的表达，导致体外脑膜瘤的增殖率降低，但未诱导细胞凋亡（Graillon et al.，2017）。

Simpson 分级

1957 年 Donald Simpson 描述了脑膜瘤切除程度的原始分级方案（Simpson，1957）。该量表由 5 个等级组成，并将手术切除程度与症状复发相关联（**表 14.3**）。手术切除的完整性始终被确定为重要的预后因素（Kallio et al.，1992；Condra et al.，1997；Stafford et al.，1998；Pollock et al.，2012；Heald et al.，2014），尽管其相关性受到质疑（Sughrue et al.，2010；Rogers et al.，2015）。显然，完全切除的目的必须与死亡率和发病率的风险及其对个体患者生活质量的影响进行平衡。

表 14.3 脑膜瘤的原始 Simpson 分级方案

1 级	GTR，硬脑膜附着切除	10 年复发率 9%
2 级	GTR，硬脑膜附着凝固	10 年复发率 19%
3 级	GTR，无切除或凝固硬脑膜附着	10 年复发率 29%
4 级	部分肿瘤切除	10 年复发率 44%
5 级	简单减压或活检	10 年复发率 100%

Reproduced with permission from Donald Simpson, The Recurrence of Intracranial Meningiomas After Surgical Treatment, *Journal of Neurology, Neurosurgery & Psychiatry*, Volume 20, Issue 1, pp. 22–39, Copyright © 1957 BMJ Publishing Group Ltd.

治疗：手术和放疗的作用

在治疗脑膜瘤时，需要考虑的因素包括是否存在症状、生长模式和接近敏感的神经血管结构。这些结构的压迫、侵袭或水肿一方面由肿瘤及其时间范围引起，另一方面由可用的治疗选择对这些结构的损伤引起。根据美国国家综合癌症网络指南的建议，偶发、无症状性脑膜瘤的表现较少，可通过观察进行管理（Sughrue et al.，2010；Chamoun et al.，2011）。对于较大的症状性脑膜瘤，一旦确定肿瘤分级，考虑手术或其他明确的治疗选择（包括放疗）非常重要。对于寻求确定性治疗的患者，尽管单独手术未能成功维持患者的细微亚组，标准治疗是完全切除。此外，如果脑膜瘤不能与功能区解剖结构分开，切除本身往往是不可行的。众所周知，无论是在次全切除术（subtotal resection，STR）或全切术（gross-total resection，GTR）后，均存在复发的可能性，并且已经对使用多模式治疗脑膜瘤进行了广泛探索（Stafford et al.，2001；Soyuer et al.，2004）。

在 1 级脑膜瘤中，全切除仍然是手术目标，在手术系列中有 1/2 至 2/3 的患者实现了全切除（Mirimanoff et al.，1985；Pollock et al.，2012）。在良性脑膜瘤中，次全切除的进展率较高。例如，一项研究显示，单独接受 STR 治疗良性脑膜瘤的患者的 15 年生存率为 51%，远低于 GTR 患者的 88%（Condra et al.，1997）。1 级脑膜瘤的放射疗法通常支持作为 STR 的辅助治疗，作为复发的预防措施，尤其是在肿瘤位置靠近视神经鞘或海绵窦（手术可及性可能受限）的情况下。除这些区域的较大复发肿瘤外，所有肿瘤的再次手术即使并非不可能完成，但也是一项难以完成的任务，具有相当大的风险，且完全切除的可能性较低。资深作者放弃了视神经周围（前床突、结核、膈肌）小复发再次手术的想法。研究显示，在这些病例中，术后 5 年和 10 年，放射疗法在 68%～100% 的 WHO 1 级脑膜瘤中实现了长期控制（Pollock et al.，2012；Santacroce et al.，2012）。

对于 2 级脑膜瘤，神经外科医师一致认为单纯 STR 治疗不足。一项研究报告，STR 后非典型性脑膜瘤的 10 年局部控制率仅为 17%（Goyal et al.，2000）。建议在 STR 后进行放疗或立体定向放射外科（stereotactic radiosurgery，SRS）以治疗 2 级脑膜瘤的残留肿瘤。在对 619 例次全切除的非典型性脑膜瘤的系统分析中，接受辅助 SRS 的患者的 5 年复发率为 53.3%，仅进行连续监测的患者为 89.9%，该显著性差异表明辅助治疗的潜在获益（Lagman et al., 2017)。目前大多数北美和英国神经外科医生在Simpson 1级和2级GTR后观察到非典型性脑膜瘤。但是，必须承认2级脑膜瘤复发的临床影响通常比1级脑膜瘤更显著（Marcus et al., 2008）。STR后2级脑膜瘤可实施多种形式的放射疗法，如SRS和分次外照射放射疗法（EBRT）。研究表明，放疗时机可能对改善局部控制起关键作用。例如，Choi等在6个月内再次证实次全切除术后放疗显著控制了局部肿瘤生长（Choi et al., 2010）。多段SRS也被推荐用于非典型脑膜瘤，尤其是位置敏感的肿瘤（Choi et al., 2010）。Kaur等进行了一项系统研究以检查放疗在2级和3级脑膜瘤中的作用（Kaur et al., 2014）。尽管他们已经观察到辅助放疗的临床获益趋势，但缺乏统计学显著性，可能是由于样本量小，限制检测组间任何差异的统计能力。进一步阐明放射治疗2级脑膜瘤的试验正在进行（Jenkinson et al., 2015）。

对于新诊断的WHO 3级（恶性）脑膜瘤复发性脑膜瘤患者，手术后大剂量EBRT是一线治疗。复发已显示与切除范围相对关，因此，当肿瘤和正常周围组织之间有清晰的界限，对这些恶性肿瘤通常进行渐进性GTR手术（Sughrue et al., 2010；Sughrue, et al., 2010）。最近的一篇论文回顾性分析了37例患者接受间变性脑膜瘤治疗，并得出结论，扩大全切除术具有总生存期优势（Moliterno et al., 2015）。尽管不存在记录手术和放疗治疗恶性脑膜瘤的疗效信息的随机试验，回顾性研究报告了3级脑膜瘤的多模态治疗（Moliterno et al., 2015）。此外，在这些肿瘤类型中，已证实如果使用放疗，较高剂量可能显著改善局部肿瘤控制（Milosevic et al., 1996; Rogers et al., 2015）。Magill等报告了他们使用^{125}I近距离放射治疗的经验，治疗14例非典型和28例恶性脑膜瘤用尽了其他治疗方法（Magill et al., 2016）。该类型患者诊断后的中位生存期分别为11.1年和9.1年。各自的组织学类型。尽管存在相关并发症包括放射性坏死（16%）、伤口破裂（12%）和感染（6%），这些结果与历史队列结果相比有利，并构成高级别脑膜瘤患者的有效治疗选择。

特殊种类（类型）脑膜瘤

脑膜瘤的常见位置是矢状窦旁、蝶骨翼和凸面。

矢状窦旁脑膜瘤

矢状窦旁脑膜瘤起源于上矢状窦硬脑膜（superior sagittal sinus, SSS）。它们是最普遍的群体，约占所有颅内脑膜瘤的1/4。中间1/3的SSS含有超过50%的矢状窦旁脑膜瘤，而前1/3略多于后1/3。按部位列出的脑膜瘤发生率最有可能反映体内蛛网膜帽细胞密度的分布。对SSS、桥静脉、导静脉及其侧支的解剖和血流动力学的理解患者的眼底管理及术前评估是矢状窦旁脑膜瘤患者手术的关键。因此，不仅需要静态结构成像，往往需要数字减影血管造影。手术造成的静脉受损后果从暂时性无症状至症状性脑水肿，从可逆性出血性静脉梗死引起的神经功能缺损到静脉梗死转化为恶性脑肿胀可能导致严重的永久性神经功能缺损，甚至死亡。在某些情况下，治疗症状可能是适当的以及与静脉流出道阻塞相关的体征支架植入术（Higgins et al., 2008；Ganesan et al., 2008）。

与其他部位脑膜瘤患者相似，矢状窦旁脑膜瘤患者的治疗应基于与患者相关的考虑（例如，社会功能、职业、爱好、年龄）、肿瘤（例如，解剖学方位、大小、生长速度、是否存在钙化）及其对周围组织（例如脑水肿、SSS狭窄/闭塞、存在静脉侧支循环），以及所有其他可用的治疗选择（手术、分次放疗、SSS和静脉支架植入术）。

最常见的是达到Simpson 2级，但在某些情况下侵入矢状窦硬脑膜壁或管腔的肿瘤术中可能出现肿瘤残留。对于这些患者，在后续治疗中是否进行辅助放疗放射学监测开始或进展后应根据个体情况进行考虑。虽然SSS打开至切除腔内脑膜瘤的扩展部分，然后进行缝合，或修补是可能的，它容易失败与血栓形成，并有严重不良后果，特别是在后1/3处尝试时的SSS。大多数外科医生，包括作者，主张切除-仅在矢状窦完全闭塞的情况下调整静脉回流。这些可能包括静脉通道镰刀和触手以及使者脉。仔细的术前侧支循环及其在手术中保留的初步评估是必需的。导致逐渐和均匀的再生长或复发，SSS完全闭塞应更积极在第二次手术时切除。

大脑镰旁脑膜瘤

约9%的颅内脑膜瘤起源于大脑镰。与矢状窦旁脑膜瘤不同，大脑镰旁脑膜瘤往往有桥静脉向深部延伸，一些恶性脑膜瘤延伸至大脑半球，并压迫胼胝体周围动脉和胼胝体，桥静脉在其上方延伸。事实上，在大多数情况下，在硬脑膜打开时，肿瘤是不可见的，相反，人们可以看到覆盖它的凸面大脑。镰旁脑膜瘤可为单侧或双侧，肿瘤体积在各自一侧的比例不同。对于完整的手术切除，当需要时，建议切除镰状起点，但需要确保保留重要的硬膜静脉通道，特别是当SSS也受到损害时。鉴于这些肿瘤倾向于“生长到大脑”，在某些单侧病例中，从对侧靠近可能是有利的，以避免过度的脑回缩和操作，干扰上覆桥静脉，及早控制镰血供。肿瘤邻近辅助运动皮层的患者术后可能会出现短暂的偏瘫和缄默症。

凸面脑膜瘤

15%的颅内脑膜瘤起源于凸面。压迫邻近的大脑，其血液供应主要通过脑膜动脉。与其他位置一样，大的、生长迅速的Ⅱ级和Ⅲ级以及分泌型脑膜瘤通常伴有病灶周围水肿，通常表明软脑膜表面破裂。这些肿瘤倾向于重新形成额外的皮质血供（Alvernia and Sindou，1994）。拉伸或压迫邻近皮质静脉造成的静脉回流障碍可能是其周围水肿的原因。

在造影后成像中，大多数脑膜瘤可见“硬脑膜尾”，即造影剂沿远离其附着处的脑膜的锥形延伸。显示成簇的脑膜间皮瘤细胞聚集物延伸到周围硬脑膜上，距离主脑膜瘤附着处不同（Borovich and Doron，1986）。由于复发往往出现在切除边缘，Kinjo等人提倡0级切除，在肿瘤周围切除2 cm环状硬脑膜的附加袖带（Kinjo et al.，1993）。考虑到凸面脑膜瘤比例较高时达到Simpson 1级甚至0级切除的相对容易程度，该组脑膜瘤的手术治愈可能性高于其他位置的脑膜瘤。然而，这并不意味着每个凸面脑膜瘤在首次就诊时都应该接受手术治疗。例如，老年人的偶发小脑膜瘤经常变得静止和非进行性，不需要治疗。

蝶骨翼脑膜瘤

蝶骨翼脑膜瘤（sphenoid wing meningiomas，SWM）占颅内脑膜瘤的10%~20%。它们通常被讨论为外侧（LSWM）或内侧蝶骨翼脑膜瘤（MSWM），与每组相关的考虑完全不同，尤其是与手术和预后相关。一组以骨内成分为主，累及蝶骨大翼的特殊脑膜瘤，称为蝶眶脑膜瘤（SOM），将单独讨论。

外侧蝶骨翼脑膜瘤

起源于外侧蝶骨翼的脑膜瘤的处理和手术与凸面脑膜瘤相似。骨受累和斑块状肿瘤在该组脑膜瘤中似乎相对常见，需要特别考虑。有些沿中颅窝有广泛的斑块延伸，切除可能具有挑战性，尤其是在颅底神经出口孔附近。在大多数情况下，潜在的骨质增生性骨显示在骨板层内含有肿瘤细胞，为了实现完全切除，必须切除骨内板，甚至扩大至整层颅骨，如果外板也受到影响，应在切除开始时在硬膜外钻孔。为了将复发风险降至最低，需要非常大的开颅皮瓣，并应切除受累的脑膜。

内侧蝶骨翼和床突脑膜瘤

作为一个群体，内侧SWM更难处理，特别是由于其接近和潜在累及神经血管结构以及海绵窦侵袭。延伸到中颅窝有时可通过神经孔和颅底向颅外连接到颞下窝。海绵窦受累从外侧壁到广泛至窦内不等（“全海绵窦”）。为了避免手术并发症，肿瘤最好使用立体定向放疗扩展（即，改善症状或控制肿瘤生长）。在某些情况下，需要更广泛的颅底入路，如额颞眶颧入路（手术入路另见**第21章**和**第27章**）。

主要起源于前床突（anterior clinoid process，ACP）的脑膜瘤称为床突脑膜瘤，可延伸至鞍上区和（或）通过小脑幕前裂孔延伸至脑桥前池和周围池。它们有包绕颈内动脉起始部的倾向。在大多数情况下，肿瘤和周围神经血管结构之间存在蛛网膜平面，但一些脑膜瘤与外膜粘连，一些残留肿瘤可能不得不留下。同样，其他结构，如颈内动脉（internal carotid artery，ICA）分支、大脑前动脉和大脑中动脉的近端A1和M1段、视神经和视交叉、动眼神经和垂体柄可与脑膜瘤融合，少数病例甚至在肿瘤内走行。在这些病例中，通过广泛裂开侧裂识别脑膜瘤上极的远端大脑中动脉分支将以逆行方式安全识别动脉走行。重要的是要限制和保留豆纹分支，因为这些是最脆弱的。经常有延伸至视神经管上外侧段的情况，即使在术前成像中不容易看到，在视力受损的病例中也应进行探查。如果同侧视神经和视交叉被肿瘤包绕，额下轨迹识别对侧视神经，有助于我们以逆行方式进行视交叉和视神经减压，从而有利于保留其通过垂体上动脉供血的血供。

蝶眶脑膜瘤

SOM约占颅内脑膜瘤的5%，但文献中发表的数量在很大程度上取决于该组的确切定义。SOM通常是惰性的，如果视力得到保持、未生长或已经确定视神经萎缩的重度视力损害，则不需要干预。手术的主要适应证是潜在或早期视神经受损、眼球突出或出于美容原因。

尽管肿瘤的范围差异很大，但倾向局限于蝶骨，其大翼形成大部分眶外侧壁，并延伸至中颅窝底及其椎间孔（圆孔、卵圆孔和棘孔）以及眶上裂。这位于小翼和大翼之间，并通过连接ACP与蝶骨体的光学支柱向内侧与视神经管分离。鳞状颞骨也可受累。软组织成分可累及颅内室以及眼眶，可向下生长至颞下窝或深部生长至颞肌。颅内成分是可变的，从斑块扩展到明显的颅内肿块。骨窗设置的图像引导有助于彻底切除受累骨（Marcus et al.，2013）。切除阶段为硬脑膜外切除，随后为硬脑膜内切除。目的是在涉及视神经管和眼眶时减压，这可能需要“定制”的床突切除术。眶尖或累及海绵窦的残留肿瘤如果进展，可能需要放射治疗。

前颅窝脑膜瘤

嗅沟脑膜瘤

10%~15% 的颅内脑膜瘤被归类为嗅沟脑膜瘤（olfactory groove meningiomas，OGM）。它们起源于帽状嵴和额蝶骨缝之间的中线，前颅窝底延续至蝶骨平台处。OGM 在诊断时可达大体积，大多数患者为嗅觉丧失型，表现出不同程度的认知障碍。偶尔可表现为典型的 Foster—Kennedy 综合征，包括嗅觉丧失、一只眼视神经萎缩和另一只眼视盘水肿。对于大病变，额部经基底入路联合眶上截骨术或其改良可早期控制其血供，血供主要来自筛前动脉，在额窦骨化并在其起始处钻骨骨质增生骨后，放置颅周皮瓣修复颅底。前外侧入路允许早期识别和保护后神经血管结构，如大脑前动脉和视神经（手术入路另见**第 21 章**和**第 27 章**）。

蝶骨平面和鞍结节脑膜瘤

5%~10% 的颅内脑膜瘤分为蝶骨平面（PSM）或鞍结节脑膜瘤（TSM）。任意，起源于蝶骨缘前方的肿瘤称为 PSM，而起源于蝶骨缘后方的肿瘤称为 TSM。TSM 的起源可在鞍结节本身、视交叉沟或鞍膈处，后者有时单独称为鞍膈脑膜瘤。不能总是确定大脑膜瘤的确切起源，但考虑到其起源部位与视器的关系，TSM 倾向于升高，而 PSM 则抑制视交叉。计算机断层扫描（CT）上骨质增生的位置也可提示起源部位。

手术的主要指征是保留视力。尽管与垂体和垂体柄非常接近，但术前几乎总是保留垂体功能，这与该区域的其他病变相反。无论术前放射学外观如何，了解延伸至视神经管的频率非常重要（Sughrue et al.，2015；Nimmannitya et al.，2016）。MRI 显示病变较小或延伸至蝶窦且无血管包绕且未向颈动脉外侧延伸的病变可考虑采用内镜下鼻内入路延长手术，尤其是当病变质地较软时。在某种程度上，这可以通过 T2- 加权 MRI 序列上的明亮信号来预测。翼点入路能够处理进一步延伸至脚间池和颈内动脉周围，病变组织可能涉及同侧视神经的一定程度操作，神经内侧区域可能是一个盲点。前半球间入路而不是额下入路可以更容易地保留嗅觉，避免操作视神经，但斜坡后延伸，尤其是有前固定视交叉的斜坡后延伸，是一个盲点（另见**第 21 章**和**第 27 章**中的手术入路）。

小脑幕脑膜瘤

根据广泛的部位和延伸的脑膜瘤，需要不同的手术入路。只要可能，切除小脑幕附着是可取的，以实现完全切除，但必须考虑来自脑深部结构的潜在重要静脉引流及其变异性。

这在镰幕交界区和环形区周围尤其重要（见下文）。位于前方的幕上脑膜瘤通过经侧裂或颞下入路进入，尽量减少脑回缩。尽早打开脑池和脑脊液出口是可取的，但在暴露的最开始时可能不容易实现。插入腰椎引流管通常不安全，尤其是对于存在脑水肿的大病变。应特别注意保留小脑幕裂孔处滑车神经的完整性。

枕半球间入路暴露大脑镰幕肿瘤，枕经幕入路用于延伸至松果体区和后中央幕裂孔者（手术入路另见**第 37 章**。）大病变可能需要幕上和幕下联合入路，尽可能对横窦进行保护。保留通畅的直窦和深静脉是最重要的，可能需要留下残留的肿瘤。颅后窝病变为小脑上，可扩展至桥小脑角，岩幕脑膜瘤经枕下开颅入路。它们倾向于移位而不是直接累及脑神经。

岩斜区脑膜瘤

尽管相对罕见（约 2% 的颅内脑膜瘤），但这些是最具挑战性的病变之一。其中一些脑膜瘤是静态的或表现出缓慢的生长速率，尤其是在老年患者中，大多数患者在临床治疗中、表现为症状极轻或完全无症状，仅在进展时进行手术。岩斜区脑膜瘤的起源以内听道内侧的岩斜交界处为中心，向后至梅克尔腔。真正的斜坡脑膜瘤起源于第 6 对脑神经内侧，可扩展至海绵窦。

斜坡和岩斜区脑膜瘤在出现症状前均可生长为相当大体积。在此期常延伸至海绵窦和小脑幕，侵入梅克尔腔。根治性切除术的发病率与脑神经功能障碍有关，第六对脑神经特别脆弱。术前 MRI 的 FLAIR 序列上脑干的信号变化表明软脑膜表面破坏。在这些病例中，预判病变（肿瘤）与脑干及其血管供应粘连，建议进行次全切除。可能来自颅神经、血管和脑干的神经功能缺损的严重性使实践转向更保守的手术，尽可能减少神经功能缺损并维持生活质量（手术入路另见**第 24 章**。）

枕骨大孔区脑膜瘤

枕骨大孔区脑膜瘤（foramen magnum meningiomas，FMM）罕见，仅占所有颅内脑膜瘤的约2%。最常见的定义将其起源于脑膜置于颈2椎弓上缘与下、中交界处之间斜坡1/3，外侧延伸至颈静脉结节。早期表现为神经压迫引起的神经功能缺损，但诊断通常是延迟的。这主要是因为与该区域肌肉骨骼和神经系统受累的常见症状相似。交叉轻瘫又称交叉偏瘫，常在放置较靠前的FMM的背景下提到，但在实践中很少遇到。

脑膜瘤的位置，从外周（后侧 *vs*. 后外侧 *vs*. 前外侧 *vs*. 前侧）以及颅-尾侧（颅内伸展 *vs*. 脊柱伸展）决定了手术入路。对于更靠前的位置，远外侧入路是理想的。然而，髁突切除（经髁入路）的需要和程度应根据病变的位置和大小量身定制。即使是中等大小的脑膜瘤，也经常通过置换髓质和脊髓创建足够的手术通道，从而排除了髁突切除的需要。然而，对于较小的前倾角，可能需要经髁入路。对于主要延伸至上颈椎管和C1结节水平枕骨大孔的患者，不需要切除髁。向上延伸至颈静脉孔的肿瘤常有颈静脉结节遮挡肿瘤的视野。恰好位于椎动脉（VA）硬脑膜入口内侧的附件给VA观察该附件带来了另一个困难。当脊髓副神经进入硬膜内间隙时，松解将其与VA分离的第一小齿韧带，打开更宽的手术窗进入位于前方的脑膜瘤。在许多硬脑膜来源未被切除的病例中，术后MRI上持续增强的硬脑膜基底部在长期内趋于稳定（手术入路也可参见**第31章**）。

脑室内脑膜瘤

脑室内脑膜瘤非常罕见，占所有颅内脑膜瘤的1%~3%。它们被认为起源于脉络丛内的脑膜细胞。许多罕见报告的儿科脑膜瘤是脑室内的。在**第35章**中对其进行了讨论。

颅盖脑膜瘤

尽管这些脑膜瘤可以是纯骨内的，但许多脑膜瘤的颅内扩展是轻微的硬脑膜病变。手术指征通常是美容和诊断性的（与其他病理，如转移瘤相鉴别）。术中定制或预形成的图像引导颅骨成形术通常在切除时完成。位于静脉窦上方的颅盖脑膜瘤（如上矢状窦）是比较疑难的，治疗具有挑战性。

多发性脑膜瘤

这些可见于1%~9%的脑膜瘤，女性发生率更高，不一定表明与NF2综合征相关（Terrier and François，2016）。它们可能在不同的时间出现。多发性病灶可见于放射或诱导而形成的脑膜瘤。

脑膜瘤术前栓塞的病例和对照

在过去的几十年中，微导管和栓塞治疗的快速技术进步使我们能够把这些技术纳入脑膜瘤的术前管理和准备，以达到更安全的切除目标。目前这是一个有争议的问题，对已发表文献的分析为脑膜瘤的术前栓塞提供了依据。

随着时间的推移，症状性脑膜瘤生长的一线治疗是手术切除。然而，如果靠近功能区或结构以及可及性有限，切除可能受到肿瘤位置的阻碍。可能妨碍充分切除肿瘤的其他因素包括肿瘤血管丰富和硬脑膜静脉窦受累。栓塞可以通过减少肿瘤管腔血供来减少术中失血，缩短手术时间，使肿瘤易于切除（Gruber et al.，2000；Dowd et al.，2003）。但是，一些外科医生认为术前栓塞的受益没有超过风险。例如，存在脑膜瘤栓塞后大量失血、蛛网膜下腔出血和视网膜栓塞的报告（Hayashi et al.，1987；Raper et al.，2014）。其他潜在并发症包括通过ECA分支与CA吻合意外栓塞脑动脉（Raper et al.，2014）。在2000年，比较了两组各30例患者，一组进行了术前栓塞，第二组没有进行术前栓塞（Bendszus et al.，2000）。得出的结论是在切除的过程中对失血量和止血没有任何影响，并且存在一例栓塞造成的永久性神经功能缺损。

关于颅内脑膜瘤的术前栓塞的作用已经达成了有限的共识。2013年最近的一项系统性回顾分析了36项研究，包括459例在脑膜瘤切除术前接受该手术的患者。在这些患者中，有4.6%（21/459）报告的并发症是栓塞的直接结果。这21例患者中严重并发症的发生率为4.8%（1/21），死亡率9.5%（2/21），发生率是并发症率的2倍。因此，可以说脑膜瘤的术前栓塞存在显著的发病率和死亡率的风险。但是，这些风险可能会受到精心选择该手术受益最大的患者的限制。分析术前栓塞作用的进一步前瞻性研究将可能阐明该手术在某些脑膜瘤类型中的受益和风险。

预后

残留肿瘤、组织学分级和可能的生物学（基因组、转录组和甲基化组）因素决定复发风险。当考虑脑膜瘤的预后时，分析 WHO 肿瘤分级以及进行何种治疗方式，以及是否仅进行手术或同时进行放疗是至关重要的。良性脑膜瘤生长缓慢，全切除后 5 年复发率为 5%（Riemenschneider et al.，2006）。非典型脑膜瘤 5 年复发率为 40%。间变性 WHO 3 级脑膜瘤的复发率为 80%，是 2 级的两倍，是 1 级脑膜瘤的 16 倍（Choy et al.，2011）。在接受多模式治疗的患者中，非典型和间变性脑膜瘤的 5 年和 10 年生存率分别为 95% 和 79%，64% 和 35%（Palma，1997）。复发的一个主要临床因素是切除范围。患者年龄、位置和其他肿瘤因素将影响与切除程度相关的决定。同样，根据年龄和许多其他因素、个体情况决定是否进行影像学监测或辅助放疗，包括局部残留或复发的 SRS。

争议：偶发脑膜瘤的处理和随访

偶发脑膜瘤治疗的决策取决于多种因素，如年龄、大小、位置、治疗的潜在发病率及其在诊断时和之后的有效性，以及诊断的知识对患者的心理影响。尽管有良好的意图，但应根据个人情况考虑适应证，指南可能是向后迈出的一步，提供粗略的治疗包，而不是定制、精炼和灵活的个人治疗计划。例如，肿瘤与重要结构（如脑神经）的接近程度可能是 1 例患者发生潜在不可逆缺陷前治疗的重要因素，但也可能是另 1 例患者采用保守治疗的原因，此时手术的潜在发病率不可接受。生长速率是可变的，在许多情况下是非线性的。因此，对于影像学随访管理的患者，理想情况下，应采用一种长期的可靠的体积评估方法。

血管外皮细胞瘤（HPC）– 孤立性纤维瘤（SFT）

虽然不是脑膜瘤，但本章讨论了血管外皮细胞瘤纤维瘤（haemangiopericytoma-solitary fibrous tumour，HPC-SFT），因为这些肿瘤表现为脑膜瘤，因此，过去将其中一些肿瘤归类为脑膜瘤和血管外皮细胞瘤（HPC）。事实上，直至 1954 年 Begg 和 Garret 报告了首例脑膜 HPC 时，HPC 通常被归类为血管母细胞性脑膜瘤（Begg and Garret，1954）。在身体的其他部位，HPC 被越来越多地归类为孤立性纤维性肿瘤（SFT），然而直到最近在 CNS 中，它们仍被分开，尤其是因为预后不同。自 2013 版 WHO 软组织和骨肿瘤分类（Fletcher et al.，2013）以来，HPC 和 SFT 被视为一种疾病。HPC 一词已被放弃，现在这两个实体都被称为 SFT。这是因为它们具有相同的 NAB2-STAT6 融合基因。对硬脑膜 / 脑膜 HPC 的分子研究发现了相似的遗传畸变，最近的 WHO CNS 肿瘤分类（Louis et al.，2016）也认为血管外皮细胞瘤纤维瘤是相同的实体瘤（**图 14.3**）。

SFT 通常累及胸膜、腹膜、脑膜和下肢，但可见于任何身体部位。发现 12%~22% 为恶性（DeVito et al.，2015）。脑膜 SFT 几乎总是良性的，但存在非常罕见的恶性变异。HPC 通常为 WHO 2 级和 3 级。尽管脑膜 HPC 和 SFT 通常彼此不同，但存在重叠。总体而言，将脑膜 HPC 和 SFT 视为相同疾病谱的一部分可能是最实际的。尽管最终的诊断试验是 NAB2-STAT6 融合基因的鉴定，但这作为第一步并不实际。相反，使用免疫组化方法对 STAT6 核染色进行鉴定是一种好的替代检阅方法（Schweizer et al.，2013）。影像学表现与脑膜瘤相似，在位置和信号特征方面。这些特征使 SFT/HPC 的诊断更有可能包括：异质性 T2 加权像上的信号强度；低信号区域的存在注射钆后 T2 信号强度明显增强；与肿瘤相邻的硬膜尾缺失；颅骨缺失骨骼增厚；在磁共振波谱上，肌醇峰值升高（Clarençon et al.，2011）。少数没有硬脑膜附着脑实质内或很少在脑室内（Bisceglia et al.，2011）。

血管外皮细胞瘤 - 孤立性纤维瘤的治疗与临床管理（包括手术切除和组织诊断）与脑膜瘤是一致的。如果诊断为 HPC，身体分期为全身转移瘤较高（25%~50%）。主要潜在困难手术时可能出血过多，因为许多 HPC 血管丰富。

术后 HPC 的复发率为 60%~75%，总体 5 年生存率在 65% 至 95%，中位生存率为 7~16 年（Guthrie et al.，1989；Kim et al.，2003；Rutkowski et al.，2012；Melone et al.，2014）。肿瘤复发时易出现恶变（Apra et al.，2017）。尽管根据最新 WHO 对 SFT 和 HPC 的分类，这些临床结局之间存在明确的区别历史上不同的条件。Champeaux 等分析了 SFT 和 HPC，

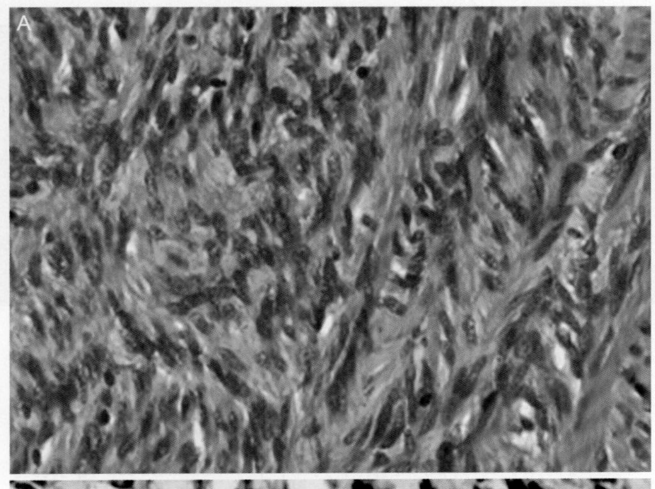

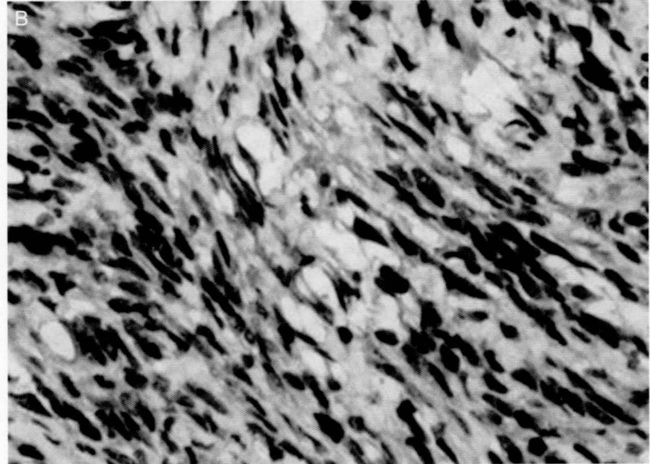

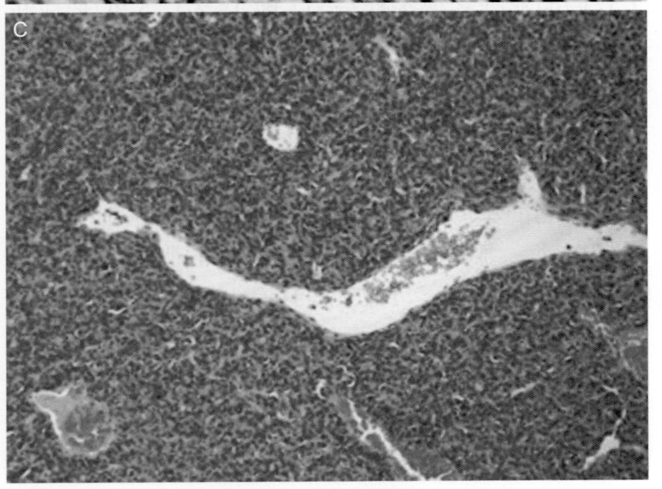

图 14.3 （A）孤立性纤维瘤——梭形细胞束是这种肿瘤的特征，影像学上常酷似脑膜瘤。这种肿瘤的组织学可误认为成纤维细胞性脑膜瘤或神经鞘瘤。免疫组化将解决这种差异。（B）孤立性纤维瘤 STAT6 免疫反应性——SFT 和相关肿瘤血管外皮细胞瘤的中心和（迄今为止）特异性基因异常是 NAB2 和 STAT6 基因之间的融合。这导致 STAT6 的核定位被免疫组化很好地证明。（C）血管外皮细胞瘤——一种高度细胞性肿瘤，由无模式的梭形细胞组成，具有特征性的扩张的薄壁血管。与相关孤立性纤维瘤一样，STAT6 的核表达将被免疫组化预期

Courtesy of Dr Kieren Allinson, Department of Pathology, Addenbrooke's Hospital, Cambridge.

但在多变量分析中组织学类型（SFT *vs*. HCP）是独立的预后因素之一（Champeaux et al., 2017）。其他显著预后因素在同一分析中包括静脉窦浸润和完全切除度。放疗对总生存期的影响不清楚（Trifiletti et al., 2017）。鉴于高复发率和转移潜能，统一使用术后放疗。

结论

脑膜瘤是 30 岁以上成人最常见的原发性脑肿瘤，目前实现治愈或长期控制肿瘤的现代外科治疗和医疗技术是我们应继续坚持的努力方向。良性脑膜瘤的自然病程是长，患者应了解每一种干预措施都有风险，应了解与观察相关的风险及其随时间的可能发展。如果在肿瘤最小的时候进行手术，许多最终生长的肿瘤可能可以通过手术治愈，围术期的内科和神经疾病发病率较低。手术和放疗等物理治疗方式可能已经达到了顶峰，我们期待靶向药物治疗和免疫治疗的进展，以帮助我们延长和改善患者的生活，尤其是复发性脑膜瘤患者。血管外皮细胞瘤（HPC）现在被认为是孤立性纤维性肿瘤（SFT）的一个实体。因此，HPC-SFT 形成了一个病理实体，具有从良性到恶性的一系列行为，具有复发倾向并形成远处转移。

参考文献、EBRAIN 的相关链接

扫描书末二维码获取。

第 15 章　颅底脊索瘤和软骨肉瘤

Rami O. Almefty・Ossama Al-Mefty 著
薛湛 译，伊志强 审校

引言

脊索瘤和软骨肉瘤由于在好发部位、临床表现和影像学特点等方面的相似性而经常被成对比较。然而，它们代表了两种独特的病理特点以及完全不同的临床预后。本章将回顾这两种疾病并着重介绍它们的主要不同。

流行病学

颅底脊索瘤和软骨肉瘤属于少见肿瘤，占全部脑肿瘤的 0.1%，合计的发病率为 0.02/100000（CBTRUS，2012）。软骨肉瘤比脊索瘤更少见。

脊索瘤位于颅底、可活动的脊椎，以及骶骨。McMaster 等利用国家癌症研究所（NCI）的监测、流行病学和最终结果（SEER）的项目，计算出基于人口的发病率为 0.8/10 万人。在他们的研究中，脊索瘤在颅底（32%）、脊柱（33%）和骶骨（29%）中的发生率几乎相同（McMaster et al.，2001）。Heffelfinger 等发表了梅奥诊所的 155 例脊索瘤的诊疗经验，其中 76 例（49%）发生在骶骨，55 例（35%）发生在颅底，24 例（15%）发生在活动的脊椎（Heffelfinger et al.，1973）。由于这项研究是基于单一机构的经验而非基于人口，其结果可能会受到机构的专业特色和转诊模式的影响。

脊索瘤一般以男性为主，男女比例可能高达 2∶1（Heffelfinger et al.，1973; McMaster et al.，2001），然而，对于颅底脊索瘤却不是这样，其在不同性别的发病率几乎相同（McMaster et al.，2001，AlMefty et al.，2007）。颅底脊索瘤也比其他部位脊索瘤的发病年龄更早。根据 McMaster 等的研究，颅底肿瘤的发病中位年龄为 49 岁，其中 1/4 的患者出现在 35 岁之前（McMaster et al.，2001）。本文资深作者（OA）发表的 89 例颅底脊索瘤的研究中，平均发病年龄为 37.7 岁（Almefty et al.，2007）。脊索瘤在儿童中更罕见，特别是在 5 岁以下的儿童中。在一项全国性的横断面数据库分析中，Chambers 等报道了 594 例颅底脊索瘤，其中 30 例发生在 10~19 岁的患者中，26 例发生在 10 岁以下的儿童中（Chambers et al.，2014）。与此同时，Borba 等总结了 76 例儿童颅底脊索瘤病例，其中 21 例是 5 岁以下儿童（Borba et al.，1996）。脊索瘤在非裔美国人中极为罕见（McMaster et al.，2001；Almefty et al.，2007）。

病理

脊索瘤起源于蝶枕软骨联合处的原始脊索残余（图 15.1）。它们通常被描述为生长缓慢，但这掩盖了它们的恶性和侵袭性行为（图 15.2）。它们形成灰色、胶状、分叶状的肿块，被覆软组织成分，可见浸润性骨受累。镜下可见均匀的泡状细胞，体积小、卵圆形、核偏心化、染色质致密、胞浆中有许多空泡。假包膜呈现由纤维束形成的厚的透明隔或带有薄间隔的小叶。小叶的外观可以是浆状细胞片或粘蛋白池。细胞薄片含有不同程度的胞浆内黏蛋白（Heffelfinger et al.，1973）。Heffelfinger 等描述了同样具有软骨成分的脊索瘤软骨样变异（Heffelfinger et al.，1973）。软骨样脊索瘤和软骨肉瘤在组织学上进行区分可能较为困难，需要通过免疫组化来加以区分，因为软骨样脊索瘤的行为与非变异脊索瘤相同（Rosenberg et al.，1994; Almefty et al.，2007）。除了典型和软骨样亚型外，脊索瘤的另一种亚型是去分化型或非典型型。非典型脊索瘤罕见，但细胞学和临床上具侵袭性。

软骨肉瘤起源于原始间充质细胞或颅骨软骨基质层的胚胎残存。它们通常发生在长骨和骨盆，很少发生在颅骨。大体上，它们是由多个相互连接的软骨状或黏液状黏稠物组成。这些肿瘤可分为典型肿瘤、间充质肿瘤和黏液样肿瘤。典型肿瘤是最常见的，包含在不同软骨基质中的单核或多核的大细胞。

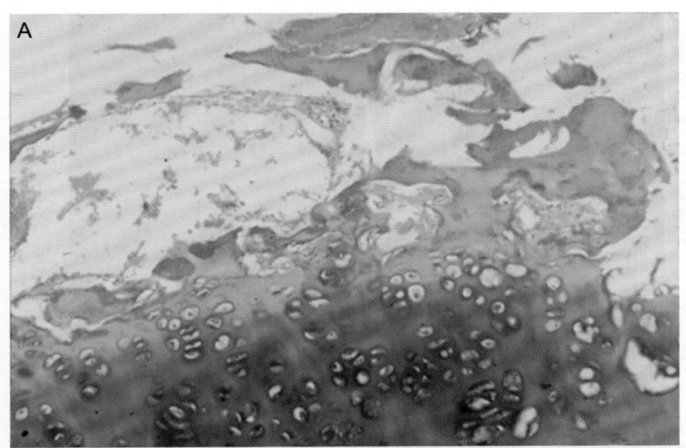

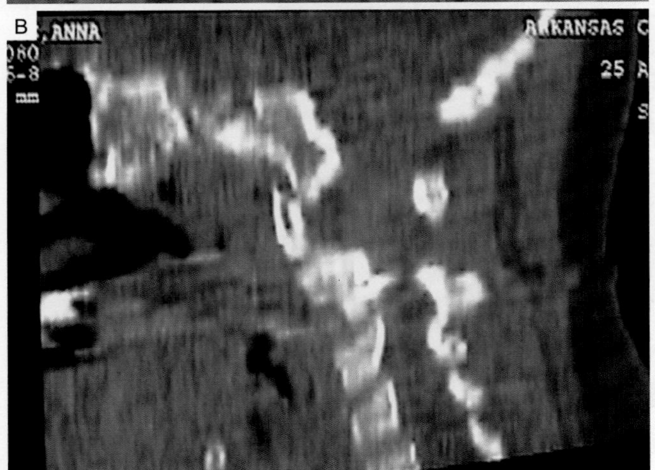

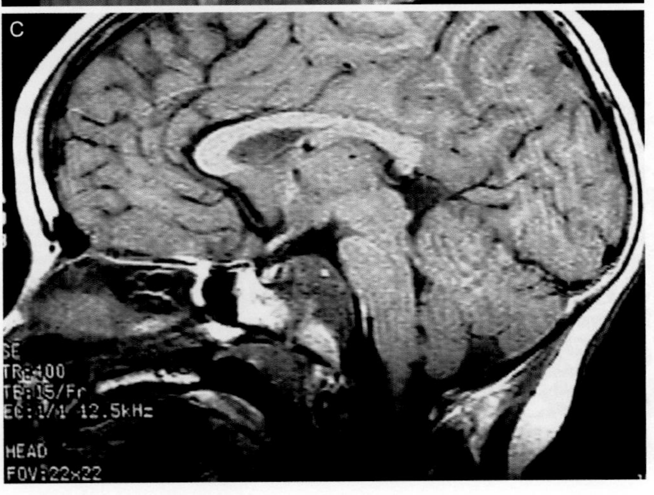

图 15.1 H&E 染色（A）、矢状位 CT（B）和矢状位 MRI（C）显示脊索瘤起源于蝶枕软骨联合处

根据有丝分裂率、细胞数量和细胞核大小，典型软骨肉瘤可分为Ⅰ级、Ⅱ级或Ⅲ级。在高级别肿瘤中，软骨基质有丝分裂增加，软骨基质减少（Evans et al.，1977）。间充质型肿瘤包含相对分化良好的软骨区域和未分化的圆形或梭形细胞，而黏液样型肿瘤有黏液样基质，包含一串圆形细胞（Korten et al.，1998）。

关于脊索瘤和软骨肉瘤之间必须研究的主要病理区别是它们的免疫组化特性（图 15.3）。脊索瘤细胞的角蛋白、EMA、S-100 和波形蛋白呈阳性，包括软骨样变异。软骨肉瘤的细胞角蛋白和 EMA 呈阴性，而 S-100 和波形蛋白呈阳性（Rosenberg et al.，1994）。Brachyury 是一种核转录因子，有助于脊索瘤的诊断以及与软骨肉瘤的区别。脊索瘤外的短线染色是罕见的，通常不表现在考虑鉴别诊断的病变中。当加入 S-100 和上皮标志物作为免疫组化检测手段时，可达到 100% 的敏感性（Oakley et al.，2008；Jo et al.，2014）。

遗传学

迄今为止的研究结果表明，脊索瘤是一种遗传异质性肿瘤，常出现大染色体区域失衡，不伴有复发性结构重排（Hallor et al.，2008）。Scheil-Bertram 等在 33 个病例的研究中发现了 166 个独特的畸变，证明了其遗传异质性（Scheil-Bertram et al.，2014）。当脊索瘤核型异常时，表现出第 1、3、4、9、10、13、18 条染色体的全部或部分丢失、第 7 条和第 20 条染色体获得，以及同位染色体 1q 的形成（DeBoer et al.，1992；Bridge et al.，1994；Sawyer et al.，2001；Scheil et al.，2001；Tallini et al.，2002；Sandberg and Bridge，2003；Kuzniacka et al.，2004；Brandal et al.，2005；Bayrakli et al.，2007）。1p36 被认为是散发性脊索瘤的肿瘤抑制基因位点（Dalpra et al.，1999；Miozzo et al.，2000；Riva et al.，2003），7q33 是家族病例的位点（Kelley et al.，2001）。Hallor 等运用阵列比较基因组杂交技术（aCGH）发现 70% 的病例中伴有 CDKN2A 和 CDKN2B 缺失（Hallor et al.，2008）。更先进的技术如 aCHG 和全基因组单核苷酸多态性微阵列分析（SNP）已经发现 91%~100% 的脊索瘤染色体出现异常（Scheil et al.，2001；Hallor et al.，2008；Le et al.，2011；Kitamura et al.，2013；Scheil-Bertram et al.，2014）。

Al-Mefty 等能够明确脊索瘤细胞遗传学异常的临床意义。具有正常核型的脊索瘤在新发病例中复发率为 3%。另一方面，核型异常的新发脊索瘤，其复发率为 45%。他们在 75% 的复发病例中发现了异常核型，而在新发病例中这一比例为 24%。染色体 3、4、12、13 和 14 异常的肿瘤显示复发频繁和生存率下降。13 号染色体异常具有最高的进展优势比（OR 24），中位无复发生存率仅为 4.5 个月，明显短于不涉及 13 号染色体的异常核型肿瘤。值得注意的

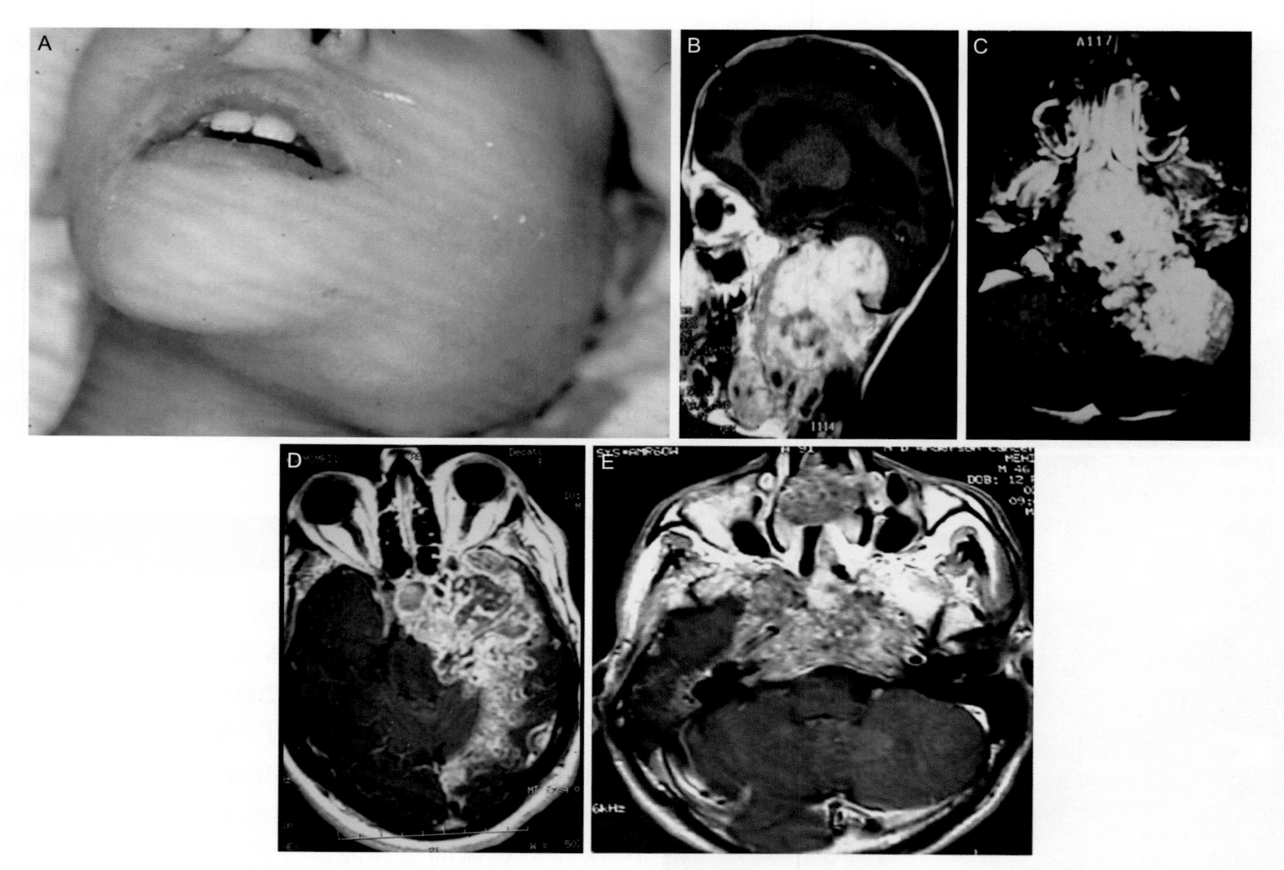

图 15.2 （A、B）患者面相和增强 MRI 显示脊索瘤广泛侵蚀颅底及颈部。（C、D、E）轴位 MRI 显示脊索瘤的侵袭性

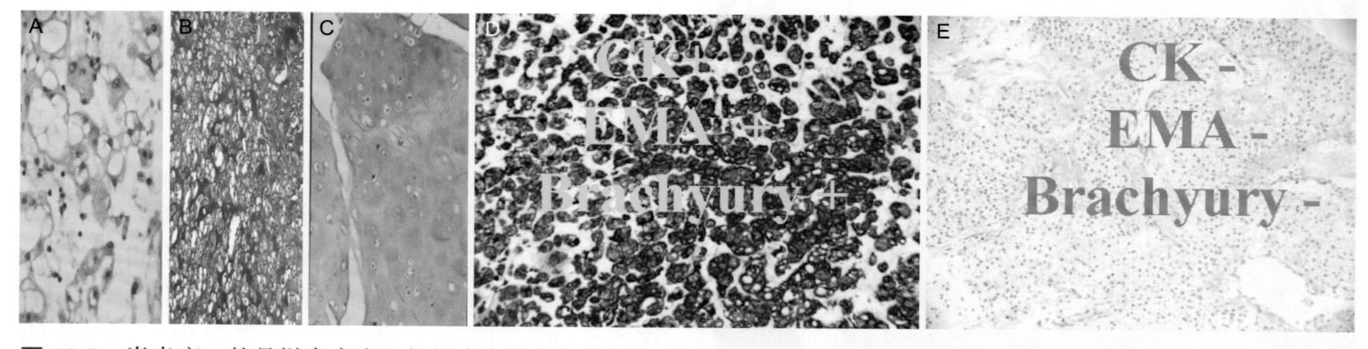

图 15.3 脊索瘤、软骨样脊索瘤和软骨肉瘤的 H&E 染色；脊索瘤及软骨肉瘤的免疫组化染色

是，核型是使用 G 显带技术进行的，比较基因组杂交可能会发现 G 显带技术未检测到的异常（Almefty et al.，2009）。其他作者发现 2p 获得（Kitamura et al.，2013）、9p21 缺失（Horbinski et al.，2010）和 p53 过表达（Naka et al.，1996）与较差的预后相关。SMARCB1 位点缺失与低分化病例相关（Mobley et al.，2010），CDKN2A 和 CDKN2B 纯合子缺失与转移性病例相关（Hallor et al.，2008）。脊索瘤证明了肿瘤进展的经典理论，即额外积累的基因突变与更有侵略性的临床行为相关。

术前检查和计划

脊索瘤患者的术前评估应包括 MRI、CT 和血管成像。对全部现有的影像学资料进行全面回顾，对于了解肿瘤的扩展以及与重要的神经血管结构的关系，从而制定最佳的根治性切除和术后放疗方案至关重要。脊索瘤在CT上表现为位置居中、边界清楚，主要为斜坡上的高密度肿块。CT检查的最大价值在于显示广泛的溶解性骨受累，其可扩散到整个颅底，必须被去除以达到真正的根治性切除。可能存在瘤内钙化，这很可能代表骨分离。脊索瘤在增强序列显示强化。MRI和CT是互补的，MRI能更好地描述肿瘤组织的范围和良好的解剖细节。典型的脊索瘤表现为T1低至中等信号，T2高信号，中度或明显强化。如果出现坏死或大量黏液物质，强化可减弱或消失。血管成像可用于勾画肿瘤边界或脑血管的移位，并用于研究静脉解剖以进行入路规划（Erdem et al.，2003）。这通常可以通过无创检查来完成，我们发现动态CT血管造影尤其有帮助（Bi et al.，2015）。有时，如果血管狭窄严重，需要血管造影术来评估侧支血流，或者对于之前接受过放疗的患者，需要评估放疗导致的血管病变，因为这些情况可能会使动脉周围的任何分离变得非常危险。

对术前评估有帮助的其他研究还有垂体功能测试和神经眼科检查。脊索瘤常累及鞍区，可能发生垂体功能低下，应予以诊断和纠正。许多脊索瘤患者以视力障碍为主诉，肿瘤经常扩散到与视觉相关的器官。基线检查对于随访这些患者很重要。

治疗

了解脊索瘤的行为和自然病史至关重要，以便更好地管理患者的疾病。虽然它们在组织学上是良性的，但它们的自然病史和侵袭性行为是恶性的。脊索瘤不治疗生存期较短，复发率高（Forsyth et al.，1993；Gay et al.，1995；Al-Mefty and Borba，1997；Ammirati and Bernardo，1999），并且具有转移倾向（Markwalder et al.，1979；Fagundes et al.，1995）和手术种植（Arnautovic and Al-Mefty，2001；Fagundes et al.，1995）。考虑到脊索瘤的恶性行为，早期、积极的治疗是明确的。脊索瘤必须在诊断时开始治疗，没有观察期。

对于在诊断初期实施根治性切除并给予高剂量放疗的病例，已有长期生存的报道（Al-Mefty and Borba，1997；Almefty et al.，2007）。任何治疗不足都会导致复发。复发脊索瘤的预后较差，3年和5年生存率分别为43%和7%（Fagundes et al.，1995）。为此，必须尽一切努力在最初治疗时控制脊索瘤。

手术切除对无进展生存率的影响已经得到了很好的证实（Forsyth et al.，1993；Fagundes et al.，1995；Gay et al.，1995；Al-Mefty and Borba，1997；Colli and Al-Mefty，2001；Tamura et al.，2015）。颅底和显微外科技术的进步使根治性切除颅底脊索瘤变得安全。在讨论脊索瘤的手术切除时必须考虑几个因素。其中的关键是脊索瘤作为岛屿存在于周围的骨骼中，而不仅仅是清晰可见的软组织肿块。因此，为了达到根治性切除，除了完全切除软组织块外，还必须对周围骨进行广泛的磨除。由于脊索瘤有蔓延至整个颅底的趋势，术前必须仔细阅读CT影像，以了解骨受累情况，并制订相应的手术计划。

我们将脊索瘤分为三种类型来描述这种现象。Ⅰ型肿瘤局限于单一解剖区域，较为少见。Ⅱ型肿瘤侵犯两个或多个相邻解剖区域，可以通过单一手术方式进行彻底切除，而Ⅲ型肿瘤扩展到多个区域，需要多种手术方式。我们发现60%的肿瘤累及海绵窦，50%累及岩尖，25%累及枕髁，50%累及硬膜下（Al-Mefty and Borba，1997）。这些肿瘤累及情况必须在入路选择时加以预测、研究和计划。事实上，通常需要多个手术入路从而实现根治性肿瘤切除，并提供长期控制的最佳机会。

脊索瘤的所有入路都应考虑到脊索瘤起源于硬膜外这一事实，因此应首先采用硬膜外入路。如果肿瘤尚未侵犯到硬膜下，则应尽一切努力保持手术在硬膜外进行。如果肿瘤已在硬膜下扩散，则可以选择从硬膜外入路进行硬膜下切除的方式。

由于大多数脊索瘤广泛累及斜坡，通常采用经前方中线入路。我们发现唇下经上颌窦入路、经蝶窦入路和经斜坡入路可以提供良好的暴露（Al-Mefty et al.，2008）。斜坡全长可以暴露，其提供了一个广泛的工作区域，适合显微镜和内镜技术。我们推荐使用显微镜来磨除斜坡，因为它提供了重要的三维视角。神经内镜是一种非常价值的设备，它可以显示显微镜看不到的区域。显微镜与内镜的联合使用是一种很好的策略，我们发现其对于所有类型的肿瘤都适用（Abolfotoh et al.，2015）。所有的颅底外科医生都应该掌握这两种技术，因为它们是互补的。

由于常累及海绵窦，脊索瘤根治性切除包括移除海绵窦部分，这可以从经中颅窝入路安全完成（Al-Mefty，1998）。当枕骨髁受累时，需要采用经髁入路，这可能需要枕骨-颈椎融合，这可以在同一暴露中完成（Al-Mefty，1998）。由于脊索瘤根治性切除常涉及广泛的颅底切除，肿瘤常侵犯至硬膜下，因此需考虑脑脊液漏的可能性，并准备带血管蒂的颞肌或皮瓣。

由于根治性切除非常重要，我们应尽一切可能达到最大程度的切除肿瘤。作为这个策略的一部分，我们认为术中成像是必不可少的。我们推荐所有的脊索瘤手术都应在多模态手术室（AMIGO）进行。这个手术室配备了术中MRI、CT扫描、PET-CT、超声和血管造影，使得术者在离开手术室时知道所有可能的肿瘤已被切除（**图** 15.4A~C）。

脊索瘤手术中另一个需要考虑的是手术播散的潜在风险（**图** 15.5A~C）。手术中应采取一切措施避免潜在播散的可能性。所有斜坡病变的术前计划都应该考虑到脊索瘤的可能性。如果考虑脊索瘤，必须采用尽可能减少肿瘤播散风险的方法和技术。采用可以提供最佳视野的手术入路。开颅完成后、肿瘤

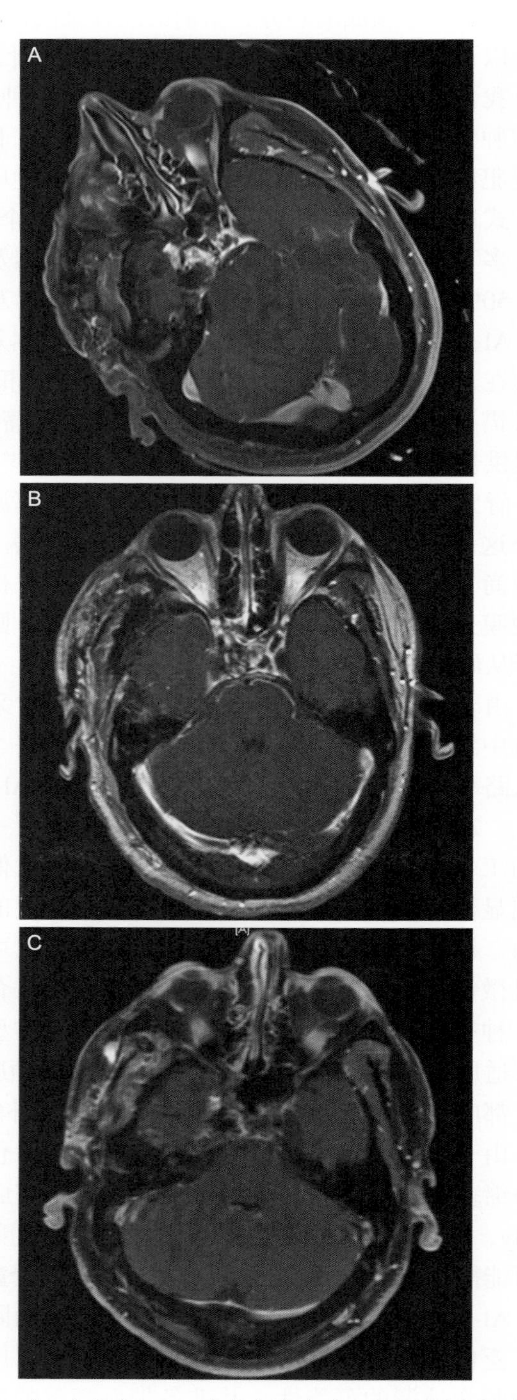

图 15.4 （A）术中MRI示残余脊索瘤。（B）再次切除后，术后MRI未见肿瘤残余。（C）3个月随访MRI未见肿瘤残余

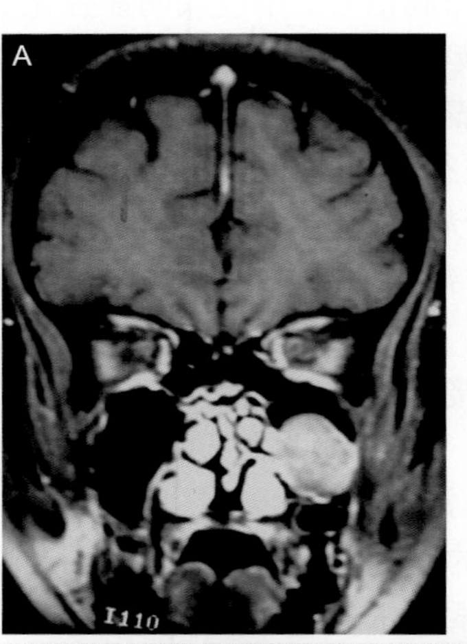

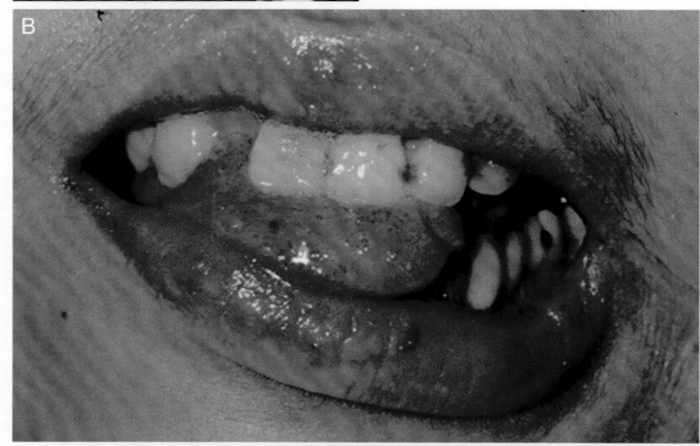

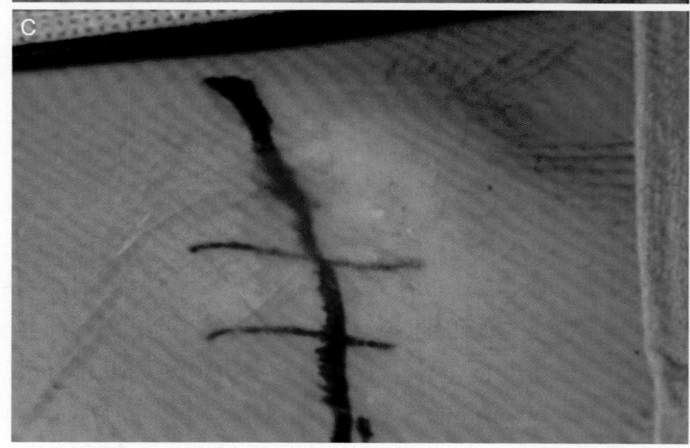

图 15.5 脊索瘤手术播散的案例。（A）冠状位MRI提示经上颌窦入路后脊索瘤的上颌骨播散。（B）患者照片显示经唇下入路后脊索瘤在齿龈播散。（C）患者照片显示在腹部取脂肪处出现腹部播散

切除开始之前，术野和手术通道应覆盖纤维蛋白胶和棉条。在肿瘤完全切除后，放入清洁的移植物之前，先去除明胶和棉条。在关颅之前，所有被污染的治疗巾都要更换，并使用干净的器械和手套。如果脂肪或筋膜是从其他部位采集的，需使用干净的器械和手套，并在清洁的区域完成（Arnautovic and Al-Mefty，2001）。

应秉承脊索瘤是恶性的，复发后预后不佳的理念，因此长期控制的最佳机会是在初次发病时给予最大限度的治疗。因此，根治性切除后应给予大剂量放疗。脊索瘤是相对放疗抵抗的肿瘤，然而，大剂量辐射（如粒子治疗）已被证明可以改善局部控制和生存期（Hug et al.，1999；Munzenrider and Liebsch，1999；Igaki et al.，2004；Noel et al.，2005；Weber et al.，2005）。由于脊索瘤具有局部复发率高和浸润性的特点，以及播散的倾向，放疗区域应包括整个手术术区、手术通道和相关解剖结构。

与脊索瘤相比，软骨肉瘤预后良好。软骨肉瘤的根治性切除可以实现肿瘤长期控制和可治愈的可能性，应予提倡。放疗已被证明对肿瘤长期控制是有效的，但这可能缘于肿瘤的侵袭性较低，因此在完全切除后放疗可能不是必要的。我们提倡根治性切除肿瘤，不做术后辅助放疗，对任何微小残留都进行影像学监测。

预后

影响脊索瘤预后的因素包括年龄、组织学分型和所接受的治疗。性别的影响将不做详细讨论，只是说已经报道了相互矛盾的结果。不幸的是，由于脊索瘤较为罕见，且经常与软骨肉瘤混合，以及缺乏统一的治疗，脊索瘤患者的真正预后难以确定。然而，我们将讨论这些因素如何影响预后，并强调长期控制的最佳机会是根治性切除，包括受累的骨岛，然后在最初诊断时进行高剂量放射治疗。

年龄对预后的影响已经产生了相互冲突的结果，除了那些不到5岁的侵袭性脊索瘤患者。在5岁以下的儿童中，65%的肿瘤是非典型的，而典型亚型的肿瘤细胞更多。此外，近60%不到5岁的患者发生转移（Borba et al.，1996）。然而，总的来说，在儿童人群中，我们很高兴地看到一些使用根治性切除和高剂量放疗策略的患者获得长期的无瘤生存（未发表的数据）。

非典型脊索瘤的预后比典型或软骨样脊索瘤差（Ouyang et al.，2014；Yakkioui et al.，2014）。在他们关于脊索瘤和软骨肉瘤的开创性工作中，他们引入了软骨样亚型，Heffelfinger等认为，软骨样亚型有一个更良性的过程，其他作者也支持这一主张（Heffelfinger et al.，1973；Rich et al.，1985）。然而，关于这种类型的预后意义的争论随之而来，我们在一项109例免疫组织化学染色病理证实的患者的研究中令人信服地表明，软骨样肿瘤确实是脊索瘤的一种亚型，其预后无差异，而且两种脊索瘤亚型的预后都明显比软骨肉瘤差（Almety et al.，2007）。其他研究也支持这一发现（Forsyth et al.，1993；Colli and Al-Mefty，2001；Bohman et al.，2014）。这些发现强调了通过免疫组化染色确认病理诊断的重要性。

对于颅底脊索瘤患者，根治性手术切除与大剂量放疗相结合已被证明是最佳的治疗策略。然而，这一管理方式并不是统一遵循的，所以在一些文献中可能低估了脊索瘤患者的生存期。有两个关键点是明确的，首先，任何不积极的治疗方法注定会复发，以及导致复发后预期寿命缩短。其次，根治性切除加上预先的大剂量放疗提供了延长控制的机会。事实上，当完全切除肿瘤并使用辅助质子束治疗时，无复发生存率为74%，而当存在残留肿瘤时，这一数字降至40%（Almefty et al.，2007）。

尽管软骨肉瘤经常被和脊索瘤归为一类，但一再显示其预后比脊索瘤好得多。在我们对20例软骨肉瘤患者的研究中，没有一例复发或死亡。其中一半患者接受了质子束治疗（Almefty et al.，2007）。质子束治疗已被证明有极好的控制率，5年和10年生存率在90%~100%范围内（Hug et al.，1999；Munzenrider and Liebsch，1999；Ares et al.，2009）。然而，很有可能这些优秀的控制率更表明了肿瘤对于预后有利的生物学特性。因此，我们的做法是尝试完全切除软骨肉瘤，避免放射治疗。小的残余软骨肉瘤可随访。

争议

脊索瘤的最佳放射方式

我们在本章中已经阐述了大剂量放疗对脊索瘤的好处。基于粒子的治疗，已经显示优于传统的基于光子的治疗（Cummings et al.，1983；Fuller and Bloom，1988；Catton et al.，1996；Hug et al.，1999；Munzenrider and Liebsch，1999；Zorlu et al.，2000；Igaki et al.，2004；Noel et al.，2005；Weber et al.，2005；Ares et al.，2009），其中经验最多的是质子治疗。脊索瘤的放疗必须考虑到脊索瘤与重要结构密切

相关，相对放疗抵抗，需要大剂量放疗，有较高的局部复发率，有较高的手术播散率，显微镜下的肿瘤岛屿分散在整个颅底，局部控制是整体生存的关键问题。基于这些特征，质子治疗有诸多优势，非常适合颅底脊索瘤。质子治疗的主要优势之一是它没有出口剂量，使正常组织接受辐射的体积比光子小。脊索瘤的特点使得分步质子治疗比单次放疗更有优势。单次放疗通常针对肿瘤的大体体积和有限的微观体积。任何超出目标范围的微小肿瘤都会获得急剧下降的放射剂量。相反地，正如Hug等所描述的，脊索瘤质子照射使用的临床靶体积的概念定义为"显微镜下疾病的任何危险区域，一般包括整个手术区域和最初延伸的解剖结构"（Hug，2001）。临床靶体积的形状和大小明显不同于肿瘤的大体体积，因此脊索瘤并不适合单次放疗。

使用碳离子作为粒子治疗是一项发展中的技术，已经获得了一些作者的关注（Schulz-Ertner et al.，2007；Takahashi et al.，2009）。碳离子提供了一些与质子治疗相同的优势，虽然它们的剂量急剧下降，但有更高的生物等效剂量。较高的生物等效剂量和强度调节能力可以允许在较低剂量时产生相同的肿瘤效应，进而降低毒性。Schulz-Ertner等报道，手术加碳离子治疗的3年和5年局部控制率分别为80%和70%，总生存率分别为92%和89%（Schulz-Ertner et al.，2007）。Takahashi等报道了3年和5年无复发生存率为70%和70%，但只有9例患者被纳入（Takahashi et al.，2009）。碳离子疗法可能成为脊索瘤辅助治疗的一个令人感兴趣的选择，但需要更多的患者和更长的随访研究。

经鼻切除脊索瘤

随着前颅底经鼻入路的发展和日益普及，该技术在脊索瘤的治疗中得到越来越多的应用。我们已经提到了内镜技术的优点以及外科医生学习这项技术的重要性。内镜切除脊索瘤的争议不是利用这项技术，而是将其作为唯一的手术方式使用。由于脊索瘤是起源于斜坡的硬膜外肿瘤，通常需要前中线入路。然而，脊索瘤并不局限于可见的软组织肿块，而是以岛状存在于周围的颅骨中。因此，根治性切除脊索瘤需要切除受累的骨质。通常，为了达到这一目标，需要多种入路，而单独经鼻入路的病例无法达到期望的根治性切除。此外，斜坡通常涉及广泛，需要大量的磨除。为了在这样的关键区域进行磨除，最好使用手术显微镜提供的三维视野。最后，脊索瘤有手术播散的风险，因为需要保持视野深度的感觉，内镜需要持续运动，不断通过一个不包含肿瘤的区域，可能增加植入的风险。

参考文献

扫描书末二维码获取。

第 16 章　皮样囊肿和表皮样囊肿

Andrew McEvoy 著
王拓 译，伊志强 审校

引言

皮样囊肿和表皮样囊肿是颅内常见的发育性良性肿瘤。它们通常来源于神经管闭合时两个融合的神经外胚层，也称为先天性外胚层囊肿。目前对于它们产生的具体原因，是由于胚胎发生的第 3~5 周神经管闭合失败引起的，还是由于早期的原肠发育失败导致中胚层的异常引起的（Dias and Walker，1992）还存在一些争论。有时，表皮样囊肿是由于表面外胚层医源性植入而引起的获得性病变（称为皮样植入）。

流行病学

皮样囊肿很少见，约占颅内肿瘤的 0.3%；而颅内表皮样囊肿发病率约为皮样囊肿的四倍，占颅内肿瘤的 0.5% ~1.5%（MacCarty et al.，1959; Gormley et al.，1994）。两者都表现为缓慢的线性生长，但皮样囊肿通常出现在较早的年龄，症状持续时间较短。

病理

皮样囊肿往往发生在中线附近。颅内最常见的部位是靠近前囟的硬膜外部位，以及鞍区、鞍旁，和硬膜内的脑室区域。最常见的椎管内部位在马尾附近，可与真皮窦道相关，增加了细菌感染的风险。

皮样囊肿由上皮细胞碎片和角蛋白组成，也包括毛囊、皮脂腺和汗腺等真皮成分（**图 16.1**）。腺液的活跃分泌以及随后的生长和破裂被认为是其早期表现的可能原因（Osborn and Preece，2006）。

大体上，皮样囊肿界限分明，分叶状，珍珠状包块，有厚的部分钙化的囊。囊肿的内容物可能包括腺体产生的黄色、恶臭的液体，也可能包含头发和牙齿。组织学上，皮样囊肿同时表现出真皮和表皮成分，尽管与表皮样囊肿相比，上皮细胞内衬的分化可能较差。

表皮样囊肿主要在颅内，远离中线。最常见的部位是桥小脑角（40%~50%），是该区域成人第三大最常见的颅内病变，仅次于前庭神经鞘瘤和脑膜瘤。也见于第四脑室、鞍区和鞍旁区、大脑半球和脑干。脊柱的表皮样囊肿少见，胸椎层面较多。

表皮样囊肿仅由上皮细胞碎片组成，包括胆固醇和角蛋白，呈板层状分布，不涉及真皮（**图 16.1**）。这导致了一个不规则和分叶的肿块，其表面有光泽，沿着卵裂面包围周围的神经和血管。囊肿包含由进行性上皮脱屑引起的软角膜玻璃化物质，术中常被描述为具有典型的“蜡烛蜡”外观。

表皮样囊肿和皮样囊肿表现方式不同。首先是局部占位效应，它与肿瘤的位置和缓慢的线性增长速度相关。颅中窝囊肿通常无症状，故一旦发现往往体积较大，可合并三叉神经麻木等非典型表现。

其次，急性起病的影像学表现往往继发于囊肿破裂（**图 16.2**）。病因可能是外伤性的、医源性的或自发性的，从而导致囊肿内容物渗漏至蛛网膜下腔并伴有化学性脑膜炎。这应与由真皮窦道引起的椎管内皮样囊肿的感染性脑膜炎相区别。囊肿破裂可导致多种神经功能障碍表现，包括头痛、癫痫发作、血管痉挛、神经系统缺陷和死亡。

最后，皮样囊肿可能与其他先天性发育异常相关，这些先天性异常可能是其最初表现的原因。在椎管内（McLaughlin et al.，2013）和颅内（Pai et al.，2007）皮样囊肿中均有与 Klippel-Feil 综合征相关的报道。间充质发育异常的存在支持了 Dias 和 Walker 提出的概念，即皮样囊肿发生的关键性胚胎事件发生在神经管关闭之前，大约在神经管的三椎板形成的时候（Dias and Walker，1992）。**表 16.1** 展示了皮样囊肿和表皮样囊肿的特征。

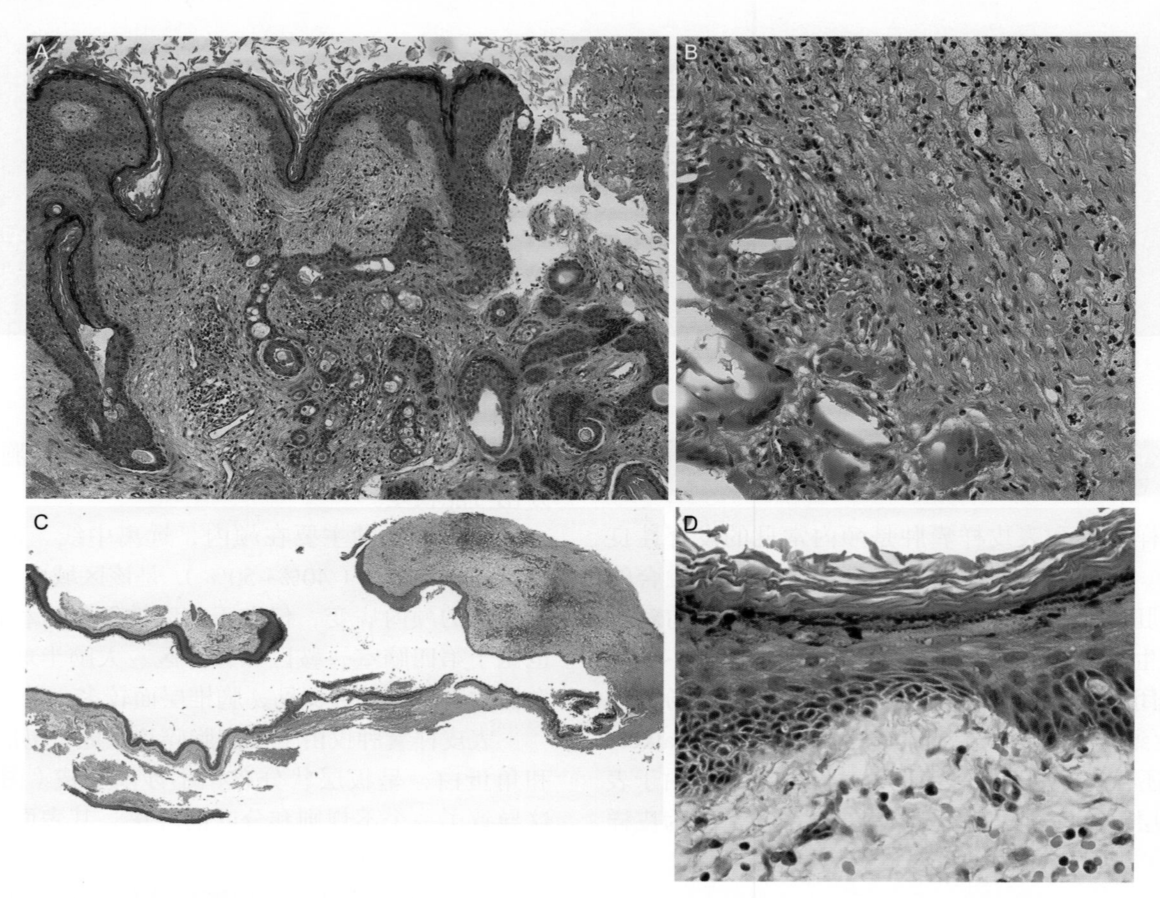

图 16.1　皮样囊肿和表皮样囊肿的组织病理学。（A）皮样囊肿的壁，有层状鳞状上皮，表面角化明显。囊肿壁显示成熟的附件结构，包括毛囊皮脂腺，属于皮样结构。（B）有巨噬细胞和血黄素色素的局灶性异物巨细胞反应提示以前的囊肿破裂。（C）低倍镜下表皮样囊肿显示单房囊肿，有鳞状上皮和纤维胶原壁，但没有附件结构。（D）上皮内衬为单层鳞状上皮并角化

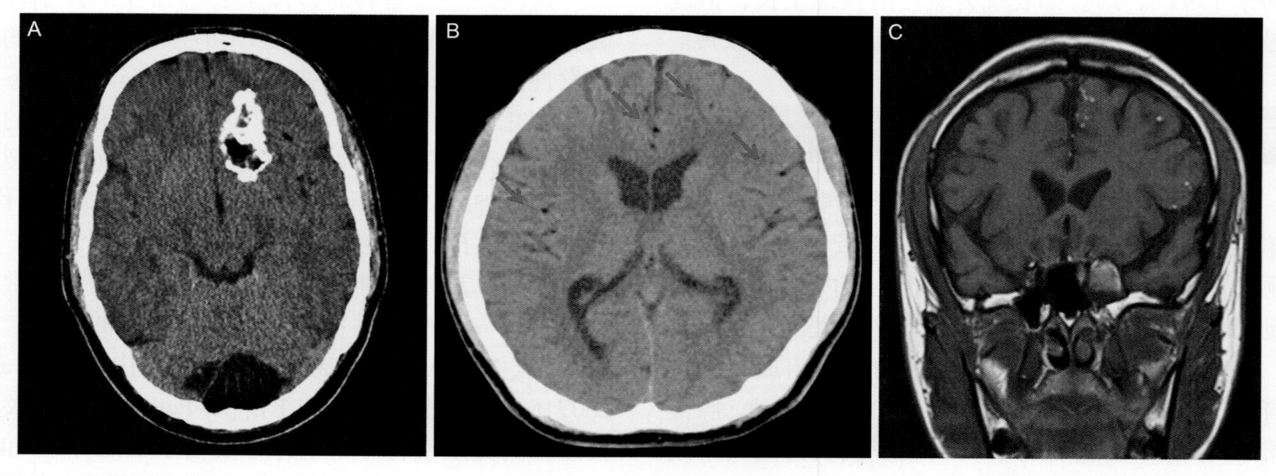

图 16.2　皮样囊肿破裂。（A）CT 显示左侧额部钙化样皮样囊肿破裂。（B）CT 示蛛网膜下腔弥散性脂肪室。（C）冠状位 T1W MRI 显示左侧鞍旁皮样囊肿破裂

表 16.1　皮样囊肿和表皮样囊肿的特征

	皮样囊肿	表皮样囊肿
发病频率	罕见	常见
部位	中线部位	远离中线
表现	早期	晚期
内容物	真皮内容物	无真皮内容物
囊肿破裂	常见	少见
合并发育异常	可能出现	无
手术切除	容易	困难

影像学特点

典型的表皮样囊肿和皮样囊肿的影像学表现见**表** 16.2。

磁共振成像液体衰减反转恢复序列（fluid attenuated inversion recovery，FLAIR）和扩散加权成像（DWI）有助于区分表皮样囊肿和蛛网膜囊肿。与表皮样囊肿不同（**图** 16.3），蛛网膜囊肿 FLAIR 表现为信号衰减，DWI 表现为自由弥散不受限（**图** 16.4）。

皮样囊肿（**图** 16.5）在磁共振成像上表现各异，取决于脂肪、毛发、皮脂和牙齿含量的比例。它们与脂肪瘤的不同之处在于，在所有序列上，脂肪密度并不一致。囊肿内出血可导致 CT 上的高密度，有时可掩盖潜在的病变（Sanchez-Mejia et al.，2006）。

手术

手术目的

手术切除任何占位性病变的主要目的包括：诊断、缓解症状和改善预后。在 MRI 多模态序列的辅助

表 16.2　皮样囊肿和表皮样囊肿的影像学特点

影像序列	皮样囊肿	表皮样囊肿
CT	低密度，与脑脊液密度相似 分叶状 细线状表现 无强化	低密度，稍高于脑脊液密度 33% 病例合并骨质破坏 无强化
T1W MRI	典型高信号，与脂肪密度相似 无强化	等信号，与脑脊液信号相似 边缘有时可见高信号 无强化
T2W MRI	多变	等信号，与脑脊液信号相似
FLAIR	多变	高于脑脊液信号
DWI	弥散受限，信号高于脑脊液	弥散受限，信号高于脑脊液
脂抑制序列	T1 加权的高信号受到抑制	无变化
局部效应	占位效应明显 相关异常（颈椎先天融合畸形、皮毛窦）	沿神经血管间隙生长

诊断下，手术主要目的并不是明确诊断。手术的目的是缓解疾病的症状，这通常与肿块的占位效应相关。

目前，疾病未来发病风险很难预测，关于保守治疗的利弊将在后面的章节中进行更广泛的讨论。

术前评估

患者应接受全面的 MR 诊断成像，并由经验丰富的神经放射科医生进行阅片。对于颅后窝囊肿，应特别注意颅颈交界区存在的发育异常，包括 C1 枕骨化、颅底凹陷、寰枢椎半凸、Klippel-Feil 综合征和 Chiari 畸形（Chandra et al.，2005）。

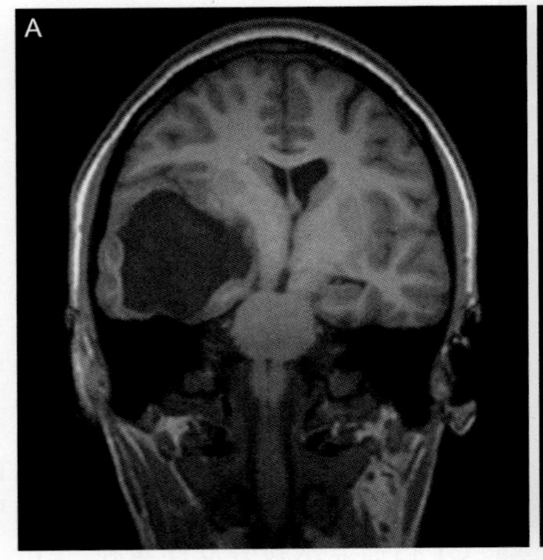

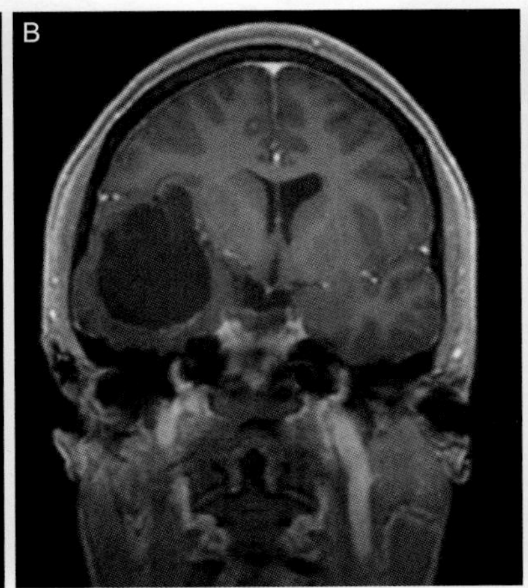

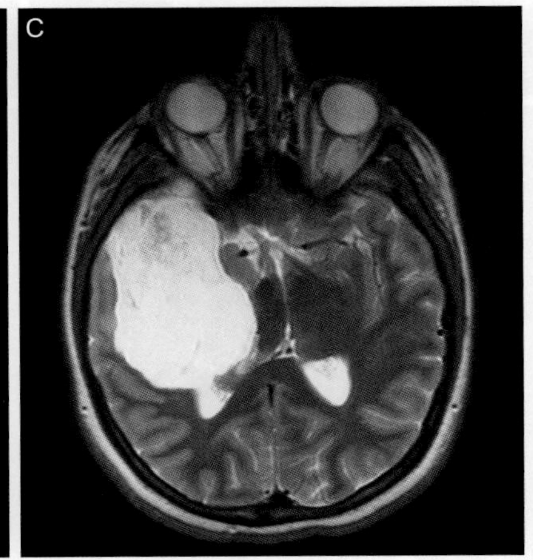

图 16.3　表皮样囊肿。（A、B）冠状位 T1W MRI，平扫和增强显示右侧外侧裂区表皮样囊肿。（C）轴位 T2W MRI 显示右侧外侧裂区表皮样囊肿

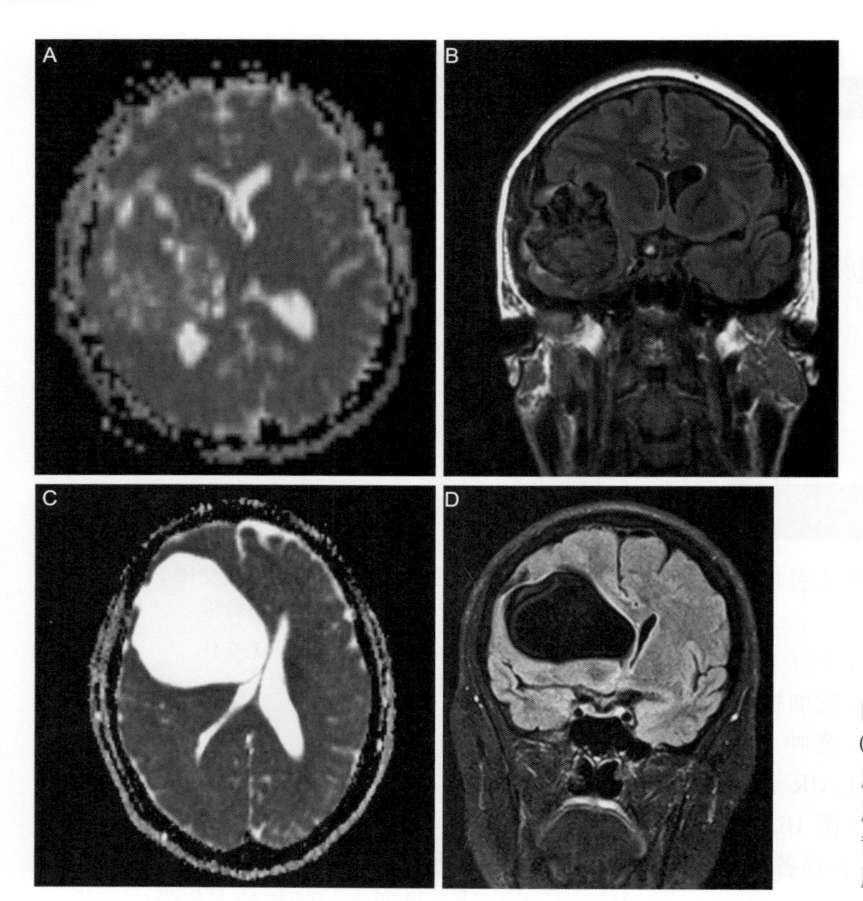

图 16.4 表皮样囊肿（A、B）与蛛网膜囊肿（C、D）的鉴别。（A）ADC 图显示表皮样囊肿弥散受限，（B）冠状 FLAIR 表现表皮样囊肿持续高信号，（C）ADC 图显示蛛网膜囊弥散不受限，（D）冠状位 FLAIR 表现蛛网膜囊肿信号较低

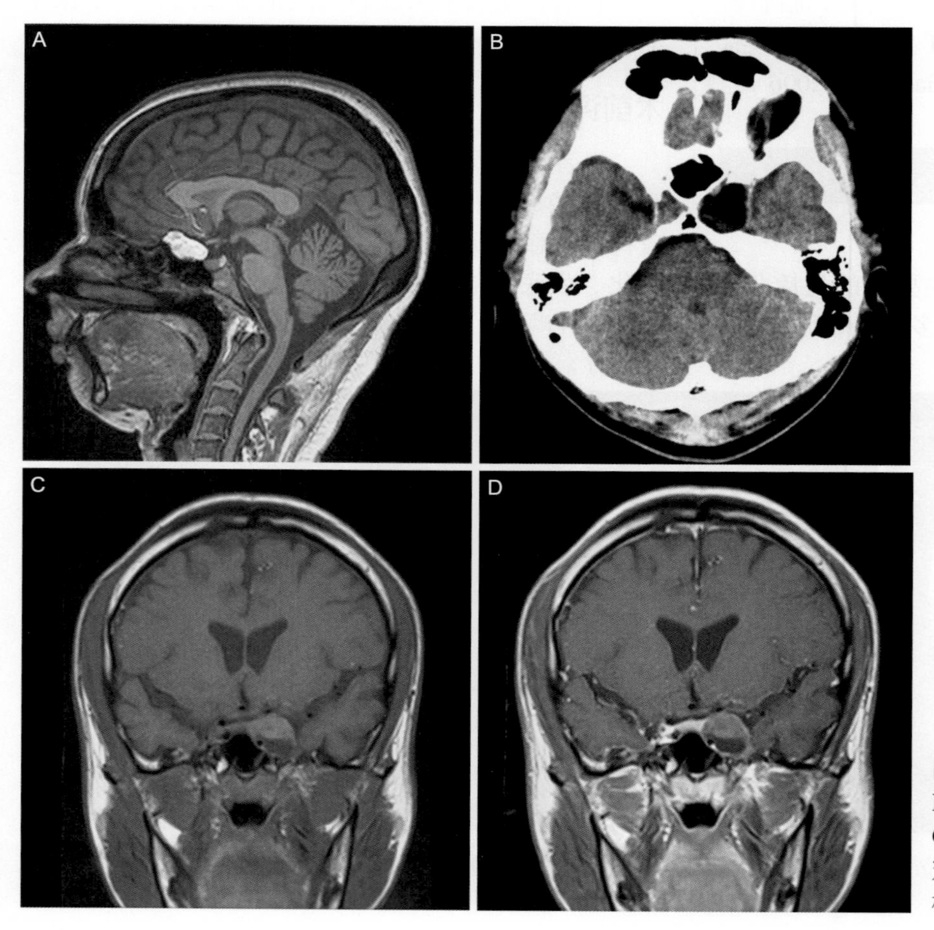

图 16.5 皮样囊肿（A）矢状位 T1W MRI 显示鞍旁皮样囊肿，（B）水平位 CT 扫描显示鞍旁皮样囊肿，（C、D）冠状位 T1W MRI 强化前后显示鞍旁皮样囊肿

所有的患者都应该检查是否有皮肤窦道的迹象，这可能会导致细菌感染。在这种情况下，囊肿的手术切除应包括窦道的完全切除。

囊肿呈缓慢的线性生长，意味着几乎没有肿瘤相关性的血管源性水肿。由此，术前使用皮质类固醇是没有必要的。然而，当囊肿破裂或术后囊肿内容物泄漏时，皮质类固醇被认为可以减少化学性脑膜炎的严重程度和持续时间，可以考虑应用。

外科手术理念

手术目标是尽可能完整切除囊肿，包括囊肿的上皮内衬，以缓解症状并消除囊肿复发的风险。然而，由于肿瘤的位置深在而关键，以及肿瘤与周围神经血管结构的复杂关系，对手术技术的要求较高。鉴于这是一种良性的囊性病变，术前评估过程中，当手术会有较高风险导致术后发生严重的神经功能缺失时，保留功能的次全切除比全切更为可取。

由于肿瘤比较罕见，很少有大型病例系列的研究报道。Yasargil 报道了单一中心接受治疗的 43 例患者（包括 35 例表皮样囊肿和 8 例皮样囊肿），其中 41 例（34 例表皮样囊肿和 7 例皮样囊肿）采用显微颅底外科手术入路完成了囊肿的完整切除，并取得了良好的结果（Yasargil et al.，1989）。此类肿瘤全切除被定义为完全切除囊肿内容物和囊壁。Lynch 等报道的全切除率较低，从 0~75% 不等（Lynch et al., 2014）。这反映了手术具有一定的困难，需避免造成神经功能受损。Chivukula 等指出微创颅底技术的发展可能会改变此类肿瘤的治疗方式，但是否能够提高全切率还有待观察（Chivukula et al., 2013）。

除了手术入路外，手术切除技术也有很高要求。肿瘤常与颅底邻近结构和周围脑组织粘连紧密，尤其皮样囊肿更为明显，并且经常引起蛛网膜和软脑膜肉芽肿反应。此外，表皮样囊肿的又一特点是能够在正常解剖间隙内生长，质地柔软或稍韧，也可侵犯蛛网膜下腔。最后，肿瘤长时间持续生长可导致周围正常结构受压移位，例如基底动脉受压后可能从脑干腹侧移位。无论何时都应严格执行显微手术原则，充分暴露，轻柔牵拉，保存正常的蛛网膜和精准地止血。手术切除的原则包括使用超声吸引器进行囊内减压，然后通过在囊壁和蛛网膜之间形成的间隙切除囊壁。尽量避免囊肿的内容物渗入蛛网膜下腔，因为其具有强烈的刺激性，可能引起化学性脑膜炎。这就需要在切开囊肿壁之前，对周围正常结构进行准确的分层。如果囊壁与脑实质或重要的神经血管粘连紧密，可以选择残留部分囊壁，虽然这样增加了肿瘤复发的风险，患者必须长期随访，但避免了重要的神经血管损伤，后者对于患者来说可能是灾难性的。

大部分学者会把表皮样囊肿和皮样囊肿手术放在一起报道，导致二者极易混淆。目前没有证据表明表皮样囊肿的预后比皮样囊肿更差。在肉芽肿生长的部位，皮样囊肿的囊壁和蛛网膜之间的分离比较困难，而表皮样囊肿的切除难点则为正常组织间隙内的肿瘤。

目前，皮样囊肿和表皮样囊肿的术后治疗未涉及放疗或化疗，除非个别患者发生恶变。

并发症

皮样囊肿和表皮样囊肿手术切除的一个常见的并发症是囊肿内容物“溢出”到周围的脑脊液，导致囊肿内容物在蛛网膜下腔和脑室内扩散，引起化学性脑炎（图 16.2）。Liu 等报道常见的临床后遗症包括：头痛、癫痫和脑积水等（Liu et al., 2008）。也有无不良反应报道（Carvalho et al., 2020）。通过锐性分离，对手野进行大量的冲洗，以及用棉垫保护周围脑组织等措施均可以降低术囊肿内容物溢出的风险。虽然类固醇药物可以用来治疗化学性脑膜炎，但临床中大部分选择保守治疗，如果发生脑积水则应采取脑脊液分流治疗。

复发

提倡肿瘤全切，以减少复发的风险，因此第一次彻底切除肿瘤至关重要。皮样囊肿和表皮样囊肿的复发率可能与次全切除后残留肿瘤的体积有关。然而肿瘤的生长速度是线性的，这样一来患者会长时间没有临床症状。Yamakawa 报道在一组 29 名接受表皮样囊肿切除术并长期随访的患者中，7 名患者在平均 8 年 10 个月后出现原位复发，而在第一次切除后平均 12 年 6 个月后出现二次复发（Yamakawa et al., 1989）。由于第一次手术增加了肿瘤粘连的程度，因此再次手术切除时更加困难。但患者如果出现临床症状，应积极推荐再次手术治疗。

恶变的风险

皮样囊肿和表皮样囊肿发生恶变是罕见的、确定的颅内鳞状细胞癌病因，经常在颅底发生转移和侵袭。Hamlat 等发表综述报道发现 52 例囊肿恶性转化，中位生存期为 9 个月（Hamlat et al., 2005）。放疗可以有效延长生存期，中位生存期由 3 个月延长为 26 个月。脑膜癌只出现于表皮样囊肿的恶变，且预后特别差。尽管极其罕见，但对于那些手术后恢复较差，且没有脑积水、没有肿瘤复发但肿瘤部位出现增强灶则应考虑恶变。

影像学随访的争议

确诊后保守治疗期间，影像学检查可以作为常规复查方案，手术次全切或全切后影像学复查同样重要。

影像学复查的好处是可以密切监测肿瘤的生长和复发，这样患者和外科医生都可以很好地了解肿瘤的变化。如果肿瘤开始侵犯重要结构或侵犯远隔部位，就会使肿瘤全切更加困难。尽管恶变罕见，在文献中仅有数例报道，影像学随访在早期发现恶变方面具有优势（Hamlat et al., 2005）。

影像学复查主要缺点是有可能增加患者心理负担。影像学进展但没有临床症状，则不是明显的手术指征。因此，更合适的方法是当患者出现新的症状或体征时再进行影像学检查。

目前还没有关于表皮样囊肿和皮样囊肿的随访指南，从外科医生的角度来看，术后立即进行磁共振扫描可以建立残留肿瘤的基线。定期影像学检查可以为患者提供复发风险或手术风险的信息。个别患者没有新的临床症状，但有明显的影像学进展，可能即将发生神经功能损伤时，可以积极手术治疗。总之，术后随访及影像学复查的频率应与患者讨论，制订个体化的随访方案。

延伸阅读、参考文献、EBRAIN 的相关链接

扫描书末二维码获取。

第 17 章　嗅神经母细胞瘤

Georgios Klironomos・Lior Gonen・Fred Gentili 著
鲁润春 译，伊志强 审校

引言

嗅神经母细（esthesioneuroblastoma，ENB）临床罕见，起源于鼻腔顶部，是一种来源于神经外胚层的恶性肿瘤。1924 年由 Berger 和 Richard 首次报道，随后该肿瘤有多个命名，目前最常用的英文术语为 esthesioneuroblastoma 和 olfactory neuroblastoma。组织学和分子学研究表明 ENB 最可能起源于筛板、鼻中隔上 1/3 和上鼻甲处嗅觉上皮的基底细胞。人类的嗅觉上皮基底细胞保留了分裂和分化再生的能力。ENB 是一种侵袭性、能够发生转移的肿瘤，局部可透过筛板向颅内生长或复发。有时很难与其他鼻腔及鼻旁窦肿瘤相鉴别。

流行病学和临床表现

ENB 约占上消化道肿瘤的 0.3%、鼻腔恶性肿瘤的 3%~6%（Broich et al.，1997）。男性略多见（男性 55%，女性 45%），多个种族均可发病。文献报道其好发年龄呈双峰分布，第一个高峰约 20 岁，第二个高峰约 50 岁（Klepin et al.，2005）。然而，最近一篇综述显示 ENB 发病年龄呈单峰分布，在 50~70 岁（Platek et al.，2011）。目前尚未发现 ENB 的好发因素。

ENB 患者的临床表现是隐匿性的、非特异性的，类似其他良性和恶性鼻腔肿瘤。多数肿瘤较小者并无症状，常偶然发现。最常见的症状是鼻塞后伴随单侧鼻出血，病程常为 6~12 个月。随肿瘤大小和侵袭周围结构的程度的不同可能出现不同的症状，如头痛、面部疼痛、鼻窦炎、嗅觉减退或丧失，若累及眼眶可导致视力障碍、复视和眼球突出。肿瘤也可累及颅内导致相关症状，如颅高压导致的恶心及呕吐，下丘脑和垂体累及导致的垂体激素紊乱，视路累及导致视力障碍。ENB 相关的副肿瘤综合征已有报道，最常见的是抗利尿激素异常分泌综合征（syndrome of inappropriate secretion of antidiuretic hormone，SIADH）和 ACTH 异常分泌（Gabbay et al.，2013）。异位 ENB 见于口腔、鼻窦、上颌窦和颅内（Purochit et al.，2015）。ENB 的症状在多数是非特异性，类似鼻腔良性肿瘤。因此类似症状者应考虑 ENB 以便早期诊断。

诊断

任何患有持续性鼻部症状的患者都应由耳鼻喉科医生进行全面检查。除了详细的全身查体和脑神经检查，还应该用软镜进行全面的鼻腔和鼻咽部检查。镜下 ENB 表现为鼻腔内鲜肉样、红黄色肿物，表面被覆黏膜，可能合并溃疡。

一旦确诊肿瘤应进行高分辨率（3 mm 层厚）计算断层扫描（CT）的平扫和增强，范围应包括颅底、鼻旁窦和颈部。肿瘤由于细胞密度高 CT 平扫呈高密度，增强显示不均匀强化。CT 主要优点在于对骨性结构的评估。冠状位和矢状位薄扫可显示筛板、纸样板和蝶窦侧壁的骨质破坏（**图 17.1**）。所有 ENB 患者应进行颈部 CT 扫描以评估区域淋巴结转移。

MRI 的优势是软组织成像清晰，是评估肿瘤生长范围的重要方法。T1 相显示为较灰质低的信号，增强为不均匀强化。T2 相显示为稍高信号，该序列能够显示肿瘤的囊变，并能够鉴别黏液潴留和肿瘤。MRI 是评价肿瘤侵犯眼眶、硬膜和颅内的最好的方法。ENB 尤其是高级别者因细胞密度高，在 DWI 上表现为弥散受限。

脑血管造影不作为诊断常规推荐。部分病例可用来评估肿瘤与颈动脉关系以及肿瘤血供。富血运肿瘤做术前栓塞也有意义。

影像学评估后下一步就是活检。ENB 因血供丰富，我们推荐在手术室全麻下进行活检。

若怀疑转移，应行颈部 CT 或者 PET-CT。

分期

诊断时 ENB 可以表现为局限于鼻腔内的肿物，更多表现为侵犯鼻窦、眼眶和颅内（图 17.1）。首诊时约有 10% 的患者合并颈部淋巴结转移。原发病例远处或者血行转移罕见，复发者可出现。常见的转移部位是肺部、骨骼和脑，罕见有迟发的远隔硬膜转移。准确评估肿瘤侵犯的范围对治疗方案选择和预后评价至关重要。有若干个关于 ENB 的分期系统。第一个也是最常用的是 1976 年由 Kadish 等提出（Kadish et al.，1976）。该系统定义如下：肿瘤局限于鼻腔为 A 期，侵犯鼻旁窦为 B 期，延伸至鼻旁窦外为 C 期。上述系统并未描述区域淋巴结和远处转移。Morita 于 1993 年进行改良，将区域淋巴结和远处转移定义为 D 期（Morita et al.，1993）。

第二个常用的分期方法由 Dulguerov 提出（Dulguerov and Calcaterra，1992）（表 17.1）。该分期更为详细，将肿瘤累及鼻腔、鼻窦和筛板进行区分，同时将累及前颅底、硬膜及脑组织分类。该分期还增加了区域淋巴结及远处转移，并应用传统的 TNM 分期进行分类。

目前哪种分期方法最能精确地指导治疗和评估预后尚无定论。Jethanam 等报道一组 261 例 ENB 患者的回顾性分析，结果显示 Kadish 4 个分期患者预后差别显著。合并淋巴结和远处转移的患者预后较差。显而易见的是淋巴结和远处转移显著影响预后，因此应纳入分期判断中。

大体表现、组织学和病理分期

肿瘤表现为鼻腔内被覆完整黏膜的肿物，偶尔分化差的肿瘤可合并溃疡。切面显示为鲜肉样，因肿瘤血供丰富表现为鲜红色。

组织学上 ENB 细胞为黏膜下巢样或片状排列。肿瘤巢之间为透明样、纤维状、富血管或者炎性基质。某些情况下，可能会看到肿瘤细胞呈局灶性或完整的片状排列，间隔少量基质。肿瘤细胞片状排列多见于、但并非仅限于高级别的肿瘤。ENB 细胞的核通常很小，呈圆形及“盐胡椒”征，核仁小。核多态性通常是轻度的，但偶尔会出现较大的细胞，

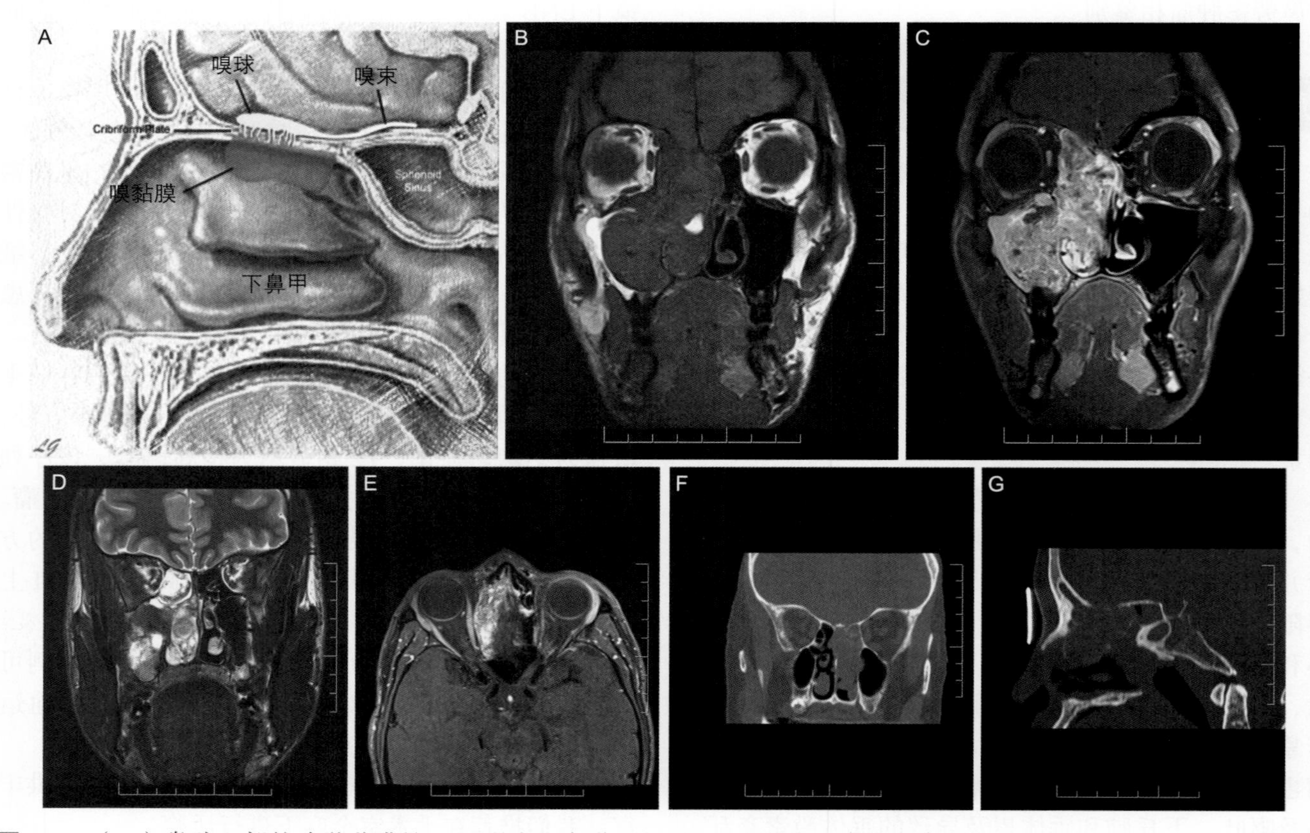

图 17.1 （A）鼻腔上部的嗅觉黏膜是 ENB 的起源部位。（B）21 岁男性，鼻塞加鼻出血 6 个月，MRI T1 平扫冠状位。（C）增强显示不均匀强化。（D）T2 冠状位显示高信号病灶，额叶硬脑膜完整。（E）T1 增强轴位显示纸样板受压。（F）冠状薄扫 CT 显示纸样板和筛板完整。（G）另一例 ENB，55 岁女性，伴有嗅觉丧失和鼻塞，CT 显示筛板受侵蚀

表 17.1　Dulguerov 分期和 Biller 分期

	Dulguerov 分期	Biller 分期
T1	肿瘤局限于鼻腔和（或）鼻旁窦内，未累及蝶窦或筛窦气房	肿瘤局限于鼻腔和鼻旁窦内，未累及蝶窦
T2	肿瘤累及蝶窦和（或）筛板	肿瘤累及眼眶和（或）颅内
T3	肿瘤累及眼眶或前颅窝，未侵犯硬脑膜	肿瘤侵犯脑组织，但可切除
T4	肿瘤累及脑组织	肿瘤广泛累及脑组织，无法切除
N0	无淋巴结转移	无淋巴结转移
N1	有淋巴结转移	有淋巴结转移
M0	无远处转移	无远处转移
M1	有远处转移	有远处转移

Source data from Pavel Dulguerov, Thomas Calcaterra, Esthesioneuroblastoma: The UCLA experience 1970–1990, *The Laryngoscope*, volume 102, issue 8, pp. 843–9, 1992 and Hugh F. Biller, William Lawson, Ved P. Sachdev, et al. Esthesioneuroblastoma: Surgical treatment without radiation, *The Laryngoscope*, volume 100, issue 3, pp. 1199–201, 1990.

其胞核突出，类似于神经节细胞。细胞质可能极少，如“小圆形蓝细胞肿瘤”，或轻度嗜酸性或两亲性（如类癌或垂体腺瘤细胞）。有丝分裂活动通常较低，但是高度未分化的肿瘤的特征是高有丝分裂率、富核多态性、间质少和内有坏死区域。肿瘤基质主要两部分构成：一是相互交叉的细胞突起，后者呈为嗜酸性、纤维状（神经纤维）；二是丛状或者球状毛细血管构成的血管床。肿瘤细胞可围绕基质形成栅栏样形成 Homer-Wright 样假玫瑰花环结构，这是分化良好肿瘤的特征。

鼻腔肿物活检中，神经纤维包绕的假玫瑰花环几乎是 ENB 的病理标志。低分化的肿瘤常见真正的 Flexner-Wintersteiner 型玫瑰花结，后者肿瘤细胞排列呈腺样结构。有时可见血管周围玫瑰花结。部分 ENB 可见钙化、坏死（较高级别肿瘤）、囊变、肿瘤细胞包绕的鳞状或腺样上皮区。极少数情况下 ENB 表现为向黑素细胞或成肌细胞的分化，或显示局灶性腺样结构，上述情况增加了鉴别诊断的难度。

最常用的 ENB 分级系统是 Hyams 开发的 ENB 分级系统（Hyams et al.，1998）。该系统分级内容包括：肿瘤发育程度、神经纤维的数量、玫瑰花结的类型和密度、有丝分裂活跃度、坏死、核多态性程度（**表 17.2**）。已有几项研究表明 Hyam 分级与预后有良好的相关性（Miyamoto et al.，2000；Dulguerov et al.，2001）。

免疫组织化学特征

所有拟诊 ENB 病例均应行免疫组织化学检查。病理鉴别诊断非常重要，病理直接指导治疗并确定预后。应谨慎对待复发肿瘤，其免疫组织化学特征可能有变化。ENB 可以表达非特异性烯醇酶、嗜铬粒蛋白和突触素。ENB 的诊断需大部分肿瘤细胞突触素或嗜铬粒蛋白阳性。其他神经内分泌或神经元标志物（例如 CD56 和 CD57）也呈阳性。肿瘤细胞巢周围的支持细胞呈 S-100 染色阳性，该细胞对正常嗅上皮中的嗅觉细胞具有支持作用，且有类似施万细胞的超微结构。S-100 阳性细胞对于 ENB 诊断非常重要，应同黑色素瘤区分开来。在高级别肿瘤不会表现为 S-100 阳性。偶尔肿瘤细胞也会呈 S-100

表 17.2　Hyams 分期

分级	小叶状排列	分裂指数	核多态性	坏死	玫瑰花环	纤维基质
Ⅰ	+	无	–	–	HW	++
Ⅱ	+	低	+/–	–	HW	+
Ⅲ	+/-	中	+	罕见	FW	+/-
Ⅳ	+/-	高	++	常见	无	-

HW, Homer Wright; FW, Flexner-Wintersteiner

Source data from Hyams et al., *Tumours of the upper respiratory tract and ear*, 2nd edition. Washington: Armed forces institute of Pathology; Copyright (c) 1998.

阳性。胶质原纤维酸性蛋白（glial fibrillary acidic protein，GFAP）、b-微管蛋白和微管相关蛋白表达程度不固定。30%~40%的ENB显示出角蛋白和低分子角蛋白的局部染色。上皮标志物在ENBs中通常是阴性的，尽管在某些情况下可能会看到散在阳性染色。间质标志物（如结蛋白、肌生成素、波形蛋白和肌动蛋白）的染色也为阴性。尽管有一些黑素细胞分化和黑色素沉着的报道，黑素细胞细胞标志物（如HMB-45）还是阴性的。尤因肉瘤和PNET的标志物如MIC2（CD99）、FLI1均为阴性。常见的白细胞抗原和其他造血标志物也是阴性的，参见**图**17.2。

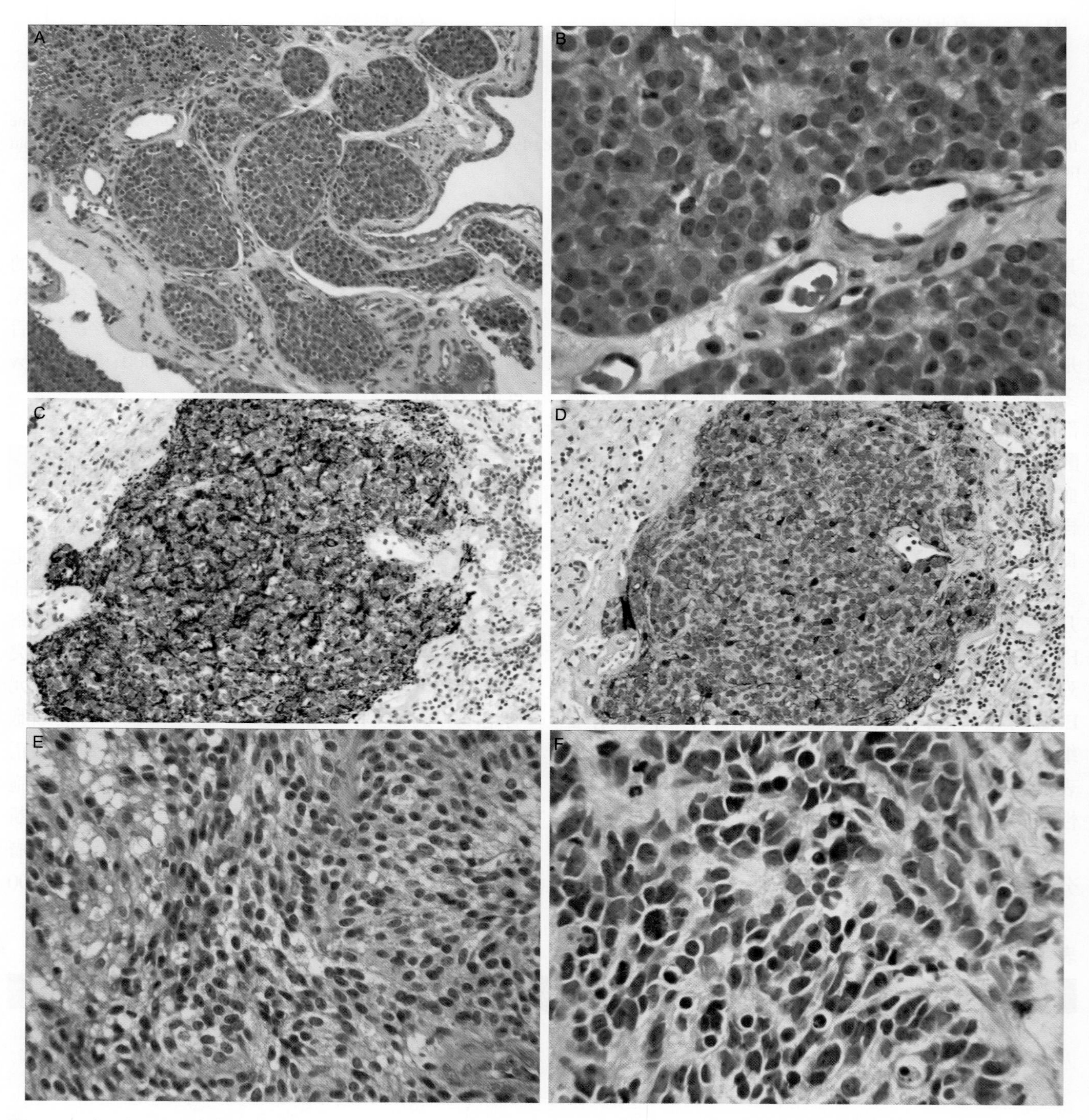

图 17.2 （A）H&E染色，低倍显微镜，显示了Ⅰ级ENB典型的小叶样排列。注意完整覆盖的鼻黏膜。（B）H&E染色，高倍显微镜，Ⅰ级ENB，显示肿瘤细胞具有相对一致的、圆形至卵圆形的细胞核，细颗粒细胞质，周围包绕神经原纤维基质。可见Homer-Wright样假玫瑰花环。（C）ENB嗜铬粒蛋白染色呈阳性。（D）支持细胞S-100染色呈阳性，此为ENB的特点。（E，F）Ⅳ级ENB，H&E染色，注意其高核多态性和有丝分裂活跃

鉴别诊断

ENB 的鉴别诊断谱较广泛，所有鼻窦肿物均应纳入鉴别。ENB 必须与上皮分化的神经外胚层起源的其他肿瘤（神经内分泌肿瘤）区分开，例如分化差的小细胞或非小细胞肿瘤［鼻窦未分化癌（sinonasal undiff erentiated carcinoma，SNUC）］。带有神经分化的神经外胚层肿瘤，如副神经节瘤、恶性黑色素瘤、尤因肉瘤 / PNET、神经纤维瘤和神经鞘瘤也必须进行鉴别。其他需要鉴别的是淋巴瘤、横纹肌肉瘤、腺癌、腺样囊性癌、鼻窦鳞癌、鼻咽癌、骨肉瘤和软骨肉瘤。可能在该区域生长的良性肿瘤包括内翻乳头状瘤和垂体腺瘤。

鉴别诊断对于治疗选择、患者的随访和总体预后至关重要。神经内分泌肿瘤侵袭性更高，具有更高的局部和远处复发风险。高级别 ENB 可能难以与神经内分泌肿瘤鉴别。通常 SNUC 具有较高的有丝分裂率。神经内分泌癌细胞角蛋白染色呈阳性，但 ENB 通常呈阴性。神经内分泌癌中不存在 S-100 染色，但在 ENB 中具有特征性的阳性。

治疗

ENB 需手术、放疗和化疗三者不同形式组合或者单独治疗。最常见的治疗策略是对可切除者行手术切除加术后放疗；对于较晚期、转移性或无法手术者采用化疗。

手术的主要目标是全切除加切缘干净。传统的手术方法是经颅面部切除病变，包括使用双额开颅和侧鼻切开术、Weber-Ferguson 切口或面部脱套入路。经眉间颅底入路是另一种传统的入路。累及硬脑膜的肿瘤需要切除硬脑膜和嗅束。如果发生脑部侵犯，需行安全范围内的脑组织切除，以保证切缘干净。通过面部入路尚可进行部分或全部的上颌切除，并行眼球摘除。

近二十年来内镜经鼻入路得到了空前发展，可单独或者与传统入路联合治疗 ENB。Kadish A 期、B 期和无明显侧向生长的 C 期肿瘤是单纯内镜手术的最佳适应证，可实现切缘干净。已有研究显示单纯内镜下切除 ENB 的结果比较满意（Hanna et al.，2009）。随着经验的积累和内镜颅底重建技术的日益成熟，手术并发症的发生率逐渐降低。对于掌握好适应证的患者，内镜手术是一种出色的、微创的治疗方法。

放射治疗是 ENB 的重要治疗选择。它可以单独使用，也可以在术前或术后应用，也可以与化学疗法联合使用。对于无法手术或者无法完全切除的局部或区域性病变，放疗可单独或者与化疗联合应用。几项研究表明，手术切除联合放疗比单纯手术或放疗效果更好（Jethanamest et al.，2007）。术后放疗的目标是治疗微小残留病灶，通常以适形调强放疗的方式进行，疗程为 1.8~2 Gy，总剂量最多可达 70 Gy。多项研究对术前放射治疗效果进行了评估。术前放疗的目的是减少肿瘤体积并增加肿瘤的可切除性。Bachar 等的报道显示接受术前放疗和术后放疗的两组患者在生存期和复发率方面没有差异（Bachar et al.，2008）。

ENB 化疗的数据非常有限，其治疗策略是基于治疗其他头颈部恶性肿瘤的经验。通常，化疗是在术前或术后与放疗一起使用。化疗常应用于局部或远处进展病例中。

预后和复发

ENB 的局部复发率取决于首次治疗。Demiroz 等的研究（2011）显示，单纯手术治疗者 5 年局部复发率为 71%，手术加术后放疗者 6 年局部复发率为 17%。复发病例治疗能否成功取决于复发的程度，因此鼻内镜和 MRI 的密切随访很重要。局部复发通常是可以治疗的，可以进行进一步的手术（内镜或开放），如果可能的话再加上抢救性放疗。对 33 篇文章的 meta 分析显示，有 20.2%的患者发生了颈部转移，这其中 61.7%的患者在初始治疗后 6 个月发生了转移。这些复发者的挽救率（定义为无疾病生存期为 1 年）为 31.2%，与单独使用任一疗法相比，联合手术和放疗的挽救率更高（Gore and Zanation，2009）。多达 10%的患者发生远处转移，这部分患者预后较差。尽管预后较差，抢救治疗仍可缓解症状并延长生存期。McElroy 等（1998）的报告显示，基于顺铂的治疗对晚期疾病有效。

结论

嗅神经母细胞瘤是一种罕见且侵袭性强的肿瘤，其治疗仍具有挑战性。使用统一的分期系统有助于判断生存期和复发率。多模态、多学科治疗是大多数患者的首选。虽然筛板下方的小肿瘤单纯手术治疗即可，但绝大多数 ENB 患者需行手术加放疗。复发转移灶可能需要化疗。ENB 的复发较常见，可能在初次治疗后很多年出现，因此需对患者进行长期的密切随访。

内镜手术单独或者联合开放颅鼻手术对于ENB的治疗是一个积极的补充。早期的研究结果显示内镜的效果比较满意，对于选择性的病例其效果优于传统入路。

争议

ENB中颈部淋巴结转移性的治疗方法尚未确立。文献显示初诊时淋巴结受累的发生率可能约为10%，但最终20%～30%的患者会发生淋巴结转移。在就诊时或在随访期间出现临床或影像学淋巴结转移的患者适合进行颈淋巴结清扫和术后颈部放疗。颈淋巴结清扫的程度取决于受累淋巴结的范围。选择性或预防性颈淋巴清扫术不是标准的，也没有研究显示具有明确益处。尽管其他数据支持颈部淋巴结的选择性照射（Monroe et al.，2003），但尚无研究表明颈部选择性放疗能降低淋巴结复发的发生率（Noh et al.，2011）。尽管如此，对于接受放疗的患者，颈部通常被预防性地包含在治疗区域中。

延伸阅读、参考文献

扫描书末二维码获取。

第 18 章 颅底恶性肿瘤

Benedict Panizza · Adel Helmy 著
鲁润春 译，伊志强 审校

引言

颅底外科肿瘤多数是良性的。这些肿瘤治疗的策略如下：选择合适的手术入路（内镜经鼻、前方、侧方、后方中线）、保护周围的神经血管结构、内部减瘤和包膜外分离。颅底恶性肿瘤（malignant skull base tumours，MSBT）是一组更为罕见且组织学上更为多样的肿瘤，其治疗起来更加复杂，需要一套独特的治疗原则。因此，尽管病理、结果和预后差异很大，但它们仍被归为一类病变。为了达到最好的治疗效果，需要真正的多学科合作：外科专科联合（神经外科、头颈外科、耳科、整形修复外科）、放射科和肿瘤科。几种较常见的颅底恶性肿瘤，如脊索瘤、软骨肉瘤和嗅神经母细胞瘤在单独的章节中阐述，在此不再赘述。

颅底可以见到众多的病理类型，这反映了头颈部和颅内交界区域的解剖复杂性。这些肿瘤可能来自皮肤、黏膜、唾液腺、软骨、骨骼或肌肉。最实用的临床分类是分为前颅底和侧颅底肿瘤（**表 18.1**）。从病理学角度可将肿瘤分类为：起源于颅底肿瘤，周围区域肿瘤侵袭颅底（鼻腔、颞下窝，远处转移）。

关于颅底肿瘤的确切流行病学数据很少。但是此类肿瘤均非常罕见，其中最常见的鳞状细胞癌（squamous cell carcinoma，SCC），发病率仅为每年 0.5~1/1 000 000 人，它起源于鼻腔、鼻窦并延伸至前颅底。这些肿瘤在日本、印度尼西亚和亚洲的某些地区更为常见。原发性颞骨鳞癌的发病率估计为每年 6/1 000 000 人，实际上进行颞骨切除的病例中，90% 是皮肤鳞癌转移至颞骨。

原则上，颅底恶性肿瘤的最佳治疗方法是整块切除加切缘干净。分块切除可能造成术腔种植，并降低切缘干净比例。一些情况下无法整块切除：如大的肿瘤会阻挡深方重肿瘤边缘的处理；肿瘤毗邻重要结构（如颈静脉孔区或颈内动脉），这时整块切除会合并较高的病死率。在这些情况下，可采用分块切除结合大体清扫。这通常需要进行广泛的颅面部切除，并需进行挑战性的硬脑修补以避免脑脊液漏和气颅，同时需行整形外科修复以保证创面有足够的组织覆盖。

放疗是最常见的辅助治疗，范围需包括肿瘤边缘。部分肿瘤的化疗日渐增多。

美国癌症分期联合委员会（American Joint Committee of Cancer Staging，AJCC）已发布了针对几种颅外肿瘤的分期系统，这些系统依据三项内容：T（肿瘤范围）、N（区域淋巴结受累）和 M（区域淋巴结外远处转移）。TNM 分期系统见**表 18.2**，并非所有的肿瘤都有完整的数值。TNM 分期的意义：预

表 18.1 常见恶性颅底肿瘤病理类型

前颅底肿瘤	侧颅底肿瘤
鳞状细胞癌	
唾液腺恶性肿瘤（腺癌、腺样囊性癌、腺泡性癌）	
肉瘤（例如骨肉瘤、纤维肉瘤、横纹肌肉瘤、脂肪肉瘤、尤因肉瘤）	
恶性黑色素瘤	基底细胞癌
鼻腔鼻窦未分化癌	
嗅神经母细胞瘤	

表 18.2 颅外肿瘤 TNM 分期方法

T：肿瘤大小范围	N：淋巴结转移	M：远处转移
Tx：无法评价	Nx：无法评价	
Tis：原位癌	N0：无区域淋巴结转移	M0：无远处转移
T0：无原发肿瘤	N1：邻近区域淋巴结转移	M1：远处转移
T1~T4：肿瘤的大小和（或）范围	N2~N3：侵犯更多的淋巴结或者远处淋巴结转移	

Source data from *AJCC Cancer Staging Manual*.

后判断；治愈性手术或姑息性手术的选择；是否处理头颈部淋巴结。美国国家综合癌症网络（National Comprehensive Cancer Network，NCCN）提供了详细的依据 TNM 分期系统（Network，2019）治疗头颈部恶性肿瘤的方法。

前颅底肿瘤

临床评估

前颅底恶性肿瘤最常就诊于耳鼻喉科，主诉为嗅觉丧失、老年化（如味觉减退）、疼痛、鼻塞、流鼻涕和鼻出血。局部侵袭严重者，海绵窦侵犯可导致复视或眼肌麻痹，眼眶直接受累导致眼球突出、球结膜水肿或疼痛，视神经通路的直接受压导致视野损害或视力下降。额叶直接浸润可引起癫痫发作，颅内压升高可引起头痛，但很少作为首发症状。

门诊体格检查结合鼻内镜检查有时可以发现鼻腔内的肿瘤。增强 MRI 仍然是诊断和确定肿瘤累及范围的首选方法。薄扫 CT 加多维度重建可提供有关肿瘤骨质侵犯的详细信息，这对手术计划至关重要，尤其能指导颅底重建。

任何新诊断考虑为恶性颅底肿瘤者均应行 TNM 分期，必要时进行颈淋巴结检查和全身成像以评估淋巴结转移和远处转移。

根据病变的程度和范围，还可能需头颈外科医生联合眼科或牙科进行评估。

完善临床评估后，获得病理诊断是决定治疗方案的关键因素，常需进行经鼻活检。但富血运肿瘤如青少年鼻咽纤维血管瘤等为活检禁忌。

肿瘤位置和病理类型

尽管病理类型多种多样，但肿瘤的恶性程度和侵袭范围是治疗策略选择的决定因素。中度恶性肿瘤，如低级别腺样囊性癌、软骨肉瘤、嗅神经母细胞瘤，可进行保守的切除以避免神经功能缺损，术后辅助放疗控制残留病变。对于尚未全身扩散的恶性程度更高的肿瘤，如鳞状细胞癌、黑色素瘤、恶性程度高的肉瘤，应在肉眼下进行更广泛的切除，以期治愈。通常很难作出治疗选择，要取决于患者的意愿、伴随疾病、外科团队的技术特点。

手术治疗

过去 10 年，内镜技术在前颅底肿瘤中的应用大大增加。然而目前的证据并不支持内镜技术对前颅底恶性肿瘤有确切的疗效（Rawal et al.，2012），其中嗅神经母细胞瘤除外。内镜是就是实现手术目标的一个方法，如可证明其治疗肿瘤效果等同于传统方法，那么内镜入路或者联合入路应用将更加广泛，因其并发症发生率较传统颅面入路显著降低（Castelnuovo et al.，2014）。

放射疗法

术后放疗是手术切除的重要辅助治疗，其目的可以是姑息性亦可是治愈性。临床上此类肿瘤常距切缘非常近，应常规建议患者术后进行放疗会诊。因常需要在重要的神经血管区域给予较大剂量放疗，所以常采用直线加速器而非放射治疗。常采用分次以降低正常组织的剂量，如总剂量 60 Gy 分 30 次进行。

其他辅助治疗

化疗也是一个治疗手段，常治疗肿瘤切缘阳性或者肿瘤出现包膜外扩散的情况。但也有特殊情况。一方面，于鼻腔鼻窦未分化癌的患者，许多头颈外科中心仅给予放疗加化疗，也达到了与手术类似的效果。另一方面，皮肤恶性肿瘤合并神经扩散目前尚无化疗有效的证据。

结局

颅底会遇到多种多样的恶性肿瘤。行颅面部入路切除的患者 5 年无疾病生存率为 60%、5 年无复发生存率为 53%。1/3 的患者出现术后并发症，伤口问题最常见。围术期死亡率约为 4%（Patel et al.，2003）。黑色素瘤的围术期并发症率相似，但长期预后较差，其 3 年无疾病生存率为 30%，无复发生存率为 26%（Ganly et al.，2006）。内镜手术能达到类似的疾病控制率，且围术期并发症较少。对于所有头颈部恶性肿瘤，切缘阴性者生存期较长。

侧颅底肿瘤

临床评估

侧颅底病变最常累及颞骨，但也可从颞下窝延伸至中颅窝。临床表现多种多样，但最常表现为原发性的皮肤肿物或者局部治疗后的皮肤病变。肿瘤向深方生长可导致各种症状：颞骨侵犯导致听力下降、耳痛、面瘫及平衡障碍，海绵窦及岩尖受累导致复视及面部麻木，脑干及后组脑神经症状，颞下颌关节受累引起的张口受限。

首先应确定肿瘤的起源部位：皮肤最常见；少见者起源于颞下窝，如唾液腺恶性肿瘤、原发性间充质肿瘤。须评估区域淋巴结转移。MR 和 CT 成像对于确定肿瘤的部位和范围至关重要。

肿瘤位置和病理类型

需神经外科干预的最常见的病变是侵犯颞骨的鳞状细胞癌，后者是侵袭性恶性肿瘤，主要起源于外耳道皮肤，5%起源于中耳表皮。因肿瘤常起源于皮肤并扩散到颞骨并累及耳前颞下颌沟区域，通常需行颞骨切除以达到切缘干净。文献报道一组病例中，T4 期肿瘤（侵犯岩骨内侧或广泛的软组织累及）最常见于耳前区域，该区域的预后较差（Essig et al., 2013）。其他类型肿瘤包括：基底细胞癌（耳郭上最常见的肿瘤）、唾液腺恶性肿瘤（腺癌、腺样囊性癌、腮腺腺癌）、肉瘤。颞骨解剖较复杂，肿瘤一旦突破中耳，可能经多种途径扩散：向前方侵犯颈动脉和咽鼓管，向内侧侵犯前庭、耳蜗和内耳道，向下方侵犯颈静脉球和后组脑神经，向上方突破鼓室盖进入中颅窝。

关于鳞状细胞癌已经有几种分期方法。无论哪种方法，下列因素均被认为预后不良：骨质浸润，中耳侵犯，面神经麻痹，硬脑膜受累，沿神经扩散和局部淋巴结肿大。

手术治疗

侧颅底恶性肿瘤应力求整块切除以获得最佳效果，这一要求较前颅底肿瘤更强。鼻腔内肿瘤的活检或切除正好位于空气和肿瘤的界面上，覆盖正常组织的完整黏膜是阻断肿瘤细胞种植的屏障。然而侧颅底肿瘤手术中，深部的切缘常有富血管床，再加上高速磨钻的使用，易出现肿瘤种植。

图 18.1 是一例侵袭性颞骨鳞状细胞癌 合并 House-Brackmann 6 级面瘫患者的影像和手术照片。针对鳞状细胞癌有若干种颞骨切除的方法，所有均包含浅表腮腺切除术。外侧岩骨切除术包括外耳道切除，骨质切除至鼓膜环，须保留面神经。颞骨次全切术需进一步切除鼓室和内听道及其内神经，仅保留岩尖和颈动脉。岩骨全切除术需进一步切除颈动脉和岩尖，可能损伤海绵窦结构，故很少应用。此例患者进行了根治性腮腺切除、下颌骨切除、外侧颞骨切除，并结合颞部开颅将影像学上受累的硬脑膜一并切除。应尽量避免切除硬脑膜，以免增加肿瘤脑脊液播散的风险，除非硬膜确实受累且手术能够完整切除。保留硬脑膜不仅能阻断病变播散，而且能使放疗照射范围更集中。

虽然已经有各种方法来尽量降低牺牲颈动脉的风险，其致残率仍较显著。术前球囊闭塞试验常用来预测颈动脉闭塞后的脑缺血并发症风险，其预测准确性各异，术后卒中的风险为 2%~16%，血栓栓塞和低灌注均为致病因素（van Rooij et al., 2005; Whisenant et al., 2015）。因此，经验丰富的医生均主张尽量保留颈动脉（例如，**图 18.2** 和**图 18.3**），考虑到术后放疗的获益，颞骨全切术带来的并发症难以接受。

侵袭性肿瘤切除至颈动脉外膜后，应分别在术后 2~3 天和 2~3 周进行血管造影，以除外血管损伤、夹层或假性动脉瘤。颈静脉孔受累的肿瘤预后较差，颈静脉球切除和后组脑神经麻痹的并发症难以接受。因此上述情况应首选颞骨次全切除再结合辅助治疗。

颞骨切除术需整形外科医生参与以提供术区软组织覆盖。最常应用的是带蒂游离瓣，从颈外动脉供血。这可能会影响颈部淋巴结清扫。

放射疗法

切缘干净加术后放疗的患者预后是最好的。切缘阳性者也建议术后放疗以治疗残留病变。对于部分侵袭性的病例（如颈静脉球或颈动脉受累），应避免大范围手术切除，行姑息性切除辅以术后放疗。

其他辅助治疗

免疫疗法如 PD-1 和 PDL-1 抑制剂可能会显著改变晚期皮肤恶性肿瘤的治疗策略。在晚期皮肤鳞状细胞癌的残留和复发病例治疗中，其短期（1~2 年）效果较好。新的治疗方法如何同目前治疗融合仍然需要进一步临床试验来研究。

结局

对于外侧颞骨切除术，疾病特异性 5 年生存率为 62%，无疾病生存率为 59%。

争议

皮肤恶性肿瘤累及神经是一个特别复杂的问题。部分亚组表现为易侵犯神经，可累及三叉神经或面神经分支（Panizza et al., 2014; Warren et al., 2016b）。三叉神经受累为麻木或者蚁行感，面神经累及表现为面瘫。肿瘤可向颅内发展侵犯脑干，也可经分叉处蔓延累及邻近神经。因肿瘤累及范围广需进行广泛切除。另一策略是姑息性切除后给予受累神经放疗，这样能降低手术风险。既往已经有诸多中心报道无脑干累及者手术预后良好（70%的根治性切除）

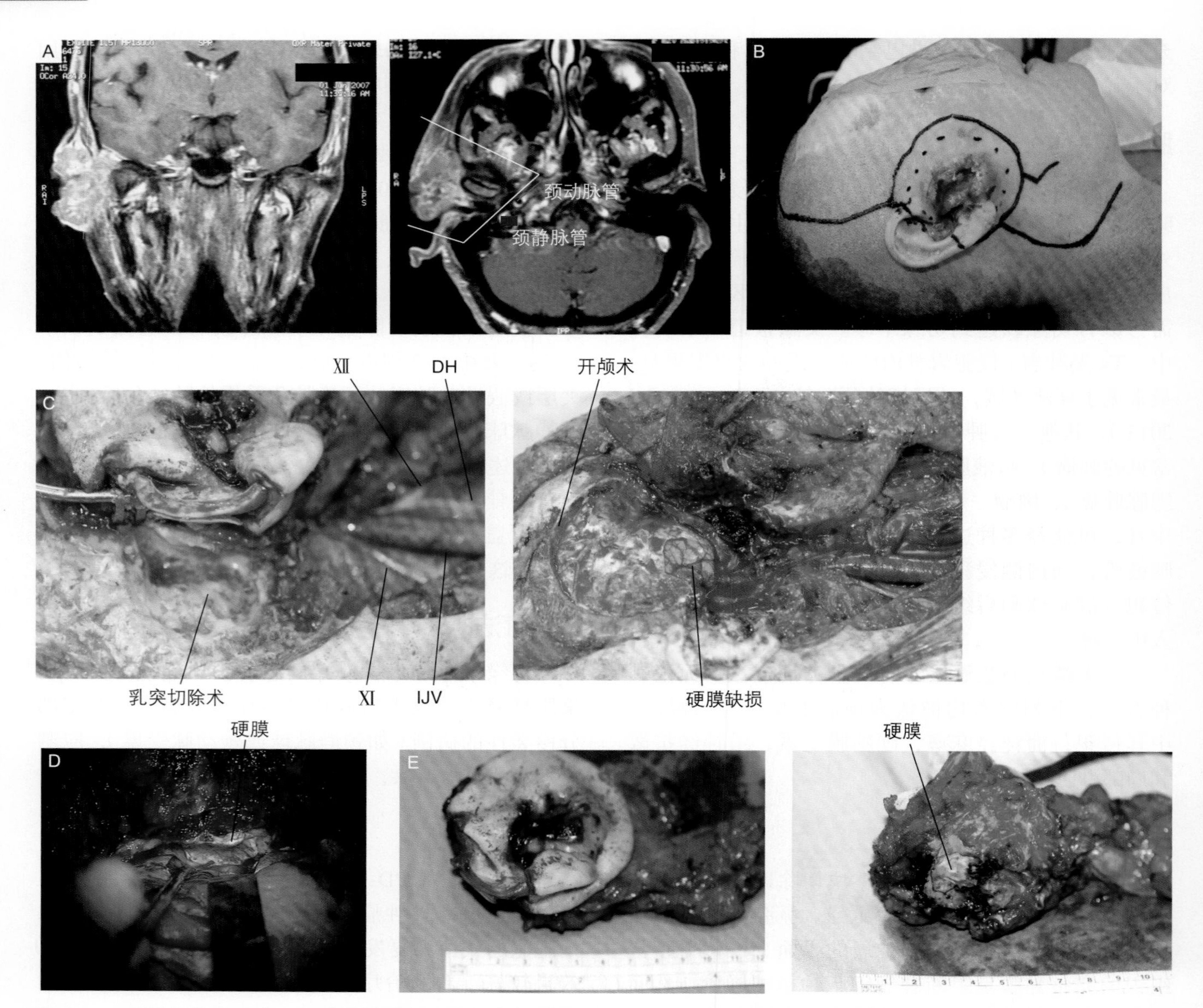

图 18.1 颞骨鳞状细胞癌。该患者表现为耳郭前方的溃疡性病变。（A）术前 MRI T1 增强矢状位和轴位。手术切除的范围限于轴位上的白线内，紧贴颈动脉管和颈静脉球。（B）手术计划切除部分耳郭，切口向上下延伸以便进行开颅、显露颞下窝、切除颈部病变。（C）术中大体照片显示从颞下窝切除肿瘤、颞部开颅、分离肿瘤深方边界并切除受累硬脑膜。（D）术中显微镜下照片，显示开颅并离断肿瘤深方。硬膜与颅底骨质粘连。需磨除颅底骨质以便整块切除病变。（E）肿瘤的浅层和深层边缘（染色的硬脑膜）（Ⅺ，副神经；Ⅻ，舌下神经；IJV，颈内静脉；DH，舌下神经降支）

（Warren et al.，2016a）。

图 18.4 是一位 55 岁患者的手术前后影像，该患者主诉为三叉神经第三支支配区域的疼痛和感觉丧失。活检证实为腺样囊性癌，术前 MRI T1 增强显示病变通过卵圆孔延续生长至三叉神经半月节。对于此类广泛生长的肿瘤，首先要考虑肿瘤是否可以完全切除，并且肿瘤完全切除结合放疗能否达到满意的肿瘤控制。如考虑进行大范围切除，则只有在完全切除肿瘤才可是使患者获益，其范围包括下颌神经位于半月结的部分及其颞下窝的分支。手术具体细节本章不赘述，需要者可参考文献（Redmond and Panizza，2016；Solares et al.，2016）。

需要平衡全切除肿瘤（可能是治愈性切除）带来的生存获益和手术风险，后者包括整块切除颞下窝和半侧下颌的风险、下颌神经损伤导致的眼外肌麻痹。

患者术前状态良好，经过讨论患者选择手术彻底切除病变。行颞下耳前入路显露颞下窝，结合半下颌切除术以完全去除下颌骨槽中的下牙槽神经。在咬肌深面进行操作以保留面神经。然后行颞下开

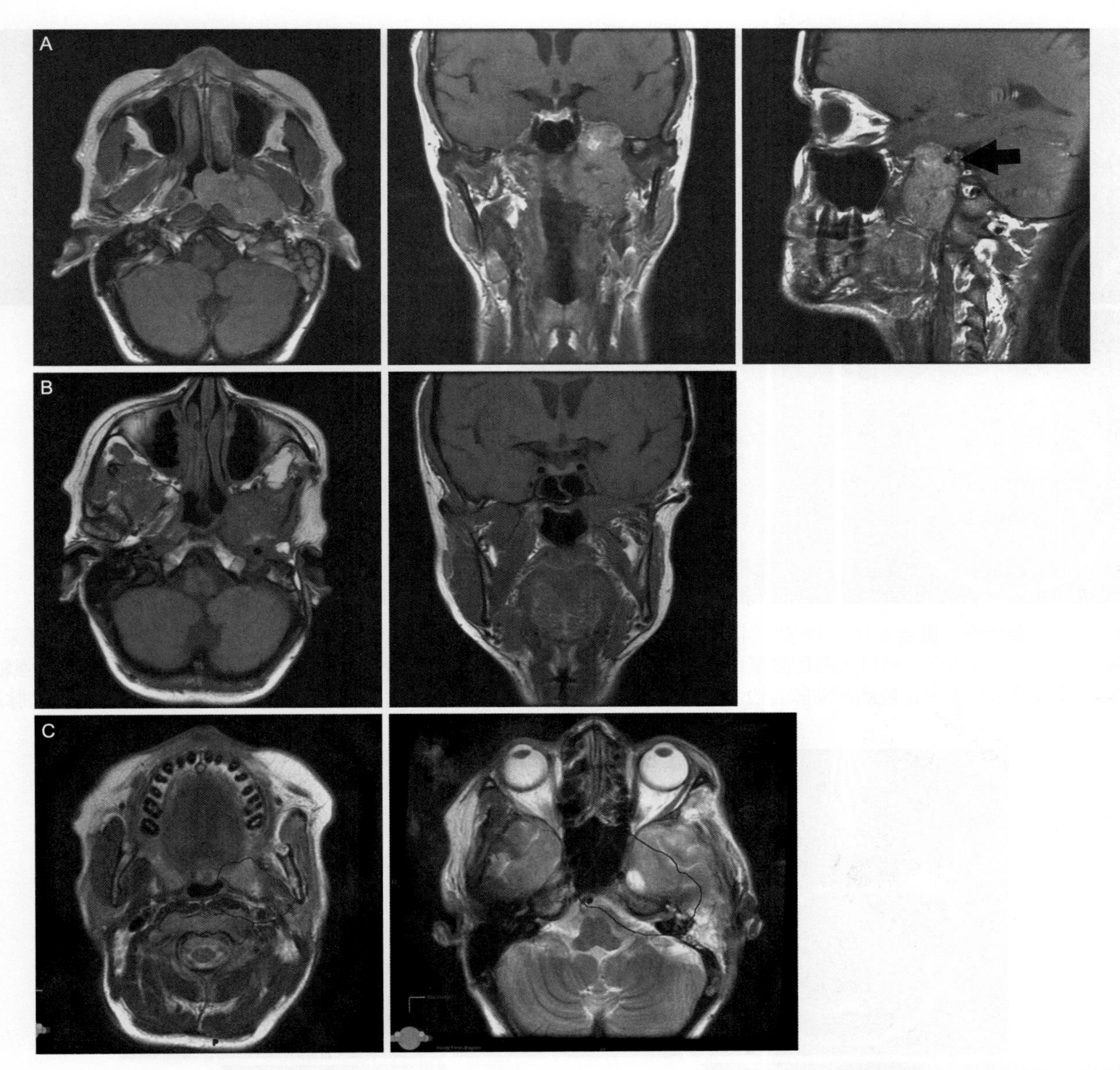

图 18.2　低级别腺癌。患者女性，52 岁，因左中耳积液导致耳聋，内镜检查发现鼻腔后部光滑的血管性肿块。活检显示低级别腺癌。患者行颞下窝病变切除和中颅窝开颅手术。术后放疗剂量为 60 Gy，分割为 30 次。（A）T1 增强轴位、矢状位、冠状位。矢状位显示肿瘤包绕颈动脉（箭头）。（B）术后 T1 轴位、冠状位。（C）术后放疗范围覆盖术前肿瘤生长范围

颅经硬膜外入路显露三叉神经半月节。颞下颅骨开颅之前，先从下面显露圆孔和卵圆孔，以便从颅内硬膜下牵拉颞叶和在三叉神经 2、3 支之间切开并分离两层硬膜。沿此层次逐步解剖可暴露海绵窦，类似于 Dolenc 入路。须保留 V1 以避免角膜感觉丧失。V2 的上部用于划定半月神经节切除的上界。一旦神经分离出来，即从圆孔取 V2 送冰冻以确认切缘干净，使病变同 V3 安全分开并进行硬膜下分离最终将病变与颞下窝部分一同整块切除。V2 切缘阳性者需进一步向远端磨除进入翼腭窝。根据影像学制订手术计划可降低术中切缘意外阳性的概率。

图 18.4C 显示患者术后面神经功能完好、下颌神经麻痹。术后 7 年患者仍然良好存活。即使对于这些困难病例，详细的术前计划、颅底和神经外科多学科联合也可以带来满意的结果。

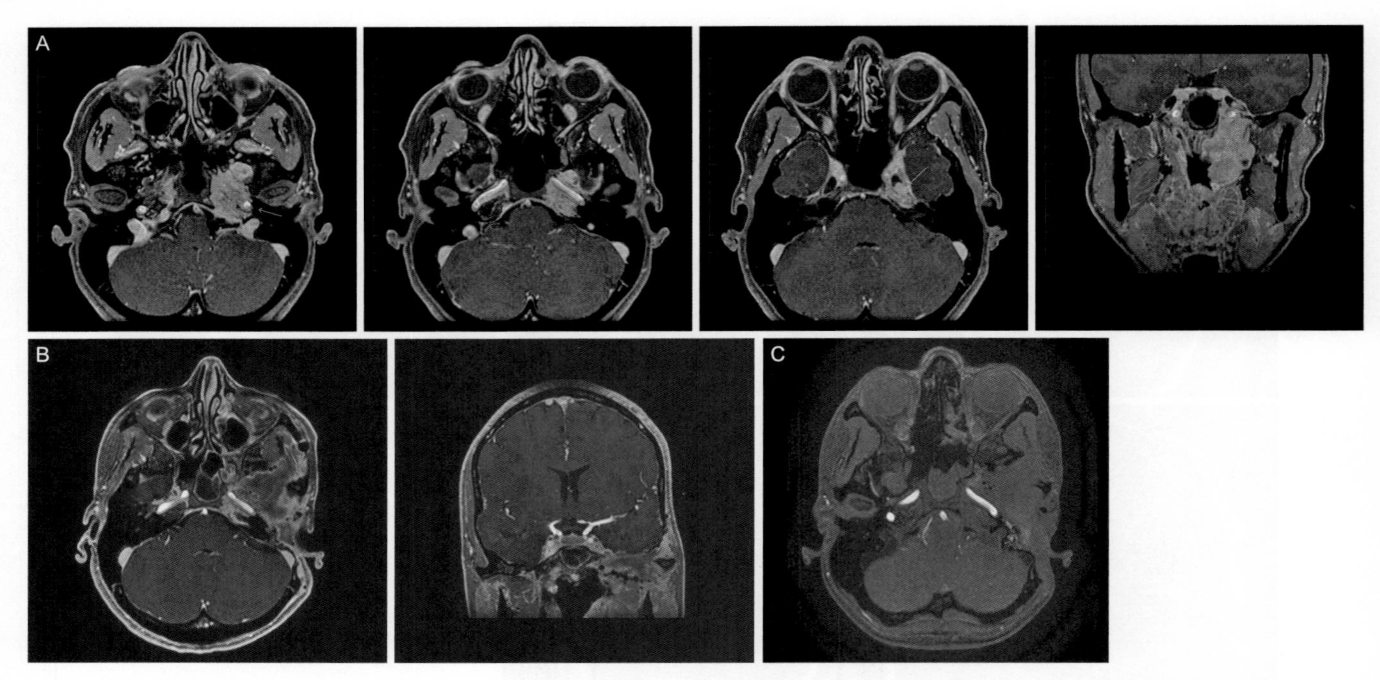

图 18.3 腺样囊性癌。患者女性，37 岁。主诉为左侧耳痛和咽鼓管功能障碍 18 个月。活检证实为腺样囊性癌。患者采用经鼻内镜切除至鼻咽部边界、经口入路切除至口咽部边界，并接受了颞下窝入路以及中颅后窝开颅手术。（A）术前 T1 增强轴位、冠状位。肿瘤紧贴海绵窦并包绕颈动脉岩段（箭头）。（B）术后 T1 增强。（C）术后时间飞跃法 MR 血管成像确认颈动脉通畅

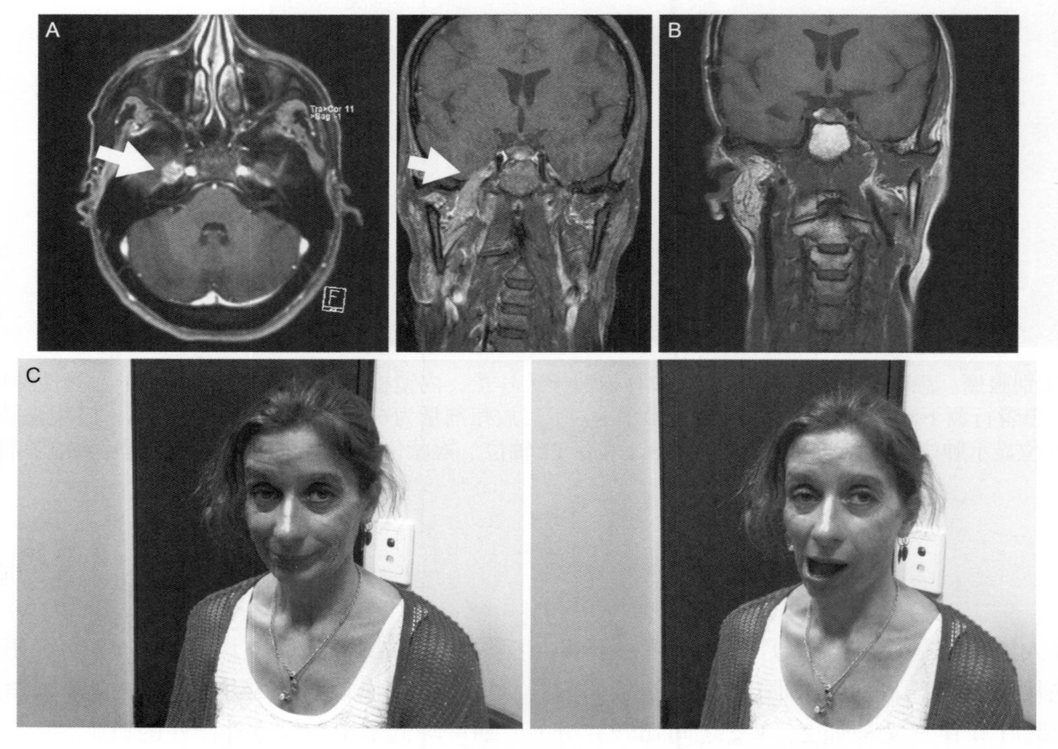

图 18.4 腺样囊性癌合并沿神经播散。该患者表现为下颌神经支配区的蚁行感和感觉异常。（A）术前 T1 增强轴位和冠状位，显示颞下窝强化病变，通过卵圆孔侵犯海绵窦（箭头所示）。（B）术后 7 年 T1 增强冠状位显示三叉神经下颌支切除。（C）术后复查。左图为嘱患者“微笑”和“抬眉”，显示面神经功能完好。右图为嘱患者伸下颌，因行颞下窝和下颌骨切除患者下颌偏向患侧

延伸阅读、参考文献

扫描书末二维码获取。

第 19 章　眼眶肿瘤的手术治疗

Joseph D. Chabot · S. Tonya Stefko · Paul Gardner 著
鲁润春 译，伊志强 审校

引言

眼眶病变多种多样，应依据病变位置和病理类型选择入路和治疗策略。眼眶毗邻鼻窦、前颅窝和中颅窝，需神经外科医生、耳鼻喉科医生和眼科医生多学科合作。

对于原发性眶内病变和邻近病变累及眼眶者，经典的开眶术、开颅显微镜手术和内镜经鼻入路能够进行 360° 的活检或切除。

本章阐述眼眶病变相关解剖、临床表现和手术技术。

解剖

在 Albert Rhoton 博士关于眼眶解剖的文章中，描述了一个"七法则"：由七块骨骼组成的金字塔内包含七根神经和七块肌肉（Martins et al.，2011）。金字塔的底部是眼睛和眼睑的前面，向后逐渐变细延续为眶尖。这个金字塔的体积大约为 30 ml，由脂肪、肌肉、神经、血管、腺体、结缔组织和眼球（约 7 ml）组成。

构成眼眶的七块骨头是额骨、筛骨、泪骨、腭骨、蝶骨、上颌骨和颧骨。眶顶主要由两部分构成：前部是额骨，将眼眶与额叶分开；后部是蝶骨小翼，分隔眼眶和鞍旁区域。

额骨在下内侧与筛骨相连，筛骨构成眼眶内侧壁。后方的蝶骨体、前方的泪骨和上颌骨连接筛骨和额骨共同形成眼眶内侧壁，将眼眶与鼻腔分开。

在下方，腭骨的眶突和上颌骨的眶面形成三角形的眶底，其外侧界为眶下裂。该壁将眼眶与翼腭裂和上颌窦隔开。

颧骨向上方与蝶骨大翼共同构成眼眶外侧壁，并将眼眶与颞肌和颞叶分开。

七条神经穿过眶尖的两个开口。内侧为视神经管，是 4.5 mm 宽、5~10 mm 长骨管，走行于蝶骨小翼内，视神经和眼动脉其内穿行。硬脑膜返折形成镰状韧带覆盖视神经管内口。颅内硬脑膜穿过视神经管并分成两层：视神经鞘和眶周筋膜。眼动脉在视神经的外下方进入视神经管，在眶内终止于视网膜中央动脉。后者是视网膜的主要血供来源。颈内动脉发出穿支供应视交叉前部和管内视神经（Hendrix et al.，2014）。

其余 6 条神经穿行眶上裂：分别为动眼神经、滑车神经、展神经以及三叉神经眼支分出的泪腺支、额支和鼻睫支。视柱分隔眶上裂与视神经管。

在视神经管的外口，四块直肌起源于总腱环并形成一个圆锥形结构，其顶部为眼球，视神经位于中心（**图** 19.1）。上斜肌起源于眶内侧壁的后上方。上睑提肌起自眶顶，下斜肌起至眶底前内侧。

眼上静脉（superior ophthalmic vein，SOV）是主要的引流静脉，由内侧属支汇合而成。眶下静脉由外侧属支汇合而成。这些静脉与眼眶前部（金字塔底）的面静脉和角静脉形成吻合，SOV 通过眶上裂向后与海绵窦交通。

临床表现

眼眶病变的症状取决于病变与眼外肌和视神经的关系。圆锥外病变可位于眶筋膜外（眶外）或眶筋膜内（眶内）。早期多为突眼和复视，晚期因病变压迫眼球和视神经导致视力障碍。圆锥内病变位于直肌和视神经之间，多早期出现视力丧失，并有轴向眼球突出和多个方向的复视。

视神经管内病变表现为早期视力丧失、视盘水肿和视神经睫状分流血管，复视或眼球突出少见。

眼眶肿瘤分为两大类：原发眼眶内肿瘤，邻近的颅内或鼻窦病变侵犯眼眶。邻近病变累及眼眶者最常见是脑膜瘤和鼻窦癌（Gardner and Stefko，2014）。眼眶原发肿瘤及其位置见**表** 19.1（Tailor et al.，2013）。

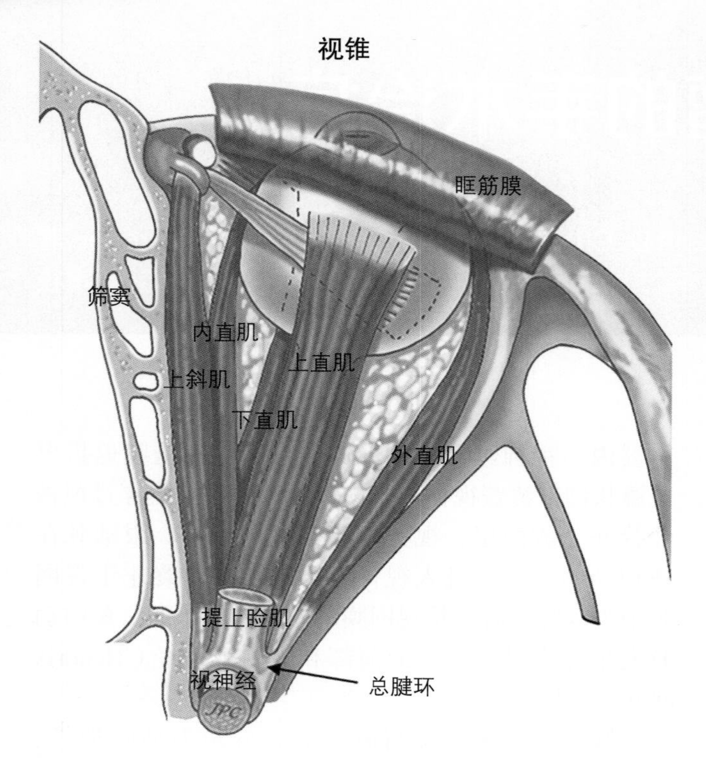

图 19.1　眼眶内视锥：眼眶上面观，眶顶被切除，眶筋膜翻向前方。提上睑肌（LP）自起点处切除。起自总腱环并构成视锥的肌肉是上直肌（SR）、外直肌（LR）、下直肌（IR）。上斜肌（SO）向上内侧走行。下斜肌未显示。视神经（ON）位于锥体的中心

©Jon Coulter, MA, CM1.

表 19.1　眼眶肿瘤部位分类

视锥内	视锥外
海绵状血管瘤[a]	血管外皮细胞瘤[b]
视神经胶质瘤	淋巴样增生[b]
视神经鞘脑膜瘤	不典型增生[b]
原发眼眶黑色素瘤	淋巴瘤[b]
转移瘤	多形性腺瘤
	腺样囊性癌
	泪腺淋巴瘤
	神经鞘瘤[b]
	神经纤维瘤[b]
	转移瘤

[a] 偶可位于视锥外

[b] 偶可位于视锥内

Data from Tailor, T.D., Gupta, D., Dalley, R.W., Keene, C.D., & Anzai, Y., Orbital neoplasms in adults: clinical, radiologic, and pathologic review, *Radiographics*, Volume 33, pp. 1739–58, Copyright © 2013

手术策略

把眼眶看作为以视神经为中心的时钟（**图 19.2**）。最安全的手术策略是避免经过视神经，通过病变在表盘上的位置选择手术方法（Paluzzi et al.，2015）。为了描述方便，本章下文中描述的都是右侧眼眶。镜像将用于左侧眼眶。

外侧入路

额颞开颅（9:00–1:00），眶颧入路（6:00–1:00）用于广泛病变

对于眼球后方、眶内上外侧的病变，可采用标准翼点切口行额颞开颅。对于眼眶下方和外侧的病变，可采用改良翼点入路（McDermott et al.，1990）。

对于眶颧入路，皮肤切口应为双额冠状或 3/4 冠状，从同侧耳屏延伸至至少对侧颞上线。采用筋膜间分离保留额肌神经。切口两端连线应穿过目标区域。从眶缘剥离颞肌可充分显露眶外侧壁。如需要更广泛的暴露，可将颞肌从颞骨上完全分离。

完成额颞开颅后将额叶和颞叶硬膜分别从眶顶和侧壁剥离。从眶下裂（inferior orbital fissure，IOF）至眶上切迹仔细剥离眶周筋膜。用脑压板保护好硬膜和眶周筋膜，在眶上切迹处或其稍外侧用摆锯切开眶顶壁，在眶下裂水平切开颧弓。磨钻连通两切口，然后取下眶顶及眶缘。

如有需要，可行硬膜外前床突磨除术以减压视神经管。应使用金刚砂钻头并持续冲洗的“蛋壳”技术磨除视神经管，然后将骨质从视神经鞘上咬除。

在眶上裂和脑膜眶韧带后方磨除骨质可显露鞍旁区域和海绵窦。

眶内病变可以通过触诊、超声或导航来定位。从前向后打开眶周筋膜，用棉片、棉签或双极处理眶内脂肪。

额眶入路（9:00–1:00）

对于眶内上外侧病变，一种微创方法是行从眶上切迹到睫毛外缘的眉毛内切口，将骨膜 U 形翻向下方，保留其内下方的蒂部。

剥离部分颞肌，锁孔处钻孔，分离额叶硬膜。然后开颅，骨窗上方至切口允许的大范围、下方平齐眶上缘及眶顶。进一步磨除额骨内板或去除眶上缘可获得最大程度显露。眼睑切口可提供稍靠下更偏外侧的显露，但此入路限制了眶外缘和上缘的切除，并且需要由眶内向眶外去除骨质。

上述入路均可使用钛板和螺钉或羟基磷灰石修

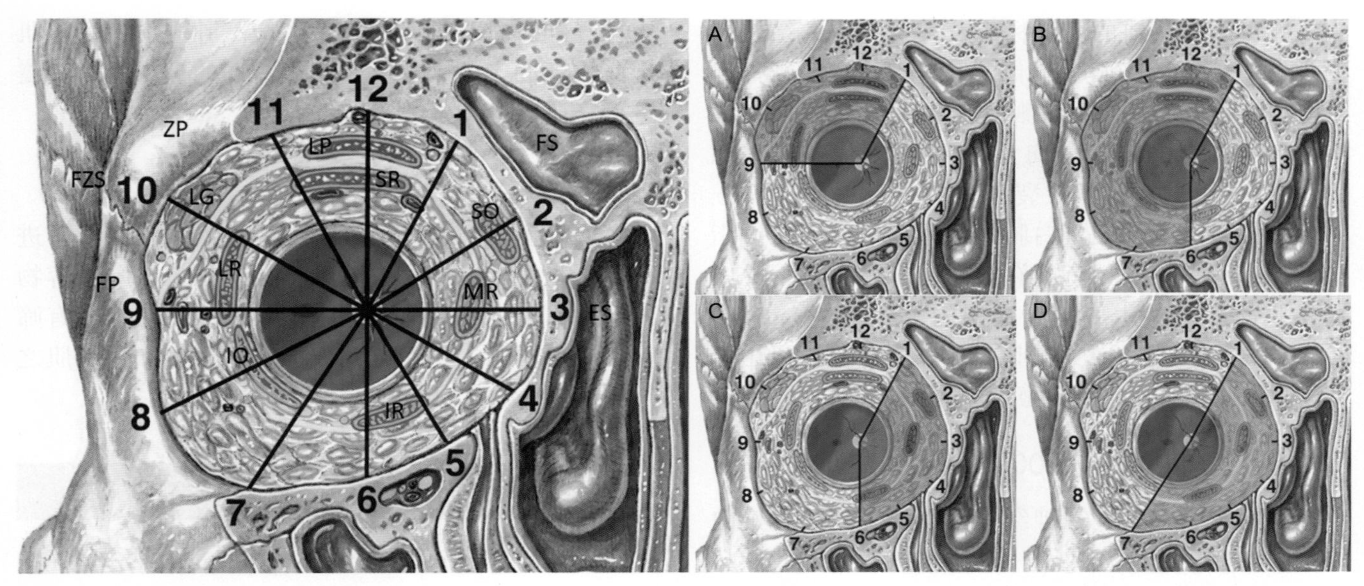

图 19.2 手术计划：以视神经为中心的“表盘”。相关的解剖结构是提上睑肌（LP）、上直肌（SR）、上斜肌（SO）、内直肌（MR）、下直肌（IR）、下斜肌（IO）和外直肌（LR）。泪腺（LG）位于上外侧。筛窦（ES）和额窦（FS）位于内侧。额骨（FP）的颧突与颧骨的额突连接形成额颧缝（FZS）。钟面的阴影部分显示了内侧和外侧入路显露的眼眶区域。额颞开颅手术（A）结合眶颧切除，可以处理更靠下方的病变（B）。内侧微眶切开术（C）是处理筛前动脉前方、1:00−6:00病变的首选方法。对于该位置筛前动脉后方病变，可单独采用内镜鼻内入路（D）或联合两种入路

补骨缺损，注意避免眼外肌卡压。

眶外侧切开术（8:00–10:00）

这是显露眶外侧肿瘤的经典入路（Maroon and Kennerdel，1976）。我们多采用外眦切开加沿眼裂的皮纹切口。上下眼睑之间的眼裂作为切口的一部分，可提供外侧眶缘的显露，而不会在面部中部形成不美观的切口。

骨膜下剥离颞肌牵拉向外侧、剥离眶周筋膜牵拉向内侧。在额颧缝和眶下裂水平分别切开眶外侧缘，然后将眶外侧壁骨折取下。

牵开器保护眶内容物，磨除蝶骨大翼显露眶尖。磨除邻近的颞骨以便分离颞叶硬脑膜，磨除蝶骨大翼平齐中颅底。

便于为眶内肿瘤创造手术通道，通过眶周的切口平行外直肌切开眶筋膜，将外直肌用缝线或者阻断带牵开，可以创造一个满意的切除眶内肿瘤的通道。采用显微技术通过减容和包膜外分离可安全地切除肿瘤。

内侧入路

前内侧微眶切开术和经结膜入路（1:00–6:00）

围绕角膜切开结膜，用双股可吸收缝线将内直肌从附着点牵开。牵开器将眼球牵向外侧。如需进一步向外侧牵拉，可行眶外侧壁切开。肿瘤切除后，将内直肌和下直肌复位于附着点，缝合结膜。该入路更适合眼眶前部病变，球后病变需增加牵拉程度，经鼻入路更为合适。

经泪阜入路用于处理视锥外病变。在泪阜和结膜半月皱襞之间切开，在泪囊和眶筋膜之间的无血管区向后内侧进行钝性分离。须识别筛前动脉和筛后动脉并电凝，以防止眶内出血威胁视力。如有需要可从前向后打开眶筋膜。

经鼻入路（1:00–7:00）

内镜经鼻入路（endoscopic endonasal approach，EEA）非常适用于病变将视神经推挤向上方和外侧的情况（Berhouma et al.，2014；Signorelli et al.，2015）。该入路成功的关键是多学科合作，包括耳鼻喉科和神经外科医生，对于视锥内肿瘤还需眼科整形医生。

单鼻孔入路需进行钩突切除、上颌窦开窗、前组及后组筛窦切除和蝶窦开放以显露整个眶内侧壁。对于视锥内病变、较大病变或眶尖占位，双鼻孔入路能够提供后方更好的操控性。需要切除同侧中鼻甲、广泛开放蝶窦，并切除鼻中隔后部。如果预期术中有脑脊液漏可能，则应在鼻中隔切除前获取鼻中隔黏膜瓣（通常取对侧）。

蝶窦后部重要的骨性标志及其所对应的结构如下：颈动脉隆起（颈内动脉海绵窦段）、外侧视神经颈内动脉隐窝（视柱）、内侧视神经颈内动脉隐窝（视神经和颈内动脉交界）。向上方、前外侧进一步去除骨质可显露视神经、眶上裂和眶尖。

多数情况下纤维蛋白胶、异体移植物或自体脂肪足以进行重建。如有脑脊液漏，可使用带蒂鼻中隔黏膜瓣来降低术后脑脊液漏的发生率（Hadad et al.，2006）。由于无法缝合眶筋膜，鼻中隔亦可用于重建眶内侧壁并防止直肌瘢痕形成。

下内侧视锥外入路（1:00–5:00）

适用于于眶尖、视神经病变以及未累及视锥内的眼眶内侧肿瘤。完成上一节所述鼻腔步骤后，从前到后轻轻地将筛骨纸样板折断，显露其深方的眶筋膜。然后在持续冲洗下磨除并小心去除眶尖和视神经表面骨质。对于眶内肿瘤，须在病变表面切开眶筋膜，然后仔细分离后将其移除。对于鞍结节和蝶骨骨平台脑膜瘤，需分离镰状韧带内侧、由内侧至外侧切开视神经管神经上表面的硬膜，以便切除肿瘤。最近的研究表明该技术可获得出色的视力保留（Gardner et al.，2008；Dehdashti et al.，2009）。

经上颌入路（1:00–7:00）

将上颌窦内侧壁切除术向前方延伸并切除部分梨状孔，可沿着眶底下方获得更多的外侧显露。该入路可以显露并分离翼腭窝及其内容物。先在圆孔处辨认 V2，然后在眶下裂深方可识别眶下神经，后者走行至眶下管。

该入路可应用于累及中颅窝、眼眶、颞下窝、翼腭窝或上颌窦的肿瘤（例如神经鞘瘤、青少年鼻咽纤维血管瘤）。须掌握三叉神经和颈内动脉咽旁段的走行以避免术中误伤。

内侧视锥内入路（4:00–7:00）

对于视锥内下内侧病变（眼球后方），内侧微眶切开术显露困难，可结合外部经结膜入路。用血管阻断带穿过内直肌和下直肌，以便牵拉和内镜下辨认解剖结构。如需进一步显露，可将缝线固定内直肌后将其从眼球上分离，将其向后内侧移位，保持其总腱环止点完整。

视神经位于术野的上外侧，而眼动脉及其分支视网膜中央动脉位于视神经的内侧，因此应沿肿瘤外侧进行分离以避免损伤上述结构。虽然双极电凝可用于收缩眶周脂肪，但应谨慎使用，以免损伤锥内神经和影响视神经的血液供应。肿瘤切除后，肌肉应重新固定于眼球上。采用前述的鼻中隔黏膜瓣进行修补。

上内侧入路（1:00– 4:00）

如要显露内直肌上方，在上述入路基础上需进一步行上内侧开眶：去除纸样板、牵拉眼眶内容物并磨除眶顶内侧部分。因内侧有眼动脉、上方有筛前和筛后动脉，这一入路仅能在内直肌和上斜肌之间创造一个狭窄的通道。

骨纤维发育不良

骨纤维发育不良（fibrous dysplasia，FD）是一种先天性疾病，未成熟的骨和纤维组织取代了松质骨。颅眶发育不良是一种常见的表现，随着病情的发展会导致眼眶面部畸形、眼球突出、眼球运动障碍和视力障碍（Amit et al.，2011）。

影像学上骨纤维发育不良分三型：硬化型（35%）、囊变型（25%）和混合型（40%）。在 MRI 上病变累及的范围可能相当广泛。MRI T2 相上骨性部通常是低信号，而囊性部分及其合并的黏液囊肿表现为高信号。CT 表现为“毛玻璃”样征象，CT 对于了解颅底骨孔受累（图 19.3）和指导术后重建至关重要。由于骨纤维发育不良通常进展缓慢，且几乎不会在成年期发生，因此常首选观察。放疗为禁忌，因其导致较高的病变恶性转化率。已报道各种药物治疗，但结果尚无定论。

对于畸形影响美容的患者，眼眶重建的方式可以是简单的骨质去除，抑或是颅眶入路辅以同种异体移植重建。急性或进行性视力丧失者应该行视神经减压术，后者对于慢性稳定的视力障碍的患者能否获益尚不确定。减压方法的选择取决于视力障碍具体因素，如前床突囊变，单纯内侧减压不能解决问题（Chen et al.，1997；Dumont et al.，2001）。

并发症

眼眶手术的并发症少见，一旦发生则后果严重。内侧入路中电凝筛动脉可避免球后血肿。对于直接累及视神经及其脑膜的肿瘤，必须保留脆弱的软脑膜血供以防止视力丧失。锥内肿瘤术后血肿的风险要大得多。

术中脑脊液漏可在内镜下用带血管蒂的鼻中隔黏膜瓣修补，以预防脑膜炎。若无法达到水密封闭，

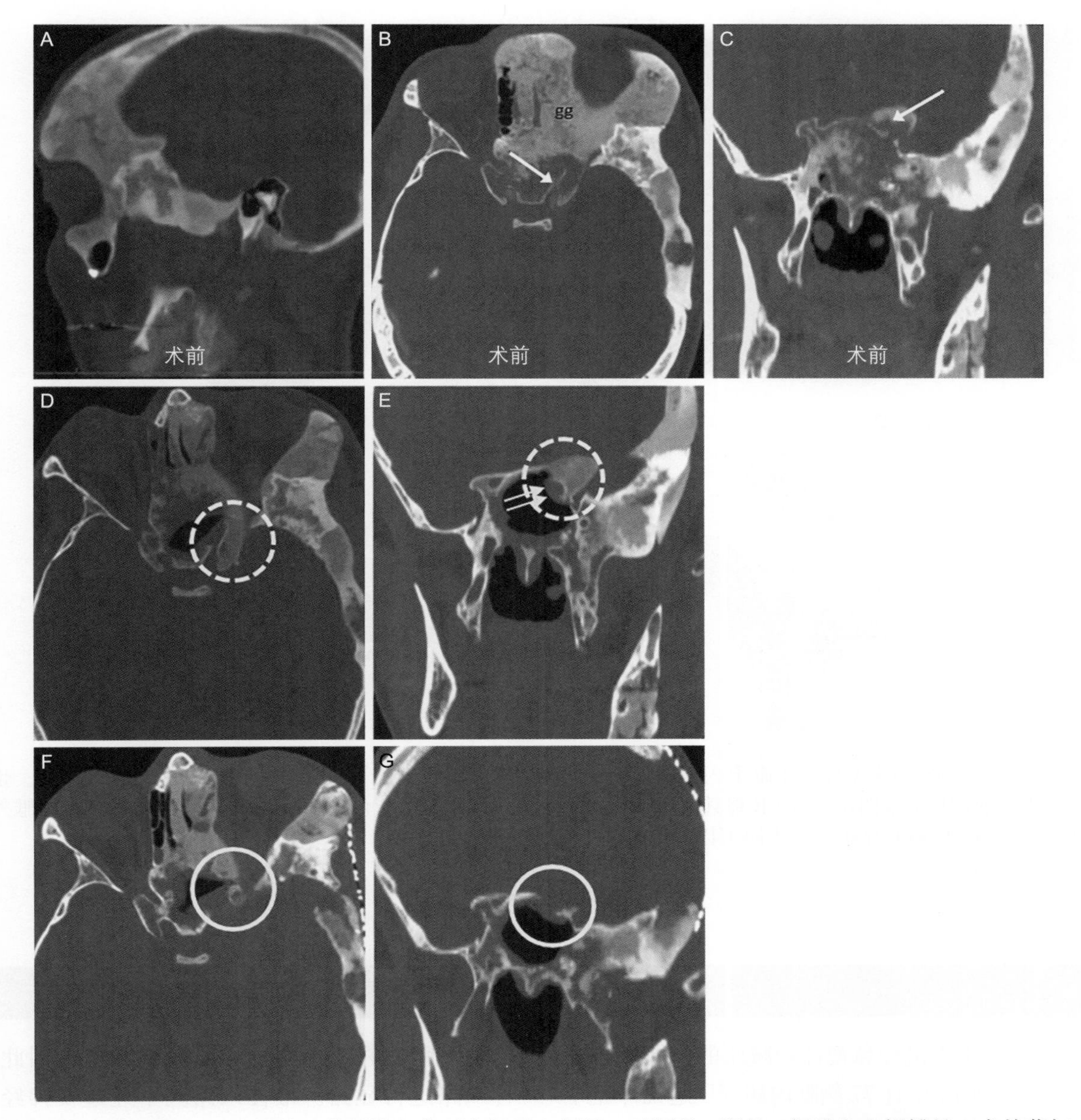

图 19.3 骨纤维发育不良：22 岁男性，骨纤维发育不良累及上颌骨、下颌骨、颞骨、额骨和左侧蝶骨。术前薄扫 CT（A、B、C）示特征性的毛玻璃外观。白色箭头（B、C）显示视神经管受压。患者表现为进行性视力丧失和视神经损害，患者接受了内镜经鼻左侧神经管减压术。术中视神经管内侧减压充分（双白箭头，E），术后症状改善。9 个月后，该患者因前床突增生（虚线圆圈，D、E）导致上方视野缺损，遂行左额颞开颅前床突切除术，行视神经管上外侧减压（白色实心圆圈，F、G）。患者的视力一直稳定，但需行眶下神经减压以及下颌骨和上颌骨磨除

则需采用显微外科技术进行多层修补、脂肪修补和腰大池引流术。眼眶手术新发复视通常是暂时性的，与眶周组织水肿有关。

争议

眶外侧切开术和眶上“锁孔”入路作为一种直接“微创”方法治疗前、中颅窝病变越来越受欢迎（**图 19.4**）。因为牵拉眶内容物的程度有限，故其缺点是手术通道狭窄。这导致控制血管和处理大的肿瘤较为困难。在尝试上述方法之前，应通过标准入路熟悉解剖结构。迄今为止，相对于标准开颅，关于微创入路处理肿瘤的大小或范围仍然没有达成共识。

对于视神经管和眶尖占位性病变，行内镜经鼻视神经减压也存在争议。蝶眶脑膜瘤和骨纤维发育不良因骨质增生造成视神经压迫，内镜经鼻入路可完成大于 180° 的视神经减压，且手术风险较低。

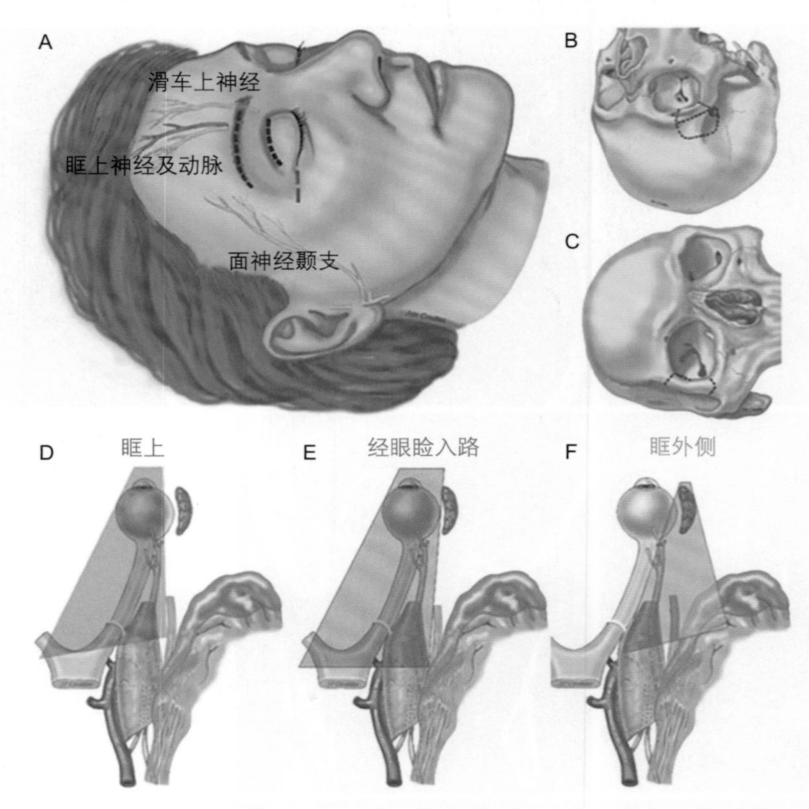

图 19.4　经眶手术入路：图 A 显示了眶上入路的微创切口：眶上（深红色）、经眼睑（蓝色）、眶外侧（橙色）。也可采用标准的翼点或耳前切口（未图示）。图 B 概述了额部开颅（红色）与眶缘（蓝色）切除的骨窗范围。图 C 显示眶外侧缘骨切除的范围。图 D、E 和 F 显示经眶入路可以显露的颅内结构

结果

我们中心关于内镜经鼻视神经减压的结果是非常满意的。2003—2015 年有 77 例眶内病变压迫视神经导致视力下降的患者进行了共 81 次内镜经鼻手术，只有 2 名患者术后视力恶化。视力改善 31 侧，稳定 48 侧。

我们还发现外侧眶切开术可处理中颅窝病变。两年中我们完成了 11 例这样的手术，其中 6 例是蝶眶脑膜瘤（未发表）。这些患者的眼球突出和复视有所改善，并且没有新的视力障碍。术中切除受累硬脑膜者难以做到硬膜水密缝合，故可能导致高危患者（如肥胖和愈合能力差者）脑脊液漏。

结论

眼眶毗邻前中颅窝和鼻腔鼻旁窦，因此可经多种入路进行显露。最佳入路应不经过视神经且尽量避免牵拉眼球。多学科团队是治疗眼眶病变的理想选择。

延伸阅读、参考文献、EBRAIN 的相关链接

扫描书末二维码获取。

第 20 章　颅骨病变

Giorgio Gioffre・Ivan Timofeev 著
刘江 译，伊志强 审校

引言

颅骨占全身骨骼的1%~2%，颅盖骨病变很少见，通常是偶然发现，或可能在其他疾病的分期检查中发现。

采用不同的分类系统可以将此病变分类如下：原发性（良性和恶性）或继发性，肿瘤性和非肿瘤性（炎症性和增殖性）。

对于许多此类病变，临床和放射学特征不具特异性，导致疾病诊断较为困难。其往往不是明确的临床表型，只是构成疾病的一部分，因而排除疾病恶性进展就至关重要。

流行病学、临床表现、影像学表现和组织病理学相结合对于鉴别疾病的病理性质是必不可少的。

本章的目的是明确每种病变的重要特征，概述其检查和治疗，根据影像学特征进行鉴别诊断。因此，将具有相似影像学表现的病理表型分组描述。

溶解性病变

转移病变

颅骨转移瘤是最常见的颅骨肿瘤，60% 的病例来源于乳腺癌和肺癌（Colas et al.，2015）。其他可转移至颅骨的原发性肿瘤包括前列腺癌、肾癌、子宫癌、结肠癌、肝癌、卵巢癌、甲状腺癌以及其他非上皮性肿瘤和骨肿瘤，而肉瘤和神经母细胞瘤是儿童最常见的原发性骨肿瘤（Mitsuya et al.，2011）。此外，在 90% 的病例中，颅骨转移与其他骨的继发性沉积有关，在 30% 的病例中与脑转移有关。

颅骨转移多发生于 60~70 岁。大多数转移病灶表现为溶解性，孤立存在，通过破坏颅骨内板或外板以侵蚀颅内或颅外组织。

常规放射和计算机断层扫描（CT）显示单个或多个溶解性病变，通常缺乏硬化边界，边缘模糊，侵袭邻近的软组织（图 20.1）。

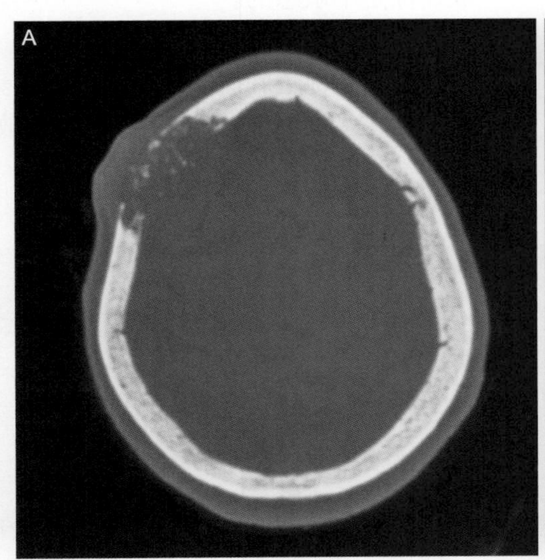

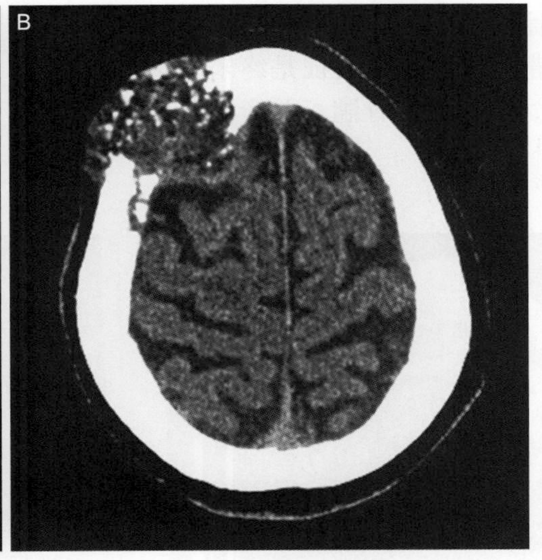

图 20.1　缺乏硬化性边界，边缘不规则，侵袭并浸润邻近软组织的溶解性病变，提示转移

增强 MRI 在颅骨转移的定性方面比 CT 和放射性核素显像更敏感，可以检测硬脑膜和软组织的浸润。典型的表现是 T1 低信号，T2 信号不均一，强化不一致。若发现肿瘤，其增强可以是均匀的、环状的或不均一的（Mitsuya et al.，2011）。骨扫描和 18FDG PET 显示高代谢，容易发现较小的颅骨转移沉积病灶。

外向性增生通常与原发性乳腺癌、前列腺癌、结肠癌和骨癌有关。其主要特征是板障双侧对称扩张，边界浸润，骨髓破坏，也可能出现混合性放射表现。

临床观察，可以是无症状的，通常在已知原发性肿瘤分期的情况下确诊，而很少是未知恶性肿瘤的初期表现。有症状的、无痛的或肿胀疼痛和头痛是最常见的症状（Stark et al.，2003；Mitsuya et al.，2011）。其他症状（神经功能缺损、癫痫和其他症状）与原发疾病有关，或可能与肿瘤颅内生长有关。

鉴别诊断为多发性骨髓瘤、其他颅骨病变、手术后或外伤后缺损。

治疗和预后取决于原发性肿瘤的性质和临床进展（**图** 20.2）。

传统的分次放射治疗仍然是主要的治疗方法。放射治疗可以在某些病例中控制肿瘤进展（Mitsuya et al.，2011），而双磷酸盐可以用于疼痛性病变的姑息治疗（Mitsuya et al.，2011）。

手术治疗的适应证包括：神经血管结构减压、疼痛性病变、周围组织和硬脑膜的广泛浸润、组织学活检（Mansfield，1977；Stark et al.，2003）。

多发性骨髓瘤

多发性骨髓瘤（multiple myeloma，MM）是一种恶性骨髓播散性疾病，其特征是终末分化浆细胞的单克隆增殖，取代正常骨髓，并产生单克隆免疫球蛋白（Colas et al.，2015）。MM 是最常见的原发性恶性骨肿瘤（el Quessar et al.，1997），发病率高峰年龄在 80 岁之后明显下降。病因尚不清楚，可能是多因素的，包括遗传和环境因素。80%~90% 的病例与细胞遗传学异常有关，最常见的是 13 号染色体缺失。

病变通常在整个长轴骨播散，60% 以上的多发性骨髓瘤患者存在多发性颅骨病变。它们通常起源于板障，推开内板并使骨膜变形，肉眼可见一个胶状红棕色组织代替骨髓。

临床表现与骨质破坏一致并伴有异常循环免疫球蛋白。颅骨受累通常是无症状的，疾病进展期发现。但是如果发生眼眶受累，可能会因颅底受累并伴有脑神经病变和眼球突出而出现症状。血清和尿液电泳是初步诊断试验的一部分。骨髓活检可确诊（Senapati et al.，2013）。

MM 也可表现为孤立的病灶，提示局限性疾病（浆细胞瘤），而无全身性表现。这在颅骨中极为罕见（Senapati et al.，2013），被认为是 MM 的早期阶段，在疾病传播之前数年就已出现（Kaur Gill et al.，2013）。

在这种情况下，只有在完成骨测量、骨髓穿刺以及血清和尿液电泳排除播散性疾病后才有可能进行诊断（Senapati et al.，2013）。

X 射线和 CT 表现具有多发、边界清楚、圆形或卵圆形溶骨性颅骨病变的特征。也可以表现为弥漫性硬化症，较少情况下表现为颅骨骨质减少。MRI 有助于显示脑膜及邻近软组织受累情况。骨髓瘤相关信号主要为 T1 低信号和 T2 高信号。增强 CT 和 MRI 显示病灶更加清晰。鉴于病变的独特的溶骨性，一般显像是不敏感的。

需与术后缺损、转移瘤、血管瘤、甲状旁腺功能亢进引起的棕色肿瘤等进行鉴别诊断。

治疗主要是通过化学疗法和局部放射疗法相结

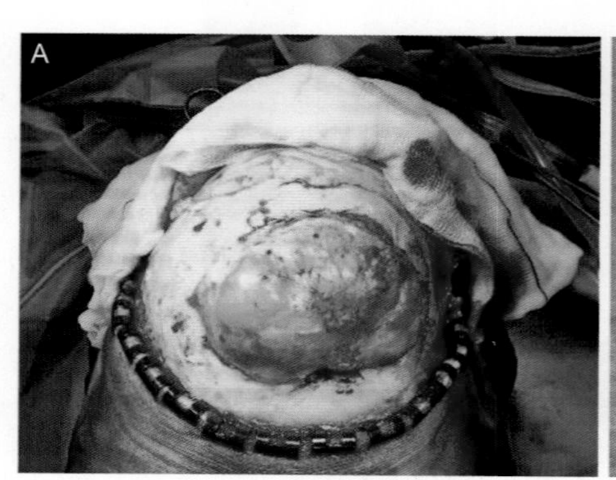

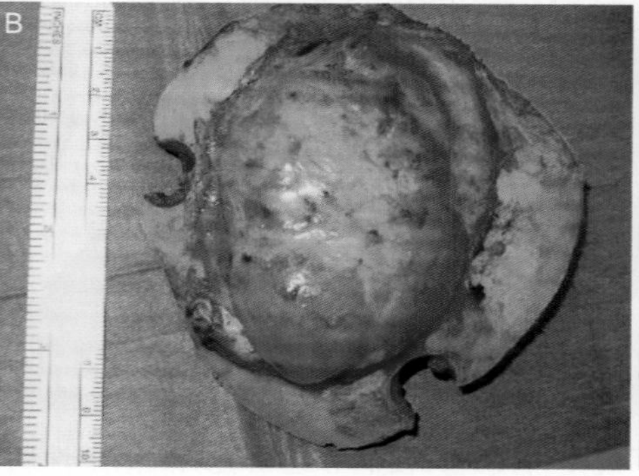

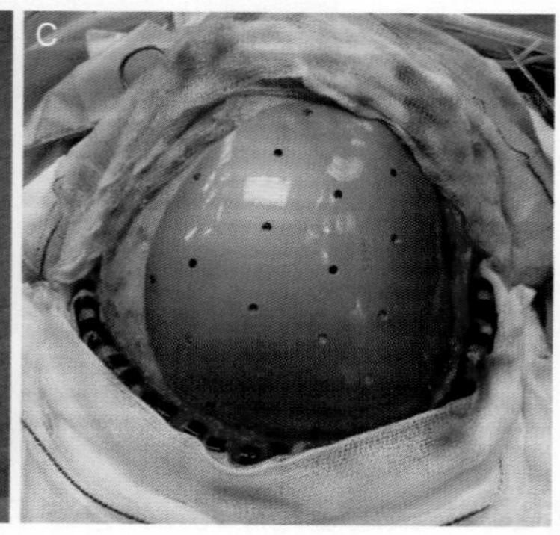

图 20.2 术中发现——切除颅骨转移灶同时行钛板颅骨修补术

合的医学方法。报道的5年生存率为20%，常规治疗方案中位生存时间为3年，如果不治疗生存时间为6个月。染色体13或11q缺失提示预后不良。

浆细胞瘤可以先行放射治疗后再行手术切除（Kaur Gill et al.，2013；Senapati et al.，2013）。

血管瘤

血管瘤是良性、生长缓慢的由间叶细胞组成的骨内血管瘤，主要成分为血管组织。

血管瘤是第二常见的原发性颅骨肿瘤，占原发性颅骨肿瘤的7%~10%。通常40岁左右发病，女性的发病率是男性的三倍。血管瘤通常是单一的（Khanam et al.，2001），但大约15%的病例可能是多发。其主要在椎体中发现，但是当它在颅骨中出现时，主要在顶骨、颞骨和额骨中（Khanam et al.，2001）。血管瘤经常作为一个单独病变发生，也可作为先天性血管瘤病的一部分出现。在某些病例中，血管瘤可能与以前的创伤有关。

肉眼可见的特征是骨膜下的棕红色病变。通常无症状且偶然发现，可伴有头痛、局部缓慢进展疼痛和肿胀触痛，有时伴有搏动感。第七和第八脑神经受压的体征可以作为颞骨的局部定位（Khanam et al.，2001；Colas et al.，2015）。

典型表现为血管瘤表面的皮肤可活动度，婴儿患病容易涉及软组织损伤，擦伤或刺激感的出现可能表明存在相关的血管畸形。

颅骨X线摄片显示界限清楚的圆形或椭圆形病变，呈放射性蜂窝状或小梁状，被薄薄的硬化边缘包围。经典的“旭日”外观并不常见（Khanam et al.，2001）。

CT通常显示边缘锐利，边界清楚的板障内溶骨性病变，周围硬化边缘较薄。在1/3的病例中，可能会出现小梁增厚并伴有放射状的突起和高密度的软组织内容物（Khanam et al.，2001；Colas et al.，2015）。MRI显示病变在T1加权影像上表现为等信号，在T2加权影像上表现为高信号。由于病变内的血流非常缓慢且体积小，通常不会显示血流流空。血管瘤通常强化明显。

血管造影可以显示出血供丰富的病变，主要表现为延迟的持续性“葡萄簇”外观，其主要由脑膜中动脉或颞浅动脉供血（Khanam et al.，2001）。

孤立性血管瘤的鉴别诊断主要是正常的解剖变异（血管通道、裂孔、导静脉）、手术后缺损、皮样囊肿、嗜酸性肉芽肿、转移瘤、脑膨出、板障内蛛网膜囊肿、板障内脑膜瘤、肉瘤（Khanam et al.，2001）。多发病变的鉴别涉及淋巴瘤、骨质疏松、甲状旁腺功能亢进。

血管瘤是一种良性且生长缓慢的肿瘤，几乎不需要治疗。手术适应证包括占位切除、美容和控制出血。外科手术沿正常骨质边缘整块切除。刮除可能导致大出血和复发（Khanam et al.，2001）。侵蚀较深并波及周围组织的不可切除的病变，可以通过放射疗法或超选择性栓塞治疗（Khanam et al.，2001）。恶性肉瘤转移极为罕见。

朗格汉斯细胞组织细胞增生症

朗格汉斯细胞组织细胞增生症（Langerhans cell histiocytosis，LCH）是一种多系统的、特发性的（Ralston et al.，2008）形成肉芽肿的增生性疾病，其特征是各种组织中的朗格汉斯细胞异常增殖，并包括三种相关的组织细胞病（Ralston et al.，2008；Colas et al.，2015）：嗜酸性肉芽肿（70%）是一种局部良性形式，其特征是组织细胞的局部浸润，大多数病例涉及颅骨（De Angulo et al.，2013）；Hand-Schuller-Christian综合征（20%），是一种多发慢性传播形式；而Letter-Siwe综合征（10%），是一种急性、恶性、弥散性类型（Ralston et al.，2008）。

LCH最常影响年轻人，其中70%的患者年龄在20岁以下，并且最常见于白人男性（90%）。嗜酸性肉芽肿的特有发病率是0.4/100 000。

LCH主要涉及中轴骨，其中颅骨经常受到影响，特别是在额叶和顶叶区域（Colas et al.，2015），其次是乳突、下颌骨和面骨。

嗜酸性肉芽肿是一种自限性的、逐渐扩大的、柔软的单灶性颅骨占位，通常有数月的病史，而Hand-Schuller-Christian和Letter-Siwe综合征则多系统受累，预后较差。

在嗜酸性肉芽肿中，常规影像学检查和CT表现为边缘切锐的“穿凿样”病变，周围硬化层稀少，边缘呈斜角，内外边缘均累及（**图20.3**；另请参见Ralston et al.，2008）。乳突部位的特征是明显的骨破坏。溶解缺陷内的软组织通常显示明显增强。MRI表现为局灶性溶解性T2高信号软组织肿块，通常具有皮质外延伸，外观呈“香槟软木塞”或“衣领纽扣”，具体取决于它们的单皮质或双皮质延伸。18-FDG PET显示增生性病变中的摄取增加（Ralston et al.，2008）。应该与其他原因引起的颅骨溶解性病变（表皮样脓肿、皮样囊肿、术后缺损、转移、颅骨结核）进行鉴别诊断。涉及颞骨的病变必须与严重的乳突炎和横纹肌肉瘤鉴别。

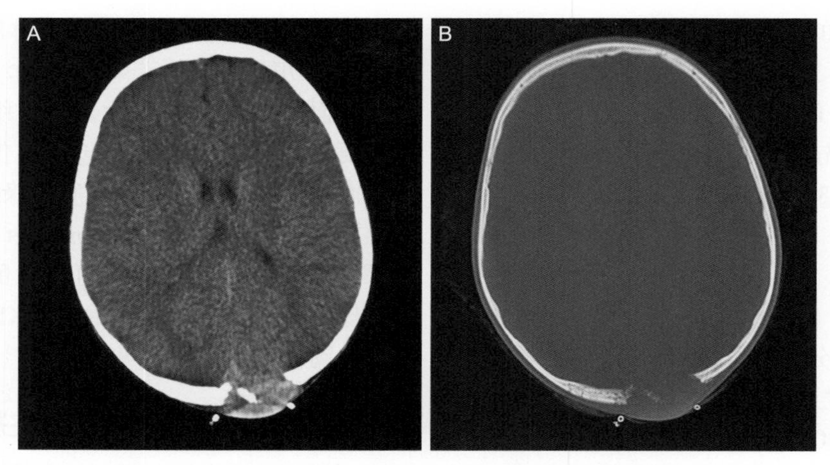

图 20.3　LCH——“穿凿样”病变，边缘锐利，没有明显的硬化，且软组织增强较弱

自然病史是可变的，取决于诸如发病年龄、受累程度、多器官功能障碍的存在和复发等因素。在多灶性疾病中死亡率达到 18%。治疗取决于疾病的程度；嗜酸性肉芽肿可自发消退，但据报道有 30% 的病例复发，通常发生在不同的部位，主要是儿童。治疗手段包括单纯观察（De Angulo et al.，2013），局部手术切除，针对复发病灶的放疗治疗以及在多灶性颅盖受累情况下联合放疗和化疗。

尤因肉瘤

颅骨原发性尤因肉瘤（Ewing’s sarcoma，ES）非常少见（不到所有病例的 4%），而其他地方的继发性异源性扩散则更为多见（Salunke et al.，2011）。发病高峰在 15~25 岁，男性高发（Desai et al.，2000；Salunke et al.，2011）。它通常累及顶骨和额骨，而很少影响颅底（Desai et al.，2000；Salunke et al.，2011）。

组织起源不确定，可能起源于间充质干细胞（Desai et al.，2000；Salunke et al.，2011）。

主要肉眼特征是与骨膜下骨异常沉积相关的骨破坏模式。

临床表现包括局部肿胀、颅内压升高和伴有局灶性神经功能缺损的体征和症状（Desai et al.，2000）。

尽管颅内原发性肿瘤似乎表现出很弱的侵袭性（Salunke et al.，2011），但在发病前两年中的转移病例占 80%，通常发生在肺部和其他骨骼上（Desai et al.，2000）。

可能不表现出“洋葱皮”或“旭日样”病变的典型影像学特征。最常见的是，颅骨的尤因肉瘤表现为非特异性溶解性病变，具有骨膜反应和强化的内容物，MRI 显示软组织效果更好，软组织成分的信号表现不一（Desai et al.，2000）。

鉴别诊断主要涉及成骨肉瘤、原始神经外胚层肿瘤、横纹肌肉瘤、转移性神经母细胞瘤和淋巴瘤（Desai et al.，2000）。

与中轴骨相比，颅骨原发病变预后往往更好。

局部复发性疾病患者的预后较差，复发后 5 年生存率为 10%~15%（Salunke et al.，2011）。

根治性手术切除加术后放疗和化疗可使 2 年无病生存率达到 55%~60%（Desai et al.，2000）。

成骨肉瘤

成骨肉瘤是一种非脑膜上皮性恶性肿瘤，起源于血管周围鞘的多能间充质细胞。

尽管它是多发性骨髓瘤之后第二常见的原发性骨恶性肿瘤，但在颅骨病变中极为罕见。最常见于 20~40 岁的男性，通常继发于以往的放射治疗、佩吉特病、纤维异常增生、巨细胞瘤和慢性骨髓炎（el Quessar et al.，1997）。肉眼特征与出血性软组织的坏死和钙化相一致。

通常表现为快速增长的肿块，伴有明显的疼痛（el Quessar et al.，1997）。相关的临床特征取决于肿瘤的位置而表现出多样性。不幸的是，高度侵袭性的过程通常伴随着主要发生在肺部的快速远处转移。

X 线平片和 CT 显示一个透光的、界限不清的病变，邻近硬化（无骨膜反应）常伴有轴向和非轴向成分大部强化。MRI 显示 T1 低信号，T2 不均匀一致高强度信号变化，增强后明显强化。影像学特征取决于组织学类型。成骨细胞型可表现为典型的“旭日”外观，延伸至软组织，伴有相关的皮质增厚，但也可表现为非特异性强化溶骨性病变，伴有周围骨增厚和散在钙化。鉴别诊断包括转移瘤、软骨肉瘤、骨软骨瘤以及良性和恶性脑膜瘤（el Quessar et al.，1997）。

全切除加扩大切除并与放疗和化疗相结合是外科治疗的目标，以达到局部控制肿瘤和减少局部复发和转移扩散（el-Quessar et al.，1997）。尽管进行治疗，但预后很差，只有少数患者获得了长期生存。

纤维肉瘤

纤维肉瘤是一种非脑膜瘤性恶性间质肿瘤，起源于骨髓的结缔组织。它是一种罕见的肿瘤，多继发于佩吉特骨病、既往放疗、骨纤维结构异常、巨细胞瘤、骨梗死或慢性骨髓炎，好发于中年人（Mansfield，1977）。颅骨受累通常是临近原发部位（鼻窦、面部、头皮、硬脑膜）浸润的结果。

临床上表现为病变快速增长、局部侵袭和迅速转移至肺和骨骼。

在普通的X射线和CT上，纤维肉瘤表现为不确切的不同强化软组织含量的非特异性溶解性病变，（Mansfield，1977）。MRI显示T1低信号和T2非均一高信号变化。鉴别诊断主要是转移瘤、良性和恶性脑膜瘤。

外科治疗目标是通过广泛全切除结合放疗和化疗达到对该病的局部控制。

破骨细胞瘤（巨细胞瘤）

被认为是起源于巨噬细胞来源的单核细胞，是一种非常罕见的颅骨肿瘤，通常发生在长骨的骨骺（Leonard et al.，2001；Harris et al.，2004）。

发病通常在30~40岁，女性占多数（Harris et al.，2004）。可以罕见地继发于佩吉特病：这种情况通常与肿瘤的多骨形式有关，通常出现在老年人群，颅面骨受累，与原发灶相比，转归更有利（Leonard et al.，2001）。

当局限于颅骨时，破骨细胞倾向于颞骨和蝶骨（Leonard et al.，2001；Harris et al.，2004）。

破骨细胞瘤往往表现为疼痛并逐渐增大的肿块，有时可能与先前的外伤有关。

恶性变性发生在5%~10%的病例中（Leonard et al.，2001），而假恶性行为并不少见，多与肺转移有关（Harris et al.，2004）。

放射学特征是具有均匀增加的软组织含量的非特异性溶解性病变（Harris et al.，2004）。多房病变可类似于甲状旁腺功能亢进中的动脉瘤性骨囊肿或棕色肿瘤。单房病变在放射学上可类似于巨细胞肉芽肿、软骨母细胞瘤和软骨黏液样纤维瘤（Harris et al.，2004）。此外，影像学检查也不能与黏膜下鼻咽癌的溶解性转移或直接浸润区分开来。

根治性切除术是金标准，但是由于其位置和浸润方式，并非能够达到全切。术前动脉栓塞可控制术中出血。当部分切除时，这些肿瘤倾向于在相对较短的时间内（1~2年）复发。

巨细胞瘤通常是放射线耐受的，放射治疗时可能发生恶性转化（Harris et al.，2004）。放射疗法仅提倡针对无法切除的复发病变以及表现出明显的恶性行为的病变。NF-κB配体（RANKL）信号通路的受体活化剂调节破骨细胞的分化和激活，其在巨细胞瘤的发病机制中起着关键作用，在外科手术无法干预时，成为有希望的治疗靶点。

动脉瘤性骨囊肿

动脉瘤性骨囊肿（aneurysmal bone cyst，ABC）是由许多薄壁血管空间组成的病变，被纤维化和矿化的组织小梁隔开，缺乏正常的内皮细胞。

它很少发生在颅盖（占颅骨病变病例的1%~6%）（Colas et al.，2015），文献中仅报道了60例。性别分布均等，通常会发生于20岁以下的患者。也沿头颅穹顶骨骼均匀分布，对称性波及颅骨内外面。

ABC的病理生理学尚不清楚，并且是否确实提示肿瘤性病变尚有争议。通过局部血流动力学紊乱来解释该现象的发生。

尽管一种主要涉及颅内生长并伴有颅内出血的形式已经报道，但ABC通常表现为可触及的肿块。ABC也可以继发于纤维发育不良、巨细胞瘤和成骨细胞瘤。

常规放射学检查和CT成像显示清晰可见的溶骨性病变，呈肥皂泡样外观，被菲薄的内外骨板环绕的多腔结构罕有增强。MRI表现为多分隔病变，含有液-液水平和血液降解产物。血管造影显示富血运病变。发现实性成分可能提示是转移所致（Colas et al.，2015）。

ABC的肿瘤性质尚有争议，其进展通常是不可预测且易变的。完全的手术切除是可以治愈的。在这方面，刮除术和次全切除术与出血和高复发率有关。可以考虑进行术前选择性动脉栓塞术，以避免过多失血。

如果由于位置或出血风险被认为不可切除，则建议进行放射治疗。实施冷冻手术和酒精栓塞术以降低部分切除病灶的复发率。

骨内脂肪瘤

板障内脂肪瘤是已知的最罕见的骨肿瘤之一（Kaneko et al.，2011），文献中只有很少的病例报道。它是一种良性病变，由薄骨小梁基质中的成熟脂肪细胞组成，起源于促成成熟大脑分化的间充质干细胞的异常分化（Kaneko et al.，2011）。它们在临床上表现为缓慢生长的病变，可累及骨膜。

成像与骨内充满脂肪的空腔一致，周围骨无强化、浸润或侵蚀特征。

鉴别诊断为皮样囊肿，表现为高密度，并来自骨折或骨梗死后的修复过程，可见周围骨渗透。纤维发育不良和脑膜瘤也应考虑在内。

尚未见复发，恶性转化少见。考虑到良性病史，根治性切除术可能是不合理的，在无症状的情况下，宜继续观察随访（Kaneko et al.，2011）。

板障内表皮样和皮样囊肿

这些是良性颅骨病变，组织学上表现为包涵体囊肿，包涵体囊肿是由于胚胎发育过程中神经管闭合时外胚层或真皮成分进化中断引起的，很少是由于外伤性植入引起。表皮样囊肿仅包含表皮组织和角质化碎片，而皮样囊肿可能包含真皮成分，如毛囊、皮脂腺和牙齿。

最常见于10岁内的儿童，也可以在出现在年龄较大的儿童和成人，可影响颅骨和颅底。它们通常比硬膜内病变少见。临床上可以表现为无痛、活动性差、生长缓慢。皮样囊肿多发于中线及前囟门周围的颅骨缝隙，表皮样囊肿多见于顶骨、额骨、枕骨或眶旁。囊肿可以影响颅骨内板或外板，或两者都影响。CT表现为无强化的低密度病灶，边界清楚，常有钙化边缘和其他钙化化区域（**图**20.4）。在T1 MRI上，病灶呈现比脑脊液略高信号，T2等信号，FLAR高信号，DWI显示弥散受限。超声也可以用于诊断和监测表皮样和皮样囊肿（Riebel et al.，2008）。出于美容原因和预防潜在的但罕见的颅内内容物破裂等并发症，通常涉及内板的较大且生长较快的囊肿时考虑采用外科手术治疗，手术选择包括开放式和内镜切除及刮除术。

总体预后良好，通过非手术治疗也可自发消退。

表20.1 溶解性病变

增生型病变

骨瘤和良性成骨细胞病变

骨瘤是一种良性间叶性肿瘤，肉眼上类似于成熟的片状骨。起源于成熟的皮质骨，并向外生长形成坚固的穹顶状肿块，主要分布在膜性骨化形成的区域。它是最常见的原发性颅骨肿瘤（Haddad et al.，1997），占颅面部骨肿瘤的30%，在一般人群中患病率为0.4%，在女性中发病率更高，女：男比大约为3：1，并且40~50岁人群发病率达到峰值（Colas et al.，2015）。通常位于鼻旁窦，较少累及颅骨和下颌骨。主要发生于额骨，但也可能发生在颅骨的任何地方，多起源于颅骨外板（Haddad et al.，1997），但也可能起源于板障或颅骨内板上，并经常发生于颅骨骨缝附近，正常情况下一般不会发生在此位置（Colas et al.，2015）。

无临床症状多见，表现为孤立、无痛、生长缓慢、坚硬的颅骨病变，通常仅被视为外观问题。

如果是多发性病变，则应考虑诊断Gardner综合征（常染色体显性遗传的胃肠道息肉病，其特征是伴

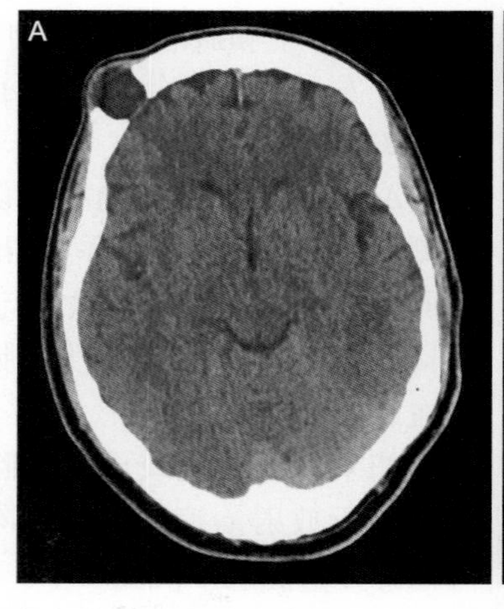

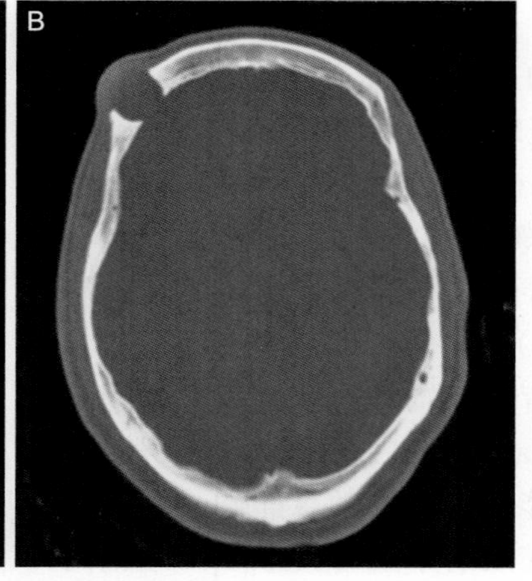

图 20.4 非增强型低密度病变，具有表皮样囊肿特征性的明确的骨质边缘

表 20.1　主要溶解性病变

转移	转移细胞浸润显示原发病灶的特征
多发性骨髓瘤	多形性的，增大的浆细胞，常呈片状，核椭圆形，核偏心，染色质团块，核周晕，核分裂，细胞质内含物（Russell 小体）
血管瘤	海绵状：头盖骨最常见的亚型，由大量充满血液的由内皮细胞排列成的窦状通道构成，由于骨重塑导致纤维隔膜和骨小梁重构；毛细血管：椎体中最常见的亚型，由毛细血管团和相关坏死组成；静脉：由厚壁静脉通道组成，由于小梁增厚，呈放射状反应性骨形成。
朗格汉斯组织细胞增多症	朗格汉斯细胞的单克隆增殖，存在特征性 Birbeck 颗粒，“网球拍”形细胞质细胞器，具有中心线密度和条纹外观
尤因肉瘤	片状细胞，细胞核小，圆形深染，细胞质稀少，核质比高，常形成假菊形团
骨肉瘤	成骨细胞：50% 的病例表现为单核或多核非典型多角形细胞，在大量的未成熟类骨中有明显的间变性和高分裂。其他亚型：软骨母细胞、成纤维细胞、毛细血管扩张
纤维肉瘤	细胞密度高，恶性胶原成纤维细胞，呈“人字形”片状或束状排列，细胞核呈梭形，轻度深染，有丝分裂活性高
破骨细胞瘤	具有多面体和多核巨细胞的血管基质，核仁突出。圆形单核区细胞和梭形基质细胞通常共存
表皮样和皮样囊肿	包涵体囊肿包含角化和复层鳞状上皮。皮样囊肿真皮成分（皮脂腺、汗腺、毛囊等）

有良性软组织肿瘤、甲状腺癌、颅骨和下颌骨多发性骨瘤）。

在 X 射线和 CT 成像中，骨瘤通常表现为等密度，增强不明显，界限分明的多变的中心不均匀病灶（图 20.5）。MRI 表现为均匀的低信号 T1 加权信号和 T2 多变信号加权图像，不累及周围的软组织或骨骼，也没有增强效应（Colas et al.，2015）。骨扫描可以显示不同的摄取，主要取决于病变的骨合成阶段。鉴别诊断需注意骨内良性和恶性脑膜瘤（图 20.6），以及恶性非脑膜瘤。

完全手术切除是治疗的目标（Haddad et al.，1997），主要是出于美容的原因而实施。如果病变很小并且起源于外板，则可以通过钻孔或刮除术将其去除，避免损伤内板。对于较大的病灶或起源于内板的病灶，可能需要进行规范的开颅手术，同时进行颅骨重建。

其他良性成骨细胞病变：

- 骨样骨瘤：良性成骨细胞瘤，在颅骨病变中不常见，因为它最常见于长骨。典型表现为夜间疼痛，阿司匹林缓解。
- 成骨细胞瘤（也称为成骨纤维瘤）：在颅骨病变中极为罕见，仅蝶骨位置发生的有过报道。与骨样骨瘤相似，但通常不会引起疼痛。病变往往比骨样骨瘤和肉瘤性病变血供更丰富，虽然非常罕见，但也有过报道（Figarella-Branger et al.，1991）。

骨样骨瘤和成骨细胞瘤在组织学上是无法区分

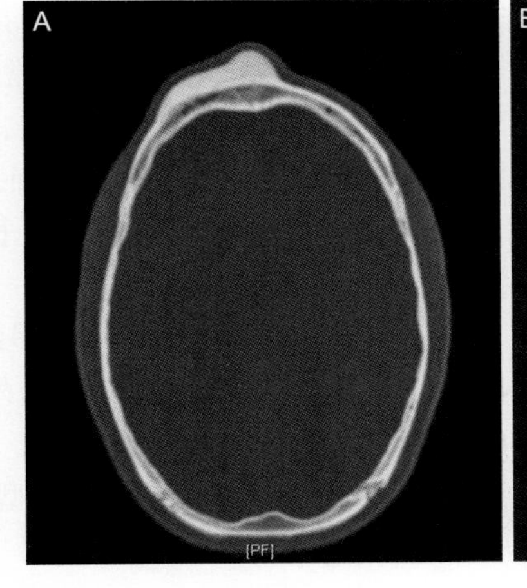

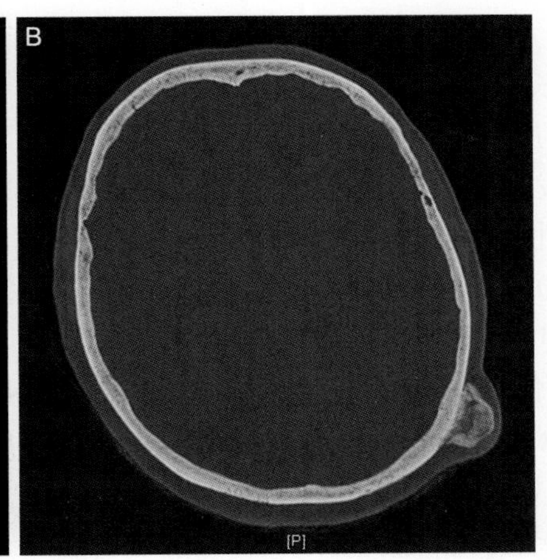

图 20.5　破骨细胞病变——骨瘤（A）和骨软骨瘤（B）

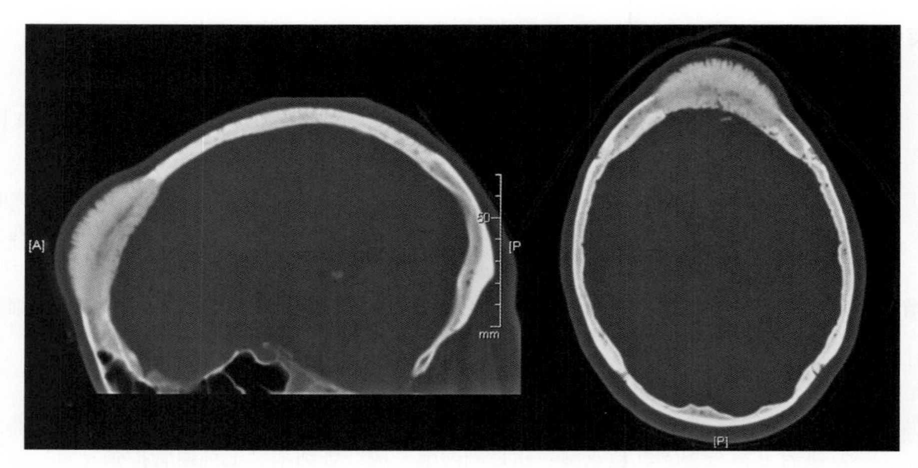

图 20.6 骨内脑膜瘤——成骨细胞膨胀性病变

的，常规的鉴别是基于前者的大小，其测量值小于 1 cm，而成骨细胞瘤是更大的病变，易导致组织受压。

软骨瘤（骨软骨瘤）

软骨瘤是良性骨软骨瘤，肉眼上类似于软骨或骨化软骨。软骨瘤是最常见的良性骨骼骨软骨肿瘤，占所有骨肿瘤的 9%~10%。主要好发于 20~50 岁女性，通常发生在由软骨内骨化形成的骨骼中，颅面骨几乎是唯一的膜内起源，而相对的斜坡和颅底是软骨内骨化形成的，软骨瘤非常罕见，占颅内肿瘤的比例低于 0.5%（Rathore et al.，2005）。因此，它主要发生在颅底的蝶骨（蝶骨 - 枕软骨结合）、枕骨（岩 - 枕软骨结合）和筛骨（蝶骨 - 筛骨软骨结合）区域。据报道，也可发生在脉络丛和脑膜，当不是发生在颅底时，额顶骨是最常见的位置（Rathore et al.，2005）。

根据类骨质和软骨样元素之间的比例，在肉眼上表现为无蒂的软骨样肿块或无柄外生骨疣，有或没有软骨帽。

临床上表现为生长缓慢的颅骨肿块。当出现在颅底时，会出现脑神经压迫相关的症状。多发性病变可能与 Ollier 病（多发性内生软骨瘤病）或 Maffucci 综合征（多发性内生性软骨瘤伴皮下血管瘤病）有关（Fountas et al.，2008）。

这些病变具有小叶状软组织肿块的放射学特征，其中包含曲线形的钙化斑，并伴有圆齿状的骨内膜的骨吸收（Fountas et al.，2008）。在 CT 扫描上显示中等程度的高密度（**图** 20.5），在 T1 加权 MRI 上表现为高信号，其多样模式取决于脂肪、纤维组织、血管和矿化骨的数量。软骨帽可以轻度增强。骨骼扫描可以显示出不同的吸收，具体取决于骨骼的合成阶段。主要与良恶性脑膜上皮肿瘤、骨内或骨侵犯、恶性非脑膜上皮肿瘤（肉瘤）鉴别诊断。

治疗的主要手段是外科完全切除（Fountas et al.，2008）。当不能完全切除时，神经结构减压是主要目标。很少转化为软骨肉瘤（1%），但在综合征性内生软骨瘤病的情况下转化为软骨肉瘤的可能性更高（25%~30%）。

额骨内板增生症

由于新骨的特发性沉积（通常呈结节状），额骨内增生症包括不规则增厚的内板、板障和额鳞。通常是双侧的，在镰的结合处远离中线生长（She and Szakacs，2004）。一般人群中的发病率为 1.4%~5%，最常见于老年白人女性，女：男高达 9：1（She and Szakacs，2004）。

该病几乎都是无症状的，关于其病理意义存在争议。

该病的病因仍然未知，但是可能与内分泌失衡有关。通常发现它与内分泌异常（肢端肥大症、高泌乳素血症）、代谢异常（肥胖症，DM）、高血压、头痛、脑神经损伤症、癫痫、痴呆症和抑郁症有关，表现为数年缓慢的进行性增长（She and Szakacs，2004）。

CT 和 MRI 显示额叶内板呈结节状对称增厚，厚度可达 4 cm。关于这种情况的外科治疗，很少有文献报道，尚无重要的病例研究。

表 20.2 总结了主要的增生型病变。

表 20.2 主要增生型病变

骨瘤	• 致密的：类皮质骨，有很少的纤维组织，几乎完全来自外板 • 松质骨（或小梁）：包括致密的、小梁状的、纤维状的和脂肪状的成分，通常起源于板障或内板 • 纤维状的：由板层骨构成，细胞较多的基质通常最终演变成“致密”型
骨软骨瘤	• 软骨瘤：在大量透明软骨基质内散在陷窝中的良性软骨细胞，s100 和波形蛋白免疫组化阳性 • 骨软骨瘤：覆盖外生骨疣的良性软骨细胞，有皮质、小梁和正常骨髓

混合溶细胞性病

神经母细胞瘤

神经母细胞瘤是一种起源于神经嵴细胞的肿瘤，在成为交感神经节细胞之前，其发育在神经母细胞阶段被阻止。这就解释了其有向颅面骨骼转移的趋势，因为颅面骨骼具有相同的神经外胚层起源（D'Ambrosio et al.，2010a）。这是儿童最常见的颅骨转移（D'Ambrosio et al.，2010a）。50% 的病例原发病变来自肾上腺髓质，而其余病变影响交感神经链。

0~10 岁的儿童最普遍，没有表现出性别优势。

转移发生在 50% 的患者中，通常主要通过血液传播到肝、肺和骨骼。在多达 25% 的病例中发现了颅骨的转移（D'Ambrosio et al.，2010b）。当颅面骨骼受累时，常见表现包括眼眶扩张时容易出现面部挫伤和突眼，或颅骨单个或多个肿块迅速增大，这可能与脑神经功能缺失有关（D'Ambrosio et al.，2010b）。尽管脑膜作为脑侵犯的保护屏障，但颅底受累和颅内扩张也时有发生。

颅骨转移性受累可产生多种不同的影像学表现，包括骨质增厚、“头端”骨膜反应、溶解性缺损、骨缝分离。CT 通常显示中度高密度病变，并伴有邻近骨的渗透性改变。MRI 显示 T2 低信号和 T1 高信号改变，软组织浸润常表现为较厚的“斑块样”硬膜外延伸。大多数病变均增强显著。

鉴别诊断主要是横纹肌肉瘤、朗格汉斯细胞组织细胞增生症、尤因肉瘤和成骨肉瘤（D'Ambrosio et al.，2010b）。

考虑到疾病的放射敏感性，放射疗法是治疗的主要手段，如果存在神经血管结构的局部受压，则放射疗法可与化疗和外科手术结合应用。

佩吉特病

骨的佩吉特（Paget）病是一种慢性代谢性疾病，其特征是异常的过度骨转换（Ralston et al.，2008），定位于单一骨骼或延伸至相邻节段，引起破骨细胞异常激活，导致骨吸收率增加，伴随成骨细胞活性亢进和产生较薄弱的编织骨（Ralston et al.，2008）。Paget 病涉及活跃的溶解期到修复期 / 静止期；这些可能共存，也可能不共存，个别部位的进展速度不同。

发病率随年龄增加而增加，在 40 岁以上的成人中患病率为 3%，在 80 岁以上的成年人中患病率为 10%。性别分布是平等的，最常见于高加索人和德系犹太人。

颅骨受累存在于 30%~65% 的病例中，大部分发生在额骨和枕骨中（Colas et al.，2015）。

病因不明。与 HLA-DR2 有基因连锁的基因通过增加基因表达抑制凋亡，其中最重要的是 SQSTM1，它是核因子 κB（NF-κB）配体信号通路中的支架蛋白（Ralston et al.，2008）。

通常无症状，经常偶然因血清碱性磷酸酶升高后发而现（Ralston et al.，2008; Colas et al.，2015）。也可以表现为疼痛，弥漫性颅骨增厚。如果出口变窄，则可能发生神经卡压病变，最常见的是第八脑神经伴搏动性耳鸣和听力损失（纯感音神经性或混合性）。约有 33% 的患者存在扁平颅底，有或不伴有颅底凹陷，多见于女性，存在发生脑干压迫可能。根据疾病的严重程度，由于病变中血管的高度密集和骨骼的积极重塑，高输出量心力衰竭和继发性甲状旁腺功能亢进可能随之发生。据报道，肉瘤转化发生在不到 1% 的病例中（Hansen et al.，2006），主要是骨肉瘤（50%~60%）、纤维肉瘤（20%~25%）和软骨肉瘤（10%）。巨细胞瘤也与佩吉特症有关，在多发性骨疣的情况下常常是多发的，几乎只累及颅面骨。与原发性破骨细胞瘤相比，该肿瘤在老年人中存在，侵袭性行为倾向相对较差（Leonard et al.，2001）。

根据疾病的阶段，概述为三种放射学形式：早期破坏阶段，以溶骨性、放射状病变为特征（“颅骨局限性骨质疏松症”，额骨受累占优势）。增强明显反映了该阶段血供增加。中间过渡期，表现为溶解和硬化并存。在此阶段，常规放射线影像显示出边界清楚的“斑驳”骨区域，而 CT 显示“棉絮”样的板障扩张。硬化模式盛行的晚期，导致皮质骨和小梁的均匀增厚。

MRI 显示溶骨期 T2 高信号，以及硬化期的可变的 T1 高信号，与骨髓替代的状态有关（Colas et al., 2015）。

骨扫描显示放射性核素的吸收与成骨细胞过度活跃有关。

持续的溶解性病灶，不会随时间而转变为硬化，内容物增多而无骨膜反应是肉瘤或巨细胞瘤转化的可疑表现。

鉴别诊断是颅骨转移，硬化性的（前列腺、乳腺、淋巴瘤）或溶骨性的（肺、肾、甲状腺），纤维发育不良以及所有导致颅骨增厚的原因（额骨内增生病变，脑膜瘤）。治疗的主要手段是药物，以控制疼痛为目标，主要通过破骨细胞抑制剂来实现。密切监测疾病分期和影像学随访发现恶性退行性变是必要的保证。由于该病血供丰富，外科治疗极具挑战性，大出血较常见。

纤维发育不良

纤维发育不良是一种间质前体骨的先天性非遗传性良性疾病。这是由 GNAS 基因编码的 Gsα 蛋白在成骨祖细胞中突变，导致成骨细胞的异常分化和突变，正常骨逐渐被与纤维结缔组织混合的不成熟编织骨（Colas et al., 2015）替代（Bowers et al., 2014; Wu et al., 2014）。

纤维发育不良占所有骨肿瘤的 2.5%（Bowers et al., 2014），其中发病率为 1:4000~1:10000。男性和女性发病情况相同，通常是在 13 岁前。

在 75%~80% 的病例中为单骨型，但年轻患者更常见的是多发性骨疣。颅骨受累多骨疣形式多见，主要累及蝶骨、额骨、筛骨、上颌骨、枕骨和颞骨（Bowers et al., 2014）。

临床表现包括：眶颅区域无痛性局限性骨肿胀，眼球突出，脑神经（通常为视神经）病变卡压症，头痛，癫痫发作，自发性头皮出血（Bowers et al., 2014）。在多骨体形式中，这些发现与长骨骨折和畸形有关。

恶性变性很少见，仅不到 1%的病例可见。在单骨位置风险更大，尤其是在上颌骨和下颌骨以及放射治疗之后（Bowers et al., 2014）。骨肉瘤是最常见的恶性肿瘤，其次是纤维肉瘤和软骨肉瘤。

病变通常在儿童时期生长，并且不会发展到青春期以后（Colas et al., 2015），随着骨骼成熟结束（Wu et al., 2014）。

这种疾病的多骨形成可能是部分 McCune-Albright 综合征，以三联征为特征：多骨性疾病、咖啡斑、多发性内分泌功能障碍。

三种主要的放射学表现：变形性骨炎样的（占病例的 35%），具有交替的硬化和溶解特征，硬化主要累及颅底，而溶解性病变以“虫蚀”的外观影响颅顶（**图 20.7**）。硬化的“致密”型（占病例的 50%），其特征是骨骼均匀增厚，被认为是最不活跃的形式。CT 显示主要在颅骨底部出现磨砂玻璃外观（Bowers et al., 2014）。囊性或“溶解性”（占病例的 15%）类型，被认为是最活跃的形式，在 CT 上表现为非均匀的膨胀骨模式，放射状病变被类似蛋壳的薄硬化区域包围。囊性变在 T2 加权像上呈高信号 MRI，而硬化区域显示明显低信号（Bowers et al., 2014）。增强给药后病灶有不同程度非均匀一致的强化。

鉴于疾病的多态性，鉴别诊断涉及多种疾病，包括佩吉特症、神经皮肤疾病、脑膜瘤、棕色肿瘤、骨硬化症、额内骨质增生、地中海贫血和颅干骺端发育不良。

手术指征取决于进行性神经损伤的存在、疾病的程度和患者的年龄。当符合手术指征时，完全手术切除是治疗的目标。如果无手术指征，目标是达到神经结构减压（Bowers et al., 2014）。单期骨重建是必要的。肿瘤对放化疗有耐受，据报道放疗会增加肉瘤转化的风险。

表 20.3 总结了混合性溶解 - 增生性病变。

外伤性和先天性病变

颅骨膜血窦

这种情况由静脉跨板障静脉通道组成，连接颅内静脉系统与颅外或帽状腱膜下静脉（Bouali et al., 2015）。这是一个非常罕见的发现，通常从儿童期到 30 岁被确诊。

颅骨膜血窦主要位于矢状窦旁，在中线额叶区

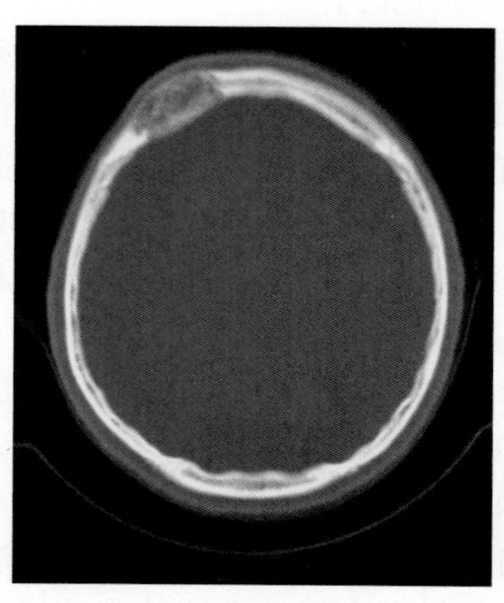

图 20.7 纤维不典型增生，显示出骨质疏松的非均匀模式，并伴有射线可透过的病变，周围有薄薄的硬化区域

表 20.3　混合性溶解－增生性病变

佩吉特（Paget）病	疾病不同阶段的显微特征不同；在早期的溶解破坏阶段，巨大的多核破骨细胞占优势，引起严重的吸收和纤维血管组织骨髓替代；向晚期硬化阶段的过渡包括一个中间阶段，随着成骨细胞活性增加，导致最后阶段成骨细胞活性下降，血管基质消失，留下硬化、易碎的骨和萎缩的骨髓。这种硬化骨由增厚的小梁组成，缺乏结构强度（"浮石骨"）
纤维发育不良	成纤维细胞、未成熟的编织骨和软骨的轮匝－骨小梁漂浮在纤维基质中形成"中国字母"形状

域，但也可能发生在更外侧。两种类型为："封闭"型，其中血流来自硬脑膜窦并汇入硬脑膜窦；"引流"型，血液经板障引流（Bouali et al.，2015）。

临床表现为中线附近的柔软可复位的肿块，随着 Valsalva 动作和头部位置的变化而波动（Bouali et al.，2015）。神经功能障碍很少见，但沿上矢状窦的血流紊乱被认为是引起非特异性症状（如头痛，呕吐和心动过缓）的潜在原因（Bouali et al.，2015）。不同的病因包括：先天性，与其他血管异常有关，尤其是 VHL 综合征；先天性－创伤混合，提示大量的导静脉被 ICP 的短暂增加（咳嗽、劳损）所撕裂，最终使静脉曲张逐渐侵蚀颅骨；创伤性，当颅骨骨折撕裂导静脉或硬脑膜窦，引起静脉硬膜外血肿。

动脉造影显示跨板障血管通道增强，与可能异常且缓慢充盈的颅内静脉连通。

鉴别诊断包括头皮血管畸形（海绵状血管瘤），经 CT 和 MRI 血管造影排除，表明缺乏颅内循环的参与。还应考虑假性脑膜膨出、颅裂症、增长颅骨骨折、头皮皮样囊肿（Bouali et al.，2015）。

手术指征主要包括美容，预防大面积颅内出血和发生空气栓塞的风险，并且主要通过开颅／颅骨切除术进行，闭合颅外静脉与颅内静脉窦之间的连系以及切除颅外组织并实施颅骨成形术。血管内闭合已有报道（Bouali et al.，2015）。这种情况的预后相对较好的。

头颅血肿

根据定义，骨膜下出血，在颅缝处终止。它是由于出生创伤造成的，占活产婴儿的 1%，但如果凝血障碍存在，也可能是非创伤性的。最常见于顶叶凸面，可能在出生后 24~48 小时明显；持续数天，通常在 4 周内消退，甚至可能需要更长时间（Kaufman et al.，1993）。如果一个月后不愈合，骨膜被抬起的部位可能会出现钙化，并伴有外板重塑。

需要与头皮水肿进行鉴别诊断，头皮水肿穿过颅缝并在几天后消退，伴有帽状腱膜下出血，类似地穿过颅缝，向颈部延伸。可能需要进行 CT 成像以排除凹陷性颅骨骨折和脑膜膨出。

头部包扎可能促进吸收。包裹前针头抽吸液体是有争议的，因为它可能会导致感染。如果发生钙化，由于美容原因，可能需要通过钻孔进行手术切除（Kaufman et al.，1993）。

软脑膜囊肿

这是一种板障内假囊肿，没有上皮质，几乎完全由颅骨骨折引起的，主要发生于三岁以下的儿童。当与颅骨骨折无关时，出现上皮质（"真正的网膜内软脑膜囊肿"），病因可能是先天性的，也可能是外伤后增大的 Pacchioni 肉芽肿（Menkü et al.，2004）。顶叶最常见（50%），其次是额叶和枕叶。

此结果通常与对颅骨的打击有关，可以认为是生长性骨折的一种保留形式，内板和外板破裂合并硬膜和蛛网膜撕裂，与实质损伤和脑膜裂口疝相关／不相关。由于蛛网膜和脑组织通过缺损本身搏动引起骨缘重塑（Açikgöz and Tekkök，2002），随后骨折扩大形成骨内缺损（Menküet al.，2004）。相反，生长性骨折与内、外板的机械性损伤有关，囊肿可能经过或超过板障形成软脑膜假性囊肿（假性脑膜囊肿）（Açikgöz and Tekkök，2002）。

软脑膜囊肿表现为一个柔软的、脉动的、波动的肿块，患者仰卧时更突出，一年内发生 50% 的病例原发性损伤，偶尔伴有癫痫发作或局灶性神经功能缺损。

CT 和 MRI 显示脑膜和大脑疝。MRI 对评估脑实质受累和硬脑膜状态有较高的特异性。鉴别诊断主要是表皮样囊肿和先天性蛛网膜板障内囊肿（Menküet al.，2004）。

外科治疗包括切除囊肿，保留或切除疝的脑组织。硬脑膜缺损的闭合对于防止复发是必要的（Açikgöz and Tekkök，2002），当然颅骨重建也是必不可少的。

参考文献、EBRAIN 的相关链接

扫描书末二维码获取。

第 21 章　前外侧颅底病变的手术治疗

Michael D. Cusimano・Michael P. Meier 著
刘红杏 译，冯恩山 审校

引言

本章概述治疗前外侧颅底病变的主要注意事项。介绍包括鼻窦区和前颅窝区在内的相关解剖特点，重点描述如何选择合适的手术方式以及术前检查原则和围术期管理方案。

本章节重点描述前外侧病变的手术前决策和术中技巧。详细阐述以下几种术式：前纵裂入路（anterior interhemispheric approach）、眶上微创开颅术（supraorbital minicraniotomy）、内镜下经鼻扩大入路（extended endoscopic endonasal approach）、眶颧入路（orbitozygomatic approach）以及颞下窝入路（Fisch approaches）。最后，我们选择了四个案例，通过对手术相关问题的讨论，来阐述手术入路的选择原则及争议。

神经解剖

神经外科医生熟练掌握解剖，不仅有利于定位诊断，还有利于手术入路的选择。对前外侧颅底病变的手术式而言，外科医生应该熟悉病变上方、下方和穿经前外侧颅底的相关解剖结构。为了选择合适的手术入路，医生还必须掌握鼻和眶，颅骨和经颅骨的解剖。

蝶骨是颅底解剖的核心部位，包括蝶骨体、蝶骨小翼和蝶骨大翼、翼突，贯穿颅底的各骨孔，以及裂隙和蝶窦。蝶骨还为颈内动脉、脑膜中动脉和第Ⅰ～Ⅵ对脑神经提供自然通道。神经外科医生应该重视由前到后、由后到前、由外到内、由内到外、从上到下及从下到上等不同的视角，理解头部处于不同位置时各解剖结构相对应的旋转视角情况。蝶骨不仅是中颅窝的核心，还联系额骨、眶和鼻的复合体结构组成前颅窝及其上下区域的结构。

额骨是构成前颅窝的主要骨性结构，额窦的大小和位置变化很大，涉及眶上外侧脊和眶顶。术前需仔细研究这些骨性结构的影像特征，特别关注开颅和颅底重建过程中可能涉及的额窦、蝶窦和筛窦。由于眶顶部骨质非常薄且有很多隆起，手术中进行简单的磨骨就容易使其移动。额部硬脑膜向前颅窝底延伸，将前颅窝底隆起的骨质磨除后，硬脑膜变得相对松弛，额叶下部的手术通道被广泛打通，可以在牵拉额叶相对较轻的情况下充分显露病灶。

尽管蝶骨和额骨构成眶壁的主要骨性结构，但在理解前外侧颅底病变时，熟悉包括颧骨在内的其他参与眶壁的骨性结构也很重要。

硬脑膜在中线部位折叠后形成大脑镰，分离海绵窦外侧壁与硬脑膜层，可以显露走行于硬脑膜与海绵窦壁之间的脑神经，其中第Ⅲ、Ⅳ、Ⅵ脑神经进入眶上裂，V2 神经穿过圆孔至颅外。

手术前相关问题

前外侧颅底病变的检查

详细的病史有助于对病变作出初步诊断，以及明确是否需要进一步的手术干预，甚至紧急手术。完整的神经系统检查包括眼科检查如视力、瞳孔对光反射、相对性传入性瞳孔障碍、色觉以及眼底镜下检查视盘血流灌注等。标准的认知评估，例如蒙特利尔认知评估（Montreal cognitive assessment）（Nasreddine et al., 2005）对于监测患者的疾病进展非常有效。尽管额叶病变一般不会引起局灶性运动症状，除了嗅觉检查外，关注这些症状也非常重要。多学科综合团队，包括神经外科专家、神经眼科专家、内分泌科专家以及耳鼻喉科专家等，对患者进行评估。如果有需要，应由专科医师完成视野检查、光学相干层析成像、血液激素水平检查等。还可能需耳鼻喉科、肿瘤内科、神经放射和肿瘤放疗科等学科的医师一起参与术前讨论，综合的评估有助于最佳治疗方案的选择。

影像学特征

我们常规利用计算机断层扫描（computed tomography，CT）来观察骨性结构的正常解剖、病理改变（如骨肥大）、鼻窦标志（如蝶窦间隔）等，如果有必要明确血管解剖，还应检查CT血管造影（CT angiography，CTA）。常规利用增强或非增强MRI的T1和T2加权像扫描来确定肿瘤和脑组织的关系、是否侵犯颅底、眶内结构、血管走行和其他局部结构。在MRI检查中，需特别注意蛛网膜界面及局灶瘤周水肿情况，这对手术过程及预后评判均很重要。

对于肿瘤性病变，我们很少采用传统的数字减影血管造影。但对于CTA检查仍然不明确可能涉及重要血管的病变，可以采用DSA。对于血管丰富的病变，例如青少年鼻咽血管纤维瘤，术前可采用血管栓塞控制出血。如怀疑来自其他器官的恶性转移病灶，可以进行全身CT甚至正电子发射断层扫描（positron emission tomography，PET）检查。

鉴别诊断

如果病史短，症状进展快，特别是多发脑神经病变，应怀疑为感染性病变或恶性肿瘤。因世界各地的流行病学情况不同，前外侧颅底病变的种类繁多，为了便于记忆，可以使用“肿瘤”“感染”或“血液”来鉴别诊断。肿瘤包括原发性良性肿瘤（如脑膜瘤、垂体腺瘤、颅咽管瘤）、原发性恶性肿瘤（如嗅神经母细胞瘤、脊索瘤、软骨肉瘤）、继发性肿瘤（如鼻窦癌的直接扩散或远处转移的血源性扩散）；感染（如真菌、细菌、结核杆菌或其他）以及其他炎性病变；血管性病变如动脉瘤等。肿瘤也可以根据细胞来源分类（如骨骼、软骨、脑膜、神经、内皮细胞等）。

手术计划

手术前要重点关注病史、体格检查以及有鉴别诊断意义的特殊检查，切除肿瘤对进展缓慢的病变，体弱的以及老年患者，手术可能不是主要的治疗方法。如果需要组织病理诊断、以颅内减压或神经结构减压（如视力丧失或颅内压升高），且能耐受手术的患者应考虑手术治疗。手术前需要考虑预期的病理以及病变是否可以完全切除。其他一些情况下，如有些肿瘤可次全切除联合放疗，单独活检继之放疗或化疗作为辅助治疗。保护重要功能，维持手术后生存和生活质量是制订手术方案的核心。除此之外，在选择手术方案时不但要考虑肿瘤的位置，还要结合外科医生的经验和手术熟练程度。

在开始手术前，外科医生应该充分考虑到手术中每个环节。专业技术精湛的外科医生会在手术后再次思考手术步骤，反思每个患者成功或失败的因素，仔细记录每个病例。术前简要汇报病史对手术方案的制订是必不可少的。手术过程包括术前准备和麻醉准备（如成分备血、致痫性病变准备抗癫痫药）、患者体位、手术入路、肿瘤切除程度、结构重建等。外科医生需要了解手术的每一步以及相关的风险、特殊设备或材料的准备。如神经导航、选择特定模式的神经电生理监测、术中超声、显微器械、超声吸引装置、光学合适的内镜、纤维蛋白胶等。告知麻醉医生预估的手术时长、出血量、特别危险的手术阶段以及所需的额外药物（如抗生素、糖皮质激素等）及降低颅内压的方法如甘露醇、过度通气和手术体位等。

一般情况下，应在摆手术所需的体位之前放置腰大池引流管。如果手术中可能出现颅底脑池与鼻腔的沟通、严重的脑脊液（cerebrospinal fluid，CSF）漏的以及需要对漏口进行多层封闭，为了防止CSF搏动对漏口的冲击，常规在术前放置腰大池引流管。对于部分硬膜外或硬膜下手术，特别是部分锁孔手术，为了减少脑组织的牵拉，也可以在术前放置腰大池引流管，这种情况下引起脑疝的可能性很小。

确定好手术入路后，下一步需要注意的是患者的体位和体位固定技巧。保证患者始终保持同一个体位，所有的压力点都得到保护。当患者处于一个舒适的体位时，将其安全地固定在手术台上，就可以安全旋转，依靠重力的作用来拓宽术野，从而进入更深的解剖位置，最大限度地减少对脑组织的牵拉。患者体位应该头高脚低，利于静脉引流。根据病变的位置，头部保持中立或旋转，用三个或四个颅骨钉的头架固定头部。利用重力作用，结合足够的移除骨瓣，在最大限度减少对脑组织牵拉的情况下，实现对深部结构的显露。颈部进行充分伸展，可以获得更宽广手术视野。

在决定手术入路时应充分考虑缺损结构的重建问题。同种异体组织，如阔筋膜和脂肪是理想的修复材料，人工合成材料或动物制品也可以接受，但一般价格更高。我们会尽量保留骨膜以备重建，但有的情况下骨膜难以保留，如存在与消化呼吸道相通的大面积破损，需要用带血管蒂的皮瓣进行修复。我们已经见过许多病例，一些简单的硬膜缺损，采用了分离的骨膜进行修补，如果选择阔筋膜或合成的移植物，会得到同样好或更好的效果。如果患者需要再次手术或放疗，或两者都需要，头皮受损会是预后不良的原因，有时甚至是致命的。一般来说，如果不准备使用骨膜当做带血管蒂的瓣（例如封闭鼻腔），那么最好将保留在头皮上。应该尽量避免把它留在颅骨上，这样会失去血运或神经支配。

在包括额颞部开颅术的病例中，我们常规进行筋膜间入路进行分离。切开颞肌筋膜的浅层，使之与颞浅筋膜一起保留在皮瓣上，然后在脂肪层与颞肌深筋膜之间进行分离，以防止面神经额支的损伤。

患者及治疗方案的选择

颅底病变的治疗一般包括保守治疗、手术治疗、放射治疗以及综合治疗。在前外侧颅底病变中，对于良性肿瘤，患者的症状主要由肿瘤组织压迫引起，并非侵袭导致，这种病变一般能做到完全切除，应积极进行手术治疗。颅底恶性且放疗敏感的病变或病情危重患者的病变，建议放射治疗。对于不典型病变需要进行活检，然后根据组织诊断决定下一步治疗方案。影像学提示为良性、无临床症状的病变，可定期复查影像学。然而，最终治疗方案必须由经验丰富的神经外科医生决定。

前外侧入路具有多种优势，比如显露颅底解剖结构好、在不同角度下提供广泛的操作空间、上下视角空间大、理想的重建条件（如额窦）和脑组织牵拉少等。

在决定手术入路方式时应该考虑到病变的解剖和最可能的病理这两个问题。

前外侧及眶颧入路的相关解剖：眶（眶上裂、视神经管上侧或外侧、眶后壁、眶上壁、眶侧壁）、蝶骨、鞍旁、小脑幕切迹、基底池、视神经、视交叉、Willis 动脉环、颞叶内侧部、额叶基底部、中脑前外侧以及颞下窝等。

前外侧及眶颧入路的疾病类型：血管病变，如前交通动脉瘤、颈内动脉起始段动脉瘤，后交通动脉或基底动脉上部动脉瘤；肿瘤性病变，包括脑膜瘤、神经鞘瘤、颅咽管瘤、垂体腺瘤、脊索瘤、软骨肉瘤、不同类型的骨肿瘤以及继发在脑膜上的肿瘤；颅内感染，例如曲霉菌病等。总之，需要切除或减压而非组织活检的病变应采用这种手术方法。

手术入路

前纵裂入路

前纵裂入路是治疗前颅底病变的常用术式。常用于切除病变主体位于中线且没有向两侧广泛生长的肿瘤。如果病变位于颅底较低位置、肿瘤位置较深以及不在前纵裂表面的病变，骨窗位置可以偏低，鞍上病变则需要较高的骨窗，部分深部病变可以行对侧中线旁开颅以到达病变区。

手术体位：采用仰卧位，抬高背部及头部约 10°，使头部位于心脏水平上方，头取正中位或者略微偏向一侧，目的是依靠重力作用使额叶远离颅底，在最低限度牵拉脑组织的同时获得最佳的显露效果。

手术切口：通常沿双侧冠状缝至耳郭顶部或耳屏。一定不要用所谓的“soutar”式切口，我们认为这种切口没有任何优势。如前所述，为了避免牺牲带血管蒂的骨膜，头皮切口不易太低。但对于非常小的病变或其他无需保护骨膜的手术，可在前额发际线后或额纹处作直切口。对于单侧病变，特别是需要显露颞窝区的病变，可以做问号式切口。包括帽状腱膜和骨膜在内的皮瓣尽可能单层提起，以确保其在手术过程中的血液供应。如果计划用带血管蒂的骨膜瓣重建，我们倾向于将骨膜从颅骨上剥离，与头皮各层也分离，这样就可以将骨膜单独提起并保存，避免骨膜基底部血管和神经受损。

开颅要求：在中线上钻两个或两个以上的骨孔，将上矢状窦（superior sagittal sinus，SSS）从颅骨上剥离，避免损伤。在关键孔处钻一骨孔，可以开双额颅骨骨窗，也可以将骨窗向健侧延伸，跨过上矢状窦 1~1.5 cm，以便于沿双侧大脑镰旁进行手术显露。

硬脑膜和硬膜下：硬脑膜的剪开方式取决于所需的手术入路。为了充分显露，可以缝合结扎 SSS 的基底部，沿离断的 SSS 处剪开大脑镰，形成完整的中线通路，常用于前交通动脉瘤夹闭术或中线脑膜瘤切除术。硬脑膜剪开方式可以是一个底部朝向上矢状窦的半圆形，可以是朝向眶缘的半圆形，也可以是十字形剪开，具体采用何种方式取决于具体的手术入路。为了防止脱水后挛缩，尽量将剪开的硬脑膜平铺在脑组织表面。引流到上矢状窦的桥静脉要尽量显露出来并加以保护。到达前纵裂后，需充分释放 CSF，使脑组织充分塌陷，在尽量避免牵拉脑组织的情况下，充分显露病灶。

重建问题：完成颅内操作及缝合头皮前，使用桥式颅骨成形术（Cusimano et al.，2012）封闭骨孔，也可以使用价格较高、兼容 MRI 的钛，以及低轮廓的微型钢板，以保证前额开颅手术的面部修复效果。如果额窦开放，则需要硬脑膜不透水缝合，并覆以有血运的组织，或切除额窦，使其丧失功能。在额窦开放的情况下，由于感染风险高，应避免使用甲基丙烯酸甲酯、硅橡胶及其他类似的人造重建材料。

眶上微创开颅术

眶上额下入路可以较好地显露同侧前颅底、鞍上及鞍旁区域，在极少数情况下，还可显露对侧上述区域及后床突区。自1908年Fedor Krause(Krause，1908) 第一次报道这种术式以来，经后续逐渐改进，使开颅手术更加微创，同时兼顾美容效果。Perneczky 小组(van Lindert et al.，1998；Reisch et al.，2003) 报道了经眉弓切口进行眶上锁孔开颅术的手术技巧，可在最低限度牵拉脑组织的同时，对颅底深层病变充分显露。

体位：为了充分利用此入路的优势，需要将患者的头部进行旋转和伸展，以准确到达病变部位。对于同侧病变，头部旋转至15°，对侧病变旋转至30°~60°。

切口：考虑到额窦解剖的个体差异，皮肤切口位于眉毛内，眶上孔的外侧，并向外侧延伸几毫米。

开颅：在眼轮匝肌和枕额肌之间牵开肌肉，在颞上线前缘处将颞肌向下牵拉，并在此处钻一骨孔，铣刀头紧贴前颅底且平行于眉弓方向，从钻孔处向内侧铣开颅骨，退出铣刀后，再从钻孔处沿切口上缘铣一“C”形线，与之前的切割线结合，最终形成一小骨瓣。为了提高术中的可操作性，在骨窗内侧可做适当磨除，以扩大显露。

硬脑膜和硬膜下：做一个弧形硬脑膜切口，根部朝向眼眶。通过打开视交叉池和颈内动脉池或过度牵拉使用前面提到的放置腰大池来引流 CSF，以避免脑组织。切除颅底病变后，相反的顺序进行关颅。需要注意的是，该入路无法保留骨瓣，如果病理要求切除颅底的同时进行带血管蒂的骨膜重建，应选择另一种入路。

内镜手术

1996 年 Cusimano 和 Fenton 首次报道了使用全内镜双鼻孔入路(Cusimano and Fenton，1996)。此手术技术在 1993 年第一次应用，包括双鼻孔显露、鼻中隔后部切开术以及包括蝶窦、筛窦以及上颌窦在内的广泛的颅底显露。学术会议上经常报道此方法，并获得广泛的认同(DiIeva et al.，2014)。由于经蝶窦入路进入至鞍区和鞍上间隙的内容将在另一章中介绍，下面将讨论扩大经鼻内镜入路(endoscopic endonasal approach，EEA) 治疗前颅底病变的具体特点。

对于体积大、质地坚硬的病变，越过中线较远的病变或包绕重要动脉的病变，EEA 有一定的局限性。由于从前颅底下方移动视神经的操作难度大，限制了前颅底的开放。我们采用双鼻孔和四个内镜进行手术，这通常需要与有鼻窦手术经验的医生合作下(Cusimano and Fenton，1996；Cusimano et al.，2012；Cusimano et al.，2013)。此外，对于扩大入路，基底池可能会大面积开放，从而导致高流量 CSF 漏，我们通常在手术前做腰大池引流，并且用带血运的鼻中隔黏膜瓣进行重建。这是我们从 1996—1997 年一直沿用的方法，并且取得了巨大成功。

术前准备和体位：放置腰大池引流管后，患者仰卧，背部抬高 10°。当接近蝶鞍时，头部处于中立位置，使前额与地面平行，如果病变在蝶窦侧较多，则需要将头部后仰。在铺单时要将腹部和右腿预留出刀口部位，以获取用于颅底重建的脂肪和筋膜。用浓度为 1：100,000 的肾上腺素浸泡脱脂棉填充鼻腔。我们使用 0° 内镜进行鼻腔检查，30°、45° 和 70° 内镜进行颅底手术。我们常规准备神经导航和微多普勒来定位小脑下动脉和大脑前动脉。

手术入路：去除双侧中鼻甲，保留鼻中隔黏膜瓣，通常只在一侧鼻孔进行。为了更好地了解患者的解剖结构，即使不需要切开蝶窦，也要寻找并探查蝶窦开口。根据需要将梨骨和筛骨垂直板的后部从蝶窦取下，取下的骨片储存在杆菌肽中，以备颅底重建。如果需要，可以在两侧行蝶窦切开术。对于更多位于嘴侧的病变(例如在鞍结节、蝶骨平台交界区或筛状板区)，应打开筛窦的后(或前) 室并从侧面取下，如果显露至筛后动脉的前方，嗅觉可能受到损害。对于此部位肿瘤，通常会侵袭并破坏了嗅丝，多数患者在术前就已出现嗅觉障碍，术前应做详细的评估。一般用磨钻磨开前颅底，必要时要用 Kerrison 咬骨钳咬除，或用骨刀辅助磨除。骨刀取下的骨质较完整，有利于颅底重建。

通过双极电凝烧灼双侧后组筛动脉，阻断肿瘤下部的血供。广泛打开硬脑膜以暴露肿瘤的基底部、前部、后部以及尽可能显露肿瘤外侧缘。活检并明确诊断后，根据其病变大小，在中心部位去容减压，减压后的肿瘤变得松动，仔细探查边缘和毗邻的蛛网膜界面，在肿瘤和蛛网膜之间锐性分离，仔细切除肿瘤，切除过程中要尽量保留蛛网膜结构，这样可以保留蛛网膜下的重要结构，如大脑前动脉等。

重建问题：为了避免术后 CSF 漏等并发症，在腰大池引流下进行逐层重建至关重要。一般采用筋膜和脂肪填塞，也有一些国家的医生习惯使用硬脑膜替代品。脂肪可用于无效腔填塞，也可用于阔筋膜硬脑膜成形术。理想情况下采用“嵌入式”(in- lay)，放置在游离硬膜边缘下方(Cusimano and Suhardja，

2000）。在阔筋膜充分放置前，保持腰大池引流管关闭状态，在缝合阔筋膜时打开引流管，随后将先前保存好的骨片放于缺损处，骨片与缺损缘重叠并楔形嵌入，再通过一些组织胶来固定，这些组织胶会附着在带血管蒂的鼻中隔膜黏膜瓣上，起到固定作用。用聚乙烯醇缩醛海绵填塞鼻腔来支持重建，填塞水平和后鼻孔一致，这样既能保持填塞物的稳定，又利于呼吸的通畅性。术后第二日夹闭腰大池引流管，术后第三日拔除填塞物。

眶颧入路

在 20 世纪 80 年代中期，Pellerin 等（1984）和 Harbuka 等（1986）首次描述了眶 - 颅 - 颧入路（OCZO），或简称眶颧入路（OZY 或 OZO），该术式可以到达颅后窝的前、中、上部。OZY 入路是经典额颞开颅术的延伸，结合了颅底通路宽、手术距离短、可操作性强及脑组织牵拉小等优点。自 1991 年以来，我们广泛使用该方法来治疗各种病变（van Furth et al.，2006）。

眶颧入路的术式有多种变异。最常见的是额颞开颅加颅眶骨切开术，只包括带颧骨的眶上壁和外侧壁，不包括颧弓。该入路对于累及前颅窝至动眼神经三角区的病变，如前循环动脉瘤非常有效。对于动眼神经三角区后部的病变，则摘除颧弓后手术效果更好。对于中线结构的病变，既可以行单侧眶上缘和眶壁切除，也可以经鼻额缝双侧操作。我们常规先下骨瓣，再取眶壁骨，即所谓的“两步走技术”，在直视下操作手术则更加安全、有效。另外，如 Al- Mefty（Al-Mefty，1987）和其他学者（Jane et al.，1982；Ikeda et al.，1991）报道过“一步走”技术，即将颅骨和眶壁骨作为同一个骨瓣去除，也是可行的。

体位：类似于额颞开颅，根据不同病变的显露范围，患者的头向对侧旋转 10°~45°。颈部略微伸展，在重力作用下，使额叶和颞叶远离颅底。

切口：如同创伤手术中的小皮瓣，从耳屏前部开始，向上达中线与发际的交界点附近，刀口呈弧形切口或问号状。采用筋膜间入路分离皮瓣，连同骨膜一起向前翻转至眶缘，用小骨刀将眶上神经及其伴随的血管从眶上孔分出，小心剥离眶壁内骨膜，深 2.5 cm~3 cm，开颅之前显露颞肌和颧弓。

开颅和骨瓣成型：我们倾向于采用桥式颅骨切开术（bridge cranioplastic technique of craniotomy）（Cusimano and Suhardja，2000），根据手术需要决定额颞区的显露范围。眶颧骨离断分五步完成，由一名外科医生负责切割，另一名医生负责保护眶内容物。为了防止挤压眶内容物造成严重的三叉 - 迷走神经反射，术中操作要轻柔，最好用长棉条覆盖于硬膜之上，并用脑压板阻挡，以防误伤脑组织，此时麻醉医生也应该提高警惕，预防严重的心动过缓。第一步，轻抬额底硬膜，用铣刀从眶上切迹的外侧开始，向后铣开眶顶约 2.5 cm。第二步，继续向外侧铣眶顶，达距离眶下裂一半的位置。第三步，铣刀从颞下窝处放入眶下裂，铣向上、后方，直到与第二步对接。第四步，铣刀从眶腔进入，放入眶下裂，沿着颧骨或所谓的“颧骨隆起”向外下铣开。在本步操作中，首先要在眶下裂处用铣刀的尖端向深部切割，然后向上、后方反复切割到颧骨的中点。最后将铣刀置于颧骨的后缘，向上铣至前一切口的末端，切口保持在颧骨面部孔上方，以避免开放上颌窦。最后用骨凿轻敲剩余的骨桥，最终游离眶颧骨。根据手术显露的需要，开颅范围可做适当的调整，如果病变较大，可以通过扩大骨窗来增加显露范围，例如，通过下颌关节的关节盂和头部半脱位，并移除髁突窝，来实现颈内动脉岩段的显露。通过去除中颅窝底部的骨质，可以切除颅底或颞下窝的病变。

硬脑膜和硬膜内：硬膜剪开的部位取决于病变的起源部位，以及对前颅窝或中颅窝的需求程度。海绵窦和 Meckel 囊区病变应尽量经硬膜外显露。如果需要硬膜内显露，通常在以外侧裂为中心 C 形剪开硬脑膜，将硬脑膜呈帐篷状向上伸展，以拓宽手术视野。

重建问题：病理类型和手术切除程度决定重建方法。如果前外侧颅底的骨质被移除，要尽量将硬脑膜复位。如果出现鼻窦开放，需要去除窦内黏膜并用带血管的组织覆盖。仔细将取下的骨片放回至原来的解剖位置，避免周围骨片边缘卡压脂肪组织。若破损非常小，则打开的眶周筋膜无需缝合。骨片通常用微型钛板或打小孔后用粗的不可吸收缝线固定于原来的颅骨上，也可以采用桥接技术连接起来，用不可吸收缝线缝合，再用自体骨屑填充钻孔。如果资金允许，可以使用预制的钻孔覆盖物或骨替代材料。

颞下窝入路

颞下窝入路虽然不是前外侧入路，但可用于切除延伸至中颅窝及眶后区的病变。这些部位的手术是神经外科医生和耳鼻喉科医生最具挑战性的手术之一。Fisch 等（Fisch，1978；Fisch and Pillsbury，1979）首次描述了三种不同的入路治疗岩尖、斜坡和蝶骨旁的肿瘤，此入路涉及基本的神经血管结构，如颈内动脉、颈静脉和第Ⅴ～Ⅻ对脑神经。这些是从颅底和颅底下方向上看的下外侧入路，非常适合颞骨区域的病变以及前至中颅窝底和翼上颌裂的病变。Fisch A、B和C型入路的关键点如下所述。

A型入路的**适应证**包括累及颞骨迷路下部及岩尖区病变，包括颈静脉球瘤、脑膜瘤、脑神经鞘瘤、胆脂瘤和下斜坡脊索瘤。

手术方法A型：将颞-颈部皮肤切开，识别面神经及其主要分支。沿着外耳道的皮肤、鼓膜以及下至镫骨底板的听小骨都必须移除。尽管会导致传导性听力损失，但保留了内耳功能。其后切开乳突以显露面神经管，然后在膝状神经节和颧骨顶部之间的上鼓室前面磨一个凹槽，移入面神经。必须显露颈动脉，如果手术需要且患者能够耐受，可以在发出舌动脉分支水平以远结扎颈动脉。如果肿瘤已经阻塞静脉窦（如颈静脉球），乙状窦也可以结扎，并将颞下颌关节向前移位。岩骨次全切除术可以看到颈动脉壁、迷路下骨质、颅后窝硬脑膜和延续至颈静脉孔的乙状窦。肿瘤剥离后，必须阻塞咽鼓管，将外耳道封闭为盲管，用腹部脂肪和颞肌封闭无效腔。

手术方法B型：位于斜坡、枕骨大孔、蝶窦和咽上部的病变则最好采用B型入路。颞骨次全切除后，向下翻转颧弓、颞肌和面神经。将颞下颌关节脱位，切除下颌髁突，显露卵圆孔和棘突。切除咽鼓管、中颅窝硬脑膜和三叉神经的分支。肿瘤切除后，将外耳道封闭为盲管，用钢丝连接颧弓，颞肌复位。

手术方法C型：B型入路可扩展为C型入路，可显露鼻咽部、翼腭窝和鞍旁区。将眶突与眶外侧缘一起向下翻转，切除翼状突。为了增加显露，还需要临时性切断汇合入V3的面神经分支，通过抬高中颅窝硬脑膜来暴露颈内动脉海绵窦段下部，外科医生可以切除此部位病灶，如广泛的青少年鼻咽血管纤维瘤或放射失败的鳞状细胞癌。

术后相关问题

在进行任何手术前，都应该仔细考虑潜在的术后并发症，并与患者和手术团队讨论。手术计划必须考虑到潜在的并发症和预防这些并发症的方法。外科医生应该亲自和团队一起演练计划，公开讨论预防感染。术后也要进行反思，提供详细的术中情况，与外科团队进行术后讨论。

外科手术的关键目标之一是保障患者的安全并防止并发症的发生。例如，应该尽量避免脑组织牵拉，可以通过去除遮挡通路的骨质、适当调整头部位置、过度通气、使用高渗药物等来减少脑组织水肿。通过术前置入腰大池外引流管持续引流CSF的方法，拓宽手术视野，减少对脑组织的牵拉。如果硬脑膜无法修补或修补不理想，术中行CSF引流则有助于避免术后CSF漏。在三叉神经和（或）面神经受累者中，可以对部分患者进行睑缘缝合术来避免术后角膜炎和溃疡。所有眶周手术、三叉神经、面神经或岩浅大神经受累的患者应每2~4 h常规使用角膜润滑膏，并定期进行眼科评估。

在围术期每4~6 h时重复使用一次抗生素，配合术中细致的组织处理及缝合，有助于降低感染的风险，特别是开放鼻窦的手术。存在腰大池引流和鼻腔填塞物时，应继续应用抗生素预防感染。尽量在回重症监护病房前拔除气管插管，这样有利于尽早评估神经系统功能，以便及时发现可能存在的神经功能缺失并积极处理。

常规在术后6~12 h进行CT检查，最好是增强扫描。在部分出现术后并发症的病例中，需要行其他影像学检查，如CTA、MRI。一般来说，为了防止术后空气及血液等对影像的干扰，特别是腔填充自体物质（如脂肪）时，MRI扫描最好在术后一段时间后进行。

神经外科团队和其他专业医生在术后至少每日评估两次。患者出院后，护士要与其联系。由术前见过患者的团队人员常规进行MRI评估和术后临床评估，以便为患者定期行门诊评估。

案例分析与争议讨论

案例1

31岁，男性，左眼眼压增加，眼球活动受限。头部CT显示中颅窝巨大占位性病变，延伸至左侧眶内，有明显的骨质增生（图21.1）。神经体格检查显示左眼突出，眼球运动受限，受限程度为上0、下60%、外80%和内90%。轻度瞳孔传入障碍，三叉神经所有分支的感觉均下降约10%。MRI扫描显示中颅窝占位，大小7.4 cm×6.6 cm×5.3 cm，囊性，部分实性，病变不均匀强化，向眶内生长，向下至颞下窝。肿瘤位于上直肌下部，推断肿瘤可能起源于动眼神经上支。

如前所述，我们决定实施左侧额颞开颅-眶颧骨离断及颞下减压术。术前行持续腰大池外引流，手

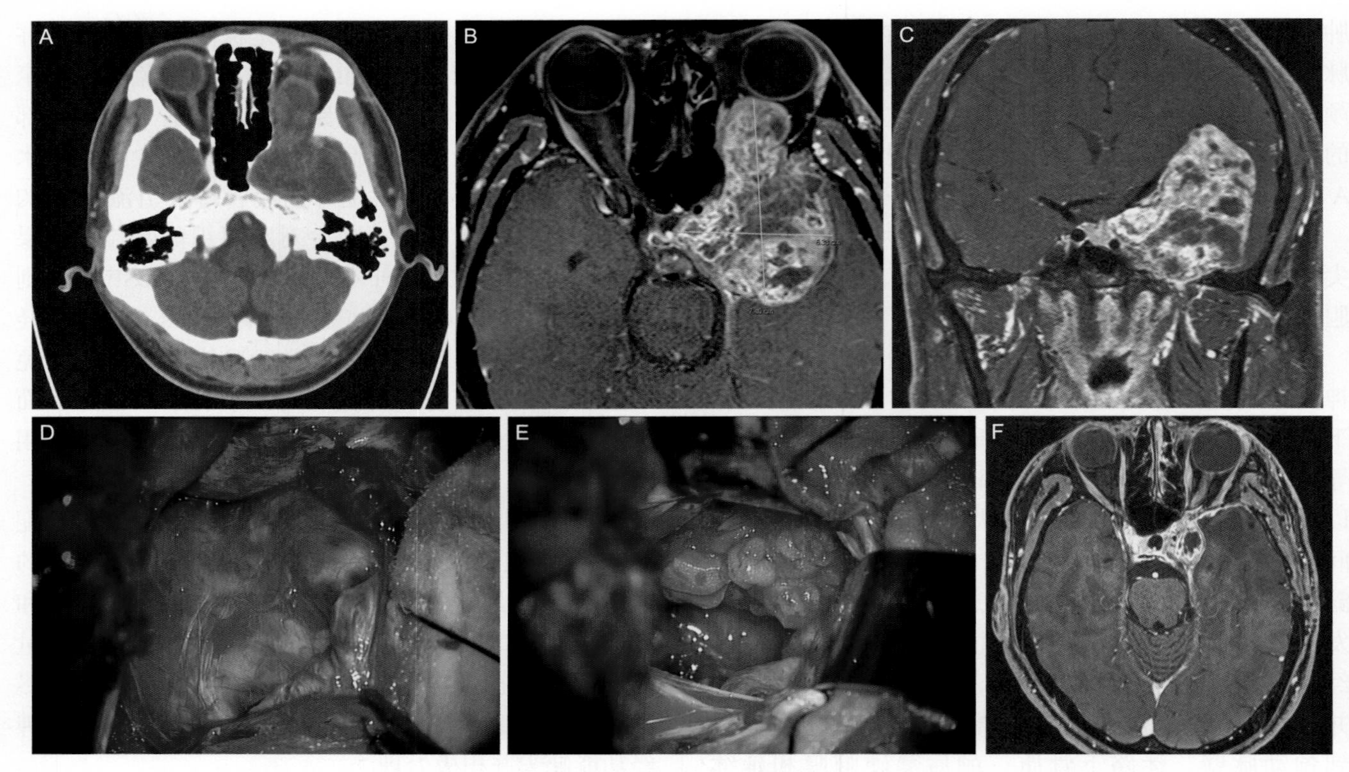

图 21.1 （A）轴位头颅 CT 扫描：显示广泛的颅底病灶，骨质侵袭。（B）轴位 MRI 增强 T1 加权像：显示部分实性、部分囊性病变长入眼眶，将海绵窦向右侧推移。（C）冠状位 MRI 增强 T1 加权像：显示左侧 ICA 向内侧下脱位，大脑中动脉被向上推。（D）术中显微镜下：显示肿瘤位于海绵窦硬脑膜内壁下。（E）术中显微镜下：能看到脂肪样肿瘤。（F）术后 6 个月轴位 MRI 增强 T1 加权像：显示小残留病变内的脂肪植入物

术在神经导航、超声以及神经生理监测下进行。由于眶上裂（SOF）变宽，第二步眶骨切开较容易。显露完全后，可见眼眶、SOF 和蝶骨小翼的移位。首先从硬膜外分离直达中颅窝，电凝后切断脑膜中动脉。自眶上裂开始，从海绵窦外侧壁的两层膜之间进入海绵窦外侧壁，一直游离至圆孔，向后小心地将外侧硬膜层和内侧神经束膜层分开。在平行于 V2 走行的方向切开神经束膜，暴露出黄色的肿瘤，用镊子配合吸引器将后部的肿瘤及眶内肿瘤完全切除，但在海绵窦前部纤维分隔中的肿瘤难以切除，复查 MRI 显示残余肿瘤的存在。最后用超声和内镜检查瘤腔，确认肿瘤已基本全切除。采用硬脑膜进行重建，将脂肪移植在眼眶及左侧海绵窦区域，然后用钛板固定颅骨。术后病理证实为神经鞘瘤。术后 18 个月随访，患者恢复良好，Karnofsky 评分为 100 分，无神经功能缺失及复发。

案例 2

71 岁，男性，反应迟钝伴短暂记忆缺失进行性加重 6 个月。患者仅表现为认知功能障碍及嗅觉减退，第 Ⅱ 到 Ⅻ 对脑神经均无异常，无视盘水肿。影像学显示前颅窝底占位性病变，增强扫描显示肿瘤明显强化，肿瘤基底部可见骨质破坏，疑似嗅沟脑膜瘤（**图** 21.2）。行开颅显微镜下肿瘤切除术。尽管肿瘤起源于中线部位，但病灶体积较大、基底宽且附着于颅底，横向延伸超过双侧瞳孔中线位，故采用经眶额入路。

在双冠状皮肤切口后，将附有骨膜的皮瓣前翻，保留皮瓣。为了减少脑组织的牵拉，首先去除额眶骨，以实现尽可能低的前颅底通路，因肿瘤向右侧生长较多，所以在右侧进行眶骨切开并移除整个眶顶，左侧眶顶仅部分显露。分离硬膜外至肿瘤基底部，电凝后切断供血动脉（如筛前和筛后动脉分支），再行硬膜下分离并分块切除肿瘤，手术过程中无需牵拉脑组织。完全切除肿瘤后，用预先保存的骨膜进行颅底重建，并用骨蜡和组织胶封闭。病理证实为脑膜瘤，WHO 1 级。

此病例可以选择的开颅方式还有很多种，可以是单侧开颅也可以是双侧开颅或微创开颅，但必须考虑到筛板的深度、双额的显露、显露的高度，以

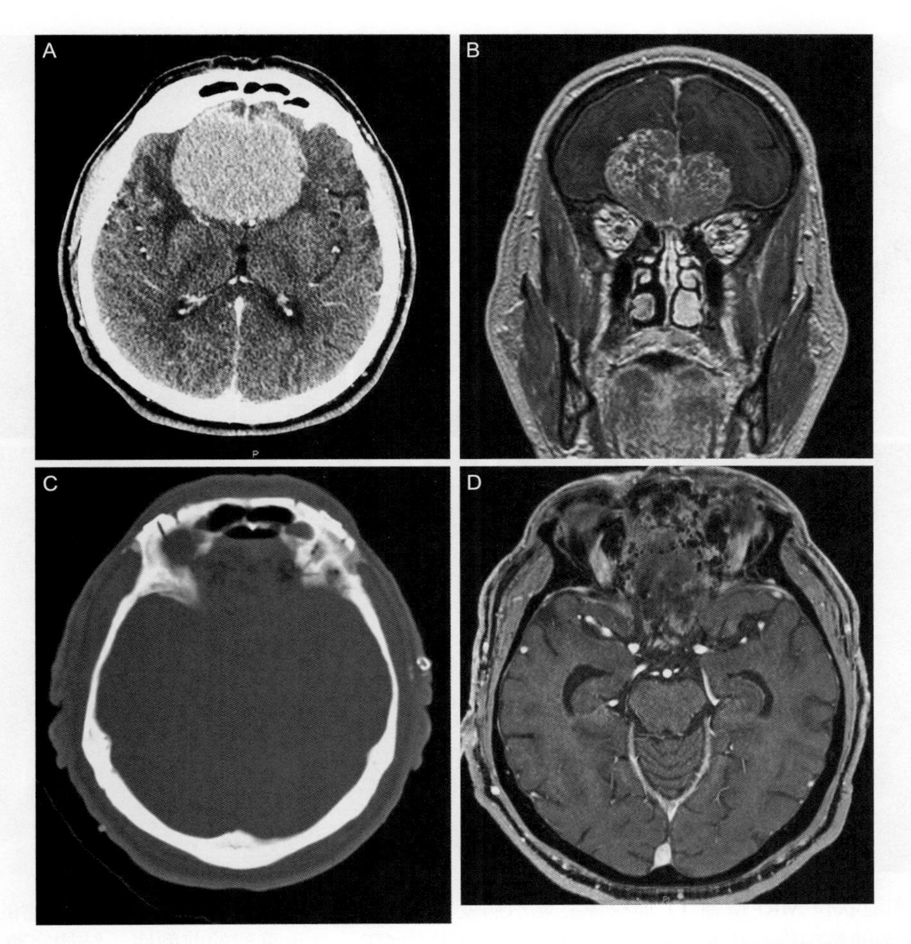

图 21.2 （A）轴位头颅 CT：显示前颅底病变，均匀强化，双侧 A2 段向后移位。（B）冠状位 MRI 增强 T1 加权像：显示病变附着在筛板上。（C）术后轴位 CT 骨窗：显示颅底重建。可以看到经前颅底行低位开颅并移除了眶骨。（D）术后 6 个月轴位 MRI 增强 T1 加权像：显示肿瘤完全切除。可以看到位于筛窦气房水平硬膜外的小气泡，未见明显的肿瘤残余

及颅底重建时骨膜瓣长度等问题。对此患者来说，微创开颅不是最佳选择。可以采用经典的翼点入路，但不利于颅底重建，肿瘤残留的可能性也很大。也可以采用低位颅骨开窗，切或不切眶顶的单侧额下入路，由于肿瘤基底部宽广，可能需要双侧的颅底重建，操作起来难度很大，特别是额窦发育较大时，重建难度更大。通过前纵裂入路显露病变区比较容易，保留骨膜瓣后也可以进行颅底重建，但脑组织难免会受到牵拉及损伤，对病变的暴露、切除及颅底重建并无优势。也可以通过内镜行病灶切除，但难以做到完全切除肿瘤，相对很容易到达病灶而无脑组织牵拉的额眶入路来说，也没有优势，肿瘤切除后颅底缺损严重，内镜手术也不能提供足够的修复材料，甚至会因为大量出血和残留肿瘤而使手术变得更加复杂。我们采用的双侧额 - 眶 - 颅入路可以方便有效地全切肿瘤，比较容易处理受累的硬脑膜和颅底骨质，无需过度牵拉脑组织，并可提供有血运的修复材料。

案例 3

一位 62 岁的女性患者，随访 5 年。由于偏头痛持续加重，检查发现前颅窝占位性病变。随访发现病灶逐渐变大，影像学显示为脑外病变，增强扫描显示肿瘤明显强化、基底部位于颅底硬脑膜（**图 21.3**）。最终，在讨论了包括继续随访观察、伽玛刀治疗和分次放射治疗在内的所有治疗方案后，患者要求手术治疗。我们认为病变可能是起源于筛板的脑膜瘤，最好的手术方法是通过内镜扩大入路切除肿瘤。常规放置腰大池引流管后，夹闭引流管，摆放体位，行内镜下肿瘤切除术。在神经导航的辅助下，利用 70° 内镜开放蝶窦前壁，显露蝶骨平台及筛板，在肿瘤下方的前颅窝底钻孔，硬脑膜水平可见骨质增生，表明这是肿瘤的起源。充分磨除骨质，完全显露肿瘤基底部，切开肿瘤基底部，先进行瘤

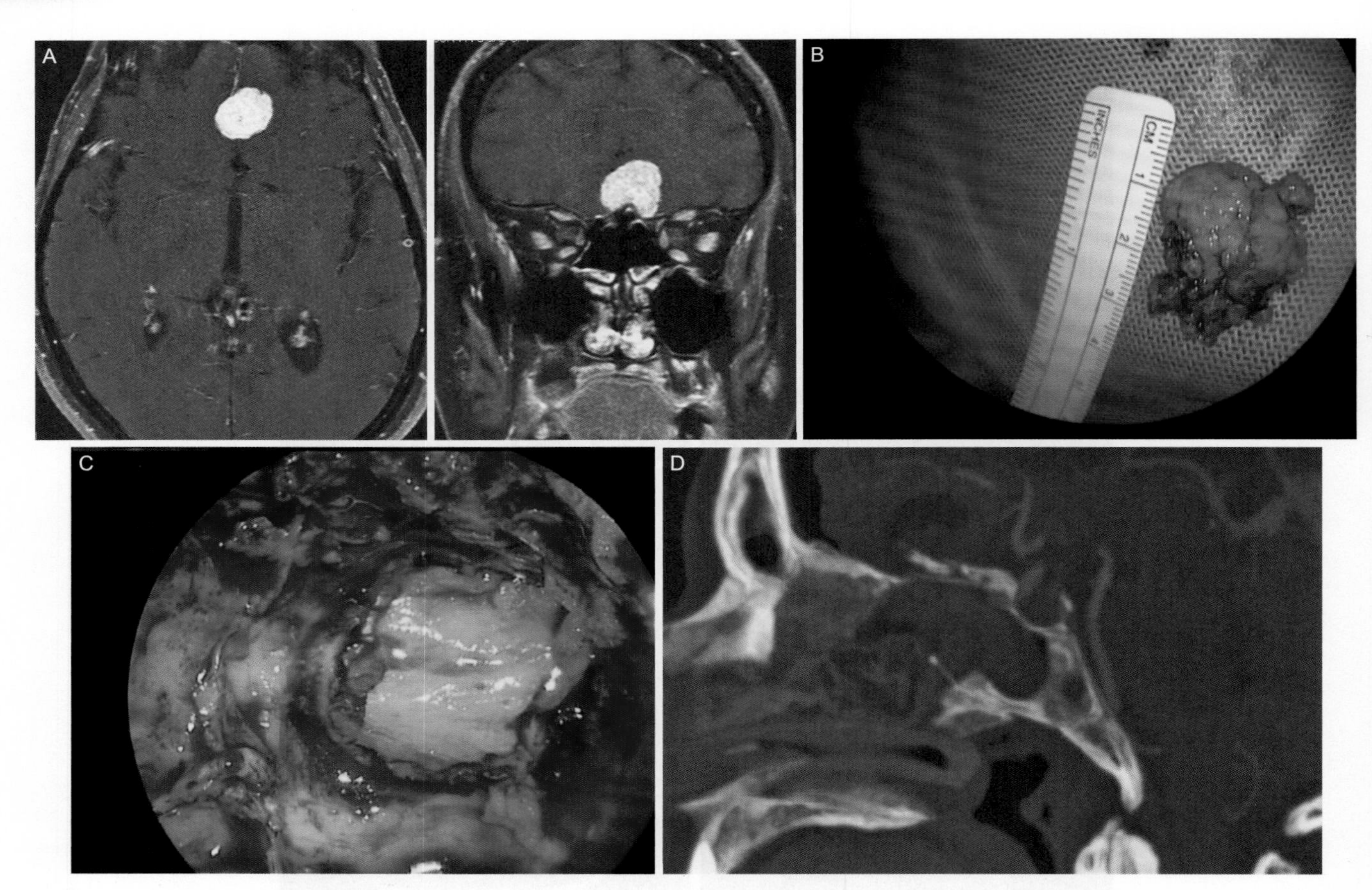

图 21.3 （A）轴位和冠状位 MRI 增强 T1 加权像：显示病变位于筛板之上。（B）术中图片显示肿瘤的大小。（C）内镜下见颅底重建（带血管蒂的鼻中隔黏膜瓣置入前）。（D）术后矢状位 CT：显示重建的前颅底，结构完整

内切除，然后在蛛网膜界面处逐渐剥离，保护周围正常脑组织，完全切除肿瘤，保留完整的蛛网膜，双极电凝肿瘤周边的硬脑膜。右侧嗅束完整，虽然左侧嗅束被推挤移位，但仍保持完整。完全切除肿瘤后行颅底重建，先打开腰大池外引流，然后在硬脑膜开口处放置小的脂肪块，将阔筋膜平铺于脂肪块表面，阔筋膜周边位于硬脑膜下，用两块小骨块覆盖于阔筋膜表面，再用组织胶粘接带血管蒂的鼻中隔黏膜瓣。术后病理证实为脑膜瘤，WHO 1 级。术后 18 个月随访，患者状态良好，右侧嗅觉正常，Karnofsky 评分为 100 分，肿瘤无复发。

案例 4

此病例是一位 56 岁的女性患者，因贝尔麻痹（Bell’s palsy）入院，头部 CT 扫描偶然发现前颅窝底占位性病变。当时无症状而未手术治疗。MRI 扫描显示病变基底位于筛板硬膜，肿瘤明显强化，随访发现病灶逐渐变大，大小达 4.0 cm × 2.5 cm × 3.5 cm（图 21.4）。

我们讨论了所有可能的治疗方案后，患者要求手术治疗。我们认为开颅手术切除指征明确，为安全、有效的治疗方法。

常规放置腰大池引流管后，做双冠状皮肤切口，将头皮皮瓣和骨膜前翻，保留皮瓣。在正中线上打开左额大于右额的骨窗，额窦开放，黏膜予以去除。为了减少脑组织的牵拉，首先去除额眶骨，以实现尽可能低的前颅底通路。左侧进行了眶骨切开并移除整个眶顶，右侧眶顶仅部分显露，在中线部位鼻额缝以下去除部分骨质，咬除鸡冠并双极电凝上矢状窦的前极，首先行硬膜外分离并逐步切断肿瘤的供血动脉（如筛前和筛后动脉分支），再行硬膜下肿瘤切除。嗅束完全被肿瘤浸润，先行瘤内切除，然后在蛛网膜界面上逐渐将肿瘤剥离。筛板后部和蝶骨平面前部可见明显的骨质侵袭，说明肿瘤起源于此。切除肿瘤与受累的大脑镰下部以及受侵袭的骨质，双极电凝去除肿瘤、骨质及硬膜后的区域，彻底止血。我们进行了阔筋膜和脂肪移植，用骨蜡和组织胶封闭前颅底，然后再进行颅骨成形术。手术在超声和

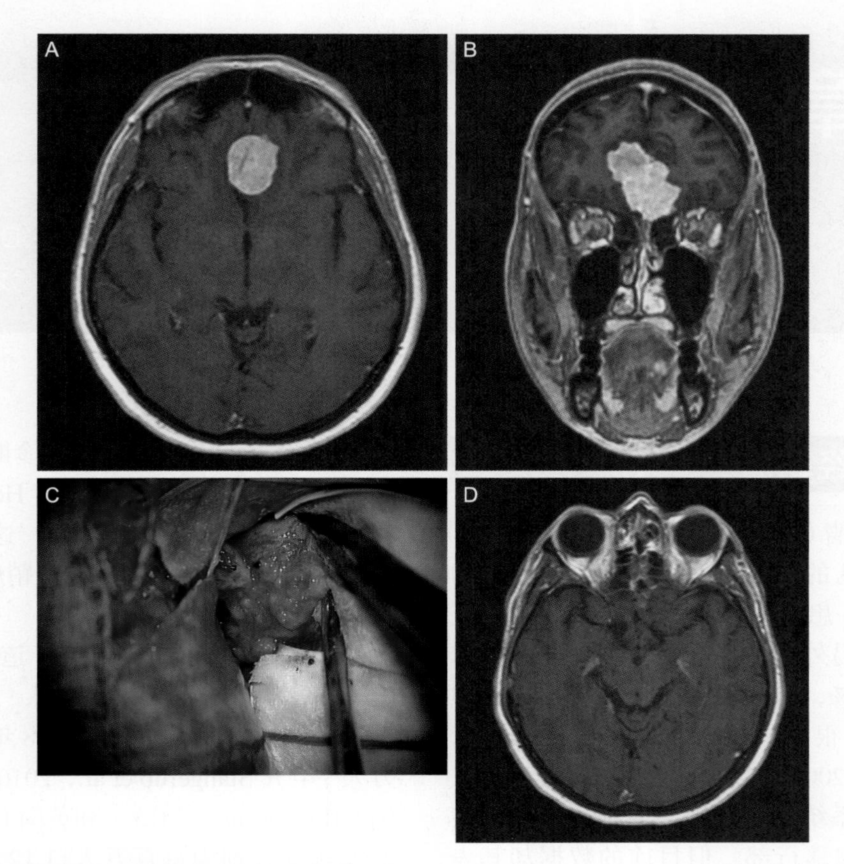

图 21.4　（A）轴位和（B）冠状位 MRI 增强 T1 加权像：显示起源于筛板，巨大分叶状前颅窝占位。（C）术中镜下视野：从额下及前外侧显示肿瘤。（D）术后轴位 MRI 增强 T1 加权像：显示肿瘤切除完全

神经导航引导辅助下进行，病理显示为 WHO 1 级脑膜瘤。患者预后良好，认知功能未受损，Karnofsky 评分为 100 分，嗅觉丧失。20 个月随访，无复发。

颅底内镜为不同类型的病变提供了不同的手术入路。通过对案例 3 和 4 的分析，我们讨论了内镜的适应范围及局限性，特别是向侧方生长的病变，局限性更明显。在大多数情况下，筛板限制了前颅窝侧面的显露，如果将视神经移位，筛板的限制会明显改善。尽管带角度的内镜能很好地显示肿瘤的侧位或前位，但鉴于内镜手术空间有限，操作有一定难度。相比之下，开颅手术可以更加有效、完全地切除肿瘤。另外，对于基底较宽的病变，由于内镜器械长度有限，影响了手术操作。而质地坚硬和部分钙化的病变，以及血供丰富的病变（如脑膜瘤），不会因肿瘤内减容而塌陷，也限制了内镜的使用。

内镜手术的一个潜在挑战是如何通过充分的颅底重建来预防颅内感染，特别是那些需要多次手术和放疗的患者。对于上述类型的肿瘤，制订手术计划时就需重视颅底重建问题。与大面积的颅底缺损相比，小面积骨质缺损的重建更容易，特别是使用前述的逐层颅底重建方法。尽管我们认为病例 4 中横向生长的筛板脑膜瘤可以通过内镜进行手术，但因为病变明显向上生长，我们决定进行开颅手术，最终手术效果很好。总之，外科医生应该使用那些能为患者取得最好结果的方法实施手术。

参考文献

扫描书末二维码获取。

第四篇　肿瘤和颅底——桥小脑角病变

第22章　神经鞘瘤

Tiit Mathiesen · Petter Förander · David Pettersson 著
汤可 译，卜博 审校

散发性前庭神经鞘瘤

前庭神经鞘瘤（vestibular schwannoma，VS）是桥小脑角最常见的肿瘤，占所有颅内肿瘤的6%~8%。65%~75%患者的肿瘤起源于第八脑神经中的前庭下神经。另外一些作者报告说，起源于前庭下神经的高达90%，其余的起源于前庭神经上神经；耳蜗神经起源的很少（Komatsuzaki and Tsunoda，2001；Khrais et al.，2008）。前庭神经鞘瘤最初被认为起源于中枢神经系统和周围神经系统之间的少突胶质细胞-施万细胞移行部，但目前的数据却其表明与内耳道内前庭神经的感觉神经节有关（Xenellis and Linthicum，2003；Roosli et al.，2012；Tryggvason et al.，2012）。

历史上，只有大的、危及生命的肿瘤才能得到诊断和治疗。在20世纪20年代，与VS切除相关的手术死亡率超过70%。历史上的神经外科先驱们在治疗方面取得了跨越式的改进和提高。使用囊内切除技术，Cushing将手术死亡率降低到30%（Cushing，1917），但复发肿瘤的高死亡率成为一个问题（Olivecrona，1950）；Dandy再次进行了根治性手术，代价是更高的面神经损伤风险（Dandy，1934）。Olivecrona开创了保留面神经的根治性手术（Olivecrona，1950）。接下来的发展是House的显微外科和Leksell的放射外科（Norén et al.，1993）。今天，因治疗而死亡的情况很少。治疗选择包括观察和扫描、显微外科、放射外科和放射治疗。个人治疗选择取决于肿瘤大小、症状学和预期的自然史（图22.1）。

散发性前庭神经鞘瘤的流行病学

检查指征放宽和更容易地获得MRI图像，使神经鞘瘤检出率大大提高。Stangerup和同事发现，在丹麦，MRI扫描仪的数量与前庭神经鞘瘤的发病率呈线性关系（Stangerup et al.，2004）。在美国，前庭神经鞘瘤在1991年被诊断为10人/（100万人·年）（National Institutes of Health, 1991）。然而，尸检材料中的人口研究发现，这种疾病的发病率在0.8%~2.4%，表明大多数神经鞘瘤并没有被诊断出来（Schmidt et al.，2012）。

Tos和Thomsen小组报道，丹麦1976年的发病率为3.1人/（100万人·年），2004年增至22.8人/（100万人·年），2008年降至19.8人/（100万人·年）（Stangerup et al.，2010）。最近，据估计美国（Babu et al.，2013）和英国（Evans et al.，2005）的发病率分别为每百万人口12例和14例。丹麦的最新发病率估计为每年35人/（100万人·年）（Sass et al.，2018）。各国之间的差异可能很好地反映了当地的诊断流程和患者登记数量，但群体之间也可能存在生物差异；美国数据发现显示，在监测流行病学和最终结果（SEER）数据库中登记的患者中，高加索人占主导地位（Gal et al.，2010）（图22.2）。

最常见的诊断年龄仍在50~64岁，性别分布均等。与1980年代相比，近几十年来，神经鞘瘤的平均大小有所下降，诊断时听力方面表现更好（Gal et al.，2010；Stangerup et al.，2010）。

病因学、电离辐射和手机

神经鞘瘤是WHO Ⅰ级的良性肿瘤（图22.3）。恶性神经鞘瘤是罕见的，但在所有影像诊断的神经鞘瘤中，应该包括这个重要的鉴别诊断。如果有侵袭性的临床表现，则应该怀疑恶性的可能，并最终需要组织病理学评估和诊断。神经鞘瘤的遗传学特征已得到广泛的研究。突变通常存在于22q12.2号染色体上的神经纤维蛋白（NF2）基因中，该基因在大多数散发性前庭神经鞘瘤中被双向灭活，就像在2型神经纤维瘤病相关神经鞘瘤中一样。散发性肿瘤的突变通常是小缺失。该基因产物是一种590氨基酸蛋白，名为merlin（神经膜蛋白）（Lee et al.，2012；Lassaletta et al.，2013），其为一种肿瘤抑制基因。神

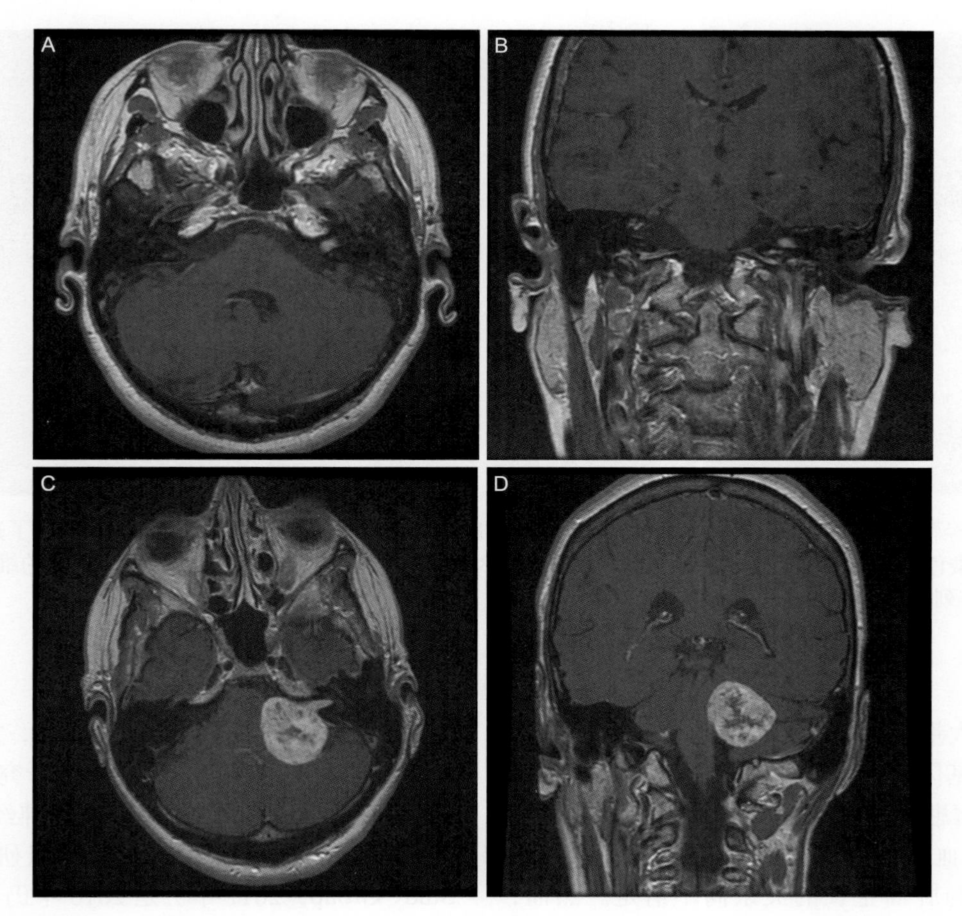

图 22.1 前庭神经鞘瘤 MRI。轴位（A）和冠状位（B）T1 加权 MRI 钆剂增强，可见内听道内前庭神经鞘瘤。轴位（C）和冠状位（D）T1 加权 MRI 钆增强，显示大型前庭神经鞘瘤伴脑干压迫

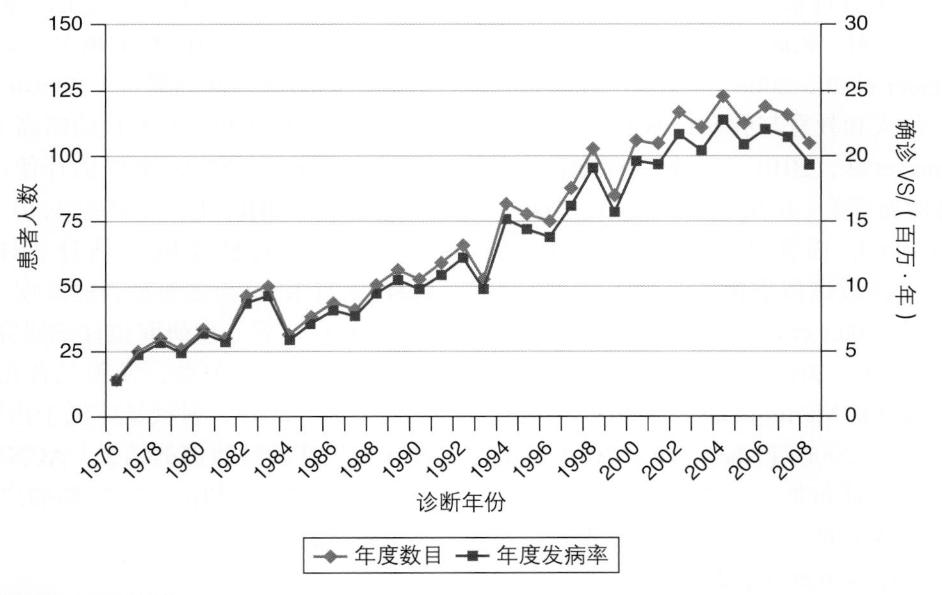

图 22.2 前庭神经鞘瘤的流行病学

Reprinted from *Otolaryngologic Clinics of North America*, Volume 45, issue 2, Sven- Eric Stangerup, Per Caye-Thomasen, Epidemiology and Natural History of Vestibular Schwannomas, pp. 257– 8, Copyright (2012), with permission from Elsevier.

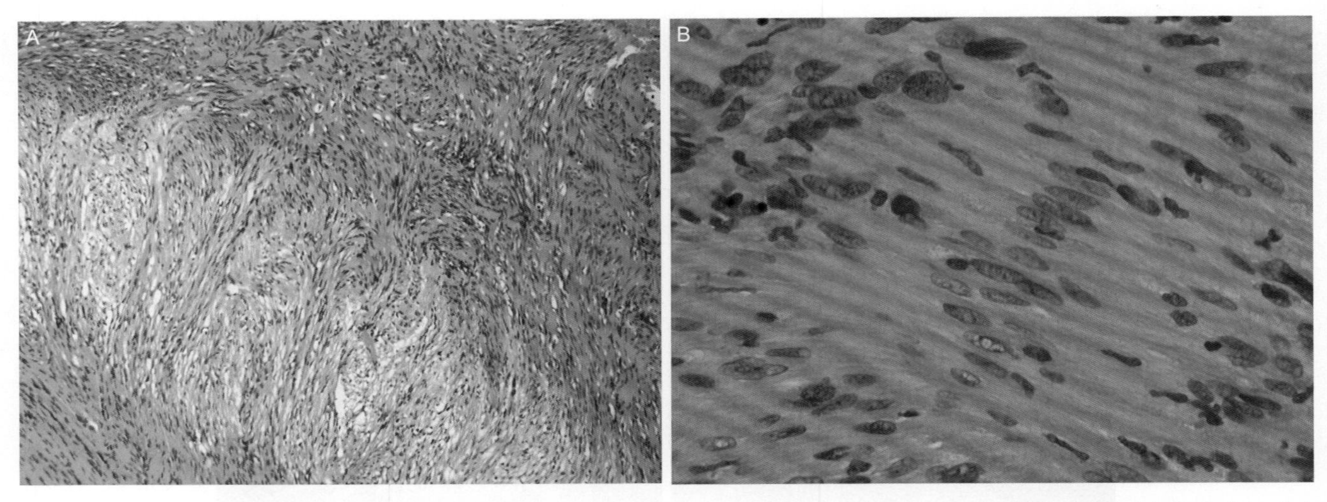

图 22.3 前庭神经鞘瘤的组织病理学。(A)神经鞘瘤(H&E，×100)。两种不同的组织学模式表征了这些肿瘤。致密、高细胞区和苍白染色的低细胞区分别称为 AntoniA 和 AntoniB 组织。神经鞘瘤(H&E，×400)。同名的维罗凯体(Verocay body)，由成排排列的肿瘤细胞核构成，为这些神经鞘瘤的一个特征

经膜蛋白抑制大量不同的细胞内生长促进信号，这可以解释单一基因缺陷增加了致瘤概率(**图 22.4**)。在前庭神经鞘瘤患者中，5%~10% 的患者在 9q34 或 17q 上有增加。血管生成是肿瘤生长不可缺少的，但血管生成因子与肿瘤生长的关系尚不清楚。然而，一些小型的研究发现，VEGF 抑制剂贝伐珠单抗可延缓神经鞘瘤的生长。

尽管其他环境和生物因素，如射频场、噪声、吸烟、化学品、社会经济地位、分娩和激素替代等已经进行了研究，散发性前庭神经鞘瘤唯一公认的危险因素是电离辐射(Ron et al.，1988；Preston et al.，2002；Schneider et al.，2008)。出乎意料的是，在两项研究中，收入和教育与肿瘤诊断有关(Inskip et al.，2003；Schuz et al.，2010)。分娩和激素替代治疗也与肿瘤风险增加有关(Schoemaker et al.，2007；Benson et al.，2010b)，而在两个病例对照和一个队列研究中目前正在吸烟似乎保护吸烟者免于发生神经鞘瘤(Schoemaker et al.，2007；Benson et al.，2010a；Palmisano et al.，2012)。噪声在 1985 年被报告为病因因素(Preston-Martin et al.，1989)，但无法证实(Edwards et al.，2006；Fisher et al.，2014)。化学暴露是难以回顾性评价的。石棉和甲苯显示出矛盾的结果，但众所周知的致癌物苯被反复报道与神经鞘瘤有关联(Pettersson et al.，2014)。

射频场和手机使用是否会导致神经鞘瘤属于一个有争议的领域(Pettersson et al.，2014)。Hardell 及其同事进行的病例对照研究表明，手机使用与患前庭神经鞘瘤风险之间存在剂量依赖性相关性(Hardell et al.，1999；Hardell et al.，2005；Hardell et al.，2013)。相比之下，更大的研究和前瞻性设计的研究未能证实手机使用与前庭神经鞘瘤之间的任何关联。INTERPHONE 病例对照研究(Interphone Study Group，2011 年)是 2016 年仍在进行的研究，对移动电话和前庭神经鞘瘤相关性进行的最大研究，发现经常使用移动电话的优势比为 0.85(95% CI，0.69~1.04)，≥10 年的移动电话使用的优势比为 0.76(95% CI，0.52~1.11)。在丹麦进行的一项队列研究发现，11 年或 11 年以上的手机用户的相对风险为 0.87(95% CI，0.52~1.46)(Schuz et al.，2011)。最近更新的英国队列研究(Benson et al.，2013)发现，任何使用手机的相对风险略高于 1(RR，1.19；95%CI，0.81~1.75)，类似估计使用 10 年或更长时间手机者(RR，1.17；95%CI，0.60~2.27)，以及 5~9 年使用的最高风险估计(RR，1.46；95%CI，0.94~2.27)，这与瑞典最新的发现一致(Petersson et al.，2014)。后一项研究也仔细研究了肿瘤侧别和首选打电话侧耳的关系，发现二者在发病概率上没有任何关联。此外，射频暴露低于指导限值的情况下，并未发生实验性致癌的结果(AGNIR，2012)。综上所述，使用手机和前庭神经鞘瘤之间并无强烈病因学关系支持证据。

自然历史

人们不再相信所有新诊断的肿瘤患者都会受益于手术。随后，MRI 随访期间的自然史数据已经可供参考使用。在许多患者中检测到肿瘤生长缓慢或

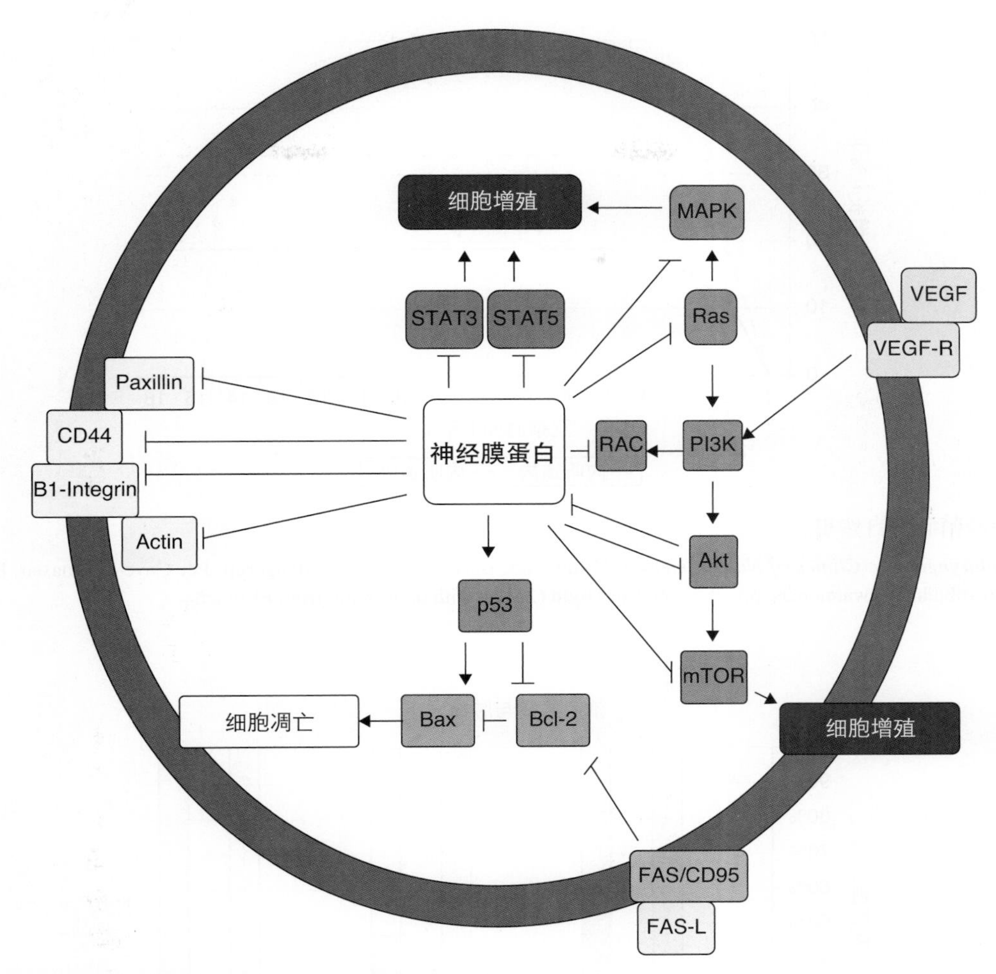

图 22.4　显示神经膜蛋白与细胞内级联分子相互作用的示意图

Reproduced from Sughrue, M. E., Yeung, A., Rutkowski, M. J., et al., Molecular biology of familial and sporadic vestibular schwannomas: implications for novel therapeutics, *Journal of Neurosurgery*, Vol. 114, No. 2 (2011) with permission from JNS Group.

无生长。对 26 项研究和 1340 名患者的 meta 分析（Yoshimoto，2005）显示，在 38 个月的平均随访期间，46% 的肿瘤变大（95%CI，43%~48%）和 8%（95%CI，6%~10%）的肿瘤变小。生长中的肿瘤的平均年增大 1.2 mm。许多进展中的肿瘤生长非常缓慢，只有 40% 得到治疗。自然史主要选择进行保守治疗的较小肿瘤进行研究，但也包括了一些较大肿瘤的患者；其中许多老年患者的肿瘤有回缩变小。因此，最初的保守治疗是可能的，特别是在老年患者，假如没有什么症状，尽管肿瘤很大，仍然可以保守治疗。

对良性肿瘤来说，38 个月是短期随访，但也有更长的随访研究。Stangerup 和 Caye Thomasen 等（2012）发现，在对小于 20 mm 的内听道内外肿瘤进行长期随访期间，增大者为 29%，缩小者为 1%（图 22.5）。对于内听道内肿瘤，Kirchmann 等（2017）发现经过 9.5 年的随访，肿瘤有生长的占 37%，其中 61% 的肿瘤生长到颅后窝。Stangerup 和 Kirchmann 在随访第五年之后，发现后续肿瘤都没有进展。

治疗目标

大多数前庭神经鞘瘤的生长缓慢，在放射影像学监测下，能得到安全管理，而不需要都进行手术。前庭神经鞘瘤手术例数已经有所减少。最近，美国 17% 登记的前庭神经鞘瘤患者进行影像扫描和随访观察，21% 的患者接受了放射外科治疗（Gal et al.，2010）。治疗目标已从彻底切除肿瘤转变为肿瘤控制和维持神经功能（Kemink et al.，1991；Park et al.，2006；Seol et al.，2006）。许多小肿瘤通过放射外科治疗，或者影像学随访监测，以选择生长较快的病变进行治疗。较大的肿瘤更多地使用大部切除或部分切除（图 22.6）。通常，外科手术的一个目标是消剪残余肿瘤至最大程度，为伽玛刀放射外科创造条件。次全切除肿瘤减少了分离肿瘤 - 神经界面时，使已

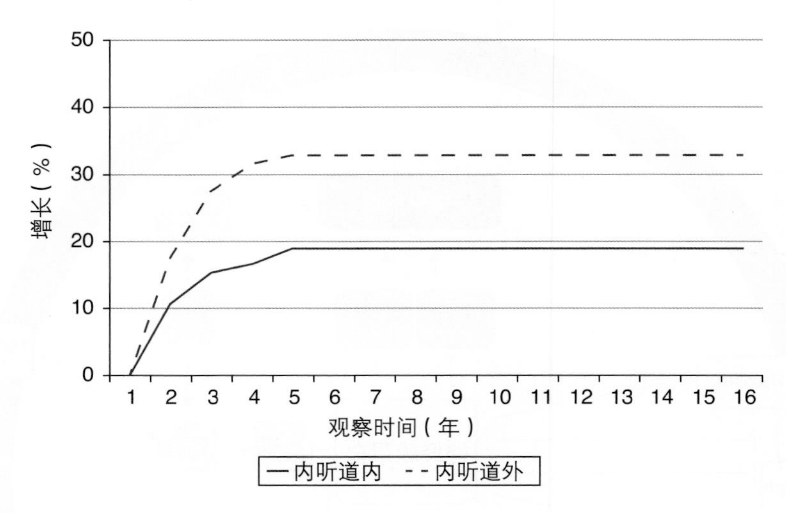

图 22.5 前庭神经鞘瘤的自然史

Reprinted from *Otolaryngologic Clinics of North America*, Volume 45, issue 2, Sven-Eric Stangerup, Per Caye-Thomasen, Epidemiology and Natural History of Vestibular Schwannomas, pp. 257– 68, Copyright (2012), with permission from Elsevier.

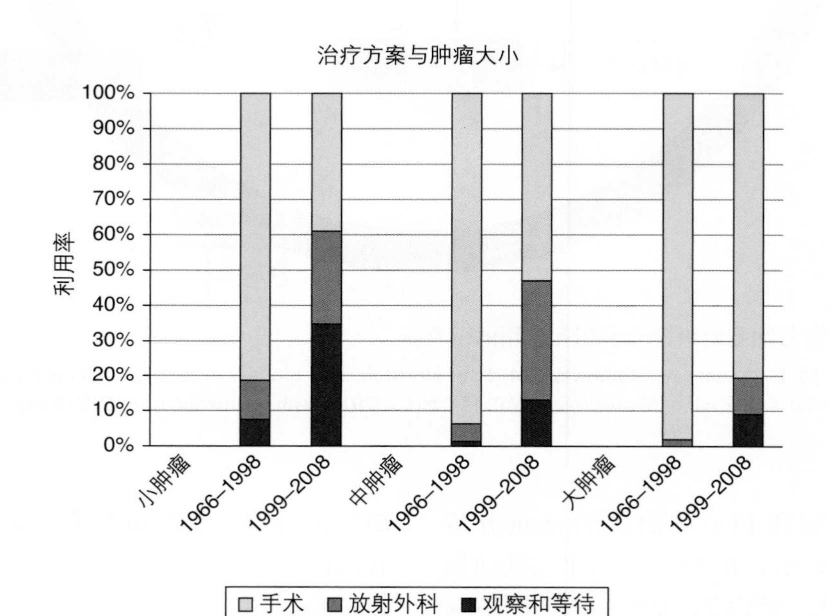

图 22.6 前庭神经鞘瘤的处理措施的改变。在这个图中，肿瘤大小被定义为小（<1.5 cm）、中（1.5~2.5 cm）和大（>2.5 cm）

Reproduced with permission from Jaymin Patel, Rohit Vasan, Harry van Loveren, et al, The changing face of acoustic neuroma management in the USA: Analysis of the 1998 and 2008 patient surveys from the acoustic neuroma association, *British Journal of Neurosurgery*, Volume 28, Issue 1, 2014 © The Neurosurgical Foundation, reprinted by permission of Taylor & Francis Ltd, www.tandfonline.com on behalf of The Neurosurgical Foundation.

经受损神经功能变差的概率，并且与更佳的面神经结果相关（Park et al.，2006；Schwartz et al.，2013）。对于较大肿瘤，大部切除时听力保存的概率更高（Iwai et al.，2015）。虽然所有已知前庭神经鞘瘤患者的并发症比例可能有所下降，但实际并发症数量有所增加（Patel et al.，2013）。这一矛盾结果反映了由于对不同的病例进行混合分析研究，增加了大肿瘤的比例，但也有手术经验不足的问题存在。持续关注主要的临床神经功能的结果和外科技术是很重要的（Rahimpour et al.，2016）；非彻底切除肿瘤的手术比例也将随之增加。

残余神经鞘瘤的生长

较低的根治性切除会转化为较高的肿瘤复发率。切除程度与复发风险之间的关系可能取决于手术技术、肿瘤生物学特征和病例的选择。此外，不同外科医生和医学中心之间随访策略可能会有差异。Bloch 等描述了近全切除后 5 年内 3% 的复发率和次全切除后 32% 的复发率（Bloch et al., 2004）；Schwartz 等平均随访 3.7~3.9 年，发现复发率为 21%~22%，（Schwartz et al., 2013）。几个后续的患者系列报道中，未能证实这种近全切除和大部切除之间复发率的差异，取而代之，他们描述了 5 年的复发率为 7%~9%。在近全切除和大部切除的患者之间，肿瘤复发率没有重大差异（Sughrue et al., 2011; Chen et al., 2014b; Syed et al., 2017）（**图 22.7**）。回顾性复发数据也很难评估，因为放射学显示的进展并不一定意味着治疗失败，也并未提示达到需要额外进一步治疗的程度；在大多数系列报道中，只有大约一半已显示复发的患者接受了额外的治疗（Sughrue et al., 2011; Syed et al., 2017）。所有残瘤在生物学上并不相等。内听道内残留肿瘤的血供丰富，其潜在复发概率更高，而脑干上孤立的残余肿瘤具有更低的能量和营养供应。在小的偶然发现的神经鞘瘤中，通常在保守治疗的 3~5 年内可以检测到生长（Stangerup and Caye-Thomasen, 2012），但偶然发现的有惰性的肿瘤，其生物学行为与曾经是大病变的残余肿瘤可能有所不同。实际上长期随访的数据是缺乏的，我们不知道即使进行更长的随访，残瘤的复发率将如何增加。

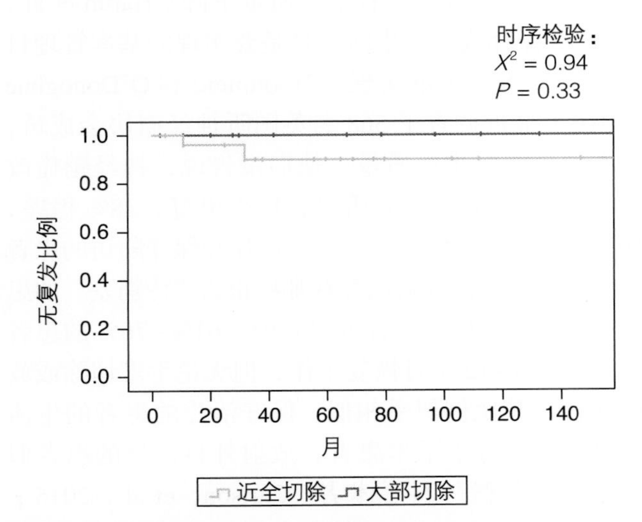

图 22.7 前庭神经鞘瘤大部切除和近全切除术后复发

Reproduced with permission from M.I. Syed et al., The behaviour of residual tumour after the intentional incomplete excision of a vestibular schwannoma: is it such a bad thing to leave some behind?, *Clinical Otolaryngology*, Volume 42, Copyright © 2016 John Wiley and Sons.

初次伽玛刀放射外科治疗和肿瘤控制

放射外科利用多个聚焦光束可以实现边界剂量锐利的梯度下降，只有在较小的治疗体积情况下在几何上是可能实现的。因此，小肿瘤是最常见适应证。初期，在大多数患者中都能看到肿瘤皱缩，这是预期的治疗效果。1969 年至 1974 年，最初有 9 个病例进行了放射外科治疗。1993 年，Norén 等报告了最早一组 254 名患者（Norén et al., 1993）。他发现 55% 患者肿瘤缩小，33% 患者肿瘤大小稳定和 77% 的患者听力保留，但暂时性的面部不适和三叉神经障碍发生率较高。随后，将照射剂量减少，没有发现肿瘤控制率的降低，从而将放射的并发症最小化。治疗的目标从皱缩转向"控制"，其定义为长期随访时间至少超过 1~2 年而肿瘤无进展。重要的是，成功的治疗包括治疗后高达 30% 的患者出现肿瘤肿胀。最近有文献（Boari et al., 2014）报道，患者接受的边缘剂量约为 13 Gy，肿瘤控制率为 97%，平均随访 6 年；平均随访 9 年的肿瘤控制率为 92%（54）；平均随访 12.5 年（最低 10 年）肿瘤控制率也是 92%（Hasegawa et al., 2013）。如果患者有可用听力，则将边缘剂量从 12 Gy 减少到 11 Gy（Régis et al., 2013a）。怀疑早期治疗失败而选择再治疗，或者只选择 Koos 1 级肿瘤的患者，肿瘤长期控制率为 98%~99%（Régis et al., 2013a）。前庭神经鞘瘤 Koos 分级见**表 22.1**。然而，在文献报道的病例系列中，控制率确实并不一定能反映真实治疗效果。控制率可以调整，以示放射外科对肿瘤生长控制作用，而自然史不会导致大多数肿瘤的进展。Miller 等（2014）估计，实际上放射外科取得的 10 年控制率为 78%~87%，他们还讨论了放射外科的控制作用在稳

表 22.1 Koos 分级量表

等级	说明
1	肿瘤仅局限于内耳道
2	肿瘤延伸到桥小脑角，但不侵犯脑干
3	肿瘤充满整个桥小脑角
4	肿瘤压迫推移脑干和邻近的脑神经

Source data from Koos, W. T., Day, J., Matula, C., & Levy, D. I. (1998). Neurotopographic considerations in the microsurgical treatment of small acoustic neurinomas, *Journal of Neurosurgery*, 88(3), 506–512.

定的肿瘤和治疗前再生长的肿瘤之间是否存在差异。然而，调查人员分别研究这些队列的数据，发现之前的肿瘤的生长速度对后续肿瘤长期控制没有任何影响（Meijer et al.，2008；Niu et al.，2014；Wangerid et al.，2014）（图 22.8）。文献报道分次放疗对前庭神经鞘瘤的治疗获得了成功，但由于病例选择的标准不同以及时间有限的随访，使我们很难得出其长期效果的结论（Combs et al.，2005；Choy et al.，2013；Litre et al.，2013）。

联合显微外科、放射外科、补救性放射外科的肿瘤控制

该治疗计划的理论基础在于能接受次全切除后高达 30% 的复发风险，包括随后的放射外科手术和相信后续的放射外科能够控制肿瘤。Hori 等报道对残留肿瘤，不论稳定的肿瘤或继续生长的肿瘤共 11 例实行放射外科手术，11 例肿瘤均得到控制（Hori and Maruyama，2013），而其他人报道的肿瘤控制率约为 90%，结果与最初进行治疗的神经鞘瘤的长期随访数据类似。van de Langenberg 等（2011）报告说，在对大神经鞘瘤有意进行次全切除手术后，随访不到 3 年，肿瘤控制率为 90%。Rowe 等（2007）和 Iwai 等（2015）选择伽马刀放射外科手术，发现 10 年期肿瘤控制率为 86%，95% 患者的面神经功能为 House-Brackman 1~2 级，42% 的患者听力保留。对于已手术的神经鞘瘤，肿瘤体积大（>6 cm^3）是治疗失败的一个危险因素，需要在少数患者中进行补救性救手术。电离辐射是发生肿瘤的一个既定危险因素，一些病例报告描述了放射外科治疗的患者中肿瘤出现迅速增长，甚至发生了胶质瘤。然而，事实上其绝对风险很低。对已治疗患者的回顾性综述和对恶性神经鞘瘤的评估分析，并不支持放疗造成肿瘤恶变或以某种可检测到的特定速率诱导形成继发性恶性肿瘤（Demetriades et al.，2010）。大量文献报道支持对残留和复发肿瘤选择放射外科或显微外科治疗（Jeltema et al.，2015；Nonaka et al.，2016；Samii et al.，2016b；Wise et al.，2016；Huang et al.，2017）。

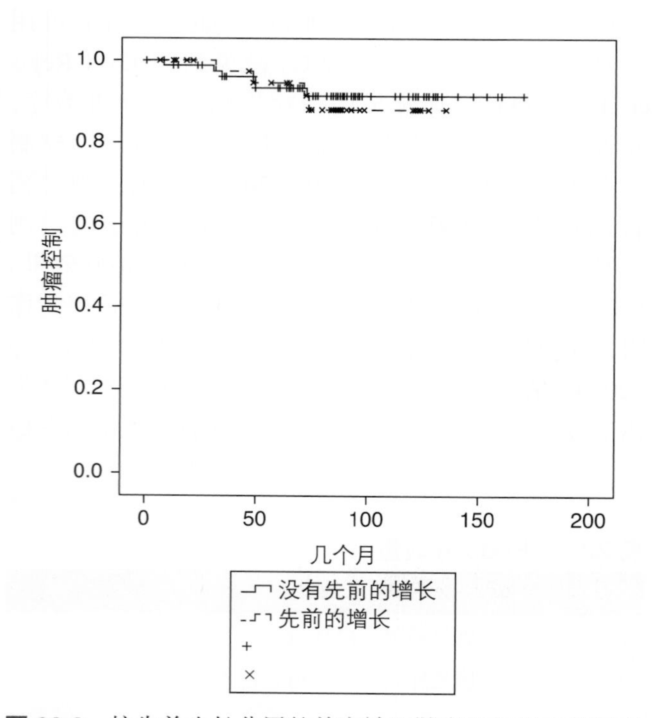

图 22.8 按先前生长分层的前庭神经鞘瘤的伽玛刀控制率

Reproduced with permission from Theresa Wangerid, Jiri Bartek, Mikael Svensson et al., Long- term quality of life and tumour control following gamma knife radiosurgery for vestibular schwannoma, *Acta Neurochirurgica*, Volume 156, Issue 2, pp. 389– 96, Copyright © 2013 Springer Nature.

症状和生活质量

在诊断时，大多数患者有典型的三联征中的一个或多个症状：听力障碍、眩晕和耳鸣。Harun 等在连续 1200 例患者中，报告了这三个症状发生率分别为 93%、67% 和 84%（Harun et al.，2012）。面部神经和三叉神经也可能受到影响，但更多的是通过治疗受到影响；头痛可能是治疗前的一种症状，但在手术后仍然存在或发生。神经系统症状的核心是主观上的不适和痛苦，因为只有一小部分患者的肿瘤会有潜在危及生命的可能。与参照人群相比，前庭神经鞘瘤患者确实有生活质量下降（Harun et al.，2012）。保存或恢复生活质量是要实现的基本管理目标，但事实上很难实现。Broomfield 和 O'Donoghue（2016）最近调查了 568 名英国听神经瘤协会成员，调查的核心是生活质量，他们报告说，神经鞘瘤改变了他们整体的生活质量，18% 更好，38% 稍差，19% 特别差。"稍差"在接受治疗和保守随访的患者中分布平均，而外科治疗在那些报告"特别差"的患者中占主导地位。在各种研究中，61%~76% 的患者在治疗后 6~12 个月恢复工作，但无论手术切除或放射外科，其比例似乎相似。保守治疗的患者的生活质量似乎略好于手术患者，放射外科治疗的患者似乎略好于显微外科手术者（Carlson，et al.，2015；Golfinos et al.，2016）。综上所述，治疗效果和治疗之间的差异很难评估。生活质量是一个不可靠的术语。医生更关心与健康相关的问题，特别是那些受到特定疾病及其治疗影响的问题。最常见的仪器 SF-36 实际上是测量健康相关因素，而不是实际生活质量。

尽管患者健康状况良好，治疗并发症很低，但生活质量可能依然很低，反之亦然。我们要优先处理的事项是疾病的具体症状及其对健康的相对影响（**图22.9**）。即使如此，这个话题仍然是复杂的，并受到个人处理方式、神经功能障碍的持续性、持续时间、患者期望值以及护理者如何实际处理不同症状的影响。教科书知识包括对面神经功能、耳鸣和单侧听力丧失的关注，但 Carlson 和同事的前瞻性研究却将头晕和头痛描述为长期生活质量下降的最强预测因素（Carlson et al.，2015a；Carlson et al.，2015b）。将经常出现的缺陷如听力损失和面神经功能与间歇性功能障碍如头晕和头痛进行比较是十分困难的。持续的症状可能被列为不那么麻烦，因为它们是可预测的并可以调整的。护理人员能意识到这些问题可能更好，在治疗前有意识地处理这些神经功能障碍，在治疗期间并在随后的康复中尽量避免这些问题。

观察和扫描、显微手术或放射外科：伴随听力障碍和听力恶化

根据美国耳鼻咽喉头颈外科协会（AAO-HNS）A 类或 B 类和 Gardner-Bobertson 分类的Ⅰ类或Ⅱ类，保留听力和有用听力通常被定义为纯音测听（pure-tone audiogram，PTA）下降小于 50 dB，言语分辨率（Speech Discrimination Score，SDS）评分大于 50%。Gardner-Bobertson 分类在**第 25 章**中描述。在 538 名患者的前瞻性研究中，11% 的患者有 A 类听力，12% 的患者有 B 类听力（Tveiten et al.，2015）。一个由 128 名患者组成的亚组仅观察了 7 年，A 类听力从 32% 下降到 22%，B 类听力从 32% 下降到 23%，C 类听力从 8% 上升到 11%，D 类听力从 30% 上升到44%。Sughrue 发现在随访的26~52个月期间，50% 的功能性听力丧失（Sughrue et al.，2010），而 Stangerup 等（2008）跟踪 334 例听力良好和言语分辨率超过 70% 的患者，适合“观察和扫描”，持续随访 10 年。在那些患者身上，听力只保留了 31%。然而，纳入的 SDS 很好（100%）的患者随访 10 年听力的保存率为 88%。内听道内神经鞘瘤包括一个亚组肿瘤特别小，未经治疗，随访 9.5 年，听力学测量的可用听力平均保存率为 34%，言语分辨保存率为 58%（Kirchmann et al.，2017）。在平均 44 个月的随访中，Régis（Régis et al.，2013a）发现 38% 的患者听力损失超过 10 dB，其中 5% 的人耳聋。对大多数患者来说，未治疗患者的听力结果是令人沮丧的。

在治疗后，选择显微手术的病例显示，在回顾性系列报道中，8%~51% 的患者保持了可用听力（Samii et al.，2006；Tveiten et al.，2015）。在显微外科亚组中，包括 539 名前瞻性队列研究中的 139 名患者，14% 的患者保留了可用听力（Tveiten et al.，2015）。显微手术系列的结果变异范围较大，这也反映了他们选择手术患者的标准不同和手术时机各异。

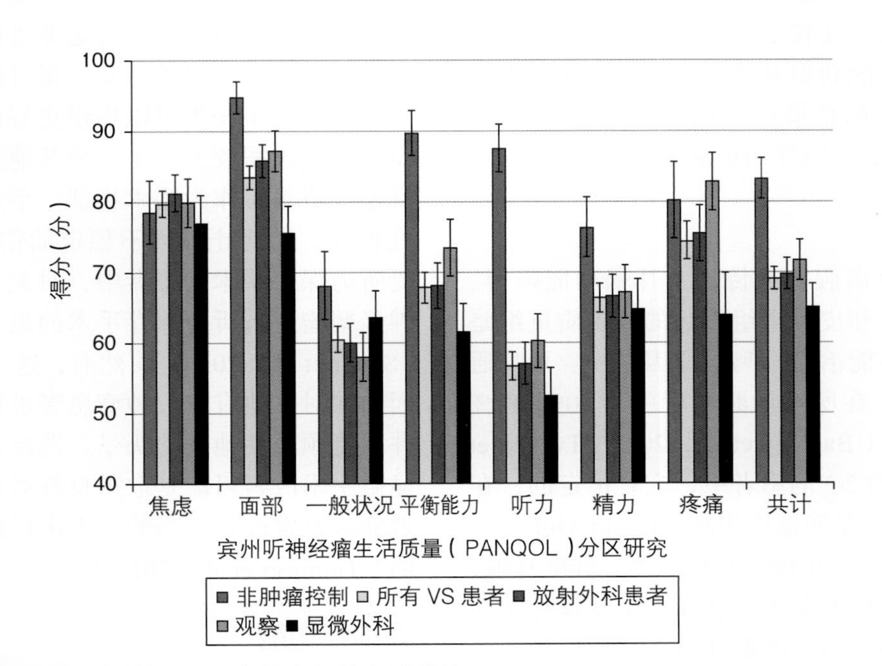

图 22.9 前庭神经鞘瘤特定疾病结果的长期健康相关生活质量

Carlson, M., Tveiten, O., and Driscoll, C., et al, Long-term quality of life in patients with vestibular schwannoma: an international multicenter cross-sectional study comparing microsurgery, stereotactic radiosurgery, observation, and nontumor controls, *Journal of Neurosurgery*, Vol. 122, No. 4 (2015) with permission from JNS Group.

然而，最重要的是，个人手术技能和患者选择经验对于显微手术结果至关重要，经验丰富的外科医生一贯报告选定特定患者，并能预测术后可获得良好听力（Samii et al.，2006；Rahimpour et al.，2016）。系列研究报道，根据患者的选择，显示听力保存从10%~70%。然而，在最初有利的听力结果之后，15%~20%的患者可能会进一步丧失最初保留的听力（Wang et al.，2013）。

在放射外科手术后，听力将进一步下降，在头两年，听力下降5.9 dB/年，此后听力下降1.9 dB/年（Yomo et al.，2012），并可能发生突发性耳聋。Carlson等（Carlson et al.，2013）描述了10年后可用听力23%保存，这与肿瘤自然发展史相近。关于放射外科潜在益处的比较数据结果互相冲突。在一项公开的前瞻性比较研究中，Régis等发现放射外科治疗后听力的保留率为60%，而在5年后未经治疗的对照组中听力保留率为14%（Régis et al.，2013b）。Boari声称在治疗前听力良好的年轻患者中取得了特别好的效果（Boari et al.，2014）。相反，Tveiten等在两个中心的前瞻性实验中并未发现其优势。他们的放射外科队列研究包括240名患者，随访7年；其中A级听力患者从25%下降到7%，B级听力患者从22%下降到12%，C类患者从12%下降到11%，D类从41%增加到70%。放射外科与自然史之间的听力保护的明显差异无法断言，放射外科手术后的结果实际上更糟（Tveiten et al.，2015）。两项正在进行的随机对照研究比较了最初的放射外科和最初的保守治疗，希望能获得对放射外科的潜在听力保护效果让人有信心的结果（https://www.clinicaltrials.gov：NCT 02249572 和 NCT 01938677）。

耳鸣

耳鸣被推测是由假突触传递、耳蜗功能障碍、前庭传出纤维丧失和皮质重组引起的。皮质重组是耳蜗神经切断术不能治愈耳鸣的原因之一。耳鸣通常具有高频音高，在所有诊断患者中有70%~80%的患者发现耳鸣（Baguley et al.，2006；Tveiten et al.，2015）。在大约2/3的患者中，它是恒定的，在其余的1/3的患者中是间歇性出现。David Moffat小组将耳鸣归类为轻度、中度、重度三型。轻度耳鸣，这种耳鸣只在静默状态下才能感知，中度耳鸣在环境背景噪声也能感知到；严重耳鸣甚至能干扰患者的睡眠（Quaranta et al.，2007）。他们发现患者中度耳鸣占2%~26%，重度耳鸣占11%~24%。耳鸣的治疗效果是变化不定的，而且其效果不能充分复制。一些作者认为，耳鸣可以通过在手术中保留听力得到改善或耳蜗神经切断来改善，而不是保留一个无功能的神经。然而，耳鸣的结果是不可预测的，在保守治疗、显微外科和放射外科之间没有统计学差异。在平均随访3年期间，大多数患者报告耳鸣没有变化，改善了6%，恶化了16%（Quaranta et al.，2007）。耳鸣本身并不是外科治疗的适应证，在较大的人群中也没有发现耳鸣明显地影响患者生活质量，尽管个别患者可能会经历被描述为灾难性的不适。耳鸣引起的残疾与严重程度没有直接关系。随着时间的推移，大多数患者似乎适应了存在的耳鸣。

眩晕和头晕

头晕是前庭神经鞘瘤患者生活质量的最重要的听-前庭预测指标，无论保守治疗还是积极治疗，其与散发性前庭神经鞘瘤患者的长期生活质量下降密切相关（Gauden et al.，2011；Jufas et al.，2015）。超过50%的前庭神经鞘瘤患者有头晕，通常步态不稳和眩晕仅占8%，而且在诊断后8年症状仍然存在（Carlson et al.，2014）。一项前瞻性队列研究（Andersen et al.，2015）报告，在初始阶段，旋转性眩晕占11%，严重头晕占9%。在70%以上的被调查患者中，能检测到对水平半规管的冷热水试验（“管性瘫痪”）反应丧失。管性瘫痪和体位不稳与中重度头晕有关，而与听力和肿瘤大小的关系则不太清楚。中枢性补偿允许调整和适应，随后，尽管前庭功能丧失，特别是当前庭丧失是渐进的，大量神经鞘瘤患者并不会有头晕的感觉。很可能较大的肿瘤和前庭功能的逐步丧失可以提供更好的补偿和调适。在没有肿瘤体积较大、生长或其他症状的情况下，通常不能将头晕作为手术指征。手术确实允许切断前庭神经，以终止任何不稳定的信号。在17/19名接受听力保存手术的患者中，对无其他症状的小前庭神经鞘瘤进行听力保存手术的患者解决了眩晕障碍（Samii et al.，2016a）。然而，这一说法是有争议的，因为在对其他有较大肿瘤患者进行的研究中，手术并不能预测性地改善头晕。选择合适的患者和通过显微手术改善可能是取得良好效果的关键。许多患者症状自发改善，当然，手术后前庭康复也是必要的（Thomeer et al.，2015）。

面神经功能

面神经麻痹与听力障碍被细化并分级，二者被列为前庭神经鞘瘤治疗后最明显的损害（Carlson，Tveiten et al.，2015）。**表** 22.2 为 House-Brackmann

表 22.2 House-Brackmann 评分

等级	总功能	动作
1 正常	各区域正常对称功能	
2 轻度功能障碍	眼睑闭合时检查时轻微无力 可能有轻微的同步运动 静止，正常对称	前额 - 中等到良好的功能 眼睛 - 最小的努力即可完成关闭 嘴 - 轻度不对称
3 中度功能障碍	两侧明显的，但不是毁容的差异 明显的（但不严重的）同步运动、挛缩或面肌痉挛 静息时，正常的对称和张力	前额 - 轻到适度的运动 眼睛 - 努力完全关闭 嘴 - 最大的努力，轻度力弱
4 中度严重的功能障碍	明显的无力和（或）不对称变形 静息时，正常的对称和张力	前额 - 无运动 眼睛 - 没有完全关闭 嘴 - 最大努力仍不对称
5 严重的功能障碍	只有几乎看不到的运动静息时，不对称	前额 - 没有 眼睛 - 不完全关闭 嘴 - 轻微运动
6 完全瘫痪	无运动	

面神经功能评分系统表。面神经功能障碍会引起角膜失去保护，饮水、进食、说话等方面都出现困难。此外，心理困扰会导致自尊心下降、焦虑和抑郁，这是面瘫患者社会交往能力障碍的最重要的预测因素（VanSwearingen et al.，1998）。但出乎意料的是，面神经功能障碍对长期生活质量评分的影响很小（Carlson et al.，2015b）。Lassaletta 等（2013）表明，明显可见的面神经麻痹导致外科医生过度地强调面瘫，而不是其他术后症状，此点获得很多临床医生一致同意。

前庭神经鞘瘤患者很少（<5%）出现面神经功能障碍，有面瘫则提示面神经鞘瘤的可能性大大增加。面神经受累主要见于肿瘤比较大的患者。因此，在随访观察非生长的肿瘤时，预计不会发生新的面神经功能障碍。显微手术后，面神经结果能反映手术的技能和目标是否达成。风险随肿瘤大小、切除程度和手术经验而变化。对于较大的肿瘤来说，暂时的面肌无力是相当常见的，而永久性的面神经障碍发生率为 20%，基本是在大肿瘤完全切除术后；而在较小或次全切除的肿瘤中永久性面瘫发生率要低得多。放射外科手术采用低辐射剂量、高分辨率 MRI 和更先进的手术计划系统，使面神经障碍发生率更低；它们发生在不到 1% 的患者中（Yang et al.，2009；Régis et al.，2013a；Wangerid et al.，2014）。

中间神经损伤可能发生在 50% 以上的显微外科手术患者中，但只有在特别探究时才能经常注意到（Yang et al.，2009；Noonan et al.，2016）。症状包括眼睛干燥和味觉改变。当伴发角膜感觉缺失或眼睑不能覆盖角膜时，泌泪缺乏会带来更多问题。如果味觉对他们工作来说很重要，味觉障碍可能严重影响其生活质量。

头痛

在回顾性研究（Carlson et al.，2015a）和前庭神经鞘瘤手术后的调查中，0~77% 的参与者报告了持续性头痛。头痛通常是紧张型的头痛。在三个月后，头痛经常是最严重的时候，但随后疼痛程度下降，许多患者在进一步的随访中，头痛变得不那么明显。乙状窦后开颅术后头痛不适的主诉较多，随后按因果关系的推测分析，可能与切口愈合后硬脑膜的牵张、无菌性脑膜炎、脑脊液假性囊肿、磨钻形成的骨末刺激以及静脉窦狭窄引起颅内压轻度升高有关。每一种理论分析都需要验证，且均已通过临床的案例得到证实，例如通过使用超声骨刀去骨代替磨钻磨除骨质，以减少骨末量的措施确实降低了头痛的发生率。直到最近，Carlson 等前瞻性地对随访观察、显微外科或放射外科治疗神经鞘瘤患者的头痛（Carlson et al.，2015a）进行了研究。在报告中头痛的发病率为60%，这与一般人群一生中头痛的估计发病率一致。观察后头痛改善10%，放射外科治疗后头痛改善14%，显微外科治疗头痛后改善19%；观察后10%头痛恶化，放射外科治疗后14%头痛恶化，显微外科治疗后25%头痛恶化。尽管显微手术在治疗后第一年与更多的头痛有关，长期结果并不显示两组之间有统计学上的显著差异。发病时比较年轻，以前有偏头痛，既往有头痛史和严重的焦虑和抑郁预示治疗后更糟糕的头痛，这也是一般人群头痛的常见因素。在所有患者中，6%~9%的患者，无论治疗如何，1年后头痛仍然严重，其是生活质量下降的重要原因。保守治疗的前庭神经鞘瘤患者头痛的发生率是对照组的两倍（Breivik et al.，2012）。

非前庭神经鞘瘤

在生物学和病理学上，非前庭神经鞘瘤与前庭神经鞘瘤非常相似。它们生长缓慢，似乎也对放射外科有反应（Pollock et al.，2002）。流行病学数据来源于专科中心的外科患者系列，可能反映了一定的选择偏差。然而，很明显，非前庭神经鞘瘤是罕见的，占颅内神经鞘瘤的6%~10%，或不到所有颅内肿瘤的1%。其中最常见的是三叉神经鞘瘤，其次是颈静脉孔鞘瘤和面神经鞘瘤。

依此顺序，在动眼、滑车、舌下神经和展神经上发现了十分罕见的神经鞘瘤。耳蜗或前庭也可能发生肿瘤。在第三脑室、垂体或额叶基底部发现了与脑神经无关的偶发神经鞘瘤。神经鞘瘤也发生在脑外的头颈部，在眶内和身体的其他地方，但不在本章讨论范围内。

三叉神经鞘瘤

三叉神经鞘瘤占颅内神经鞘瘤的1%~8%（MacNally et al.，2008；Chen et al.，2014a）（图22.10）。最常见的症状是面部感觉减退，其次是头痛、头晕和共济失调。肿瘤可以起自三叉神经根、神经节和神经的任何部分，尽管集中在神经节周围是最常见的。肿瘤最初是由Geofrey Jefferson（Jefferson，

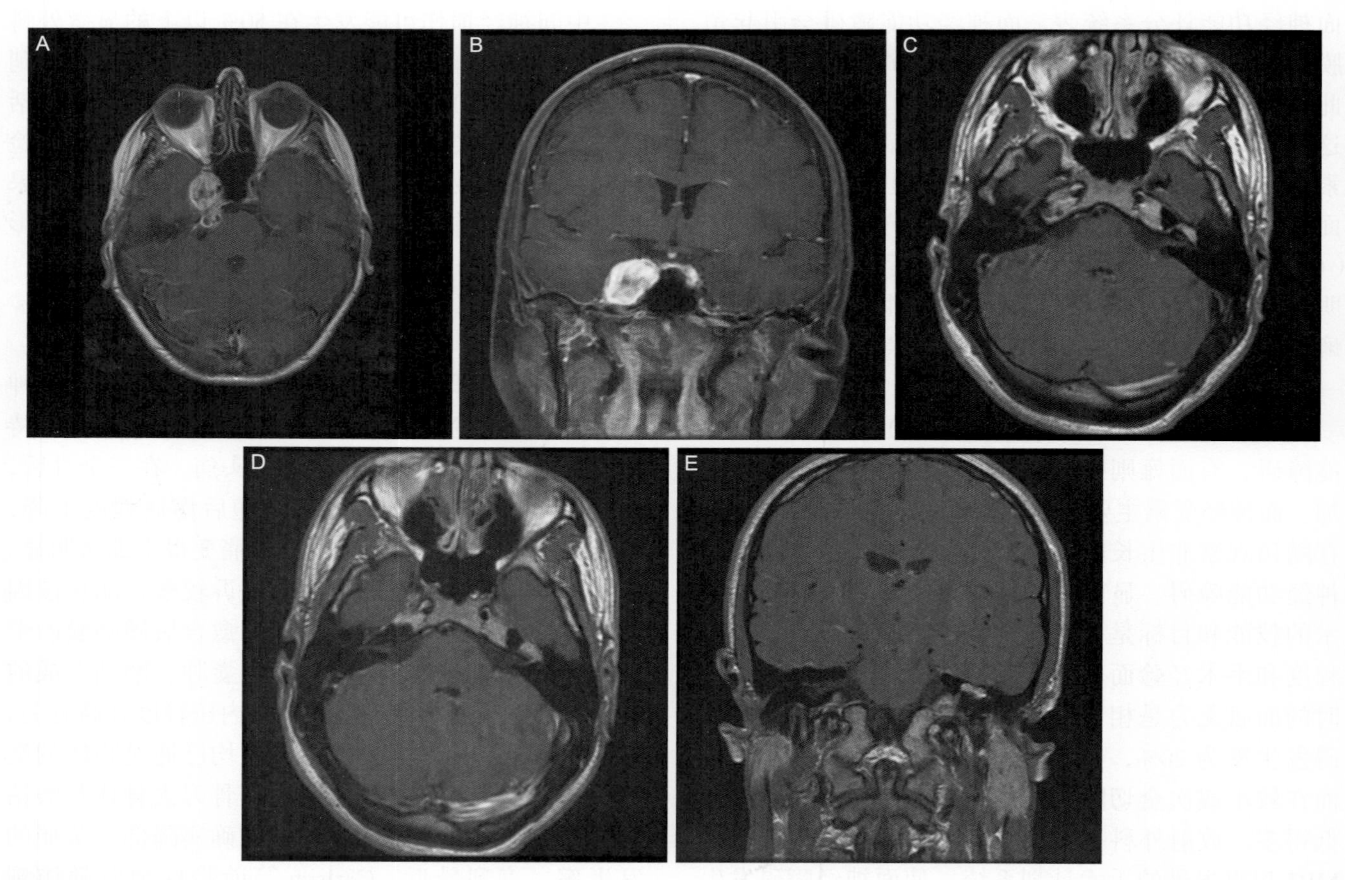

图 22.10 三叉神经和面部神经鞘瘤。轴位（A）和冠状位（B）T1加权MRI与钆强化扫描提示三叉神经神经鞘瘤。轴位图像表现为典型的哑铃形，其中一部分从Meckel腔延伸到颅后窝，一部分从海绵窦延伸到中颅窝。轴位（C、D）和冠状位（E）T1加权MRI钆增强成像，提示左侧增强神经鞘瘤沿膝状神经节两侧的迷路和鼓室段延伸

1953）根据其位置分类为 A~C，而“D”则是后来添加的（**表** 22.3）。最常见的位置是 C，它表现为一个哑铃肿瘤骑跨在岩骨上，通过三叉神经孔从中颅窝延伸到颅后窝。

与前庭神经鞘瘤相似，处理的重点目标已经从根治性切除转变为功能的保留和肿瘤的长期控制。因此，三叉神经鞘瘤显微外科目的是切除肿瘤主体和保留完整的神经根，除非临床行为或组织病理学表明为侵袭性肿瘤。显微外科手术和颅底技术的发展增加了三叉神经神经鞘瘤的全切率，这些肿瘤在显微外科手术发展之前很少被彻底切除。主体位于海绵窦的神经鞘瘤，可以优先采用 Dolenc 技术的额颞入路（Dolenc，1994），包括硬膜外切除前床突和海绵窦外侧壁两层硬脑膜分离技术，即将颞底的硬膜自海绵窦外侧壁的内层上解剖分离下来。在肿瘤向颅后窝中度扩展的患者中，颅后窝的肿瘤可以通过扩大的三叉神经孔彻底切除或者几乎完全去除。颅后窝部分的肿瘤较大时，需要切开小脑幕并磨除岩骨嵴前部或采用第二个入路（枕下乙状窦后入路），才能完全切除（Yoshida and Kawase，1999）。枕下入路的通道对颅后窝肿瘤是足够的，可以在硬膜下磨除部分岩骨（尖），从颅后窝进入 Meckel 腔。显微手术切除小三叉神经鞘瘤是可行的而且并发症很低。放射外科对小神经鞘瘤通常也能理想控制，肿瘤过大或者接近视路结构是放射外科的禁忌。放射外科治疗三叉神经鞘瘤失败的病例，或者为了保留功能而行保守治疗无效而肿瘤继续增长的病例，手术并发症并没有增加。对于那些主要向颈动脉内侧扩展的患者，可以考虑采用扩大的经鼻内镜下经翼突入路。进入上颌窦后，磨开上颌窦后壁进入翼腭窝和颞下窝。在岩尖，三叉神经节骑跨岩骨段颈内动脉水平段的两侧。

表 22.3　三叉神经鞘瘤改良的 Jeffersson 分类

类型	主要部位	发生率
A	颅中窝	40%
B	颅后窝	22%
C	哑铃瘤；颅中窝、颅后窝	32%
D	起自节后神经	6%

Reproduced with permission from S. P. MacNally, S. A. Rutherford, R. T. Ramsden, et al, Trigeminal schwannomas, *British Journal of Neurosurgery*, Volume 22, Issue 6, 2008

手术后三叉神经功能的结果取决于手术技术和优先要处理的事项；通过精微的颅底显微手术技术和近全切除或大部切除术，可以有较高程度的手术根治性，术后有 10% 的感觉改善和不到 10% 的恶化（Chen et al.，2014a），而早期或更多的根治性系列报道报告了较高的三叉神经功能丧失率。较大肿瘤和海绵窦延伸的手术可能导致复视，死亡病例发生在较早的报道中。尽管视觉缺损较小，三叉神经功能障碍是非常麻烦的。Westerlund 研究了颅底脑膜瘤患者新出现的三叉神经症状（Westerlund et al.，2012），大多数患者似乎适应了麻木或轻微的神经病理性疼痛，而眼部症状和罕见的痛性感觉缺失是主要并发症。

第三、第四和第六神经鞘瘤

第三、第四和第六神经鞘瘤非常罕见，最常见于 2 型神经纤维瘤病患者。偶发性动眼神经神经鞘瘤占颅内神经鞘瘤的不到 1%，是偶然的或在工作期间发现的头痛或复视时发现；部分性动眼神经麻痹是常见的症状；现有文献总共有 40~100 例的报告。它们可以沿着神经走行出现在任何地方，发生在硬膜间腔、海绵窦壁（动眼和滑车神经）、海绵窦（外展）或眼眶内，并且具有缓慢的生长速度，在许多症状轻微的患者中应有条件进行“观察和扫描”。如果肿瘤小和远离视器，症状性肿瘤或生长的肿瘤可以通过放射外科治疗，而显微手术对所有肿瘤都是可行的。非彻底切除的手术其主要目的是保持神经功能，而且需要与随后的放射外科手术结合，以达到控制肿瘤的目的。根治性手术在技术上是可行的，但不能保留神经功能。神经移植的结果尚未见报道。移植较小的神经（滑车和展）在理论上是可能的，而动眼神经移植后其运动功能恢复很差，证明神经吻合是徒劳无益的。

面神经神经鞘瘤

面神经神经鞘瘤占颅内神经鞘瘤的不到 2%。与其他神经鞘瘤一样，它们生长缓慢，对立体定向放射外科治疗敏感，控制肿瘤通常是可行的。面部神经鞘瘤可以发生在神经的任何地方。膝状神经节和鼓室段最常见（**图** 22.10）。根据发生部位，将面神经肿瘤分为三类。一个常见的位置是内听道，在那里其类似前庭神经鞘瘤，并延伸到桥小脑角。这些肿瘤不能和面神经分离开来。第二类肿瘤生长在面神经管中（fallopian canal），可能表现为对比增强（MRI），增厚的神经段。第三个典型的位置是在岩浅大神经和膝状神经节周围，在岩骨的颞下表面产生外生性的硬膜外肿瘤。

在发生面瘫之前，可发生广泛的轴突功能丧失。因此，如果位于内听道内，许多面神经神经鞘瘤患者也可以出现耳鸣和听力损失，或如果位于颞下会有占位效应。位于岩骨内的面神经鞘瘤通常引起面神经功能障碍，除非它们是偶发的。面神经鞘瘤的根治性手术包括牺牲神经的完全切除和随后的移植。因此，手术目标必须有先见之明而且决策透明。神经移植不可能提供比 House-Brackman 3 级更好的面部功能，因此通常在明显的高级别面神经麻痹患者才会使用。对于大肿瘤和面神经功能良好的患者，在肿瘤有进展的情况下，大部切除肿瘤附加放射外科手术是一个很好的选择。由膝状神经节产生的颞下肿瘤完全用颞下硬膜外入路切除，这样才能保留面神经功能（Ichimura et al.，2010）。小肿瘤可能生长非常缓慢，可以通过影像学监测进行观察。如果小肿瘤临床有进展或影像学检查增大，可行伽玛刀放射外科治疗。

颈静脉孔后组脑神经鞘瘤

颈静脉孔神经鞘瘤包括起源于舌咽、迷走神经和副神经的肿瘤；它们占所有颅内神经鞘瘤的不到 3%（图 22.11）。舌咽神经肿瘤可能是最常见的，但通常很难识别起源的神经。最初，许多肿瘤因为颅内压增高常规检查才发现。这种情况依然在发生，但特定的神经功能障碍更常见。在所有患者中，约有一半患者存在部分或全部颈静脉孔综合征和吞咽困难，而 30%~60% 的患者表现为前庭耳蜗症状。

肿瘤可以位于神经走行的任何地方。Kaye 和 Samii 根据起源和生长模式将颈静脉孔鞘瘤分为 A、B、C 和 D 四类（Kaye et al.，1984；Samii et al.，1995）。颈孔 A 型神经鞘瘤占据桥小脑角；B 型为孔内，硬膜内延伸；C 型为颅外（此处不进一步讨论），D 型哑铃状颅内外均有生长。对于根治性切除，颅内 A 型肿瘤采用乙状窦后入路，而 B 型和 D 型肿瘤则需要乙状窦后 / 经岩骨入路。经岩骨面神经移位的入路在过去经常使用，因为并发面神经瘫痪，现在很大

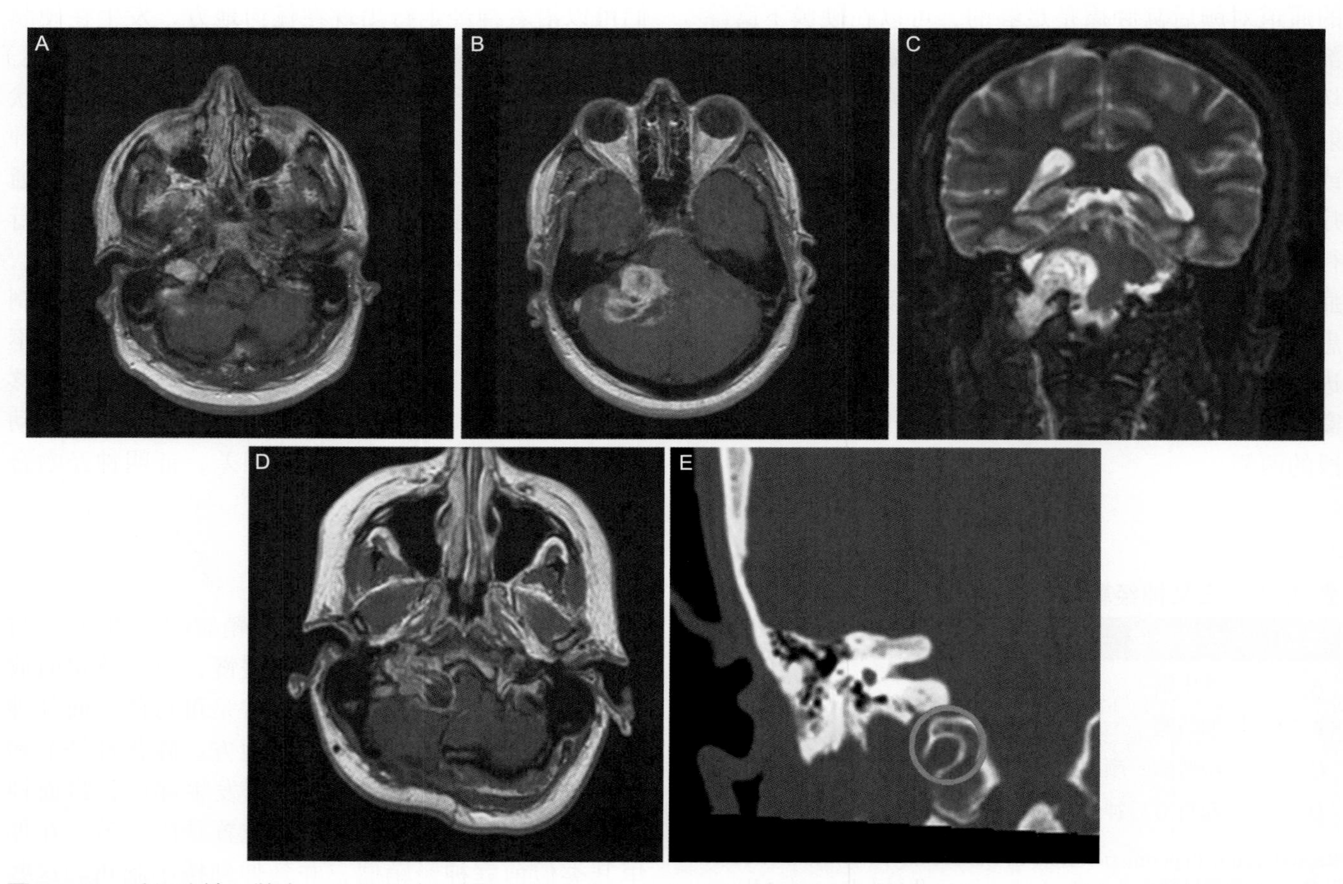

图 22.11　后组脑神经鞘瘤。后组脑神经鞘瘤的轴位（A，B）T1 加权 MRI 钆增强和冠状 T2（C）短 T1 翻转恢复（STIR）MRI 序列。可见肿瘤自颈静脉孔发出。复发性舌下神经鞘瘤（D）T1 加权 MRI 与钆增强。舌下管可以很容易地在冠状 CT（CT）扫描（E）上识别为鹰喙（红色圆圈）。舌下神经鞘瘤造成舌下神经管扩大，并破坏鹰喙的外观。此点这有助于区分舌下神经鞘瘤和其他后组脑神经鞘瘤

程度上已经被放弃。后组脑神经鞘瘤全切除或近全切除术后，后组脑神经功能障碍发生率高达100%，面神经障碍发生率为11%~80%，前庭耳蜗神经障碍发生率为4%~45%（Park et al.，2016）。颈静脉孔肿瘤的根治性手术具有后组脑神经功能受损的高风险，伴随着声音嘶哑、吞咽困难或带管生存。后组脑神经功能障碍可能需要较短或较长时间的管饲、胃造口术或气管切开，这对生活质量有很强的负面影响（Mathiesen et al.，2007）。肿瘤生长缓慢，功能保存已成为颈静脉孔肿瘤的主要目标。通过手术行肿瘤的硬膜内减压和修剪肿瘤以创造条件进行放射外科治疗，能得到中期生长控制，并保留舌咽、迷走神经和副神经功能（Park et al.，2016）。然而，超过10年的长期数据还没有被评估或发表，并且前庭神经鞘瘤放射外科治疗得到长期控制的结果被泛化。脊副神经鞘瘤手术可获得理想切除，除同侧脊副神经轻瘫外，其他并发病症发生率很低。

舌下神经鞘瘤

颅内舌下神经鞘瘤是很罕见的，仅在小的临床系列和个案病例报告中有描述，共约100例。它们似乎比其他神经鞘瘤更常出现囊性变，肿瘤进展快速而且容易复发（**图22.11**）。半侧舌肌萎缩和舌下轻瘫是典型症状。多达一半出现单侧舌下轻瘫患者，会在舌下神经孔附近的颅底周围发现良性或恶性肿瘤。通过侧方部分经髁入路可以切除舌下神经管内的神经鞘瘤，继而通过舌下神经管到达硬膜下。根治性切除神经鞘瘤后，随即行神经移植，舌下功能能得到迅速恢复（Mathiesen et al.，2009）。目前尚未对移植的功能益处，以及手术大部切除肿瘤后是否进行辅助放射外科治疗的可行性进行评估。随访有限的病例报告表明，对舌下神经鞘瘤来说，肿瘤大部切除后辅助放射外科治疗也同样是可行的。据报道单侧舌下神经麻痹并不影响言语功能；因此，几位作者认为这种神经功能障碍能得到很好的容忍。然而，其对吞咽和生活质量的影响尚未进行批判性分析。

争议：小的散发性听神经鞘瘤

小的散发的前庭神经鞘瘤的处理备受争议。“观察和扫描”被推荐给许多患者。

在技术上，小肿瘤可以通过显微或放射外科治疗，因此许多患者选择其中一种治疗。争议在于是否应该对患者进行治疗或跟踪随访？如果选择积极的治疗，哪种治疗更好？

1. “积极治疗”是基于症状进展或肿瘤生长的风险，再加上病理的不确定性。大约1/3的听力良好的患者在3年的随访中失去功能听力。肿瘤可能会扩大到并发面神经功能障碍的风险，实际中此点对于较小的肿瘤几乎可以忽略不计。肿瘤生长到一定的大小时，无法实施放射外科手术，余下的选择就会很少。最后，在肿瘤不太可能是恶性的情况下，早期切除是优选的方案。理想情况下，早期治疗肿瘤，可保存听力和面神经功能。

   “最好尽早冒更大的风险，以获得治愈和保持听力”

2. “观察和扫描”是基于良性肿瘤的自然病史。主要的论点是，只有1/3小的散发前庭神经鞘瘤在5年的随访中生长，晚期生长是可能的，但不是预期的。对于有稳定肿瘤的患者来说，治疗很可能是徒劳的，因为无论是手术还是放射手术都无法预测能改善听力、眩晕或耳鸣。此外，显微外科手术和较少采用放射外科治疗使患者面临疾病本身固有的治疗不适和致残率，此外还使患者面临发生治疗并发症的随机性风险。影像检查显示肿瘤生长或症状进展是治疗的指征。

   “最好避免不必要的治疗，在最终治疗结果没有统计学上更差的情况下，治疗可以推迟。这是“最好的保留长期听力的方式”

   2.1 “不要采用积极的放射外科治疗”是基于：①认为放射外科的目标是“肿瘤控制”，但在大约70%的患者没有任何治疗，5年的结果也是“肿瘤控制”（未变化）；②放射外科可能有并发症。对面神经和前庭耳蜗神经的辐射可能损害功能。面神经麻痹的治疗风险为1%~2%，在放射手术后的随访中，尽管相反的数据已经发表，听力预计会缓慢恶化。众所周知，电离辐射有染色体损伤和随后的诱导新发肿瘤或已有肿瘤恶变的风险。

   “为了治愈肿瘤，应该切除肿瘤，肿瘤恶变的风险虽然低，但无法控制”

   2.2 “没有积极的显微外科治疗”是基于以下信念：①手术需要住院治疗，没有规律的生活，固有的致残率和疼痛；②严重的并发症，包括死亡，虽然很少，但对遇到该情况的少数人来说是真实存在的；③大多数手术系列表明显微外科手术后面神经并发症和短期听力损失的发生率高于放射外科手术。

   “应该治疗肿瘤，而显微手术可能发生的急性严重并发症是不可接受的”或“放射外科是保

持长期听力的最佳策略”

这些争议反映了医学证据和个人价值观的差异。在文献数据方面有普遍的共识，但大量的研究和meta分析只为大量的不同患者和外科医生的并发症发生率和结果提供了平均值。因此，患者个人治疗风险并不能盲目地从大型临床研究中推断出来。治疗风险随外科医生个体的技能和经验而不同；外科医生和患者也可以根据复发和致残的风险而就治疗目标达成一致。电离辐射在人群水平上增加了肿瘤的发病率，但就个别患者来说，只是一个边际效应。文献报道中有极少数肿瘤有快速生长和组织学上的恶性变，但文献没有将之描述为高风险从而建议避免进行放射外科手术。在随访期间，肿瘤可能会生长，听力可能丧失，但病情进一步严重恶化是非常罕见的。放射外科的最佳理由是文献支持放疗后能长期维持更好听力；然而，不同的研究有不同的结果和结论。科学的挑战是评估患者是否与大宗病例报道的人群一样从治疗中获益，而不是文献报道的其他亚组不理想的治疗结果。

最重要的是，每个患者个体对结果和可接受风险的价值观各不相同。通过透明的风险评估，对于相同的肿瘤，不同的患者可能选择等待和扫描、放射外科或显微外科治疗的其中一种。外科医生有责任以透明的方式分享知识和经验，而不隐藏个人经验和治疗结果，并与患者共同决定；该决定应能反映患者的价值观、外科医生的专业知识和职业道德。

参考文献、EBRAIN的相关链接

扫描书末二维码获取。

第 23 章　血管球瘤

Omar Pathmanaban・Andrew King 著
汤可 译，卜博 审校

引言

血管球瘤是一种生长缓慢、血管丰富的肿瘤，发生在解剖复杂的颈鼓区内，位于侧颅底。它们通常是良性的，但局部行为是侵入性的，在某些情况下侵犯到邻近的岩骨、桥小脑角（cerebellopontine angle，CPA）和颈部。肿瘤通过低阻力途径扩展，如乳突气房、血管周围和血管内间隙、咽鼓管和颅底骨孔，并可以直接侵蚀破坏骨质。

临床表现

血管球瘤通常是比较惰性的，由于缺乏症状或症状轻微，并不被关注，因此在诊断前可以发展到相当大的体积。当症状变得明显时，它们代表了球瘤的生物学特征，由于肿瘤富于血管，90% 的患者有搏动性耳鸣；由于肿瘤有局部侵袭性生长，导致 80% 的患者出现传导性听力丧失（Fayad et al.，2010）。约 10% 的患者出现耳痛和耳部充盈感（Fayad et al.，2010）。其他解剖学上定位的神经症状与外侧颅底的侵袭路径有关（**表 23.1**）。迷路受侵入可发生眩晕，耳蜗受累可出现感觉神经性听力丧失。脑神经麻痹的发生率在已经发表的文献报道中各不相同，由于肿瘤缓慢进展引起的功能代偿，在没有术前功能障碍表现的情况下，肿瘤可能已经侵犯了神经（Makek et al.，1990）。因为舌咽和迷走神经在颈静脉孔受累，吞咽困难和（或）构音障碍可能是就诊时最明显的表现；因为病变位置的不同，使任何后组脑神经综合征都成为可能（**表 23.2**）。在一定比例的患者中可出现明显的面部运动功能障碍（Fayad et al.，2010；Jackson et al.，1990；Makek et al.，1990）。患者有时也可见面部感觉障碍和复视，通过颈静脉孔扩展到桥小脑角，或沿岩骨后面扩展，分别侵犯了三叉神经和展神经。在颅内肿瘤相当大的情况下，由于可能发生脑干压迫，会出现局灶症状 / 单侧长束神经功能障碍和（或）梗阻性脑积水。霍纳（Horner）综合征可继发于脑干受压的大肿瘤，或者更有可能是由于颈内动脉被肿瘤包裹和侵袭而对交感神经的损伤。用耳镜在外耳道可见经典的红色肿块（**图 23.1**），在 90% 以上肿瘤侵犯中耳病例中均可见此征，其表现称为“落日征”（Fayad et al.，2010）。

表 23.1　解剖定位症状

症状	所涉及的解剖结构
耳聋	中耳 / 耳蜗
头晕 / 眩晕	迷路 /CPA- 脑神经Ⅷ
构音障碍	颈静脉孔 - 脑神经 X
吞咽困难	颈静脉孔 - 脑神经Ⅸ /X
面肌无力	岩骨 /CPA- 脑神经Ⅶ
面部麻木	岩尖 /CPA- 脑神经 V
复视	岩尖 /CPA- 脑神经Ⅵ
头疼	脑干 / 第四脑室 - 脑积水
舌肌萎缩	舌下神经管 - 脑神经Ⅻ

表 23.2　后组脑神经综合征

综合征	神经麻痹
Vernet 综合征	Ⅸ、X、Ⅺ
Collet-Sicard 综合征	Ⅸ、X、Ⅺ、Ⅻ
Villaret 综合征	Ⅸ、X、Ⅺ、Ⅻ、交感神经（Horner 综合征）

临床解剖及分类

血管球瘤根据解剖位置描述大致分类三种：

- 鼓室球瘤：局限于中耳。
- 颈静脉球瘤：局限于颈静脉孔。
- 颈鼓球瘤：累及颈静脉孔和中耳。

鼓室球瘤起源于沿 Jacobson 神经（脑神经Ⅸ鼓下支）中耳走行的副神经节。颈静脉球瘤（**图 23.2**）

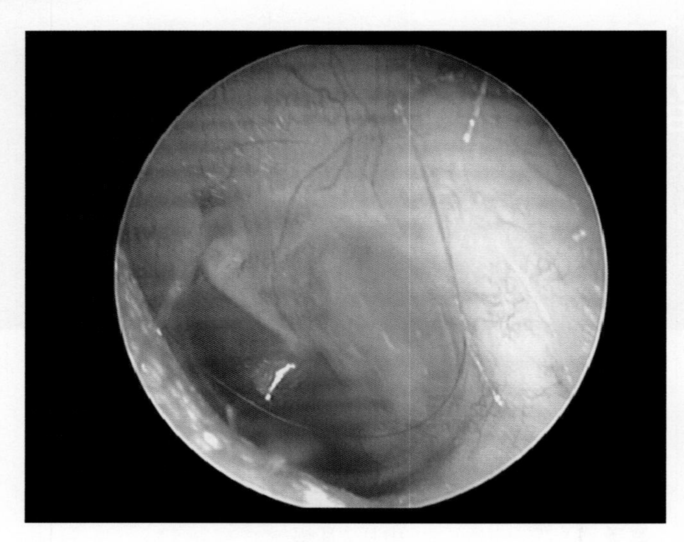

图 23.1 耳镜照片，显示落日征。中耳可见特征性血红色血管球瘤

可能产生于与颈静脉球外膜相关的副神经节，沿 Arnold 神经（脑神经 X 的耳支）或 Jacobson 神经的颈静脉窝段（Forbes et al.，2012）发展。中耳底部脆弱的颈静脉骨板（菲薄皮质骨，将下鼓室与下内侧颈静脉球部隔开）是颈静脉和中耳腔肿瘤扩展的途径，是定义肿瘤名称和起源的解剖标志。对于大的颈静脉瘤，起源点的判断只能是学术性的，只能推断。然而，确定球瘤的解剖阶段在临床上是很重要的，因为仅限于中耳的肿瘤可以由耳科医生通过经鼓室入路切除，致残率最低，而扩展范围大的肿瘤则需要更多的侵袭性颅底入路。最常用的两个放射学分类系统是 Jackson-Glasscock 分类（**表** 23.3）和 Fisch 分类（**表** 23.4）（Jackson et al.，1982；Fisch and Mattox，1988）。

影像特征

CT 和 MR 结合成像是颞骨球瘤诊断和分型的首选方法。轴位和冠状薄层 CT 成像可以清楚展示骨侵犯的程度，其边缘通常不规则。磁共振可进一步揭示肿瘤与颅底神经血管结构的关系，以及肿瘤扩展到 CPA 的程度（**图** 23.3）。T1 加权和 T2 加权 MR 图像的特征是混合信号强度，称之为“盐和胡椒”征，反映了富血管流空信号（高流量的肿瘤血管），以及肿瘤局灶区域内血液代谢产物引起的高强度信号（Rao et al.，1999）。T1 加权钆增强提示肿瘤对强化剂摄取率高，图像显示明显增强信号，可见平滑的肿瘤轮廓。

在现代诊断中，通常不需要导管造影，但在某些诊断不明确的情况下和在所有选择外科治疗的病例（术前进行栓塞 - 见本章后面的治疗部分）中是有用的）。造影可见致密的富血管肿瘤染色（**图** 23.4），由于瘤内动静脉分流，常有早期静脉充盈，通常有多个颈外动脉供血血管（特别是咽升动脉），在巨大肿瘤中，颈内动脉和（或）椎动脉也有血供（Rao et al.，1999）。

其他检查和会诊

应进行听力测量以确定听力损失程度。喉镜检查是为了评估声带的功能。所有患者都需要内分泌学会诊，血浆和 24 小时的尿液收集，生化检查项目包括甲基肾上腺素和儿茶酚胺，即使没有儿茶酚胺过度分泌症状的病例也要检查。这是因为只有一小部分颅底副神经节瘤是分泌性的，也有多灶的可能性，瘤中混有额外的未检测到的分泌性副神经节瘤。最近新出现的 3- 甲氧基甲胺（多巴胺衍生物）试验，最好在所有患者中进行检查。它可以作为治疗后肿瘤是否恶性变和复发的生物标志物，以及是否会出现血流动力学不稳定的危险因子（Eisenhofer et al.，2012）。遗传基因咨询应成为日常管理的一部分，即使在没有家族史的情况下，也应为所有病例提供遗传基因咨询和检测。基因检测的目的是确定个体肿瘤是否进展，以及同时发生和异时发生肿瘤方面的风险。它还能识别高危家庭成员，并就养育子女的选择提供咨询，包括胚胎着床前诊断。关于其他部位肿瘤的放射学检查，各医疗机构方案各不相同，包括磁共振成像和 123 碘苄基胍（MIBG）放射性同位素成像。我们首选的方式是全身 MRI，包括冠状 T1 加权和 STIR 序列和轴向脂肪饱和 T2 加权序列。一些中心也使用生长抑素受体显像和正电子发射断层扫描进行筛查。

病理学

起源

血管球瘤产生于肾外自主神经副神经节。副神经节储存和分泌儿茶酚胺，并被认为起着稳态作用，但它们在健康个体中的生理目的仍然很大程度上是未知的（颈动脉体的氧化学感受器除外）。它们是胚胎发育过程中从神经嵴衍生出来小的神经内分泌主细胞簇（Heth，2004）。来自这些细胞的肿瘤，包括血管球瘤，被正确地命名为副神经节瘤，其与嗜铬

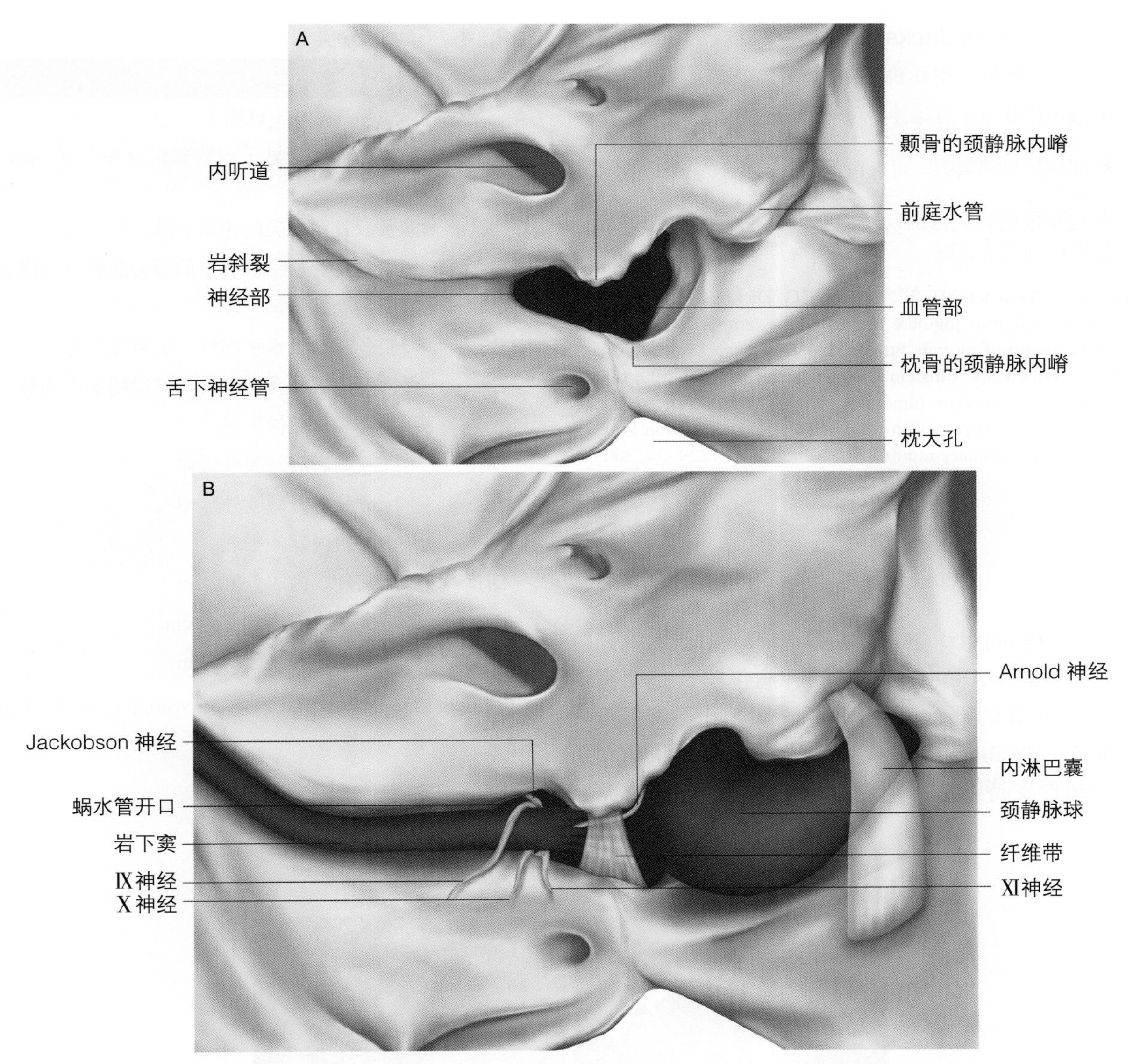

图 23.2 （A）颈静脉孔的两种分类。传统将颈静脉孔分为血管部和神经部，血管部包括乙状窦和第Ⅹ和Ⅺ脑神经。神经部包含有第Ⅸ脑神经。一些作者提出了将血管部细分出一个额外的间腔，其中包括单独位于后面的乙状窦和一个额外的中间部（颈静脉内间隙），由后方的岩枕韧带（连接枕骨和颞骨内嵴的纤维或骨带）和前方的硬膜返折之间的空间构成。这个颈静脉内间隙含有第Ⅹ和Ⅺ脑神经。颈静脉孔的三个腔隙，乙状窦部位于后外侧，为血管部。较小的岩前内侧部分收集下岩窦的回流 - 此部为“岩部”；颞骨和枕骨的颈内嵴由纤维连接，有时是骨带形成颈内分隔。第三个腔隙是颈内嵴 -“神经部”，位于乙状窦部和岩部之间 [神经部包括与岩下窦相邻的第Ⅸ、Ⅹ和Ⅺ脑神经，后二者走行于乙状窦、颈内静脉交界处的血管壁的前方]。
（B）岩下窦通过颈静脉球内侧壁开口连接乙状窦。该开口位于前方的第Ⅸ脑神经和后方第Ⅹ、第Ⅺ脑神经之间。这些神经穿过颞骨颈内嵴内侧缘的硬脑膜，并通过颈内静脉的内侧。耳蜗导水管开口位于第Ⅸ脑神经附近的岩部上方。上咽和枕动脉的脑膜分支、第Ⅸ脑神经的鼓室分支 Jackobson 神经的进入鼓室，到达鼓室，脑神经Ⅹ的分支 Arnold 神经的耳支进人位于乙状窦前壁的乳突管，从鼓室缝处穿出，是颈静脉孔内与血管球瘤相关的结构

细胞瘤具有相同的谱系；它们可能保留功能性儿茶酚胺的产生和分泌（De Lellis，2004）。这些肿瘤大致可分为三个亚组：

- 嗜铬细胞瘤：肾上腺内部的副神经节瘤（功能性）。
- 交感神经副神经节瘤：肾上腺外部，从颅底到骨盆沿交感链任何部位均可发生（通常是功能性的，也称为嗜铬副神经节瘤）。
- 副交感神经副神经节瘤：肾外副交感神经支配的肿瘤，出现在颅底和颈部与第Ⅸ和第Ⅹ脑神经分支（很少功能性；也称为非嗜铬性副神经节瘤）鼓室球瘤属于副交感神经非嗜铬性副神经节瘤亚组。

表 23.3 Glasscock-Jackson 分类 [a]

Ⅰ	累及颈静脉球、中耳和乳突的小肿瘤
Ⅱ	肿瘤向内耳道下方延伸；可能沿颅内骨管扩展
Ⅲ	肿瘤瘤扩展到岩尖；可能沿颅内骨管扩展
Ⅳ	肿瘤扩展到岩尖范围以外，到达斜坡或颞下窝；可能有颅内骨管扩展

[a] Adapted from, Glasscock ME 3rd, Jackson CG, Dickins JR, Wiet RJ: Panel discussion: Glomus jugulare tumors of the temporal bone–The surgical management of glomus tumors. *Laryngoscope* 89: 1640–51, 1979 (16) and Willen SN, Einstein DB, Maciunas RJ, Megerian CA: Treatment of glomus jugulare tumors in patients with advanced age: Planned limited surgical resection followed by staged gamma knife radiosurgery— A preliminary report. Otol Neurotol 26:1229–34, 2005 (41).

组织学

副神经节瘤的组织学切片（**图 23.5**）用苏木精和伊红染色（H&E），可见一个薄的肿瘤包膜，一个富含薄壁毛细血管的纤维血管间质，围绕圆形或多角形主细胞（Zellballen），形成有诊断意义的巢状球和周围的纺锤形支持细胞。免疫组织化学显示，针对突

表 23.4 Fisch 分类

分类	说明
A	限于中耳（鼓室球瘤）
B	限于中耳 / 乳突，颈静脉板完整，无迷路下受累
C	涉及颞骨和岩尖的迷路下部
C1	颈动脉孔受累，但有限的颈动脉管垂直段破坏
C2	侵犯颈动脉管垂直段
C3	侵犯颈动脉管水平部分，破裂孔幸免
C4	侵入超过破裂孔，到海绵窦段的颈内动脉
De	颅内硬膜外延伸扩展
De1	<2 cm 颅后窝硬膜外延伸
De2	>2 cm 颅后窝硬膜外延伸
Di	颅内硬膜内延伸扩展
Di1	颅后窝硬膜内成分 <2 cm
Di2	颅后窝硬膜内成分 2~4 cm
Di3	颅后窝硬膜内成分 >4 cm

From Fisch, U. & Mattox, D. 1988. *Microsurgery of the skull base*, Thieme.

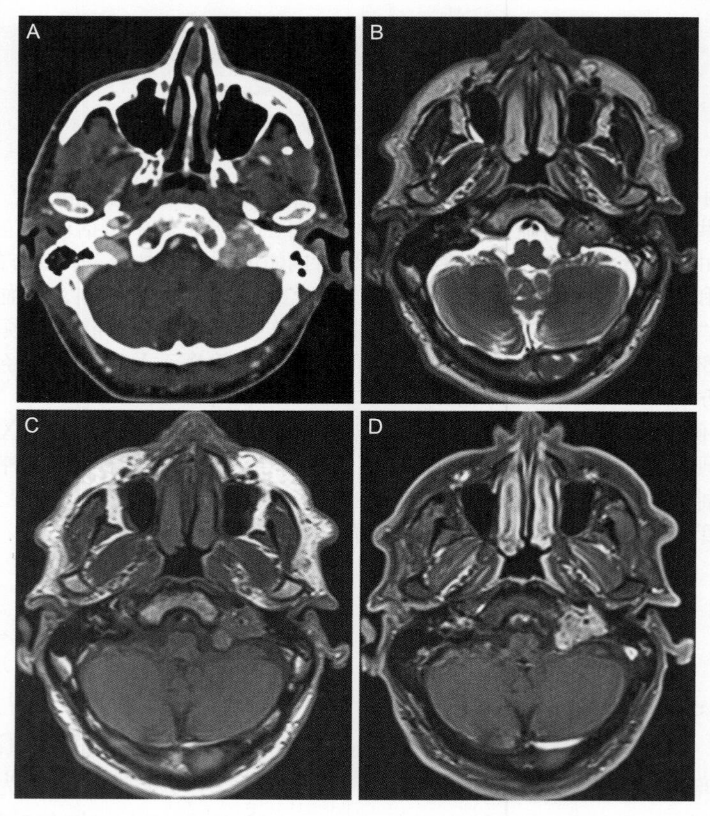

图 23.3 颈静脉孔水平横断面成像：对比增强后轴位 CT 扫描（A），T2 加权轴位 MR（B），增强前 T1 加权轴位 MR（C）和增强后 T1 加权轴位 MR（D）图像显示左侧典型的可强化的颈静脉球瘤，有骨质破坏和血管流空

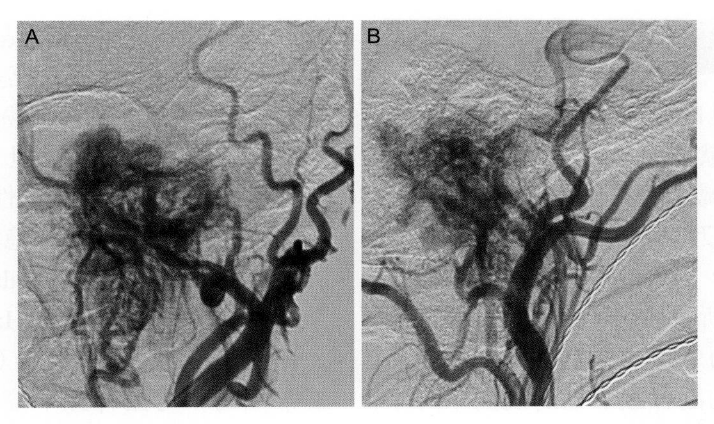

图 23.4　动脉内数字减影血管造影：选择性左颈外动脉导管造影显示正位（A）和侧位（B）的颈静脉球瘤，具有特征性的富血管外观

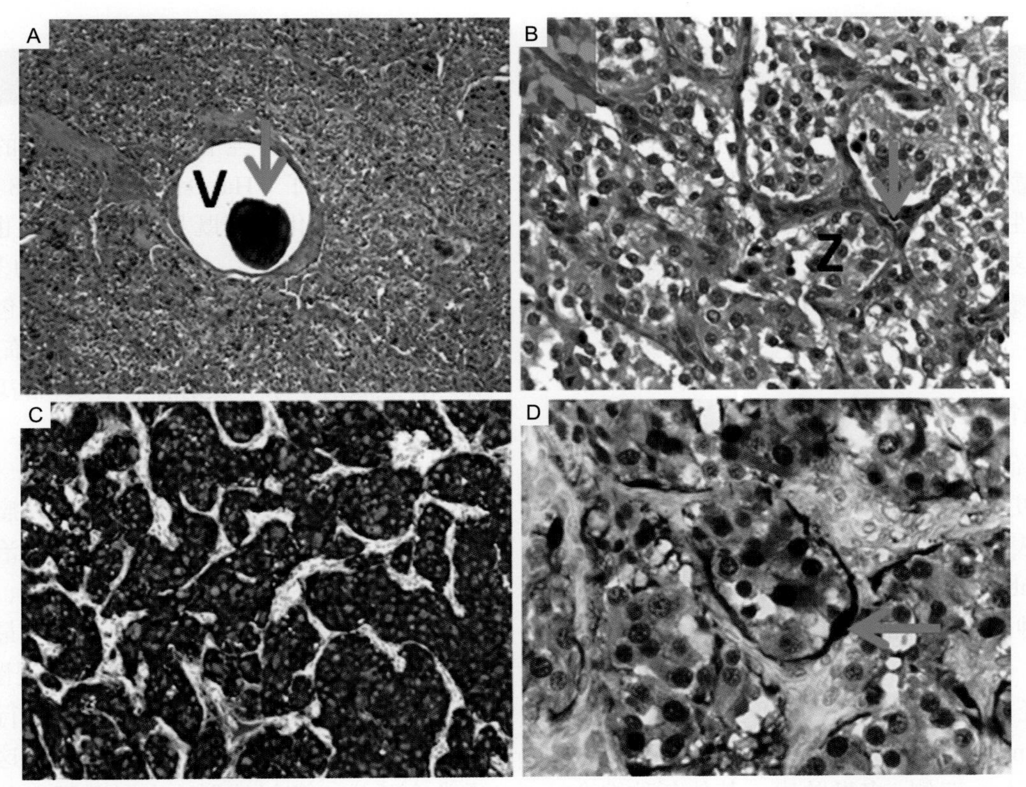

图 23.5　颈静脉球瘤的组织学：颈静脉球瘤的H&E染色切片（A，×100原始放大）显示血管血管内栓塞材料明显（箭头）。高功率 H&E 显微照片（B，×400 原始放大倍数）显示肿瘤细胞（Z）与周围丰富的毛细血管网络（箭头）的“Zellballen”排列。免疫组织化学使用抗突触素抗体（C，×200 原始放大）显示肿瘤细胞的弥漫性强免疫反应，证实神经内分泌细胞血统。S100 免疫染色（D，×630 原始放大）显示强烈的抗 S100 染色的支持细胞周围的肿瘤细胞巢（核和细胞质染色代表非特异性染色）。双极密集染色的黄斑细胞（箭头）清楚地看到与中心细胞巢相关的是一个密集的棕色染色细胞，双极投射包围细胞球

Photomicrographs courtesy of Dr Daniel du Plessis

触素的抗体在主细胞中呈阳性反应，S100 和 GFAP 在支持细胞中呈阳性反应（Branica et al.，1993）。电子显微镜不是一项常规的诊断检查，但证实了神经分泌颗粒在主细胞中的存在（Warren et al.，1985）。在组织学上是不能确定肿瘤的分级。在有转移的高级别肿瘤中支持细胞明显丢失（Kliewer and Cochran，1989），但恶性肿瘤的其他显微特征，如有丝分裂性相和坏死并不可靠，世界卫生组织（WHO）分类认为转移是恶性肿瘤的唯一诊断标准（DeLellis，2004）。

流行病学

这些肿瘤是相当罕见的，因此，其准确发病率是未知的，已发表的文献中发病率数字差异较大。神经内分泌肿瘤嗜铬细胞瘤 - 副神经节瘤谱的合并发病率为每年 0.8 例 / 每 10 万人（Beard et al.，1983）。女性患者更多见，女性：男性比为 4：1（Reddy et al.，1983）。由全身转移所致的恶性血管球瘤极其罕见，目前尚不清楚恶性血管球瘤的具体发病率是多少；据估计，所有部位的副神经节瘤的发病率每年不到 100 例 /4 亿人（Welander et al.，2011）。零星散发的血管球瘤通常在生命的第五个十年被诊断出来，而遗传性肿瘤往往更早得到诊断。

危险因素

环境

值得注意的是，颈动脉体增生见于高海拔地区，此部位散发性副神经节瘤多见于高海拔地区，尤其是女性。在这种情况下，颈静脉球瘤也更常见，这可能是由于慢性缺氧，但这仍有待证实（Saldana et al.，1973）。

遗传学和遗传性综合征

有副神经节瘤家族史和女性性别使副神经节瘤发生的风险更高。血管球瘤是散发性或家族性的，最近的数据表明，多达 50% 的肾外副神经节瘤是家族性的（Fishbein et al.，2013）。此外，副神经节瘤也是其他几种遗传综合征的一部分：多发性内分泌肿瘤 2 型（RET 基因）、von Hippel Lindau 综合征（VHL 基因）、神经纤维瘤病 1 型（NF1 基因）和 Carney 三联症 /Carney-Stratakis 综合征（Galan and Kann，2013）。年轻人、双侧 / 多发肿瘤、其他各种综合征的痕迹和家族史可能指向遗传综合征的诊断，但重要的是，所有副神经节瘤患者都被转介到临床遗传学服务进行全面检查。目前至少有 15 个已知的易感基因，现在下一代子女的基因检测可以选择测序的方法。最近的一份共识文件建议哪些基因应该包括在测试序列中（Toledo et al.，2017）。家族性副神经节瘤是常染色体显性遗传，具有可变外显性，有些是由于母体遗传印迹而通过父系突变传播的。遗传的副神经节瘤与琥珀酸脱氢酶（SDH）的亚基的编码基因突变有关，SDH 在 Krebs 循环和线粒体呼吸链中起着重要作用。有四个基因（SDHA、SDHB、SDHC、SDHD）编码单独的酶亚基，另一个基因编码是一种有利于（flavinate）第一亚基（SDHAF2）的蛋白质。SDHx 基因被认为具有抑癌功能。虽然这方面的机制和介质尚不完全清楚，但 SDHx 突变可能干扰细胞氧传感，导致琥珀酸和活性氧离子和过氧化物积累，导致缺氧诱导因子 1α 的稳定，从而激活缺氧信号级联反应（Heth，2004；Galan and Kann，2013）。迄今已发现五种遗传性 SDHx 副神经节瘤综合征，每一种都有不同的基因突变（**表 23.5**）。SDHD 突变是最常见的，与副神经节瘤综合征 1（paraganglioma syndrome 1，PGL1）有关，这在荷兰家族性颅底 / 头颈部副神经节瘤患者中特别普遍，这是由于单一的基础基因突变造成的（Hensen et al.，2011）。

治疗和预后

虽然颅底副神经节瘤通常是良性的，但患者的生活质量降低了（Havekes et al.，2008）。对血管球瘤肿瘤的最优化处理既具有挑战性，也有争议（见“争议”部分），需要一个由经验丰富的多学科管理团队，提出个性化最佳方法，这个团队包括神经外科医生、神经肿瘤学家、内分泌学家、临床遗传学家、介入神经放射学家、放射肿瘤学家和病理学家。

保守治疗

血管球瘤通常进展缓慢，有些肿瘤在长期随访中是静止的。因此，在某些情况下，治疗的风险可能超过无所作为的风险，因此，观察、等待和重新扫描方案通常是最基本的管理策略。最初，在 6 个月时进行重复扫描。静态肿瘤和生长缓慢的小肿瘤可以保守管理，并每年一定时间间隔进行临床和影像学检查。一旦确定肿瘤的惰性行为，这种监测间隔通常会延长。类似的方法有时适用于肿瘤较大的老年人和那些手术可能产生明显并发症的患者。较大的肿瘤、较小（特别是在较年轻的患者中）但生长快速的肿瘤和分泌性肿瘤可能需要手术和（或）放射治疗。已经出现肿瘤同侧后组脑神经功能缺损则降低了治疗的阈值（标准），因为它减少了患者对医源性损伤的恐惧，并且这些临床表现发出了肿瘤表型更具侵袭性的信号。治疗决定必须结合患者的遗传状况和伴发肿瘤作出。当双侧有脑神经缺损的风险时，这一点是极其重要的。在这种情况下，医疗团队的决定必须尽量减少永久性气管切开术和肠内喂养的风险。治疗的目的是为了保留功能，同时控制肿瘤。

表 23.5 家族性副神经节瘤综合征

综合征	染色体	基因	说明
PGL1	11q	*SDHD*	• 副神经节瘤 / 嗜铬细胞瘤 • 副神经节瘤更常见 • 一半以上的病例是多发的 • 通常是副交感神经 • 有不良报道，但不常见 • 母体传播（基因母体印迹） • 高的外显率 • 最常见的家族性副神经节瘤综合征
PGL2	11q	*SDHAF2*	• 副交感神经神经节瘤 • 一般是多发的 • 母体传播（基因母体印迹） • 高的外显率
PGL3	1q	*SDHC*	• 副神经节瘤 • 主要是副交感神经 • 在 1/5 的情况下是多发的 • 有不良报道，但不常见 • 低外显率
PGL4	1p	*SDHB*	• 副神经节瘤 / 嗜铬细胞瘤 • 副神经节瘤更常见 • 在 1/5 的情况下是多发的 • 最常见的是交感神经分泌肿瘤 • 最常见于盆腔 / 腹部 / 胸腔 • 有见于颅底的报道，但少见 • 与肾细胞癌有关 • 恶性肿瘤风险较高 • 高的外显率 • 诊断年龄相对较小，典型 • 预后相对较差 • 第二常见的家族性副神经节瘤综合征
PGL5	5p	*SDHA*	• 副神经节瘤 / 嗜铬细胞瘤 • 副神经节瘤更常见 • 交感神经或副交感神经 • 未见多发者 • 未见恶性者 • 低外显率

手术

过去几十年来，随着多学科团队的广泛协作、术前栓塞、术中脑神经监测以及先进的显微外科技术的应用，针对血管球瘤的手术进展迅速，鼓室球瘤可以通过神经 - 耳科经外耳道完全切除，从而达到听力保存和最低致残率。因此，手术是这些病例的首选治疗，放疗的作用有限。根据肿瘤大小和侵入结构的不同，也可以通过经乳突 - 经颈部和颞下窝入路来彻底切除颈静脉球瘤和颈静脉鼓室球瘤。当检查（包括喉镜检查）表明肿瘤一侧已存在后组脑神经缺损时，这一方案是合适的；而部分切除（辅助放射治疗或进一步观察）是在后组脑神经功能正常时与患者讨论的一种选择。根据 Fisch 分类有助于确定手术方案，但每个患者都是独特的，手术方案必须量身定做。**第 24 章**详细介绍了手术解剖、入路和技术细节。这些肿瘤含丰富血管，因此术中出血可能是灾难性的，因此强烈建议所有患者都应该进行术前介入导管栓塞治疗。在有颈内动脉受累的病例，应该进行颈动脉球囊闭塞试验。如果准备牺牲患侧的静脉时，也应该充分的研究对侧静脉窦的发育和回流情况。在一个经验丰富的团队手中，要准备好所有的治疗方式和辅助治疗措施。手术有可能治愈，但术后致残率很高，特别是脑神经功能障碍。在大约 80% 的患者（即使是大肿瘤患者）中，能实现肿瘤大体切除，并且可以预期在 85% 以上的病例肿瘤能得到长期的控制。值得注意的是，大体全切除的患者有多达 7% 的报告复发，但不到 1% 的手术治疗患者继续死于肿瘤进展（Suárez et al., 2013）。手术最显著的缺点是新的脑神经障碍发生率高（20%~60%，尽管有些是暂时的）。尽管围术期死亡率较低，在 1%~3% 的区间（Makiese et al., 2012），但后组脑神经麻痹最终可能产生致命后果。由于手术后脑神经的致残率，许多医疗中心治疗策略正在从为大多数患者选择手术治疗（不包括鼓室球瘤）转向选择放射治疗（见“争议”部分）。

放射治疗 / 放射外科

放射治疗可作为一线治疗，部分切除后的辅助治疗，或作为二线治疗复发或残余肿瘤再长的情况。可选择适形分割放射治疗、立体定向放射外科或低分割立体定向放射治疗，主要根据单个肿瘤特征、患者的选择和医院可提供的资源。一般情况下，放射外科适用于直径小于 3cm 的较小病变，较大病变需要分割放疗。照射的目的是阻止肿瘤生长（控制肿瘤生长），而不是根除肿瘤，在大多数系列报道中，对所有形式的放射治疗都观察到肿瘤控制率超过 90%，在某些系列中进行了长达 10 年的随访。脑神经致残率与手术相比是有优势的，有些患者在治疗后脑神经功能甚至有所改善（Tran Ba Huy，2014）。在接受常规放射治疗的病例中，约 3% 的病例因随后的肿瘤进展而死亡。治疗相关死亡率也低于 2%。急性毒性症状常见，但持续时间短暂，包括头痛、恶心、呕吐、黏膜炎和体重减轻。对一些患者来说，长期口干、吞咽困难和感染性中耳炎 / 外耳炎也是存在的问题，在多达 5% 的病例存在医源性感音神经性耳聋（Suárez et al.，2013；Tran Ba Huy，2014）。在过去的外束放疗时代，骨坏死和脑坏死是严重的并发症，在使用新的调强适形和立体定向技术后，这些并发症已基本上消除。血管后遗症，包括颈动脉狭窄和缺血性并发症可能发生，但似乎并不常见，然而，对于接受治疗且预期生存期较长的年轻患者，需要评估晚期血管并发症的发生率。同样，辐射后诱发恶性肿瘤的发生率被认为很低（不到千分之一），但对于尚有几十年生命的年轻患者，也需要长期随访观察（Tran Ba Huy，2014）。

药物治疗

α- 受体阻滞剂通常用于有分泌功能的肿瘤患者，应在计划手术干预前几周开始用药，以降低血压危险起伏波动和心律失常的风险。由于这些肿瘤产生去甲肾上腺素而不是肾上腺素，β- 受体阻滞剂的使用频率较低。对于孤立性血管球瘤体患者，全身化疗没有作用，但化疗在某些转移性副神经节瘤中可以缓解或稳定病情（Patel et al.，1995）。

治疗后管理

所有患者，无论治疗方式如何，都应间隔 MR 扫描跟踪随访。治疗后如果存在相应的脑神经功能障碍，应设法解决。如果后组脑神经已牺牲，通常需要气管造口和鼻胃 / 胃造口术喂养。发音困难和吞咽问题可以通过语音训练治疗得到改善，如果发声问题持续存在，喉科医生可以提供各种药物注射和手术治疗来改善。面瘫需要理疗、眼科会诊，有时还需要做面部表情肌修复手术，最好通过面部功能专科诊所进行管理。听力丧失和平衡问题可以分别用助听器和前庭康复来解决。由于副神经功能障碍导致的肩关节活动减少和随后的肩痛，应采用理疗运动治疗。舌肌萎缩和构音障碍需要语言治疗支持。

争议

颞骨血管球瘤的治疗差异性较大。特别是选择放射治疗抑或手术治疗作为初始治疗方案一直存在争议。基本上在身体的所有其他部位，手术是良性肿瘤管理的支柱。然而，因为复杂的解剖和精微的神经血管结构，颅底是极其独特的部位。尽管手术技术取得了显著进展，但切除术伴有相对较高的脑神经并发症。如果接受肿瘤部分切除的策略，脑神经功能可在一定程度上得到保护，也就是说如果必要的话，可在脑神经上留下少量的肿瘤（Wanna et al.，2014）。虽然这点曾经有争议，但现在被大多数颅底学会视为一个很好的策略。同时，有针对性的放射治疗和放射外科方法已经发展起来，以尽量减少风险，同时在大多数情况下实现肿瘤控制。严重的并发症，如骨坏死和脑坏死，过去因此而加强了外科治疗模式，现在则是非常罕见的。因此，放射治疗已经成为近年来许多单位的主流。然而，在某些情况下，仍应选择特定的病例进行手术治疗：

- 放疗 / 放射手术后持续生长
- 肿瘤有 CPA 或岩骨扩展和脑干压迫
- 症状性儿茶酚胺分泌性肿瘤（主分泌细胞对辐射抵抗）

此外，在以下情况下，对初始治疗方式仍有争议：

- 年轻患者
- 小型有生长变化的肿瘤
- 治疗前已有脑神经障碍的患者

因此，医生应该为年轻患者提供手术或放射外科手术的选择，并讨论两者的风险，包括可能出现的放射晚期效应和目前仍缺乏十年后高质量随访的数据。手术后脑神经损伤的风险与肿瘤的大小成正比（Moe et al.，1999），因此，与体积小但有生长的肿瘤患者进行这种讨论也是合适的，因为术后脑神经缺损的风险很可能很低。最后，对于在治疗前已经有脑神经障碍的患者，与手术相关的主要并发症——脑神经损伤，在一定程度上不再考虑，但也不应低估诸如面肌瘫痪等新的功能障碍。此外，术前发现的明显的后组脑神经功能障碍往往是不完全的，手术过程中的牺牲神经可能会变为完全损伤而产生意想不到的吞咽问题。然而，虽然有一部分患者在放射治疗后神经功能可能得到一些主观改善，但大多数人的神经功能障碍不会改善，放射治疗使患者无手术治疗的机会，同时仍然使他们暴露在标准剂量的放射风险之下。因此，在某些情况下，手术无疑仍有作用，但大多数患者将接受放射治疗。

不可能进行随机对照试验来回答这些问题，因为该病罕见，需要超过几十年的长时间随访，复杂的肿瘤解剖变异性和混合人群，包括患有共患病的老年人、有或者没有多种系瘤源性突变的患者。因此，对已发表的病例系列文献报告、专家意见和选择患者的标准等的回顾性综述，在后续管理中有指导作用，在可预见的将来，这些复杂的情况很可能仍然存在争议。

结论

颅底血管球瘤（副神经节瘤）是生长缓慢的良性神经内分泌肿瘤，其具有局部侵袭性，但表现出较低的恶性转化率。它们是散发性或家族性的，家族性的肿瘤通常提示 SDHx 突变。在管理方面，多数患者可以进行观察并行连续的影像学复查。当需要治疗时，可选择放射治疗和手术治疗，最近大多数病例都转向放射治疗。

参考文献

扫描书末二维码获取。

第 24 章　桥小脑角及岩骨病变的手术治疗

Nicholas Hall · Yuval Sufaro · Andrew H. Kaye 著
赵博、卜博 译，卜博 审校

引言

二十世纪之交，神经外科之父 Harvey Cushing 将桥小脑角（cerebellopontine angle，CPA）区域描述为“神经外科的阴暗角落”，将这个解剖区域形象地比喻为“盖茨堡血腥的栅栏角”。由于当时放大倍数和照明条件的限制，现代颅底亚专科神经外科医生可以理解，那个年代像 Cushing 这样的先行者在治疗此部位大肿瘤，而且已有神经功能障碍时，手术所面临艰巨的技术挑战。在那个阶段，Cushing 提倡肿瘤次全切除作为唯一安全合理的手术策略，然而，在那之后不久，Dandy 开始提倡安全地全切 CPA 区肿瘤。

从那以后，引入了更高端的麻醉技术、围术期预防性应用抗生素、手术显微镜和脑神经监测技术，CPA 区域手术取得了长足的发展。病例向亚专科中心集中，大家认识到经验和精细技术的重要性，从而使得颅底外科转变为亚专科，进而降低了手术的死亡率和致残率。由于此部位脆弱而微细的解剖组织具有重要的神经功能，使得该部位病变的治疗颇具挑战。现在，这个部位病变的治疗效果通常可以做到极低的致残率。

本章旨在概述 CPA 的解剖和病理，描述了患者的临床表现和不同疾病诊断所需的检查，以及治疗这些病变的外科技术、入路和结果。

解剖

术者对此处复杂的解剖关系、解剖变异和病变造成的解剖扭曲变形都应该有详尽了解，进入这个美丽但危险的角落里进行手术，对术者的能力是极大的考验。

桥小脑角裂是由小脑岩面在脑桥和小脑中脚周围折叠而成，在桥小脑角中，小脑上下脚向上下延伸。

在此角又分为三部：上、中、下部。每个部分都包含供血动脉、脑干的一部分、脑裂的一部分和一系列脑神经。

桥小脑角上部（腔）包括小脑上动脉（superior cerebellar artery，SCA），中脑表面，脑神经Ⅲ、Ⅳ和Ⅴ，小脑上脚和小脑中脑裂。神经血管复合体穿过小脑中脑池。

桥小脑角中部（腔）内含小脑前下动脉（anterior inferior cerebellar artery，AICA）、第Ⅶ和Ⅷ脑神经复合体、脑桥前外侧表面、小脑中脚、桥小脑裂。Lushka 孔位于中腔的尖端，内侧是第四脑室的外侧隐窝。小脑绒球位于外侧隐窝脉络丛发出处的头侧稍偏后方。

桥小脑角下部（腔）包括后组脑神经Ⅸ ~ Ⅻ、小脑后下动脉和延髓外侧面、小脑下脚和小脑延髓裂。第六脑神经在裂的底部附近，沿着一条包含裂的上下肢的连线走行。脑神经、动脉、静脉和脑脊液蛛网膜池的复杂解剖，以及这些结构的解剖变异，Albert Rhoton 在他的专著中有详尽的描述（Rhoton，2007）。

脑神经穿过蛛网膜池进入各自的颅骨孔洞。舌下神经起自延髓，在与脊神经腹侧根连线相续的沟中自橄榄前方发出，进入枕髁的舌下神经管（孔）。副神经是由脊髓根和颅内根构成的，颅内根起自延髓下 1/3、橄榄前面，脊髓根起自上颈髓。迷走神经神经根束从迷走神经下根下方自脑干发出，它们之间难以区分，因为它们都是以多个根丝向前走行，进入颈静脉孔的血管部。舌咽神经由一个或两个相对比较粗大的神经根构成，从橄榄体后方的脑干发出，在脉络丛腹侧走行，与迷走神经和副神经分开，进入颈静脉孔的神经部。面神经在前庭蜗神经进入脑干处前方 1~2 mm 的地方自桥延沟外侧端发出。在脑干部位，面神经和前庭蜗神经大部分情况下是明显分开走行，但在小脑延髓池部位几乎一起走行。AICA 经常在Ⅶ和Ⅷ脑神经的脑干起源下方或两者之间穿过。Ⅴ脑神经从脑桥中点发出，从脑桥外侧倾斜向前向 Meckel 腔方向走行，走行（坐）于颞骨前端的三叉神经压迹中。三叉神经轴向旋转的变异性相当大，其在穿过脑池时与小脑上动脉关系密切。

桥小脑角病变的表现

不同的性质、大小的病变其临床表现差别很大。较小的病变可能是偶然发现的，作为对头痛等常见疾病的筛查的一部分，或者与病变的位置及其周围结构有关的特定症状，如前庭神经鞘瘤引起的听力损失和的共济失调，从而得到诊断。发病的缓急和特定的神经症状，为查明病变类型和部位提供了重要的线索。血管性病变（缺血和出血疾病）表现为几秒钟和几分钟内出现超急性症状。快速增长的病变，如转移瘤，可能导致急性脑积水，通常出现在数天至数周，但绝大多数 CPA 区病变生长缓慢，并在几个月甚至几年后出现症状。

特征性的神经功能障碍为病变的位置和类型提供了重要的线索。CPA 上部的病变常伴有三叉神经感觉减退或偶尔面部疼痛 / 复视。岩前病变可表现为第六神经麻痹所致的复视。CPA 中部病变表现为第Ⅶ和第Ⅷ脑神经复合体的症状，更常见的是平衡失调和听力损失，而不是面肌无力，面肌无力可能是面神经瘤的一个迹象。CPA 下部病变可能出现声音嘶哑、呛咳或误吸所致的反复胸部感染。较大的病变表现出与脑积水一致的症状，从头痛、恶心、呕吐、视力下降到记忆和步态障碍。特别大的病变压迫脑干和小脑，可能表现为进行性步态不稳、乏力和肌肉痉挛，最终导致昏迷和死亡。

在 CPA 内最常见的病变是听神经瘤，在多个病例组中，占 CPA 病变的 78%~85%（House，1964；Moffat and Ballagh，1995）。该部位第二常见的肿瘤是脑膜瘤，在 Moffat 1993 年的 305 例来自剑桥 Addenbrookes 的肿瘤中占 6.5%（Moffat et al.，1993），在 Revilla1947 年系列报道中占 6%。第三常见的病变是表皮样囊肿，分别占 4.6% 和 6%。在这个位置的其他病变也有报道，但总共只占病变的 2.7%。罕见鉴别诊断包括颈静脉球部病变 1.7%；其他神经鞘瘤：面神经鞘瘤 1%，三叉神经鞘瘤 1%，蛛网膜囊肿 0.7%，转移瘤 0.7%。其他极其罕见的诊断包括：动脉瘤、动静脉畸形、脉络丛乳头瘤、脂肪瘤、淋巴瘤、室管膜瘤、髓母细胞瘤、脊索瘤、软骨肉瘤、内淋巴囊瘤和胆固醇肉芽肿。在 MRI 和 CT 上的影像学特征可以为许多鉴别诊断提供相当大的帮助，许多病变具有特征性的表现。Bonneville 优雅地描述了一种节段性的方法来对罕见 CPA 部位病变进行影像学诊断（**图** 24.1 和**表** 24.1）（Bonneville et al.，2001）。

不同表现特征可以为查明病变类型提供线索，例如对于脑膜瘤和其他脑神经鞘瘤，常表现为听力完好，而面神经或三叉神经受累。病变鉴别的其他

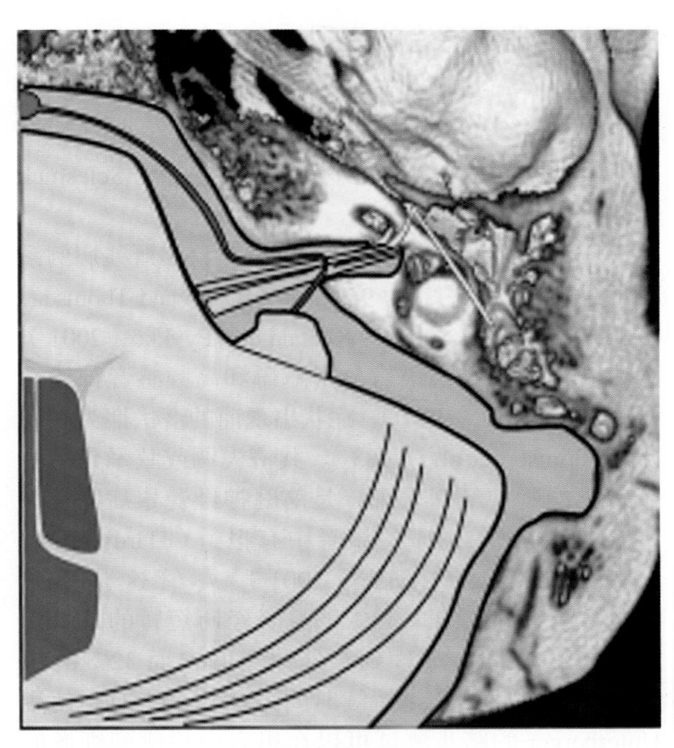

图 24.1　颅后窝成分的解剖表现。颜色与**表** 24.1 相关

表 24.1　基于起源部位的 CPA 区病变的分段鉴别诊断方法

脑池	表皮样囊肿 皮样囊肿 脂肪瘤 神经管肠源性囊肿 神经上皮囊肿	脑膜	脑膜瘤 蛛网膜囊肿 转移瘤
动脉	动脉瘤 动脉扩张	神经	听神经瘤 面神经瘤 中枢神经系统神经瘤
颅底	胆固醇肉芽肿 副神经节瘤 腺皮炎 软骨肉瘤 内淋巴囊瘤 垂体腺瘤	脑实质 / 脑室	毛细胞星形细胞瘤、胶质瘤、转移瘤、血管母细胞瘤、室管膜瘤、髓母细胞瘤、淋巴瘤、乳头状瘤、DNET

Reproduced from Bonneville, F., Sarrazin, J.L., Marsot-Dupuch, K., et al, Unusual Lesions of the Cerebellopontine Angle: A Segmental Approach, *RadioGraphics*, Vol. 21, No. 2, March 2001 with permission from RSNA.

影像学特征包括Ⅶ/Ⅷ神经复合体神经鞘瘤引起的内耳门（internal auditory meatus，IAM）的扩张和重塑，脑膜瘤中有硬脑膜尾征和平坦基底，以及表皮样囊肿中存在脑脊液样信号，即T1低信号、T2高信号（DWI高信号、ADC低信号）（Bonneville et al.，2001）。

前庭神经鞘瘤患者的表现

虽然听神经瘤的典型表现症状是单侧听力损失、耳鸣和共济失调，但有越来越多的患者在MRI检查时偶然发现，5%~12%的为无症状肿瘤（Selesnick et al.，1999）。

听力丧失是最常见的表现症状，许多既往病例系列报告听力丧失率为94%~96%（Tos and Thomsen，1984；Hardy et al.，1989；Kentala and Pyykkö，2001）。通常，患者会经历语言分辨障碍和高频感音神经性耳聋（Johnson，1977）。症状出现前的潜伏期为3~8年（Thomsen et al.，1983）。共济失调或眩晕是另一个常见的听神经瘤表现，是前庭神经受累症状。这种症状在50%~77%的患者中有报道（Hardy et al.，1989；Kentala and Pyykkö，2001），尽管这是不常见的主要表现特征。47%的患者经历短暂的眩晕发作，持续时间在2秒到5分钟之间，而32%的患者的发作时间更长，持续时间可达几个小时。使用Unterberger的踏步测试可以在患者中检测到细微的平衡异常。在这个测试中，患者被要求直立，闭着眼睛，手臂前伸与躯干成90°，并在现场行走。如果患者偏离现场超过指定线路50 cm或偏离角度超过30°，则判定为阳性。更严重的共济失调可能与肿瘤较大以及小脑功能障碍有关。

耳鸣是另一个常见的特征性表现，见于57%~83%的患者。耳鸣很少单独出现，在3%的患者中，耳鸣是唯一的主诉。在Samii报道的1000名听神经瘤患者中，他评估了术前症状，发现在单纯内听道肿瘤中，肿瘤增大的情况下86%耳鸣反而变少，在肿瘤增大压迫脑干时，51%的患者变为无耳鸣（Matthies and Samii，1997）。

小脑功能障碍是较大肿瘤的一个常见表现特征，如果肿瘤直径超过4 cm，58%的患者中都会出现小脑症状。小脑功能障碍通常表现为指鼻试验和步态异常。

眼球震颤是症状表现时的一个常见体征，根据肿瘤压迫部位表现出不同的类型。大肿瘤引起脑桥凝视中枢的明显压迫，可能出现视动性眼球震颤或Bruns眼球震颤。Bruns眼球震颤包括宽幅的同侧水平眼球震颤和对侧凝视的高频小幅眼球震颤。小肿瘤引起的前庭眼球震颤表现为远离病变侧的小幅水平眼球震颤（Kaye and Laws，2012）。

脑神经功能障碍更为少见，在Samii研究系列报道中，18%的患者表现为轻微的三叉神经感觉减退，通常在V2分布区。随着肿瘤的扩大，发病率增加到32%（Matthies and Samii，1997）。面肌无力也很少见，但可以表现出瞬目反射消失或延迟，这一表现见于多达17%的患者中（Matthies and Samii，1997）。外耳道后部的感觉丧失是常见的，继发于中间神经受累。

头痛是另一个常见的特征性表现，见于20%~85%的患者（Stucken et al.，2012）。头痛通常是MRI或CT脑扫描偶然发现听神经瘤的原因。

颅内压升高在听神经瘤的早期报告中很常见，导致头痛、恶心、呕吐、视力下降、复视、视盘水肿和意识改变等症状。在Cushing1917年病例系列中，66%的患者有复视（Cushing，1917），而在UCSF最近发表的一项研究中，复视只有3%（Selesnick et al.，1993）。

展神经受累产生向侧方注视时复视并不太常见（1.8%）（Matthies and Samii，1997）。听神经瘤时表现为三叉神经痛、面肌痉挛和突发性听力丧失的情况十分罕见（Matthies and Samii，1997）。

桥小脑角病变的进一步评估

影像学评估

临床医生可用的影像学工具的进展无疑改变了颅底和CPA部位病变的诊断视角。从1910年使用平片成像“颞骨岩锥部”的早期开始，跨过气脑造影和增强脊髓造影的时代，我们已经开始将CT和MRI作为金标准工具。在诊断方面，MRI诊断听神经瘤的敏感性和特异性高达100%（Brackmann and Kwartler，1990；Newton et al.，2010）。增强钆对比序列和薄层采集序列，如重度饱和T2快速自旋回波和3DFTCISS，使前庭神经鞘瘤检测得以小至3 mm，灵敏度和特异性率分别为97%和96%（Stuckey et al.，1996；Naganawa et al.，1998）。

前庭神经鞘瘤的典型MRI表现是在IAM内的肿瘤，通常造成IAM扩大，肿瘤进而不同程度扩展到CPA。肿瘤在T1序列上为低信号，在T2序列上与脑脊液相比为低信号，与脑干相比为高信号。与神经鞘瘤相比，脑膜瘤具有广泛的硬脑膜基底，更有可能在T1和T2图像上与大脑呈等信号强度，钆剂可明显增强。CPA部位脑膜瘤很少以IAM为中心生长，即便它们长在IAM也不扩张IAM。相比圆形的前庭神经鞘瘤，脑膜瘤的形状通常被认为是更椭圆形，而且也有硬脑膜尾征，此点不存在于神经鞘瘤。表皮样肿瘤具有特征性的MRI表现，在T1和T2序列上与CSF相同，没有钆增强，但在DWI和ADC图像序列有很强的弥散限制。

虽然在诊断方面没有必要，但CT扫描可能有助于评估CPA部位病变。与MRI相比，IAM的扩大在CT上表现得更好，CT上钙化能很好识别，而大约25%的脑膜瘤有钙化。我们通常使用CT作为外科计划的辅助手段，因为它提供了关于颞骨岩部气化程度、内听道周围气房的存在和颈静脉球的骨解剖的有价值的信息。我们利用这些信息来确定是否适合经迷路入路，以及在乙状窦后入路中磨除内耳道外侧的程度，以利切除长入内听道内的肿瘤。侵及颞骨岩部的CPA部位肿瘤，如胆脂瘤或颈静脉瘤，有关面神经管、颈静脉孔内侧壁和中耳的解剖信息，对于术中计划如何显露也至关重要。

听力测量

鉴于前庭神经鞘瘤占CPA部位病变的75%~85%，其特征性表现为听力丧失，故听力测试是术前评估CPA部位病变的重要手段。由于所有CPA区手术都有听力恶化的风险，因此进行听力基线评估也很重要。此外，一些可理想显露和切除肿瘤的方法，如经迷路入路，会导致单侧耳聋。显露的改善和手术致残率降低可能使这一入路成为一种首选的方案，但必须确定对侧听力是否正常，以确保该方法不会使患者全聋。

听神经瘤患者的纯音听力（pure-tone audiogram，PTA）阈值范围为5~130 dB，平均阈值为66.5 dB。约16%的患者完全丧失听力，无法测试。65%的患者有高频段听力丧失，22%的患者有广泛频段听力丧失（Johnson，1977; Stucken et al.，2012）。言语辨别能力差是耳蜗后病变的典型特征。在Johnson的1977年研究中，500例听神经瘤患者中有24%没有言语分辨障碍，56%的患者有60%或更低的言语分辨率（speech discrimination scores，SDS）。

PTA和SDS的结合构成了“可使用”和“可挽救”听力的几个定义的基础，这些定义用于评估听神经瘤患者术中听力保留的潜力。Gardner Robertson听力功能量表将患者的听力分为很好、有用、无用、差和完全丧失（**表**24.2），0~30 dB PTA和70%~100%SDS的病例最有机会保存听力。

表 24.2　Gardner Robertson 听力分级

Gardner Robertson 听力分级	描述	言语分辨率（SDS）	最大纯音听力（PTA）
Ⅰ	很好	70%~100%	0~30 dB
Ⅱ	有用	50%~69%	31~50 dB
Ⅲ	无用	5%~49%	51~90 dB
Ⅳ	差	1%~4%	91 dB 至最大值
Ⅴ	完全丧失	0	测不到

Reproduced with permission from Gardner G, Robertson JH, Hearing preservation in unilateral acoustic neuroma surgery, *Annals of Otology, Rhinology & Laryngology*, Volume 97, pp. 55–66, Copyright © 1988, SAGE.

听觉脑干反应（auditory brainstem responses，ABRs）测量下听觉通路神经元对刺激的同步反应。在Selters和Brackmann于1977年将其应用从研究扩展到临床应用后，ABR成为筛选听神经瘤患者的成熟方法（Selters and Brackmann，1977）。ABR包括发出刺激和测量记录随后的诱发反应。最常用的是100 μs的短声刺激。这种反应是从头皮电极记录下来的，并显示为一系列可预测的波，分别标记为波Ⅰ到Ⅴ。波Ⅰ和Ⅴ是最稳定的，分别代表耳蜗、神经和下丘神经元（核团）的活动。最可靠的波间潜伏期是Ⅰ到Ⅴ波间潜伏期差值，称为IT5。波间潜伏期差大于0.2 ms提示异常（Selesnick and Jackler，1992）。文献报道，根据ABR诊断听神经瘤的测试灵敏度为优秀，灵敏度报告在93%~100%，特异性为90%（Stucken et al.，2012）。自从引入MRI以来，这些数据被证明是不太准确的，灵敏度为63%~95%；特别是1 cm以下的小肿瘤，其准确率为58%（Schmidt et al.，2001）。发现ABR不像以前认为的那样敏感，导致了堆叠ABR的发展。堆叠ABR基本上测量了所有的Ⅷ神经纤维，而不仅仅是一部分神经纤维，因此不太受肿瘤的大小和位置影响。2005年，Don等发表了一组54例小肿瘤患者的研究，显示堆叠ABR 95%的敏感性和88%的特异性（Don et al.，2005）。

面神经功能

术前面神经功能评估是诊断评估的重要内容。尽管17%的前庭神经鞘瘤患者存在轻微的肌无力，仅有1/3的患者有自觉症状（Matthies and Samii，1997）。导致脑干和第四脑室移位的较大肿瘤报告面肌无力的发病率为26%（Matthies and Samii，

1997）。轻微的面肌无力可能会表现出瞬目反射（传出弧）减缓，一小部分患者有味觉改变，而更大比例的患者会表现出外耳道后部感觉减退。

术前和术后面神经功能应记录在案，并有大量的量表可供评估面神经功能。由 House 于 1985 年设计的长期公认的评价系统得到了广泛的接受，到目前为止，大多数术后结果都是根据这个量表报告的（House and Brackmann，1985；也见**第 22 章**）。这个量表受到了广泛的批评，因为它无法对面部的每个区域进行单独的评估。在 19 种得到验证的面神经评估方法中，只有 Sunnybrook 系统（Ross et al.，1996）对每个面神经区域进行评分，检查静态和动态活动以及连带运动，因而具有良好的观察者间可靠性（Fattah et al.，2015）。

术前面部无力和 CPA 部位病变的患者可能有面神经鞘瘤。面部神经瘤通常横向延伸到内耳道以外，进入或跨过 IAM 的底部。

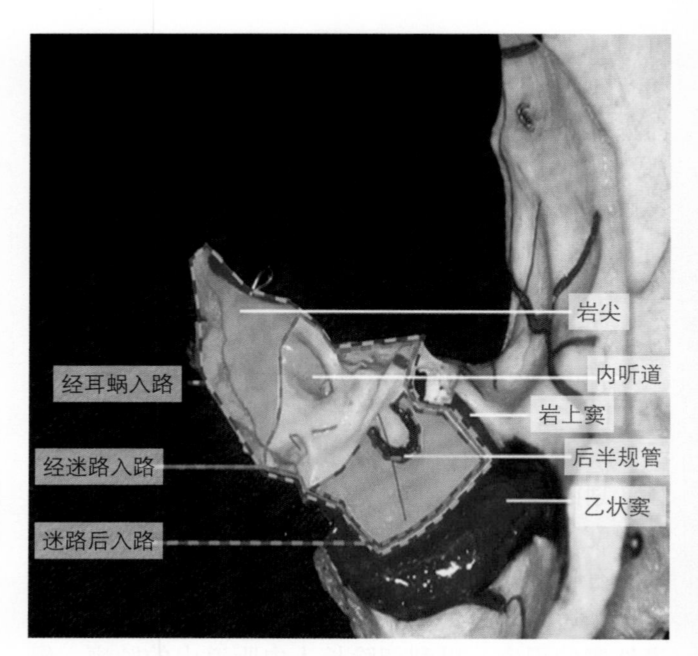

图 24.2 经岩骨入路骨切除术的三维演示

手术治疗 CPA 区肿瘤

必须进行复杂的分析和研究，才能确定 CPA 区和岩部病变的最佳手术入路。要考虑到多种因素，如病变的解剖位置、大小、患侧的听力状态、患者的骨质和静脉窦解剖以及病变的影像学特征。

手术入路可分为乙状窦前入路和乙状窦后入路。乙状窦后入路涉及枕骨开颅手术，包括枕骨切开术和枕骨切除术。而乙状窦前入路要求磨除岩骨，显露硬脑膜和颅后窝病变，在乙状窦前操作对脑组织牵拉很轻。乙状窦前通常是指岩后入路，它们都是基础乳突切除术的扩展。在这一类手术中，岩骨切除术从后到前依次包括迷路后、经迷路和经耳蜗入路，骨质切除依次增多。这些入路使得手术可达 CPA 区，具体说就是斜坡的中、上 2/3。岩骨切除术越靠前，手术进入颅后窝的通道越宽（**图 24.2**）。迷路后入路，几乎从未单独使用，避开前庭器官，因此是三种入路中最不容易致残的，而经迷路入路涉及切除前庭器官，因此不可避免地导致听力损失。进一步切除耳蜗需要面神经移位，有至少部分面神经损伤的可能性，从而显著增加入路相关的致残率。已有对经岩骨入路的一些改良的报道，目的是降低相关的脑神经致残率，同时改善手术暴露。在经颅入路中，选择性切除从壶腹到总脚的后半规管和前半规管，允许在接近经迷路入路的范围内暴露，同时有可能最大程度上保留听力。使用这种方法保留听力结果的文献报告很少，主要是由于它很少使用，同时需要术者具备特定的高超手术技巧。然而，据报道，此方法保留听力比例为 58%~100%（Sekhar et al.，1999；Horgan et al.，2001；Kaylie et al.，2004；Brandt et al.，2010）。在经耳囊入路中，通过完全切除半规管和面神经骨管化，进入耳囊。与经耳蜗入路一样，听力丧失，但面神经受损率降低。与经壶腹入路相似，经耳蜗入路临床结果资料很少。面神经功能保留的报告往往模棱两可。大多数可用的研究都认为 HB Ⅰ ~ Ⅱ是良好的面部功能结果。长期随访的 HB Ⅰ ~ Ⅱ报告从 27%~90% 不等。当然也与病变类型有关。当采用经耳蜗入路切除岩斜区脑膜瘤时，面神经的功能保留结果差异较大（De la Cruz and Teufert，2009；Gurgel et al.，2012；Miller et al.，2015）。

一般情况下，乙状窦后入路的 CPA 区暴露范围很广。通过这种方法，可以切除在整个 CPA 区的病变，上至小脑幕，下至枕大孔。如果较小的病变位于岩枕软骨结合部的内侧，乙状窦后入路的显露受到一定限制，但不用牵拉脑干，可避免无法接受的副损伤。较大的斜坡和岩斜病变采用该入路可以先暴露肿瘤的前部，因为肿瘤在其缓慢生长过程中通过挤压脑干有效地打开了解剖走廊。乙状窦后入路受小脑幕的限制，对于位于幕切迹以上或跨过岩尖进入中颅窝的肿瘤，仅用这种入路难以完全切除。在这种情况下，无论是分期的或中颅窝 - 乙状窦前联合入路，均可以到达小脑幕和岩尖上方。

在以 IAM 为中心的较大病变中，如大的前庭神经鞘瘤，我们更喜欢使用经迷路入路。它的优点是通过旋转手术台调整入路的角度，显露陷入小脑半球内的肿瘤，使小脑牵拉最小化，它还缩短了术者与肿瘤之间的工作距离，便于更好地操作器械。有经验的外科医生在充分暴露的情况下，经迷路入路甚至能切除巨大的神经鞘瘤。某些解剖因素可能使这种方法不太可取，包括高位的优势的颈静脉球、乳突气化不佳和乙状窦前置。这些因素都减少了这种入路的工作空间，减少了可视的角度，特别是较大肿瘤的下表面和脑干面。

联合乙状窦前中窝入路为位于脑神经前方的病变提供了极好的暴露，但与入路相关的并发症随之增加。最常见的是迷路后中颅窝联合入路开颅，术者可以直视肿瘤的前外侧、脑桥上部和中脑下部，特别适用于延伸到中颅窝的肿瘤。

对于主要位于岩尖和中颅窝内的病变，如许多三叉神经神经鞘瘤，最广泛的最佳切除途径通常主要是通过中颅窝、颞下入路，并有可能通过 Kawase 入路等方法进一步去除岩尖。Kawase 三角的边界是三叉神经的 V3 支在前方，岩浅大神经在外侧，弓状隆起位于后方，内侧为岩上窦。这种方法也被称为岩前入路。在这些病变中，许多骨质已被肿瘤侵蚀，这是很常见的。对于主体局限于内听道内的肿瘤，如果 CPA 区扩展较少而听力完整，采用经中颅窝入路到达 IAM 也能比较容易地肿瘤切除。

虽然肿瘤的解剖位置和大小在选择入路的决策中起着重要的作用，但必须有所限制。在有明显并发症或高龄的患者中，最佳的选择可能只是侵袭性最小的入路。在这种情况下，手术的目标可能会从肿瘤的完全切除转变为脑干和小脑的减压，通过乙状窦后入路进行有限的减瘤手术。外科医生盲目追求完整肿瘤切除必须受到限制，因为并发症很高，例如在面神经或后组脑神经鞘瘤或 NF2 患者中，听力保护是首要的。

此外，预估肿瘤的质地和血供在确定理想的入路中起着一定的作用。T2 高信号的肿瘤可能韧性更小，允许囊内切除减压和更容易从周围的神经血管结构中剥离。相反，血供丰富或质地坚韧的肿瘤可能需要一种更精细的入路来最大限度地暴露肿瘤，并为手术者提供更短、更好的切除肿瘤的角度。

在某些情况下，特别是当肿瘤从前向颅后窝广泛扩展时，需要分期使用多种入路切除肿瘤。

乙状窦入路

乙状窦后入路是理想的前庭神经鞘瘤的保留听力的术式。对于许多其他主体在颞骨岩部的肿瘤，我们也倾向这种方法。这种入路也能显露更大的前方病变，如岩斜脑膜瘤，并且特别适用于老年人和更虚弱的人群，因为他们不能耐受麻醉时间延长或颞下入路中对颞叶的长时间牵拉操作。对于大多数表皮样囊肿，这种入路可以安全地切除肿瘤，结合使用成角内镜，可以完全切除肿瘤。

体位：虽然描述了许多体位，我们倾向侧卧或公园长椅位。患者侧卧在手术台上，手术侧向上。对侧腋部垫有腋卷，腋部在手术台的最前端，对侧臂保持在与同侧手臂的臂沟相连的托槽上。两条腿都弯曲，两个枕头横向放置在它们之间。臀部固定在手术台上，背部支撑托放置在躯干中部，同侧肩膀被轻轻地绑在上面。三钉头架固定头部，头部屈曲并转向地面 10°~15°。此时通常放置腰大池引流。术中对面神经功能的持续电生理监测是必不可少的。对于 CPA 范围内的肿瘤，我们也倾向于使用气管内导管监测后组脑神经，主要是声带监测，另外通过软腭电极和斜方肌电极监测对应的脑神经。对于颈部粗短的患者，我们偶尔使用半坐位。

切口和暴露：S 形切口，从乳突后 1 cm，横窦乙状窦交界处上方约 2.5 cm 到乳突尖端水平以下。切口的下端远离乳突尖端向内弯曲，以避开在 C1 横突周围深在的椎动脉（**图 24.3**）。肌肉和筋膜向枕下翻转，外侧到二腹肌沟。然后在星点的水平上钻孔，孔加宽以暴露横窦乙状窦交汇点。进一步向后钻孔并暴露横窦，向下在菲薄的枕骨鳞部钻孔，开颅完成。必须注意保护硬脑膜，并确保在暴露过程中不要损坏位于上方的静脉窦，并且骨管化经常遇到的乳突导静脉，远离静脉窦电凝和离断导静脉。我们使用 5 mm 糙面金刚石磨钻安全地蛋壳化静脉窦。硬脑膜以不对称的 Y 形打开，以乙状窦和横窦为基底翻开硬膜瓣。在打开硬脑膜之前，通过腰大池引流出 5~10 ml 的脑脊液。这减轻了硬脑膜和颅后窝的内容物的张力。对于非常大的肿瘤，未经治疗的脑积水将是腰大池引流的禁忌，在这种情况下，需要通过一个小的硬膜切口打开枕大池引流脑脊液。打开硬脑膜后，可利用手术显微镜进入基底池，进一步引流脑脊液。

在此阶段，连接 Greenberg 牵开器系统，在必要时，使用脑压板牵开器非常轻柔地牵开小脑。在确认肿瘤后，识别并打开肿瘤后方囊壁上的蛛网膜界面。此操作有利于分离肿瘤包膜，使肿瘤远离周围重要且必须保护的结构。在下方，确认并保护Ⅸ ~ Ⅺ脑神经复合物和 AICA 袢，AICA 的分支经常与前庭神经鞘瘤的后壁和 CPA 区中部的肿瘤相关，这些都

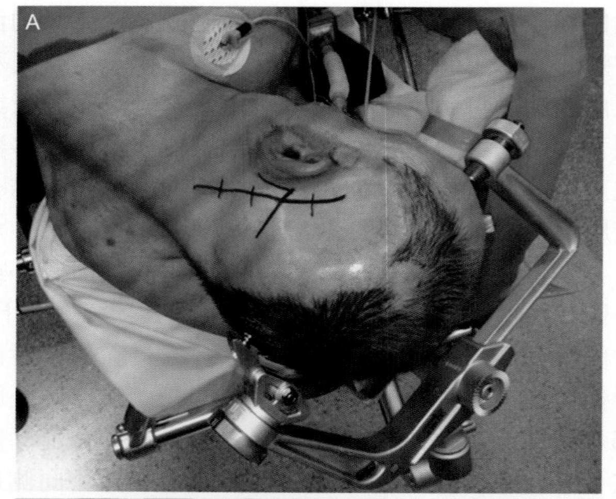

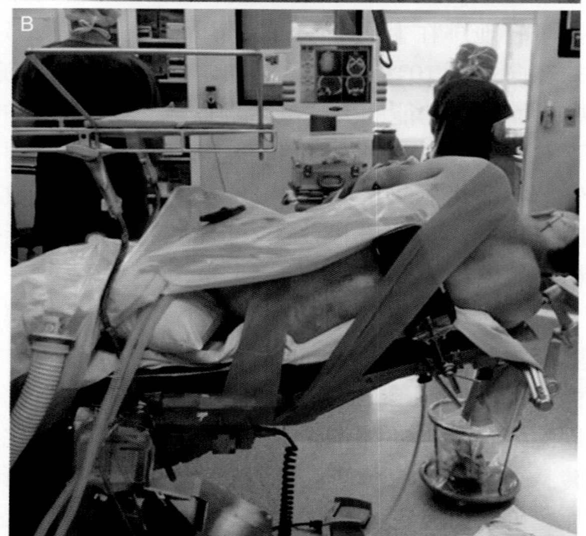

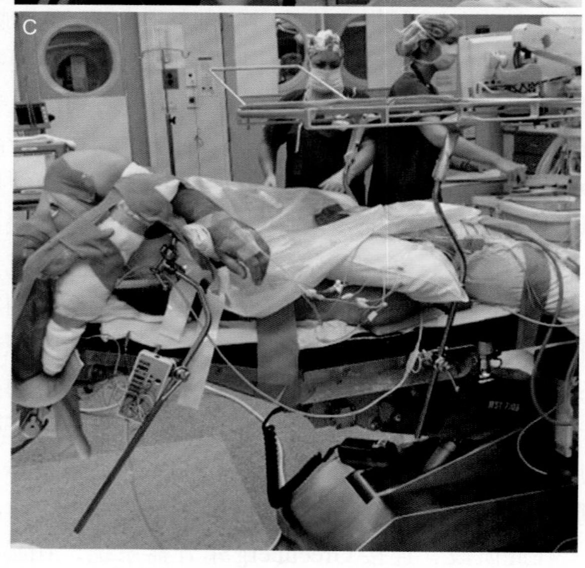

图 24.3 乙状窦后开颅手术的体位和切口。(A)皮肤切口;(B)侧卧位;(C)侧卧位，注意腋窝垫卷的位置、对侧上臂和同侧手臂悬挂和布袋托槽的排列

必须保存。然而，如果确认较小的血管分支进入肿瘤包膜，可以将之电凝切断。上方，首先辨认第Ⅴ和Ⅳ脑神经以及 Dandy 静脉。可能的情况下尽量保留 Dandy 静脉，但偶尔可能需要电凝切断之，特别是有可能从岩上窦上撕脱的危险时。应注意确保此时 SCA 的分支不要被无意中电凝。这是文献报告中该静脉电凝相关的一些并发症的原因。

在大多数 CPA 区肿瘤中，可以进入肿瘤包膜和小脑之间的蛛网膜界面，沿此界面解剖分离，可直视脑干和各自的脑神经根进入区（root entry zones, REZ）。在较大的肿瘤中，因为脑干严重受压，在分离肿瘤和脑干的界面之前，首先要使用双极电凝、锐性分离和吸引器来进行肿瘤内减压。双极电凝必须在最低电压设置下使用，以尽量减少热传递和损伤神经的风险。在前庭神经鞘瘤的情况下，充分内减压后，可将肿瘤向下牵拉，然后从肿瘤包膜上方解剖分离第Ⅴ脑神经，并在侧方充分显露第八脑神经根进入区（REZ）和 AICA。如果不尝试保护听力，可将前庭和耳蜗纤维锐性切断，并注意确保保留旁边的Ⅶ脑神经。AICA 经常在两个神经之间走行。面神经也可以通过其白色和接近舌咽神经根入脑干区（REZ）来识别，并通过温和的电刺激来识别。在确定了Ⅶ脑神经的位置后，可以进一步内减压切除肿瘤，锐性仔细地打开肿瘤 - 脑干界面。使用显微剪刀或锋利的蛛网膜刀，沿侧侧方向（a side-to-side direction）将Ⅶ脑神经从包膜上分离下来。在手术目的是保留听力的情况下，不要切断耳蜗神经，而是用一种细致的锐性分离技术，将耳蜗神经自肿瘤的包膜上游离下来。

对于其他 CPA 区肿瘤，原则保持不变，内减压为将肿瘤包膜从周围血管、脑神经以及小脑和脑干面剥离创造了空间。前庭神经鞘瘤周围有蛛网膜界面，面神经位于肿瘤包膜表面，并受到肿瘤的牵拉。相反，脑膜瘤通常表现出一层蛛网膜之间的包膜和上覆的神经血管结构，这有助于识别细致的解剖平面。当肿瘤延伸到 IAM 或颈静脉孔时，可能需要进一步磨除骨质以安全地切除瘤体。一旦打开 IAM 的硬脑膜，分离肿瘤包膜和 IAM 边缘之间的蛛网膜界面，进一步瘤内减压切除，以移动肿瘤。在切除肿瘤后，使用 70° 内镜检查 IAM 的外侧部，以确保没有小块肿瘤残余物残留在磨开的 IAM 内。

经迷路入路

该入路可导致听力丧失，因此特别适合于治疗较大的前庭神经鞘瘤，特别是听力已经丧失的病例。它对这些肿瘤特别有用，因为暴露打开 IAM 的后壁和上壁，允许显露 IAM 底部的面神经，从而可以很好地显示肿瘤的最外侧部分，以便进行大体全切。此外，该入路提供了一个更直接的CPA区暴露，并避免了牵开小脑。该方法与中颅窝开颅和切开小脑幕相结合，提供了对CPA区前部高处并延伸到中颅窝的肿瘤的全景性视角。在这种方法中，必须注意评估和保留Labbe静脉的汇入点，并尽量减少对颞叶的牵拉，对这些结构的任何损害都会导致明显的并发症。

在典型的经迷路入路中，在Trautmann三角区打开颅后窝硬脑膜，该三角以乙状窦、颈静脉球和上岩窦为界。前置乙状窦或高位颈静脉球的存在可能会限制该入路的应用。高位颈静脉球可见于9%~18%的颞骨，可能与颞骨气化不良有关。

我们进行大多数CPA区手术，需要颅底专家组建一个颅底团队，包括经验丰富和熟练的神经耳科医生。我们更喜欢在手术中使用仰卧位，三钉头架固定头部，并旋转大约45°。侧屈可以拓宽肩部与术区之间的角度，以便在处理较大的、靠上部的肿瘤时，更好地显露肿瘤上极和小脑幕。床头应抬高至30°，以改善静脉回流，颈部应稍牵引过伸，使面神经管与地面平行。取腹部脂肪，如果需要重建小脑幕，可从大腿外侧获取脂肪和阔筋膜。我们使用一个大的C形切口，在乳突和乙状窦后面。在翻开皮瓣后，T形切开骨筋膜并将之剥离，显露乳突皮质骨，然后由神经耳科医生进行广泛的乳突皮质切除术。

完成乳突切除术，前方暴露外耳道后壁薄层皮质骨。上方显露中颅窝底硬膜和岩上窦的硬脑膜，后显露乙状窦，乳突骨质蛋壳化，显示二腹肌嵴，然后向下方显露颈静脉球。打开乳突窦和鼓窦入口，移除砧骨，显露上鼓室隐窝内侧壁上的外侧半规管，面神经水平段位于外侧半规管的深面和前部。确认并开放半规管，移除外侧管，打开前庭和后、上管，以显示位于面神经第二膝深面的总脚。骨管化面神经管。在前庭深处，270°磨开内听道（internal auditory canal，IAC），在内听道底部确认横嵴。通常可以通过耳蜗水管引流部分脑脊液，使小脑得到一定程度的松弛。我们认为特别实用的相关技术，包括移除乙状窦后的枕骨约1 cm，这样可以向后牵拉乙状窦，从而增加暴露。我们还努力尽量减少对乙状窦的压迫，或在主侧静脉窦的情况下，尽量向下推移压低高位颈静脉球，以增加手术空间。在某些情况下，这会影响到术者的决策，采用此入路抑或乙状窦后入路。我们还认为最大限度地暴露IAM是有帮助的，特别是在肿瘤特大、前部肿瘤更多的情况下，其中270°开放IAM能更好地显露这部分肿瘤（**图24.4**）。

在前庭神经鞘瘤的情况下，打开IAC硬脑膜，在IAC底部刺激并辨认面神经、前庭和耳蜗神经。在我们的团队中，神经外科医生打开硬脑膜，释放脑脊液，并识别肿瘤周围的蛛网膜界面。刺激肿瘤包膜以排除面神经，安全地打开包膜。使用剪刀、吸引器和超声碎吸对病变进行内减压切除。这种切除后，可将肿瘤边缘从小脑、岩上静脉、后组脑神经和SCA的穿支上翻卷下来。一旦肿瘤被切除到足以识别自脑干发出的Ⅷ和Ⅶ脑神经，再进一步内减压切除并向侧方剥离这些神经。解剖蛛网膜界面和去除菲薄的包膜，术者通常可以向侧方牵拉和切除肿瘤，直到神经粘连最严重的IAM口。在内听道口，面神经散开来且变得菲薄，必须十分小心仔细地剥离以保留面部功能。IAM内肿瘤的成分通常会越来越少，直到最后仅有这部分残瘤。然后，我们沿着自内侧到外侧方向切除IAM内的残瘤肿瘤，目的是实现完全切除肿瘤。如果面神经特别粘连紧密且十分菲薄，我们可以选择在这一点上单独留下少量的残余肿瘤包膜，尽管这种情况很少见但是十分必要。在肿瘤切除和面神经解剖分离过程中，持续的肌电图（EMG）监测是减少神经损伤的关键。无论是在解剖分离过程中还是肿瘤切除完成后，近心端电刺激可以评估功能完整性。

经过细致的止血，打开的硬脑膜在显微镜下缝合，一直到内听道口。然后将中耳腔填充小块脂肪和肌肉的组合体，用冲洗液将CPA区填充后，将抗生素脂肪移植物放置在乳突腔中。颞肌筋膜以水密的方式闭合，皮肤分层闭合，以乳突绷带和敷料加压包扎。

迷路后入路

迷路后入路可以到达中斜坡区域。就其本身而言，对岩斜区和CPA暴露量有限。然而，在听力有用（serviceable hearing）的患者中，作为经小脑幕颅中窝联合入路的一部分，这项技术在切除跨越颅后窝和中颅窝病变中起着重要的作用。该入路的详细描述可在外科文献中找到（Brackmann，1979；McElveen et al.，1988；Glasscock et al.，1991；Ortiz Armenta，1992）。患者的体位类似于经迷路入路。在完成乳突切除术后，使用高速钻进一步向内侧切除颞骨，以暴露Trautmann三角，其对应于小脑区域的硬膜：下方为颈静脉球硬脑膜、上方为中颅窝硬脑膜、后方为岩上窦和乙状窦，前方为耳囊。沿Trautmann三角

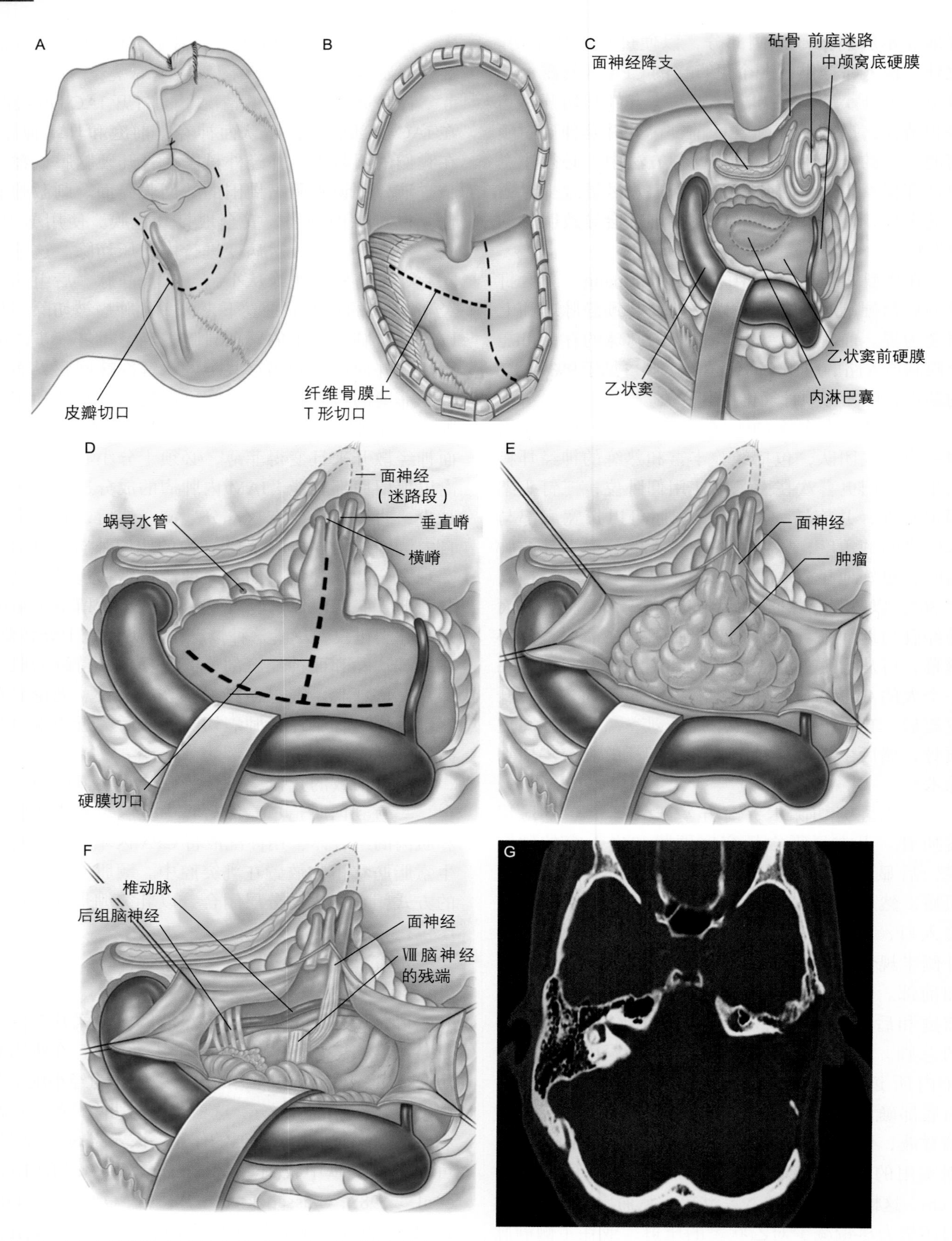

图 24.4 （A）经迷路入路的皮肤切口。（B）纤维骨膜切口，暴露乳突皮质。（C）扩大的乳突切除术，骨管化半规管和面神经降支。（D）完成颞骨和内耳道解剖。显示硬膜切口线。（E）切开硬脑膜，并向各方牵开，初步暴露肿瘤。（F）切除完成时肿瘤床。面神经在它最常见的位置，向内和向上移位。（G）经迷路入路切除一大体积神经鞘瘤术后。术后CT显示左侧颞骨缺损。经迷路入路对桥小脑角和内耳道的暴露比枕下入路更直接

的下部可见内淋巴囊，在后半规管的下方。应注意不要解剖内淋巴囊或磨钻磨入半规管，因为这很可能导致永久性听力损失。然后，平行于耳囊，以之为基底将硬脑膜瓣翻起。

经耳蜗入路

在经岩后入路中，该入路最大限度地去除岩骨，以获得最大程度的前方暴露。该入路提供了一条宽阔的通路，到达斜坡的中上部以及脑干前方。这种方法对听神经瘤的切除不太有用，而且有入路相关的固有的并发症，如面瘫和潜在的脑脊液漏。经耳囊时根据需要手术入路可做相应的变化，其中保持骨性面神经管完整，其作为一个骨桥位于入路的视野中。经耳蜗入路有两种方法。经典的正如 House 和 Hitselberger 所描述的，涉及面神经移位（Hisselberger，1966；House and Luetje，1979）。它涉及面神经的完全骨化，向后移位面神经，以获得平坦的暴露。将岩浅大神经自膝状神经节发出处切断，以便释放游离并移位面神经。一旦面神经后移，就可进入耳蜗。在 Fisch 描述的经耳囊入路中，没有移位面神经，但阻断和切除了外耳道。沿岩下窦继续磨除直到岩尖。颈内动脉的岩骨段位于所暴露视野的外侧面。

联合中颅窝和经岩骨入路

涉及岩斜区的肿瘤，延伸到中脑周围或脑桥周围结构，可以采用经岩入路。对于更广泛延伸到前床突和颈动脉池前方的病变，应考虑扩大经岩骨入路。为了到达这些区域，经岩骨方法具有许多优点。术者到这些区域的手术距离比乙状窦后入路短，对小脑和颞叶的牵拉程度最小，神经结构（即脑神经Ⅶ和Ⅷ）得到保护，耳科结构（即耳蜗、迷路和半规管）得到保留，主要的静脉窦（即横窦和乙状窦），连同 Labbe 静脉和其他颞叶和基底静脉均被保留下来。

患者的体位方式与经迷路的大致相同。切口在耳屏前始于颧骨，向后上围绕耳郭上 2~3 cm 向后上延伸，然后下降到乳突后面。从颅骨骨膜和筋膜上锐性剥离皮瓣。将颞肌筋膜锐性切断翻开，并与胸锁乳突肌保持连续性，然后将颞肌本身锐性切开并自骨面剥离，然后向前下翻转。钻孔四枚，横窦两侧各两个。第一孔位于星点的内下方，它正好位于横窦和乙状窦交界处的下方。第二孔位于颞骨鳞部和乳突交界处，在颞上线延长线上，该孔开口在幕上区。后续两孔位于前两孔内侧 2~3 cm 的位置。位于横窦两侧，两孔距离更近一些。在不连通跨窦骨孔的情况下，进行颞顶开颅和枕外侧开颅。然后连通跨窦的骨孔。细致分离窦壁后，抬起骨瓣。术者接下来进行颞骨后部切除，根据肿瘤的程度和患者的术前听力状况，可以选择迷路后或经迷路入路切除骨质。一旦骨质切除完成，即可打开颅后窝的硬脑膜，然后打开颞叶的硬脑膜，结扎岩上窦，将上下两处硬膜连通，在 Labbe 静脉注入横窦和岩上窦之前结扎岩上窦，Labbe 静脉一定要保留。然后，用蛇形牵开器轻轻牵开颞叶，在显微镜下剪开小脑幕，在小脑幕切迹处，在仔细完全切开小脑幕之前，在小脑幕切缘深部合 1~2 针，牵开小脑幕，扩大显露，然后向内在第Ⅳ脑神经进入小脑幕后方剪开幕缘。在这一步之前，可以看到Ⅳ脑神经穿过蛛网膜下的中脑周围池。向前牵拉小脑幕缘，显露该部位全景式解剖结构（图 24.5）。

CPA 区病变的手术结果

前庭神经鞘瘤

为了评估前庭神经鞘瘤的切除效果，我们对乙状窦后和经迷路的手术结果进行了比较。这两种方法都有优点和缺点，实际上，大多数团队都开发了一种他们最熟悉和最舒服的方法。

在多个系列的文献报道中，在死亡率、面神经功能和听力保存方面，决定结果的最大单因素是肿瘤大小（King and Morrison，1980；Ruth et al.，1985；

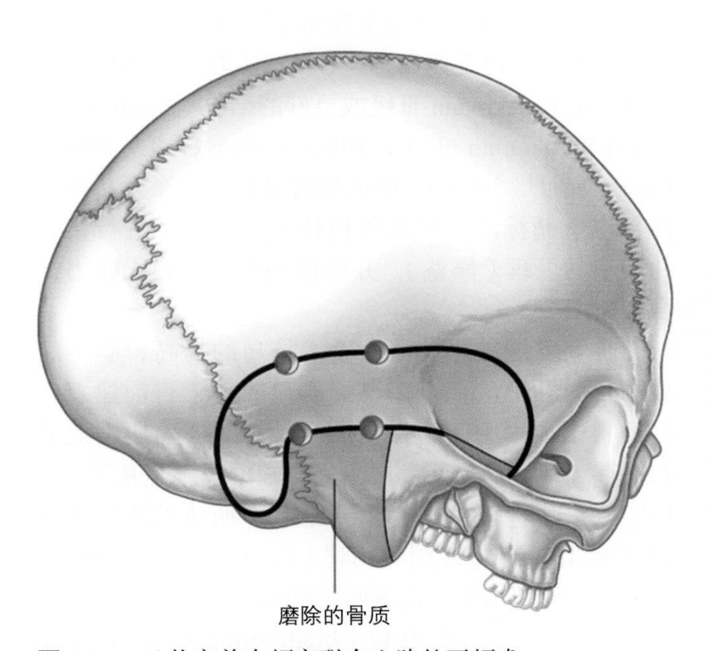

图 24.5　乙状窦前中颅窝联合入路的开颅术

This article was published *in Brain Tumors: An Encyclopedic Approach*, Third edition, Kaye, Andrew H. II. Laws, Edward R., pp. 535 to 553, 614, Copyright Elsevier 2012.

Hardy et al.，1989；Anderson et al.，2005；Samii et al.，2010；Sughrue et al.，2011）。尽管有关入路相关的致残率最低的辩论仍在继续，已经有许多研究强调了每一种入路各自的良好结果。

在考虑特定病变的入路选择时，我们认为，除了双侧肿瘤或先前存在的对侧听力损失外，大多数患者的主要关切是术后面部无力和病变是否全切，而不是保留听力（Kaye and Laws，2012）。术后面肌无力对患者心理影响不应低估，也是术后生活质量的主要决定因素（Ryzenman et al.，2005；Nicoucar et al.，2006；Browne et al.，2008）。

来自 UCSF 的 Sughrue 最近全面回顾了听神经瘤文献中面神经保存的结果，评估了 296 项研究，25 000 名患者，并在 79 项研究中报告了 11 873 名患者（Sughrue et al.，2010b）。这一分析将术后 House-Brackmann 评分Ⅰ或Ⅱ分作为面神经保存的标准，面神经保留率在中颅窝入路为 85%，经迷路入路为 81%，乙状窦后入路为 78%。小于 2 cm 的肿瘤患者面神经保留率为 90%，大于 2 cm 的肿瘤患者为 67%。小于 65 岁的患者面神经保留率低，为 71%，相比大于 65 岁的面神经保留率是 84%，而且发现术中监测有助于面神经保留。术前存在面肌无力是术后面肌无力的独立预测因子，其发生率高达 33%。术前面部无力多见于大肿瘤，也可能因为神经被肿瘤包裹，而不是推移（Lye et al.，1982）。

如果术前存在严重无力，或手术中面神经被切断，应考虑术中面神经重建方案。使用腓肠神经或耳大神经移植修复的面神经在 45%~75% 的病例中具有 House-Brackmann Ⅲ级或更好的结果（Fisch et al.，1987；Stephanian et al.，1992；Gidley et al.，1999；Bacciu et al.，2009）。在这种情况下，显微外科神经修复应遵循标准的显微外科技术，对神经进行精细和最小的处理（修整），并要做到神经外膜无张力缝合的原则。

听觉监测技术：随着手术技巧的提高，脑神经Ⅶ的功能和解剖保存率已经明显改善，目前注意力已经集中在术中听力保留的目标上来。为协助监测和保存Ⅷ神经功能而发展出来的辅助技术是基于"远场"或"近场"电位技术。"远场"听觉监测技术在 1978 年由 Levine 使用和描述（Levine et al.，1988）。目前有几种技术用于监测听觉功能。

脑干听觉诱发电位（brainstem auditory evoked potentials，BAEPs）是一种生物电神经活动，它是对前庭耳蜗神经刺激的反应的记录。将听觉刺激器（声刺激）放置在监测侧的耳部，通过放置在头皮和耳部电极记录和监测平均所获得的电生理信号。为了获得 BAEP 信号，必须要将之与背景噪声区分开来，平均需要几千个波形，以滤过背景噪声，因此得到的波形响应具有明显的时间延迟。这种几秒到几分钟的延迟意味着确定波形变化的实时原因比较困难。BAEPs 的预后意义仅基于波形的保存，因此其应用价值有限（Oh et al.，2012）。设置设备参数和监测工作需要专业知识，应该由专业的技术员实施。

耳蜗电图（EcoG）和直接复合近场动作电位（direct compound near action potentials，dCNAPs）记录了接近耳蜗神经刺激起源的电反应。这意味着监测刺激获得的电反应所需的平均次数减少，能实现了对神经功能的更快速评估。在该技术中，参考电极和接地电极分别放置在同侧耳垂和前额上。泡沫给声耳塞不仅能将电极固定在适当的位置，而且减少了外部声音干扰。给一个短声刺激，通过平均计算得到一个波形。在 dCNAP 中，在靠近肿瘤的神经上放置电极后，直接从听神经本身即可记录并测量到动作电位。这些近场技术的优势是获得更快，从而能更及时反映术中改变。随着敏感性和特异性的提高，dCNAP 在术后功能中的预测价值也有所提高（Yamakami et al.，2009）。近场技术确实有具体的缺点，EcoG 只提供关于听觉通路外侧部分的功能信息。使用这种技术可能无法识别神经近端的分支（Colletti et al.，1998）。在中、大肿瘤中，将 dCNAP 的记录电极放置在第Ⅷ脑神经上有一定的技术难度，因此，这种监测技术一般仅限于切除较小的肿瘤中使用。有些文献报告在使用该监测技术后，听力保留方面的结果有所改善（Danner et al.，2004），小肿瘤的听力保留率可高达 71%。

听力保护的结果：以听力保护为目标的手术效果已有广泛报道，这一入路听力保留的成功率在整个专业内有明显的差异。文献报道听力保留率从 17%~100% 不等，肿瘤的大小与听力保护率之间有明确的关系。虽然许多学者认为，在较大的肿瘤中，听力保存率可以忽略不计，但一些作者发表了数据，显示在非常大的肿瘤中，听力保存率为 43%（Matthies and Samii，2002）。Sughrue 最近回顾了有关听力保存率的文献，并确定了 123 项研究，其中 49 项可以提取详细数据（Sughrue et al.，2010a）。在对 998 例患者的分析研究中，听力保留率明显地取决于肿瘤的大小、术前听力水平和患者的年龄。在随访 6 个月至 7 年期间，总听力保留率为 52%。30 岁以下患者的听力保留率为53%，60岁以上患者保留率为29%。肿瘤小于1 cm的患者，听力保存率为64%，而大于3 cm的肿瘤的听力保存率为32%。

听力保留的长期持续性也仍然是一个有争议的问题，House小组报告说，56%的患者患有延迟性听力损失（Shelton et al.，1990）。延迟性听力损失机制的理论包括耳蜗周围的疤痕组织形成或耳蜗血液供应的微血管损伤（Chee et al.，2003）。此后，一些其他研究表明，长期听力保存的持续存在，维持率为85%~96%（Betchen et al.，2005；Woodson et al.，2010；Mazzoni et al.，2012）。

对侧耳的急性听力损失已被报道为听神经瘤手术的并发症，以及在颅后窝手术后轻度听力下降是常见的。这一现象背后的机制尚不清楚，但可能与导致淋巴周围脑脊液压力降低和外淋巴低张力有关。这些情况也可能自发改善（Clemis et al.，1982；Walsted et al.，1991）。

脑干和耳蜗植入

在耳蜗神经和耳蜗的解剖和功能完整的情况下，可以植入电子耳蜗。在前庭神经瘤手术中，如果采取经迷路入路，可以植入电子耳蜗，术中要进行技术方面的考虑，并保留耳蜗神经。

听觉脑干植入物（auditory brainstem implants，ABI）通常用于双侧听力受到威胁的情况。这种情况最常见于神经纤维瘤病2型（NF-2）患者，其中患者有双侧前庭神经鞘瘤。在第一次肿瘤切除后，如果预期在这一侧的听力已经明显减弱或丧失，可以放置植入物；或者在第二次神经鞘瘤切除后，听力已经丧失的情况下再植入。保留听力的患者从ABI中获得的好处很少，因为它很少获得比环境声音和封闭集词汇更多的听力质量。如果在第一侧手术后植入ABI，听力完整，它通常不会启用，直到对侧听力已经丧失。虽然详细的讨论超出了本章的范围，但如果可能的话，我们赞成在NF-2患者中切除肿瘤，尝试保留听力并尽量减少耳聋的发病率。通过乙状窦后入路或经迷路入路，ABI的放置是可行的。手术技术已有详尽的描述（Toh and Luxford，2008），但本质上涉及在腹侧耳蜗核上放置电极。该核不能直视，因此必须使用间接的表面标志：放置在第四脑室侧隐窝附近的背核和面神经和舌咽神经根之间腹核的下侧。一旦放置，电极阵列被用来测试植入体和邻近神经和结构的响应。该阵列使用Teflon或脂肪固定在第四脑室侧隐窝侧开口处，电极引线位于乳突腔，接地电极置于颞肌下。

结果表明，85%的患者感受到听觉信号。结合唇读，93%的患者在3~6个月时表现出更好的句子理解。大多数患者有环境声音的意识，以及封闭集单词、辅音和元音。听力结果持续改善直到8年之后（Ebinger et al.，2000；Maini et al.，2009）。

岩斜脑膜瘤

岩斜脑膜瘤产生于斜坡的上2/3，第Ⅴ脑神经的内侧。这些肿瘤通常挤压脑干，但也可能推挤或包绕基底动脉、Ⅲ~Ⅺ脑神经，并延伸到Meckel腔、海绵窦、Dorello管、内听道或颈静脉孔。手术切除通常很具有挑战性，因此，手术并发症发生率可能相应地增加。

对该部位肿瘤切除的程度和并发症发生率，已发表的文献报道有很大的差异，主要取决于治疗团队的理念。岩斜脑膜瘤切除后切实存在的致残率肯定使术者权衡侵袭性与保守性切除所带来的后果。包括显微镜技术的改进、术前成像和放射外科技术的发展在内的因素，使患者的预后有所改善。在较大的肿瘤中，显微手术仍然是唯一可行的治疗方案。切除这些肿瘤无疑与明显的致残率有关。Feng Xu等回顾840例接受岩斜脑膜瘤手术切除的患者，死亡率为0~9%，新脑神经障碍的发生率为20.3%~76%。总切除率为28%~85%（Xu et al.，2013）。Almefty等报告64例患者的结果，其中54例有长期随访，39%有持续性脑神经缺损，主要是Ⅴ~Ⅷ脑神经。值得注意的是，Ⅴ和Ⅷ脑神经更有可能从术前状态中改善，而Ⅵ脑神经最有可能发生永久性障碍（Almefty et al.，2014）。脑干压迫常见于体积大的肿瘤。解剖有脑干软脑膜受累或基底动脉包裹的肿瘤可能导致灾难性的脑干梗死。可能有助于确定的术前指标是T2信号测量的肿瘤质地（软硬度）、MRI上肿瘤与脑干之间的CSF裂隙的存在或脑干水肿的MRI证据，这些信息提示肿瘤与脑干的粘连严重（Uede et al.，1996；Carvalho et al.，2000）。

切除程度确实对肿瘤复发起重要作用。全切除术后，复发率为6%~9.8%。据报告，次全切除后复发高达26%~41%（Seifert，2010；Li et al.，2013；Almefty et al.，2014）。对于预估会发生严重神经功能障碍的患者，应该排除全切除的可能性，在获得肿瘤可能会进展的证据之后，应着手放射治疗。

三叉神经鞘瘤

随着现代显微外科技术的发展，三叉神经鞘瘤死亡率大大降低。Chen对459例患者的回顾性综述描述了5例手术死亡和1%的死亡率(Chen et al., 2014)。其他并发症包括脑神经损伤、脑脊液漏、脑膜炎和脑积水。许多患者将留下一定程度的永久性三叉神经功能障碍，最常见的是持续存在的三叉神经感觉减退(Fukaya et al., 2010)，应该在术前告知患者这些症状可能永远无法缓解。伴发的面神经损伤往往需要眼睑缝合来预防神经源性角膜炎。新出现的术后脑神经功能障碍，如展神经和动眼神经麻痹，通常在4个月内缓解。其他一些术前即存在的神经功能缺损，如小脑和脑干受压综合征、复视、面部疼痛和面肌无力、听力下降术后可能改善。脑脊液漏和(或)脑积水可能需要安放分流装置。

颈静脉孔区神经鞘瘤

手术切除这些肿瘤后的并发症包括吞咽困难、声音嘶哑、误吸和喘鸣。最近的报告显示，严重吞咽困难和误吸的发生率非常低(Bakar, 2008; Bulsara et al., 2008; Cavalcanti et al., 2011)。对一些严重吞咽困难持续存在的病例，可能需要气管切开术或声带内(移)置技术。然而，许多患者可以通过临时鼻饲和精心的肺清洗来管理，以减少发生吸入性肺炎的概率。大多数人最终会适应和耐受有规律的饮食。

皮样和表皮样肿瘤

随着显微外科的发展，皮样和表皮样肿瘤手术的死亡率和致残率都有了明显的下降。Yaşargil 等报道86%的患者都有改善，有9%的致残率和5%的死亡率。在同一系列报道中，脑膜炎(包括化学性)的发生率为19%，19%的患者存在脑积水(Yaşargil et al., 1989)。

这些病变的主要并发症是无菌性脑膜炎、化脓性脑膜炎、脑积水和与病变位置相关的神经功能障碍。神经障碍是由于后组脑神经受累，继而出现吞咽困难、吸入性肺炎和甚至死亡。

皮样囊肿和表皮样囊肿在多年后都可以复发，但症状性复发是罕见的。复发概率与未切除的包膜体积有关。这种包膜将以正常的细胞转化速度产生细胞(Alvord, 1977)，因此症状性复发比较少见。复发的肿瘤仍然可能是良性的，但在皮样囊肿和表皮样囊肿中都有恶性变化的报道。

只有当囊肿内容物破裂进入脑脊液间隙时，才会发生播散。Maravilla(1977)描述了这种传播模式，其沿蛛网膜下腔播散然后继发多个卫星灶。

争议

小的前庭神经鞘瘤的管理：观察、立体定向放射外科与显微外科切除

对于在中老年患者中许多小于1.5 cm的病变，最初的管理措施(观察和密切的影像学和临床随访)是合适的。这些患者肿瘤的生长即触发下一步的干预。

治疗小于2 cm大小的肿瘤可以是显微外科或放射外科。小肿瘤手术应该在大型医院的亚专科中心进行，全切除率极高，面神经良好率通常超过90%。对于小肿瘤而言，放射外科是一种可行的替代方案，可以很好地控制肿瘤生长，面神经功能障碍发生率极低。但是，放射手术失败后的抢救性显微外科手术，相比之下，通常需要进行更具挑战性的神经解剖分离工作，因而面瘫发生率更高。

服用抗凝药物的患者，放射外科手术为相对禁忌，因其可明显增加瘤内出血率。

NF-2 患者干预的时机和肿瘤切除程度

鉴于这一组患者听力保存的高度优先性，前庭神经鞘瘤的治疗本质上更保守。肿瘤进行性生长，伴有听力极差或已经失聪，应行显微手术切除肿瘤。在听力保持完整的情况下，我们采取了一种最大限度的内减压策略，同时将术中的优先事项转为保留耳蜗神经上。这种情况经常意味着残留的肿瘤仍然存在，患者可能需要多次乙状窦后开颅手术。对NF-2患者，我们通常采用保守的治疗措施，除非病变大到压迫小脑。在这组患者中，放射外科在控制生长方面不太有效，通常不建议，除非作为一种挽救策略。

大肿瘤且有可用听力患者的入路选择

除了NF-2患者人群，以及一小部分特发性原因导致肿瘤对侧听力差的患者，我们通常主张，在大肿瘤的情况下，手术的主要目标仍然是脑干和小脑的安全。我们认为，采用经迷路入路能最大限度地减少小脑牵拉，让术者有最大角度安全地将肿瘤从脑干上分离下来，而且手术结果更佳。在大肿瘤中，我们认为在任何入路中有用听力保存的可能性都很低，因此我们通常选择经迷路入路。

延伸阅读、参考文献、EBRAIN 的相关链接

扫描书末二维码获取。

第五篇 肿瘤和颅底——鞍区和鞍上区肿瘤

第25章 垂体肿瘤

Kanna Gnanalingham・Zsolt Zador・Tara Kearney・Federico Roncaroli・H. Rao Gattamaneni 著
戚其超、冯子超 译，倪石磊 审校

垂体：基础解剖

垂体位于蝶鞍之中，在颅底中线距鼻尖后方约5 cm处（图25.1A）。其上方与下丘脑和第三脑室、前上方与视交叉和终板、前下方与蝶窦、侧方与海绵窦和颈内动脉海绵窦段、后方与后床突和斜坡紧密相连。

垂体有两个不同的组成部分，分别是起源于外胚层的前叶和起源于神经外胚层的后叶（图25.1B）。垂体前叶占腺体体积的80%，并在水平面上延伸至两个侧翼。垂体前叶产生的激素有促肾上腺皮质激素（adrenocorticotropic hormone，ACTH）、催乳素（prolactin，PRL）、生长激素（growth hormone，GH）、促甲状腺激素（thyroid-stimulating hormone，TSH）、卵泡刺激素（follicle-stimulating hormone，FSH）和黄体生成素（luteinizing hormone，LH）。正常状态下内分泌细胞有明确的分区，产生GH和PRL的细胞分别集中于侧翼的前部和后部；而多数产生TSH和ACTH的细胞分别位于中央楔形叶的前部和后部；促性腺激素细胞则散布于前叶各处（图25.1C）。

垂体的血液供应对其激素分泌功能是不可或缺的（图25.1D）。垂体上动脉和垂体下动脉作为颈内动脉床突上段和海绵窦段的直接分支，各自供应垂体及下丘脑腹侧。垂体上动脉围绕下丘脑腹侧和垂体柄形成初级毛细血管丛，构成垂体门静脉系统。该血管丛汇集成数条门静脉引流前叶，并在前叶周围组成次级毛细血管丛。次级毛细血管丛随后汇集成垂体前静脉并引流汇入海绵窦。此血管丛的重要性在于它将下丘脑弓状核释放的下丘脑促垂体激素与垂体前叶联系起来，并调节其激素分泌。后叶由垂体下动脉供血，引流进入垂体后静脉。垂体通过垂体柄向上与下丘脑联系，而垂体柄包含下丘脑室旁核和视上核的轴突。这些轴突将催产素和加压素运送到垂体后叶，并释放入垂体后静脉（图25.1）。

垂体肿瘤的流行病学

垂体疾病相对常见，多数为垂体腺瘤。一项基于影像学和尸检研究的meta分析提示，偶发垂体腺瘤的预估患病率约为17%，无性别差异（Ezzat et al.，2004）。然而大多数垂体病变很小且偶发，不需要临床干预。

有症状垂体腺瘤的发病率为19~28/（百万·年），发病率高峰年龄段在30~60岁，总体上更常见于绝经前妇女。确切的患病率在不同研究人群之间存在差异；外科手术相关研究因聚焦于产生占位效应的病变易导致偏倚，而药物治疗相关研究可能纳入了更多的功能性垂体腺瘤，如通常需药物治疗的催乳素型腺瘤。综合不同病例组，多达20%的垂体腺瘤是偶然发现的，并且很多为无症状。

需要临床干预的垂体腺瘤占所有颅内肿瘤的10%~15%，是仅次于胶质瘤和脑膜瘤的第三常见的肿瘤类型。垂体腺瘤分类基于病理和免疫组化特征。目前，世界卫生组织（WHO）内分泌器官肿瘤分类明确了7种类型和13个亚型（WHO，2017）。这些类型主要包括催乳素细胞腺瘤（催乳素免疫染色阳性，39%）、促性腺激素细胞腺瘤（LH/FSH免疫染色阳性，27%）、生长激素细胞腺瘤（GH免疫染色阳性，16%）、促肾上腺皮质激素细胞腺瘤（ACTH免疫染色阳性，16%）和促甲状腺激素细胞腺瘤（TSH免疫染色阳性，1%），其他包括零细胞腺瘤和多激素细胞腺瘤（WHO，2017）。

儿童垂体腺瘤的发病率约比成人低十倍，占所有儿童颅内肿瘤的2%~6%（Keil and Stratakis，2008）。只有3.5%~8.5%的垂体腺瘤在20岁之前被诊断。儿童垂体腺瘤在发育关键时段往往对儿童发育产生重要影响。

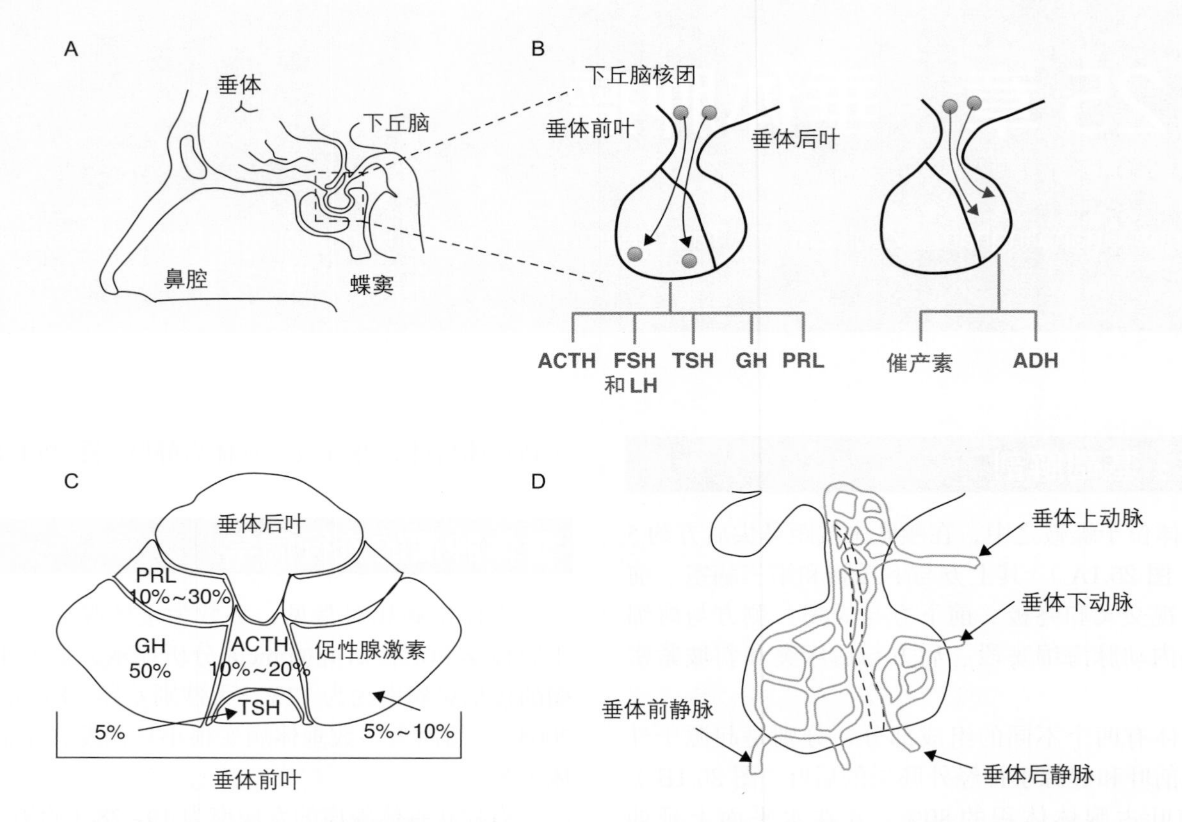

图 25.1 （A）垂体局部解剖。（B）垂体结构和激素分泌。（C）垂体内激素分泌细胞的分布。（D）垂体血供，垂体门脉系统

遗传学

癌基因 - 原癌基因平衡失调导致肿瘤细胞克隆增殖的经典概念可能解释了垂体肿瘤发生的一部分原因，但垂体腺瘤的发病机制仍不完全清楚（Daly et al.，2009；Marques and Korbonits，2017）。有多个研究支持垂体肿瘤是单克隆起源的，然而也有证据提示其为多病灶的单克隆扩增。

大多数垂体肿瘤为散发性（95%）。少数为家族性（5%），表现为家族性垂体腺瘤或为孤立性（即家族性孤立性垂体腺瘤，FIPA），或作为一种家族性遗传综合征的一部分，包括多发性内分泌腺瘤病 1 型（MEN 1）、多发性内分泌腺瘤病 4 型（MEN 4）、McCune-Albright 综合征、Carney 综合征（CNC）、X 连锁肢端肥大综合征（XLAG 综合征）、SDH 突变和 DICER 基因突变（Vandeva et al.，2010；Marques and Korbonits，2017）。

散发性垂体腺瘤

已发现多种致癌基因可促进垂体肿瘤的形成（Daly et al.，2009；Marques and Korbonits，2017）。最早确定的是 *gsp* 癌基因，在 40% 的生长激素细胞腺瘤中可检测到 *gsp* 癌基因的功能性突变。该基因编码 GTPase 的 Gα_s 亚单位，突变后导致 cAMP 水平持续升高，促使细胞受到生长激素释放激素（growth hormone release hormone，GHRH）持续刺激，继而导致生长激素细胞腺瘤的发生。其他相对常见的突变基因还有编码 USP8（泛素特异性蛋白酶 8）和 PI3K（磷脂酰肌醇 3- 激酶）的基因。高达 80% 的垂体腺瘤被发现有细胞周期蛋白异常表达，包括细胞周期蛋白依赖激酶（cyclin-dependent kinases，CDK）、垂体肿瘤转化基因 1（*PTTG1*）和多种生长因子。

家族性垂体腺瘤

家族性孤立性垂体腺瘤（familial isolated pituitary adenomas，FIPA）：本病定义为在一个家族中发生 2 例或 2 例以上的垂体腺瘤，但与其他肿瘤无关联。大部分（约 60%）FIPA 是大腺瘤，类型以生长激素细胞腺瘤和催乳素细胞腺瘤为主。芳基烃受体相互作用蛋白基因（*AIP*）突变已被确定为 15%~30% FIPA 家族患病的病因（Marques and Korbonits，2017）。*AIP* 基因位于染色体 11q13.2 区，突变后不能与其配位结合，从而失去了其作为抑癌基因的作用。*AIP* 突变阳性携带者发生垂体腺瘤的概率为 12%~30%。

MEN1（多发性内分泌瘤1型）：MEN1的发病率为1~10/（10万·年）。该综合征是由染色体11q13上的*MEN1*抑癌基因功能缺失突变引起的（Balogh et al.，2006；Daly et al.，2009；Marques and Korbonits，2017）。该突变为显性遗传，外显率高达90%。MEN1基因编码的蛋白Menin与一系列其他的蛋白和基因表达之间存在复杂的调控互作效应。该疾病表现包括原发性甲状旁腺功能亢进、胰腺神经内分泌肿瘤和垂体腺瘤，其中40%的突变病例会罹患垂体腺瘤。组织学分型的分布特点与散发性腺瘤相似。MEN1中催乳素细胞腺瘤对多巴胺激动剂的应答率较低（约40%可控制至正常），且侵袭性更强。大多数MEN1相关性垂体肿瘤是大腺瘤，因此这些患者临床表现出占位效应的比例是非MEN1患者（散发性患者）的2倍（大约为80% *vs.* 40%）。

MEN4（多发性内分泌瘤4型）：这是一种非常罕见的常染色体显性遗传综合征，由编码细胞周期蛋白依赖性抑制因子p27的*CDKN1B*基因突变引起。这种综合征首先在大鼠中被发现，因移码突变合成不稳定蛋白（MENX）所致（Pellegata et al.，2006）。纯合子和杂合子动物均患有促性腺激素细胞腺瘤和嗜铬细胞瘤，即外显率为100%。患者可表现有肢端肥大症、原发性甲状旁腺功能亢进症、肾血管平滑肌脂肪瘤、睾丸癌和宫颈类癌等。

McCune-Albright综合征：该综合征于1937年被首次提出，其特征有牛奶咖啡斑、骨纤维异常增殖症、激素异常（如性早熟、生长激素分泌过多和催乳素分泌过多）（Albright et al.，1937；McCune and Bruch，1937）。McCune-Albright综合征是由合子后体细胞染色体20q13.2-q13.3上的*GNAS1*基因（鸟嘌呤核苷酸结合蛋白，α-刺激活性多肽1）突变引起的，该突变产生了典型的嵌合样表型，也造成了由受累细胞系决定的不同临床表现。特定的受累组织类型包括垂体，尤其是形成生长激素和催乳素分泌性腺瘤，以及皮肤、股骨近端和面部骨骼。

Carney综合征（CNC）：这种罕见的综合征于1985年被首次提出，特点为黏液瘤（皮肤和心脏）、斑点状色素沉着及内分泌高活性，包括垂体腺瘤（Casey et al.，1998）。仅10%的CNC患者有垂体腺瘤，而其中75%有生长激素、IGF-1和催乳素水平亚临床升高。Carney综合征的遗传机制多变，相关突变位点包括17q22-24的CNC1基因，该基因编码蛋白激酶A调节亚基Ia（PRKAR1A），以及位于2p16的CNC2基因。

X连锁肢端肥大巨人症（XLAG）：约10%的巨人症是Xq26.3上GPR101基因散发性或遗传性的微重复所致。巨人症患者在出生后的前四年会出现异常生长。催乳素-生长激素细胞增生或混合性催乳素细胞/生长激素细胞腺瘤是XLAG患者的病理基础。XLAG的临床特征虽然显著，但基因诊断具有挑战性，特别是体细胞嵌合体患者。手术治疗可使XLAG治愈（Marques and Korbonits，2017）。

琥珀酸脱氢酶突变：琥珀酸脱氢酶的四个亚单位之一及其相关组装因子发生突变的患者可发生垂体大腺瘤，更常见于家族性腺瘤，且比散发性腺瘤更具侵袭性，对药物治疗常具有抵抗性（Marques and Korbonits，2017）。

DICER1基因突变：杂合子*DICER1*基因的突变可导致家族性胸膜-肺母细胞瘤和发育不良综合征，其特征是发生多种肿瘤，包括囊性肾肿瘤、睾丸间质细胞瘤、甲状腺肿和肉瘤。尽管外显率较低，*DICER1*突变后的儿童也可患垂体母细胞瘤。

放射学

颅骨X线

X线目前应用较少（**图25.2A**）。在计算机断层扫描（CT）和MR出现之前，X线平片有助于发现蝶鞍扩大，颅咽管瘤引起的后床突和斜坡侵蚀破坏，鞍结节脑膜瘤引起的蝶窦扩大，以及视神经胶质瘤造成的“J”形蝶鞍。颅骨异常增厚是肢端肥大症的特征性改变。

颅脑CT

CT扫描可显示鞍区扩大和垂体占位（**图25.2B**），也有助于识别钙化灶，这更常见于颅咽管瘤和鞍结节脑膜瘤。垂体卒中在颅脑CT上表现为蝶鞍内高密度病变。垂体的血管特点可通过增强CT或CT血管成像来辨识。然而，CT最广泛的应用是评估鼻窦特点，有助于设计经鼻手术的入路和（或）制订术中神经导航的计划。冠状位和矢状位重建可用于评估颅底/鼻窦的解剖结构。

颅脑MR

颅脑MR是评估不同层面垂体病变肿瘤大小、强化特点以及神经血管关系的标准检查（**图25.2C，D**）。由于缺乏血脑屏障，应用钆对比剂后脑垂体信号较正常脑组织明显强化（**图25.2D**）。造影剂先在垂体后叶浓聚，然后是垂体前叶。

正常垂体的大小随年龄和性别而异，上限为

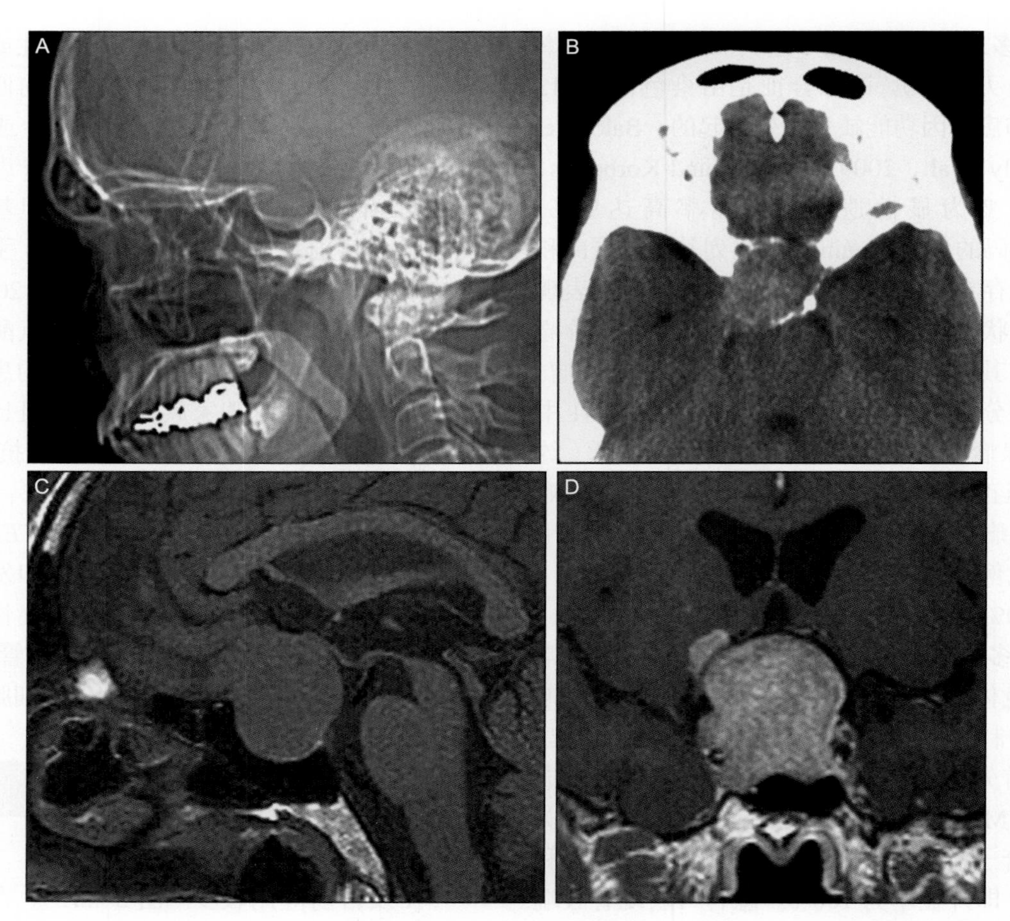

图 25.2 颅骨侧位 X 线片（A）显示继发于腺瘤的垂体窝扩张。轴位 CT 扫描（B）显示垂体肿物。矢状位 T1 加权 MR 扫描（C）和冠状位 T1 加权 MR 增强扫描（D）显示垂体巨大腺瘤伴视交叉压迫

9~10 mm。然而需注意的是，垂体在青春期或孕期会出现生理性增大，在 MRI 冠状像上呈球状外观，大小可达 12 mm。

在 T1 加权成像上，垂体后叶显示为高信号，也被称为“亮点”。MRI 评估邻近神经血管结构较 CT 更好，尤其是视神经、颈内动脉与垂体瘤的关系。垂体微腺瘤可导致单侧腺体肿大，同时垂体柄向对侧移位。

动态 MR

大多数垂体腺瘤可由常规 MR 检查发现，然而小腺瘤却显示不清。动态 MRI 可识别出垂体微腺瘤相对于正常腺体的对比增强改变（**图** 25.3A~C）。这项技术需要从静脉注射造影剂 2~3 分钟后开始，快速连续地获取 T1 加权 MRI 图像。与正常垂体相比，微腺瘤通常在较晚（有时较早）的时间点强化。强化时间点与肿瘤大小、血管分布、血脑屏障的完整性以及个体差异相关（Kanou et al.，2002）。

其他特殊 MR 序列，如扰相梯度回波（spoiled gradient echo，SPGR），也可用来发现传统 MR 序列难以观察到的微小腺瘤。

岩下窦静脉采血

岩下窦静脉采血（inferior petrosal vein sampling，IPSS）是一种确定库欣病过量 ACTH 产生部位的有效检测方法（Deipolyi et al.，2011）（**图 25.3D，E**）。其虽为侵袭性操作，但卒中、出血及穿刺部位血肿等风险较小，因此目前常规用作辅助诊断方法。该检查需将静脉导管置入岩静脉，直接从采集的静脉血中检测应用促肾上腺皮质激素释放因子（CRF）前后的 ACTH 水平。岩静脉内测得的激素水平可与外周血激素水平作比较分析。IPSS 的敏感性可达 80%~90%，但 IPSS 的诊断价值更多体现在确定 ACTH 的中枢性（即垂体）来源而不是判断垂体内微腺瘤的侧别。

垂体腺瘤分级体系

垂体腺瘤的分级体系通常以解剖和影像学信息为基础，一种广泛使用的方法是按肿瘤大小分级，

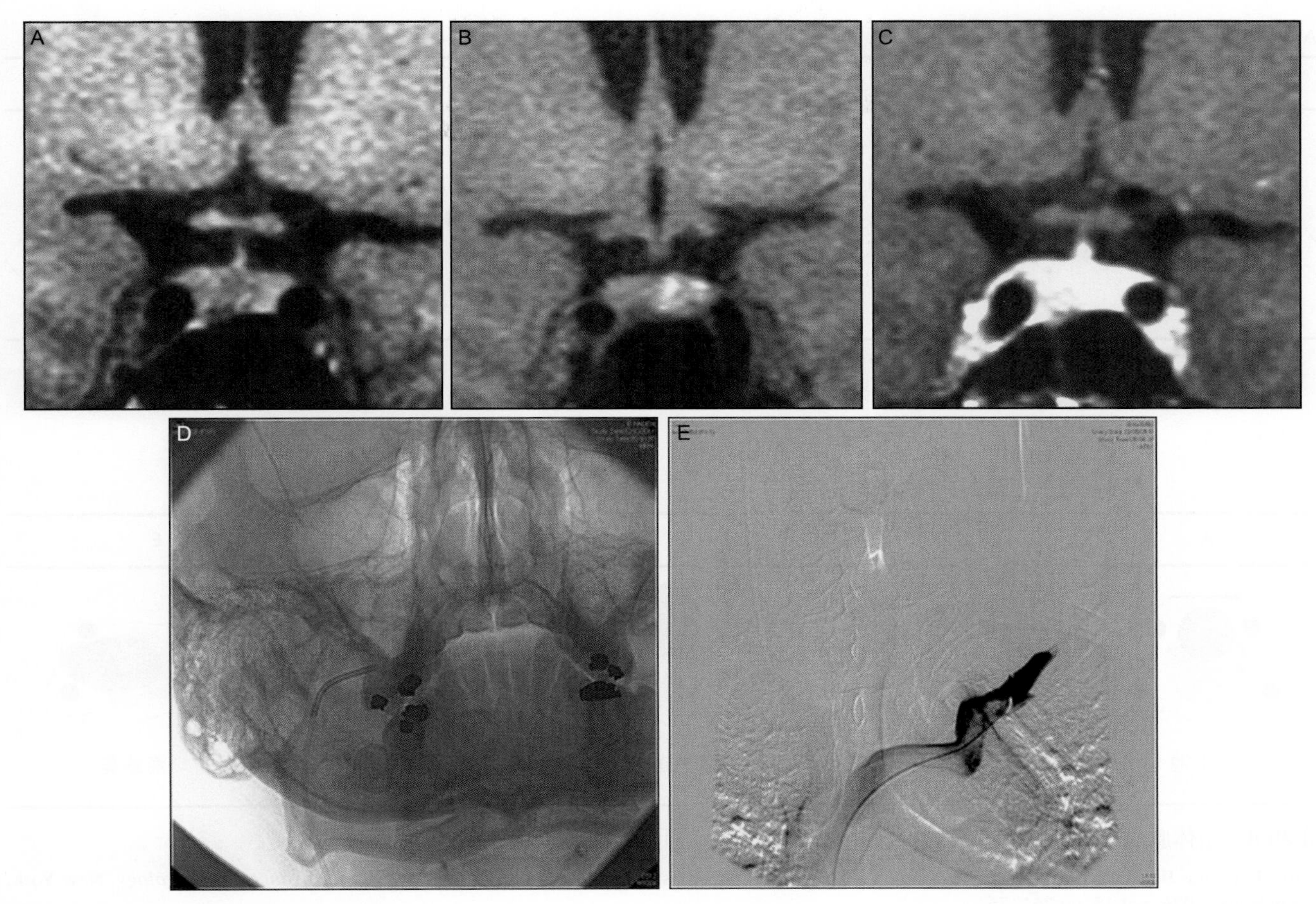

图 25.3　动态 MRI 扫描的不同阶段（A~C）显示库欣病患者的右侧微腺瘤，在 5 秒（B）时显示比左侧正常垂体增强弱，但在 3 分钟后（C）差别消失。正位（AP）颅骨 X 线片显示血管内导管（箭头，D）插入右侧岩下窦，然后通过对比剂（E）显影

最大直径大于 1 cm 称为大腺瘤，小于 1 cm 称为微腺瘤。较复杂的分级方法常常根据邻近结构的受累情况来分级，例如肿瘤向鞍旁或鞍上区扩展，向鞍底、蝶窦及远处侵袭的程度，分级的目的是评估肿瘤切除的困难程度、肿瘤残留的可能性，以及预测复发率和生化缓解率。

垂体腺瘤分级的放射学概念最初是在 20 世纪 70 年代由 Hardy 和 Wilson 建立（Hardy and Vezina，1976；**图** 25.4）。在该分级体系中，不突破鞍底的垂体腺瘤被归为非侵袭性垂体腺瘤，破坏蝶鞍的腺瘤被归为侵袭性垂体腺瘤（**图** 25.4A），另外，按肿瘤的鞍上扩展程度，分为硬膜内病变和硬膜外侵犯（**图** 25.4B）。

Knosp 分级（Knosp et al.，1993）主要评估肿瘤侵犯海绵窦的程度，关注点为肿瘤与海绵窦段颈内动脉的关系（**图** 25.5）。

病理学

组织病理学

以往垂体瘤根据其细胞质的着色特性分为嗜酸性、嗜碱性和嫌色性（Kernohan and Sayre，1956）。着色性与腺瘤的功能相关：嗜酸性细胞腺瘤通常产生 GH，与巨人症和肢端肥大症有关；嗜碱性细胞瘤一般分泌 ACTH；嫌色性细胞腺瘤则无激素活性（**图** 25.6）。电子显微镜的使用促进了腺瘤分类的发展，可识别致密颗粒型和稀疏颗粒型的生长激素腺瘤亚型，随着免疫组织化学的发展，垂体腺瘤的分类谱系和亚型得以建立（Kovacs et al.，2001）。

形态功能学分类

垂体腺瘤目前的分类主要包括 7 种形态功能类型（WHO，2017），每种类型又分为具有不同组织学和超微结构特征、免疫表型和功能的亚型。垂体激

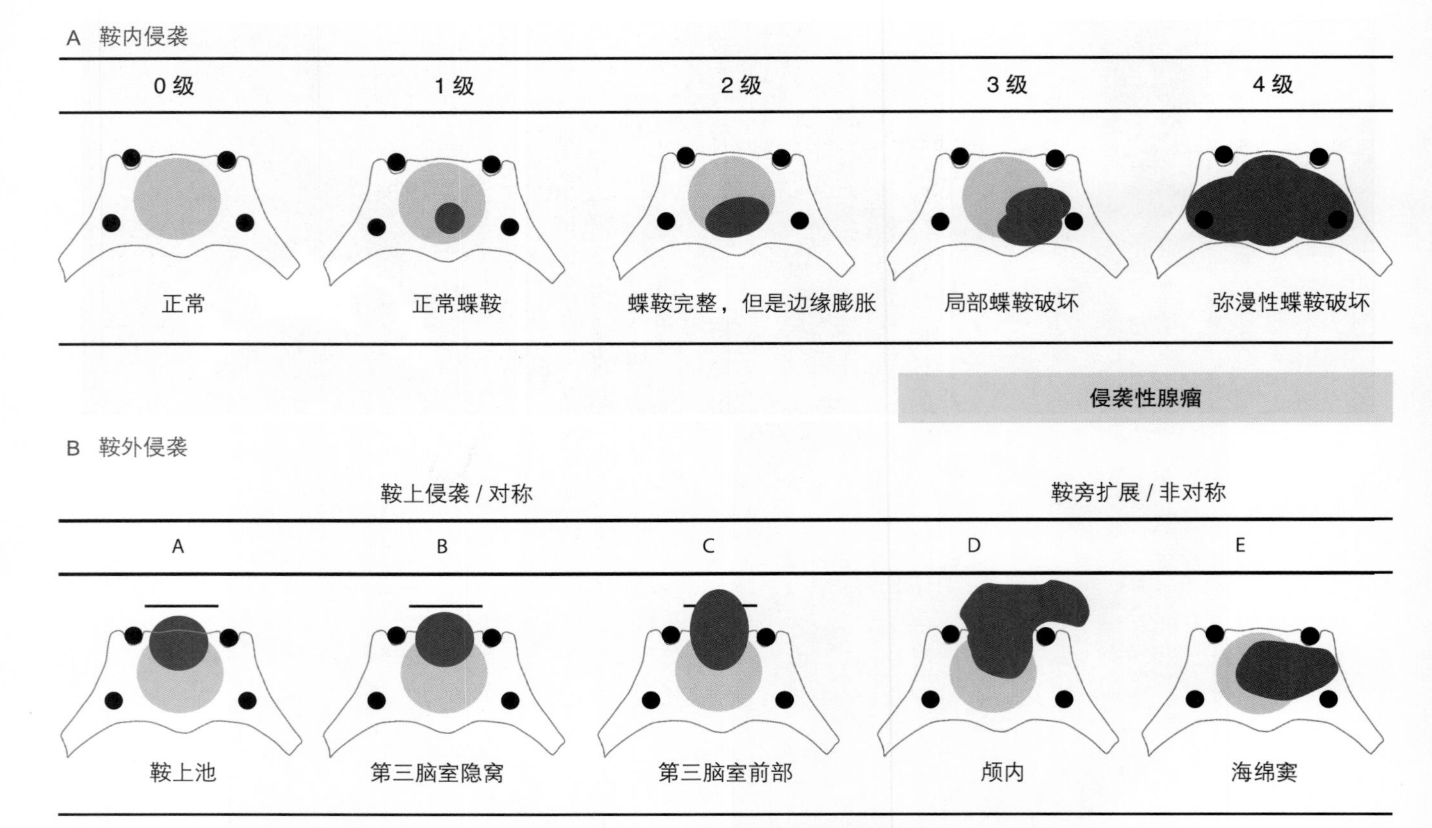

图 25.4 垂体腺瘤改良 Hardy 分级。3 级、4 级、D 和 E 说明可能存在海绵窦侵袭

Hardy J, Vezina JL: Transsphenoidal neurosurgery of intracranial neoplasm, in Tompson RA, Green JR (eds): *Advances in Neurology*. New York, Raven Press, 1976, vol 15, pp 261–75.

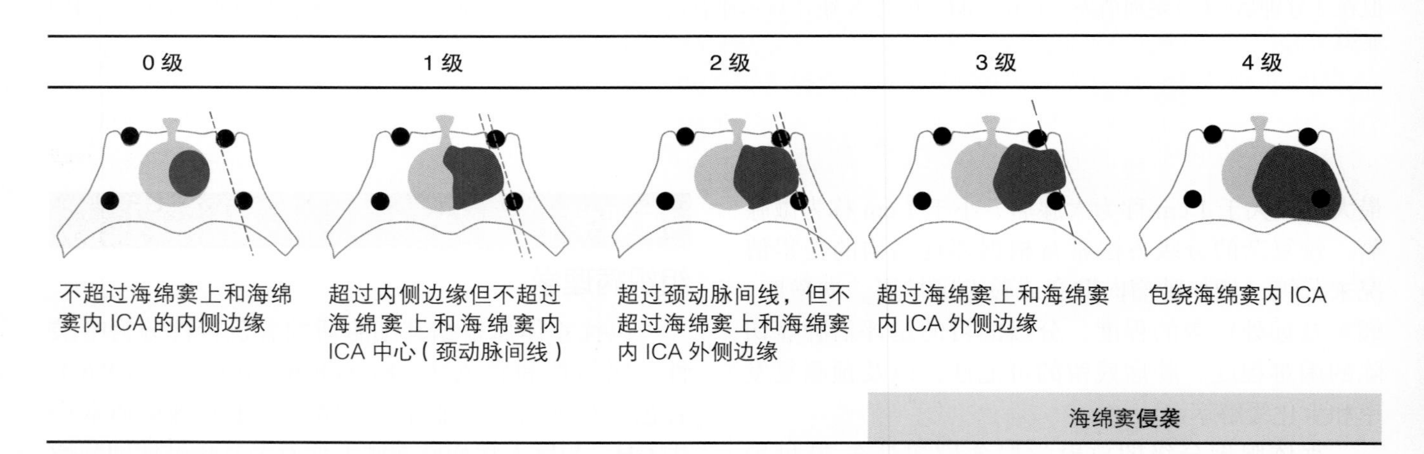

图 25.5 垂体腺瘤 Knosp 分级。3 级和 4 级说明海绵窦侵袭

Reproduced with permission from Knosp, Engelbert; Steiner, Erich, Pituitary Adenomas with Invasion of the Cavernous Sinus Space: A Magnetic Resonance Imaging Classification Compared with Surgical Findings, *Neurosurgery*, Volume 33, Issue 4, pp. 610–17; discussion 617–18.

素的免疫组化是腺瘤的主流分类技术；对细胞角蛋白和转录因子 SF1、pit1 和 T-pit 的免疫组化染色也有助于进一步明确腺瘤类型。针对垂体腺瘤表皮生长因子受体（EGFR）、雌激素受体、e- 钙黏着蛋白、VEGF 和线粒体的染色也有少量应用。当鞍区肿瘤的光镜特征不提示典型的垂体腺瘤，且病变必须与其他原发、非腺瘤性肿瘤或转移性肿瘤相鉴别时，需使用更多其他的抗体染色。

垂体腺瘤的病理特征需与激素过度分泌的临床表现和生化证据相关联。一种或多种垂体激素免疫

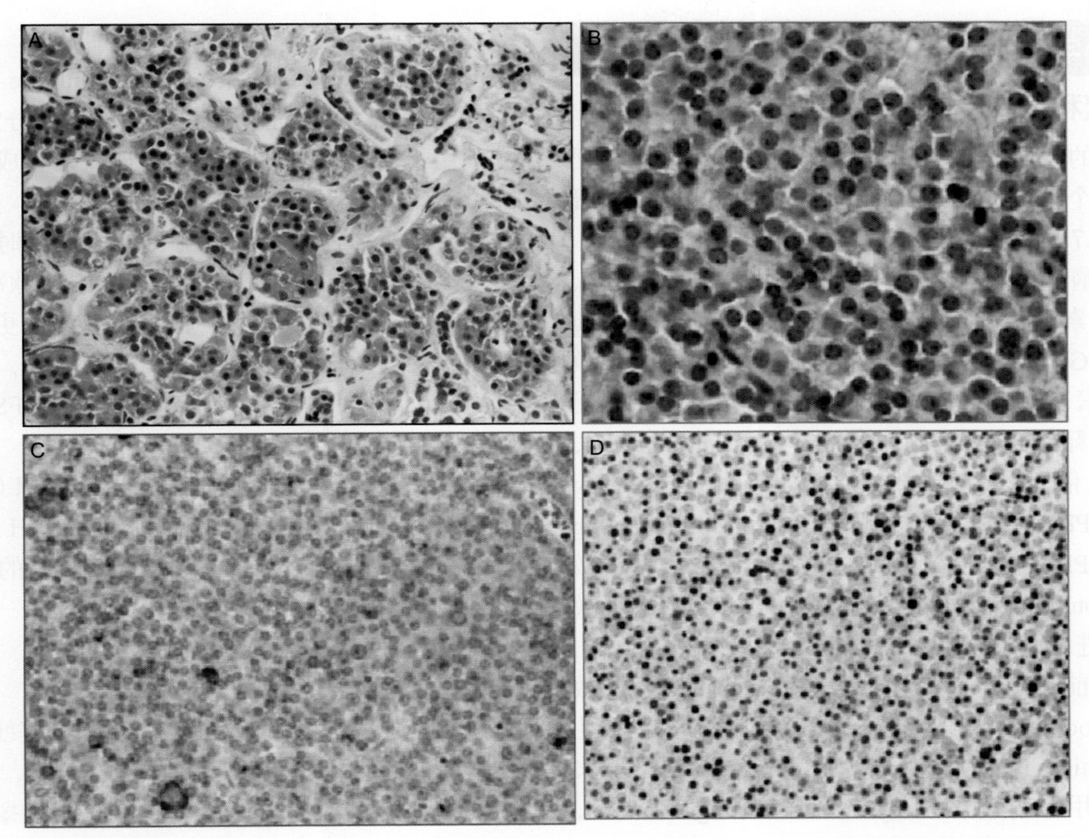

图 25.6　正常垂体苏木精伊红染色（A，×10）。稀疏颗粒型生长激素腺瘤（B~D），显示苏木精 - 伊红（B，×10）、生长激素（C，×10）和细胞角蛋白免疫染色（D，CAM5.2，×10）

组化阳性，但临床上无激素高分泌的腺瘤被定义为临床静默型或临床无功能型腺瘤。功能缺乏可能来自多种因素，包括激素释放缺陷或无生物活性激素的合成。事实上，免疫组化检测的是肿瘤细胞胞质中激素的存储，而不指示其分泌活动。最后，如催乳素腺瘤和促性腺激素腺瘤，虽然可释放活性激素，但因发生在绝经后妇女，临床也表现为无功能性，只表现为肿块压迫症状。

电镜仅应用于光镜特点和免疫表型不能诊断的罕见病例。超微结构特征，如分泌颗粒的数目、位置和大小，中间丝聚集与否及位置，以及核包体是否存在，都是诊断时考虑的因素。

肿瘤行为和治疗反应的预测

影响垂体腺瘤预后的因素包括组织类型、增殖活性和肿瘤侵袭性。欧洲内分泌学会的最新指南中提出了一种综合性的临床 - 病理方法来定义侵袭性腺瘤，包括侵袭性、快速生长、治疗抵抗性和高增殖性（Raverot et al.，2018）。WHO 2004 版分类中提出的对非典型垂体腺瘤的定义，在 2017 版中不再使用（WHO，2017）。

评估有丝分裂活性有助于预测复发，特别是扩展到鞍外和不能全切的腺瘤。

鉴于免疫染色的实验室间差异性和定量分析缺乏一致性，Ki-67 增殖指数的评估预后价值未被广泛接受。尽管如此，Ki-67 值≥3% 应引起重视，因为这可能提示侵袭性行为。

应用免疫组化评估腺瘤 O6- 甲基鸟嘌呤 -DNA 甲基转移酶（MGMT）表达，可帮助预测替莫唑胺（TMZ）的疗效。低水平的 MGMT 免疫表达与良好疗效相关，但 MGMT 的免疫表达水平并不总是与 MGMT 基因启动子甲基化水平相一致。免疫组化中 DNA 错配修复蛋白（MSH6）的核表达也有助于评估化疗疗效。

生长抑素受体 2、3 和 5 的免疫染色水平在预测生长抑素类似物疗效上的价值仍存在争议。

垂体癌的定义仍限于发生颅脑 - 脊柱轴内或外部转移的腺垂体肿瘤。垂体癌极为罕见，德国国家垂体肿瘤登记垂体癌约占垂体腺瘤 0.12%，占 SEER（监测、流行病学和最终结果计划）数据库中侵袭性腺瘤的 6%。儿童垂体癌非常罕见。

内分泌学

垂体激素和稳态反馈回路

垂体的激素分泌功能是通过下丘脑、垂体和靶器官等多个反馈回路来调节的。这些反馈回路的概要如图 25.7 所示。

下丘脑弓状核分泌生长激素释放激素（GHRH）、生长激素抑制激素（growth hormone- inhibiting hormone，GHIH，通常称为生长抑素）、促甲状腺激素释放激素（thyrotropin releasing hormone，TRH）、促性腺激素释放激素（gonadotropin- releasing hormone，GnRH）、催乳素释放激素（prolactin- releasing hormone，PRH）、催乳素抑制激素（prolactin-inhibiting hormone，PIH，多巴胺）、促肾上腺皮质激素释放激素（corticotrophin- releasing hormone，CRH）。这些激素被分泌进入垂体门脉系统，然后转运到垂体前叶。

垂体前叶产生六种激素：促肾上腺皮质激素（adrenocorticotrophic hormone，ACTH）、催乳素（prolactin，PRL）、生长激素（growth hormone，GH）、促甲状腺激素（thyroid stimulating hormone，TSH）、促卵泡激素（follicle stimulating hormone，FSH）和黄体生成素（luteinizing hormone，LH）（图 25.1 和图 25.7）。

催产素和抗利尿激素（anti-diuretic hormones，ADH，也称为血管加压素）是垂体后叶分泌的激素。它们由下丘脑室旁核和视上核神经元合成，经轴突穿过垂体柄进入后叶。

有的垂体激素是动态分泌的，周期时长从几天至几个月不等。例如，GH 在一天内以脉冲式释放，刺激肝中 IGF-1 的产生，后者血液浓度更稳定（图 25.7B）。皮质醇的释放在早晨达到高峰，在午夜达到低谷（图 25.7C）。其他激素如 LH 和 FSH 遵循每月一次循环模式。

垂体激素的主要靶器官有肾上腺（ACTH）、甲状腺（TSH）、生殖器官（FSH 和 LH）和乳房（PRL）。其他激素如 GH 对骨骼、肌肉的生长及全身各系统有更广泛的影响。

基线、激发和抑制内分泌试验

垂体激素检查可作为内分泌评估的基线检查。基本内容包括催乳素、甲状腺功能、IGF-1、9 am 或随机皮质醇、ACTH、LH、FSH、雌二醇及睾酮。催乳素检测对于垂体瘤患者是一项重要的检查，因为绝大多数催乳素分泌型腺瘤可通过药物手段进行治疗，

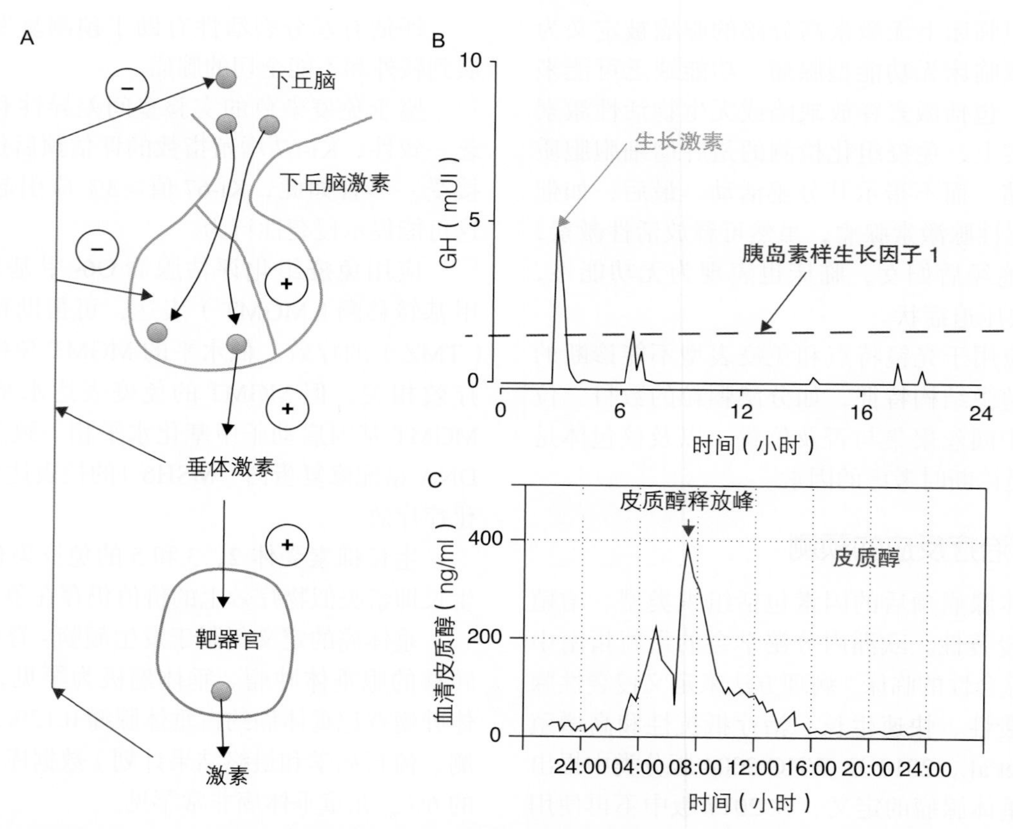

图 25.7 激素反馈回路（A）脉冲式生长激素释放（B）和血清皮质醇释放的昼夜节律的示意图（C）

从而避免手术。

激发试验可用于研究垂体或靶器官是否存在功能减退。一个常见案例是胰岛素应激试验，利用低血糖刺激血糖负向调节激素 ACTH、皮质醇或 GH 产生的特点（**图 25.8A**），通过诱导低血糖来评估皮质醇或 GH 的缺乏程度。胰高血糖素应激试验是该试验的替代方法，患者对这种试验的耐受性更好。胰高血糖素应激试验将葡萄糖上调至高于正常水平，然后逐渐恢复到正常水平，从而刺激血糖负向调节激素 GH 和 ACTH 变化。

抑制试验用于探究激素是否过度分泌。例如，地塞米松抑制试验通过抑制 ACTH 和皮质醇的产生，从而证实库欣综合征（**图 25.8B**）。口服葡萄糖耐量试验用于生长激素分泌过量的诊断。在肢端肥大症患者，升高血糖并不能引发生长激素分泌的抑制。这些试验的临床应用将在后面的特定章节中详细说明。

有时短时二十四肽促皮质素试验（Short Synacthen Test，SST）可作为评估垂体分泌 ACTH 的替代指标。二十四肽促皮质素可评估肾上腺对外源性 ACTH 的反应，但不能确定患者有内源性 ACTH 分泌。然而，如果患者长期缺乏 ACTH，则有可能出现肾上腺萎缩，因此 SST 可作为慢性 ACTH 缺乏的间接评估办法。换言之，它不能用于评估新近发生的 ACTH 缺乏，因为时间不足以导致肾上腺萎缩，当内源性 ACTH 缺乏时肾上腺仍然会对外源性 ACTH 应答。

治疗方式选择

手术治疗

手术可解决肿瘤相关的占位效应并使激素异常分泌恢复正常。在神经影像特点不明确的情况下，可进行诊断性活检。

具体手术技术详述见随后章节。手术入路的设计通常由正常垂体的中心位置决定。因此，暴露垂体区域虽有多种入路，但绝大多数病例是通过内镜经鼻入路治疗的，参见**图 25.9**。

药物治疗

药物治疗有多个应用层面。简单来说，它分为补充缺乏的激素来治疗激素分泌不足和通过药物抑制垂体肿瘤分泌过量激素。

垂体肿瘤造成垂体功能低下的常见原因有：①肿瘤对正常垂体组织的压迫效应；②术后垂体功能损害；③放疗后垂体功能减退。ACTH 和 ADH 缺乏可能危及生命，需要尽快替代治疗。其他激素缺乏可缓慢补充。

在一些功能性腺瘤中，激素过量和占位效应可通过药物手段成功控制。最常见的示例是使用多巴胺激动剂治疗催乳素腺瘤。对其他激素分泌活跃的腺瘤来说，药物治疗虽然没有那么有效，但同样不失为一种选择（例如，生长抑素治疗 GH 分泌型腺瘤）。

放射治疗

放射治疗主要作为一种辅助性治疗，用于控制

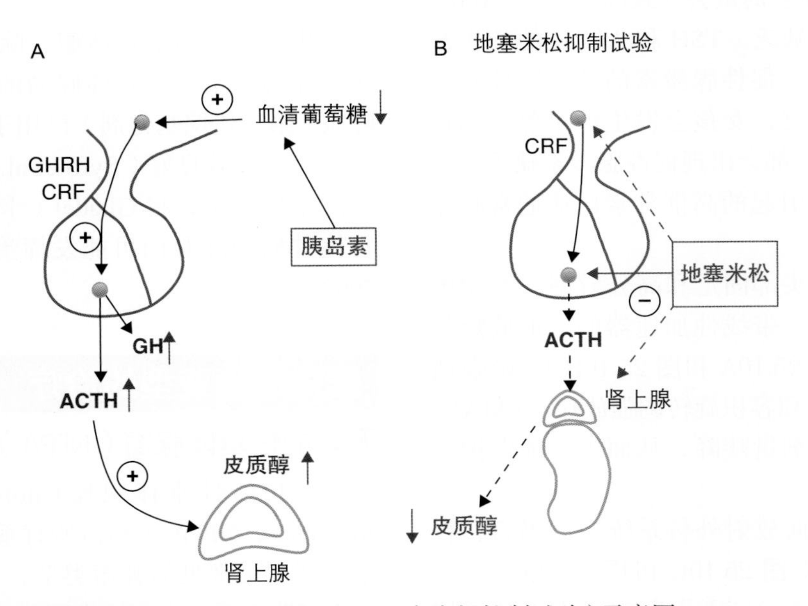

图 25.8　刺激试验（A- 胰岛素应激试验）和抑制试验（B- 地塞米松抑制试验）示意图

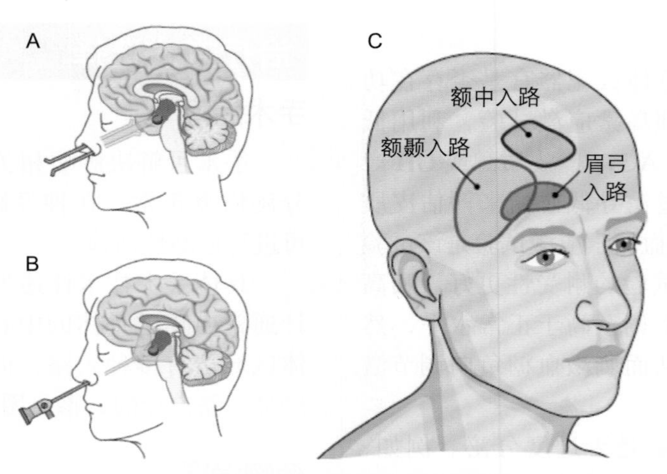

图 25.9 垂体瘤手术入路示意图。显微镜（A）和内镜（B）技术下经鼻蝶入路。经颅手术（C）包括眉弓、翼点和额部开颅手术

因不能安全切除而残留的肿瘤生长。在少数情况下，它可作为有手术禁忌或不适合手术患者的一线治疗。

放射治疗的模式包括传统的直线加速器，在5~6 周的时间内，每天从多个端口发出射线进行放射治疗，总剂量为 40~50 Gy。分割放疗的优点是允许邻近正常神经组织在放射间隙得以恢复（Kanner et al.，2009）。据报道，在 10 年的随访期间，93% 的患者疾病得到有效控制（Darzy and Shalet，2009）。

放疗并发症包括治疗后几年内垂体功能逐渐减退。鞍区放射治疗后的垂体功能减退是进行性的和不可逆的，因此需要定期监测和调整治疗。风险受辐射剂量影响，并且每种激素系统的敏感性存在差异（Darzy and Shalet，2009）。GH的产生最容易受影响，即使在辐射剂量低于 24 Gy 的情况下也会出现分泌不足，40~50 Gy 的辐射剂量会导致高达 50%~100% 的病例出现 GH 分泌缺乏。TSH 和 ACTH 的产生对放射治疗相对不敏感。促性腺激素的缺乏因性别而异：剂量低于 30 Gy 时，女孩会发生性早熟；剂量在 30~50 Gy 时，男女都会出现促性腺激素缺乏。由下丘脑抑制功能损害引起的高催乳素血症通常临床表现不明显。

放疗中采用面罩头部固定和高分辨率三维 MRI 引导能使靶区更准确。带线性加速器的适形放疗是现代的标准流程（图 25.10A 和图 25.10B）。调强适形放射治疗（IMRT）和容积旋转调强放疗（VMAT）有助于调控靶区外的剂量陡降，从而更好地保护正常组织。

最常用的立体定向放射外科系统是伽玛刀和直线加速器（LINAC）（图 25.10C 和图 25.10D）。常采用单剂量（15~20 Gy），或分为 2~5 次。肿瘤控制率为 88%~97%，视神经功能的损伤率为 0~12%，影响垂体功能的比例为 0~41%。

这些放疗模式的选择取决于残余肿瘤的大小和形状：立体定向放射外科推荐用于距视神经 3 mm 以上的较小的、局部的病变，而较大的病变可能更适合常规分割放射治疗。

质子束是一种治疗某些颅底病变的新型方式，具有辐射剂量陡降的优点（即“布拉格峰”效应）。可对肿瘤进行更高剂量放疗的同时，相对保护邻近正常组织。质子束不是垂体腺瘤常规推荐的治疗方法，它更适用于残余颅底脊索瘤和软骨肉瘤的治疗，这些肿瘤需要较高剂量的放射治疗，同时保护正常脑干组织和视交叉。

化疗

化疗很少用于垂体瘤，除非其他治疗方法无效时，作为强侵袭性垂体腺瘤的挽救治疗。口服替莫唑胺（第二代烷基化剂）已用于垂体腺瘤和垂体腺癌的治疗，疗效良好（Syro et al.，2011）。一项 I 期试验的结果表明，将 Gliadel（卡莫司汀膜片）放置在垂体肿瘤切除腔内可能发挥治疗作用（Laws et al.，2003）。

垂体腺瘤亚型的治疗

无功能性垂体腺瘤（NFPA）

无功能性垂体腺瘤（non-functioning pituitary adenomas，NFPA）约占所有垂体肿瘤的 20%，是手术病例中最常见的肿瘤类型，大约 80% 属于促性腺激素细胞谱系。它们通常不分泌具有活性的激素。因

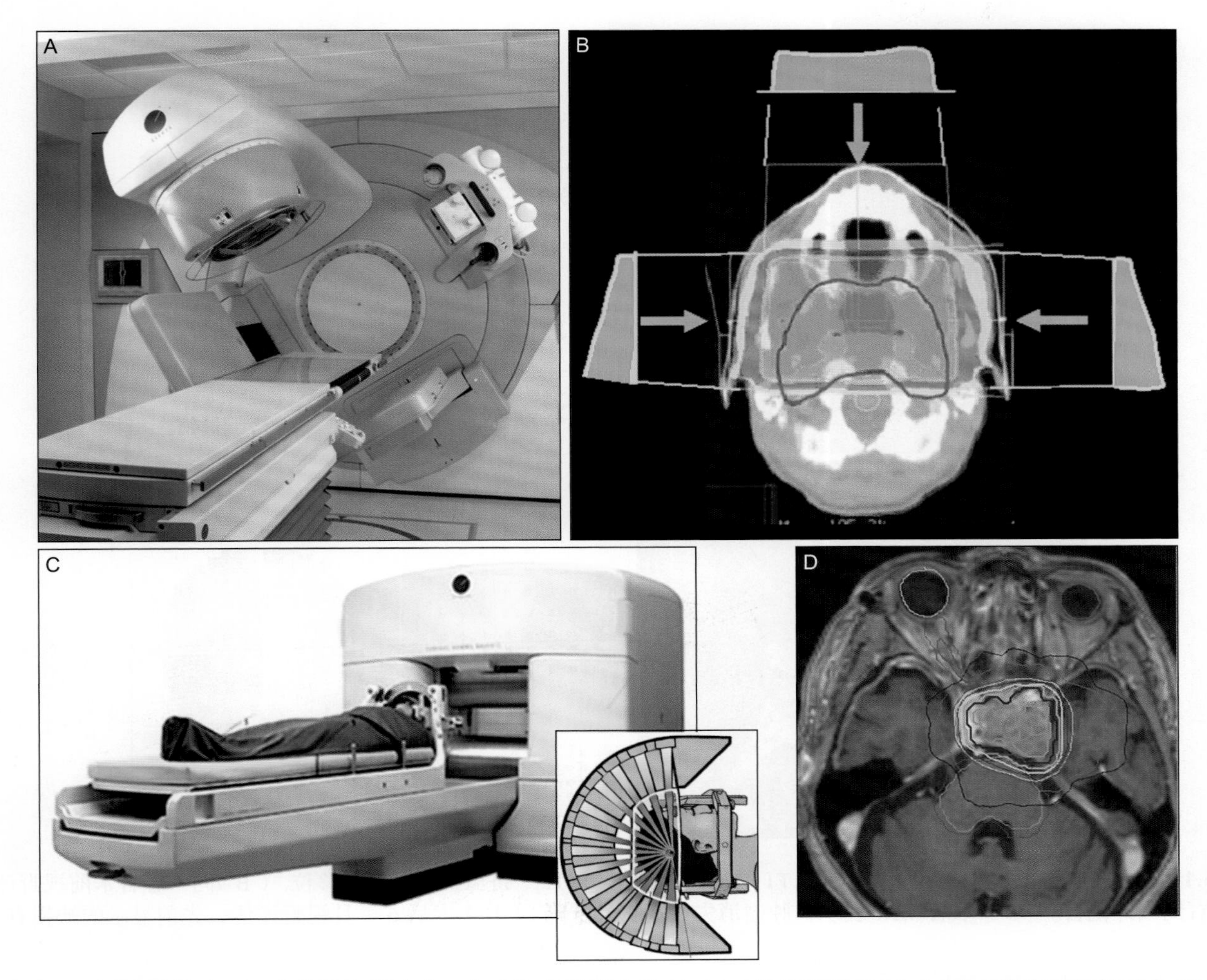

图 25.10　不同放疗模式。（A）常规放射治疗，多叶准直器瞄准光束。（B）放疗剂量计划。（C）立体定向放射手术（Leksell 伽玛刀）。（D）放疗计划计示意图

此，它们在临床上保持功能静默，直到它们因继续生长压迫正常腺体而引起垂体功能低下或局部占位压迫的临床表现。出于同样的原因，NFPA 主要是大腺瘤。

NFPA 最常见的临床表现是视野缺损，可在 60%~80% 的病例中检出。视交叉通常从正中线的下方开始受压迫，最初累及颞上象限，然后进一步发展为双眼颞侧偏盲（图 25.11B）。如果病变位置靠后，近侧视束受压较重，并累及 Wilbrand 膝，也有可能发生对侧同向偏盲。高达 70% 的病例表现为头痛，8%~20% 的病例表现有内分泌失调，2%~7% 的病例出现肿瘤卒中，而脑神经麻痹较少见（3%）。

随着 MRI 和 CT 检查的日益普及，NFPA 越来越多地被偶然发现。全套垂体功能检测应被作为常规筛查。

主要的治疗是外科手术，以减轻对周围结构的压迫。最常用的手术方法是内镜经蝶入路垂体肿瘤切除术。

术后大多数患者的视力得以改善，完全恢复正常的占 35%，部分改善的占 60%，只有 5% 左右的患者没有视力改善，甚至发生视力恶化（Gnanalingham et al.，2005）。术后视力的改善通常是渐进式的，且持续数年，但最终视力改善的患者中约 50% 在最初的 6 个月内恢复（图 25.11D）。

非手术治疗的垂体瘤约有 10% 会出现自发性消退，但也有 50% 将持续进展最终需要手术治疗。残余肿瘤可通过分割放疗或立体定向放疗治疗。

催乳素型腺瘤

催乳素腺瘤的发病率在 6~8/100（万·年），且存在性别差异。育龄妇女患泌乳素微腺瘤的频率要高于男性 20 倍，可能是因为催乳素微腺瘤对生育能力和月经周期的影响促使早期检查。然而，男性和女性的催乳素大腺瘤发生的频率相同。此外，对于患有微腺瘤的女性来说，常见的症状是肿瘤激素分泌引起的少经或闭经、不孕和溢乳，而不是占位效应。

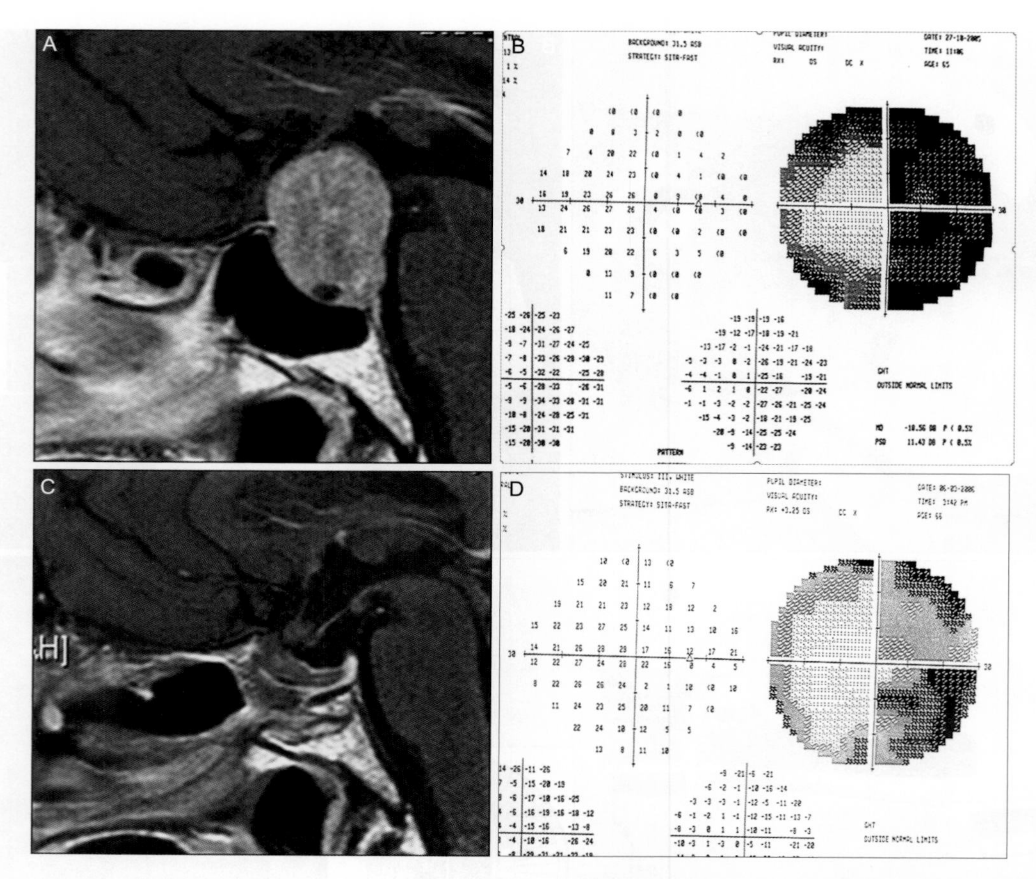

图 25.11　无功能垂体瘤案例。（A）矢状位 T1 增强 MRI 扫描 NFPA，挤压视交叉向上移位。（B）同一患者术前视野评估，显示右侧颞部偏盲。（C）术后 MRI 表现，肿瘤消失后视交叉下降。（D）术后 6 个月视野评估，先前显示的缺损有显著改善

男性高催乳素血症可引起性欲下降、勃起功能障碍及乳腺发育，溢乳少见，参见**图** 25.12。

催乳素基线水平测定是诊断的第一步，但有几个因素会影响血清催乳素水平。例如，静脉穿刺所致的应激可能会引起催乳素升高，因此从导管中采集的血液样本更准确。高泌乳素血症的其他外部原因包括神经源性刺激类药、抗抑郁药、抗精神类药等药物，以及继发于肾或肝功能不全的血浆清除率降低。非分泌性垂体病变压迫垂体柄也可导致血清催乳素一定程度增加（通常为 500~1000 mU/L），孕期和哺乳期的血清催乳素数值为 3000~6000 mU/L。一般来说，催乳素水平大于 2000 mU/L 很可能与催乳素腺瘤有关，催乳素水平与肿瘤大小也有相关性。

两个需要注意的生化特点是钩状效应和出现巨催乳素。在钩状效应中，由于非常高的泌乳素水平的信号猝灭效应，高泌乳素水平被错误地检测为低水平。这种假象可用连续样品稀释法校正（St-Jean et al.，1996）。巨催乳素是一种生理上不活跃的催乳素形式，存在于少数人群中。事实上是催乳素与 IgG 结合后形成，一些实验室将其误测为催乳素，导致

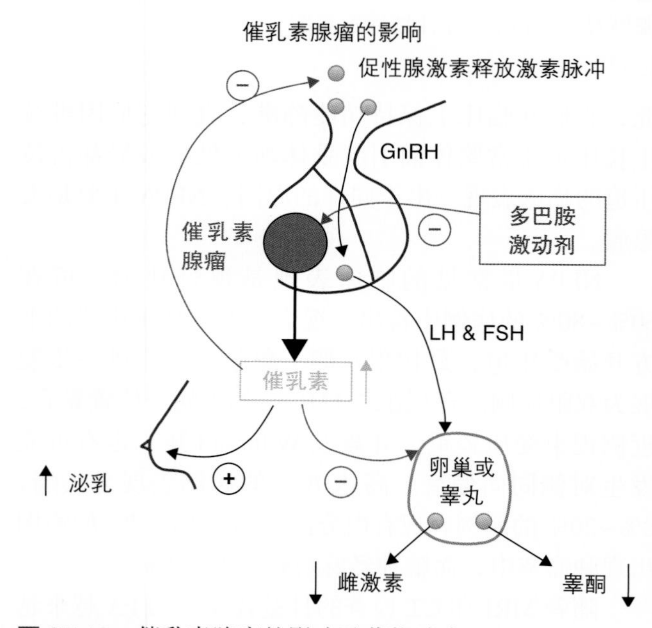

图 25.12　催乳素腺瘤的影响及药物治疗

结果假性升高。

大多数催乳素腺瘤可用多巴胺激动剂如卡麦角林、溴隐亭或培高利特等药物进行治疗。这些药物

可使约90%患者的血清高催乳素水平有效降低并使肿瘤缩小。应用多巴胺激动剂类药物的患者推荐长期临床随访。有研究报道，当磁共振检查不到肿瘤，且高泌乳素分泌被完全抑制时，一些患者的多巴胺激动剂可成功地长期停用，但这种情况并不普遍（Schlechte，2007）。

卡麦角林的一个罕见但严重的副作用是心脏瓣膜病变，它继发于多巴胺刺激的瓣膜内成纤维细胞增殖。因此，建议在开始服用卡麦角林之前进行超声心动图检查，并监测这种副作用。多巴胺激动剂，尤其是卡麦角林，因其诱发自然流产和先天性畸形的风险最小，可用于治疗怀孕期间的催乳素瘤。

约10%的患者对治疗无反应或无法耐受多巴胺激动剂的副作用，如恶心、抑郁等。因此，只有少数不能耐受各种多巴胺激动剂或没有治疗效果的患者需要手术治疗。手术治疗对80%~90%的泌乳素微腺瘤有效，但仅对50%的泌乳素大腺瘤有效。高泌乳素血症可持续存在，甚至在初始正常化后复发。如果无法药物治疗，也可考虑对不能手术的肿瘤进行放射治疗。

生长激素型腺瘤

生长激素型腺瘤约占所有垂体腺瘤的20%，发病率为3百万/年~4百万/年。99%的病例中过量的生长激素来源于垂体腺瘤，异位来源极为罕见（内分泌学会指南，Giustina et al.，2010）。

该肿瘤的临床表现通常是过量生长激素引起的相应症状和（或）肿瘤的占位效应（表现为头痛和视觉障碍）（图25.13B，C）。儿童和青少年的骨骺生长较活跃，生长激素过量会导致巨人症；而在成人中，生长激素过量则会导致肢端肥大症。肢端肥大症的体征和症状包括软组织及内脏器官肿胀、下颌突出和前额高起。此外，过量的生长激素对身体的生理功能有广泛影响，涉及下列多个系统：70%的病例有肌肉骨骼系统疾病（如关节病、退行性骨关节炎、椎体骨折和压迫性神经病变），60%的病例有心血管疾病（如心肌病、心律失常、高血压和瓣膜病），50%以上的病例有呼吸系统疾病（如阻塞性睡眠呼吸暂停和鼻息肉）。此外，生长激素过量对内分泌系统也有明显影响，可引起糖尿病、高血压、血脂异常和痛风等。肢端肥大症患者患结肠癌的风险是普通人的两倍。总体上来说，由于上述心血管、呼吸系统和肿瘤的影响，未经治疗的肢端肥大症患者的死亡率是一般人群的两倍。

性别和年龄匹配的IGF-1水平是检测的一线指标。由于生长激素以一种脉冲式的模式分泌，所以很难解读随机生长激素水平的临床意义。IGF-1被用作反映GH分泌水平的替代标志物，在肢端肥大症

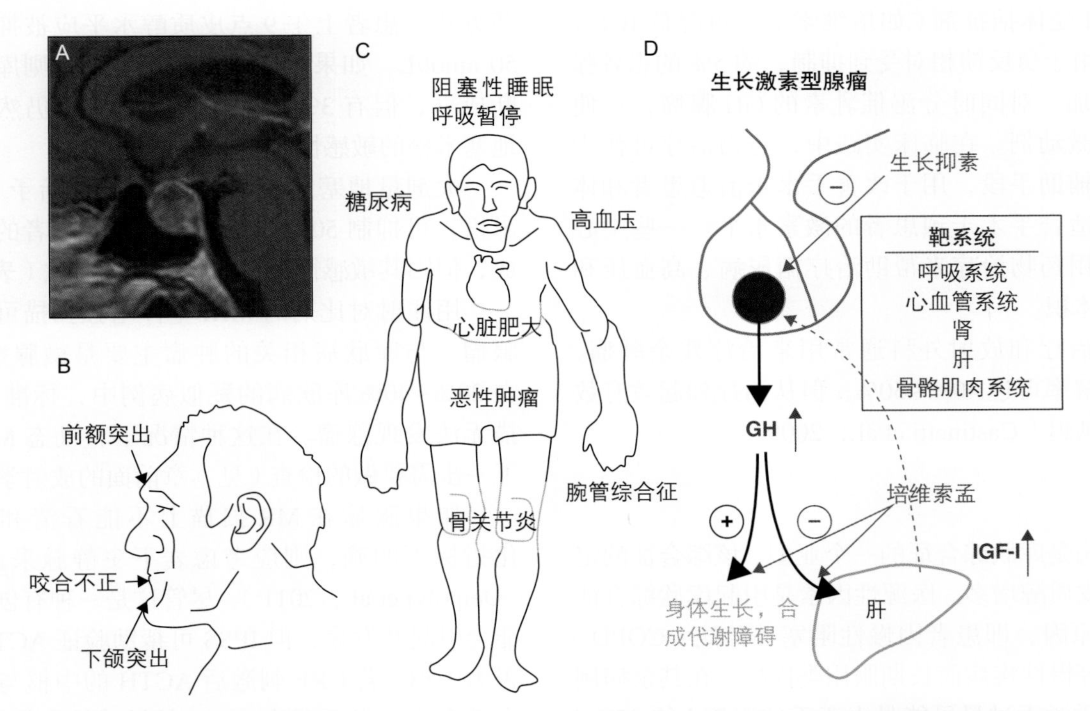

图25.13 （A）MRI T1像上一个生长激素型大腺瘤。肢端肥大症的特征（B）累及多个器官系统的症状（C）。治疗生长激素型腺瘤的药物的反馈通路与靶点（D）

患者中，该指标通常升高。口服葡萄糖耐量试验可确认患者是否有生长激素分泌过量，该试验评估了血清生长激素水平对葡萄糖是否有充分的反馈机制。如果 GH 谷值低于 0.4 μg/L 且 IGF-1 水平正常，则可排除肢端肥大症（Giustina et al.，2010）。在生长激素日曲线中，平均生长激素水平升高且大于 1 μg/L 可进一步证实上述结论。在 30%~50% 的病例中，催乳素的分泌量也随之明显升高。

在术前，医生应通过颅脑 MRI 明确垂体腺瘤的存在。如果 MRI 结果为阴性，则应通过进一步影像学检查来寻找产生 GH/GHRH 的垂体外来源（如胸腹部 CT）。

外科手术是治疗肢端肥大症最有效方法，目标是使激素水平（即 GH 和 IGF-1）正常化，并解除肿瘤对周围结构的压迫。经鼻蝶手术的预后较好，平均缓解率可达 50%~90%（Giustina et al.，2010）。然而，治疗效果取决于外科医生的经验、肿瘤大小、肿瘤侵袭性和术前生长激素水平等多方面的因素。预测良好预后的因素包括微腺瘤（即小于 1 cm 的肿瘤）、MR 提示非侵袭性腺瘤和术前 GH 水平低于 10 μg/L。对于术后肿瘤有残余和首次手术后病情未缓解的患者，可考虑尽早行二次手术探查以降低手术瘢痕的影响。

药物控制包括生长抑素类似物（如奥曲肽），对大约半数患者可有效降低其 GH 水平，对约 30% 患者可部分缩小肿瘤体积（**图** 25.13D）。在 95% 的病例中，GH 受体拮抗剂（如培维索孟）可降低 IGF-1 水平，但由于负反馈相对受到抑制，约 5% 的患者腺瘤体积增加。对同时分泌催乳素的 GH 腺瘤，可使用多巴胺激动剂。在临床实践中，药物治疗可作为一种术后辅助手段，用于改善手术未治愈患者和体格因素不适合手术干预患者的激素水平。一些中心在术前使用药物治疗来帮助治疗糖尿病、高血压和缩小肿瘤体积。

放射治疗和放射外科通常用来治疗残余肿瘤，治疗的缓解率可达 40%~50%，但从治疗到起效有数年的时间延迟（Castinetti et al.，2009）。

库欣病

库欣病是库欣综合征的一个亚型，该综合征的定义是血清皮质醇增多。医源性因素是引起库欣综合征最常见的原因，即患者因慢性阻塞性肺病（COPD）或脑肿瘤等慢性疾病而长期服用类固醇。在其余病例中，糖皮质激素过量可能是由于垂体腺瘤（约 85%）或其他异位来源（约 1%）导致 ACTH 分泌过多所致。肾上腺腺瘤导致产生的皮质醇过多约占 15%。

导致库欣病的垂体腺瘤少见，其发病率约为 1 百万 / 年 ~2 百万 / 年。糖皮质激素过量所引起的症状包括向心性肥胖、满月脸、性欲减退、皮肤薄、身高增长迟缓、高血压、多毛症、情绪障碍、容易淤血、葡萄糖耐受不良、虚弱、骨量减少和肾结石（**图** 25.14B~D）。库欣病的诊断常被延误，患者通常有难以控制的糖尿病、高血压或肥胖等，在经过漫长的临床就诊后才被最终诊断为库欣病。

诊断库欣病的方法很复杂，因为没有一种诊断方法具有绝对的敏感性和特异性。血清皮质醇水平遵循昼夜节律模式，同时还受到压力、抑郁、酗酒、神经性厌食症或怀孕等多种因素的影响。

首先要做的筛查包括清晨皮质醇和 ACTH 水平，24 小时尿游离皮质醇或午夜和上午 9 点唾液皮质醇水平。夜间唾液皮质醇测量的敏感性和特异性为 95%~98%，可用于门诊。午夜一次法地塞米松抑制试验即在 23:00 给予患者 1 mg 地塞米松口服，次日上午 9 点测量血清皮质醇。若血清皮质醇低于 50 nmol/L 可排除库欣综合征。总的来说，垂体和异位来源的库欣综合征，其皮质醇和 ACTH 水平都升高。在肾上腺肿瘤导致的库欣综合征中，皮质醇水平高，但 ACTH 水平不高（**表** 25.1）。

随后需行诊断性动态试验，包括小剂量地塞米松抑制试验（LDDST），即按一定剂量给予地塞米松（每 6 小时给药 0.5 mg，持续 48 小时），通过这种给药方式，患者上午 9 点皮质醇水平应被抑制到低于 50 nmol/L。如果未能达到这一水平，则库欣病的诊断成立，但有 3%~8% 的库欣病患者仍然保持着对地塞米松的敏感性。

大剂量地塞米松试验是在 23:00 给予 8 mg 地塞米松，可抑制 50% 垂体源性库欣病患者的皮质醇生成，但因其敏感性低，不作为常用方法（**表** 25.1）。

用注射对比剂的 MRI 垂体增强扫描可检测垂体腺瘤。与库欣病相关的肿瘤主要是微腺瘤。然而，在 20%~40% 库欣病的疑似病例中，标准的 MRI 扫描无法发现腺瘤。在这种情况下，动态 MR 扫描是下一步需要做的检查（见本章前面的放射学部分）。

如果腺瘤在 MR 扫描上不能看清和（或）生化指标不明确，则应考虑岩下窦静脉采血（IPSS）（Deipolyi et al.，2011）。尽管这是一种有创检查，可能会引起并发症，但 IPSS 可帮助验证 ACTH 来源是否为中枢（若 CRF 刺激后 ACTH 的中枢与外周比例大于 3∶1，几乎具有 100% 的敏感性和特异性）。此外，通过岩下窦静脉采血（IPSS），若 CRF 刺激后

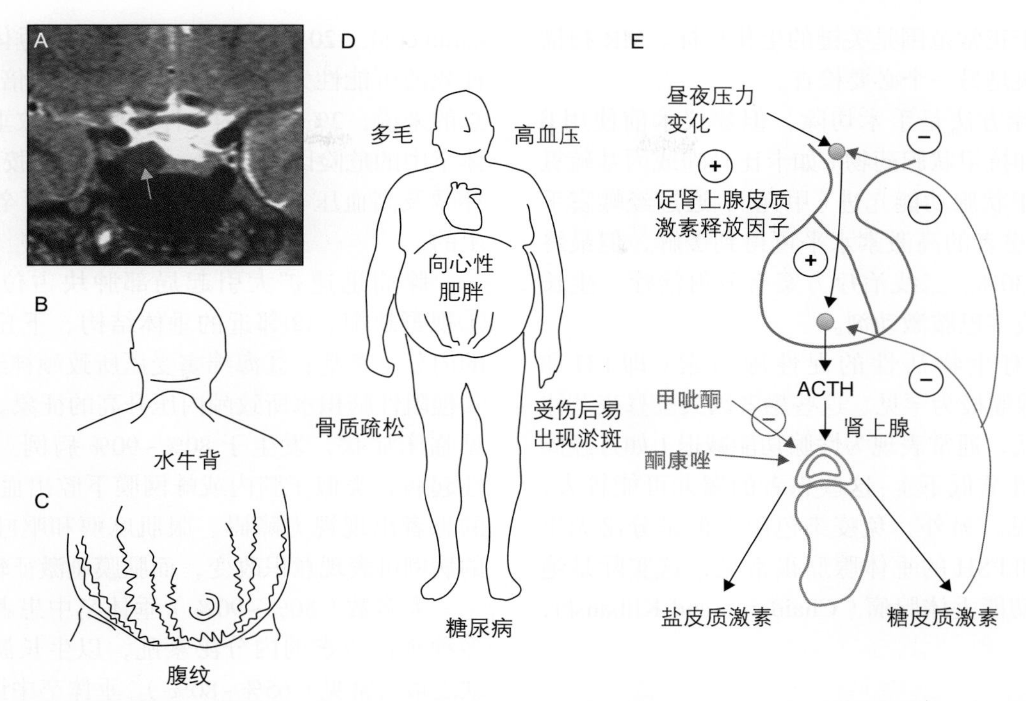

图 25.14　MRI 显示右侧垂体微腺瘤引起库欣病（A）。库欣病的临床特征包括水牛背（B）、腹纹（C）、向心性肥胖和累及多器官的症状（D）

表 25.1　不同原因引起库欣综合征的患者的血清基础 ACTH 和皮质醇水平比较。库欣病的诊断方法很复杂，因为没有单一检查有绝对的灵敏度和特异度。低剂量地塞米松抑制试验 (LDDST) 和大剂量地塞米松抑制试验 (HDDST) 的典型变化如图所示

肿瘤	ACTH	皮质醇	LDDST	HDDST
正常	→	→	↓	↓
垂体腺瘤	↑	↑	↑	→或↓
异位 ACTH	↑↑	↑	↑	↑
肾上腺肿瘤	↓	↑	↑	↑

左右侧岩下窦中 ACTH 水平差异大于 1.5 倍时，可正确判断约 70% 的病例垂体病变的侧别。

对于怀疑异位肿瘤或肾上腺腺瘤的病例可行胸部、腹部及盆腔 CT 检查。

对于垂体腺瘤所致库欣病，经鼻手术切除仍然是最有效的治疗方式。对于非侵袭性肿瘤，选择性微腺瘤切除术的初始缓解率可达 70%~80%，但长时间的随访发现，复发率高达 20%。大腺瘤的缓解率较低，尤其是侵袭性大腺瘤。

药物治疗包括抑制肾上腺类固醇合成的药物（如甲吡酮、酮康唑、氨鲁米特和米托坦）（图 25.14E）。药物治疗适用于术前改善病情，也适用于手术治疗不能治愈的患者。垂体放射治疗 / 放射外科通常也用于手术不能完全缓解的病例。

在垂体手术后病情仍在进展的患者中，双侧肾上腺切除术是治疗糖皮质激素过量的一种挽救性选择。这种治疗可导致 Nelson 综合征，由于缺乏糖皮质激素的负反馈作用，促肾上腺皮质激素（ACTH）分泌上调并伴随促黑素细胞刺激激素（MSH）水平升高，因为二者来自相同的前体——前阿片黑素皮质素。MSH 水平升高会刺激黑素细胞，导致皮肤过度色素沉着。此外，残余的垂体瘤可增大继而引起占位效应。

临床上“静默型”促肾上腺皮质激素腺瘤可由于占位效应而出现症状，在更为少见的一部分患者中也可转为库欣病。

其他功能型腺瘤

促甲状腺激素腺瘤更为罕见，约占所有垂体腺瘤的 0.5%~1%，每年发病率为百万分之一，因此只有相对较少的病例系列研究报道（Sanno et al., 2001）。这些肿瘤大多数是大腺瘤，表现为占位效应所致的体征和（或）甲状腺素过量引起的症状，包括体重减轻、心悸、睡眠障碍和疲劳。TSH 腺瘤在临床上与其他引起甲状腺功能亢进的病因难以区分。

血清 T4 升高合并 TSH 水平升高或 TSH 未被有

效抑制而处于正常范围是关键的生化指标。MR 扫描确定垂体肿块是另一个必要检查。

主要治疗方法是手术切除，但建议术前使用β受体阻滞剂和抗甲状腺药物（如卡比马唑或丙基硫氧嘧啶）控制甲状腺功能亢进（甲亢）。通过经蝶窦手术，约 80% 患者的高激素水平可得到缓解，但最终治愈率约为 30%。二线治疗方案有放射治疗、生长抑素类似物或多巴胺激动剂。

分泌具有生物活性的促性腺激素（即 LH 和 FSH）垂体腺瘤极为罕见。这些患者因失去昼夜节律和睾酮水平低，通常表现为性腺功能减退（如月经周期不规则或性欲低下）。这些患者的睾丸可能较大，尽管极为罕见。另外，免疫染色阳性但是分泌无生物活性 LH 和 FSH 的垂体腺瘤很常见，这实际是绝大多数的无功能垂体腺瘤（Chaidarun and Klibanski，2002）。

垂体卒中

垂体卒中是一种继发于垂体腺瘤梗死和（或）出血的急性临床症状（英国内分泌学会指南，Rajasekaran et al.，2011）。由于血供丰富，垂体肿瘤出血或梗死的可能性大约是其他脑肿瘤的 5 倍（**图 25.15**）。总的来说，2%~7% 的垂体腺瘤可导致垂体卒中。垂体卒中的危险因素包括：抗凝、多巴胺激动剂治疗、怀孕及高血压等，尽管大多数情况下卒中是自发发生的。

腺瘤迅速扩大引起局部肿块占位效应，伴有①视野缺损；②邻近的垂体结构、下丘脑受压引起的内分泌紊乱；③海绵窦受压所致颅神经功能障碍；④梗阻性脑积水所致颅内压升高的征象。头痛是最常见临床症状，发生于 80%~90% 病例。头痛相对急性起病，类似于脑内或蛛网膜下腔出血。30%~40% 的患者出现视力障碍、眼肌麻痹和呕吐。大约 20% 的病例可表现意识改变，而脑膜刺激征较少见。

大多数（80%~90%）垂体卒中患者存在一种或多种垂体激素的内分泌紊乱，以生长激素和 ACTH 缺乏最为常见（65%~80%）。垂体卒中评分（0~10）是基于意识障碍水平、视力、视野缺损和眼肌麻痹的分级标准（Rajasekaran et al.，2011）。

垂体卒中的治疗方案取决于症状的严重程度。

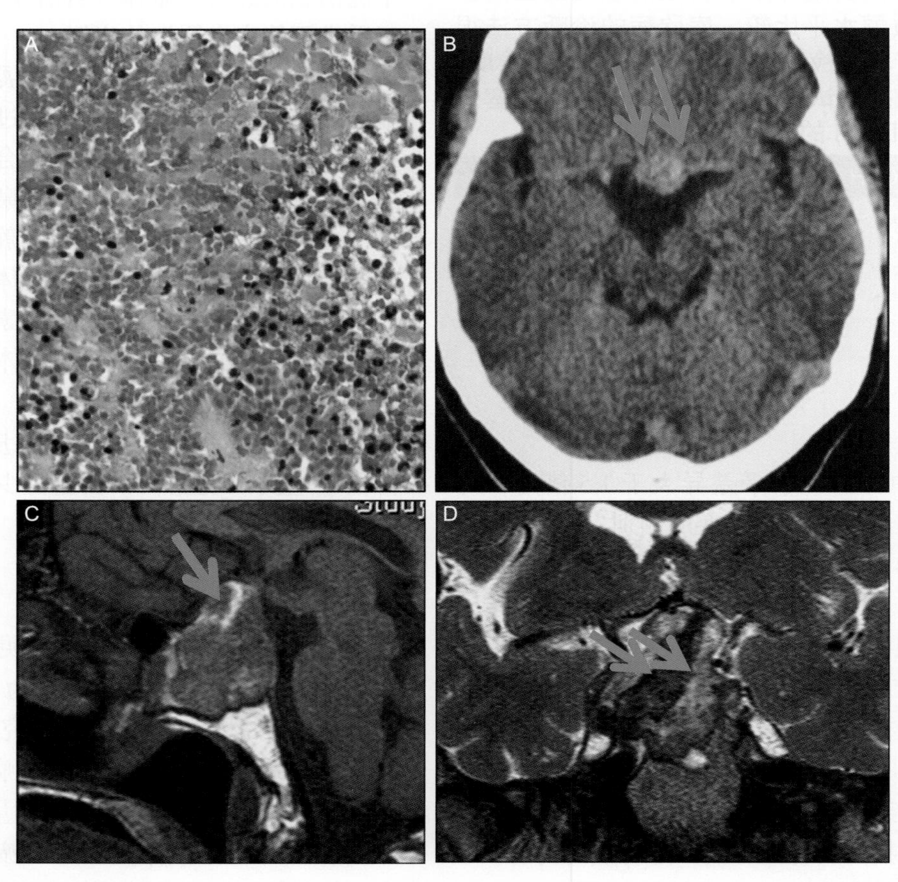

图 25.15　一个垂体卒中病例颅脑 CT（B）和 MR 的 T1 矢状位（C）和 T2 冠状位（D）显示垂体大腺瘤内的出血（箭头所指）。苏木精—伊红染色证实出血和炎症细胞浸润（A）

需要考虑的因素包括意识水平下降、视力损害的严重程度、MR 表现、内分泌和电解质紊乱等。最基本的治疗应该包括类固醇替代疗法（如静脉注射氢化可的松）和补液。

对大多数有视力障碍并伴相应占位效应及 MR 表现有视交叉受压的患者建议进行紧急手术，而手术减压的时机仍无定论。一般来说，早期手术治疗适用于那些有严重视力缺陷或视力缺损程度较轻且已经过保守治疗的患者。一般情况下，一旦患者经保守治疗后病情稳定，手术减压应在 1~2 天内进行。经蝶窦入路是大多数患者的首选手术方案，脑积水的患者则需置入脑室外引流。术后患者视力一般会得到改善。然而，大多数起病时有垂体功能减退的患者其激素缺乏无法恢复。此外，有研究发现，单纯采用保守治疗，肿瘤也可能随时间推移而缩小，视力也会有所恢复。

颅咽管瘤

颅咽管瘤是一种少见的鞍上区肿瘤，发病率为 0.5 百万 / 年 ~2.5 百万 / 年。这是一种起源于颅咽管和（或）拉特克裂残余部位的鳞状上皮样、常伴有钙化的囊性肿瘤。组织学上可分为造釉型和乳头型，术中深棕色的机油状囊液伴钙化斑和胆固醇结晶是其特征性表现。

80%~90% 的病例出现内分泌功能障碍，有时伴有占位效应的体征，如视野缺损（20%~25%）。8%~35% 的病例可表现为尿崩症。

MR 和 CT 通常根据钙化（80%~90%）、位于鞍上、囊性成分和斑片状强化来鉴别颅咽管瘤和垂体腺瘤（**图** 25.16A）。病灶可起源于鞍区、垂体柄和鞍上区，并突入第三脑室。

治疗原则包括安全前提下最大限度切除肿瘤并行视交叉减压，同时注意将手术并发症发生率降到最低，尤其是下丘脑损伤。囊性复发处理较为棘手，通常通过置入 Omaya 囊来处理。放射治疗和立体定向放射外科只适用于肿瘤有残余和不适合手术的患者。通过这些措施，肿瘤控制率可达到 80%。

拉特克囊肿

是一种由鞍区或鞍上拉特克囊胚胎残留形成的非肿瘤性上皮性囊性病变。大多数拉特克囊肿是无症状的，患者常因偶然发现就诊。囊性内容物通常为蛋白性液体，在 MR 的 T1 像上呈高信号（**图** 25.16B）。

如果囊性病变很小，而且影像学检查提示病变较稳定，可先行保守治疗。如果病变相对较大特别是当囊肿持续增大时，手术的目标是引流囊液并对视交叉进行减压。囊肿复发可能需要进一步行手术引流（如经蝶窦或经颅入路）和（或）置入 Omaya 储液囊，以便于以后复发时经皮引流。

垂体炎症

淋巴细胞性垂体炎：这是一种少见的自身免疫性炎性疾病［发病率 1/（百万·年）］。最常发生在围产期妇女，可分为急性、亚急性和慢性三种亚型。在急性垂体炎中，最常见的临床表现与快速扩张的炎性肿块引起的占位效应有关。在亚急性或慢性炎症中，占位效应和激素紊乱的症状相对较轻微。

通过临床病史和 MRI 表现可疑诊该病，但若无法确诊，可行手术活检明确诊断。MR 表现为腺体对称增大，垂体柄增厚并均匀强化（**图** 25.16C）。

治疗方式取决于症状发展的速度：对于症状急剧恶化且对药物治疗无反应的病例，需手术减压。如果肿块占位效应较轻，保守疗法（包括类固醇和激素替代疗法）可成功地逐步缩小病灶体积（Falorni et al.，2014）。

神经结节病：这是系统性结节病的罕见表现。该病 5%~15% 的患者会累及中枢神经系统，死亡率达 10%~20%。脑神经、下丘脑、脑膜和垂体是中枢神经系统最常见的受累部位。垂体结节病只占所有鞍内病变的不到 1%。最常见的激素不足是性腺功能减退，其次是 TSH、ADH 不足。

辅助检查包括颅脑 MRI（鞍区和硬脑膜强化）、血清 ACE 水平升高和脑脊液分析。通常需要手术活检行组织学确诊。药物治疗包括激素替代、类固醇或其他免疫抑制剂（例如强的松龙、甲氨蝶呤、环磷酰胺和硫唑嘌呤），也可行低剂量放射治疗。虽然异常的 MRI 表现可通过类固醇消除，但激素缺乏在大多数病例中仍长期存在（Langrand et al.，2012）。

垂体感染

垂体感染较为罕见。该病发生可源自腺体的无菌性坏死、脑脓肿或结核瘤的血行播散或直接扩散（Zhang et al.，2012）。垂体脓肿约占垂体病变的 0.5%，最常见的表现是头痛和视觉障碍。最常见的病原体是链球菌和葡萄球菌。垂体结核瘤常发生于免疫抑制患者和其他部位有结核病灶的患者。

典型的影像学表现为周边强化的鞍区肿块、弥散像受限（**图** 25.16D）。治疗方案包括经鼻蝶或经颅入路手术引流。最重要的是行组织学和微生物学分析以明确诊断，其次是长期应用抗生素（至少 6 周或

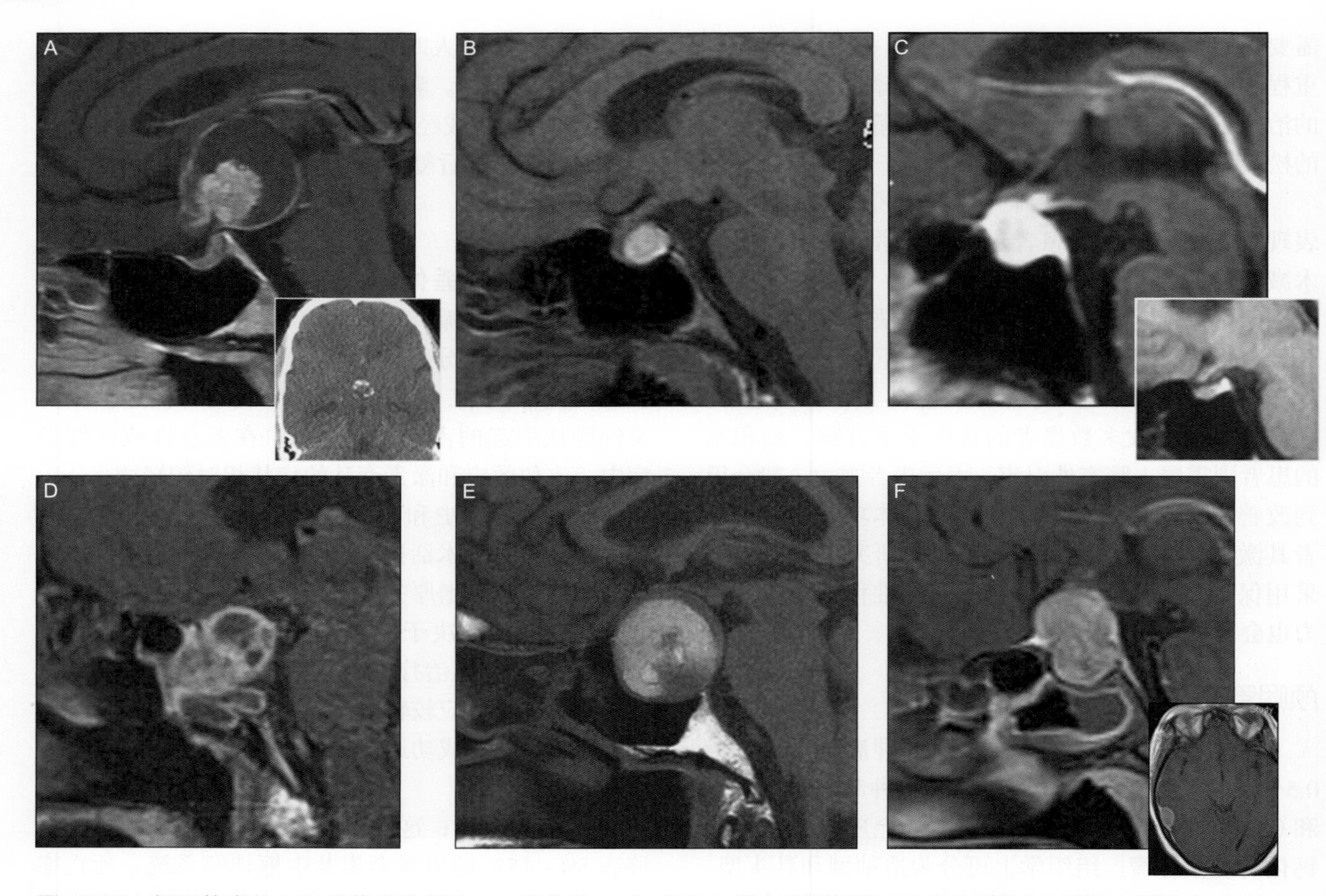

图 25.16 颅咽管瘤的 MR 影像学实例（A：强化的 T1 矢状位，插入的图显示 CT 上的钙化）；拉特克囊肿（B：MR T1 矢状位）；淋巴细胞性垂体炎（C：强化的 T1 矢状位，插入的图显示 8 个月后病灶的缩小）；垂体脓肿（D：强化的 T1 矢状位）；原发于肠腺癌的垂体转移瘤（E：MR T1 矢状位）和垂体癌（F：强化的 T1 矢状位，插入的图显示右侧颞部硬脑膜转移）

更长时间）并进行多次 MRI 增强扫描确定治疗效果。

继发性恶性肿瘤

根据尸检研究，垂体转移瘤的发病率在 1%~3.6%（Fassett and Couldwell，2004）。几乎所有肿瘤都能转移到垂体。最常见的转移方式是血行传播，很少通过周围骨组织直接转移。最常见原发恶性肿瘤是乳腺癌和肺癌（图 25.16E）。垂体转移瘤仅在 7% 的病例中有症状，以尿崩、眼肌麻痹、头痛和垂体前叶功能障碍为最常见的表现。

手术活检 / 切除是主要的治疗方式，并根据原发恶性肿瘤种类及疾病分期，术后辅以肿瘤局部放射治疗及全身系统性肿瘤治疗。大多数患者在发现垂体转移时原发疾病已经全身性扩散，因此预后很差。

其他鞍旁病变

还有其他几种病变，如脑膜瘤、脊索瘤、软骨肉瘤、骨纤维结构不良、朗格汉斯细胞组织细胞增生症和血管性病变，这些病变可发生在鞍旁并扩展至蝶鞍。垂体腺瘤的鉴别诊断是颇具挑战性的，但大多数可根据病史和影像学（MR/CT）表现做出准确诊断。这些疾病在本书的其他章节有介绍。

术后内分泌管理

垂体功能减退的发生率

术后垂体功能减退的概率取决于多个因素，包括所用内分泌检查是否准确得当，术前垂体功能损害的程度，以及肿瘤的类型和大小。总体而言，经蝶术后新发垂体激素缺乏的概率为 10%~20%。而且，50%~70% 的垂体腺瘤患者术前已确定有垂体功能低下，LH/FSH 缺乏是最常见的（Jahangiri et al.，2014）。发生一过性尿崩的概率为 16%~25%，尽管永久性尿崩的概率低于 5%，但也取决于肿瘤的类型，颅咽管瘤的风险相对较高。

类固醇替代治疗

一般来说，接受垂体手术的患者有皮质醇不足的风险，并可危及生命。在诱导麻醉和术后应给予患者氢化可的松，直到其内源性皮质醇可满足机体需要。

围术期和术后的氢化可的松替代方案有所不同。一个典型范例如下：在手术时静脉注射 100 mg（8 小时后追加一次剂量），在随后两天逐步减量，给予口服药物 20 mg（8:00）、10 mg（12:00）、10 mg（18:00），然后维持口服药物剂量在 10 mg（8:00）、5 mg（12:00）、5 mg（18:00）。2~3 周后，患者需要基线检测（09:00 时皮质醇水平）和动态试验（如胰岛素或胰高血糖素应激试验）来确定是否需要长期类固醇替代。如果患者术前没有服用类固醇，可在术后几天内评估上午 9 点皮质醇水平，当上午 9 点皮质醇水平较低（即 <400 nmol/L）时，患者应行类固醇替代治疗。术后几个月后，也需要对患者皮质醇轴做进一步检验，因为随时间推移垂体功能可能恢复。术后长期类固醇替代的需求各不相同，大多数患者不需要。

术后高钠血症和低钠血症

高钠血症：尿崩（diabetes insipidus，DI）是引起术后高钠血症的最常见原因。诊断 DI 的典型生化标准是多尿（即尿量 >200 ml/h，持续 3 小时或以上），伴有高钠血症（即血清钠 >145 mmol/L）和血清渗透压增高并尿渗透压降低。垂体手术后立即出现的一过性 DI 很常见，对于经鼻入路手术的患者，这种一过性 DI 的发生率在 10%~30%。永久性 DI 很少见，发生在 0~7% 的病例中（Schreckinger et al.，2013）。DI 更常见于颅咽管瘤（尤其是术后）、神经结节病和垂体转移瘤的患者。

除了一过性和永久性 DI，还有一种少见的三相模式（占术后病例的 1%~3%）。包括一个 DI 急性期，在手术后最初几天出现，与 ADH 释放突然停止有关；随后退变的下丘脑核团引起 ADH 激增，通常出现在术后 1~2 周，导致低血钠（即抗利尿激素异常分泌综合征，syndrome of inappropriate ADH release，SIADH）。此阶段之后，由于 ADH 耗尽，又回到永久性 DI 阶段。

DI 的一线处理方法是补液（口服或静脉注射，视情况而定），并定期多次重复生化检验。根据治疗效果的不同，可能需要 DDAVP 替代治疗（静脉注射，口服或鼻腔喷雾剂）。在纠正血清钠水平时应相对平缓（即每天不超过 10 mmol/L）。

低钠血症：术后低钠血症是垂体手术少见并发症（10%~15% 的病例），发生原因可能有抗利尿激素分泌异常综合征（SIADH）或脑盐耗综合征（CSW）。因为它们的治疗方案差别很大，因此应将这两种疾病鉴别开来。垂体手术后，SIADH 比 CSW 更常见。它的特点是 ADH 分泌过多，导致水通过远端集合管在肾潴留。这会导致尿量减少、低钠血症和身体内水含量增加。

治疗是每天限制液体摄入在 500~750 ml 范围内，每 24 小时重复生化监测（或根据低钠血症的严重程度而更频繁），直到血清钠正常。一定要平缓纠正血钠（即每天血钠变化小于 10 mmol/L），以避免脑桥中央髓鞘溶解的风险。偶尔需应用地美环素，更少情况给予高渗盐水和（或）托伐普坦（一种血管加压素受体 2 拮抗剂，需密切监测）治疗。

垂体手术后 CSW 较少见，它更常见于颅脑损伤或蛛网膜下腔出血后。该病与肾尿液中钠的过度流失，血容量减少，尿钠含量升高有关。治疗方法是用盐片补充治疗（可能对胃有刺激作用），静脉注射生理盐水，和（或）使用氟氢可的松。

区分 SIADH 和 CSW 或有困难，最有用的鉴别要点是评估体液容量状态（如中心静脉压等）和对生理盐水补液的反应（即 SIADH 低钠会恶化但 CSW 低钠会改善）。

热点问题

残余肿瘤的处理

残余肿瘤的治疗方案取决于多种因素，因此，最好是在垂体多学科诊疗团队（MDT；图 25.17）的参与下，为患者制订个体化的医疗管理决策。

大多数患者在术后 4~6 个月进行 MRI 复查，以确保肿瘤腔的血液和其他止血材料被吸收。是否进一步手术、放疗或继续观察取决于 MR 扫描结果（如残余肿瘤的大小和侵袭性）和其他的一些因素，如组织学特征、持续存在的与肿瘤相关的症状（如视力障碍）、年龄、并发症、垂体功能、生育状态（是否想要生育）和患者意愿。

通常，有症状并且肿瘤相当大或逐步增长的患者，可经鼻或经颅入路进行二次手术。放射治疗和立体定向放射治疗对于控制难以切除的残余小肿瘤非常有效。早期放射治疗适用于已确定的垂体功能低下和有其它并发症的患者。年龄是放射治疗的另

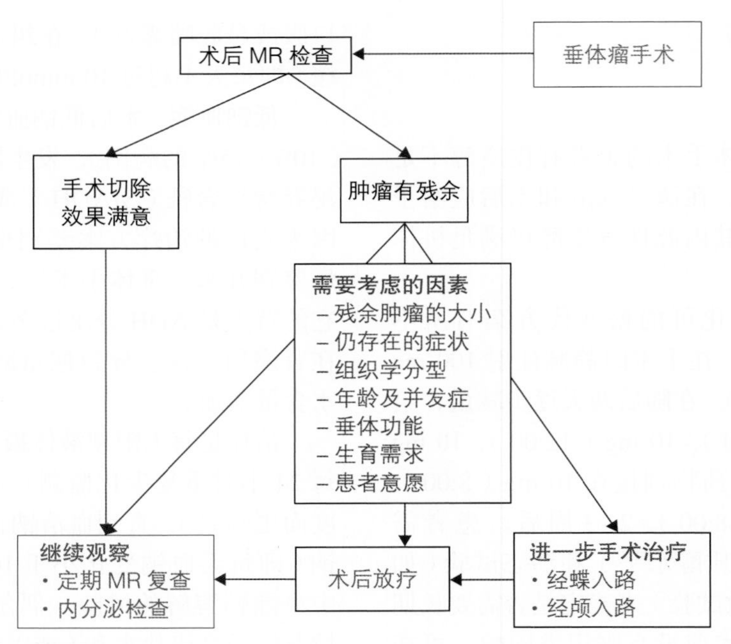

图 25.17 残余肿瘤的临床决策流程图

一个考虑因素，因为较年轻的患者更可能因为放疗而承受长期并发症（例如神经认知后遗症、继发性肿瘤等）。术后 MR 扫描上有可疑小肿瘤残留，但没有明显相关症状，可定期行 MR 复查（通常 1 年 1 次），确定后可在后期行手术干预，对于垂体功能相对完好的患者尤其如此。

偶发垂体瘤的治疗

随着 MR 检查的普及，更多的垂体瘤被偶然发现。在因垂体疾病以外的原因而接受颅脑影像学检查的成人中，MRI 发现偶发瘤的比例在 10%~38%，尽管只有不到 1% 的患者是大腺瘤（即最大直径 > 1 cm）。

一般建议意外发现垂体瘤的患者进行内分泌检查，包括评估垂体功能是否减退和激素是否分泌过多（Freda et al., 2011）。

垂体偶发瘤的治疗取决于多个因素，包括病变大小、内分泌状况、视力情况，还要考虑其他因素，如患者年龄、并发症和患者意愿。一般来说，对于造成视交叉压迫、病变已引起视力缺陷和（或）激素分泌异常的偶发瘤患者，应考虑手术，但催乳素瘤除外，通常可采取药物治疗方式（图 25.18；Freda et al., 2011）。

对于无相关症状的微腺瘤患者，可采取保守治疗。通常在前 3 年需要每年进行一次 MR 扫描，如果病变在影像学上保持稳定，则逐步增加扫描的时间间隔。如果在观察期间病变明显增大，可考虑手术。这种情况更可能发生在大腺瘤，一项近期研究显示 24% 的大腺瘤患者肿瘤会增加，尽管在所有偶发瘤，这种风险每年约为 8%（Freda et al., 2011）。选择保守治疗的患者也需知情病变仍存在较小的垂体卒中（约 2%）及引发视力障碍的潜在风险，这种情况需要紧急手术减压。

创伤性脑损伤（TBI）和动脉瘤性蛛网膜下腔出血（SAH）后垂体功能减退

近年来，对脑外伤或蛛网膜下腔出血后引起垂体功能减退的认识不断增加。据报道，脑外伤后垂体功能减退的发生率在 15%~68%（系统回顾中平均为 27.5%）（Agha et al., 2007；Schneider et al., 2007）。的确，一些特征性的垂体功能低下症状，如疲劳、情绪低落、注意力不集中和其他神经认知问题，经常被归因于脑损伤本身，因此垂体功能损害始终未被认识。据报道，外伤后出现的垂体激素分泌异常可涉及多种激素；最常受影响的是促性腺激素（13%）、生长激素（12%）和促肾上腺皮质激素（8%）。50%~70% 的病例可自行恢复。急性期 DI 可出现在约 20% 的病例和 7% 的长期存活者中。研究发现，颅脑损伤的严重程度可能是垂体功能低下的一个预测因素，重度、中度和轻度颅脑损伤垂体功能低下的发生率分别为 35%、11% 和 17%（Schneider et al., 2007）。

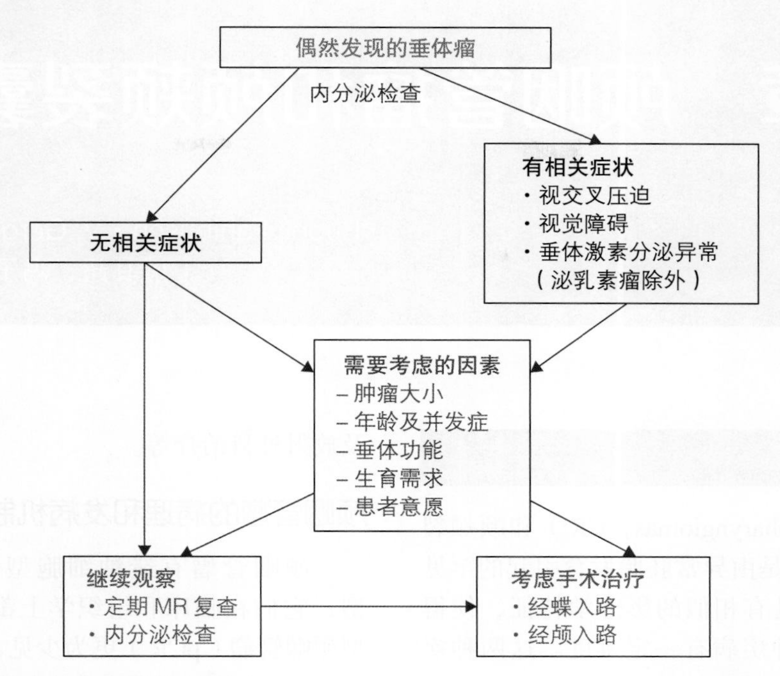

图 25.18　偶然发现的垂体瘤的临床决策流程图

关于蛛网膜下腔出血术后垂体功能减退的文献很少。SAH 后 38%~55% 的患者发生急性垂体功能障碍（系统回顾中平均为 47%），但该数据是基于多个相对例数较少的病例研究（Schneider et al.，2007）。最常受影响的激素是促性腺激素（25%）、生长激素（6%）和促肾上腺皮质激素（21%）。此外，对文献的系统回顾显示，随时间推移，损伤 6 个月后 26% 的患者垂体功能会逐渐恢复，只有 7% 在 14 个月后仍有垂体功能障碍（Schneider et al.，2007）。

了解脑外伤和蛛网膜下腔出血后引起垂体功能低下非常重要，因为一些临床症状（疲劳、神经精神症状）常被归因于原发疾病，而未想到是由于激素缺乏。补充缺乏的垂体激素对治疗神经认知症状的效果尚不明确，仍需进一步研究。

参考文献、EBRAIN 的相关链接

扫描书末二维码获取。

第26章　颅咽管瘤和颅颊裂囊肿

Rudolf Fahlbusch · V. Gerganov · H. Metwali 著
戚其超、冯子超 译，倪石磊 审校

引言

颅咽管瘤（craniopharyngiomas，CR）和颅颊裂囊肿（拉特克囊肿）都是由异常胚胎发育引起的罕见垂体病变。有时它们具有相似的影像学特征，使得在影像学上鉴别这两种疾病有一定难度。这两种疾病，尤其是颅咽管瘤的外科治疗颇具挑战性。

颅咽管瘤完全切除可提高无复发生存率，但同时也伴随术后并发症及垂体功能不全的风险增加。在大多数情况下，颅咽管瘤被认为是一种“慢性疾病”。这两种疾病外科治疗原则的主要区别在于，对于颅咽管瘤而言，必须切除增厚的囊壁以实现肿瘤全切，而拉特克囊肿几乎不可能也不建议尝试囊壁完全切除。对大多数拉特克囊肿患者来说，清除囊肿内容物通常足以达到治愈效果。与颅咽管瘤相比，拉特克囊肿很少复发。

颅咽管瘤

颅咽管瘤的发病率相对较低，其人群发病率约为0.13人（10万人·年）。据统计，美国每年新增颅咽管瘤340例（Bunin et al.，1997）。其发病年龄分布表现为双峰模式，第一个高峰出现在5~14岁的儿童，第二个高峰出现在50~60岁的成人（Nielsen et al.，2011）。颅咽管瘤占儿童原发性脑肿瘤的5%~10%（Hussain et al.，2013）。颅咽管瘤非常罕见，根据已报道的病例系列，即使是“该领域专家”每年也仅有6~10个新患者。

颅咽管瘤在组织病理学上属于颅内良性肿瘤，但可能会与邻近结构包括垂体柄、灰结节或下丘脑等紧密粘连，这使得完全切除肿瘤具有挑战性。然而近期许多研究证实，在大多数情况下手术切除是可行的且不会导致严重的并发症。其他治疗措施主要包括非根治性手术切除后分割放疗、囊内容物吸除及Ommaya囊植入术、腔内放疗或化疗药物灌洗及放射外科治疗等。

颅咽管瘤的病理和发病机制

颅咽管瘤有造釉细胞型和乳头型两种主要亚型，它们在临床和组织学上都有所不同。其中乳头型颅咽管瘤（pCR）更为少见，仅占所有颅咽管瘤的11%~14%，主要见于成人。乳头型颅咽管瘤目前被认为是由垂体前叶或垂体柄上皮细胞化生形成的（**图26.1**）。造釉细胞型颅咽管瘤（aCR）可出现于任何年龄，但主要见于儿童。造釉细胞型颅咽管瘤是由拉特克囊发育过程中异位胚胎残留的肿瘤样转化引起。造釉细胞型颅咽管瘤与一些牙源性肿瘤类似，这表明其有共同的胚胎起源。造釉细胞型颅咽管瘤大体病理通常为小叶状，边缘尖锐不规则，常黏附于周围结构并具有侵袭性。组织学上由成熟的鳞状上皮和假乳头组成（**图26.1**）。造釉细胞型颅咽管瘤有实性或囊性成分。囊性内容物通常是黏稠的，颜色可为黄色、深棕色或黑色（“机油样”外观），颜色的不同反映了胆固醇晶体含量的不同。与之相反，乳头型颅咽管瘤通常外覆包膜，实性成分为主，与周围邻近结构无粘连。如果存在囊性成分，则囊内液体是清亮的（Crotty et al.，1995；Shin et al.，1999；Larkin and Ansorge，2013）。

除临床及组织病理学上的差异外，目前认为这两种亚型还具有不同的遗传来源。颅咽管瘤的发生是由单个已确定的癌基因突变驱动，与年龄无关；这些癌基因是造釉细胞型中的连环蛋白β-1基因（CTNNB1）和乳头型中的BRAF基因，两者均为克隆性突变。除这两种突变外，在这两种亚型中均未检测到其他的频发突变或基因畸变（Brastianos et al.，2014）。

近年来，颅咽管瘤的发病、进展及复发的分子机制得到广泛研究。随着比较基因组杂交技术、基因测序技术及靶向基因分型技术等分子生物学技术的发展及基因工程动物模型的不断开发，颅咽管瘤

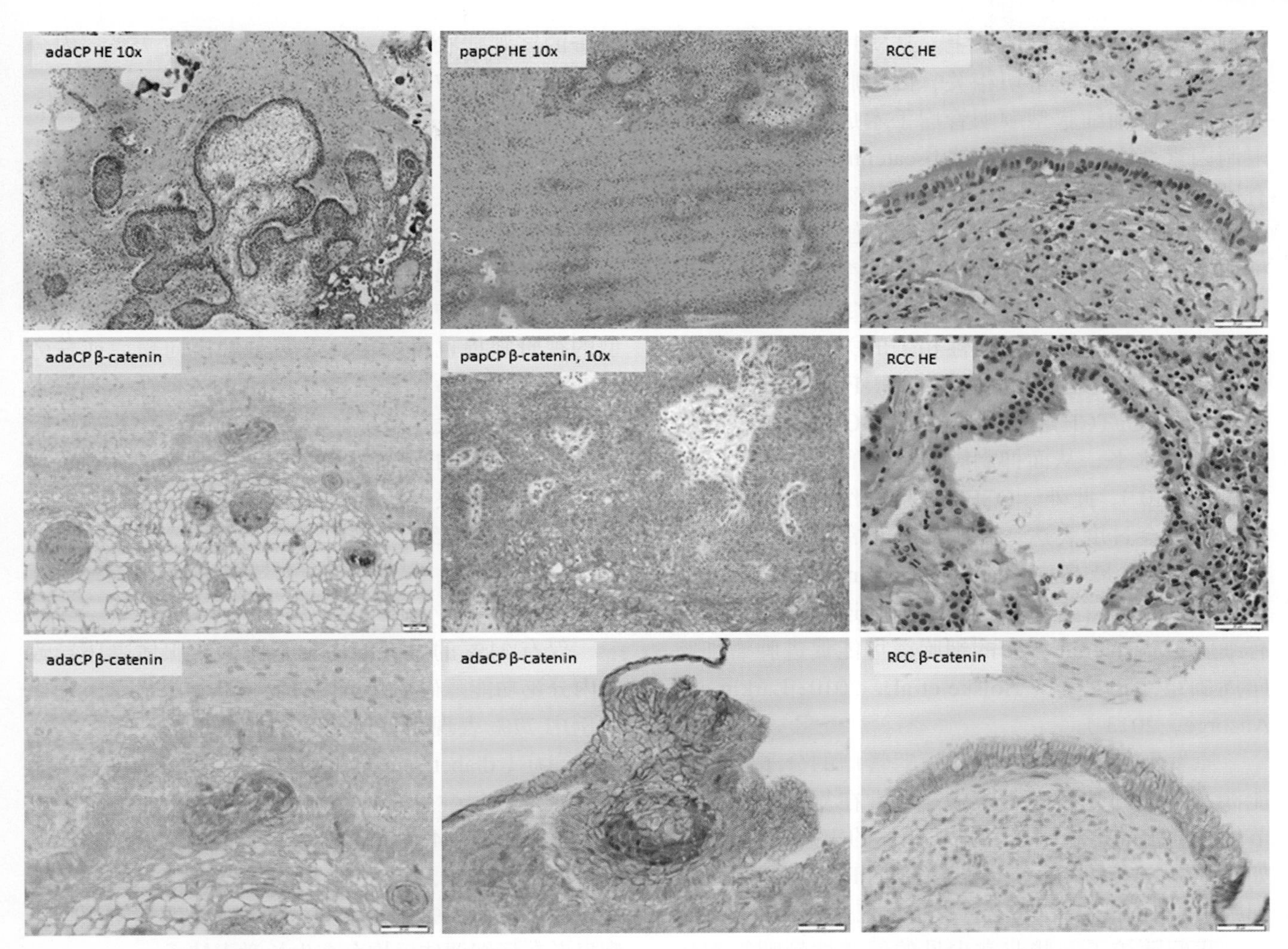

图 26.1　左侧一列显示了造釉细胞型颅咽管瘤的组织学特征，上方切片是为 HE 染色，中间切片和下方切片是采用 β-catenin 染色。中间列上方两图显示了乳头型颅咽管瘤的组织学特征，其中上方切片为 HE 染色，中间切片为 β-catenin 染色。中间列下方切片显示了造釉细胞型颅咽管瘤与脑组织的 β-catenin 染色。右侧列图片显示了拉特克囊肿的组织学特征，上方切片和中间切片显示了部分假复层柱状上皮，下方切片显示拉特克囊肿不被 β-catenin 染色，有助于将其与颅咽管瘤鉴别

Courtesy of Dr Kieren Allinson, Department of Pathology, Addenbrooke's Hospital, Cambridge.

一些致病机制已经被阐明。

造釉细胞型颅咽管瘤致病的分子水平异常或驱动因素主要与 Wnt/β-catenin 信号通路密切相关。该信号通路在脊椎动物胚胎发生时神经管发育形成背腹侧轴的过程中发挥重要作用。但在乳头型颅咽管瘤中并未发现 β-catenin 突变（Crotty et al.，1995；Prabhu and Brown，2005；Holsken et al.，2009；Larkin and Ansorge，2013）。

3 号染色体上 β-catenin 基因的 CTNNB1 突变和 β-catenin 表达的异常也与其他癌症的发生密切相关，如结直肠癌、肝细胞癌和髓母细胞瘤等（Hussain et al.，2013）。

约 70% 的造釉细胞型颅咽管瘤可发现 CTNNB1 突变。而新近研究证实，几乎在所有造釉细胞型颅咽管瘤中均存在 CTNNB1 突变，在采用全外显子组测序时 CTNNB1 突变的阳性率为 92%，应用靶向基因分型时为 96%（Brastianos et al.，2014）。

CTNNB1 突变导致 β-catenin 蛋白结构稳定，引起 Wnt 信号通路处于持续性激活状态（Holsken et al.，2009；Holsken et al.，2010；Larkin and Ansorge，2013）。大多数 CTNNB1 突变发生在 3 号外显子上（Sekine et al.，2002）。基因工程动物模型实验已证实 Wnt/β-catenin 通路在颅咽管瘤发病机制中的重要作用。仍有一些未发现 CTNNB1 突变的造釉细胞型颅咽管瘤，其发病机制尚不确定。但很可能与 Wnt 通路激活相关。

随着对颅咽管瘤发病机制的研究进展，近年来很多研究主要集中在肿瘤行为的潜在分子机制及与

周围邻近结构的解剖关系上。从实用神经外科的角度来看，这些问题密切相关，因为肿瘤对邻近结构的侵犯是造釉细胞型颅咽管瘤手术成功切除的重要限制因素。有趣的是，虽然β-catenin突变存在于所有肿瘤细胞中，但细胞核β-catenin突变仅在造釉细胞型颅咽管瘤浸润边缘的一小簇细胞中发现。因此，推测Wnt信号通路通过β-catenin突变而激活参与造釉细胞型颅咽管瘤的肿瘤迁移行为。此外，造釉细胞型颅咽管瘤中与细胞移动性相关的关键细胞骨架蛋白fascin（FSCN1）的浓度也升高。FSCN1的表达与Wnt/β-catenin/TCF通路有关。下调CTNBB1可降低FSCN1的水平，从而抑制肿瘤细胞的迁移（Holsken et al.，2010）。此外，EGFR在造釉细胞型颅咽管瘤细胞中也会过度表达，在肿瘤与正常脑组织之间的浸润区表达最高。β-catenin、fascin和EGFR在造釉细胞型颅咽管瘤中参与肿瘤细胞迁移行为，提示有细胞核β-catenin突变的细胞簇可能促进肿瘤细胞向周围组织的浸润（Holske et al.，2010；Larkin and Ansorge，2013）。

原发和复发造釉细胞型颅咽管瘤的分子机制可能涉及不同的基因表达模式。通常在复发肿瘤中调节细胞增殖的生长因子和相关受体的表达均会上调，如血小板源性生长因子受体a（PDGFR-a）及成纤维细胞生长因子-2（FGF-2）（Sun et al.，2010）。

我们随访了一些非常少见的侵袭性颅咽管瘤病例，有很高的的复发倾向。其中一名年轻的12岁女性患者，因颅咽管瘤复发在一年内数次手术。最终肿瘤已经浸润到整个鞍上区、鞍旁区以及基底节，增殖率很高（MiB 20%）。患者在13岁时去世，也是在最后一次手术加放疗6个月之后。

乳头型颅咽管瘤发病的分子机制最近才被阐明（Brastianos et al.，2014）。通过全外显子组测序技术，在所有乳头型颅咽管瘤中均检测到BRAF（V600E）频发突变；通过靶向基因分型技术，95%的肿瘤可检测到此种突变。

充分理解颅咽管瘤发病的分子机制对颅咽管瘤的诊断具有重要意义，并可能为将来的分子靶向药物治疗提供靶点。

临床表现

根据资深专家的文献报道，在1983—2005年期间的291例（83%成人，17%儿童）手术患者中，47%表现为视力损害，31%表现为内分泌激素缺乏，17%表现为脑积水和头痛，5%表现为神经功能障碍。检查的客观症状表现为视交叉综合征占75%，内分泌功能障碍占77%。尿崩症发生率为30%。

成人

视力障碍

根据肿瘤位置和侵犯范围不同，颅咽管瘤可引起不同类型的视野缺损。典型的双眼颞侧偏盲是由于鞍内或鞍上肿瘤从下方压迫视交叉引起。其他类型的视野缺损也可发生，尤其是肿瘤向鞍后或鞍旁进展时。约47%的患者在就诊时自述存在主观视觉症状，但眼科检查结果显示75%的患者存在视力障碍。40%~70%的患者在就诊时可发现视神经通路功能障碍。视野缺损后常伴随视力下降，进展到晚期则引起视神经萎缩。

内分泌表现

仅有31%的患者会出现垂体柄或腺体受压导致的内分泌功能障碍症状。内分泌检验结果显示，确诊病例中77%表现为垂体前叶功能减退症，30%表现有尿崩症（diabetes insipidus，DI）。近80%患者自述性欲减退，男性患者中约90%有阳痿，而绝大多数女性出现闭经。40%的患者在就诊时存在甲状腺功能减退的相关症状，25%的患者出现肾上腺功能不全的症状和体征，20%的患者有尿崩症。几乎所有颅咽管瘤患者在仔细评估后均存在生长激素缺乏。

下丘脑自主神经功能表现

颅咽管瘤患者也可出现睡眠-觉醒节律改变、肥胖、电解质紊乱和体温调节异常。但是目前尚缺乏定义自主神经功能障碍的客观标准。此外，由下丘脑引起的垂体功能障碍也可表现为内分泌紊乱（三级垂体功能不全）。

神经系统相关表现

颅咽管瘤的首发症状多为头痛。通常发生在前额，晨起时较重。尤其是在较小的颅咽管瘤中，头痛可能是手术治疗的唯一指征。头痛的原因也可能是由体积较大的肿瘤压迫室间孔或导水管所致的脑积水引起。

动眼神经麻痹常见于肿瘤向鞍旁生长压迫动眼神经。听力减退及三叉神经症状多见于向桥小脑角生长的肿瘤。癫痫多见于压迫颞叶内侧的鞍旁颅咽管瘤，肿瘤压迫穹隆则会引起短期记忆缺陷。

儿童的特殊临床表现

视觉障碍

儿童的视觉障碍通常很晚才被发现。即使已经存在明显的视力减退，可能也无自觉症状，但这种视力障碍在20%~60%的儿童颅咽管瘤患者中存在。视力障碍的具体表现取决于肿瘤对视觉通路的侵犯情况。眼底检查显示20%的颅咽管瘤病例存在视盘水肿（Poretti et al.，2004；Yosef et al.，2015）。

内分泌表现

因生长激素缺乏而引起的身材矮小和因促性腺激素缺乏而引起的青春期延迟是儿童颅咽管瘤患者的常见临床表现。也可表现为促肾上腺皮质激素缺乏或甲状腺功能减退的症状（Poretti et al.，2004；Halac and Zimmerman，2005）。肥胖性生殖无能综合征（弗勒赫利希综合征）表现为性腺功能减退和肥胖，这是由下丘脑性垂体功能减退引起。

儿童颅咽管瘤患者也可表现为尿崩症，而渴感缺乏。这种情况非常危险，因为损失过量液体的同时却无充足补充。

自主神经症状

主要是下丘脑功能不全的表现，如肥胖、睡眠节律改变、电解质紊乱和内分泌功能障碍等。

影像学表现

主要的影像学诊断方法是磁共振平扫和（或）增强。MRI可评估肿瘤生长的范围及其与神经血管的关系。评估时应注意视神经和视交叉的解剖特点、颈内动脉的长度、前交通动脉的位置、第三脑室底以及肿瘤是否真性突破进入脑室内。

CT可用于发现钙化，这是颅咽管瘤一个典型的影像学标志。CT扫描对于确定颅底骨质的解剖结构也是至关重要的，尤其是计划行颅底入路手术治疗时。此外，CT也是脑积水引起急性意识障碍时的急诊诊断方法。

分类

颅咽管瘤有多种分类系统（Yasargil et al.，1990），以下是常用的分类方法。

根据肿瘤的生长位置，颅咽管瘤可分为鞍上型和鞍内型；根据肿瘤与鞍膈的关系，颅咽管瘤也可分为膈上型和膈下型；此外，肿瘤可位于视交叉的前方或后方，也可抬高第三脑室的底部，甚至某些情况下会突破脑室生长即存在脑室内成分。肿瘤可向各个方向延伸，主要是侵及外侧的鞍旁区或后方的鞍后间隙。此外我们也发现有异位生长的颅咽管瘤（如桥小脑角、蝶窦或咽部等）。

形态学上，颅咽管瘤通常为囊实性，较少有纯实性或纯囊性，肿瘤的实性钙化也很常见。

术前评估

术前必须对垂体前叶进行全面的内分泌功能评估，包括T3、T4、TSH、LH、FSH、睾酮或雌激素、促肾上腺皮质激素、皮质醇、催乳素、生长激素和IGF-1，并应行动态测定。视力评估应包括视敏度、视野及眼底检查。这些评估对于后续治疗和作为随访的基线参考至关重要。

治疗

颅咽管瘤患者手术的方式及时机取决于许多因素，包括肿瘤相关因素（肿瘤大小、生长范围、粘连或对邻近重要结构的侵犯）和患者自身因素（年龄及内分泌功能状况）（图26.2）。某些情况下需尽快手术，而在其他情况下保守治疗或放射治疗可能会更佳。

对症治疗

合并脑积水的患者可行脑室-腹腔分流术，此外肿瘤切除时可同时行囊腔脑室分流术或更少用到的囊腔腹腔分流术。有根治术禁忌或进行性视交叉综合征的患者若存在严重的自主神经症状适合行减瘤术，必要时可行放疗。

外科干预的指征

手术指征在于减轻垂体受压并保留其内分泌功能，以及解除肿瘤对视交叉或视神经及动眼神经的压迫。脑积水是手术治疗的绝对适应证。

根治性切除的禁忌证

术前评估时禁忌证主要包括严重瘤周水肿和双侧下丘脑浸润。伴有不可逆的下丘脑功能障碍的患者表现为极度肥胖或睡眠/清醒节律改变，影像学表现为严重下丘脑受压或肿瘤周围水肿。对于这些患者，我们推荐使用地塞米松治疗以确定下丘脑功能紊乱是否可逆。若下丘脑功能恢复，则可考虑手术治疗；如果其功能障碍不可逆，则仅建议对症治疗（见下文）。

手术中的主要限制因素包括严重的肿瘤钙化、

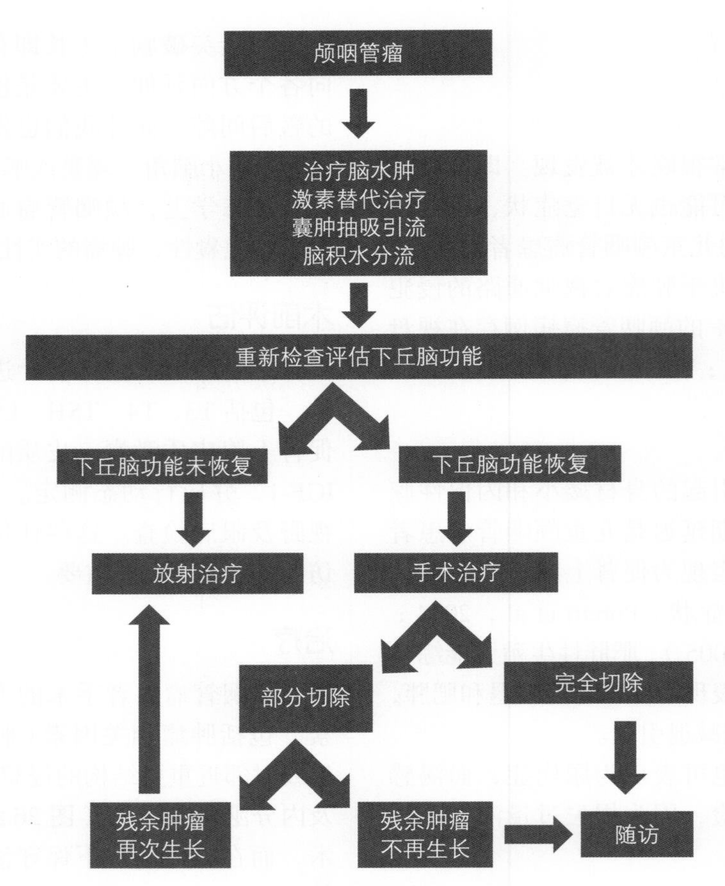

图 26.2 颅咽管瘤的治疗流程图

肿瘤附着于下丘脑或小穿支血管以及术中反复出现的心动过缓等。

外科治疗

颅咽管瘤的手术治疗理念自 1982 年以来不断发展，但始终以安全和根治性切除为目标。在 1982—1996 年的初始阶段，共有 168 例患者接受手术，经颅手术的患者中有 45.7% 实现肿瘤全切，而经鼻蝶手术的患者中有 85.7% 实现肿瘤全切。未完全切除的主要原因是下丘脑黏附或浸润、肿瘤主体钙化及血管附着（Fahlbusch et al.，1999）。在 1996 年至 2005 年间，由于技术进步，颅咽管瘤手术安全且根治性切除的比例提高，经鼻蝶手术的全切率达到 88.5%，经颅手术的全切率达到 79.5%（Fahlbusch and Hofmann，2008）。

作者自 2005 年起采用个性化治疗理念。患者筛选和治疗方案主要取决于患者的临床情况，特别是内分泌功能和自主神经功能状态。

临床病例

一位巨大囊性颅咽管瘤男性患者，自述存在短期记忆缺陷，但无内分泌功能及视觉障碍。在给予囊腔 - 脑室分流术后随访，记忆障碍较前明显改善，并不需要根治性手术。

一位囊性颅咽管瘤女性患者，因其有生育需求，因此先行囊腔 - 脑室分流术，在她成功怀孕和生育后再行根治性肿瘤切除手术。

一名最初被误诊为大麻性精神错乱的 18 岁男性，影像学检查显示一个较大囊性颅咽管瘤继发严重脑积水。考虑到他严重的认知障碍，决定先行脑室 - 腹腔分流术，随后置入囊肿腹膜分流装置。只有在他的认知功能改善后，我们再行根治性肿瘤切除。

手术治疗注意事项

Hoffmann 等（1992）和 Yasargil 等（1990）最先报道了颅咽管瘤的根治性手术切除。随后，陆续完成了通过多种入路进行颅咽管瘤全切手术，其中完全切除巨大颅咽管瘤极具挑战，出现了多种改良或联合手术入路用于切除此类颅咽管瘤，其安全并全切除肿瘤的前提是充分暴露肿瘤的各个部分。

经额外侧小骨窗开颅切除颅咽管瘤的第一个先决条件是，缓慢生长的肿瘤引起神经血管结构的持续性稳定性移位，从而提供一个潜在的且足够大的切除通道。重要的是，这些经过视交叉下方、视神经 - 颈内动脉、颈内动脉 - 动眼神经和经终板的手术通道在肿瘤切除过程之中及之后能够或多或少地保持稳定。肿瘤床在肿瘤切除开始后不会坍塌并保持开放以暴露深部肿瘤，这也是该入路手术的优势。最开始该入路是在一侧额部行开颅手术，随着手术骨窗逐步缩小，发展为目前的额外侧入路。其主要目的是保护额叶，因为在肿瘤体积较大时额叶尤其脆弱。此外，大骨窗开颅并没有提高我们切除深部病灶的能力，只要达到充分的瘤内减压，即可通过轻微牵拉使得周边肿瘤的部分进入视野。

任何手术入路的第二个要求便是手术入路相关并发症的风险不应很高。额外侧入路即符合这一要求，即使是那些主要向鞍上区域发展而在鞍内几乎没有的巨大颅咽管瘤（图 26.3），我们也倾向采用该入路。部分颅咽管瘤即使体积较大也可由经鼻蝶显微镜、内镜或联合入路成功切除。

脑室内颅咽管瘤可经大脑半球间经终板入路或经胼胝体入路切除。经胼胝体入路局限于脑室和中线，不能切除存在鞍旁受累的颅咽管瘤；经大脑半球间终板入路既可暴露肿瘤脑室内部分，也可暴露部分鞍旁肿瘤。

肿瘤的鞍旁侵犯程度会影响手术入路侧别的选择。位于床突上段颈内动脉和后交通动脉及其穿支外侧的鞍旁部分需要经同侧颈内动脉 - 动眼神经间隙进入。因此存在肿瘤鞍旁侵犯的情况下，应在患侧开颅。

对于存在视交叉前置或肿瘤向斜坡后生长的病例，一些学者描述了经岩骨入路从下到上、从后到前地显露肿瘤。

应特别注意穹隆的走向和位置，尤其是侵犯第三脑室的肿瘤（图 26.4）。

常用手术入路的详细介绍

经蝶入路

经典的经蝶入路适用于所有鞍膈下颅咽管瘤包括鞍内型和鞍上型（图 26.5）。对于鞍膈上肿瘤可应

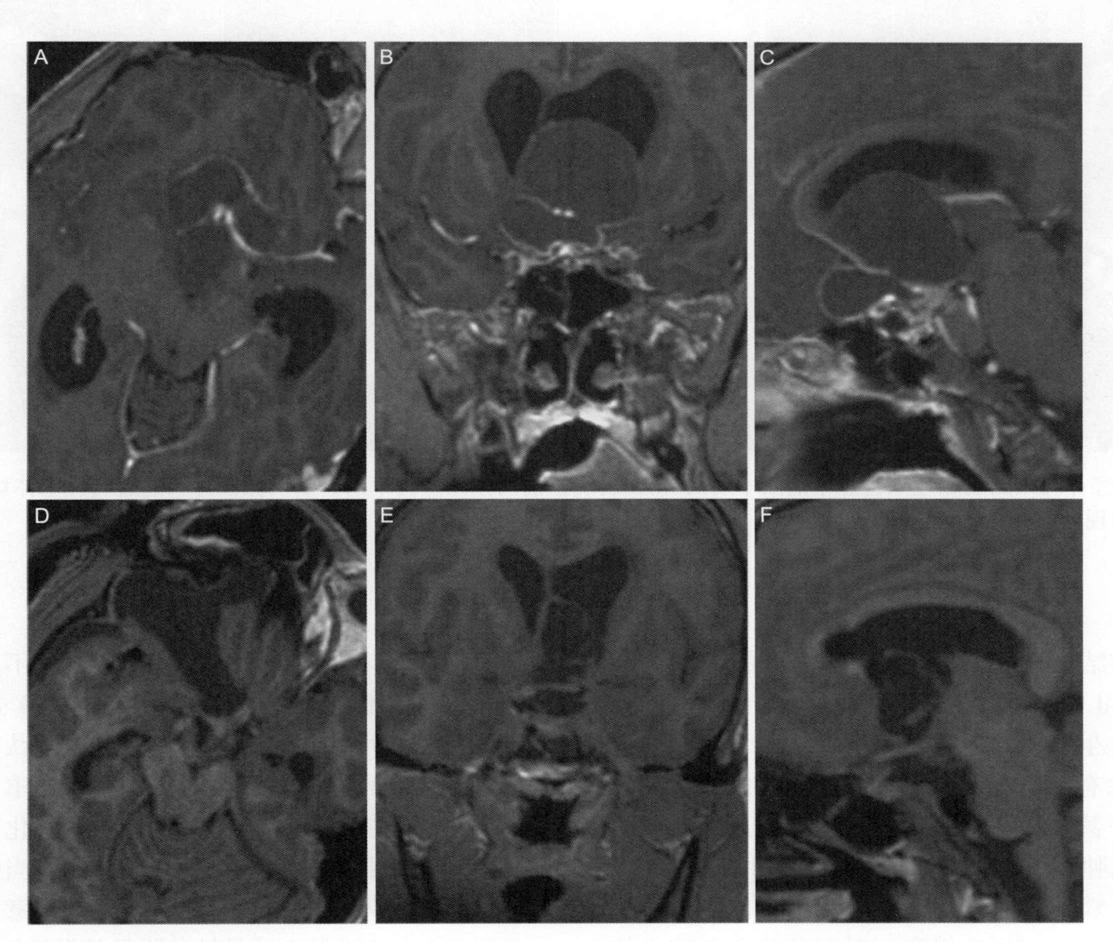

图 26.3　额外侧入路开颅切除大颅咽管癌术前及术后 MR 表现，应用术中 MRI 对患者进行手术

Source data from Gerganov, et al. *J Neurosurg*. 2014 Feb; 120(2): 559–70.

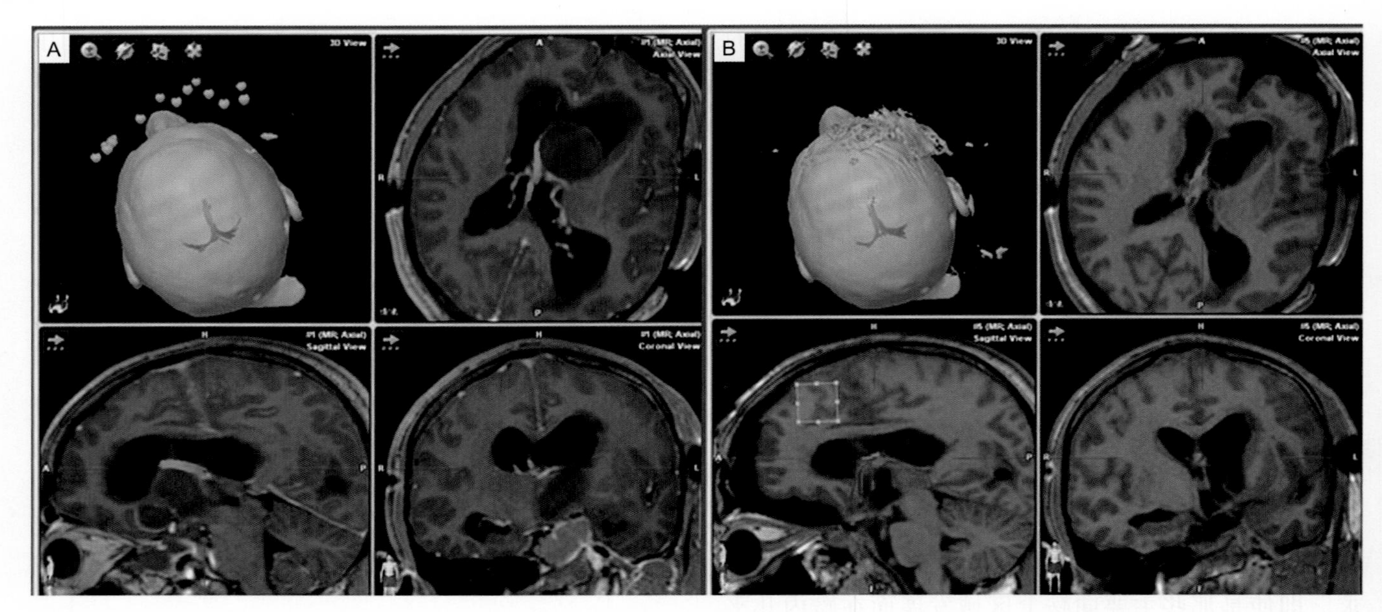

图 26.4 对穹隆进行导航定位，特别是肿瘤在第三脑室中、存在较大的脑室内成分时的纤维束成像。A 为穹隆术前影像，B 为额外侧开颅切除颅咽管瘤保留完好的穹隆影像

Source data from Gerganov, et al. *J Neurosurg*. 2014 Feb; 120(2): 559–70.

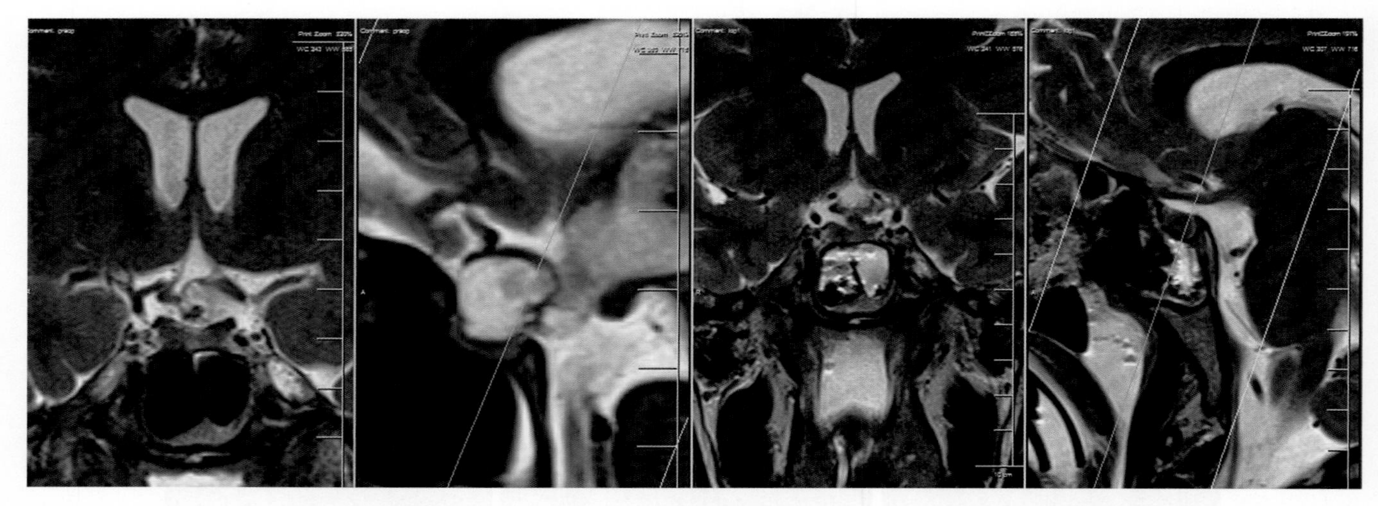

图 26.5 经鼻蝶入路切除颅咽管癌术前及术后的 MRI 表现，前两张图片为术前，后两张图片为通过切开垂体切除肿瘤术后 MRI 表现

用切除鞍结节（经鞍结节）的扩大经蝶入路（最初由 Weiss et al. 发表）。但是其局限性在于当肿瘤向蛛网膜间隙外生长或与周围脑结构关系密切时，安全地完全切除有一定难度；对于主要在鞍内而鞍膈上较小侵犯、甚至鞍上型颅咽管瘤，可通过切开鞍膈以完全切除肿瘤（资深术者的经验）。

经鼻蝶入路通常是在显微镜下、内镜下或显微镜内镜联合应用抵达蝶窦。对于鼻腔开口较小的儿童首选唇下切口，肿瘤偏外侧时，少数情况下会联合经上颌窦入路。当蝶窦未气化或气化不充分抑或是蝶鞍结构不可见时（小于 3~4 岁的儿童），神经导航或 C 形臂可提供帮助。虽然有些学者认为这种情况是经鼻蝶入路的禁忌证，但经验足够丰富的垂体外科医生仍能够安全地磨开鞍底。在气化充分的鼻窦中颈内动脉隆起有定位中线的作用。当蝶窦内的骨性分隔嵌入颈内动脉隆起时要特别注意，因为这些覆盖在颈内动脉上的骨性分隔是其保护屏障。

正常蝶鞍大小约为 10 mm × 6 mm × 8 mm，磨

钻磨除鞍底骨质至最大范围后，由中线向两侧剪开硬脑膜至海绵窦内侧壁，后方到达后海绵间窦，前方至与鞍膈的连接处。半数病例的正常垂体位于前方（不同于垂体腺瘤）。在这种情况下，鞍膈需切开1 mm甚至更多才能暴露出较厚的颅咽管瘤囊壁。

肿瘤内容物无论是囊性、实性抑或钙化均应首先从蝶鞍内各肿瘤部分开始切除，术者应从中线或外侧开始，然后移向鞍上区域，以期抬高的鞍膈有所下降。

切除增厚的肿瘤包膜虽然费时且有挑战性，但为了防止复发必须将其切除（这与拉特克囊肿的薄壁不同）。建议首先切除易辨认的肿瘤壁，然后沿鞍膈下方由前向后、由内向外分离后方解剖结构。垂体柄通常可保留。有时质硬的肿瘤部分必须在其垂体柄的起源位置锐性切除，如果有残留肿瘤不能完全切除，可选择应用双极仔细电凝。

在一些病例中，若要实现肿瘤全切，脑脊液（CSF）鼻漏难以避免。脑脊液漏的位置多位于较薄的前方鞍膈，可从上肢或腹部取小块脂肪修补漏口，用纤维蛋白胶封闭。有些医生倾向采用更复杂的鞍底重建方式。扩大经鞍结节入路的所有患者均会有脑脊液漏，这也是这种入路的主要缺点和术中需解决问题，尽管最近有经验的内镜外科医生报道使用黏膜瓣覆盖可明显改善这一现状，但仍有多达一半的患者需行二次手术。

额外侧入路

视神经较长和视交叉后置病例的肿瘤切除

在这种情况下，视交叉通常移位到后上方，为视交叉下方和前方区域提供了一个较大的操作空间。外科医生可逐步进行肿瘤内减压。首先将对侧视神经的内侧面与肿瘤分离，注意保护视神经表面的小血管。随后切除肿瘤鞍上区域的中央部分，并使对侧视神经下方的肿瘤进入手术视野。将对侧视神经下部的肿瘤逐步减压并与视神经下表面、颈内动脉（ICA）和后交通动脉分离。切除视神经下部肿瘤后可见对侧动眼神经进入动眼神经三角。将显微镜移至中央视野径路可观察鞍后区域。由于该区域通常存在完好的Liliequist膜，肿瘤可相对容易地从基底动脉及其分支上分离。Liliequist膜被肿瘤拉伸，将位于脑桥前或桥小脑角池的肿瘤下垂部分与临近结构相隔离，尽管这种情况在以前的手术病例中并不明显。

通常不能直接看到同侧视神经下部肿瘤，该部分肿瘤可通过颈动脉膜内侧切口打开颈动脉池，利用同侧视神经和颈动脉之间的空间（视神经颈内动脉三角）切除肿瘤。

视神经较短和视交叉前置病例的肿瘤切除

在这些病例中，视交叉前方和下方空间非常狭窄，无法暴露鞍上区域的肿瘤部分。在这种情况下，需在终板池中进一步解剖蛛网膜。暴露双侧A1和A2，将A1与双侧视神经和视交叉分离，并保持其与额叶紧贴，以减少穿支动脉的损伤风险。大脑前动脉复合体随额叶抬起，显露出终板。为切除肿瘤的脑室内部分，在中线处打开终板，需牢记肿瘤与视交叉及走向下丘脑的大脑前动脉和前交通动脉分支的关系。

垂体柄周围手术

只有在垂体柄被广泛侵犯时，为了根治肿瘤而切除垂体柄才是合理的。在肿瘤侵犯垂体柄较轻时，可尝试行垂体柄部分切除（其直径的1/3至1/2）来保持其连续性和血液供应。打开视神经管顶部并切除鞍结节外侧部分后将视神经内移可更好地暴露垂体柄。

鞍旁部分的切除

肿瘤突向颈内动脉和后交通动脉外侧的部分可通过切开颈内动脉膜、分离钩回和颈内动脉来切除。切除这部分肿瘤时应考虑脉络膜前动脉的走行。

囊内容物吸除

囊内容物吸除是一种可暂时缓解周围结构受机械压迫之相关症状的治疗方法。由于囊肿往往会再次复发，一种可行的方法是在囊肿中放置Ommaya或Rickham储液器，这样就可实现重复囊肿抽吸。为使引流导管到达最佳位置，应用导航控制很有帮助。囊肿抽吸引流适用于一般情况较差患者的暂时处理或复发囊性颅咽管瘤不适合手术切除的患者。

儿童颅咽管瘤

长期患病儿童的生活质量常会受影响，主要是因为内分泌紊乱、代谢失衡和视力障碍。由内分泌科医生发表的一组病例中，不同经验水平外科医生完成的根治性切除使近50%长期生存患者的生活质量降低（Muller，2013）。尤其成问题的是青春期发育和整体生长发育以及病态下丘脑性肥胖。有些作者认为由于手术可引起下丘脑损害且即使是全切术后复发率也很高，所以儿童不应尝试根治性切除。

对于学步年龄以上的儿童患者，应尝试完全切除并保留所有功能以减少复发风险。延长治疗前的观察时间可使有些儿童早期获益。对于囊性大颅咽管瘤且临床情况较差或年龄很小的儿童患者，经囊内导管引流或植入 Ommaya 储液器可能是一种有价值的治疗措施。随着患者生长发育，该治疗方式可不断减压并改善症状。对于囊肿体积较大引起占位效应的患者，囊肿引流减压后尽早行肿瘤切除的分期手术方式也是一种可供选择的治疗策略（Fahlbusch et al.，1999）。

对于学步期儿童患者以及肿瘤生长侵犯重要结构如下丘脑时，有计划的部分切除可能是最佳的临时治疗选择，如果肿瘤还在生长，则可在患儿成熟后再行治疗。尽管成人和儿童行肿瘤次全切除后辅以术后放疗均可获益，但应用于低龄患者时应极其谨慎。目前一项多国家参与的随机试验正在调查次全切除辅以放疗的预后情况（Muller，2013）。

手术治疗情况及护理

激素

术后激素评估为必需的。术前皮质醇不足的患者应在术中及术后早期接受大剂量氢化可的松治疗。随后减少到正常的每日维持剂量。基础激素状况评估通常在术后 6~10 天后进行。如果存在激素缺乏，应予以补充。要特别关注儿童和青少年激素状况，以支持正常的生长发育和青春期（Honegger et al.，1999）。

在作者经蝶入路手术行安全切除的第一组病例中，有 10% 表现出继发性甲状腺功能减退，也有 10% 存在促肾上腺皮质激素缺乏。在采用相同理念经蝶入路手术的患者中，20% 有继发性甲状腺功能减退，40% 有促肾上腺皮质激素缺乏。在积极的手术切除组中，新发内分泌缺陷比例更高。约 20% 有继发性腺功能减退，30% 有继发甲状腺功能减退，60% 有肾上腺功能减退。内分泌功能障碍的发生率在经蝶入路治疗的病例中要更少一些。

电解质

颅咽管瘤切除术后患者更易发生尿崩症，从而导致电解质紊乱。尿崩症发生率从术前的 16% 增加到术后的 59.4%（在积极手术切除的情况下高达 70%）。尿崩症一般在术后早期出现，或在术后 5~7 天延迟出现。尿崩症的特点是多饮、多尿和高钠血症。意识清醒的患者可通过饮用液体补偿多尿损失的液体，从而使血钠水平保持在正常范围内。意识不清或者不能自主喝水的患者，其治疗更加困难。尿崩症通常用去氨加压素治疗。我们一般根据尿量、尿比重和钠含量来判断是否需要开始使用去氨加压素治疗。使用去氨加压素后，缓慢调整其剂量至所需的最后固定剂量。有些患者仅为短暂的尿崩症，可在 1~2 周内恢复。我们倾向于主要在晚上给予患者去氨加压素，在白天非必需不用，这样可使患者有无间歇的连续睡眠。

少数情况下，有些患者会在术后出现低钠血症。若此类患者皮质醇水平正常或替代充分，则应对患者进行液体限制。有些患者可能需要临时的静脉补钠。如果低钠血症持续存在，可给予氟可的松甚至托伐普坦（抗利尿激素拮抗剂）治疗（Ichimura et al.，2015）。纠正低钠要缓慢而避免波动。血钠水平波动可引起脑水肿和桥脑髓鞘溶解。

视力

术后要检查视力和视野。文献报道经颅手术后，大约 1/3 患者的视交叉综合征完全消退，另外 1/3 的患者视力部分恢复。14.7% 的患者在经颅手术后视力下降。而经蝶入路手术后，46.7% 的患者交叉综合征完全消退，另外 40% 的患者视力部分恢复。术后没有患者出现视力恶化（Fahlbusch et al.，1999）。

认知功能

由于肿瘤对穹隆的压迫，认知功能障碍在术前和术后都可出现。部分患者术后出现好转（5/8）。这些患者在认知驱动力减少（2/4）、注意力丧失（2/2）、昼夜节律消失（2/2）和注意力持续时间减少（1/1）方面有改善。在我们的手术病例中，没有出现认知功能恶化的病例，但手术后儿童的认知发育和学业表现可能会下降（Honegger et al.，1998）。

切除程度

在最早一组 168 例患者的报告中（Fahlbusch et al.，1999），经颅手术和经蝶手术的肿瘤全切除率分别为 45.7% 和 85.7%。肿瘤全切后 5 年无复发生存率为 86.9%，10 年为 81.3%。另一方面，次全切除后 5 年无复发生存率为 48.8%，部分切除后为 41.5%。初次手术后，10 年总生存率为 92.7%，其中肿瘤全切的治疗效果最好。此外，在 148 例接受初次手术的患者中，117 例（79%）患者术后无功能损伤，生活可自理。

随后，该作者又报道了进一步 73 例的经验（Hoffmann et al.，2012）。88.5% 的经蝶入路病例与 79.5% 的经颅入路病例完成肿瘤全切。整个病例系列肿瘤全切率达到 83.1%（作者之前的病例系列为 49.3%）。并发症发生率 13.8%，无死亡病例。经颅入路治疗的患者新发内分泌功能障碍的比例更高（16.3%~66.7% *vs*. 2.6%~50.0%），而经蝶入路术后出现的比例较低（5.2%~19.2% *vs*. 2.9%~45.7%）。

手术并发症

经蝶手术后，2% 的病例出现脑脊液鼻漏。应及时处理脑脊液漏，以避免继发脑膜炎。如果手术中出现脑脊液漏并有较大蛛网膜破口，可在术后立即置入腰大池引流作为预防措施。发生迟发脑脊液鼻漏时，可首先行腰大池引流作为试验性治疗，在某些情况下可直接采用手术修补。

经颅手术后，有 2 例（176 例经颅手术）出现下丘脑功能失调。其他非特异性并发症如伤口感染、硬膜外血肿和癫痫也有报道。

争议

全切除 *vs*. 部分切除

近期文献报告，平均有 53% 的病例可实现肿瘤全切除（Yang et al.）。在最近报道的大宗病例系列中（**表** 26.1），其肿瘤全切率从 13%（Lo et al., 2014）到 83%（Hoffmann et al., 2012）不等。87.5% 的巨大颅咽管瘤患者可实现全切（Gerganov et al., 2014）。部分切除仅适用于缓解症状的减压治疗，从而避免对重要结构的损伤。全切手术的禁忌证包括不可逆的下丘脑功能障碍，但肿瘤全切率也取决于医疗机构和个人经验。

虽然肿瘤全切与更高的总生存率和较低的复发率相关，但它禁用于存在不可逆下丘脑功能障碍或瘤周水肿的患者。保留功能是手术的主要目的之一，如果肿瘤黏附于下丘脑或小血管，或有严重钙化，则不应尝试全切手术。这类患者应继续随访，直到肿瘤残余部分增大到再次手术为首选治疗方案时。如果残余部分由于无法接受的高致残风险而不能手术，则建议放疗（**表** 26.2，**图** 26.6，**图** 26.7 和**图** 26.8）。

手术入路

我们采用内镜辅助经蝶入路的方法对鞍膈下颅咽管瘤（鞍内或鞍内及鞍上）进行手术。经颅入路用于鞍膈上颅咽管瘤。对于鞍膈上方颅咽管瘤，作者以前也曾使用半球间和翼点入路。不过最近我们更倾向于额外侧入路。

单纯内镜下扩大经蝶入路切除鞍膈上颅咽管瘤也被详细描述。这种方式脑脊液漏比例高，全切率低。Kassam 团队在 2008 年报道了一组 16 例患者的病例，其中 50% 完全切除，但术后脑脊液漏的发生率很高，需要再次手术（58%）（Gardner et al., 2008）。同一团队近期报道中脑脊液漏发生率在 15%~23%，尿崩症 48%~67%，垂体功能低下发生率 25%~58%。肿瘤全切率介于 37%~69%（Koutourousiou et al., 2013；Cavallo et al., 2014）。

表 26.1 颅咽管瘤和拉特克囊肿之间的重要区别

	颅咽管瘤	拉特克囊肿
位置		
• 鞍内	++	+++
• 鞍内和鞍上	++	+
• 鞍上	++	(+)
临床症状		
• 下丘脑紊乱	+++	-
• 视力	+++	+
• 垂体功能不全	+	+
• 头痛		+++
影像学特点		
• 钙化	+++	(+)
• 囊肿形成	++	+++
• 脑水肿	++	-
囊壁	厚	薄
组织学		
• β 连环蛋白	++	-
手术		
• 经蝶手术	++	+++
• 经颅手术	+++	(+)
• 分流术	+	-
囊壁切除	+++	(+)

颅咽管瘤的放射治疗

分割放射治疗用于治疗残余或复发性颅咽管瘤患者，以及因并发症发病率过高而被认为不适合完全手术切除的病例。计划性不完全切除肿瘤后使用放疗是有争议的。采用这种策略的根据是，若尝试根治性手术，有报道其病死率很高。

另一个有争议的理念是在颅咽管瘤切除术后立即进行放疗，或者在之后不考虑再次手术直接放疗。其理由在于再次手术的手术难度更大。一些研究表明，采用此种治疗策略的颅咽管瘤患者 10 年控制率（75%~90%）优于单纯不完全切除（30%~50%）。然而，目前还没有前瞻性的随机研究比较不同治疗策略的优劣。

放疗的主要缺点其是对照射局部产生的副作用，这些区域往往由对辐射高度敏感且脆弱的结构组成，

表 26.2 近期聚焦全切率、并发症率、死亡率和复发率的颅咽管瘤手术大型系列研究列表

	年份	数量	全切率	并发症率	死亡率	复发率
Van Effenterre & Boch	2002	122	59% 全切，29% 次全切，12% 部分切除	85% 极佳，9% 良好，5% 一般	2.5%	29/122
Mortini, 2011	2011	112	71.6%	8.8% 的患者术前日常生活需要部分或全部依赖他人	2.7%	24.5%
Karavitaki, et al., 2005	2005	121	16/121			部分切除的患者仅有 38% 的无复发生存率，而全切患者为 100%
Zuccaro, et al., 2005	2005	153	69%	术后内分泌症状几乎在所有患者中恶化，但视力情况却显著改善	NA	全切患者为 0
Caldarelli, et al., 2005	2005	52	40/52	即使有 60% 的患者依赖于激素替代治疗，部分患者表现为肥胖，长期随访结果显示所有存活患者临床状态良好。约 80% 的尿崩患者症状减轻；视力视野缺损情况改善或保持稳定，除 1 例患者外，所有患者术后神经系统症状减轻	2/52 早期 1 例迟发	术后 1~8 年，9 例需要手术治疗的复发病例（3 例为真性复发，6 例是由于未完全切除肿瘤残留的再生长）。12 例患者接受了放疗，其中 6 例为初次手术肿瘤未完全切除，6 例为复发后治疗
Duff, et al., 2000	2000	121	69/121	总体“良好疗效”率为 60.3%		29 例（24%）复发
Maira, et al., 2004	2004	92	63%	所有患者均治疗效果良好。10 例患者出现术后脑脊液漏，仅有 1 例需要行鞍区修补手术	2/92	8/92
Puget, et al., 2007	2007	66	20%	在本前瞻性研究中，无病例术后新发多食、病态肥胖及行为异常	NA	NA
Shi, et al., 2006	2006	284	83.5%	176 例患者（62.0%）保留了垂体柄，52 例（18.3%）中断，56 例（19.7%）难以辨认。 63 例（80%）患者重新获得日常生活的正常活动能力，29 例（14.2%）独立生活，9 例（4.4%）日常生活需要辅助	一月内 12 例 4 例迟发	随访中，23 例（14.1%）患者在肿瘤全切后 1.0~3.5 年（平均 1.8 年 ±1.6 年）内复发，24 例（64.9%）患者在肿瘤次全切或部分切除 0.25~1.5 年（平均 0.5 年 ±0.4 年）后复发
Yang, et al., 2010	2010	442	58%		五年总生存率全切为 98%、次全切 + 放疗为 99%；十年总生存率全切为 98%、次全切 + 放疗为 95%	两年无进展生存率全切为 88%，全切 + 放疗为 91%；五年无进展生存率全切为 67%，全切 + 放疗为 69%
Lo, et al., 2014	2014	123	15%	Kaplan-Meier 法提示由于治疗、而非肿瘤进展引起视力恶化、垂体前叶功能减退、尿崩、癫痫和脑血管事件的发生率分别为 27%、76%、45%、16% 和 11%	疾病相关生存率为 88%，总生存率为 80%。初始治疗方式不影响疾病相关生存率或总生存率，而高龄为总生存率的负向预后因素、但与疾病相关生存率无关	患者接受次全切 + 放疗或者 CD+ 放疗无进展生存率最高（分别为 82% 和 83%）。辅助放疗和挽救放疗之间无进展生存率无显著差异（84% *vs*. 74%，$P = 0.6$）
Hofmann, et al., 2012	2012	73	83.1%	13.8% 新发内分泌系统损害症状在经颅入路中更为常见（16.3%~66.7% *vs*. 2.6%~50.0%），而经蝶入路较少见（5.2%~19.2% *vs*. 2.9%~45.7%）	0	NA

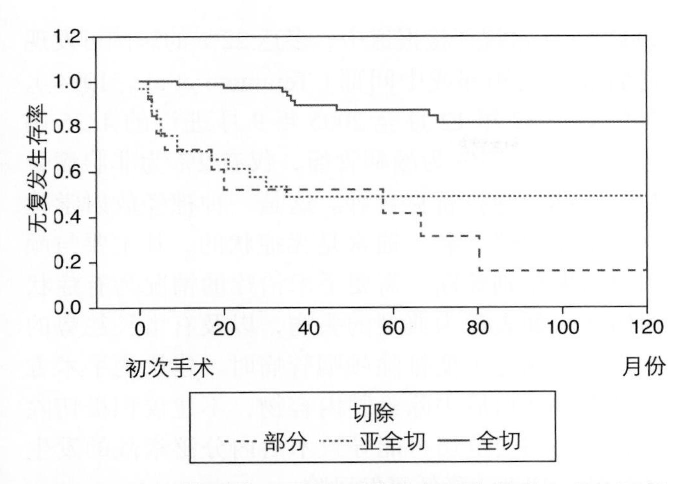

图 26.6　颅咽管瘤患者术后不同肿瘤切除程度患者的无复发生存期

Fahlbusch et al.

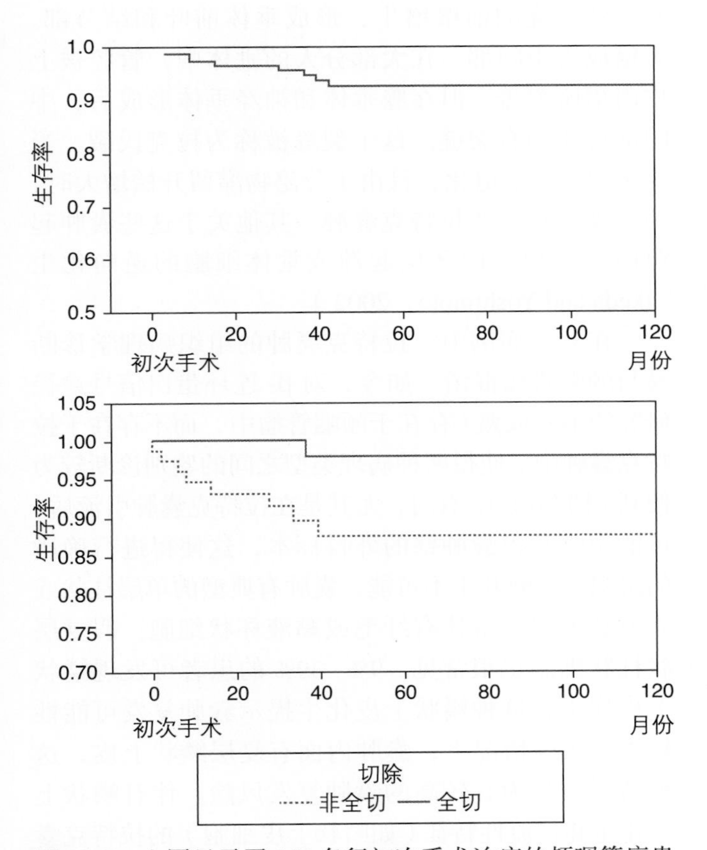

图 26.7　上图显示了 148 名行初次手术治疗的颅咽管瘤患者的精确生存率曲线，下图展示了行初次手术治疗后肿瘤切除程度不同的颅咽管瘤患者的生存时间

Fahlbusch, R., Honegger, J., Paulus, W., Huk, W., & Buchfelder, M. 1999. Surgical treatment of craniopharyngiomas: experience with 168 patients. *J Neurosurg*, 90, 237–50.

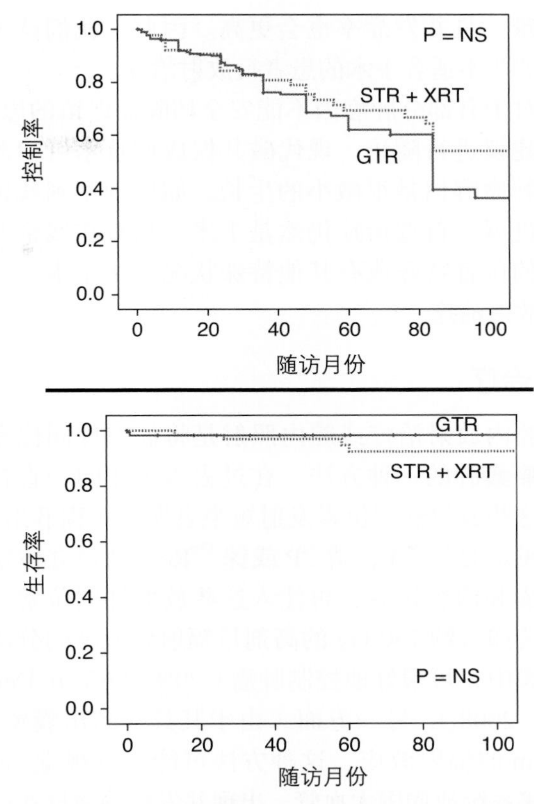

图 26.8　行全切术和行部分切除术后放疗患者之间的总体生存率和复发率比较

Reproduced from Yang, I., Sughrue, M. E., Rutkowski, M. J., et al. 2010. Craniopharyngioma: a comparison of tumour control with various treatment strategies. *Neurosurg Focus*, 28, E5, with permission from JNS Group.

照射这些区域会造成迟发垂体功能不全和癫痫。对于 6 岁以下的儿童，会导致认知障碍。即使最近分割放射治疗方面已经取得了进展，可提高放射治疗的精确度并减少对正常脑组织的辐射暴露，但放疗相关并发症的发生率仍然很高。早期囊性成分增大发生在放射治疗完成后的几个月内，虽然没有疾病进展，但仍可能导致视神经受压和脑积水。据报道，颅咽管瘤囊性成分增大的发生率在 10%~20%。

放射治疗的主要副作用常为迟发性，包括脑血管异常、放射性坏死、神经认知功能障碍和放射性神经病变。已有研究表明，接受放射剂量高于 50 Gy 的患者中，1%~2% 会发生放射性视神经病变。最常见的晚期并发症是垂体功能障碍，30%~50% 的患者在 5~10 年后出现新发垂体激素缺乏，需要补充（Brada and Thomas，1993）。颅咽管瘤行放射外科治疗的临床结果不如分割放疗，肿瘤控制更差且放射毒性也没有降低（Aggarwal et al.，2013）。

现代颅咽管瘤显微手术可在手术并发症发生率较低和几乎无死亡率的情况下实现肿瘤全切（Gerganov et al.，2014）。正如文中其他部分所提到的，肿瘤控制的最佳长期预后是在没有残余肿瘤的患者中观察到的。一些作者甚至建议在完全切除肿瘤后行放射治疗。有放疗史的患者，再次手术会更加困难，且并发症率也会更高。因此，我们认为应只给那些不适合手术的患者行放射治疗。

对于有部分肿瘤因不能安全切除而保留的患者，我们建议进行随访。现代磁共振成像技术可检测到残余肿瘤哪怕是很微小的生长。如果观察到残留肿瘤的进展，首选治疗仍然是手术。只有在残余肿瘤生长的位置特殊或有其他特殊状况无法手术，才会考虑放射治疗。

腔内治疗

腔内放射治疗或腔内照射是将放射性同位素注入肿瘤囊肿的一种方法，在过去六十年间一直在使用。这些放射性同位素发射短半衰期的短程 β 射线，最常见的是钇 ^{90}Y，磷 ^{32}P 或铼 ^{186}Re。通过立体定向抽吸囊肿内容物后，再注入这些放射性同位素。它们可传递大约 150 Gy 的高剂量辐射到囊肿的分泌上皮内膜中，可很好地控制肿瘤（70%~96%）（Derrey et al.，2008）。另一方面，由于其具有超出囊壁 3~3.5 mm 的辐射效应，这种方法可能影响视觉功能、内分泌系统或周围大血管。出现并发症的数据在已发表文献中差异很大。因此，该技术尚未被广泛接受。

另一种过去应用的方法是将博来霉素立体定向灌注到囊肿腔内（Hukin et al.，2007）。报道的有效率差异很大，从 57% 到 100% 不等；并且，由于博来霉素的毒性或其可能溢出囊肿腔，对周围结构产生损伤的风险可能很高。

未来发展

颅咽管瘤治疗的未来发展基于对下丘脑形态结构的新认识，包括具有特定内分泌和植物神经功能的神经核团。先进的 7T 磁共振成像技术可为手术治疗的决策提供更客观的标准。传统的治疗可通过发展包括抗激素治疗在内的分子治疗得以加强。

下丘脑性肥胖症目前主要通过 Baretić 疗法暂时控制，总体仍很难治疗（Rottembourg et al.，2009）。以瘦素为主的治疗方法效果欠佳（Trivin et al.，2009；Roemmler-Zehrer et al.，2014）。最近关于重氮嗪和二甲双胍的临床试验仅处于探索阶段（Aubert et al.，2011；Hamilton et al.，2011；Malin and Kashyap，2014）。

拉特克囊肿

拉特克囊肿是由位于垂体中间区域的拉特克裂中腺体残余形成的非肿瘤囊性结构（Saeger et al.，2007）。在常规尸检报道中，多达 22% 的病例可发现它们位于远侧部或中间部（Teramoto et al.，1994）。在作者 1982 年 12 月至 2005 年 9 月进行的 4335 例鞍区手术中，7% 为颅咽管瘤，仅有 2% 为非腺瘤囊肿，大部分为拉特克囊肿。这是一种神经放射学检查中常见的偶发病，通常是无症状的。其主要与颅咽管瘤做鉴别诊断。需要手术治疗的情况为有症状的病变，如表现为典型的头痛，以及有增长趋势的病变，特别是不能排除颅咽管瘤时。建议的手术方式是囊肿开窗后去除囊肿内容物，不建议积极切除囊肿壁。病变全切可能导致术后内分泌紊乱的发生率升高，却无法降低复发风险。

拉特克囊肿被认为在脑垂体的发育过程中发生。在妊娠第三或第四周，原始口腔头侧的隆起与间脑（漏斗部）向下的突出相互吻合，形成垂体腺体的两叶。然后囊的前壁增生，形成垂体前叶和结节部。后壁成为中间部。在大部分人的垂体中，管腔被上皮内褶所覆盖。但在腺垂体和神经垂体形成后，中间部可能仍有裂缝。这个裂缝被称为拉克氏裂。当这条裂缝未能退化，且由于分泌物潴留开始增大时，即出现症状性的拉特克囊肿。其他关于这些囊肿起源的理论包括内胚层起源或垂体细胞的逆向化生（Ikeda and Yoshimoto，2002）。

在某些病例中，拉特克囊肿的组织病理学诊断易与颅咽管瘤混淆。如今，对 β- 连环蛋白信号途径研究的不断成熟（存在于颅咽管瘤中，而不存在于拉特克囊肿中）使得两种病理类型之间的鉴别诊断较为便利（图 26.1）。有时，尤其是在拉特克囊肿引流后，可能很难获得囊肿壁的外科标本，这使得进行确凿的组织学诊断几乎不可能。囊肿有典型的单层柱状或立方状上皮，常伴有纤毛或黏液杯状细胞。假复层状柱状细胞也很常见。9%~39% 的患者可发现鳞状上皮化生，这种鳞状上皮化生提示囊肿复发可能性较大。极少情况下，囊肿内面有复层鳞状上皮，这种情况被认为有较高的囊肿复发风险。伴有鳞状上皮化生和过渡性特征（如鳞状上皮细胞）的拉特克囊肿，在组织病理学检查和影像学检查上类似囊性颅咽管瘤。一些作者指出拉特克囊肿和颅咽管瘤之间可能存在联系。Ikeda 等回顾了 42 例拉特克囊肿患者，发现 3 例囊肿壁有鳞状上皮，与颅咽管瘤表现类似（Ikeda and Yoshimoto，2002）。

拉特克囊肿通常起源于鞍内的中间部。囊肿可能很大，也可能延伸到鞍上池。孤立的鞍上拉特克囊肿很少见。在鼻咽、蝶窦、斜坡和桥小脑角生长的异位拉特克囊肿则更为少见。

临床特征

根据 Weiss 团队发表的关于拉特克囊肿病例最多的一组研究（Aho et al.，2005），偶然发现的拉特克囊肿患者约 70% 无症状。约 30% 的患者由于局部占位效应和压迫视路、垂体导致出现垂体功能不全等症状。最常见的症状是头痛。在少部分患者中，表现有全垂体功能低下、进行性视力减退和类似脑膜炎或垂体炎的症状。

无症状的病变

Aho 等（2005）报道了 160 例拉特克囊肿。其中 42 例是在做其他目的 MRI 检查中偶然发现的，囊肿并未生长或引起内分泌、视觉体征和症状（Aho et al.，2005）。在 Teramto 团队的另一个病例系列研究中（Sanno et al.，2003），随访期间仅有 5.4% 的病例囊肿体积增加（Sanno et al.，2003）。

有症状的病变

症状性病变最常出现在 40 到 50 岁，女性占比略高。与拉特克囊肿相关的典型症状包括头痛、垂体功能不全和视觉障碍。头痛存在于所有症状性病变中，可作为手术的唯一指征。鞍内病变常在前囟周围引起疼痛感觉。在压迫海绵窦的病变中，患者可能有眶周疼痛。

举例来说，一名 17 岁的学生患有拉特克囊肿，只有严重头痛的症状，这影响了他在学校的表现。手术后，他的头痛完全消失，恢复了成功的校园活动。一位 57 岁的女士表现为间歇性头痛，之后进行了数周的持续抗顽固疼痛治疗，她决定接受手术。手术后她的头痛症状彻底而永久性消除。

据报道，35%~50% 接受手术治疗的患者术前存在视力障碍，包括视野缺陷及视力下降。Jahangiri 等报道，41% 的成人和 45% 的儿童患者术前出现垂体功能低下。最常见的内分泌功能障碍是高催乳素血症和生长激素缺乏，其次是肾上腺功能减退和性腺功能减退。尿崩症约在 7%~20% 的患者中出现，比其在颅咽管瘤中的发病率低。其他罕见的表现包括化学性脑膜炎或囊内出血（Harrison et al.，1994；Jahangiri et al.，2011；Neidert et al.，2013）。一些病例表现为症状突然发作，并伴有囊内出血的影像学证据。这种情况被描述为拉特克囊肿卒中（Neidert et al.，2013）。

影像学特征

磁共振成像是术前评估拉特克囊肿和鉴别拉特克囊肿与其他鞍区囊性病变如颅咽管瘤的主要影像学方法（Zada et al.，2010）。囊肿的信号强度各不相同，根据其内容物的成分，可为低信号、高信号或等信号。尽管大多数囊肿显示均匀的信号强度，但高达 40% 的囊肿内有一个由蛋白质和细胞碎片组成的结节，通常在注射造影剂后不会增强（Brassier et al.，1999；Byun et al.，2000；Binning et al.，2005）。薄边缘强化可归因于囊肿壁的炎症或鳞状上皮化生，或垂体的环样移位（Brassier et al.，1999；Byun et al.，2000；Kim et al.，2004；Zada，2011）。菲薄的囊壁即使本身被增强，也可能低于 MRI 的分辨能力。所有病例中，对比增强的模式和强度并不恒定。这可能是由于囊肿内容物的偶尔溢出而引起的周围组织（即垂体或鞍区硬脑膜）炎症反应。垂体常被囊肿压迫移位，有时囊肿仍被包裹在腺体内部。囊肿通常单纯位于鞍内或位于鞍内、鞍旁或鞍上。单纯鞍上囊肿很少见。

计算机断层扫描可用于发现颅咽管瘤中较常见的钙化。尽管如此，仍有报告显示拉特克囊肿也会有钙化，但钙化很少见，且程度较轻。进一步鉴别诊断是鞍区脓肿和淋巴细胞垂体炎。

治疗

无症状的拉特克囊肿（通常小于 1 cm）可通过定期 MRI 影像、内分泌及眼科检查随诊。

有症状的拉特克囊肿是手术治疗的指征。头痛可能是唯一的症状。手术目的是局部减压，如果可能的话，获取组织进行组织学诊断。清除囊肿内容物是最常用的策略。在最佳的手术情况下，当囊肿位置较浅且与鞍底硬脑膜直接相连时，可在不切开垂体的情况下开窗，并取部分囊壁行组织学检查。鞍内或鞍上囊肿可引流，囊壁会塌陷，而垂体功能得以保留（**图** 26.9）。在某些情况下，囊肿位于垂体内部，外科医生需要切开垂体。在这种情况下，手术者仅清除囊肿，但不应冒险取囊肿壁进行活检。尝试完全或积极切除囊肿壁可导致包括尿崩症在内的内分泌缺陷的发生率升高。然而据一些文献报道，囊壁残余与较高的囊肿复发率相关。经验表明，并不提倡为了降低潜在的复发风险而积极囊肿切除，从而使相关并发症发生率上升。

单纯的鞍上囊肿应采用经颅入路，尤其是不能排除颅咽管瘤时。

结果和随访

术后 MRI 显示拉特克囊肿手术引流的有效率

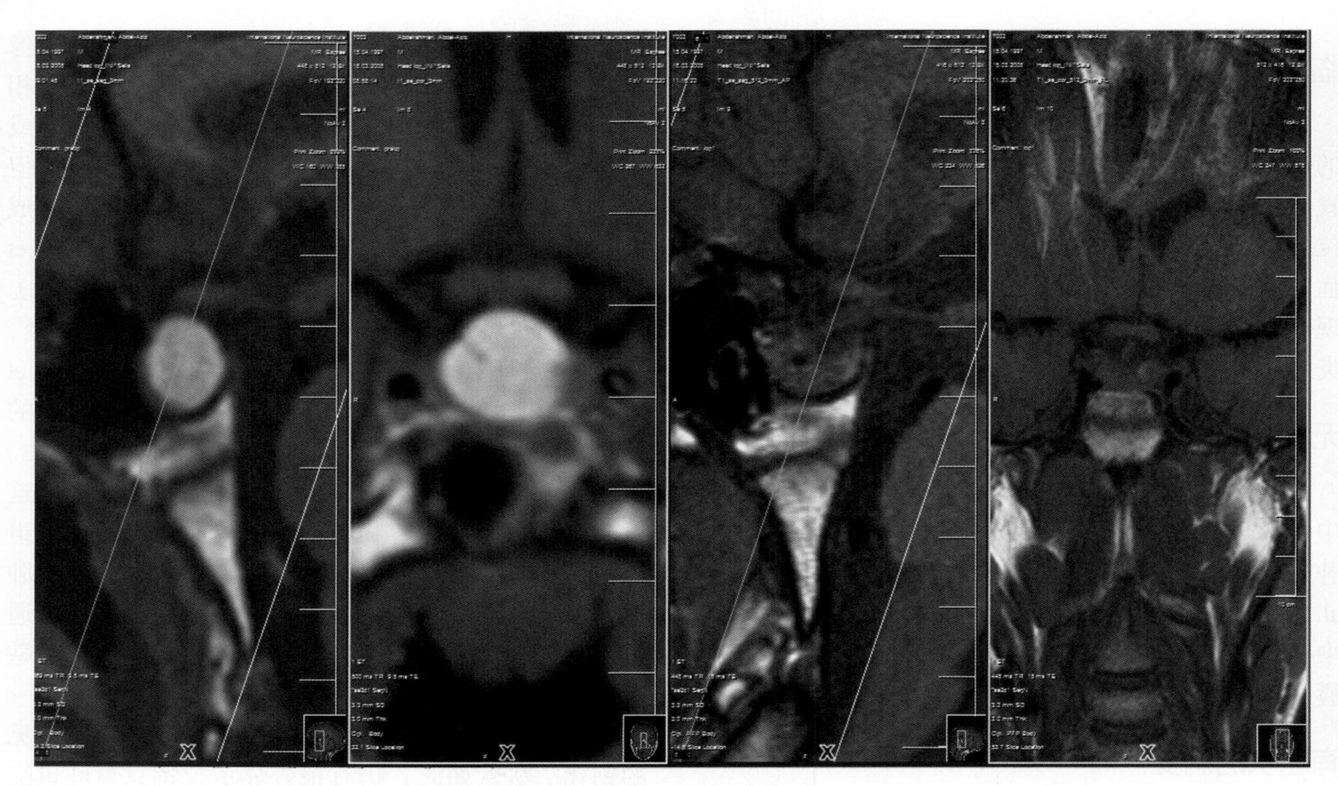

图 26.9 术前和术后 MRI 显示经蝶手术后完全排空的拉特克囊肿

达 90% 以上。所有病例术后头痛均立即改善，手术引流后视力改善达 80% 以上。Weiss 团队（Aho et al.）展示的成人拉特克囊肿大宗手术病例，初次手术全切率为 97%，5 年复发率为 18%（Aho et al., 2005）。头痛、视觉症状和高催乳素血症通常在手术治疗后改善，但由于垂体受到慢性压迫，全垂体功能减退和尿崩症较少得到改善。积极切除囊肿壁后，尿崩症更易发生。我们经历过一些患者术后出现暂时性低钠血症，限制液体摄入可控制症状。

拉特克囊肿开窗或切除术后总体长期复发率在 3%~33%。复发风险可能与术前影像学检查中囊肿壁的强化方式、鳞状上皮化生、慢性炎症或复层上皮、积极的囊肿壁切除和腹部脂肪组织的植入有关。

拉特克囊肿手术治疗后，建议 3 个月后进行磁共振成像，然后每年进行一次，持续 5 年。之后每 2~3 年一次，如果临床稳定，则再持续 10 年。

拉特克囊肿的症状性复发是罕见的，据报道复发率在 5%~18%。复发通常在 MRI 随访时被发现，伴随或不伴随症状再现。放射学证据发现复发本身并不意味着需要再次手术。症状性复发是行再次充分引流手术的指证。如果复发是不伴症状的，则应进行定期的磁共振成像检查以及眼科和内分泌检查。

争议

如何评价切除程度是治疗拉特克囊肿的讨论重点之一。可由外科医生的印象描述，或根据术后 MRI 表现。外科医生的印象是主观的，在许多情况下很难从正常的垂体组织中安全地观察和切除囊肿的薄壁。囊肿壁在 MRI 上通常不可见，只有囊肿内容物才能显示出拉特克囊肿的放射学特征。术后 MRI 不能确定是否切除囊肿壁，但能证实囊肿内容物的完全清除。因此，“拉特克囊肿全切除术”这个术语是非常有争议的。

我们建议经蝶入路开窗及清除囊肿内容物。蛛网膜应保持完整。如果术中有脑脊液漏证据，我们从大腿或腹部皮下组织取小脂肪块来密封。经颅入路可用于孤立性鞍上症状性拉特克囊肿，特别是当囊肿较大或颅咽管瘤不能排除时。

致谢

作者要感谢德国埃尔兰根大学神经病理学研究所 Rolf Buslei 教授提供的组织学切片。

延伸阅读、参考文献、EBRAIN 的相关链接

扫描书末二维码获取。

第 27 章　鞍区及鞍上区肿瘤的外科治疗

Jayson A. Neil · William T. Couldwell 著
戚其超、冯子超 译，倪石磊 审校

引言

尽管鞍区和鞍上肿瘤的位置相近，但它们有多种起源极为广泛的疾病谱。这些肿瘤可能是先天性病变，如脂肪瘤、拉特克囊肿、蛛网膜囊肿和错构瘤，也可能是从周围结构发展而来，引起垂体腺瘤、脑膜瘤、颅咽管瘤、脊索瘤、视神经胶质瘤等。非肿瘤性病变，如海绵状血管畸形、骨纤维结构不良以及结节病等炎症性病变也可发生于此，来自远隔部位的肿瘤以转移瘤的形式可出现在垂体和海绵窦。极大的病种多样性使治疗这些肿瘤病例更加复杂，因为可能会遇到各种各样的病理类型。

该区域有许多重要结构，包括垂体、重要血管和多个脑神经，导致治疗鞍区和鞍上肿瘤尤为复杂。避免损伤这些重要结构是治疗计划的关键组成部分。

在本章中，我们将讨论鞍区和鞍上区域的解剖，也会讨论这些肿瘤的诊断检查、治疗、手术策略、术后护理和并发症处理，然后详细阐述与这些主题相关的争议问题。

手术解剖

充分了解鞍区和鞍上解剖对肿瘤发病机制和发展方式的理解以及对手术入路的规划至关重要。尽管该区域的许多病变可涉及多个区域，为了简化讨论，我们将解剖分为鼻腔和蝶窦以及鞍区、鞍旁区和鞍上区。

鼻腔和蝶窦

鼻腔是一对结构，向前通过鼻孔开放，向后通过后鼻孔向鼻咽部开放。它由位于中间的鼻中隔隔开。骨性鼻中隔由下方的犁骨和上方的筛骨垂直板构成，附着在蝶窦的窦口或前壁，是可靠的中线标志。侧壁有下鼻甲、中鼻甲和上鼻甲，筛窦、额窦和上颌窦以及鼻泪管的开口。上缘为筛板，后缘为蝶骨。在后上面，鼻腔通过位于上鼻甲内侧上方的蝶窦开口与蝶窦相通。下鼻甲是一块独立的骨，也是最大的鼻甲。

蝶窦为单一的中线结构，通过成对的蝶窦开口向蝶窦前下方与成对的鼻腔相通。它被蝶骨包围，可被多个偏心分隔所隔开。蝶窦的血供来源于蝶腭动脉和筛后动脉。蝶腭动脉的后隔分支为鼻中隔黏膜瓣提供血管蒂，走行于蝶窦开口下缘下方，向前进入鼻中隔黏膜。颈内动脉和视神经紧靠蝶窦上外侧壁，蝶窦本身常围绕这些结构形成轮廓，并且在蝶窦内可能形成无骨质覆盖区。水平的岩骨段颈内动脉延续至海绵窦段，在内镜领域文献称为“斜坡旁”颈内动脉，垂直于后外侧蝶窦。其继续延伸为海绵窦内段，这段动脉在更远处于后外侧成环状，在蝶窦内不可见。它在鞍区两侧重新形成“鞍旁”颈内动脉。很重要的一点是鞍旁颈内动脉表面骨质可能菲薄或缺如。

鞍旁颈内动脉和视神经压痕之间的交界处称为视神经颈动脉隐窝（optico-carotid recesses，OCR）。外侧 OCR 标志着视柱和前床突的位置，可能气化较明显，从内镜视野观察显示为中空。内侧 OCR 位于中床突和内侧海绵窦附近。蝶鞍位于蝶窦的上、后两个面（图 27.1 和图 27.2）。

鞍区

蝶鞍是位于蝶骨体部的鞍形凹陷。垂体窝位于凹陷的中心，前上缘是鞍结节，后缘是鞍背，侧缘是海绵窦，前下缘及下缘是蝶窦，上缘是鞍膈和鞍上池。垂体位于垂体窝，由前叶（腺垂体）和后叶（神经垂体）组成。腺垂体起源于原始口腔的拉特克囊，沿颅咽管上升进入鞍区。神经垂体是第三脑室底部的内凹，下降进入鞍区。

鞍旁区

鞍旁区由双侧海绵窦组成，海绵窦由扩张的静脉通道组成，颈内动脉海绵窦段和脑神经Ⅲ、Ⅳ、

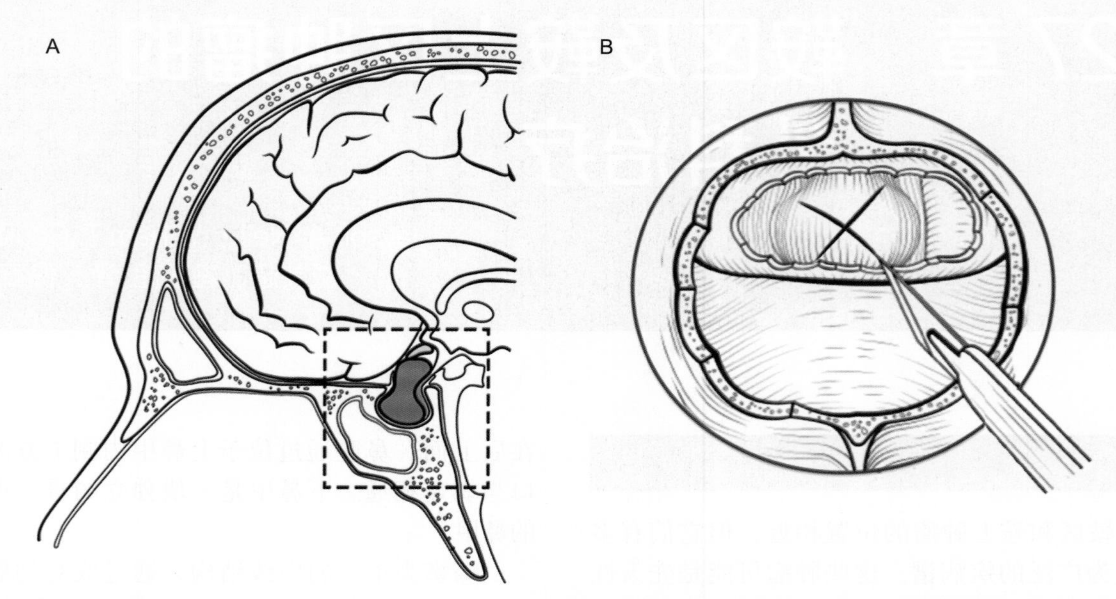

图 27.1 （A）垂体腺瘤标记为紫色，黄色标记的视交叉推挤向上移位，蓝色标记的正常垂体推挤向后或向上移位。（B）通过显微镜从下方观察前颅底，显示鞍区脑膜的切口，蝶鞍位于该切口的后部和上部

V1、V2、Ⅵ通过其中。海绵窦内侧为单层骨膜；来自蝶鞍底、中颅窝底和斜坡的硬脑膜与骨膜汇合，在海绵窦其余部分周围形成双层硬脑膜（图 27.2）。

鞍上区

鞍上区主要由鞍上池组成。鞍上池是位于蝶鞍正上方第三脑室下方的脑脊液腔。它其中的结构有漏斗柄、视交叉和 Willis 环（图 27.1 和图 27.2）。它在轴位像上呈五边形。

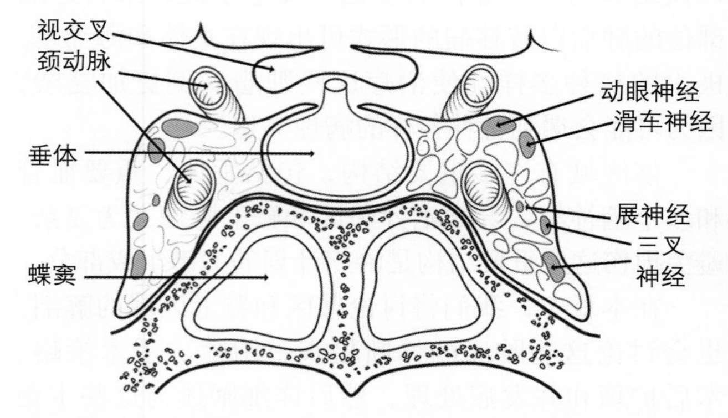

图 27.2 鞍区的冠状位截图示意图，描绘出了蝶鞍、双侧海绵窦（含内容物）、鞍上池

术前准备

临床评估

患者的临床症状和体征取决于病变性质、病变的大小、位置和生长时间。应结合详细的体格检查获取完整的临床病史，包括头部、颈部和脑神经（尤其注意第Ⅰ～Ⅵ对脑神经）的检查。鞍区和鞍上肿瘤常表现为头痛、视物模糊或重影、视力丧失及与内分泌疾病相关的症状（如闭经、溢乳、肢端肥大、库欣综合征、垂体功能减退），以及血管性损害（如短暂性缺血发作、卒中），若肿瘤体积较大，还可能出现脑积水。如果肿瘤侵犯鼻旁窦，患者还可出现与鼻窦闭塞相关的症状，如鼻塞、鼻窦炎等。

常规的神经眼科评估包括视力、视野评估和眼底镜检查，可据此判断是否有视盘水肿、静脉充血或其他提示颅内压升高的表现。其中，眼底镜检查还能够提示是否有视神经损伤和萎缩。规范的视野检查有利于进一步评估神经损伤，能够提示我们视神经是否受到鞍上肿瘤的压迫。同时，视交叉受损引起的典型双颞侧偏盲以及包括视神经管受压在内的多种形式的压迫都可通过眼科检查来鉴别。光学相干断层成像（optical coherence tomography，OCT）可用于获得高分辨率视网膜图像，有助于更好地评估视神经萎缩的程度和轴突的完整性。在视神经通路减压术后，若观察到视网膜神经纤维层（retinal nerve fibre layer，RNFL）能维持在一定的厚度，对于视力改善而言，是积极的预后因素。

实验室检验评估

标准的实验室检验评估，包含全血细胞计数、基本的代谢检查和凝血功能评估。如果患者有恶性肿瘤、淋巴瘤、感染或肉芽肿病史，则还应行与这些疾病相关的专门检查，如腰椎穿刺脑脊液分析等。此外，还需行全面的内分泌检查，这在**第 25 章**有详细介绍。

影像学评估

磁共振成像（MRI）仍然是评估鞍区和鞍上病变的最佳检查方法。尤其是薄层 T1 平扫加强化磁共振成像应作为一项常规检查，这也是脑垂体评估流程的一部分。此外，磁共振压脂序列和薄扫 T2 矢状位及冠状位重建有助于明确病变的范围及其与海绵窦、视神经和其他脑神经、颈内动脉的关系。计算机断层扫描（CT）可显示蝶鞍和颅底的骨性结构，有助于评估一些肿瘤如颅咽管瘤、脊索瘤或软骨肉瘤等的钙化情况，也可提供出血相关信息，如脑垂体卒中。此外，CT 在鉴别病变是否累及骨质方面，要优于 MRI，如脑膜瘤是否有颅骨骨质增生或鼻旁窦过度气化，或其他伴有骨破坏的病变。如果怀疑有血管性病变如大动脉瘤、血管包裹或破坏，则在任何干预实施前都应行 CT 血管成像或常规脑血管造影以明确病变性质。

手术计划

暴露鞍区及鞍上病变有多种手术入路，包括但不限于经鼻蝶入路、翼点入路和额下入路及相应的改良入路。所有这些入路均可在手术显微镜、内镜或双镜联合下进行，多种入路联合应用可用于切除体积较大的病变或复杂病变。在选择入路时，应考虑病变的预期病理、病变位置及与周围组织的关系。同时，关注垂体、垂体柄、视神经和其他脑神经移位的方向有助于确定入路的侧别和特征。术前应有明确的手术切除和关颅计划以避免脑脊液漏等术后并发症。在手术开始之前，准备必要手术设备，相关人员也需要具备一定经验。

术中

经颅入路

翼点入路

翼点入路有若干优点，首先是被大多数神经外科医生所熟知；其次，此入路可在手术早期即观察到视神经、视交叉、垂体柄、颈动脉和大脑前动脉。另外，这种方法也提供了进入鞍上池的最短距离，并使术者早期可从视神经后方观察术区，从而更方便地控制颈内动脉及其分支。此外，此入路可较早地释放脑脊液，有利于脑组织减压，并且较少侵犯额窦，减少脑脊液漏和感染的风险。但如果病变导致显著的前颅底受累，或预期有广泛的颅底重建，那么这种情况下双侧额下入路相对于翼点入路更具优势。

采用翼点入路时，患者取仰卧位，同侧垫肩，手术台稍抬高使头部位于右心房上方的水平面。头部用 Mayfield 三钉头架固定，旋转 30°~40°，稍微后仰。头部可灵活地调节以提供一个由低到高的径路，便于暴露向上延伸的病变。进一步后仰有利于上方视角，并有助于额叶在重力作用下自然下垂。皮肤切口为沿发际线后方的平缓曲线，从颧骨水平的耳屏前方到正常发际线最前端的中线。直线切开颞肌筋膜和颞肌，多数情况下将皮肌瓣一同掀起并向前下方牵拉（**图 27.3**）。颅骨钻孔位置在关键孔、颞上线后方及颞窝下方。将硬脑膜与颅骨分离，并使用带足板的高速钻头铣开骨板，这可根据手术入路而调整。

使用咬骨钳和高速钻将蝶骨小翼的外侧面切除至眶脑膜动脉。C 形剪开硬脑膜，并向前悬吊。及早分离外侧裂可释放脑脊液、使脑组织松弛，有利于暴露嗅神经、视神经和动眼神经，以及颈内动脉和大脑前动脉。此时，可见鞍上池及大多数鞍上肿瘤（**图 27.4**）。肿瘤减压将有助于分离周围神经血管结构（**图 27.5**）。优先以水密方式缝合硬脑膜，用钛板和螺钉复位固定骨瓣。使用 Medpor 聚乙烯植入物对切除的蝶骨翼进行颅骨修补以避免颞肌功能受影响。以标准方式缝合颞肌、筋膜及其浅部软组织。参见**专栏 27.1**。

额颞入路的改良：额眶入路和眶颧入路

将标准额颞入路扩展至额眶入路（去除眶缘）或眶颧入路（去除眶缘和颧骨）的主要目的是提供更佳的从下到上的视野径路，同时减少对额叶和颞叶的牵拉。具体使用哪一种变式取决于肿瘤的具体特点。在大多数情况下，使用额眶入路，骨瓣包括一段前外侧眶缘（从眶上切迹的外侧延伸到眶缘的外侧）。铣刀小心操作以避免损伤眶周筋膜。当需要更广泛的上方径路时，可使用眶颧入路。这种变式需要通过向下和向后牵开颞肌，采用单骨瓣或双骨瓣法开颅，具体技术细节在其他章节中介绍。

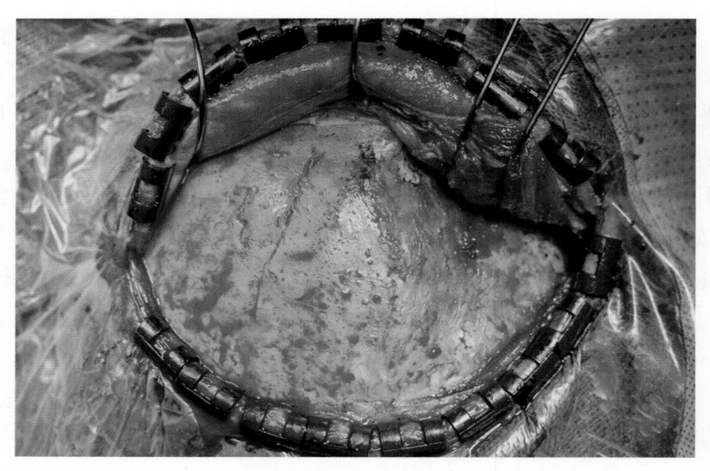

图 27.3 皮肤切口、皮肌瓣抬起及右侧翼点开颅术的手术照片

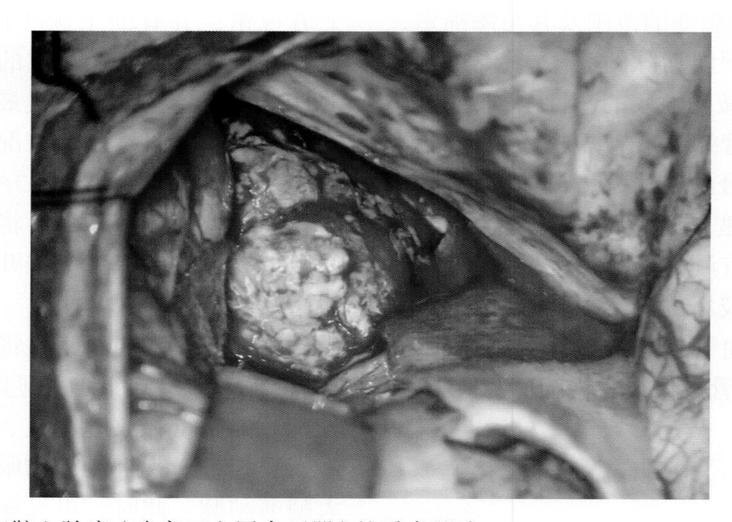

图 27.4 右侧翼点入路观察鞍上肿瘤（略高于金属牵开器）的手术照片

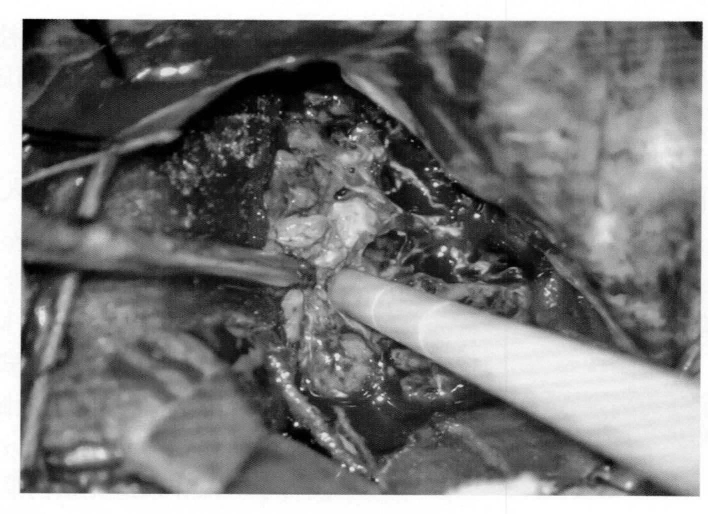

图 27.5 经右侧翼点入路观察鞍上肿瘤和超声吸引器减压的手术照片

额下入路

经额或额下入路可根据需要进行单侧或双侧开颅，必要时可向颅底下方延伸（**图** 27.6）。在单侧额下开颅术中，患者的体位类似于翼点入路，但头部旋转较小，距中线 10°~20°。双冠状皮肤切口一般止于正中线或对侧颞上线。将头皮皮瓣和骨膜向前翻起，以显露眶上血管和神经并辨认眶缘。通常在关键孔的位置钻孔（将颞肌翻向前部以显露关键孔）。根据是否暴露矢状窦确定中线上的钻孔位置。骨瓣位置较低，应刚好在眼眶上方，该骨瓣几乎都会进入额窦。我们通常选择将额窦颅骨化（切除后壁）并磨除黏膜，随后鼻额开口由肌肉或筋膜堵塞。通常 C 形剪开硬脑膜，基底位于下方。

在双侧额下开颅术中，患者应严格仰卧，抬高手术床至头部位于右心房上方水平。用 Mayfield 三钉头架固定头部，并略微后仰使双侧上颌突置于最高点，以促进脑下垂（**图** 27.7）。皮肤切口在两侧耳屏前，从一侧颧骨至另一侧颧骨。向前仔细解剖，保留骨膜用于颅底重建。沿双侧关键孔附近的上面进行必要的最小限度颞肌分离。在关键孔、颞上线后缘及上矢状窦后方两侧钻孔（**图** 27.6）。从骨瓣分离矢状窦时要小心，如果矢状窦与颅骨紧密附着，可在矢状窦两侧钻孔之间用金刚钻磨出骨槽，再用 Kerrison 咬骨钳咬除之间的骨脊。无需在前额上钻孔。将硬脑膜从颅骨上剥离，并使用带足板的高速

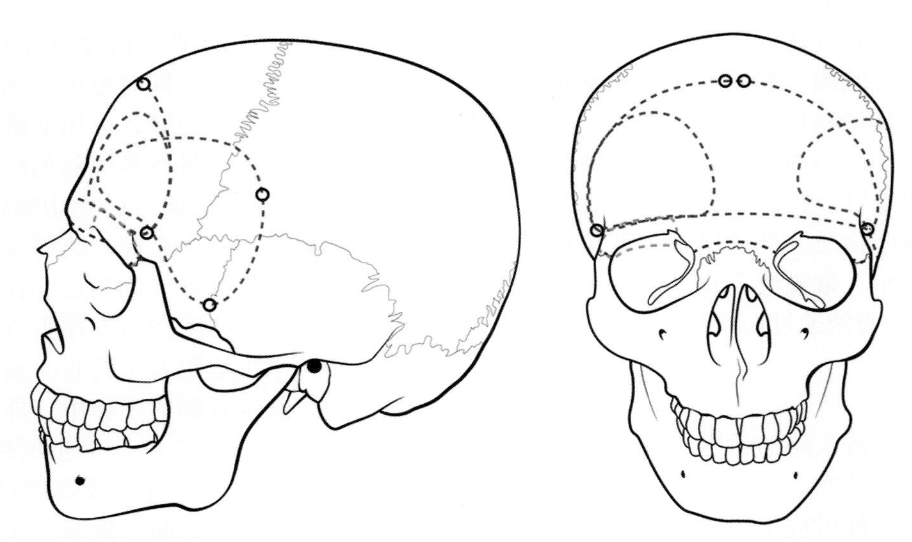

图 27.6　基于手术入路的开颅路径图。图示为单侧经额（红色）、翼点（绿色）和双侧经额（蓝色）入路。另外还可联合经眶和额下扩大骨切除

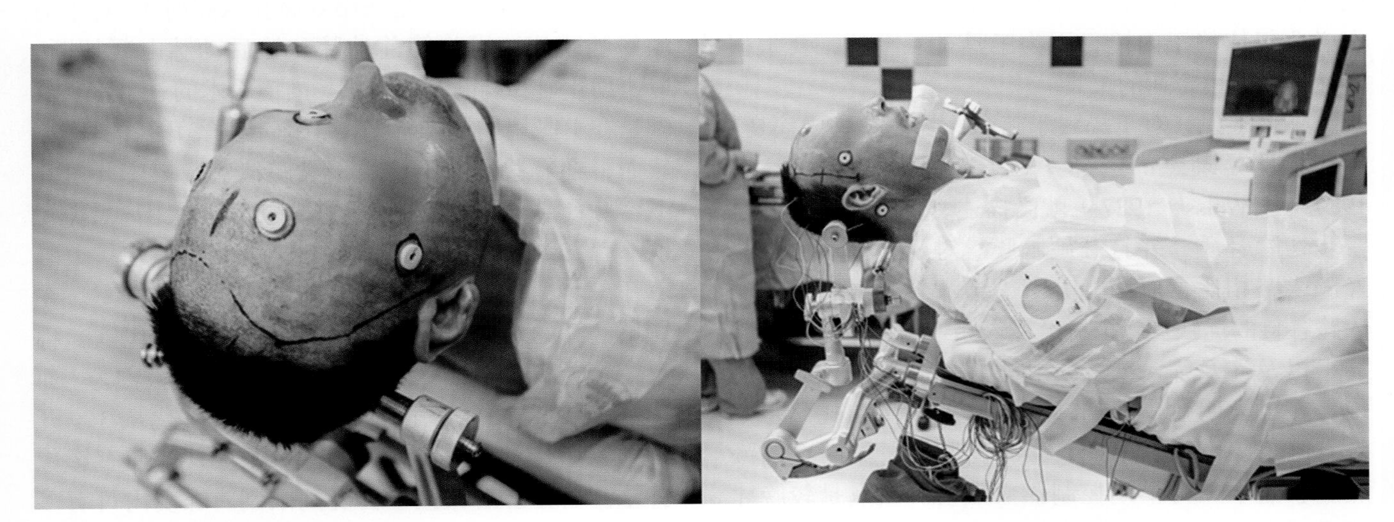

图 27.7　患者体位和标记的皮肤切口的手术照片

钻头进行开颅操作。用高速钻和咬骨钳去除额窦后壁，将额窦颅骨化。并完全去除额窦黏膜，用筋膜和颞肌堵塞额窦开口。切开硬脑膜至上矢状窦外侧，即病理学允许范围内的前方（通常在矢状窦的前 1/3 处）。通过大脑镰用 2-0 丝线双环结扎矢状窦，并在结扎线之间切开。

无论是单侧额下入路还是双侧额下入路，大脑均被轻轻抬起，嗅神经可在其与视神经交叉处查见。如果可能的话，应尽量松解嗅球和嗅神经上方的蛛网膜，以避免损伤这些神经。沿前颅底或在鞍上池内可见到肿瘤。肿瘤切除是按照从前到后的方式进行。按常规如果肿瘤基底位于硬脑膜（如脑膜瘤），早期离断肿瘤基底可阻断其血供并有助于切除肿瘤。肿瘤内减压至关重要，因为大多数神经血管位于病变的后外侧，肿瘤内部减压将有助于肿瘤与周围的神经血管分离。硬脑膜首选以水密封方式缝合，必要时需用补片修补硬脑膜。如果需要重建颅底，可用自体脂肪及筋膜移植物填充前颅底缺损。手术开始时收集的带血管蒂的颅周筋膜移植物可用于进一步重建。用钛板和螺钉复位固定骨瓣，同时避免在前额上放置任何硬体物质，并确保颅周移植物有足够的血供、避免绞窄。常规缝合皮肤软组织。腰大池引流有助于防止脑脊液通过伤口漏出。

内镜入路

本节主要叙述内镜入路的手术方法，内镜入路通常指经鼻入路至前颅底、蝶窦、鞍上池和鞍旁区域。事实上各种入路都可应用内镜。无论是经颅入路还是经鼻入路均可使用显微镜、内镜或两者联合应用。即使大部分手术操作在显微镜下进行，内镜也能提供极大帮助，如用角度镜观察术腔周围查找残余肿瘤。同样的，在经鼻手术中，外科医生也没有必要仅依赖于内镜，因为工具是互补的，要根据实际情况选用合适的工具。

一般来说，对于局限于筛窦、蝶窦及鞍内病变，经鼻入路是理想的选择。对于鞍外病变，Weiss 在 1987 年（Weiss，1987）就已描述，需要沿前颅底进一步切除骨质，并打开硬脑膜。对于这些病例，与经颅入路相比，应该充分考虑扩大经鼻入路与经颅入路各自的优缺点。扩大经鼻入路最适用于中小型肿瘤，以及涉及筛窦、蝶窦和蝶鞍的肿瘤。该方法的优势在于无明显皮肤切口，无上矢状窦结扎，基本没有脑组织牵拉，早期直接暴露肿瘤，同时在前颅底脑膜瘤中，可早期控制供血血管。缺点是较晚才能看到鞍上病变的神经血管结构，同时脑脊液漏的发生率较高，如果肿瘤在眶上向外侧、向额窦前上方或向颈内动脉后上方生长，则可能难以全切。尤其是对于脑膜尾征延伸到前颅底之外的脑膜瘤，应用此入路具有一定的挑战性。在前颅底脑膜瘤中，如果需开放筛板区域或肿瘤侵犯筛板，使用这种入路时保留嗅觉是有困难的。

手术开始前给予患者鼻喷雾血管收缩剂，患者采取仰卧位，气管插管置于左侧。调整床的位置，使头部位于右心房上方水平。头部用 Mayfield 三钉头架固定，稍微向左偏头并向右旋转，便于外科医生站在患者右侧，在观察患者头部时处于中立位。使用浸泡黏膜收缩剂棉片填塞鼻腔，注册神经导航并将内镜显示屏及导航显示屏置于手术床床头位置。准备右下腹或大腿外侧作为切取脂肪和筋膜修补的部位。

移除棉片，用 0° 内镜探查鼻孔，观察上、中、下鼻甲的解剖结构，同时也可看到鼻中隔、鼻后孔和蝶窦开口。如有必要，可用麻醉剂和肾上腺素浸润鼻腔黏膜止血。虽然鼻中隔偏曲的发生率大于不偏曲，但对于明显的成角（“鼻中隔骨刺”）仍需磨平，以便不受阻挡地进入鼻腔。值得注意的是，中鼻甲通过水平基板与筛骨外侧相连，在更前面，垂直附着在筛板上。中鼻甲在前方在垂直方向附着，在后方逐渐转向水平地附着于腭骨。通常情况下，如果不需完全切除术者侧的中鼻甲，那么就需要将鼻甲移位（外侧化），以扩大手术通路便于放置内镜。在中鼻甲移位时，鼻甲垂直板爆裂可导致筛板骨折，进而发生难以治疗的脑脊液漏。在有些病例，可在术前薄层 CT 上看到中鼻甲中有气房（气泡中鼻甲），这种情况可导致中鼻甲肥厚，须予以切除。

根据病变的位置，需进行蝶窦前壁切除及鼻中隔后上部切除（特别是采用双鼻孔入路时）。对于前颅底脑膜瘤，可将筛前动脉和筛后动脉电凝切断，以协助止血和离断肿瘤血供。内镜手术的一个重要步骤是在上鼻甲内侧蝶筛隐窝中确定蝶窦开孔的位置。然而，在有些情况下，由于黏膜覆盖，蝶窦开口并不容易看到。当神经剥离子进入蝶筛隐窝距离后鼻孔顶部后方约 15 mm 处，即可进入蝶窦口。在扩大蝶窦开口后，切除或磨除蝶窦前壁，可开放蝶窦。在气化良好的蝶窦中，蝶鞍底部完全被气房包围，称为“蝶鞍型”蝶窦。如果只是部分气化，被称为“前鞍型”。如果没有气化，如幼童（蝶窦气化从 3 岁开始），则为“甲介型”，对于这种类型，即使有影像引导，经鼻暴露蝶鞍也会受到限制。蝶窦内可有多个分隔，且很少在中线。这些分隔附着的后方可能与颈内动脉毗邻，因此应磨除以防止骨折撕裂血管。在手术中，内镜一般位于视野的上方，吸引器位于下方，显微器械在两者之间。如果有必要进行侧方暴露，可切除纸样板，但需保留眶周筋膜。所有骨质切除均应使用带有金刚钻头的高速磨钻。如需打开硬脑膜，应首先电凝硬脑膜，然后切开。随后采用标准的显微外科技术切除肿瘤，包括肿瘤内减压和自神经血管结构分离。当分离囊壁时，应避免牵拉神经血管结构，因为直到手术结尾，这些结构都常处于暴露不佳的状态。

许多经鼻病例存在较高的脑脊液漏风险，需行多层颅底修补。肿瘤切除形成的无效腔可由明胶海绵或脂肪移植物填充。硬脑膜缺损边缘嵌入自体筋膜移植物或异体脱细胞真皮移植物（AlloDerm），在少见的较大缺损中，可用自体犁骨、鼻中隔骨或Medpor加强。最后，将带血管蒂的鼻中隔黏膜瓣旋转覆盖于颅底缺损表面，并可用脂肪移植物或硬膜密封胶固定。鼻中隔黏膜瓣以蝶窦开口下的蝶腭动脉后鼻中隔支为蒂，常用单极从鼻底开始分离制作，前方可至鼻孔，上方沿保留嗅黏膜（鼻中隔黏膜上方1~1.5 cm处）的蝶窦开口上部线性切开。但不适当地在鼻中隔上方使用单极也会损害黏膜、损伤嗅觉。腰大池引流脑脊液用于缺损较大的病例，通常在术后应用2~3天以促进移植物愈合。

内镜经鼻蝶垂体切除术（EETSH）

垂体腺瘤是最常见的经鼻内镜切除的病变。磨除蝶窦前壁骨质暴露蝶窦。鞍底骨窗范围取决于肿瘤的位置，尽管不常用，有时可能还需要在上下方分别暴露出海绵间窦。同样，对于中线部位较大的肿瘤，也不要求显露海绵窦，但可通过辨认颈内动脉内侧的蓝色区域来识别。鞍底硬膜X形切开并避免误入静脉窦，对硬脑膜的边缘电凝处理有利于更好地进入蝶鞍。

绝大多数大腺瘤质地柔软，在获得足够的病理标本后，可轻易地使用刮匙和吸引器将其清除。建议首先清除鞍内下侧面，因为鞍膈过早下降可能会使切除后方的肿瘤受到阻挡。在某些情况下，腺瘤质地允许"包膜外切除"，从切开的硬膜边缘开始，用剥离子在肿瘤外缘和蝶鞍硬脑膜之间环形分离出界面。在这些情况下，应注意分离上极时避免撕破鞍膈的蛛网膜层，以防脑脊液漏，同时防止损伤受压的正常垂体。清除肿瘤上部后鞍膈会完全下降，也表明减压充分。通常正常垂体可保留，因为它比肿瘤质地更坚韧，并且可根据术前MRI上垂体柄偏移方向预测其位置。

在肿瘤减压后，用30°镜检查术腔，可进一步确定角落部位的肿瘤残余。使用0°内镜进行手术，视野为锥状，因此鞍区病变向前延伸至前颅窝的部分位于盲区；为了暴露充分，可磨除鞍结节骨质。如计划更广泛的切开硬脑膜，则需电凝切开上海绵间窦，并通过角度镜补充视野。

微腺瘤切除术需要在周围"正常"垂体内确认病变。微腺瘤的侧别可通过术前影像（MRI和PET，如^{11}C-甲硫氨酸）和生化分析（如岩下窦采血）预测，但在手术时可能位于蝶鞍深部。可通过不同的颜色和柔软度来辨认正常垂体及肿瘤。由于微腺瘤切除最常见的适应证是过度分泌型内分泌病变，因此需要完全切除以达到治愈目的，切除范围应超出软性边界，以确保切除"假包膜"以外的浸润性肿瘤细胞。有一些学者推荐"垂体半切术"，以确保切除充分。

导致脑脊液漏的术中鞍膈裂口可以是一个针尖样小孔，也可以是向鞍上池的较大缺损，根据具体情况采用单纯脂肪、人工材料移植物或鼻中隔黏膜瓣进行修补。

扩大内镜经鼻经蝶骨平台手术（EEETS）

对于鞍上病变，在选择扩大内镜经鼻经蝶骨平台手术时，磁共振的支持因素包括：①血管未被包裹，表现为肿瘤和血管之间的脑皮质袖套；②在冠状面，没有肿瘤向外侧侵犯到颈内动脉或瞳孔中线以外；③T2加权像呈明亮高信号表明肿瘤质地软。另一个重要的考虑因素是肿瘤侵犯视神经管。该入路不易操作视神经管上外侧角，但可磨除、开放并减压视神经管的下缘和内侧缘。

蝶骨平台对应的是两侧的直回，因此经蝶骨平台径路到达鞍上池由前下向后上倾斜。因此，对于像颅咽管瘤这样的病变，蝶骨平台磨除不必向前扩展得太远，而磨除鞍结节处增厚的骨质甚至切开上海绵间窦更为重要。

辨认OCR和视神经管，并在两侧视神经管之间V形磨除蝶骨平台骨质。游离骨碎片时需谨慎，可采用从前向后的方向剥离，以避免其边缘倾斜损伤视神经。控制上海绵间窦出血，剪开后可扩大通路。

在对压迫视交叉的病变进行颅内分离时，应保留起源于下方和沿垂体柄走行的垂体上动脉供血分支，以避免视神经缺血。同样，在磨除视神经管骨质时应保护眼动脉。对于由第三脑室底部延伸到第三脑室的病变，经鼻内镜入路可提供良好的视野和直接的操作通路。位于漏斗后位置的颅咽管瘤比漏斗前位置的颅咽管瘤更具挑战性，特别是在需要保留垂体柄完整性的情况下。

扩大经鼻内镜入路治疗鞍旁病变

如果考虑采用内镜经翼突入路治疗鞍旁病变，第一步是切除中鼻甲，通过钩突后的中鼻道进入上颌窦。需辨认中鼻道的结构，如筛泡和半月裂，在蝶腭动脉孔处电凝蝶腭动脉，其位置与翼管神经有时会交叠。如果计划做鼻中隔黏膜瓣，应在另一侧鼻孔。重要的解剖标志是：翼管神经位于蝶窦底部平面外侧，三叉神经 V2 支起源于圆孔，位于翼管 45° 向上外侧指向的位置。翼腭窝与颞下窝通过翼上颌裂相连，上颌动脉终末支位于其中。翼腭神经节发自 V2，它有包括腭大和腭小神经在内的多个分支，而 V2 延续为眶下神经。副交感和交感神经纤维均通过翼管进入翼腭神经节，尽管只有副交感神经突触。三叉神经节在深部自上外侧骑跨岩骨段颈内动脉。打开上颌窦后壁可查见该神经节。磨除骨质时翼管指示水平的岩骨段颈内动脉及垂直的海绵窦段颈内动脉的连接处。三叉神经鞘瘤可侵蚀周围骨质，形成通往岩尖自然扩大的手术通路。该入路也可用于治疗岩尖区胆固醇肉芽肿。

术后

结果

术后结果因疾病种类和肿瘤位置的不同而有很大差异。对于无功能垂体腺瘤，一项大型 meta 分析显示总体死亡率、并发症发病率和复发风险分别为小于 1%、小于等于 5% 和 18%（Murad et al.，2010）。一项颅咽管瘤的 meta 分析显示，37% 的患者在手术后新发内分泌功能障碍，与接受放疗或不接受放疗的次全切除相比，全切除后的内分泌功能障碍发生率是后者的 2.5 倍（Sughrue et al.，2011）。最近的另一项综述指出，次全切除后再进行放疗可获得最佳的无进展生存结果，5 年和 10 年生存率分别为 93% 和 82%（Lo et al.，2014）。对于前颅底脑膜瘤，最近一项综述表明，开颅手术（92.8%）比内镜手术（63.2%）更容易实现肿瘤全切除，内镜下脑脊液漏发生率（31.6%）高于开颅手术（6%）（Komotar et al.，2012）。

并发症管理

经颅手术相关的并发症通常包括脑软化和术后癫痫、感染、术后血肿、脑神经或血管损伤。通过做足够的骨窗暴露从而尽量减少脑组织牵拉和细致的硬膜内手术技术，可降低术后脑软化和癫痫发作的风险。术前、术中使用抗生素和严格的无菌技术可降低感染风险。术后血肿可通过术前停用抗凝和抗血小板等药物和良好的止血来预防；术后血肿若有明显临床症状应积极清除。术前充分研究每个患者独特的解剖特点和影像，包括血管成像（如果适用），可避免脑神经和血管损伤。肿瘤内减压，包括使用超声吸引器，可改善手术视野和增加分离的安全性。如果大动脉被肿瘤包裹，留下一小部分残余肿瘤比行复杂的血运重建术或造成血管损伤更为可取。最后，如果怀疑有血管损伤，则应考虑术中或术后行血管造影。

经鼻手术的并发症通常与肿瘤切除不充分或脑脊液漏有关；偶尔可见神经血管损伤。通过术前影像的仔细评估，以及寻找肿瘤侵犯及附着点的范围，可降低肿瘤切除不充分的风险。肿瘤切除不充分通常是由骨窗暴露不充分引起的。骨窗暴露应至少足以包括肿瘤的附着部位，且不限制暴露。如果这难以实现，那么所选择的入路可能不适用于该病变。严密的硬膜封闭可降低脑脊液漏的风险。有多种手术方法，但通常建议多层封闭，硬膜下嵌入筋膜或其他硬膜替代物、脂肪、鼻中隔黏膜瓣及鼻腔填塞。多层封闭加硬膜下嵌入植入物，再联合 3~7 天的脑脊液腰大池引流，可显著减少术后脑脊液漏。最后，合理的术前计划和基于影像学了解患者的个体化解剖结构，可降低神经血管结构损伤的风险。由于手术操作空间又长又窄，外科医生的经验也将在手术中发挥重要作用。此外，角度内镜会产生很好的视觉效果，但手术可能会受到工作角度或显微操作不方便的限制，参见**专栏 27.1**。

争议

经颅入路与扩大内镜入路治疗脑膜瘤的比较

外科医生应该同时掌握用于切除肿瘤（如前颅底脑膜瘤）的经颅术式和扩大的内镜技术，因为这两种技术不仅有用，而且对于一些肿瘤（如大型嗅神经母细胞瘤）是同时需要的。然而，决定使用何种方法可以而且应该是一个非常个体化的决定，这取决于许多因素，尤其是手术医生的经验和术中舒适度。

根据肿瘤的位置和大小，经鼻扩大或扩展的内镜经筛板入路对某些肿瘤具有特殊的优势。此入路可直接暴露并切除前颅底增厚的骨质附着，任何生长在鼻旁窦的肿瘤都更适合通过这种方法切除。同

专栏 27.1　病例

男：21 岁，复视、左眼外展受限 1 个月。详细的神经检查显示为单纯性左侧第Ⅵ脑神经麻痹。增强磁共振成像显示蝶窦、鞍区、鞍上、颅底及左侧海绵窦病变。CT 显示病灶内有大的钙化灶（图 27.8）。左侧翼点开颅经硬膜外入路通过 Parkinson 三角进入海绵窦，使用超声吸引器、普通吸引器和经蝶窦环形刮匙切除。在整个手术过程中，使用显微镜和内镜作为观察工具。在同一手术区域，采用经鼻入路进入蝶窦、鞍区和颅底内以处理肿瘤。借助吸引器和环形刮匙等手段切除该肿瘤，并使用金刚石钻头磨开颅底。同样，在这部分手术中手术显微镜和内镜都被广泛使用。用自体脂肪移植物填充海绵窦和蝶窦，用纤维蛋白胶封闭蝶窦内移植物，并在 6 天后夹闭并取出脑室外引流管。术后 MRI 显示在后上侧有微小的残留肿瘤。无并发症，也无新发神经功能缺损。病理分析显示该组织符合软骨肉瘤，患者将进一步接受放射治疗。

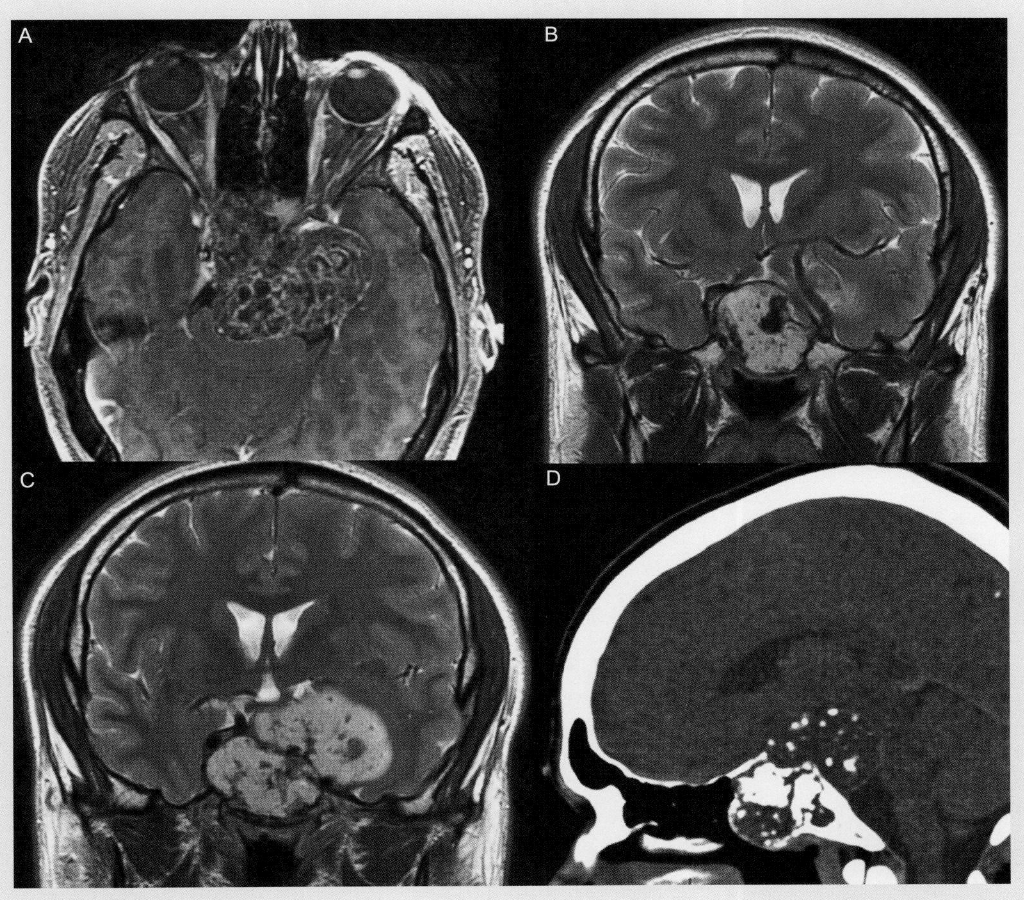

图 27.8　轴向 T1 加权 MRI 显示肿瘤累及蝶窦、左侧海绵窦和桥前池（A）。冠状位 T2 加权 MRI 显示左侧颈内动脉向前、上移位（A），视交叉抬高，侵犯左侧海绵窦（C）。矢状位 CT 显示病灶内有大的钙化灶，填充蝶窦、蝶鞍和鞍上区域（D）

样，肿瘤在手术的早期就被阻断血流，甚至筛前和筛后动脉也可在肿瘤切除前电凝并切断。此外，这种入路减少了对大脑的牵拉和对神经血管结构的操作。

上述内镜入路的缺点与中线暴露固有的局限性和术后脑脊液漏的风险有关。向眶内侧壁或眶顶外侧延伸，向视神经管外侧延伸，或向蝶骨嵴延伸的肿瘤或脑膜尾征，很难通过中线暴露完全切除，但更容易通过经颅入路切除。与经颅入路相比，内镜入路中神经血管结构往往较晚才可见，而且如果操作不当容易对其造成损伤。因此，对于明显包绕脑神经或颈内动脉、前交通动脉或大脑前动脉的肿瘤，最好通过经颅入路，这样上述血管在病灶的近端和远端都可看到（必要时可控制）。需要修补的脑脊液漏在内镜入路中比经颅入路更常见，因为与经颅入路相比，经鼻入路的封闭难度更大，而且内镜入路造成的支撑性骨质的缺损更大。然而，现代外科技术包括使用异体脱细胞真皮移植物（AlloDerm）等材料进行多层封闭和带蒂鼻中隔黏膜瓣联合脑脊液腰大池引流，可显著降低这些手术的脑脊液漏发生率。

结论

鞍区和鞍上肿瘤仍然是最具挑战性的神经外科疾病之一，因为周围解剖结构复杂，重要的神经血管结构高度集中。此外，病理类型的多样性使基于病理特点的治疗方法和临床预后都存在很大差别。然而，外科技术的不断进步，包括经颅手术和经鼻入路中都在使用内镜设备和内镜技术，也在使治疗效果不断提高。

延伸阅读、参考文献、EBRAIN 的相关链接

扫描书末二维码获取。

第六篇 肿瘤和颅底——颅后窝肿瘤

第 28 章 髓母细胞瘤

James Rutka 著
吴越、钟东 译，钟东 审校

引言

1925 年，Bailey 和 Cushing 开创性地描述了一类“好发于儿童的小脑中线部位的胶质瘤”，并命名为髓母细胞瘤（Bailey and Cushing，1925）。他们推测这种肿瘤起源于第四脑室室管膜的胚胎性未分化细胞，描述了其细胞结构和核分裂象增多的典型组织学特征。后来的研究发现其他一些幕上肿瘤也具有这些特征及相似的不良预后。这类异质性的“小而圆的蓝色细胞”肿瘤被命名为中枢神经系统原始神经外胚层肿瘤（primitive neuroectodermal tumours，PNET）。根据 2007 年世界卫生组织分类（Louis et al.，2007），这类肿瘤由未分化或分化不良的神经上皮细胞组成。根据各自最突出的细胞特点，被命名为神经母细胞瘤、室管膜母细胞瘤、髓上皮瘤、节细胞神经母细胞瘤和松果体母细胞瘤。髓母细胞瘤归类为幕下原始神经外胚层肿瘤。然而，新的分子生物学研究证据表明，髓母细胞瘤是一种具有独特生物学行为的恶性肿瘤。此外，研究分析表明，相对组织病理学分类而言，根据肿瘤的生物学特征对中枢神经系统原始神经外胚层肿瘤进行分类更加简明和实用（Picard et al.，2012）。

近期美国脑肿瘤注册中心（Central Brain Tumor Registry of the United States，CBTRUS）（Ostrom et al.，2013）援引 WHO 胚胎性肿瘤的分类（髓母细胞瘤和中枢神经系统原始神经外胚层肿瘤）显示，0~14 岁年龄组最常见的大脑和中枢神经系统肿瘤是毛细胞性星形细胞瘤（17.5%）和胚胎性肿瘤（15.7%）。而 15~19 岁年龄组的胚胎性肿瘤比例降至 4.3%。5~9 岁年龄组数据经年龄校正后的髓母细胞瘤发病率为 0.66/10 万。患者中男性比例较女性稍高（1.4/1）。

病因、发病机制、分类

现已证实多种多瘤病毒可在大鼠和仓鼠中诱发与人类髓母细胞瘤（medulloblastoma，MB）类似的肿瘤。然而，目前尚未发现人类胚胎性肿瘤的确切致病因素。有学说认为，髓母细胞瘤来源于发育中小脑的外颗粒层（external granular layer，EGL）所在区域。另一些学说则关注脑室和背侧脑干的神经祖细胞区域。外颗粒层（EGL）中神经元前体细胞的增殖受 Sonic Hedgehog（SHH）信号通路的调控（Wechsler-Reya and Scott，1999）。髓母细胞瘤基因组学和分子生物学研究的类似发现加深了我们对其发病机制和生物学行为的认识和理解。目前，已证实至少存在四种在遗传学和临床表现上各不相同的髓母细胞瘤变异型（Taylor et al.，2012）。对髓母细胞瘤按这些亚型进行分类在预测患者预后和生存期方面已显现出重要价值。

1. WNT（Wingless）亚型表现为 CTNNB1 基因突变导致的 WNT 信号通路的激活，引起细胞核内 β 联蛋白的增加。另一个常见现象为 6 号染色体缺失。该亚型约占髓母细胞瘤的 10%，常见于大龄儿童和成人，男女性别比为 1∶1。大部分患者组织学类型为经典型，预后很好。
2. SHH（Sonic Hedgehog）亚型表现为 SHH 信号通路的激活，并常合并 PCTH1、SMO 和 SUFU 基因突变，同时可以有 GLI2 和 MYCN 基因扩增。常见的染色体异常为 9q 和 10q 缺失。该亚型占髓母细胞瘤的 30%，好发年龄呈双高峰分布，常见于婴儿和成人，男女性别比为 1∶1。此亚型常见的组织学类型为促纤维增生型，婴儿患者预后较好，而其他 SHH 激活的髓母细胞瘤预后一般。
3. 亚型 3 尚未发现有主要信号通路的激活。该亚型的特征为 MYC 基因扩增。重要的细胞遗传学变异为 17q 等臂染色体。约 25% 的髓母细胞瘤属于这一亚型，常见于儿童和婴儿，性别比例男性稍多。常见的组织学类型是大细胞间变型（large cell anaplastic，LCA）肿瘤。此亚型患者的预后不良。

4. 亚型4是目前认识最不清楚的一型。常见的异常扩增基因是MYCN，常见的结构改变为SNCAIP复制（亚型4α）。和亚型3患者类似，亚型4的大多数患者存在17q等臂染色体。亚型4是最常见的髓母细胞瘤亚型（占35%），儿童常见，性别比例男性居多（3：1）。组织学类型主要为经典型，少部分病例为大细胞间变型（LCA）。与SHH亚型患者一样，亚型4的患者预后差异较大。

如**表28.1**所示，髓母细胞瘤常合并家族性癌症综合征。Gorlin综合征（痣样基底细胞癌综合征）常合并的髓母细胞瘤组织学类型为促纤维增生型，属于SHH亚型。Turcot综合征合并的髓母细胞瘤见于10岁以下的儿童。Li-Fraumeni综合征患者约5%合并髓母细胞瘤。

原始神经外胚层肿瘤（PNET）的发病机制认为髓母细胞瘤和幕上PNET来源于室管膜下基质细胞，这类细胞可分化成为神经元和胶质细胞。因此推测它们可能存在共同的前体细胞。然而，越来越多的研究表明髓母细胞瘤（也即幕下PNETs）和幕上PNETs存在不同的遗传学改变。另外两类胚胎性组织来源的实体肿瘤包括非典型畸胎样/横纹肌样瘤（atypical teratoid rhabdoid tumour，ATRT）和富含神经毡和真菊形团的胚胎性肿瘤（embryonal tumour with abundant neuropil and true rosettes，ETANTR）。ATRT好发于幼龄儿童，与髓母细胞瘤的鉴别特征是INI1/hSNF5染色阴性。ETANTR原称为“室管膜母细胞瘤”，预后很差。根据转录特征可将中枢神经系统PNET分为3个分子亚型（Picard et al.，2012）：

1. 亚型1：染色体19q13.41-42位点的C19MC基因扩增及LIN28阳性。该亚型富含神经干细胞基因。临床特点为发病年龄低、中线部位肿瘤（小脑、脑干、脊髓）、预后不良。
2. 亚型2：表达更多的少神经标志物［一种区分运动神经元和少突胶质细胞分化的标志物，少突胶质细胞转录因子2（OLIG2）呈阳性］。
3. 亚型3：迄今为止尚未发现该亚型的确切标志物，仅被描述为LIN28/OLIG2阴性。该亚型的基因存在间充质分化。与其他两种亚型相比，该亚型患者更易出现肿瘤转移，但总体预后实际上更好（Adamski et al.，2014）。

组织病理学

典型的髓母细胞瘤起源于小脑蚓部并长入第四脑室，为粉红色、灰色或紫色肿块。肿瘤可见小灶性坏死，与幕上PNET有相似的大体特点。实质性肿瘤生长更快，并更常伴有囊变、出血和坏死（Louis et al.，2007）。主要有3种组织学类型：

1. 经典型（**图28.1A**）最常见（占70%）。由紧密排列的细胞构成，具有圆形、卵圆形或更多长而深染的细胞核，周围有稀疏的细胞质。少于40%的病例可见到神经母细胞菊形团（Homer-Wright）。肿瘤常见神经元分化，表现为神经元标志物突触素阳性。
2. 促纤维增生型（**图28.1B**）在婴儿和成人中更常见，通常与SHH分子亚型有关。该亚型表现为结节状和无网织纤维区（“白岛”）两种形式，周围有高度增生的、具有多形性细胞核和致密细胞间网状纤维的肿瘤细胞。结节内突触素表达阳性，而结节外细胞的Ki-67增殖指数更高并且GFAP表达阳性。该亚型的一种变异型为伴有广泛结节的髓母细胞瘤（medulloblastoma with extensive nodularity，MBEN），原命名为小脑神经母细胞瘤。促纤维增生型婴儿患者预后较好（Rutkowski et al.，2005）。

表28.1 髓母细胞瘤相关的家族性综合征

综合征	外显率	基因	位点	其他表现
Gorlin	AD	PTCH	9q31	BCCs、掌跖皮肤点状凹陷、颌骨囊肿、硬脑膜钙化、分叉肋、卵巢纤维瘤、巨头畸形
Turcot	AD	APC	5q21	多发性结肠肿瘤、其他脑肿瘤（星形细胞瘤、室管膜瘤）
Li-Fraumeni	AD	TP53	17p13	肉瘤、绝经前乳腺癌、急性白血病、其他脑肿瘤（星形细胞瘤、脉络丛肿瘤）
Bloom	AR	BLM1	15q26.1	侏儒症、光过敏、面部皮疹
范科尼贫血	AR	多基因		骨髓衰竭、白血病、实体肿瘤

AD，常染色体显性；AR，常染色体隐性；BBC，基底细胞癌

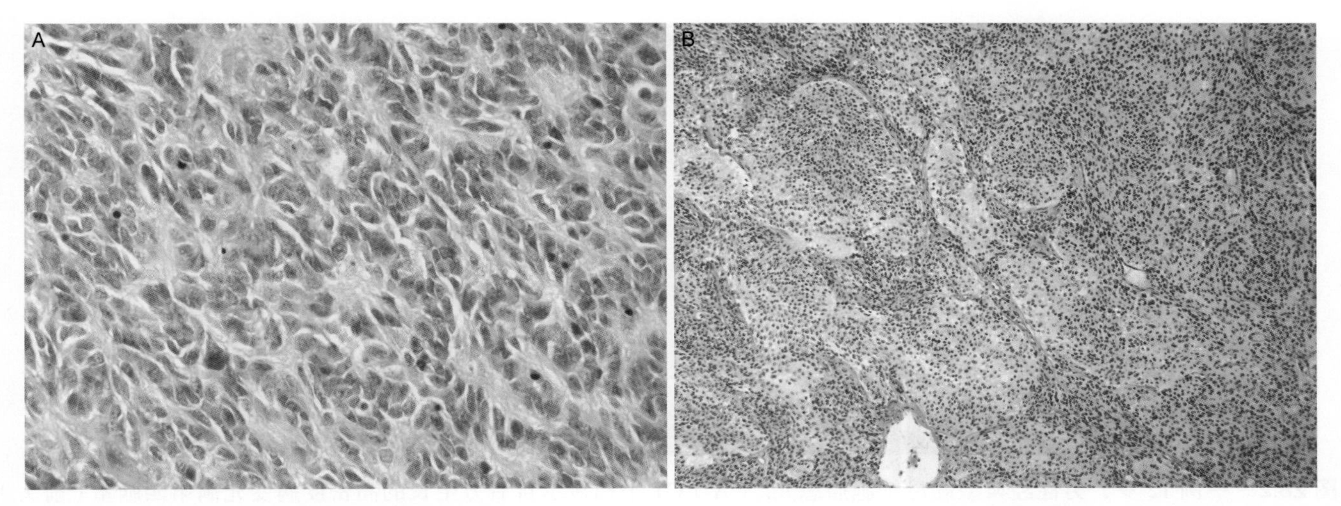

图 28.1 （A）经典型髓母细胞瘤，神经母细胞菊形团（Homer-Wright）在这种Ⅳ级肿瘤中虽不常见，但具有高度特征性。（B）促纤维增生型/结节型髓母细胞瘤中有分化更好的苍白色结节样组织，为髓母细胞瘤较好预后的特征。该组织学特点在促纤维增生型/结节型中多见

Courtesy of Dr Kieren Allinson, Department of Pathology, Addenbrooke's Hospital, Cambridge.

3. 大细胞型和间变型在细胞学上有明显的重叠，目前认为是同一类型。这类变异型见于4%的髓母细胞瘤中，更多常见于分子亚型3，预后最差。该类型细胞黏附性差，有丝分裂和凋亡现象多见。

以往认为髓肌母细胞瘤和黑色素性髓母细胞瘤是两种独立的亚型，现在认为这两种亚型分别是髓母细胞瘤的肌源性分化和黑色素性分化。

中枢神经系统原始神经外胚层肿瘤与胚胎性肿瘤的显微镜下"小而圆的蓝色细胞"特征类似。确切而言，这些分化程度低的细胞的细胞核/细胞质比例高。而分化较好的亚型可见神经元的组织学特征。神经母细胞菊形团（Homer-Wright）的出现频率各异。肿瘤钙化常见，也可见到血管内皮细胞增殖。Ki-67增殖指数在各亚型间存在差异，但总体较高。

临床表现

临床症状和体征取决于患者的年龄。颅后窝中线部位肿瘤常引起梗阻性脑积水和颅内压增高。前囟未闭的婴幼儿可导致巨头畸形和囟门膨隆，常伴有进食差、易怒、发育迟缓及呕吐。这类患儿往往被诊断为牛奶过敏和胃肠道疾病。严重病例的急性表现为昏睡、呼吸暂停、心动过缓和痫样发作（"脑积水危象"导致的强直状态）。巨大原始神经外胚层肿瘤的低龄患儿可因瘤内出血病情迅速恶化，并伴有脑疝表现。

大龄患儿通常表现为晨起头痛和呕吐，呕吐后头痛可缓解，其原因可能是睡眠过程中CO_2的积累引起脑血管扩张，从而导致颅内压（ICP）升高。症状持续时间从几周到两个月不等。后期可出现预警体征，如第Ⅵ对脑神经麻痹导致的斜视和（或）复视。肿瘤的直接压迫症状取决于肿瘤的部位。中线病变引起躯干共济失调和长束体征。侧方的病变见于较大的儿童和青少年，表现为脑神经麻痹、眩晕和共济失调。儿童突发的斜颈也提示需进一步检查。

30%~40%的髓母细胞瘤在诊断时即发生转移，主要由诊断影像学检查发现。亚型3和亚型4的特点是早期播散。脊髓转移瘤可表现为（下肢）轻瘫、膀胱功能障碍或神经根症状。

影像学特点

对于前囟未闭的儿童，头部超声可用于初步影像诊断颅后窝肿瘤引起的脑积水。计算机断层扫描（CT）可显示小脑中线病变以及病变周围血管源性水肿和阻塞性脑积水（**图 28.2**）。髓母细胞瘤是富细胞肿瘤，CT扫描上呈高密度。22%的病例可见钙化，59%的病例可见囊性变（Poretti et al.，2012）。所有颅后窝肿瘤患者都应进行详细的头部和脊柱磁共振检查（MRI）。幼龄儿童可能需要全身麻醉才能完成MRI扫描。如果患者由于颅内压增高病情迅速恶化，则不能因为要做MRI检查而延误及时的外科治疗。和脑组织相比，T1加权像上肿瘤表现为低等信号，T2加权像上肿瘤信号呈多样性。富细胞的病变T2加权呈低信号。像髓母细胞瘤这种富细胞的高级别肿瘤，其细胞核/细胞质比高，游离水较少，在弥散加

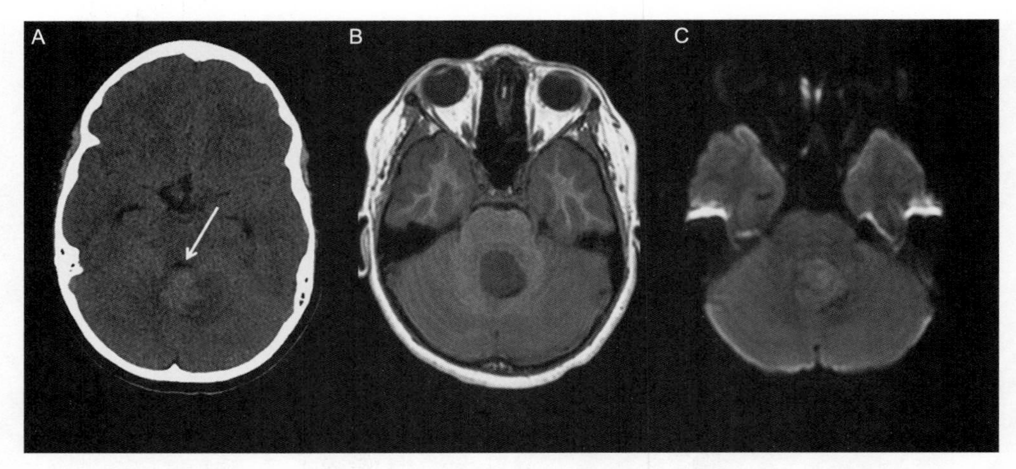

图 28.2 一例 12 岁、男性经典型髓母细胞瘤患儿。（A）CT 平扫显示自后方生长的高密度病变充满第四脑室（箭头）并引起三室脑积水。（B）在轴位 T1 加权 MRI 上，肿瘤呈低信号。（C）DWI 成像呈高信号（弥散受限）。CT 高密度和 DWI 弥散受限是富细胞性和高度恶性的标志

Courtesy of Dr Kieren Allinson, Department of Pathology, Addenbrooke's Hospital, Cambridge.

权像（DWI）上表现为高信号（弥散受限）（Jaremko et al.，2010）。这个特点可用于鉴别髓母细胞瘤与其他常见颅后窝肿瘤，如毛细胞星形细胞瘤（pilocytic astrocytoma，PA）和室管膜瘤。此外，髓母细胞瘤通常起源于第四脑室顶部，而室管膜瘤则起源于第四脑室底部。室管膜瘤表现为“可塑性”生长方式，肿瘤可从第四脑室出口长出。约 14% 的髓母细胞瘤也可见长出第四脑室出口。约 40% 的初诊髓母细胞瘤可见脑室系统和脑脊髓蛛网膜下腔的种植转移（**图 28.3**）。术前应行全神经轴的磁共振平扫或钆增强扫描以发现转移性病灶。术后为了肿瘤分级而进行的神经轴扫描应推迟到 2 周以后，以减少残腔和血液降解产物引起的假阳性可能（Meyers et al.，2000）。

中枢神经系统原始神经外胚层肿瘤可能具有相似的影像学特征。幕上中枢神经系统原始神经外胚层肿瘤的 MRI 特点是肿瘤大而瘤周水肿较轻（**图 28.4**），增强 MRI 扫描呈不均匀强化。DWI 一般呈弥散受限表现，相应的表观弥散系数（ADC）值较低（富细胞特点）。常见钙化和瘤内出血，两者在梯度成像（gradient imaging，GE）上都表现为磁敏感区。鉴于肿瘤常沿软脑膜扩散，因此应行全神经轴的影像学检查。

治疗

儿童髓母细胞瘤和中枢神经系统 PNET 患者应在有治疗经验的儿科中心进行多学科协作治疗。患者表现为梗阻性脑积水导致的颅内压增高的症状和体征。在患者病情允许的情况下，详细的术前评估至关重要。通常静脉输注地塞米松可通过减轻血管源性脑水肿来改善症状。各中心根据情况完善相应序列的全神经轴 MRI 检查（“肿瘤处理流程”）。如时间允许，可完善听力和肾功能检查作为治疗基线评估，因为辅助化疗和放射治疗有相应的毒理作用。需患儿的家长同意治疗方案、参与临床研究和输血治疗。

对于脑积水的处理尚存在争议。如患者病情危急，可急诊行脑室外引流（external ventricular drain，EVD）以挽救生命，但需特别小心避免发生小脑幕切迹上疝。仅 10%~40% 的患儿术后需行永久性脑脊液分流，因此不推荐常规行脑室腹腔分流术（ventriculoperitoneal shunts，VPS），因为行 VPS 的患者将终生面临分流相关并发症的风险（Lee et al.，1994）。术后需行永久性分流手术的危险因素有幼龄、术前严重脑积水、肿瘤体积大、肿瘤播散。巴黎的一项研究发现，术前行内镜下第三脑室造瘘（endoscopic third ventriculostomy，ETV）显著降低了术后脑积水的风险（Sainte-Rose et al.，2001），但该研究作者也承认常规行 EVT 会增加一些不需造瘘治疗患儿的手术风险。术前获得的脑脊液标本都应行细胞学检查。

手术治疗

多数外科医生倾向于俯卧位中线枕下开颅手术。术中神经监测尤为重要。术中持续性出血通常提示肿瘤残留。神经内镜是探查“角落里”残余肿瘤的有力工具。手术目标是在最大安全性的前提下全切肿瘤（gross total resection，GTR）。术后 MRI 复查肿瘤残余体积大于 1.5 cm^3 和患者不良预后相关（Zeltzer et al.，1999）。如肿瘤侵入第四脑室底或与后组脑神经粘连紧密，则应避免过度切除肿瘤，避免导致

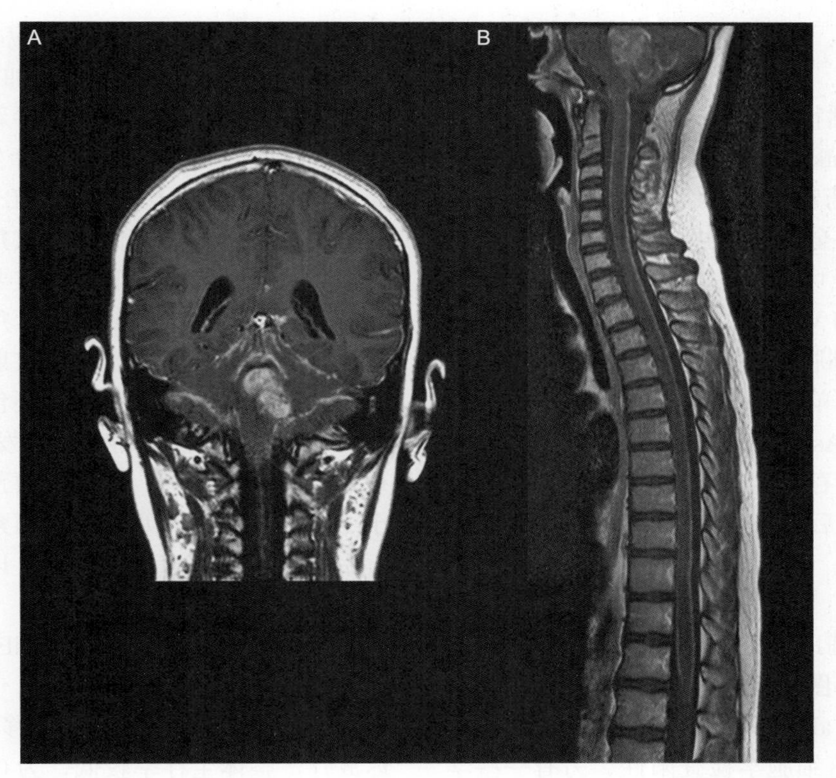

图 28.3　一例 10 岁男性患儿、髓母细胞瘤播散。（A）冠状位 T1 加权增强扫描见第四脑室内原发肿瘤呈均匀强化及小脑软膜弥漫性强化。（B）全脊柱正中矢状位 T1 加权增强扫描见全脊髓表面薄层状软膜强化，呈"糖衣"征

Courtesy of Dr Kieren Allinson, Department of Pathology, Addenbrooke's Hospital, Cambridge.

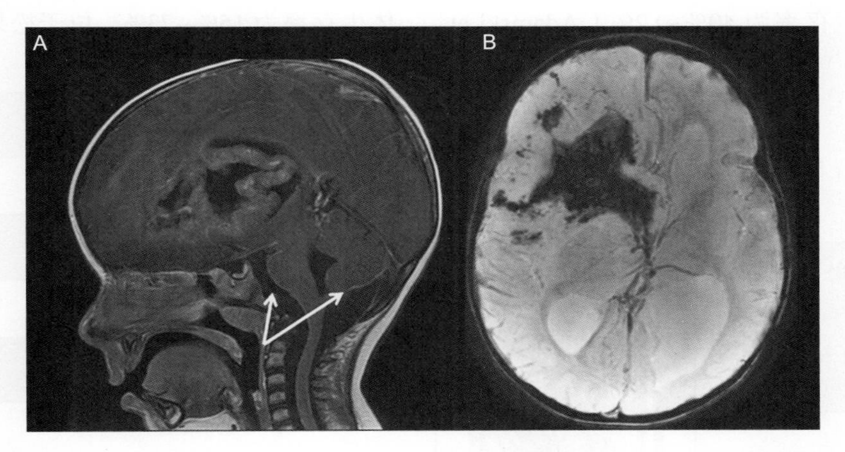

图 28.4　一例 2 岁男性患儿、幕上 PNET。（A）正中矢状位 T1 加权增强扫描见一巨大分叶状肿瘤，内有巨大的囊性成分，边缘较厚呈均匀强化。箭头示沿脑干和小脑下表面的软脑膜薄层强化。（B）轴向梯度回波序列显示肿瘤中央明显磁敏感区（暗区），以及周边小片状磁敏感区（出血和钙化）

Courtesy of Dr Kieren Allinson, Department of Pathology, Addenbrooke's Hospital, Cambridge.

大大降低患者生活质量的术后瘫痪。一些中心利用术中 MRI 来实现肿瘤全切，取得了令人鼓舞的效果（Avula et al.，2013）。术后应在 72 小时内或 2 周后复查 MRI，以避免血液降解产物导致的假阳性。腰穿脑脊液可行细胞学检查和了解肿瘤分期，结合全神经轴 MRI 扫描，可提高敏感性（Fouladi et al.，1999）。腰穿脑脊液标本比 EVD 或术中脑脊液标本更可靠（Gajjar et al.，1999）。

非手术治疗

患儿的年龄很大程度上决定了首次髓母细胞瘤切除术后的后续治疗方案。3 岁以下的儿童，应避免放射治疗（放疗），因为放疗可导致神经认知功能损害的后遗症。

3 岁以下

即使对于肿瘤播散的病例，现有的治疗方案也不推荐放射治疗（Rutkowski et al.，2005）。通常，先进行系统性的铂类药物化疗，然后再进行清髓化疗和自体干细胞移植。全身化疗也可联合脑室内甲氨蝶呤化疗。脑室内化疗可通过头皮下贮液囊（Ommaya 囊）或已经放置了的 VP 分流系统完成，需特别注意避免甲氨蝶呤扩散到腹腔内（如分流阀）。局灶放疗可用于复发患者，与单纯化疗相比其疗效尚存在争议（Grill et al.，2005；Ashley et al.，2012）。3 岁以下患儿预后很差，5 年生存率为 50%~70%。组织学亚型为促纤维增生型者预后较好，5 年生存率近 90%。

3 岁以上

这一年龄组的辅助治疗可根据临床标准分为一般风险组和高危组（**图 28.5**）。预后不良的因素包括肿瘤转移（Chang et al.，1969）、肿瘤残余体积大于 1.5 cm^3、脑脊液脱落细胞学检查阳性，另有一些学者认为是大细胞 / 间变型组织学亚型也是预后不良因素。高危组患儿放疗剂量为 3600 cGy 的颅脑脊髓照射再追加瘤床照射和局部转移灶照射。放疗后辅助全身化疗。5 年生存率为 40%~82%（Adamski et al.，2014）。一般风险组患者应行减量颅脑脊髓放疗（2340 cGy），对肿瘤床再追加 5400 cGy~5580 cGy 的补量照射，通常同步行长春新碱化疗。放疗后行全身化疗（以顺铂为基础），5 年生存率为 85%（Gajjar et al.，2006）。质子放疗优于光子放疗，虽然二者对靶区放射剂量相同，但质子放疗对瘤周正常组织的影响更小。目前质子放疗的重要不足是费用更高以及可获得性差。提高放射治疗疗效的策略包括超分割放疗和使用放疗增敏剂。放射治疗的重大风险除了对幼儿认知功能损害以外还包括耳毒性、内分泌障碍（甲状腺功能障碍和生长发育不良）、放射性坏死、继发恶性肿瘤。复发肿瘤预后极差，生存率低于 10%。预后相对好一点的因素包括局部复发并可行手术切除、化疗敏感性高，以及可再次行放射治疗（Pizer et al.，2011）。

目前婴儿中枢神经系统 PNET 的治疗方案基于与髓母细胞瘤治疗相类似的方案。剂量密集化疗方案包括大剂量化疗联合自体干细胞移植用于试图避免或推迟放疗。整体生存率较低，为 0~49%。大龄儿童中枢神经系统 PNET 较少见，尚无高强度循证医学证据的治疗方案。大龄儿童被视为高危组患者。目前尚不清楚肿瘤残留或转移是否为不良预后的强力因素。总体生存率为 15%~73%，位于松果体区的 PNET 比其

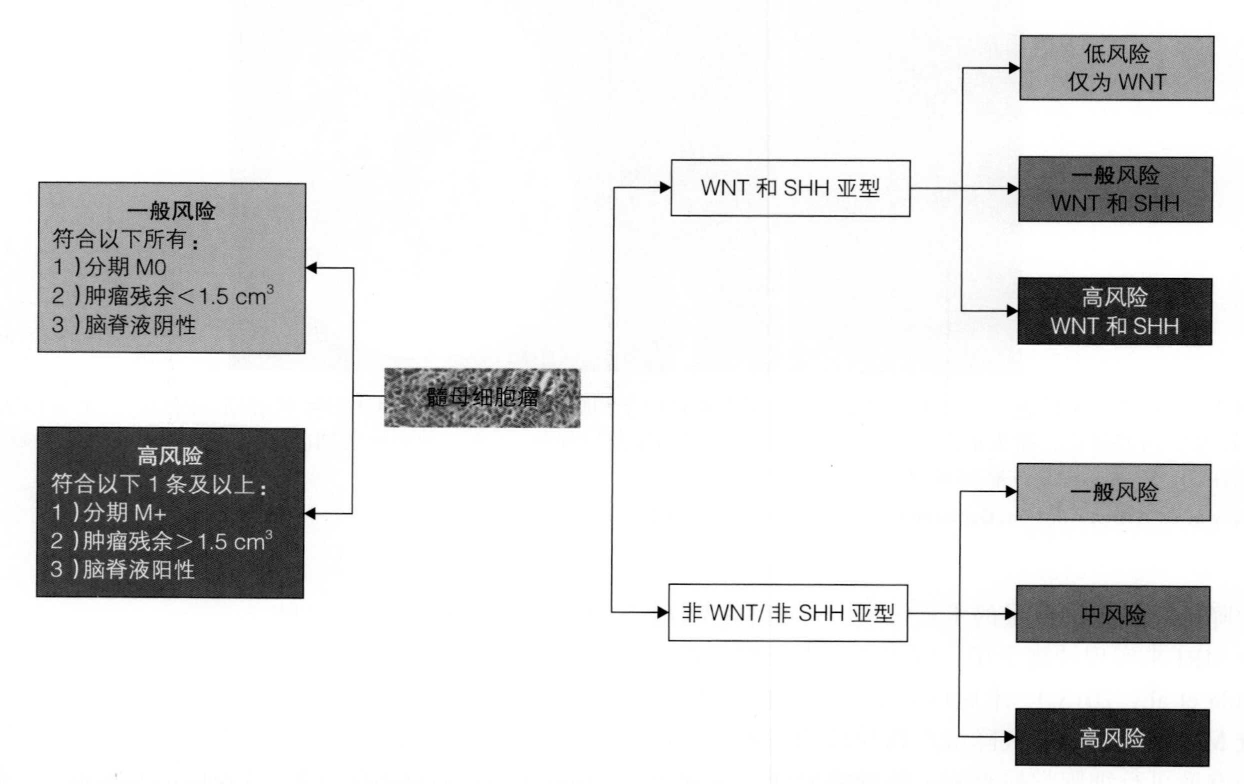

图 28.5 左图所示为年龄大于 3 岁的髓母细胞瘤患者临床分型，分为一般风险组和高风险组。右图所示基于分子特征的髓母细胞瘤分型（Gottardo et al.，2014）。高风险标准包括肿瘤转移（M+）、MYC 扩增、非全切 / 近全切除和组织学为大细胞 / 间变型

他部位预后更好（Chintagumpala et al., 2009）。

胚胎性肿瘤将来的治疗策略是一个值得深入研究的领域。根据细胞遗传学生物标志物对患者进行分组可以预测生存期，并为改进治疗策略提供依据（Shih et al., 2014）。WNT亚型的患者生存率较高提示这类患者可能接受了过度治疗（Adamski et al., 2014）。新型分子靶向药物smoothened抑制剂LDE225和GDC-449用于治疗SHH亚型患者正在研究中并已取得了令人鼓舞的疗效（Kool et al., 2014）。研究发现转移性病变之间极其相似而与其相应的原发肿瘤显著不同，据此转移性病变的治疗策略可能发生巨大变化（Wu et al., 2012）。生物学预后因子有重要意义，目前已证实与髓母细胞瘤不良预后相关的因子包括非WNT/SHH亚型、FSTL5过表达、MYC/MYCN扩增和17q染色体获得。中枢神经系统PNET的不良预后预测因子包括C19MC扩增和LIN28阳性。

病例报告——争议

图28.6所示为一例2.5岁女性患者。主诉为进行加重的下肢无力和膀胱功能障碍2周（**图28.6A**）。矢状位T1加权增强MRI显示第四脑室内肿瘤呈不均匀强化，合并三室脑积水（**图28.6B**）。脊髓MRI显示多发性结节状转移灶，胸2和胸9水平脊髓受压，腰段脊髓巨大占位病变压迫马尾神经。可见膀胱扩张。该患者需优先处理的问题有三个：神经功能障碍的治疗、肿瘤的治疗、脑积水的治疗。优先处理哪个问题存在争议。神经肿瘤学多学科决策认为先进行颅后窝原发肿瘤手术治疗，并尽快对脊椎病变进行放射治疗。由于不能确定其症状由哪个脊髓转移灶引起，所以不先行脊椎手术治疗。原发病灶（髓母细胞瘤）在24小时内全切（**图28.6C**）并在术后第一天开始脊髓放疗。患者5天内接受了2000 cGy的下胸段和腰段脊髓照射。患者术后脑积水仍存在，治疗方案在脑室外引流术和脑室腹腔分流术之间存在争议。最终方案选择行脑室腹腔分流术，其原因是基于患者急需辅助治疗，以及需要尽可能减少脑脊液分流术后并发症（Kulkarni et al., 2010）。患者术后乏力症状缓解，并根据髓母细胞瘤高危组方案进行进一步治疗。

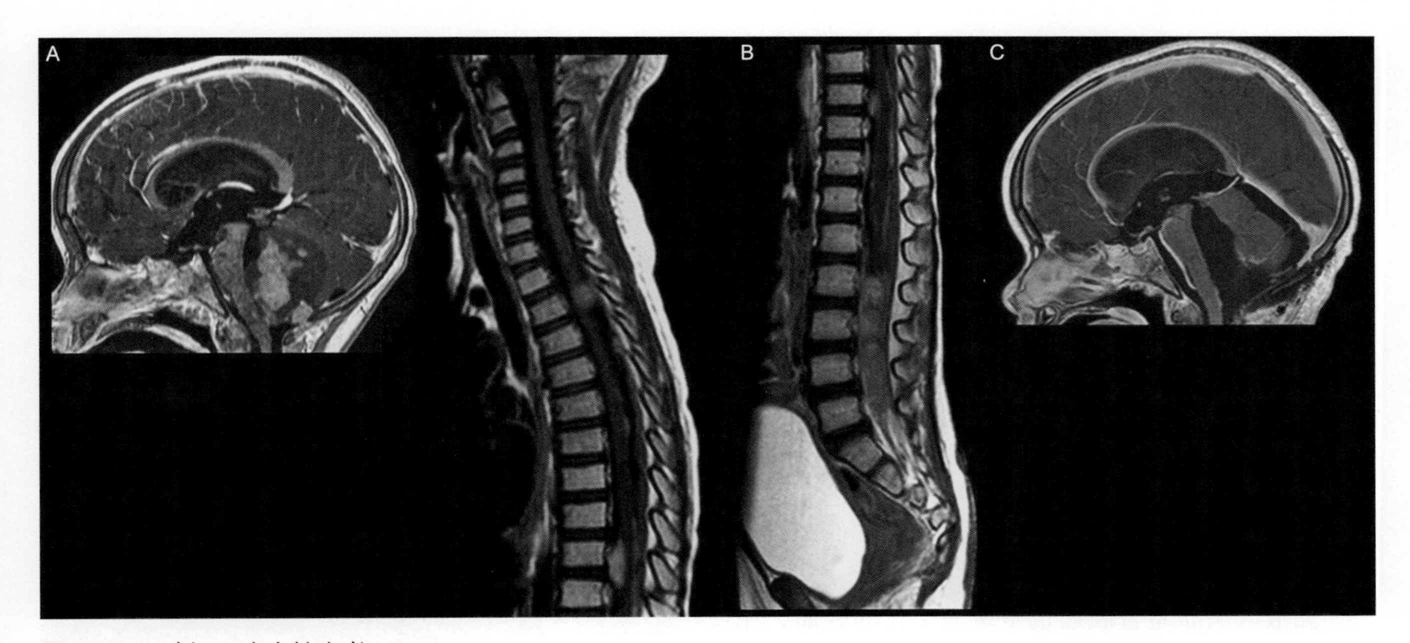

图28.6　一例2.5岁女性患者

Courtesy of Dr Kieren Allinson, Department of Pathology, Addenbrooke's Hospital, Cambridge

参考文献、EBRAIN的相关链接

扫描书末二维码获取。

第 29 章　室管膜瘤

Christopher Chandler 著
吴越、钟东 译，钟东 审校

流行病学

室管膜瘤是一种生长缓慢的神经胶质瘤，起源于中枢神经系统（central nervous system，CNS）室管膜表面的放射状胶质干细胞，包括室管膜下瘤和黏液乳头状室管膜瘤。因而，室管膜瘤的发生与脑室表面最相关，主要见于第四脑室。大部分室管膜瘤发生于儿童，约占儿童中枢神经系统肿瘤的 10%，发病率仅次于星形胶质细胞瘤和原始神经外胚层肿瘤（primitive neuroectodermal tumours，PNET），其发病率无性别差异。大部分儿童室管膜瘤发生于颅内，约半数患儿年龄为 5 岁以下（Foreman et al.，1996）。有趣的是，大多数（超过 2/3）的儿童室管膜瘤发生于颅后窝，而成人颅内和脊髓室管膜瘤的发病率几乎相同，且成人颅内室管膜瘤发生于幕上和幕下的概率几乎相同。成人室管膜瘤非常少见，其中多发生于椎管内，如脊髓圆锥的髓内或髓外。

室管膜瘤有两种罕见的亚型：室管膜下瘤和黏液乳头状室管膜瘤。室管膜下瘤是一种生长缓慢的良性肿瘤，其确切发病率尚不清楚，许多患者终生无症状，而在尸检中偶然发现。有症状的病例多见于中老年人。与其他室管膜瘤亚型一样，室管膜下瘤与脑室表面相关，主要见于第四脑室，其次是侧脑室。许多偶然发现的室管膜瘤可能不会进展，也不需外科手术切除。手术常可治愈肿瘤，但肿瘤切除不完全除外。

黏液乳头状室管膜瘤也是缓慢生长的肿瘤，相对而言好发于青年成人，并且几乎只发生在椎管内（髓外）圆锥区，但也有中枢神经系统其他部位发生的报道。黏液乳头状室管膜瘤很少发生转移，与室管膜下瘤类似，手术常可治愈肿瘤，但肿瘤切除不完全除外。

病理学

原世界卫生组织（WHO）分级将室管膜瘤分为四个亚型：室管膜下瘤（WHO Ⅰ级）、黏液乳头状室管膜瘤（WHO Ⅰ级）、经典型室管膜瘤（WHO Ⅱ级）和间变型室管膜瘤（WHO Ⅲ级）。经典型室管膜瘤还有几种形态学变异类型：细胞型室管膜瘤、乳头状室管膜瘤、透明细胞型室管膜瘤，伸长细胞型室管膜瘤，但这些变异型分类对预后并无预测价值。

除了罕见的亚型（室管膜下瘤和黏液乳头状室管膜瘤），儿童室管膜瘤多为经典型和间变型两种类型。本章后续内容将讨论这两种室管膜瘤亚型的特点和治疗。

经典型室管膜瘤（图 29.1）细胞密度中等，核分裂象罕见或缺如。细胞大小均匀，异型性小，胞核 /

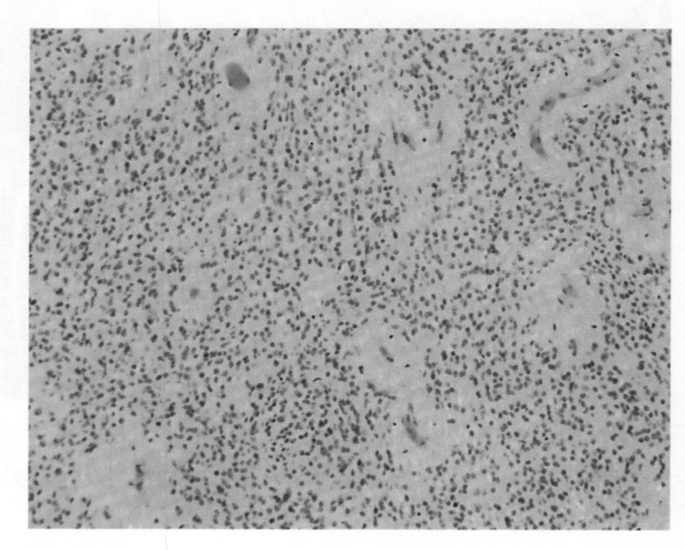

图 29.1　室管膜瘤，WHO Ⅱ级。细胞密度中等，血管假菊形团，分裂象少见。61 岁男性患者，腰 1 水平髓外硬膜下病变。上皮膜抗原（epithelial membrane antigen，EMA）在核周成点状分布，GFAP 阳性，Ki67 2%，RELA 阴性

Courtesy of Dr Kieren Allinson, Department of Pathology, Addenbrooke’s Hospital, Cambridge.

胞质比例高。典型的结构特征包括血管周围假菊形团和更少见的室管膜菊形团。血管周围假菊形团是由围绕血管放射状排列的肿瘤细胞形成，而室管膜真菊形团是由柱状排列的肿瘤细胞本身形成的中央腔隙。大部分室管膜瘤，特别是血管周围假菊形团附近的纤维区呈 GFAP 染色阳性。肿瘤偶可见坏死区，但不一定表明肿瘤发生间变。虽然室管膜瘤的组织学诊断标准已十分明确，但根据室管膜瘤的组织学特征来划分其亚型一直以来都具有挑战性，且不同组织学亚型对患者预后的预测是十分重要的。由于肿瘤内部异质性、不同观察者间的差异、定义的变化、不同组织学标准的应用、不同病理学家对间变肿瘤标准掌握不同、小样本特殊病例等综合因素导致了室管膜瘤病理分级的争议。这导致室管膜瘤特别是间变型肿瘤的分类存在困难，解决这一问题的针对性工作正在进行中（Tihan et al.，2008；Ellison et al.，2011）。

间变型室管膜瘤（**图** 29.2）是一种总体预后较差的恶性肿瘤。细胞密度高，生长速度快，分裂活性高，有扩散的倾向。组织学上表现为假栅栏状坏死、微血管增生和血管周围假菊形团。遗憾的是，目前间变型室管膜瘤的神经病理学标准尚无可靠的广泛接受的共识，虽然大多数神经病理学家认为的重要指标有：分裂指数、Ki67、细胞密度和分化程度。Ki67 增殖指数与患者生存率有明显相关性，Ki67 指数大于 5% 的患者生存率明显降低。

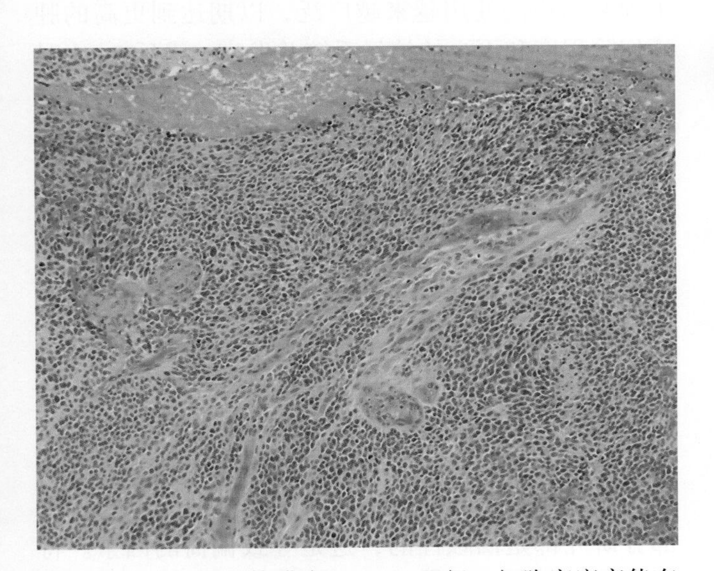

图 29.2　间变型室管膜瘤，WHO Ⅲ级。细胞密度高伴有坏死（顶部），内皮细胞增生，分裂象活跃。5 岁患儿，幕上肿瘤。EMA 在核周点状表达，GFAP 阳性，Ki67 40%，RELA 阳性

Courtesy of Dr Kieren Allinson, Department of Pathology, Addenbrooke's Hospital, Cambridge.

由于缺乏共识，医生面临严峻的挑战（Robertson et al.，1998），因为经典型室管膜瘤和间变型室管膜瘤的治疗方案有明显不同，患者的预后也不尽相同，因此医生应当谨慎决策。

肿瘤分子遗传学

已发现室管膜瘤存在一系列细胞遗传学异常，但这些改变与影响肿瘤分级或决定治疗策略的因素并不一致（**表** 29.1）。高达 30% 的室管膜瘤存在 22 号染色体的异常，包括单倍体、缺失或易位（Hamilton and Pollock，1997）。

有趣但并不意外的是，研究发现脊髓髓内室管膜瘤多见于神经纤维瘤病Ⅱ型患者，因此有理由认为 NF-2 基因以某种方式参与室管膜瘤肿瘤发生（Slavc et al.，1995）。其他遗传学异常包括 6q、9q、3p、10q 和 11q 的缺失。透明细胞型的组织学特征可与少突胶质细胞瘤类似，不存在 1p、19q 共缺失。这些细胞遗传学改变未来可能在诊断和个体化、生物学驱动的治疗模式发挥重要作用。

尽管到目前为止尚无生物学标志物的显著性得到验证，室管膜瘤的生物学标志物也是值得深入研究的内容（Andreiuolo et al.，2013）。其分子表达谱巨大进展已经促进了新的室管膜瘤 WHO 分类（**专栏** 29.1），未来可能会引导室管膜瘤的治疗方法的改变。

治疗

外科治疗

放射治疗的作用

室管膜瘤是需要外科治疗的肿瘤。长期以来，人们一直认为所有年龄组和不同中枢神经系统部位的室管膜瘤的预后关键取决于手术切除的程度（Healey et al.，1991；Perilongo et al.，1997）。对于神经外科医生而言，最大的困境是由于肿瘤倾向于与颅后窝的脑干、脑神经以及脊髓组织、神经根（髓内和黏液乳头状室管膜瘤）粘连，因此全切肿瘤可能导致严重而明显的神经功能障碍。全切肿瘤这样激进的外科治疗需要谨慎地和次全切除肿瘤的策略相权衡，因为次全切手术后即使完成后续多模态神经肿瘤治疗总体预后也不佳（Merchant，2002；Merchant et al.，2009）。

室管膜瘤患者初始检查需行颅脑 - 脊髓全神经轴的 MRI 检查以明确肿瘤部位、肿瘤和邻近结构（脑

表 29.1 室管膜瘤亚型的分子病理学和遗传学总结

解剖部位	分型	遗传学	病理学	年龄组
幕上	ST-EPN-RELA	*RELA* 融合基因	经典型 / 间变型	婴儿→成人
幕上	ST-EPN-YAP1 ST	*YAP1* 融合基因	经典型 / 间变型	婴儿 / 儿童
幕上	ST-SE	平衡基因组	室管膜下瘤	成人
颅后窝	PF-EPN-A	平衡基因组	经典型 / 间变型	婴儿
颅后窝	PF-EPN-B	全基因组多倍性	经典型 / 间变型	儿童→成人
颅后窝	PF-SE	平衡基因组	室管膜下瘤	成人
脊柱	SP-EPN	NF2 突变	经典型 / 间变型	儿童→成人
脊柱	SP-MPE	全基因组多倍性	黏液乳头型	成人
脊柱	SP-SE	6q 缺失	室管膜下瘤	成人

专栏 29.1 关键点

- 室管膜瘤是儿童主要肿瘤
- 大多数发生于颅后窝
- 手术全切是唯一的最重要的预后因素
- 在组织学上区分经典病例和未分化亚型有明显的困难
- 适形辅助放射治疗可提高术后生存率
- 化疗主要用于 3 岁以下儿童以控制疾病，且需延迟放射治疗
- 大部分肿瘤局部复发
- 儿童的 5 年生存率为 36%~64%

干、脑神经）的关系，以及是否存在转移。室管膜瘤的 MRI 可能表现多样，但最常表现为 TI 序列的等 / 低信号、T2 序列高信号，增强扫描显著强化（**图** 29.3 和**图** 29.4）。FIESTA 序列（稳态进动快速成像）对于脑神经和血管结构的显示有更精确的分辨率，弥散加权成像（DWI）和表观弥散系数图（ADC）现被常规用于高级别肿瘤的鉴别。MRS 序列也有助于诊断室管膜瘤，表现为低 NAA/ 胆碱比值，介于 PNET 和胶质瘤之间。室管膜瘤也可见钙化、囊变和出血。室管膜瘤的典型影像学特征是肿瘤占据第四脑室外侧隐窝或分别由第四脑室中间孔和外侧孔长入桥小脑角区和椎管内。术前和围术期，特别是伴有脑积水的患者使用大剂量类固醇激素可有效减轻脑肿胀。幕下室管膜瘤患者常出现症状性的脑积水，外科医生的首要决策是脑积水的处理。迄今为止，对于这类脑积水尚无共识或进展规定采用何种方式治疗。内镜下第三脑室造瘘术、脑室外引流术、分流术都有支持者，还有的主张肿瘤切除术前不行脑脊液引流处理。鉴于只有小部分患者术后发生脑积水，术前分流是最不常用的选择。

最佳的手术入路取决于肿瘤的部位。幕下肿瘤可以通过标准枕下正中入路颅骨切开 / 颅骨切除开颅，而对于更侧方的肿瘤可采用乳突后入路颅骨切开 / 颅骨切除开颅。如术前未做脑脊液引流，可在开颅前行枕部钻孔脑室外引流术（external ventricular drain，EVD）。许多外科医生采用小脑延髓裂入路切除第四脑室肿瘤，可避免或减轻小脑蚓部的损伤，以减少术后发生颅后窝缄默症或综合征的风险。

手术目的是全切肿瘤，这对于疗效和预后十分重要。由于室管膜瘤常和脑干、桥小脑角的脑神经粘连紧密，因此即使对经验丰富的外科医生而言避免这些结构的损伤仍具有挑战性。因此，术中神经生理和超声的使用越来越广泛，以期达到更高的肿瘤切除程度和更少的神经系统并发症。术后 24 小时内进行磁共振检查是十分必要的，以准确记录肿瘤切除程度，这将影响治疗方案和预后。术中磁共振有助于即时发现肿瘤残余。如果术后发现肿瘤残留并仍是可切除的，则应准备再次手术并争取全切。为了全切肿瘤而采用的愈加激进的手术策略是有代价的，常导致患者明显的神经功能障碍，并可能需气管切开术和胃造瘘术。尽管采用激进的手术策略，也只有不到 50% 的儿童室管膜瘤能达到全切。

室管膜瘤很难有统一的治疗策略，其原因包括以下几个因素：发病率较低、肿瘤的病理分级不一致，以及比较不同亚型患者间的疗效的困难性。大部分研究都是回顾性的，这是导致偏倚的因素。特别是研究样本小，跨度时间长，治疗方法和分类标准可能已经发生变化。影响室管膜瘤治疗的重要因素是外科手术切除程度和磁共振检查的普及。

颅内室管膜瘤的综合治疗尚有争议，包括手术联合放疗和化疗。较低的 5 年生存率导致缺乏一致

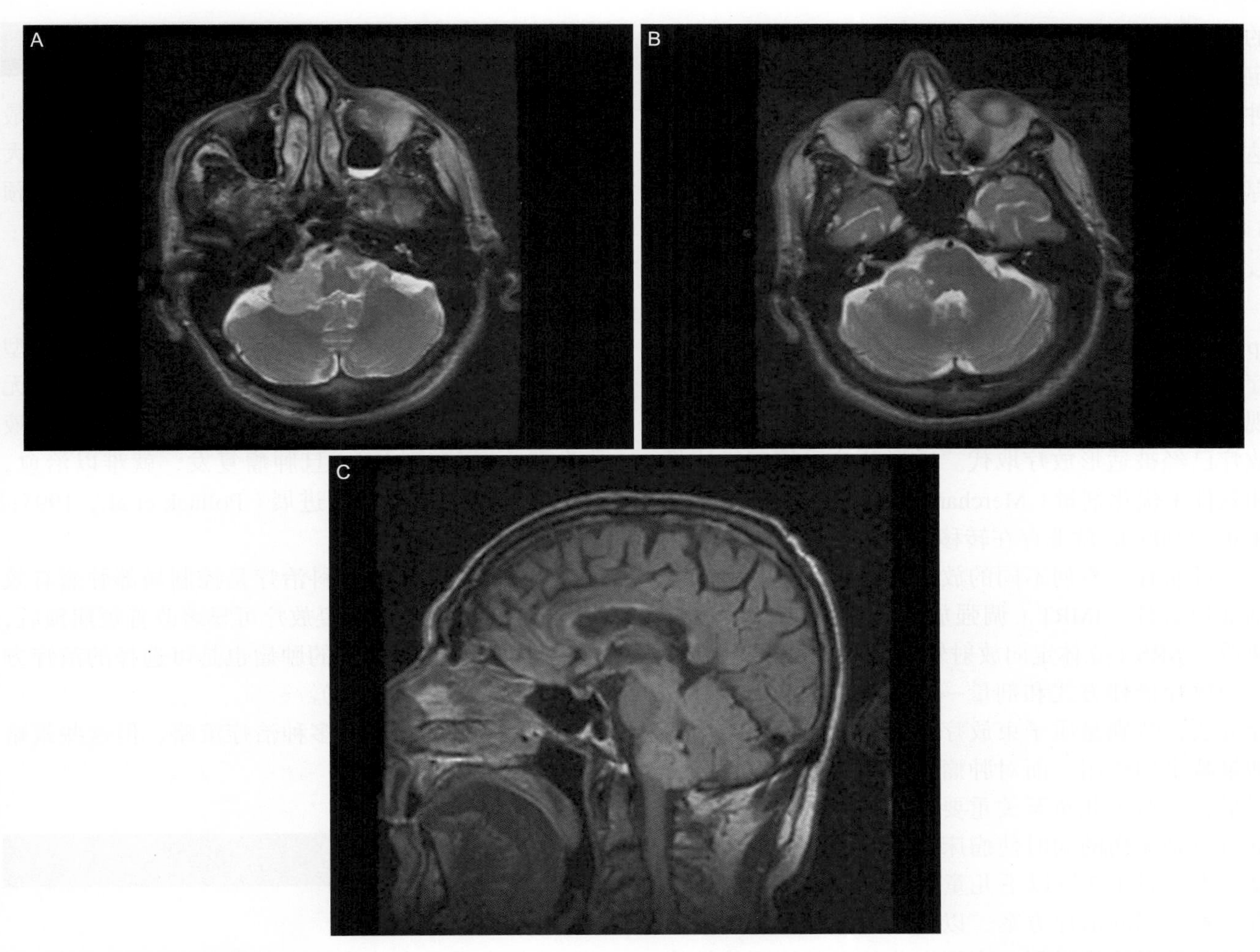

图 29.3 磁共振影像显示颅后窝室管膜瘤通过第四脑室外侧孔长入桥小脑角，形态和桥小脑角施万细胞瘤类似。（A、B）轴位 T2 加权成像。（C）矢状位 T1 加权成像钆对比剂增强

Courtesy of Dr Kieren Allinson, Department of Pathology, Addenbrooke's Hospital, Cambridge.

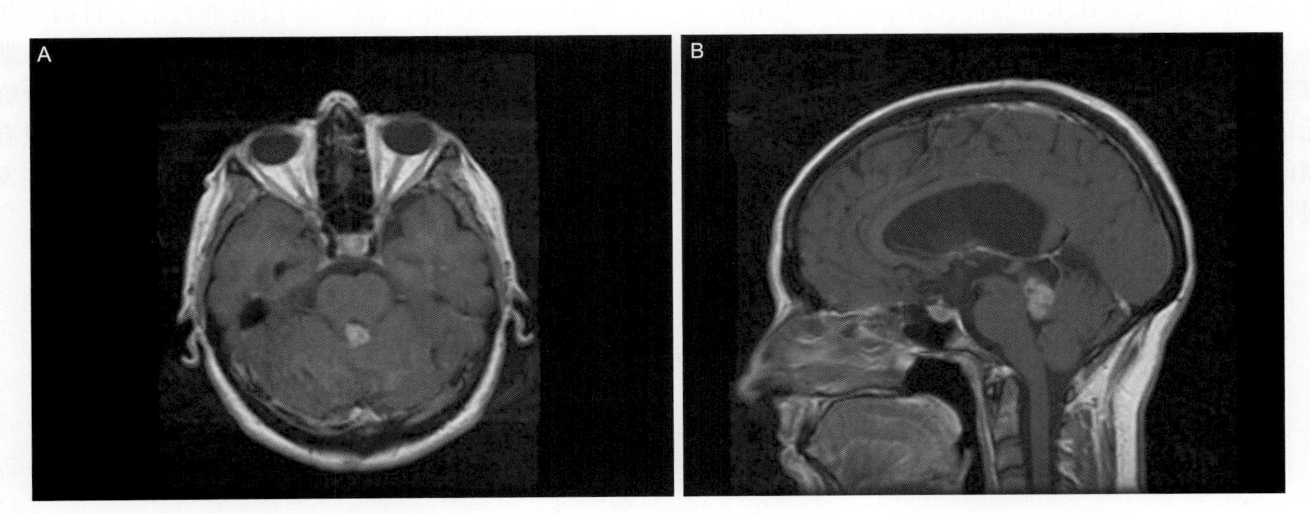

图 29.4 磁共振 T1 加权钆对比剂增强显示第四脑室室管膜瘤阻塞中脑导水管。（A）轴位；（B）矢状位

Courtesy of Dr Kieren Allinson, Department of Pathology, Addenbrooke's Hospital, Cambridge.

的治疗方案。局部复发是治疗失败的主要原因。决定患者是否采取放化疗的因素包括：患者的年龄、肿瘤分级、切除程度，以及是否存在转移灶。已经达成共识的是接受放疗的患者比化疗的患者无病生存率更高，因此放疗被认为是必须完成的辅助治疗，3岁以下儿童除外（Shuman et al.，1975；Mork and Loken，1997）。

在相当长的一段时间内，全脑脊髓放疗（craniospinal radiation，CSI）曾是髓母细胞瘤的标准辅助治疗，直到在室管膜瘤中发现肿瘤初诊时和复发时出现播散性病灶的概率比预计的要低得多。全脑脊髓放疗已经被适形放疗取代。适形放疗采用三维成像和软件来优化剂量（Merchant et al.，2004；Merchant et al.，2009），除非存在转移性病灶。

目前有一系列不同的放疗方案可供选择：超分割加速放疗、IMRT（调强放疗）、LINAC（直线加速器）、SRS（立体定向放射外科），以及质子束放疗。关于放疗最佳方式和剂量一直存在着争议。新的放疗方法，特别是质子束放疗，通过降低周围结构的剂量减少副作用，而对肿瘤或瘤床又能稳定在致死剂量，这对于儿童至关重要。放疗策略的核心是尽量减少副损伤的同时使瘤床达到致死剂量以减少肿瘤复发。对于3岁以下儿童或存在转移灶的患者也有多种不同的治疗方案，以化疗为基础，控制肿瘤进展并推迟放疗时间，直到患儿的年龄达到能够接受放疗（Zacharoulis and Moreno，2009）。然而研究表明，3岁以下患儿接受放疗后无病生存期延长，功能预后良好，这种治疗方案有可能在未来更加普及（Merchant et al.，2004）。目前放射外科治疗只用于复发病例，但可能在未来与传统的放疗联合使用。

化疗的作用还不是很清楚，其治疗方案和药物也多种多样（Bouffet and Foreman，1999）。目前尚无证据表明单用或联合用药化疗能显著影响室管膜瘤的临床病程。化疗辅助残余肿瘤的切除作用较局限，其主要作用是推迟患儿的放疗时间。

预后

室管膜瘤的总体预后取决于多种因素，其中最关键的是手术切除的程度（Healey et al.，1991）。大部分研究表明，所有年龄组中肿瘤全切的患者预后显著好于次全切除的患者（Bouffet et al.，1998；Merchant，2002）。

儿童患者预后不良的指标包括：年龄小于3岁、肿瘤不完全切除、肿瘤转移和组织学类型为间变型肿瘤。影响老年患者预后的因素包括：年龄、有无转移、位置（颅后窝 *vs.* 脊柱）和组织学类型（黏液乳头型 *vs.* 间变型）。一旦肿瘤复发，就难以治愈，治疗的重点是控制肿瘤进展（Pollack et al.，1995；Robertson，1998）。

多次逐级扩大的外科治疗是控制局部肿瘤有效的姑息性治疗手段。重复放疗可显著改善短期预后，这对于肿瘤学特性变化的肿瘤也是可选择的治疗方案（Bouffet et al.，2012）。

复发室管膜瘤也有多种治疗策略，但这些策略的有效性证据较少。

争议

质子束 *vs.* 放疗

近年来质子束放疗的应用越来越广泛，可能改善室管膜瘤的总体预后。质子束放疗与标准的光子放疗相比，放射剂量和疗效一致而对周围结构的剂量更低。质子束放疗显而易见的优势是放疗相关副作用的减少，对于儿童患者可能显著降低远期致残率（MacDonald et al.，2008）。放射外科治疗目前仅用于复发肿瘤，但未来可能与传统放疗联合使用。遗憾的是，质子束放疗和放射外科治疗都没有充分临床评估，在行全脑脊髓质子束放疗的儿童中，只有一项临床试验报道质子束放疗可减少全身并发症发生率（Yock et al.，2016）。

参考文献

扫描书末二维码获取。

第 30 章　血管母细胞瘤

Ammar Natalwala・Donald MacArthur 著
程崇杰、钟东 译，钟东 审校

病史与流行病学

血管母细胞瘤（haemangioblastomas，HBLs）是一种少见的、高度血管化的良性肿瘤，约占所有颅内肿瘤的 1%~2.5%。这种特殊的肿瘤最早于 1872 年由 Hughlings 和 Jackson 首先发现，而直到 1928 年才被 Cushing 和 Bailey 正式命名为“血管母细胞瘤”，用来描述以前被称为“血管胶质瘤”的中枢系统的血管性肿瘤，并以此与中枢神经系统毛细血管扩张、海绵状血管瘤和静脉性血管瘤相区别（Weil et al.，2003）。1895 年，德国眼科医生 Eugen von Hippel 首次提出了视网膜血管瘤病；1926 年，瑞典病理学家 Arvid Wilhelm Lindau 描述了结合视网膜血管瘤和小脑 HBLs 的临床综合征（现称为 von Hippel-Lindau 综合征或 VHL），并提出了一系列诊断标准，包括“明确的肿瘤特征”“血管成分的组成”和“囊肿形成的趋势”（Hussein，2007）。

大约 30% 的中枢神经系统的 HBL 病例与 VHL 有关，另外 70% 的病例则为散发性。VHL 临床上具有异质性，可伴发的其他相关肿瘤包括视网膜血管瘤、肾囊肿、肾细胞癌（renal cell carcinomas，RCC）、胰腺肿瘤、嗜铬细胞瘤、中耳内淋巴囊肿瘤和附睾囊肿（Bründl et al.，2014）。VHL 相关性 HBLs 的发病年龄，较散发性的 HBLs 更小（通常在 20~30 岁，而散发性的 HBLs 通常好发于 40~50 岁）。

临床表现

肿瘤的症状多由肿瘤本身的压迫作用，偶尔因肿瘤卒中或副肿瘤效应（如红细胞增多症）引起。据既往报道，从发病到诊断的平均时间从 7 周到 13 个月不等，其主要取决于 HBL 的类型，通常 VHL 病例能更快诊断。HBL 同时含有实性和囊性成分，通常是囊性部分引起肿瘤的压迫症状。实性部分一般生长缓慢，患者可以发病多年仍无症状。无症状的 VHL-HBLs 患者往往在影像学体检时被无意间发现。

95% 的累及小脑和脑干的 HBLs 患者以头痛为首发症状，随后出现呕吐、共济失调、眩晕、复视和眼球震颤等伴随症状。少数患者出现颈部疼痛、恶心、构音障碍或脑神经损伤。累及椎管的 HBLs 患者常有锥体束征并伴疼痛症状，其中 50% 的患者伴有脊髓空洞症（Hussein，2007）。椎管内 HBLs 更好发于年轻男性，部位常位于胸段脊髓内。尽管 HBLs 本身生长缓慢，却可能发生危及生命的并发症（Richard et al.，2000）。例如，肿瘤可压迫阻塞脑脊液循环通路导致脑积水，以及瘤体自发破裂引起大出血。

HBLs 异常分泌红细胞生成素（EPO）可导致红细胞增多症，实际上 HBLs 是唯一一种与红细胞增多症相关的脑部肿瘤（在 9%~20% 的脑内 HBLs 中可见，椎管内 HBLs 中没有发现）（Hussein，2007）。这一过程中涉及的分子遗传学机制将在本章后面讨论。

病理机制

好发部位

HBLs 可发生在中枢神经系统的任何部位，但幕下更好发，约占所有成人颅后窝肿瘤的 7.5% 和椎管肿瘤的 4%（Bründl et al.，2014）。**图 30.1** 概述了所有 HBLs 和 VHL 患者的常见发病部位。幕下型 HBLs 常见于小脑背侧、延髓闩和脊髓背根起始部。幕上 HBLs 比较少见。Mills 及其同事系统回顾了 132 例 HBLs 病例，发现有 60% 为 VHL（Mills et al.，2012）。HBLs 的其他位置包括脊髓神经根，可以为髓外硬膜下和（或）硬膜外，但都位于神经束膜内，因此完全切除会损伤神经根。外周神经系统的 HBLs 也有文献报道，包括眼眶、肠道和腹膜后。

影像学和大体表现

HBL 通常与周围组织有清楚的界限，但包膜

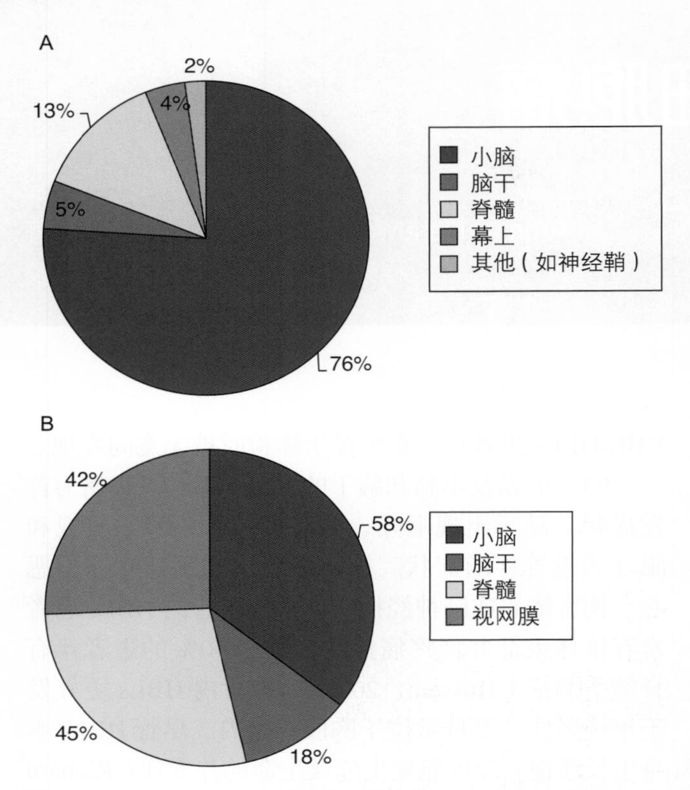

图 30.1 （A）HBL 在中枢神经系统中最常见的位置和（B）HBL 在 VHL 患者中的分布（肿瘤通常发现位于多个位置）。百分比基于文献中报道的平均值（Ammerman，2006；Gläsker，2005；Hussein, 2007；Kanno，2014；Padhi et al.，2011）

并非总是完整。因此，肿瘤有时会侵及邻近脑组织，在 CT 和磁共振 T1 加权相中可表现为明显强化，而 T2 加权相及 FLAIR 序列可以帮助评估瘤周水肿（Wind and Lonser，2011）。Sun 和他的同事报道了几种不同的影像学表现：囊壁和结节均有强化或囊壁无强化但结节均匀强化的囊性 HBL，实性 HBL 由多个小的实性肿瘤组成，且实性肿瘤内可包含单个或多个囊肿（Sun et al.，2015）。如图 30.2 所示，了解这些影像学特点有利于准确诊断。

囊性 HBLs 常见于小脑，其内由黄 / 灰色蛋白液和致密的红色结节组成，直径通常为 0.5~2.5 cm（Richard et al.，2000）；囊性结构可位于瘤体内或瘤周（Hussein，2007），有研究报道瘤内囊肿的形成主要是由肿瘤内坏死引起的，而瘤周囊肿则是源于肿瘤间质化过程中产生的水肿（Jagannathan et al.，2008）；一般囊性 HBLs 均能发现肉眼可见的壁结节。实性 HBLs 和伴有瘤内囊肿的实性 HBLs 通常位于椎管内（Richard et al.，2000）。

实性 HBLs 体积更大，血供更为丰富，更容易累及脑干。该类型 HBLs 的生长模式被描述为“跳跃式”生长，其特征是经历 2.1 年 ±1.6 年的静止期后进入快速生长期（1.1 年 ±1.3 年）。Lonser 等人报道了 VHL 相关 HBLs 呈现线性和指数增长模式（Lonser，2014）。

组织学表现

HBLs 均为良性，WHO 分级为Ⅰ级（图 30.3）。内部含有丰富的毛细血管网，以及散在的、充满脂质的基质细胞（Richard et al.，2000）。根据两种成分的相对比例，HBLs 可分为血管网型（毛细血管占优势）和细胞型（基质细胞占优势）；据报道，细胞型（25%）的复发率比血管网型（8%）更高，可能与后者富含肥大细胞有关（Hussein，2007）。肿瘤内的血管间隙大小不一，病灶中心的血管可能发育不良。基质细胞通常处于静止期，但也可能出现显著的胞核不均一性，但有丝分裂现象很少，这被认为是退行性改变，对预后影响不大。髓外造血灶少见，可能是由于基质细胞产生 EPO 所致。与 HBLs 相邻的脑组织可能表现出明显的胶质增生，可能有类似星形细胞的突起（内部包含有大量的 Rosenthal 纤维），这容易导致误诊，尤其是在活检组织较小时，不要误诊为毛细胞型星形细胞瘤。

基质细胞并不是中枢神经系统的正常组分，且 HBLs 的发生机制仍存在争议。目前认为这些基质细胞来源于血管间充质细胞。这些基质细胞缺乏特定的细胞器或细胞表面分子，可分化为红细胞和血管内皮细胞。

病理学上，HBLs 主要与转移性肾透明细胞癌相鉴别，后者也可见于 VHL（Hussein，2007），其他少见的鉴别诊断包括副神经节瘤和血管瘤性脑膜瘤。除了形态学上的差异，特异的免疫组化标志物包括 CD10、D2-40、上皮膜抗原、抑制素 α 和 S100，可以帮助做出明确的诊断。

分子肿瘤遗传学与危险因素

VHL 以常染色体显性方式遗传（Asthagiri et al.，2010），在 65 岁时有超过 90% 的外显率。VHL 基因是一种位于 3 号染色体短臂上的抑癌基因，广泛表达于胎儿和成人组织中。它编码 VHL 蛋白（pVHL），这是一种靶向作用于缺氧诱导因子 α（HIF-α）的 E3 泛素连接酶，从而调节许多缺氧诱导相关基因的表达，包括负责血管再生的基因（血管内皮生长因子 VEGF）和促红细胞生成素（EPO）。pVHL 还可以通过 HIF 非依赖激活途径，参与一系列肿瘤抑制调节

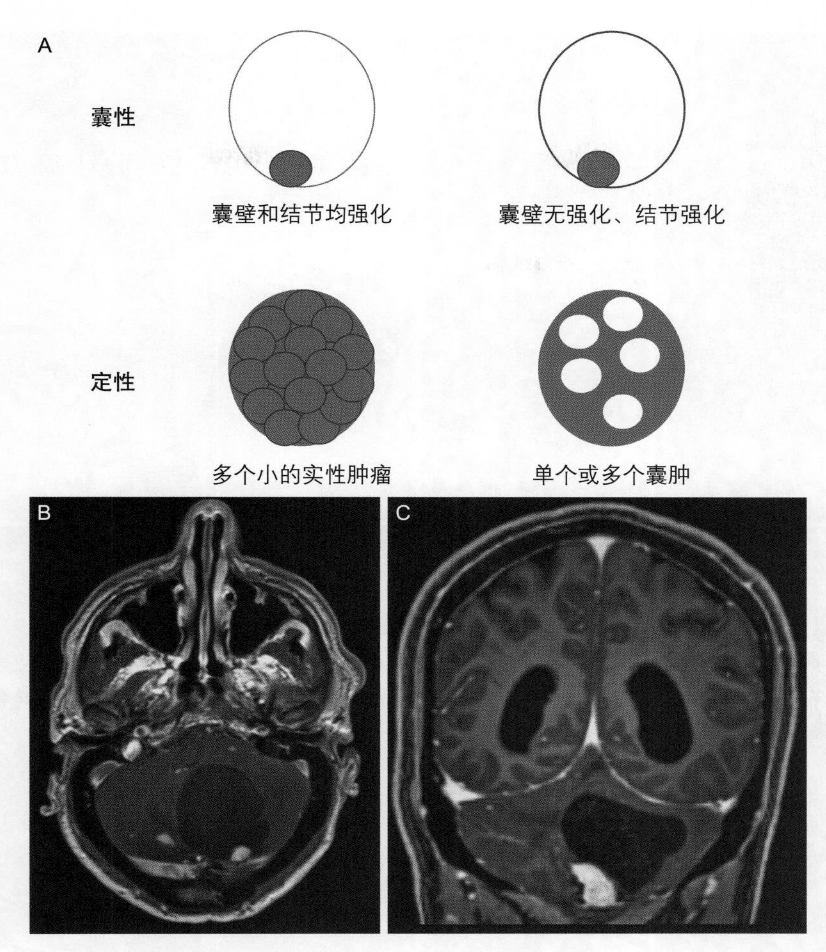

图 30.2 （A）描绘了 HBL 的不同形态学亚型和增强 MRI 成像上的区别（基于 Sun et al.，2015 年报道的描述）。（B 和 C）轴位和冠状位图像，分别显示 1 例 52 岁男性 VHL 患者的颅后窝 HBL 的典型 MRI 表现（T1 增强）。图像 B 显示左侧增强的壁结节和相关的囊肿（无强化的囊壁），以及右侧邻近的孤立性结节（以及其他较小的结节）

过程，如细胞外基质、细胞凋亡、微管稳定性、纤毛形成和基因转录等（Hsu，2012）。VEGF 蛋白的表达诱导大量的反应性血管相关细胞进入肿瘤，这可能是导致肿瘤高度血管化的原因（Hussein，2007）。

VHL 患者存在 VHL 基因的种系突变或单拷贝缺失。据推测，家族性聚集性 VHL 起源于那些因 VHL 基因体细胞突变而导致双等位基因失活的细胞（Gläsker，2005），在一小部分散发 HBLs 病例中也发现了 VHL 基因突变（10%~44%）。Shankar 等人还发现 3p 染色体上基因位点的复发性体细胞突变（50%）和杂合度丢失（LOH）（72%）的发生率明显较高。这些改变共同导致 VHL 病例的双等位基因失活（47%），以及散发 HBLs 病例一个以上等位基因失活（72%）（Shankar，2014）。基因型 - 表型研究已经确定了几种不同的 VHL 亚型具有不同的肿瘤特征，这将在一个单独的章节中进行更详细的讨论。

治疗原则

目前治疗 HBL 的方法包括手术切除（可行术前血管内栓塞）、立体定向放射外科（stereotactic radiosurgery，SRS）和放射治疗。手术要尽量做到完全切除，对于位置可达的肿瘤，能以最小的致残率和死亡率让患者获得根治（Hussein，2007）。最佳的治疗时机尚存在争议，但有神经症状进展、肿瘤或囊肿生长、瘤卒中时，应考虑积极干预。

手术治疗

HBLs，尤其是实性 HBLs，常被拿来与动静脉畸形（arteriovenous malformations，AVM）相比较，两者的手术原则相似，即避免瘤体出血的情况下争取全切。医生应避免进入瘤体内操作或进行活检，因为即使轻微的肿瘤组织切除都可能引起大出血（Hussein，2007）。在实性 HBL 手术中我们应沿

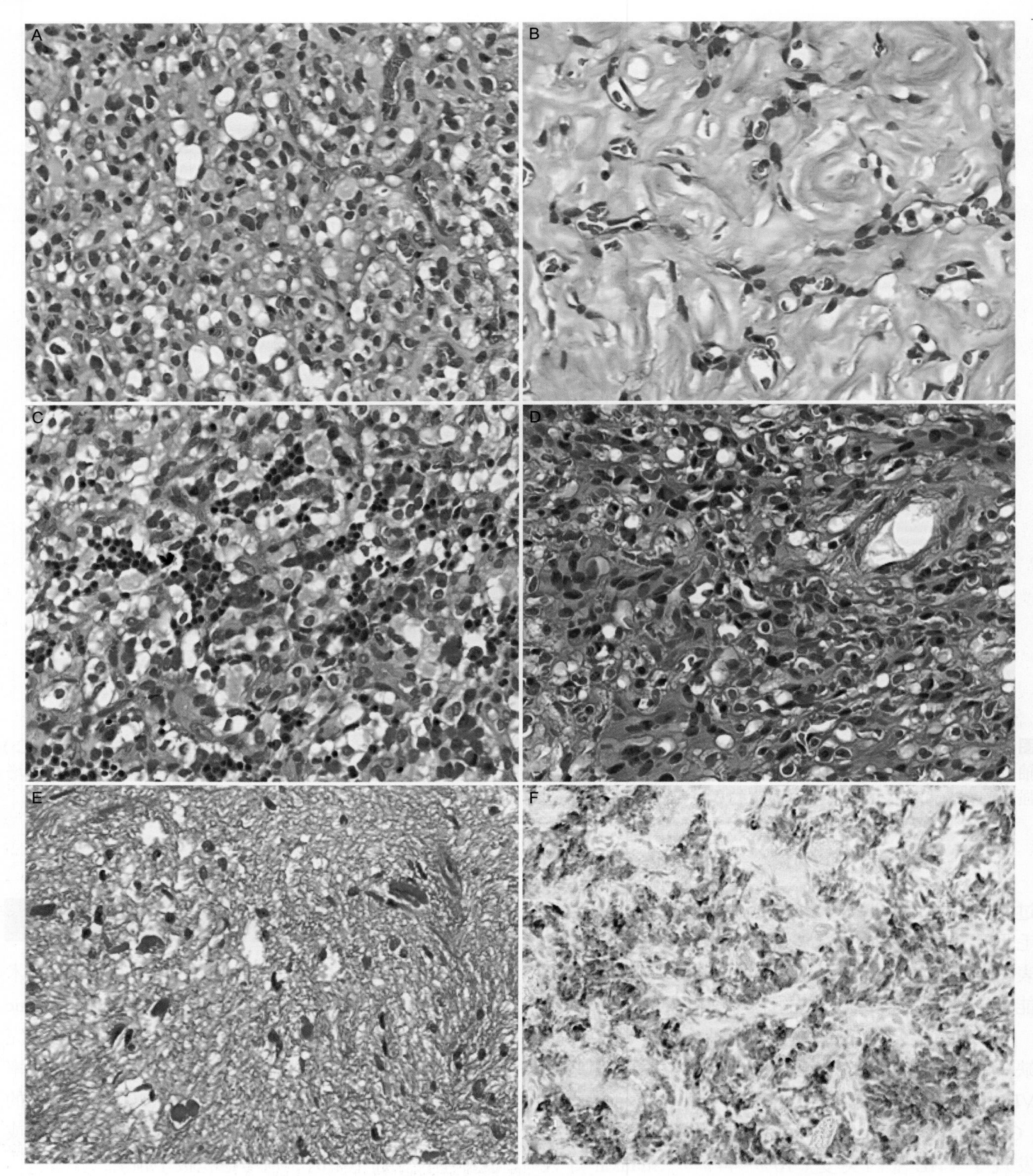

图 30.3 （A）HBL（WHO Ⅰ级）由毛细血管和间质细胞组成，胞浆内有不同程度的空泡化（H&E，×20）。（B）这两种成分的比例差异很大，常见胶原化的乏细胞区（H&E，×20）。（C）髓外造血病灶可见，认为是基质细胞产生 EPO 所致，可能与继发性红细胞增多症有关（H&E，×20）。（D）核异质性考虑是退行性改变，即使有时很明显也不影响预后（H&E，×20）。（E）邻近脑组织内可能有毛状胶质细胞增生，伴有明显的深色 Rosenthal 纤维（H&E，×40）。（F）基质细胞对抑制素 -α 的免疫反应有助于区分 HBL 与转移性肾癌（抗抑制素 -α 免疫组织化学，×10）

瘤体和肿瘤周围胶质组织之间进行暴露和切除，这样操作能达到广泛暴露、边界清楚和整块切除的效果。与动静脉畸形一样，术中应在处理引流静脉前切断供血动脉，以避免引流静脉阻断导致高灌注出血。有多根供血动脉时常和异常粗大的引流静脉难以辨别。囊性 HBLs 的囊壁结节通常呈红色或橙色，可在术中辨认，必须完全切除囊壁结节以防止复发。对于影像学有强化的囊肿壁也应尽量切除；而无强化的囊壁，Gläsker 认为它们不含有肿瘤细胞，只是单纯反应性的胶质增生，可以不处理（Gläsker et al., 2010）。对于一些位置深的实性 HBLs，可能还需要扩大的颅底手术路径（Dow，2002）。最常见的手术入路包括枕下正中和乳突后入路，C1 椎板也可考虑在术中切除。对于脑干的 HBLs 应非常小心地处理，因为其与软脑膜有粘连，手术操作可导致严重的出血和神经功能损伤（Hussein，2007）。术中电生理监测可增加在脑干、桥小脑角和脊柱脊髓进行 HBLs 切除手术的安全性。**图** 30.4 展示了 HBL 手术的术中所见和被切除的囊壁结节。

一些手术团队主张术前栓塞供血动脉以减少肿瘤血供和术中出血，尽管这些操作本身有导致出血、梗死和肿胀的风险，甚至引起继发性脑积水。可供选择的栓塞材料较多，液体材料如氰基丙烯酸正丁酯（NBCA）胶和 Onyx 胶因具有最好的持久性和渗透性，通常作为首选。然而，这些材料可能在血管中移位，有时导致静脉阻塞，从而引起梗死或出血（Shin et al., 2014）。Cornelius 及其同事们报道了这种事件的发生率，相对于脑干或椎管 HBLs（5.6%），在小脑 HBL（43%）中更为常见（Cornelius et al., 2007）。**图** 30.5 显示了 HBL 栓塞前后的血管造影图像。

此外，术中吲哚青绿造影术也是一种实用的手术辅助手段，可以帮助术者更好识别与肿瘤相关的血流和靶血管。同样，术中超声检查也被推荐用于帮助识别肿瘤与脑实质或脊髓之间的界面，特别是在肿瘤包膜不清时。

非手术治疗

当无法进行手术时，也可以考虑其他治疗方案，包括 SRS、普通放射治疗和一些挽救性全身治疗。

SRS 通常用于复发或多发 HBL 病例，或当它们位于功能区或高风险区域难以全切时。如果是多发病灶，通常很难知道是哪个病变引起了这些症状。囊性成分可能会影响 SRS 治疗的效果（Matsunaga et al., 2007）。Kano 等最近随访了北美和日本的 19 个中心，接受了 SRS 的 186 名 HBLs 患者共 517 个病灶，剂量为 15~18 Gy（Kano et al., 2015）。在平均 5 年的随访时间中，20 例死于肿瘤进展，另有 9 个因其他原因死亡。存活时间延长的预测因素有年龄较小、无神经症状、病灶较少和高 Karnofsky 表现评分（KPS）。肿瘤 5 年控制率为 89%，10 年控制率为 79%。约 41% 的 VHL 相关 HBL 患者有新发肿瘤，16% 的散发 HBL 病例在原部位复发，其 5 年复发率分别为 43% 和 24%。13 例（7%）患者有放射不良效应，其中 1 例死亡。也有研究报道将 SRS 作为术前辅助手段，可显著减少血管数量，有利于手术安全切除（Kamitani et al., 2004）。

外照射放疗（external beam radiotherapy，EBRT）

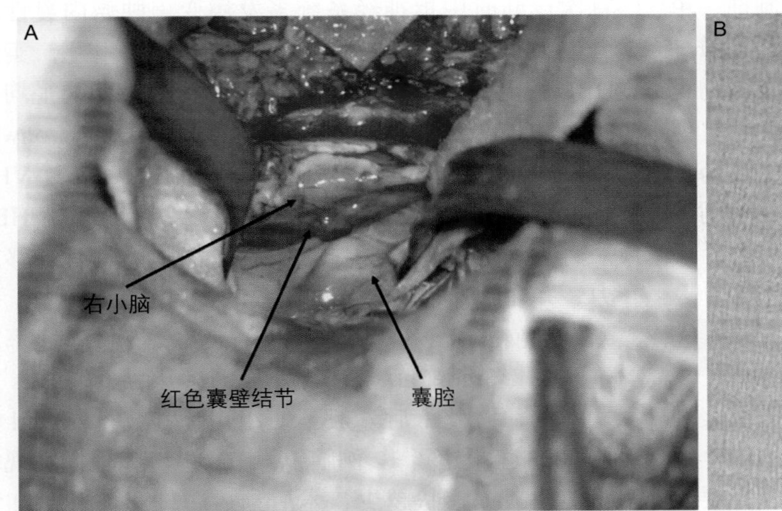

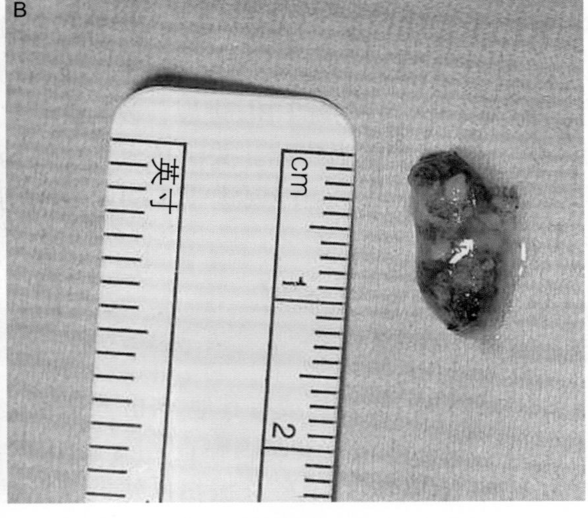

图 30.4 （A）术中图像显示被打开的右侧小脑囊腔内的囊壁结节。（B）囊壁结节整块切除

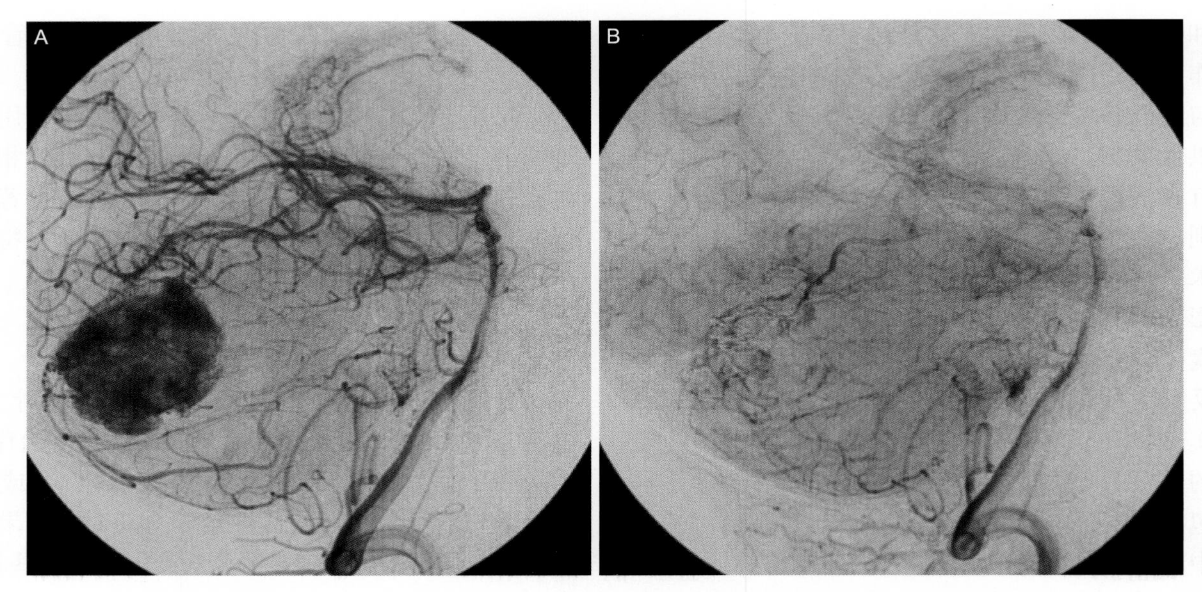

图 30.5 一例 53 岁患者左侧小脑 HBL 的术前血管内治疗。肿瘤内侧部分由右侧小脑后下动脉（PICA）供血，外侧部分由左侧小脑上动脉（SCA）供血。（A）在栓塞前注射造影剂后可见血管红晕。（B）用 NBCA 闭塞右侧 PICA 远端蚓部分支，栓塞后图像显示肿瘤血管减少。感谢 Dr.Robert Lenthall（诺丁汉大学医院介入神经放射主治医师）提供介入放射学建议和影像

也被用于治疗 HBLs，一项研究调查了 20 年来 EBRT 在 HBL 中的使用情况，发现总剂量 50 Gy 的局部控制率达到 57%，而低于 50 Gy 的局部控制率为 33%（Smalley et al.，1990）。Simone 等探讨了幕下脑脊髓照射对晚期 VHL 相关 HBL 的疗效，共治疗 7 例 HBL 患者共 84 个病灶（总剂量 43.2 Gy 分，24 期），平均随访时间 73.8 月。治疗后肿瘤体积平均增加 25%，肿瘤总数增加到 91 例（增加 8.3%）（Simone et al.，2011），但总体肿瘤生长率低于 HBL 自然进程。

挽救性全身治疗已被尝试用于手术和放疗后仍复发的患者。Capitanio 等描述了包括化疗药物（IFN-2a）、酪氨酸激酶抑制剂、选择性 VEGF 抑制剂、单克隆抗体（贝伐珠单抗）和酞胺哌啶酮（沙利度胺）。根据病例报道和Ⅱ期试验的结果，显示这些药物可以帮助控制中枢神经系统 HBL 进展，改善症状，但在影像学表现没有明显影响。关于抗血管生成药物在治疗 HBLs 中的作用还需要进一步的研究来阐明（Capitanio et al.，2013）。

基因检测

多发病变、低龄发病或有其他 VHL 疾病的表现时建议进行种系 VHL 突变基因筛查。除了脑和全脊柱脊髓扫描、腹部超声或磁共振扫描外，还需要监测 24 小时尿儿茶酚胺、视网膜眼底照相和荧光血管造影。Melmon 和 Rosen 诊断标准要求在 VHL 家族史基础上至少发现 1 个视网膜、中枢神经系统或内脏病变；若无家族史者，要求至少 2 个中枢神经系统病变或 1 个中枢神经系统病变 +1 个内脏病变，同时排除单侧附睾乳头状囊腺瘤、普通肾囊肿和阔韧带乳头状囊腺瘤。

预后

文献报道 HBL 的复发率一般在 20%~33%，与肿瘤复发相关的临床病理因素包括：低于 30 岁发病、首次诊断时中枢神经系统多发病变、肿瘤内囊性成分以及间质细胞比例较低（Hussein，2007），实性 HBL 的复发率也较高。VHL 患者在随访期间平均每 2.1 年即出现一个新的中枢神经系统 HBL（Conway et al.，2001）。与散发 HBL 病例相比（44%），VHL 患者出现新肿瘤的比例要高得多（93%）。虽然 HBL 一直被认为是良性肿瘤，但肿瘤细胞仍具有迁移能力，并在脑外远隔部位复发。

小脑 HBL 完全切除后预后良好，5 年生存率超过 50%（Sun et al.，2015）。完全切除后，HBLs 复发率低，因此术后一般不使用化疗和放疗。Weil 等在 2003 年报道了 12 例脑干 HBLs 患者，他们发现术前神经缺损症状越少，术后预后越好，而肿瘤和囊肿大小不影响预后。12 例患者术后短期神经功能均

有好转或稳定，长期随访（>36 个月）中只有 1 例病情恶化。

Jagannathan 等人在 2008 年报道了 VHL 相关 HBL 患者的手术结果，其中 88% 的患者术后症状稳定或改善，12% 患者出现新的小脑体征，但在平均 9 天后消失；长期随访（平均 84 个月）结果显示 7.5% 病例病情恶化，10% 病例死亡；94% 的脑积水术后得到缓解，6% 的患者仍需要性脑脊液分流手术。Mills 及其同事们报道在 77% 的幕上 HBLs 病例中实现了完全切除，术后 5 年无进展生存的比例分别为 100%（全切）和 53%（次全切）。

最近的一个单中心研究调查了 92 例椎管 HBLs 患者术后 5 年的随访情况（60 例散发性，32 例 VHL 相关）。这些患者接受了 102 次手术（共切除 116 个 HBLs 肿瘤），其中 41% 为髓内肿瘤，全切率高达 94%。平均随访时间 50 个月，术后 41% 的患者功能改善，44% 的患者病情稳定，15% 的患者病情恶化。与预后相关的主要因素是是否全切肿瘤。77% 的患者术前伴有空洞，这些患者中有 83% 术后空洞减少。从临床预后来看，腹侧和髓内肿瘤总体上恢复更差（Deng et al.，2014）。

对于接受 SRS 的患者，中枢神经系统 HBL 的 5 年无进展生存比例在 63%~85%，其他研究报道 SRS 的 5 年肿瘤控制率在 71% 到 96% 之间，但放射性坏死可能导致严重的副作用，特别是在脑干部位（Rachinger et al.，2009）。SRS 术区的肿瘤控制率在 10 年时下降到 61%，在 15 年时下降到 51%（Wind and Lonser，2011）。Kano et al.（2008）报道 SRS 后 3 年的总体生存率为 94%，5 年为 90%，10 年为 74%，局部肿瘤控制率分别为 92%、89% 和 79%。改善肿瘤控制率的因素有 VHL 相关 HBL、实性小肿瘤，以及较高的边缘剂量。14 例患者（7%）出现不良放射反应，1 例死亡。

所有中枢神经系统 HBLs 分次放疗的无进展生存比例从 33% 到 90.5% 不等，高剂量放疗的预后更好（剂量≥50 Gy，57% vs. 剂量<50 Gy，33%）（Mills et al.，2012）。Koh 等人报道了接受体外放射治疗的患者中，VHL 相关 HBL 的 5 年无进展生存比例为 80%，散发性 HBL 为 48%（Koh et al.，2007）。

多个中心报道的死亡率范围从 4%~8% 不等（Conway et al.，2001；Padhi et al.，2011；Bründl et al.，2014）。Bründl 及其同事的 10 年生存比例显示全切患者为 83%，而次全切患者仅为 17%，其中 75% 的患者术后症状稳定或改善。术后并发症包括出血（17%）、脑积水（4%~11%）、脑脊液感染（13%）、缺血（8%）、脑脊液漏（8%）、新发复视（4%）、新发偏瘫（4%）、延髓综合征和四肢瘫（8%），脑干 HBLs 预后最差（Bründl et al.，2014）。San Pedro 及其同事们观察了 44 例 HBL 标本后发现，相对于无症状轻微瘤内出血（显微镜下），自发性肉眼出血少见。肿瘤大小、脊神经根位置和实性 HBLs 与出血率相关。Gläsker 等人报道了直径小于 1.5 cm 的 HBLs 几乎没有出血的风险。

争议

单发血管母细胞瘤筛查 VHL 的年龄限制

对于没有 VHL 家族史的 HBL 患者，低龄发病（VHL 相关 HBL 的平均年龄为 29 岁，散发性 HBL 的平均年龄为 48 岁；见 Maher，2011）、病灶位于小脑以外（散发性病例中非常罕见，但在高达 50% 的 VHL 病例中可见）和病灶多发（在高达 90% 的 VHL 病例中可见）时，可临床诊断为 VHL。

绝大部分 VHL 患者（97%）在 60 岁之前发病（Maher et al.，1990），但第一例 VHL 患者确诊时已有 73 岁（Kanno et al.，2014）。法国 VHL 研究小组（Richard et al.，1998）认为，所有散发性 HBL 的患者都应接受 VHL 的诊断筛查，这一建议得到较广泛认同。据报道，单发病灶 HBL 的患者中 VHL 基因突变的频率仍有 4%~14%（Catapano et al.，2005）。然而，体细胞嵌合体突变，特别是对于具有新发突变的患者，可能外周血白细胞并未携带该突变基因，从而导致基因检测出现假阴性（Butman et al.，2008）。因此，即使突变分析结果为阴性，也应对早发性 HBL 患者进行密切监测；即使对于初筛结果为阴性的中老年 HBL 患者（>50 岁），家族性 VHL 疾病的风险也不能完全排除（Woodward et al.，2007）。

血管母细胞瘤的放射治疗

对于多发病灶，特别是累及脑干的病例，放射治疗有其独特优势，避免反复多次外科手术，还可以干预那些外科手术难以处理的高风险区域。然而，当评估治疗方式“控制肿瘤进展”的效果时需更谨慎地得出结论，因为大多数情况下该肿瘤本身具有公认的跳跃生长模式，即生长期平均持续 13 个月，静止期持续 2 年或更长时间（Ammerman et al.，2006）。

HBL 的 SRS 疗法有 7%~20% 的并发症发生率，其不良反应包括顽固的瘤周水肿，需要长时间使用皮质类固醇，甚至需要手术切除（Asthagiri et al.，2010）。约 25% 的 HBL 病例在 SRS 早期即出现病灶缩小，随后又进展扩大（Asthagiri et al.，2010），大部分病例起始扩大，后面病灶逐渐缩小。因此，SRS对病灶的远期影响仍不确定。

相比之下，对于常规部位的病灶，外科手术能更好地解除占位并缓解症状。有症状的HBLs应首选手术治疗，只有在手术效果不理想或患者不接受时，才选择SRS；而对于体检偶然发现的无症状病变，应谨慎考虑采用SRS干预。在一项为期10年的观察性研究中，虽然97%的HBLs表现为影像学生长，但此时只有50%的病例出现症状并需要治疗（Ammerman et al.，2006），其中45%的肿瘤初次检查时没有症状，随着时间的推移最终出现症状。

延伸阅读、参考文献

扫描书末二维码获取。

第 31 章　颅后窝肿瘤的手术入路

Jacques J. Morcos・Osaama H. Khan・Ashish H. Shah 著
程崇杰、钟东 译，钟东 审校

引言

第四脑室和枕骨大孔的病变和脑干关系密切，手术难度大。了解第四脑室、后组脑神经和基底池的解剖结构对于决定手术入路至关重要。而详细的术前检查和计划，则可以尽量减少手术并发症，同时最大限度地切除肿瘤。

本章概述了颅后窝病变（特别是第四脑室和枕骨大孔区域）的相关解剖和外科手术技巧。本章将分为两个部分，分别对第四脑室的显微外科手术入路和枕骨大孔的颅底手术入路进行介绍。

术前准备

当发现颅后窝病变后，详细了解其病理和毗邻结构是基本要求。术前影像学检查（CT/MRI）可以评估神经、血管关系以及是否存在脑积水。合并脑积水可能需要在手术前行脑室造瘘或脑室 - 腹腔分流术处理（Tamburrini et al.，2008）。如果评估肿瘤切除后阻塞性脑积水有望逆转，或脑脊液转流后能在术中减轻小脑压力，可考虑行脑室造瘘术。如果评估术后脑积水不易缓解，则选择脑室 - 腹腔分流术。如果怀疑是血管母细胞瘤或其他血管性病变，术前可行血管造影进行确诊。对于某些血管病变，术前栓塞供血动脉有利于外科手术的进行。但血管母细胞瘤有时不易完成栓塞，因为其供血动脉可能很细导致难以完成选择性插管（Standard et al.，1994; Sakamoto et al.，2012）。

手术入路主要取决于病变的大小和位置。对于第四脑室附近的病变，有两种主要的手术入路：枕下经蚓部入路和经膜髓帆入路。经蚓部入路不太理想，因为需要切开皮质才能进入第四脑室，可能会破坏小脑间传导束。该入路更适用于病变没有形成足够的空间和手术通道，又需要从第四脑室的上极进入的情况（Tanriover et al.，2004）。相比之下，经膜髓帆入路可能更适合于 Luschka 孔和 Magendie 孔附近的病变，或者更大的、更靠近颅骨的，已形成了手术通道的病变。

第四脑室解剖

对于神经外科医生来说，第四脑室内的病变具有高度挑战性，因为病变周围几乎没有无功能的结构（Lassiter et al.，1971；Alvisi et al.，1985；Liu et al.，1998）。对第四脑室解剖的熟悉掌握对于处理肿瘤尤为关键，这里我们要强调该区域解剖的一些关键点。

第四脑室病变最常见的手术方式是从枕下正中后入路。在暴露视野的上端，小脑后切迹在小脑半球之间形成裂缝，延伸到小脑蚓部。蚓面位于第四脑室顶部的背侧，分为两个主要部分：锥体和蚓垂（位于小脑扁桃体之间）。就在蚓垂的深面，第四脑室从中脑导水管延伸到 Magendie 孔。Rhoton 将第四脑室顶分为上下两个主要部分。第四脑室顶的下部由两层结构（脉络膜和下髓帆）组成。小脑延髓裂是在小脑腹侧和延髓背侧之间延伸的复杂裂缝，四脑室顶的下部可以通过小脑延髓裂的上半部分进入。下髓帆形成一层薄膜，从小结侧向延伸至绒球小叶，下髓帆和小结形成第四脑室顶下半部的颅侧，而脉络膜末端形成尾端。下髓帆在头侧与上髓帆相连，在尾侧与脉络膜端相连。

脉络膜是将脉络丛的血管传输到第四脑室的蛛网膜。脉络膜在 Luschka 孔和 Magendie 孔的蛛网膜下腔存在开窗。这一解剖结构在讨论经膜髓帆入路时尤为重要。

手术操作

枕下开颅

枕下后正中入路是处理第四脑室和颅后窝病变

的主要手术入路。推荐选择俯卧位，只有在特殊情况下才使用坐位。Mayfield 头架用于头部屈曲和枕颈部后移，以便暴露病变，但需确保没有因过度屈曲而影响颈静脉回流。在俯卧位时，患者身体下面应小心垫上垫子，以避免重力引起压力性损伤，手术床平面通常设置头部向上倾斜大约 10°，以促进静脉回流。

通常切口范围从枕外隆凸上方 2 cm 处到 C2 棘突水平。注意不要破坏枕外隆凸以上的骨膜，因为关颅时它经常被用作硬脑膜补片。皮下深部的解剖在上项线水平以下进行侧向分离。这样做的具体目的是创造空间，允许在上项线横向切割，并确保肌肉的水密缝合，宽度不超过 5~10 mm。皮下组织和深部肌肉之间没有必要一直向下方分离，因为这种分离并不能增加暴露，相反它还会造成组织无效腔，有引起假性脑膜膨出的风险。下一步寻找肌肉中线无血管区，并沿其走行切开直至 C1 平面，两侧肌肉组织按 T 形分离。然后使用拉钩将肌肉向两边特别是向下方牵开。这样就压缩了肌肉和皮肤的边缘，因此最大限度地减少了暴露的深度，在显微操作时具有增加暴露角度的极大优势。沿 C1 后弓小心地剥离骨膜，注意不要使用单极电凝进行操作，以尽量避免损伤椎动脉沟内的 V3 段椎动脉。这种偏离中线区域的暴露最好用剪刀反复钝性扩张后切开筋膜，或者在骨膜剥离子尖端用纱布推开骨膜，而不损伤椎动脉。在沿着 C1 后弓暴露之前，还需要明确是否存在椎体发育异常（如寰椎后弓融合不全），以免误伤脊髓。枕骨大孔的后唇用成角的刮匙显露出来。开颅的范围和确切位置因病变本身的差异而有所不同，典型的骨瓣大小约 3 cm × 3 cm，打开枕骨大孔向两侧暴露至枕髁附近。骨瓣可以钻单孔或两个小孔，或者当硬脑膜很容易剥离时可不钻孔，从利用暴露良好的枕骨大孔边缘作为铣刀的起始点。开颅完成后，若病变延伸至枕骨大孔以下，还需切除 C1 后弓，操作时同样需要注意椎动脉和椎旁静脉丛。静脉出血用混有凝血酶的明胶海绵很容易止血。对于硬脑膜粘连较轻的年轻患者，通常需要悬吊硬膜以减少术后硬膜外血肿的风险。硬脑膜呈 Y 形剪开，纵行切口可略偏向中线一侧，以避免枕窦出血。若术前预计到枕窦发达，可以血管夹夹闭控制。枕大池释放脑脊液减压后，开始显微镜下操作。

经膜髓帆入路

当完成止血并牵开硬脑膜后，小脑扁桃体可以从蚓部向侧方移位，暴露出第四脑室顶下部、脉络膜丛和下髓帆。用自动牵开器来增加暴露往往适得其反，我们提倡广泛地锐性松解蛛网膜，包括保护和分离双侧小脑后下动脉（posterior inferior cerebellar arteries，PICA）的远端。仔细解剖分离从四脑室正中孔到髓帆水平的脉络丛后，就可以看到整个四脑室。沿着下髓帆向上解剖可以暴露第四脑室上部和顶部的肿瘤（Tanriover et al.，2004）。而若从上髓帆进入则很容易损伤小脑上、中脚，因为它们构成了四脑室的侧壁。随着颅内解剖分离层次的深入，将 PICA 动脉的分支（脉络丛支）被分开，以便松解小脑。膜髓帆入路通常从肿瘤较大的一侧开始操作。一旦术区充分暴露，可以利用自动牵开器通过扁桃体向上和侧面的移位来“保持”（而不是“创造”）暴露空间。因此，在手术过程中，我们提倡适当屈曲头部。图 31.1 展示了经膜髓帆入路。

经小脑蚓部入路

经蚓部入路是第四脑室肿瘤手术的传统入路，包括横切下蚓部。切开蚓部就能暴露小结及其下方的髓帆表面。中线切口可以从小结和脉络膜的内侧进行，注意避免损伤双侧 PICA 动脉的扁桃体段。经蚓部入路可以充分暴露整个第四脑室底，从闩部到中脑导水管开口上下径约 4 cm（Tanriover et al.，2004）。然而，该入路对于侧隐窝和 Luschka 孔的暴露有限，而且还造成一定程度的神经损伤。

我们应当看到小脑蚓部入路和膜髓帆入路相比，虽然经膜髓帆入路对于病变腹侧的暴露可能有限，但是造成神经损伤更小，总的说来更有优势。有报道，由于更好地保留了蚓部和小结，膜髓帆入路降低了术后小脑缄默症和共济失调的发生率（Tanriover et al.，2004；Deshmukh et al.，2006）。

第四脑室肿瘤

Matsuchima 于 1992 年首次描述了第四脑室的经膜髓帆入路，以避免横切小脑中线结构（Matsushima et al.，1992）。自那时起，该手术入路被广泛采用，以获得侧隐窝和第四脑室底的良好暴露。然而，经膜髓帆入路对体积较大的第四脑室病变的疗效却存在争议。最近，Tomasello 等回顾了第四脑室大型病变的切除程度，他的团队能够实现大多数肿瘤约 90% 的切除率（Tomasello et al.，2015）。使用经膜髓帆入路暴露对于 Luschka 孔和上侧隐窝附近的病变，如室管膜瘤和脉络丛乳头状瘤，具有明显的优势（Lee et al.，2012；Tomasello et al.，2015）；而对于靠近第四脑室底的大型肿瘤和累及脑干的肿瘤，其工作角

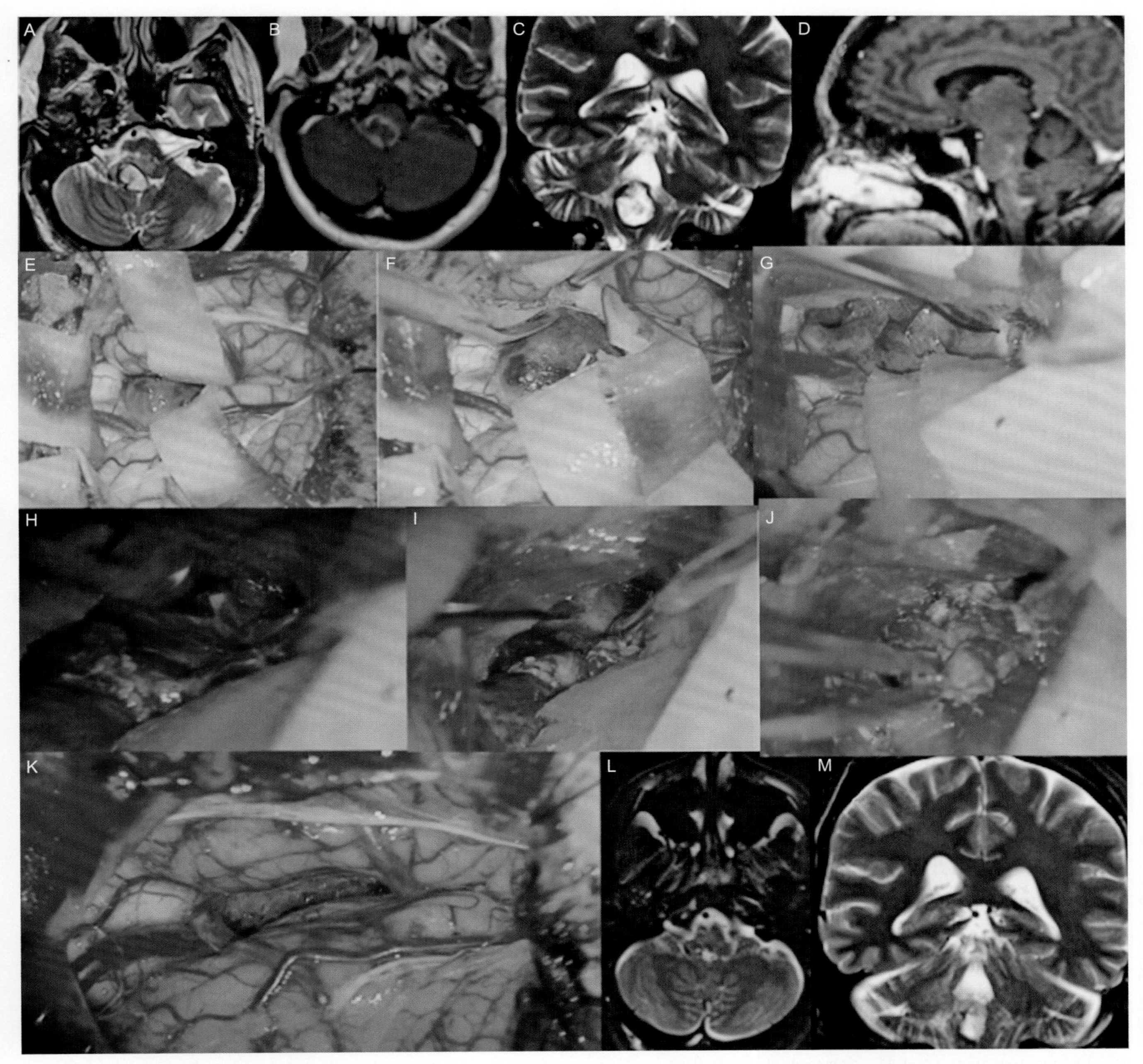

图 31.1 经膜髓帆入路切除脑干海绵状血管畸形。35 岁女性，症状为新近出现的吞咽困难、复视、右侧辨距不良。MRI（A- 轴位 T2，B- 轴位 T1 增强，C- 冠状位 T2，D- 矢状位增强）显示第四脑室海绵状血管畸形。手术采用枕下开颅右侧膜髓帆入路（F）广泛打开硬脑膜（E）。可见海绵状血管畸形突出于双侧小脑扁桃体之间。面神经刺激器不仅用于标记面神经丘（G），也可作为解剖工具使用（I）。锐性分离（H）整体（K）切除病变（J）。术后轴位（L）和冠状位（M）MRI 证实海绵状血管畸形全切

度则不如经小脑蚓部入路理想。然而，若有明显脑干浸润或病理提示高级别肿瘤的情况下，过分积极的手术切除也不值得提倡（El-Bahy，2005）。总的来说，我们的经验是首选经膜髓帆入路，如果术中暴露不足，可以适当切开下蚓部。

枕骨大孔区解剖

枕骨大孔（foramen magnum）（起源于拉丁语，意为“大洞”），位于枕骨的底面。其中有硬脑膜、延髓、副神经脊髓支、椎动脉、脊髓后动脉、齿突尖韧带和覆膜穿过。

舌下神经管位于颈静脉孔的下方和内侧。舌下神经管的底面由枕髁组成，前内侧壁由斜坡构成，后外侧壁由枕骨鳞部构成，顶面由颈静脉结节构成。舌下神经管走行有舌下神经、咽升动脉的脑膜支和舌下静脉丛。此外，还存在乳突导静脉和髁导静脉通过的骨孔。

椎动脉起源于锁骨下动脉，共有四段：V1 段从起始部至 C6 横突孔，V2 段从 C6 至 C2 横突孔，V3 段从 C2 横突孔至硬脑膜环，V4 段穿过硬脑膜后汇入基底动脉。V1 颈段向上、向后方走形于颈长肌和前斜角肌之间，到达 C6 横孔；V2 椎间孔段穿过上六块颈椎的横突孔上行，向上、向外进入寰椎横突孔；V3 段向后弯曲，位于寰椎侧块后内侧，走行于寰椎后弓椎动脉沟的上表面，这段动脉正好也位于枕下三角范围内（周围有静脉丛），发出分支供应枕下肌肉，然后进入寰枕筋膜下的硬脑膜；V4 的分支是脑膜后动脉、脊髓前动脉和小脑后下动脉。从外科角度来看，必须警惕 PICA 动脉可能发生的解剖变异从硬膜外段发出（从 V3 而不是 V4 段发出），因此在入路过程中有电凝导致损伤的风险。

V4 段沿Ⅸ、Ⅹ、Ⅺ和Ⅻ脑神经起始处腹侧向上走行，通常与对侧 V4 汇入基底动脉前在脑桥下缘水平发出 PICA 动脉。PICA 从近端到远端分为五个主要节段：延髓前段、延髓外侧段、扁桃体延髓段、带帆扁桃体段和皮质段（Lister et al.，1982）。基底动脉形成后再发出小脑前下动脉（anterior inferior cerebellar arteries，AICA），走行于小脑下表面，与桥小脑角的Ⅶ、Ⅷ脑神经密切相关。随后，基底动脉还发出小脑上动脉（superior cerebellar arteries，SCA）和大脑后动脉（posterior cerebral arteries，PCA），PCA 构成了 Willis 动脉环的后环。此外，基底动脉还能发出脑桥动脉，偶尔发出迷路动脉。

在决定手术入路时，了解枕下区肌肉的解剖是很重要的，因为该区域受到强有力的肌肉保护。胸锁乳突肌和二腹肌分别附着于乳突尖和乳突尖深部。枕动脉向后延伸至乳突尖深部。头夹肌和头最长肌位于胸锁乳突肌的深处。正后方有斜方肌位于中线，深部是头半棘肌。当把这些肌肉从上项线游离后，就可暴露出枕下三角了，枕下三角以头上斜肌、头下斜肌和头后大直肌为界。第一颈神经背支和椎动脉及其静脉丛位于枕下三角内，枕大神经从该三角穿过。

在这个三角区进行解剖，可以使椎动脉移位，暴露枕髁，必要时可以磨除枕髁，进入枕骨大孔和脑干前部。

枕骨大孔区肿瘤

过去，暴露颅颈交界区腹侧病变曾非常困难。在二十世纪早期，神经外科医生多次尝试从后路安全切除该部位病变均未成功（Elsberg and Strauss，1929；Flores et al.，2013）。然而，在 20 世纪 80 年代，Heros 和 George 分别独立采用了一种新的手术方式（远外侧开颅术），安全地到达了该区域，有助于切除这类病变（Heros，1986；George et al.，1988）。在过去的三十年里，远外侧开颅术一直是进入该区域的主要手术入路。

远外侧入路主要用于切除枕骨大孔区脑膜瘤，其全切效果已被广泛报道。最近的研究表明，近 60%~90% 的病例采用远侧开颅术可以达到全切除。Komotar 等最近总结了影响手术切除范围的因素包括：大型肿瘤、神经或血管侵犯、肿瘤质地坚硬和术前曾接受放疗（Komotar et al.，2010）。对枕骨大孔区肿瘤进行激进的外科手术也可能增加手术致残率。对于那些小的残留肿瘤，伽玛刀照射瘤床防止复发可能是更安全的辅助治疗方式。

手术技巧

远外侧入路

远外侧入路是治疗斜坡下 1/3、枕骨大孔或 C1 水平脑外腹侧、腹外侧病变的理想入路，也适用于位于延髓和脑桥下部腹外侧的脑内病变。**图 31.2** 展示了远外侧入路。

枕骨大孔背侧或背外侧的病变不需要这种入路，因为通过比较简单的枕下入路或乙状窦后入路即可切除。对于远外侧入路，其主要目的就是找到合适角度避开小脑遮挡，向内侧及上方暴露（Elhammady et al.，2012）。这就是为什么我们将患者置于 3/4 侧俯卧位，病变侧朝上的原因。摆放头部有四个步骤：颈部屈曲，向地平面旋转，向地平面倾斜，最后枕颈部向上或向后移位。这四个动作的结合增加了肩膀和头部之间的角度，并有助于寰枕关节的部分开放，使得枕髁的暴露更容易。该体位使同侧小脑半球因为重力作用与病变分离。切口呈曲棍球棍状，在中线从 C2 椎体水平至枕外隆凸，然后向侧方拐至乳突尖。软组织分离技术与枕下后正中开颅类似，尽管这里远外侧入路是偏向一侧的。在上项线处保留一个肌肉袖带以便缝合，头皮拉钩将肌肉及皮下组织向两侧牵拉。一般来说，骨瓣呈泪滴形状，因为枕骨大孔区骨瓣较上部窄。通常骨瓣长度 3 cm 已足够，

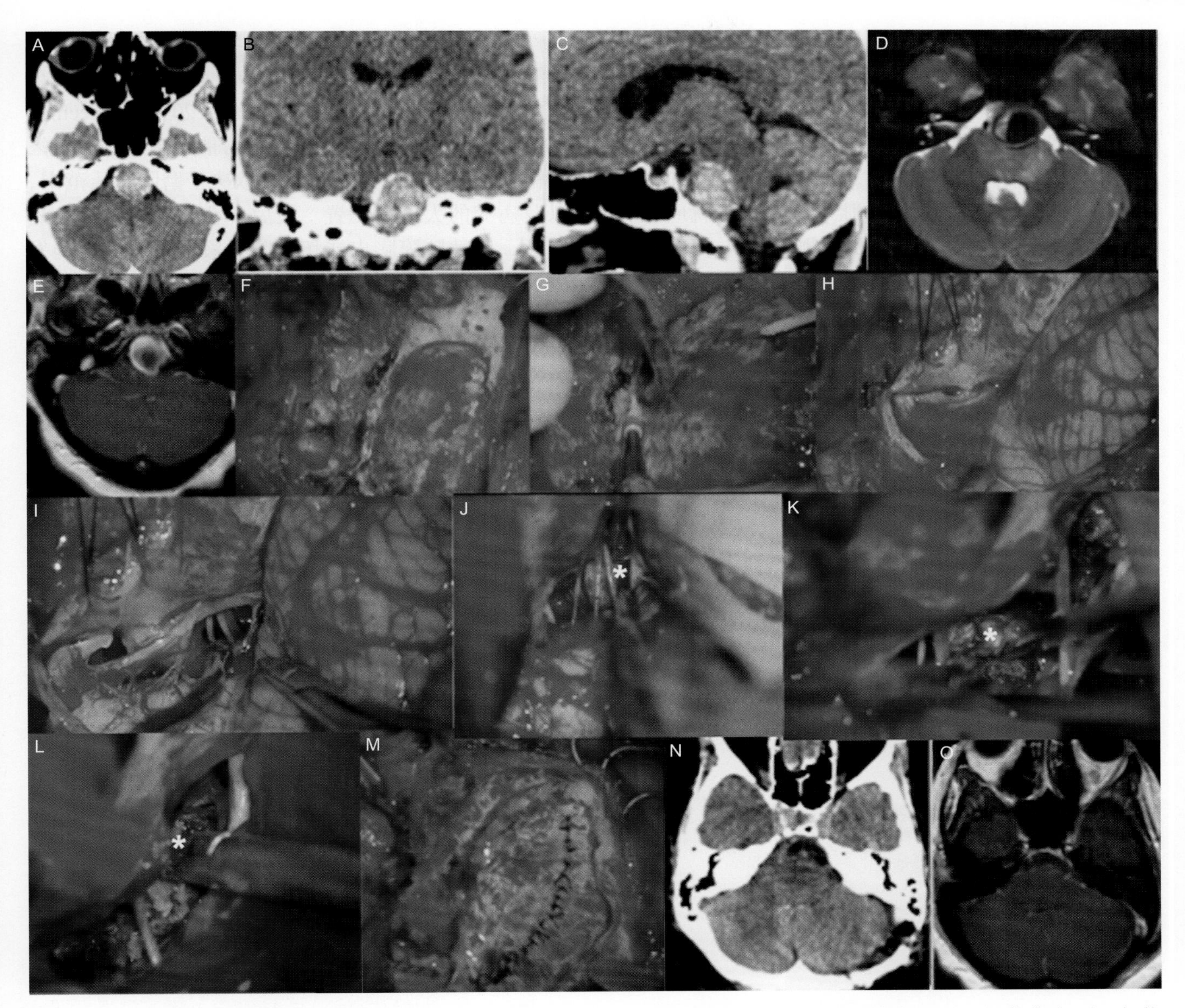

图 31.2　远外侧入路切除颈静脉结节脑膜瘤。54 岁女性，症状为展神经麻痹。CT 扫描［轴位（A）、冠状位（B）、矢状位（C）］显示病变部分钙化，MRI［轴位 T2（D）和 T1 增强（E）］可见液平和强化。采用右侧 3/4 侧俯卧位乙状窦后开颅（F），磨钻扩大骨窗为“远外侧”入路（G）。悬吊硬脑膜（H）扩大术野并广泛解剖蛛网膜（I）。可见肿瘤（*）位于后组脑神经深面（J），先行瘤内分块切除肿瘤减压（K）后分块切除肿瘤（L）。切除肿瘤后硬脑膜水密缝合（M）。术后轴位 CT（N）和轴位 MRI 增强（O）显示肿瘤全切

当然可以根据实际手术需要作具体调整。如果需要暴露乙状窦后的关键部位，骨瓣可以更贴近乙状窦。骨瓣游离后，再用火柴头或圆形磨钻磨除枕骨大孔边缘直至枕骨髁。由于枕髁位于枕骨大孔的前侧方，磨除骨质时不需要延伸到髁内，因此这种入路的“远外侧”标志意味着髁突没有磨除。在特殊情况下，如病变浸润髁突，可能需要一个真正的“经髁”入路。彻底的骨质磨除之后，需要切除同侧的 C1 后弓，手术操作和注意事项同枕下开颅术。硬脑膜随后 U 形切开（以侧方为基底）并悬吊。当悬吊起来的硬脑膜底部没有骨质突起时，说明骨质暴露充分。硬膜瓣的底部应尽可能平坦，否则显微手术视角的暴露则不够靠外侧。

打开硬脑膜、释放脑脊液松弛脑组织的主要目的之一是正确识别显微解剖结构，包括穿过硬脑膜的椎动脉（VA）、上两根齿状韧带及后组脑神经。XI 脑神经位于齿状韧带后方，椎动脉 V3 段在最上齿状韧带处穿过硬脑膜。分开前方齿状韧带，以便更好地显露腹侧基底在前方的肿瘤，如枕骨大孔区脑膜瘤。随后彻底解剖开小脑延髓裂的蛛网膜，以便

松解小脑半球。一旦肿瘤周围解剖清晰显露，应尽可能阻断血供并切除肿瘤。值得注意的是，枕骨大孔脑膜瘤应根据其与椎动脉 V3 段的关系进行治疗（Flores et al.，2013）。如果脑膜瘤起源于椎动脉的上方，那么应该从肿瘤上方开始解剖分离；同样的道理，如果病变起源于椎动脉下方，那么就应该从肿瘤下方开始解剖。术中需要监测后组脑神经功能、体感诱发电位和运动诱发电位。如果肿瘤和血管结构之间没有明显的蛛网膜界面，最好残留一小块肿瘤以保护血管。硬脑膜必须水密闭合，以降低术后脑脊液漏和假性脑膜膨出的风险，如有必要可使用自体骨膜代替（Flores et al.，2013）。

远外侧入路术后最常见的并发症是脑神经麻痹、假性脑膜膨出或脑积水。30%~40% 的患者术后出现后组脑神经麻痹，但大多数（80%）在术后最初几个月内症状有所改善（Komotar et al.，2010；Talacchi et al.，2012）。枕髁磨除 >50% 还可能发生颅颈交界区失稳。术后是否需要枕颈融合取决于磨除骨质范围，以及病变的大小和位置。最后，在切除枕骨大孔病变后，假性脑膜膨出或切口脑脊液漏也有潜在的发生风险，细致严密的组织缝合和硬脑膜水密缝合有助于避免这些并发症。

延伸阅读、参考文献、EBRAIN 的相关链接

扫描书末二维码获取。

第七篇　肿瘤和颅底——脑室肿瘤

第 32 章　脑室肿瘤

Paul Grundy・Vasileios Apostolopoulos 著
戴缤 译，胡志强 审校

引言与治疗原则

根据美国中央脑肿瘤登记处（CBTRUS 2006—2010 统计报告，*n*=326 711；Ostrom et al.，2013）统计，约 1.2% 的原发性脑肿瘤位于脑室内。它们代表了一组不同组织来源的肿瘤，但大多数是低级别肿瘤。影像学鉴别较为困难，但通常通过考虑肿瘤的影像特征、患者年龄、肿瘤在脑室内的位置、临床表现和相关的疾病（如结节性硬化症）来缩小范围。即使继发于脑积水的颅内压升高是脑室肿瘤常见的临床表现，但越来越多的脑室肿瘤是被偶然发现的。我们观察到其特征性的生长模式，并被认为是各种类型的脑室肿瘤的典型特征。根据其生长方式和肿瘤大小，脑室内肿瘤可以局限在一个脑室内，也可以延伸到邻近的脑室（如中枢神经细胞瘤），或通过流出孔进入邻近的脑池（如第四脑室室管膜瘤）。大型肿瘤可以穿过室管膜壁延伸到脑实质内（例如巨大脑膜瘤或脉络丛肿瘤）。事实上，对于极大的肿瘤，有时很难区分它们是延伸到脑室的实质性肿瘤，还是相反的情况（**图** 32.1）。脑室内肿瘤的治疗需个体化，但通常情况下，首要考虑的是脑积水的治疗。对于第三脑室肿瘤，神经内镜可以同时进行脑脊液分流和活检。脑脊液分流应该先进行，因为活检可能会导致肿瘤出血以致能见度降低。如果怀疑是生殖细胞肿瘤，应检测脑脊液和血浆肿瘤标志物。通过脑脊液播散的肿瘤需行全颅脊髓轴成像（**表** 32.1）。除非延误会对患者造成伤害，所有病例都应该在神经肿瘤学 MDT 会议上讨论，然后再计划明确的手术方案。如果患者没有症状，肿瘤没有生长，或者患者不适合手术，保守治疗和影像学随访可能是最好的选择。对于年龄较大、身体状况不佳的患者，如果肿瘤级别较低，且临床病程缓慢，则仅行脑脊液分流术可能是最佳选择（例如，老年人第四脑室室管膜下瘤）。

分类（解剖学、病理学、局部解剖学）

不同的脑室内肿瘤往往发生在脑室系统的特定部位，很大程度上是因为它们起源的细胞群体先前就存在于脑室系统的某些部位（**表** 32.1）。这一认识有助于脑室内肿瘤的影像学鉴别诊断。脑室内肿瘤可能起源于脑室系统、透明隔膜或脉络丛内的室管膜或室管膜下。胶样囊肿与胚胎端脑 / 间脑界面内胚层成分错位有关。许多脑室内肿瘤是脑实质内肿瘤外生至脑室的，例如，大型星形细胞肿瘤可以从额叶、

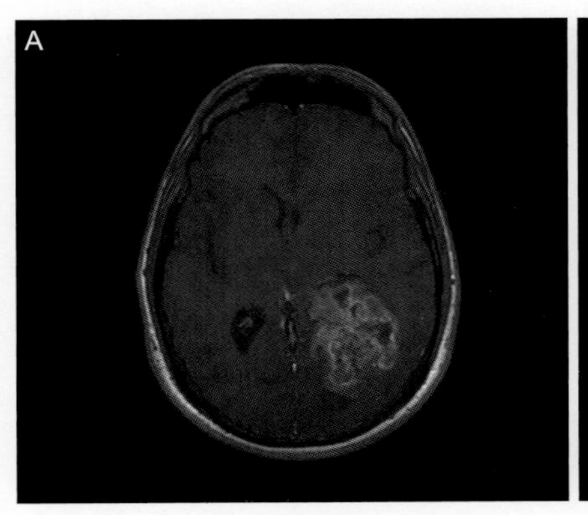

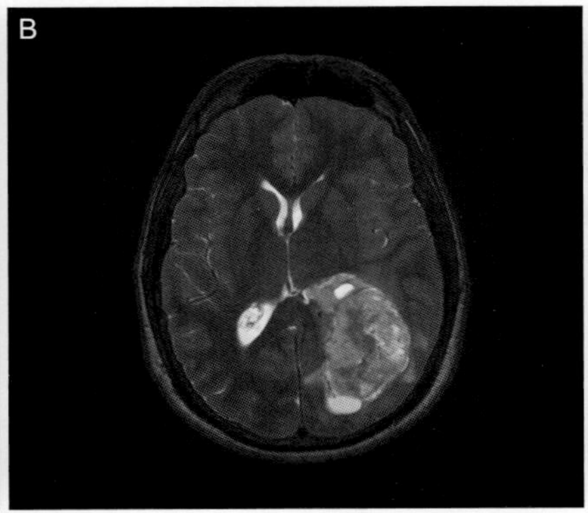

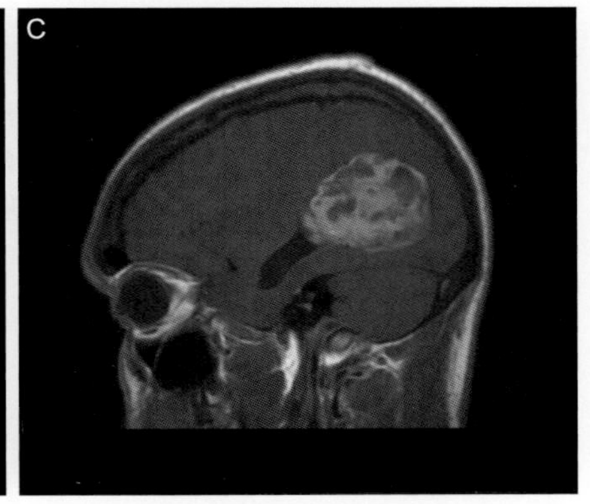

图 32.1　神经节细胞胶质瘤，其外观提示脑室内位置，术前认为是脑膜瘤。外生性内在胶质瘤可生长到邻近脑室。轴位（A）和矢状位（B）T1MRI 钆增强像，轴位 T2 像（C）

表 32.1 脑室内肿瘤快速鉴别表

位置	附着物	起源细胞	肿瘤	WHO	MRI 特征	最常见的位置、相关条件、患者人群	脑脊液播散，复发的可能性
侧脑室	脑室壁	室管膜细胞（神经胶质细胞室管膜分化）	**室管膜瘤**	Ⅱ、Ⅲ	边界清楚，分叶状，不均匀（+-）有钙化，出血，囊肿，T1 像等信号，T2 像高信号，强化明显	第四脑室如果是幕上边可以在脑室外、神经纤维瘤病 2 型患者	有可能，如果切除不完全可以复发
		室管膜下胶质细胞	**室管膜下瘤**	Ⅰ	边界清楚，分叶状，T1 像低信号，T2 像高信号大多数都是不强化的，可能会有一些表现强化	通常位于第四脑室，老年室管膜瘤患者多欠	不会播散，彻底切除可以治愈
		室管膜下结节内混合的神经元和巨细胞星形胶质细胞	**室管膜下巨细胞星形细胞瘤**	Ⅰ	边界清楚，其他室管膜下结节，T1 像呈低等信号，T2 像高信号，强化明显	侧脑室靠近室间孔区域，结节性硬化症儿童常见	不发生
	透明隔	前体神经元细胞	**中枢神经细胞瘤**	Ⅱ、Ⅲ	广泛附着在透明隔上，边界清楚，呈分叶状，可含囊肿、钙化，极少出血，T1、T2 像都是等信号，不均匀强化	侧脑室靠近室间孔，青年人	不可能，彻底切除可以治愈，非典型具有高复发率
		星型胶质细胞	**星型细胞瘤**	Ⅱ、Ⅲ、Ⅳ			不可能播散，可能复发
	三角区	脉络丝、蛛网膜帽细胞	**脑膜瘤**	Ⅰ、Ⅱ	分叶状，均匀强化	左侧常见	不可能
		脉络丝	**脉络丝肿瘤（CPP Ⅰ、Ⅱ、Ⅲ）**	Ⅰ、Ⅱ、Ⅲ	结节状明显强化	三角区，青年人	CPP Ⅰ型少见 CPP Ⅲ型常见，推荐做全脊柱 MRI
		淋巴细胞	**淋巴瘤**			少见，通常多发	不可能
第三脑室	室间孔	室间孔脑旁体成分	**胶体囊肿**	Ⅰ	T1 像高信号，T2 像等低信号，没有强化	第三脑室前部，室间孔	没有播散，彻底切除可以治愈，没有彻底切除可复发
		脉络丛	**脉络丛乳头状瘤，脉络丛癌**		T1 像高信号，T2 等低信号，没有强化	少见	CPP Ⅰ、Ⅱ型少见，CPC Ⅲ型多见，建议做全脊柱 MRI

（续表）

位置	附着物	起源细胞	肿瘤	WHO	MRI 特征	最常见的位置、相关条件、患者人群	脑脊液播散，复发的可能性
		蛛网膜颗细胞 - 中间帆	**脑膜瘤**			少见	不发生
	鞍上区	鳞状细胞 - 颅颊裂	**颅咽管瘤**		参考第 26 章		不可能，如果切除不彻底容易复发
		生殖细胞	**生殖细胞肿瘤（生殖细胞瘤和非生殖细胞瘤）**		T1、T2 像等信号或稍高信号，均匀强化	松果体 / 鞍上区，儿童 / 青年人	有可能
	第三脑室后部	来自丘脑的肿瘤可发生进入第三脑室后部，但这个区域最常见肿瘤起源于松果体区（可参见相关章节），梗阻性脑积水是最常见的临床表现，需要首先处理					
第四脑室	脑室壁 / 底部	室管膜细胞	**室管膜瘤**	Ⅱ、Ⅲ	边界清楚分叶状，有异物成分 +-，钙化出血，囊肿 T1 像等信号，T2 像高信号，强化表现	第四脑室幕上也可以在脑室外神经纤维瘤病 2 型	有可能，不彻底切除可以复发
		室管膜下细胞	**室管膜下瘤**	Ⅰ	边界清楚分叶状 T1 像低信号，T2 像高信号，大部分没有强化，部分可强化	通常在第四脑室，室管膜瘤老年人群	不发生播散，彻底切除可治愈

胼胝体或丘脑生长到脑室，脑干胶质瘤可以外生到第四脑室。

髓母细胞瘤通常是小脑蚓部肿瘤（年轻人也可以在小脑半球内生长），但通常表现为充满第四脑室大部的大肿瘤。鞍区和鞍上较大的肿瘤向上生长到第三脑室的情况并不少见。同样，松果体区肿瘤可以从松果体区生长到第三脑室后部。接下来将介绍脑室特定部位肿瘤生长的更多细节。

前体和后角

肿瘤通常来源于脑室壁（室管膜瘤、室管膜下瘤）或透明隔（中枢神经细胞瘤）。原发性透明隔肿瘤（星形细胞瘤、淋巴瘤和生殖细胞瘤）极为罕见。透明隔转移性黑色素瘤已有报道（Cipri et al.，2009）。

大的、高级别的实质内星形细胞肿瘤可以外生进入脑室，许多肿瘤会堵塞室间孔，或隔断后侧脑室而造成梗阻，导致整个脑室积水或导致脑室后部增大——囊状脑室。

中枢神经细胞瘤（central neurocytomas）起源于透明隔内的神经细胞前体。T1、T2 像与灰质等信号，强化不均匀。通常，肿瘤以宽基底与透隔附着，可以在侧脑室内生长到相当大（**图 32.2**）。偶尔，也可以通过室间孔生长到第三脑室。肿瘤边界清楚，可分叶状，含有囊肿，有不均匀的信号和流空影，也可有钙化。肿瘤偶尔会包围穹隆柱，在这种情况下，为了保存记忆，可能不会进行完全的手术切除。这一肿瘤的细节将在本章后面讨论。

室管膜下瘤（subependymomas）是一种边界清楚的无强化良性肿瘤，最常见于第四脑室，但也可见于侧脑室内，表现为附着在侧脑室侧壁的无强化或低强化肿瘤。如果出现症状或在影像上出现进展，就需要手术切除。在侧脑室内，通常可以完全切除，做到手术治愈。该肿瘤需要根据患者的年龄和一般健康状况实施个体化治疗。对于高龄和无症状患者，

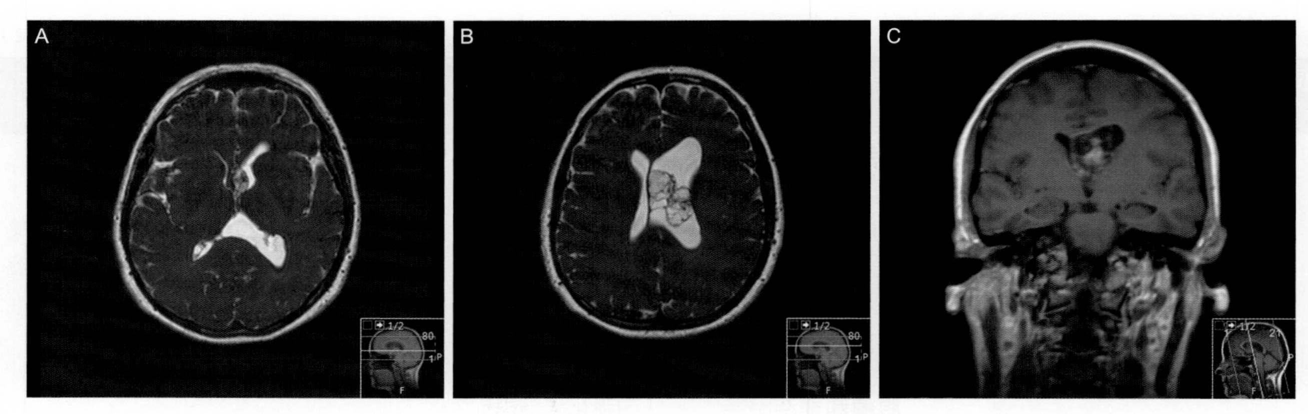

图 32.2 侧脑室中枢神经细胞瘤，轴位 T2（A）和冠状位 T1（B）增强像表现典型，累及透明隔和穹隆柱，突入第三脑室，左侧侧脑室扩张

保守治疗是一种合理的治疗选择。

室管膜下巨细胞星形细胞瘤（subependymal giant cell astrocytomas，SEGA）是起源于室管膜下结节的胶质和神经元混合分化的肿瘤，常见于结节性硬化症患者。它们在 T1 上呈等或低信号，在 T2 上呈高信号，并显示强烈强化。它们通常在室间孔的区域生长缓慢，而上面的室管膜则完好无损。如果达到一定大小会导致梗阻性脑积水。如果患者没有症状，通常的做法是密切监测，并进行系列成像和临床随访。如果连续扫描显示持续生长或患者发生脑积水，则需手术切除。部分学者还建议对较小的病变进行立体定向放射外科治疗。

在接受 mTOR 抑制剂治疗的患者中，术后 SEGA 的复发率较低。这些药物下调了在许多癌症中被发现过度活跃的细胞周期中的 mTOR 信号通路。在 SEGA 中，这些药物不仅可以降低 SEGA 的复发率，还可以使其他与结节性硬化症相关的肿瘤缩小，如血管纤维瘤和血管平滑肌脂肪瘤。然而，应仔细权衡这种治疗的益处与显著的、潜在的副作用，包括免疫抑制和反复感染、严重贫血、血小板减少症相关性疲劳、恶心和腹泻（Campen and Porter，2011）。

成人室管膜瘤（ependymomas）多见于第四脑室（60%），但也可见于侧脑室。从理论上讲，它们可以生长在颅脑脊髓轴（第三脑室、导水管）内的任何脑脊液间隙中，也是最常见的脊髓内肿瘤之一。它们是边界清楚的肿瘤，增强并且经常含有钙化。它们通常在 T1 与白质呈等信号或低信号，在 T2 呈高信号。

星形细胞瘤（astrocytomas）可以从周围的脑实质生长进入脑室。然而，它们很少能以原发性室间隔肿瘤的形式生长。

颅后窝三角

脑膜瘤是侧脑室三角区最常见的脑室内肿瘤，但仅占所有颅内脑膜瘤的 4%。更常见的是成人，女性发病率较高，原因还不完全清楚，同时左侧发病率高于右侧。它们被认为起源于胚胎期间困在脉络丛内的蛛网膜帽细胞。它们可能会长到很大，并引起高颅内压的症状，但也可能是偶然的。影像上呈现的是大的均匀强化的肿瘤，通常有一个重要的供血血管，MRI 上可以看到它进入肿瘤，这根血管通常是脉络膜动脉的一个分支（**图** 32.3）。脑室内脑膜瘤也可以发生在第三脑室后部（中间膜的蛛网膜细胞）或第四脑室（脉络丛内的蛛网膜细胞）。治疗方案（取决于肿瘤大小和临床情况）包括手术、SRS 或监测。

脉络丛肿瘤起源于脉络丛，最常位于儿童的侧脑室和成人的第四脑室。最常发生在 15 岁以下儿童中，但也可能发生在出生早期。在组织学上，可以被分为脉络丛乳头状瘤（CPP-WHO Ⅰ）、不典型脉络丛乳头状瘤（CPP-WHO Ⅱ）或脉络丛癌（CPC-WHO Ⅲ）。所有这些类型的脉络丛肿瘤的放射学表现相似，但预后明显不同。大多数肿瘤表现为边缘分叶状和流空的急切强化的肿瘤，而且常常可以达到很大的体积。当它们长到很大时，可以穿过室管膜进入周围的实质。患者倾向于出现脑积水，这既是由于脑脊液产生的增加，也是由于梗阻。无论 WHO 分级如何，最好的治疗方法是大体全切除。术前应考虑栓塞术，因为它可以减少术中出血，而术中出血可能是灾难性的。CPC 术后采用放射治疗，但最重要的预后因素是肿瘤残留物的存在与否。CPC 的

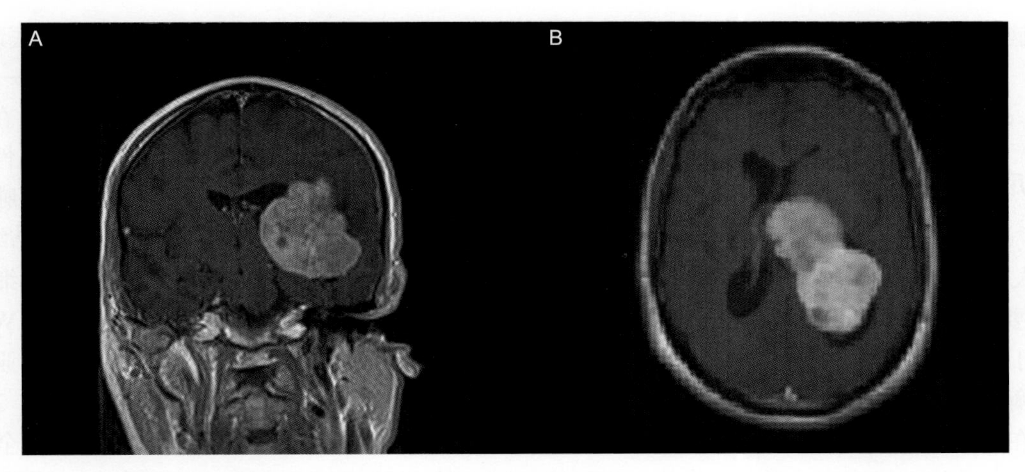

图 32.3 侧脑室三角区的脑室内脑膜瘤。冠状面（A）和横断面（B）T1WI

预后一般被认为是很差的。CPP 可以被完全切除后治愈。脉络丛肿瘤的位置、大小和增强特征有时会使其难以与该区域的脑膜瘤相鉴别。脑脊液播散在 CPP Ⅰ、Ⅱ很少见，但已有个别病例报道。脑脊液播种是 CPC 的常见播种方式。因此，在做出任何明确的诊断之前，必须进行全脊柱磁共振检查。

第三脑室

第三脑室前部

室间孔

胶样囊肿（colloid cysts）是最常见的第三脑室肿瘤。胶样囊肿的真实发病率不能被准确计算，因为这些肿瘤中有很大一部分是无症状的，因此报道不足（Pollock and Huston，1999）。它们是良性病变，由上皮衬里的囊肿组成，囊内充满含有黏蛋白、胆固醇和透明质的凝胶密度物质。不同病例所含物质成分的相对比例可能不同，从而导致影像上的不同表现和手术时的不同浓度。

在 CT 上，它们典型表现为高密度和部分表现为等或低密度单眼病变，填充在前第三脑室，伴或不伴脑积水。在 MRI 上，它们可以是低信号或高信号，T1 无强化，但最常见的是 T2 低信号。它们可以被偶然发现或表现为急性、间歇性或慢性梗阻性脑积水（间歇性头痛、跌倒发作）。虽然这些囊肿的起源尚不完全清楚，但人们认为它们起源于原始神经上皮的异常折叠，在该区域，原始神经上皮将端脑与间脑分隔开来。虽然猝死罕见，但已有报道。传统上认为这与活动肿瘤引起的急性梗阻性脑积水（“球瓣机制”）有关，但继发于急性下丘脑功能障碍的心脏受累的理论已变得越来越突出（Turillazzi et al.，2012）。

作为一般原则，有症状的胶体囊肿应切除。根据Ⅱ级证据，98% 的无症状胶体囊肿在长期随访中临床上将保持无症状状态（Pollock and Huston，1999）。对于 50 岁以下的患者和囊肿大于 1cm 的患者，观察到无症状囊肿的概率也较高（Pollock et al.，2000）。

手术选择包括经皮质或经胼胝体入路的开放手术、内镜切除或无框架立体定向抽吸术。每种方式都有利弊。开放入路有更高的机会完全切除囊肿，但也可能有更高的癫痫发作或穹隆损伤的风险。脑室的大小可能是内镜手术的一个限制因素。囊肿内容物的黏度也可能是立体定向或内镜抽吸的限制因素。如果抽吸不完全，胶样囊肿会复发。

鞍区肿块的扩展，很可能是大型垂体腺瘤，在 MRI 上具有典型的垂体瘤、双颞叶视野障碍和内分泌激素紊乱的表现。

鞍上肿瘤（suprasellar tumours）延伸至脑室，最常见的是颅咽管瘤，但也有生殖细胞瘤——请参见**第 27 章**。

视路和下丘脑**胶质瘤**（optic pathway and hypothalamic gliomas），最常影响儿童人群。更多细节见**第 38 章**和**第 88 章**。

脑膜瘤从颅底向上延伸。更多细节见**第 14 章**。

第三脑室后部

1. **松果体区肿瘤**（pineal region tumours）可生长至第三脑室后部。请参阅有关这些肿瘤的章节。
2. **小脑幕边缘脑膜瘤**（meningiomas from the tentorial edge）（包括松果体区肿瘤的鉴别诊断）。
3. 蛛网膜囊肿（arachnoid cysts）较难发现。它们会导致第三脑室积水。如果有症状，可以通过内镜开窗治疗。

4. **皮样囊肿**（dermoid cyst）罕见。

第四脑室（成人）

1. **室管膜瘤**（ependymomas）强化的分叶状肿瘤更多见于年轻人，倾向于通过脑室流出孔向外生长（**图 32.4**）。主要的治疗方法是手术治疗，但是当这些肿瘤起源于第四脑室底部时，行根治性切除需要谨慎地平衡脑神经麻痹的重大风险。在这种情况下，如果在肿瘤和第四脑室底部之间保持良好的解剖平面，术后脑神经麻痹（很可能发生）很可能随着时间的推移而逐渐改善（尽管不能保证完全恢复）。所有这些都应该在手术前与患者仔细讨论。由于存在脑脊液肿瘤播散的风险，术前必须对整个颅脑脊髓轴进行成像。室管膜瘤的组织学分级和临床意义之间的非相关性是有据可查的。2016 年新的世卫组织中枢神经系统肿瘤分类没有进一步阐明这一点。然而，一个新的实体，RELA 融合阳性室管膜瘤（儿童常见的幕上室管膜瘤）被包括在内。此外，以前细胞室管膜瘤实体从分类中被删除，因为它被认为与标准室管膜瘤相同。
2. **室管膜下瘤**（subependymomas）——无强化（或有时含有强化成分）的分叶状肿瘤多见于中老年患者，常为偶发发现。如果小而无症状，或者患者不适合接受手术，可以保守治疗。偶尔脑脊液分流可能是必要的，但由于这些肿瘤的临床病程缓慢，患者通常被保守治疗。对于有较大或有症状的肿瘤年轻患者应该考虑切除，但通常选择慎重的次全切除，以避免损伤第四脑室底部。
3. **髓母细胞瘤**（medulloblastomas）——起源于小脑蚓部，最常见于儿童，但很少发生在年轻人（可能发生在小脑半球）。通常表现为急性梗阻性脑积水。2016 年世卫组织中枢神经系统肿瘤分类提供了这些肿瘤成熟的组织学亚型（促结缔组织 / 结节型、髓母细胞瘤伴广泛结节型、大细胞型和间变性型）和四种现已建立的遗传亚型（WNT 激活型、SHH 激活型、第 3 组亚型和第 4 组亚型）的通常组合非常有力的说明（Louis et al.，2016）。治疗应优先考虑：急性脑积水的处理、全脑脊髓轴成像和脑脊液取样、MDT 讨论、原发肿瘤的手术（力求最大限度地切除肿瘤、建立组织学和分子亚型）以及根据疾病的分期和患者的年龄进行进一步的肿瘤学治疗。当地建立的协议通常适用。在表现时，相当大比例的患者已经在脊柱有继发性沉积。预后不良的公认因素包括就诊时继发沉积或脑脊液肿瘤播散、原发肿瘤次全切除和年龄较小等（更多细节见第 28 章）。
4. **脉络丛肿瘤**（choroid plexus tumours）——第四脑室对于这些肿瘤来说是一个不寻常的位置，但它们可以在这里发生，并极易分化为分叶状肿瘤。主要治疗方法是外科手术。如果次全切除，它们可能会复发。
5. **外生性脑干胶质瘤**（exophytic brain stem gliomas）——通常是脑桥胶质瘤。在儿童中更为常见（更多细节见第 7 章）。
6. **囊虫病**——如果患者来自流行区或曾到流行区旅行，则仔细加以鉴别。

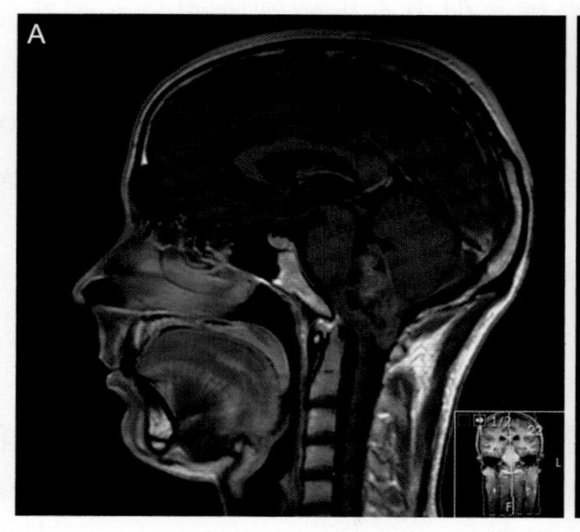

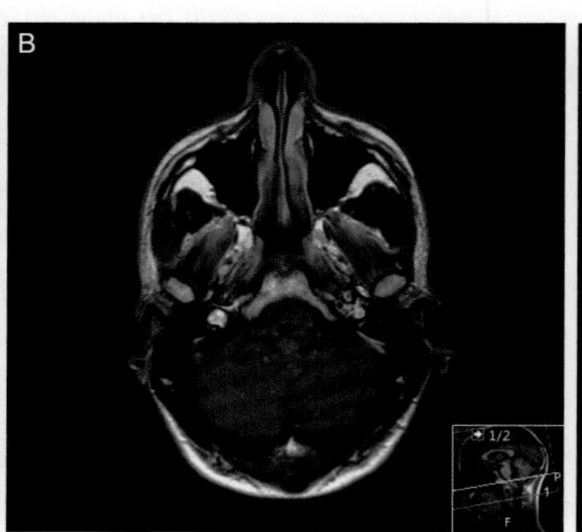

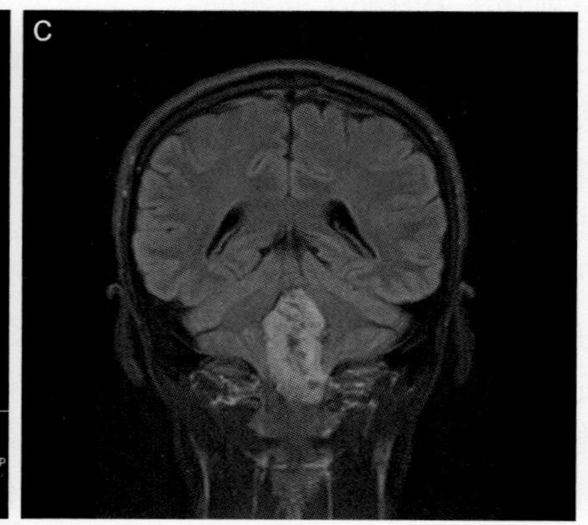

图 32.4 第四脑室室管膜瘤，矢状位（A）和轴位（B）T1 像和冠状位（C）FLAIR 表现典型，呈片状强化，压迫脑干，沿大脑孔生长，累及小脑后下动脉分支

临床表现

脑室内肿瘤的临床表现取决于其位置、大小和进展速度。快速发展可导致急性脑积水（严重头痛、嗜睡、恶心和呕吐），需要在明确治疗肿瘤之前进行脑脊液分流。然而，生长缓慢的肿瘤在出现症状之前会有很长一段时间没有症状，通常表现为慢性的、NPH 样的临床表现（认知功能下降、步态障碍和大小便失禁）。这些患者的治疗应该集中在肿瘤的外科治疗上，因为这也可以解决由此导致的脑积水。由于影像的广泛应用，偶然性诊断尤其是低级别脑室内肿瘤，如今已变得越来越容易。某些脑室内肿瘤可以达到很大的尺寸，并且可以引起脑室周围神经结构的后位效应而带来的症状。左侧脑室的大肿瘤与记忆和语言障碍有关。两侧的大肿瘤都可能导致运动障碍，如果它们从脑室外侵犯到实质，也可能导致癫痫。视力障碍可能是由于长期的高颅内压造成的，也可能是由于直接压在视觉通路上而导致的各种视野缺陷。后第三脑室和松果体区的肿瘤也可以表现为 Parinaud 综合征和急性脑积水。大的颅后窝肿瘤通常表现为急性梗阻性脑积水，并取决于其大小和范围，并伴有平衡障碍。低级别肿瘤的症状缓慢且渐进出现和发展，很少因瘤内出血而发展加快，这会导致病情突然恶化（Ogbodo et al., 2012）。

治疗

如果脑室肿瘤导致梗阻性脑积水，并伴有神经状态恶化，脑脊液分流术应优先考虑。对于第三脑室肿瘤，如果肿瘤阻塞了两个室间孔，应该考虑双侧脑室引流。可以通过插入脑室外引流管引流，或者根据诊断，可以先进行内神经镜下第三脑室造瘘术，然后进行肿瘤（如后第三脑室 / 松果体区肿瘤）的内镜活检。当脑室阻塞发生在后第三脑室或以下时，神经内镜第三脑室造瘘术有可能成为脑脊液分流的一种选择。

对于患有慢性脑积水的生长缓慢的肿瘤的患者，肿瘤的处理可以放在首位。然而，在这些情况下，如果决定对患者进行保守治疗，可以用脑室腹腔分流术来治疗脑积水。对于被诊断为较低级别的脑室病变且不适合接受脑室肿瘤切除的老年患者，这是一个被普遍认可的治疗方案。

对于那些有脑脊液播散潜在性的肿瘤（**表** 32.1），术前对整个脊柱和脑脊液进行增强 MRI 检查是必要的，这样才能对肿瘤进行分期。

松果体区肿瘤应送检血液和脑脊液中的肿瘤标志物。如怀疑转移瘤，应考虑全身 CT 扫描。

中枢神经细胞瘤

低级别肿瘤，最常见于年轻人。1982 年首次描述时（Hassoun et al., 1982）被列为 WHO Ⅰ级肿瘤，但由于某些组织学亚型复发率高，随后被升级为 WHO Ⅱ级肿瘤。通常出现逐渐发作的症状，提示脑积水引起的颅内压升高。除了头痛外，慢性脑积水的临床表现还包括认知功能减退、步态障碍和大小便失禁。当肿瘤很大时，由于肿瘤对脑室周围结构的直接影响，患者也可能出现症状。肿瘤内出血可能导致症状突然恶化，从而明确诊断。它们通常预后良好，但如果不完全切除，可能会复发。它们通常位于侧脑室，起源于透明隔，偶尔延伸到第三脑室。它们表现为轻度至中度强化，可含有囊肿、钙化和流空。

流行病学

罕见，在不同的文献中报道，占脑肿瘤的 0.5%。

病理学

具有神经元分化的高分化肿瘤。由于细胞质透明，与其他透明细胞肿瘤鉴别较为困难。突触素和神经元核抗原的存在通常被用来确认诊断。肿瘤的细胞质空泡化使肿瘤呈“煎蛋”状，与少突胶质瘤相似。

当 MIB-1 标记指数超过 3% 时，局部控制和生存预后较差（Rades et al., 2004）。这些肿瘤被称为非典型中枢神经细胞瘤。

尽管中枢神经细胞瘤的性质通常是良性的，但已有中枢神经细胞瘤恶变的报道（Amagasa et al., 2008）。

治疗

由于这些肿瘤的发生率很低，没有足够的数据来支持大型前瞻性研究。有关中枢神经细胞瘤治疗的最高水平证据来自 meta 分析。关于中枢神经细胞瘤治疗的最大 meta 分析报告（n=438）得出结论，在所有病例中，如果评估结果为安全，应该尝试大体全切除（Rades and Schild, 2006）。在该研究中，根据 MIB-1 标记指数大于 3% 和有无不典型组织学特征，将肿瘤分为典型和非典型中枢神经细胞瘤。在

351 例典型神经细胞瘤患者中，大部切除后加放疗获得了相同的 5 年生存率，但局部控制率略高（100% *vs.* 87%）。然而，考虑到放射治疗的风险，一般不建议这样做。然而，放疗对接受大部切除的典型神经细胞瘤患者是有益的，因为它提高了 5 年生存率和局部控制率，几乎达到了大部切除（gross total resection，GTR）的效果（见**专栏** 32.1）。

次全切除的 5 年生存率和局部控制率很低，但术后放疗显著改善（生存率 43%~78%，局部控制率 7%~70%）。

可采用大脑半球间 - 胼胝体或经皮质入路手术切除这些肿瘤。大脑半球间 - 胼胝体入路可以方便地进入脑室，无癫痫发作的风险，而且发生断流综合征的风险非常低。

中枢神经细胞瘤的治疗总结见**专栏** 32.1。典型中枢神经细胞瘤的组织病理学特征见**图** 32.5。

预后

预后这在很大程度上取决于肿瘤的增殖潜力和肿瘤被切除的程度。

专栏 32.1 中枢神经细胞瘤（典型和非典型）的处理

1c 级建议
- 如果安全可行，可尝试 GTR（适用于典型和非典型中枢神经细胞瘤）
- STR+RT=GTR 控制率 / 生存率，适用于 GTR 被认为高风险的典型中枢神经细胞瘤
- 典型神经细胞瘤 STR 后放疗建议剂量为 50~54 Gy
- 不推荐不典型中枢神经细胞瘤 GTR 后放疗
- 不典型中枢神经细胞瘤 STR 后放疗剂量建议为 55~60 Gy

2c 级建议
- 典型中枢神经细胞瘤 GTR 后不要使用放疗
- 活组织检查、脑脊液分流和放疗有时对典型中枢神经细胞瘤有效

CSF，脑脊液；GTR，大部分切除；RT，放疗；STR，次全切

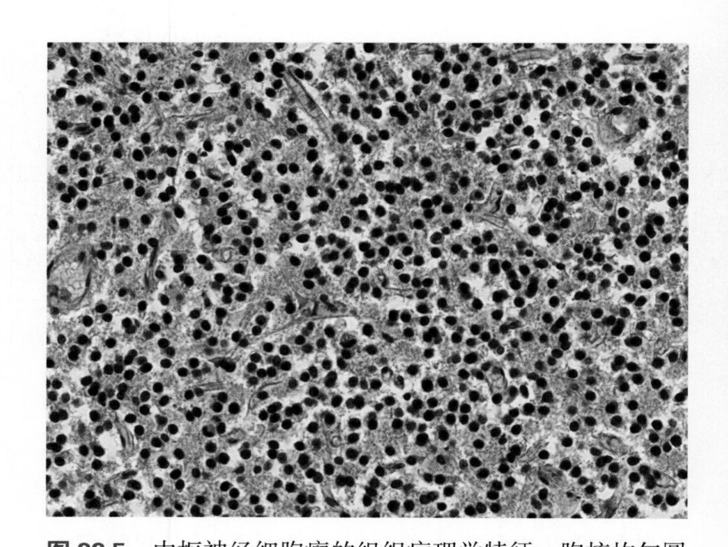

图 32.5 中枢神经细胞瘤的组织病理学特征。胞核均匀圆形的神经细胞是典型的特征。偶尔可能会出现形状不佳的玫瑰花环，如本例所示。推测突触素有很强的免疫反应性

Courtesy of Dr Kieren Allinson, Department of Pathology, Addenbrooke's Hospital, Cambridge.

参考文献、EBRAIN 的相关链接

扫描书末二维码获取。

第 33 章 胶样囊肿

Asim Sheikh · Paul Chumas 著
戴缤 译，胡志强 审校

引言

胶样囊肿（colloid cysts）是良性的，多为脑室肿瘤，占所有颅内肿块病变的 0.5%~2%。最常见于第三脑室前部的室间孔水平，如果有症状，通常表现为侧脑室梗阻性脑积水。最初的描述将它们与 CT 出现之前时代的猝死联系在一起。它们也被称为神经上皮囊肿（**图** 33.1、**图** 33.2、**图** 33.3 和**图** 33.4）。

治疗方案包括单独治疗脑积水，抽吸囊肿内容物，通过内镜或显微外科方法摘除囊肿。

流行病学

库欣（Cushing）描述了一例胶样囊肿的无症状病例。有趣的是，据报道，在哈维·库欣（Harvey Cushing）本人的尸检中发现了一个胶样囊肿（Fulton，1946）。由于大多数胶样囊肿没有症状，所以很难确定这种良性病变的确切发生率（Fulton，1946）。随着现代影像技术的日益普及，越来越多的无症状胶体囊肿被诊断出来。根据尸检和磁共振成像，患病率估计为每 8500 人中有 1 例（de Witt Hamer et al.，2002）。芬兰的一项研究计算出，在 14 年的观察期内，症状性胶质囊肿的发病率为每年 3.2/ 百万，占所有颅内肿瘤的 2%（Hernesniemi and Lievo，1996）。Vandertop 估计，每百万人 1 年仅有 1 例出现症状（de Witt Hamer et al.，2002）。确诊年龄从妊娠期胎儿到 76 岁不等（Gaertner et al.，1993；Romani et al.，2008），但最常见的确诊年龄在 20~50 岁。虽然胶样囊肿被认为是先天性的，但在儿童中很少有报道（Macdonald et al.，1994；Maqsood et al.，2006）。

发病机制

胶样囊肿通常在冠状面上位于第三脑室室间孔

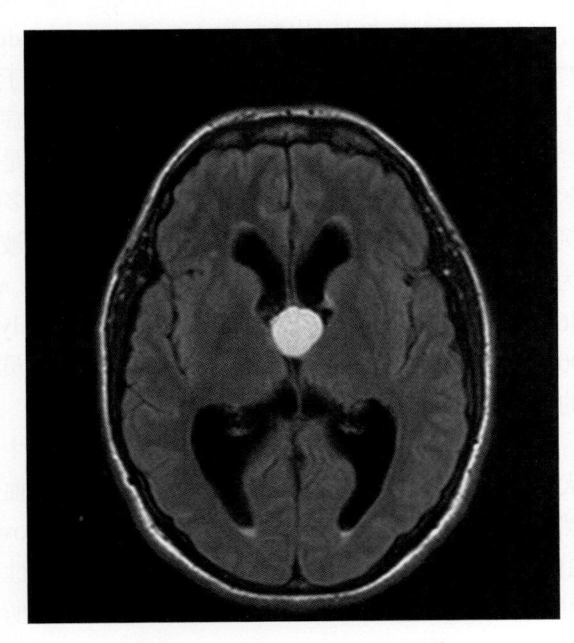

图 33.1 胶体囊肿的 MRI T2W FLAIR 图像

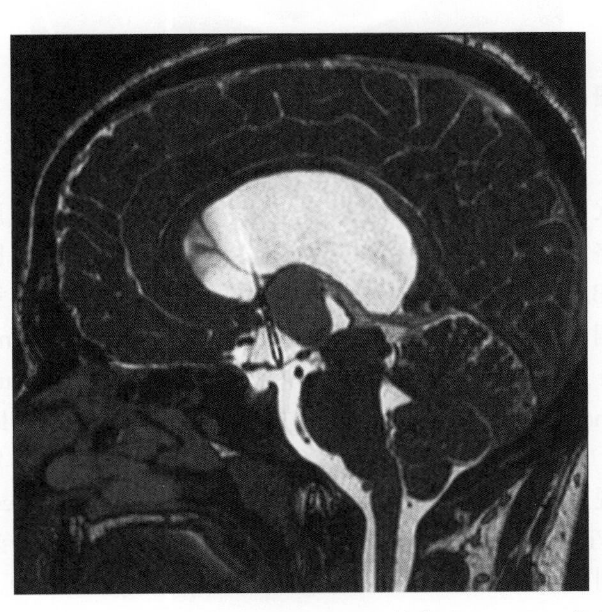

图 33.2 胶样囊肿及脑室外引流的矢状位 T2W CISS 序列

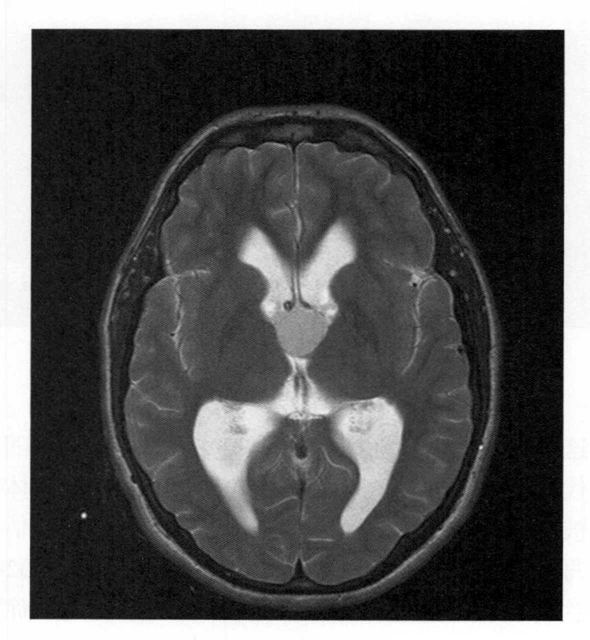

图 33.3 胶样囊肿 T2W 轴位图像

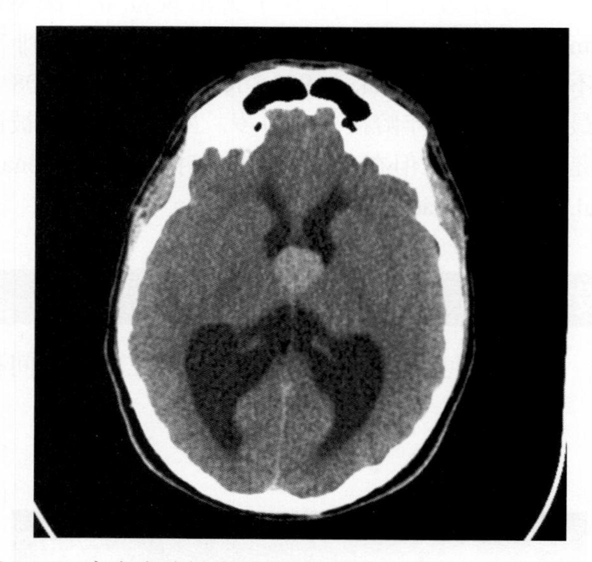

图 33.4 高密度胶样囊肿的 CT 轴位图像

水平的前方，但也可以位于第三脑室、穹隆柱或脉络丛更后面的位置（Fries and Perneczky，1994）（**图 33.5**）。其他罕见的部位包括侧脑室、透明隔、第四脑室和脑桥前区（Ciric and Zivin，1975；Shima et al.，1976；Jan et al.，1989；Maurice-Williams and Wadley，1998；Jeffree and Besser，2001；Killer et al.，2001；Jaskólski et al.，2003）。大多数被发现为孤立病变，但也有多个囊肿的描述（Maurice-Williams and Wadley，1998）。它们的大小从几毫米到 9 cm 直径不等（Shuangshoti and Netsky，1966）。

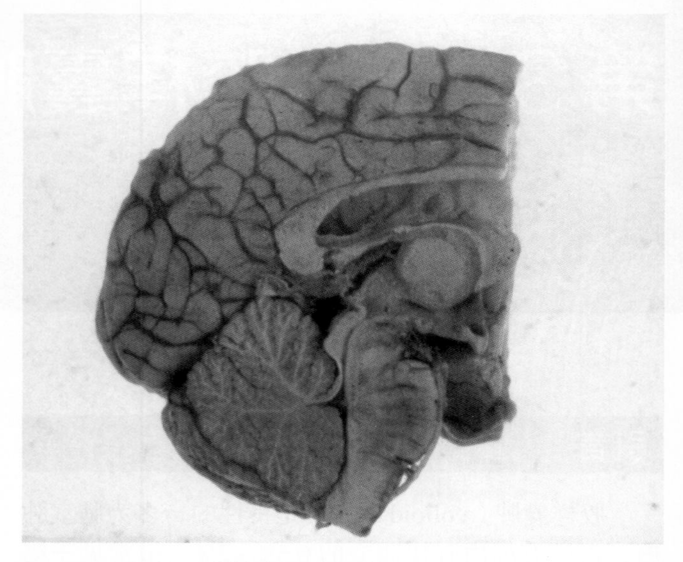

图 33.5 矢状面胶样囊肿的尸检图

Acknowledgment: Dr Azzam Ismail, Consultant Histopathologist, Leeds General Infirmary.

组织学上，囊肿由单层假复层柱状上皮和立方低柱状上皮组成（**图** 33.6、**图** 33.7 和**图** 33.8），其中单层假复层柱状上皮有或没有纤毛（Leech et al.，1982）。黏液杯状细胞也很常见，高碘酸希夫染色黏液呈阳性。上皮和包膜一起构成囊壁。囊壁的厚度可以是可变的，囊肿的内容物是一种无定形物质，被认为是上皮细胞分泌的黏液和细胞脱落。含量的稠度也很不稳定，从液体到黏液，可以是半固体或固体。这是规划治疗方案时的一个重要考虑因素（Bosch et al.，1978）。

胶样囊肿既往有很多名称，包括神经上皮细胞、神经肠性囊肿和原发性放线肌瘤（Power and Dodds，1977；Graziani et al.，1995）。它们被认为起源于神经上皮细胞，包括脉络丛、室管膜和胚胎异位症的神经上皮细胞。最近的一个假说表明它们可能是非神经起源的（Takahiro et al.，1992）。虽然大多数病例是零星和孤立的，但也有几个家族性病例被描述为提示的常染色体隐性遗传模式（Ibrahim et al.，1986；Akins et al.，1996；Nader-Sepahi and Hamlyn，2000；Joshi et al.，2005）。在两个或更多家庭成员发病的情况下，筛查可能是有价值的。

病理上，胶样囊肿可以由于胶样物质的产生而增大，导致梗阻性脑积水，或者由于晶体内出血而突然增大，进而它们可能压迫邻近的结构。Sjovall 在 1910 年提出，脑脊液在室间孔水平的间歇性阻塞可能是由于囊肿附着在 Tela 脉络膜上的摆动所致

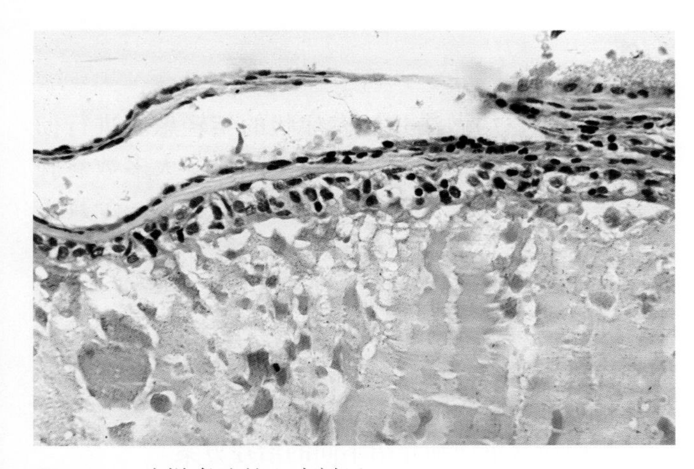

图 33.6 胶样囊壁的上皮衬里

Acknowledgment: Dr Azzam Ismail, Consultant Histopathologist, Leeds General Infirmary.

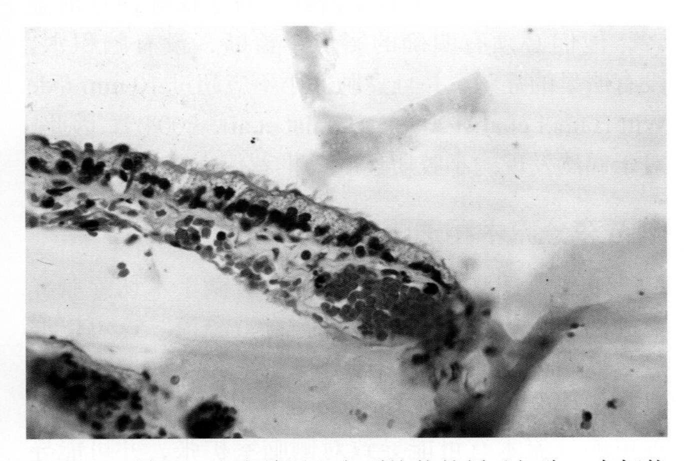

图 33.7 衬里上皮为单层立方到柱状的纤毛细胞，有杯状细胞，壁呈纤维状。染色为苏木精 - 伊红染色（H&E）

Acknowledgment: Dr Azzam Ismail, Consultant Histopathologist, Leeds General Infirmary.

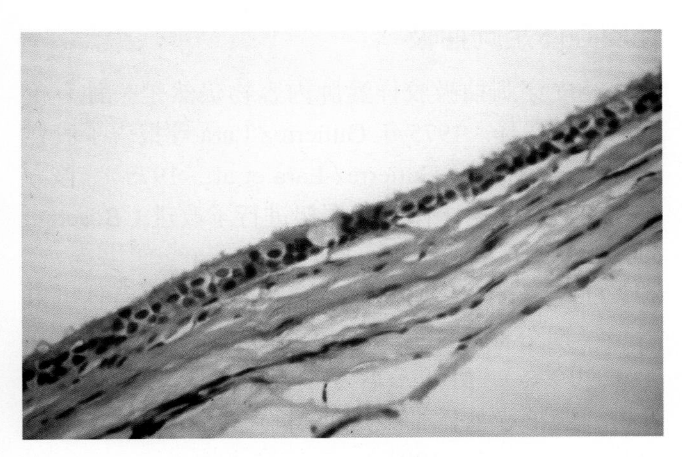

图 33.8 立方上皮衬里

Acknowledgment: Dr Azzam Ismail, Consultant Histopathologist, Leeds General Infirmary.

（Sjovall，1910）。胶样物质的产生既会导致囊肿大小增加，又会导致局部炎症。体积的突然增大可能是由于囊肿内的急性出血引起的，并可能导致迅速且往往严重的神经功能缺损（Malik et al.，1980；Beems et al.，2006）。附近的结构也可以通过囊肿扩大来压缩，例如，穹隆的局部压力会导致长期记忆问题（Aggleton et al.，2000）。直接压迫第三脑室侧壁并由此损害下丘脑心血管调节中心被认为是急性恶化的原因（de Witt Hamer et al.，2002）。体位的改变可能会直接压迫大脑内静脉，并导致颅内静脉压升高（Hamlat et al.，2004）。腰椎穿刺后也可能出现急性恶化。

表现

患者可能会出现各种各样的症状，但没有一种是特定的症状。症状可能是由于急性间歇性颅内压升高，推测可能是带蒂囊肿的活动导致脑脊液循环的间歇性梗阻，也可能是由于长期的部分脑脊液流出梗阻而导致的（永久性）脑积水。也有越来越多的患者出现偶然发现的囊肿。

最常见的症状是头痛（68%）、步态障碍（47%）和短期记忆力丧失（37%）。恶心、呕吐（37%）和视力模糊（24%）也很常见（Little and MacCarty，1974）。最常见的体征是视盘水肿（47%）和步态障碍（32%）。1/4 的患者在检查中没有明显的症状（Little and MacCarty，1974）。

头痛的持续时间、部位和性质各不相同。最近的一项研究将患者分为三组。一组以头痛为主要症状（72%），另一组伴有或不伴有颅内压升高迹象的记忆力丧失，最后一组出现阵发性症状，但两次发作之间没有症状（Pollock et al.，2000）。然而，这种区分较困难，而且症状的组合有很多种。

值得讨论的是，既往胶样囊肿导致猝死的风险被高估。在 CT 出现之前，胶样囊肿与猝死高风险相关，因为推测囊肿的移动性会导致急性脑脊液流出阻塞。这很可能与腰椎穿刺和脑室造影等干预措施有关。然而，慢性脑积水患者也有可能出现失代偿和死亡。囊肿可直接压迫下丘脑心血管反射中枢，导致病情急性恶化（de Witt Hamer et al.，2002）。

影像学诊断

在 CT 等技术出现之前，气脑造影（pneumoencephalography）是诊断第三脑室肿瘤的主要手段。随着CT和MRI的出现，胶样囊肿的诊断变得更加容易。CT上的等密度病变会给诊断带来挑战（Powell et al.，1983）。

急性脑脊液阻塞时，CT表现为室间孔水平边界清楚的胶样囊肿，并伴有脑积水和脑室周围透明影。囊肿通常是高密度的，但也可能是等密度或低密度的（Ganti et al.，1981；Hine and Chui，1987）。CT上呈低密度的囊肿通常有液体内容物，因此可以选择抽吸治疗（El Khoury et al.，2000）。一些囊肿表现为中度周边强化，但这并不常见。

在MRI上，大多数囊肿在T1加权像上呈均匀高信号，在T2加权像上呈低信号（Maeder et al.，1990）。胆固醇酯的存在可能会导致T2加权图像上中央部分的信号强度较低。较少见的情况，密集的碎片可能会形成一个待定位置的结节，可以在CT和MRI扫描上看到。

脑室内出血在CT扫描和MRI上偶尔类似胶样囊肿。在影像学检查中，室管膜下瘤、中枢神经细胞瘤和室管膜下巨细胞星形细胞瘤可能与胶质囊肿发生在同一区域，但这些实体瘤可以根据其形状、对比度增强和信号强度来区分。

自然发展过程

胶样囊肿在颅内病变中所占比例不到2%（Little and MacCarty，1974）。因此，对这种罕见肿瘤的长期随访并不常见。Pollock发表了一系列跨越24年观察的155名患者的文章（Pollock et al.，2000）。发现有4个因素与症状相关，分别是年龄（44岁以下）、较大的囊肿（大于13 mm）、脑室扩张和MRI T2加权像上的信号增加。

胶样囊肿的自然病史与囊肿生长速度、脑脊液梗阻的发展以及囊肿大小随年龄增长而趋于稳定有关。自然生长史可以分为三类。第一类是在脑脊液阻塞和脑室扩张之前，囊肿就停止生长的无症状患者。第二类，也是无症状的，囊肿最初的快速增长导致脑室扩张，但随后囊肿趋于稳定和生长不足维持了一个无症状的过程。最后，第三类囊肿增大会导致脑脊液阻塞和脑室扩张，进而引发症状，这类患者在MRI上通常具有高信号的T2特征。

囊肿可以自发破裂（Motoyama et al.，2002），并且可以自发缩小（Hattab et al.，1990）。

治疗

目前成熟的做法是对有症状的年轻患者进行彻底的胶样囊肿显微切除手术。实际上，大多数囊肿是在头疼扫描后偶然被发现的。这造成了一个真正的两难境地，要确定这些是真的囊肿导致的偶发症状还是囊肿导致的复杂症状的表现。

在一小部分老年患者或者那些不适合长期麻醉的患者中，脑脊液分流是有效的措施。而保守放射学监测方法可能适用于无症状的小囊肿。

我们在这里详细介绍不同的治疗方案。

保守治疗

大多数胶样囊肿要么出现症状，要么在发现后不久就有症状，因此需要治疗。对于保守治疗的患者，他们必须有明确的影像学诊断，没有脑积水，没有明显的症状，并且囊肿大小不应超过10 mm（de Witt Hamer et al.，2002；Hamlat et al.，2004）。因此，对于偶然发现的小胶质囊肿，推荐保守治疗。

脑脊液分流术和透明膜切开术

出现急性脑室扩张且不适合显微手术切除胶样囊肿的患者，可能需要紧急脑脊液分流。这可以通过放置双侧脑室外引流或分流来实现。或者，也可以采用内镜下透明膜切开术的单侧分流术。单独放置单侧分流术有可能导致对侧脑室扩张，并可能导致神经状况恶化。

位于第三脑室后1/3的胶样囊肿很少见，可能会导致第三脑室扩张。在这些情况下，可以进行内镜第三脑室造瘘术（Hopf et al.，1999）。

经皮立体定向抽吸

经皮穿刺抽吸胶样囊肿内容物仍然是一种有价值的治疗选择。1975年Gutierrez-Lara等报告了胶样囊肿的徒手抽吸（Gutierrez-Lara et al.，1975）。该方法随后通过使用立体定向框架进行了改进（Bosch et al.，1978）。

抽吸的优点是操作简单且相对安全，而且可以用于早期分流手术后脑室正常或小的患者（Bosch et al.，1978）。虽然术后复发率较高，但在某些患者中，全抽吸或次抽吸可能是唯一需要的治疗方法（Mathiesen et al.，1993）。

抽吸的缺点包括较高的复发率（Mathiesen et al.，1993），复发可发生在术后6年内。抽吸手术并不是万能的，因为囊肿内容物可能太黏稠，高黏滞性在CT上表现为高密度，在2/3的病例中可见（Rivas and Lobato，1985；Kondziolka and Lunsford，1992）。此外，囊壁可能太硬或小体积囊肿可能导致抽吸针的偏离（Kondziolka and Lunsford，1992）。因为操作中产生血管损伤和机械创伤，早期尝试抽吸有较高的死亡率。抽吸时内容物溢出可能导致脑室炎或导水管堵塞（Antunes et al.，1980）。由于以上原因，经皮穿刺抽吸现在仅限于非常有限的患者。

内镜下抽吸

囊肿内容物的内镜抽吸最早是由Powell等在1983年描述的。Deinsberger在1994年指出，内镜下抽吸胶样囊肿是安全的，即使囊壁开得很大，复发率也很低（Deinsberger et al.，1994）。

内镜下囊肿切除术

许多已发表的文献都提倡内镜下切除胶样囊肿。

与开放手术相比，内镜手术的优点是手术时间更短（平均时间为110分钟 *vs.* 显微手术切除的平均206分钟），由于皮质切口较小，并发症发生率较低，因此术后癫痫发作的风险较低（Lewis et al.，1994）。一项内镜下切除胶样囊肿的13年随访显示复发率仅为6.3%（Levine et al.，2007）。两组的死亡率和分流依赖率相似。因此，一些中心将这种技术作为治疗的首选。

然而，最近的另一项研究回顾了关于内镜和显微外科手术切除胶样囊肿的现有文献（Sheikh et al.，2014）。这项研究的结论是，显微手术切除胶样囊肿似乎比内镜切除的完全根治率高得多，复发率低，再次手术少。这可能与用双手显微剥离关键粘连结构的囊壁以实现真正的大体全切除的优势有关。**表33.1**和**表33.2**提供了有关这些技术的比较数据。

内镜下切除胶样囊肿的技术是在全身麻醉下进行的，患者仰卧，头部支撑在马蹄形头架下。使用大约15°的仰视位置。在中线冠状缝线正前方做一个直切口，并进行钻孔。打开硬脑膜，用14号法式剥离导入器和针头进行脑室插管。硬质或软质内镜通过剥离导管插入。当囊肿附着在更靠后的位置或检查第三脑室和导水管是否有碎片时，显微镜手术更有利于胶样囊肿的切除。

室间孔（Monro孔）通常被胶样囊肿阻塞。血管囊壁用内镜双极或单极电极凝固。一些中心还利用磷酸钛酸钾（KTP）600 μc激光纤维凝固和穿孔囊肿包膜。然后抽出内容物，以脉冲或连续的方式使用乳酸林格氏溶液维持充分的冲洗。可使用一对1 mm穿孔活检钳去除囊肿包膜和胶体物质。在手术结束时，检查第三脑室和导水管是否有碎片或堵塞。

在神经内镜置入脑室留下的穿刺通道中，并连接到Ommaya囊，如果需要，即可以将其转换为分流器。在皮质开口处放置凝胶海绵，以帮助防止脑脊液渗漏。

表33.1　显微手术与内镜手术在胶样囊肿治疗中的比较

参数	显微手术	内镜手术	*P*值
平均年龄	40.0	40.5	
性别	3.1：1	1：1.4	
囊肿大小（mm）	13.2	14.3	
大部切除率	96.8%	58.2%	<0.0001
复发率	1.48%	3.91%	0.0003
死亡率	1.4%	0.6%	0.2469
再手术率	0.38%	3.0%	0.0006
分流依赖率	6.2%	3.9%	0.1160
随访平均数（月）	49.7	36.7	
随访范围（月）	11~144	10~76	

Adapted with permission from Ahmed B. Sheikh, Zachary S. Mendelson, James K. Liu., Endoscopic Versus Microsurgical Resection of Colloid Cysts: A Systematic Review and Meta-Analysis of 1278 Patients, *World Neurosurgery*, Volume 82, Issue 6, p. 1187, Copyright © 2014 Elsevier.

表33.2　术后并发症比较

疗法	癫痫	记忆缺陷	术中出血	静脉梗死	脑内血肿	硬膜下血肿	动脉梗死	偏瘫	脑膜炎	总体发生率
内镜 *n*=666	0.3%	5.0%	1.2%	0	0	0.2%	0.3%	0.9%	2.7%	10.5%
显微手术 *n*=552	4.3%	5.1%	0	2.1%	0.05%	0.018%	0.07%	1.6%	1.6%	16.3%
经胼胝体 *n*=446	2.9%	4.9%	0	2.7%	0	0.2%	0.9%	1.1%	1.1%	14.4%
经皮质 *n*=106	10.4%	5.7%	0	0	2.8%	0	0	3.8%	3.8%	24.5%

Adapted with permission from Ahmed B. Sheikh, Zachary S. Mendelson, James K. Liu., Endoscopic Versus Microsurgical Resection of Colloid Cysts: A Systematic Review and Meta-Analysis of 1278 Patients, *World Neurosurgery*, Volume 82, Issue 6, p. 1187, Copyright © 2014 Elsevier.

囊肿摘除的显微手术入路

经皮质、经脑室入路

大多数胶样囊肿位于第三脑室的前 1/3，可以通过 Dandy 在 20 世纪 30 年代描述的经皮质、经脑室入路将其切除（Dandy，1933）。

第三脑室前部病变通过冠状前缝开颅进入，而更多的脑室后部病变是通过更多的额部开口进入，允许更倾斜的后部轨迹通过室间孔。在 20 世纪 30 年代，Dandy 切除了部分额叶以进入第三脑室。这现在被细化到只有切开 10~15 mm 的皮质，无论是经脑回的，还是最好是经脑沟的。较大的肿瘤可以通过同侧入路接近，而较小的囊肿可以通过对侧入路接近。虽然这可以用于脑室正常的患者，但在出现脑积水时更理想。

常见的术后并发症包括癫痫（9.3%）、脑膜炎（3.3%）、伤口感染和穹隆损伤导致的记忆问题。88 例报告病例中有 87 例可以全切除（98.8%）。Charalampaki 等已经描述了用内镜辅助的经皮质 - 脑室技术 100% 切除胶样囊肿（Charalampaki et al.，2006）。

大脑半球间经胼胝体入路

此入路的优点是可以在没有脑积水的情况下使用，通过中线相对无创的通路和小的胼胝体切开术进入胶样囊肿，这是一条直接到达胶样囊肿的途径。

然而，这项技术在技术上要求更高，附近的血管结构很容易受损。这些动脉包括上矢状窦、皮质桥静脉、大脑前动脉和足周动脉。之后可以出现一过性偏瘫。通过将胼胝体切开的前后向长度保持在 2 cm 以内，可以避免断流综合征。缄默症可由双侧扣带回内的辅助运动区后退引起，穹隆损伤导致记忆障碍是一种持续的风险。

大脑半球间、经胼胝体入路在全身麻醉下进行，头部用精确导航装置固定。颈部应弯曲，手术台应放置在 15° 仰视位置。神经导航通过定位远离皮质桥静脉的无血管通道，有助于计划开颅手术的切口位置和轨迹。典型的开颅瓣穿过中线，位于冠状缝前 4 cm 和后 2 cm。胼胝体的入路位于胼胝体下方和扣带回之间。确定了踝缘动脉和足周动脉，并注意避免将牵引器直接放在血管上，可以轻轻地回缩，两侧是同侧半球。作 2 cm 或更小的胼胝体前部切开术以进入侧脑室。脑室的偏侧性由脉络丛、丘纹静脉和室间孔的方向决定，然后使用以下轨迹之一。

对于通过室间孔出现的较小病变，可采用穹隆旁入路，经室间孔直接入路，无需进入第三脑室即可切除。

穹隆间入路可用于较大的病变和位于较后的病变，或存在相关的透明隔。入路在透明隔的两大脑半球和两个穹隆之间进行，通过大脑内静脉之间的间隔膜进入第三脑室。这项技术最大的缺点是穹隆易受双侧损伤，这可能导致严重的顺行性遗忘（Sweet et al.，1959）。对于较大的囊肿患者，穹隆可能会被囊肿撑开，这样更容易通过这种途径进入（**图** 33.9、**图** 33.10 和**图** 33.11）。

采用脉络膜下入路可避免穹隆损伤。经丘脑带腱膜下剥离可扩大室间孔的后方。这是由 Lavyne 和

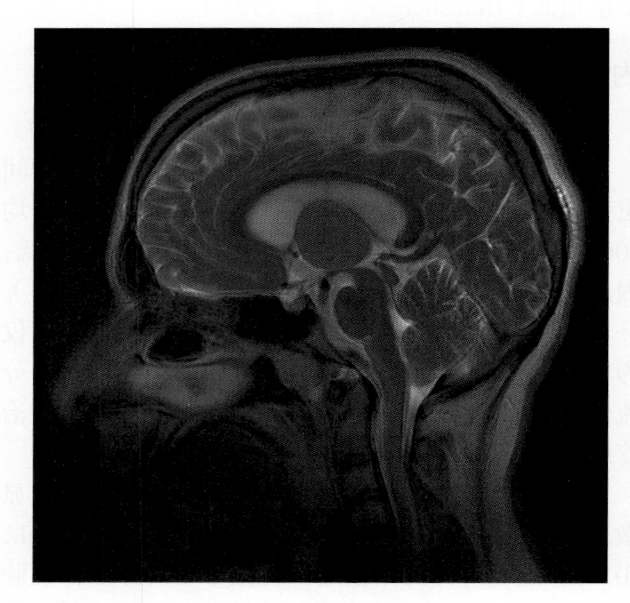

图 33.9 大的胶样囊肿，穹隆柱被推开

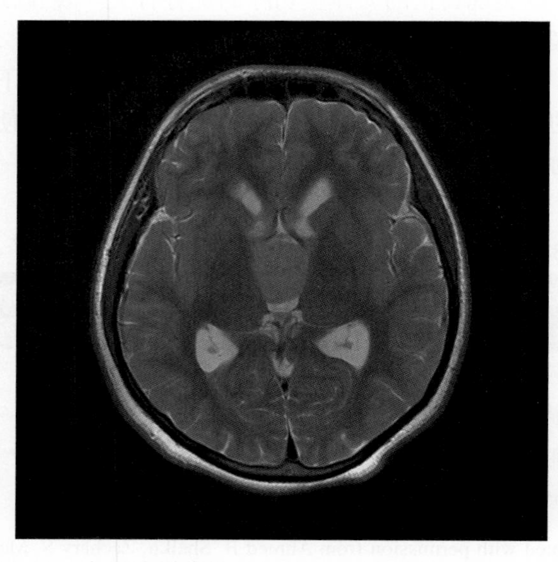

图 33.10 大型胶样囊肿的矢状位 T2 加权成像

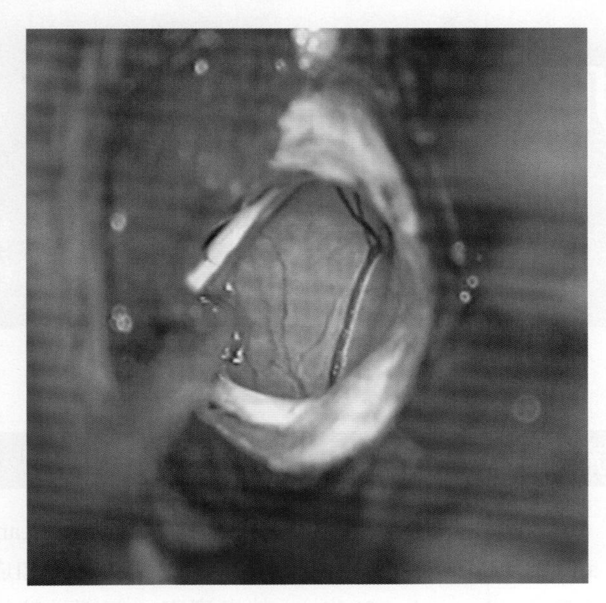

图 33.11 大脑半球间经穹隆入路。左侧脑室被切开，然后透明隔裂开以观察胶样囊肿，术前扫描结果如**图** 33.9 和**图** 33.10 所示。请参阅链接中的视频：https://drive.google.com/open?id=0B3x_xC0sImigajQxYTBTUWoyZ1E

Patterson（1983）推广的。这一入路受到丘脑纹状静脉末端的限制，尽管部分学者描述了丘脑纹状静脉的分离，但这存在丘脑内静脉梗死的风险，因此不推荐使用。

经脉络膜入路，类似于穹隆保留穹隆，可以通过穹隆带解剖穿过内侧脉络丛（Wen et al.，1998）。这避免了丘状纹状静脉流入大脑内静脉，但大脑内静脉在中间膜内仍有危险。穹隆也必须用这种方法来保护。

脉络膜下入路和经脉络膜入路的主要缺点都是对丘脑纹状静脉和大脑内静脉产生潜在危险。然而，对于较大的肿瘤，脉络膜裂隙可被下面的囊肿撑开，这便于进入。

额部终板入路

该入路采用额下解剖或旁正中入路至终板。对于第三脑室前区的第三脑室胶样囊肿或侵犯视交叉上隐窝的第三脑室胶样囊肿，采用该入路是有利的（Desai et al.，2002）。

目前还没有关于内镜辅助囊肿切除与经终板入路相结合的文献，尽管这在解剖研究中已被证明是可行的（Abdou and Cohen，2000）。这可能是未来发展的一个趋势。

治疗中存在的争议

偶然发现的囊肿大小不到 1 cm，这造成了临床上的两难境地。很大一部分是因为临床中头痛行 CT 检查时偶然发现的。需要仔细地临床评估，有时可能包括一段时间的颅内压（intracranial pressure，ICP）监测。当患者的头痛严重到足以实施神经成像的时候，可能很难建议他们报告头痛的重要性，将其作为早期脑积水的迹象。这可能会降低手术干预的门槛，这取决于患者的心理状态。

保守治疗的囊肿患者所需的影像学监测频率尚不清楚，例如无症状的非常小的偶发囊肿、无关的头痛或典型的偏头痛。

在内镜和显微外科手术之间进行选择也是一个有争议的话题。如前所述以及**表** 33.1 和**表** 33.2 中所述，这两种技术各有优缺点。内镜手术可提供较小的开颅和切开皮质束范围，但需要充分扩大脑室，可能很难去除所有囊膜，因此复发率较高。一般来说，手术类型（内镜还是显微外科）的选择取决于外科医生的经验 / 专业知识以及医患交流。至于显微手术入路（经皮质或经胼胝体），这在很大程度上取决于外科医生的偏好。虽然一些外科医生认为，经皮质入路为治疗大多数胶样囊肿提供了更好的切入角度，但脑室需要充分扩大，因此癫痫的风险增加。相反，大脑半球间入路可用于小脑室或大脑室的患者。考虑到患者的特点，年轻的健康患者通常行显微手术，这些患者可能对大手术有更多的耐受性，而且对于长期的病情控制更为重要。在囊肿解剖和形态有利的情况下保留内镜手术入路，适用于手术并发症可能不能很好耐受的稍大年龄组。最后，囊肿抽吸术或脑脊液分流术通常用于身体状况差的患者或老年人，因为长期控制不是一个重要的因素。然而，选择这些方法中最重要的因素是术者的操作经验。

延伸阅读、参考文献、EBRAIN 的相关链接

扫描书末二维码获取。

第 34 章　脉络丛肿瘤

Jonathan Roth・Rina Dvir・Shlomi Constantini 著
戴缤 译，胡志强 审校

引言

脉络丛肿瘤（choroid plexus tumours，CPT）是一种罕见的起源于脉络丛上皮的脑室内肿瘤。根据世界卫生组织 2007 年和 2016 年的分类，有三种肿瘤亚型（Wrede et al.，2009；Menon et al.，2010；Dudley et al.，2015；Louis et al.，2016）:

- 脉络丛乳头状瘤（choroid plexus papilloma，CPP）是良性的，占 CPT 的 40%~60%
- 脉络丛癌（choroid plexus carcinoma，CPC）是恶性的，占 CPT 的 30%~50%
- 非典型脉络丛乳头状瘤（atypical choroid plexus papilloma，ACPP）是一种中间亚型，占 CPT 的 10%~30%

通常，CPT 被认为在婴儿期更为普遍；然而，CPT 也可能出现在成年期。

在本章中，我们将讨论脉络丛肿瘤的主要诊断、遗传和治疗相关方面的内容。

流行病学

脉络膜肿瘤主要发生在 2 岁之前的婴儿（Lam et al.，2013）；然而，也可能发生在较大的儿童和成人（Turkoglu et al.，2014）。其患病率、病理学特征和解剖位置分布在不同年龄组之间存在差异（Lam et al.，2013）。CPT 占儿童脑肿瘤的 2%~5%，而在成人脑肿瘤中所占的比例为 0.4%~0.8%。CPT 通常表现为先天性 / 新生儿肿瘤，占出生第一年诊断的脑肿瘤的 10%~20%。（Serowka et al.，2010；Lang et al.，2012；Sun et al.，2014b）.

不同年龄段患者，肿瘤病理也不尽相同。CPC 和 ACPP 在婴幼儿年龄组中更为常见，CPC 的中位年龄为 3 岁。男性略占优势，可能是 CPT 与 X 连锁突变有关（Menon et al.，2010；Dudley et al.，2015）。

CPT 通常发生在脑室系统，因为它们起源于脉络丛。在儿童患者中，它们通常位于侧脑室，大部分位于脑室（**图** 34.1）。第三脑室 CPT 很少见，多见

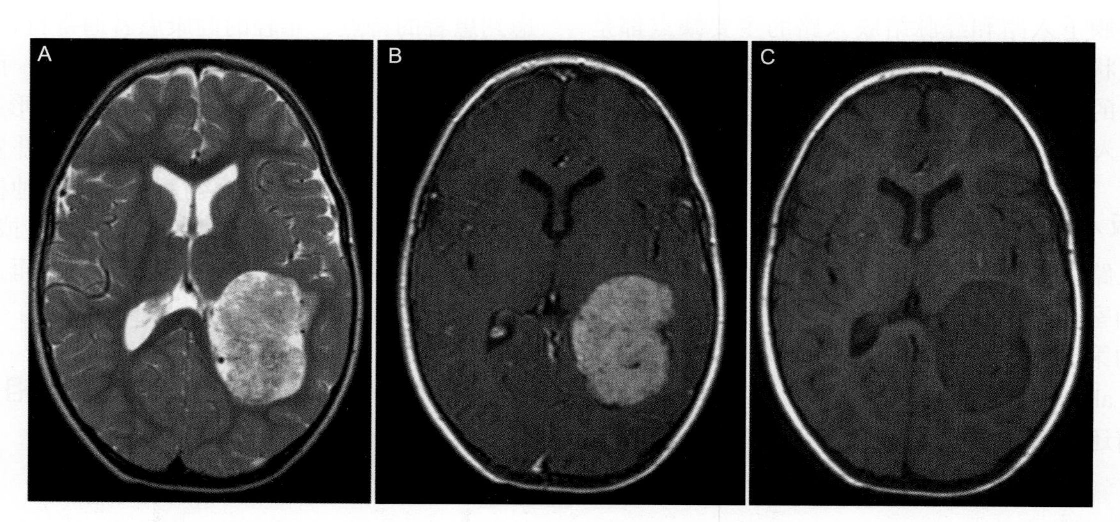

图 34.1　图示为一个 2 岁半的 CPP 患儿。轴位 T2（A）、T1- Gad（B）和 T1（C）MRI 扫描，显示脑室肿瘤。肿瘤被完全切除

Courtesy of Dr Kieren Allinson, Department of Pathology, Addenbrooke’s Hospital, Cambridge.

于婴儿（Gupta et al.，2013）（图 34.2）。在成人中，大多数 CPT 发生在颅后窝，大部分发生在第四脑室（Bostrom et al.，2011）。虽然 CPP 的发生发展与脑室系统密切相关，但 CPC 并不会限制于脑室系统。CPC 可能生长达到非常大的体积，在婴儿中表现为巨大的半球肿瘤。

与 CPP 和 ACPP 相比，CPC 预后是最差的（Lam et al.，2013；Dudley et al.，2015）。肿瘤完全切除后 CPP 患者 5 年的总生存率（overall survival，OS）为 84%～100%（Wrede et al.，2009；Lam et al.，2013；Dudley et al.，2015）。相比之下，CPC 是一种高度恶性肿瘤，尽管采用多种模式治疗，但预后不佳，5 年总生存率为 26%～70%（Wrede et al.，2009；Lam et al.，2013；Dudley et al.，2015）。大多数 ACPP 的 OS 与 CPP 相似，但少数亚组显示与 CPC 的生物学行为和预后相似（Wrede et al.，2009）。

症状表现

CPP 是导致脑脊液过多的两种实体瘤之一，另一种是脉络丛增生（choroid plexus hyperplasia，CPH）。CPP 患者的脑脊液量可达 5 L（Fujimura et al.，2004；Cataltepe et al.，2010；Nimjee et al.，2010），并伴随脑脊液蛋白水平升高。因此，CPP 可导致继发于以下几种原因的脑积水：脑脊液分泌过多、脑脊液循环通路梗阻和脑脊液吸收障碍。许多 CPT 患者表现为脑积水（Pencalet et al.，1998；Bettegowda et al.，2012；Sun et al.，2014b）（见图 34.2、图 34.3、图 34.4 和图 34.7）。

婴儿继发脑积水颅内压增高的体征和症状包括头围增大、向上凝视受限“落日征”、全身肌张力减退、囟门膨出、呕吐和发育不良（failure to thrive，FTT）。在年龄较大的儿童和成人中，症状通常包括

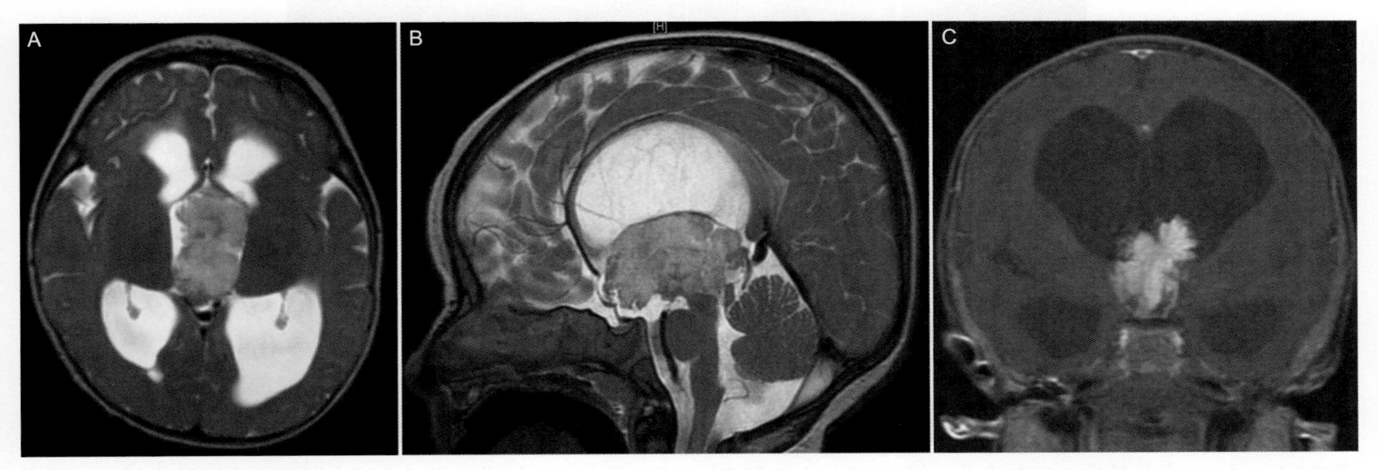

图 34.2 5 个月龄的 ACPP 患儿。轴位 T2（A）、矢状 T2 和冠状 T1-Gad（C）MRI 扫描显示第三脑室病变。肿瘤被完全切除，并对儿童进行了随访

Courtesy of Dr Kieren Allinson, Department of Pathology, Addenbrooke’s Hospital, Cambridge.

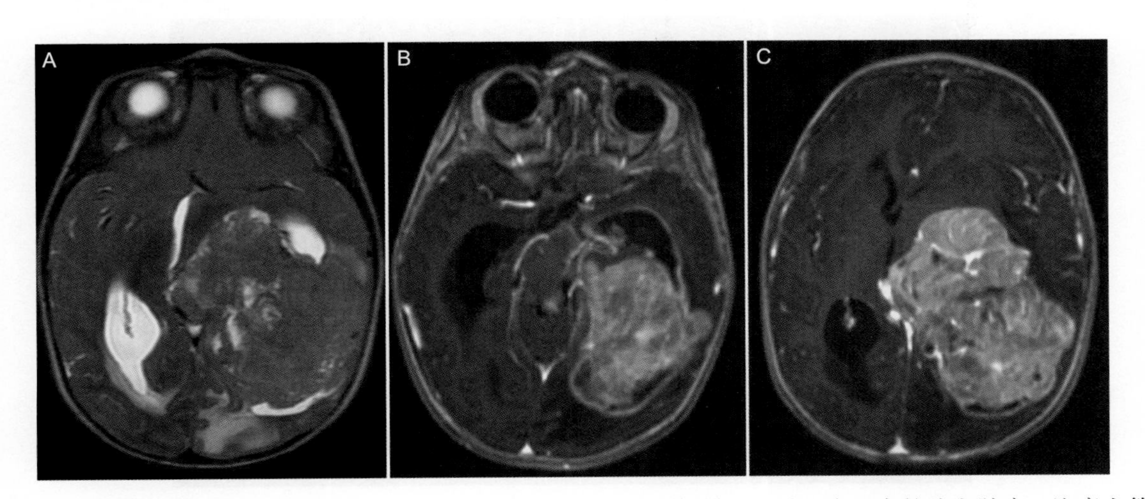

图 34.3 20 个月龄的 CPC 患儿。轴位 T2（A）和 T1- Gad（B&C）MRI 扫描，显示一个巨大的脑室肿瘤。注意室管膜增强。肿瘤被完全切除，然后进行化疗。该患儿在确诊后一年内死于肿瘤

Courtesy of Dr Kieren Allinson, Department of Pathology, Addenbrooke’s Hospital, Cambridge.

头痛、恶心呕吐、视力下降和取决于确切位置的局灶性体征（Lang et al.，2012）。

由于CPC通常是大的侵袭性肿瘤，它们可能表现出半球肿块效应的继发症状（颅内压升高和癫痫发作）（图34.3）。与CPC相比，APCC与CPP的关系更为密切（图34.2和图34.4）。它们往往中等大小，位于脑室内，一般不侵犯周围半球。它们在婴儿年龄组更为普遍，但也可能出现在成年期。

诊断

CPT大多位于脑室系统内。如前文所述，儿童患者的CPP多发生在侧脑室，瘤体主要位于脑室，而成人患者的CPP多发生在第四脑室（图34.1、图34.3、图34.4、图34.6和图34.7）。CPT也可起源于第三脑室（Mishra et al.，2014）和桥小脑角区（CPA）（Menon et al.，2010；Prasad et al.，2014）的局部脉络膜丛（图34.2和图34.5）。CPP也可能发生在颅内外，如松果体区（Sasani et al.，2014）、脑干（Xiao et al.，2013）、鞍区或鞍上区（Bian et al.，2011）和脑实质（Imai et al.，2011）。

典型的CPP影像学表现为菜花样病变，MRI T1像呈等信号，呈明显均匀强化（图34.1）。然而，在极少数情况下，病变可能不会增强（Pratheesh et al.，2009）。T2像常呈等高信号（图34.1、图34.5、图34.6和图34.7）。CT上通常表现为为等密度，伴有轻度钙化。CPP很少呈囊性或伴有壁性结节（Emami-Naeini et al.，2008）。ACPP在影像学上的表现与CPP大体相似（图34.2和图34.4）。

CPC通常具有一个大的，非均匀强化外观。软

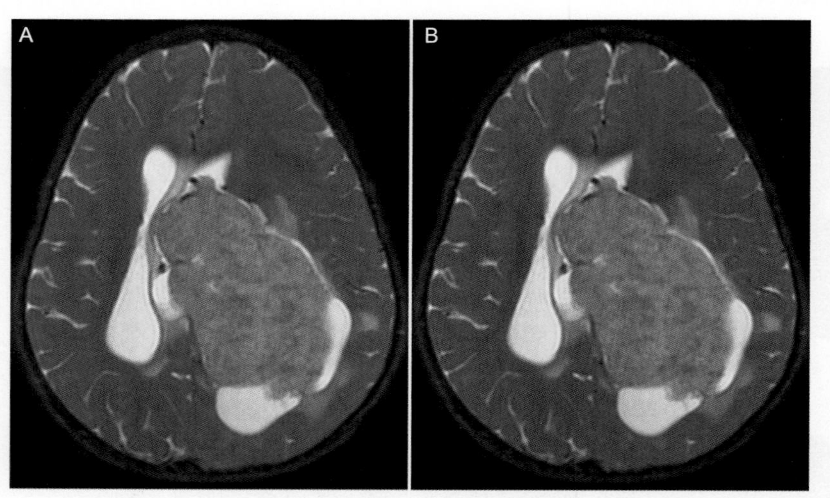

图34.4 一个11个月龄的ACPP患儿。轴位T2（A）和T1-Gad（B）MRI扫描，显示室性大肿瘤。由于肿瘤复发，肿瘤被完全切除并接受化疗

Courtesy of Dr Kieren Allinson, Department of Pathology, Addenbrooke's Hospital, Cambridge.

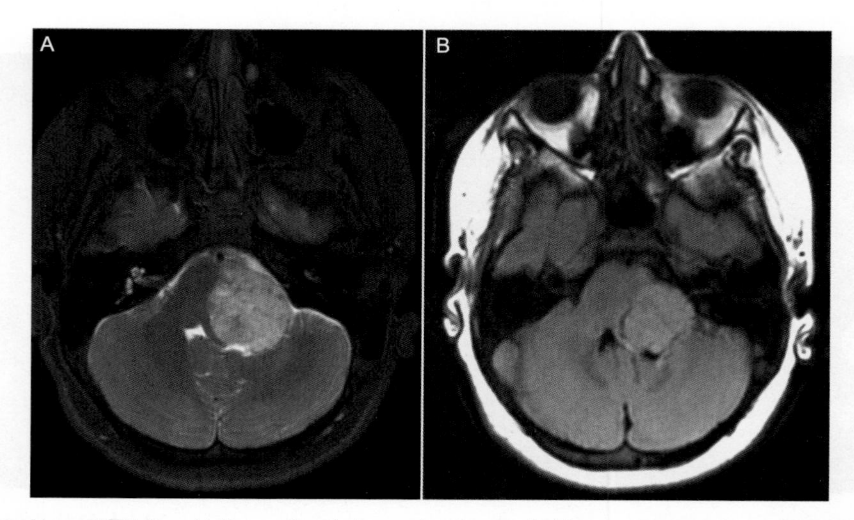

图34.5 一个患有CPP的12岁患儿。轴位T2（A）和T1（B）MRI扫描，显示CPA病变。病灶完全切除

Courtesy of Dr Kieren Allinson, Department of Pathology, Addenbrooke's Hospital, Cambridge.

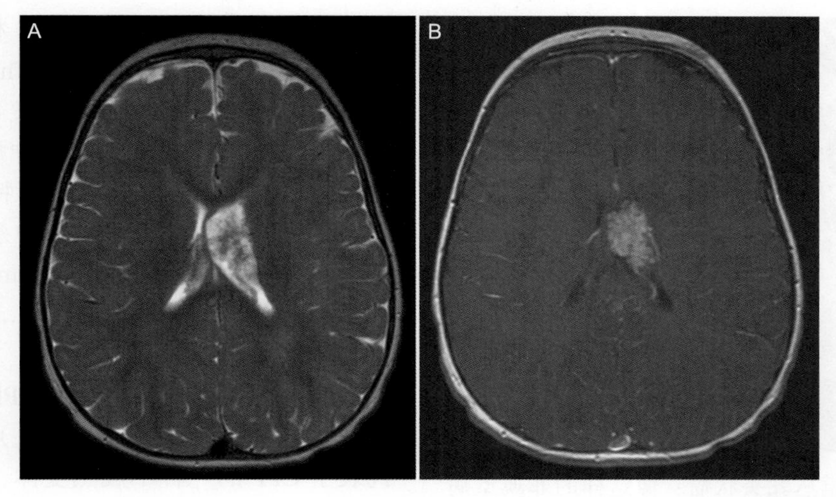

图 34.6　一个患有 CPP 的 15 个月龄患儿。轴位 T2（A）和 T1- Gad（B）MRI 扫描，显示侧脑室病变。肿瘤被完全切除
Courtesy of Dr Kieren Allinson, Department of Pathology, Addenbrooke's Hospital, Cambridge.

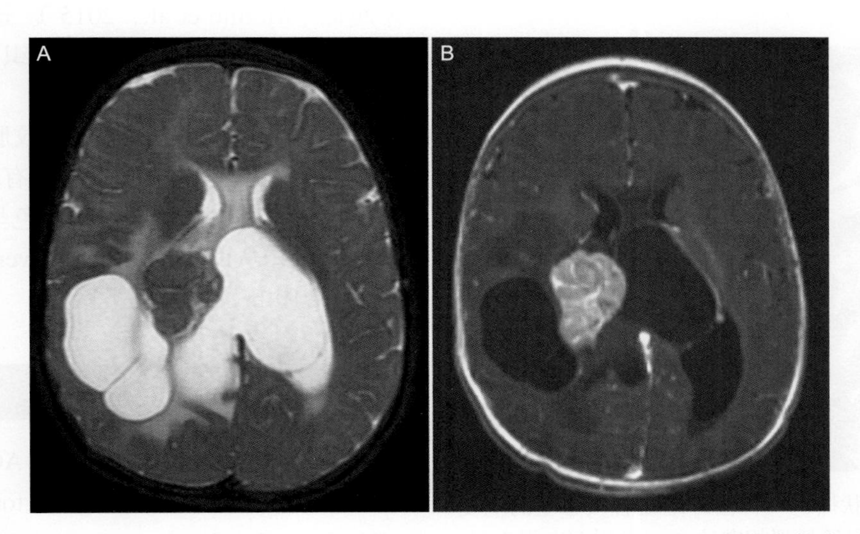

图 34.7　患有 CPP 的 5 个月龄的儿童。轴位 T2（A）和 T1-Gad（B）MRI 扫描显示脑室肿瘤伴囊肿。肿瘤被完全切除
Courtesy of Dr Kieren Allinson, Department of Pathology, Addenbrooke's Hospital, Cambridge.

脑膜扩散（或转移）在 CPP 中很少见（约 5%）。然而，在多达 50% 的 ACPP 和 CPC 病例中可能出现这种情况，因此需要进行脊髓 MRI 检查（Menon et al.，2010，Wrede et al.，2009）（**图** 34.3）。目前还不清楚手术是否是转移的危险因素（Sun et al.，2014b）。

最重要的是血液供应。脉络膜血管经常充血，导致大的深部静脉，包括丘脑静脉、心房静脉、大脑内静脉和盖伦静脉。这些动静脉通常位于肿瘤的内侧或深部。外周引流室管膜静脉也很常见，特别是在较大和高级 CPT 患者。早期数字减影血管造影（digital subtraction angiography，DSA）可见肿瘤的显影，脉络膜动脉突出明显。

脑积水通常继发于前面所述的各种机制。

病理

CPC 具有恶性肿瘤的典型组织病理学特征，如高核分裂指数、细胞异型性和脑组织侵犯（**图** 34.8）。相反，CPP 是类似于非肿瘤性脉络膜丛的良性乳头状肿瘤（**图** 34.9）。然而，尽管存在明显的组织学差异，脉络膜丛增生（choroid plexus hyperplasia，CPH）、CPP、ACPP 和 CPC 之间存在组织学连续性（D'Ambrosio et al.，2003）。然而，对于 CPT 的遗传学和分子研究还很有限。虽然少见，但 CPP 和 ACPP 转化为 CPC 的情况已有报道（Jeibmann et al.，2007）。

CPH 是一种没有生长潜力的非肿瘤病理形态，但是 CPH 和 CPP 之间的鉴别诊断是比较困难的

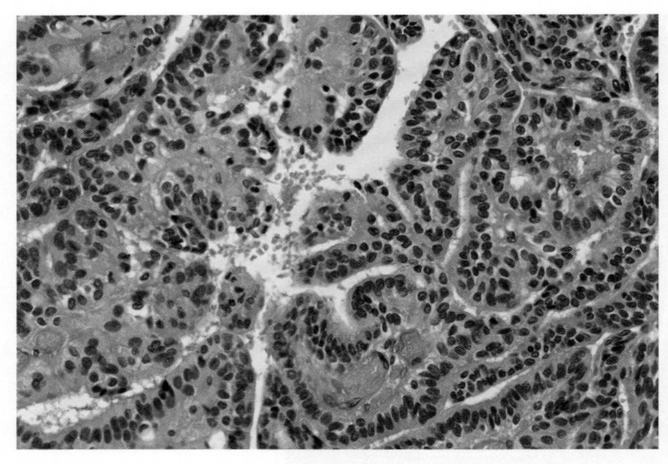

图 34.8 非典型脉络膜丛乳头状瘤：像这样的非典型病例，有丝分裂活动增强，乳头状形态改变

Courtesy of Dr Kieren Allinson, Department of Pathology, Addenbrooke's Hospital, Cambridge.

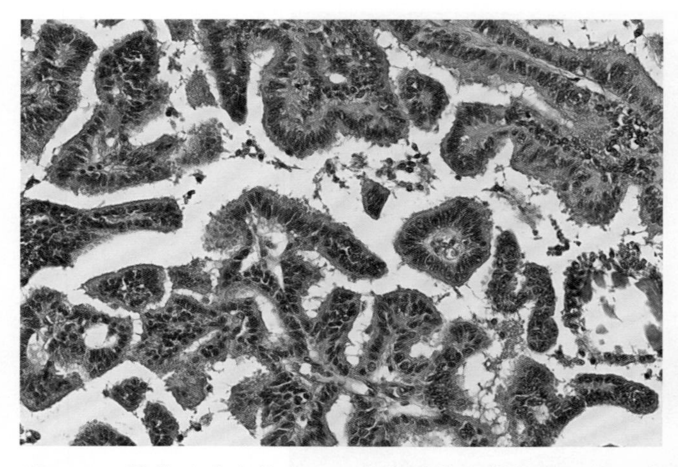

图 34.9 脉络丛乳头状瘤：一种由纤维血管核心上的上皮构成的乳头状结构。有丝分裂相在这个一级病例中很少见

Courtesy of Dr Kieren Allinson, Department of Pathology, Addenbrooke's Hospital, Cambridge.

（D'Ambrosio et al.，2003；Cataltepe et al.，2010）。区分两种病理可以有很多方法，包括 MIB-1 增殖指数（在 CPH 中接近 0，而在 CPP 中介于 0.2~17）。组织学上，EAAT-1 的表达将 CPP 与正常脉络膜丛相鉴别。EAAT-1 是一种神经胶质谷氨酸转运蛋白，常见于 CPT，在正常脉络丛中不存在（Beschorner et al.，2009）。

自 2007 年以来（同时在 2016 年版本中），世界卫生组织描述了一个中间组，即非典型 CPP（ACPP）（Louis et al.，2016）。这些肿瘤类似于 CPP，但有丝分裂活性增加（≥2 个 / 10HPF）（Jeibmann et al.，2006）。与 CPP 和 CPC 相比，ACPP 往往发生在年轻患者中（Wrede et al.，2009；Lam et al.，2013）。ACPP 的 OS 与幼儿 CPP 的 OS 相似，但被认为是 3 岁以上儿童预后不良的因素（Thomas et al.，2015）。

CPC 是 Li-Fraumeni 综合征（Li-Fraumeni syndrome，LFS）的典型儿童肿瘤之一，LFS 是一种家族性癌症易感性综合征，其特征是在年轻时发生恶性肿瘤的频率较高。TP53 种系突变是 LFS 的遗传标志。CPC 患者应筛查 Li-Fraumeni 综合征相关突变（TP53 种系突变）（Gozali et al.，2012；Giacomazzi et al.，2013）。

遗传学和分子研究显示 CPP 和 ACPP 之间存在相似之处（Merino et al.，2015）。有研究表明 ACPP 代表了 CPP 的一种不成熟变体，其特征是增殖活性增加，而 CPC 似乎代表了一种基因上不同的肿瘤（Japp et al.，2015）。CPC 与 TP53 突变高度相关，突变的 TP53 拷贝数越多，CPC 的侵袭性越强，生存率越低（Merino et al.，2015）。这些突变要么是种系 LFS 的一部分，要么是肿瘤组织本身的体细胞 TP53 突变。

CPC 和非典型畸胎瘤 - 横纹肌瘤（atypical terato-rhabdoid tumour，ATRT）可能有相似的组织学表现。然而，在 CPC 中 INI1 蛋白染色呈阳性，而在 ATRT 中呈阴性，从而区分两者（Stevens et al.，2009；Sun et al.，2014b）。

治疗

儿童和成人患者的 CPP、ACPP 和 CPC 的治疗基础是完全手术切除（gross total resection，GTR）（Wrede et al.，2009；Safaee et al.，2013；Koh et al.，2014；Sun et al.，2014a；Dudley et al.，2015）。各种研究表明完全切除、总生存率和无进展生存率之间存在显著相关性（Sun et al.，2014a；Dudley et al.，2015）。与 ACPP（63%）和 CPC（47%~62%）相比，CPP（80%~100%）更容易实现 GTR（Pencalet et al.，1998；Wrede et al.，2009）。GTR 后肿瘤的复发率，在 ACPP 中估计约为 30%，在 CPP 中约为 6%（Jeibmann et al.，2007）。

由于 CPT 在婴儿中更常见，而且往往血运非常丰富，因此需要解决几个技术要点，以提高患者的安全性，减少失血和患者的复发率。

术前栓塞

术前栓塞术（preoperative embolization，PE）已经在少数系列报道中介绍了较好的疗效。经前或后脉络膜动脉对供血动脉进行超选择性栓塞，使用如微球束、NBCA、对 onyx 胶和组织丙烯酸胶等各种材料，已被证明可显著减少术中出血，降低了手术难度，同时提高了肿瘤切除程度（Takahashi et al.，2009；Trivelato et al.，2012；Haliasos et al.，2013b；Wang et al.，2013）。有趣的是，PE 可以减少手术后脑脊液的产生；然而，它并不能减少对永久性脑脊液分流的需求（Haliasos et al.，2013a）。在一个病例报道中，对一个三个月龄的婴儿进行了栓塞治疗术前考虑第三脑室 CPP（Wind et al.，2010）。栓塞治疗后后，肿瘤被完整切除。

年龄并不是行 PE 的限制因素，甚至有研究表明，在新生儿期和月龄几个月就进行了 PE（Otten et al.，2006；Hartge et al.，2010；Wind et al.，2010）。

手术切除

麻醉相关因素包括术前准备足够的血液制品。手术时，应放置静脉通路（必要时也可以考虑中心静脉置管）和有创性动脉通路。大量失血和大量输血是需要解决的主要问题，特别是在婴儿手术中（Piastra et al.，2007）。

患者的体位应该适合良好的静脉回流，而不会压迫颈静脉。头部应该高于心脏的高度。手术环境应该舒适。该肿瘤的切除手术可能极易出血，过小的“微创”入路可能会影响外科医生的手术舒适度和患者的安全。

外科医生必须尝试及早识别和控制滋养血管。然而，通常情况下，尤其是体积较大的肿瘤，只有在肿瘤进行一定的减容后，血管才能够显露出来。因此，在这种情况下，应该采用有效的手术技术，包括肿瘤分块切除，根据术中出血情况及时输血，并每隔几分钟填塞压迫止血一次，以减少失血。在这种情况下，外科医生和麻醉师的配合是最重要的，一旦患者出现低血容量体征麻醉师就应该提醒外科医生注意大出血。巨大的肿瘤（尤其是 CPC）手术切除可能需要大量输血。氨甲环酸（TXA）是一种抗纤溶药物，已被推荐用于减少 CPT 患儿的手术失血量（Phi et al.，2014）。

大多数 CPP 质地偏软，比较容易被吸除。因此，可以实现相对快速的肿瘤切除，暴露肿瘤供血血管，并进行阻断和止血。重要的是要“保护”脑室周围组织（特别是室间孔的区域）以避免脑室系统血液铸型形成。肿瘤切除后，用清洗液对脑室系统进行充分冲洗很重要，避免血性脑脊液可能引发硬膜下血肿和积液（Pencalet et al.，1998）。一些外科医生主张用纤维蛋白胶“封闭”皮质造瘘口（Pencalet et al.，1998）。

脑室系统的手术入路选择取决于肿瘤的大小和脑室的确切位置关系以及滋养血管。一般情况下，位于脑室内的病变通常位于后外侧，因此限制了大脑半球间入路。考虑到光辐射纤维和弧形纤维（尤其是在优势侧），可以通过低位顶枕交界处或经顶上小叶经皮质入路。另一种进入脑室的入路是经对侧大脑半球间跨语言区入路。其他经颞 / 顶入路取决于肿瘤的主体和所覆盖的皮质。位于侧脑室体部的肿瘤可经胼胝体入路处理。第三脑室肿瘤可以通过有或没有脉络膜延伸的室间孔入路，也可以通过后方入路，就像到达松果体区一样。最近，神经内镜下切除第三脑室脉络丛肿瘤已有报道（Santos and Souweidane，2015；Sufianov et al.，2015）。CPA 病变可经乙状窦后入路，第四脑室病变可经膜髓帆入路。

第四脑室的 CPT 可能侵犯脑干（Kumabe et al.，2008），因此，这些病例应该在术中监测的同时进行手术，尽可能进行次全切除，并联合辅助治疗。

已有研究表明，即使在肿瘤完全切除后，脑积水也可能持续存在。除了对手术中血性脑脊液的反应外，也可能是继发于先前的脑脊液吸收障碍。梗阻性脑积水可能源于室间孔或导水管的局部粘连。此外，继发于脑室受累和血性脑脊液的刺激，术后发热很常见，这需要与术后方案相鉴别。因此，肿瘤切除后，需要对脑室系统进行冲洗以清除血块和置换血性脑脊液。通常需放置脑室外引流，以便在术后数天内置换更新脑脊液。

在出现严重脑积水的病例中，肿瘤切除前早期 EVD 可以控制颅内压。然而，尤其是在儿童身上，可能引起严重的电解质失衡（Phi et al.,，2011）。

放疗和化疗

CPP 通常被认为是良性肿瘤，在肿瘤全切除后不需要其他辅助治疗。CPC 是一种高度增殖的恶性肿瘤，可沿神经轴转移，通常预后较差。CPC 治疗的主要手段是手术配合辅助化疗。在合适的病例中，可以在手术前实施新辅助化疗。年龄较大的儿童和成人通常采用化疗联合放疗的治疗方案。CPC 的化疗方案，包括 ICE 方案（异环磷酰胺、卡铂和依托泊苷）（Berrak et al.，2011）和包含多药化疗方案（卡铂、环磷酰胺、依托泊苷、阿霉素和甲氨蝶呤）（Passariello et al.，2015）。ICE 还被用作肿瘤切除前的新辅助治疗，增加了 GTR 的发生率，并减少失血量（Lafay-Cousin et al.，2010；Schneider et al.，2015）。一些机构采用干细胞支持的清髓性大剂量化疗作为前期治疗（Zaky et al., 2015），或作为复发病例的补救性治疗（Mosleh et al., 2013）。GTR后CPC的5年和10年总生存率分别为70%和67%（Dudley et al., 2015）。

放射治疗在CPC治疗中仍然是一个有争议的问题。在最近的一项基于人群的研究中，放射治疗未能改善CPC患者的OS（Cannon et al., 2015；Dudley et al., 2015）。然而，在2014年发表的另一项meta分析中，放射治疗为接受完全或不完全切除CPC的患者提供了生存优势（Sun et al., 2014b）。在与Li-Fraumeni综合征相关的CPC中，放疗与较差的OS率有关（Bahar et al., 2015）。

立体定向放射外科已选择性地应用于难治性肿瘤（Kim et al., 2008）。它也可以应用于手术后复发的小肿瘤和（或）远处肿瘤。

ACPP的辅助治疗存在争议。在较年轻的患者中，ACPP不被认为是一个不良的预后因素。完全切除后随访观察是公认的治疗方案（Thomas et al., 2015）。对于3岁以上的儿童，由于ACPP对预后有影响，建议在GTR后密切随访（Thomas et al., 2015）。

对于未完全切除的ACPP，辅助化疗是公认的治疗方法。与CPC治疗方案类似，包括各种治疗方案，如大剂量化疗和干细胞治疗（Mosleh et al., 2013；Zaky et al., 2015）。根据儿童的年龄和肿瘤残留情况，该方案推迟了放射治疗的使用。

CPC的有利预后因素包括幕上位置、肿瘤的GTR、无TP53突变（无论是体细胞突变还是生殖细胞突变）、年龄大于3岁、无肿瘤扩散、无肿瘤复发和辅助治疗（Sun et al., 2014b）。

参考文献、EBRAIN的相关链接

扫描书末二维码获取。

第 35 章　脑室病变的外科治疗

Eduardo C. Ribas · Guilherme C. Ribas · Ramez W. Kirollos 著
戴缤 译，胡志强 审校

侧脑室和第三脑室的解剖学研究

侧脑室的解剖学研究

侧脑室位于大脑半球的深处，环绕着丘脑，丘脑的形状为卵圆形。侧脑室被细分为多交通部分，根据它们与丘脑的位置关系而有不同的名称，额角对应于位于丘脑前面的脑室部分，体部是位于丘脑上方的部分，三角区 atrium 位于丘脑后方部分，脑室的颞角位于丘脑下方，枕角对应于脑室的一个可变的后伸，后者逐渐缩小到一端（Timurkaynak et al.，1986；Rhoton，2003）（**图** 35.1、**图** 35.2、**图** 35.3 和**图** 35.4）。在额角与脑室体部之间可见室间孔，连接侧脑室与第三脑室。

这五个部分中的每一个都有顶部、底部、侧壁和内壁，前角和颞角以及中庭也有前壁（Timurkaynak et al.，1986；Ribas，1999；Rhoton，2003）。除丘脑外，界定侧脑室部分的其他结构有胼胝体、尾状核、海马、穹隆、杏仁核、终纹和透明隔。

海马由阿蒙角和齿状回组成，前者以海马旁回在脑室内的旺盛突起为特征，后者沿海马旁回的上、内侧和平面分布，称为下丘（Williams and Warwick，1980；Wen et al.，1999）。海马体由分配皮质构成，以三层细胞为特征，覆盖着与这些不同细胞层的神经元轴突形成的白质相对应的海马槽（Williams and Warwick，1980；Heimer，1995；Duvernoy，1998）。有趣的是，正如脊髓和脑干等其他系统发育古老的神经结构一样，海马体的白质是在外部而不是内部分布的。

从宏观上看，海马体在前方由头部和躯体组成，它们共同构成颞角底部的内侧部分，并由尾部构成，尾部终止于脑室的内侧壁（Timurkaynak et al.，1986；Rhoton，2003）。

穹隆沿着海马体生长，形成穹隆的纤细海马伞，构成颞角底部最内侧的结构。穹隆继续向后延伸，它围绕着丘脑的最后部，称为穹隆，形状类似于穹隆的脚。穹隆的两个脚通过穹隆或海马连合连接在一起，然后连接到胼胝体压部的下表面。穹隆的海马伞继续向前和向内，穹隆脚变成穹隆体，穹隆与对侧穹隆的主体并列在一起，穹隆的海马伞与对侧穹隆的躯体并列在一起，穹隆的海马伞继续向

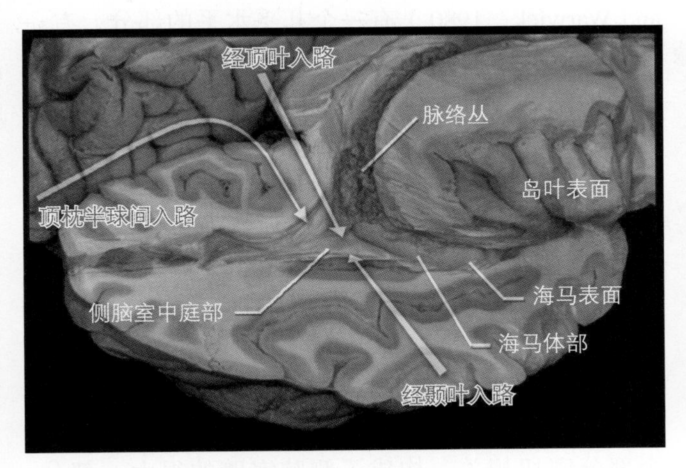

图 35.1　通过丘脑后方的冠状面切开和颞角水平的轴向切开显露侧脑室，图中显示了三种通向该区域的常用入路（黄色箭头）

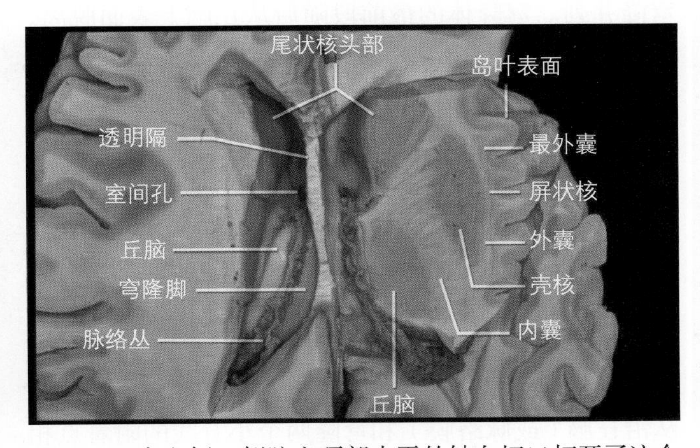

图 35.2　在左侧，侧脑室顶部水平的轴向切口打开了这个腔。在右侧，一个更靠近尾部的轴向切面横跨大脑的中央核心，揭示了它的结构：基底节、丘脑和白质被膜。注意内囊膝部与室管膜表面在室间孔水平的接近

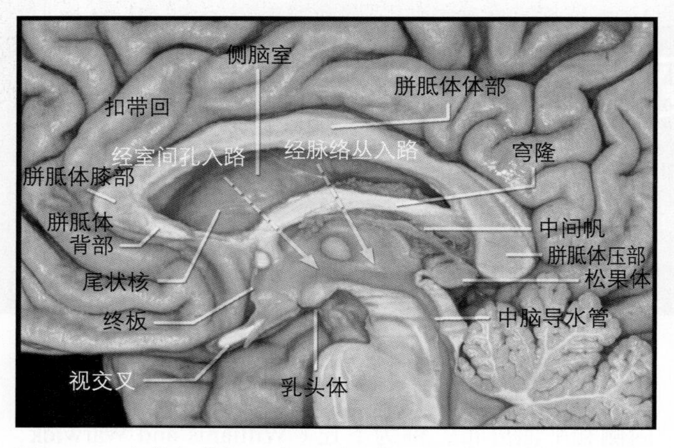

图 35.3 中线矢状切口穿过胼胝体，露出第三脑室和侧脑室（前角和体部）。黄色箭头描绘了这些空洞可能的手术方法

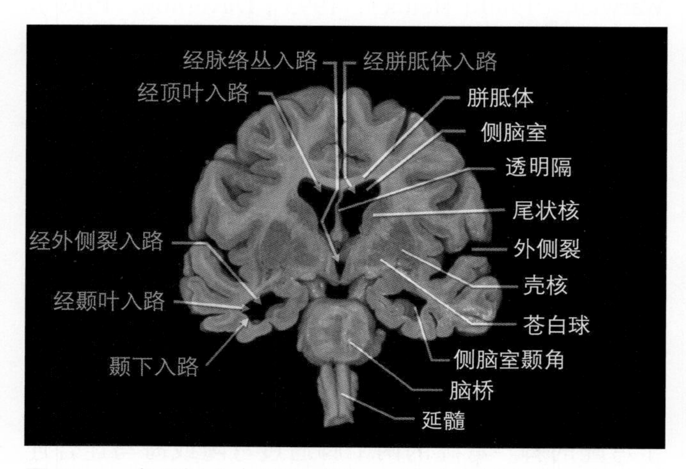

图 35.4 在室间孔水平穿过两个半球的冠状切面，描绘了侧脑室和第三脑室的不同入路（黄色箭头）

前和向内延伸，穹隆的脚变成穹隆体，穹隆与对侧穹隆并列。穹隆体的最前段随后从丘脑上表面脱离，再次远离对侧穹隆，形成前外侧和下突，成为穹隆柱。它的大部分纤维向后延伸到前连合，穿过下丘脑实质，最终到达同侧的下丘脑乳头体（图 35.2 和图 35.3）。从丘脑分离时，穹隆柱成为室间孔的前缘，其后缘由同侧丘脑的最前缘形成（Timurkaynak et al.，1986；Nagata et al.，1988；Rhoton，2003）。根据穹隆的位置，穹隆脚对应于脑室前壁的最内侧，穹隆体对应于室体下极的最内侧。

脉络膜裂是位于丘脑和穹隆之间的裂隙，与脉络丛沿丘脑（或脉络膜）和穹隆两个小脊线的附着点相对应。它延伸到脉络膜下点（位于外侧膝状体水平的海马头部和体部交界处的旁边）和室间孔之间，后者对应于穹隆柱从丘脑分离而导致的裂隙扩大（Nagata et al.，1988；Rhoton，2003）（图 35.3）。由于脉络膜裂环绕丘脑，额角和枕角没有脉络丛（Nagata et al.，1988；Wen et al.，1998）。

尾状核与穹隆平行，外侧环绕丘脑，由头部、体部和尾部组成，分别构成前角外侧壁、室体外侧壁、房部前壁最外侧和颞角顶板内侧部分。尾状核的尾部与杏仁核在前方汇合，杏仁核构成颞角的前壁（Wen et al.，1999）。

沿着尾状核的内侧，终纹横跨丘脑和尾状核之间的丘脑 - 纹状沟，也呈 C 形。这种结构由起源于杏仁复合体的一束细小的纤维束构成，终止于尾状核头部之下的一个被称为“终纹床核”的核（Williams and Warwick，1980；Heimer，1995）。在脑室体内，终纹在丘脑纹状静脉下方运行。

丘脑的上表面构成脑室体底，其后表面称为枕部，构成脑室前壁的中间部分，位于尾状核的外侧尾部和穹隆的内侧脚之间。两个丘脑的内侧表面构成第三脑室的侧壁（Yamamoto et al.，1981）。其最后和最下表面位于两个脉络膜裂的内侧，构成了大脑横裂两侧的上极，其中有环池和部分四叉池。

胼胝体是最大的大脑连合，由连接两个半球几乎所有皮质的纤维组成（图 35.3）。例外的是由前连合连接的颞叶的前部，主要的视觉区域，以及大多数不是半球间连接的躯体感觉区域（Brodal，1981）。沿着正中矢状面，胼胝体与大脑的关系大致类似于一个向前向下的钩。它的前部较厚，有一条曲线，有一个前凸，称为胼胝体膝部，里面有小钳子，一束连接两极和额叶前部的纤维束。膝部下方有一个较薄的水平和基底部分，称为胼胝体吻部，向后终止于前连合处，并与额眶表面相连。膝后，胼胝体的躯干（Heimer，1995；Rhoton，2003）或躯干（Williams and Warwick，1980）有一个几乎水平的部分，有一个略高的曲线，并连接大多数额部和顶部凸起。胼胝体的主干与胼胝体的压部相连，压部是胼胝体最后面和最厚的部分，里面有大钳，这是一束连接顶叶和枕叶的纤维束（Williams and Warwick，1980）。

在形态学上，胼胝体可以理解为一组横跨中线的纤维，并向几个方向散开，以便散布在两个半球。胼胝体的纤维可以看做是一只拍打翅膀的蝴蝶，蝴蝶的身体对应于胼胝体的中线部分，每只翅膀的拍打对应着它的纤维在每个半球的分布。

根据胼胝体的纤维形态，胼胝体与侧脑室的五个部分密切相关，构成了侧脑室壁的很大一部分，与其他脑室表面一样，室管膜排列在胼胝体的内侧。

在前方，吻部和膝部分别构成两个额角的下极和前壁，而躯干则构成额角和脑室体的上极。

当胼胝体压部的纤维向外侧和后方张开时，它们在两侧构成脑室和后角的上极和侧壁。当它们向内侧和下方延伸至脑室和后角时，它们也构成这些脑室部分的内侧壁和下壁。因此，压部的纤维包围了整个脑室和后角，并参与了它们所有壁的组成。

在每个脑室的内侧壁上，可以看到一个明显的压部突起，被称为胼胝体的球状突起，在更后面的后角的内侧壁上，通常也可以看到另一个突起，被称为距骨裂，对应于距骨裂深部的脑室内膨出。

透明隔由两层薄薄的白质膜组成，夹杂着散在的神经元和胶质细胞，形成脑室前角和小体的内侧壁（Williams and Warwick，1980）。在每个额角中，各自的透明隔膜上附着在胼胝体的上干上，前部附着在胼胝体的膝部，下部附着在胼胝体的吻部。在脑室体处，透明隔膜上附着在胼胝体的主干上，下附着于穹隆的每一个躯干，并向内侧排列在一起（**图 35.2** 和**图 35.3**）。

由于穹隆的身体向后延伸，最终与压部的下表面相连，透明隔沿前后方向逐渐降低，最后形成斜面。透明隔的后端决定了室体的后界和脑室的前界（Timurkaynak et al.，1986；Rhoton，2003）。

每个脑室和枕角的底部由一个称为侧支三角的平坦的三角形区域组成，这个三角的前部延伸变得突出，构成了颞角底部的侧方隆起。颞角底部的内侧半部分由海马体形成，海马体对应于海马旁回的脑室内突起，其后方宏观上的附着点位于脑室的内侧壁上（Timurkaynak et al.，1986；Wen et al.，1999；Rhoton，2003）。

尽管侧支三角和隆起对应于大脑基底表面深侧支沟的脑室内投影，但脑室和颞角的底部大多位于梭形回之上。梭形回位于颞下回的内侧、海马旁回的外侧，外侧与枕颞沟相连，内侧与侧支沟相连（Ono et al.，1990）。在梭形回与脑室底部和颞角之间，可见下纵束。

主要的白质纤维束可以通过纤维解剖来识别（**图 35.5**）。上纵束位于额叶、顶叶和后颞叶的深处，位于侧脑室的外侧。两极的、外部的和内部的包膜由几条白质通路组成，这些通路在岛状表面下运行，但当它们的纤维继续向脑叶移动时，从岛状极限沟下面通过。极囊是由短的连合纤维形成的，这些纤维将相邻的岛状回相互连接，并继续向两端的盖部延伸。外囊位于屏状核的内侧，主要由钩状束、额枕下束和闭孔纤维三大纤维束组成；内囊位于壳核的内侧，由投射纤维（主要是锥体纤维和皮质桥小脑纤维）组成。前连合穿过苍白球前下极下方，其纤维连接颞叶的内侧两侧。

构成脑室和颞角侧壁的白质构成所谓的矢状层（Ludwig and Klinger，1956），它位于颞叶皮质下白质（u纤维、颞桥小脑纤维）下面，由额枕下束、前连合纤维和含有光辐射纤维的丘脑后脚组成。

视辐射纤维起源于外侧膝状体区。虽然其前束最初指向前方，形成一条名为 Meyer 袢（Ebeling and Reulen，1988）的曲线至后弯，但其中束、后束和后束的走行则更为笔直和后方。最后，这些纤维将继续向后延伸到距骨裂的上岸和下岸（Párraga et al.，2012）（**图 35.5**）。在视觉辐射纤维下面，发现了被称为绒毡层的胼胝体纤维（Williams and Warwick，1980），它们构成了与脑室腔更内部、更直接相关的纤维。丘脑下茎的纤维特别由听觉辐射组成（Türe et al.，2000；Williams and Warwick，1980），因为它们走向 Heschl 回，所以被发现比颞角更靠前和更靠上。与每个侧脑室相关的大脑结构见**图 35.6**。

第三脑室的解剖学研究

第三脑室是一个位于大脑中心、丘脑之间的单腔（Yamamoto et al.，1981；Rhoton，2003）。它从两侧脑室接收脑脊液，通过位于其上极前部的两个相邻的室间孔，并通过大脑侧裂的导水管流入第四脑室，导水管的开口位于下极的后部。一些脑脊液也是由位于顶端的两个小的脉络丛产生的。

第三脑室的前壁主要由终板形成，终板是一层薄膜，从前连合（上和后）延伸到视交叉（下和前），后者已经在下极的前缘形成了一个突起（Yamamoto et al.，1981）（**图 35.3**）。终板与视交叉之间的小隐窝称为视隐窝。终板的上 1/3 隐藏在胼胝体吻部后面，下 2/3 位于容纳前交通动脉的终板池内。

第三脑室的侧壁主要由两个丘脑组成，其中两个室间孔位于该脑室腔的最前方和最上方，彼此毗邻。

在两侧，浅上凹的下丘脑沟从室间孔向导水管的开口延伸，将丘脑与同侧下丘脑隔开，同侧下丘脑与对侧下丘脑基本连续，所有这些表面都呈 U 形。U 的侧臂与侧壁相对应，上部 2/3 由丘脑构成，下部 1/3 由下丘脑构成。U 的底部由下丘脑构成，对应于第三脑室底部的一部分。

每个侧壁的上界是由丘脑延髓纹沿每个丘脑的上内侧缘，从室间孔到缰核连合。这个连合连接两个缰核，缰核是位于两个丘脑背内侧表面的小隆起，高于后连合。

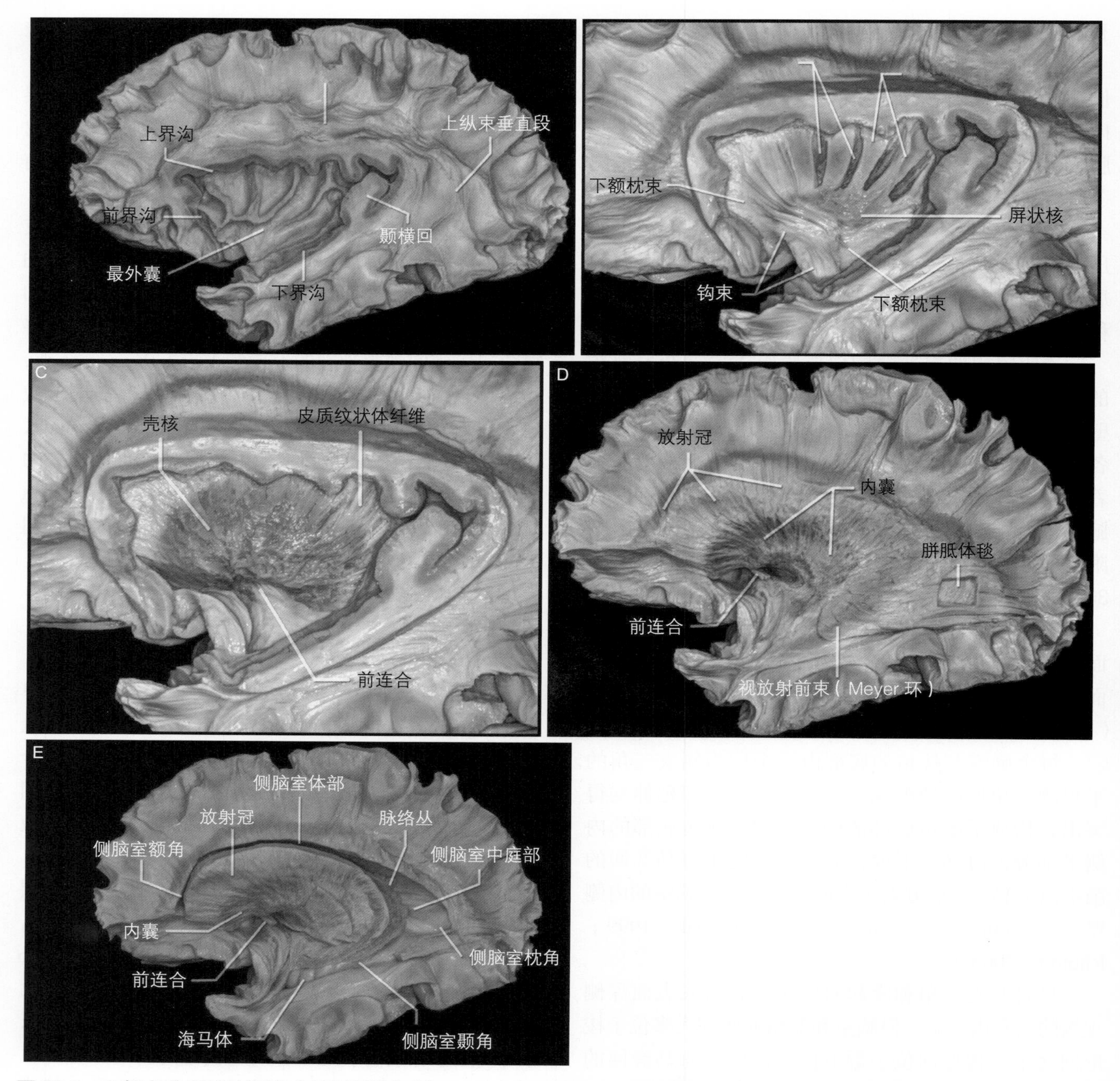

图 35.5 左侧大脑半球的渐进式外侧纤维解剖，显示与侧脑室相关的岛状和岛周白质束。（A）最外囊是由短的缔合纤维组成，在切除岛叶皮质后露出。上纵束（SLF）位于岛区外，在剥离和去除较浅的短联合纤维后可见。（B）在岛区解剖过程中发现额枕下束和钩状束（IFOF、UF），并可辨认其至其他脑叶的轨迹。（C）移除先前的白质纤维会导致壳核以及下面的前连合纤维暴露。（D）摘除豆状核后可见内囊；绒毡层由胼胝体纤维形成，位于岛区后方深处。（E）沿岛区外缘作深圆形切口，广泛暴露侧脑室腔，包括前角、体部、脑室、枕角和颞角

在大约 2/3 的大脑中，马萨中间层连接两个丘脑内侧上半表面（Yamamoto et al.，1981）。

第三脑室底部从视交叉延伸至 Sylvius 导水管开口，后连合为其上缘，中脑被盖为其下缘，可分为下丘脑前部和中脑后部。前部从前到后由视交叉、漏斗、灰结节和乳头体组成，后部已经对应于脚间窝的顶部，由中脑被盖形成（**图** 35.3）。漏斗与垂体柄连续，通过视上室 - 垂体束将下丘脑与垂体后叶（神经垂体）相连，该束运输含有催产素和加压素激素的胶体液滴（Nieuwenhuys et al.，2007）。

当从脑室上方和内部观察底部时，可以很容易地辨认出视交叉突起和灰结节之间的漏斗状隐窝，

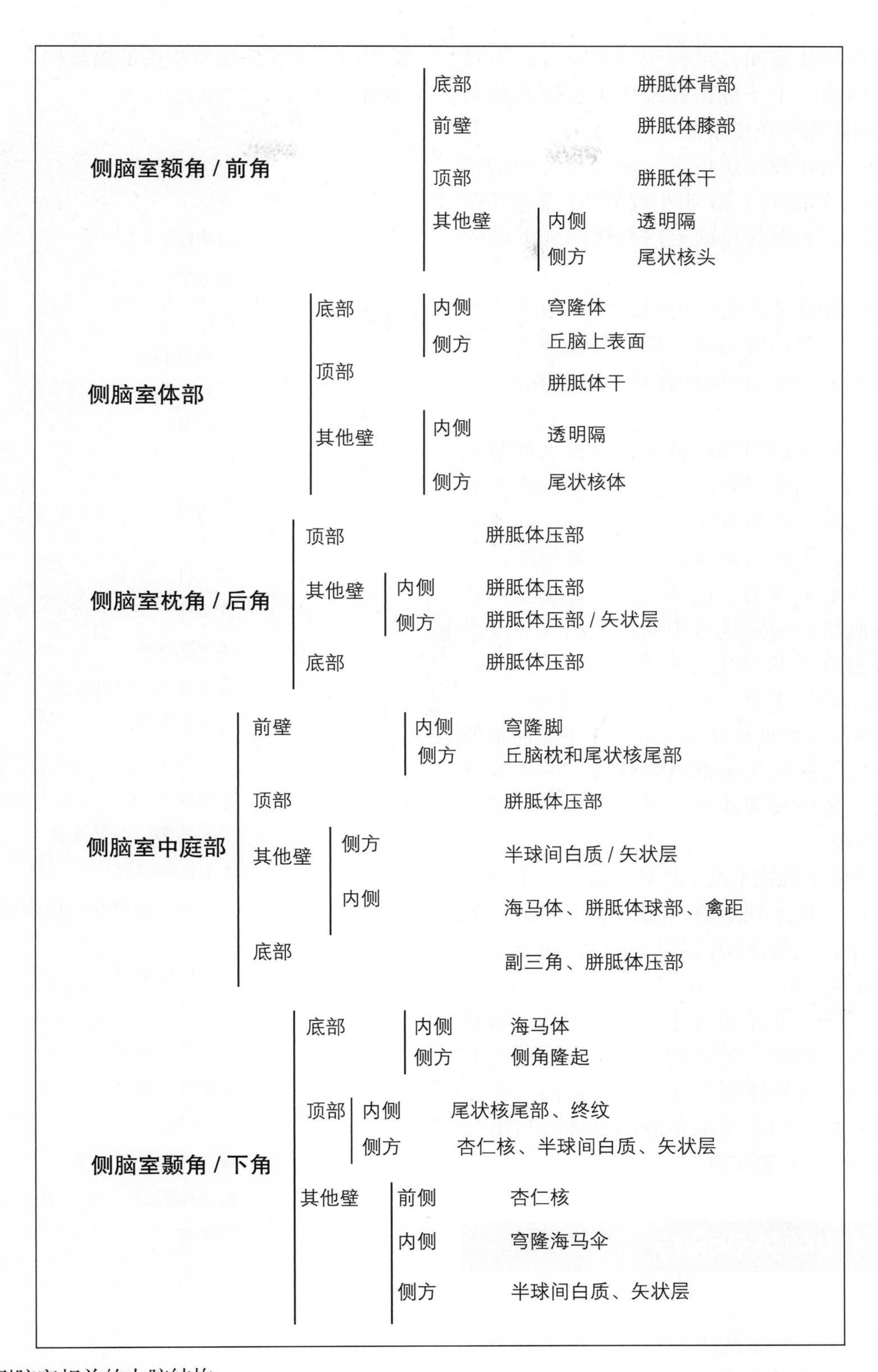

图 35.6　与各侧脑室相关的大脑结构

乳头体在漏斗状隐窝后面显示为两个突起。内镜下第三脑室吻合术应切开漏斗窝和乳头体之间薄且通常为半透明的区域。在乳头体的后面，第三脑室的底部是凹面和光滑的，以更后面的导水管的三角形开口为标志。

第三脑室的底板位于视交叉的正后方，位于视束和大脑脚之间，脚间窝的顶板与第三脑室底板的中脑部的前侧相对应。当前穿孔物质沿基底区向前扩散至两个视束时，后穿孔物质沿第三脑室底部的整个下侧扩散。

第三脑室顶端从室间孔延伸至缰核连合，由穹隆构成的上层结构、上下脉络膜组成的层以及这两层薄膜之间的间隙构成正中膜池。

第三脑室上层和神经层位于前部，由并列的穹隆两体构成。tela 脉络膜上瓣与两侧穹隆下缘密切接触，而 tela 脉络膜下瓣与丘脑上内侧缘两侧的髓纹相连。

位于 tela 脉络膜层之间的中间膜池在前终止于两个室间孔水平，向后开口进入四叉神经池或松果体池。小梁内有脉络膜后内侧动脉和大脑内静脉（**图 35.3**）。

大脑内静脉是由前间隔静脉和丘脑纹状静脉交界处形成的，当它们穿过穹隆下方，穿过脉络膜裂隙，靠近室间孔时，通常发生在它们进入中间薄膜池的入口点附近。大脑内静脉是由前间隔静脉和丘脑纹状静脉交界处形成的，通常发生在靠近室间孔的穹隆下通过脉络膜裂隙进入中间膜池的入口点附近。大脑内静脉在松果体上方向后流出中间膜池，与 Rosenthal 基底静脉汇合，形成 Galen 大静脉。

两条脉络丛沿正线两侧从 tela 脉络膜下层向下伸入第三脑室。每条脉络丛束都沿着其蒂与同侧侧脑室的脉络丛通过脉络膜裂连续，脉络膜裂界定了第三脑室顶部的外侧。

后壁从松果体上隐窝（位于缰核连合上方）延伸到导水管的开口，从上到下包括松果体上隐窝、缰核连合、松果体、松果体隐窝和后连合，即导水管开口的上方（**图 35.3**）。

松果体位于三叉神经池的外侧，位于第三脑室外，由双柄附着于后壁，该双柄突出于缰核连合上方，低于后连合。松果体隐窝在松果体前面，构成松果腺上下附着物之间第三脑室腔的延伸。与第三脑室相关的大脑结构见**表 35.1**。

表 35.1 与第三脑室相关的脑结构

前壁		室间孔
		穹隆
		前连合
		终板
		视凹陷
		视交叉
侧壁		丘脑
		丘脑延髓纹
		下丘脑沟
		下丘脑
底部	下丘脑	视交叉
		漏斗窝
		漏斗
		三叉神经结节
		乳头体
		后穿孔物质
	中脑	中脑被盖 / 脚间窝顶
		后穿孔物质
		中脑导水管口
顶部		室间孔
		穹隆体脚、海马连合
		上 tela 脉络膜
		间隔池（脉络膜后内侧动脉、大脑内静脉）
		下 tela 脉络膜
		脉络丛
		松果体上隐窝
后壁		松果体上隐窝
		松果体缰
		缰核连合
		松果体隐窝
		松果腺
		后连合

幕上脑室肿瘤的外科治疗

术前计划

一旦诊断明确，要做的决定包括：是否有手术切除的适应证，如果具备适应证，目标是否是大体全切除。最后，可以计划选择合适的手术入路。

影像学

术前检查包括 MRI 成像，以确定病变的特征及其解剖来源和范围。典型的表现有时可作为诊断性征象，如第三脑室胶样囊肿或具有特征性扩散受限的表皮样瘤。T2 加权序列上的高信号可能表示高含水量和低密度，而计算机断层扫描（CT）可能显示钙化。

对于一些有脑脊液种植倾向的病变（如原始神经外胚层肿瘤、室管膜瘤、生殖细胞肿瘤），应完成包括脊柱在内的整个神经轴的成像以计划处理。

肿瘤标志物

若最初在血清中检测到阳性肿瘤标志物，随后在脑脊液中也检测到阳性肿瘤标志物，这就需要进一步的治疗。对于第三脑室附近的生殖细胞肿瘤，甲胎蛋白（alpha-fetoprotein，AFP）或人绒毛膜促性腺激素（human chorionic gonadotropin，HCG）水平的升高将诊断限制在少数几个类别，这些类别都至少在最初通过放疗或化疗得到控制。请参阅**第 36 章**。

内镜手术

在切除一些脑室内病变之前，内镜手术可以作为紧急治疗，以缓解脑脊液阻塞，获得活检，或开窗切除囊性病变。同时可采集脑脊液进行肿瘤标志物和细胞学检查。对于阻塞导水管的病变，推荐进行第三脑室造口术。如果病变浸润到第三脑室底部，阻塞了室间孔，那么内镜下透明隔切开术和插入单个脑室腹膜分流术可以简化脑脊液分流。如果除了解除梗阻性脑积水的手术外还计划进行内镜活检，建议首先进行脑室造口术，因为活检部位的出血可能会遮盖完成手术所需的内镜检查。使用柔性内镜可以方便两种手术通过相同的骨孔。

决策

手术切除的适应证取决于患者和病变因素。患者因素包括年龄、并发症和预期预后。肿瘤因素考虑了转移和脑脊液扩散的存在，以及是否有可供选择的非手术治疗，如淋巴瘤或生殖细胞瘤。在某些情况下，例如肿瘤标志物阳性的生殖细胞肿瘤，开始放射或化疗的初步治疗，之后保留手术切除任何残留的肿瘤。

手术入路的规划是重要的，并依赖于对复杂和多因素的评估。该入路必须量身定做，以达到预定的切除目标，并需要了解预期的手术“盲点”和每种入路的潜在发病率。一般情况下，手术入路的选择取决于计划切除的范围，而切除范围又取决于患者的因素，包括神经功能缺损的存在、病变的类型和预后，以及是否有有效的辅助治疗来处理残留病。病变的大小、形态、范围和一致性等技术特征有助于决定最合适的手术入路。

幕上脑室病变的手术入路

表 35.2 显示了幕上脑室病变的手术入路。

体部和额角入路

经胼胝体入路

患者仰卧，颈部屈曲，头部抬高。要么是冠状切口，要么是基于侧向的 U 型皮瓣。传统上，横穿中线的双额开颅手术在上矢状窦（superior sagittal sinus，SSS）上直接有一个或两个骨孔，或者如果愿意，在上矢状窦的两边各有一个骨孔，并在暴露的冠状缝的后面 1/3 和前面 2/3 延伸。正是基于这样一个事实，即胼胝体切开术必须放在前面，因为穹隆位于胼胝体（corpus callosum，CC）的后面，然后才能向前向下扫，形成透明隔（Rhoton，2002）。颅脑关系表明，室间孔位于冠状缝水平，中央沟位于冠状缝后 5 cm（Ribas et al.，2006），这表明中央前回和中央后回的位置应该受到保护，以防操纵或回缩。开颅手术的前后尺寸应该足以让外科医生选择一个没有桥静脉的区域，从而在不破坏这些关键血管的情况下进行大脑间入路。虽然任何一个侧脑室都可以通过这个入路进入，但更容易暴露出要进入相应脑室的半球的更多部位。一些作者主张术前对引流

表 35.2 幕上脑室病变的手术入路

	侧脑室体 + 额角	侧脑室三角 + 房部	第三脑室	第三脑室后部	第三脑室前部
入路	经胼胝体 / 经皮质入路	经皮质 / 经沟上颞顶内	经孔脉络膜 / 脉络膜下	枕部经小脑幕	经颅终板经颅 EEETS
盲区	对侧侧脑室顶 FM	血管蒂尖端	第三脑室顶	第三脑室顶盖同侧壁	第三脑室脚间池（漏斗后）顶
	桥静脉 SMA 胼周动脉	视辐射上纵束 / 弓状束	穹隆、丘脑 / 静脉	深静脉 视觉皮质	嗅 ACoA 穿支 垂体柄
	穹隆、丘脑 / 静脉	↓	穹隆 深静脉 下丘脑	顶盖 深静脉	下丘脑 穹隆

ACoA，前交通动脉；EEETS，经蝶窦扩展鼻内镜；FM，室间孔；SMA，补充运动区

静脉进行详细的成像，如 CT 静脉造影（computed tomography venogram，CTV）或磁共振静脉造影（magnetic resonance venogram，MRV），然后可以在图像引导下量身定做，避免桥静脉。

大脑半球间入路（**图 35.4**）需要仔细解剖，因为内侧额叶可以粘连，所以必须保留更深于镰刀下缘的软膜表面。矢状面上的轨迹是由室间孔的表面标记在与上颞线相交的冠状缝对应的平面上引导的，因此，在开颅手术中检查部分暴露的冠状缝的倾斜度和使用图像引导使入路变得容易。虽然脑部牵引器放置不当会造成后退损伤，但过度的“动态后退”也同样有害。因此，需要一种大脑放松和温和操作的策略。在出现严重脑积水的情况下，在开始时先放置脑室引流管，而不会完全塌陷脑室，这有利于手术入路，如果外科医生愿意的话，还可以将脑牵引器作为一个“夹持器”放置。

CC 显露出来，并通过其闪亮的白色和表面的血管图案来识别。理想的方法是辨认两条足周动脉，这些动脉都是侧方分离和活动的，每条动脉都有相应的半球，这样就不会破坏到软膜表面的供应分支。根据经验，特别是在脑室扩张的情况下，可以辨认透明隔附着处中线矢状面的中央白色间隔。这样可以将胼胝体切开术放置在足以进入所需侧脑室的侧面。只要显示脑室内病变的轨迹是正确的，一般不需要大的胼胝体切开术。重要的是胼胝体切开的位置，而不是大小，以避免损伤穹隆。CC 纤维的分离显示了潜在的紫色室管膜，一旦被刺穿，它就允许脑脊液出口。

一旦进入脑室，需要辨认脉络丛，脉络丛跟随到室间孔。一旦丘脑纹状静脉被识别，脑室的偏侧性就建立起来（Rhoton，2002）。如果没有脉络丛可见，这很可能是前角，如果向后改变轨迹仍然显示腔内没有脉络丛，则应怀疑进入透明隔腔。

最好进行透明隔切开术，避免鼻中隔静脉出血，特别是当病变阻塞室间孔时，如果脑脊液流量不能恢复，以后可以使用单一导管进行脑脊液分流。在许多情况下，病变可能会遮挡脑室间标志物的视线，因此可以通过透明切开术检查对侧脑室，并以此为参照来确定穹隆和深静脉的相对深度和位置。

在切除病变之前，要么确定穹隆和重要静脉的位置，要么至少知道它们的相对位置。如果可能，在术前影像的辅助下确定病变的起源。病变可能主要发生在透明隔（如中枢神经细胞瘤和一些室管膜下瘤）、脉络丛（如乳头状瘤或脑膜瘤）或室管膜壁（如胶质瘤或巨细胞星形细胞瘤）。在大型或双侧病变中，解剖起源可能无法确定。如果可能，首先将脉络丛与病变表面凝固并分离，以控制可能的血供来源。根据病变与间歇性止血的一致性，进行分段切除，进行抽吸或 CUSA 手术抽吸，因为过多的出血将妨碍脑室内的可视化。切除的范围考虑了患者的因素，如年龄、病变的性质、是否有辅助治疗以及术前是否存在神经功能障碍。这可能需要在穹隆附近留下一小部分残留物或粘连在主要静脉上。对于发生在脑实质的外生性进入脑室的病变，必须注意不要扩大切除范围，以免损伤周围的尾状核、丘脑或位于室间孔附近水平的内囊膝部。

在大多数情况下，建议脑室外引流几天，直到脑脊液引流清。它可以通过胼胝体切开在手术开始或结束时放置，穿过硬脑膜，远离切口。然后仔细缝合硬脑膜，用骨孔盖替换骨瓣，并缝合伤口。

这种方法的缺陷包括牵引器对 SSS 的压迫，如果延长可能会导致血栓形成。主桥静脉的牺牲可能导致静脉梗死和术后癫痫，矢状面轨迹过后有损伤穹隆的风险。如果该结构被误认为 CC，则可能发生扣带回损伤，进入的是跟骨周血管和胼胝体边缘血管之间的区域，而不是两条跟骨周动脉之间的走廊，扣带回的挫伤和周围肿胀可能导致术后补充运动区（supplementary motor area，SMA）综合征。足周动脉损伤或其相应半球分支断裂可能导致偏瘫，特别是影响下肢。进入透明隔腔而不是进入侧脑室和混淆进入哪个脑室可能会导致严重的损伤，例如尝试中隔吻合术损伤尾状核或丘脑。应避免通过入路或在切除过程中损伤穹隆，如果病变是粘连的或部分浸润穹隆，则建议进行次全切除。最后，如果透明膜切开术没有清晰的视野和方向，可能会导致隔静脉出血，如果放置不当，可能会损伤穹隆的一部分。

该入路的盲点包括对侧侧脑室的顶端，肿瘤可能不易完整切除。需要注意的是，对于较大的脑室内病变，室间孔、穹隆静脉和丘脑纹状静脉最初可能会被病变遮挡。

经皮质入路

另外，体部和前角可以通过额叶皮质入路进入（Rhoton，2002）。额上沟通常很深，最初的经额沟入路或经额中回入路可以提供通向脑室的轨迹。这种方法在脑积水的病例中更容易使用。影像引导有助于规划穿过白质束的轨迹（Szmuda et al. 2014）。

一旦进入脑室，随后的手术步骤与上述描述的步骤相似，但要记住手术切面的方向是从更外侧到更内侧的轨迹。

侧脑室房部入路

虽然侧脑室的主体位于中线附近，但房部或三角区位于两个丘脑后面的中线空洞之外，因此它们的进入需要离中线入路。关于房部，要记住的一个关键解剖学特征是，虽然压部在中线两端的最后端覆盖松果体或四分叉池，但其侧向延伸覆盖两侧和后方，覆盖丘脑枕窝，并包围构成枕角的两个脑室及其可变的后部延伸，这些后部已经在脑实质内，因此位于沿中线可见的压部最后部的后面。

鉴于这一解剖位置，只有房部最上方和最前面的肿瘤可以通过已描述的经胼胝体前入路到达额角和每个侧脑室的体部，而其他房部肿瘤根据其主要位置、范围和血管供应需要不同的经皮质入路。进入脑室房部的主要途径是经顶入路、经颞入路和顶枕半球交替入路（**图 35.1**）。

计划入路不仅要考虑避开运动语言中枢的大脑皮质进入部位，还要考虑穿过白质束的轨迹。由于神经元的可塑性，皮质损伤所致的神经功能障碍通常会恢复，但白质束损伤会导致永久性的功能障碍。必须说明的是，应该采用最安全的轨道，而不是最短的轨道。图像引导的使用在优化轨迹指向目标方面非常有用，但外科医生应该根据经验，选择最短的路径。

经顶入路

虽然顶内沟有时被打断，但它是一个非常明显的沟，横跨顶叶的上外侧表面，通常与中央后沟的下段和下行段连续。这些沟的实际或投影的交汇点或过渡点构成顶面到房部最近的点（Harkey et al.，1989；Ebeling and Steinmetz，1995；Ribas et al.，2006）。然而，经顶骨显微神经外科入路（**图 35.4**）必须通过这两个沟之间的移行点为起点，沿顶内沟向后移动可以进入房部的更后面部分，特别是在不扩大的情况下。

对于这种入路，患者最好是半坐位，开颅手术应该以顶内沟和中央后沟的实际或投影的转换点为中心，沿矢状缝在 λ 上方约 6 cm，在其外侧约 5cm（Ribas et al.，2006）。

术前通过仔细研究 3D-MRI 图像，可以估计出双侧脑沟的形状、断端及其接合部位，融合 CT 和 MRI 图像可以更好地估计其接合部位在颅骨表面的投影。

术中确定顶内和中央后沟可见段的位置后，考虑到它们在 MR 图像上通常或已知的走行，其实际或计划的汇合点或转折点的识别通常可以被识别为蛛网膜下腔的可变性扩大，如果有的话，也应该借助神经导航来确认。经常会发现静脉沿着或紧挨着两个脑沟延伸。

经顶骨入路可经脑沟、软膜下或经脑回入路，但始终考虑到中央后沟和顶内沟之间的交界处是更安全地到达房部的最近和最容易的表面部位，手术入路必须遵循脑沟的方向，它总是通向最近的脑室腔（Harkey et al.，1989；Ebeling and Steinmetz，1995；Ribas et al.，2006）。该入路必须沿着向后倾斜 30° 的径向入路（Ribas et al.，2006）。神经导航和术中超声对确定通往房部的路径都有很大帮助。

通常需要一个宽的沟开口来暴露和允许坚固病变的零星输送，因此能够在术前影像上计划使用深沟并在手术中解剖定位是有利的。

一旦遇到脑室腔，手术走廊可以扩大，如有必要，可以沿着顶内沟方向向后切除更多的脑组织，最好是从顶上小叶内侧切除更多的脑组织，以避免进一步损害上纵向和弧形束，这些束主要从顶下小叶内的顶内沟外侧延伸。

经顶叶入路进入房部后沿顶内沟水平，即在躯体感觉皮质之后，总是会损伤顶叶 U 形纤维、顶叶投射纤维（主要是顶脑桥 - 小脑纤维）以及覆盖房部并向距骨裂楔缘延伸的最上端纤维，从而造成对侧同名下象限缺损。

虽然非显性顶叶损害更多地与左侧忽视和失认、空间定向障碍、建筑和穿衣失用有关，但显性顶叶损害可导致言语困难、阅读困难、计算困难、失用、触觉失认，并可能导致 Gerstmann 综合征（书写困难、计算困难、手指失认和右 / 左定向障碍）。

后颞入路

经颞上沟远端入路适合于更多的下房肿瘤（Harkey et al.，1989；Ebeling and Steinmetz，1995；Ribas et al.，2006），特别是当这些病变向颞角延伸或从脉络膜前动脉获得大量血液供应时。这种方法可能会损害沿房部侧壁运行的光辐射。Wernicke 区及其潜在的语言相关纤维也处于危险之中，因为它主要位于颞上回的后侧和优势半球的边缘上回内。在可行的情况下，清醒开颅手术可以将这些风险降至最低。

颞上沟的最远端，在其通常的三叉点之前，位于后侧裂点（侧裂末端）后方 2~3 cm 处（Ribas et al.，2006）。就开颅手术而言，该区域位于水平顶乳突缝合点和鳞状缝合的上升后侧交会点上方约

3 cm 处，这通常是一个可以触摸到的位置，在乳突上部上方有轻微的凹陷（Ribas et al.，2006；Ribas and Rodrigues，2007）。一旦确定了侧裂末端正下方和后方的水平沟段，就可以采用横沟、软膜下或横脑沟入路，向前和放射方向 30°~40°（Ribas，2005；Ribas et al.，2006）（**图 35.1**）。使用神经导航和术中超声可以增强脑室路径。如有必要，可进一步切除脑组织以获得足够的暴露。

由于 Heschl 回位于三角形颞面的前方，其内端紧挨着房部，因此侧裂最后方的开口也可以通向心房。然而，由于这个水平的裂缝是平的，所以这个开口在技术上是困难的。此入路需要进一步切除颞上盖内表面（听觉初级皮质区）和缘上回的底部。

在大的病变中有一个盲点，在缩小一些肿瘤肿块之前，在脉络丛附着处的血管蒂可能不会暴露。

可供选择的入路

完全避开视觉白质束的侧脑室躯体和三角区的解剖学手术入路包括大脑半球间经胼胝体入路、经内侧顶枕沟或经扣带回峡部的后半球间入路（下文描述）以及最近描述的小脑上下 / 小脑幕上入路，然后再经侧支沟入路。

顶枕沟的半球间部分与枕角有关，而与三角区无关。后方入路和在扣带回楔前或峡部区域进行皮质切除术可以进入三角区，但对于这种深部入路来说，如果不是必要的话，有一定冗余空间的大脑是可取的，如果存在巨大的肿块，可能会妨碍其使用。

顶枕半球间入路 Yaşargil（Yaşargil，1996）提出的顶枕半球间入路（**图 35.1**）是独特的，因为它是唯一不损害光辐射的入路。然而，这并不是一条直达的入路，手术走廊也受到枕骨后退程度的限制。在存在深厚的实心半球肿块的情况下，通过半球间入路获得进入所需的松动和回缩可能是有问题的。

由于入路沿着楔骨是半球间的，理想情况下患者应该处于半坐位，所以沿中线的开颅手术应从顶枕沟最远端对应的 λ 延伸到枕窝最突出的颅点和距骨裂最远端对应的后枕骨上脑点斜颈通常位于斜颈上方 3~4 cm，而 λ 通常位于斜颈上方 2~4 cm（Ribas et al.，2006）。

枕半球间入路是因为皮质顶枕静脉在加入窦之前通常有平行于上矢状窦几厘米的上升路线（Oka et al.，1985；Yaşargil，1996）。入路应在镰状 - 天幕交界处和楔面朝向压部之间进行，楔骨的前尖部是顶枕沟与距骨裂的连接处，也是它们各自的动脉通常汇合的地方。如有必要，可以通过牺牲小的引流静脉来帮助枕骨外侧后退，主要是通过打开脾旁脑池和释放脑脊液。发现了非常白的压部和 Rosenthal 静脉，很容易看到扣带回的同侧峡部与紧随其后的楔前底部一起包裹在压部周围，这些都构成了经大脑进入房部的位置。

由于房腔位于侧面，这样的窗口必须沿侧方和前方方向开，直到找到构成房部前壁的丘脑肿瘤或白色枕骨，以及附连的脉络丛球体。

这种入路的主要限制是枕骨后退的程度，对于任何其他的脑室入路，如果有脑室扩大，它是容易的。由于该入路需要大量的脑回缩，而且是通过间接途径完成的，神经导航和术中超声不如其他入路有帮助，它的成功依赖于对解剖标志及其方向的识别。

其他入路 更基本的颞叶入路，通过切除颞下回后部及其内侧邻近梭形回的窗口（对应于颞角后侧和房部的底部），可以避免优势半球内的视神经辐射和语言区，但更适合于已经占据颞角的下部病变（**图 35.4**）。对于这些入路，重要的是要记住，颞下回虽然宽，但高度短，暴露在外面需要非常低的颞骨开颅手术。由于梭形回主要位于岩骨上表面，开颅手术的基础应包括颧弓根部远侧和上侧的耳前凹陷、水平顶乳突与位于乳突上部的鳞状缝合的后部和上缘交汇处（Ribas and Rodrigues，2007）。

采用巧妙的小脑上入路，切开小脑幕，显露侧脑沟，然后经小脑沟入路进入三角区下方 10 mm 处的侧脑室下侧。对于大小和位置合适的病变，该入路将是完美的。可以想象，通过这种方法可能不能充分暴露较大的固体块，特别是具有较高伸展的固体块。包括海马体在内的内侧结构需要用这种方法保护。

颞角入路

参见**第 81 章**和**图 35.4**。

第三脑室入路

主脑室

初始入路与前面描述的经胼胝体入路进入侧脑室相同。必须注意的是，胼胝体切开术将在通常的位置进行，因为轨迹仍将允许进入整个第三脑室。将胼胝体切开术放在更靠后的位置，不仅有损伤穹隆的风险，而且即使通过 CC 的压部，最终也可能进入四叉池，而不是第三脑室。此外，后部脱节综合征的视觉成分可能对患者产生毁灭性的影响。

一旦进入侧脑室，在经孔入路和经脉络膜入路之间的选择将取决于病变的形态及其与室间孔的关系和大小（Rhoton et al.，1981）。穹隆间入路从分离透明隔叶开始，打开穹隆间间隙，穿过第三脑室顶部，有双侧穹隆损伤的高风险。

经椎间孔入路　这对于出现在扩张的室间孔的病变是理想的。适用于绝大多数胶质囊肿和其他一些前第三脑室或“哑铃”病变。对于那些可以进入侧脑室的移动性病变，手术是很方便的（**图** 35.3）。深静脉的形态多种多样，在切除过程中必须加以保护（Türe et al.，1997）。需要温和牵引以避免第三脑室顶部的血管附着物撕裂，这是一个盲点。在切除病变的前下部时需要注意，以避免下丘脑的损伤。

解剖学观察表明，大多数胶样囊肿实际上出现在间置膜内，因此由脉络膜内侧后动脉的分支供应，这也解释了那些位于透明隔部分叶片内的胶样囊肿通过间置膜的延伸而形成的原因（Morris and Santoreneos，2012）。在一些胶样囊肿中，尤其是偶发的，穹隆带的前部仍然完好无损，并延伸到囊肿的包膜上。抓住这层膜来操纵囊肿可能会导致囊肿附着的穹隆变形和随后的功能障碍。因此，在放大的情况下，切开上面的这一层会使囊肿移动，使其能够通过室间孔输送，并在凝固和分离其血管蒂后完整切除。

经脉络膜入路　室间孔实际上是脉络膜裂的前部扩张的开放部分，然后经脉络膜入路打开穹隆和丘脑之间的间隙，在丘脑纹状静脉后面进入第三脑室（**图** 35.3 和**图** 35.4）。这部分被脉络丛覆盖，一旦脉络丛被轻轻地从裂隙送出，就会明显地通过一层膜（穹隆带）附着在穹隆的正中上方，而通过丘脑带连接到丘脑的下侧。由于后一层膜可能包含几条从丘脑到丘脑纹状静脉的引流静脉，因此最好切开穹隆带，这是一种“经脉络膜穹隆下”入路，而不是丘脑带，以避免损害丘脑的静脉引流（Rhoton，2002）。然而，在实践中，大多数需要手术的病变都是如此之大，以至于脉络膜裂隙的这一部分是“张开的”，这些膜被拉伸并容易打开。这将获得进入并可视化整个第三脑室，从它的前部范围到会阴上隐窝（Ulm et al.，2009）。

盲点

- 第三脑室顶端和对侧大脑内静脉。

第三脑室前部

这种病变从鞍上脑池延伸到第三脑室。如果主要位于脑室内，则可经胼胝体、经孔或脉络膜入路。其余的可经终板、额部、大脑半球间或翼点开颅，或经鼻内镜扩大入路。参见**第 27 章**。

第三脑室后部

这些是松果体肿瘤或其他病变，发生在四叉脑池并延伸到脑室。最好是通过幕下小脑上入路，它可以很好地显示第三脑室顶板，并可以仔细地从深静脉中剥离病变。然而，尾部延伸到顶盖区域可能是一个盲点。或者，可以采用枕部经小天幕入路，它能更好地显示病变的尾部范围。巨大的压部可能会使病变沿第三脑室顶部的延伸变得模糊。见**第 37 章**。

内镜手术入路

除了获得活检和解除脑脊液阻塞外，内镜手术在切除脑室内病变方面也有新的作用。脑室内囊肿，如有症状的大型松果体或侧脑室蛛网膜囊肿，或与肿瘤相关的囊肿，可在内镜下开窗进入脑室，如果需要，可从脑室壁取活检。通过第三脑室蛛网膜囊肿的“双极”开窗（即内镜下开窗将上穹顶送入室间孔，进入侧脑室并穿过囊肿），下极与桥前池连通，建立脑脊液循环，并可能降低复发风险（Kirollos et al.，2001）。

内镜下切除胶样囊肿在许多情况下是可以实现的，但不是所有情况下都可以实现。在脑室扩大的情况下，含有容易抽出的内容物的可移动囊肿适合内镜技术（见**第 33 章**）。

在专家手中，一些实实在在的脑室病变可以通过内镜途径切除（Barber et al.，2013；Selvanathan et al.，2013）。

特殊并发症

除了早先描述的手术技术导致神经血管损伤的技术并发症外，还存在特定的手术风险（Hassaneen et al.，2010；Milligan and Meyer，2010；Symss et al.，2014）。

记忆障碍

这可能是由于前叶操作造成的（Villani et al.，1997；Friedman et al.，2008）。

下丘脑功能障碍

这可能会发生，尤其是涉及第三脑室底部的病变。最常见的是暂时性的，如低钠血症或尿崩症。

视觉和凝视功能障碍

松果体区病变可延伸至后第三脑室并累及顶盖。垂直凝视的限制可以在功能上得到补偿，但其他功能障碍，如偏斜、远 / 近调节障碍和包括吻侧内侧纵束在内的几条通路参与的动态性复视，对功能结果和生活质量有显著影响（Hart et al.，2013）。

分离综合征

虽然在经典情况下，这会导致失读症，但没有失写、异手综合征、触觉障碍和左 / 右失用症。然而，这种情况很少见于人类，尤其是在前胼胝体切除术后的较长时间内（Villani et al.，1997；Symss et al.，2014）。例外情况是破裂涉及压部。在这些情况下，视觉结果，如匹配和理解不同视野中的物体，对日常活动（如驾驶）具有重要意义。

争议

在颞上入路和经顶入路之间的选择是有争议的。

颞上沟的后部通常很深，很容易辨认，但在优势半球，上唇是隐藏语言区域的颞上回。因此，在裂开沟的过程中，如果需要的话，松动或退缩应该转向下唇而不是上唇。同样，顶沟的上唇后上松动术更好，以避免过度操作顶下小叶，顶下小叶起着位于边缘上和角回的语言功能，而顶下小叶的语言功能位于缘上回和角回，这是一种较好的顶沟上唇后上松动术。

在深部解剖中，白质束最浅的是从额叶定向的上纵束或弓状束，其重要的语音功能联系是深至颞上沟（尽管也可能延伸到颞中沟）和顶下小叶，深至缘上回和角回。因此，从颞上沟或顶内沟到三角区的轨迹的方向应该避免切断这些重要的连接，前提是意识到这一区域与入路的距离很近。通过这两条沟中的任何一条入路都相当远离内囊或放射冠更深的后肢。然而，在横断的情况下，不可避免地要横切两个更深的层，即具有重要功能的光辐射和没有可识别的神经缺损的绒毡层。额枕下束（IFOF）的破坏可能导致语义性失语。在与房部侧壁相关的矢状层，IFOF 位于弓状束的内侧，位于光辐射纤维的外侧。在更后面，这两个入路的轨迹所在，IFOF 纤维更多地张开，到达枕叶、顶上叶和颞基底区的凸面（Martino et al.，2011）。

在通过颞上沟入路时，光辐射方向与颞沟方向平行，因此分离术可能会分离纤维，避免大量束纤维分裂。可能导致的高级象限视野缺陷通常对患者的日常活动影响不大，这些患者往往会很快适应这种缺陷。

相反，通过顶内沟入路，白质解剖的方向必须改变，以保持“对齐”，而不是穿过光学辐射纤维。从解剖学上讲，一种“高位”的顶内入路通过到视觉辐射的上方是有利的，因为它对白质纤维的破坏最小，白质纤维在中庭的顶部上密度最小。然而，由此产生的累及下视野的暗点通常可以被患者注意到。如果出现较大的下象限暗点，可能会影响患者的活动能力和日常活动（如爬楼梯）。

尽管颞上沟入路提供了早期进入脉络丛的通道，脉络丛为脑室脑膜瘤提供血液供应，但是大多数病变似乎没有过多的血管，任何一种入路都不会造成出血的特殊问题。

参考文献、EBRAIN 的相关链接

扫描书末二维码获取。

第八篇　肿瘤和颅底——松果体区肿瘤

第36章　松果体肿瘤

Mueez Waqar · Samantha Mills · Conor L. Mallucci · Michael D. Jenkinson 著
王镔 译，许海洋 审校

引言

松果体区位于中脑顶盖和第三脑室顶部之间的中线区域。松果体肿瘤很少见，儿童患者较成人患者多（Louis et al.，2016）。松果体肿瘤有多种组织学类型，包括生殖细胞肿瘤（germ cell tumour，GCT，60%）、松果体实质肿瘤（pineal parenchymal tumour，PPT，30%）和胶质瘤（5%）（见图36.1）。其他组织学亚型较少见，包括松果体区乳头状肿瘤（papillary tumour of the pineal region，PTPR）、室管膜瘤、脑膜瘤、淋巴瘤和转移瘤（Al-Hussaini et al.，2009）。既往治疗时，由于开放性手术的死亡率极高，所以许多松果体肿瘤患者在不进行组织学诊断的情况下，直接进行放射治疗。而当下神经外科和神经肿瘤学的治疗方案由肿瘤类型决定，包括组织活检、开放手术、分次放疗和化疗。松果体肿瘤治疗的最新进展主要是由儿科患者的临床试验推动的。

临床表现和术前检查

松果体肿瘤患者常见临床表现有颅内压升高（87%）、帕里诺（Parinaud）综合征（76%）和小脑体征（52%）（Konovalov and Pitskhelauri，2003）。其中帕里诺综合征是由于中脑受压所致，表现为上视受限、调节反射丧失、对光反射丧失和辐辏性眼球震颤。术前需要对全脑和全脊髓进行增强磁共振成像，以确定脑积水存在与否、外科手术入路中的解剖结构以及是否存在转移播散（Awa et al.，2014）。检测血清和脑脊液中的肿瘤标志物也是必要的。如人绒毛膜促性腺激素β（β human chorionic gonadotrophin，β-HCG）和甲胎蛋白（α-fetoprotein，AFP）升高可不经活检直接诊断为GCT的亚型。在没有肿瘤标志物升高的情况下，需要通过内镜、立体定向或开放手术的方法进行组织活检。如存在脑积水，首选的治疗方法是内镜第三脑室造瘘术（endoscopic third ventriculostomy，ETV）进行脑脊液分流手术，该方法在分流手术中即可对肿瘤进行活检。

生殖细胞肿瘤

流行病学

松果体区是颅内GCT最常见的部位（Arora et al.，2016）。超过90%的病例发生在20岁之前，发病高峰出现在出生后和青春期早期，男性更易患病（Louis et al.，2016）。

病理学和遗传学

大多数颅内GCT是散发的。这些肿瘤细胞中可能有一个额外的X染色体，与克兰费尔特（Klinefelter）综合征相关。其他常见的染色体变异还有1q、8q或12p的增加，以及较少发生的11q、13和18q的丢失。GCT与唐氏综合征和1型神经纤维瘤病有关（Louis et al.，2016）。

颅内GCT最常见于松果体区，而鞍上或双病灶（松果体区和鞍上同时存在）较少见。GCT在病理学上分为生殖细胞肿瘤（生殖细胞瘤，占70%~80%）和非生殖细胞瘤性生殖细胞肿瘤（non-germinomatous germ cell tumour，NGGCT）（Al-Hussaini et al.，2009）。

生殖细胞瘤的肿瘤细胞与原始生殖细胞相似，而NGGCT的肿瘤细胞则具有与胚胎发育阶段相关的特征（例如畸胎瘤细胞的多能性）。有些GCT同时包含这两种亚型的细胞类型，这种情况在世卫组织分类中仍被归类为NGGCT（Louis et al.，2016）。通常，除成熟畸胎瘤外，所有GCT的亚型都被认为是恶性的。

生殖细胞肿瘤

生殖细胞瘤

生殖细胞瘤可随神经轴播散，由核仁突出且胞

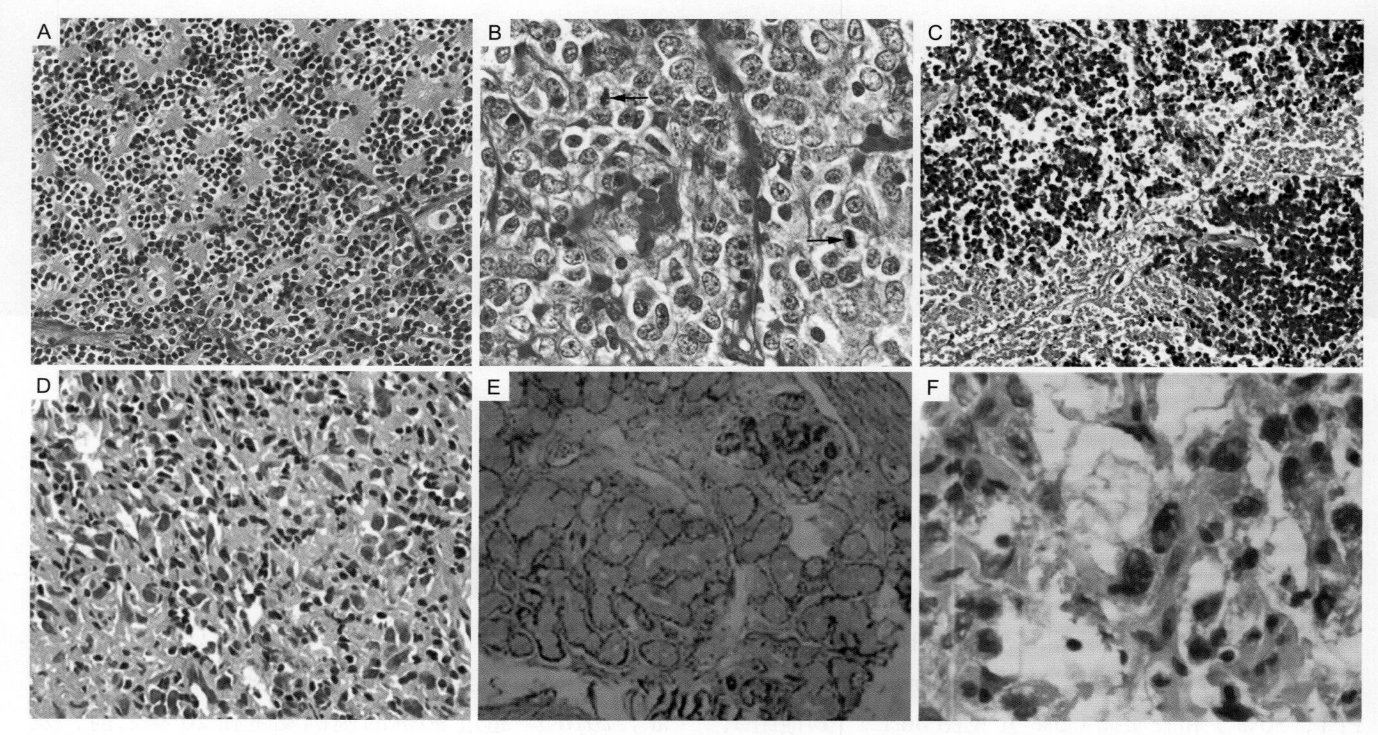

图 36.1 松果体肿瘤组织病理。（A）松果体细胞瘤：肿瘤细胞密度适中，具有类似松果体细胞的分化良好的细胞；通常细胞以单个细胞核为特征。（B）PPTID：虽然缺乏绝对的诊断标准，但这些肿瘤的特点是中等程度的细胞密度、细胞成熟度、核异型性和有丝分裂指数（箭头显示有丝分裂灶）。（C）松果体母细胞瘤：具有高等程度的细胞密度且含有原始细胞的肿瘤，核质比高，有丝分裂指数高。（D）生殖细胞瘤：具有特征性细胞，表现为细胞核大、核仁突出、富含糖原且清晰的胞质。（E）成熟畸胎瘤的黏液腺：这些肿瘤还可以有其他几种细胞形态。（F）未成熟干细胞表现为胚胎干细胞；肿瘤细胞体积大，核仁突出，胞质丰富

浆清晰的巨核细胞组成，具有有丝分裂旺盛、增殖指数高的特征（**图** 36.1D）。免疫组化方面，肿瘤细胞的细胞膜呈 c-kit 阳性，细胞核呈 OCT4 阳性（Louis et al.，2016）。含有合体滋养层巨细胞的生殖细胞瘤可以分泌低水平的 β-HCG（**专栏** 36.1）。

非生殖细胞瘤性生殖细胞肿瘤

NGGCT 包括畸胎瘤、胚胎性癌、卵黄囊瘤和绒毛膜癌。大约 13.5% 的松果体区 GCT 表现出混合组织学特征（Al-Hussaini et al.，2009）。与生殖细胞瘤不同，NGGCT 含有细胞角蛋白，表明包含上皮细胞系细胞，这是两种主要 GCT 类型之间的主要组织病理学区别。

畸胎瘤

畸胎瘤是最常见的单纯 NGGCT（占松果体区 GCT 的 7%）（Al-Hussaini et al.，2009）。其包含来自三个胚层的组织成分。如果肿瘤各组分完全分化，肿瘤被称为成熟畸胎瘤，而如果任一组分未完全分化，肿瘤被称为未成熟畸胎瘤（**图** 36.1E 和**图** 36.1F）。畸胎瘤内的实体成分很少会发生肿瘤性改变，若发生，则肿瘤被归类为畸胎瘤伴恶变。免疫组化结果取决于肿瘤中存在的组织成分，可呈 c-kit 阳性。未成熟畸胎瘤中分化不完全的肠腺也可以分泌 AFP（Louis et al.，2016）。

胚胎性癌

肿瘤由类似于胚胎干细胞的未成熟干细胞组成。肿瘤细胞体积大，核仁突出，包浆丰富，呈紫红色（嗜酸性）或透明。细胞呈片状、腺样或乳头状生长。免疫组化阳性标志物除细胞角蛋白外，还包括 PLAP、OCT4 和 CD30（Louis et al.，2016）。

卵黄囊瘤

卵黄囊瘤细胞类似卵黄囊的内胚层细胞。肿瘤细胞小，核仁不明显，细胞质稀少，AFP 呈阳性（Louis et al.，2016）。

绒毛膜癌

绒毛膜癌含有转化的胎盘成分，主要为两

种细胞——细胞滋养层细胞和合体滋养层巨细胞（syncytiotrophoblastic giant cell，STGC）。二者免疫组化均呈细胞角蛋白阳性，而 STGC 中 β-HCG 和人胎盘催乳素也呈阳性（Louis et al.，2016）。

生殖细胞肿瘤的治疗流程

图 36.2 展示了疑似松果体区 GCT 的术前检查和治疗的流程图。通过检测血清和脑脊液中的肿瘤标志物，肿瘤可被分为分泌型和非分泌型，这直接决定了治疗路径。腰椎穿刺术和脊椎 MRI 通常被用来检查颅脊播散的存在与否，有时肿瘤播散仅能通过显微镜下脑脊液细胞学检查才能确定。这样，这些患者就可以得到更积极的治疗。ETV 结合内镜松果体区活检被认为是治疗松果体肿瘤伴脑积水的最佳技术，约 80% 的松果体肿瘤可不行分流手术（Shono et al.，2007），也可同时将由于分流术造成的医源性肿瘤播散风险降至最低（Kumura et al.，1986）。

肿瘤标志物

应检测血清和脑脊液中 AFP 和 β-HCG。若检测结果升高可作为确定 GCT 亚型的标志（**表** 36.1）。非生殖细胞性混合性 GCT 可能含有卵黄囊或绒毛膜癌成分，分别与 AFP 和 β-HCG 升高有关。多达 1/3 的生殖细胞瘤（含有 STGC）可以分泌 β-HCG，导致 β-HCG 上升，但 β-HCG 上升量通常低于 NGGCT。肿瘤标志物也被用作衡量治疗反应和预后的监测指标。

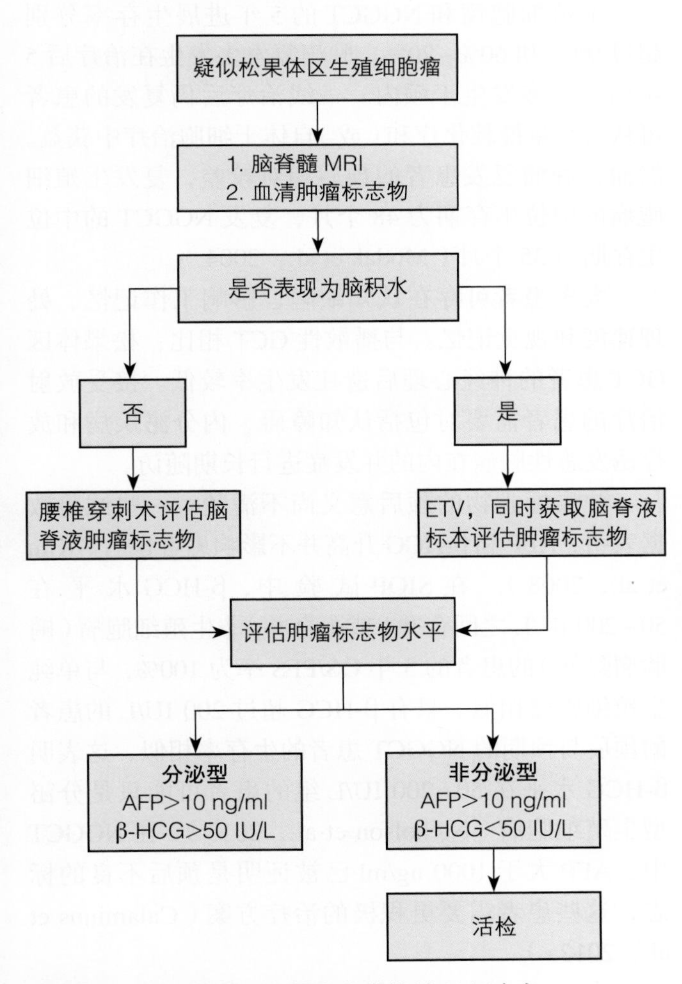

图 36.2 松果体区生殖细胞肿瘤的处理和治疗

肿瘤活检

非分泌性肿瘤应进行活检。对于伴发脑积水的患者，ETV 和活检可以同时进行（Pettorini et al.，2013）。在不伴发脑积水的情况下，可以使用立体定向活检。立体定向活检诊断率较高（94% *vs*. 81%），但其活检相关死亡率更高（1.3% *vs*. 0.3%）。这两种松果体区活检方法均有 4%~5% 的出血风险，由于均需靠近深静脉操作（Balossier et al.，2015a）。具有典型影像学特征的双病灶和尿崩症符合生殖细胞瘤诊断标准，不需要活检。

治疗

生殖细胞瘤

单纯的生殖细胞瘤可以仅通过放疗治愈。具有高 β-HCG 特征的生殖细胞瘤亚型（通常 >50 IU/L，由于含有 STGC 成分），可能需要更积极的治疗。

- **手术**：细胞减灭术并不能改善患者预后（Sawamura et al.，1997），然而，含有生殖细胞瘤成分的混合型非生殖细胞瘤，如果放疗后仍残留肿瘤，应考虑需要手术治疗（Oya et al.，2014）。国际中枢神经系统 GCT 研究小组的数据显示，残留肿瘤小于 1.5 cm^3 的生殖细胞瘤患者预后较好（平均 6 年随访的复发率为 38%，优于更大残余的 65%）（Souweidane et al.，2010）。然而，这一数

表 36.1 肿瘤标志物和生殖细胞肿瘤

肿瘤类型		AFP	β-HCG	PLAP
生殖细胞瘤	生殖细胞瘤	-	+/-[1]	+
NGGCT	混合型	+/-	+/-	+/-
	畸胎瘤	+/-[2]	+/-[2]	-
	胚胎性癌	-	-	+
	卵黄囊瘤	+	-	+/-
	绒毛膜癌	-	+	+/-

[1] 含有 STGC 的生殖细胞瘤可以分泌 βHCG。

[2] 不成熟畸胎瘤中极少部分含有分泌 AFP 或 β-HCG 的组织；然而对于含有卵黄囊成分或绒毛膜癌成分的混合型生殖细胞瘤的鉴别诊断也应给予充分考虑。

据需要进一步验证，因为它与国际儿科肿瘤学会（The International Society of Paediatric Oncology，SIOP）试验结果不符。

- **放射治疗**：生殖细胞瘤对放疗敏感。颅脊放射治疗（craniospinal irradiation，CSI）实现了5年无进展生存率（PFS）和总生存率（OS）超过90%（Bamberg et al.，1999）。放射治疗可能导致迟发不良反应，包括神经和认知障碍、继发性恶性肿瘤和内分泌病（Bamberg et al.，1999），儿童中更多见。降低放疗不良反应的措施包括：
  1. 减少照射体积：建议对局部肿瘤行局灶性放射（Rogers et al.，2005）。
  2. 减少总剂量：5年生存率与旧方案相当（Bamberg et al.，1999; Calaminus et al.，2013）。
  3. 诱导化疗结合包括脑室的局部放射：最大限度地降低肿瘤播散风险（Calaminus et al.，2013）。诱导化疗的患者获益正在ACNS 0232中进行评估，这是一项Ⅲ期随机对照试验。
  4. 依据放疗反应降低放射剂量：诱导化疗后放射剂量的降低取决于肿瘤对放疗的反应性（Legault et al.，2013）。
- **化疗**：国际中枢神经系统GCT研究（**表36.2**）显示，由于预后极差（5年PFS<50%），化疗不能单独使用（da Silva et al.，2010）。诱导化疗的作用仍在评估中。SIOP在多个机构中开展异环磷酰胺、卡铂和依托泊苷（ifosfamide，carboplatin and etoposide，ICE）方案，该方案以铂为基础，使用卡铂替代顺铂降低化疗毒性（Calaminus et al.，2013）。

非生殖细胞瘤性生殖细胞肿瘤

依据患者预后，肿瘤可分为三个亚型：低危（成熟畸胎瘤）、中危（以生殖细胞瘤为主伴有畸胎瘤的混合GCT）和高危肿瘤（胚胎性癌、绒毛膜癌、卵黄囊瘤及以上述成分为主的混合GCT）。中危组10年OS率为70%，而高危组10年OS率为10%以下，凸显了准确的组织学分类的重要性。

- **手术**：NGGCT的切除原则如下。
  1. 成熟畸胎瘤：切除通常可治愈。
  2. 化疗后残留：二次探查手术可改善NGGCT的预后，最近的临床试验鼓励采取这种方法（Czech et al.，2012）。残留通常为成熟畸胎瘤（多数）、与原肿瘤不同类型的非生殖细胞瘤或坏死/瘢痕。若肿瘤标志物正常而残留病灶增大则应行二次探查手术。
  3. 对辅助治疗无效的肿瘤：如果一线和（或）二线治疗无效，患者可能会从手术中受益。
- **放射治疗**：对于NGGCT，放射治疗的预后较差，5年无进展生存率不到50%。对于播散性肿瘤，建议进行全面的CSI。对于局灶性肿瘤，可以考虑仅对肿瘤和脑室进行放射治疗。SIOP试验5年PFS和OS率低于儿童肿瘤组试验（**表36.2**，5年PFS分别为67%~69%和84.3%），由于SIOP试验中没有在局灶性肿瘤中进行CSI（Calaminus et al.，2012b；Goldman et al.，2015）。
- **化疗**：单纯化疗方案的预后极差（5年PFS为50%，第3次国际CNS GCT试验，**表36.2**）（Marec-Berard et al.，2002；da Silva et al.，2010）。MAKEI 89试验采用三明治化疗（化疗、放疗-化疗方案），如果治疗反应充分，该方案患者预后与不接受第二次化疗方案的试验相当（Bamberg et al.，1999）。因此，诱导化疗后放疗伴（或不伴）手术治疗残留肿瘤，已成为NGGCT治疗的标准。

预后

生殖细胞瘤和NGGCT的5年进展生存率分别超过90%和60%~70%。肿瘤复发多发生在治疗后5年内，且多发生于颅内。一线治疗后仍复发的患者可从大剂量挽救化疗和（或）自体干细胞治疗中获益。然而，肿瘤复发患者的预后相对较差，复发生殖细胞瘤的中位生存期为48个月，复发NGGCT的中位生存期为35个月（Modak et al.，2004）。

大多患者可存在认知缺陷，影响工作记忆、处理速度和视觉记忆。与播散性GCT相比，松果体区GCT患者的神经心理后遗症发生率较低。接受放射治疗的患者需要对包括认知障碍、内分泌疾病和放疗诱发恶性肿瘤在内的并发症进行长期随访。

肿瘤标志物的预后意义尚不清楚。一些试验数据表明，AFP和β-HCG升高并不影响患者预后（Kim et al.，2008）。在SIOP试验中，β-HCG水平在50~200 IU/L之间合并（或不合并）非生殖细胞瘤（畸胎瘤除外）的患者的5年OS/PFS率为100%，与单纯生殖细胞瘤相似。只有β-HCG超过200 IU/L的患者的预后与预期的NGGCT患者的生存率相似，这表明β-HCG水平在50~200 IU/L组的患者可能只是分泌型生殖细胞瘤（Nicholson et al.，2013）。在NGGCT中，AFP大于1000 ng/ml已被证明是预后不良的标志，这些患者需要更积极的治疗方案（Calaminus et al.，2012a）。

表 36.2 评估颅内生殖细胞肿瘤辅助治疗的临床试验

研究	分组	肿瘤类型	转移情况	平均年龄（范围）	病例数	一线辅助治疗			5 年生存率	
						放疗	化疗（诱导）	化疗（放疗后）	PFS	OS
第三次国际 CNS GCT 试验，非随机（多个）	低危	生殖细胞瘤（β-HCG<2.2 IU/ml）	0	15（8~24）	11	无	4 疗程 +/- 基于反应性的追加		27.3%[1]	88.9%[1]
	中、高危	NGGCT 或生殖细胞瘤（β-HCG>2.2 IU/ml）	+/-	10（0.3~19）	14	无	至多 6 疗程的环磷酰胺、依托泊苷和大剂量卡铂联合化疗		50.0%[1]	58.3%[1]
POG 9530，非随机（美国），反应依赖辐照剂量	低危	生殖细胞瘤（β-HCG<50 IU/ml）	0		8	局灶 CR：30.6 Gy <CR：50.4 Gy	2 疗程顺铂、依托泊苷、长春新碱、环磷酰胺	无	87.5%	100.0%
			1	15.1（9.5~17.7）	4	CR 后进行 CSI：30.6 Gy <CR：36 Gy		无	100.0%	100.0%
MAKEI 83/86/89，非随机（德国），非一线化疗	MAKEI 83/86	生殖细胞瘤（β-HCG<100 ng/ul）	非相关[2]	13（6~31）	11	CSI：36 Gy 加量照射：14 Gy	无	无	100.0%	100.0%
	MAKEI 89				49	CSI：30 Gy 加量照射：15 Gy	无	无	88.8%	92.0%
MAKEI 89，NGGCT 组	N/A	NGGCT	+/-	11（2~24）	27	CSI：30 Gy 加量照射：20 Gy	2 个疗程的顺铂、依托泊苷、博来霉素	2 个疗程的顺铂、异环磷酰胺、长春新碱	74.0%	59.0%
SIOP CNS GCT 96，非随机（多个），颅内 GCT 最大型的报道数据	仅放疗	生殖细胞瘤（β-HCG<50IU/L）	0	13（4~42）	125	CSI：24 Gy 加量照射：16 Gy	无	无	97.0%	95.0%
			0		65	局灶 40 Gy	2 个疗程的卡铂、依托泊苷、异环磷酰胺	无	88.0%	96.0%
	放化疗		1		45	CSI：24 Gy 加量照射：16 Gy	无	无	100.0%	98.0%
	未转移	NGGCT（未发表数据）	0	12（0~30）	146	局灶照射 54 Gy	4 个疗程的顺铂、依托泊苷、异环磷酰胺	无	69.0%[4]	78.0%[4]
	转移		1		43	CSI：30 Gy 加量照射：24 Gy			67.0%[4]	70.0%[4]
儿童肿瘤组 NGGCT 试验，NGGCT 非随机（美国）试验	N/A	NGGCT 或生殖细胞瘤（β-HCG>50IU/L）	+/-	12（3~23）	102	CSI：36 Gy 加量照射：18 Gy（原发），>9 Gy（转移）	最多 6 个疗程的卡铂、依托泊苷、异环磷酰胺	如果无反应（+/- 二次探查手术）。噻替哌和依托泊苷	84.3%	93.0%

[1] 在第三次国际 CNS GCT 试验中为 6 年生存率，此处为无事件生存率，而不是 PFS。[2] 15.2% 的患者在初治时即存在播散，仍使用相同的方案治疗。[3] 此处为无事件生存率，而不是 OS。[4] 中位随访时间 36~55 个月

松果体实质肿瘤

流行病学

PPT约占所有松果体区肿瘤的30%，发病时的平均年龄为21岁（Al-Hussaini et al.，2009）。男女患者发病率相当。松果体母细胞瘤在较小的儿童中更常见，而低级别肿瘤在老年人中更常见（Selvanathan et al.，2012）。

病理学和遗传学

大多数PPT是散发的。基因改变包括4q2和12号染色体的增加，以及10号和22号染色体的丢失（Von Beuren et al.，2012）。松果体母细胞瘤很少见，与双侧视网膜母细胞瘤（5%~13%）和家族性双侧视网膜母细胞瘤（5%~15%）相关。PPT被认为起源于松果体细胞，世界卫生组织将其分为四级：松果体细胞瘤（WHO Ⅰ级）、中分化松果体实质瘤（pineal parenchymal tumours of intermediate differentiation，PPTIDs）（Ⅱ级和Ⅲ级）（见**专栏**36.2）和松果体母细胞瘤（Ⅳ级）。松果体乳头状肿瘤（papillary tumor of the pineal region，PTPR）相当于Ⅱ级或Ⅲ级。与PPT不同，PTPR可能起源于室管膜周室下连合体细胞。原发松果体区肿瘤的组织学诊断具有挑战性，应由有经验的神经病理学家进行。

松果体细胞瘤

松果体细胞瘤占PPT的14%~30%，边界清楚，生长缓慢，不经脑脊液播散（Fevre-Montange et al.，2010）。肿瘤细胞密度适中，细胞分化良好，类似松果体细胞（**图**36.1A）。肿瘤细胞呈片状或小叶状生长，可围绕细胞质突起排列，形成典型的松果体细胞瘤花环。通常，细胞含有单个规则细胞核，但也可以看到多核巨细胞且细胞核形状奇特（多形性亚型）。坏死罕见，有丝分裂指数低。免疫组化染色中神经元标志物（突触素、神经纤维和神经元特异性烯醇化酶）和光感觉分化标志物（视网膜S抗原和视紫红质）可呈阳性。间质细胞可以对胶质标志物呈阳性反应（例如GFAP）（Louis et al.，2016）。

松果体母细胞瘤

松果体母细胞瘤占原发性松果体区肿瘤的24%~50%（Fevre-Montange et al.，2010）。其被认为是松果体区的原始神经外胚层肿瘤（primitive neuroectodermal tumour，PNET）。肿瘤中富含未成熟细胞，边界不清（**图**36.1C）。细胞可能聚集成玫瑰花环：荷马-赖特（Homer-Wright）玫瑰花环和弗莱克斯纳-温特斯坦纳（Flexner- Wintersteiner）玫瑰花环（表明存在视网膜母细胞分化）。有丝分裂指数高，核质比高；由于核染色突出，胞质稀少，被称为“小蓝细胞”。松果体母细胞瘤具有局部侵袭性，边界不清，有通过脑脊液扩散的倾向。免疫组化类似于松果体细胞瘤（Louis et al.，2016）。

中分化松果体实质肿瘤

PPTID占原发性松果体区肿瘤的20%~62%（Fevre Montange et al.，2010）。诊断标准尚不明确，但“中度”是关键词——描述细胞密度、细胞成熟度、核异型性和有丝分裂指数（**图**36.1B）。生长呈弥散样（神经细胞瘤样）、小叶样（内分泌样）或混合样。过渡亚型也以松果体细胞瘤花环为特征。同时含有松果体细胞瘤和松果体母细胞瘤成分的肿瘤也可以归为这一类。坏死、软脑膜受累和血管增生均可出现。MIB-1标记指数可能是比组织学分级更重要的预后因素（Louis et al.，2016）。

松果体乳头状肿瘤

PTPR是一种罕见的肿瘤，以上皮样和乳头样为特征，常有坏死灶。有丝分裂指数和MIB-1标记指数中度升高（Louis et al.，2016）。有些患者有复发的倾向，需要反复手术（Santarius et al.，2008；Fauchon et al.，2013）。

诊断

诊治流程如**图**36.3所示。影像特征不具有特异性，与GCT的差异为其更有可能存在周围钙化。松果体细胞瘤往往边界清楚，而松果体母细胞瘤边缘不清晰，且15%出现转移（Gaillard and Jones，2010）。尽管缺乏确诊特征，PPTID通常比松果体细胞瘤更具局部侵袭性和异质性。多模态成像可能有助于肿瘤分级的预测，但组织诊断仍十分重要。

治疗

松果体细胞瘤

- **手术**：完全切除可治愈，应考虑用于有症状的肿瘤患者。组织学证实的小肿瘤（<1 cm）生长缓慢，由于手术并发症发生率很高，可以进行定期MRI监测。全切的5年总生存率（84%）要好于次全切除加放疗的5年总生存率（17%）（Clark et al.，2010b）。
- **放疗**：英国神经肿瘤学会的指南建议在残留肿

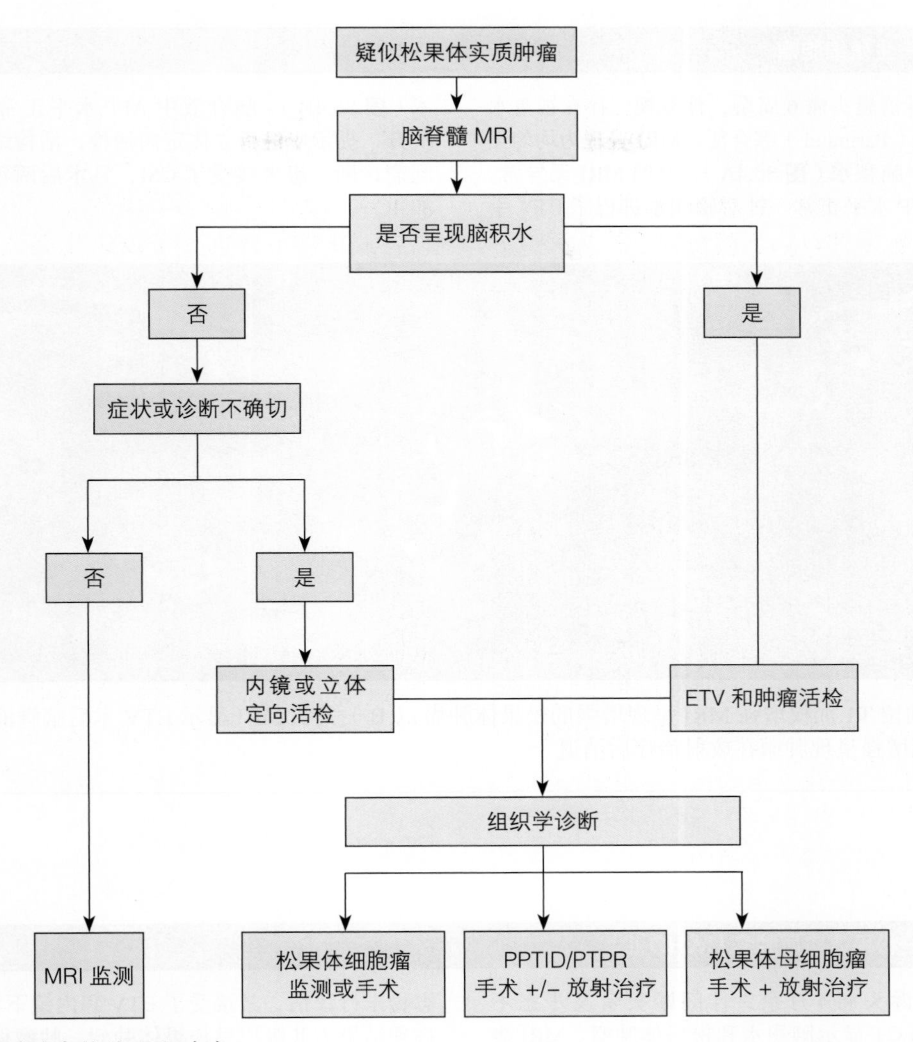

图 36.3 松果体实质肿瘤的处理和治疗

瘤的情况下进行放射治疗（英国神经肿瘤学会，2011b），但还没有证明它会影响 OS/PFS 的证据（Clark et al.，2010a；Clark et al.，2010b）。

- **立体定位放疗**：作为主要治疗手段时，30 个月的 PFS 率超过 85%（Balossier et al.，2015b）。由于缺乏关于长期预后的研究，高达 50% 的肿瘤不生长可能只是反映了小的松果体细胞瘤的自然病史。它对残留肿瘤的有效性可能更高，在这方面研究报道 5 年 PFS 为 100%（Mori et al.，2009）。
- **化疗**：无论针对首诊还是复发，都没有有效的化疗方案。

松果体母细胞瘤

- **手术**：切除范围（extent of resection，EOR）已被证明影响患者生存（Lutterbach et al.，2002），但数据仍然有争议（Lee et al.，2005；Selvanathan et al.，2012）。在一项系统综述中，全切较大部切除或活检显著提高了患者生存期——5 年 OS 分别为 84%、53% 和 29%。尽管大部切除组加放疗改善了患者生存期（5 年 OS 64%），但仍低于全切（Tate et al.，2012）。一般情况下，残留肿瘤体积小于 1.5 cm^3 可以提高 PNET 患者的预后（Zeltzer et al.，1999）。
- **放疗**：患有松果体母细胞瘤的成人和年龄较大的儿童应用辅助 CSI（British Neuro-Oncology Society，2011a）。由于有造成神经认知缺陷的可能，其在非常小的儿童中的应用是有争议的。即使采取正常照射剂量，在仅使用化疗方案的研究中患者预后结果仍较差（Duffner et al.，1995；Hinkes et al.，2007）。
- **立体定位放疗**：由于缺乏高质量数据，不应常规使用立体定向放射治疗（Balossier et al.，2015b）。
- **化疗**：化疗与改善预后有关。在一项 meta 分析中，手术 / 放疗和手术 / 放疗 / 化疗的 5 年 OS 率分别

专栏 36.1 病例 1—生殖细胞瘤

21 岁男性患者主诉清晨头痛 6 周余，伴复视。存在视盘水肿，但存在帕里诺（Parinaud）综合征。MRI 表现为均匀强化的松果体肿瘤伴脑积水（图 36.4A）。脊髓 MRI 无异常。血清 β-HCG 和 AFP 水平正常。针对脑积水进行了 ETV 手术（图 36.4B）。脑脊液中 AFP 水平正常，β-HCG 仅轻度上升，提示应进行立体定向活检，活检结果确定了生殖细胞瘤诊断。患者接受了 CSI，且术后两年仍无病生存（图 36.4C）。

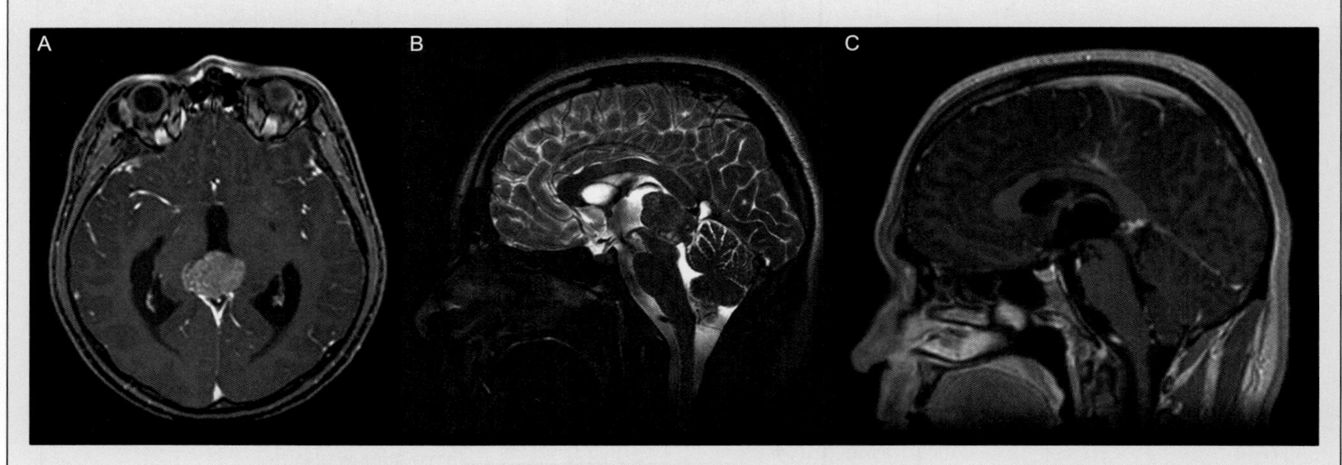

图 36.4 （A）轴位 T1 加权增强 MRI 呈现增强的松果体肿瘤；（B）矢状 MRI 显示 ETV 术后脑脊液行脑桥前流动；（C）矢状 T1 加权增强呈现肿瘤在放射治疗后消退

专栏 36.2 病例 2—松果体实质肿瘤（WHO Ⅱ）

59 岁女性患者主诉头痛 4 月余，伴间断头晕及步态不稳。摔倒后，头部 CT 显示脑积水和松果体肿瘤。MRI 表现为部分实体部分囊性的增强的松果体肿瘤伴脑积水（图 36.5A）。脊髓 MRI 无异常。鉴于患者年龄和性别，肿瘤标志物未行评估，其接受了 ETV 和内镜下活检（图 36.5B）。病理结果为Ⅱ级原发松果体肿瘤。肿瘤得到完全切除（图 36.5C），患者已被建议进行适形分割放射治疗。

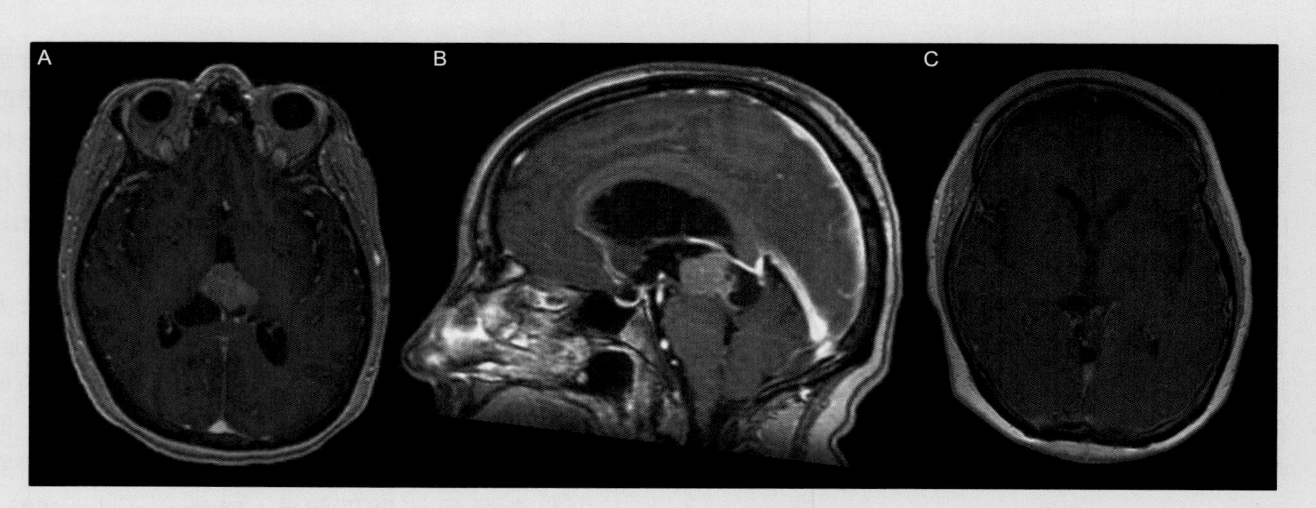

图 36.5 （A）轴位和（B）矢状位 T1 加权增强 MRI 呈现了增强的松果体肿瘤，（C）肿瘤全切后的轴位 T1 加权增强 MRI

为 45% 和 52%（Tate et al.，2012）。以铂为基础的化疗方案似乎是最有效的，结合常规放射治疗的Ⅱ期试验报告 5 年 OS 率为 71%~83%（Pizer et al.，2006；Hinkes et al.，2007）。对于非常小的儿童来说，大剂量化疗可能有助于推迟放射治疗。成人对化疗方案的耐受性很差，不推荐使用。

中分化松果体实质肿瘤和松果体乳头状瘤

PPTID 和 PTPR 的最佳治疗策略尚没有明确的标准，也没有前瞻性的证据来指导治疗决定。

- **手术**：回顾性分析表明，EOR 影响 PPTID 和 PTPR 的预后。在对 PPTID 的 meta 分析中，没有肿瘤残留的患者的 10 年 OS 为 100%，而有肿瘤残留少于 50% 和多于 50% 的患者的 10 年 OS 分别为 40% 和 15%（Lutterbach et al.，2002）。PTPR 的预后较差，5 年 OS 为 73%（Louis et al.，2016）。
- **辅助治疗**：并非所有 PPTID 患者都需要接受辅助治疗（Villa et al.，2012）。在有残留肿瘤的情况下可以采用放射治疗。Ⅲ级肿瘤的患者有高脊髓复发率，这些患者应行 CSI（Fauchon et al.，2000）。对于Ⅱ级肿瘤，对瘤床的局部放射治疗可能就足够了。有丝分裂指数可以作为指导治疗决策的有力指标，如果有丝分裂指数特别高，则患者可以采用松果体母细胞瘤的治疗方案进行治疗（Fukuoka et al.，2012）。对这些肿瘤还需要进一步的前瞻性研究。放疗在 PTPR 中的作用尚未确定（Fauchon et al.，2013）。

预后

松果体肿瘤的预后差异性大，且取决于治疗手段。在松果体细胞瘤中，全切患者的 5 年 OS 为 84%，患者没有明显的放射治疗获益（Clark et al.，2010a）。松果体母细胞瘤患者的预后较差，预后很大程度上取决于患者的年龄。在儿童中，使用当下的放射治疗方案和以铂为基础的化疗方案可以实现 5 年 OS 率超过 70%。PPTID 和 PTPR 患者的预后尚不明确，介于松果体细胞瘤和松果体母细胞瘤之间。一个重要的限制似乎是这些肿瘤的诊断标准，应该更加明确，以便在未来的临床试验中对患者进行适当的分组。通过多变量分析确定的非治疗相关预后因素包括肿瘤范围，与预后较差相关的转移表现、肿瘤分级和年龄小于 5 岁，对较高级别的 PPT 影响更明显（Lutterbach et al.，2002）。

手术要点 / 争议

- MRI 不能准确识别肿瘤类型，但对手术计划是必不可少的。
- ETV 是脑脊液引流的首选方法，且不需要分流。
- 肿瘤标志物升高不需要活检，即可提示为 NGGCT。
- 在没有肿瘤标志物升高的情况下，需要进行病理诊断以确定适宜的治疗路径（注：生殖细胞瘤也可能出现 β-HCG 轻度升高）。
- EOR 是所有 PPT 的预后指标，松果体细胞瘤可以通过全切治愈。
- 化疗后存在残留肿瘤的 NGGCT 应在放疗前进行二次探查手术
- PPTID 和 PTPR 完全切除后辅助放射治疗的作用尚不清楚。

延伸阅读、参考文献、EBRAIN 的相关链接

扫描书末二维码获取。

第 37 章　松果体区病变的外科治疗

Christoph M. Woernle · René L. Bernays · Nicolas de Tribolet 著
王镔 译，许海洋 审校

引言

松果体区病变位于大脑中央的间脑 - 上丘脑区。该区域腹侧为四叠体、中脑顶盖，两侧为左右上丘，背侧为胼胝体压部，尾侧为小脑蚓部和喙侧为第三脑室后部。主要的解剖学和手术挑战是位于背侧的盖伦（Galen）静脉、位于尾侧的小脑中央前静脉、位于前方的大脑内静脉和位于外侧的基底静脉。

根据外科医生的经验，大多数松果体区肿瘤都可以通过以下两种入路安全切除：枕部经小脑幕入路适用于合并脑积水或直窦陡升而肿瘤位置低的情况，对于第三脑室后部肿瘤则推荐采用幕下小脑上入路。

历史回顾

20 世纪初，Harvey Cushing、Feudor Krause 和 Sir Walter Dandy 首次发表了关于松果体区肿瘤手术经验的精彩报道（Krause，1926; Dandy，1936 ; Cushing，1983）。在没有显微外科技术的情况下，在这些脑深部且解剖困难的区域进行手术往往死亡率极高，受到一些同时代人的反对（Schmidek，1977）。现如今，采用幕下小脑上入路或枕部小脑幕入路切除这些位于颅内最复杂区域之一的病变（Ringertz et al.，1954; Poppen and Marino，1968; Stein，1971; Reid and Clark，1978; Stein，1979; Sawamura et al.，1997; Sawamura and de Tribolet，2002）。

松果体区和第三脑室的显微解剖

松果体区的病变位于大脑中央的间脑 - 上丘脑区。肿瘤起源于松果体本身或松果体周围结构，被重要的解剖结构所包围（Guest and Kleriga，1979）。该区域腹侧为四叠体、中脑顶盖，两侧为左右上丘，背侧为胼胝体压部，尾侧为小脑蚓部和喙侧为第三脑室后部（Stein，1971; Schmidek，1977; Guest and Kleriga，1979）。松果体是间脑中线尾端的附属器，位于第三脑室的松果体隐窝。松果体的茎在背侧与缰联合相连，在腹侧与后连合相连。

松果体的血运主要由大脑后动脉分支通过脉络膜后内侧动脉供应。除了松果体，其还供应第三脑室的下丘、上丘和脉络丛。通常情况下，松果体肿瘤会使脑池中的这些动脉发生侧向移位。脉络膜后外侧动脉供应丘脑后结节，其通常因松果体肿瘤而向外侧移位。小脑上动脉被认为是重要的动脉标志物，因为松果体肿瘤常使其向下移位。此外，枕内侧动脉起源于大脑后动脉，其分支至距状沟动脉，应铭记在心（Poppen，1966; Poppen and Marino，1968; Page，1977; Guest and Kleriga，1979）。

主要的解剖学和手术挑战是 Galen 静脉系统。Galen 静脉有数条流入静脉：上蚓静脉和小脑前中央静脉在中线处汇入 Galen 静脉的腹尾部。大脑内静脉和松果体静脉自腹侧汇入。在松果体肿瘤中，大脑内静脉的后部自喙部隆起，有时静脉可不汇合。在 Galen 静脉外侧，枕内侧静脉、基底静脉第三段和中脑后静脉汇入。松果体静脉是松果体区肿瘤的引流静脉，引流到大脑内静脉的后部或 Galen 静脉。松果体区肿瘤可以紧密邻着在大脑内静脉和（或）Galen 静脉上。基底静脉或大脑内静脉的损伤会导致严重的并发症。离断或压迫枕内侧大静脉可能导致同向偏盲或视觉癫痫（Lazar and Clark，1974; Guest and Kleriga，1979; Sawamura et al.，1997; Sawamura and de Tribolet，2002）。

临床症状和术前准备

松果体区病变且有症状的患者出现的临床症状各异，有时是非特异性的。可以出现头痛、步态障碍、精神变化、锥体束征、小便失禁和听力障碍（少见）。

松果体区病变且有症状的患者的特异症状有失代偿性脑积水和神经-眼科疾患，如帕里诺（Parinaud）综合征或复视（Schmidek，1977；Sawamura et al.，1997；Sawamura and de Tribolet，2002）。

影像

一旦出现神经系统症状，应进行CT或MRI初步检查。这些检查可以快速且可视地确定有无梗阻性脑积水或出血。如出现这些情况，可能需要进行脑室外引流（external ventricular drain，EVD）或内镜下脑室脑池造瘘术（endoscopic ventriculocisternostomy，EVT）。其次，应进行增强MRI检查。一些中心还建议行血管造影术对病变处动脉和静脉解剖进行了解。3T MRI和MRA可极好的显示血管解剖。因此，我们认为将血管造影术作为常规是没有必要的。

肿瘤标志物

松果体区GCT中可以使血清和脑脊液中的肿瘤标志物升高。β-HCG升高通常与绒毛膜癌和10%的生殖细胞瘤有关。在畸胎瘤、胚胎性癌和卵黄囊瘤中可以观察到AFP的升高。肿瘤标志物可以用来监测患者的治疗结果和复发情况（见**第36章**）。

鉴别诊断

大多数松果体区肿物起源于幕下并扩展到第三脑室的后部。这些病变向丘脑延伸或向下延伸至四叠体。恶性胶质细胞肿瘤侵袭丘脑和中脑，是影响肿瘤可切除性的决定性因素。

应考虑以下鉴别诊断。

生殖细胞肿瘤：生殖细胞瘤、畸胎瘤、胚胎性癌、卵黄囊瘤和绒毛膜癌。

松果体实质瘤：松果体细胞瘤、中分化松果体实质瘤和松果体母细胞瘤。

胶质瘤、转移瘤和海绵状血管瘤

镰幕脑膜瘤：从外科角度看，镰幕脑膜瘤或中间帆脑膜瘤可被认为是松果体肿瘤。该部位脑膜瘤非常罕见，仅占所有颅内脑膜瘤的1%，文献中只有100例报道。

决策和手术流程

GCT和恶性PPT需要综合治疗，包括化疗、放疗和手术（Lutterbach et al.，2002）。单纯生殖细胞瘤可以在不进行手术，仅靠化疗和放疗治愈（见**第36章**）。

依据外科经验，大多数松果体肿瘤都可以通过以下两种入路安全切除：枕部经小脑幕入路适用于合并脑积水或直窦陡升而肿瘤位置低的情况，对于第三脑室后部肿瘤则推荐采用幕下小脑上入路。

对于梗阻性脑积水合并中脑导水管受压的病例，肿瘤切除前应进行EVT或EVD。

内镜手术和活检

目前，内镜下微创肿瘤活检联合EVT可用于组织病理分析和（或）治疗梗阻性脑积水。它是一种良好的诊断和治疗工具，在有经验的术者手中处理简便（Ellenbogen and Moore，1997；Azab et al.，2014）。

EVT多于开放手术之前进行（见**第33章**）。如果骨孔位于Kocher点前外方2~3 cm处，则之后可以在同一位置进行内镜活检。有些术者使用两个骨孔。

联合入路的第一步是收集CSF进行肿瘤标志物和细胞学检查，第二步是ETV，第三步是病变活检。活检手术最后进行是因为脑脊液中的血液可能会掩盖漏斗隐窝和乳头体之间的脑室造瘘术最佳位置（Al-Tamimi et al.，2008）。

利用神经导航和（或）术中MRI可使手术更安全、有效，且提高诊断率（O'Brien et al.，2006）。

内镜辅助的幕下小脑上入路由Cardia等人于2006年首先提出。该技术用于探明肿瘤残留和清除中脑导水管中的血块，以预防术后梗阻性脑积水（Cardia et al.，2006）。

Uschold等人于2011报道了仅使用内镜切除PPT和松果体囊肿的经验。对于血运丰富、有浸润性、跨中线或位于天幕上方的肿瘤可考虑进行开放手术（Broggi et al.，2010）。

立体定向活检常受限于有限的活检组织量。松果体肿瘤和GCT通常在同一病变内表现出不同细胞群体中的基因异质性。

因此，神经病理学家喜欢尽可能多的组织来进行详细诊断。

最近一篇关于松果体区病变的立体定向活检的综述汇报该技术有1.3%的并发症率和8.1%的死亡率。诊断准确率为94%。如今，该手术并不常用，已被内镜联合手术所取代（Zacharia and Bruce，2001；Al-Tamimi et al.，2008）。

幕下小脑上入路

幕下小脑上入路可以被认为是一种中线入路，

通过自下而上的手术通道直视病灶整体。分离 Galen 深静脉系统及相关的静脉是手术成功且不发生并发症的关键。

幕下小脑上入路的适应证包括松果体区上部病变、第三脑室后部病变、松果体区中线病变和四叠体中脑背侧病变。

为了避免术中颅内压升高，可以考虑行 EVT 或放置 EVD，来引流脑积水。

患者取坐位，躯干和颈部微曲，胸骨和下颌之间保持两指宽。坐姿时，小脑幕应与地面水平，重力可以让小脑下垂而不回缩。文献亦报道可使用 3/4 俯卧位、半侧卧位或协和式飞机体位进行替代。

常规行神经导航、消毒和术前准备。采取正中切口，自枕外隆起到 C4 的中线进行标记。对标记的切口使用局部麻醉剂和肾上腺素进行渗透麻醉。皮肤切开后，置入 Raney 夹。重要的是保持在中线筋膜平面，将肌肉从上颈线的附着处分离出来。这样可以避免肌肉损伤，并最大限度地减少失血。

对于开颅手术，建议使用高速钻头。骨孔可以为两个位于两侧横窦的上方，也可以为 1 个位于中线处窦汇上方。小心地将窦从骨瓣上剥离，以避免损伤窦。使用微型多普勒探头确认硬脑膜窦内血流充足是很重要的。使用骨蜡封住骨边缘，以降低空气栓塞的风险。应避免行颅骨切除术。

在打开硬膜前，为防止颅后窝充盈，应给予甘露醇，如果有 EVD，可直接行脑脊液引流。硬脑膜瓣应该按曲线打开，从外侧开始，穿过中线，以控制中线枕窦出血，该步骤很重要，之后向上反折。为了进一步减压，可以开放枕大池。中线桥静脉可以电凝，但应避免牵拉引起的侧方静脉牺牲。在剥离粘连并打开蛛网膜后，小脑会因重力而下移。天幕下和小脑之间的通道被打开后，确定静脉走行非常重要且极具挑战性。应分离小脑上和四叠体池中较厚的蛛网膜组织。在两侧对称地进行分离，小脑轻度向下移位，暴露出松果体区。分离上蚓静脉和小脑中央前静脉后，可使小脑蚓部进一步向下回缩。彻底切断所有桥静脉、上蚓静脉和中央前静脉，偶尔会引起小脑蚓部上面静脉梗死。如果可能，应分离并保留半球桥静脉。在桥静脉较粗的情况下，为了获得中间手术通道，应牺牲内侧桥静脉，保留外侧桥静脉（图 37.1）。

应避免损伤、撕裂或压迫回缩的小脑中央前静脉、蚓静脉、大脑内静脉和基底静脉，防止发生静脉充血和梗死。如果需要剥离或电凝小脑中央前静脉，应尽可能远离基底静脉汇合处。

幕下小脑上入路可形成经中线的直接视野，易于为松果体区周围复杂的解剖结构提供定位。该入路可以很好地辨认所有中线结构，同时暴露第三脑室的两壁和顶部，Monro 孔及中脑背侧四叠体的病变。粘连严重的肿瘤可在直视下从大脑内静脉或大脑大静脉上分离出来。然而，在某些情况下，使用该入路从中脑导水管周围组织和四叠体中剥离肿瘤可能比使用枕部小脑幕入路更困难。如果小脑幕陡升及尾侧和外侧夹角较小，则幕下小脑上入路具有一定

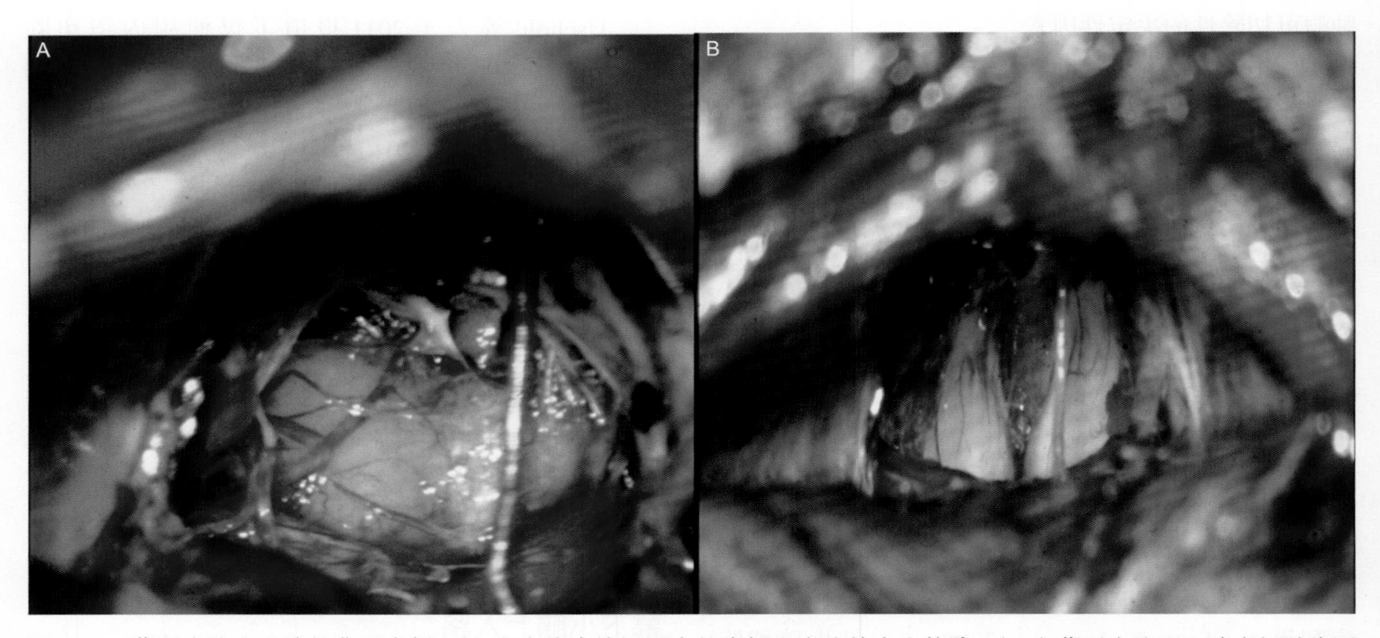

图 37.1 幕下小脑上入路的典型病例。（A）中线直接视野中的病损和小脑前中央静脉。（B）幕下小脑上入路全切肿瘤后的中线直接视野，小脑前中央静脉得到保留

局限性。

幕下小脑上外侧入路避免了蚓静脉和小脑中央前静脉的回缩（Kodera et al.，2011）。

在外科医生要求麻醉师压迫颈静脉并处理所有静脉渗漏之后，应使用连续或间断缝合对硬脑膜进行水密缝合。相关主要方法的摘要，请参见**专栏 37.1**。

枕部小脑幕入路

枕部小脑幕入路最早由 Horax 于 1937 年提出，并于 1962 年由 Poppen 改良，因此该入路现多称为 Poppen 入路。这种具有侧方视野的外侧入路的主要原则是避免蚓静脉和小脑中央前静脉回缩（Clark，1983）。

枕部小脑幕入路的适应证为松果体区肿瘤，肿瘤向下延伸，肿瘤自四叠体向上延伸、后部大脑镰旁或仅位于幕上的天幕脑膜瘤，肿瘤延伸至丘脑枕和侧脑室内侧以及侧脑室三角区肿瘤。

患者的体位有数种选择。3/4 俯卧位有助于内侧枕叶由于重力向外侧移位，避免回缩且降低同向偏盲的风险。通过使用非优势叶侧入路，可以避免语言功能异常。其他体位还有俯卧位或协和式飞机体位（Lozier and Bruce，2003）。该入路也可以采用坐位，但需要将枕叶移位（Azab et al.，2014）。入路左右侧选择由肿瘤的延伸方向、窦汇的形状及主要枕桥静脉的位置来决定，尽管通常枕部很少出现大的皮质桥静脉。考虑以上因素，通常更偏爱选择右方入路。

如果导水管没有堵塞，腰大池引流可能有助于大脑减压。有关麻醉和手术原则，请参阅前面的“幕下小脑上入路”部分。

一些术者建议使用 U 型皮肤切口。以我们的观点来看，正中线旁 1 cm 的直切口就足够了。这两种切口中都要小心避免损伤枕小神经、枕大神经和枕动脉。开颅手术应根据术前 MRI 和枕桥静脉位置进行个体化设计。骨孔置于窦汇上方 2 cm 和 7 cm 的中线右侧处。钻孔应遵循先远离矢状窦，最后朝矢状窦方向进行。如果出现窦损伤，迅速去除骨瓣，处理静脉出血会更容易且可控。

硬脑膜开口呈 C 形或三角形，向上矢状窦反折。应考虑到枕叶的移位幅度较小。可以行同侧侧脑室枕角穿刺来释放脑脊液，以获得足够的大脑移位。大脑大静脉和 Labbé 静脉必须保留，这两条静脉都汇入横窦。如前所述，通常不存在较大的枕部桥静脉，然而，当遇到这类静脉时，可能会显著限制暴露。这样的静脉应该被保留，因为牺牲它们可能会导致枕叶出血性静脉梗死。

手术通道位于枕叶和大脑镰之间，4~5 cm 深。枕部小脑幕入路具有良好的视野，是切除向下延伸至小脑 - 中脑池肿瘤的首选入路。这是幕下小脑上入路的盲点。与直窦平行，从后向前切开天幕 1 cm，可以看到病变、其周围的深静脉结构以及小脑蚓部。枕部小脑幕入路的解剖学优势在于展现幕上和幕下之间的宽阔视野（Lozier and Bruce，2003）（**图 37.2** 和**图 37.3**）。

在外科医生要求麻醉师压迫颈静脉并处理所有静脉渗漏之后，应使用连续或间断缝合对硬脑膜进行水密缝合。枕部小脑幕入路的主要原则见**专栏 37.2**。

典型病例

一名 21 岁男性患者在过去数月出现轻度步态共济失调和眩晕，GCS 15 分。MRI 和 CT 扫描显示小脑蚓旁增强的囊性病变（**图 37.4A**、**图 37.4B** 和**图 37.4C**）。选取左侧 3/4 俯卧位，对患者行枕部小脑幕入路显微手术完全切除肿瘤。为了在手术中行大脑充分减压，行腰大池引流术。术后 GCS 依然为 15 分，有一定程度的眩晕和平衡障碍，术后第 8 天症状完全消失。MRI 显示无肿瘤残留，无脑积水、静脉充血或脑梗死的症状。神经病理学结果为毛细胞性星形细胞瘤（WHO Ⅰ级）。随访 2 年，无肿瘤复发和神经功能缺失（**图 37.4D**、**图 37.4E** 和**图 37.4F**）。

镰幕脑膜瘤手术

从手术角度来看，镰幕交界处脑膜瘤或中间帆脑膜瘤是极具挑战性的病变，兼具松果体区手术入路和深部脑膜瘤切除的复杂性。而且，脑膜瘤的特殊特征使手术变得更加困难，例如附着于深部而难探及的硬膜，以及侵犯静脉窦，危及引流重要大脑区域的深静脉血流。

在设计这些病变的手术时，应仔细考虑其特殊

专栏 37.1　幕下小脑上入路的主要事项

1. 坐位
2. 分离较厚的蛛网膜（注意其后的静脉）
3. 识别并保护 Galen 静脉
4. 识别并保护小脑中央前静脉
5. 识别并保护基底静脉和肿瘤旁的大脑后动脉
6. 大脑内静脉位于肿瘤前上方
7. 四叠体位于肿瘤下方

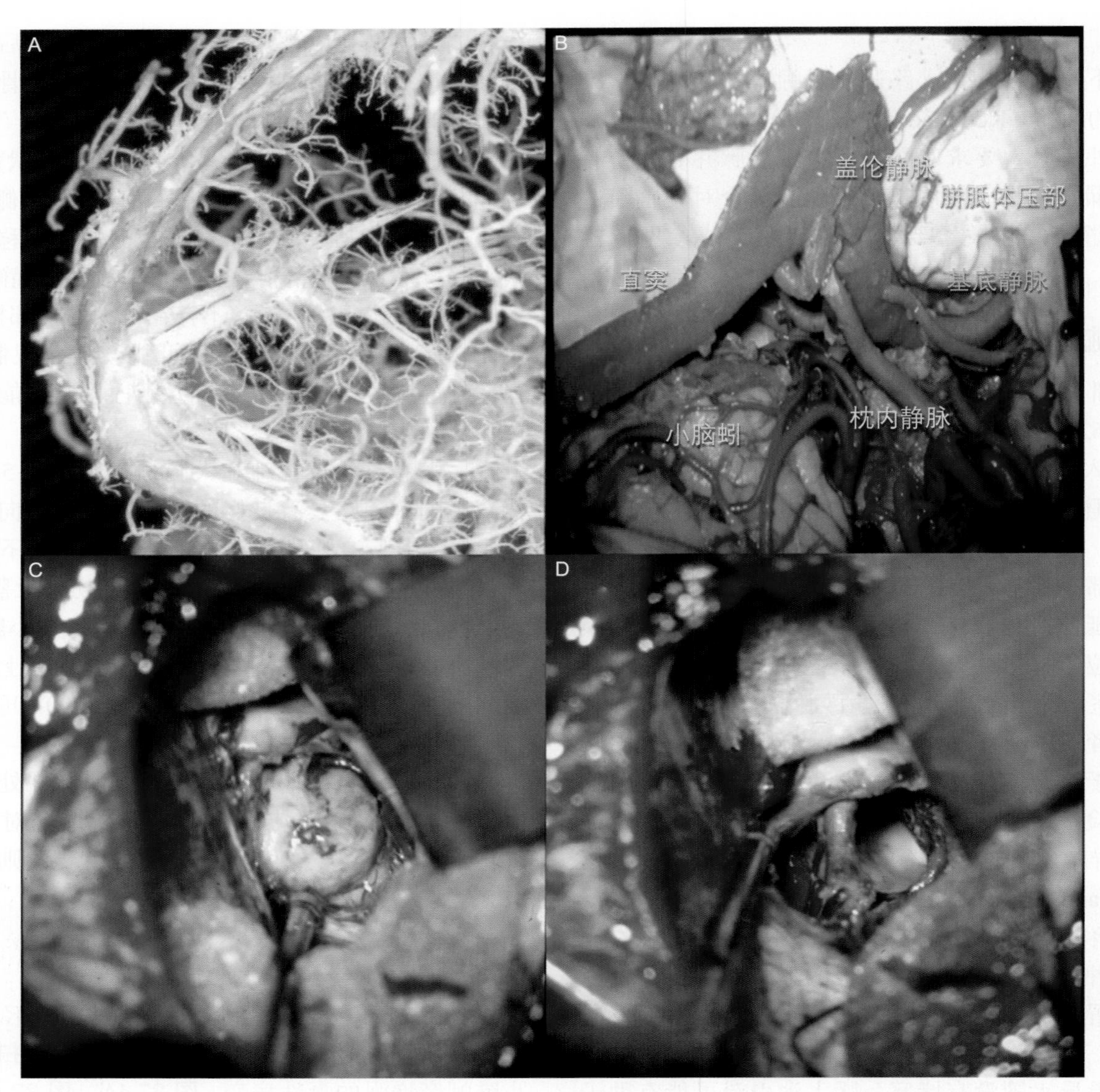

图 37.2 坐位枕部经小脑幕入路。（A 和 B）枕部经小脑幕入路的静脉解剖。（C）切开小脑幕暴露肿瘤。（D）肿瘤切除后，盖伦（Galen）静脉 / 小脑中央前静脉、基底静脉

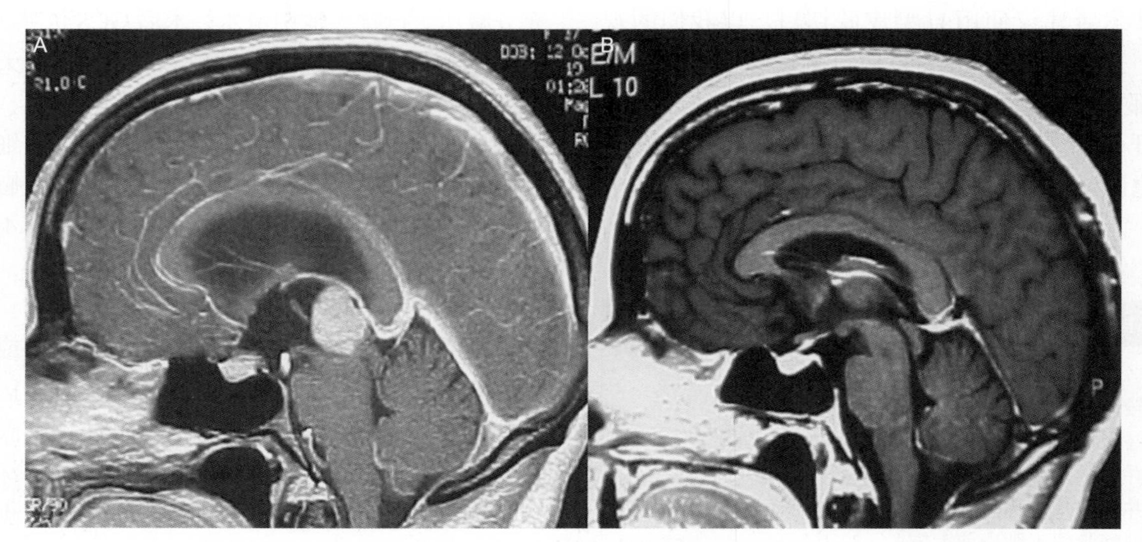

图 37.3 枕部经小脑幕入路典型病例。（A）术前病损在四叠体后，存在陡升的直窦。（B）枕部经小脑幕入路全切肿瘤后的图像

专栏 37.2　枕部经小脑幕入路的主要原则

1. 公园长椅位
2. 识别并保护枕内侧静脉
3. 切开大脑镰
4. 识别并保护小脑蚓部
5. 识别并保护盖伦（Galen）静脉
6. 识别并保护基底静脉
7. 识别肿瘤
8. 识别并保护大脑内静脉
9. 识别并保护四叠体

点。它们附着在大脑镰和天幕的硬膜处，与两侧直窦相邻。部分或全部窦可被持续压迫或彻底闭塞。

应特别注意深静脉结构和侧支循环，并不惜一切代价保护它们。

如果直窦闭塞，则可以切除，但如果是部分闭塞的，就必须保留，即使是以留下一小块肿瘤为代价，小块肿瘤之后可以行放射治疗。

在镰幕脑膜瘤的病例中，肿瘤通常包裹直窦和镰幕交界处。小脑幕切开应于肿瘤的外侧，并向后向前延伸到游离的天幕边缘，切断其血供。小脑幕的静脉血管和静脉池可以引起大量出血，但通常可以被双极电凝很好地控制。然而，天幕血管可以参与本已稀薄的侧支静脉回流，因此应尽可能多地保留天幕。天幕瓣向外侧方反折。然后，术者可以看到小脑上动脉和围绕脑干的展神经。在镰幕脑膜瘤手术中，用同样的方法切开大脑镰，露出左侧的肿瘤。然后切开左侧的天幕。此时可以结扎和切断直窦的后部。在减少肿瘤体积后，即可在所有面上进行肿瘤离断。肿瘤离断中最危险的部分为前极，有深静脉连接肿瘤。切除肿瘤后，对 Galen 静脉上的剩余部分进行分离、修剪和切除。然而，如果 Galen 静脉和大脑内静脉被严重侵及，残存这些静脉周围的肿瘤并再进行放射治疗更好。

在手术结束时，外科医生可以检查胼胝体压部、大脑内静脉、小脑上动脉、四叠体、小脑上脚以及小脑中脚（**图** 37.5）。镰幕脑膜瘤手术的主要原则见**专栏** 37.3。

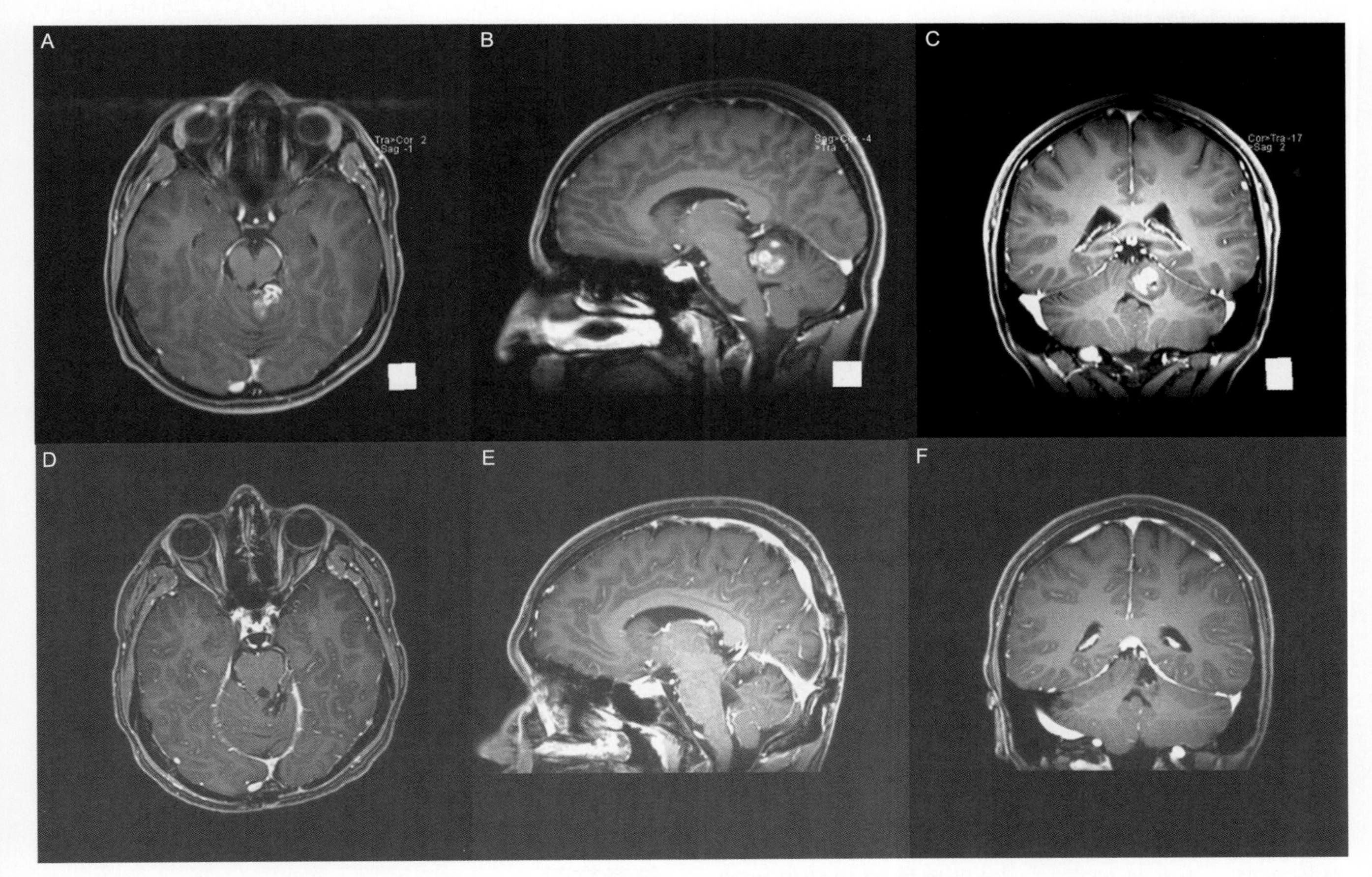

图 37.4　枕部经小脑幕入路的典型病例。（A、B、C）伴有症状的左侧小脑蚓部病变的术前轴位，矢状位和冠状位 MRI。（D、E、F）术后六个月随访枕部经小脑幕入路全切左侧小脑蚓部毛细胞型星形细胞瘤的 MRI

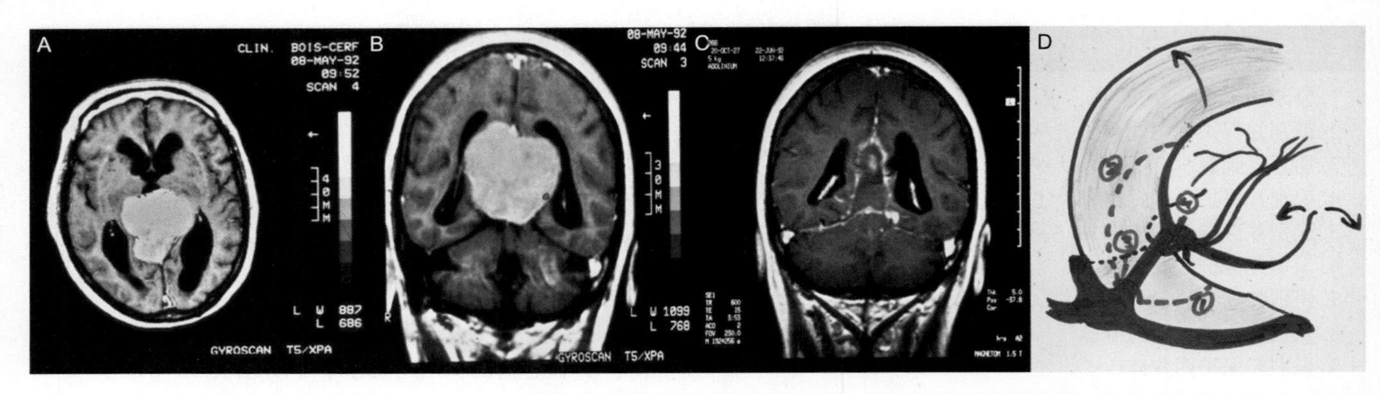

图 37.5　镰幕脑膜瘤的典型病例。（A、B）镰幕脑膜瘤轴位和冠状位 MRI。（C）镰幕脑膜瘤手术全切后的冠状位 MRI。（D）深静脉系统，小脑幕切开（1/2）和分离 / 电凝直窦与 Galen 静脉的示意图

专栏 37.3　镰幕脑膜瘤手术的主要原则

1. 公园长椅位
2. 附着在大脑镰和小脑幕的硬膜上
3. 注意窦受压和（或）闭塞
4. 识别并保护深静脉系统
5. 肿瘤包裹直窦和镰幕交界处
6. 沿着肿瘤外侧缘向前向后切开小脑幕
7. 小脑幕向侧方反折：检查小脑上动脉和展神经
8. 沿着肿瘤上缘切开大脑镰暴露另一侧的肿瘤
9. 如果肿瘤向前侵袭深部静脉，Galen 静脉或大脑内静脉，则残留部分肿瘤

幕上下联合入路治疗镰幕脑膜瘤

文献中描述了幕上下联合入路治疗大型松果体区脑膜瘤和大型松果体区肿瘤。这项技术包括显露幕下和幕上枕部硬脑膜、上矢状窦、窦汇和横窦，横窦在非优势侧可切开。枕叶和小脑较易移位，可显露出天幕，如前所述天幕可较早切开，到达肿瘤和松果体区。

术后流程和结果

在肿瘤切除后的头 24 小时内，患者应在重症监护病房接受监护。一些同行建议常规使用甘露醇和地塞米松。应在接下来的七天内逐步减量。在头 48 小时内，应行 MRI 评估切除率、脑梗死或脑积水。如果患者出现急性脑积水或神经功能变差的迹象，应立即进行 CT 扫描。

术后相关并发症包括小脑性共济失调、一过性视物变形、永久性偏盲、一过性展麻痹和帕里诺综合征。同向偏盲是枕部小脑幕入路手术的一种罕见并发症，但一般为一过性发生。文献中描述的总死亡率在 5%~10%。

并发症处理

为了预防肿瘤切除术中和术后的并发症，了解患者病变处的解剖，特别是静脉解剖是非常必要的。主要目标是避免静脉梗死。进行术前和术中检查以防止空气栓塞，必要时给予抗水肿治疗和脑脊液引流。

坐位松果体区病变手术中涉及一些麻醉注意事项。麻醉师应使用胸前多普勒监护仪，并注意呼气末二氧化碳分压，以诊断空气栓塞。如果栓塞恶化，患者应该有动脉和中心静脉通路以便在空气栓塞发生时同时压迫两条颈静脉并吸去气体。必要时可以使用地塞米松和甘露醇。

为了检查急性脑积水或静脉充血或梗死导致的术后神经功能变差，患者应该在重症监护病房接受至少 24 小时的监护。

松果体囊肿的处理和随访

松果体囊肿可在 4% 的 MRI 上出现，通常被认为是松果体区偶发的良性病变。松果体囊肿的治疗和随访在文献中存在争议。在我们看来，对于大小为 2 cm 左右的无症状囊肿，应行随访。如果 MRI 检测到囊壁增强，应与神经肠源性囊肿行鉴别诊断。

如果有病变扩大、导水管受压症状或持续压迫导水管并发展为脑积水的迹象，应考虑手术治疗（Berhouma et al.，2015）。对于脑积水的病例，可以考虑 EVT 而非开放手术切除囊肿。

参考文献

扫描书末二维码获取。

第九篇　肿瘤和颅底——肿瘤综合征

第 38 章　神经纤维瘤病

Fay Greenway · Frances Elmslie · Timothy Jones 著
李晔 译，汤劼 审校

引言

斑痣性错构瘤病一词最早于 1920 年首次被用来描述一组常见的神经皮肤表现的多系统疾病，这些疾病都合并有晶状体样的视网膜肿瘤（phacomata）。另一些人则引用希腊词根 phakos，意为“斑痣”或胎记，因为组织的异常生长或肿瘤的形成在这些情况下也会出现。首先被认为是斑痣性错构瘤病的三种疾病是：神经纤维瘤病（neurofibromatosis，NF）、结节性硬化症（tuberous sclerosis complex，TSC）和希佩尔 - 林道综合征（von Hippel- Lindau syndrome，VHL）。其他疾病，如斯特奇 · 韦伯（Sturge-Weber）综合征和 PHACE（颅后窝畸形、血管瘤、脑动脉性血管异常、心脏缺陷、眼部异常）综合征也可能包括在内。每一种疾病均由不同的遗传缺陷所引起，在蛋白质表达方面有某些重叠。这些疾病有着共同的发病机制——抑癌基因的表达紊乱。本章详细介绍了在临床实践中的斑痣性错构瘤病，并重点关注了其神经系统的后遗症以及对神经外科实践的影响。

1 型神经纤维瘤病

1 型神经纤维瘤病（neurofibromatosis type 1，NF1）是最常见的斑痣性错构瘤病，发病率为 1/3000（Walker et al.，2006）。其显示出的常染色体显性遗传，是由于位于染色体 17q11.2（基因产物神经纤维瘤蛋白，Ras 癌基因调节器）上的 1 型神经纤维瘤病抑癌基因突变引起的（Viskochil et al.，1990）。大约 50% 的病例表现出新的种系突变（Jett and Friedman，2010）。临床异质性以神经纤维瘤、咖啡牛奶斑、腋窝和腹股沟雀斑样色素沉着斑、视神经胶质瘤以及虹膜错构瘤等为特征。神经纤维瘤是一种由施万细胞组成的良性肿瘤，其中的一些细胞与轴突分离，支持细胞（成纤维细胞和肥大细胞）的组织增殖不如正常的神经束，会有神经周围层破裂。

诊断标准

1 型神经纤维瘤病需要以下两种或两种以上标准的临床诊断（National Institutes of Health Consensus，1988）：

- 六个或多于六个的牛奶咖啡斑（儿童 >0.5 cm 或成人 >1.5 cm）
- 两个或多于两个的皮肤 / 皮下神经纤维瘤或一个丛状神经纤维瘤
- 腋窝或腹股沟雀斑样色素沉着斑
- 视神经胶质瘤
- 两个或多于两个的虹膜结节（裂隙灯检查可见的虹膜错构瘤）
- 骨发育不良（蝶骨翼发育不良，长骨假关节弯曲）
- 有 NF-1 的一级亲属

基因分析可能会明确不符合诊断标准的幼儿患者，并有助于受影响的个体作出生殖决策。

病例

病例 38.1

一名表现为广泛的皮肤神经纤维瘤，体重减轻 3 个月，L3 皮节麻木，膝关节力量和反射为 3/5 级的 24 岁女性。磁共振成像发现腹膜后肿块侵入 L3 椎体，伴有椎体压缩、椎管受侵犯和硬脊膜受压。成功地对她进行了 L1~L5 椎板切除减压术和椎弓根螺钉固定。组织学已证实了恶性周围神经鞘瘤（图 38.1）。

病例 38.2

一名 5 岁的女孩，表现出了发育延迟、多个咖啡牛奶斑和头围增加。磁共振成像发现了视交叉和视神经病变（图 38.2）。

筛查

建议在儿科医师的关注下定期进行儿童临床检

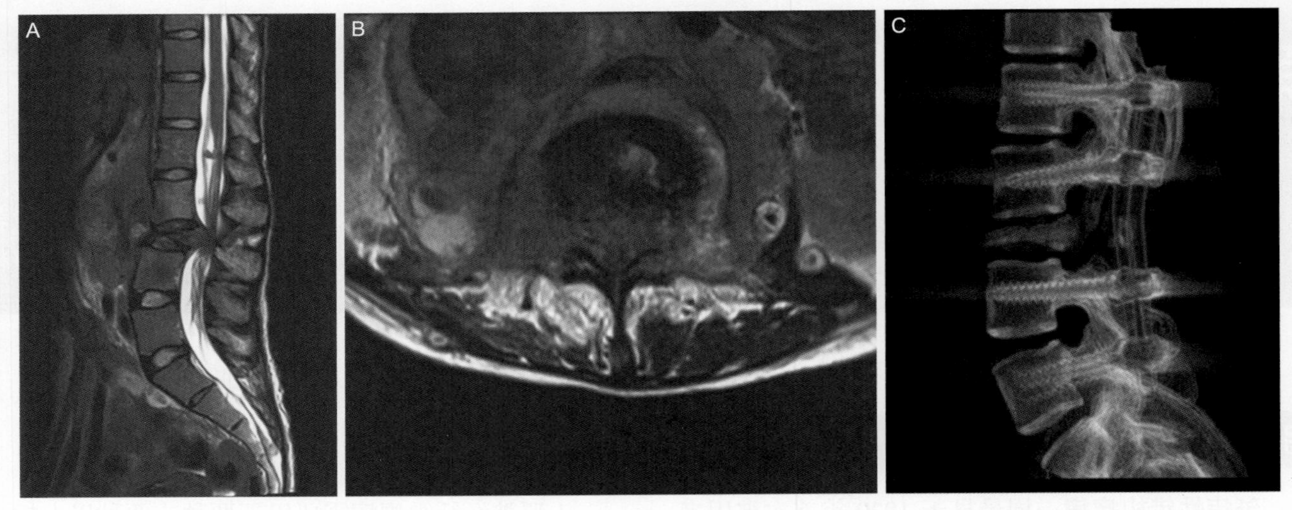

图 38.1 （A）矢状位 T2 加权磁共振成像，和（B）轴位 T2 加权磁共振成像显示腹膜后肿块侵入 L3 椎体，伴有椎体压缩、椎管受侵犯和硬脊膜受压。（C）术后 CT 重建

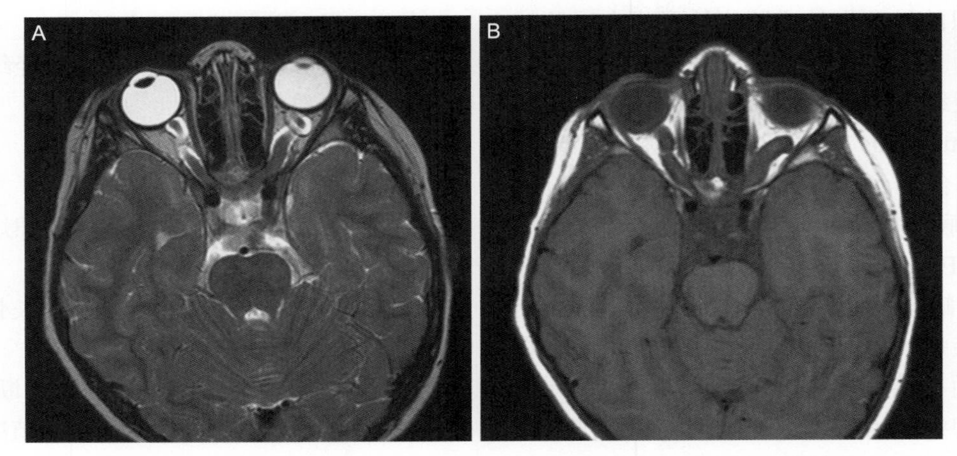

图 38.2 （A）轴位 T2 加权磁共振成像显示视神经增厚、盘曲；第四脑室后不明确的高信号病变。（B）眼眶轴位 T1 加权磁共振成像显示视神经增厚、盘曲，左侧较右侧粗

查，必要时转诊至 1 型神经纤维瘤病专科诊所。不提倡脑成像监测。应为受影响患者提供 1 型神经纤维瘤病的基因检测，并应要求进行产前诊断基因检测（Ferner et al.，2007）。

临床特征

皮肤表现通常是 1 型神经纤维瘤病的首个症状。咖啡牛奶斑是躯干上浅棕色且边缘清晰的斑块，通常在出生时出现，且数量会在出生后的头几年增加。1 型神经纤维瘤病临床表现的发病率和发病年龄参见**表** 38.1。

神经纤维瘤

神经纤维瘤是良性周围神经鞘瘤。其表现为局灶性皮肤或皮下、弥漫性或结节性丛状病变。典型的无痛、进展缓慢，遵循良性过程，发展至十几岁与二十岁早期。可能会出现美观问题，但可切除，有复发和增生性疤痕风险。皮肤触诊时很明显的皮下神经纤维瘤，可能会有触痛或在受累神经分布中引起感觉异常。其很少发生恶变。丛状神经纤维瘤沿神经长轴生长，且可能累及多个神经分支和神经丛。多发性病变可在神经干上发展并呈结节状，导致肿块增厚、潜在的巨大肿块、浸润软组织并导致骨骼肥大。累及多个脊髓神经根时，患者可能出现继发于脊髓压迫的脊髓病表现。

中枢神经系统肿瘤

毛细胞型星形细胞瘤（WHO 1 级）是 1 型神

表 38.1 1 型神经纤维瘤病主要临床表现的发生率和发病年龄

临床表现	发生率（%）	发病年龄
咖啡牛奶斑	>99	出生至 12 岁
皮肤褶皱处雀斑样色素沉着斑	85	3 岁至青春期
虹膜结节	90~95	>3 岁
皮肤神经纤维瘤	>99	>7 岁（通常为青春期晚期）
丛状神经纤维瘤	30（可见）~50（成像）	出生至 18 岁
面部丛状神经纤维瘤	3~5	出生至 5 岁
恶性外周神经鞘瘤	2~5（8%~13% 的终身风险）	5~75 岁
脊柱侧凸	10	出生至 18 岁
脊柱侧凸需要手术	5	出生至 18 岁
胫骨假关节	2	出生至 3 岁
肾动脉狭窄	2	终身
嗜铬细胞瘤	2	>10 岁
严重认知障碍（智商 <70）	4~8	出生
学习问题	30~60	出生
癫痫	6~7	终身
视神经胶质瘤	15（仅有 5% 有症状）	出生至 7 岁（最多 30 岁）
脑胶质瘤	2~3	终身
蝶骨翼发育不良	<1	先天
中脑导水管狭窄	1.5	终身

经纤维瘤病中最常见的儿童颅内肿瘤，发病率高达 15%。大多为视路胶质瘤（optic pathway gliomas, OPG）（Listernick et al., 2007），其中 20% 发生在脑干。其通常比散发性的同类肿瘤进展更为缓慢。视路胶质瘤可累及视神经、视交叉或下丘脑。大多数患者无症状，但可导致视力损失、眼球突出、内分泌紊乱，且这些症状多见于儿童。1 型神经纤维瘤病患者脑干或小脑胶质瘤的发生率高于普通人群，且在儿童期接受视路胶质瘤放疗的 1 型神经纤维瘤病患者中更为常见（Kleinerman, 2009）。

超过半数的 1 型神经纤维瘤病患者在 T2- 磁共振成像上可见高信号病变（不明确的高信号病变），最常见于 8~16 岁儿童。其为此疾病的病理学特征，且极可能由髓鞘形成异常或胶质增生所引起。

恶性外周神经鞘瘤

恶性外周神经鞘瘤 (malignant peripheral nerve sheath tumours, MPNST) 起源于先前存在的结节状或丛状神经纤维瘤；虽罕见（2%~5% 的频率），但其是与 1 型神经纤维瘤病相关的最常见的恶性肿瘤。既往有丛状神经纤维瘤的患者罹患恶性外周神经鞘瘤的风险为 8%~13%，通常发生于 20~30 岁（Evans et al., 2002）。恶性外周神经鞘瘤的预后比散发性肿瘤患者差。发生在儿童和青少年中时的恶性程度往往很低，且可能难以与非典型的丛状神经纤维瘤区分。疼痛或肿块扩大为典型的初始症状。

恶性肿瘤

英国最近的一项研究表明，1 型神经纤维瘤病患者罹患癌症的相对风险为 2.7，估计 70 岁时罹患恶性肿瘤的总风险为 36%（Walker et al., 2006）。尤其值得注意的是乳腺癌风险的增加（年龄 <50 岁），因此建议从 40 岁起对受影响女性进行早期乳腺筛查（Sharif et al., 2007）。

管理

1 型神经纤维瘤病患者应由多学科专家团队管理，包括神经学、儿科学、遗传学、眼科学、神经外科学、整形外科学、骨科、软组织肿瘤外科、精神病学、皮肤科、放射科以及病理学。管理的主要内容是对疾病表现进行针对年龄特异性的积极监测、对患者进行教导、每年在专科诊所做复查，且在疾病表现出症状或有进展迹象时进行外科干预。

视路胶质瘤可通过化疗（长春新碱和卡铂）进行治疗（Rosser and Packer, 2002），手术通常用于美容目的或治疗角膜暴露。由于存在神经血管、内分泌、神经心理学后遗症，以及继发高级别恶性胶质瘤以及恶性外周神经鞘瘤的风险，因此不再提倡放疗（Sharif et al., 2006; Lee, 2007）。视路胶质瘤治疗时机的决策仍具挑战性，对于何为该疾病的渐进性表现（影像学进展与视力退化）尚无普遍共识。

脊柱丛状神经纤维瘤的手术目的是治疗引起神经功能缺损的病变。由于血管生成和累及周围结构，手术可能会有挑战。由于病变多发性的特点，因此不可治愈，因此建议减压（椎板切除和减压）并考虑融合，以预防渐进性后凸畸形。恶性外周神经鞘瘤的手术应以无肿瘤边缘的完全切除为目标，并对未完全切除的肿瘤进行辅助放疗。

其他中枢神经系统肿瘤应进行连续的磁共振成像观察，并对局灶的、可切除的、有症状的肿瘤予以切除。

影响肿瘤性分子途径的药物，如雷帕霉素（西罗莫司）和依维莫司、哺乳动物雷帕霉素靶点（mTOR）途径的抑制剂，可能在今后 1 型神经纤维瘤病的研究中发挥作用。雷帕霉素已在小鼠模型中被证明能抑制哺乳动物雷帕霉素靶点（mTOR）途径，尤其是在恶性外周神经鞘瘤和胶质瘤中（Gottfried et al.，2010），而在 1 型神经纤维瘤病中进行性的低级别胶质瘤中使用依维莫司的试验结果则尚未公布（NCT01158651，2010）。

争议

关于视路胶质瘤的最佳处理有几种观点（Listernick et al.，2007）。包括监测、眼科检查的选择（视力、视野、色觉、视觉诱发电位）、定期监测的年龄限制、使用监视成像（磁共振成像）、复查频率、进展定义（放射和临床），以及最佳的最终管理。有依据表明，卡铂和长春新碱具有包括减缓肿瘤进展并改善或稳定视力等良好的化疗疗效（Mahoney et al.，2000；Fisher et al.，2012；Dodgshun et al.，2015）。文献表明放疗弊大于利，一项研究报告称，视路胶质瘤放疗后的继发性中枢神经系统肿瘤的相对风险增加了三倍，其中儿童的风险最大（Sharif et al.，2006）。有了如此之好的化疗依据，手术在视路胶质瘤中的作用就受到了限制。仅在出现第三脑室梗阻性脑积水（典型的下丘脑或视交叉病变）、明显的突眼畸形、失明、近盲，才考虑行眶内视神经部分切除。

2 型神经纤维瘤病

每 25000 人中就有 1 人受 2 型神经纤维瘤病（neurofibromatosis type 2，NF2）影响，估计发病率约为 1/60000（Evans，2009）。由于染色体 22q12.2 上 2 型神经纤维瘤病肿瘤抑制基因的突变（基因产物 merlin，又称 schwannomin，细胞增殖的接触依赖性抑制的关键调节器），NF2 呈现常染色体显性遗传（Rouleau et al.，1993；Trofatter et al.，1993）。这种显性遗传基因型——表型相关性强，60 岁时的外显率达 99%。2 型神经纤维瘤病的特征是双侧前庭神经鞘瘤（vestibular schwannomas，VS）（WHO Ⅰ级，由新生施万细胞组成）。其他表现包括脑膜瘤（颅内、脊柱和视神经管）、其他部位的神经鞘瘤（脑神经、脊髓、外周神经）、眼部体征（晶状体后囊混浊）、室管膜瘤，罕有皮肤表现（咖啡牛奶斑）。

诊断标准

已提出了多项诊断标准（美国国立卫生研究院标准 1987 年，1991 年修订；曼彻斯特标准，1992 年）（Evans et al.，1992；Evans et al.，2018）。根据磁共振与分子遗传学检测，2011 年提出了新的诊断标准（Baser et al.，2011），但大多数仍使用曼彻斯特诊断标准（**专栏** 38.1）。

病例

病例 38.3

一名 33 岁女性出现跌倒，头痛，恶心，步态不稳，右侧耳鸣。检查发现视盘水肿，计算机断层扫描（CT）发现右侧桥小脑角区增强明显的肿块，伴有梗阻性脑积水。磁共振成像（**图** 38.3）证实了双侧前庭神经鞘瘤和脑膜瘤，因此被诊断为 2 型神经纤维瘤病。她接受了较大的右侧前庭神经鞘瘤切除术，同时持续观察左侧前庭神经鞘瘤和脑膜瘤。

筛查

临床诊断为 2 型神经纤维瘤病的患者应进行基因检测。如发现一个突变，受影响父母的孩子应从出生起就接受基因检测，并开始对高危个体进行临床筛查。在英国，并无标准筛查方案，建议的筛查指南见**专栏** 38.2（Evans et al., 2005）。

专栏 38.1 2 型神经纤维瘤病诊断标准——曼彻斯特（Manchester）标准

A. 双侧前庭神经鞘瘤

B. 患有 2 型神经纤维瘤病和单侧前庭神经鞘瘤或以下“任意两个”* 的一级亲属：
脑膜瘤、神经鞘瘤、胶质瘤、神经纤维瘤、晶状体后囊混浊

C. 单侧前庭神经鞘瘤和以下两种：
脑膜瘤、神经鞘瘤、胶质瘤、神经纤维瘤、晶状体后囊混浊

D. 多发性脑膜瘤（两个或以上）和单侧前庭神经鞘瘤或其中任意两个：神经鞘瘤、胶质瘤、神经纤维瘤、白内障

* “任意两个”是指两个单独的肿瘤或白内障

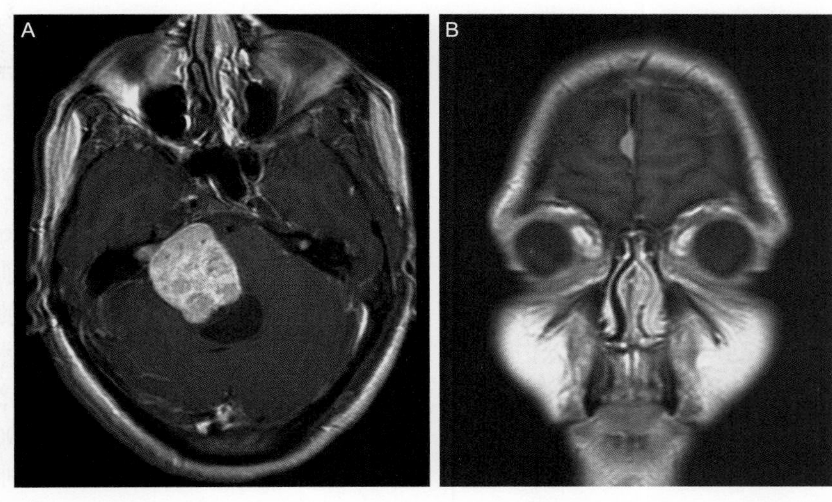

图 38.3 （A）增强 T1 加权磁共振成像显示右侧桥小脑角增强前庭神经鞘瘤和左侧小的管内神经鞘瘤。（B）增强 T1 加权磁共振成像显示增强的硬膜下大脑镰旁脑膜瘤

其他有 2 型神经纤维瘤病风险的人群包括（Evans et al.，2005）：有一级家族史、30 岁以下单侧前庭神经鞘瘤或脑膜瘤的患者（约 10% 的儿童孤立性脑膜瘤最终将被诊断为 2 型神经纤维瘤病）、多发性脊髓瘤（神经鞘瘤或脑膜瘤）、皮肤神经鞘瘤患者。孤立性单侧前庭神经鞘瘤患者罹患 2 型神经纤维瘤病的风险较低（如年龄 >30 岁，则 <1%）（Mohyuddin et al.，2002）。症状出现前进行基因检测可用于受影响的家庭成员，它可以指导临床筛查，能够在早期发现肿瘤并改善预后。

临床特征

90%~95% 的患者通常在 30 岁时发生双侧前庭神经鞘瘤（Parry et al.，1994）。他们会表现出听力下降，发病时通常是单侧，但大多数患者会进展为耳聋。他们也可能出现前庭症状；耳鸣、眩晕和失衡。与神经纤维瘤不同，神经鞘瘤是由生长在神经周围的纯施万细胞组成的包裹性肿瘤，发生于有施万细胞的神经处。2 型神经纤维瘤病好发于第八对脑神经的原因尚不清楚，但其他脑神经神经鞘瘤也会发生。

大约有一半的 2 型神经纤维瘤病患者会出现脑膜瘤，40% 的患者为多发性，而且可能发生于颅内（包括视神经鞘），也可能发生于脊髓。髓外硬膜下肿瘤（最常见的为背根神经鞘瘤），发生在 26%~90% 的患者中，取决于病例系列（Evans，2009）。低度恶性室管膜瘤和胶质瘤也以 2 型神经纤维瘤病为特征，主要发生于颈椎和脑干。60%~80% 的患者会有 2 型神经纤维瘤病的眼部表现，包括后囊混浊。皮肤病灶和咖啡牛奶斑也会发生在 2 型神经纤维瘤病中，但比 1 型神经纤维瘤病少且不明显。

管理

2 型神经纤维瘤病患者应由多学科专家团队管理，配备神经外科、耳鼻喉科、神经科、遗传学、听力学、儿科以及听力治疗方面的专家（考虑在早期即可教授患者与家人唇读与手势）。2 型神经纤维瘤病的管理旨在保护听力并最大限度地提高生活质量。人们对 2 型神经纤维瘤病 - 前庭神经鞘瘤的自然历史知之甚少，因此使得此项管理具有挑战性。外科医师需具备耳蜗、脑干听觉植入物来管理前庭神经鞘瘤与听觉康复的经验。患者应接受常规的临床与放射检查，如**专栏** 38.2 所述。如出现肿瘤生长、渐进性听力损失或有症状的肿瘤迹象，则应进行治疗。

贝伐珠单抗是血管内皮生长因子受体的单克隆抗体抑制剂，在 50% 的 2 型神经纤维瘤病患者中被证实了听力改善和前庭神经鞘瘤的肿瘤消退，但对 2 型神经纤维瘤病相关的脑膜瘤则影响甚微（Plotkin et al.，2012）。目前正在进行试验，以进一步评估其在儿童和青少年，以及在 2 型神经纤维瘤病相关脑膜瘤中的应用（NCT01767792，2013），（Nunes et al.，2013）。

立体定向放射外科治疗在外科手术中具有一定作用，然而关于它的使用存有争议，显微外科仍为公认的主要治疗方式。2 型神经纤维瘤病 - 前庭神经鞘瘤比散发性肿瘤患者更难治疗——通常表现为年龄较小、肿瘤更大、多灶性，且复发和面神经损伤的风险更高。手术时机非常关键，多项因素在决策过程中起着重要作用：

专栏 38.2 建议筛选指南

最初的颅骨（头颅）和脊柱磁共振成像年龄为 10~12 岁，除非受到严重影响的家庭

白内障和其他眼部异常会影响早期视力，其他肿瘤（尤其是颅内脑膜瘤）可能会发生在生命的前 10 年。最初的磁共振成像可能在 10~12 岁，或早期受严重影响的家庭；在此年龄段之前肿瘤出现症状很罕见。

年度听力测试

每年进行一次听力测试，包括听性（听觉）脑干反应（从青少年早起开始可能有用），但所有患者均应使用磁共振成像来监测，因为通常（经常）会出现肿瘤生长而听力却无退化。

无肿瘤：年龄 <20 岁，磁共振成像每 2 年筛查一次；年龄 >20 岁，每 3 年筛查一次

直径小于 6 mm 的肿瘤手术，不太可能比较大的肿瘤更成功，但前庭神经鞘瘤生长在年轻患者中的比例更高，因此 20 岁以下的患者，每 2 年进行一次磁共振成像筛查，年龄较大的患者，每 3 年进行一次磁共振成像筛查，对于无肿瘤无症状的有风险个体而言应足矣。

肿瘤：每 1 年做一次磁共振成像筛查

一旦出现肿瘤，磁共振成像检查应至少每年进行一次，直至确定个体的生长速度。

脊柱肿瘤常在磁共振成像上被发现。仅有 30% 的脊柱肿瘤患者出现有症状，需行脊柱手术，但每年进行一次完整的神经系统检查是明智的预防措施，每 2~3 年进行一次脊柱磁共振成像检查，除非在初次扫描中未发现肿瘤。

- 听力和面神经功能的保护
- 肿瘤的大小和生长模式（磁共振成像序列可用于评估进展情况）
- 听力状态和及其退化程度
- 考虑使用耳蜗植入物，或脑干听觉植入物的听觉康复装置，如果这么做的话，何时植入（首次手术比翻修手术更容易，即使听力可用，也可植入，并可在以后激活）
- 肿瘤的切除范围——仅在肿瘤易发生时才能完全切除（磁共振成像可用于监测任何残余肿瘤）

其他中枢神经系统肿瘤——脑膜瘤、室管膜瘤以及其他神经鞘瘤，包括颅内和脊柱肿瘤的治疗，遵循积极监测的标准原则，直至有迹象表明病情进展或出现症状时才考虑手术切除。

争议

立体定向放射外科治疗（stereotactic radiosurgery，SRS）已被证明是治疗散发性前庭神经鞘瘤的一种有效方法，大量研究表明，即使 SRS 的治疗效果并没有改善，但是结果与显微手术切除也具有可比性（肿瘤控制率介于 92% 和 98% 之间，听力保留率为 60%~90%，面神经保留率为 90%~95%）（Golfinos et al.，2016）。其效果对于 2 型神经纤维瘤病则较差。SRS 治疗所担心的是恶性转化的风险、继发性肿瘤的发展，以及对周围结构的有害影响（听力下降和面神经损伤）。尽管对散发性前庭神经鞘瘤治疗后的放射外科结果进行了研究，但对 2 型神经纤维瘤病的立体定向放射外科治疗文献仍相当贫乏。2 型神经纤维瘤病 - 前庭神经鞘瘤则更难治疗，由于其更容易侵犯或浸润第八对脑神经，而散发性前庭神经鞘瘤则更容易压迫第八对脑神经使其移位；因此无论选择哪种治疗方式，听力和面部保护均为一项挑战。目前尚无直接比较 2 型神经纤维瘤病 - 前庭神经鞘瘤的显微外科结果和立体定向放射外科治疗结果的研究。在决定 2 型神经纤维瘤病 - 前庭神经鞘瘤的最佳治疗时应考虑几个因素。

有利于立体定向放射外科治疗的因素包括：

- 避免手术死亡、脑脊液漏（cerebrospinal fluid，CSF）、出血、脑膜炎、静脉血栓栓塞等并发症
- 技术上难以手术切除的肿瘤；通常是不能完全切除且复发风险较高的肿瘤
- 多发性中枢神经系统肿瘤患者避免多次手术
- 立体定向放射外科治疗可用于不适合麻醉的患者
- SRS 在散发性前庭神经鞘瘤的良好疗效

影响立体定向放射外科治疗的因素包括：

- 前庭神经鞘瘤新的恶性转化风险
- SRS 理论上有导致继发性恶性肿瘤的风险（Plowman and Evans，2000）。数据有限，但有人认为这种风险非常低（Rowe et al.，2007）（18 例随访时间 >900 年的患者中仅发现了 2 例恶性肿瘤（1.7%）。其他人认为（Evans et al.，2006），大多数研究的随访期都很短，因此延迟报告可能会错过（真正的结果难以得知）。一项研究表明，接受放疗的 2 型神经纤维瘤病患者的恶性肿瘤风险为 10 倍（Baser et al.，2000）
- 缺乏长期随访和结果数据

研究立体定向放射外科治疗的肿瘤控制率、听力和面部保护的少数研究因为随访持续时间不同（Subach et al.，1999；Rowe et al.，2003；Mathieu et al.，2007；Phi et al.，2009；Sharma et al.，2010）（26~96个月），使得研究之间的比较变得困难；局部控制率的结果介于66%~98%，可用听力保护介于33%~66%（Mallory et al.，2014）。显微外科和立体定向放射外科治疗的结果没有比较。由于2型神经纤维瘤病是一种罕见的疾病，患者登记和前瞻性结果收集可能有助于确定最佳治疗。

结节性硬化症

结节性硬化症的发病率为6000~10 000例活产中的1例，人群患病率为2万分之一（Sampson et al.，1989；O'Callaghan et al.，1998）。由于两种不同的肿瘤抑制基因[染色体9q34上的TSC1基因（Fryer et al.，1987）和染色体16p13.3上的TSC2基因（Kandt et al.，1992），编码hamartin和tuberin蛋白]的突变，因此表现出了常染色体显性遗传。其形成复合体，通过mTOR（哺乳动物雷帕霉素靶点）途径调节细胞生长与增殖（Tee et al.，2002）。结节性硬化症的特征是错构瘤以及良性肿瘤病变，影响中枢神经系统以及皮肤、肾、心脏和肺等。中枢神经系统主要表现为皮质错构瘤（结节）、皮质下胶质细胞错构瘤、室管膜下胶质结节和室管膜下巨细胞瘤（subependymal giant cell tumours，SGCT），请参见**专栏38.3**。

诊断标准

结节性硬化症（TSC）的诊断标准请参见**专栏38.3**。

产前诊断可通过显示心脏及脑部病变的胎儿超声检查和磁共振成像（MRI）进行（Curatolo et al.，2008）。

病例

病例38.4

1例无明显家族史，经胎儿超声心动图确诊为心脏横纹肌瘤的3岁女孩。出生时的脑部磁共振成像（**图38.4A**）发现了与结节性硬化症一致的病变。她因局灶性强直性癫痫发作、单发性肾囊肿、单发性肾血管平滑肌脂肪瘤而发育迟缓、3岁时退行性心脏横纹肌瘤，磁共振成像扫描显示出了结节性硬化症的发展特征（**图38.4B**）

专栏38.3　结节性硬化症的诊断标准

A. 遗传诊断标准

正常组织DNA中TSC1基因或TSC2基因致病性突变的鉴定。

10%~25%的结节性硬化症患者未发现突变。

B. 临床诊断标准

明确诊断：两个主要特征或一个主要特征及≥2个次要特征。

可能诊断：一个主要特征或≥2个次要特征。

主要特征

1. 色素脱失斑（≥3个，直径至少5 mm）（最好使用伍兹灯进行观察）
2. 血管纤维瘤（≥3个），或头部纤维斑块（90%的患者在4岁时会出现；皮肤神经元错构瘤通常发生在颧骨，少量分布于上唇）
3. 指/趾甲纤维瘤（≥2个）
4. 鲨鱼皮斑
5. 多发性视网膜错构瘤
6. 皮质发育不良*
7. 室管膜下结节
8. 室管膜下巨细胞瘤（SGCT）
9. 心脏横纹肌瘤
10. 淋巴管平滑肌瘤病（LAM）†
11. 血管脂肪瘤（≥2个）†

次要特征

1. 斑斓皮损
2. 牙釉质小凹（>3个）
3. 口腔纤维瘤（≥2）
4. 视网膜脱色斑块
5. 多发性肾囊肿
6. 非肾错构瘤，如错构瘤性直肠息肉

*包括结节和脑白质放射状移行线。

†无其他特征的两个主要临床特征（淋巴管平滑肌瘤病和血管平滑肌脂肪瘤）组合不符合明确诊断的标准。两者同时出现时的诊断还需要其他特征。

Data from Krueger, D.A. & Northrup, H., Tuberous sclerosis complex surveillance and management: Recommendations of the 2012 international tuberous sclerosis complex consensus conference, *Pediatric Neurology*, Volume 49, Issue 4, pp. 255–65, Copyright © 2013 Elsevier.

病例38.5

一例于产前36周超声检查发现多发性心脏横纹肌瘤的6岁男孩。由于对结节性硬化症的怀疑，因此对新生儿进行了磁共振成像检查，发现了室管膜下结节和一个较大的右侧室管膜下病变，疑似室管膜下巨细胞瘤（**图38.5**）。他在22周时出现婴儿癫痫。

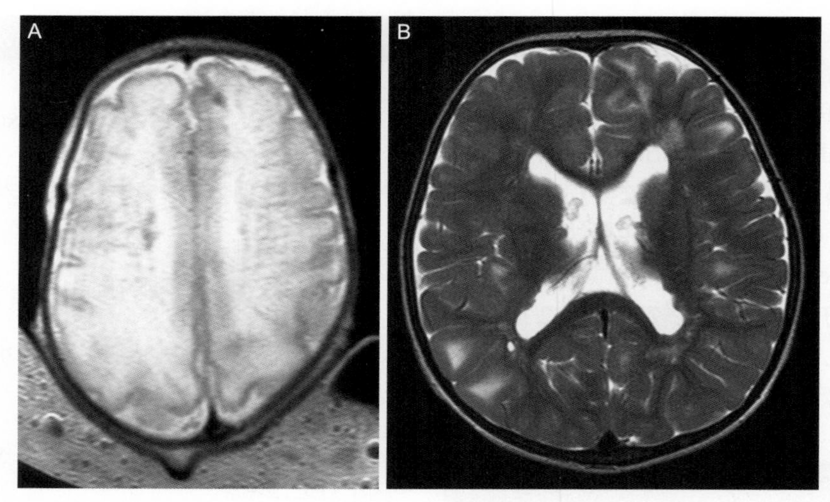

图 38.4 （A）轴位 T2 加权磁共振成像，年龄 3 天，显示放射状移行线，左额叶（低信号）结节。（B）轴位 T2 加权磁共振成像，年龄 3 岁，显示多个结节（高信号），室管膜下结节沿侧脑室壁散发

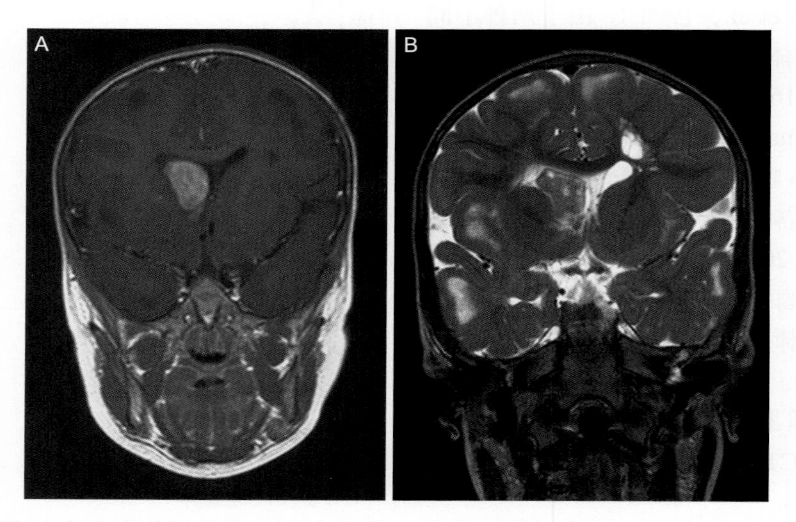

图 38.5 （A）冠状位增强 T1 加权磁共振成像和（B）冠状 T2 加权磁共振成像显示右侧脑室和多个皮质下结节的室管膜下巨细胞瘤

4 岁时由于成像序列上的渐进性增大而接受了室管膜下巨细胞瘤切除术。他的学习困难与之有关联。

筛查

疑似结节性硬化症患者应接受脑磁共振、脑电图（如疑似癫痫发作或患者在出生前已被确诊为儿科患者）、结节性硬化症相关神经精神疾病障碍评估、肾和腹部成像、肾功能血检、成年女性以及有症状成年男性的肺功能测试、皮肤科检查是否有严重的皮肤损伤、儿科患者的心脏超声心动图和心电图（ECG）检查、眼科和牙科检查。一旦确诊，建议定期进行监测成像和临床复查；如患者无症状，则从出生至 25 岁，每 1~3 年应接受一次脑部磁共振成像（Northrup and Krueger，2013）。对受影响者的家庭应进行全面的临床评估，并提供基因检测与咨询。

临床特征

德国神经学家 Heinrich Vogt（1875—1936）描述了结节性硬化症临床症状的三联征：癫痫发作、学习障碍和皮肤损害。仅有 29% 的患者出现三联征，6% 的患者无此三种症状（Schwartz et al.，2007）。结节性硬化症是一种具有多种临床特征的多系统疾病，如**专栏** 38.3 所述。非中枢神经系统病变包括皮肤表现（参见**专栏** 38.3）、肾囊肿、血管平滑肌脂肪瘤、肾细胞癌、肺淋巴管平滑肌瘤病、心脏横纹肌瘤和视网膜错构瘤。

90% 的结节性硬化症患者发现有中枢神经系统病变（Curatolo et al., 2006）：

- 皮质结节——良性错构瘤的特征是胶质细胞和神经元细胞增殖，皮质结构损失——神经元发育异常、巨细胞和畸形的星形胶质细胞；大小不一且数量众多。
- 室管膜下结节（subependymal nodules，SENs）——错构瘤，常见于侧脑室室管膜下壁；一些突入脑室内（呈现特有的“烛泪征”）；典型钙化。
- 室管膜下巨细胞瘤（SGCTs）（又名室管膜下巨细胞星形细胞瘤，SEGA）——WHO 1 级肿瘤，显示混合的胶质 - 神经细胞排列；其与室管膜下结节的区别在于成像序列上的渐进性生长或是否引起脑积水；这些会发生在大约 10% 的结节性硬化症患者中。
- 白质线性移行线——呈放射状，从室周白质向皮质下区域辐射。
- 皮质发育不良。

管理

应在与当地服务相关的专业多学科诊所对结节性硬化症患者进行随访。80%~90% 的患者有癫痫发作；1/3 的患者可通过药物成功治疗。难治性癫痫患者可行手术或进行迷走神经电刺激。当特定的病灶被确定为致痫灶时可考虑手术治疗。需要在术前对致痫区进行彻底识别，且考虑手术的切除范围（Fallah et al., 2015）。Jansen 等（2007）表明，57% 的儿童术后达到了癫痫发作消失，另外 18% 的儿童在一年的随访中癫痫发作频率降低（>90%）。对于导致梗阻性脑积水、颅内压升高、影像学肿瘤进展，或出现新的局灶性神经功能缺损的肿瘤，应予以考虑手术切除。

争议

结节性硬化症相关肿瘤中 mTOR 通路上调的发现为治疗策略提供了新的可能性。西罗莫司（又名雷帕霉素）为一种结合并抑制 mTOR 磷酸化下游靶点的免疫抑制剂。自 2001 年以来就被批准为免疫抑制剂，并被发现可用于治疗结节性硬化症（Jozwiak et al., 2006）。依维莫司是西罗莫司的衍生物，可有效减少肾血管平滑肌脂肪瘤、室管膜下巨细胞瘤（Franz et al., 2006），以及散发性淋巴管平滑肌瘤病患者的病变体积。已于 2010 年被美国食品及药品管理局批准用于治疗无法接受手术切除的结节性硬化症相关的室管膜下巨细胞瘤（Krueger et al., 2010）。2013 年，依维莫司治疗结节性硬化症相关室管膜下巨细胞星形细胞瘤的双盲、安慰剂对照试验结果发表于 EXIST-1 试验中（Franz et al., 2013）。研究还表明，与安慰剂相比，肿瘤体积至少减少了 50%（Franz et al., 2013）。外科手术可能不再是与结节性硬化症相关肿瘤的首选治疗方案。

希佩尔 – 林道综合征

希佩尔 - 林道综合征（von Hippel-Lindau syndrome，VHL）的发病率估计为 36 000 例活产中的 1 例，患病率为 39 000~53 000 例中的 1 例（Melmon and Rosen, 1964; Maher et al., 2011）。由于染色体 3p25 希佩尔 - 林道综合征（VHL）抑癌基因突变，其具有常染色体显性遗传（Latif et al., 1993）。蛋白质产物通过 HIF（缺氧诱导因子）途径调节细胞增殖。20% 的病例由新生突变引起。希佩尔 - 林道综合征在 65 岁时具有显著的表型变异性以及超过 90% 的外显率（Maher et al., 1990）。希佩尔 - 林道综合征是一种多系统疾病，以中枢神经系统、视网膜以及其他内脏的多发性血管母细胞瘤（HGBs）为特征。希佩尔 - 林道综合征与其他神经皮肤综合征不同，通常与皮肤表现无关。血管母细胞瘤由血管细胞和间质细胞组成。

诊断标准

希佩尔 - 林道综合征的诊断标准请参见**专栏 38.4**。

专栏 38.4 希佩尔 - 林道综合征的诊断标准

有家族史

单个希佩尔 - 林道综合征肿瘤的存在足以确诊（例如：视网膜或中枢神经系统血管母细胞瘤、透明细胞肾癌、嗜铬细胞瘤、胰腺内分泌肿瘤或内淋巴囊肿瘤）。

无家族史

通常在希佩尔 - 林道综合征中发现的所有肿瘤都可能是散发性的。

因此，诊断需要存在两种肿瘤：

- 两个中枢神经系统血管母细胞瘤；
- 或一个中枢神经系统 - 血管母细胞瘤和一个内脏肿瘤（在一般人群中很常见的附睾和肾囊肿除外）。

在不确定的情况下，可采用对管理更广泛家庭有用的基因检测。完成评估需进行磁共振脑成像、肾部超声、腹部 CT 扫描和尿素氮的评估。

病例

病例 38.6

一例表现为头痛、眩晕和步态不稳的 33 岁男性患者。影像学检查发现了有局部占位效应的颅后窝病变（**图** 38.6）。他接受了手术切除；组织病理学证实了血管母细胞瘤和血清突变的希佩尔 - 林道综合征。他还接受了视网膜血管母细胞瘤的冷冻疗法和肾细胞癌的肾切除术。他的胰腺和附睾囊肿正在观察中，同时也正在进行中枢神经系统监测。

筛查

1/3 的中枢神经系统血管母细胞瘤与希佩尔 - 林道综合征相关。希佩尔 - 林道综合征患者的血管母细胞瘤往往比散发性病例患者的诊断早 10 年。新诊断为中枢神经系统 - 血管母细胞瘤的患者应具有完整的家族史和希佩尔 - 林道综合征相关表现的临床回顾，并进行完整的神经系统成像。如怀疑患者是希佩尔 - 林道综合征，则应转诊至专科中心进行进一步评估。一旦确诊，即可开始监测筛查。筛查可能包括从童年早期开始的视网膜血管瘤的年度眼科评估，青少年时期开始的血管母细胞瘤的颅脑磁共振成像和肾细胞癌、胰腺肿瘤的腹部磁共振成像，以及对嗜铬细胞瘤的年度血压监测和泌尿系统检查（Maher，2004）。

临床特征

60%~80% 的希佩尔 - 林道综合征患者（Richard et al.，2000；Wanebo et al.，2003）会出现中枢神经系统 - 血管母细胞瘤，最常见于小脑、椎管，脑干和神经根较不常见。视网膜血管母细胞瘤发生在 50% 以上的患者中，通常会出现此疾病最早期的表现，并可致突然失明。其他相关病变包括内脏囊肿（常见但罕有损害器官功能的肾、胰腺和附睾囊腺瘤）、肾细胞癌、肾上腺和肾上腺外嗜铬细胞瘤、无功能性胰腺内分泌肿瘤、内淋巴囊肿瘤，偶尔还有头颈部副神经节瘤。肾细胞癌是最常见的恶性肿瘤及致死原因，其次是中枢神经系统血管母细胞瘤（Maher et al.，1990）。

管理

希佩尔 - 林道综合征具有发展多器官肿瘤的终生风险。患者应由希佩尔 - 林道综合征专家团队管理。应进行监测，以便早期发现以更好治疗病变。完全手术切除有症状的中枢神经系统血管母细胞瘤是治疗的主要手段。一项针对 80 例患者的研究显示，随访 61 个月后无复发（Jagannathan et al.，2008）；其他研究则认为在 53 个月时的复发率为 17%（Conway et al.，2001）。影响行手术决策的因素包括神经系统症状、影像上显示的生长迹象（这将使得手术切除术更困难），或存在增大的囊肿或空洞（Lonser et al.，2003；Weil et al.，2003）。

围术期检查应包括整个神经系统磁共振成像，

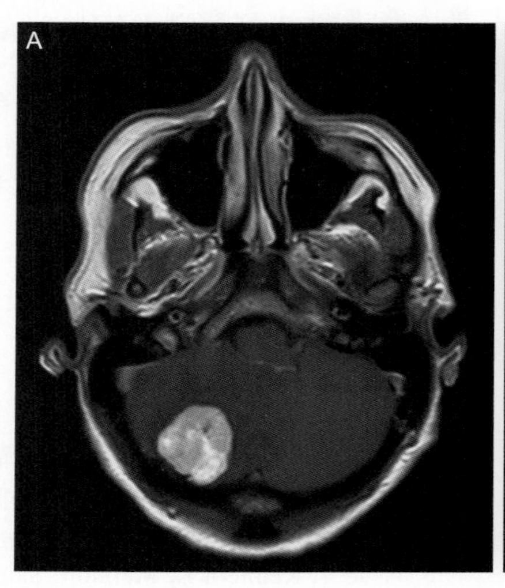

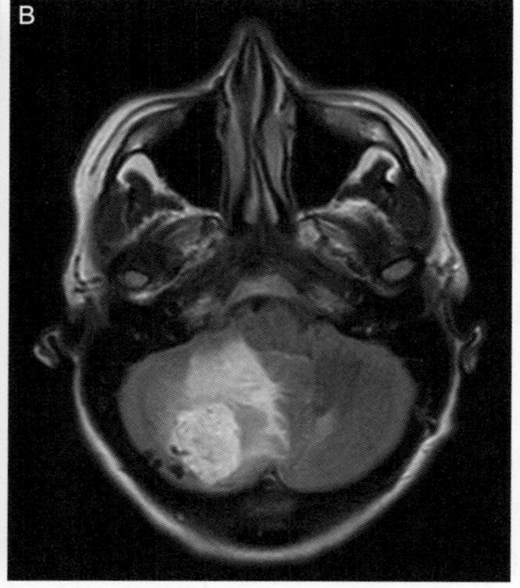

图 38.6 （A）对比增强，T1 加权磁共振成像显示右小脑半球血管母细胞瘤实质性增强；（B）T2 加权磁共振成像显示实质性病变、相关的血流空洞和病灶周水肿，以及局部占位效应

由于围术期麻醉期间高血压危象的风险，应该对嗜铬细胞瘤进行术前检查，并考虑在切除手术前进行栓塞肿瘤。

计划手术治疗颅后窝血管母细胞瘤时，应考虑脑室外引流、释放脑脊液，打开枕大池进一步降低脑脊液压力，超声引导下瘤周或瘤内囊肿引流，静注甘露醇和（或）速尿（呋塞米），以及使用经颅超声引导下以确定最佳骨瓣去除范围，以充分暴露肿瘤。囊性血管母细胞瘤的切除原则是切除壁结节防止肿瘤复发。囊肿壁本身无需切除，除非在磁共振成像上或行手术时的直视下发现囊壁有肿瘤的成分（Jagannathan et al.，2008）。应用显微外科的标准原则对肿瘤进行解剖（确定肿瘤和小脑之间的边界平面），并逐步分层深入解剖肿瘤边缘。使用不粘连双极电凝镊，在血管进入或离开肿瘤包膜时需电凝后锐性分离。在血供中断时肿瘤会变软，使得轻柔的牵拉肿瘤成为可能，以增加肿瘤的暴露并进行切除。

血管内皮生长因子是VHL蛋白的下游靶点之一。舒尼替尼（sunitinib）是一种血管内皮生长因子受体抑制剂，已获准用于晚期转移性肾细胞癌，并已被用于与希佩尔-林道综合征相关的肾细胞癌。舒尼替尼对中枢神经系统血管母细胞瘤的作用尚未得到证实，但研究仍在进行中（Jonasch et al.，2011）。立体定向放射外科治疗（SRS）可考虑用于手术无法切除的病变。很少有研究可确定此种治疗的长期安全性与有效性（Asthagiri et al.，2010）。

争议

立体定向放射外科治疗可用于治疗与希佩尔-林道综合征相关的血管母细胞瘤（体积小于3 cm^3，肿瘤未完全切除或无法切除）。立体定向放射外科治疗可最小化（减少）患有多个血管母细胞瘤个体的手术切除次数。立体定向放射外科治疗术后的肿瘤控制率分别为5年83%、10年61%、15年51%（20例希佩尔-林道综合征患者，44例血管母细胞瘤患者）（Asthagiri et al.，2010）。另外一组研究为5年控制率93%，10年时82%（80例希佩尔-林道综合征患者，335例血管母细胞瘤患者）（Kano et al.，2015）。如果手术切除肿瘤后无并发症，可以达到治愈的效果。手术切除后的神经功能状态保持稳定或改善（98%患者在小脑血管母细胞瘤切除术后的3个月有改善）（Lonser et al.，2003；Weil et al.，2003；Jagannathan et al.，2008）。

对80例希佩尔-林道综合征患者的回顾性分析数据显示，41%的患者在立体定向放射外科治疗后67个月的随访中出现了新的肿瘤生长（1年7%，3年21%，5年43%，10年84%）（Kano et al.，2015）。与未接受立体定向放射外科治疗的希佩尔-林道综合征中形成新肿瘤的情况无明显差异（Wanebo et al.，2003；Ammerman et al.，2006）。

目前尚无放疗后的继发性恶性肿瘤或恶性转化的报告，但应予以关注。在一项针对186例接受立体定向放射外科治疗的血管母细胞瘤患者研究中，仅有13例（7%）出现了放射治疗不良反应，其中一例患者由于这些副作用而死亡（Kano et al.，2015）。然而这些现象并未在希佩尔-林道综合征或散发性血管母细胞瘤的患者中发现。希佩尔-林道综合征患者有多发性血管母细胞瘤风险，因此重复放疗并非始终可取的。

共济失调毛细血管扩张症

共济失调毛细血管扩张症（ataxia telangiectasia，AT）不再被归类为神经瘢痣错构瘤病之一。由于其病例报告与某些中枢神经系统肿瘤以及血管造影学上的隐匿性毛细血管畸形有关，因此在历史上被囊括于神经外科文献中。与其他神经错构瘤不同，共济失调毛细血管扩张症与皮肤或眼部表现无关，且表现为常染色体隐性遗传。由于其导致小脑退化与进行性共济失调，因此与神经科医师最为相关。

延伸阅读、参考文献

扫描书末二维码获取。

第 39 章　少见的脑病变

Yizhou Wan · Hani J. Marcus · Thomas Santarius 著
李晔 译，汤劼 审校

引言

我们将在本章中讨论一些神经外科少见肿瘤，这些肿瘤并不常见，在其他地方也没有涉及。

由于这些肿瘤的少见性，本章回顾了关于它们的已知情况，并主要对它们的诊断进行讨论。文中对治疗的描述主要来源于已发表的病例报告。

迷芽瘤

迷芽瘤是由异常位置中的正常组织组成的（即“正常”组织）肿块（Lee and Roland，2013）。在组织学上表现为正常组织，这与错构瘤不同，一个例子是小脑发育不良性神经节细胞瘤（L'hermitte-Duclos 病）。表皮样和皮样囊肿是大家最熟悉的的颅内迷芽瘤，其为单独一章的主题。已在神经系统中发现了某些较少见的迷芽瘤，如颅内胰腺（Heller et al.，2010）、唾液腺（Hintz et al.，2014）以及神经肌肉组织肿块（Hebert-Blouin et al.，2012）。位于鞍区的唾液腺迷芽瘤已得到了很好（完整）的描述（Hintz et al.，2014）。其他常见部位包括主要外周神经，如神经肌肉迷芽瘤的臂丛神经和坐骨神经（Hebert-Blouin et al.，2013）。

神经迷芽瘤极为少见，最常见于头颈部，尤其是鼻子（**鼻神经胶质瘤**）。其他区域包括躯干和背部，通常表现为孤立性的无症状肿块（Downing et al.，1997）。患者可从儿童早期开始发病，神经迷芽瘤的平均发病年龄约为 10 岁（Hebert-Blouin et al.，2012）。

病理学

迷芽瘤的组织学取决于其来源组织。神经迷芽瘤可能是由纤维组织中无序排列的胶质细胞组成，或是类似于大脑或小脑皮质的成熟神经组织（Downing et al.，1997）。神经肌肉迷芽瘤（neuromuscular choristomas，NMC）由成熟的横纹肌细胞和平滑肌细胞与神经纤维混合而成，通常是坐骨神经和臂丛神经，但也会累及脑神经，如视神经、上颌神经、动眼神经、面神经以及前庭蜗神经（Hebert-Blouin et al.，2012）。

治疗

临床表现取决于解剖部位。例如，鞍区唾液腺迷芽瘤可导致激素缺乏，而肿瘤向蝶鞍上延伸可导致头痛或视力障碍（Hebert-Blouin et al.，2012）。神经肌肉迷芽瘤沿外周神经生长巨大时，导致感觉、运动功能障碍，可能会引起疼痛、无力和感觉改变。颅内神经肌肉迷芽瘤常见于内听道或桥小脑角，在影像学上类似前庭神经鞘瘤的表现（Boyaci et al.，2011）。神经肌肉迷芽瘤的放射学表现无特异性，可能会与神经鞘瘤难以鉴别（Boyaci et al.，2011）。术前的影像学检查对于确定神经迷芽瘤与中枢神经系统之间的关系至关重要（Downing et al.，1997）。神经迷芽瘤的恶性转化从未有过报道（Newman et al.，1986）。

预后

这些肿瘤的少见性意味着它们的自然史并未被很好地阐释。一般认为它们的病变“生长缓慢”，可进行保守治疗（Boyaci et al.，2011）。一些作者则主张进行完全切除（Awasthi et al.，1991）。

错构瘤

错构瘤是一种由正常组织成分构成的肿瘤，但组织结构紊乱。囊肿和假性囊肿将在其他章节中描述，本节描述的是在中枢神经系统中发现的其他病变，包括小脑发育不良性神经节细胞瘤（L'hermitte-Duclos 病）、皮质胶质神经元错构瘤和下丘脑错构瘤。所有这些病变的共同点是它们可能表现为发育畸形，但其可能会被误认为是更常见的肿瘤或囊性病变。

流行病学

自1920年首次描述L'hermitte-Duclos病（LDD）以来，文献已描述过超230多例病例。此疾病可以在从出生至六十岁期间发现，无明显性别差异。有人认为小脑发育不良性神经节细胞瘤和Cowden综合征（多发性错构瘤综合征）之间存在遗传联系。Cowden综合征为一种常染色体显性遗传错构瘤综合征，表现为乳腺、甲状腺、泌尿生殖道和子宫内膜的肿瘤和错构瘤（Nowak and Trost，2002）。

在结节性硬化症（tuberous sclerosis complex，TSC）的中枢神经系统表现中，一个重要的诊断标准是皮质胶质神经元错构瘤。结节性硬化症为一种多系统受累的常染色体显性遗传病，由结核菌素和编码harmaline（参与细胞增殖和分化的蛋白质）蛋白基因突变引起。它们会在任何器官系统中引起良性非侵袭性病变（Curatolo and Maria，2013）。新生儿发生率为1/6000（Kwiatkowski and Manning，2005）。

下丘脑错构瘤的发病率为1/50 000至1/100 000（Weissenberger et al.，2001）。

病理学

小脑发育不良性神经节细胞瘤的特征是小脑叶的局部增厚，是由发育不良的神经节细胞替代了小脑的浦肯野细胞和颗粒细胞，以及肥大神经节细胞的错构瘤过度生长所致（Wei et al.，2014）。显微镜下颗粒细胞层有异常神经节细胞，分子细胞层增厚、过度髓鞘化，浦肯野细胞减少或消失（Ozeren et al.，2014）。组织病理学上也可见钙化和血管扩张，但无多形性或有丝分裂（Wei et al.，2014）。

结节性硬化症的特征是皮质结节中的胶质细胞和神经元细胞增生，六层皮质结构丧失。在皮质结节内发现各种异常细胞，主要是形状畸形的星形胶质细胞、巨细胞和发育异常的神经元。室管膜下结节的另一个特征性发现是可伸入室间孔附近侧脑室壁的错构瘤生长。这些细胞可慢慢成长为室管膜下巨细胞星形细胞瘤（subependymal giant- cell astrocytomas，SEGAs），其为结节性硬化症中最常见的脑肿瘤（Curatolo and Maria，2013）。

下丘脑错构瘤为一种发育异常，影响漏斗和乳头体之间下丘脑区域的肿瘤（Striano et al.，2012）。

治疗

小脑发育不良性神经节细胞瘤的患者最初无症状，但随着肿瘤的逐渐增大，通常会出现长达15年之久的与单侧小脑功能障碍相关的不确定的神经功能症状（Ozeren et al.，2014）。患者有时可表现为梗阻性脑积水急性失代偿（Nowak and Trost，2002）。

磁共振成像用来诊断小脑发育不良性神经节细胞瘤具有相当的特异性，尤其是在合并Cowden综合征时。增大的小脑叶失去脑沟回，导致小脑半球不对称增宽。病变在T2加权像（**图**39.1）上不增强，显示的特征为低信号互不相连的等信号带（条纹征）。表明了扩大的小脑皮质中脑回变宽，脑沟结构位移（Nowak and Trost，2002）。

由于病变与正常小脑实质界限不明显，因此有症状的小脑发育不良性神经节细胞瘤很难被切除。术中磁共振成像和（或）术中组织学显示组织病理学上的转换区可能有帮助。

结节性硬化症的临床表现多种多样，为多系统受累的疾病。从神经学角度来看，治疗重点是控制癫痫。其通常发生在1岁以内，从局灶性癫痫发展至婴儿痉挛。室管膜下巨细胞瘤可用哺乳动物雷帕霉素（西罗莫司）靶点途径抑制剂或手术治疗（Franz et al.，2006）。

下丘脑错构瘤的典型特征为痴笑性癫痫、发育迟缓和性早熟。磁共振成像通常显示病变位于第三脑室内的垂直附着面和（或）下丘脑下方的水平附着面（**图**39.2）。

这些病变似乎具有内在的致痫机制（Maixner，2006）。据报道，手术切除可改善症状并控制癫痫发作（Palmini et al.，2002）。完全切除病变有挑战性，

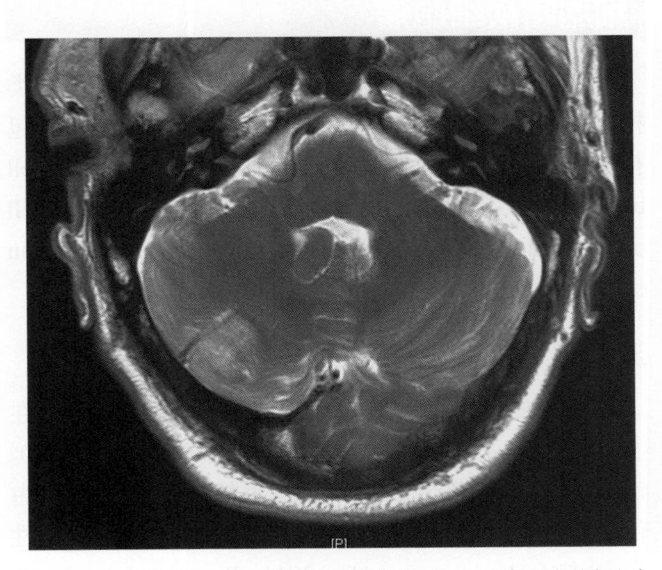

图39.1　小脑发育不良性神经节细胞瘤。异常组织累及小脑皮质，T2高信号，小脑叶增宽

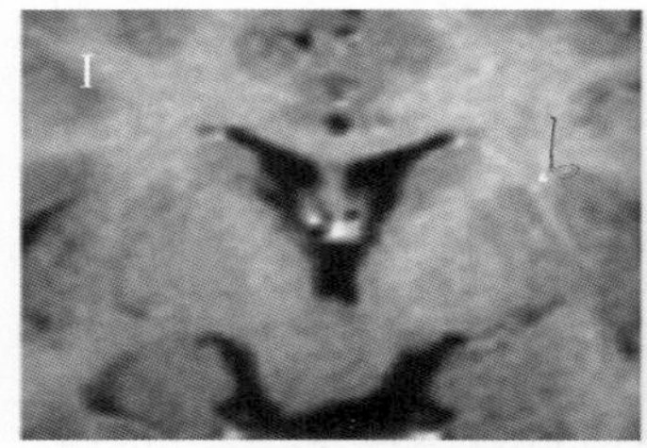

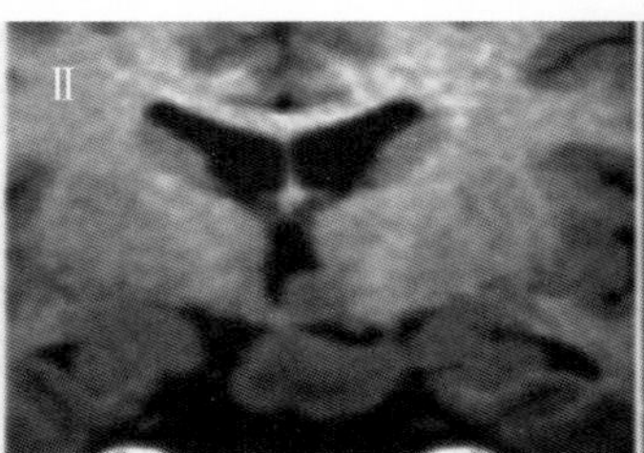

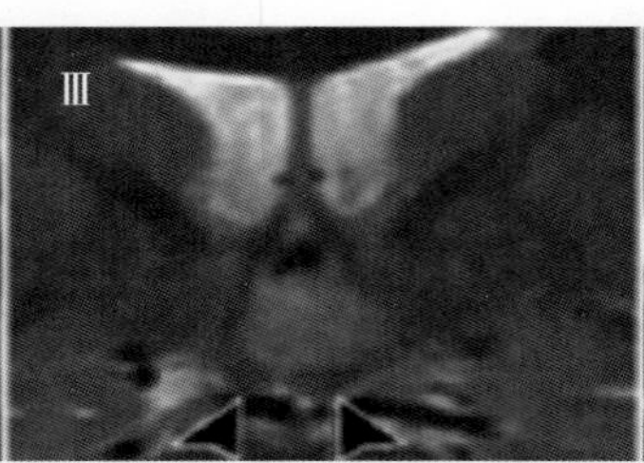

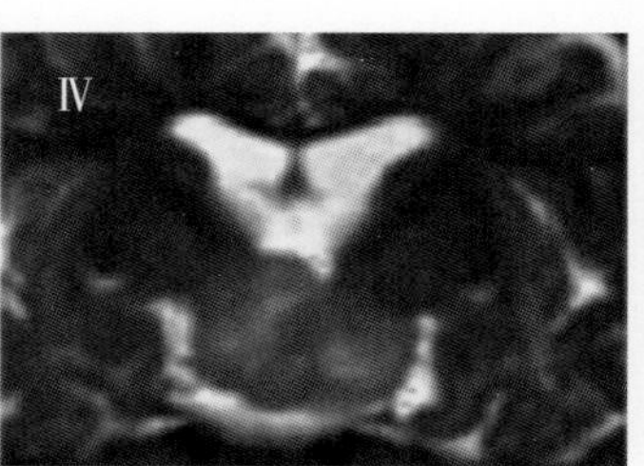

图 39.2 下丘脑错构瘤的 Delalande 分类：Ⅰ型为水平方向；Ⅱ型为垂直方向；Ⅲ型为水平和垂直；Ⅳ型为巨大错构瘤

Adapted from Endoscopic Treatment of Hypothalamic Hamartomas. *J Korean Neurosurg Soc*. 2017; 60(3): 294–300. doi: 10.3340/jkns.2017.0101.005, which is published under a Creative Commons License.

由于很难预测患者癫痫病程的严重程度，因此手术的最佳时机尚不清楚（Maixner，2006）。

预后

由于小脑发育不良性神经节细胞瘤病变的进行性生长，因此通常需要手术切除，但由于难以实现完全切除，所以复发很常见（Ozeren et al.，2014）。

结节性硬化症的肾并发症，如血管平滑肌脂肪瘤、肾囊肿和肾细胞癌为最常见的死亡原因（Curatolo and Maria，2013）。

Harvey 等在他们 29 例下丘脑错构瘤患者的病例系列中报告称，在 1~6 年（平均 2.5 年）的随访中，15 例患者获得了癫痫发作的控制，7 例患者随访 1~6 年（平均 2.5 年）的癫痫发作减少了 90%。手术并发症包括视束损伤、脑膜炎、交通性脑积水和缺血性丘脑梗死（Harvey et al.，2003）。

垂体细胞瘤、垂体颗粒细胞瘤和梭形细胞嗜酸细胞瘤

2007 年世卫组织对中枢神经系统肿瘤的分类描述了良性（WHO Ⅰ级）非腺瘤性垂体肿瘤，包括垂体细胞瘤、垂体颗粒细胞瘤（granular cell tumour，GCT）和梭形细胞嗜酸细胞瘤（spindle cell oncocytoma，SCO）（Louis et al.，2007；Covington et al.，2011）。

流行病学

非腺瘤性垂体瘤非常少见，最近的 meta 分析在文献中发现了 112 例病例（Covington et al.，2011）。诊断的平均年龄在 50~60 岁，垂体细胞瘤男性略占优势，垂体颗粒细胞瘤和梭形细胞嗜酸细胞瘤女性占优势（Covington et al.，2011；Pirayesh Islamian et al.，2012）。

病理

垂体细胞瘤起源于垂体细胞、垂体后叶及垂体柄部的特殊胶质细胞（Zygourakis et al.，2015）。组织学上，垂体细胞瘤的特征为由伸长的双极梭形细胞构成（Brat et al.，2007）。

垂体颗粒细胞瘤起源于垂体颗粒细胞，由多边形嗜酸性颗粒状细胞组成，由于胞浆内溶酶体丰富，PAS 呈强阳性（Orning et al.，2013）。梭形细胞嗜酸细胞瘤也来源于垂体细胞，其特征是梭形细胞与上皮样细胞交织成束状，超微结构分析显示线粒体聚集（Zygourakis et al.，2015）。

治疗

非腺瘤性垂体肿瘤患者最常见的症状是视觉障碍（例如双颞侧偏盲）（Covington et al.，2011）。其他症状包括头痛、疲乏以及与垂体机能减退有关的症状（如性欲减退）。尿崩症很少见。

磁共振成像上的几个特征有助于诊断（**图 39.3**）（Covington et al.，2011）：如为单纯鞍内病变且与垂体明显分离，则可考虑为垂体细胞瘤；如病变为鞍上，或鞍上与鞍内混合病变，且与垂体明显分离，则可考虑为垂体颗粒细胞瘤；如病变为鞍上与鞍内混合，但与垂体边界不清，则可考虑为梭形细胞嗜酸细胞瘤。与垂体颗粒细胞瘤和梭形细胞嗜酸细胞瘤相比，垂体细胞瘤在 T1 加权像中表现为同质而非异质性增强（Covington et al.，2011）。

实际上，这些病变可能很难与垂体腺瘤区分开，经蝶切除手术通常被认为安全有效（Zygourakis et al.，2015）。然而由于这些病变质地坚硬，且可能高度血管化，一些作者主张在选定手术的病例中进行术前栓塞（Wolfe et al.，2008）。辅助（药物）治疗的作用尚不清楚（Zygourakis et al.，2015）。

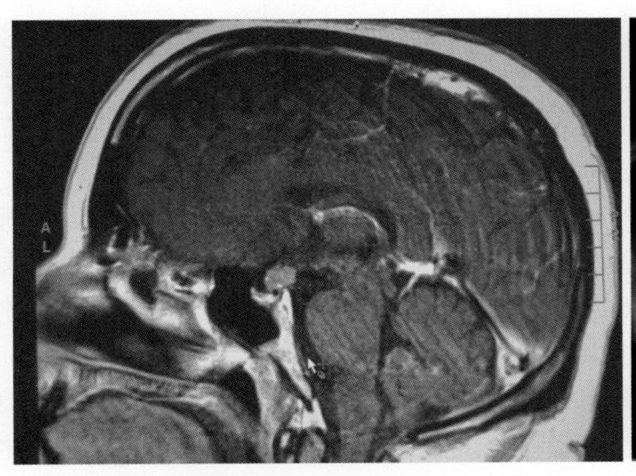

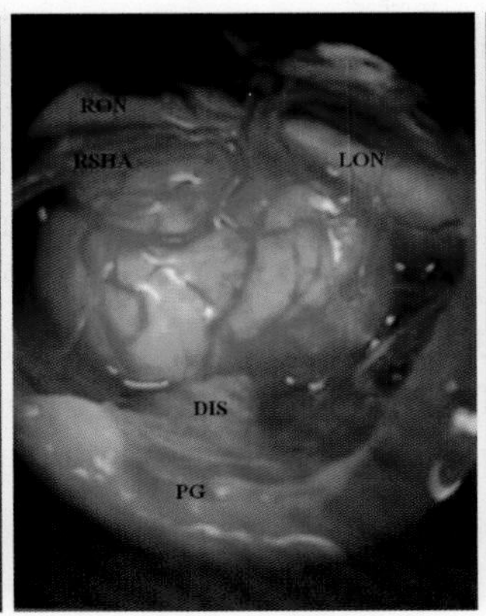

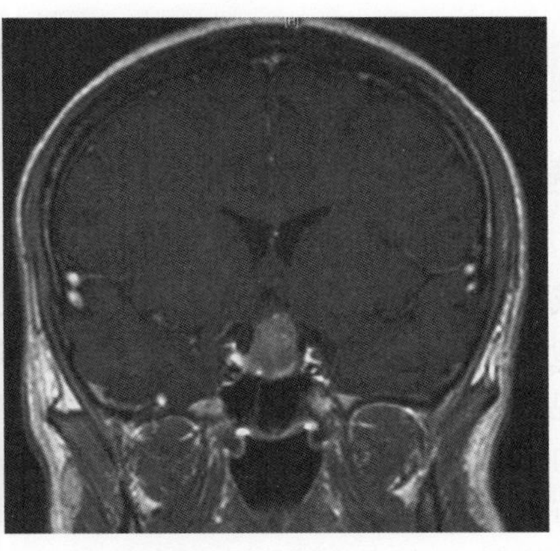

图 39.3　垂体颗粒细胞瘤（GCT）。（A）磁共振成像（T1 对比）显示垂体柄垂体颗粒细胞瘤。在这种情况下，肿瘤与垂体分离，并应考虑诊断。（B）经蝶骨内镜入路— 术中照片显示肿瘤与垂体分离，如磁共振成像所示。（C）垂体颗粒细胞瘤——在这种情况下无法与更常见的垂体腺瘤或更少见的原发性非腺瘤性垂体瘤（即垂体细胞瘤和梭形细胞嗜酸细胞瘤）区分开

预后

非腺瘤性垂体肿瘤通常为良性，手术切除可治愈。

神经节细胞瘤

神经节细胞瘤通常和神经节胶质瘤都被认为是起源于灰质的肿瘤。神经节细胞瘤与神经节胶质瘤的不同之处在于其缺乏胶质成分，由异常成熟的神经节细胞组成（WHO Ⅰ级）。

流行病学

其占所有脑瘤的 0.1%~0.5%，多发生于儿童和青年人中（Koeller and Henry，2001）。

病理

颅内不同部位发生率依次下降：颞叶、小脑、顶枕区、额叶、比邻三脑室的下丘脑区域、脊髓（Koeller and Henry，2001）。

术中涂片组织学显示神经节细胞内有泡状核以及显著的核仁。可通过大小不一、形成簇状并具有异常树突分支的肿瘤神经节细胞的存在来区分神经节细胞瘤和浸润性神经胶质瘤。

治疗

其表现为占位效应或癫痫发作。可能有相当长的病史，因为其术后预后良好，尤其要考虑该诊断。

非增强 CT 扫描显示高信号，无血管源性水肿。磁共振成像表现为 T1 加权像低信号强度，T2 加权像混合信号强度（Shin et al.，2002）。这些特征使神经节胶质瘤和神经节细胞瘤的鉴别变得困难。

预后

恶性转化并不常见，更容易在神经节胶质瘤中发现，这是由于胶质 / 星形细胞成分显示出细胞增多、有丝分裂和坏死（Adesina and Rauch，2010）。

副神经节瘤

来源于嗜铬细胞（自身来源于神经嵴细胞）的肿瘤被称为副神经节瘤，无论其解剖位置如何。肾上腺内副神经节瘤被称为嗜铬细胞瘤。肾上腺外副交感神经副神经节瘤最常见的部位是头颈部。最常见于颈内静脉和颈外静脉分支处的颈动脉体，其被称之为化学感受器瘤。颅内副神经节瘤发生在颈静脉孔区域，颈静脉球瘤是最为常用的描述。颈静脉球瘤由一个或多个主体组成，在骨性颈静脉球的内部。颈静脉球瘤可见于颈内静脉任何部位。

流行病学

副神经节瘤的发病率低于 1/3000（Gad et al.，2014）。生活在高海拔地区的人中更为常见，发病率为普通人群的 10 倍（Athanasiou et al.，2007）。可能与低氧诱导分泌儿茶酚胺的主要细胞增生有关（Knight et al.，2006）。平均发病年龄为 45 岁左右（Kotelis et al.，2009）。

颈静脉球瘤很少见，占头颈部肿瘤的 0.6%。女性是男性的 2~3 倍（Lee et al.，2002）。

病理

副神经节瘤具有遗传异质性。其可偶尔发生，或作为如多发性内分泌肿瘤Ⅱ型、神经纤维瘤病Ⅰ型和希佩尔 - 林道综合征等肿瘤综合征的一部分出现（Knight et al.，2006）。副神经节瘤具有四个不同的遗传基因易感性位点。其表明常染色体显性遗传与年龄以及低氧相关的外显率。其中三个基因的突变编码为琥珀酸脱氢酶复合体的亚基（Knight et al.，2006）。

副神经节瘤的组织学表现为主细胞，呈典型的被称为“细胞球”的假肺泡模式排列（Zellballen）（Athanasiou et al.，2007）。

颈静脉球瘤的组织学特征是由高血管性的间质中的上皮样细胞或主细胞组成，周围被薄层包膜包绕（Guild，1953）。

治疗

化学感受器瘤患者通常表现为颈部外侧肿块，伴有或不伴有后组脑神经受累（8~12 对）（Knight et al.，2006）。

颈静脉球瘤生长缓慢，诊断前可能有明显的潜伏期。体征和症状包括单侧耳聋、耳鸣、声音嘶哑、吞咽困难、头痛以及后组脑神经麻痹（Watkins et al.，1994）。10%~20% 的病例可能为多发，虽然通常为良性，但肝、肺、淋巴结和脾的局部侵袭和转移均已被报道。术前检查应包括磁共振成像和 CT 扫描，以确定骨受累程度。

与嗜铬细胞瘤和肾上腺外交感神经副神经节瘤相比，头颈部副神经节瘤很少产生大量儿茶酚胺（Chen et al.，2010）。从神经内分泌角度来看，这使得这些患者的手术选择变得不那么具有挑战性。

影像学检查之所以是手术成功之关键，是由于化学感受器瘤的定位在技术上具有挑战性，且活检具有危险性。肿瘤增大通常会挤压颈内与颈外动脉，但不会导致其管腔变窄（Wieneke and Smith，2009）。鉴别诊断包括迷走神经鞘瘤和神经纤维瘤、迷走神经球瘤以及淋巴结肿块。淋巴结不是典型的高血管性，迷走神经球瘤好发于头侧，迷走神经肿块趋向于将两条颈动脉血管挤压到一起而非分开（图 39.4）。

直径高达 10 cm 的大肿瘤更有可能包裹颈动脉。辅助放疗在这种情况下则可用于缩小肿瘤以提高肿瘤的切除率。术中可进行颈内动脉重建，并进行端到端吻合（Gad et al.，2014）。

历史上，颈静脉球瘤的治疗方法始终是显微外科切除。据报道，肿瘤生长的平均倍增时间为 4 年或更长，但肿瘤侵袭性及老年患者处理效果则可能较差（Kemeny，2009）。切除方法取决于肿瘤大小和部位，且可能包括耳科和神经外科共同切除（Watkins et al.，1994）。

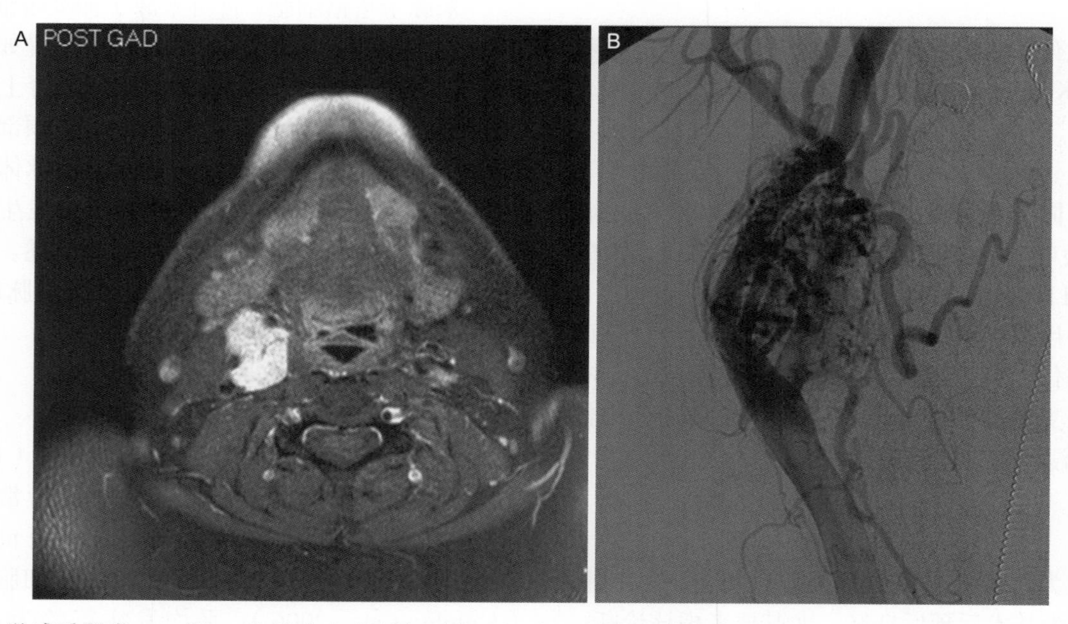

图 39.4 化学感受器瘤。一例 59 岁的女士出现右耳痛。（A）磁共振成像轴位 T1W 显示出可将副神经节瘤与神经鞘瘤和神经纤维瘤等病变相区分的颈内与颈外动脉扩张。（B）术前栓塞证实右咽升动脉分支粗大，向肿瘤有广泛供血，切除后无并发症。ECA，颈外动脉；ICA，颈内动脉；IJV，颈内静脉

立体定向放射外科疗法在降低对颅底关键结构辐射损伤方面的明显优势，必须基于与其局限性之间的相互平衡。放射外科疗法的相对禁忌证包括 3~4 cm 的大肿瘤、颅底边界不清的大肿瘤。目前尚无直接比较放射外科疗法与显微外科疗法的随机对照试验，但对 19 项回顾性研究的 meta 分析表明放射外科疗法有效，在 335 例患者的联合样本中有 95% 的患者实现了临床控制（Guss et al.，2011）。

预后

与化学感受器瘤切除术相关的死亡率和发病率分别为 1% 和 33%（Gad et al.，2014）。脑神经损伤、切口血肿和缺血性卒中均可能发生。虽然淋巴结远处转移的风险较低，但仍有必要对可能的淋巴结转移进行随访。残留病变也可通过放疗加以控制。

颈静脉球瘤为典型的惰性肿瘤，由于治疗目标是长期肿瘤控制使其复发率降低，因此果断使用立体定向放射疗法和现代显微外科疗法可实现此目标（Fayad et al.，2009）。

朗格汉斯细胞组织细胞增生症

朗格汉斯细胞组织细胞增生症（Langerhans cell histiocytosis，LCH）的前身为组织细胞增多症 X，其为一组异质性肿瘤，通常影响骨骼，特征为病理细胞的克隆性增殖，具有朗格汉斯细胞的特征（Abla et al.，2010）。朗格汉斯细胞源于骨髓的树突状细胞（抗原递呈细胞），通常存在于淋巴结和皮肤中。

术语“嗜酸性肉芽肿”已用于描述单个朗格汉斯细胞组织细胞增生症病变，“Hand-Schüller-Christian 病”用于描述一个系统内的多个朗格汉斯细胞组织细胞增生症病变，“Abt-Letter-Siwe 病”用于描述多个系统内的多个朗格汉斯细胞组织细胞增生症病变（Arico et al.，2003）。

流行病学

朗格汉斯细胞组织细胞增生症通常见于儿童，估计发病率为每年每百万 4~4.5 例（Chaudhary et al.，2013）。

病理

朗格汉斯细胞组织细胞增生症的病因尚不清楚。有数据表明，种系突变可能使某些患者易患朗格汉斯细胞组织细胞增生症。大约 1% 的朗格汉斯细胞组织细胞增生症患者有一名受影响的亲属。此外，对双胞胎的研究发现，单卵双胞胎与双卵双胞胎的一致性比率较高（分别为 92% 和 10%）（Abla et al.，2010）。也有数据表明，如 HHV6 病毒可能导致朗格汉斯细胞组织细胞增生症，然而大多数研究均未能证实此种病毒的相关性（Abla et al.，2010）。

朗格汉斯细胞组织细胞增生症在组织学上的诊断取决于病变内是否存在朗格汉斯细胞伴随巨噬细胞、T 淋巴细胞、嗜酸性粒细胞以及多核巨细胞。这些朗格汉斯细胞可通过免疫组织化学上的 CD1a 或电子显微镜下的伯贝克（Birbeck）颗粒来确定（Abla et al.，2010）。后者现可能更容易通过一种诱导伯贝克颗粒形成的内吞受体 langerin（CD207）的免疫组织化学染色来鉴别（Valladeau et al.，2000）。

与朗格汉斯细胞组织细胞增生症相关的病变最常见于骨内，尤其是颅骨。中枢神经系统内已对三种病变模式作了描述（Grois et al.，2010）：

1. 脑结缔组织内界限分明的肉芽肿，趋向于脑室周围器官。
2. 非肉芽肿性神经退行性病变主要影响脑干和小脑。
3. 垂体柄的肉芽肿，侵犯下丘脑，表现为周围脑弥漫性浸润。

治疗

临床症状和体征取决于朗格汉斯细胞组织细胞增生症病变的部位及性质。颅骨单一病变是朗格汉斯细胞组织细胞增生症最常见的表现。累及下丘脑 - 垂体轴可导致 25% 的患者尿崩症（Grois et al.，2010）。非肉芽肿性神经退行性病变可导致高度易变的表现，从轻微反射异常和轻微认知缺陷，到明显的共济失调或行为障碍。

CT 扫描和磁共振成像分别用于检查颅骨与脑病变（Grois et al.，2010）。头颅 CT 扫描可显示具有特征性的边缘倾斜的颅骨内病变。脑部磁共振成像可显示垂体柄增大，并可能延伸至下丘脑（图 39.5）。磁共振成像也可显示放射性退行性变，T2 加权像呈对称性高信号改变，T1 加权像呈低或高信号，有时基底节和脑干也有信号改变。

指导朗格汉斯细胞组织细胞增生症决策的依据是有限的。单灶性颅骨病变通过简单的病灶刮除术甚至组织活检都可以提供诊断结果，且通常可治愈（Abla et al.，2010）。中枢神经系统病变导致尿崩症的治疗可能包括类固醇或化疗（Grois et al.，2010）。手术切除和放疗也被用于下丘脑 - 垂体轴以外区域的病变。

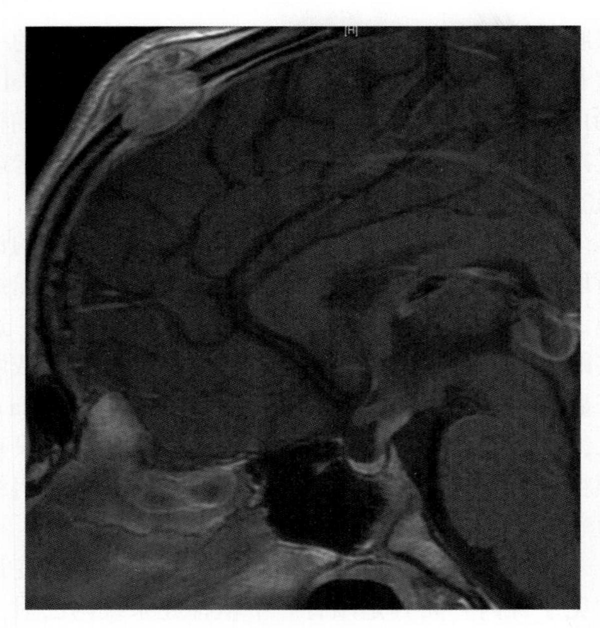

图 39.5 朗格汉斯细胞组织细胞增生症（LCH）。一例前额有肿块并伴有慢性便秘的 14 岁男孩。随后被诊断为尿崩症和生长激素缺乏症，磁共振成像（T1 钆增强造影）显示垂体柄增厚、增强，颅骨溶解性病变伴增强。头骨病变的活检诊断为朗格汉斯细胞组织细胞增生症。根据朗格汉斯细胞组织细胞增生症 4 期方案，进一步检查发现了肠道和化疗的关系

预后

朗格汉斯细胞组织细胞增生症的预后高度可变。病变局限于单系统的患者，通常具有较高的自发缓解率和良好的预后。多系统受累患者的预后可能非常不理想；累及高危器官（肝、脾或骨髓）的患者在最初的 6 周内治疗无效，死亡率高达 35%。

结节病

结节病为一种多系统炎症性肉芽肿疾病，通常会影响肺部（Joseph and Scolding,, 2007）。这种涉及中枢神经系统的症状，被称为神经鞘瘤病，是此疾病少见但严重的并发症。

流行病学

每 10 万人中就有 40 人患有结节病（Joseph and Scolding,, 2007）。仅有不到 10% 的结节病患者表现出神经系统疾病的症状和体征，尽管尸检研究表明有相当比例的患者患有亚临床的症状。其通常于 20~40 岁被诊断出，某些种族群体，如北欧人和西非人，罹患此种疾病的风险要高得多。

病理

结节病的确切病因尚不清楚。遗传学研究表明，Ⅰ类人类白细胞抗原（HLA）-B8 抗原和由 HLA-DRB1 和 DQB1 等位基因编码的Ⅱ类人类白细胞抗原可能使某些患者易患此病（Vargas and Stern，2010）。某些环境诱因也被提出，包括真菌、金属、燃木火炉、复印机墨粉以及传染病，如结核分枝杆菌和痤疮丙酸杆菌。

组织学上结节病以非干酪性肉芽肿为特征。神经系统结节病最常见于大脑底部的软脑膜。脑实质扩张可能会发生，通常与周围星形胶质细胞活化和胶质增生有关。

治疗

神经系统结节病最常见的症状为脑神经麻痹，50%~75% 患者中可见。此种麻痹通常可能由基底脑膜炎引起，但也可能是由于神经肉芽肿或颅内压升高所致。癫痫发作是神经系统结节病的另一种常见的表现形式，通常反映存在肿块性病变，发生于约 10% 的患者中（Joseph and Scolding，2007）。

增强磁共振成像可能会显示软脑膜钆强化。约 40% 的患者可见多发性脑白质病变（Joseph and Scolding，2007）。也可以是大的肿块，可以是类肿瘤病变。腰椎穿刺可显示蛋白升高（>2 g/L），轻度淋巴细胞增多，可能还有寡克隆区带。全身检查也可提供结节病依据，包括血液检查（血清血管紧张素转化酶、红细胞沉降率和钙升高），以及胸部 X 射线或胸部 CT 扫描检查（肺门和纵隔肿大）。

结节病的一线治疗方法是皮质类固醇（Joseph and Scolding，2007; Vargas and Stern，2010）。相当高的发病率与长期使用皮质类固醇有关，尤其是在糖尿病、高血压或骨质疏松症患者中。为此，包括甲氨蝶呤和羟氯喹的“节约类固醇”免疫抑制剂也被用于治疗结节病，尽管这些制剂也存在并发症风险。耐药结节病患者的一系列病例报道了放疗的成功（Bruns et al.，2004）。手术的作用仅限于可疑病例的活检，以及如脑积水等并发症的治疗。

预后

神经系统结节病的自发缓解已被报道，但非常少见；疾病恶化时，大多数患者需要长期随访并接受治疗。

肿瘤样多发性硬化

多发性硬化症（multiple sclerosis，MS）是一种影响中枢神经系统的自身免疫性疾病，以脱髓鞘和轴突损失为特征。肿瘤样多发性硬化（tumefactive multiple sclerosis，TMS）描述了直径大于2 cm的多发性硬化病变的存在，通常为孤立性，可能被误认为是其他占位性病变，如影像学上表现为脑肿瘤（Hardy and Chataway，2013）。

流行病学

肿瘤样多发性硬化的患病率估计为每1000例多发性硬化症中的1~2例（Hardy and Chataway，2013）。通常于20~40岁被诊断出。

病理

肿瘤样多发性硬化的确切病因尚不清楚。肿瘤样脱髓鞘病变在多发性硬化症以外的疾病中也有报道，包括人体免疫缺陷病毒等病毒感染，以及他克莫司等药物治疗的副作用。肿瘤样脱髓鞘病变在组织学上与其他多发性硬化症变无明显区别。活动性病变包括脱髓鞘区域的反应性星形胶质细胞以及含髓鞘的泡沫巨噬细胞（Hardy and Chataway，2013）。宏观上，病变通常边界分明，好发于额叶与顶叶（Altintas et al.，2012）。

治疗

肿瘤样多发性硬化的表现通常类似于危险性高的占位性病变，包括颅内压升高、癫痫发作和局灶性神经功能缺损的症状和体征。头痛和呕吐在儿童中尤为常见（Altintas et al.，2012）。

增强磁共振成像可用于研究肿瘤样多发性硬化。直径可达12 cm的病变已有报道，但大多范围在2~6 cm（Lucchinetti et al.，2008）。其通常伴有脑水肿，但通常少于恶性肿瘤。大多数病变在钆剂的作用下增强，且环形强化，环形强化反映了远离更慢性非强化核心的活动性炎症（Hardy and Chataway，2013）的环状（**图**39.6）（通常为闭合，但对于肿瘤样多发性硬化，开环征具有高度特殊性）。

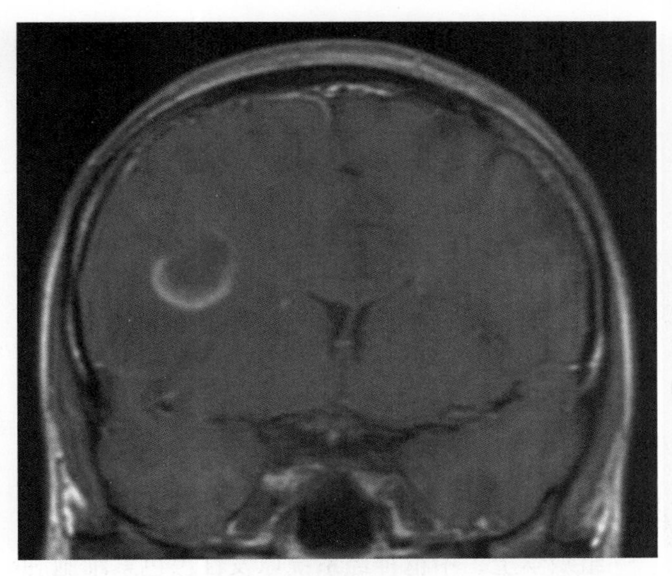

图39.6 肿瘤样多发性硬化斑块。“开环征”对多发性硬化症相对特异。增强部分被认为代表脱髓鞘的推进前沿，因此多位于病变的白质侧。因此，环的开口部分通常指向灰质。立体定向活检证实了多发性硬化症的诊断

非增强头颅CT平扫可能有助于区分肿瘤样多发性硬化和恶性肿瘤；增强磁共振成像大脑中的高信号区域、非增强头颅CT平扫的低密度区域更可能代表肿瘤样多发性硬化（Kim et al.，2009）。腰椎穿刺可显示不匹配的寡克隆区带（存在于脑脊液，但不存在于血清中）。全身性检查对于排除脉管炎、肉芽肿、感染或恶性肿瘤等其他病状也很重要。其中包括血液检查和胸部、腹部以及骨盆CT扫描（Hardy and Chataway，2013）。

治疗采用大剂量皮质类固醇（Altintas et al.，2012）。血浆置换对皮质类固醇无效的患者而言似乎不失为一种合理的二线选择。抗CD20 B细胞单克隆抗体（利妥昔单抗）也已获得了一些成功使用（Fan et al.，2012）。“对症治疗”如β干扰素、醋酸格拉替雷也可能有助于降低复发的风险，但必须考虑不良反应的风险。手术的作用仅限于在诊断不确定的情况下进行活检，以及治疗如脑积水并发症。

预后

总体来说，肿瘤样多发性硬化患者的预后似乎并不比其他多发性硬化症患者差。事实上，在最大的肿瘤样多发性硬化患者队列中，长期预后优于与典型多发性硬化症匹配的对照组（Lucchinetti et al.，2008）。

原发性中枢神经系统黑色素瘤和黑色素细胞瘤

中枢神经系统原发性黑色素细胞肿瘤是一系列以软脑膜黑色素细胞克隆性增殖为特征的肿瘤，这些黑色素细胞衍生于胚胎早期的神经嵴（Liubinas et al.，2010）。这些肿瘤包括弥漫性软脑膜黑色素细胞

增多症或黑色素瘤病、黑色素细胞瘤以及原发性恶性黑色素瘤；目前的讨论仅限于黑色素细胞瘤和原发性恶性黑色素瘤。脑膜黑色素细胞浓度分布最多处为脊髓和颅后窝，而这些部位肿瘤正是肿瘤最常见的部位（Goldgeier et al.，1984）。

流行病学

黑色素细胞瘤的发病率约为一千万分之一，原发性中枢神经系统黑色素瘤的发病率为两千万分之一。发病高峰出现在第五个十年，且轻微肥胖女性发病率略高（Liubinas et al.，2010）。

病理

组织学上，中枢神经系统原发性黑色素细胞肿瘤的诊断依赖于肿瘤细胞或相关巨噬细胞中黑色素的识别（Liubinas et al.，2010）。黑色素细胞瘤虽是一种不侵犯周围大脑的低级别病变，但也有人认为黑色素细胞瘤是中度级别（Bra t et al.，1999；Navas et al.，2009）。原发性中枢神经系统黑色素瘤与其他部位的黑色素瘤相似，可表现为侵袭性、出血或坏死。宏观上，黑色素细胞瘤和原发性中枢神经系统黑色素瘤通常为轴外的孤立性病变。

治疗

黑色素细胞瘤和原发性中枢神经系统黑色素瘤的表现是包括颅内压升高、癫痫发作和局灶性神经功能缺损的症状与体征的其他占位性病变。必须进行皮肤科和眼科检查以及 CT 扫描分期，以排除远处病灶的主要来源。

神经影像学显示存在可疑病变。脑部 CT 扫描通常显示等密度或高密度病变，伴有或不伴有异常钙化（图 39.7），对比增强。磁共振成像可显示异常的肿瘤病变，T1 加权像高信号，T2 加权像低信号，均匀增强。

黑色素细胞瘤和原发性中枢神经系统黑色素瘤的治疗是完全手术切除。不完全切除的黑色素细胞瘤可能需要放疗，但恶性黑色素瘤相对而言具有抗辐射性。化疗的作用尚不清楚，但已被用作辅助治疗以及复发患者的治疗（Cornejo et al.，2013）。

预后

黑色素细胞瘤通常为良性，手术切除可治愈。而原发性中枢神经系统黑色素瘤则预后差。尽管原发性中枢神经系统黑色素瘤的严重程度不如转移性黑色素瘤，但可能容易局部复发或全身扩散，平均生存期约为 6 年（Cornejo et al.，2013）。

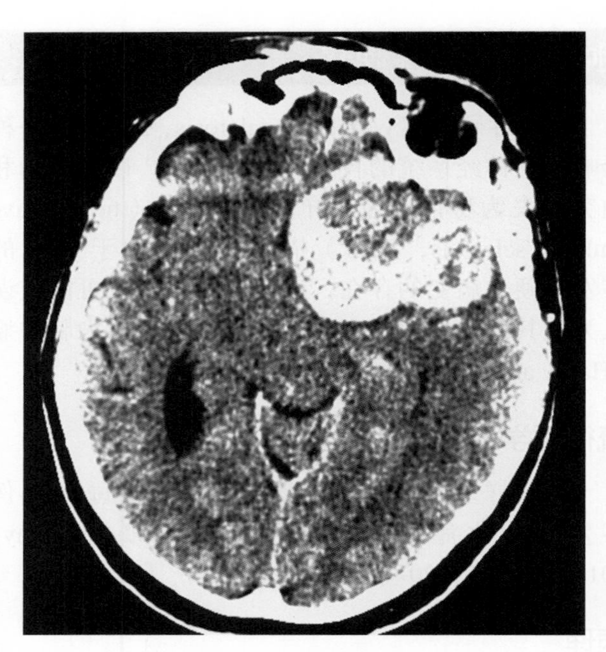

图 39.7 黑色素细胞瘤。一例表现为头痛的中年女性。皮肤科和眼科检查均无显著变化。非增强 CT 扫描显示一个混合密度的病变，并伴有异常钙化，表明了病变长期存在。分期 CT 扫描未显示其他部位的病变，该女性接受了完整的手术切除。组织病理学证实为黑色素细胞瘤，且术后 5 年情况良好

颅内脂肪瘤

流行病学

这些肿瘤极为少见，发病率估计为所有颅内肿瘤的 0.06%~0.46%（Truwit and Barkovich，1990）。然而，由于成像技术的日益广泛应用，早期的研究可能低估了其真实发病率。其分布似乎无任何年龄或性别差异（Eghwrudjakpor et al.，1992）。已报道的最小年龄病例为 3 天大的儿童，最大年龄病例为 91 岁妇女（Cascino et al.，1958；Yalcin and Fragoyannis，1966）。

病理

颅内脂肪瘤是 Rokitansky 在 1856 年尸检后意外发现并首次描述（Rokitansky，1856）。Harvey Cushing 于 1922 年任命 Merrill Sosman 为 Brigham 医院的放射科医生，他首次用气脑造影术对患者进行了诊断（Sosman，1946）。这些病变被认为是由蛛网膜下池发育过程中胚胎脑膜原发性分化不良导致的先天性畸形（Verga，1929）。它们可能会干扰其所在位置附近的皮质发育（Yildiz et al.，2006）。最常见的是它们与胼胝体发育不良或缺失有关（Macpherson et al., 1987)。报道的其他异常包括，囊状或梭形动脉瘤、动静脉畸形、矢状缝和镰状窦未闭（Futami et al., 1992；Sasaki et al., 1996）。宏观上看，它们不会产生占位效应，因此神经和血管可以穿过（Yildiz et al., 2006）。

治疗

45% 病例的脂肪瘤位于脑半球间、胼胝体周围。它们也常位于中脑背侧。很少有人在与癫痫相关的外侧裂中报道过这种疾病（Yildiz et al., 2006），参见**图** 39.8。

偶发性病变最为常见，在 CT 扫描上呈低密度，在 T1 和 T2 加权像上都呈高信号。将其与常出现在中线的皮样囊肿相鉴别很重要（Yildiz et al., 2006）。

预后

脂肪瘤是进展缓慢的病变，因此，即便是保守治疗也预后良好。对于药物难治性癫痫发作的患者可考虑手术，但由于肿瘤与周边神经关系密切，全切除肿瘤手术是有危险的（Yilmaz et al., 2006）。

争议

及时准确的诊断是脑瘤患者治疗的指导原则（Omuro et al., 2006）。对于少见的脑部病变进行诊断本身就具有挑战性，但本章强调了在研究此类病变时的几个非常重要的因素（**专栏** 39.1）。鉴于此类病变的少见性，其治疗手段也始终存在争议。并不

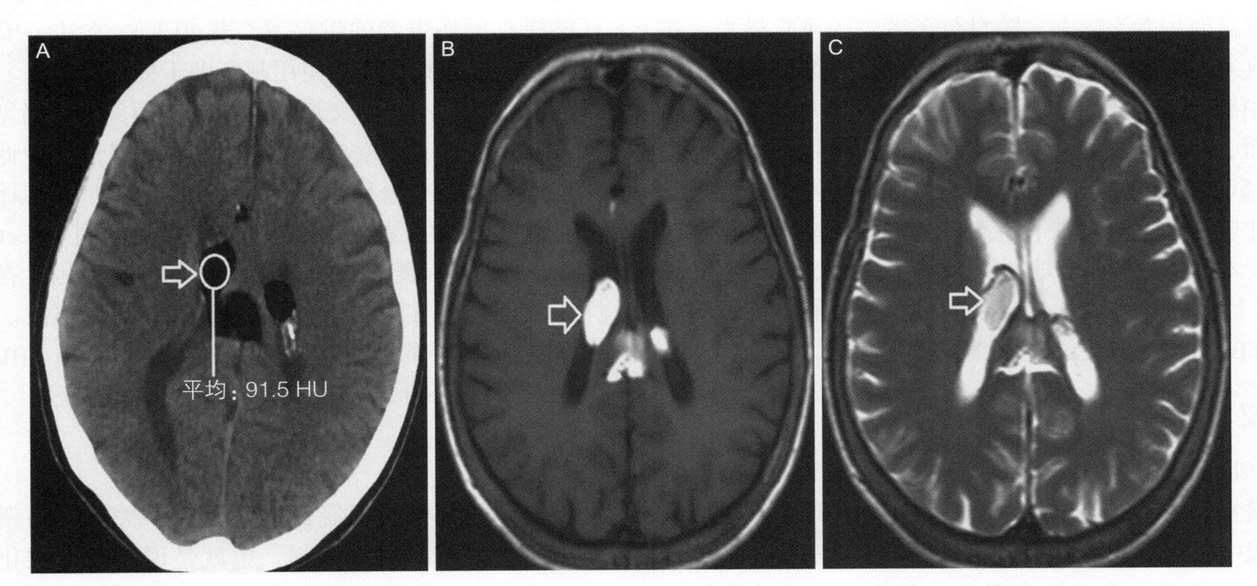

图 39.8 颅内脂肪瘤。（A）CT 扫描显示侧脑室与第三脑室的同质低密度病变，约 100 个 Hounsfield 单位。（B）T1 加权磁共振成像显示高强度肿块病变。（C）T2 加权磁共振成像也显示高强度肿块病变

专栏 39.1	治疗少见脑占位时应考虑的因素
病史	年轻人发病 有轻微或短暂的神经系统症状史、有家族史 自身免疫或炎症性疾病的个人
检查	皮疹 裂隙灯检查结果
研究	避免凭经验使用类固醇，除非有显著的肿块效应 脑、脊髓磁共振成像 腰椎穿刺，无禁忌状况下 HIV 抗体和梅毒血清学 全身 CT 扫描 活检

意外的是缺乏随机对照试验来指导手术决策，因此建议主要是基于病例系列报道。

延伸阅读、参考文献

扫描书末二维码获取。

第十篇　神经创伤和重症监护

第40章　颅脑损伤的流行病学及预后

Nabeel Alshafai・Andrew Maas 著
刘伟明 译，吴量 审校

引言

创伤性脑损伤（traumatic brain injury，TBI）是造成死亡和残疾的主要原因。在中、低收入国家，随着机械化的增加，TBI 发病率逐渐增加。然而，弱势道路使用者（行人、骑自行车者）的风险最大。在高收入国家，儿童、青年和老者的 TBI 发病率最高；其中跌倒是老年患者 TBI 发病率显著增加的原因。然而，TBI 是一种影响所有年龄段的疾病，被称为"沉默的流行病"。了解 TBI 的流行病学对制订医疗保健规划和适当开展有针对性的预防活动至关重要。

本章将总结全球 TBI 流行病学状况，并反思 TBI 给健康经济和社会带来的负担。我们将回顾当前的 TBI 分类系统、预后评测及预测模型。

定义

目前 TBI 有多种定义。这对精准诊断带来混淆和模糊，导致在患者队列对比中产生困难。在临床实践中，可能很难从症状上区分轻度 TBI、酒精中毒或药物滥用。在老年患者中，跌倒伴头皮挫伤可能继发于原发性心脏事件，这种情况很难在短暂性意识丧失、心脏事件引起的眩晕或轻度 TBI 之间进行鉴别。此外，有些患者因症状出现较晚，会在确立诊断的病史中引入主观因素。因此，迫切需要客观指标来确认 TBI 的诊断或排除标准。各种各样的新手段，包括生物标志物、眼球运动和平衡能力，都显示出潜在应用价值，但仍需要在队列研究中验证。

世界卫生组织将 TBI 定义为除非法药品、酒精及其类似物、药物或其他治疗有关的损伤外（Andelic et al.，2012），由外部机械能对头部造成的急性损伤（Carroll et al.，2004）。

TBI 也被定义为："由外力引起的脑功能改变或有其他脑病理学证据"（Menon et al.，2010）。TBI 已经取代了旧的术语"头部损伤"，除了单纯影响头皮、颅骨和面部的损伤，它强调了脑损伤的重要性（Roozenbeek et al.，2013）。

病因学

机动车是最常见的"杀手"。现已证明采取预防措施，可有效地减少道路交通事故相关的 TBI 数量，并能提高创伤患者的生存率（**表 40.1**）。立法、安全带、安全气囊和头盔的使用都有助于提高安全性。预防活动应针对不了解交通风险的弱势道路使用者（例如体弱多病者或儿童）以及车辆司机。虽然在中低收入国家，道路交通事故仍然是脑创伤最常见的原因，但在欧洲，跌倒是目前脑创伤更为常见原因（Peeters et al.，2015）。**表 40.1** 概述了 TBI 的常见原因。在美国，火器伤害在 1990 年首次超过道路交通事故。在战争情况下，简易爆炸装置造成的爆震伤是 TBI 的常见原因。**表 40.2** 列出了减少 TBI 影响的方法。

发病率

当我们分析当前流行病学研究中关于发病率的研究时，发现了很多限制，也就是说缺乏标准化的流行病学报告、年龄标准化的发病率、针对轻度和中度 TBI 的数据，以及较低和中等收入国家的数据。

表 40.1　TBI 常见原因

TBI 的主要原因
道路交通事故（44%~80%）
跌倒[$]（12%~55%）
暴力[@]（7%~17%）、火器伤（>50% 自杀）（Aarabi et al.，2001）
工作和运动（4%）
其他

[$] 最近，这是北欧、美国和澳大利亚等地致伤的主要原因，特别是在儿童和老年人（>75 岁）中。

[@] 高风险人群：男性、年轻人、非白人（56% 为非裔美国人）、受伤时失业、未婚、非法药物使用史、曾受法律制裁、贫困和低教育水平。

表 40.2 减少 TBI 的影响

减少 TBI 的影响
严格限定血液酒精浓度
使用安全带
独立的儿童约束法律
严格执行车速限制
摩托车驾驶员强制佩戴头盔
更快沟通以提升临床诊治
更好的创伤救治系统
提高 CT 扫描可及性
改善重症监护病房（ICU）设施和救治
其他

这些挑战需要在未来的研究中加以解决。需要记住的是，同一个患者多发性创伤和反复头部创伤（初次和后续多次头部创伤）经常被忽视，这对于理解此类患者的晚期预后至关重要。

在对过去 24 年发表的 28 项欧洲研究系统回顾发现，每年住院的总发病率为每 10 万人 262 例（Peeters et al.，2015）。最近新西兰一项基于人群的研究发现有较高的发病率，为每 10 万人 790 例（Feigin et al.，2013）。这个研究报告的高发病率与基于住院数据的低发病率之间差异表明后一种方法严重低估了 TBI 总负担。各国间报告的发病率差异不太可能反映实际差异，相反可能是由于病例确定、使用定义变量以及在某些情况下侧重于不同人群所造成的。

患病率

患病率是指某一特定时间点（点患病率）或某一特定时期（期患病率）存活的脑创伤患者总数（现有和新病例）。在 2013 年的一项对 15 项流行病学研究进行的系统评价中（Frost et al.，2013）（25134 成人），作者发现有 12% 的患者经历过伴发意识丧失的 TBI（男性的风险是女性的两倍）。McKinlay 等观察儿童年龄组（高风险），发现超过 30% 的人在 25 岁之前至少经历过一次 TBI（McKinlay et al.，2008）。这些数字与美国疾病控制中心（Center for Disease Control，CDC）报告的估计数字相比似乎偏高，美国目前生活着 530 万人 TBI 患者。

死亡率

欧洲的平均死亡率为 10.5~11.7/10 万人，变化范围较大，从 3.0~21.8/10 万不等，主要由病例组合决定（Peeters et al.，2015；Majdan et al.，2017）。**表 40.3** 概述了美国和欧洲报告的死亡率。尽管世界范围内的脑创伤发病率上升，但一些研究表明，在发达国家，由于遵循循证指南和建议，TBI 的死亡率有所下降（Lu et al.，2005；Gerber et al.，2013）。然而，在比较过去 30 年的观察性研究报告的死亡率时，并没有发现生存率的提高（Rosenfeld et al.，2012）。

另一个重要的问题是，“急性期死亡率”并不是 TBI 患者唯一的影响：TBI 患者过早死亡的长期风险显著升高。这包括：自杀，随后的伤害和攻击，甚至在伤后 6 个月对社会人口学和家庭因素进行调整之后（Fazel et al.，2014）。TBI 住院患者康复后，平均预期寿命缩短 9 年（McMillan et al.，2011）。这取决于患者年龄和受伤严重程度。研究发现，经历 TBI 后，至少在 13 年内，每年的死亡率增加 7 倍（McMillan et al.，2011）。

TBI 的分类

TBI 的分类方法多种多样，包括根据机制、临床严重程度、损伤负担、结构损伤程度、初始预后风险和预期预后进行分类。**表 40.4** 列出了这些可以用于分类的不同领域。我们建议 TBI 的分类不应局限于单一的领域，而应纳入多维视角。目前，没有这样的多维综合分类系统存在，但这一目标正在进行

表 40.3 全世界 TBI 后的死亡率

区域	死亡率 /10 万	参考文献
美国	17.1（2010）	CDC，2015；Rutland-Brown et al.，2006
西弗吉尼亚州	23.6（1989—1999）	Adekoya and Majumder，2004
欧盟	10.5~11.2	Peeters et al.，2015；Majdan et al.，2016
- 奥地利	12.6	Majdan et al.，2016
- 丹麦	7.3	Majdan et al.，2016
- 法国	11.5	Majdan et al.，2016
- 德国	8.3	Majdan et al.，2016
- 意大利	7.6	Majdan et al.，2016
- 挪威	10.4	Sundstrøm et al.，2007
- 瑞典	9.2~9.5	Sundstrøm et al.，2007；Majdan et al.，2016
巴西	5.1~26.2	De Almeida et al.，2016；Koizumi et al.，2000
中国	12.99	Cheng et al.，2017；Jiang et al.，2019

大规模观察研究（Maas et al.，2017）。

损伤机制

不同机制造成不同类型损伤。在闭合性 TBI 中，道路交通事故中的加速和减速力可能导致患者出现典型的弥漫性轴索损伤。摔倒时，头部撞到坚硬表面，通常会导致局灶性脑挫裂伤。高速子弹造成的穿透伤，通常会沿弹道造成大面积损伤，转化的动能会引起远距离脑实质损伤。在挤压伤中，能量在很大程度上被颅骨吸收，并不是所有的能量都传递到大脑。因此，颅骨损伤可能是广泛性的，而脑损伤可能不那么严重。在爆炸损伤中，几种机制共同损害大脑。这些伤害包括原发性伤害（由于压力波），次级伤害（被爆炸物碎片和其他物体碰撞），第三级伤害（被爆炸抛落时头部撞到物体）或第四级伤害（热和有毒伤害）。

临床严重程度

TBI 临床表现多样，如头部撞击后迅速出现定向障碍或意识改变，可伴有或不伴有遗忘，直至完全失去意识和昏迷。格拉斯哥昏迷量表（Glasgow Coma Scale，GCS）是世界上常用的评估意识水平的工具（Teasdale and Jennett，1974）。在 GCS 评估中，记录观察到的三个部分（眼、运动、言语量表）反应。为方便分类及研究，总分由 3~15 分不等；但是，就单个患者而言，分离 GCS 的各维度的重要性再怎么强调也不过分。GCS 量表由完全不同的几个部分（E、V、M）组成，每个“分数”都是定性的和不连续的（例如，从 M2 到 M3 的变化与从 M4 到 M5 的变化没有任何关系，更不用说从 E3 到 E4 了）。值得注意的是，特别是在损伤早期，GCS 可能会随着时间而改变，可作为复苏或早期恢复的指标。对 GCS 一个或多个部分的准确评估可能会被酒精或药物使用、院前镇静、麻醉和插管情况所掩盖（Balestreri et al.，2004；Stocchetti et al.，2004）。事实上，文献综述揭

表 40.4 TBI 分类的不同方法

损伤机制	临床严重程度
• 闭合性 • 穿透性 • 挤压 • 爆炸 • 组合性	• GCS 3~8：重度 • GCS 9~13：中度 • GCS 14~15：轻度
损伤负担（AIS 和 ISS）*	**结构损伤：CT 分类**
1：轻微 2：中度 3：重度不危及生命 4：重度危及生命 5：危重 6：几乎不可存活	• 弥漫性损伤 I • 弥漫性损伤 II • 弥漫性损伤 III • 弥漫性损伤 IV • 可去除占位病变 • 不可去除占位病变
预后风险	
CRASH 和 IMPACT 预测模型	

* 每个身体部位的 AIS：外部（皮肤）、头部 / 颈部（包括脑损伤）、胸部、腹部 / 骨盆内容物、脊柱和四肢

ISS：损伤严重程度评分（Baker et al.，1974）

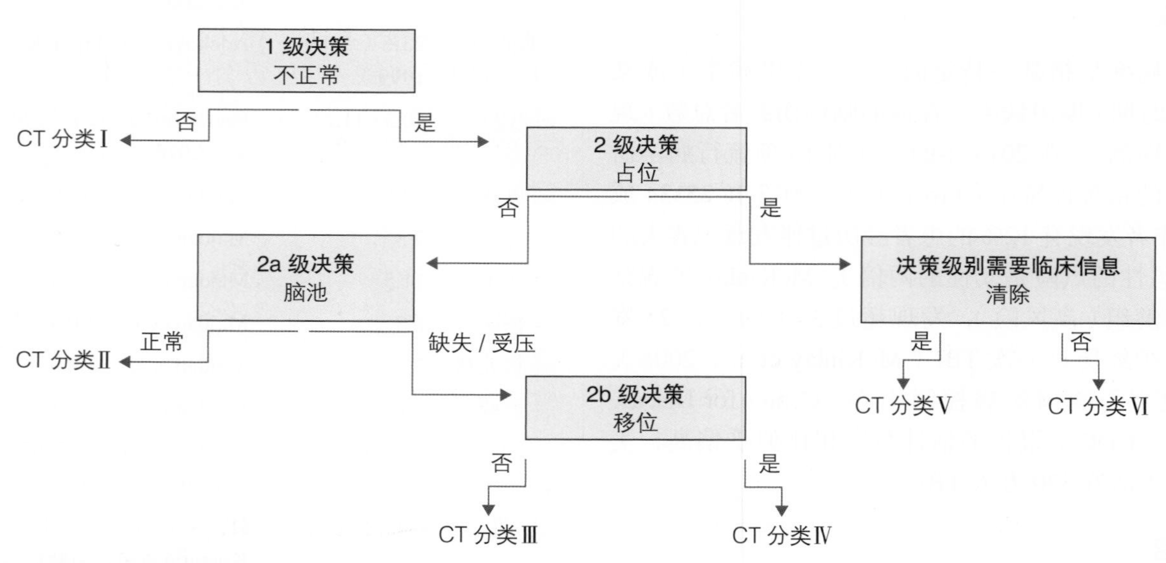

图 40.1 马歇尔（Marshall）CT 分类以树状结构表示

Prediction of outcome in traumatic brain injury with CT characteristics: A comparison between the CT classification and combinations of CT predictors. Maas AIR, Hukkelhoven CWPM, Marshall LF, Steyerberg EW. *Neurosurgery* 2005, 57, 6, 1173–82.

示了超过 25 种不同的 TBI 严重程度分类方法。尽管 GCS 有上述局限性，但根据 GCS 总分，TBI 分为轻度、中度和重度（**图 40.1**）。

除了 GCS，对 TBI 严重程度有多种临床分类方法。其中许多针对特定亚群，但没有一个有说服力地证明优于 GCS。然而，我们应该认识到，GCS 并不能提供轻度 TBI 的程度分类，因为它并不能捕捉细微的变化，如"大脑功能的改变"。伤后轻微和短暂的症状可能与创伤后应激障碍（post-traumatic stress disorders，PTSD）和（或）脑震荡后综合征引起的症状重叠。目前这仍是一个模糊的领域，需要进一步的研究来区分不同的诊断和对患者结果的影响（Maas et al.，2017）。

颅外损伤（损伤负荷）

约 35% 的 TBI 病例和颅外损伤有关。根据简要损伤评分（Abbreviation Injury Score，AIS），对人体六个部位的损伤严重程度进行统一评分。在 AIS 中，身体分为六个区域：外表（皮肤）、头 / 颈部（包括脑损伤）、胸部、腹部 / 盆腔内容物、脊柱和四肢。严重性评分从 1 到 5（1 为轻微；2 是中度；3 是重度不危及生命；4 重度危及生命；5 是危重；6 是可能无法存活）。损伤严重程度评分（Baker et al.，1974）的目的是通过将得分最高的三个身体区域的二次得分相加，总结出总的损伤负荷。

结构损伤程度（CT 分类）

通过神经影像学可以很好地评估结构损伤程度。虽然 MR 检查比计算机断层扫描（CT）更敏感，但 CT 仍然是诊断性成像的主要手段，因为它对检测颅内血肿有足够敏感性，以及检查的速度、可用性和安全性。CT 上结构损伤程度通常采用马歇尔分类法进行分类（**图 40.1**）（Marshall et al.，1991）。这提供了一个描述性系统，主要区分可见的结构损伤存在与否，区分弥漫性损伤（包括亚分类）和占位病变。Marshall 分类法的局限性在于，分级不是按顺序排列的，即在弥漫性损伤患者中可以发现颅内压升高迹象，但在占位损伤患者中却不能体现颅内压。虽然马歇尔 CT 分类法并没有从预后的角度出发，但许多研究表明，CT 分类与预后之间存在明显的联系。鹿特丹（Rotterdan）和赫尔辛基（Helsinki）CT 评分代表了从预后角度开发的分类系统（Maas et al.，2005；Raj et al.，2014）。

预后风险

另一种不同的分类方法是根据基线预测进行分类。目前已有多种预后模型预测 TBI 患者死亡风险或不良预后。两个最大的预后模型，CRASH 和 IMPACT，已经得到了广泛验证，表现良好，并且目标是预测死亡率和不良预后（https://www.crash2.lshtm.ac.uk 和 https://www.tbi-impact.org）（Perel et al.，2008；Steyerberg et al.，2008；Lingsma et al.，2013；Han et al.，2014；Majdan et al.，2014）。IMPACT 模型建立主要针对中重度 TBI 患者；而 CRASH 模型还包含了轻度 TBI 患者。它们基于患者入院，提供住院护理之前的可用数据进行开发的。因此，它们非常适合用于在基线计算预后风险。这两种方法都证实，最大的预后信息包含在三个核心预测因子中：年龄、运动得分和瞳孔反应情况。IMPACT 研究组进一步评估了结构成像（CT 特征如占位病变、脑水肿、创伤性蛛网膜下腔出血）、继发性损害（缺氧、低血压）和实验室数据（葡萄糖、血红蛋白）等因素的额外获益。虽然在这个更复杂的模型中也发现了额外预测能力，然而该模型只能解释结果中 35% 的方差。许多其他因素可能具有判断预后的重要作用，但没有在多变量模型中对 IMPACT 和 CRASH 模型发现的严谨性进行研究，这些因素包括损伤的 MRI 表现、并发症、损伤严重程度评分、开颅前时间超过 4 小时、ICP 增高和自身调节指数。

尽管预测模型对于更可靠地告知亲属预后结果是有用的，但应该认识到预测模型是基于人群的估计，产生的收益不过是风险评估值，有大量不确定性因素，这在置信区间中有所表示。出于这个原因，预后分析的最大应用不是在患者个体水平上，而是在"组"水平上量化和分层脑损伤严重程度上，为评价治疗质量、临床试验分层和协变量调整提供参考（Maas et al.，2017）。

值得补充的是，最近研究显示早期 MR 成像作为 TBI 预后工具有优越性，但其预测价值、急性期病变模式与长期预后之间的相关性仍不确定（Haghbayan et al.，2014）。尽管大量证据表明，在检测大多数类型的创伤性病变方面，MRI 优于 CT，但目前是常规使用 CT，而 MRI 在急性期的使用不常见（Haghbayan et al.，2014）。

有几项研究强调生物标志物作为预测工具的价值，如 S-100β 蛋白和 ApoE4 等位基因。

S–100

S-100β 蛋白是一种有应用前景的生物医学标志

物，用于诊断、监测和预测 TBI 严重程度。TBI 患者术前血清 S-100β 可以作为术后生存和神经系统预后的预测因子（Goyal et al.，2013），并可以反应继发损伤。测量 S-100β 水平对评估 TBI 的严重程度和确定中重度损伤患者的长期预后是有用的（Mercier et al.，2013）。

ApoE4

最近的一项 meta 分析表明，ApoE4 等位基因可能与严重脑创伤患者预后不良有关，可以作为预测脑创伤患者预后的生物标志物（Zeng et al.，2014）。存在 ApoE4 等位基因对严重脑损伤恢复率的影响不受其他共变量影响（Alexander et al.，2007），也可能与随后的认知能力下降风险有关。

结果评估：格拉斯哥预后评分（Glasgow Outcome Scale，GOS）及其他

从临床和研究的角度来看，准确描述 TBI 预后的结果是至关重要的。历史上，大多数 TBI 研究使用格拉斯哥预后评分或扩展版 GOS 来提供 TBI 术后功能结局的整体评估（**表 40.5**）。

GOS 最初于 1975 年被提出，用来描述 TBI 预后的整体功能评估（Jennett and Bond，1975）。虽然适用于于较重的 TBI，但人们认识到该量表在较高水平上不敏感，因此引入了 Glasgow 预后扩展评分（Glasgow Outcome Scale Extended，GOSE）。研究者需要评估主要角色改变、生活独立性以及社会和休闲活动参与等方面，用以总结伤害引起各种变化影响。但是，应当认识到，GOSE 仍然是一种对预后整体分类的办法，并且存在着“天花板效应”。TBI 可引起许多方面的问题：各种各样的神经精神障碍与功能障碍和生活质量低下相关。神经心理后遗症包括：情绪障碍（Bombardier et al.，2010；Tanev et al.，2014）、认知障碍、人格改变，以及对社会和家庭影响。

轻度 TBI 后遗症与创伤后应激障碍症状之间可能存在重叠。在轻度 TBI 和（或）创伤后应激障碍的退伍军人中，轻度 TBI 和创伤后应激障碍中认知障碍的重叠反映了神经、心理和生理因素复杂相互作用，这需专门评估和管理（Benge et al.，2009；Brenner，2011）。

长期以来，人们一直认为生活质量评估不适用于 TBI，因为神经认知后遗症可能会妨碍对患者生活质量感知的准确评估。然而，事实证明这是错误的。患者报告的生活质量、结果评估与 TBI 测量高度相关。生活质量（Quality of life，QOL）评估可能是通用的，例如健康调查简表（Short-Form-36，SF36），但也要考虑到疾病特异性。由多学科工作组进行的疾病特异性的生活质量测量，并开发了脑损伤后生活质量量表（Quality of Life afer Brain Injury，QOLIBRI）。该量表提供了典型脑损伤造成影响的健康相关生活质量（health-related quality of life，HRQOL）概况。然而，更佳的整体评估，似乎使用 QOLIBRI-OS 更可取，它采用了简短的六项评估。QOLIBRI 发现与 QOLIBRI-OS、GOSE、SF36、医院焦虑和抑郁量表中到高度相关（Ware et al.，1993；Truelle et al.，2010；von Steinbüchel et al.，2010a；von Steinbüchel et al.，2010b）。一个重要方面是了解患者自己对生活质量的看法（Dijkers，2004）。迄今为止，预后的评估多是单维的，集中在单一领域。另一种方法可能是采用多维结合的评估方法，不过还需要进行更多的工作，以确定哪些工具最适合于某种具体情况，并确定不同因素的权重。根据损伤严重程度区分预后的历史数据显示，重度脑损伤患者的死亡率为 36%，5% 为植物生存状态，15% 为重度残疾，15%~20% 为中度残疾，25% 为良好恢复。根据报道，中度损伤患者的死亡率为 7%，植物生存状态为 1%，重度致残率为 7%，中度致残率为 25%，良好恢复率为 60%。轻度损伤患者的死亡率很低，

表 40.5 格拉斯哥预后评分（GOS）和格拉斯哥预后扩展评分（GOSE）

分值	GOS	分值	GOSE
1	死亡	1	死亡
2	植物生存	2	植物生存
3	严重残疾（有意识但依赖）	3	低级别重度残疾
		4	高级别重度残疾
4	中度残疾（独立但残疾）	5	低级别中度残疾
		6	高级别中度残疾
5	良好恢复（可恢复正常活动）	7	低级别良好恢复
		8	高级别良好恢复

GOS:

GOSE:

绝大多数患者可恢复良好，但仍有较高频率的持续症状，包括头痛、视觉障碍、头晕、疲劳、记忆力下降、注意力集中和较高执行功能受影响，从而导致家庭、社会生活和就业困难。随着医疗进步，有证据表明，在专科重症监护下接受治疗的中度和重度损伤患者，6 个月预后有所改善（中度残疾和良好恢复从 40.4% 增加到 59.9%）（Patel et al.，2002）。

卫生经济成本

管理 TBI 的经济成本是巨大的，对社会来说是一个巨大负担，但不幸的是，很少有研究量化这一成本。由于长期的经济影响和残疾对家庭、工作和社会的负担，美国 TBI 的人均终生费用估计为 396 000 美元。在美国，疾病控制和预防中心估计，TBI 的直接和间接费用总计超过 580 亿美元。

在大多数研究中，根本没有考虑到非住院性脑损伤的费用。Feigin 等进行了一项基于人群的 TBI 研究，发现 30% 的病例来自非住院患者（Feigin et al.，2013）。虽然众所周知，脑损伤的费用会随着严重程度的增加而增加（见**表** 40.6），但在人群中，轻度脑损伤（占所有脑损伤病例的 95%）的患者数量非常大，这意味着治疗这些病例的总费用几乎是中度 / 重度脑损伤的 3 倍。通过针对高成本损伤的管理和以人群为基础的旨在减少低成本轻伤发生率的项目，可以减少经济负担和改善预后结果。

表 40.6　众所周知，创伤性脑损伤的费用会因严重程度而增加，特别是那些需要住院治疗和对康复服务要求较高的患者

TBI 等级	轻度	中度	重度
每人直接医疗费用（美元）	21 160 (Farhad et al., 2013) 至 35 954	25 271 (Farhad et al., 2013) 至 81 153 (McGregor and Pentland, 1997)	57 637 (Farhad et al., 2013) 至 >100 000 (Faul et al., 2007)

结论

我们只是发现了 TBI 的冰山一角。迫切需要进行进一步标准化的流行病学研究，特别是在低收入国家中。从长远来看，这将对重新分配资源、制订更好的经济计划以减轻社会医疗负担产生重大影响。脑创伤研究中需要注意的关键领域是危险因素和预后预测因子的作用。目前，一些前瞻性多中心研究正在进行中。最大的两个研究：TBI 科研和临床知识转化研究（Transforming Research and Clinical Knowledge in TBI study，TRACK-TBI）将招募 3000 例患者；欧洲 TBI 神经创伤有效性合作研究（Collaborative European Neuro-Trauma Effectiveness Research in TBI study，CENTER-TBI）（Maas et al.，2015），在未来 5 年内招募 5000 名患者，都将使用一组广泛的标准化变量。

延伸阅读、参考文献、EBRAIN 的相关链接

扫描书末二维码获取。

第 41 章 创伤性脑损伤的病理生理学

John K. Yue · Hansen Deng · Ethan A. Winkler · John F. Burke · Catherine G. Suen · Geoffrey T. Manley 著
杨程 译，刘伟明 审校

原发性脑损伤的病理生理学

头部创伤被分为两个病理生理阶段，其机制不同，需要的临床治疗方式也不同。原发性创伤是由机械负荷转化为脑组织（例如神经元、神经胶质、轴突和血管）变形所致，然后开启细胞反应，导致自主调节和代谢紊乱。创伤最初的表现差异很大，从脑震荡中皮质神经元快速不连续的去极化，钝器撞击造成的局灶损伤，直至严重损伤如弥散性轴索断裂、急性血管破裂形成血肿。

继发性损伤发生在更长的时间段里，包括脑缺氧、低血压、肿胀和颅内压（intracranial pressure，ICP）增高。在 2007 年的一项 meta 分析中，作为 TBI 临床试验预测和分析研究国际行动（International Mission for Prognosis and Analysis of Clinical Trials in TBI，IMPACT）中的一部分，McHugh 和他的同事对 9205 例中重度创伤性脑损伤患者进行统计，发现入院时观察到缺氧、低血压和低体温的患病率分别为 20%、18%、10%（McHugh et al.，2007）。继发性损伤，尤其是在急性损伤期和住院期间，与不良预后相关，需要立即引起足够重视、稳定病情，并给予外科和（或）药物治疗。

闭合性颅脑损伤的生物机械学

闭合性颅脑损伤是指撞击后颅骨和硬脑膜未受损的情况，患者会出现一系列神经病学体征和症状。机械负荷到 5% 的凝胶会在颅骨造成局部凹陷或骨折（生物力学实验结果，译者注）；在旋转过程中，整个皮质下会发生弥漫性剪切（Holbourn，1994）。大量的动物模型研究、人类尸体解剖、计算模拟以及影像学，可表现出创伤性脑变形特征，但是作为临床研究的一部分，直接进行人体测量具有挑战性。

脑创伤初级阶段是通过机械负荷属性、导致脑组织移位类型以及撞击持续时间和速度来定义的。力沿着不同轴线在头部产生独特应力模式（例如伸长、压缩、弯曲、剪切和扭转）（Ommaya et al.，2002）。脑创伤造成的伤害不能归因于任何单一原因。外力通常转化为头部撞击力或者冲击载荷，在现实世界里两者可以并存。头部运动是平移或旋转的，这取决于两轴排列的情况：即力轴作用方向与头部重心和寰枕关节连线轴的关系。头部是固定不动还是颈部可以自由伸展 / 屈曲，这对决定损伤机制是非常重要的。

撞击负荷

撞击负荷发生在碰撞时，在低速跌倒时能测量到 3~7 ms 的短持续时间。撞击可以导致颅骨骨折、硬膜外血肿以及局灶性脑损伤。脑挫伤可以观察到冲击伤（直接在撞击下方）和对冲伤（与撞击完全相反）。可以在着力点观察到高正压，力传导通过脑实质在对冲伤部位产生拍击效应。在细胞水平上，对冲伤部位为高负压、空泡化（称为对冲空泡化）形成和随后塌陷，以及脑实质对后部颅骨内壁的反弹，都与对冲伤形成有关。颅骨弹性回弹会导致脑脊液（cerebrospinal fluid，CSF）压力显著升高并加剧组织损伤。脑挫伤常伴发颅内血肿。创伤后早期阶段，挫伤是出血性的，脑回顶部挫伤比脑沟挫伤更严重，它和脑肿胀会随着时间推移消退，但依然有组织颜色改变。

尸检发现冲击伤和（或）对冲伤高发部位是额颞部和脑基底区，与原发撞击部位无关。枕部减速过程中的拉格朗日（Lagrangian）应变张量场显示额底附近解剖学约束破坏后，大脑才能压迫枕骨，因而这些区域易于损伤。对冲伤与颞部、枕部撞击有关。撞击时脑部扭转也被认为是造成对冲伤的重要因素，但还没有确凿证据来证实这个理论。

脉冲载荷

在平移或旋转运动中，脉冲载荷由惯性力产生。

正常的生理环境下，脑脊液（CSF）压力对大脑运动时移位有相当大抑制作用，脑脊液的缺乏也表明能增加脑卷积滑动和剪切应变（Pudenz and Shelden，1946）。由于大脑的惯性，大脑移位滞后于颅骨及附着的硬膜，在大脑不同区域发生不同程度卷积滑动，包括弥散性白质束损伤。相对于蝶鞍区和鞍上间隙附近的颅底区域，脑实质更易移动。白质比灰质更硬，因此，更多的应力会分布在界面区域。将大脑固定在颅底的血管、神经和硬脑膜结构（如远端颈内动脉、视神经、嗅束、动眼神经和垂体柄）由于惯性效应在弥漫性轴索损伤（diffuse axonal injury，DAI）中更易受到影响。胼胝体压部和脑干背外侧更容易遭受急性弥散性轴索损伤，因为相对于顺应性更好的大脑皮质，其运动轨迹与颅底相似。

不同强度的平移和旋转运动可以同时发生。即使直线加速度高达 1000 g，单纯的头颈平移运动通常不会产生急性硬膜下血肿（subdural haematomas，SDH）、弥散性点状出血或颈髓损伤。而当直线加速与头颈部角运动结合时，就会产生上述损害。在角加速期间，除弥漫性轴索损伤外，基底节区深层血肿发生率更高。旋转损伤经常发生在车祸伤中，轴索和血管会被拉伸或压缩超过生理极限，引起剪切应变，并经常因硬膜下桥静脉撕裂而引起急性硬膜下血肿。

当单个惯性负荷与较小的末端冲击相结合时引起的损伤很常见，如严重的伸展 / 屈曲挥鞭损伤、硬膜下血肿、滑动性挫伤和脊髓损伤。在角加速度过程中，旋转轴位于枕髁或颈底部，从而扩大旋转负荷以及剪切作用。车辆突然碰撞时，在座椅上进行水平运动，会诱导对头部和颈部产生惯性力。当从后面施加的力使头部在颈底部向后旋转时，会发生后部负荷，而当从前面施加的力使头部向前旋转时，会发生前部负荷。

静态或准静态负荷

一种比较少见的机械负荷是静态或准静态的，其发生在可以忽略不计的速率和加速度的逐渐挤压中，机械机理类似于正在关闭的电梯门。稳定负荷会导致颅骨骨折和脑损害，脑损伤一般比撞击负荷造成的皮质挫伤位置更深。相比于持续时间较短和速度较快的钝器击打创伤，挤压伤产生的能量往往传递到颅中窝的孔和裂隙，引起相关的脑神经、交感神经和血管内膜损伤。

脑创伤形态学分类

传统脑创伤分类法主要关注损伤的范围（局灶与弥散）和损伤解剖学位置与脑膜关系（硬膜外 / 轴外与颅内 / 轴内）。下面部分采用后一种分类方案进行，从最靠近颅骨的轴外层开始，向内延伸至脑内组织。

硬膜外血肿

硬膜外血肿（epidural haematoma，EDH）在硬脑膜外侧，典型的原因是部分菲薄的颞骨鳞部骨折，会撕裂脑膜中动脉。由此产生的血肿将硬脑膜从颅骨内板剥离，形成一个卵圆形团块，并压迫邻近的脑组织。血肿受骨膜约束，骨膜穿过颅缝，因此血肿一般不会越过骨缝。静脉性硬膜外血肿较少见，其形成原因是颅顶、颅后窝或颅前窝的硬脑膜静脉窦破裂。硬膜外血肿发生在额部、颅顶部或者颅后窝者少见，但也占全部硬膜外血肿的 25%。

硬膜外血肿发生率远低于硬膜下血肿，约占脑损伤的 2%。虽然硬膜外血肿可出现在所有年龄段，但多发生于 50 岁以下患者中，尤其在儿童患者，其主要原因是脑膜和板障静脉出血，在儿童中硬脑膜与颅骨紧密粘连。相对较低的静脉压和较紧密硬脑膜和颅骨粘连，是儿童硬膜外血肿出现变异和偶尔出现亚急性表现的原因。在影像学表现中，根据计算机断层扫描影像（computed tomography，CT）将硬膜外血肿分为 3 个类型：Ⅰ型（急性）、Ⅱ型（亚急性）和Ⅲ型（慢性），发生率分别为 58%、31% 和 11%（Zimmerman and Bilaniuk，1982）。Ⅰ型特征是密度较高的血肿，伴有低密度“漩涡”，提示正在出血（即从撕裂血管活动性出血形成致密组织团块的低密度区）。最终，升高的压力使出血点闭塞，形成Ⅱ型血肿，为等密度，高密度团块。Ⅲ型以血管周围组织血液再吸收而形成低密度聚集为主要特征，并伴随新生血管和肉芽组织形成的可增强包膜。

硬膜外血肿的典型症状见于 15%~20% 的病例，表现为头部创伤后出现短暂意识丧失，进展到中间清醒期，然后神经系统症状恶化至昏迷。中间清醒期表示从脑震荡中恢复，在此期间，患者可能会诉受伤同侧严重头痛，伴恶心、呕吐和昏睡，随后由于硬膜外血肿扩张，颅内压继发增高，造成失代偿而进入昏迷状态。清醒间歇期不是硬膜外血肿独有的，其最初用于描述急性硬膜下血肿病例。硬膜外血肿的神经功能恶化可能会伴随对侧偏瘫、同侧动眼神经麻痹、去大脑强直、动脉血压增高、心律失常、呼吸紊乱，如不纠正，就会导致呼吸暂停和死亡。

硬膜下血肿

硬膜下血肿（subdural haematoma，SDH）来源于硬膜下间隙与静脉窦连接的桥静脉撕裂，或是由脑表面软脑膜浅表动脉破裂。硬膜下血肿不受硬脑膜附着的限制，它以典型的双凹形在皮质表面延伸，越过小脑幕或进入纵裂。硬膜下血肿可分为急性、亚急性和慢性。急性硬膜下血肿表现为新月形高密度聚集区。亚急性硬膜下血肿为等密度，症状通常较轻，出现在伤后的7~21天。慢性硬膜下血肿（发生在伤后21天以上）是低密度的，在血肿聚集和扩展出现压迫迹象之前可能不会有任何症状（Sambasivan，1997）。

急性硬膜下血肿可有以下症状：刻板运动障碍、动眼反射受损、小脑幕切迹疝、单侧瞳孔固定和扩大。动脉出血常导致侧裂附近血凝块。术后并发症包括血肿再聚积和手术部位感染（如骨髓炎、脑膜炎、脑室炎）。

据报道，急性创伤性硬膜下血肿有高达22%~66%的死亡率。病变在4个小时内手术清除可降低致残风险，而对于临床状态良好的薄层血肿可以考虑保守治疗。脑创伤基金会的指南根据血肿厚度、中线偏移和GCS评分推荐了具体标准以便进行干预。然而，这些标准必须结合患者状况、伤前状态、病史长短和伴随损伤等情况综合评定（Chesnut，1997）。回顾以往，在伤后4个小时内减压的患者死亡率为30%，相比之下，伤后4小时后接受外科治疗的患者死亡率为90%（Seelig，1981）。早期一系列快速外科治疗干预结果显示，整体死亡率低至8%~10%（Bajsarowicz et al.，2015）。其他预测指标包括神经功能障碍程度、性别以及术后颅内压增高。急性硬膜下血肿的快速诊断和手术清除病变仍是最重要的预后因素。硬膜下血肿清除时是否去骨瓣减压的问题目前正在进行一项随机对照试验（RESCUE-ASDH）。目前，在手术时是否去除骨瓣的决定（一期去骨瓣减压术）是基于对大脑损伤的负担（如存在大的脑挫伤）、临床评估损伤的严重程度和损伤机制，最重要的是观察术中脑肿胀程度。

慢性硬膜下血肿

慢性硬膜下血肿（chronic subdural haematoma，CSDH）是一种独特的病理类型，它在特定人群（老年患者或脑萎缩患者）中表现为一种特殊的临床综合征。假定的病理变化是轻微头部创伤，导致横跨硬膜下间隙的桥静脉撕裂而产生小血肿，但这在脑萎缩患者中不明显。最初血肿容量很少，患者并无症状，初始往往被忽略。在一部分患者中，新生的炎性膜通过血液产物和跨膜渗透梯度发展，加重了血肿包裹、潜在持续出血和聚集。其病程缓慢，在创伤几周后会出现明显临床表现，并出现颅内低密度的硬膜下血肿。尽管如此，血肿仍可能有反复急性出血表现，出血可能来自炎性新生膜。

慢性硬膜下血肿的临床特征为头痛、偏身轻瘫、言语障碍（优势半球）或者行为紊乱（例如情绪爆发、注意力不集中、躁狂和抑郁状态），如果病情恶化不进行治疗，最终会导致昏迷。双侧慢性硬膜下血肿更可能快速地进展为昏迷，即便血肿量较少也应积极治疗。慢性硬膜下血肿普遍发生在大脑凸面，也可以发生在纵裂和小脑幕上方，但较少发生在颅后窝。

治疗可以用钻孔引流术（一个或两个孔可帮助血肿冲洗）、小骨瓣开颅术或通过闭式引流系统。干预风险包括硬膜下间隙感染、癫痫和复发。由于内皮细胞具有明显的有丝分裂潜能和血管通透性，硬膜下血肿包膜内增生的微血管出血和复发有关。有1级证据表明，在硬膜下腔内放置软性引流管48小时可以减少复发率（Santarius et al.，2009）。

蛛网膜下腔出血

蛛网膜下腔出血（subarachnoid haemorrhage，SAH）多在闭合性脑损伤中发现，来源于皮质血管的直接损伤。它与较差预后和更严重的损伤相关。尽管在大多数情况下，它似乎反映了受伤时受到更大暴力，而和继发性脑损伤没有直接关系，然而，在一部分创伤性蛛网膜下腔出血患者中，可能会造成继发性损伤（如脑肿胀、血流动力学上明显血管痉挛，以及由于大脑对额外生理变化的适应阈值降低而导致代谢和自动调节紊乱）。创伤后血管痉挛可以早在伤后两天发现，在5~7天时到达最重程度（Weber et al.，1990）。

皮质蛛网膜下腔出血与邻近脑挫伤病程进展相关，提示颅盖骨下蛛网膜下腔出血是皮质微出血和脑实质内明显损伤的早期征兆。钝性创伤性脑损伤患者在与GCS评分、年龄、性别和存在颅内占位病变相匹配后，创伤性SAH患者停留重症监护室（intensive care unit，ICU）时间更久，患者出院回家的可能性较低，在急性住院期间死亡的可能性高出1.5倍。在穿透性TBI中，SAH与不良预后之间存在显著相关性。

脑室内出血

脑室内出血（intraventricular haemorrhage，IVH）占所有头部创伤病例的1.5%~3.0%，主要发生在严重TBI。原发性脑室内出血患者尸检中可见穹隆内透明隔、脉络丛和室管膜下静脉受损。原发性脑室内出血（指局限于脑室系统的孤立性出血）的发生率很低。由于IVH伴随其他颅内损伤，估计仅有21%患者达到功能恢复（GOS为中度残疾或良好恢复）。在不常见的孤立性脑室内出血病例中，GOS可能有更大改善。一般来说，小的样本量使得解释脑室内出血与其他脑创伤相关联系时变得困难。

脑挫伤

脑挫伤是局灶性或多灶性的，位于皮质或皮质下区域，是由直接撞击或加速/减速损伤造成。挫伤表现为来自受损的小动脉、静脉或毛细血管造成的表面损伤。脑疝性挫伤是指当脑组织从一个颅腔移位到另一个颅腔时，通常是沿着大脑镰、小脑幕或枕大孔边缘，导致突出组织受压而产生挫伤。中间结构挫伤是指胼胝体、基底节、下丘脑和脑干的皮质下组织损伤。

小鼠皮质撞击模型表明，大脑水肿在创伤后24小时达到峰值，同时挫伤皮质的大脑血流（cerebral blood flow，CBF）显著减少。CBF在创伤后第七天恢复正常，在此期间，局部充血区域周围出现低血流量区。对人脑进行的非穿透性头部损伤研究表明，额叶和颞叶挫伤更为严重，且患者无清醒间歇期（Adams et al.，1985）。对急诊开颅手术切除的挫伤组织进行细胞分析证实，坏死是主要发现，细胞凋亡是继发性级联损伤反应的一部分。在急性神经元变性期间，脑脊液中肿瘤坏死因子迅速增加，并在数小时内逐渐减少。中性粒细胞和巨噬细胞通过提高趋化因子聚集来维持脑炎症的级联反应。脑肿胀和挫伤周围迟发性血肿可造成颅内压增高，因此，不管是否需要手术干预，都要监测颅内压。单侧病变的预后较好，而双侧病变的临床表现可能延迟发作。这种临床表现的二次恶化可延迟至伤后10天，需要在出院时向患者及其亲属仔细交代。低钠血症可加剧这种风险，在出院前必须监测血清钠，因为抗利尿激素分泌失调综合征可与TBI共存。

弥漫性轴索损伤

弥漫性轴索损伤（diffuse axonal injury，DAI）是因为角加速度而引起的整体性轴索损害。弥漫性脑损伤占脑创伤的50%，产生包括从脑震荡到昏迷和植物人状态的一系列后果。过去，弥漫性轴索损伤被定义为大脑半球、胼胝体、脑干和小脑弥漫性损伤（Gennarelli et al.，1982）。长束结构（轴突和血管）尤其危险。MR分级为：Ⅰ级（大脑半球矢状窦旁白质）、Ⅱ级（Ⅰ级+胼胝体局灶性病变）和Ⅲ级（Ⅱ级+大脑脚局灶性病变）（**表41.1**）。Ⅰ级和Ⅱ级一般在2周内表现出GCS的显著改善，而Ⅲ级需要2个月才能恢复，这表明DAI累及脑干会导致长期意识丧失或昏迷。

严格来说，弥漫性轴索损伤的明确诊断需通过尸检中β-淀粉样前体蛋白（β-APP）的免疫染色和识别深部白质中轴突回缩来确定的。因为它需用显微镜显示，故体内诊断具有挑战性；此外还会合并一种或多种类型的脑损伤，包括挫伤、缺氧和颅内出血。尽管有大量数据表明弥漫性轴索损伤与中重型脑创伤有关，但因为患者很少死于轻型脑创伤，因此很难从组织学上证明弥漫性轴索损伤与轻型脑创伤有关。轻度轴索损伤可能为轻型脑创伤（mTBI）/脑震荡期间和之后的损伤提供了病理生理学基础；或者，功能和代谢障碍可能与较少的结构性轴突损伤有关（Vespa et al.，2005）。

轻型创伤性脑损伤/脑震荡

美国疾病控制和预防中心将轻型脑创伤（mild TBI，mTBI）/脑震荡定义为由快速线性和（或）旋转的加速减速运动，导致大脑结构或血管生理破

表41.1　弥漫性轴索损伤分级

DAI分级	病理
Ⅰ	灰白质界面（通常为额叶、脑室周围颞叶的矢状窦旁白质）
Ⅱ	胼胝体局灶性病变（通常为体部和压部），外加Ⅰ级损伤
Ⅲ	脑干（通常为中脑头部、小脑脚、内侧丘系和皮质脊髓束），外加Ⅰ级和Ⅱ级病变

Data from Tong KA, et al, Hemorrhagic shearing lesions in children and adolescents with posttraumatic diffuse axonal injury: improved detection and initial results, *Radiology*, Volume 227, Issue 7, pp. 332–9, 2003

坏而引起的一过性神经功能障碍。美国康复医疗协会（American Congress of Rehabilitation Medicine，ACRM）将轻型脑创伤定义为以下一项或多项症状：意识丧失（loss of consciousness，LOC）、在事故发生前后记忆丧失、精神状态改变或者是短暂或非短暂的局灶性神经功能缺陷。美国退伍军人事务部和国防部（The U.S. Department of Veterans Affaers and Department of Defense，VA/DOD）提供了类似的临床指南，同时明确了若有颅内病变存在，至少将患者归类为中型脑创伤。

估计有 75% 脑创伤患者被归为“轻型”，但这个数值很可能低估，因为这些患者中的大多数都没有去急诊室就诊。目前对脑震荡的分类主要关注点为神经功能损害，如视觉、记忆、平衡障碍和意识改变（alteration of consciousness，AOC）和（或）意识丧失。脑震荡诊断在很大程度上适用于非穿透性颅脑损伤所导致以下一种或多种情况：定时 / 定向障碍、意识丧失小于 30 分钟或创伤后遗忘症（post-traumatic amnesia，PTA）持续时间小于 24 小时、短暂性局灶性神经功能缺陷和（或）癫痫、急诊评估 GCS 评分为 13~15 分；然而，目前存在的多个脑震荡分级量表并没有明确共识。轻型脑创伤 / 脑震荡可能是由于缺乏敏感性，所以缺乏影像研究证据，故对其进行临床诊断而言是一个挑战。最近利用磁共振成像（magnetic resonance imaging，MRI），包括磁共振波谱，识别一些轻微脑创伤后患者的脑结构改变，这给轻型脑创伤诊断带来了希望。

轻微脑创伤 / 脑震荡病理生理始于头部动量的突然改变，导致部分栓系的大脑对颅盖产生机械拉伸或压缩，引起弥散性神经元活动、放电和轴突剪切。神经认知缺陷往往随时间恢复，极少检测到病理情况。然而，即使 GCS 评分在 13~15 的患者在正电子放射层扫描术（positron emission topography，PET）上也存在急性和亚急性葡萄糖代谢紊乱，需要仔细评估脑震荡后的风险（Giza and Hovda，2001）。轻微脑创伤 / 脑震荡后立即进行脑微透析检查，在大脑半球、海马和脑干的兴奋性氨基酸和离子通量水平升高。尤其是细胞外钾离子通过电压门控通道急剧升高。脑电图（electroencephalogram，EEG）研究表明，脑震荡后的脑电图具有兴奋性和癫痫样特征，性质上与全身性癫痫发作相同。此外，在这期间，感觉诱发电位完全消失（Shaw，2002）。轻微脑创伤 / 脑震荡后的早期，葡萄糖利用率和糖酵解的增加以维持神经元随意的去极化和放电，也可以恢复受干扰的膜电位。随后，弥漫性神经元抑制（如扩散性抑制）生效。扩散性抑制的特征是离子梯度完全破坏、电活动丧失和血管收缩，可以触发梗死发展和引发级联反应导致细胞凋亡（Dreier，2011）。

mTBI/ 脑震荡后生理紊乱持续存在，并增加进一步损伤的易感性。在最初的高代谢之后，低代谢和 CBF 降低可能持续 4 周。额外的刺激（如直接的皮质刺激或反复的脑震荡）延长了细胞恢复时间并诱导细胞死亡，这是由于脑震荡后神经元激活和 CBF 之间去耦连导致无法匹配增加的代谢需求。根据影响严重程度，细胞内 Ca^{2+} 的积累也升高，这会损害线粒体代谢并引发程序性细胞死亡。在存活的细胞中，细胞可塑性降低，这与神经传递改变有关，特别是 N- 甲基 -D- 天冬氨酸（NMDA）受体亚单位。

穿透性脑损伤

与钝性脑创伤相比，穿透性脑创伤（penetrating brain injury，PBI）较少见并且预后很差，发生在非钝性投射物撞击颅骨和硬脑膜时。常见表现为脑脊液漏，可能需要手术干预。投射物体在经过路径上会挤压脑组织，并在撞击时产生骨碎片，这需要外科清创术治疗。物体形状和动能 $E=1/2\ mv^2$（E= 能量，m= 质量，v= 速度）与组织损伤程度相关。高速投射物会产生压迫和再膨胀波（空化波），造成局部剪切损伤、脑实质挫伤和血肿。CT 可以清楚地看到内部骨碎片、创道、组织损伤程度、血肿和占位等征象。由于血管损伤的高风险，建议行脑血管造影术。高风险因素包括创道经过脑室、累及双侧半球、穿过大脑中心部位或伴随血管损伤。穿透性脑损伤后癫痫控制是临床治疗的一个重要部分。

脑代谢和自主调节

大脑是静止时能量消耗最大的器官，约占 22%，相比较肝占 21%、心脏占 9% 和肾占 8%。大脑只占整个体重的 2%，然而却占了心输出量的 20% 和静息氧耗量的 20%。脑的氧代谢率（cerebral metabolic rate of oxygen，$CMRO_2$）在健康成人中保持相对平稳，约为 3.5 ml/（100 g · min)，而在 3~12 岁儿童中，可能会高达 5.2 ml/（100 g · min）。葡萄糖是脑主要的三磷酸腺苷来源，大脑代谢产生的大约 50% 能量用于突触活动（即神经传递素的产生、释放和摄取）；25% 用于维持电化学梯度，其余 25% 用于分子运输、生物合成和其他过程。

有氧代谢是大脑的主要程序，通过糖酵解、柠檬酸循环和有氧氧化，葡萄糖有效地转化为36~38个ATP分子，脑创伤后会造成葡萄糖代谢紊乱。当神经元和星形胶质细胞将葡萄糖转化为2个ATP分子和2个乳酸分子时，脑循环中无氧糖酵解周转显著增加，细胞外乳酸水平升高。高糖酵解通过钙介导干扰，导致乳酸/葡萄糖比例升高、脑脊液乳酸中毒和线粒体功能受损。高糖酵解和乳酸积聚的持续时间可以反映损伤程度和较差预后，见**图41.1**。

$CMRO_2$、大脑葡萄糖代谢率（cerebral metabolic rate of glucose，CMRG）以及脑血流量（CBF）是神经生理学最常用的测量指标。在健康成人中，大脑氧代谢率为3.3 ml/（100 g · min）、大脑葡萄糖代谢率为5.5 mg/（100 g · min）和脑血流量为54 ± 12 ml/（100 g · min）。在脑创伤后昏迷的患者中，脑氧代谢率降至1.2~2.3 ml/（100 g · min），并与GCS评分和预后相关。神经元和星形胶质细胞储存葡萄糖和氧气是有限的，因此，持续的脑血流量对于其存活至关重要。直径30~300 μm的小动脉可以改变阻力来控制脑循环。大脑氧代谢率和脑血流量之间存在线性关系，这与氧气输送扩散理论一致。血流-代谢耦合是指血流随脑组织代谢需求而变化的过程，主要受组织中二氧化碳变化的影响。除了在那些动脉血氧分压急剧低于50 mmHg以下的患者之外，PaO_2不影响CBF。脑创伤后脑代谢下降，脑血流量相应降低。

葡萄糖代谢

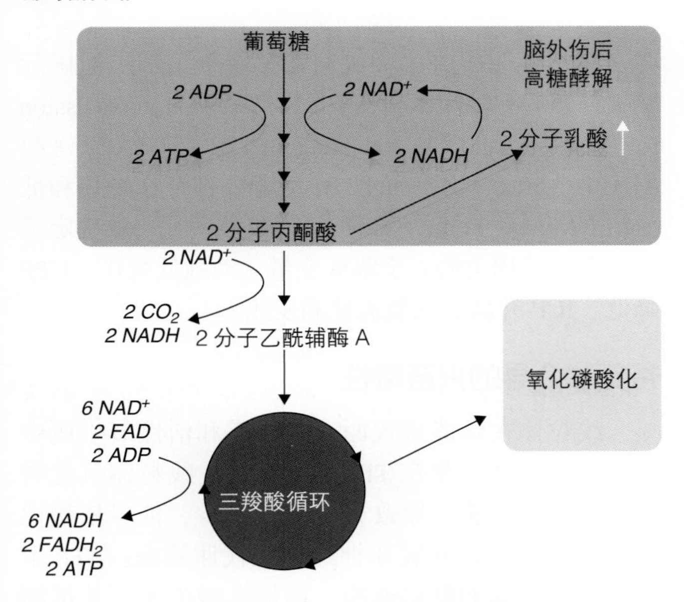

图41.1　葡萄糖代谢可分为三个不同过程。糖酵解是将葡萄糖转化为丙酮酸。这会产生两个ATP分子（净生成），丙酮酸若转化为乳酸（无氧呼吸），则不需要氧气。三羧酸循环是一个生化循环途径，消耗乙酰辅酶A的碳骨架，产生还原当量［烟酰胺腺嘌呤二核苷酸（NAD）-H和黄素腺嘌呤二核苷酸（FAD）-H］、二氧化碳和两个ATP分子。氧化磷酸化的最后一步利用前面步骤中产生的还原当量，在线粒体膜上产生氢离子梯度，从而驱动质子ATP酶，从而产生额外的34个ATP分子，使每个葡萄糖分子（有氧呼吸）总共产生38个ATP分子

压力和黏度

圆柱管内层流动的Hagen-Poiseuille定律被用来描述脑血流与脑灌注压（cerebral perfusion pressure，CPP）、血管直径和血液黏度的关系。CBF=k[CPP × d（4）]/（8 × l × v），其中k为常数，d为动脉直径，l为动脉长度，v为血液黏度。如果脑灌注压在60~160 mmHg范围内，成人的CBF维持在50 ml/（100 g · min），以维持大脑的恒定代谢供应（Cipolla，2009）。其中，脑灌注压通过计算平均动脉压（mean arterial pressure，MAP）和颅内压的差值获得。

脑血流量可通过自主调节来维持（**图41.2**）。脑血管具有肌源性能力，可以扩张或收缩，以抵消血管壁张力（反应脑灌注压）的偏差，从而维持恒定的血流。在正常脑灌注压60~160 mmHg外，血管会扩张至最大化或经历强迫扩张（即“压力突破”）。大多数严重脑创伤患者在临床过程中某个时候，存在自主调节受损或缺失。当自主调节功能丧失时，大脑容易受到全身血压紊乱影响，造成继发性损伤（如脑血流量减少所致局部贫血或脑血流量快速增加造成的血肿）。严重脑创伤患者更易受到低脑灌注压造成的继发性损害。因此，血流代谢和自动调节是不同的机制，允许大脑循环满足局部代谢需求，并稳定对抗系统性血压紊乱干扰。

全血黏度的变化在很大程度上由红细胞压积和血清纤维蛋白原决定，在正常生理环境下会影响血流量并诱导自主调节反应。血液黏度增加会降低脑代谢和引起动脉舒张，而血液黏度的降低会增加代谢对脑的供应并引起动脉收缩。急性脑梗死后，血细胞比容和纤维蛋白原增加与脑血流量减少相关，因此，急性应激时，血液黏度的变化可能对脑循环有重要的血流动力学影响。

二氧化碳反应性

二氧化碳反应性是动脉二氧化碳分压（partial pressure of arterial CO_2，$PaCO_2$）影响脑血流量和脑血管系统的过程。动脉二氧化碳分压的正常范围在20~60 mmHg，每1 mmHg的波动会造成脑血流量

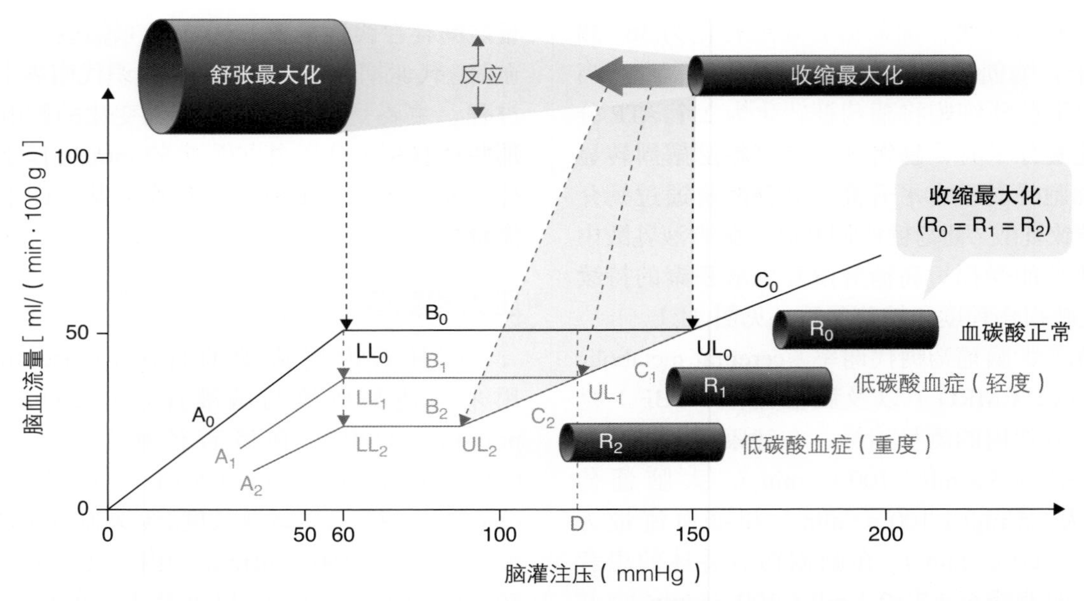

图 41.2 脑血管自动调节(A,自动调节)是在系统血压变化时保持恒定血流量(B,血流量)的机制。在一定的血压范围内,脑血流量是恒定的,但高于这个范围(UL,上限)和低于这个范围(LL,下限),血管最大限度地收缩或舒张(分别),血压的变化传递至脑血流量变化。这可能导致下限以下的缺血,并加剧上限以上的颅内高压。治疗性过度通气(C_0~C_2)以降低颅内压导致血管收缩(R_0~R_2)。这有两个潜在的破坏性影响。首先,降低脑血流量,增加脑缺血的风险。这可以通过测量颅内氧合来缓解。其次,自动调节范围缩小,更难针对适当的脑灌注压。这可以通过使用诸如脉冲反应性指数(pulse reactivity index,PRX)的自动调节度量来缓解

2%~3% 的变化。高碳酸血症(肺换气不足)会引起血管舒张和脑血流量增加,而低碳酸血症(肺通气过度)则有相反的效应。这是通过碳酸酐酶改变血管周围间隙的pH值来调节的,且是乙酰唑胺激发的基础。静脉注射乙酰唑胺(如 1 g)的正常反应是血管扩张,在 10~15 分钟内脑血流量增加到 30%~60%。乙酰唑胺不能扩张血管意味着血管已扩张至最大,通常是由慢性缺血引起。脑创伤急性阶段一般会有充血和脑脊液代谢性酸中毒,若在最初 24 小时,患者持续丧失对二氧化碳反应,会增加死亡率或严重神经功能损害风险。当二氧化碳反应性引起脑血流量和脑动脉 - 静脉氧含量差(arterio-venous oxygen content difference,$AVDO_2$)变化时,自主调节影响 CBF 而保持 $AVDO_2$ 相对恒定。过度换气和控制 $PaCO_2$ 是治疗 ICP 升高的重要干预措施,但需要监测脑氧合,以确保过度动脉血管收缩不会造成缺血。

严重头部创伤后的继发性损害

TBI 后复杂的神经生物化学途径会破坏脑血管循环,造成持续数分钟到数周的继发性损伤,而继发性损伤的治疗对于最大限度地提高患者预后至关重要。虽然并非所有这些机制都被完全了解,但国际脑损伤预后和临床试验任务(the International Mission for Prognosis and Clinical Trials in TBI,IMPACT)数据库中,20% 和 18% 的 TBI 患者分别存在缺氧和低血压(Murray et al.,2007)。经反复研究一致确定了和不良预后相关的五个临床变量:动脉低血压、CPP 降低、ICP 升高、低氧血症和发热。

谷氨酸介导的兴奋毒性

线粒体在脑能量代谢、钙稳态和活性氧生成中起着重要作用。早在 TBI 后 1 小时,线粒体氧化磷酸化就可能失能,导致 ATP 生成减少,能量依赖性膜离子泵失效,并破坏神经细胞代谢稳态。ATP 生成降低会增加糖酵解速率,增加乳酸生成,并可能在受损脑的脑脊液和细胞外液中积聚。高乳酸水平可导致酸中毒、膜损伤、血脑屏障通透性改变和脑水肿,从而进一步导致神经元功能障碍。细胞内消化酶(即过氧化物酶、蛋白酶、磷脂酶)和半胱天冬酶的激活导致亚细胞水平结构损伤、DNA 降解和神经元死亡(即坏死和凋亡)。

钙离子内流过多与谷氨酸引发的损伤之间的关系得到了很好理论支持,导致线粒体电子转移 ATP

合成和钙蛋白酶过度激活脱钩。谷氨酸介导的兴奋毒性激活 NMDA 受体，通过未经检查的钙流入线粒体触发神经元去极化。由于离子泵不能恢复膜电位，线粒体功能紊乱成为受损组织不能获取能量的主要原因。实验表明，L 型电压敏感通道上的钙例子负荷是无毒的，而 N- 甲基 -D- 天冬氨酸受体上的钙离子负荷是具有神经毒性的。有毒活性氧（例如一氧化氮、超氧化物和过氧化氢）的产生也取决于 NMDA 的激活，因此 NMDA 在损伤后是兴奋性中毒的关键驱动因素。这些细胞改变导致脑水肿、颅内压增高、血管受压、最终形成脑疝（Lucas and Newhouse，1957）。在评估缺血和异常血氧测量（如脑灌注压和颈静脉血氧饱和度）的原因和治疗此类疾病时，应考虑线粒体失能，由于潜在的线粒体损伤，维持充分的灌注可能不会改善临床预后。线粒体功能紊乱的实质是在充足的氧气和代谢底物的情况下，不能有效地进行 ADP 的氧化磷酸化。

细胞外谷氨酸含量增高在介导创伤性和局部缺血性脑损伤中都起着重要作用。间质谷氨酸升高有如下几种机制：血脑屏障（blood-brain barrier，BBB）损害和谷氨酸外渗到撞击区；细胞膜损伤以及微穿孔、complexin 蛋白Ⅰ和 complexin 蛋白Ⅱ上调促进细胞外分泌；谷氨酸转运体受损。B- 内酰胺类抗生素（如头孢曲松）是谷氨酸转运蛋白（GLT1）的有效刺激物，GLT1 是负责灭活突触谷氨酸的星形胶质蛋白。B- 内酰胺可以提升脑中 GLT1 表达以及 GLT1 的功能活性，还可以减少谷氨酸的神经毒性并在局部缺血损伤和神经变性中提供神经保护潜能（Rothstein et al.，2005）。钙介导的线粒体基质肿胀和线粒体外膜破裂使呼吸链解离，并进一步损害 ATP 的产生。不受控制的钙离子内流和膜破裂也会引起线粒体通透性转换孔（mitochondrial permeability transition pore，mPTP）的开启，导致细胞凋亡的级联反应。环孢素 A 是一种免疫抑制剂，已被研究能够抑制脑创伤患者线粒体通透性转换孔的开放，且被证明对线粒体肿胀、膜破裂和离子稳态失衡具有神经保护作用（Okonkwo et al.，1999）。

大脑代谢的扰动

脑创伤损伤线粒体功能，导致神经退化和限制神经再生。重度脑创伤后，有氧代谢突然向高糖酵解 / 无氧代谢转变，并伴有高葡萄糖转换，导致大脑酸中毒。在脑创伤一周内，即使在氧气充足的情况下，通过正电子放射断层扫描术仍发现有 56% 的患者表现出高糖酵解。酸中毒将血红蛋白氧解离曲线右移并可能会增加受损脑组织的氧气供应。创伤性脑损伤后，升高的脑脊液乳酸水平通常在伤后 12 小时内恢复正常，而脑缺血和弥散性脑肿胀仍存在。乳酸在受损的大脑能量学中的作用颇有争议，从代谢废物变成补充燃料、具备神经保护作用和皮质神经元中的信号分子。脑内微透析导管（**图 41.3**）允许对脑创伤第二阶段细胞外神经递质和代谢物变化进行生化分析。微透析测定的乳酸 / 丙酮酸比值是无氧代谢标志，并与颅脑损伤后的预后相关（Timofeev et al.，2011）。乳酸 / 丙酮酸比值（lactate/pyruvate ratio，LPR）可因为脑缺血和线粒体功能紊乱而升高。在大脑乳酸 / 丙酮酸比值升高的患者中，微量透析显示，外源性乳酸治疗可显著提高大脑葡萄糖水平。这与先前的证据相关联，即乳糖在神经元和星形胶质细胞的线粒体中直接氧化为丙酮酸（Lazaridis and Andrews，2014）。

严重脑创伤后，磷酸戊糖途径（pentose phosphate pathway，PPP）的活性提高会导致大脑葡萄糖摄取增加，超过脑代谢率和乳糖产生（**图 41.4**）。颅脑损伤后输注同种异型葡萄糖可使磷酸戊糖途径活性增加 19.6%，而对照组为 6.9%。磷酸戊糖途径的产物（NADPH、核糖 5- 磷酸和赤藓糖 -4- 磷酸）可上调脂肪酸合成、促进 DNA 修复和复制以及增加氨基酸和神经递质的产生，这是脑损伤后受刺激的过程（Dusick et al.，2007）。NADPH 被用来生成还原性谷胱甘肽和硫氧还蛋白、谷胱甘肽过氧化物酶的辅助因子，以及在急性损伤后对抗氧化应激的过氧化还原蛋白。磷酸戊糖途径不会利用氧作为底物也不生成 ATP，但作为一种抗氧化剂，有助于缺血脑组织中的葡萄糖代谢从糖酵解转到磷酸戊糖途径。

创伤性脑损伤患者中，发现有 30% 的患者在没有缺血情况下脑代谢率值明显下降，由正常值 3.3 ml/（100 g · min）降至 1.2~2.3 ml/（100 g · min）。虽然脑创伤后脑代谢率与 GCS 紧密相关，也是神经预后的一个重要预测指标，但脑代谢率降低并不一定是脑缺血的结果，也不会直接导致患者病情恶化。造成患者病情加重的原因包括严重的原发和继发损伤以及意识水平下降。在平均 GCS 为 6 分的重型 TBI 研究报告中，尽管没有缺血，但氧化代谢降低和持续代谢危象（LPR>40）的发生率为 25%，这表明 LPR 是 TBI 后广泛线粒体功能障碍导致代谢抑制的指标，进一步削弱大脑在应对继发性损伤时满足代谢需求的能力。虽然极低的 $CMRO_2$ 表示不可逆的细胞损伤，但 LPR 仍可作为无明显组织损伤区域可逆性线粒体功能障碍的敏感标志物。使用 ^{15}O PET 的已发表研

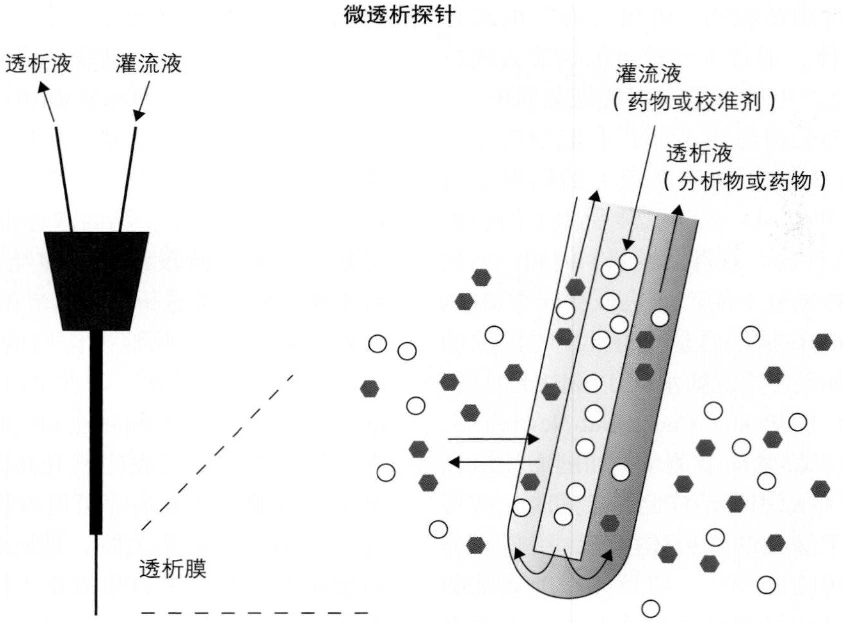

微透析探针

透析液

灌流液

灌流液
（药物或校准剂）

透析液
（分析物或药物）

透析膜

图 41.3 微透析是一种对脑细胞外间隙取样的技术。将侵入性探针插入脑实质，以超低流速（通常为 0.3 μl/min）注入液体（灌流液）。导管末端的半透膜允许物质扩散到导管内，并回收流出的液体（微透析液）。在临床上，最常见的分析是葡萄糖、乳酸、丙酮酸、谷氨酸（一种兴奋性神经递质）和甘油（一种衡量细胞膜破裂的指标）。乳酸和丙酮酸之间的比率（LPR，乳酸 - 丙酮酸比率）提供了无氧呼吸和有氧呼吸之间的平衡的量度（图 41.1）。在 TBI 中，乳酸 / 丙酮酸 >25 被认为是病理性的，与不良的临床结局相关

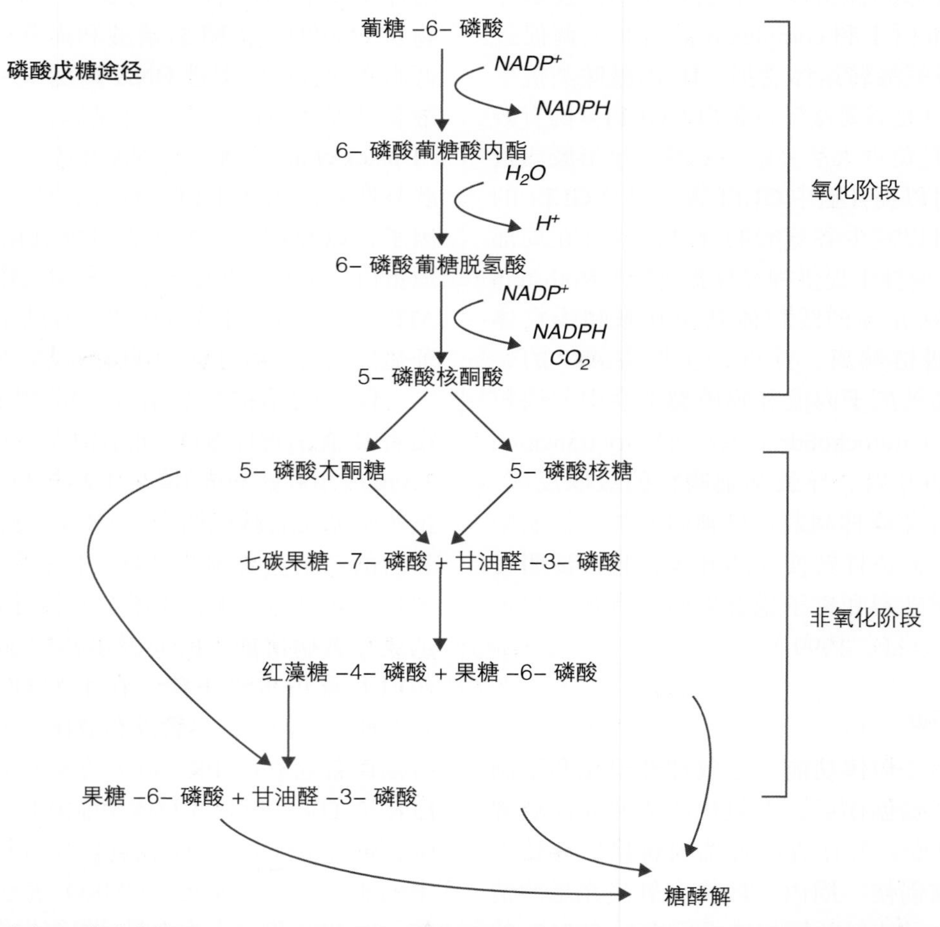

图 41.4 磷酸戊糖途径。磷酸戊糖途径（PPP）是葡萄糖利用的替代途径，在颅脑损伤后被发现上调。它提供了几种具有潜在保护作用的生化底物，这是一个积极探索的研究途径

究表明，代谢阈值为 37.6 μmol/（100 ml · min），超出则导致不可逆损伤。

自主调节丧失和压力反应性指数

如前面所述，血管的自主调节是一种肌源性机制，血管壁紧张会直接引起血管平滑肌收缩。平均动脉压升高会引起血管收缩，并在 5~15 s 内降低大脑血容量（cerebral blood volume，CBV）和颅内压，而平均动脉压降低则会导致血管扩张和颅内压升高。严重损伤后数天自主调节功能可能会被干扰，干扰的风险取决于损伤严重程度。当脑血管系统反应性变差时，量化血管反应性在脑创伤后具有重要临床意义。在脑损伤后机械通气患者中，平均动脉压和颅内压的慢波波动持续 30 秒到几分钟是很常见的。持续监测这些变化，并将它们的关系计算为 -1 和 +1 之间的压力反应指数（pressure reactivity index，PRx）（Czosnyka et al.，1997），负相关表明血管反应性良好（当平均动脉压升高时，由于动脉血管收缩导致颅内压下降）和能自主保护，而正相关则提示自我调节的丧失和较差的预后。在大宗病例患者中，PRx 小于 0.3 与 GOS 良好预后相关。

PRx 在脑创伤后第一天常受到损害，在伤后最初 48 小时内自主调节丧失预示着更多的继发性损害，包括大脑缺氧和进一步缺血损伤。保留的自我调节是重要保护机制，防止平均动脉压瞬间紊乱。PRx 除了是一个强有力的预后预测因子外，还是指导创伤后治疗和 CPP 管理的重要临床工具。PRx 随 CPP 动态变化，从而有可能定义 CPP 阈值，在该阈值下，PRx 以最小化来保护最大化自动调节：这被称为"CPP 最优"（CPP_{opt}）。TBI 患者持续 PRx 监测，根据损伤严重程度确定实时的 CPP_{opt}，CPP 调整若小于 CPP_{opt} 似乎会增加死亡率风险，而 CPP 大于 CPP_{opt} 似乎会二分为 GOS 良好和不良两种结果。靶向 CPP_{opt} 是否是有效的治疗靶点尚待确定。

颅内压升高

Monro-Kellie 假说解释，在正常情况下，颅腔的总体积保持不变，由三种主要成分构成：血液（CBV，动脉和静脉）、液体（CSF）和脑实质。一个成分增加通常会导致另一个成分代偿，通过脑脊液和静脉血的移位来维持恒定的 ICP。当代偿机制耗尽时，ICP 呈指数增长。颅内压低于 20~25 mmHg 的患者预后明显更好。颅内压升高（>20~25 mmHg）可通过降低 CPP（MAP–ICP）诱发缺血和缺氧；由于 CBF 与 CPP 成正比，TBI 后低血压、ICP 升高和缺氧可严重限制脑的供给。

脑创伤后水肿很常见，可归因于三种不同的机制：血管源性、细胞毒性和渗透性。第一，BBB 内皮细胞破裂引起的结构损伤导致富含蛋白质的渗出物流入脑间质，增加细胞外体积而不引起细胞肿胀。第二，细胞容量可以在不破坏 BBB 情况下累积。离子流入和神经细胞膜通透性增加导致细胞毒性水肿和细胞肿胀。而细胞毒性水肿是最常见脑水肿，导致间质体积减小。第三，坏死组织具有高渗性，导致细胞内渗透梯度造成液体积聚。毫不奇怪，水肿会导致 ICP 增加和继发缺血事件，进一步加剧破坏结构完整性和组织损伤。

在创伤后脑水肿治疗中，高渗药物例如甘露醇和高渗盐水可降低颅内压。然而，需要重点注意的是一旦血脑屏障受损，甘露醇可能会恶化血管源性脑水肿。在 86% 自主调节完整患者中，甘露醇快速滴入可以降低颅内压 10% 以上，而在自主调节受损患者中，只有 35% 的患者观察到颅内压下降（Muizelaar et al.，1984）。当丧失自主调节时，渗透性药物可能会增加 CBF，而此时无代偿性血管收缩，因此可能无法实现预期的 ICP 降低。甘露醇作用的其他潜在机制包括作为自由基清除剂，通过使内皮细胞脱水改善微血管血流，降低红细胞压积和渗透负荷。尽管采取了密切的治疗措施，难治性 ICP 仍是 46%TBI 死亡的主要原因。

脑血流障碍

在未受损的大脑中，在 60~160 mmHg 的脑灌注压对脑血流量仅有轻微影响。在脑创伤和自我调节受损后，CBF 变得越来越依赖 CPP，轻微的波动可能引发进一步缺血损伤。如前所述，CPP=MAP-ICP 和 CBF=CPP/CVR，其中 CVR（cerebrovascular resistance）是指脑血管阻力。颅内压继发性升高可能恶化 CPP，降低 CBF。CBV 定义为每 100 g 脑组织的血液毫升数，可使用稳定氙气测量 CBF 和注射对比剂后的平均通过时间来计算。在正常情况下，CBF 是 CBV 的反映，但在创伤后，由于生理障碍，CBF 和 CBV 之间存在分离。由于严重颅脑损伤后代谢降低，因此确定 $AVDO_2$ 对于准确解释 CBF 和诊断低灌注或高灌注是必要的。CBF 通常在受伤后的前 6 小时内较低，并在前 24 小时显著增加。低 CBF 通常与高 $AVDO_2$ 无关，更可能是低氧化代谢的标志，而不是缺血。高 CBV 并不总是与严重 TBI 患者的脑肿胀相关；除充血外，还有其他因素导致脑肿胀和难治性高血压 ICP。在没有急性充血的患者中，CBF 始终与功能恢复相关（即，最严重残疾患者的 CBF 最低）。

最近的研究结合氧 15 标记的正电子发射断层扫描（oxygen 15-labelled positron emission tomography，^{15}O PET）和氟 18 标记的氟咪唑（fluorine 18-labelled fluoromisonidazole，^{18}F FMISO），进一步描述了早期脑创伤中的大血管和微血管缺血特征（Veenithet al., 2016）。缺血脑容量（ischaemic brain volume，IBV）和缺氧脑容量（hypoxic brain volume，HBV）的比较表明，HBV 中弥散性缺氧边界与微血管塌陷有关，而 IBV 代表大血管缺血和不可逆损伤。创伤性挫伤显示 CBF 和 $CMRO_2$ 降低，但 CBV 和氧摄取分数（oxygen extraction fraction，OEF）与对照组相似。在挫伤周围无明显组织功能障碍区域，$CMRO_2$ 较低，但 CBF、CBV 和 OEF 与对照组相似。经典推理表明，随着 $CMRO_2$ 的减少，增加 OEF 以进行补偿。然而，最近使用 DTI 的研究表明，挫伤周围经常出现与细胞毒性水肿一致的低扩散系数边缘，这可以解释由于广泛的微血管衰竭和选择性神经元丢失导致的 OEF 最小变化。

充血

充血，也称为血管充血或过度灌注，是由于 CBF 超过 $CMRO_2$ 需求时，血流 - 代谢耦合中断引起。CBV 升高通常表明创伤后充血，伴随 ICP 升高预示着恢复不良。急性充血通常与颅高压（ICP>20 mmHg）相关，但低于正常血流通常表明完整的血流 - 代谢耦合，而不代表缺血。充血性高 ICP 患者通常较年轻，平均 GCS 较低（≤6），存在基底池消失和难治性高血压，并表现出明显的自动调节功能丧失。值得注意的是，CBF 在功能上与 CMRG 耦合，而不是与 $CMRO_2$ 耦合，因此富足灌注可能是对损伤后高糖分解的适当代谢反应。从历史上看，过度换气是为了降低 CBF 和随后的 ICP 升高，但诱发缺血风险限制这种方法应用。脑损伤后，由于正常生理的破坏，CBF 可能不再准确反映 CBV，在急性 SDH、ICP 升高和缺血患者中，CBV 为正常值的一半。因此，多种病因可能导致严重头部创伤后颅内高压和脑肿胀。

脑缺血

缺血性损伤包括梗死核心和半暗带。缺血核心经历缺氧诱导的细胞内稳态丧失和坏死，而半影区的凋亡过程可以作为治疗靶点。当 CBF 不能满足大脑代谢需求（例如低 CBF 和高 $AVDO_2$）时，就会发生脑缺血。假设血流 - 代谢耦合是完整的，ICU 经常使用颈静脉球血氧饱和度从其与 $AVDO_2$ 的反向关系来评估 CBF 是否充分。正常的 $AVDO_2$ 范围为 4~9 ml/100 ml，低 CBF 和缺血状态会增加氧提取，导致 $AVDO_2$ 增加。经颅多普勒非侵入性地测量大脑基底动脉的血流速度，以估计 CBF，同时要注意出血可导致血管痉挛，从而增加血流速度，而与 CBF 无关。缺血通常见于急性 SDH 和弥漫性脑肿胀，TBI 后大脑代谢供应不足预示着高致死率和致残率。PET 已经证明，以前基于 CBF 和血氧定义缺血是不准确的，维持氧气输送可能不足以防止继发性损伤。TBI 后的线粒体功能障碍降低了需氧量，向高糖分解的转变增加了乳酸积累。因此，CBF 降低可能被误解为缺血，维持足够的灌注（CPP>70 mmHg）可能不会改善由于线粒体 ATP 合成受损导致的脑灌注异常。

如前所述，在正常生理情况下，$AVDO_2$ 保持相对恒定，而 CBF 会根据 $CMRO_2$/CMRG 变化调整。当 TBI 后自动调节功能丧失，而 CBF 根据 $CMRO_2$/CMRG 变化调节能力丧失，且 CBF 满足代谢需求能力受损时，$AVDO_2$ 可能增加以改善脑循环中 O_2 提取。$AVDO_2$ 能够从基线值 6.7 ml/100 ml 增加到最大 13 ml/100 ml。正常状况下 $AVDO_2$ 代偿发生时的 CBF 阈值为 18 ml/(100 g · min)；由于氧化代谢降低，TBI 后可以上升到 20 ml/（100 g · min）。^{15}O PET 显示，扩散屏障缺血（从血管系统到间质的氧扩散梯度增加）是由于微血管紊乱所致，如创伤病灶周围的血管周围水肿，导致脑组织中氧分压（PbO_2）降低。

除了直接导致神经元死亡的半胱天冬酶和其他蛋白质外，三种不同的丝裂原激活蛋白激酶（mitogen-activated protein kinase，MAPK）炎症通路也参与了缺血性损伤：细胞外信号调节激酶（extracellular signal-regulated kinase，ERK）通路、c-Jun-N- 末端蛋白激酶（c-Jun-N-terminal protein kinase，JNK）通路和 p38 通路。生物标志物的应用研究已经产生了一些对神经元、神经胶质和轴突损伤具有重要意义的标志物。神经元特异性烯醇化酶是一种主要存在于神经元中的糖酵解酶。S-100B 是一种钙结合蛋白，主要存在于星形胶质细胞中。髓鞘碱性蛋白存在于白质中，是轴突损伤的标志。最近的研究发现，这些是 TBI 后脑缺血和神经炎症病理过程的重要生物标志物，反映了继发性损伤的时间进程。

皮质扩散性抑制与癫痫

皮质扩散性抑制（cortical spreading depression，CSD）是离子稳态失效导致的一种弥漫性波，可暂时中断皮质功能。它的特征是 EEG 抑制、软脑膜血管扩张以及严重头部创伤和缺血后缓慢的负电位转移（Leao，1947）。梗死周围自发性的去极化（PID）向正常脑组织传播，并呈现CSD特征。皮质脑电图（ECoG）记录显示自发的抑郁伴随着模式化的CSD以3.3 mm/min的速度在皮质表面扩散；ECoG背景活动可在2~5小时后自发恢复（Fabricius，2006）。在神经元和神经胶质细胞中传播去极化波导致氧化代谢增加，通过增加CBF和代谢活性进行补偿；因此，当血流-代谢耦联完整时，CSD不会导致正常脑神经元损伤。颅脑损伤后，血流动力学紊乱和血流代谢脱钩常见，因此CSD可能会产生额外的能量需求，这些能量需求无法由受伤的大脑代谢补偿。

CSD通过活化基质金属蛋白酶（matrix metalloproteinase，MMP）来改变血脑屏障（BBB）通透性。基质金属蛋白酶由中性蛋白酶组成，参与如下的广泛过程：BBB的开放，免疫细胞浸润神经组织，细胞因子和细胞因子受体的脱落，细胞直接损害，神经元的发育和可塑性。CSD增加MMP-9活性，导致BBB破坏和水肿形成。缺血和创伤后，MMP-9和MMP-2的神经元表达与神经毒性有关，增加了对脑出血的易感性。CSD更常发生在年轻的急性损伤患者中，并可能通过谷氨酸受体抑制剂，特别是NMDA受体拮抗剂而减弱。CSD和PID会导致梗死体积逐步增加，这是原发和继发性半暗带损伤和应激诱导变化的一部分。

癫痫发作

急性癫痫发作（包括惊厥性和非惊厥性）是有充分证据证明的继发性损伤，其可能是由于神经化学紊乱引起的，可加重组织损伤并使临床恢复过程恶化。脑电图监测表明，大多数癫痫发作并没有明显运动表现，因此需要持续监测癫痫脑电活动。ECoG记录可区分CSD标志性缓慢电位变化和癫痫发作；虽然皮质扩散性抑制和癫痫经常同时发生，但两个现象在时间、空间和强度上并无关联（Fabricius，2006）。中型至重型TBI后，超过20%的患者在第一周出现癫痫发作；发病高峰呈双峰型，早期高峰出现在伤后29小时，晚期高峰出现在伤后140小时，平均持续时间为2.8分钟，并有聚集趋势。在癫痫发作的这几个高峰，ICP继发升高，发作期ICP高于发作间期ICP。ICP升高和癫痫引起的脑肿胀风险可能归因于CBF的长期增加、细胞外水肿和间质中谷氨酸聚积。

众所周知，癫痫样活动可进一步刺激糖酵解和神经生物化学变化，从而进一步影响神经元的完整性。伴有癫痫发作的TBI患者（与无癫痫发作的患者相比）和发作期（与发作间期相比）的微透析乳酸/丙酮酸比值（LPR）较高。LPR的升高与长期代谢应激有关，因此控制癫痫发作是减少损伤后代谢应激的治疗目标。挫伤周围区域，特别是额颞叶区域，具有电活动性，能够发生癫痫样活动。重型脑创伤患者易发生癫痫。高风险因素包括脑挫伤和（或）硬膜下血肿的存在，血肿的早期清除可能与减少癫痫发作活动有关（Annegers et al.，1998）。严重脑外伤后报告癫痫的患者中，78%为继发性局灶性发作。

β-淀粉样蛋白沉积与载脂蛋白E相互作用

TBI可触发大脑皮质淀粉样-（Aβ）肽的病理性产生和积聚，尤其是挫伤和挫伤周围区域（Roberts et al.，1991）。淀粉样前体蛋白（amyloid precursor protein，APP）裂解产生载脂蛋白E（ApoE）和Aβ，而载脂蛋白E基因多态性决定了斑块沉积的风险：ApoE ε 4具有更大的风险，而ApoEε3（更常见）和ε2（罕见）都降低了Aβ负荷的风险。在三种异构体中，ApoEε4与促进轴突生长和神经保护作用的细胞骨架蛋白结合程度最低。载脂蛋白ε4多与Aβ结合，促进淀粉样蛋白纤维聚集。与局部损伤相比，颅内微透析检测到DAI患者的Aβ水平更高，因此Aβ积聚也可能取决于损伤类型。脑实质的长期轴突变性和轴突内Aβ沉积可能是由于持续的神经变性和继发性损伤所致。体外研究有支持Apo-Aβ相互作用的证据，具有载脂蛋白Eε4等位基因的脑创伤患者在海马和额叶皮质有更多的Apo Aβ沉积。

在损伤急性期，脑脊液中Aβ浓度和载脂蛋白E的ELISA测定值降低。随着时间的推移，它们的水平逐渐升高，这与神经功能改善有关。神经元损伤后，载脂蛋白Aβ的产生会立即减少，载脂蛋白E的水平降低可能是由于载脂蛋白E-脂质复合物的修复利用增加，这是回应协调神经元损伤的一部分。载脂蛋白E在脑缺血中有神经保护作用，脑室内注射载脂蛋白E可通过清除脂质和胆固醇碎片来减轻动物模型脑缺血后的神经元损伤。载脂蛋白E通过下调小神经胶质细胞和细胞因子的释放来促进抗炎效应（Kay et al.，2003）。脑创伤来源的Aβ斑块与阿尔茨海默症早期的病理特征相似。长期随访脑创伤患者也显示与阿尔茨海默症发病相关，同型载脂蛋白E是一个重要的预测因子。值得注意的是，在TBI患者6个月随访出现不良结局（GOS：死亡、植物人状态或严重残疾）中，具有ApoE ε 4等位基因有57%不良结局，而具有ApoE ε 2或 ε 3等位基因的患者为27%。

未来方向

TBI通用数据元（Common Data Elements，CDE）的成功实施，以及其在生成具有强大统计能力的新型分类方法中的效用的证明，为NIH/NINDS CDE第2版的完善提供了信息（Hicks et al.，2013），并推动了欧盟22个国家进行欧洲神经创伤有效性研究合作项目（CENTER-TBI）研究和美国11个地点的TRACK-TBI研究（Manley and Maas，2013）。其目标是使用CDEs登记近10000名患者，以提供新的多维度TBI分类方法，建立起医疗质量证据基准，并生成大型、精心策划的TBI数据库，以实现和确保后续有机会进一步研究。

结论

虽然本质上降低原发性神经损伤风险是以预防为主，但了解TBI后续情况以便临床处理和（或）预防继发性损伤在当前神经外科和神经重症中仍是至关重要的。预防“说话和恶化”的TBI患者的潜在并发症强调了一个关键概念，即原发性损伤可能很容易诱发复合继发性损伤的病理生理条件。最后，脑创伤更多的被认为是一个疾病的过程而不是单一事件；损伤类型和严重程度的内在异质性突出表明，迫切需要使用病理解剖损伤的一致定义，类似于目前心脏病、癌症和糖尿病的标准方法，验证临床、神经影像学和血清生物标志物，对损伤进行评估。目前正在进行大规模的国际TBI试验，使用经过验证的通用数据元标准来加快分类和预测方法的进展。

延伸阅读、参考文献、EBRAIN的相关链接

扫描书末二维码获取。

第 42 章　创伤性脑损伤的重症监护管理

Matthew A. Kirkman · Martin Smith 著
刘伟明 译，欧云尉 审校

引言

创伤性脑损伤（traumatic brain injury，TBI）是40岁以下成人死亡和致残的主要原因。其预后取决于原发性损伤的严重程度和继发性损伤，包括颅内高压、全身性低血压、缺氧、发热、低血糖和高血糖。监测、预防和处理可导致继发性脑损伤的因素是脑创伤重症监护管理的基础。

颅脑损伤的早期处理

处理头部损伤首先应于院前应用标准的高级创伤生命支持方案，进行及时和系统的评估和管理（**图 42.1**）。复苏和早期管理是影响严重 TBI 致死率和致残率的关键（Boer et al.，2012）。预防或立即纠正低氧血症和低血压，快速诊断和清除颅内血肿，以及治疗颅内压（intracranial pressure，ICP）升高是决定预后的关键因素。用最短时间稳定患者状态并明确治疗方案十分重要。尽管气道管理和通气是昏迷和意识水平恶化 TBI 患者的关键干预措施，但是否在院前气管插管以及该由谁进行气管插管仍然存在争议（Boer et al.，2012）。除非患者清醒并配合，否则应在等待影像和（或）正式临床评估前固定颈椎。转移前应稳定危及生命的颅外损伤。

颅脑损伤并发多发伤的处理

创伤性脑损伤通常伴随颅外损伤，包括脊柱损伤（见**第 64 章**），这会使脑损伤治疗复杂化。采用及时和适当的干预稳定或治疗颅外损伤是防止出现过长时间出血性休克、全身炎症反应综合征和多器官衰竭的关键。

多发伤患者的治疗面临的一个特殊挑战是如何平衡如下矛盾：低压复苏可以限制持续失血、缩短复苏时间，但存在使相关颅脑损伤恶化的风险。建议 TBI 患者的收缩压始终保持在 90 mmHg 以上。然而，如果在治疗危及生命的出血时需要降低血压，则低血压的持续时间应尽可能短，并改善其他生理指标，以最大限度地增加脑供氧。尤其是，必须避免低碳酸血症。

在临床评估机会受限情况下，建议在多次手术和（或）延长颅外损伤镇静期间进行 ICP 监测（Stocchetti et al.，2014）。

颅脑损伤重症监护管理通则

所有严重脑创伤患者都应在重症监护室（intensive care unit，ICU）进行治疗，多学科临床神经科学团队和其他相关专业可迅速介入，并有适当影像学和观察设备支持。轻度或中度创伤性脑损伤患者，也可能因各种适应证需要入住重症监护室（**专栏 42.1**）。

TBI 的重症监护管理是复杂的，需要细致全面的重症监护支持，以优化全身生理状态，并针对受伤的大脑进行干预（**表 42.1**）。除了对所有危重患者进行常规心肺功能持续监测和评估外，还有几种技术可用于全脑和部分脑区的监测（见下文）。

心肺功能

单次低氧血症（PaO_2<8 kPa 或 SpO_2<90%）或低血压（收缩压 <90 mmHg）与严重 TBI 不良预后密切相关，两者同时存在比单独损伤危害更大（McHugh et al.，2007）。预防或快速逆转缺氧和低血压对严重 TBI 患者至关重要。然而，治疗性高浓度氧与不良反应有关，包括自由基的形成和肺损伤，并且常压高浓度氧并不能显著改善临床脑氧代谢。尽管有一些证据表明高压氧可降低死亡率，但很少有证据表明能改善幸存者功能预后（Bennett et al.，2012）。因此，不建议常规使用超出维持关键氧合目标的高浓度氧治疗。

低血压应首先通过静脉液体复苏纠正，单靠液体复苏无法达到目标血压，则需要应用血管活性

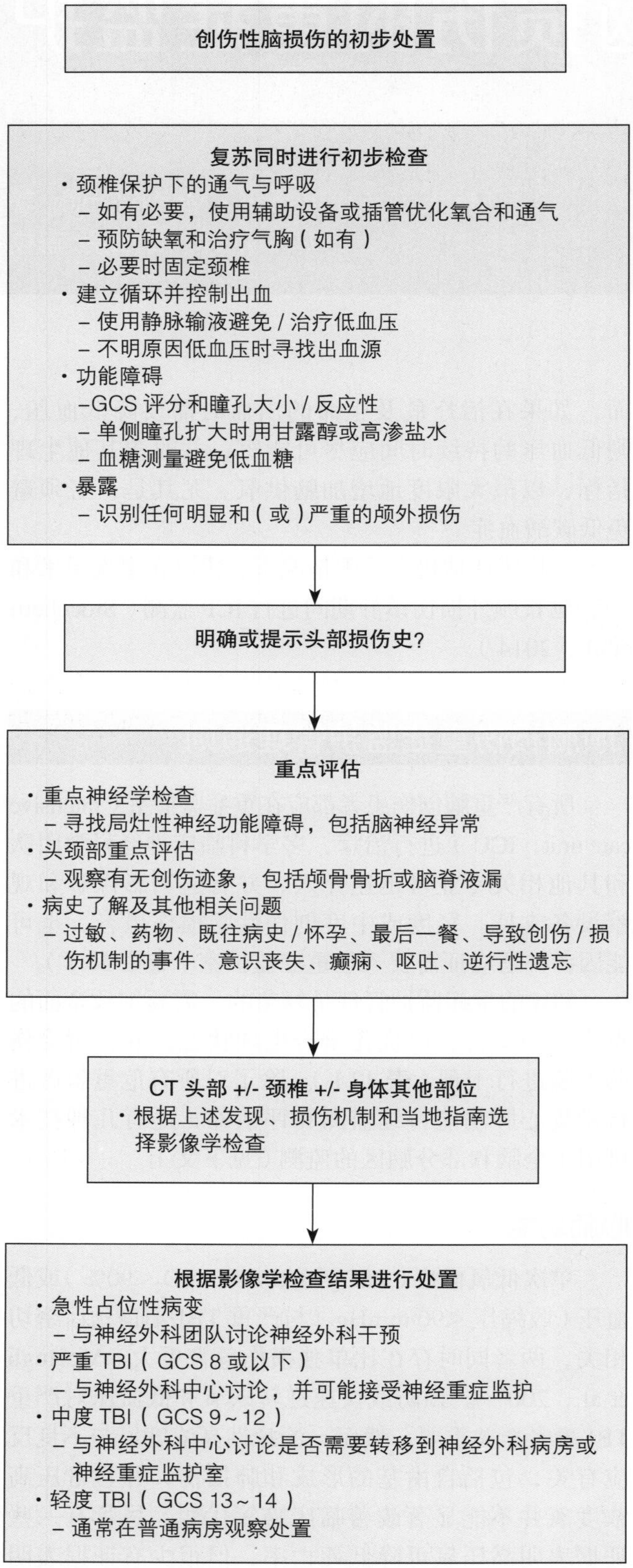

创伤性脑损伤的初步处置

↓

复苏同时进行初步检查
- 颈椎保护下的通气与呼吸
  – 如有必要，使用辅助设备或插管优化氧合和通气
  – 预防缺氧和治疗气胸（如有）
  – 必要时固定颈椎
- 建立循环并控制出血
  – 使用静脉输液避免/治疗低血压
  – 不明原因低血压时寻找出血源
- 功能障碍
  –GCS 评分和瞳孔大小/反应性
  – 单侧瞳孔扩大时用甘露醇或高渗盐水
  – 血糖测量避免低血糖
- 暴露
  – 识别任何明显和（或）严重的颅外损伤

↓

明确或提示头部损伤史？

↓

重点评估
- 重点神经学检查
  – 寻找局灶性神经功能障碍，包括脑神经异常
- 头颈部重点评估
  – 观察有无创伤迹象，包括颅骨骨折或脑脊液漏
- 病史了解及其他相关问题
  – 过敏、药物、既往病史/怀孕、最后一餐、导致创伤/损伤机制的事件、意识丧失、癫痫、呕吐、逆行性遗忘

↓

CT 头部 +/- 颈椎 +/- 身体其他部位
- 根据上述发现、损伤机制和当地指南选择影像学检查

↓

根据影像学检查结果进行处置
- 急性占位性病变
  – 与神经外科团队讨论神经外科干预
- 严重 TBI（GCS 8 或以下）
  – 与神经外科中心讨论，并可能接受神经重症监护
- 中度 TBI（GCS 9~12）
  – 与神经外科中心讨论是否需要转移到神经外科病房或神经重症监护室
- 轻度 TBI（GCS 13~14）
  – 通常在普通病房观察处置

图 42.1 创伤性脑损伤即时处理的流程

专栏 42.1 重症监护室收治头部受伤患者指征

- 严重创伤性脑损伤（定义为复苏后 GCS≤8）
- 颅内压升高的临床或放射学证据
- 由于以下原因需要机械通气：
  – 意识水平下降
  – 脑干功能障碍的证据
  – 急性呼吸衰竭（如神经源性肺水肿）
  – 呼吸暂停发作
  – 全身强直阵挛发作或癫痫持续状态
  – 任何其他导致气道受损或受到危害的原因
- 需要加强血流动力学监测和管理的心血管不稳定
- 需要有创性神经和全身监测
- 肾功能和心功能不全等全身器官的支持管理
- 神经外科干预术后
- 多系统创伤

表 42.1 重型头部损伤的重症监护处置的一般方面

通气	• PaO_2>11 kPa • $PaCO_2$ 4.5~5.0 kPa • 肺保护性通气策略（潮气量 6ml/kg 理想体重，PEEP 6~12 mmHg）作为大脑导向治疗原则 • PEEP 维持氧合（PEEP≤12~15 cm H_2O 时对 ICP 无不良影响，如果氧合改善，可能降低 ICP） • 呼吸机“整体护理”，可最大限度地降低肺炎 – 头抬高位 – 口腔卫生 – 预防消化性溃疡 – 预防静脉血栓栓塞 – 如果 ICP 允许，每日镇静
心血管	• MAP > 90 mmHg • 用等张晶体恢复正常血容量 • 如果对液体反应不足，则使用血管加压剂/正性肌力药物
ICP 和 CPP 目标	• CPP 60~70 mmHg • ICP <22 mmHg
其他	• 正常血糖 • 正常体温 • 癫痫控制 • 肠内营养 • 血栓栓塞预防

CPP，脑灌注压；ICP，颅内压；MAP，平均动脉压；PEEP，呼气末正压

药物。恢复正常血容量是心血管治疗目标的主要目标，但过于激进的液体复苏是有害的（Gantner et al.，2014）。应使用等渗晶体液维持血管内容量，尽管缺乏强力证据，0.9% 生理盐水是一个合理选择。使用白蛋白可导致死亡率增加，这可能继发于 ICP 增高（Cooper et al.，2013）。尽管人们对使用高渗盐水

（hypertonic saline，HS）溶液进行TBI后液体复苏感兴趣，但与等渗晶体溶液相比，还没有报道其对预后的获益。

没有可靠证据表明哪种血管升压药是最有效的，但去甲肾上腺素对全身血压和脑血流动力学有可预测的持续性作用，因而被广泛使用。

血糖控制

高血糖可加重继发性神经元损伤，并与严重TBI的预后恶化有关。胰岛素治疗的"严格"血糖控制可导致TBI后的低血糖和代谢危象（Vespa et al.，2012）。因此，建议适度控制血糖，将血糖浓度维持在7~10 mmol/L，避免低血糖（血糖<4.4 mmol/L）和血糖浓度大幅波动（Kramer et al.，2012）。

温度控制

发热（核心体温超过37.5~38.5℃）是预后不良的独立相关因素，50%以上重症监护病房的TBI患者都会出现发热。发热的病因有很多，包括感染和下丘脑功能障碍等。尽管有退热药、表面和血管内降温装置等治疗选择，但缺乏高质量的证据证明降温至常温后的疗效。尽管如此，以常温或轻度低温（35.5~37°C）为目标的靶向温度管理（targeted temperature management，TTM），通常被推荐用于TBI管理。

TTM具有许多潜在的神经保护作用，包括稳定血脑屏障、降低ICP、抑制炎症和细胞内钙超载等。尽管一些单中心研究显示了其疗效，在大规模随机临床试验（randomized clinical trials，RCT）中，TTM疗效的临床前证据尚未转化为积极的预后结果。与之前的系统综述不同，2014年的一项meta分析（包括RCT和观察性研究）表明，TTM在总体降低死亡率和不良预后方面有一定的益处（Crossley et al.，2014）。然而，大多数纳入试验质量较低，这可能高估了TTM对比标准治疗的有效性。特别需要指出的是研究之间存在显著的异质性，如在TTM使用时机、持续时间、目标温度以及复温的时间和速率方面。复温是TTM最危险的阶段，必须以受控的方式（每小时0.1~0.25 °C）进行，以尽量减少颅内高压反弹和高钾血症风险。令人失望的是，在最近的一项RCT中，尽管做到了伤后尽快应用TTM，维持目标温度（32~34 °C）至少72小时，缓慢复温（<1 °C/d），但未能发现TTM对单纯控制发热的益处（Maekawa et al.，2015）。TTM的其他不良反应包括颤抖，以及血糖、电解质水平和体液平衡异常。

尽管缺乏改善预后的证据，但适度的TTM可有效地降低升高的ICP，并经常被纳入ICP管理方案（见下）。最近的国际多中心Eurotherm3235 RCT，将387例对一级治疗（包括机械通气、镇静剂和床头抬高）无效的颅内高压（ICP>20 mmHg）TBI患者，随机分为标准治疗组和32~35 °C低温加标准治疗组，由于低体温组功能预后差且死亡率高，早期中止试验（Andrews et al.，2015）。因为这项研究使用低温作为第二级治疗，它没有充分解决TTM是否有利于TBI患者的难治性高ICP的问题。第三级治疗（巴比妥类药物和去骨瓣减压术）在对照组的使用率（54%）高于低温组（44%），但没有记录研究中每组使用甘露醇和高渗盐水的量。鉴于这些不足，本试验不太可能显著改变TTM在TBI中的应用，但它确实强调了TBI需要进一步高质量TTM随机对照试验。

贫血

大约50%的严重TBI患者出现贫血，这会激活缺氧细胞信号通路，并对脑供氧产生不利影响。贫血产生的确切后果和能产生脑组织损伤的血红蛋白（haemoglobin，Hb）阈值尚不确定。然而，由于脑损伤后对缺血的敏感性增加，一般重症监护中使用的限制性输血方法似乎不太可能外推到TBI患者身上。一项关于促红细胞生成素和两个输血阈值（血红蛋白浓度70 g/L和100 g/L）的RCT发现，无论是给予促红细胞生成素还是维持血红蛋白在100 g/L以上，都不能改善TBI后6个月的神经功能预后，但后者与更多不良事件相关，尤其是血栓栓塞（Robertson et al.，2014）。目前建议在TBI的急性期，血红蛋白应保持在90g/L以上，并避免过度输血（LeRoux，2013）。

凝血病

超过1/3的TBI患者出现急性创伤性凝血障碍，并与预后不良相关（Epstein et al.，2014）。低凝状态和高凝状态都可以存在，同时伴随着大量组织因子的释放、蛋白C稳态改变和血小板功能障碍。治疗上可根据当地用药习惯，应用新鲜冷冻血浆和凝血酶原复合物纠正凝血异常。对于TBI凝血障碍的逆转，目前尚无明确的指南。

在伤后3小时内给予抗纤维蛋白溶解剂氨甲环酸，可降低创伤出血患者的死亡率，而不会增加不良事件。正在进行的前瞻性RCT（CRASH-3，http://www.isrctn.com/ISRCTN15088122）正在验证该药是否对TBI也有同样好处。

癫痫发作

脑创伤后癫痫发作很常见，可引起颅内压升高、脑缺血和神经递质过度释放。创伤后癫痫（post traumatic seizures，PTS）分为早期（7天内）或晚期（7天后），并且与不良预后相关。尽管预防性抗癫痫药物（antiepileptic drugs，AED）的使用存在争议，但及时发现和治疗癫痫可改善预后。一些指南建议使用短疗程（7天）抗癫痫药物来降低早期PTS发病率，但没有证据表明这可以改善预后或降低创伤后癫痫的风险。也没有证据支持使用抗癫痫药物可预防晚期癫痫，晚期癫痫应该像任何新发癫痫一样进行管理。苯妥英钠历来是预防和治疗PTS的一线药物，但左乙拉西坦似乎疗效相同，副作用较少，不需要监测血药浓度。

脑创伤患者，尤其是颅骨凹陷骨折、穿透伤和大面积皮质挫伤/血肿患者，有发生非惊厥性癫痫（non-convulsive seizures，NCS）的风险。AED预防并不能阻止NCS的发展，治疗对预后的影响仍有待阐明。建议采用脑电图（EEG）排除不明原因持续性意识障碍的TBI患者是否有癫痫发作（Claassen et al.，2013）。

静脉血栓栓塞

严重TBI是发生静脉血栓栓塞的重要危险因素。虽然没有明确的疗效证据，建议使用分级弹力袜或间歇充气弹力袜（除非下肢创伤不能使用），直到患者可下地行走。低分子肝素或小剂量普通肝素能降低深静脉血栓形成（deep vein thrombosis，DVT）和死亡率，但其预防时机仍有争议。如果在受伤后七天内不进行药物预防，则必须权衡颅内出血相关风险与DVT显著增高风险。根据5000例以上TBI患者证据，建议中度或高度血肿扩张风险的患者在72小时后开始药物预防，对于血肿扩张风险较低且尚无血肿扩大的患者在48小时后开始预防（Abdel-Aziz et al.，2015）。

营养支持

TBI与高代谢状态和过量氮消耗有关，应在受伤后第五天，最迟在第七天，实现完全的热量替代（Carney et al.，2017）。最近的一项meta分析发现，早期饮食（在大多数研究中定义为入院后48小时内）与死亡率、不良结局和感染并发症的显著降低相关（Wang et al.，2013）。

电解质和内分泌紊乱

脑创伤后电解质钠的稳态紊乱是常见的，低钠血症和高钠血症对受伤的大脑都有不良影响。系统的诊断和治疗至关重要（**表42.2**）。

TBI后内分泌功能衰竭与下丘脑-垂体轴（hypothalamic-pituitary axis，HPA）直接损伤、颅内高压相关的下丘脑缺血和炎症相关的原发性腺体功能衰竭有关。在重型TBI患者中，HPA功能障碍导致肾上腺功能不全发生率高达50%，其影响可以是持久的，并影响伤后慢性阶段的康复。所有高危患者和不明原因的低钠血症、低血糖，或持续需要高剂量血管加压素的患者，应考虑使用标准刺激/反应试验进行垂体功能不全的急性筛查。激素替代疗法对预后的影响尚未得到很好的研究，但在出现难治性低血压的情况下应考虑使用氢化可的松，如果低钠血症持续存在，可补充盐皮质激素（Powner et al.，2006）。

非神经系统器官功能障碍

非神经器官功能障碍，特别是涉及心肺系统的功能障碍，是脑创伤后常见的疾病，也是致残和致死的独立危险因素。早期发现和及时干预是否改善预后尚不明确。系统并发症可能是由于神经性原因引起的，例如脑损伤相关儿茶酚胺和神经炎症反应，可导致神经源性心肌顿抑综合征和神经源性肺水肿；或是脑导向治疗的并发症，如继发于脑灌注压（cerebral perfusion pressure，CPP）导向治疗的急性肺损伤（acute lung injury，ALI），或TTM相关感染。TBI后肺炎特别常见，在高达80%的机械通气患者中发生。全身器官功能障碍和衰竭的管理是一个重大挑战，因为对全身器官系统衰竭的最佳治疗可能对受伤大脑产生潜在不良影响，反之亦然。关于非神经系统并发症的病因和管理的详细讨论，读者可参考其他文献（Berthiaume and Zygun，2006）。

颅内压和脑灌注压的监测和管理

ICP和CPP的监测和管理是重型TBI患者重症监护管理的重要方面。ICP监测可以获取颅内压指标，计算出CPP，识别和分析病理性ICP波形，用于预测颅内高压发展，并推导脑血管压力反应性指数。CPP是由平均动脉压（mean arterial pressure，MAP）和ICP之差计算出来的，并且可以通过这种关系进行修正。脑创伤基金会（Brain Trauma Foundation，BTF）建议在颅内压超过22 mmHg时进行干预（有些中心以>20 mmHg或>25 mmHg为阈值），并将CPP维持在60~70 mmHg（Carney et al.，2017）。

表 42.2　头部损伤术后钠紊乱特征和处理

检查	SIADH	CSWS	CDI
血浆容量	升高	降低	降低
钠平衡	阳性 / 正常	阴性	正常
水平衡	阳性	阴性	阴性
血清钠	降低	降低	升高
血清渗透压	降低	升高 / 正常	升高
尿钠	升高	升高	正常
尿渗透压	升高	正常 / 升高	降低
处置	• 限制无电解质水，最初为 1000~1500 ml/d，如果心血管状况允许 • 去甲环素，抑制肾对 ADH 的反应 • ADH 受体拮抗剂，抑制 ADH 与肾受体的结合	• 容量和钠复苏 • 氟卓可的松可限制钠的丢失	• 液体置换以维持正常血容量 • DDAVP，如果持续尿量高（>250 ml/h）

ADH，抗利尿激素；CDI，中枢性尿崩症；CSWS，脑性盐耗综合征；DDAVP，1- 脱氨基 -8-D- 精氨酸加压素；SIADH，抗利尿激素分泌失调综合征

正常值：血浆渗透压 278~305 mmol/kg；血浆钠 135~145 mmol/L；尿液渗透压 350~1000 mmol/kg；尿钠 20~60 mmol/L 或 100~250 mmol/24 h

颅内压

专栏 42.2 突出显示了 ICP 监测的适应证，强调了 2014 年专家共识建议和 2016 年 BTF 指南之间的差异。Stocchetti 等（2014 年）建议，普通 CT 扫描昏迷的 TBI 患者不需要 ICP 监测，而尽管缺乏高质量的证据支持，最新的 BTF 指南继续建议在存在特定高风险特征情况下对此类患者进行监测（Carney et al.，2017）。这种侧重点的差异可能与现代医学影像技术更能识别以前无法检测到的病变有关，从而降低继发于隐匿性病变演变而导致的颅内压升高的可能性。

技术方面

颅内压最常用测量方法是使用脑室内导管或脑实质的微换能器装置。其他测量技术如蛛网膜下腔或硬膜外的装置不甚准确，很少使用。脑室内导管测量整体 ICP（侧脑室的脑脊液压力）并可以治疗性引流脑脊液。导管相关脑室炎的风险随着导管置入时间延长而增加。使用抗生素浸渍或镀银导管可以减少（但不能杜绝）感染。脑实质微传感器 ICP 监测系统易于插入，通常通过颅骨进入装置或开颅手术时放置于脑实质内约 2 cm，也可放置于硬膜下间隙。尽管脑室内导管历来被认为是颅内压监测的“金标准”，但实质内装置提供了等效的压力测量，而且更安全，与装置相关的并发症（如血肿和感染）的风险更低（Smith，2008）。

目前已发展出几种无创性颅内压监测技术，包括经颅多普勒超声（transcranial Doppler，TCD）测出的搏动指数和超声或 CT 测量视神经鞘直径。尽管没有侵入性方法的风险，但这些技术目前无法足够准确地测量 ICP 以供临床常规使用。

颅内压升高的管理

颅内高压的负担（颅内压高于规定阈值的时间，阈值通常为 20~25 mmHg）与 TBI 不良后果相关。降低颅内压策略通常是逐步实施的，首先是一线的、更安全的干预措施，如头高位和镇静（图 42.2）。高风险的治疗方案，包括过度通气、TTM、巴比妥类药物和手术减压，适用于多模式脑监测证据的脑缺氧或脑代谢紊乱患者，或有迫在眉睫的脑疝风险的患者。

镇静

大多数镇静剂对控制 ICP 和 CPP 有益，但没有令人信服的证据表明一种药物优于另一种药物（Roberts et al.，2011）。现异丙酚被广泛应用，通常和注射短效阿片类药物联合使用。它能有效地降低脑代谢率和颅内压，并且镇静水平易于滴定，患者可被快速唤醒。α-2 激动剂右美托咪定有一定的脑损伤后镇静作用，但在脑创伤患者中没有 RCT 验证。

神经肌肉阻滞剂可以防止在气管内吸痰和其他干预过程中的 ICP 增加，但不能降低 ICP。神经肌肉阻滞剂能够增加肺炎和 ICU 获得性衰弱等颅外并发症的风险，不应经常使用。

专栏 42.2 创伤性脑损伤颅内压监测指征（脑创伤基金会指南和专家共识建议）

脑创伤基金会指南（2016）

- 所有可抢救的严重 TBI* 患者和异常头颅 CT 扫描
- 所有可抢救的严重 TBI 患者，扫描正常，有以下两种或两种以上：
  - 年龄超过 40 岁
  - 单侧或双侧运动姿势
  - 收缩压 <90 mmHg

注：这些建议是从上一版（第三版）的指南继承下来的，但没有得到现行证据标准的支持。

专家共识建议（2014）

- 昏迷 **TBI 患者，初始 CT 扫描显示轻微损伤迹象（tSAH、出血点），随后恶化（例如发展为脑挫伤、挤压或基底池缺失）
- 脑挫伤昏迷 TBI 患者，中断镇静以检查神经状态十分危险或当临床检查不可靠时
- 昏迷的 TBI 患者，双侧额叶大面积挫伤和（或）出血性占位病变邻近脑干，与最初格拉斯哥昏迷评分（GCS）无关
- 去骨瓣减压术后，评估手术对颅内压控制的有效性，并指导日常治疗
- 在可抢救的颅内高压风险增加的患者，包括：
  - GCS 运动得分≤5
  - 瞳孔异常
  - 长期 / 严重缺氧和（或）低血压
  - 压缩或闭塞的基底池
  - 中线偏移 >5 mm 或超过轴向外血栓的厚度
  - 额外的轴外血肿、实质性损伤（如挫伤）或肿胀
  - 术中脑肿胀
- 如前所述，多发伤病例中也应考虑这一点
- 不包括初始 CT 正常的昏迷性 TBI 患者 ***

ICP，颅内压；CPP，脑灌注压；GCS，格拉斯哥昏迷量表；TBI，创伤性脑损伤；tSAH 外伤性蛛网膜下腔出血。* 定义为 GCS 得分 8 分或以下。** 定义为在血流动力学和呼吸稳定后以及没有麻醉或麻痹剂的情况下，GCS 为 8 或以下。*** 在这种情况下，如果患者神经功能恶化，则建议再次进行 CT 扫描。

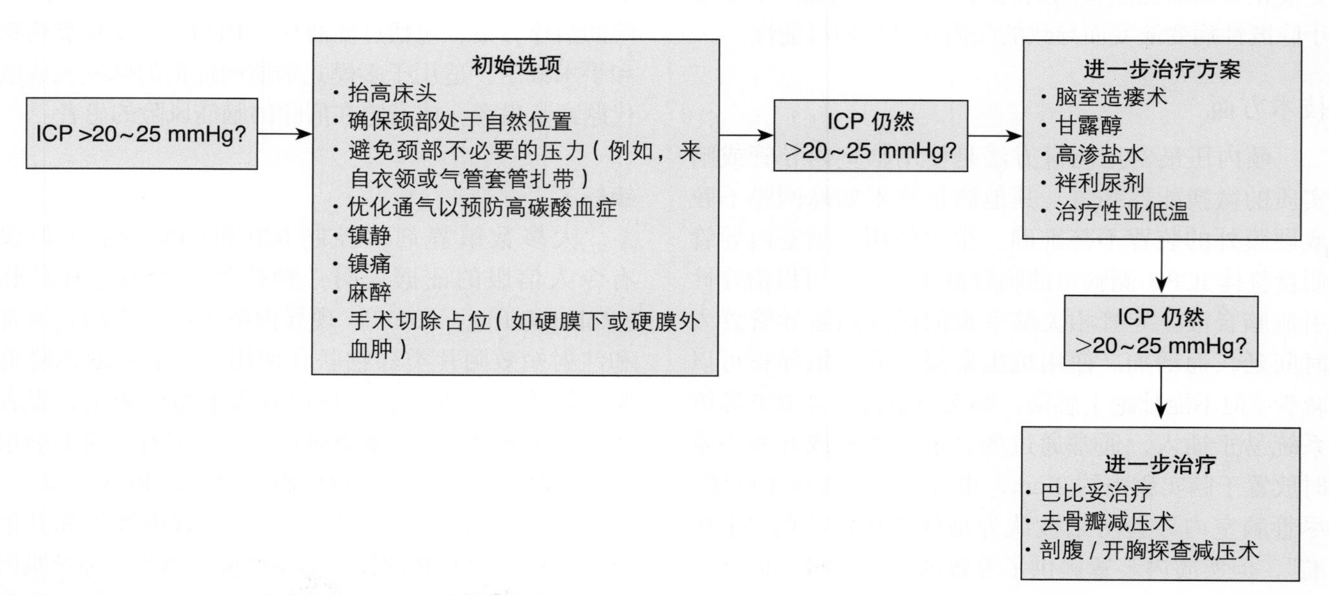

图 42.2 颅内压升高的管理流程

过度通气

过度通气可通过降低 $PaCO_2$ 引起继发脑血管收缩，有效降低ICP。但是由于脑血流量（cerebral blood fow，CBF）的严重减少，过度通气可以加重或恶化全脑和局部脑缺血（Stocchetti et al.，2005）。因此，过度通气只应作为一种暂时性措施使用，应避免在头24小时内（此时CBF常显著降低）和预防性使用。建议在过度通气期间同时进行脑氧合监测，以避免缺血发生。

渗透疗法

甘露醇（0.25~1.0 g/kg）是急性颅内压升高的标准治疗方法（Carney et al.，2017），但从未与安慰剂进行过随机比较。副作用包括最初的液体过载，随后的低血压、代谢性酸中毒和电解质失衡，所有这些都会对损伤的大脑产生不利影响。重复给药可能导致不可接受的高血清渗透压（>320 mmol/L）、神经并发症和急性肾损伤。

与甘露醇相比，HS可能对ICP产生更深远和持久的影响，但与甘露醇相比的获益尚未得到证实（Diringer，2013）。临床研究结果在HS给药的剂量、浓度、频率和方式（大剂量或持续输注）方面未达成一致，降低ICP升高的最佳渗透压负荷尚不明确。HS除了渗透作用外，理论上对受损的大脑有多种积极作用，包括血管调节、免疫和神经化学作用；它还扩大血管内容量，可能会增加CPP。

尽管先前认为乳酸只是无氧代谢的副产物，但有证据表明乳酸可以作为受损大脑的优先燃料。初步临床数据表明，高渗乳酸溶液可节省大脑葡萄糖，改善大脑能量代谢，有效降低升高的ICP（Bouzat and Oddo，2014）。在常规使用之前，还需要进一步的数据支持。

巴比妥类

Cochrane的一项系统综述证实，在TBI患者中使用巴比妥类药物并不能降低死亡率，反而会增加25%的低血压风险（Roberts and Sydenham，2012）。巴比妥类药物的心血管副作用可能会抵消降低ICP对CPP的益处。当一级和二级治疗未能控制颅内压时，可继续使用巴比妥类药物治疗难治性颅内高压，但是某些中心在这种情况下减压术优先于巴比妥类药物。

外科干预

去骨瓣减压术、脑脊液引流和其他神经外科干预治疗高颅压的作用将在**第43章**讨论。

颅内压监测和管理的证据

众所周知，高颅压是有害的，但很少有证据表明监测和管理ICP可改善预后。对包括24 792名严重TBI患者的14项研究进行meta分析得出结论：与未进行ICP监测的治疗相比，ICP监测颅内高压指导的治疗，总体上死亡率没有显著降低，然而在2012年之后发表的研究中，接受ICP监测的患者死亡率较低（Yuan et al.，2015）。目前只有一项随机研究评估ICP监测在TBI中的应用。美国颅内压研究（Benchmark Evidence from South American Trials: Treatment of Intracranial Pressure，BEST-TRIP）将ICP监测指导下治疗与无ICP监测基于影像学和临床检查的治疗进行比较，发现三个月和六个月的预后均没有差异（Chesnut et al.，2012）。ICP监测组患者接受ICP目标治疗（过度通气、HS/甘露醇和巴比妥类药物）的天数明显减少，但ICU住院时间相似。这与以往（观察性）研究结果不同，这些研究表明，通过ICP监测指导治疗的患者，这种脑导向治疗的负担会增加。

BEST-TRIP虽然在几个方面受到了批评，但它的研究结果强调了这样一种观念，即ICP监测管理对于重型TBI的管理是不可或缺的。无论是直接监测，还是通过评估临床和影像学变化间接评估，颅内高压的评估和诊断都是患者管理的基础。

脑灌注压

指南建议，通过使用液体复苏和血管升压药/强心药物来控制MAP或治疗升高的ICP，使CPP维持在60~70 mmHg（Carney et al.，2017）。有证据表明，CCP过低或过高都与不良预后相关。CPP>70 mmhg与过度液体复苏或血管加压治疗相关的ALI风险增加相关，CPP小于50 mmHg与脑灌注不足相关。另一种理论，伦德（Lund）概念，以较低的CPP（50 mmHg）为目标，尽量降低毛细血管内静水压和脑内含水量，以避免ICP继发性升高（Grände，2006），但它没有强有力证据基础，也没有被普遍接受。与CPP的单一阈值不同，使用多模态神经监测有可能在个体水平上确定“最佳”值（Kirkman and Smith，2014）。

多模态神经监测

在预测脑缺氧缺血时，监测多个生理变量比单独测量一个变量更准确（Bouzat et al.，2015）

（表 42.3）。特别强调，ICP 监测应被视为多模态神经监测策略中的一部分，而不是孤立的监测模式（Kirkman and Smith，2012）。

脑血管反应性

脑血管反应性是脑自动调节（cerebral autoregulation，CA）的一个重要组成部分，在 TBI 后常常受损，使大脑更容易受到继发性缺血损伤。监测 ABP（动脉血压）和 ICP 中自发慢波的相关性，可以计算出压力反应指数（pressure reactivity index，PRx），该指数可用于床旁持续性评估 CA。当 ABP 与 ICP 呈负相关时，PRx 的负值表示 CA 正常，正值表示无反应性脑血管循环。PRx 可用于指导治疗和确定 TBI 后最佳 CPP（图 42.3）（Aries et al.，2012）。

氧反应性指数（oxygen reactivity index，ORx）反映脑组织氧合（$PbtO_2$）和 ABP 之间相关性，可采用非侵入性替代监测手段，如 ABP、TCD 衍生血流速度和近红外光谱（near infrared spectroscopy，NIRS）衍生参数（Kirkman and Smith，2012）。

脑血流监测

TCD 是一种非侵入性技术，允许在床边实时评估脑血流动力学。虽然它测量的是 CBF 相对变化而不是绝对值，但它可以用来检测受损的 CBF 和评估 TBI 后脑血管反应性。使用热扩散流量探头可以定量测量选定区域 CBF，但应用该技术的临床数据有限。

脑氧合监测

将 ICP 和 CPP 维持在正常阈值范围内并不能保证对抗脑组织缺氧（Oddo et al.，2011）。因此，脑氧合监测通常用于评估脑氧输送和利用之间的平衡，以及脑灌注是否充分。

颈静脉血氧仪

颈静脉血氧饱和度（jugular venous oxygen saturation，$SvjO_2$）是首个床旁脑氧合监测指标，为我们了解脑损伤后脑氧合的变化奠定了基础。BTF 指南（Carney et al.，2017）建议 TBI 后 $SvjO_2$ 维持在 50% 以上，但没有任何干预性试验证实以 $SvjO_2$ 为治疗目标对预后有直接益处；并且在任何情况下 $SvjO_2$ 监测都可以被其他监测方式替代。

脑组织氧分压

脑组织氧分压（oxygen partial pressure，$PbtO_2$）监测被认为是判断脑氧合床旁监测的“金标准”，建议在严重 TBI 后使用（Le Roux et al.，2014）。$PbtO_2$ 是一个复杂的动态变量，源于影响脑氧输送和需求（氧代谢）的各种因素、感兴趣区域内动静脉血管相对比例，以及组织氧扩散梯度的相互作用。因此，它不仅仅是缺氧 / 缺血的监测指标，更是细胞功能的生物标志物。$PbtO_2$ 是一种区域监测手段，探头通常放置在血肿或挫伤周围的组织中，以监测“危险”脑区。

据报道，正常脑 $PbtO_2$ 介于 2.7~4.7 kPa（20~35 mmHg），缺血阈值通常定义为 1.33~2.0 kPa（10~15 mmHg）。然而，$PbtO_2$ 值最好看成是一个范围而不是作为一个精确的阈值，来定义缺血的缺氧持续时间和程度。指南建议采取干预措施，将 $PbtO_2$ 维持在 2.7 kPa（20 mmHg）以上（Le Roux et al.，2014）。

观察研究表明，TBI 后在 ICP/CPP 治疗导向下，$PbtO_2$ 作为补充治疗指引目标有潜在好处（Nangunoori et al.，2012）。除了体循环血压外，$PbtO_2$ 还受 PaO_2、$PaCO_2$ 和血红蛋白浓度等因素的影响，而采用何种干预手段或联合干预逆转脑组织缺氧存在争议。事实上，脑组织缺氧对特定干预的反应性似乎可以作为预测因素，如缺氧的逆转与死亡率的降低有关（Nangunoori et al.，2012）。迫切需要脑组织氧监测在创伤性脑损伤（Brain Tissue Oxygen Monitoring in Traumatic Brain Injury，BOOST2）这种 RCT 研究来确认 $PbtO_2$ 监测的好处（https://clinicaltrials.gov/ct2/ show/NCT00974259）。

近红外光谱

基于近红外光谱的脑血氧饱和度测量可提供连续和无创的局部脑血氧饱和度（regional cerebral oxygen saturation，$rScO_2$）监测，它具有较高的时间和空间分辨率，并有可能同时测量多个感兴趣部位。根据报道，$rScO_2$ 的“正常”范围为 60%~75%，但存在明显的个体内和个体间差异，因此 $rScO_2$ 值最好用作趋势监测。脑损伤后应用近红外光谱技术的研究有限，其应用受到了脑损伤后光学复杂性的影响（Ghoshet al.，2012）。近红外光谱衍生参数可以作为一种非侵入性评估大脑自动调节状态的工具，但其作用在更广泛的脑创伤监测中尚不明确。

脑微透析

脑微透析（cerebral microdialysis，CMD）允许床边分析脑组织细胞外液中的生化物质。导管探头通常放置在“高危”组织中，以便监测大脑最易受二次损伤区域的生化变化。葡萄糖、乳酸、丙酮酸、乳酸 / 丙酮酸比值（lactate：pyruvate ratio，LPR）、甘

表 42.3　TBI 神经监测技术

技术	监测指标	TBI 适应证	优势	劣势
颅内压				
脑实质或硬膜下微传感器	• ICP • CPP • 自身调节指标	• 通过 PRx 和 ORx 优化 CPP	• 相对易于植入 • 手术并发症率低 • 感染率低	• 不能体内校正 • 仅测量局部压力 • 随时间出现微小的零点漂移
脑室内导管	• 同上	• 同上，另外： • 允许对 CSF 进行治疗性引流	• 测量全身 ICP • 治疗性 CSF 引流 • 可以体内校正	• 不易植入 • 存在手术相关性大出血的风险 • 存在导管相关性脑室炎的风险
脑血流量				
经颅多普勒超声	• 血液流速 • 搏动指数 • 自身调节指标	• 可以发现脑灌注不足并有助于早期目标导向性治疗	• 无创 • 可以间歇或连续使用 • 时间分辨率好	• 测量相对（而非绝对）CBF • 依赖操作者 • 失败率 5%~10%（缺少声窗） • 在 TBI 中证据不足
脑氧合作用				
颈静脉血氧测定	• 颈静脉氧饱和 • 动静脉氧含量差异	• 评估脑灌注和供氧是否充足 • 支持 ICP/CPP 导向性治疗 • 协助内科和外科治疗滴定，指导 ICP/CPP 治疗	• 全身性评估 CBF 和代谢之间的平衡	• 脑灌注的非定量测量 • 对局部缺血不敏感 • 样本颅外污染风险
脑组织 PO_2	• 脑组织氧分压 • 氧反应	• 对于颈静脉血氧测定而言，另需： • 通过 ORx 优化 CPP	• 评估局部 CBF 和代谢之间的平衡 • 连续性 • 确定的缺血阈值	• 微创 • 在小范围感兴趣区内测量氧合 • 1 小时的"磨合期"限制其术中应用
近红外光谱（脑血氧测量）	• 脑局部氧饱和 • 自身调节指标	• 对于颈静脉血氧测定而言，另需： • 检查颅内血肿	• 无创 • 实时 • 多位置测量	• $rScO_2$ 的缺血阈值不确定 • 颅内血肿的存在和颅外组织对信号的"污染"影响读数 • 缺乏 TBI 相关证据
脑微透析	• 葡萄糖 • 乳酸、丙酮酸和 LPR • 甘油 • 谷氨酸 • 用于研究的多种生物标志物	• 用于检测脑缺血、低氧、细胞能量不足和缺糖损伤 • 在能够临床检测或用其他方式监测前预测继发性损伤的发展 • 最优化 CPP • 帮助滴定全身血糖控制等药物治疗	• 评估脑葡萄糖代谢 • 检测缺氧 / 缺血 • 评估非缺血性细胞能量障碍	• 局部检测 • 异常阈值不清 • 非连续性 • 劳动密集型
电生理学				
EEG	• 癫痫 • 诊断特异性 EEG 模式 • 部分证据表明可以检测 SDs	• 检测抽搐性或非抽搐性癫痫发作 • 诊断特征性 EEG 以预测病情	• 无创 • 检测非抽搐性癫痫发作 • 与脑缺血和代谢改变有关	• 需要熟练的解读 • 受到麻醉和镇静药物影响
ECoG	• 皮质 SDs	• 检测扩散的皮质去极化	• 目前唯一能精确识别 SDs 的方法	• 创伤大 • 没有证据表明治疗 SD 改善预后 • 基于 TBI 的证据少，因此目前只是一种研究工具

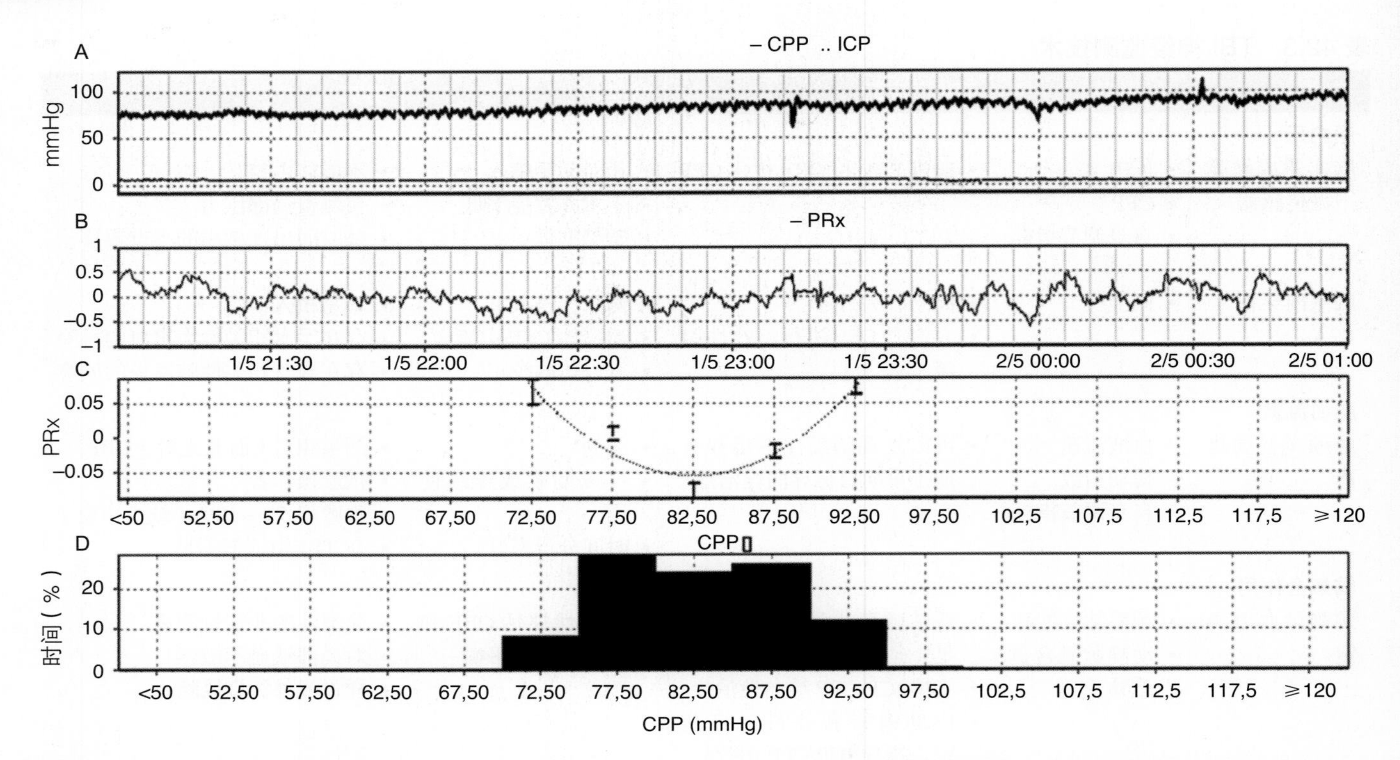

图 42.3 ICM+ 软件面板（Cambridge Enterprise，Cambridge，UK）的 4 小时趋势图截图。PRx 的确定可以指导治疗，并允许在个体水平上确定最佳 CPP（CPPopt）。图 A：CPP 和 ICP；图 B：PRx；图 C：用于评估 CPPopt 的 PRx/CPP 图；图 D：在给定的 CPP 时间间隔内 4 小时时段的百分比。图像由剑桥大学开发的 ICM+® 大脑监测软件生成

油和谷氨酸是临床上最常测量的指标，这些指标也是葡萄糖代谢、缺氧 / 缺血或细胞能量衰竭相关等特定细胞过程的标志物。CMD 能够测量底物的供应及其细胞代谢，因此它不仅可以监测脑缺血，也可以监测非缺血原因导致的细胞能量功能障碍。在临床或其他监测指标检测到脑损害之前，它可以在细胞水平上识别脑损害。

LPR 升高超过 40 并伴有脑葡萄糖低代谢（<0.7~1 mol/L）提示严重缺氧 / 缺血，与 TBI 预后不良相关（Timofeev et al.，2011）。尽管 CMD 的临床应用存在争议，但最近已经发表了相关的专家共识（Hutchinson et al.，2015）。

脑电图和皮质脑电图

EEG 用来诊断和指导治疗有癫痫或癫痫持续状态风险的患者。由于脑创伤后非惊厥发作十分常见，连续脑电图（continuous EEG，cEEG）监测被广泛应用。

扩散性皮质去极化（spreading cortical depolarizations，SD）是神经元和星形胶质细胞近乎完全的、持续的去极化，导致线粒体损伤、细胞内钙累积和兴奋毒性引起的继发性损伤。它们发生在 50%~60% 的 TBI 患者中，以前只能通过直接放置在皮质表面的电极检测到。最近的数据表明，标准头皮 cEEG 也可以检测到 SD，为常规监测急性脑损伤的这一重要病理生理学变化提供了可能。

结论

对继发性脑损伤机制的了解和对其不良后果的认识，使 TBI 的早期和重症监护管理取得了显著进展：重点是避免缺氧和低血压，控制 ICP 和维持 CPP。多模态神经监测，包括持续测量 ICP 和 CPP，可对脑生理实时变化进行个性化干预，以改善 TBI 的预后。

延伸阅读、参考文献、EBRAIN 的相关链接

扫描书末二维码获取。

第 43 章　颅脑损伤的外科治疗

Hadie Adams · Angelos G. Kolias · Adel Helmy · Peter J.A. Hutchinson · Randall M. Chesnut 著
余晓帆 译，刘伟明 审校

引言

创伤性脑损伤（traumatic brain injury，TBI）会导致残疾和生产力丧失，但其发病率和死亡率在世界各地都可控（Maas et al.，2008）。据估计，欧洲 TBI 的发病率为每年 150~300/10 万人，平均为每年 235/10 万人（Tagliaferri et al.，2006）。格拉斯哥昏迷评分（Glasgow Coma Scale，GCS）常用来划分创伤性脑损伤的严重程度，评分 8 分及以下的患者为重度，9~12 分为中度，13~15 分为轻度（CDC，2015a）。轻度 TBI 是最常见的颅脑损伤类型，TBI 在人群中的发病率数青壮年男性最高（Nguyen et al.，2016）。在西方国家，需要住院治疗的 TBI 患者的主要致伤原因是摔倒、受到暴力袭击和机动车交通事故（Lawrence et al.，2016）。创伤性脑损伤后的手术适应证包括占位病变（硬膜外血肿、急性硬膜下、脑内血肿和脑挫伤）、凹陷性颅骨骨折、弥漫性创伤性脑损伤（需行去骨瓣减压手术）。北美创伤注册登记的结果表明有 3.6% 的创伤性脑损伤患者接受了开颅手术（Esposito et al.，2005）。欧洲脑损伤联盟的一项调查显示，在有占位性病变（>25 ml）和（或）影像学表现为颅内压（intracranial pressure，ICP）升高的创伤性脑损伤患者中，有 69% 接受了急诊开颅手术（Compagnone et al.，2007）。急性硬膜下血肿是最常见需行手术清除的占位病变，约占所有急诊病例的 2/3，其次是硬膜外血肿、脑挫伤和脑内血肿。

颅内压监测

急性期重度 TBI 患者需要神经重症监护，常需要镇静和麻醉以利于气管插管和控制 ICP。该种治疗措施使神经系统体格检查的有效性受到限制，因此计算机断层扫描（computed tomography，CT）和 ICP 监测变成 ICU 指导重度 TBI 患者治疗的主要方法（Le Roux et al.，2014；Brain Trauma Foundation，2016）。控制 ICP 仍是中重度 TBI 治疗的核心原则。控制 ICP 以保证大脑有足够的血流灌注和氧气供应，避免或减轻继发性脑损伤（Valadka and Robertson，2007；Brain Trauma Foundation，2016）。脑创伤基金会（Brain Trauma Foundation，BTF）指南推荐使用 ICP 监测对重度 TBI 患者进行管理，以降低住院时间和伤后 2 周的死亡率（Brain Trauma Foundation，2016）。ICP 监测在发达国家得到了广泛应用，多项观察性研究都表明 ICP 控制欠佳可导致不良预后（Forsyth et al.，2015）。这些在 42 章（创伤性脑损伤的重症监护管理）中进一步讨论。最后，若重度 TBI 未得到及时治疗，ICP 会持续升高超过一个临界阈值，导致神经结构损伤，最终脑疝和脑死亡。

了解脑实质内的颅内压力梯度是很重要的，特别是对颅内有占位病变的患者。因为起支撑作用的硬脑膜皱褶（大脑镰）和小脑幕将颅腔分隔，常规保护脑组织不发生过度移动，这使得这些患者易产生颅内压力梯度。急性硬膜下血肿患者的大脑半球之间的压力差值大于 10 mmHg（Chambers et al.，1998）。这也为脑室内探头测量 ICP 提供了依据，不同部位脑脊液之间的压力可在一定程度上达到平衡（Brain Trauma Foundation，2016）。在临床实践中，脑室内长时间放置引流可能会出现感染的风险，从而限制了此方法的应用。因此很多单位更倾向于在脑实质内放置 ICP 探头。

先进的脑监测系统将 ICP 监测与其他的脑监测技术相结合。其他脑监测技术包括脑自我调节监测、脑化学微透析监测、脑组织氧分压监测（$PbrO_2$）和颈静脉球监测动脉 - 颈内静脉血氧含量差（Valadka and Robertson，2007；Le Roux et al.，2014；Brain Trauma Foundation，2016；Makarenko et al.，2016）。通过评估 TBI 患者的脑代谢需求和对治疗干预措施的反应，这些监测方法可作为继发性脑损伤的个体化治疗手段。一些监测设备可将多个导管和传感器放入脑实质中，以利于对患者进行床旁的持续多模态监测（Hutchinson et al., 2000）。

脑室造瘘术

针对TBI患者，脑脊液引流的作用以及最适合的引流策略（持续 *vs*. 间歇）尚不十分确定（Nwachuku et al., 2014; Brain Trauma Foundation, 2016）。即使在没有脑积水的情况下，对TBI患者行脑室外引流（external ventricular drain, EVD）或脑室造瘘术可通过减少颅内脑脊液的容积来快速控制ICP（Kerr et al., 2001; Timofeev et al., 2009; Brain Trauma Foundation, 2016）。该方法是指南推荐的一种辅助降低ICP策略的一部分。有报道称TBI患者在行脑脊液引流后出现了生命体征改善，但是如果不与其他降低ICP的治疗同时应用，还是会有相当一部分患者的ICP无法得到控制（Timofeev et al., 2009）。脑室造瘘术也会出现一系列的并发症，如EVD相关感染、引流管插入造成出血及随后的分流依赖性。

与压力传感器相连的EVD可以在引流管关闭时测量ICP（见颅内压监测部分），并在引流管打开时排出脑脊液。对于TBI患者的最佳引流策略尚未达成共识（Nwachuku et al., 2014; Brain Trauma Foundation, 2016）。EVD或脑室造瘘术在临床上的应用形式存在很大的差异，受医生和科室偏好及医疗资源影响。对于TBI患者脑脊液引流的管理应考虑到患者的年龄（Shore et al., 2004; Nwachuku et al., 2014）。脑脊液持续引流在儿童TBI患者中较为常见。值得注意的是，虽然间歇性引流可以实时显示颅内压，但患者在引流期间可能存在ICP升高的风险。持续引流有利于更稳定地控制ICP，然而，这可能会因过度引流而导致脑室塌陷。在这种情况下，EVD不再是能够测量ICP的可靠方法，因为它的测量原理依赖于传感器所在脑室腔内存在连续液体柱。

占位病灶开颅清除术

外科干预旨在减轻因（不断增大的）血肿和后续对大脑产生的伤害（Bullock et al., 2006a; Bullock et al., 2006b; Bullock et al., 2006c）。神经外科医生需要对TBI患者的神经功能缺损、瞳孔异常、中线移位程度、血肿体积和其他部位损伤是否存在及其严重程度进行初步评估，以确定是否需要行急诊开颅手术治疗。对于神经外科医生来说，对中等大小的占位性病灶进行手术清除抑或是保守治疗是最艰难的决定之一。因为手术干预可能并不总是必需的，而保守治疗则有神经功能进一步恶化的风险，对大脑造成继发性损伤，可能会进一步恶化患者预后。现有的指南和建议可行，但仅局限于专家共识层面，证据质量不高（Bullock et al., 2006a; Bullock et al., 2006b; Bullock et al., 2006c）。值得强调的是，虽然指南中必要地包含了具体的手术策略，但在实践中应考虑患者的整体临床状况，其中包括患者临床状态（GCS、瞳孔功能）、有无进一步恶化趋势、其他导致神经功能损害的原因（如代谢、药物诱导、缺氧或低血压）、相关其他部位损伤及并发症。这些因素都会影响干预措施的选择及进行干预的时间点（Bullock et al., 2006a; Bullock et al., 2006b; Bullock et al., 2006c）。

硬膜外血肿

硬膜外血肿（extradural hematomas, EDH）常见于遭遇机动车交通事故、摔倒和受到暴力袭击的青壮年（Bullock et al., 2006b）。在TBI患者中，EDH（需行手术治疗和保守治疗的病例）的发病率在2.7%~4%（Bullock et al., 2006b）。通常认为EDH是头部直接受到撞击形成，常见于受撞击部位同侧。出血来源通常为动脉，常为翼点区域的骨折导致脑膜中动脉撕裂，随后中颅窝血肿形成。EDH可发生于任何解剖部位，包括额部、枕部和顶部，这些部位的血肿分别与筛前动脉、横窦或乙状窦、上矢状窦破裂有关。与动脉破裂来源的EDH相比，静脉破裂来源的EDH血肿扩张速度更慢（Nalbach et al., 2012）。在成人TBI患者中EDH的死亡率约为10%（Bullock et al., 2006b）。手术目的是为了防止因血肿扩大、颅内压升高和脑疝引起的不可逆脑损伤或脑死亡。出现（进行性）局灶性神经系统症状或体征和（或）血肿体积扩大的患者，需紧急处置，必要时急诊手术治疗。根据临床证据和专家建议，无论GCS评分如何以及昏迷患者（GCS<9）是否存在瞳孔异常，对于血肿体积大于30 cm^3（>30 ml）EDH患者均应行手术清除血肿（Bullock et al., 2006b）。应该根据血肿位置，骨窗开颅血肿清除术，骨窗应能够达到血肿边缘，为手术提供足够视野及操作空间。如果大脑表面张力较高，检查硬膜下间隙内是否存在血凝块非常重要。当取下骨瓣之后，应该用缝线悬吊骨窗四周和中心的硬膜以消除硬膜外间隙。没有脑实质损伤的单纯EDH是典型因颅骨骨折导致颅内血肿，不同于有脑水肿倾向的脑实质损伤，单纯EDH术毕应将骨瓣还纳至原位。对于没有局灶性神经功能缺损且颅内血肿体积小（体积 <30 cm^3，血肿厚度 <15 mm，头部影像学显示中线偏移 <5 mm）的患者可行保守治疗并密切观察（Bullock et al.，2006b）。

急性硬膜下血肿

急性硬膜下血肿（acute subdural hematomas，aSDH）通常发生在摔倒、受到暴力袭击和机动车交通事故（motor vehicle accidents，MVA）（Bullock et al.，2006c）。在年轻患者（18~40 岁）中，有 56% 的 aSDH 由 MVA 引起，只有 12% 由摔倒引起。与年轻患者不同，65 岁及以上的患者中，只有 22% 的 aSDH 由 MVA 引起，56% 由摔倒引起（Bullock et al.，2006c）。出血机制因患者的年龄和受力强度不同而异。在有脑萎缩的老年患者中，中等程度的头部受力就能引起颅内出血，出血来源通常为桥静脉撕裂造成的静脉性出血。据报道，在年轻患者或头部受力强度较大患者中，有 20%~30% 的 aSDH 病例为动脉来源的出血合并有大脑表面的严重挫伤（Gennarelli and Thibault，1982；Zumkeller et al.，1996；Koc et al.，1997；Servadei et al.，1998；Maxeiner and Wolff，2007；Ryan et al.，2012）。需要行手术治疗的 aSDH 患者的死亡率在 15%~60%（Haselsberger et al.，1988；Hatashita et al.，1993；Zumkeller et al.，1996；Kok et al.，1997；Servadei et al.，1998；Bullock et al.，2006c；Ryan et al.，2012）。对于血肿厚度大于 10 mm、中线移位超过 5 mm、从受伤到入院 GCS 评分下降 2 分以上和（或）出现瞳孔异常的所有成年 aSDH 患者，临床证据及专家建议应行血肿清除手术治疗（Bullock et al.，2006c）。由于高龄可能会导致发生不良预后的概率增加，因此在决定是否行手术治疗时应综合考虑患者年龄及手术是否可以改变疾病自然进程使患者远期获益。表现为 aSDH 的 TBI 患者，影像学上常伴有明显的脑实质损伤和脑肿胀（Zumkeller et al.，1996；Bullock et al.，2006c；Li et al.，2012）。需行手术治疗 aSDH 的方式有两种，即单纯开颅血肿清除术或去骨瓣减压术（decompressive craniectomy，DC）。然而，对于是否应该去除骨瓣目前尚无定论（Kolias et al.，2012）。RESCUE-ASDH 试验纳入了成年 aSDH 患者，旨在比较单纯开颅血肿清除术和去骨瓣减压术对 aSDH 的疗效（Protocol 14PRT/ 6944）。这项试验的结果将为 aSDH 手术决策的选择提供重要参考。对于病情稳定、血肿厚度小于 10 mm、中线移位小于 5 mm、无瞳孔异常、颅内压监测无颅内高压的患者，可进行保守治疗并密切观察（Bullock et al.，2006c）。保守治疗的 aSDH 可逐渐消退，血肿通常在数周内被吸收。但仍有一部分患者的硬膜下血肿可能不会消退，逐渐形成慢性硬膜下血肿。

脑内血肿 / 脑挫伤

创伤性脑内出血（intracerebral hemorrhage，ICH）通常是指创伤性脑实质内出血和（出血性）脑挫伤。创伤后脑挫伤通常为多发性，位于额叶和颞叶的基底面（Bullock et al.，2006a）。在急性期，ICH 由（半）液态血块组成，伴随周围脑水肿。这些血块会在数天内发展演变，并在脑水肿开始消退时改变其自身密度。继发于创伤性脑出血的死亡率同病变的位置和大小有关（Bullock et al.，2006a）。外科手术旨在预防继发性脑损伤、脑干受压和脑疝。不幸的是，研究早期手术与初始保守治疗在预测和预防创伤性脑出血继发性损害中作用的唯一试验被提前终止（Gregson et al.，2012；Mendelow et al.，2015）。尽管该试验被提前终止使得样本量少、证据等级有限，但是 STITCH（创伤）试验发现早期手术可降低死亡率（Mendelow et al.，2015）。然而，需要注意，该试验中的患者大多是在医疗资源有限的情况下招募的，通常无法进行 ICP 监测。对于一侧大脑半球的创伤性 ICH，当前临床证据及专家建议应对有局灶病变和有以下指征患者行手术治疗：进行性神经功能恶化、药物难治性 ICP 增高、血肿体积超过 50 cm^3（>50 ml）、GCS 评分在 6~8 分且额部或颞部出血大于 20 cm^3（>20 ml）伴有中线移位超过 5 mm 和（或）CT 显示脑池受压（Bullock et al.，2006a）。难治性脑水肿和颅高压的弥漫性脑损伤患者，若有小脑幕切迹疝的临床表现和影像学证据，可考虑行双额 DC（Bullock et al.，2006a）。当患者出现神经功能障碍 / 恶化以及出现明显基底池、第四脑室占位效应或有梗阻性脑积水的征象时，建议行颅后窝外伤性颅内血肿清除术（Bullock et al.，2006d）。对于无局灶神经功能缺损和影像学上没有明显颅内占位效应的患者，应密切监测患者生命体征并连续多次行影像学检查。

去骨瓣减压术

重度 TBI 后的难治性颅内压增高的治疗包括药物和手术治疗（Stocchetti et al.，2008；American College of Surgeons，2015）。对于药物治疗无效的弥漫性脑肿胀或大面积脑挫伤 / 颅内血肿以及即将发生脑疝的患者，DC 是一种常规的手术治疗方式（Bohman and Schuster，2013；Kolias et al.，2013）。近年来，DC 作为重度 TBI 的主要治疗措施得到了广泛讨论。DC 是指在清除大量占位病变及坏死组织后去除骨瓣，也可作为弥漫性脑损伤和脑水肿的二级或三级治疗措施。去除骨瓣后，肿胀的大脑向颅骨外膨出，会降低颅内压并减少脑疝风险。重度 TBI 患者 DC 后的生理性改善包括大脑灌注及脑组织氧供增加、脑细胞内神经化学的改善（Yamakami and Yamaura，1993；Stiefel et al.，2004；Ho et al.，2008；Jaeger et al.，2010；Bor-Seng-Shu et al.，2012；Lazaridis and Czosnyka，2012）。并发症发生的风险也应该考虑，因为在 DC 之后可发生早期或晚期并发症（Kolias et al.，2013）。（对侧）血肿增大、伤口感染和愈合不良、硬膜下或皮下积液、脑积水、环钻综合征以及之后出现的与颅骨成形术相关的并发症均被认为是 DC 相关的并发症（Flint et al.，2008；Stiver，2009；Nalbach et al.，2012）。由于重度 TBI 患者发生严重残疾及死亡的风险仍然相对较高，一些临床试验旨在验证 DC 能否改善该类患者的预后（Protocol 14PRT/ 6944；Hutchinson et al.，2006；Cooper et al.，2011）。然而，明确 DC 的适应证、手术时机、手术技术以及最合适的预后评价标准是十分困难的，缺乏将 DC 的治疗效果与预后联系起来的高质量证据（Kolias et al.，2013）。

去骨瓣减压术的手术方法

去骨瓣减压术是一组切除部分颅骨的手术的总称。在成人重度 TBI 患者中，最常应用的 DC 术式为双额 DC 和单侧额颞顶颅骨切除术（也被称为半（球形）颅骨切除术或单侧 DC（Kjellberg and Prieto，1971；Guerra et al.，1999；Kolias et al.，2013）。对于单侧大脑半球病变所致的中线移位和（潜在）脑水肿患者（如脑实质损伤并伴有 aSDH），半颅骨切除术可能是有效的（**图 43.1**）。关于半颅骨切除术的临床证据及专家建议均表明所去除的骨瓣应足够大，骨瓣最小的前后直径应为 11~12 cm（Li et al.，2012；Tagliaferri et al.，2012），以实现颅内压的充分降低，并降低颅骨边缘脑实质损伤和皮质静脉闭塞发生率（von Holst et al.，2012；Li et al.，2013）。双额 DC 是治疗弥漫性（双侧半球）脑损伤伴难治性颅高压的一种可选择的治疗方法（**图 43.2**）（Kolias et al.，2013）。双额 DC 手术范围从前颅窝底向后延伸至冠状缝，并向两侧延伸至颞底。为了让大脑得到充分扩张，需要大面积剪开硬脑膜。关于硬脑膜处理及矢状窦结扎或保留（Bohman and Schuster，2013）有很多不同的手术技术。如用止血材料、骨膜或颞肌筋膜覆盖硬脑膜缺损处；或用硬脑膜移植物填补缺损硬脑膜（Whitfield et al.，2001；Timofeev and Hutchinson，2006；Guresir et al.，2011）。虽然目前并未对双额 DC 手术方式进行改进，但有研究表明双侧半颅骨切除术可作为弥漫性脑损伤患者的一种治疗方式（Guerra et al.，1999）。对于因颞部占位病变或水肿导致脑干受压的患者，将 DC 的手术范围延伸至中颅窝底是至关重要的。

TBI 患者行去骨瓣减压术的证据基础

DECRA 试验发现对弥漫性脑损伤患者行早期 DC 手术治疗并不能改善该类患者的功能结局（Cooper et al.，2011）。该研究同样表明接受 DC

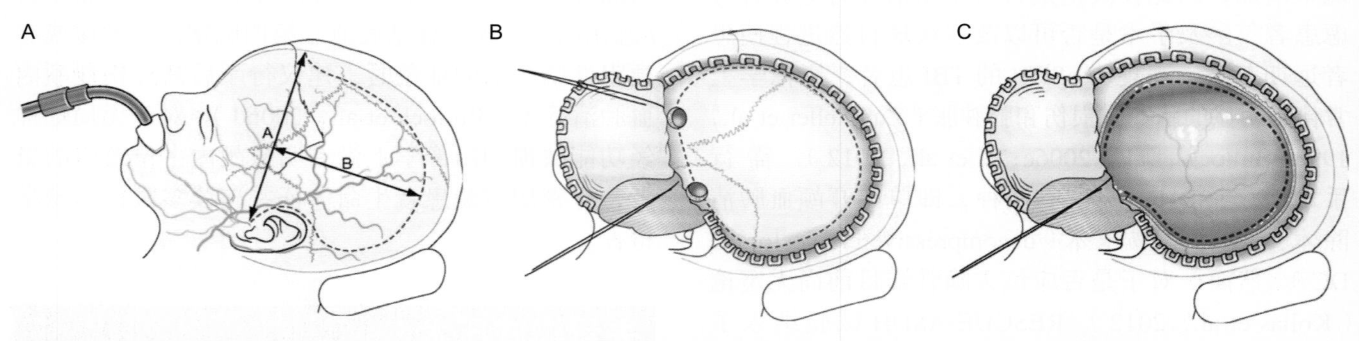

图 43.1 单侧去骨瓣减压术。（A）虚线代表单侧去骨瓣减压术中常见的皮肤切口。为了保持足够的血管供应，切口的长度（距离 B）不应超过其宽度（距离 A）。（B）肌皮瓣被掀开，虚线代表切开颅骨的一般范围。（C）硬脑膜上的虚线代表打开硬膜的最佳方法。硬脑膜呈 C 形打开，其底部毗邻蝶骨嵴。硬膜切口与颅骨切口边缘保持 5~10 mm 的距离，最大限度地降低突出的大脑受到损伤的风险

Reproduced with permission from I. Timofeev, T. Santarius, A.G. Kolias et al., Decompressive craniectomy—operative technique and perioperative care, *Advances and Technical Standards in Neurosurgery*, Volume 38, pp. 115–36, Copyright © 2012 Springer Nature.

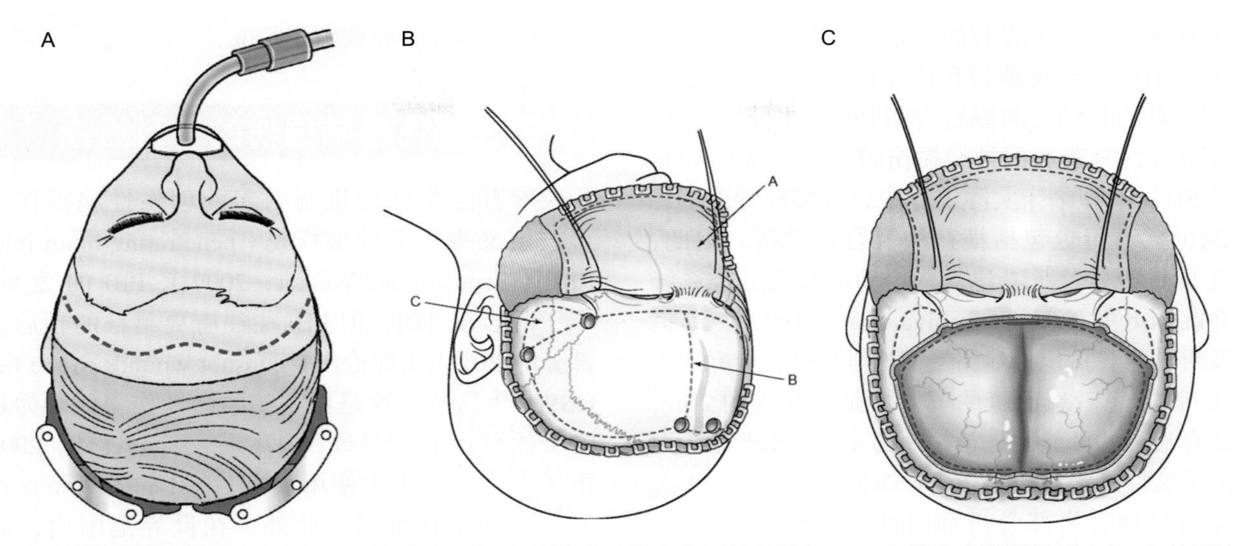

图 43.2　双额去骨瓣减压术。（A）虚线代表双额去骨瓣减压术中常用的皮肤切口，应保持在发际线后。（B）双侧冠状肌皮瓣向前掀起。颅骨上的虚线代表切开颅骨的一般范围。颞肌下减压术是可选择的手术方式。（C）骨瓣已经被去除，硬脑膜上的虚线代表打开硬膜的最佳方法。硬脑膜在中线两侧呈 C 形张开，其底部毗邻上矢状窦。前部上矢状窦及大脑镰可结扎切断（红线）

治疗的患者，机械通气时间和重症监护时间更短。RESCUEicp 试验旨在检验继发性 DC（单侧或双额 DC），作为最后一级治疗（伴有难治性颅高压的重度 TBI 患者）的临床疗效和医疗花费。408 名颅高压及难治性颅高压患者（尽管接受了标准药物治疗，但其颅内压在 25 mmHg 以上大于 1~12 小时）被随机分配到药物治疗组（可联合应用巴比妥类药物）或继发性去骨瓣减压组（Hutchinson et al.，2006）。试验表明，去骨瓣减压术显著降低了重度 TBI 患者死亡率，增加了植物状态的比例，重度残疾患者增加，中度残疾和良好预后患者的比例则变化不大。手术组患者 6~12 个月的预后有进一步改善，该组中重度残疾或良好预后患者占了很大比例。和上述试验相比，RESCUE-ASDH 是一项比较 aSDH 患者行原发单侧 DC 与单纯开颅手术（骨瓣去除 *vs*. 骨瓣还纳）疗效的随机对照研究（Protocol 14PRT/6944）。这些研究的信息将确定继发性和原发性 DC 在未来 TBI 治疗指南中的作用。根据当前可用的证据，神经外科医生和神经重症医师在决定进行 DC 时必须权衡个体患者面临的潜在风险和益处。

凹陷性颅骨骨折的外科治疗

颅骨骨折最常见于顶骨，其次是颞骨、枕骨和额骨（Cooper and Golfinos，2000）。TBI 患者通常表现为线形骨折，较少出现凹陷性骨折和颅底骨折。导致颅骨骨折所需的创伤力量很大，因此颅骨骨折患者有重大潜在的脑损伤风险。关于颅骨骨折的临床证据和专家建议，提倡对颅骨凹陷程度超过颅骨厚度或低于相邻内板 5 mm 以上的开放性颅骨骨折患者，行伤口清创及骨折复位（Bullock et al.，2006e）。其原因是希望通过早期手术降低这些患者的感染风险，特别是在硬脑膜撕裂、气颅、额窦损伤或伤口污染的情况下。急诊手术也适用于伴有潜在（增大）颅内血肿的颅骨骨折患者。骨折致颅骨明显移位，行颅骨骨折复位手术后，亦可改善患者头部的外观。通常可以使用骨折碎骨片来完成颅骨重建术；如果使用碎骨片的方法不可行，则可以使用移植物来覆盖颅骨缺损（Marbacher et al.，2008）。开放性颅骨骨折的患者应常规应用抗生素。在当前的临床证据中，并没有针对颅骨骨折患者的常规预防用药措施（Ali and Ghosh，2002；Bullock et al.，2006e；Ratilal et al.，2015）。

颅底骨折的治疗

颅底骨折可累及颅前窝、颅中窝、颅后窝，或三者的组合。本节将重点介绍颞骨岩部骨折和额窦骨折。

颞骨岩部骨折传统上根据骨折线相对于颞骨岩部长轴的方向（即从岩部底到岩部尖的连线）进行分

类。纵行骨折平行于岩骨的长轴，其最常见的并发症是听骨损伤、鼓膜破裂和传导性耳聋。横行骨折垂直于岩骨的长轴，与纵行骨折相比，横行骨折出现感音神经性耳聋和面神经损伤的风险更高（Zayas et al.，2011）。在临床实际工作中，许多颞骨岩部骨折为既包括纵行也包括横行的混合性骨折。因此，根据骨折是否累及听囊建立一个新的骨折分类系统可能在临床上更有意义（Dahiya et al.，1999）。所谓的累及听囊的骨折包括迷路受损（即耳蜗、前庭或半规管），该类患者患面瘫的可能性是正常人的 2 倍，发生脑脊液漏的可能性是正常人的 4 倍，患严重听力损害的可能性是正常人的 7 倍（Dahiya et al.，1999）。

在治疗颞骨岩部骨折和面神经麻痹的患者时，通常需要考虑有无面瘫（伤后即刻出现或迟发性面瘫）和面瘫的程度。然而，实际上很难确定面瘫发生时间及严重程度。因为很多患者存在意识障碍、或处于镇静和机械通气状态、或创伤危及生命正在接受治疗（Nash et al.，2010）。类固醇激素常被用于面瘫的患者，但近期的一项系统评价表明仅有低质量证据支持该治疗方式，尚缺乏对照研究（Nash et al.，2010）。面神经管内的面神经减压术通常只适用于立即发作的严重面瘫患者，而该类患者类固醇激素治疗无效。关于手术时机仍存在争议（Nash et al.，2010）。就自然病程而言，近期的一项系统评价纳入了 189 名接受观察的患者，其中 66% 的患者的预后可被评为 House-Brackmann Ⅰ级，25% 的患者可评为Ⅱ ~ Ⅴ级，只有两名患者为Ⅵ级（Nash et al.，2010。

高达 15% 的面部骨折累及额窦（Echo et al.，2010）。总的来说，对于额窦骨折，近年来的治疗策略转向保守，尤其在内镜技术出现之后。累及前壁的额窦骨折通常不需要干预，除非骨折是开放性或凹陷性的。累及后壁的骨折有较高的脑脊液漏的风险。对于额窦后壁骨折进行干预的适应证尚有争议，但一般来说，持续性脑脊液鼻漏或额窦后壁明显移位是可接受干预的适应证（Echo et al.，2010）。手术干预通常需行双侧冠状切口，以修复硬脑膜缺损并使额窦颅骨化。额窦的颅骨化旨在降低黏液腔形成和颅内感染的风险；它包括去除额窦后壁，剥离黏膜并填充额管。横跨于前颅窝底部的骨膜，将其用硬脑膜密封剂粘连加固于破损的硬脑膜后，可以帮助防止脑脊液漏。LeFort 骨折通常由颌面外科医生处理治疗。LeFort Ⅰ级骨折累及上颌骨和翼骨板；LeFort Ⅱ级骨折，眶壁呈金字塔形，累及眶底、眶内壁和鼻额缝；LeFort Ⅲ级骨折累及颧弓、额颧和鼻额缝以及眶底，导致颅面脱位。

穿透性创伤性脑损伤的外科治疗

所有的非钝性机制引起的创伤性脑损伤，都可被定义为穿透性脑损伤（penetrating brain injury，PBI）（Esposito and Walker，2009）。PBI 的发病率低于闭合性 TBI，但 PBI 往往有更糟糕的预后。大部分的 PBI 由头部枪伤（gunshot wounds to the head，GSWH）造成。这是典型的致命性伤害，因为超过 90% 的 GSWH 会导致致命后果（Maas et al.，2008）。由于在暴力冲突中使用火器，PBI 的发病率正在上升，特别是在美国。此外，在世界范围内，武装冲突正在造成更多的创伤性脑损伤（No authors，2001；Maas et al.，2008）。

由于大多数 PBI 由抛射物或子弹所致，因此了解弹道学是必要的。GSWH 造成的主要损伤由子弹及碎骨片或金属碎片的弹道特性（动能、治疗、速度、形状等）决定（Ordog et al.，1984）。子弹及次级金属碎片或碎骨片穿过脑实质，可形成永久性的损伤痕迹。高速的子弹将形成暂时性空腔，这是一种与动能和速度相关的现象（Aarabi et al.，2001）。当子弹减速时，子弹的动能传递到周围的脑组织。随后，暂时性空腔以波浪形的方式塌陷和扩张，对周围脑组织造成进一步的剪切力，导致出血和神经元损伤（Ordog et al.，1984；No authors，2001）。

对于 PBI 病例的放射学评估，头部 CT 平扫是首选方法。因为 CT 平扫快速，并且能够识别骨和金属碎片、显示子弹轨迹的特征、评估脑损伤的程度、检测颅内出血以及可能存在的占位效应（Aarabi et al.，2001；Tsuei et al.，2005）。建议行数字减影血管造影，特别是当子弹轨迹接近外侧裂、颈内动脉床突上段、椎基底动脉、海绵窦区、主要的硬脑膜静脉窦时，或者出现迟发性血肿或蛛网膜下腔出血进一步进展时（No authors，2001；Offiah and Twigg，2009）。PBI 后常见的血管并发症包括外伤性颅内动脉瘤、动静脉瘘（arteriovenous fistulas，AVF）、蛛网膜下腔出血和血管痉挛（No authors，2001）。

PBI 的标准外科治疗包括伤口表面的清创及硬脑膜修补，但是对于射入口小的患者，可考虑仅行简单的伤口封闭（Maas et al.，2008）。为了避免产生明显的颅内占位效应，坏死的脑组织和碎骨片应被清除。但是不建议在大脑功能区行常规的碎骨片及子弹清除术（No authors，2001）。此外，任何具有显著占位效应的颅内出血都应行手术清除。由于污染异物进入脑组织，PBI 患者极易出现中枢神经系统感染。因此建议尽早开始预防性地使用广谱抗生素（No authors，2001；Maas et al.，2008）。

脑脊液漏的外科治疗

约有 2% 的 TBI 患者发生脑脊液漏（Mendizabal et al.，1992；Brodie and Thompson，1997；Friedman et al.，2001）。那些累及额窦或筛窦以及颞骨岩部的骨折存在发生脑脊液漏的高风险（Mendizabal et al.，1992；Ommaya，1996）。大多数脑脊液漏是自限性的，可在几天内自行停止（Chandler，1983；McGuirt and Stool，1995；Brodie and Thompson，1997）。手术干预的目的是为了减少持续脑脊液漏患者症状及感染风险。有研究表明，TBI 脑脊液漏患者的感染率在 7%~30%，持续脑脊液漏会增加颅内感染的风险（Leech and Paterson，1973；Spetzler and Wilson，1978；Brodie and Thompson，1997；Savva et al.，2003；Nyquist et al.，2013；Mathias et al.，2016）。腰大池引流可作为 TBI 后脑脊液漏患者的一种治疗选择，其目的是降低脑脊液压力，从而有助于脑脊液漏的自发恢复和手术修复；同时也便于在鞘内注射荧光剂来达到诊断目的（Shapiro and Scully，1992；Mathias et al.，2016）。然而，在脑脊液漏未闭情况下，腰大池引流可能会将空气通过漏口吸入颅内，从而有颅内感染的风险。预防性应用抗生素的重要性和需行手术干预有高风险因素的患者选择标准仍有待进一步确定（Rimmer et al.，2014）。然而，疾病预防和控制中心建议对脑脊液漏患者使用肺炎球菌结合疫苗（pneumococcal conjugate vaccine，PCV13）或肺炎球菌多糖疫苗（pneumococcal polysaccharide vaccine，PPSV23）（CDC，2015b）。在英国，国立临床规范研究所建议对所有颅底骨折的患者接种肺炎球菌疫苗。

颈内动脉或椎动脉夹层的诊断和治疗

创伤后的颈内动脉（internal carotid，ICA）或椎动脉（vertebral artery，VA）夹层在年轻 TBI 患者中最为常见（Rubinstein et al.，2005）。机动车事故、摔倒、缢伤或运动相关损伤可能会造成急性血管闭塞或血栓栓塞，从而导致急性或延迟性脑卒中（Geddes et al.，2016）。损伤的机制可能是由于头部的屈曲、伸展和旋转运动使骨结构对动脉产生直接压迫或头部加速 / 减速产生的剪切力导致血管内皮损伤。在 C1~C2 水平，VA 通常因旋转力或直接受力而产生夹层，其中直接受力包括小关节面和横突关节的骨折或脱位（Blacker and Wijdicks，2004）。在临床上，夹层表现为短暂性脑缺血发作、卒中或蛛网膜下腔出血。从受伤到出现神经系统症状，通常会有一段时间的静默期。多发伤患者由于头部损伤本身或使用镇静剂而导致的意识障碍，会使临床诊断变得困难（Blacker and Wijdicks，2004）。该类患者的预后是多变的，因为夹层可能从无症状到导致严重神经功能障碍和死亡（Mohan，2014）。

夹层通常由血管壁最内侧的内膜层或中膜层撕裂所致。动脉血液在压力下不断外渗，会扩大内膜和中膜之间的夹层，造成管腔狭窄或闭塞。内膜下夹层可能会造成壁内血肿，从而导致管腔狭窄。颅腔内的动脉夹层可能也会导致动脉瘤扩张和蛛网膜下腔出血。动脉破裂后血管外的血肿被包裹，可能会导致动脉管腔狭窄（Yamaura，1994）。动脉远端栓塞是由于动脉内表面暴露的异物或脱落的血栓刺激血小板聚集而产生。由于血栓形成或附壁血肿造成的动脉管腔闭塞，也可能导致动脉远端血流减少（Mohan，2014）。

对于创伤后 ICA 或 VA 夹层的尽早识别和诊断至关重要。ICA 夹层通常造成大脑中动脉区域缺血，而 VA 夹层则可导致脑干、小脑和枕叶缺血。CT 扫描可以观察到大脑梗死或出血，而 CT 血管成像（CT angiogram，CTA）或经导管血管造影则能显示管腔的闭塞或狭窄、管腔梭形扩张、内膜瓣、近端管腔的串珠样改变、双腔征或血管扭曲（Kitanaka et al.，1994；Eastman et al.，2006；Geddes et al.，2016）。一般认为磁共振成像血管造影对于 ICA 或 VA 夹层的显示与识别没有 CTA 或经导管血管造影准确。

伴有蛛网膜下腔出血的颅内病变可经血管内治疗或行显微手术治疗（Halbach et al.，1993；Pham et al.，2011）。然而，在如今的临床实践中，外科手术治疗很少得到应用。梭形长段夹层动脉瘤无法行显微外科手术夹闭或血管内支架植入，在这种情况下，往往可以考虑行基底动脉近端 VA 栓塞治疗。由于一些患者可能无法耐受动脉完全闭塞，因此建议对优势 VA 行球囊闭塞试验（Mohan，2014）。其他的手术技术包括 VA 夹闭联合血管旁路术、VA 切除联合自体静脉原位移植术、梭形动脉瘤夹闭和包裹术（Arimura and Iihara，2016）。颅外的动脉夹层主要通过药物进行治疗，包括 6 个月的抗血小板或抗凝治疗（CADISS Trial Investigators，2015）。

创伤后脑积水的外科治疗

创伤后脑积水（post-traumatic hydrocephalus，PTH）是TBI的一种并发症，有研究报道了该类患者经永久性脑脊液分流术后出现临床症状的改善（Guyot and Michael，2000）。PTH是否出现是TBI患者随访的重要内容，PTH可表现为神经功能恶化、与颅内压力相关的头痛或正常压力脑积水综合征。伤后出现晚期脑脊液漏可能提示PTH。诊断和治疗PTH是很重要的，因为如果不治疗，它会使TBI患者的发病率和死亡率升高（Paoletti et al.，1983；Tribl and Oder，2000；Low et al.，2013）。据报道，PTH的发病率在0.7%~51.4%（Bontke and Boake，1991；Guyot and Michael，2000；De Bonis et al.，2010）。然而，通常很难确定TBI后观察到的脑室扩大与脑萎缩或是脑积水有关；电子化脑脊液输注研究报告有助于区分这两种不同的病理过程（Marmarou et al.，1996；Czosnyka et al.，2005）。正确选择能够受益于永久性脑脊液分流术的患者很重要，因为分流术后可能会出现严重并发症。对于PTH并没有明确具体的诊疗指南，但是流量可调控的脑室-腹腔分流术可减少过度引流的风险，通常作为首选的分流术。据报道，PTH是内镜下第三脑室造瘘术的相对禁忌证（Singh et al.，2008），但是这一观点受到了其他人的质疑（De Bonis et al.，2013）。很难预测PTH患者脑脊液分流术后的反应，因为这些患者通常有多种并发症及严重的潜在脑损伤。有研究还表明，DC是脑积水的一个危险因素（De Bonis et al.，2010；Kolias et al.，2013），而其他的研究并不支持这一假说（Rahme et al.，2010）。有0~88.2%的接受DC治疗的TBI患者存在脑积水（Ding et al.，2014）。通常认为脑脊液吸收不良或循环受阻是DC后脑积水的原因。然而，当前研究所纳入的一系列病例受限于研究设计本身和脑积水诊断的异质性。

颅骨成形术

颅骨成形术是对先前手术（通常是DC）或颅骨损伤所造成的颅骨缺损进行颅骨重建手术（图43.3）。对于存在颅骨缺损患者，建议行颅骨成形术，以保护容易受到损伤的大脑及恢复颅骨的外形轮廓，这可能对患者的心理和社会产生积极影响（Kolias et al.，2013）。正如在环钻综合征患者中观察到的那样，颅骨成形术可以促进神经系统康复，还可能会改善神经功能（Segal et al.，1994；Di Stefano et al.，2012；Bender et al.，2013；Honeybul et al.，2013）。然而，这种手术与严重并发症相关，最常见并发症的是伤口愈合不良和植入物相关感染（Gooch et al.，2009；Honeybul and Ho，2011；Wachter et al.，2013）。文献中讨论的各种不同的手术技术、移植物（自体骨、金属或人工合成物）和重建时间（1~12个月）尚缺乏相关共识和高质量证据（Liang et al.，2007；Beauchamp et al.，2010；Yadla et al.，2011；Glover et al.，2012；Schuss et al.，2012；Bender et al.，2013；

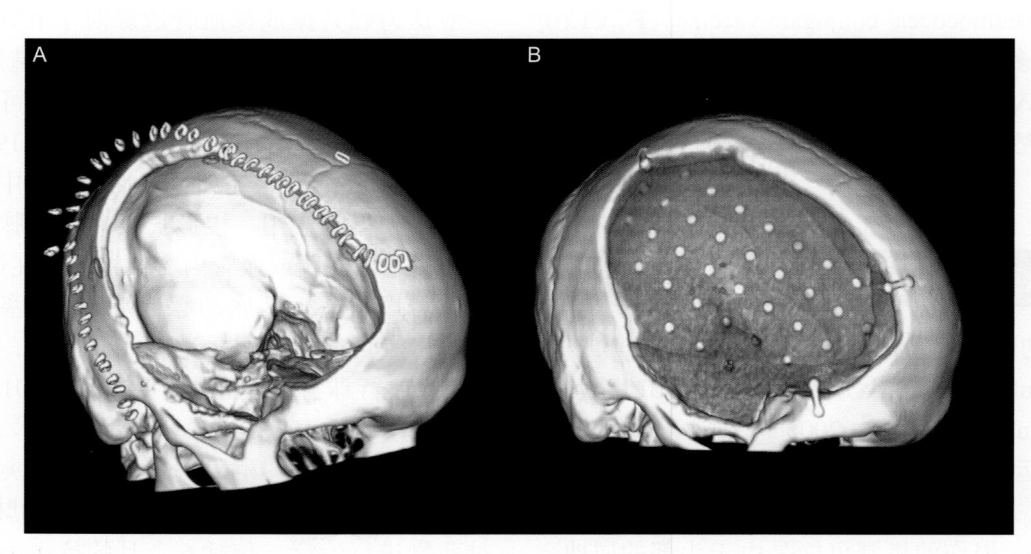

图43.3 颅骨成形术。（A）去骨瓣减压术后头部计算机断层扫描（computed tomography，CT）三维（three- dimensional，3D）重建，为治疗急性硬膜下血肿伴术中严重脑肿胀，在行单侧去骨瓣减压术后出现了大面积的颅骨缺损。（B）用定制的PEEK材料修复颅骨缺损后的CT 3D重建，颅骨成形术前的头部CT 3D重建可用于定制骨瓣的制作

Klinger et al., 2014）。关于颅骨成形术手术时机的争议主要是早期进行颅骨成形术是否会增加感染的风险，以及早期手术是否能够独立改善神经功能预后。最近一项对现有研究（全部为回顾性研究）的系统评价（包括528名患者）表明，颅骨成形术可以改善神经功能，早期行颅骨成形术能够进一步改善神经功能（Liang et al., 2007；Beauchamp et al., 2010；Yadla et al., 2011；Glover et al., 2012；Schuss et al., 2012；Bender et al., 2013；Malcolm et al., 2018）。就修补材料而言，患者自体颅骨最为常用，因为它满足了理想型材料的许多要求（即成本低、具有理想外观和轮廓、生物相容性好、质地坚固，并且还可以透过射线）。然而，近年来的一些研究表明由于自体颅骨被吸收或感染而造成手术失败率很高；最近一项自体颅骨成形术与钛颅骨成形术的单中心RCT研究证实了这一点，该研究发现，在31名自体颅骨成形术患者中，有7名患者（22%）出现了完全的颅骨吸收（Honeybul et al., 2017）。以聚甲基丙烯酸甲酯（有机玻璃，译者注）作为材料的颅骨成形术具有便宜、韧性好、重量轻的优点。然而，值得注意的是，该种材料的脆性容易致其破裂并且有发热的现象（Aydin et al., 2011）。羟基磷灰石由于具有良好的骨整合功能，近年来越来越受到欢迎。然而，它的成本仍然很高，并且有报道说这种材料在受到外伤后易断裂。钛板仍然是一种被广泛使用且相对便宜的材料，但会造成成像伪影。最近发表的羟基磷灰石对比钛板的单中心RCT研究发现，两组6个月的再次手术率相似（分别为26.9% *vs*. 29.2%），羟基磷灰石组感染的比例较低（7.7% *vs*. 20.8%），但硬膜外血肿的比例较高（34.6% *vs*. 8.3%）（Lindner et al., 2017）。用于颅骨成形术的其他材料及材料复合物还有很多，在此就不一一详述；颅骨成形术的关键步骤包括从硬脑膜仔细剥离头皮，闭合每一处的硬脑膜裂口，暴露缺损颅骨的边缘，以及牢固地固定自体骨或人工植入物。在感染的情况下，通常需取出移植物并对伤口进行清创；重要的是要等到潜在的感染被完全消除，这一过程可能需要长达1年的时间，然后重新植入移植物，以将移植物进一步感染的风险降至最低。

参考文献、EBRAIN的相关链接

扫描书末二维码获取。

第 44 章　颅脑损伤并发症

Fardad T. Afshari · Antonio Belli · Peter C. Whitfield 著
郭旭飞 译，刘伟明 审校

引言

颅脑损伤并发症可根据发生时间分为早期（1 周内）或远期（超过 1 周），也可以根据潜在的病理过程来分类（如脑脊液漏、血管并发症、癫痫和脑积水）。此外，在颅脑损伤后，通常会有许多康复方面的需求。在早期，这些需求主要集中于医疗护理（如胸部物理治疗、避免挛缩、营养和交流沟通等）。在远期，以患者为中心的目标导向治疗变得越来越重要。在本章中，我们描述了几种早期并发症，然后考虑到延迟性并发症，但根据时间分类尚不精确，并且早期和远期并发症之间有相当大的重叠。

颅脑损伤的早期并发症

血管损伤

创伤性脑损伤可能与血管损伤有关。其中，大多数发生在早期，与创伤引起的作用力传导直接相关。穿透伤（如低速子弹）很少造成血管损伤，更多是颈椎和（或）颅底的骨质损伤。

创伤性蛛网膜下腔出血

创伤性蛛网膜下腔出血是头部 CT 扫描发现蛛网膜下腔出血最常见的原因。1/3 的中重度颅脑损伤患者头部 CT 平扫可见蛛网膜下腔出血（Eisenberg et al.，1990；Servadei et al.，2002）。初次 CT 显示的创伤性蛛网膜下腔出血量与较差的预后相关（Paiva et al.，2010）。

虽然创伤性蛛网膜下腔出血后会发生血管痉挛，但这并不像动脉瘤性蛛网膜下腔出血后血管痉挛那么常见。一项系统回顾发现，没有证据表明尼莫地平可以改善创伤性蛛网膜下腔出血患者的预后（Vergouwen et al.，2006）。

颈动脉和椎动脉夹层

颈动脉夹层是最常见的血管损伤，通常发生在动脉颅外段或颅底段的栓系或骨折处（**图 44.1**）。同样，椎动脉夹层发生在 V2 和 V3 节段，也就是动脉进出横突孔处。颈动脉或椎动脉的创伤可造成内膜撕裂，导致夹层并形成假腔。假腔的扩张可能导致载瘤血管闭塞，导致远端梗死。血管的局部损伤可导致附壁血栓的形成并且会在没有夹层分离的情况下出现部分或全部闭塞。部分闭塞血管中的血栓可引起远端栓塞，常累及大脑的分水岭区域。极少有创伤性损伤引起假性动脉瘤进而导致自发性创伤后颅内出血的情况。CTA、MRA 和 DSA 是检查创伤性脑损伤后血管损伤最敏感的方法。抗血小板治疗是治疗动脉夹层损伤的主要方式，但必须考虑合并颅内或颅外出血的情况。血管内治疗在某些情况下是一种选择；然而，大多数创伤性夹层会在几周内自发愈合。创伤性夹层的处理应该尽可能以多学科的方式进行，包括神经外科、卒中医疗科和介入放射科。

动静脉瘘

动静脉瘘虽然罕见，但创伤性脑损伤后可能会形成动静脉瘘。症状可能会在第一周内出现，也可能会延迟出现。瘘管形成最常见的部位是颈动脉海绵部和海绵状静脉窦之间。颅脑创伤后颈动脉海绵窦瘘（carotico-cavernous fistulae，CCF）的发生率为 0.2%~0.3%（Fabian et al.，1999）。这些瘘管把破裂的海绵窦内颈动脉和周围静脉通道直接连接，因此流量大，容易出现症状（见**第 49 章**）。在临床上，症状表现为搏动性眼球突出、结膜充血和杂音三联征。治疗主要是血管内治疗，目的是保护视力，防止皮质静脉反流以及后续的出血后遗症。间接 CCF 通常不会在创伤后急性期发作，如果在创伤患者身上发现，可以不用紧急处理，有时会自发消退。

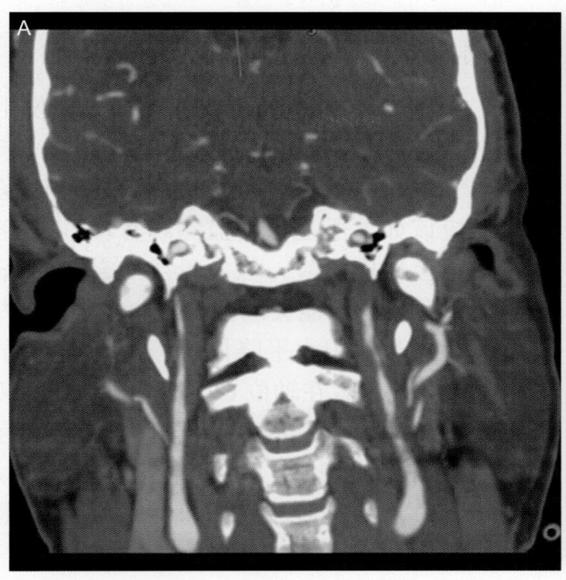

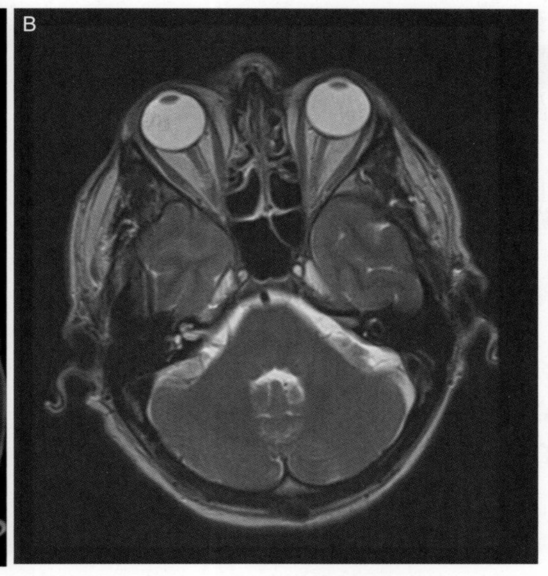

图 44.1　双侧颈动脉夹层。（A）CTA 显示双侧颈内动脉逐渐变细，显示夹层。（B）T2 加权 MRI 显示颈动脉内高信号。正常情况下，血管主要表现为流空影（低信号，如在基底动脉），但随着颈动脉闭塞，这种空洞消失了

脑神经损伤

脑神经损伤在颅脑损伤后很常见。尽管总是作为创伤早期并发症出现，但直到康复阶段，神经损伤的影响才变得突出。脑神经麻痹可能是由于创伤性脑神经损伤所致，尤其是在与颅孔出口的交界处。它们也可能是颅内压升高的结果（例如，第Ⅲ神经麻痹、第Ⅵ神经麻痹和第Ⅶ神经麻痹）。不管有没有前颅底骨折，嗅神经损伤很常见，因为脆弱的嗅神经在穿过筛板时很容易损伤。嗅神经在某些情况下可以缓慢恢复，但感觉丧失通常是永久性的；此外，由于味觉和嗅觉的感知重叠，嗅觉丧失会影响味觉。

面部和眼眶骨折引起的视神经横断或压迫，通常表现为单侧视力丧失。通常会存在传入性瞳孔（光反应）缺失。外伤后的视力损害通常需要紧急的影像学检查和眼科会诊。颅脑损伤后的复视很常见，可因动眼神经、滑车或展神经的损伤而导致，应与眼眶壁骨折或眶外侧滑车吊带损伤等非神经性、机械性的复视相鉴别。

颞骨骨折可能导致一系列损害，特别是在涉及耳囊时。在过去，这些骨折被分为纵向骨折（骨折沿着岩骨的长轴）或横向骨折。横向骨折不太常见，但更容易导致感音神经性听力障碍和面瘫。耳囊的受累现在被认为是损害脑神经功能的主要因素。这些损害包括面神经麻痹、听力丧失和脑脊液漏。面神经麻痹可以随着时间的推移恢复，但如果伴有角膜暴露必须采取保护。在创伤性面神经麻痹的治疗中，使用皮质类固醇的证据并不充分。建议及早进行语言和言语治疗以及物理治疗。面神经再生技术可以用来考虑治疗永久性致残缺陷。

听力丧失是与颞骨和岩骨骨折相关的头部损伤后的常见表现。听力障碍可能是传导性的，也可能是感音性的。传导性耳聋是由于血液堵塞耳道、鼓膜受损或听骨链断裂所致。后者应接受手术治疗，并通过高分辨率 CT 扫描检查确定诊断。建议耳鼻喉科收治以指导进一步的检查和治疗。由于耳蜗结构或蜗神经本身的损伤，会发生感音性耳聋。这可能是由岩骨骨折或继发于颅内压升高引起的神经缺血引起。

后组脑神经麻痹可以单独发生，也可以合并发生。它们通常继发于延伸至颈静脉孔的枕骨骨折。与后组脑神经麻痹相关的各种并发症在肿瘤和创伤部分都有记述，并在**表 44.1** 中进行了总结。

凹陷性颅骨骨折

创伤性脑损伤通常会导致凹陷性颅骨骨折。凹陷性骨折可在最初 CT 影像上识别出来，并且可以通过容积重建很好地显示出来。凹陷性颅骨骨折可能与潜在的脑挫伤、硬膜外或硬膜下血肿有关。此外，它们可能与硬脑膜破裂有关，并增加延迟感染、癫痫、脑膜炎或脑脓肿的风险。凹陷性颅骨骨折需手术复位的绝对指征是开放性骨折，并需要对骨折碎片进行清创，在某些情况下还需要修复硬脑膜。颅骨外膜或颞肌筋膜是硬脑膜修补的首选材料。手术

表 44.1 颈静脉孔综合征

综合征	Ⅸ	Ⅹ	Ⅺ	Ⅻ	交感症状
维拉特综合征 / 腮腺后间隙综合征	是	是	是	是	是
科莱—西卡尔综合征 / 枕骨髁—颈静脉孔连接部综合征	是	是	是	是	否
颈静脉孔综合征 / 后破裂孔综合征	是	是	是	否	否
施密特综合征	否	是	是	否	否
塔皮亚综合征	否	是	否	是	是 / 否
杰克逊综合征	否	是	是	是	否

的相对适应证包括明显碎片凹陷（+/- 血肿）引起的占位效应，凹陷大于骨厚度和影响外观。任何覆盖静脉窦的凹陷性骨折都应谨慎处理，因为骨折整复有发生大出血风险。

早期脑脊液漏

脑脊液鼻漏和耳漏是颅底骨折的常见并发症，提示硬脑膜破裂。脑脊液鼻漏可发生于突破前颅窝底硬脑膜的复杂筛骨骨折。脑脊液鼻漏也可能是由于脑脊液通过颞骨充气部分流出，进入中耳，然后通过咽鼓管进入鼻咽。脑脊液耳漏可发生于伴有鼓膜穿孔的颞骨骨折。高达 90% 的脑脊液漏在 2 周内自然愈合。其余患者可能会有持续性脑脊液漏或发展为迟发性脑脊液漏。不建议使用抗生素预防，但如果出现脑膜炎症状，应立即进行抗生素治疗。建议所有颅底骨折或确诊或疑似脑脊液漏的患者接种抗肺炎球菌疫苗（Phang et al.，2016）。对于那些持续脑脊液漏超过 2 周的患者，最佳的后续治疗还存在一些争议。通过腰椎引流排出脑脊液是非常有效的，可以最大限度地减少通过渗漏部位的流量，从而促进愈合。然而，如果瘘口很大，可能会使空气进入颅腔，任何可疑的高颅压患者都必须慎重采用，以避免发生小脑扁桃体疝。

虽然脑脊液鼻漏或耳漏在临床上症状明显，但在某些情况下，颅脑损伤后脑脊液漏可能很难与鼻分泌物区分。在这种情况下，头部前倾等动作可能会加重脑脊液漏，进一步提示脑脊液鼻漏。或者，如果可以采集脑脊液样本，可以检测脑脊液中含量较高的 β- 转铁蛋白。葡萄糖检测不太有帮助，因为鼻分泌物也可能含有葡萄糖（Baker et al.，2005）。**图** 44.2 展示了用于处理疑似脑脊液漏的流程图。

气颅

颅脑外伤合并颅顶或颅底骨折后可发生气颅（颅腔内空气）。气颅的发生率在 0.5%~1%。蛛网膜下腔内积气表明硬脑膜破裂。气颅患者脑脊液漏的风险很高，应该如上所述密切监测和管理。虽然颅内少量空气不会造成危险，但大量空气，特别是在气体有张力情况下，可能会因占位效应损伤造成中线移位。气颅可导致意识水平降低、癫痫发作或局部神经体征。仰卧位患者在轴位 CT 扫描中，由于双侧额叶前上方出现大量空气，额叶受压呈双峰状，称为“富士山征”（Michel，2004）。有时，可表现为张力性气颅，需要紧急治疗。治疗气颅通常采用高流量氧气，以降低氮气分压，促进颅内间隙空气吸收。在严重中线移位和张力性气颅的情况下，可能需要紧急头部钻孔才能让空气从硬膜下腔排出，但这种情况较为少见。

颅脑损伤的远期并发症

癫痫发作

虽然癫痫发作可能在创伤性脑损伤后早期出现，但晚期癫痫发作是康复患者最关心的问题。总体而言，高达 30% 的严重创伤性脑损伤患者可能会发生癫痫发作。癫痫发作早期会导致代谢需求增加、兴奋性毒性和颅内压升高，并可能导致严重的继发性脑损伤。尽管抗癫痫药物通常能在一定程度上控制癫痫，但这些问题在晚期也会存在。

头部损伤后癫痫发作的风险取决于几个因素。Bryan Jennett 在 CT 时代之前经典定义如下：损伤严重程度、PTA 持续时间、颅骨凹陷骨折、脑内血肿 / 挫伤。在第一周内持续癫痫发作的患者晚期发生癫痫的风险也会增加。Annegers 等根据损伤的严重程度定义了风险，主要使用 CT 前获得的数据。严重损伤的特征是脑挫伤、颅内血肿、意识丧失或创伤后 24 小时以上的记忆缺失。创伤后癫痫的 5 年累积发生概率为 10%，30 年累积概率为 16.7%。Christensen 等对儿童和青少年的研究表明，轻型脑损伤（RR，2.22；95%CI，2.07~2.38）、重型脑损伤（7.40，6.16~8.89）和颅骨骨折（2.17，1.73~2.71）增加了癫痫的风险。总体而言，晚期癫痫的风险随着时间的推移而降低，但对于风险最高的患者来说，10~15 年内仍高于普通人群的基线风险（Jennett，1973；Jennett，1975；Annegers et al.，1998；Christensen et al.，2009）。

目前有 I 类证据表明，使用抗癫痫药物可减少

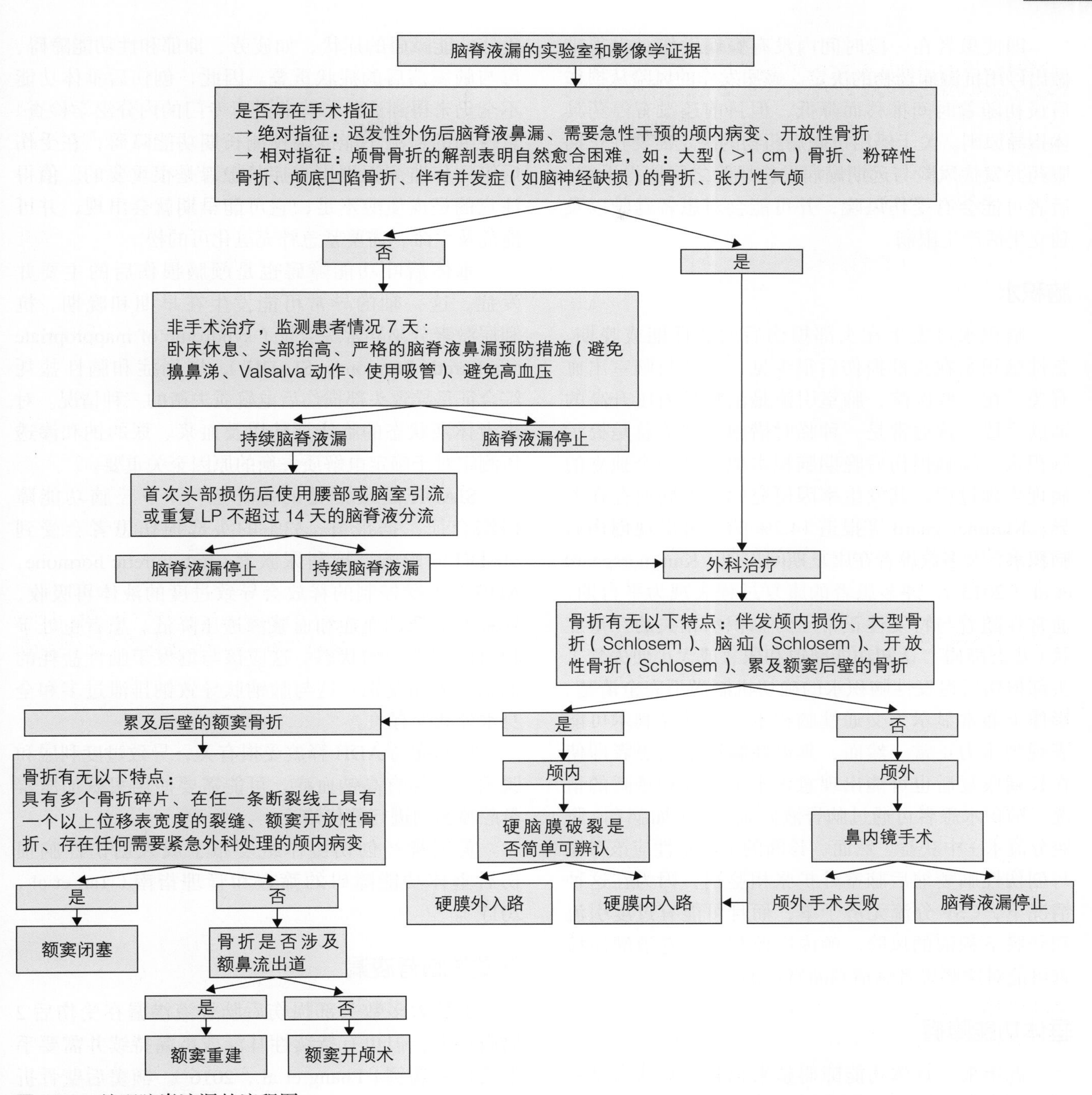

图 44.2　处理脑脊液漏的流程图

Reproduced with permission from See Yung Phang, Kathrin Whitehouse, Lucy Lee, et al., Management of CSF leak in base of skull fractures in adults, *British Journal of Neurosurgery*, Volume 30, Issue 6, pp. 596–604, Copyright © 2016 The Neurosurgical Foundation, reprinted by permission of Taylor & Francis Ltd, www.tandfonline.com on behalf of The Neurosurgical Foundation.

早期（前 7 天）癫痫发作频率，但对迟发性癫痫发作没有影响（Temkin et al.，1990）。此外，在头部损伤后早期或晚期预防性使用抗癫痫药对死亡率或神经功能障碍没有影响（Schierhout and Roberts，2001）。

传统上，苯妥英钠一直被用作颅脑损伤患者控制癫痫发作的一线药物。最近的前瞻性随机研究表明，左乙拉西坦和苯妥英钠两者也可作为有效的预防癫痫药物，且癫痫控制率没有显著差异（Szaflarski et al.，2010）。鉴于左乙拉西坦的有效性、出现症状副作用的风险低、对认知无影响、成本相对较低，现已成为首选治疗方案（Eddy et al.，2011）。

颅脑损伤的癫痫发作患者应该被告知在游泳和开放式机械上工作的风险。应建议他们避免驾驶，并通知有关驾驶管理机构。

即使患者在一段时间内没有癫痫发作，也很难做出停用抗癫痫药物的决定。癫痫发作的风险从损伤后最初随着时间推移而降低，但目前还没有停药具体指导原则。关于停用抗癫痫药物的决定需要在长期服药并发症风险与远期癫痫发作风险之间取得平衡，后者可能会有受伤风险，并可能会对患者驾驶以及独立生活产生限制。

脑积水

脑积水可发生在头部损伤后的急性期或晚期。急性脑积水在头部损伤后很少见，往往与脑室出血有关。在一些医院，脑室引流是治疗颅内压升高的辅助手段。这通常是一种临时措施，并不总是提示脑积水。颅脑损伤后晚期脑积水似乎是一个独立的病理生理过程。其发生率因研究标准不同而存在差异。Kammersgaard 等报道 14.2% 的患者出现创伤后脑积水，大多数患者在康复期间出现（Kammersgaard et al.，2013）。许多患者的康复过程表现为平台期，通常伴随着与特发性正常压力脑积水相关的三重症状（步态障碍、认知功能减退和尿急或大小便失禁）。头部损伤后迟发性脑积水的确切机制尚不完全清楚。影像上通常显示为交通性脑积水，腰椎穿刺术可能表现为压力正常。然而，延迟性脑积水的患者即使在长期康复后也可能出现意识水平下降和嗜睡的情况。脑积水患者可通过脑脊液分流手术（如脑室 - 腹腔分流术）中获益。然而，诊断的不确定性应该考虑与创伤性脑萎缩后脑室外扩张相鉴别，因为在这种情况下，CSF 分流无济于事，而且可能有过度引流和硬膜下积液的风险。颅内压监测和脑脊液灌注检查可能对这些患者病情判断有帮助。

垂体功能障碍

近年来，垂体功能障碍越来越多地被认为是一种被忽视的延迟性并发症。创伤性脑损伤可能导致垂体功能障碍，这可能导致长期的身体、认知和心理障碍。垂体功能障碍大致可分为垂体前叶功能障碍和垂体后叶功能障碍，可在颅脑损伤后早期或晚期（>6 个月）检测到。在 Bondanelli 的一项研究中，轻型、中型和重型颅脑损伤患者的垂体前叶功能障碍报告分别为 37.5%、57.1% 和 59.3%，但该研究患者队列较小（Bondanelli et al.，2004）。其他研究报告称，颅脑损伤后垂体前叶功能障碍的发生率为 20%~25%（Agha et al.，2007；Alavi et al.，2016）。垂体前叶激素最常见的改变是促性腺激素和生长激素缺乏，其次是促肾上腺皮质激素和促甲状腺激素。垂体功能障碍的症状，如疲劳、抑郁和性功能障碍，可与脑震荡后的症状重叠。因此，创伤后垂体功能不全仍未得到诊断，除非进行专门的内分泌学检查。急性期的检测不能准确预测长期功能障碍，在受伤后第一年监测识别出有症状患者是很重要的。值得注意的是皮质醇不足，它可能早期就会出现，并可能危及生命，需要紧急补充氢化可的松。

垂体后叶功能障碍也是颅脑损伤后的主要并发症。这一轴的异常可能发生在早期和晚期。抗利尿激素分泌异常综合征（syndrome of inappropriate antidiuretic hormone，SIADH）、尿崩症和脑性盐耗综合征是导致头部损伤后电解质失衡的三种情况。对患者体液状态的临床评估以及血浆、尿的钠和渗透压测定对于确定电解质失衡的原因至关重要。

SIADH 是最常见的垂体后叶 / 下丘脑功能障碍综合征，据报道，33% 的头部损伤患者会受到 SIADH 的影响。抗利尿激素（antidiuretic hormone，ADH）不受控制的释放会导致过度的液体再吸收，导致血清低钠血症和血浆渗透压降低。患者也处于相对液体超载的状态。这应该与继发于脑性盐耗的低钠血症相鉴别：这与脑钠肽导致钠排泄过多和全身水分减少有关。

尿崩症与 ADH 释放受损有关，导致过度利尿和脱水，并伴有高钠血症。可能需要使用去氨加压素鼻腔喷雾剂进行替代治疗。

英国神经创伤协作组发布了成人创伤性脑损伤后垂体功能障碍的筛查和管理指南（Tan et al.，2017）。

迟发性脑脊液漏

虽然大多数头部损伤后脑脊液渗漏在受伤后 2 周内消失，但也有持续性耳漏或鼻漏持续并需要手术治疗的病例（Phang et al.，2016）。额窦后壁骨折是脑脊液持续性渗漏最常见的损伤之一。除了伤后持续脑脊液漏外，有时还会出现迟发性脑脊液漏，这可能是由于漏口再次开放或并发的脑积水所致。薄层头部 CT 三维重建扫描为确定脑脊液漏出部位提供了必要的解剖学细节。由于脑脊液漏可导致严重的感染性并发症，建议对颅底骨折患者采取系统的治疗方法。**图 44.3** 提供了一种管理流程。

对复杂脑脊液漏进行完好的颅底修复是具有挑战性的。在前颅底，可以采用一个双冠皮瓣，并在开颅手术骨瓣上游离骨膜做一个向前的“信箱”样骨膜瓣，提供一个带血管的瓣来覆盖硬膜外或硬膜内的渗漏部位。这是一项重要的外科手术技术，但有

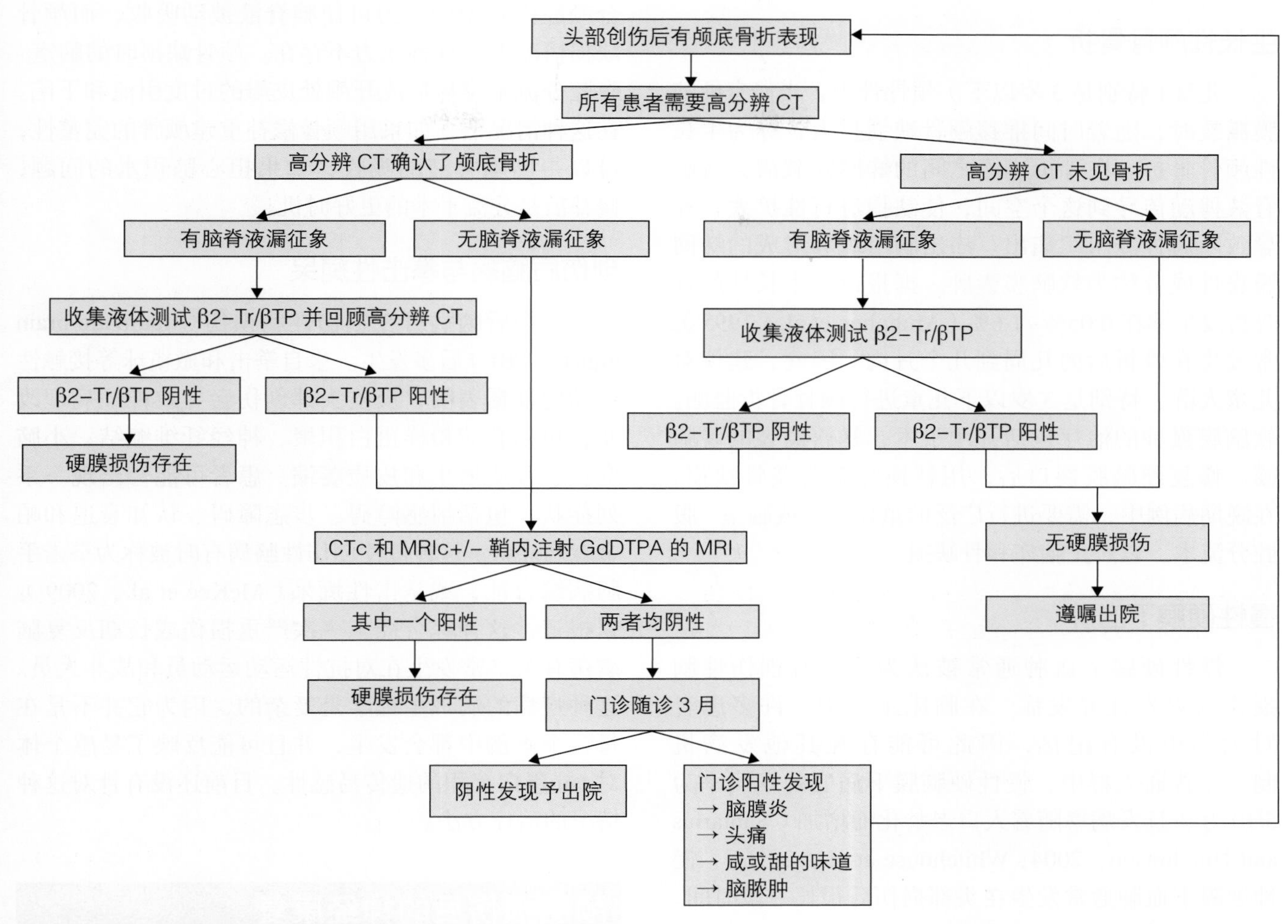

图 44.3 颅底骨折的处置和治疗流程（HRCT，高分辨率 CT）

Reproduced with permission from See Yung Phang, Kathrin Whitehouse, Lucy Lee, et al., Management of CSF leak in base of skull fractures in adults, *British Journal of Neurosurgery*, Volume 30, Issue 6, pp. 596–604, Copyright © 2016 The Neurosurgical Foundation, reprinted by permission of Taylor & Francis Ltd, www.tandfonline.com on behalf of The Neurosurgical Foundation.

嗅觉丧失的风险。另外，鼻内镜下鼻中隔皮瓣修补术提供了一种侵入性小的方法，前提是漏口有准确定位。该方法可以辅用软组织（如阔筋膜移植或带血管的鼻中隔皮瓣）、组织胶和腰大池脑脊液引流，效果良好。可通过薄层骨窗 CT 扫描、CT/MRI 脑脊液造影检查（经腰池注射碘化对比剂或钆）或向腰池内注射荧光素来确定渗漏，以方便术中定位。侧方颅底渗漏可能更具挑战性，可能需要开颅手术，如颅中窝开颅、经乳突或联合手术（Phang et al.，2016）。最后，盲囊闭合（咽鼓管闭塞）是解决脑脊液漏的最终方法，但会以听力损失为代价。

脑脊液漏和颅骨骨折后感染

颅骨骨折或头部损伤后持续的脑脊液漏会增加随后的脑膜炎或迟发性硬膜下脓肿风险。由于硬脑膜污染和破裂，穿透伤或枪伤的患者风险最高。污染伤口的处理包括清创、冲洗和硬脑膜修复。对于这种污染或感染的开放性骨折，静脉注射抗生素是必要的。

颅底骨折与脑脊液漏相关，发生脑膜炎和迟发性感染的风险也很高，需要特别注意。严重头部损伤后脑膜炎的发生率从 0.2% 到 17.8% 不等（Helling et al.，1988）。目前的文献并不支持在脑脊液漏患者中预防性使用抗生素。Cochrane 随机对照试验得出结论，无论是否有脑脊液渗漏的证据，都没有证据表明颅底骨折患者需要预防性使用抗生素（Ratilal et al.，2015）。尽管基于这种治疗的证据还不足，所有颅底骨折都推荐接种肺炎链球菌疫苗，因为肺炎链球菌是一种常见的病原体。在持续性脑脊液鼻漏或耳漏症病例中，建议修复缺损以防止延迟感染的风险。

生长性颅骨骨折

儿童（特别是3岁以下）颅骨骨折，当伴有硬脑膜撕裂时，随着时间推移颅骨缺损扩大，称为生长性颅骨骨折。在骨折边缘之间的蛛网膜皱褶会将脑脊液搏动传导到这个空间，使缺损进行性扩大，并导致随后神经组织疝出。疝出脑组织和形成的蛛网膜囊性成分称为软脑膜囊肿。据报道，生长性颅骨骨折发生率在0.05%~1.6%（Muhonen et al.，1995）。常发生在骨折后的几周到几个月内。因此，建议对儿童人群，特别是3岁以下儿童进行颅骨骨折监测。软脑膜囊肿的治疗包括开颅手术，暴露撕裂的硬脑膜。修复硬脑膜裂口后，用替换骨瓣覆盖骨缺损。在晚期病例中，需要进行广泛的重建手术或脑室-腹腔分流术，以矫正脑疝和骨缺损。

慢性硬膜下血肿

慢性硬膜下血肿通常被认为是轻微创伤性脑损伤的迟发性并发症。在临床工作中，许多患者对创伤史没有记忆，因此可能存在其他发病机制。在普通人群中，慢性硬脑膜下病变的发病率为5/10万，且发病率随着人口老龄化而增加（Santarius and Hutchinson，2004；Whitehouse et al.，2016）。慢性硬膜下血肿通常发生在头部损伤后很长一段时间。时间可能从几周到几个月不等。最初的轻微头部损伤并不会引起患者注意，但有可能导致桥静脉撕裂，引起低流量出血和急性硬膜下血肿。随着时间的推移，血肿液化导致进行性脑组织受压。患者可能会出现头痛、意识减退、癫痫发作或局灶性神经功能障碍。有症状的慢性硬膜下血肿可以通过手术钻孔引流进行治疗。对于复发或伴有明显包膜的病例可采用小骨瓣开颅手术，以便更好地越过血凝块接触到血管化的包膜。类固醇在慢性硬膜下血肿治疗中的作用仍然存在争议，文献中没有随机试验的报道。目前有正在进行的类固醇治疗慢性硬膜下血肿疗效的临床随机对照试验。

开颅手术后并发症

颅骨切除术后，有几个可能出现的问题需引起重视。颅骨缺损下方大脑区域相关的局灶性神经功能障碍称为“环钻综合征”。这可能与开颅手术骨窗边缘引流静脉扭曲或大脑血流调节紊乱所致的静脉淤血有关。随着颅腔完整性重建，这些功能障碍可能会逆转。

脑积水和开颅手术的关系很难评估，通常在闭合颅腔内积聚的压力可使脑脊液被动吸收，而颅骨缺损情况下，这种压力不存在。颅骨缺损时的脑室-腹腔分流术容易造成开颅处皮瓣的过度引流和下陷。在这种情况下，如果用颅骨修补重建颅骨的完整性，可以帮助脑脊液的吸收，如果担心脑积水的问题，修补后是分流手术的更好时机。

创伤后脑病与拳击性痴呆

创伤后脑病可在创伤性脑损伤（traumatic brain injury，TBI）后多发生。来自拳击和橄榄球等接触性运动的证据表明，反复头部创伤会导致神经病理改变，包括β淀粉样蛋白积聚、神经纤维缠结、小脑变性、胶质增生和皮质萎缩。患者可能会出现一系列症状，包括情感障碍、步态障碍、认知衰退和帕金森病症状。这种慢性创伤性脑病有时被称为拳击手脑病综合征，或拳击性痴呆（McKee et al.，2009）。据报道，这种综合征与一次严重损伤或长期反复脑震荡有关，常发生在对抗性运动运动员和战斗人员。这种疾病的病理生理学是复杂的，因为它并不是在每一个案例中都会发生，并且可能反映了易感个体对tau蛋白沉积的遗传易感性。目前还没有针对这种情况的治疗方法。

颅脑损伤后的神经康复

康复是促进患者伤后恢复的过程，旨在最大限度地提高患者的生活质量和参与日常生活、工作和休闲活动的能力。

颅脑损伤是一种异质性的疾病状态，其预后是多样的，取决于损伤的部位和严重程度。

神经康复服务应由一个涉及医疗、护理、职业治疗、言语和语言治疗、神经心理学、物理治疗、社会工作和精神病学的多学科团队提供。

康复过程始于对患者的评估，以确定认知、情绪和行为损害的性质，并明确对他们功能的影响。然后以患者为中心，设定阶段性目标，并确定短期和长期目标。这是一个动态的过程，取决于患者各阶段不断变化的康复需求（Holliday et al.，2007）。

神经康复包括急性期和急性期后期以及社区两个部分。急性期康复将重点放在患者的医疗状况上。急性期理疗的目的是优化肺功能和氧合。包括注意患者的体位、胸部物理治疗、手动胸部排痰技术、治疗前后定期吸痰和高氧。

言语和语言治疗，在急性期通常集中于吞咽困难上。TBI后吞咽障碍的发生率尚不清楚。创伤后意识水平下降和气管切开可导致吞咽困难。这些患者大多有较高的误吸风险，特别是当患者并发有胃瘫时。及早评估吞咽功能可以建立适当的喂养途径，以防止体重下降和营养不良。一旦吞咽反射恢复，就可以开始适当经口饮食。

急性期职业治疗的重点是减少损伤和预防并发症，以最大限度地保留长期功能。这包括评估患者的认知、运动和感觉功能，以便建立适当和有意义的目标。认知评估可以确定患者的意识水平，并促进他们与环境互动。运动和感觉评估可以通过设备进行适当地管理，如夹板、座椅、轮椅和各种专门的定位辅助设备和矫形器，以最大限度地发挥功能同时防止肌肉废用的长期并发症（Whitfield，2009）。

急性神经心理干预旨在处理由脑创伤引起的各种行为和心理问题。神经心理学家制订个体化的行为管理方案，并向卫生专业人员和工作人员提出改进治疗的建议，从而为患者提供最佳康复环境（Wilson and Zangwill，2003）。此外，神经心理学干预也可以为患者家属进行教育，使他们能够更好地理解患者行为，从而能够采取更好的应对策略，以使患者的各种功能得到最大限度地发挥。

在患者急性康复之后，长期康复及社区康复阶段随之而来。这一阶段的目标旨在使患者在康复过程中功能得到最大程度的恢复，与急性期相似，但更侧重于促进功能恢复，适应功能障碍，以及通过了解心理因素来制订长期补偿策略。在这一阶段的医疗中，在制订康复目标方面，患者与所处环境及与其他人的相互作用是一个重要的考虑因素。

这一阶段理疗的目标是优化并尽可能最大化肢体功能。头部创伤后痉挛状态很常见，会对患者肢体功能产生不利影响。长期固定可能导致肌肉骨骼的变形，并进一步限制患者的功能恢复。可以进行主动和被动伸展肌肉以防止挛缩的形成。通过铸型达到肌肉延长伸展以减少痉挛发生（Conine et al.，1990）。进一步控制痉挛可以通过使用抗痉挛药物如巴氯芬或使用肉毒杆菌毒素来实现。此外，物理治疗还可通过移动患者不同体位来增强本体感觉传入，以达到更好地控制肌肉运动的目的（Allum et al.，1998）。

语言和言语治疗在康复阶段起到重要作用，目的是最大限度地促进患者与他人的沟通和互动。头部损伤后，语言和非语言交流都经常会受到影响。虽然在许多情况下，这是由于语言过程障碍和言语生成障碍造成。其他情况，如认知交流障碍也会造成交流困难。有认知缺陷的患者，如注意力和集中能力受损，表现出沟通和语言技能较差。语言和言语治疗师可以找出沟通方面最严重的障碍，并采用技术手段来解决问题。在疑难病例中，补偿和适应方案可用来帮助这些患者改善沟通技能：通过技术手段是可以帮助这些患者的（Evans et al.，2009）。

这一阶段的职业治疗侧重于患者功能表现并提高其独立性，以使患者在尽可能多的日常活动中保持独立。这是通过重新学习基本技能来实现的，例如日常生活活动，包括个人卫生、着装、做饭和购物。此外，职业治疗还提供辅助设备，如专门的座椅和轮椅，来帮助他们独立生活。职业治疗师开发的恢复或适应方案包括制订个体化治疗方案，让患者进行一些通常喜欢做的活动，并改善他们的功能，使他们得以独立生活并重新回归社会角色。因此，职业治疗在从医院到社区的过渡中发挥着极其重要的作用，保证患者能够得到持续的整体康复（Evans et al.，2009）。

认知和神经心理康复是这一康复阶段的关键。脑创伤患者可能存在记忆、注意力、执行功能/计划、语言或知觉等方面的障碍。各种改善记忆、注意力、执行功能和视觉空间功能的训练模式目前正在研发和应用，这些模式有可能改善在颅脑损伤后患者认知的康复方法（Whyte et al.，2009）。

延伸阅读、参考文献、EBRAIN 的相关链接

扫描书末二维码获取。

第 45 章　脑震荡与运动相关脑损伤

Mark Wilson 著
白金月、薛钦 译，刘伟明 审校

引言

近些年来，人们对脑震荡和运动相关性脑损伤的兴趣不断增加，原因主要有三个：①它们是可预防的脑损伤类型；②越来越多的证据表明，反复的脑损伤会导致长期神经认知功能丧失；③对于运动组织机构而言，脑损伤在运动中时有意外发生，从而带来医学法律上的责任。很早以前人们已证实长期拳击运动可以导致拳击性痴呆，其他运动造成的反复性轻度脑损伤现已成为讨论的焦点。

随着时间的推移，脑震荡的定义也发生了改变。传统意义上来讲，在事件发生后立即出现持续时间不等的完全丧失意识（loss of consciousness，LOC），并伴有创伤后失忆，就可以定义为运动相关性脑震荡。将意识丧失的诊断条件取消后，神经外科医师协会将脑震荡（之后被应用于诊断运动性脑震荡）定义为：

一种由外部机械力引起的以神经功能即时和短暂性损害（如意识改变、视觉障碍、平衡障碍等）为特征的临床综合征（Gurdjian and Volis，1966）。

其他人将脑震荡定义为：

一种由生物力学因素引起的，无明显解剖学损害的脑损伤（Signoretti et al.，2011）。

脑震荡是一种由生物力学引起的以脑功能改变为主要特征的临床综合征，通常会影响记忆力和定向力，也可能包括意识丧失（美国神经病学学会）。

脑震荡可以有短期、中期和长期的后遗症。在急性期内，需要对重返赛场进行评估并作出决定。从中期来看，应对脑震荡后综合征和二次撞击综合征的风险进行管理，而长期风险则需在组织或工会层面进行管理。

最近，有人呼吁取消“脑震荡”这个术语，因为从不断演变的定义来看，这种叫法令人困惑。将其替换为反映其在创伤性脑损伤上的通用术语（例如，轻度创伤性脑损伤）更为合适，这个词通常与脑震荡交替使用（Sharp and Jenkins，2015）。然而，就本章而言，脑震荡这个术语将会继续使用。

脑震荡后综合征

轻度创伤性脑损伤（traumatic brain injury，TBI）后出现的症状通常包括头痛、头晕、疲劳、易怒、注意力不集中、睡眠障碍、记忆力减退、焦虑、对噪声和光线的敏感度升高、视力模糊和抑郁等。大部分患者的这些症状在 3 个月内消失，有大约 1/3 的患者其症状会持续 6 个月以上。

冲击性脑呼吸暂停

虽然很少考虑到这一点，但是早期对脑震荡的描述特别提到呼吸变化和呼吸暂停的发生（Koch and Filehne，1874）。John Hughling Jackson（1835—1911）了解到如果脑震荡足够严重，患者可能会因心力衰竭和呼吸衰竭而死，但在尸检时，这些病例的脑可能是正常的或接近正常的。有文献记载，轻微脑损伤后的呼吸暂停症状是常见的，而且冲击越大，呼吸暂停的时间越长（Atkinsonn et al.，1998）。这些现象发生时在影像学或尸检上很少或者几乎看不到明显的结构缺陷。这虽然不是本章的重点，但这一现象应该得到人们更多的关注，因为它可能在创伤性脑损伤致死原因中占有一定比例。

历史与运动相关损伤

波斯医生 Razes（854—925）使用脑震荡一词来描述大脑的异常生理状态，将其与严重的创伤性脑损伤区分开。在 13 世纪，Lanfrancus 将脑震荡（脑创伤造成的一过性干扰）和脑挫伤（脑损伤伴挫伤）分开。在 20 世纪初，许多人接受了这个理论，即脑震荡和脑挫伤是由于颅骨形变导致的脑缺血造成的。

在现代社会中，脑震荡已普遍与运动相关联。1893 年，一位鞋匠为一名多次头部受伤的美式橄榄球运动员制作了一顶皮头盔。1905年，美国大学橄榄球赛季有18人死亡，159人重伤，这引起了罗斯福总统的注意，他引入了能使比赛更安全的规则。从那以后，使用皮头盔的人就越来越多，分别在1935年与1939年，成为高中级别与大学级别比赛的强制规则。1931—1940年，橄榄球比赛中死亡人数从33人下降到11人。在20世纪50年代人们发明了硬塑料外壳的头盔，然而这使得头盔可以被用作攻击锤——保护装备变成了武器。因此，死亡人数增加了（1961—1970年为244人），其中75%的人因为脑出血死亡。1987—2008年，规则的改变和人们对这一问题的认识不断增强，导致所有级别的橄榄球比赛中死亡人数仅为个位数（Mueller and Cantu，2011）。在一次备受瞩目的脑损伤事件后，华盛顿和其他许多州都通过了Zackery Lystedt法（以TBI患者的名字命名）。其中的关键条款是：①对家长、运动员和教练进行教育；②在疑似脑震荡后立即停止比赛或训练，直到达到③的标准才能恢复比赛；③由一名脑震荡专家评估并书面批准后可恢复比赛；④对所有使用公共场地学校采取统一规则（Ellenbogen，2014）。

运动相关的脑损伤历来是神经外科医生的专攻领域。例如，Walter Dandy在1941年申请了第一个保护性棒球帽衬垫的专利（Fox，1984）。近几十年来，急诊医学、运动医学和其他卫生专业人员对此产生了浓厚的兴趣，他们都对这一领域的诊断和管理产生了重要的影响。而神经外科医生对各种形式头部损伤的常规治疗有独特的经验，可以了解实质性损伤的类型及其可能的后遗症。神经外科医生在这一领域起着领导与负责的作用。

鉴于运动与脑震荡之间的相关性，逐渐形成了一个运动相关脑震荡的定义。国际运动脑震荡研究协会将运动性脑震荡定义为：由创伤性力量引起影响大脑的复杂病理生理过程。几个共同的特征是：

①可由直接击打头部、面部、颈部或其他部位冲击力传递造成。

②通常会导致快速发生的短暂性神经功能障碍。

③虽然可能会发生神经病理改变，但急性期是神经功能性损害，而不是结构性的。

④可以分级，可以涉及或不涉及意识丧失。

⑤大体正常的神经影像学表现。

⑥偶尔症状会长期存在。

运动相关的脑震荡与其他机制（例如，从自行车上摔下来）造成的脑震荡没有什么特别区别，因此，重新的单独定义和分类只会增加人们更多的困惑。

当然，有些运动比轻微的头部损伤或脑震荡造成的伤害要大得多。例如，参与赛车运动涉及的力量有可能造成立即危及生命的伤害。

脑震荡的病理生理学

运动性头部损伤的病因学研究

运动中脑损伤的结果必须反映物理规律与神经解剖学细节（以及受影响区域的功能）的结合。头部突然加速或减速，会造成颅内结构的剪切伤。这种情况发生在如赛车、骑马等运动外力作用于个体的高速运动中。在橄榄球、美式足球和足球等接触性运动中，当头部在阻截时撞到地面或其他球员时，速度会变慢，同样会产生剪切力。虽然这些症状通常较轻，但更有可能反复发生，导致累积损伤。

与头部加速/减速相反，其他运动项目容易在物体撞击（相对）静止的头部时造成局灶性损伤。这种情况可能发生在如高尔夫和板球等硬球上，受伤的类型也可能会有很大的不同。

脑震荡会导致短暂性大脑功能障碍。如果允许球员返回赛场，因为相对保留了小脑和运动反射动作，球员可能看起来表现得正常（特别是职业球员）。然而，若询问问题时可能会出现记忆混乱或记忆障碍。

John Hughling Jackson描述了一个中间区域，它与中脑-间脑区域相关联，包括网状激活系统的向上投射和丘脑皮质投射系统，这些投射维持觉醒和警觉性。意识丧失很可能是在横向剪切力（由角加速度而不是线性力产生）专门破坏这一区域的情况下发生。

英国神经学病家Derek Denny-Brown（1901—1981）和W. Ritchie Russell（1903—1980）证实，在猫和猴子身上，加减速引起的脑震荡可以导致眩晕，但不会造成宏观或微观的损害。在击打时保持头部固定可以降低发生脑震荡的可能性（Denny-Brown and Ritchie Russell，1940）。此后不久，研究证明灵长类动物发生脑震荡时，会发生脑干网状激活系统内神经细胞的丢失和染色质溶解（Gurdjian，1975）。

英国神经病学家Sabina Strich描述了严重脑震荡（重度脑震荡）患者广泛的白质轴突损伤。紧急重症监护水平的提高使得这类患者得以幸存下来。很明显，以前没有意识到发生了神经元的破坏。Bryan Jennet（1926—2008）了解到这种弥漫性脑震荡损伤可能会产生累积效应，就像在拳击中发生的那样。

Ayub Ommaya验证了Holbourn的假设，即环形

（旋转）加速度通过剪切力比线性加速度和冲击力造成的破坏更大，而后者造成较小危害的压缩和拉伸（拉力）。非撞击性孤立平移线性加速度产生脑震荡的阈值要大得多，并以局灶性病变为主（Ommaya and Gennarelli，1974）。

在20世纪50年代和60年代，Richard Schneider的研究小组通过手术用透明头盖骨替代颅骨使大脑可视化，用这种方式对猴脑震荡和脑损伤类型进行了广泛研究。他证实了枕髁与C1之间的椎动脉受压可导致继发性瞬时呼吸或心脏停搏，这可能是力量直接向颅骨、颈髓交界处和高位脊髓传导力量所致，或因齿状韧带栓系上颈髓而引起剪切力损伤（Schneider et al.，1970）。

功能性损伤与结构性损伤

因为缺乏CT扫描等影像检查下肉眼可见的病理改变，脑震荡通常被认为是一种“功能性”损伤。然而，越来越多的证据表明，功能性损伤背后存在着微小结构损伤。虽然在CT上看不到，但是在应用如磁敏感加权和弥散张量成像等先进的MRI技术时，损伤通常可以被看到。在大学曲棍球联赛一个赛季的前后，对那些有脑震荡经历的球员行MRI检查，可以发现散在的微小出血和脑白质损伤（Helmer et al.，2014；Pasternak et al.，2014；Sasaki et al.，2014）。

在细胞水平上，生物力学损伤导致了钾离子的出胞、钠离子和钙离子的入胞、去极化（导致非选择性的谷氨酸释放），以及一种弥散的“扩散性抑制”状态，这些可以归因于急性脑震荡后症状（Katayama et al.，1992）。为了纠正这种细胞离子不平衡，与三磷酸腺苷（adenosine triphosphate，ATP）相关的膜离子泵超负荷工作，导致了高糖酵解、ATP的消耗与ADP的增多。在脑血流量灌注减少的背景下，导致了代谢不足。能量危机造成了自由基生成和更多损伤，这也可能是形成进一步损伤的基础。可以认为在高糖酵解期之后，这种能量代谢受损的状态会持续7~10天，而且与脑震荡后的记忆症状有关（Giza and Hovda，2014）。

在细胞骨架水平，树突和轴突这些微观结构可以被破坏，而且钙离子内流可以造成神经纤维侧支的磷酸化和轴索的崩解。轴索的拉伸可破坏微管，从而改变轴突的双向运输，进而改变轴突神经递质的释放。

弥漫性轴索损伤的轴索断裂和微出血造成“中度”和“重度”TBI。轻度TBI和脑震荡可以出现轴突的拉伸和卷曲，这会破坏轴索的微观结构。经实验证实TBI轴鞘通透性增加（Pettus et al.，1994）。液压打击损伤胼胝体的脑白质束模型显示，无髓鞘的轴突更易受到损伤（Reeves et al.，2005）。这也是除了解剖学因素造成剪切力改变外，对为什么脑部某些区域更易受到损伤的解释。有证据表明TBI改变了谷氨酸（N-甲基-D-天冬氨酸）受体亚基构成，进而改变了神经传递、钙离子内流和细胞内外信号传导。这可能造成功能（如记忆）影响（Atkins et al.，2009）。在老鼠的侧方液压打击损伤模型中，侧方液压打击会造成GABA能中间神经元的缺失（Zanier et al.，2003）。所有的这些微观病理可以解释认知功能下降。

在轻度头部创伤中也发生了细胞因子、炎症基因的上调和小神经胶质细胞浸润等炎症反应。而后者与黑质的损害有关，特别是受到TBI相关性帕金森症影响（Hutson et al.，2011）。这些位置的损伤明显影响功能性症状（海马→记忆；杏仁核→恐惧/焦虑）。

脑震荡的标志物

反复脑震荡所产生的慢性后遗症通常见于拳击手，但是现在也愈来愈多出现在其他一些对抗运动中。聚集的微管蛋白被认为是“慢性创伤性脑病”的病理标志物。虽然目前缺乏剂量-反应相关性的人体研究，但是毫无疑问的是，拳击手们身上发生的海马萎缩和脑室扩大，强烈暗示着细胞已经死亡。这种现象在老年人的TBI更明显。

N-乙酰天冬氨酸（NAA）是一种脑特异性化合物，可作为创伤后生化损伤的替代标志物，并可通过质子磁共振波谱监测脑震荡恢复情况。成人脑震荡患者的额叶NAA水平降低，30天后恢复正常，若发生第二次损伤，则恢复时间会延长至45天（Vagnozzi et al.，2008）。

基因易损性

离子通道疾病，如与家族性偏瘫偏头痛相关的CACNA1A突变，也与轻度TBI的过度反应有关（Kors et al.，2001），并可能导致不同的脑震荡后反应，甚至对二次损伤综合征易感。

在动物研究中，转基因动物（3×TG-ApoE4）显示TBI后tau蛋白积累增加（Tran et al.，2011）。ApoE4在TBI和阿尔茨海默病中的致病作用逐渐明显（Wilson and Montgomery，2007）。

脑震荡影像

传统 MRI 技术可能错误地忽视结构性损伤。梯度回波和磁敏感加权成像可以发现微小出血（**图 45.1**）。弥散张量成像可以显示特定的白质束破坏。虽然这些技术以往主要是用作研究，现在也应考虑应用于临床中，对那些存在持续脑震荡症状的患者进行检查。正电子发射断层显像可以用来证明 B- 淀粉样蛋白和 tau 蛋白的病理存在，这个技术可能在未来临床中得到应用。

脑震荡的症状

1948 年 Thorndike 首次将脑震荡分为轻度、中度和重度（Thorndike，1948），此后脑震荡的分类不断发展。包括 Schneider（Schneider and Kriss，1969）和 Kelly（Kelly et al.，1991）等提出了不同的分类系统，最新的是 Cantu 的修订版（**表 45.1**）（Cantu，2001）。

根据 LOC 和记忆缺失的持续时间对脑震荡进行分级，并不能真正反映潜在损伤的性质或严重程度，尽管从总体上看，更长时间的无意识状态可能反映了更严重的损伤。

脑震荡的管理

虽然统计数字不一，但大多数脑震荡患者受伤后几周内就会痊愈。

急性期管理

退出比赛

（运动员受伤后）在退出比赛之前，体育俱乐部应该进行赛季前计划（具体根据运动和场地）、评估

表 45.1 Cantu 脑震荡分类（修订版）

Ⅰ级	无意识丧失、创伤后失忆 / 脑震荡后体征或症状<30 分钟
Ⅱ级	意识丧失 <1 分钟，或创伤后失忆 >30 分钟但 <24 小时，或脑震荡后的体征或症状 >30 分钟但 <7 天
Ⅲ级	意识丧失≥1 分钟或创伤后失忆≥24 小时，脑震荡后体征或症状 >7 天

Reproduced from Cantu, R. C., Guidelines for Return to Contact Sports After a Cerebral Concussion. *The Physician and Sportsmedicine*, 1986, Vol. 14 No. 10, p. 75–83 with permission from Taylor and Francis.

和教育，以避免在缺少预案情况下做出退出（或不退出）比赛的决定。计划包括即时计划和长期计划，包括对立即危及生命的头部损伤紧急处理。对个体评估需要全面了解既往脑震荡病史和与脑震荡有关的既往病史或症状（如偏头痛、抑郁和焦虑）。

场边评估

最常用的评估工具是运动脑震荡评估工具，或简称 SCAT（第三版）（http://bjsm.bmj.com/content/47/5/259.full.pdf）。这是许多组织如国际足联和奥林匹克委员会等所采纳的工具。适用于 13 岁以上人群（13 岁以下使用儿童 SCAT）。在最初的评估中，如果运动员失去意识，有平衡性或协调性问题、定向障碍、失忆、茫然若失，那么就应该退出比赛并且一天都不能回到比赛。格拉斯哥昏迷量表（Glasgow Coma Scale，GCS）和 Maddocks 评分组成其中一部分。除此之外，还要进行症状评估，包括认知评估（定向、记忆和注意力）、颈部、平衡和协调检查。

返回赛场

在第四届运动相关脑震荡国际会议（2012）上，

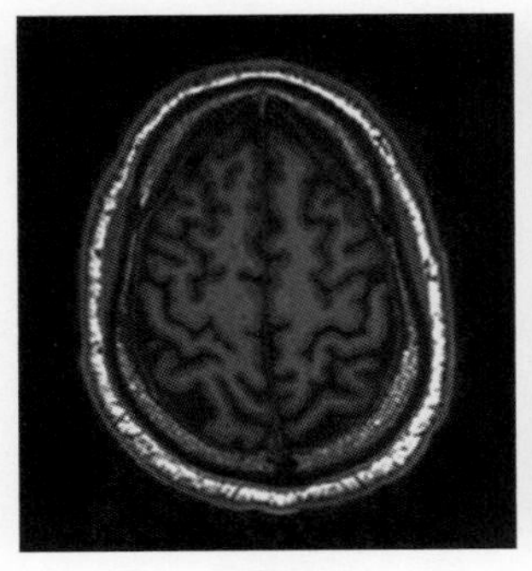

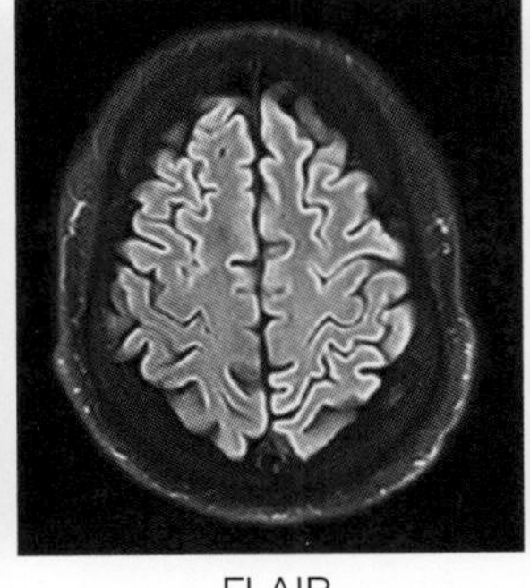

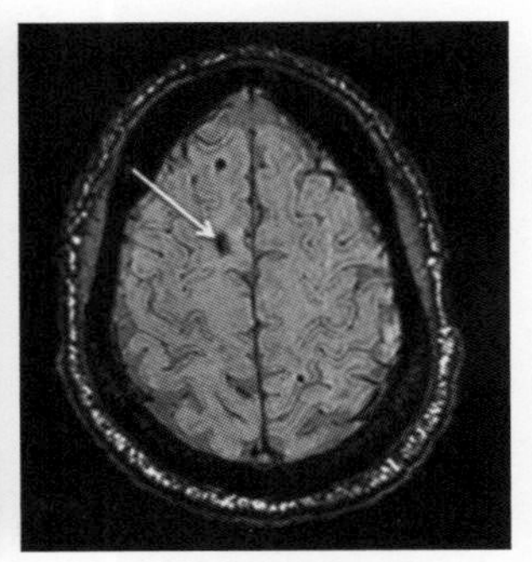

图 45.1 在磁敏感加权 MRI 上可以清楚地发现一个微出血灶，但在液体衰减反转恢复的标准 T1 序列上看不到

人们一致同意运动员在脑震荡当天不应再参加比赛（McCrory et al., 2013）。这与美国神经病学学会指南一致（Giza et al., 2013）。目前的指导方针建议循序渐进的训练计划，从没有活动（第一天），到轻度有氧运动、体育专项运动、非对抗性训练、完全对抗性练习，然后恢复正常比赛，每个阶段之间至少间隔 24 小时。

二次打击综合征

二次打击综合征是 Schneider 在 1973 年提出的一个概念，指前期脑震荡后没有恢复情况下再次受到打击导致的恶性脑肿胀。如果确实如此，二次打击综合征风险似乎在受伤后 10 天内最严重。这可能与能量危机和细胞脆弱性有关。也有可能一些二次打击损伤是和严重损伤伴随的，因为运动员在运动中经常遭受脑损伤。

后续几周内的治疗

在受伤后的几周内可以通过测试评估一些认知方面的问题，如简易精神状态评价量表（mini-mental state examination，MMSE）或 Addenbrooke 认知检查。

对于轻度 TBI 患者的家属来说，最常见的问题是他们的亲人情绪激动、脾气暴躁，且缺乏对该问题的认识。事实上，许多患者坚持认为自己很好。最好的治疗方法是家人花时间陪伴患者，并解释这是真实的、常见的，通常会在几周到几个月内解决。有些症状可药物治疗。对于认知功能障碍、注意力不集中、愤怒和攻击性，哌甲酯或金刚烷胺可能有用。多奈哌齐（用于老年痴呆症）也可能有作用。对于抑郁症，首选选择性 5- 羟色胺再摄取抑制剂（舍曲林、西酞普兰）。对于头痛，可以使用非甾体抗炎药、雷公藤多甙、普萘洛尔和阿米替林，如果合并失眠，阿米替林也有帮助。

大约 80% 的患者会出现持续性头晕。良性阵发性位置性眩晕是最常见的类型。该病可以通过变位性眼震试验（Hallpike test）进行诊断，并通过复位疗法进行治疗。如果症状持续没有改善，建议转诊到专科医生进一步诊疗。

总结

脑震荡是轻度 TBI 后的一种常见情况，而轻度 TBI 可能是一个更好的描述，因为我们开始认识到它与结构性损伤有关（即便是微观的）。轻度 TBI 会对患者及其家人造成非常严重的后果，如果把这种情况标记为通常会自行好转的脑震荡，可能会对这部分患者造成不利影响。重要的是要认识到脑震荡后遗症，并进一步研究和治疗症状持续存在的患者。

延伸阅读、参考文献

扫描书末二维码获取。

第十一篇　血管神经外科

第 46 章　正常脑血管生理学与解剖学

Diederik O. Bulters · Andrew Durnford 著
李春伟 译　伊志强 校

血管解剖学

胚胎学和 Willis 环

大脑的血液来自两组成对的动脉，即颈动脉和椎动脉，分别代表前循环系统和后循环系统。Thomas Willis 在 1664 年描述的 Willis 环，指的是这些系统的颈内动脉和椎基底动脉的分支，它们吻合在一起，在鞍上池形成一星形的环路。在功能上，随着某一支供血动脉的闭塞，Willis 环在一定程度上为其提供代偿。通常，在最初的胚胎发育过程中，颈内动脉供应大脑前、中、后动脉。后来，后交通动脉（posterior communicating artery，PComA）萎缩，基底动脉供应大脑后动脉（posterior cerebral artery，PCA）。但如果 PComA 仍大于同侧 P1，则称为胚胎型 PComA（约 25% 个体）。在大多数个体中，完全完整的 Willis 环不存在，其他常见的变异包括 PComA 发育不良或缺失、A1 发育不良和前交通动脉（anterior communicating artery，AComA）缺失。颈动脉和基底动脉之间存在胚胎性连接，可持续到成年。最常见的是永存原始三叉动脉，在颈内动脉海绵窦段之前自鞍背侧方发出与基底动脉相连。永存原始舌下动脉也可连接颈内动脉和基底动脉，从而表现为供应脑干和小脑的单一动脉。这两种变异都与脑动脉瘤的发生率增加有关。

大脑血管的结构

脑动脉血管逐渐分化为小动脉、微小动脉、穿支动脉，最终形成脑实质动脉和毛细血管。软膜动脉被脑脊液包围，形成穿支动脉。当这些动脉成为脑实质动脉时，其周围存在一个小的蛛网膜下腔延伸，称为 Virchow-Robin 空间。这些实质的血管被星形细胞的终足包裹。

脑动脉血管壁分为三层，从外到内分别称为外膜、中膜和内膜。外膜主要由胶原蛋白和纤维细胞组成。在小实质动脉和毛细血管中，相关的星形细胞末梢将其与星形胶质细胞连接。中膜主要含有平滑肌，较大的动脉一般有较多的层数。内膜由一层内皮和一层弹性组织——内弹力层组成，与中膜隔开。脑动脉与其他动脉存在结构上的差异。脑动脉的前壁较薄，它不含外弹性层，相应的内膜有较发达的内弹性层。

脑静脉的管壁较薄，与全身静脉不同，不含瓣膜，平滑肌极少，不太紧随动脉系统的走向。

颈内动脉及其分支

颈内动脉（internal arotoid artery，ICA）的起源是可变的，但通常在 C3 和 C5 之间。颈动脉窦（或称球部）在其起源处呈纺锤形扩张，其功能为主要的大动脉感受器。旁边是颈动脉体，是影响呼吸调节的化学感受器。

ICA 存在多种分段。最简单的分段是将其分为四个节段——颈段、岩段、海绵窦段和床突上段（Gibo et al.，1981）。另一种分段方法描述了七个节段（Bouthillier et al.，1996）：

1. 颈段
2. 岩段（水平）
3. 破裂孔段
4. 海绵窦段
5. 床突段
6. 眼段（床突上段）
7. 交通段（终末段）

硬膜外 ICA

颈段通常没有分支。血管造影上，如果迂曲，可能会看到一个“扁桃体环”。它通过颞骨颈动脉管进入颅底，近水平方向朝内侧走行，在破裂孔转折向上，通过岩舌韧带下方进入海绵窦。岩段有几个小分支，从血管造影上看不出来：颈鼓动脉（到内耳）和翼管动脉。破裂孔段，有人认为是多余的分类，没有分支。

海绵窦段开始于颈内动脉进入海绵窦后部，然后向前走行。它被窦内皮包围，由小梁支撑，通常包含两个重要的分支。第一支，脑膜垂体干，有三个分支：供应垂体后叶的垂体下动脉、脑膜背动脉和供应小脑幕的小脑幕缘动脉（Bernasconi 和 Cassinari 动脉）。海绵窦段的第二支为下外侧干，供应海绵窦脑神经。从血管造影上看，ICA 的 U 形部分主要由海绵窦段形成，被称为颈动脉虹吸段。

ICA 通过窦顶的硬膜覆盖物，称为近端硬膜环，其形成海绵窦顶部，并与覆盖相邻前床突的硬膜相延续。床突段是 ICA 通过远端硬膜环进入蛛网膜下腔之前及海绵窦段之间的过渡段（Rhoton，2002）。在临床上，这个区域非常重要，因为远端硬膜环可以区分引起蛛网膜下腔出血的动脉瘤与引起颈动脉 - 海绵窦漏的动脉瘤。但遗憾的是，远端环在放射学上不可见，只能估计其位置。手术中对这一区域的了解很重要，因为进入眼动脉起源处或附近的近端动脉瘤需要进行前部硬膜环的切除。远端硬脑膜环位于后内侧，与镰状韧带和覆盖前床突上内侧的硬脑膜连续。虽然这两个环在后方融合，但它们在前方有不同程度的分离，产生了内侧和外侧两个区域。外侧区域可认为是硬膜外和海绵窦外。在内侧，远端硬膜环的多余部分与 ICA 之间的空间被称为颈动脉窝。虽然通常在硬膜外，但颈动脉窝动脉瘤的破裂延伸到窝外上部，可能导致蛛网膜下腔出血。

眼段——眼动脉和垂体上动脉

眼段发出眼动脉，其起源于远端硬膜环之外，在视神经和前床突下，经视神经孔进入眼眶。眼动脉瘤起源于眼动脉起始部，向背侧或背内侧突出。小而多变的垂体上动脉从 ICA 内侧起源于眼动脉远端，环绕垂体柄。值得注意的是，床突旁、眼动脉及垂体区域的动脉瘤常被称为“眼动脉旁”动脉瘤，反映了其血管造影定位的困难。

眼动脉起源存在两种重要变异。它可起源自颈内动脉硬膜外床突部，使手术进入变得复杂。也可能起源于颈外动脉，但少见，有可能因不慎切断而失明（Geibprasert et al.，2009）。从脑膜中动脉产生的脑膜 - 眼动脉通过眶上裂进入眼眶，可取代眼动脉，如果在开放手术或介入手术中牺牲掉，会带来风险。

交通段——后交通动脉和脉络膜前动脉

交通段从后交通动脉（PComA）起源延伸至 ICA 分叉处。PComA 起源于 ICA 的背侧，约 1 cm 后连接到大脑后动脉，从而连接前循环和后循环。其走行与动眼神经接近，解释了为什么典型的后外侧突出的后交通动脉瘤可引起（累及瞳孔）动眼神经麻痹。通常 PComA 发出小的分支供应内囊膝部和丘脑，其中最大的称为乳头体前动脉。脉络膜前动脉（PComA 起点 1~3 mm 远处）通常来自 ICA 的后内侧，在其终止于 Willis 环之前，可以作为几个（1~5 个）独立的主干出现。在 ICA 起源动脉瘤的手术中必须认识到这一点。它具有重要的手术意义，因为不慎损伤可导致明显的神经功能障碍，从早期结扎动脉治疗帕金森病的研究中，有相当一部分患者出现偏瘫、偏身麻木和偏盲，这一点有充分的证据。脉络膜前动脉可分为脑池段和脑室内段。脑池段穿过视束沿其外侧向颞叶内侧走行，经过大脑脚到达外侧膝状体，然后进入脉络膜裂，成为脑室内段。其供应包括视束、内囊后缘、基底节和侧脑室颞角的脉络丛。在 ICA 分叉处，大脑中动脉（middle cerebral artery，MCA）通常向后外侧突出，因此分叉处最好带一定倾角进行血管造影观察，能很好地将其与大脑前循环分开（图 46.1A~C）。值得注意的是，血泡样动脉瘤通常发生于 ICA 非分支部分的背侧壁，当然也可能发生于其他前、后循环部位，但更为罕见。

大脑前动脉

尽管解剖学上存在着广泛的差异，但对大脑前动脉（anterior cerebral artery，ACA）的典型描述是两根动脉，每根动脉都有 A1 和 A2 段，被前交通动脉（AComA）分开（MacDonald，2009）。A1 段起自 ICA 分叉处，行向前内侧跨过视束上方，与其对应的 A1 段由 AComA 紧密相连。A1 段有时被称为前交通段或水平段。A1 与 ICA、视神经和 MCA 的关系，在经典的翼点入路分离侧裂后，清楚地显示在图 46.2A 和部分术中图 46.2B~C。

该区域有许多变异。A1 段可发育不全，由对侧 A1 经 AComA 供应，也可双干。ACA 可以不成对，双侧 A1 交汇处以远延续为单一 A2，可被认为是前交通动脉重复或开窗（Yasargil，1987）。

内侧豆纹状动脉通常起自 A1 段的后下方，穿过前穿质供应苍白球和内侧壳核（图 46.3）。A2 段从 AComA 远端延伸至胼胝体膝部，形成胼周动脉和胼缘动脉。A2 的分支包括供应额叶下部的眶额动脉（通常是第一皮质分支）和供应额上回前部的额极动脉。

前交通动脉

位于终板池，由于其动脉瘤的发生率高，所以

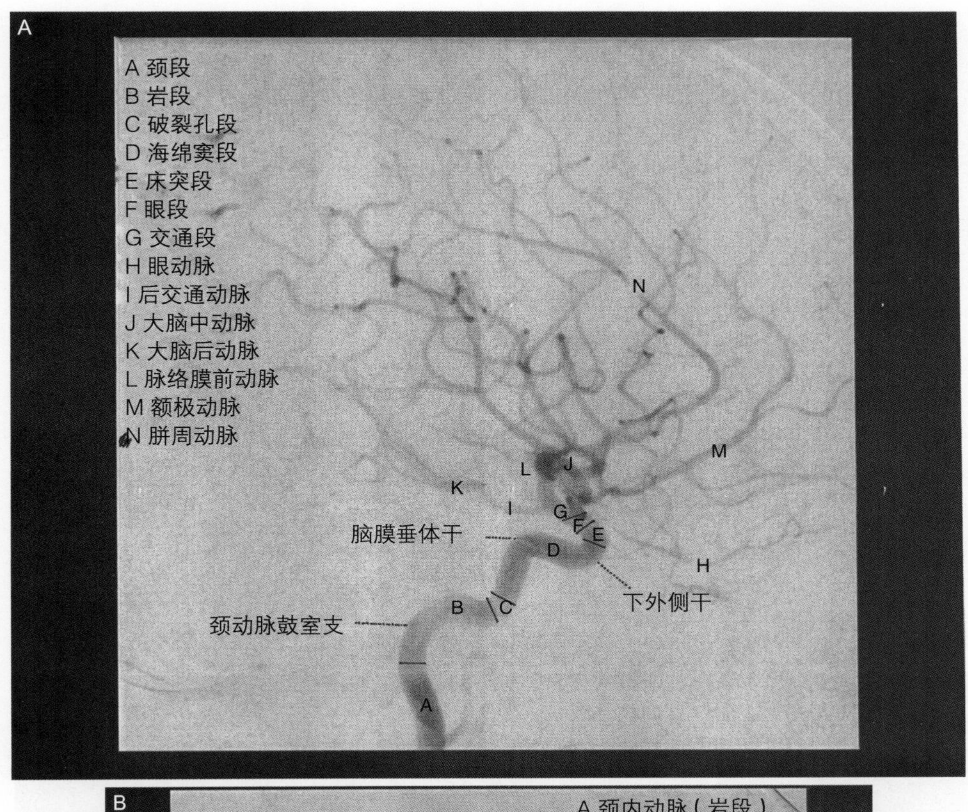

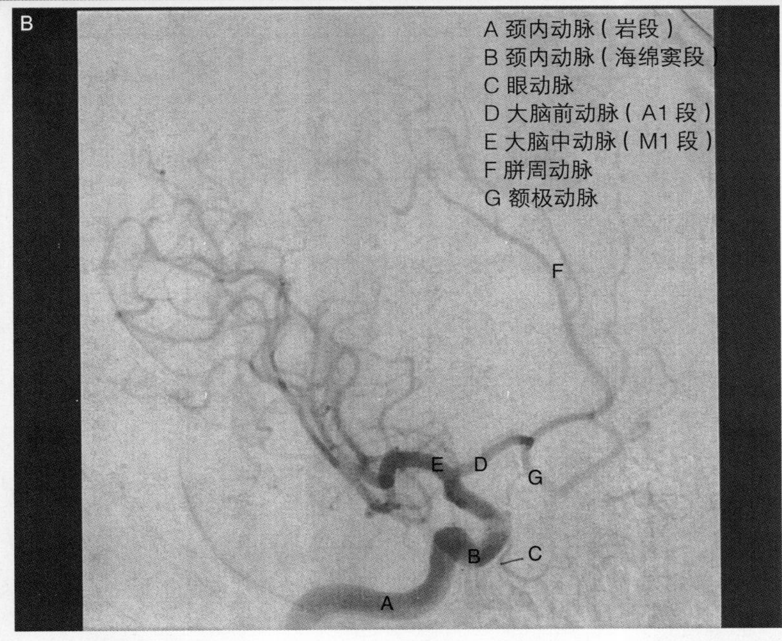

图 46.1 （A）颈内动脉侧位数字减影血管造影。注意缺失的胼缘动脉和相应的异常突出的额极动脉。虚线标记了 ICA 血管造影上看不见的岩骨段和海绵段分支的近似起源。在岛叶基部的 MCA 分叉处，分支分布差异很大，但通常包含位于裂缝深处的前（上）和后（下）干。血管造影时中动脉分叉形似烛台。前干分支，包括中央前动脉、中央（Rolandic）动脉和额叶动脉，一般供应额叶和顶叶区域，包括额叶中、下回，中央前和中央后皮质。后干一般有三个分支。顶叶后动脉和颞后动脉供应相当一部分的颞部和枕部凸部。最后，角动脉贯穿整个岛叶的长度，供应颞上回和部分顶叶和枕叶。（B）颈内动脉斜位数字减影血管造影。（C）颈内动脉前后位数字减影血管造影。注意皮质分支（M4）将与 ACA 分支吻合在内侧凸起。（D）颈外动脉侧位数字减影血管造影。主要分支依次为甲状腺上动脉、升咽动脉、舌动脉、面动脉、枕动脉、耳后动脉、上颌动脉、颞浅动脉。特别要注意的是枕动脉在此图中没有被遮挡

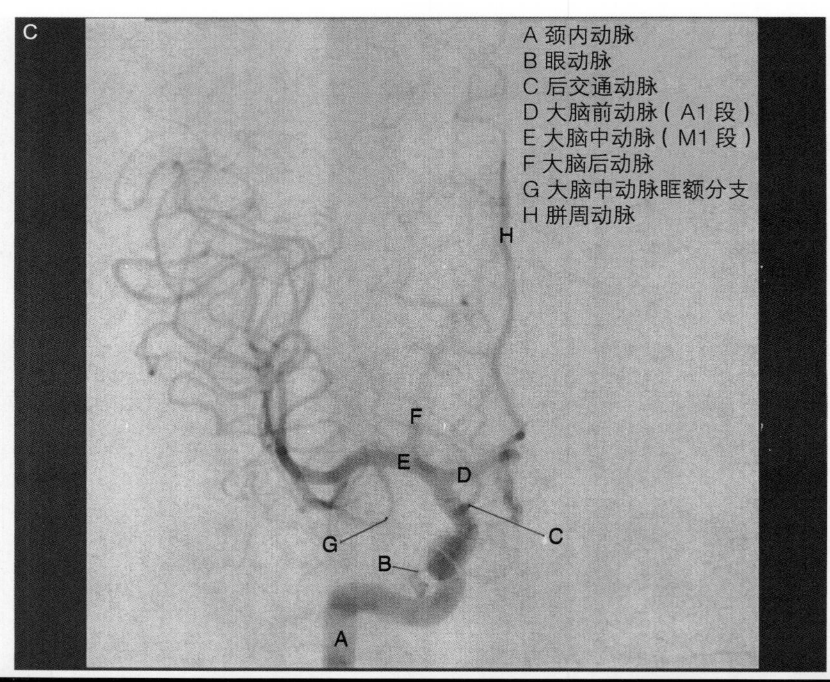

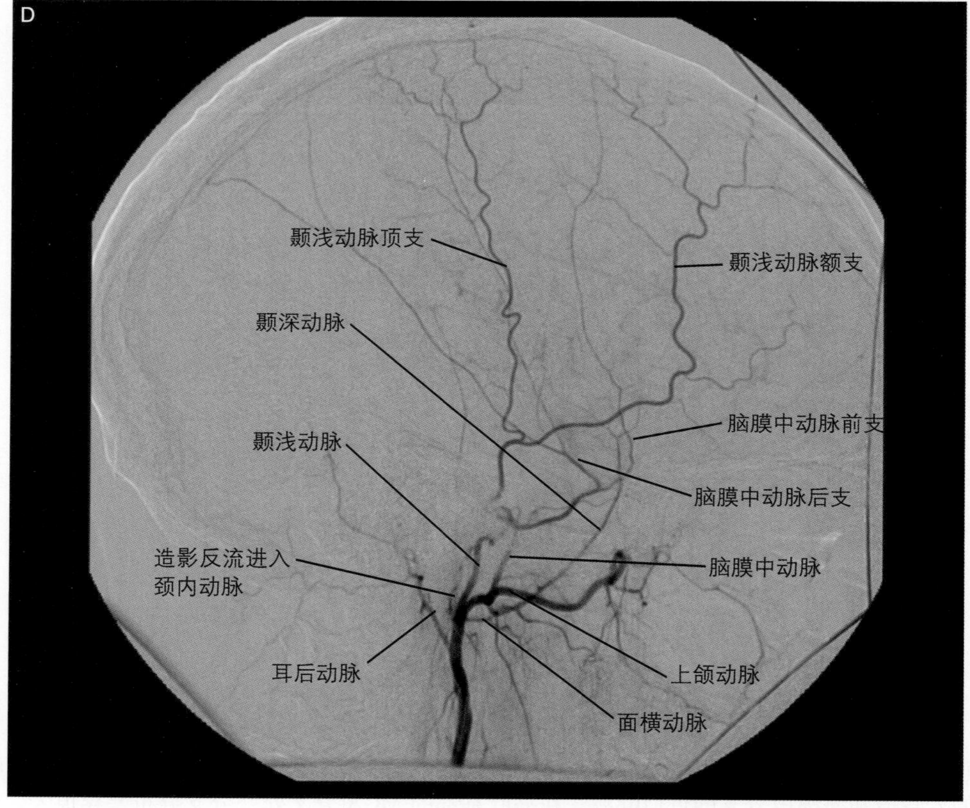

图 46.1 （续）

很重要。前交通动脉很短，长度可达 3 mm。其穿支动脉数量不一，但根据其供血区域可分为胼胝体下穿支动脉、下丘脑穿支动脉或视交叉穿支动脉。

Heubner 回返动脉

Heubner 回返动脉是 ACA 最大的穿支动脉，通常起自 A1/A2 交界处附近的 A2 段近端，但也可以起自 A1。一般沿 A1 侧方走行，供应内囊前肢及部分尾状核和苍白球。

胼缘动脉和胼周动脉

胼周（主干）动脉被认为是 ACA 的延续，紧贴

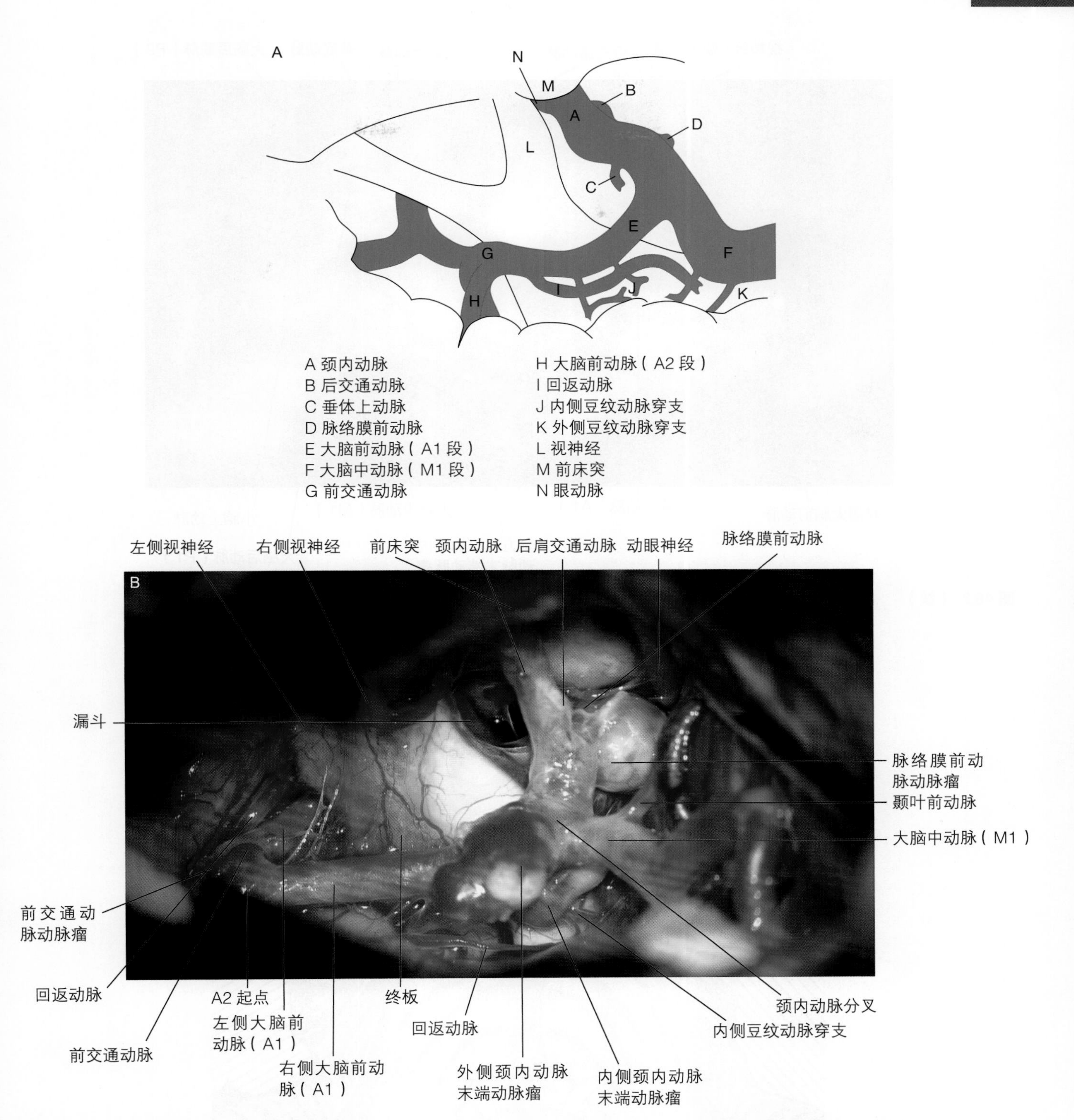

图 46.2 （A）翼点开颅术后外侧裂示意图，显示脑底部的主要动脉血管。（B 和 C）术中外侧裂打开后的照片显示 ICA、视神经、ACA、MCA 和多个动脉瘤的显露（B），以及同一患者的前脉络膜动脉动脉瘤轻轻回缩，暴露基底膜末端及其分支（C）。请注意，PCom 的方向在 ICA 深部，因此在这些示意图中没有看到。脉络膜前动脉紧密黏附在动脉瘤瘤体上，很难看清。右侧 A1/A2 交界处起源的 Heubner 回返动脉被遮挡，其漏斗部不易看清

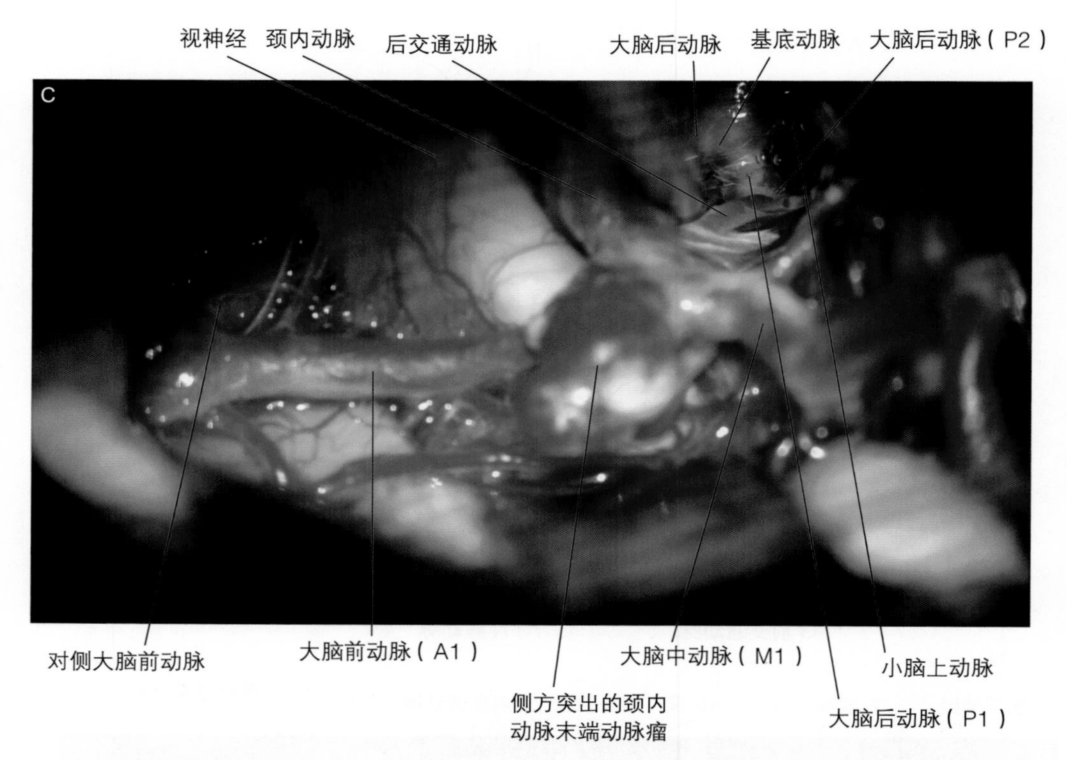

图 46.2 （续）

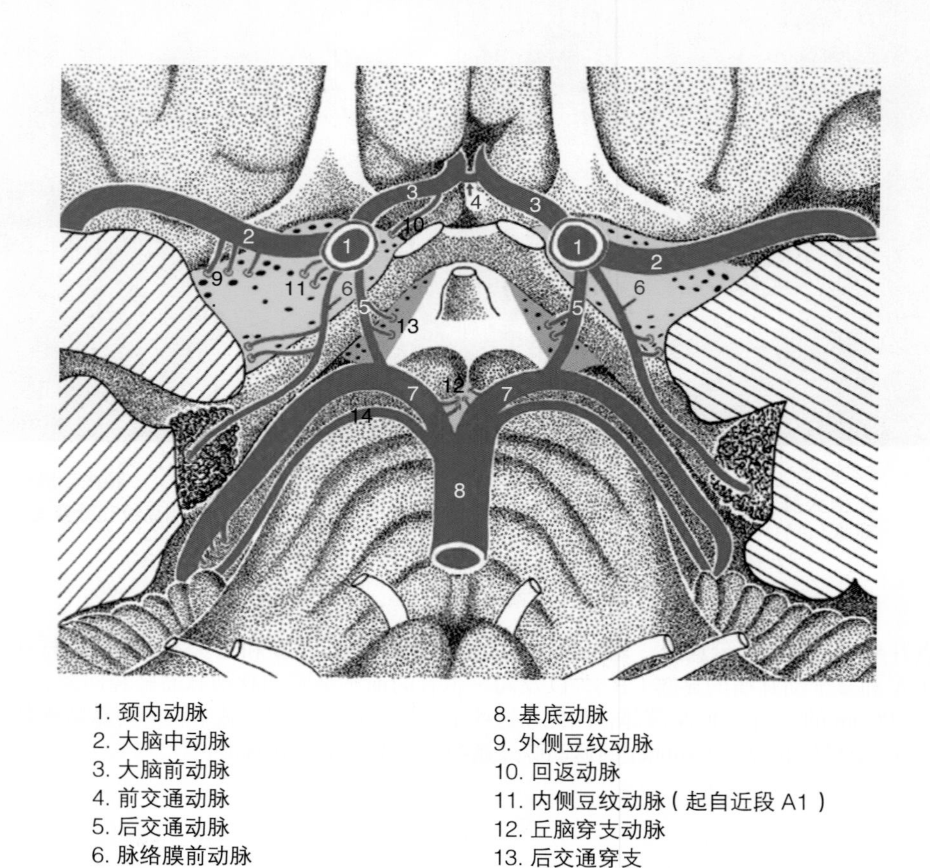

图 46.3 脑动脉的穿支通过前部（黄色）、后部（蓝色）和侧部（橙色）介质进入

胼胝体。它的分支为胼胝体及其压部、透明隔、穹隆和楔前叶供血。皮质分支与 MCA 和 PCA 的分支吻合。约 50% 的人群中存在胼缘动脉（Butler et al., 2012），它途经扣带回通过不同的分支向额上回供血。它的终点是供应中央旁小叶的中央旁动脉。

大脑中动脉

大脑中动脉（middle cerebral artery，MCA）是 ICA 最大的分支。MCA 分叉处近段为 M1，远端为 M2。M1 在额叶和颞叶之间的侧裂深部向前（或蝶骨嵴）方向走行。数目不等的外侧纹状（或豆纹动脉）动脉来自 M1 的后下方，沿其走行向后并穿透前穿质的外侧部分。它们供应基底节、内囊和尾状核。临床上，这些动脉是高血压脑出血的常见来源。M1 在其膝部处分叉，在岛叶的前部以直角向上走行。M1 唯一的大分支通常是颞前动脉和颞极支。

椎 - 基底动脉（后）系统及其分支

椎动脉作为锁骨下动脉的第一个分支出现，并通过枕骨大孔进入颅内，在延髓前侧穿过，然后在脑桥与延髓交界处连接形成基底动脉（**图 46.4A~B**）。在椎动脉汇合之前便发出了重要的分支。每条椎动脉都有一条脊髓后动脉，沿脊髓背侧下降。第二个分支，通常是最大的分支，是小脑后下动脉（posterior inferior cerebellar artery，PICA）。它有时会出现在枕骨大孔下方（约 15% 的人）。如果 PICA 发育不良，相应的小脑前下动脉（anterior inferior cerebellar artery，AICA）口径会相应增大。再一个变异是椎动脉可直接形成 PICA。PICA 从其起源处绕延髓而行，与行经橄榄体下方的舌下神经密切相关—这段 PICA 称为延髓前段（**表 46.1**）。接着延髓外侧段在延髓旁弯曲走行，扁桃体延髓段绕过小脑扁桃体的尾部，形成侧位血管造影上可见的尾袢。髓帆扁桃体段行经脉络膜和延髓之间的裂隙，上行至顶部形成颅袢。皮质段覆盖在小脑表面（Lister et al., 1982）。PICA 的分支供应延髓、第四脑室脉络丛和小脑下部和后部。最后，在双侧椎动脉形成基底动脉之前，两个很短的分支汇合形成下行的脊髓前动脉。

小脑上动脉（superior cerebellar arteries，SCA）、AICA 和 PICA 向中脑、脑桥和延髓供血，通过短或长的旋穿支动脉向前或后外侧供血，通过长旋支走行于外侧面。此外，这些血管的近段和基底动脉干也有更直接的前分支动脉。

基底动脉

基底动脉起源于脑桥延髓交界处，沿脑桥前表面桥前池上行，并在中脑处终止，分为双侧大脑后动脉。通常情况下，小的穿支动脉供应其长度范围内的脑桥。成对的小脑前下动脉来自基底动脉，靠近展神经。每条 AICA 都穿过小脑脑桥角，与面神经和前庭神经关系密切，为小脑前部和下部供血（**表 46.1**）。AICA 通常发出迷路动脉，但也可直接从基底动脉或其他部位发出。迷路动脉随着前庭蜗神经，穿过内听道，为耳蜗和前庭器供血。在基底动脉分叉前，成对的 SCA 出现，在环池中绕中脑向侧方走行。SCA 位于动眼神经下方，动眼神经将其与大脑后动脉分开。SCA 接近四叠体池的中线，以供应小脑半球上部、小脑脚和小脑蚓部。SCA 在解剖学上从近端到远端细分（**表 46.1**），也可在放射学上分为脑桥前段、环池段和四叠体段。大约 1/3 的人可有重复的 SCA。总的来说，颅后窝的三种神经血管复合体归纳在**表 46.2** 中（Rhoton，1994）。

大脑后动脉

大脑后动脉（posterior cerebral artery，PCA）的第一段，即 P1（或水平段），在与 PComA 吻合之前，位于脚间窝内。与 PComA 不同的是，穿支动脉从 P1 的后上方发出，供应内囊和丘脑。血管造影中偶见单一的较大的丘脑穿支，常被称为 Percheron 动脉，可同时供应丘脑和中脑。闭塞可导致丘脑旁正中综合征，出现意识状态改变、垂直凝视麻痹、记忆力受损三联征。P2 段形成于 PComA 远端，然后绕过动眼神经，在环池中，位于小脑幕上方，然后 P3 段开始于四叠体池。P2 分为 P2A（前段）和 P2P（后段），其交界处在大脑脚的最外侧。P2 段有多个穿支，包括丘脑膝状体动脉和侧方的脉络膜后动脉。侧方脉络膜后动脉通过脉络膜裂隙进入邻近外侧膝状体的脑室。脉络膜后动脉内侧支从近端 P2 或从环池中的 P1 段产生，并通过胼胝体压部下方进入位于大脑中帆的第三脑室顶部。P2 的分支也参与大脑脚和四叠体的供血。供应颞叶和顶叶的额外 P2 分支与动静脉畸形（arteriovenous malformations，AVM）手术有关。颞枕部的血供下方由颞后下动脉供应，前方由 MCA 的分支供血。值得注意的是，P2 在高颅压的情况下，可被压迫至小脑幕缘，导致枕叶梗死。P3 段沿颞叶内下侧穿行，发出相关皮质穿支，然后分为顶枕动脉和距状沟动脉。距状沟动脉主要供应枕叶内侧的视觉皮质，PCA 的皮质分支与 MCA 分支在枕叶和

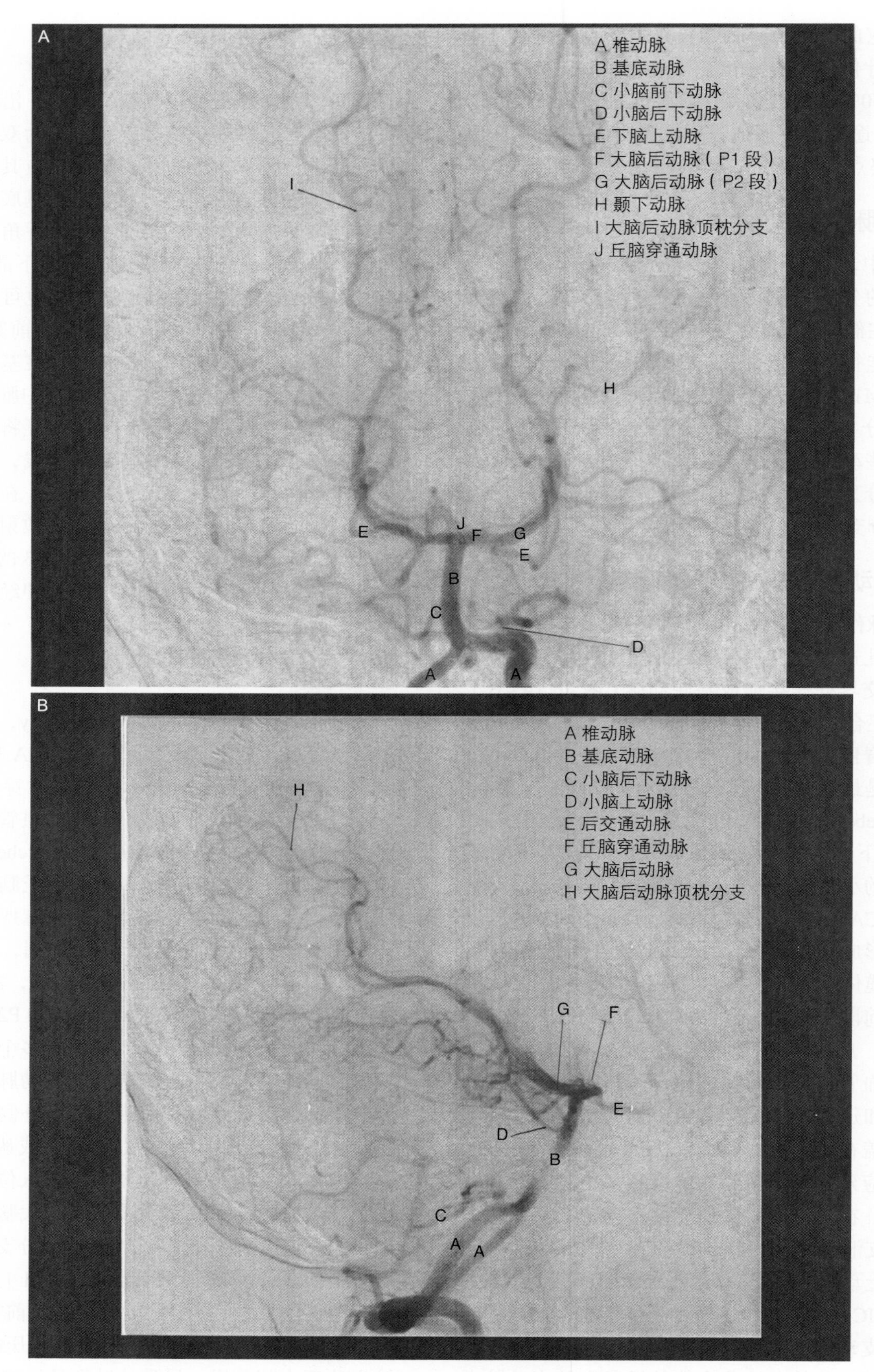

图 46.4 椎动脉前后位（A）和侧位（B）数字减影血管造影。注意左右 PICA 起源水平的不对称性

表 46.1 颅后窝动脉的血管分段

动脉	动脉分区：由近至远				
SCA	脑桥中脑前	脑桥中脑外侧	小脑中脑		皮质（上面）
AICA	脑桥前	脑桥延髓外侧	小脑绒球		皮质（岩面）
PICA	延髓前	延髓外侧	小脑扁桃体	扁桃体上段	皮质（枕下面）

表 46.2 Rhoton 在后窝的三种神经血管复合体

复合体	血管	脑干区域	裂隙	脑神经	小脑脚	小脑表面
上组	小脑上动脉	中脑	小脑中脑裂	Ⅲ、Ⅳ、Ⅴ	小脑上脚	幕面
中组	小脑前下动脉	脑桥	小脑脑桥裂	Ⅵ、Ⅶ、Ⅷ	小脑中脚	岩面
下组	小脑后下动脉	延髓	小脑延髓裂	Ⅸ、Ⅹ、Ⅺ、Ⅻ	小脑下脚	枕下面

Source data from Rhoton, A. L., JR. 1994. The three neurovascular complexes in the posterior fossa and vascular compression syndromes (honored guest lecture). *Clin Neurosurg*, 41, 112–49.

颞叶的外侧表面有吻合。人群中大约有 20%P1 段缺失，PCA 通过 PComA 由 ICA 供应（Harnsberger and MacDonald，2006）。

颈外动脉

颈外动脉（external carotid artery，ECA）通常起自 C4 水平，最初位于 ICA 的前部。经典的描述是 8 个分支（**图 46.1D**），但在实践中这可能会有很大的不同，ECA 分支与 ICA 及椎动脉分支之间存在几处吻合。咽升动脉分支与 ICA 海绵窦的分支以及椎动脉的脑膜分支有吻合；面动脉与眼动脉分支吻合，枕动脉与椎动脉分支吻合（也有颞浅动脉分支）。硬脑膜来自 ECA 分支的供血对于硬膜动静脉瘘的诊断和处理有一定的意义，如咽升动脉和枕动脉供应颅后窝硬脑膜，而上颌动脉的脑膜中动脉和脑膜副动脉供应幕上硬脑膜。

脑血管分区

图 46.5 所示为脑干、小脑和大脑的动脉供血概况。尽管传统教科书有相关描述，但脑血管的分区供应可有很大差异。这可能是由于动脉解剖变异，也可能是由于特定动脉分支所供应的皮质区域的个体差异（van der Zwan et al.，1992）。最近的 MRI 血流研究证实了这种变化，但也表明它可能与 Willis 环的解剖变异有关（van Laar et al.，2006）。同一患者的两侧半球之间也可不同。

静脉解剖学

脑静脉系统由脑浅静脉、深静脉和硬膜静脉窦组成。

浅表静脉系统

浅表静脉系统由许多不同的皮质浅静脉组成，通常伴随着动脉在脑沟内走行。这些静脉引流到一些较大的有名静脉，随后引流到静脉窦。

- 大脑中浅静脉——引流至大而深的（蝶顶窦）静脉窦
- 大吻合静脉（Trolard）——将大脑中浅静脉引流至上矢状窦
- 后吻合静脉（Labbé）——将大脑中浅静脉引流至横窦。两条吻合静脉之间常有互补，Labbé 静脉在优势半球较大，Trolard 在非优势半球较大

深部静脉系统

深静脉系统引流侧脑室和第三脑室及基底池周围的深部白质和灰质。大脑大静脉（Galen）位于胼胝体压部下方，是一条短而单一的中线血管。它是由两条大脑内静脉连接形成的，也接受两条基底静脉（Rosenthal）以及引流枕叶内侧和下部的枕静脉。大脑内静脉行至静脉汇合处，与下矢状窦连接形成直窦。基底静脉（Rosenthal）起自颞叶内侧的前穿质，向后方和内侧走行。继续绕中脑向侧方走行，通过环池，引流下丘脑、中脑、额叶和颞叶的内侧及下部，包括岛叶和岛盖。大脑内静脉位于大脑中帆（第三脑室的顶部），由脉络膜静脉和丘脑静脉结合而成。脉络膜静脉引流至侧脑室的脉络丛。丘纹静脉的属支包括尾状核横静脉、前终静脉（引流尾状核的脑室表面）和隔静脉（引流胼胝体和额叶深部白质）。

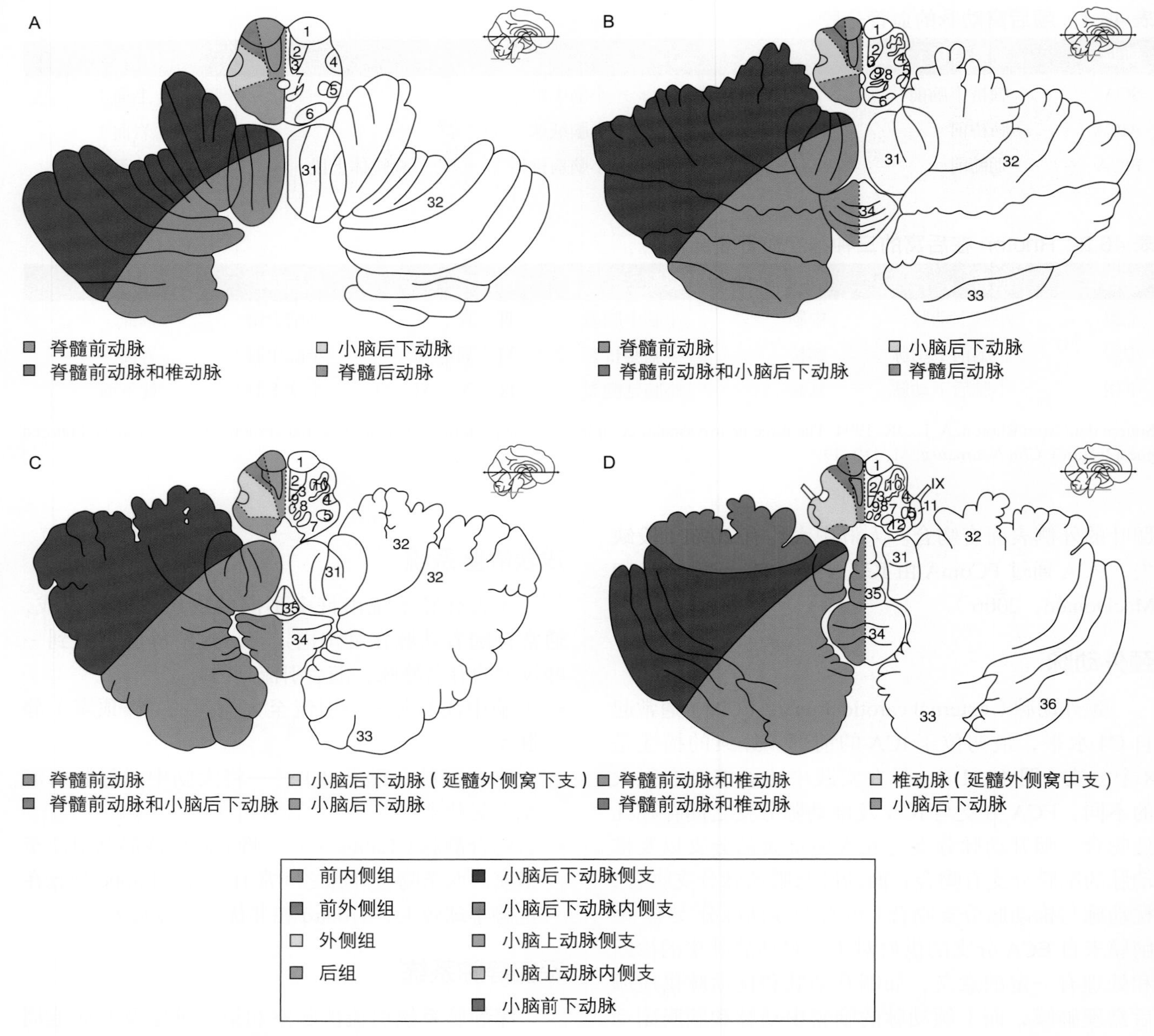

图 46.5 供应脑干、小脑和大脑的动脉血管

硬脑膜静脉窦

硬膜窦是由硬膜皱褶形成的无瓣膜的静脉通道。主要的硬膜窦有上矢状窦、横窦、乙状窦、直窦、岩上窦、岩下窦、海绵窦和蝶顶窦。上矢状窦一般起于鸡冠，止于窦汇。它也可以在窦汇之前分叉，直接与横窦相接，导致临床上误诊为上矢状窦血栓。较小的下矢状窦位于大脑镰游离缘，接纳引流胼胝体和扣带回的静脉属支，并在静脉汇合处引流至直窦。一般在放射影像上看不到。横窦通常是不对称的，多为右侧优势，它在窦汇接受来自上矢状窦大部分的血液。它们在岩骨后缘成为乙状窦，然后继续到颈静脉球部。与横窦相比，乙状窦的大小可能会有所不同，特别是当从后吻合静脉（Labbé）接受大量血液流入其近端时。

海绵窦通常接受来自大脑中浅静脉（Sylvian）、眼静脉和蝶顶窦（本身有时会引流 Sylvian 静脉）的回流。从海绵窦流出的血流经岩上窦、岩下窦（分别与乙状窦和颈静脉孔相通），也经对侧海绵窦、翼丛和斜坡静脉丛引流。枕窦的出现情况不一，在儿童

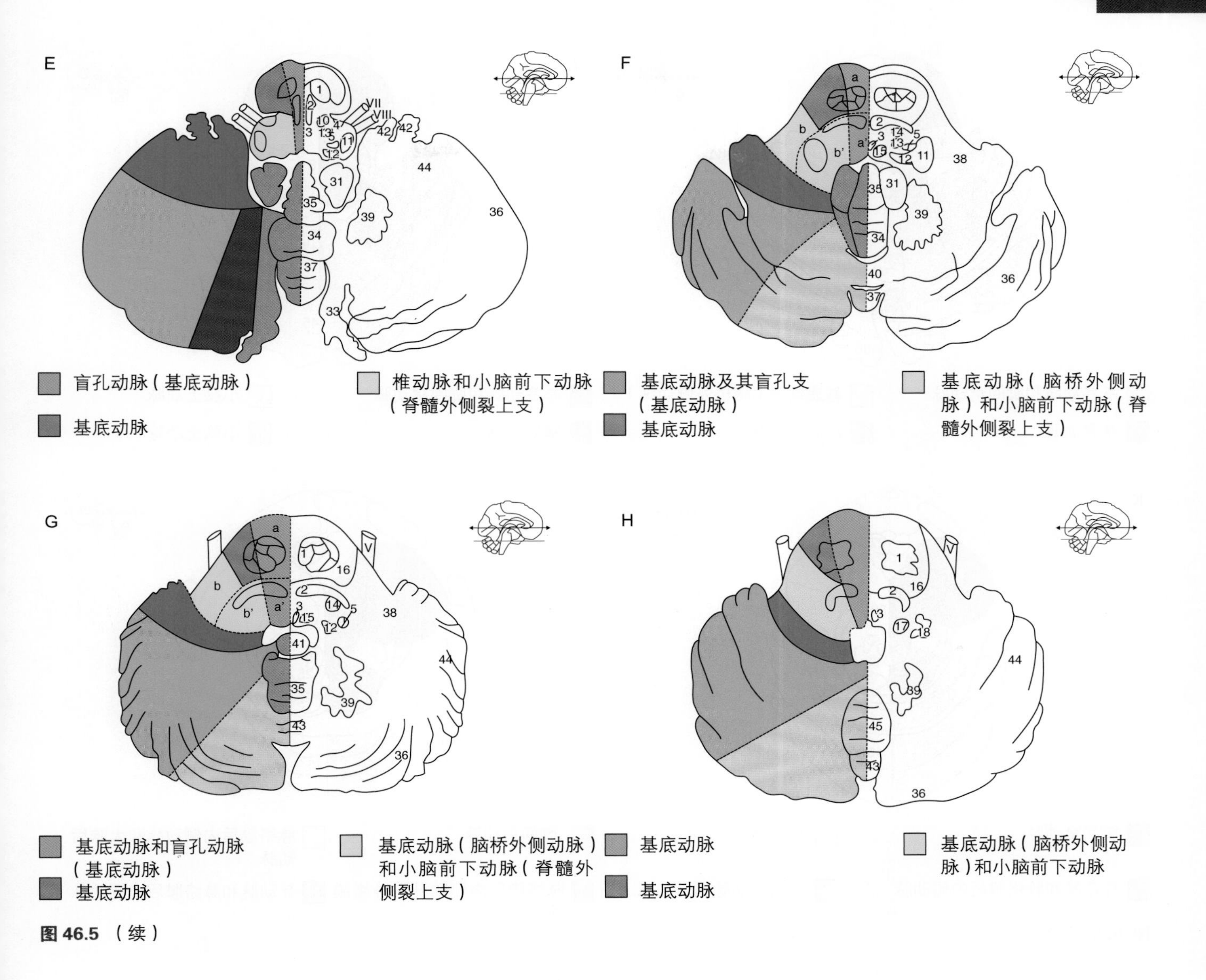

图 46.5 （续）

中更为常见，可从中线的环状沟到枕骨大孔，在原本简单的颅后窝正中入路中，枕窦可成为大量出血的来源。硬脑膜静脉窦也可通过无瓣膜的分支静脉与颅外静脉系统相通，可成为颅内感染的侵入途径（**图 46.6**）。

小脑和脑干

小脑和脑干的静脉系统有诸多变异。小脑浅表半球引流至最近的乙状窦或横窦。蚓上静脉、蚓下静脉例外，它们沿中线的小脑蚓部走行。小脑前部引流到岩上窦或岩下窦。在脑干中，静脉细小，网络广泛。中脑外侧静脉与岩静脉相邻，通常存在并沿外侧走行，上接基底静脉（Rosenthal）与岩上窦。岩上静脉或 Dandy 静脉代表大静脉，从脑桥外侧表面延伸，回流至岩上窦。它引流的范围很大，包括小脑前部、延髓后外侧以及脑桥前部。纵行于前方的静脉根据其最相邻的结构被称为间脑前静脉、脑桥延髓静脉或脊髓静脉。中央前静脉（或小脑）是一条未成对的静脉，在脑干后方走行，引流至蚓上静脉或大脑大静脉（Galen），值得注意的是其下侧标志着第四脑室的上界。它主要引流小脑血液。

AVM 手术的解剖学注意事项

由于 AVM 的动脉供血来自于正常的皮质动脉和深部动脉分支，基于血管造影了解这些血管的解剖位置对于 AVM 治疗的安全性是非常必要的。在某种程度上可由 AVM 所处脑叶位置预测其供血动脉，来自皮质动脉及其深部位置或延伸出的穿支动脉供血。大的 AVMs 可累及一个以上的脑叶，自然可由相邻血管区域（分水岭）供血。这一点在研究血管造影（DSA）时非常重要，因为意识到可能存在来自另一个血管区域的供血可避免低估病变范围。

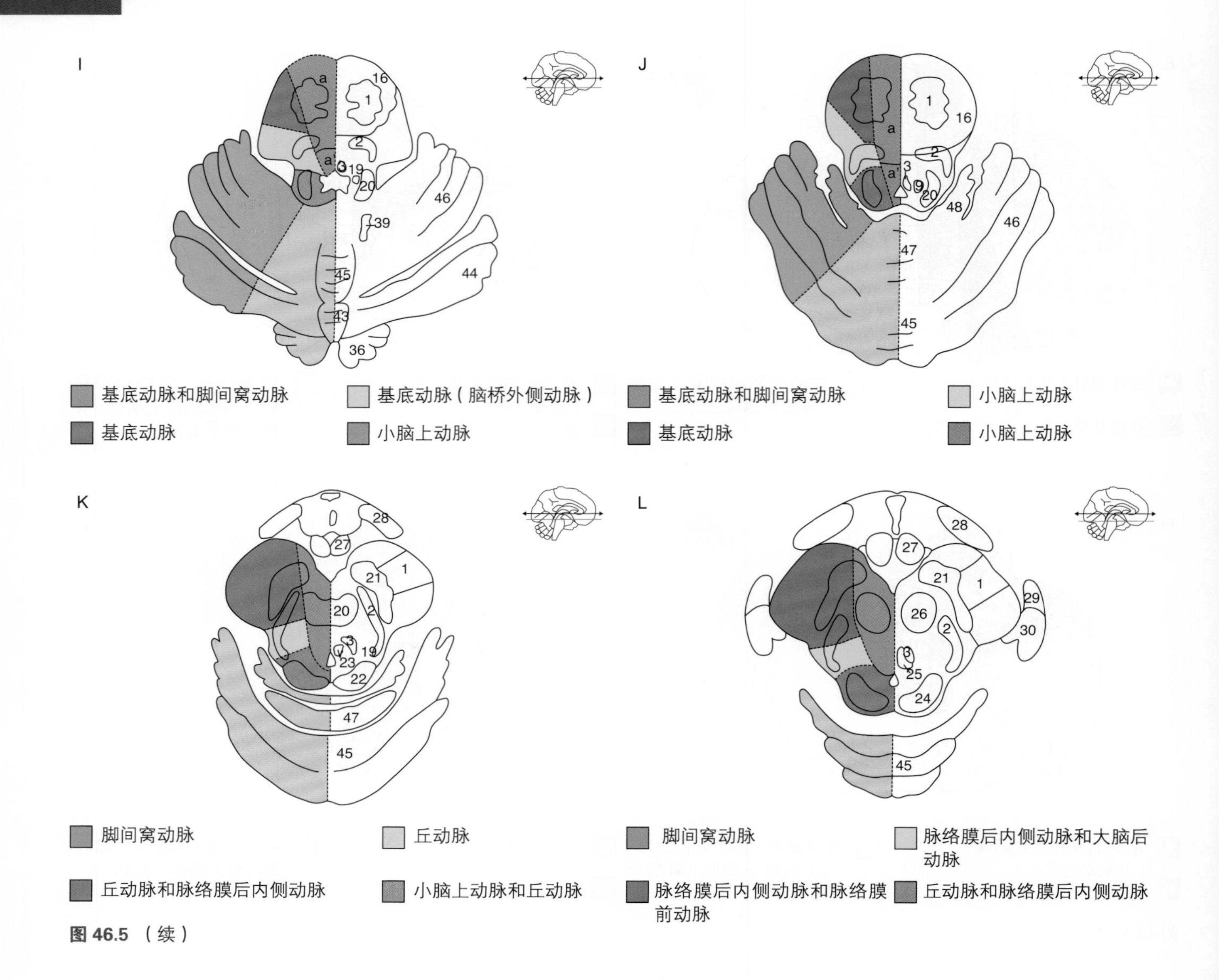

图 46.5 （续）

大脑半球外侧 AVMs

在大脑半球外侧面，AVM 分为额叶、颞叶、顶叶、枕叶和外侧裂区。向额叶上部或额极延伸接受远端 ACA 分支的供应，如前方的额极动脉、基底的额眶动脉、上方的胼缘动脉。将手术显露范围扩大到额叶内侧或基底，是达到这些血管并进行近端控制的必要手段。来自大脑中动脉 M2 上干的 M4 分支延伸至大部分额叶和中央叶（中央前回和中央后回）的皮质 / 皮质下表面，可能为运动区和语言区提供过路血管。从 M2 下干发出的相应血管向位于颞叶和顶叶的 AVM 供血，并延伸到枕叶的外表面。侧裂周围 AVM 主要累及额叶或颞叶岛盖，其供血来自岛盖段（M3）、M2 或 M1 远端。深部延伸，包括到岛叶，涉及来自豆纹动脉穿支的供血。短穿支供应岛叶皮质，而长穿支供应内囊和放射冠。通过分离外侧裂可达到并进行 MCA 供血的近端控制。颞叶 AVMs 常向下方延伸至小脑幕基底。此时，有一部分（如果不是主要的）供血来自 PCA 的 P2 段的前、中或后颞支，出现在环池近端和小脑幕缘上方，通过颞下入路可达到这些血管。

如果没有明显的深部延伸，大多数半球外侧面的 AVM 通过浅静脉引流到上矢状窦或横窦，中心位置的 AVM 可能涉及 Trollard 或 Labbé 静脉。延伸至小脑幕表面的颞叶 AVM，可能部分经 Rosenthal 静脉属支引流至深部静脉系统。

大脑半球内侧 AVMs

在前部，这些动静脉畸形由胼缘动脉分支从前上方供血，由邻近胼胝体的胼周动脉从下方供血，由额极动脉从额极部供血。该区域的皮质破坏或缺血可导致短暂性肠系膜上动脉（superior mesenteric

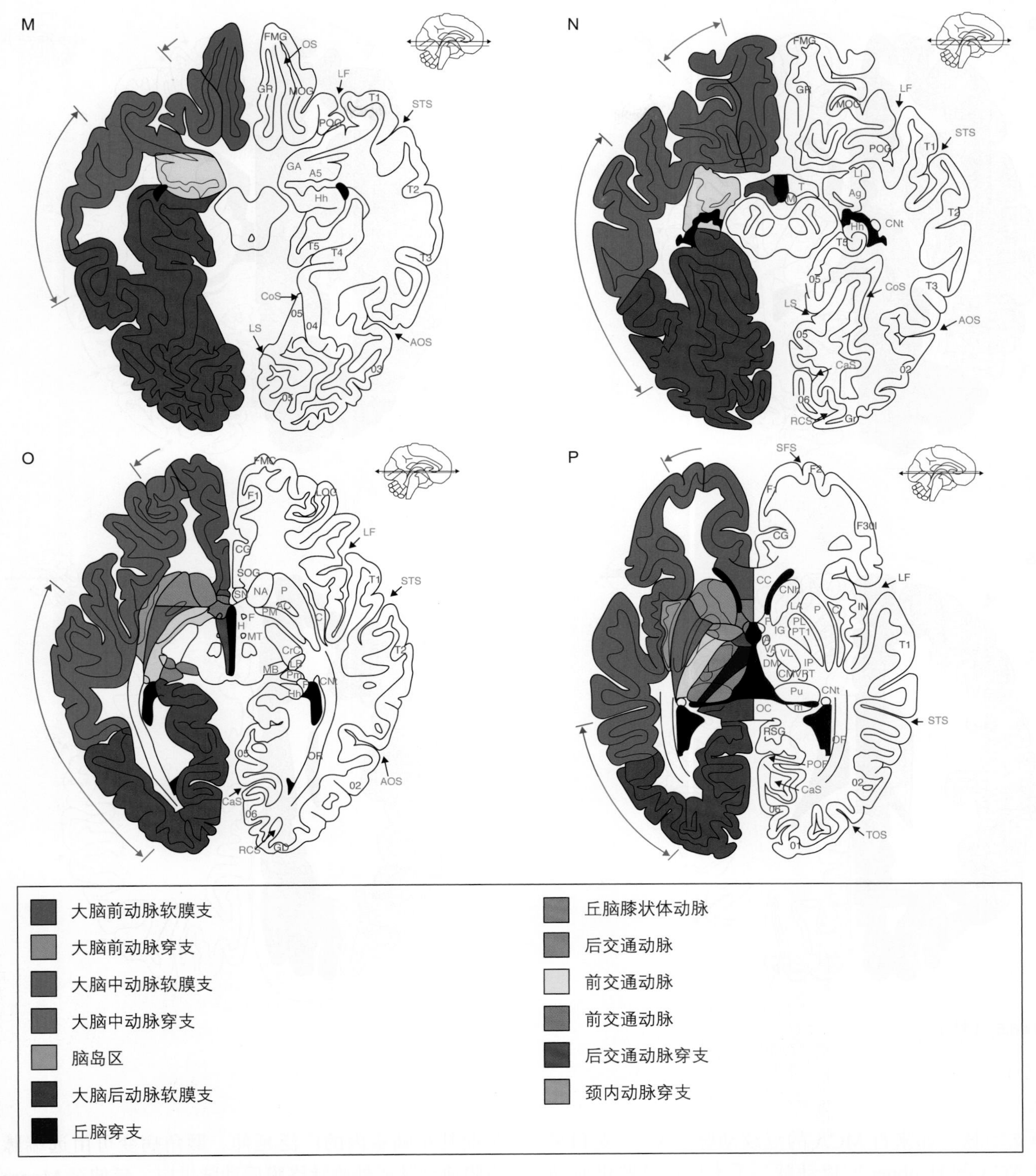

图 46.5（续）

artery，SMA）综合征。应维持远端胼周（A3 和 A4）动脉向旁中央小叶的供血。顶叶内侧和邻近胼胝体压部的 AVM 由远端 ACA 或 PCA 供血，因为 PCA 的终末支之一位于内侧顶枕沟。邻近楔回和舌回视觉皮质的 AVMs 由 PCA 另一个位于距状裂和枕叶内侧的终端分支供血。这些 AVMs 引流至上矢状窦，而涉及脑室、胼胝体压部或枕叶内侧的 AVMs 可通过室管膜、胼胝体和距状沟分支引流至 Galen 静脉。进入这些支流是通过半球间的方法。

幕上深部 AVMs

一些 AVMs 向皮质下延伸，其供血来自深部的

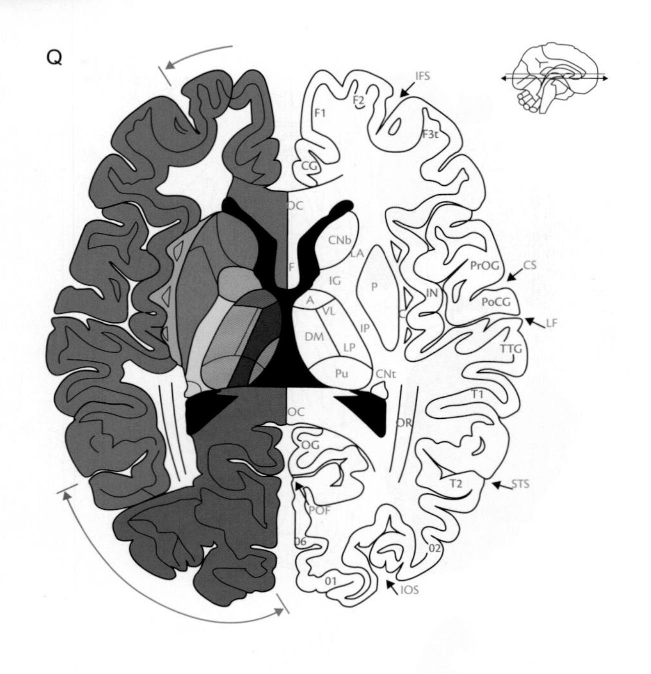

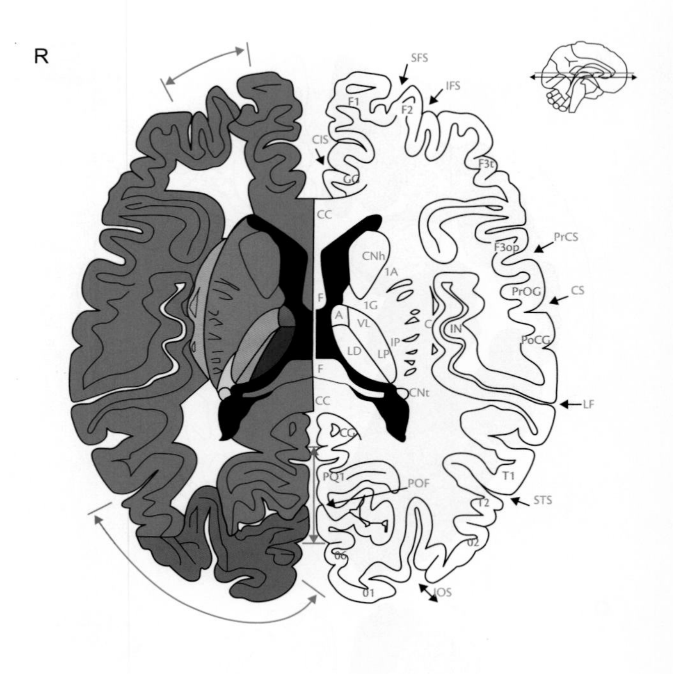

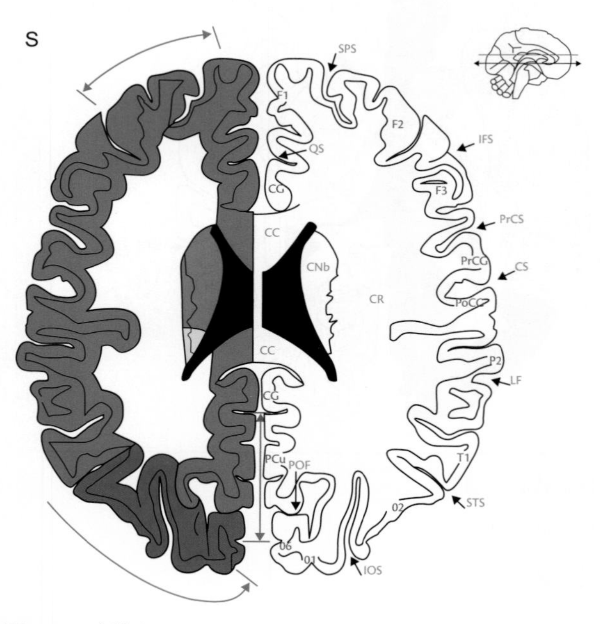

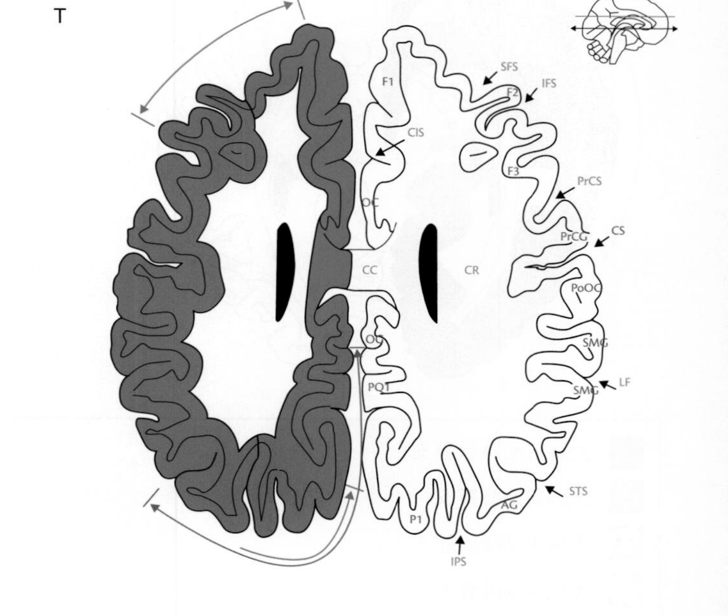

图 46.5 （续）

穿支动脉，如来自 MCA 的豆纹动脉、A1 穿支和来自 ACA 的 Heubner 回返动脉。手术接近这些供血动脉并对病变深入解剖，有可能破坏白质纤维束，如上纵束、弓状束、钩束、枕叶束、放射冠和视放射，从而导致神经功能缺损，与皮质损伤表现出的可塑性相反，这些损伤可能是永久性的。深部穿支也表明畸形团可累及基底核。AVMs 常以锥状的方式向脑室延伸，并且可能存在深部的室管膜供血动脉，即使这些供血在术前的血管造影中没有被发现。通过血管造影证实脉络膜动脉为 AVMs 供血动脉，可以预期其在脑室内的广泛延伸。颞角病变可由远端脉络膜前动脉或外侧脉络膜后动脉供应。延伸至 Monro 孔处的脉络丛，参与供应该区域的 AVM。丘脑受累的 AVMs 可以通过识别血管造影上表现为“火焰状”外观的穿支动脉，这些血管邻近基底动脉上段和近端 P1/P2。前面这些穿支是来自 P1 的丘脑穿支动脉，而后方是来自 P2 的丘脑分支。静脉引流至深部系统。

小脑 AVMs

小脑 AVMs 根据其位置由 SCA、AICA 和 PICA

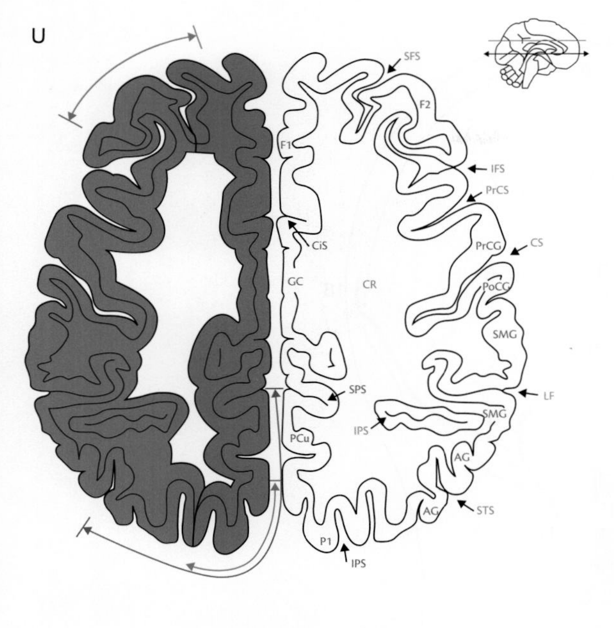

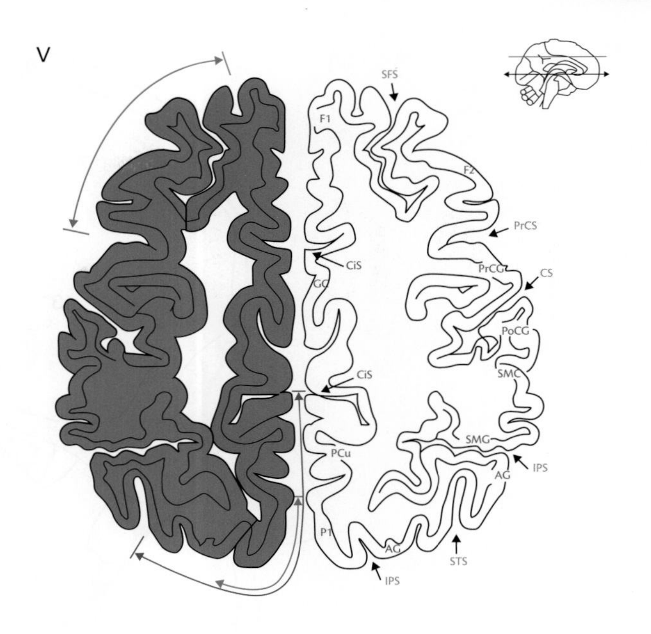

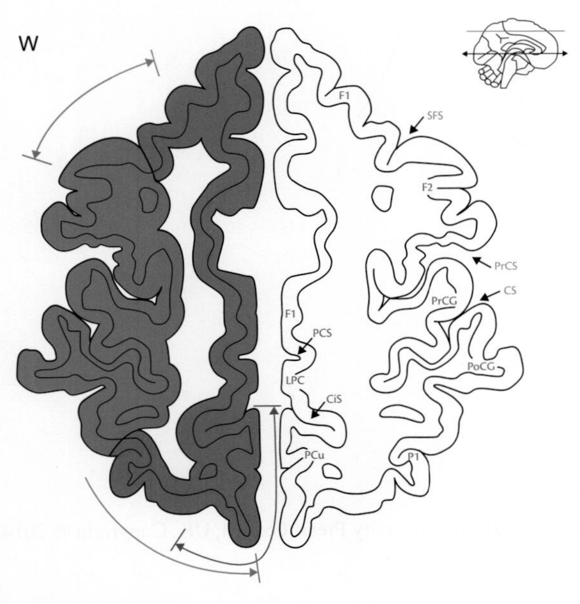

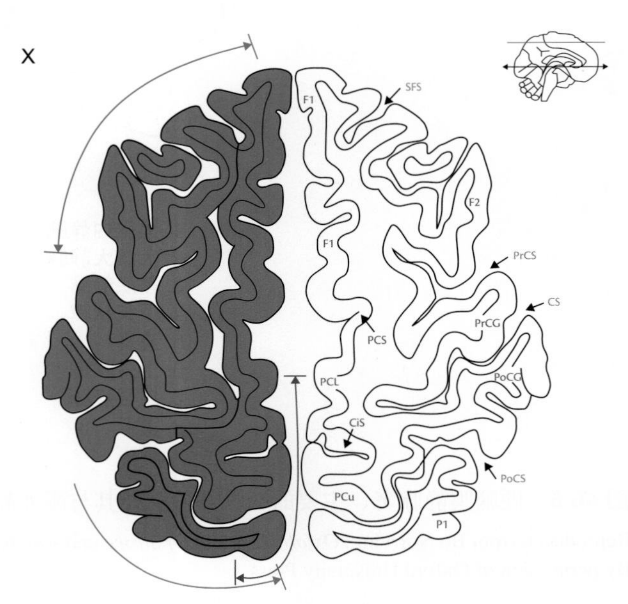

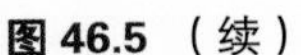
图 46.5 （续）

三个分支中的一个或多个皮质支供血。枕下表面和蚓旁的 AVMs 由 PICA "扁桃体"袢以上的分支供血，若 AVMs 延伸至第四脑室，则 PICA 脉络支也参与供血。因此，在小脑扁桃体近端控制供血或通过膜髓帆入路更为简单。此外，常常在 AVMs 供血动脉近端可见血流相关的动脉瘤。枕下和小脑幕表面，AVMs 由 SCA 远端分支供血，这些分支实际上是小脑的主要供血动脉。通过经幕下小脑上入路可以在近端控制这些供血动脉，而且可以在小脑幕裂孔和 IV 脑神经附近确认供血动脉更近端。齿状核位于小脑白质深部，由小脑上方和靠近中线的深支动脉穿过小脑供血。位于 CPA 附近的小脑岩面的 AVMs 可能有来自 AICA 皮质支的供血，并与 VII- XII脑神经关系密切。重要的是要认识到，AICA 近段或远段均有脑桥和脑干的供血穿支，因此只应闭塞为畸形团供血的穿支动脉，而不是闭塞整个供血动脉主干。AICA 动脉袢的顶点与内听道有关。静脉引流至横窦、直窦（与位于幕上的 AVMs 不同，这些引流并不作为颅后窝 AVMs 在 Spetzler-Martin 分级中的深部引流）和乙状窦。靠近深面的静脉引流是向 Galenic 深部系统引流。

血管生理学

脑灌注的自动调节和控制

尽管大脑的体积相对较小，但它需要约 14% 的心输出量，并严重依赖充足的脑血流。大脑损伤可在

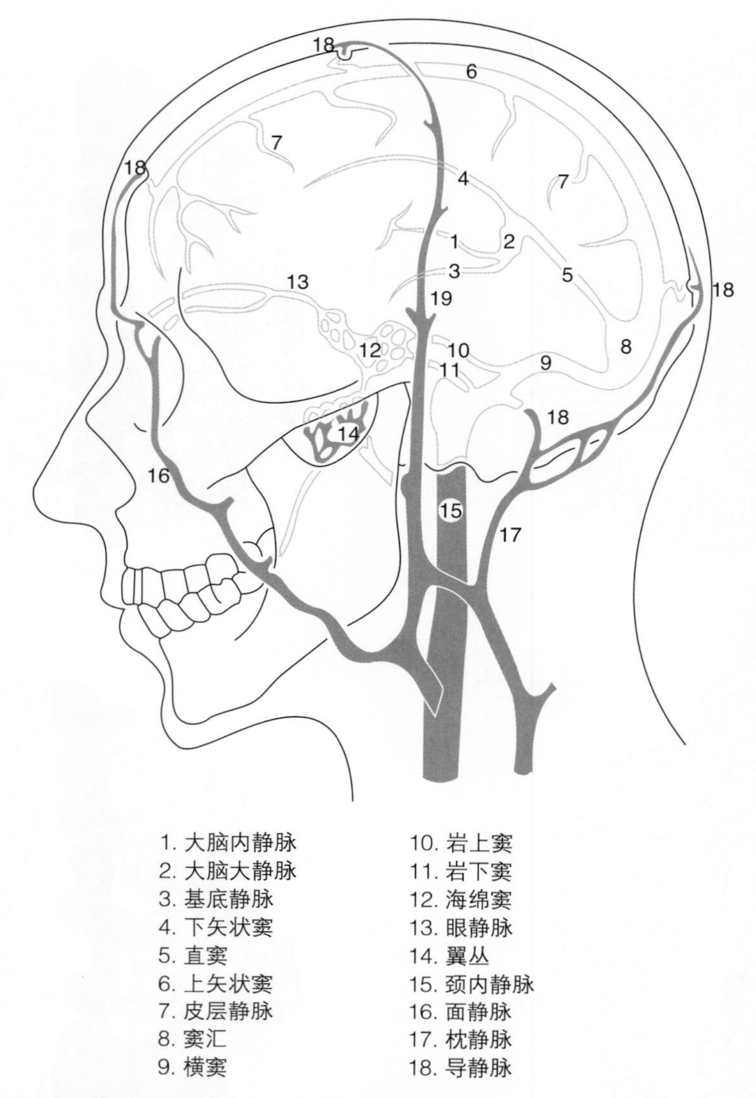

图 46.6 硬脑膜静脉窦、主要的脑深部静脉及其与颅外静脉系统的连接

一分钟内引发昏迷，如果大脑缺血时间超过 4 分钟，就会出现不可逆的神经损伤（尽管手术过程由于侧支循环通路的原因，大脑可以耐受更长的血管闭塞时间）。脑血流的自动调节是指大脑在全身血压变化的情况下仍能调节其血流的能力（Cross and Plunkett，2008）。脑灌注压（CPP）的经典定义为：

CPP=MAP－（ICP+CVP）

MAP 平均动脉压

ICP 颅内压

CVP 中心静脉压

早期对狒狒的研究表明，ICP 代表了有效的脑静脉流出压力，重要的是 ICP 在一定压力范围内矢状窦压力没有变化，反映了硬膜窦与实质静脉相比的刚性（Johnston and Rowan，1974）。CVP 通常较低，为 2~5 mmHg。因此临床上，CVP 常从方程中省略，给出：

CPP=MAP−ICP

根据 Monro-Kellie 假说，当颅内容积上升时，代偿机制最初可将 ICP 维持在正常或接近正常水平（ICP<20 mmHg）（**图 46.7**）。脑脊液（CSF）的体积通过 CSF 向椎管内的移动和增加静脉循环的吸收而减少。此外，还可能出现部分静脉窦的压迫。在临界水平上，代偿机制被打破，颅内容积的微小变化导致 ICP 显著上升。在病理生理学上，ICP 的这种上升与 CPP 和脑血流的减少有关。

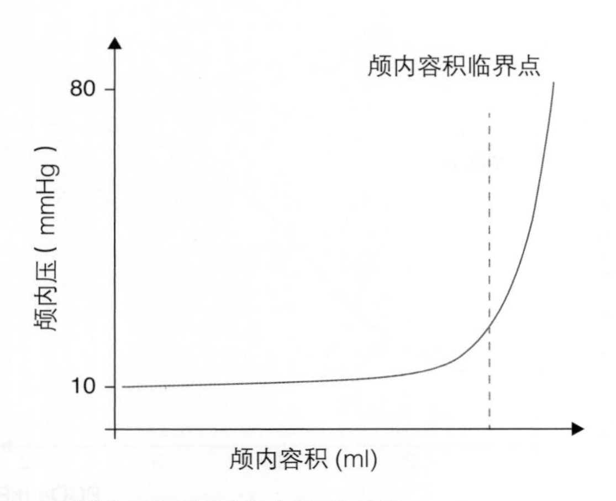

图 46.7 颅内容积和压力之间的关系

Reproduced from Catherine Spoors and Kevin Kiff, *Training in Anaesthesia*, Oxford University Press, Oxford, UK, Copyright © 2010. By permission of Oxford University Press.

大脑血流

脑血流量(cerbral blood flow,CBF)约为每分钟 700 ml[50 ml(100 g · min)]。灰质的需求量比白质大得多,每 100 g/min 接受 70 ml,而白质每 100 g/分钟接受 20 ml。总的来说,CBF 的水平对防止缺血至关重要。当血流量低于每分钟 20 ml/100 g 时,会出现脑电图变化,低于每分钟 10 ml/100 g 时,会出现不可逆的脑梗死(Yentis et al.,2013)。平均动脉压在一定范围内(50~150 mmHg),CBF 可以自动调节,并维持相对恒定(Phillips and Whisnant,1992)(图 46.8A)。高血压患者的 CBF 自主调节范围增加。在此范围外的低或高平均动脉压下,CBF 随动脉压升高而被动增加。

脑血流调节的机制

导致 CBF 自动调节的机制尚未完全清楚。目前已有一些方法用于 CBF 的测量和研究。为了测量总血流量,可以在吸入惰性气体(如 N_2O)后应用 Fick 原理测量,而放射性 133- 氙的检测、正电子发射断层扫描、功能磁共振成像和多普勒探头都被用来测量区域血流。目前已经提出三种理论来描述自动调节的机制:肌源性、代谢性和神经源性调节。参与自动调节的血管直径可能跨越 40~300 μm 的范围,但通常小于 100 μm。

肌源性调节

在 CPP 范围内保持相对恒定的 CBF 被认为涉及血管壁上的脑平滑肌的肌源性反应,特别是在曲线自动调节部分的较高压力下。经典研究表明,孤立的血管在压力升高时收缩,压力降低时扩张。

CBF 的神经源性调节——外在和内在控制

大脑血管接受颈上神经节的交感神经支配。脑实质外血管被认为是由自主神经系统调节的。但在去神经化研究中有证据显示,神经调节在脑实质内血管张力的生理调节中并不发挥主要作用。然而,当血压上升超过正常的自主调节极限时,它可能通过重置或调节正常的自主调节曲线发挥作用。这代表了一种重要的生理机制,它可以防止 CBF 的显著上升和任何相关的血脑屏障的破坏,否则就会出现血压的急性上升。脑血管系统也接受副交感神经的支配,但它被认为在正常生理条件下作用不大。慢性去神经化研究的一些证据表明,在低灌注压期间维持 CBF,从而减少缺血和梗死的潜在风险。此外,还研究了内在的或中枢的神经调节通路,以确定它们的自动调节作用,神经元性一氧化氮与所谓的神经血管单位相关,由血管周围神经节和基底膜与微血管分离的神经元组成(Talman and Nitschke Dragon,2007)。它们的确切贡献仍不清楚。

代谢性调节和血管直径的调节

代谢性调节被认为在低灌注压时影响最大。当 CBF 下降到自动调节范围以外的水平时,从血液中提取的氧气会出现代偿性上升。神经元活动的区域性增加与相应区域的脑代谢率增加有关。机制可能涉及缺氧、内在神经通路和相关代谢因子的释放。

动脉 PCO_2 和 PO_2 可以通过脑血管直径的变化影响 CBF(图 46.8B 和图 46.8C)。CO_2 对 CBF 有明显且可逆的影响。高碳酸血症可使脑动脉和小动脉血管明显扩张,从而使 CBF 增加,而低碳酸血症则相反。低碳酸血症 30 秒后,软膜动脉直径和 CBF 出现可检测的变化。由于曲线关系,在 PCO_2 的生理范围外减少会引起 CBF 的明显降低。24~48 小时后,由于生理缓冲,低碳酸血症减少 CBF 可能无法维持。在 PCO_2 数值超过 10 kPa 时,血管接近最大的扩张,因此 PCO_2 的增加对 CBF 的影响不大。高碳酸血症血管扩张的机制还不完全清楚,但被认为涉及 H^+ 对脑血管平滑肌的直接影响(Kontos et al.,1977)。最后,目前已知低碳酸血症能改善脑压调节,而高碳酸血症则会损害脑压调节。

低氧也是一种深层的血管扩张剂,以保证脑组织的充分供氧。在 8 kPa 以上的水平,PO_2 的变化对 CBF 的影响很小,CBF 接近恒定。低于 6.7 kPa 时,CBF 随缺氧程度的增加而迅速增加。同样,缺氧相

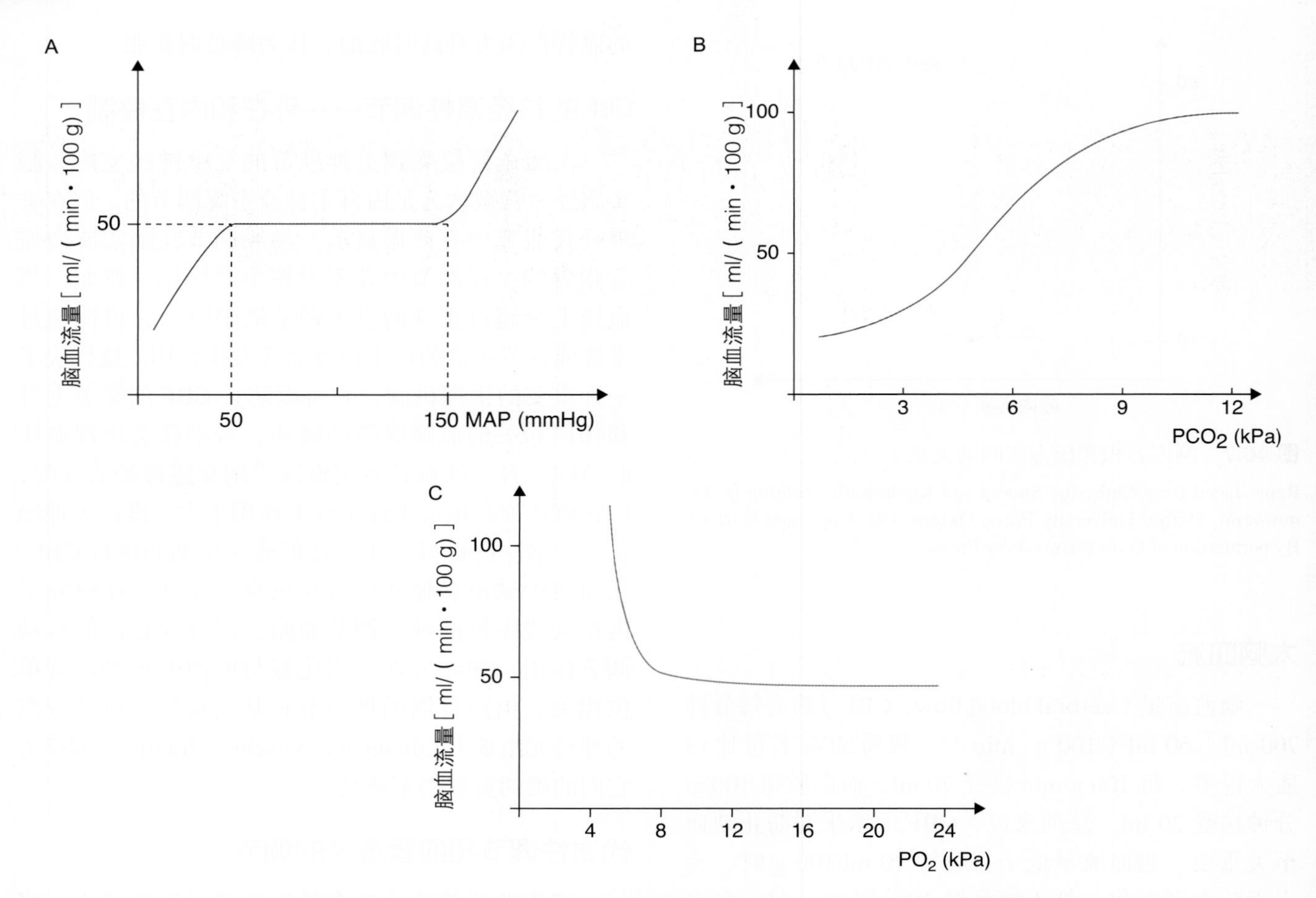

图 46.8 （A）CBF 与 MAP 的关系。（B）CBF 与 PCO_2 之间的关系。（C）CBF 与 PO_2 之间的关系

关脑血管扩张的机制也不完全清楚。一些可能的机制包括三磷酸腺苷（ATP）水平降低打开脑平滑肌上的钾通道以及一氧化氮和腺苷产生的局部变化。

争议：甘露醇与脑血流量

血液的血细胞比容水平和血液的黏度会影响 CBF。由于血细胞比容和黏度降低导致的 CBF 增加可能会通过氧气输送减少而抵消。当血细胞比容水平低于 30% 时，CBF 的增加可归因于低动脉 PO_2，可能导致脑缺血。已知甘露醇可降低 ICP，但其作用机制存在争议。传统上，甘露醇被认为是通过直接渗透作用和随后的脑水肿减少来降低 ICP（Nath and Galbraith，1986；Donato et al.，1994）。然而，包括其作用速度在内的证据更符合脑血管收缩和血管内容积减少的自动调节，以应对外周血管内容积的快速增加，从而减少脑灌注（Rosner and Coley，1987）。也有人推测脑灌注和脑血管收缩的自动调节是由于血液黏度的降低（由于红细胞流变学的改变）（Burke et al.，1981；Muizelaar et al.，1983）。然而，最近在头部受伤受试者中进行的研究并没有证明甘露醇给药后脑血流的下降（Diringer et al.，2012），还有人认为它对压力没有直接影响，而是作为一种神经保护剂。例如，它被认为是一种自由基清除剂。研究还表明，长期使用可能会通过随后的 ICP 增加而产生不利影响，最近的研究集中在高渗盐水上，它可能会类似地降低 ICP，但没有这种反弹上升（Castillo et al.，2009；Rickard et al.，2014）。总之，虽然甘露醇可快速降低脑容量和 ICP，但其确切的作用机制仍不清楚（Sakowitz et al.，2007）。

延伸阅读、参考文献、EBRAIN 的相关链接

扫描书末二维码获取。

第 47 章　动脉瘤的病理生理学

Federico Cagnazzo · Giuseppe Lanzino · Neal F. Kassell 著
李春伟 译，伊志强 审校

引言

脑动脉瘤是动脉壁的后天性病理性扩张（Sforza et al.，2009）。80%~90% 的颅内动脉瘤（intracranial aneurysms，IAs）是囊状或浆果状动脉瘤（Wiebers et al.，2004），在本章中，除非另有说明，我们讨论的均为这种特定的动脉瘤类型。在接受影像学检查的人群中，1%~2% 的人存在颅内动脉瘤，而尸检研究表明颅内动脉瘤在成人人群中的发病率在 1%~5%。颅内动脉瘤约占所有非创伤性蛛网膜下腔出血（subarachnoid haemorrhage，SAH）病例的 80%~85%。动脉瘤最常见的发病年龄是 40~50 岁，女性略多，女：男为 3：2。

动脉瘤形成和发展的学说

IAs 的病理生理学是有争议的，很可能是多因素的结果，与血流动力学、血管壁生物学、遗传易感性和外部可改变因素之间的相互作用有关（Sforza et al.，2009）。

血管壁生物学

颅内动脉瘤通常位于动脉分叉处，分叉处的胶原纤维多于弹性纤维，且肌肉层不发达。动脉平滑肌细胞（smooth muscle-cell，SMC）凋亡和弹性蛋白 / 胶原纤维重构作为血管壁重塑的一部分，可能与血管壁的质地减弱，以及随后动脉瘤的形成有关（Hara et al.，1998）。Kondo 等（Kondo et al.，1998）研究了动脉内层平滑肌细胞（SMCs）凋亡在 IAs 发生和发展过程中的作用。在这项实验研究中，通过结扎合并有肾性高血压的大鼠的左侧颈总动脉诱发其 IAs 形成。随着实验性动脉瘤的形成，动脉中层出现了 SMCs 的进行性凋亡的变化。到了凋亡晚期，大部分中层 SMCs 已消失，动脉瘤壁主要由结缔组织组成。电镜研究证实了 SMCs 的进行性凋亡变化，如染色质凝聚、细胞质和细胞核的破碎。此外，动脉瘤瘤顶表现出 SMCs 凋亡的晚期特征（高级核和细胞质的凝结，以及凋亡小体的形成）。本研究支持颅内动脉瘤的形成是由于动脉壁中层凋亡而致使颅内动脉发生复杂的动脉壁重塑的过程。

血管细胞外基质酶，如明胶酶、弹性酶（Chyatte and Lewis，1997）或基质金属蛋白酶（Bruno et al.，1998）也可能参与这一过程。

遗传因素

遗传因素与颅内动脉瘤的发生有关。颅内动脉瘤在一级亲属有 IAs 病史的患者的兄弟姐妹中发病率较高。许多研究都聚焦于分离与 IAs 相关的基因位点上，并且已经确定了几个潜在的候选基因（表 47.1）。

血流动力学因素

通过观察可以发现，在血流动力学压力增加的情况下动脉瘤形成的风险增加，如“不平衡”的前交

表 47.1　与颅内动脉瘤相关的最常见的遗传性疾病

疾病	遗传类型	基因	基因产物	患病率
ADPKD	AD	PKD1	多囊蛋白 1	>1/1000
EDS	AD	COL3A1	Ⅲ型胶原	1/100 000~9/100 000
MfS	AD	FBN1	原纤维蛋白 1	1/100 000~5/10 000
NF 1	AD	NF1	神经纤维瘤蛋白	1/100 000~5/10 000
PXE	AD 和 AR	ABCC6	ATP 结合盒	1/100 000~9/100 000

缩写：ADPKD，常染色体显性遗传性多囊肾疾病；EDS，埃勒斯 - 当洛斯综合征；MfS，马方综合征；NF1，神经纤维瘤病 1 型；PXE，弹性（纤维）假性黄瘤；AD，常染色体显性；AR，常染色体隐性

通动脉（Acom）复合体（一侧大脑前动脉 A1 段占优势，而对侧 A1 发育不良），在低压分流的患者中（例如高流量动静脉畸形、以及自发性或医源性颈动脉闭塞后沿着侧支通路形成）更容易形成动脉瘤（Matsuda et al., 1983; Kayembe et al., 1984; Redekop et al., 1998）。

最近，精密的计算机流体模型提出了动脉壁剪切应力和其他局部血流动力学因素在 IAs 的发生、发展和可能的破裂中的潜在作用。然而，这些模型大多存在缺陷，因为这种计算是基于对已破裂和未破裂的 IAs 的比较，而这是两种根本不同的病理过程。

环境（可改变）因素

为了明确各种可改变的（外部）因素与 IAs 的发展或破裂之间可能存在的相关性，已经进行了一些纵向和病例对照的流行病学研究，但只有吸烟和高血压有令人信服的证据。1983—1986 年在挪威进行的 HUNT 研究（Koskinen and Blomstedt，2006）显示，目前的吸烟者（HR，6.1）和以前的吸烟者（HR，2.7）比从未吸烟的人有更高的动脉瘤性 SAH 发病率。这种关联的原因尚不完全清楚。可能是吸烟通过各种机制引发动脉炎症反应，导致动脉瘤形成和（或）破裂（Chalouhi et al.，2012）。

动脉收缩压是与 IA 相关的另一个可改变的危险因素。在 HUNT 研究中，收缩压在 130~139 mmHg 的人群发生动脉瘤性 SAH 的风险显著高于对照人群（收缩压 <130 mmHg）。此外，收缩压超过 170 mmHg 的人群 HR 为 3.3（Koskinen and Blomstedt，2006）。有趣的是，高血压和吸烟互为促进作用：在一项前瞻性研究中，有高血压的吸烟者发生 SAH 的危险比是没有这两个因素的受试者的 13.3 倍（Lindekleiv et al.，2012）。其他可调节因素（包括饮酒、激素因素等）与动脉瘤形成和破裂之间的关系则较有争议。

位置

囊状动脉瘤通常发生在形成 Willis 环的动脉分支处。Rhoton 介绍了（Rhoton et al.，1979）关于囊状动脉瘤位置的三个基本规律：①动脉瘤产生于载瘤动脉的分叉处（如 PComA、大脑中动脉分叉、基底动脉分叉）；②动脉瘤产生于动脉的转折或弯曲处；③动脉瘤瘤体位于最大血流方向。非分支动脉瘤（位于动脉的非分支部位）较少见，往往不是浆果状动脉瘤。

约 90% 的囊状动脉瘤位于大脑前循环，其相对于各种特定位置的分布在不同人群中也不尽相同，破裂和未破裂的动脉瘤也不相同。在破裂的动脉瘤中，前交通动脉复合体动脉瘤最为常见（30%~35%），其次是颈内动脉动脉瘤（包括 PComA，30%）和 MCA 动脉瘤（20%）。在后循环中，基底动脉分叉是最常见的部位。

大小和形态

动脉瘤的大小是非常重要的，因为它与动脉瘤破裂的风险和治疗的风险相关。传统的 IA 根据瘤体的最大直径分为三组：小动脉瘤（直径不超过 10 mm）；大动脉瘤（直径在 11~25 mm）；巨大动脉瘤（直径大于 25 mm）。

囊状动脉瘤由瘤颈（动脉瘤与载瘤动脉相连的部分）和瘤体组成。随着血管内技术的发展，确定瘤颈的大小变得尤为重要。瘤颈大于 4 mm 的动脉瘤被认为是宽颈动脉瘤。瘤颈 / 瘤体比是影响血管内治疗的另一个重要形态特征。

通过计算流体动力学研究，对 IAs 的其他几个与破裂风险有关的形态学特征进行了分析，这些形态学特征包括纵横比（动脉瘤首尾尺寸除以横径）和动脉瘤角（**图 47.1**）。

动脉瘤形态不规则和继发性向外凸起（也称为血泡、子囊或分叶）的现象并不罕见。在破裂的动脉瘤中，这些子囊通常可以确定为破裂点（**图 47.2**）。动脉瘤子囊通常位于与最大流入点相对的瘤体上。在未破裂的动脉瘤中，这种不规则形态可能与破裂风险增加有关（Cebral et al.，2010），其存在与否是决定是否治疗的重要因素之一。

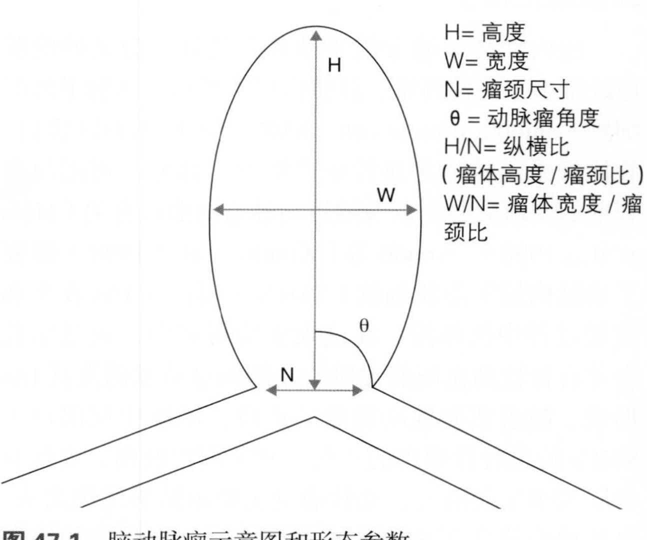

图 47.1 脑动脉瘤示意图和形态参数

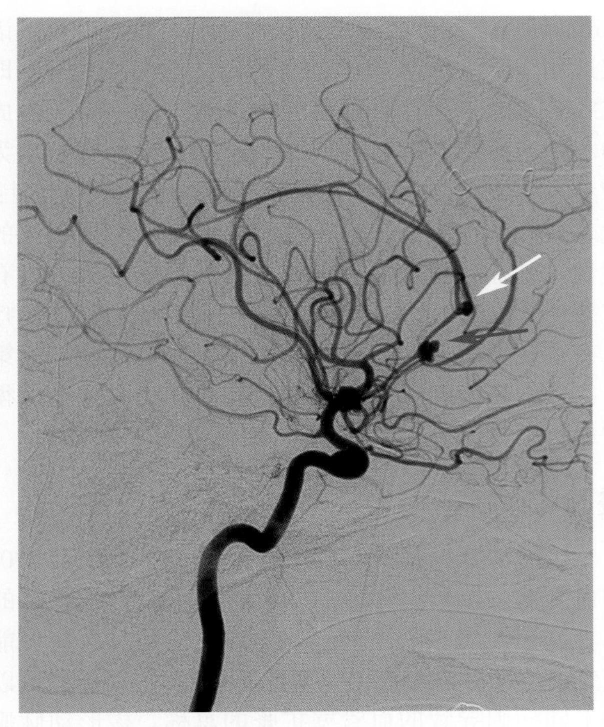

图 47.2　急性蛛网膜下腔出血（subarachnoid haemorrhage，SAH）患者。左颈内动脉（ICA）侧位血管造影动脉期显示两个大脑前动脉远端动脉瘤（红色和白色箭头）。子囊（红色箭头）考虑为破裂点

家族性动脉瘤及其相关条件

家族性动脉瘤

在有或没有动脉瘤性 SAH 病史的 IAs 患者的亲属中，患 IA 的风险会增加（Thompson et al.，2015）。IAs 患者的一级亲属、存在高血压和（或）吸烟的情况下，IAs 的风险会增加，另外，有两个或两个以上亲属受影响的人，IAs 的风险会增加 15 倍。对没有额外受影响亲属的动脉瘤性 SAH 患者的家庭成员进行筛查是有争议的。如果一个家庭有两个或两个以上亲属受影响，建议对 30 岁以上的家庭成员进行筛查（Thompson et al.，2015）。由于并非所有未破裂的动脉瘤都需要治疗，因此在筛查之前，需要就 IA 诊断的意义全面考虑。

目前已知的与 IAs 相关的可遗传和不可遗传的病理情况较多（**表 47.1**）。其中包括：

- **常染色体显性多囊肾病（autosomal dominant polycystic kidney disease，ADPKD）**：单基因病理，出现肾和其他内脏囊肿，并伴有一系列血管异常，包括脑动脉瘤（通常是多发性的）。本病 25% 的患者发现脑动脉瘤，建议多囊肾病和有 IAs 家族史的患者进行筛查。ADPKD 会使 IA 的风险增加 10~20 倍，这取决于是否还有 IAs 的家族史。在 ADPKD 中，同时存在的高血压可能进一步促进 IAs 的形成。最近的一项研究显示，与无 IAs 的 ADPKD 患者相比，有 IAs 的 ADPKD 患者（尤其是年龄大于 45 岁的患者）血压数值较高。因此，ADPKD 和高血压患者应进行 IAs 筛查（Niemczyk et al.，2014）。
- **胶原蛋白病（如 Ehlers–Danlos，Ⅳ型）**：Ⅲ型胶原蛋白存在异常，致使皮肤脆弱、关节活动度低、血管脆弱，导致主动脉夹层、颈动脉 - 海绵窦瘘和颅内动脉瘤。虽然很少见，但认识这种疾病很重要，因为这些患者由于血管脆弱，导管进行血管内诊断和治疗的风险和并发症非常高。
- **马方综合征**：由纤维蛋白（弹性组织的主要糖蛋白成分）紊乱引起的心血管系统异常。患者往往身材高大，伴有蜘蛛足样指 / 趾和关节活动度低下，并有较高的颅内和颅外动脉瘤发病风险。
- **主动脉缩窄**：主动脉管腔变窄或缩窄，最常见于左锁骨下动脉起源的远端，邻近动脉韧带。IAs 在主动脉缩窄的患者中发现较多（在 117 例主动脉缩窄患者的 MR 血管影像中，10.3% 存在 IAs）（Curtis et al.，2012）。
- **肌纤维发育不良**：特发性、节段性、非动脉硬化性、非炎症性血管疾病，主要影响肾动脉、颈动脉颅外段和椎动脉。颅内动脉肌纤维发育不良罕见。肌纤维发育不良最常见的临床表现与主要动脉的狭窄闭塞性疾病有关。与普通人群相比，肌纤维发育不良患者的 IAs 发病率更高（Cloft 等进行的 meta 分析中为 7.3%）（Cloft et al.，1998）。

颅内动脉瘤的进展和破裂风险

动脉瘤的生长反映在影像学（宏观）变化和分子水平上的结构壁变化（微观）。动脉瘤的进展取决于血管壁修复和破坏之间的平衡，在吸烟或有高血压的患者中动脉瘤的进展会被加速（Etminan and Rinkel，2016）。在最近一项对近 13 000 例 IAs 患者的 meta 分析中，Brinjikji 等发现，动脉瘤增长的总体比例为 3%/ 动脉瘤年。IAs 增长最重要的危险因素包括年龄大于 50 岁、女性性别、吸烟史和非囊状形态。动脉瘤生长似乎与高的破裂风险相关（破裂率为每年 3.1%，而稳定的 IAs 为每年 0.1%）（Brinjikji et al.，2016）。同样，Villablanca 等发现，与非生长型 IAs 相比，生长型 IAs 的年破裂率是其 12 倍（Villablanca et al.，2013），而 Mehan 等在多变量分析中发现，IAs 生长与破裂的高度相关，OR 为 55.9（Mehan et al.，2014）。

特殊情况

创伤性动脉瘤

创伤性动脉瘤（traumatic aneurysms，TAs）在所有颅内动脉瘤中占比不到1%，尽管其真正的发病率尚不清楚，许多动脉瘤可能未被发现。创伤性动脉瘤是儿童和青少年遇到的第二大常见动脉瘤类型（占儿童所有动脉瘤的5%~15%），在男性中更为常见。创伤性动脉瘤可细分为由血管壁全部三层组成的“真性”TAs。通常，它们是由直接的钝挫伤或间接的外力引起的责任血管中的“隆起”。“假性”TAs是由于血管的连续性直接被破坏进而形成血管周围血肿的结果。“假性”TAs的瘤壁仅由围绕部分机化血肿的纤维蛋白组织组成。

颅内所有主要动脉均可受累，受累血管均为外伤机制所致。最常见的位置是颈内动脉（ICA）（46%）、MCA（25%）和大脑前动脉（ACA）（22%）。

未经治疗的TAs的自然史尚不十分清楚，其破裂的风险可能很高，尤其是在连续的影像学检查中出现了进行性增大。保持一定的怀疑对于充分的诊断很重要，在高危病例中，在第一次检查阴性后重复另一次血管影像学检查可能是有意义的，因为TAs可能在创伤后几天就变得明显。创伤性假性动脉瘤是创伤性动脉瘤的一个特殊亚类，在各种外科手术后都有报道，包括经蝶手术、肿瘤和血管病变的开颅手术、第三脑室造瘘术，甚至在脑室外引流术后。

夹层动脉瘤

颅内夹层动脉瘤越来越多地被人们认识，尽管不太常见，但却是SAH的潜在病因。它们源于动脉的内膜剥离，血管壁内膜与内弹力层撕裂后血液在血管壁的不同层之间聚积。通常被称为假性动脉瘤（即在组织学切片上，它们缺乏正常的三层血管壁结构），这些病变包含正常血管壁的基本成分，因此更合适的定义是夹层动脉瘤。

夹层动脉瘤常见于椎动脉或颈动脉的颅外段，但也可累及颅内动脉。尽管到目前为止颅内夹层动脉瘤最常见于椎动脉颅内段（V4段），但其已被发现几乎可累及任何颅内动脉。前循环夹层动脉瘤发生的位置在儿童和年轻成人中更为典型。累及颅外血管的夹层动脉瘤不会引起出血，而颅内夹层动脉瘤则可表现为无症状，或是出现缺血症状、头痛或直接出血（图47.3）。

血泡动脉瘤

在过去一段时间，“血泡动脉瘤”一词被误用为Willis环分支部位的极小囊状动脉瘤。然而，该术语仅适用于从ICA床突上的背侧壁的非分支位置（即PCom和脉络膜前动脉发出的对侧，图47.4）形成的小的半球形凸起。此外，所有的血泡动脉瘤均为ICA的局灶性夹层，还是其存在两种截然不同类型：代表血管壁上的破孔的真性血泡和ICA夹层形成的假性动脉瘤，目前尚有争议。血泡动脉瘤约占所有破裂动脉瘤的1%，其特点是瘤壁非常脆弱，使治疗具有挑战性。血泡动脉瘤通常在出血后诊断，其第一次导管造影时很难识别，只有在随访时才会变得更加明显。

梭形动脉瘤

梭形动脉瘤是指动脉壁的扩张，至少累及270°的血管壁。梭形动脉瘤多见于后循环，60岁以上的患者，男性居多。病理生理学尚不清楚，有些可能与先前的动脉夹层有关，因此，“梭形”动脉瘤可以是不同病因导致的血管壁扩张的总称。梭形动脉瘤的一种特殊类型是所谓的迂曲扩张动脉瘤，其特征是整个血管段均匀的病理性扩张，通常与血管本身的扭曲有关（图47.5）。梭形动脉瘤可以是偶发的（在这种情况下常为良性的自然史），但也可出现缺血症状、与占位效应有关的症状和出血。

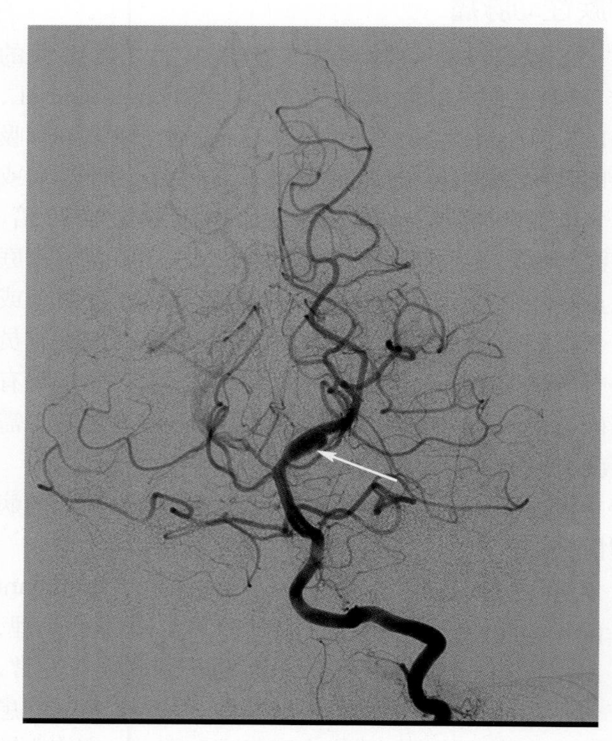

图47.3 左椎动脉血管造影显示左侧大脑后动脉夹层动脉瘤

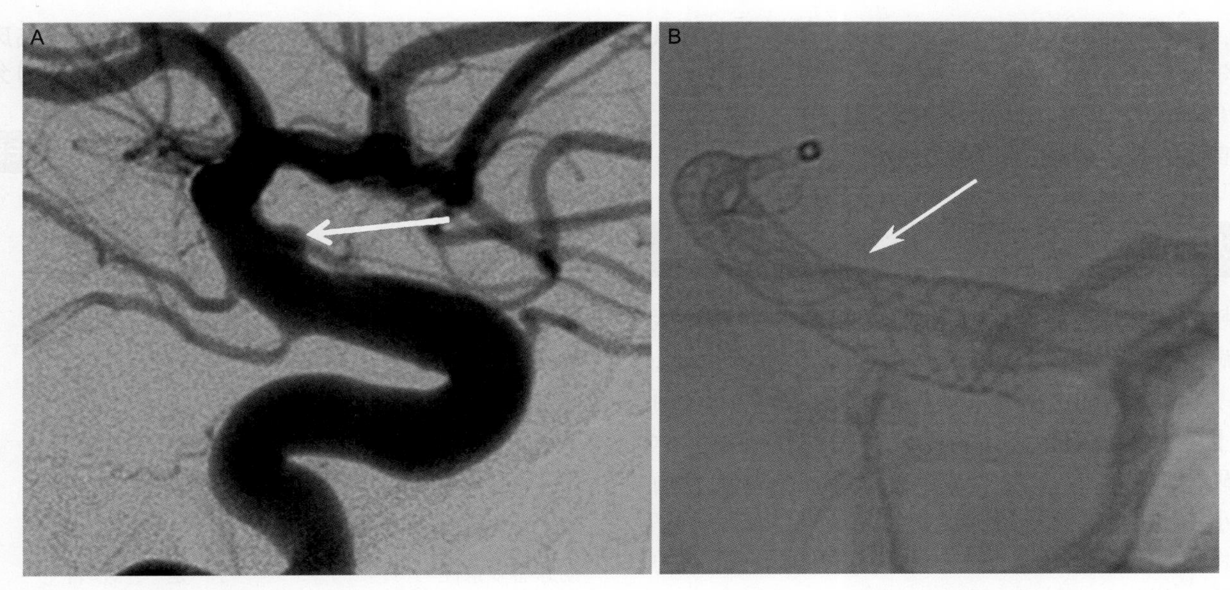

图 47.4　一个30岁的女性出现广泛SAH。血管造影显示一个血泡动脉瘤（A）累及右侧ICA的床突上段（箭头）。（B）血泡动脉瘤运用血流导向装置治疗（箭头）

细菌性动脉瘤

“细菌性动脉瘤”一词意味着存在感染和血管壁的破坏。最常见的感染源是感染性心内膜炎。细菌性动脉瘤通常累及远端分支，可发生在远离分叉的地方。针对病原体的抗生素治疗是治疗细菌性动脉瘤的主要方法，所有患者都应根据微生物病原体的敏感性进行适当的抗生素治疗。在某些临床情况下，可根据原发感染情况和相关指南，经验性地开始使用抗生素。此外，应通过一系列血培养监测全身的感染情况。细菌性动脉瘤的抗感染治疗必须持续4~6周或直到培养结果变为阴性。在特定情况下，细菌性动脉瘤也可考虑血管内治疗或手术治疗（Kannoth and Thomas，2009）。

多发性动脉瘤

多发IAs（MIAs）在不同研究中的发病率不同。日本UCAS研究中为13.9%（Morita et al.，2012），ISUIA研究中为35%（Wiebers et al.，2003）。在SAH的患者中，15%~45%的患者存在MIAs。在MIAs患者中，每个动脉瘤的破裂风险并不增加，但累计破裂风险高于只有一个动脉瘤的患者（Morita et al.，2012）。MIAs形成的确切机制尚不完全清楚。有研究表明，MIAs与吸烟、高血压、年龄和女性性别有关（Juvela，2000；Ellamushi et al.，2001；Lu et al.，2013）。然而，MIAs与这些危险因素之间的相关性仍存在争议。Ostergaard和Hog（Ostergaard and Hog，1985）对737例IAs患者（其中18%患有MIAs）进行研究发现，高血压和女性性别是MIAs的独立危险因素，而年龄没有影响。Qureshi等（Qureshi et al.，1998）研究的419例IAs患者中，30%的患者为多发IAs，研究结果显示吸烟和女性性别与MIAs相关，而高血压和MIAs的发生不相关。

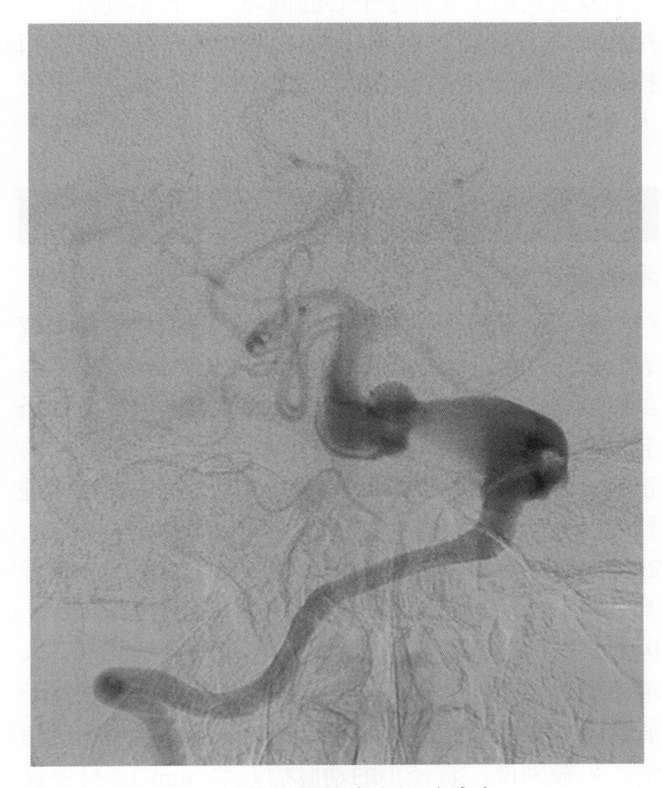

图 47.5　椎-基底动脉系统的多发性动脉瘤

最近，Lu 等（Lu et al., 2013）报道了 MIAs 破裂风险与年龄、大小和位置之间的关系。在这项研究中，中年（45~65 岁）、ACom（位置）和动脉瘤尺寸增大与较高的破裂风险相关。

颅内动脉瘤的筛查

颅内动脉瘤的筛查是有争议的，但对于某些家族性疾病，有足够的证据建议进行筛查（Steiner et al., 2013）。这些条件包括：有明确的家族史（两个或两个以上一级亲属有颅内动脉瘤）、ADPKD 和主动脉粥样硬化（见前述）。筛查应从比此家庭成员的发病年龄小 10 岁的成员开始。目前尚无明确的筛查频率和模式指南，尤其是 ADPKD，因为它们具有较高的晚期新生动脉瘤形成率（每患者年 1.4%）（Cagnazzo et al., 2017）。CT 和 MR 血管造影技术都已经发展到了很高的灵敏度，如何选择将取决于年龄（CT 的累积辐射负担）和各个中心的偏好。在开始进行一个疗程的筛查之前，必须仔细咨询患者，因为多次扫描和识别可能不需要立即干预的小动脉瘤会产生巨大的累积性心理负担。

争论

未破裂的动脉瘤的处理方法

随着无创成像技术的广泛应用，越来越多的未破裂 IAs 被诊断。对未破裂 IAs 的处理是非常有争议的。虽然绝大多数小的 IAs 将终生保持静止，但极少数仍会发生破裂，造成潜在的灾难性后果。迄今为止关于 IAs 的真实自然史数据非常少，因为即使在目前进行的两个最大的研究中，ISUIA 研究（Wiebers et al., 2003）和日本研究（Morita et al., 2012），许多患者都是根据医生和患者的选择进行手术或血管内治疗。因此，这些经常被错误地标为自然史研究的研究是未治疗患者的前瞻性队列研究。由于这种争议和相互矛盾的数据，未破裂 IAs 的治疗仍然是经验性而非科学的。一般来说，直径小的动脉瘤（<7 mm），只要没有症状，纯属偶然发现，其破裂的风险极低。动脉瘤的位置、是否存在分叶以及其他动脉瘤破裂的危险因素都会影响动脉瘤破裂，在决定积极或保守治疗时必须考虑到这些因素。此外，治疗建议还必须考虑到治疗 IAs 的风险和患者对 IAs 认识的焦虑程度。

一些研究试图根据现有信息（PHASES）（Greving et al., 2014）或专家共识（UIATS）（Etminan et al., 2015）提出治疗的算法（**表 47.2**）。IAs 的最佳治疗方式同样存在较大的争议：手术与血管内治疗。一般来说，手术能达到更高的血管造影完全闭塞率，但它的创伤性更大。血管内治疗的情况则相反。目前还没有研究直接探讨未破裂 IAs 的治疗选择。如果对未破裂 IA 患者进行保守治疗，不进行任何干预，那么就会出现随访的必要性、频率和随访方式的问题。在这种情况下，没有指南，随访必须个体化。一般来说，我们建议在诊断后 6~12 个月重复一次无创性的随访（通常是 MRA，因为无辐射）。如果无增大，那么进一步的影像学检查要根据患者年龄、危险因素、动脉瘤大小和位置等因素进行个体化选择。

表 47.2 UIATS 研究（用于管理未破裂 IA 的临床决策）和 PHASES 研究（用于预测 5 年破裂风险）分析的因素

分析因素	UIATS	PHASES
患者因素		
年龄	是	是
家族性 IAs 或 SAH	是	是
种族	是	否
吸烟	是	是
高血压	是	否
常染色体显性遗传多囊肾病	是	是
药物和酒精滥用	是	否
与 IA 相关的临床症状	是	否
动脉瘤多重性	是	否
由于害怕破裂而导致生活质量下降	是	否
预期寿命（慢性或恶性疾病）	是	否
神经精神疾病	是	否
凝血障碍	是	否
家族性 IAs 或 SAH	是	否
动脉瘤因素		
大小	是	是
形态	是	否
位置	是	是
进展	是	否
治疗相关因素		
与 IA 的年龄、大小和复杂性相关的治疗风险	是	否

延伸阅读、参考文献、EBRAIN 的相关链接

扫描书末二维码获取。

第48章 蛛网膜下腔出血的病理生理学

Jason McMillen 著
刘方军 译，伊志强 审校

蛛网膜下腔出血

大多数（85%）自发性蛛网膜下腔出血（subarachnoid haemorrhage，SAH）是由于颅内动脉瘤破裂导致。部分患者原因不明，这些患者中，大约60%的病例出血分布在中脑周围。其他非动脉瘤SAH的病因包括软脑膜动静脉畸形、肿瘤、应用抗凝剂、血管解剖变异和血管病。

中脑周围SAH是一种特殊的非动脉瘤SAH综合征，CT扫描上有出血的特征性表现。出血集中在脑桥前池和中脑周围池，可延伸到邻近的脑池，但最远不会到纵裂池和侧裂池，也不会进入脑室。

动脉瘤性SAH通常是由于颅内囊性动脉瘤壁自发性破裂所致。动脉瘤壁形成的易感原因，生长和最终破裂是多因素的，包括血管壁结构和成分的变化，以及对血管壁施压的血流动力学因素。

SAH致残率及死亡率均高，了解其生理损伤机制可以帮助提高对患者的管理水平，让患者得到较好的预后。动脉瘤性SAH的主要并发症是再出血、迟发性缺血和脑积水。

蛛网膜下腔出血及其脑损伤的病理生理学机制

颅内动脉瘤常见于血管分叉，形成的确切原因尚不清楚，被认为是继发于局部血流动力学和血管壁完整性之间的不平衡所致。没有一个单一的模型能够解释动脉瘤的形成、生长和破裂的所有方面。有多种因素参与其发病机制，包括先天性、获得性和感染。

当动脉瘤形成时，它们倾向于遵循Rhoton的动脉瘤形成规则，来自动脉的分支起点，产生于血管壁受到的剪应力最大的转弯或者凸面处。假如不存在转弯或者凸面，动脉瘤产生于血流流出的方向。

动脉瘤的破裂可能会自发发生，也会发生于运动时，如紧张或者性交。除了头痛和脑膜炎的典型症状外，患者还可能出现感觉和意识的变化，反映了早期的脑损伤。动脉瘤破裂伴随急性的颅内压增高，继发于血液外渗于蛛网膜下腔或者脑实质，血管扩张功能失调。脑灌注压的降低可以表现为意识丧失。随后的急性脑缺血和脑水肿可能会导致SAH后早期脑损伤。大量血肿和严重的早期脑损伤会使得SAH的Fisher等级升高及预后不良。脑出血可能导致脑实质的直接损伤，从而导致局灶性功能障碍。

在SAH的急性全脑缺血性损伤后，对大脑有害的病理发生相互作用（Budohoski et al.，2014）。细胞死亡机制在24小时内启动，包括坏死、自噬和细胞程序性死亡。血脑屏障崩溃和炎性机制启动，包括释放促炎细胞因子和炎性细胞的迁移。与脑损伤一样，这些都与脑血管痉挛有关。自由基释放引起氧化应激导致线粒体功能改变和其他细胞代谢紊乱，与SAH后细胞死亡增加有关。脑血流自主调节功能损害，正常的生理代偿机制受损，加重了脑缺血的程度。严重的脑代谢功能紊乱导致电生理异常，包括癫痫发作和皮质扩散去极化。这些可能导致低灌注、缺氧，即使没有血管痉挛，也会导致迟发性缺血。脑实质血管中的微血栓是由促凝活性物质的早期增加引起的，并有可能加剧大血管与微血管痉挛有关的缺血。

SAH后脑积水是常见的，可能导致进行性的神经功能损害或死亡。诊断SAH脑积水的放射学标准各不相同，但是20%的SAH患者会出现脑积水。这些患者中大约有一半会出现意识受损，需要住院紧急处理。另外一半可能会发展成慢性脑积水，需行脑脊液分流术。

SAH后脑积水是由于CSF正常的循环和吸收途径受损伤导致的。脑室内血块堵塞正常的脑脊液循环通路，如中脑导水管，导致梗阻性脑积水。血液成分，升高的蛋白质，血液分解产物如纤维蛋白，会损伤脑脊液流出后通过蛛网膜绒毛的吸收通道，导致交通性脑积水。

急性症状性脑积水通常采用脑室造瘘术和临时脑脊液外引流处理。脑脊液急性引流可能会导致动脉瘤跨壁压力的急性变化，增加再出血的风险。在处理动脉瘤之前，为了降低动脉瘤再破裂的风险，需要维持较高的颅内压。腰椎穿刺或腰大池外引流是减少脑积水的其他临时措施。在手术夹闭动脉瘤的过程中，置换血性脑脊液、第三脑室底造瘘术、终板造瘘术都能够减少慢性脑积水产生的风险。尽管采取了这些措施，有些患者还会产生永久性的脑积水，需要行脑室腹腔分流。SAH 后脑脊液中细胞和蛋白质浓度升高会堵塞脑室腹腔分流管，导致早期分流失败。所以有必要临时行脑脊液外引流，直到这些参数下降，然后植入脑室 - 腹腔分流装置。

动脉瘤的流行病学和发病率及动脉瘤破裂的危险因素

由于大多数患者在动脉瘤破裂之前无症状，所以未破裂动脉瘤的总体发病率难以准确确定。用影像学脑血管成像技术对大量人群进行准确筛查价格昂贵，并且有些技术是有创的、有辐射的。随着越来越敏感的无创影像技术的使用，检出无症状动脉瘤的数量在增加。影像学和尸检研究都表明，未破裂颅内动脉瘤的发生率 1%~9%。在芬兰和日本人口中，动脉瘤的发生率有所增加，女性、年龄增大、身体状况也会导致动脉瘤的发生率增加（Rinkel et al.，1988）。

动脉瘤破裂引起的蛛网膜下腔出血是颅内动脉瘤最具破坏性的并发症，常致残或致死。确定动脉瘤的形成、生长和破裂的风险，对于平衡干预风险及预后风险，至关重要。

据报道，一般人群动脉瘤性蛛网膜下腔出血的基线发病率为每年每 10 万人口 6~11 例。更有临床意义的是诊断为未破裂颅内动脉瘤患者的破裂和出血的风险。蛛网膜下腔出血的风险，有以下几个患者有关的因素，如年龄、女性、种族和家族史，都会增加蛛网膜下腔出血的风险。多个动脉瘤或曾破裂过的动脉瘤比单个动脉瘤再出血的风险更大——在稍后讨论的 ISUIA 的研究中所谓的 2 型动脉瘤。许多研究都认识到有些危险因素是可控的，如吸烟和高血压。许多与动脉瘤有关的特性能增加破裂的风险，如动脉瘤的解剖位置、大小、形态特征，通过影像或新发症状证实动脉瘤变大。

试图量化这些风险的最重要的研究是 ISUIA 研究（Wiebers et al.，1998；Wiebers et al.，2003）。这些前瞻性的多中心研究根据解剖位置和大小预测动脉瘤破裂的风险，得出了有用的结论。它们确定小的（<7 mm）前循环动脉瘤，1 型小的后循环动脉瘤都有较低的破裂率。所有后循环动脉瘤和直径大于 7 mm 的动脉瘤破裂率都较高。以往观点直径小于 10 mm 的动脉瘤有接近零的出血风险是不正确的。

对芬兰和日本高危人群的研究（Juvela et al.，2000；Morita et al.，2012）和其他研究确定，颅内动脉瘤的年破裂率总体在 0.95%~1.3%。在这些研究中发现的高危因素，除了大小和位置，还包括年龄、吸烟史、动脉瘤子囊。研究结果之间的差异可能是由于方法上的差异和研究的群体不同导致的。

最近的一项调查汇集了以前几项大型研究的数据，能够生成一个统计工具，根据发现具有临床意义的变量来帮助预测动脉瘤破裂风险（Greving et al.，2014）。根据 PHASES 评分（**表 48.1**）预测，来自日本和芬兰（人口）的患者，高血压、年龄超过 70 岁，动脉瘤大小、蛛网膜下腔出血史和动脉瘤的解剖位置都是动脉瘤出血的重要危险因素。吸烟和女性不是达到统计学意义的风险变量。

一些结缔组织病和其他疾病可能会增加颅内动脉瘤发生率和动脉瘤破裂导致蛛网膜下腔出血的概率。这些疾病包括常染色体显性多囊肾病（autosomal dominant polycystic kidney disease，ADPKD）、Ehlers-Danlos 综合征Ⅳ型、马方综合征、肌纤维发育不良和主动脉缩窄。20% 的肌纤维发育不良患者和 30% 的 ADPKD 患者会合并动脉瘤。相比于散发型动脉瘤，家族性动脉瘤患者在动脉瘤较小的时候、患者较年轻的时候就会发生破裂。

总的来说，未破裂颅内动脉瘤的年破裂风险约

表 48.1 动脉瘤破裂的危险因素

PHASES 显著危险因素	P- 人口，芬兰人或日本人 H- 高血压 A- 年龄 >70 岁 S- 动脉瘤大小 E- 其他位置颅内动脉瘤早期破裂出血史 S- 动脉瘤的解剖位置
其他假定的危险因素	女性 吸烟 动脉瘤家族史 影像学监测发现生长 症状性动脉瘤

Reprinted from *The Lancet Neurology*, Volume 13, issue 1, Jacoba P Greving et al., Development of the PHASES score for prediction of risk of rupture of intracranial aneurysms: a pooled analysis of six prospective cohort studies, pp. 59–66, Copyright (2014), with permission from Elsevier.

为 1%。对于具体的每个患者，要评估具体的破裂危险因素，权衡医疗机构的治疗风险，从而决定是否开颅手术或血管内治疗。

血管痉挛

血管痉挛是动脉瘤性蛛网膜下腔出血最有破坏性的并发症之一。通过医疗手段，可以预防血管痉挛的发生，降低患者神经系统损伤的致残率和患者的死亡率。血管痉挛能导致 SAH 患者 7% 的死亡，26% 的脑梗死。

血管痉挛的定义是通过血管成像能看到血管直径变窄。痉挛导致远端动脉供血延迟或减少，痉挛血管供血区缺血导致迟发性缺血性神经功能障碍。50%~90% 的 SAH 患者可以通过放射影像技术检测到血管痉挛，但只有一半的患者会表现出血管痉挛的临床症状，如缺血性神经功能障碍。相反，有些患者在放射影像上没有显示血管痉挛的动脉供血区域出现缺血表现，这表明有其他机制的作用。许多的证据显示尼莫地平有益，可以改善神经系统的功能，但几乎不改善动脉血管痉挛。相反，有些药物如内皮素 1 拮抗剂可逆转血管痉挛，但改善神经系统功能的作用有限。因此，动脉管腔狭窄并不是导致脑缺血的唯一机制。其他因素可能包括组织炎症、微血管血栓形成和线粒体功能障碍。然而，从临床角度来看，血管狭窄与缺血密切相关，预防迟发性缺血性神经功能缺损的主要策略是治疗血管痉挛。

血管痉挛病理

血管痉挛发生在蛛网膜下腔里被血块包裹的动脉。血管痉挛的病理机制是复杂的，人们对此知之甚少，血红蛋白氧化产生高铁血红蛋白、超氧阴离子自由基的形成和内皮素 1 的释放都与此有关。狭窄的血管腔有三个主要的变化。第一变化是血管壁平滑肌收缩，发生在两个阶段：一个依赖于钙和三磷酸腺苷（ATP）的急性期阶段和一个较少依赖钙和能量机制的慢性和可逆的阶段。长时间的血管收缩与血管壁的损伤有关，包括内皮细胞损伤、弹性层损伤和平滑肌坏死。第二个主要变化发生在内皮，血管扩张剂一氧化氮的合成减少，血管收缩肽内皮素 1 的产生增加。第三个变化是血管壁内炎症机制激活、细胞因子和细胞间黏附分子活性增加，导致血管壁细胞外基质和平滑肌的重塑，并直接释放炎症细胞。

血管壁的组织学改变包括内皮细胞的空泡化和紧密连接的丢失，也有内弹力层的断裂，中膜平滑肌坏死，外膜内炎性细胞和细胞外基质增多。炎症细胞和细胞外基质的增加发生在外膜。伴随慢性血管痉挛，平滑肌细胞可能在内膜增殖导致内膜增厚。

发生率

虽然在超过一半的 SAH 患者中可以检测到血管痉挛的放射学证据，但血管痉挛继发缺血的临床征象不太常见。延迟缺血性神经功能障碍（delayed ischaemic neurological deficits，DIND）发生在 30%~40% 的 SAH 患者中，并且似乎发生在出血后血管痉挛最严重的同一时期。

蛛网膜下腔出血量越多血管痉挛越常见。Fisher 放射分级与血管痉挛的发生率密切相关，从 1 级（CT 上没有蛛网膜下腔血）到 2 级（分散的蛛网膜下腔出血或出血层厚度 <1 mm），血管痉挛率增加，Fisher 3 级（蛛网膜下腔血厚度 >1 mm；23/24 例患者发生 DINDs），血管痉挛率最高。Fisher 4 级（脑内或脑室内出血，分散的或无蛛网膜下腔出血），血管痉挛的发生率较低。

据报道，SAH 临床级别增高，血管痉挛率也增加，其他危险因素可能包括年龄、高血压和脑积水。

病程和自然病史

在发病前 3 天，很少出现脑血管痉挛的临床症状，但放射影像上血管痉挛可能出现更早。在大多数情况下，临床表现是隐匿的，但偶尔可能会突然发病，发病高峰发生在 SAH 后的第 6 天至第 8 天，但也可能发生于 3 天内，或晚于 3 周后。血管痉挛的临床症状通常在放射影像学表现出现之前就消失了，这种表现可能会持续 3~4 周。血管痉挛的改变最终会消失，但如果在峰值期间不加以治疗，可能会留下永久性的缺血性神经功能障碍。

临床表现

在清醒的患者中，神经状态的改变是血管痉挛的早期临床征兆。变化的开始可以是渐进的和不易察觉的，可能包括头痛加重、轻微的精神错乱、躁动、疼痛、嗜睡或注意力减弱和认知改变。局灶性神经功能障碍最初可能很难察觉。但如果不进行有效的治疗，临床症状会从细微的发音漂移或单词模糊到更严重的神经功能障碍。这些临床变化可能有其他潜在的原因，如癫痫发作、再出血、低钠血症或脑积水，这些需要通过实验室和放射学检查排除。

血管痉挛影响大血管，受累血管的供血区会出现一系列功能受损迹象，可能是蛛网膜下腔血液最初分布的结果。大脑前动脉血管痉挛最为常见，主要影响额叶，症状包括思维混乱或躁动、嗜睡、失语、小便失禁、下肢无力。大脑中动脉受累可引起失语、单瘫或偏瘫和失用。椎基底血管痉挛更容易出现意识水平降低，而不是局灶性神经功能缺损。

其他不太明确的血管痉挛全身症状包括外周白细胞增多和发热，可能出现于发病的早期。

在昏迷或插管的患者中，血管痉挛的临床症状可能很难察觉，血管痉挛的诊断更多地依赖于辅助检查和高度的警惕。

检查方式

应排除神经功能恶化的其他原因，如电解质紊乱、脑积水、出血。高血压是对血管痉挛的初始反应，高度提示血管痉挛的诊断。

血管痉挛的诊断方法是通过直接或间接测量脑血流量和血流速度判断动脉管腔狭窄。经颅多普勒监测可在临床症状出现前检测到颅内大血管的血流速度增加（**图** 48.1）。虽然廉价和无创，但这项技术非常依赖操作者，并且只检测痉挛在前循环的大动脉。例如，血流速度超过 150 cm/s 被认为是大脑中动脉（MCA）血管痉挛的标志，其值大于 200 cm/s 表示严重的血管痉挛。由于血流速度依赖于心输出量，因此可以利用 MCA 平均血流速度与颅外颈内动脉平均血流速度的比值 Lindegaard 比值（LR），大于 3 表示血管痉挛，大于 6 表示严重的血管痉挛。

脑血流量可以直接通过放射影像学测定，如 CT 灌注成像（**图** 48.2A~F）、SPECT、氙增强 CT。利用弥散加权 MRI 成像可以早期诊断脑缺血或梗死。脑血管直接显影可以通过 CT 血管造影，或导管数字减影脑血管造影。导管造影对操作者要求高，有一定的风险，是有创检查，但却是检测小血管和大血管痉挛的最敏感的方法，检查过程中可以同时行动脉内血管扩张或球囊血管成形术等治疗措施。

脑灌注、氧合和缺氧细胞损伤的侵入性检查方法包括直接脑氧合监测和微透析技术，这些技术已经在临床中用于检测血管痉挛，但这些技术只能提供大脑某个局部区域的信息，如果没有适当的定位，会限制它们的用途。其他不常见的重症监护技术包括连续脑电图（EEG）监测，可以预测血管痉挛的发生。

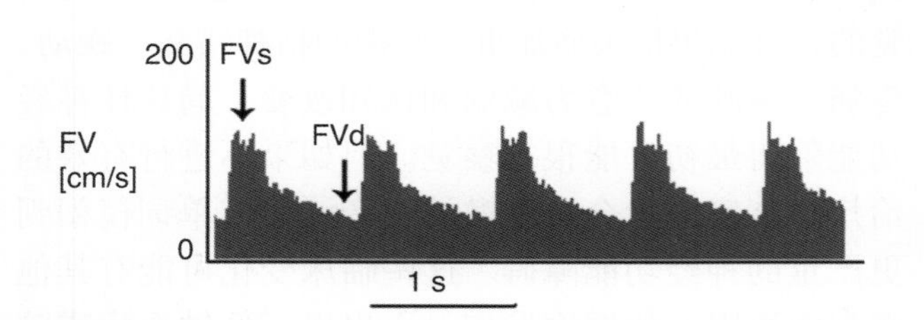

图 48.1 经颅多普勒超声。经颅多普勒显示大脑中动脉内压波形。标记收缩期和舒张期血流速度（FV）。收缩期血流速度用于测量血管痉挛的进展或量化 Lindegaard 比值（见正文）

血管痉挛的监测

早期发现和治疗脑血管痉挛是非常重要的，快速启动治疗措施，可以防止缺血性脑损伤。血管痉挛的治疗也有副作用，因此应该针对确诊的患者进行治疗。通过放射影像技术可以在患者临床症状出现之前就检测到血管痉挛，并且可能是检测无意识血管痉挛患者的唯一方法，可以对最危险的患者进行重点治疗。

血管痉挛的检测在很大程度上依赖于大量的影像学检查，这些方法各有优缺点。经颅多普勒超声无创、价格低廉，但不是每个机构都拥有这种设备，操作者水平不一，解剖学上最好的声学窗仅限于大脑中动脉，也限制它的应用。大多数神经外科中心都有导管血管造影，但为有创检查，操作复杂，需要人员多，价格昂贵，由于有一定的风险，每个患者都使用此种检查方法是不合理的。检测脑血管痉挛的方法不是唯一的，因此，每个机构应该结合现有的各种资源和知识，制订血管痉挛的检查和管理方案。

血管痉挛防治

没有一种单一的治疗或预防策略完全有效地对抗 SAH 后脑血管痉挛的不利影响。预防神经功能缺损主要依赖于通过避免低血容量和低血压来确保足够的脑灌注。每天应给 3 L 静脉补液量，如果患者贫血，可以输血。预防血管痉挛的高动力疗法不一定有用，而高血压可能增加动脉瘤再次出血的风险，因此，血压应该维持正常或者轻度升高，严格避免低血压。必须进行严密的监测，包括血压、液体平衡和神经系统功能观察。

钙通道阻滞剂尼莫地平预防继发于 SAH 脑血管痉挛导致的神经功能缺损（Pickard et al.，1989）。可以静脉注射或口服，每 4 小时 60 mg，在出现低血压的情况下，可以减少剂量或者改为每两小时 30 mg。

如果脑血管痉挛诊断明确，应尽早在神经重症监护室进行治疗，以防止 DIND。血管痉挛治疗的目的是通过增加血流速度或扩张血管管腔来改善脑灌注。“HHH”疗法包括高血压（hypertension）、高血容量（hypervolaemia）和血液稀释（haemodilution），目的是增加心输出量、改善血液流变性和改善脑灌

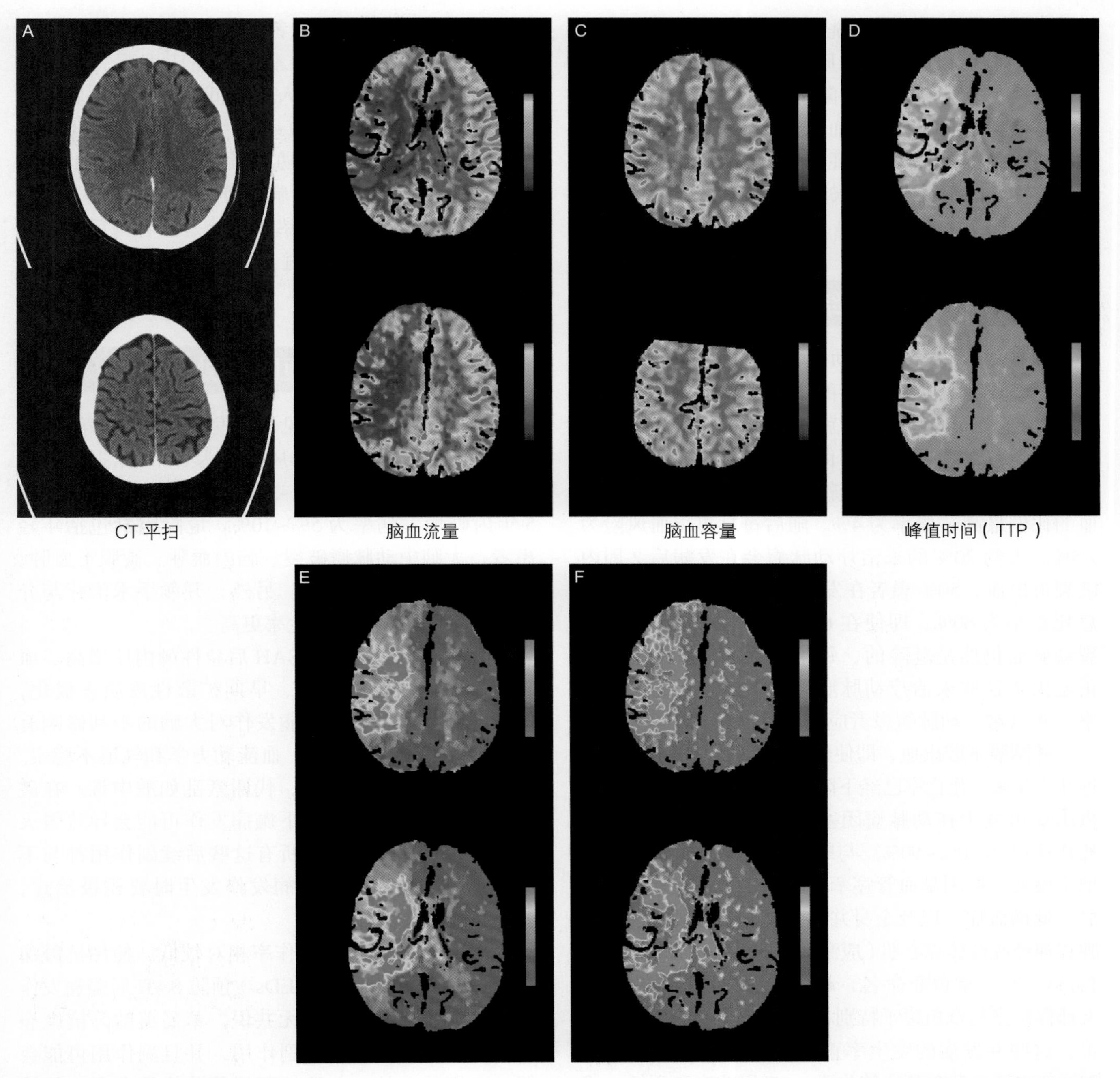

图 48.2　CT 灌注成像评价血管痉挛，右大脑中动脉区域血管痉挛的 CT 灌注成像。（A）CT 平扫未见异常，（B）脑血流量（CBF）图显示血流减少，脑血容量（CBV）正常，表示缺血。（C）CBV 降低被认为是由细胞肿胀和微血管受压引起的，提示梗死。（D）峰值时间（TTP）图显示了血管口径减小引起的对比剂累积延迟。（E）TTP 图显示了 TTP 达到后对比剂从脑血管床退出的总延迟，这是典型的血管痉挛。（F）平均通过时间（MTT）图显示了平均通过时间，即对比剂通过组织的平均时间，延迟是继发于血管痉挛的。异常参数在彩图上很明显

注。静脉输液扩大血管内体积会导致血液稀释。补液量要根据患者的临床反应进行调整，中心静脉压要维持在 8~10 mmHg。超出这个范围没有好处，并可能增加不良反应，如心功能衰竭和急性肺水肿。最有效的方法是使用强心剂和升压药物将动脉压升高到患者神经系统症状得到改善的水平。相对于高血容量和血液稀释，升高血压副作用小，有效性高。

脑血管痉挛的其他治疗方法旨在重塑动脉管腔，以改善脑灌注。诊断血管痉挛后，可以用血管造影的方式进行明确，同时可以动脉内注射血管扩张剂如维拉帕米进行治疗。通过腔内球囊血管成形术可以进行更持久的动脉重塑。因为有再次出血的风险，这两种方法都不应该在动脉瘤未治愈前进行尝试。

早期手术或介入治愈破裂的动脉瘤有助于血管痉

挛的预防和治疗。外科冲洗或者蛛网膜池引流清除颅内血凝块，可以去除痉挛原以降低脑血管痉挛的风险。此外，治愈动脉瘤后降低了再出血的风险，并为安全使用高血容量、高血压以及血管内动脉重塑提供了更大的机会。有一些证据表明，腰椎引流也可能通过将痉挛因子引入腰池来降低血管痉挛的风险（Al-Tamimi et al.，2012），但是，这仍然是有争议的。

蛛网膜下腔出血的结局

即使是经过治疗，动脉瘤导致的蛛网膜下腔出血仍病情严重，有很高的致残率和致死率。多达25%的动脉瘤破裂患者在就医前死亡。未经治疗的破裂动脉瘤的自然预后不良，继发性破裂和再出血是造成死亡的最大危险因素。发病后24小时内再出血的比例最高，概率为4%。随后每日再出血风险为1.5%。大约20%的未治疗动脉瘤会在发病后2周内破裂再出血，50%患者在发病后6个月内再次破裂，总死亡率为60%。即使在6个月后，未经治疗的破裂动脉瘤仍然是危险的，每年持续的出血率为3%。正是由于这些未治疗动脉瘤患者不良结局的高发生率，所以对于动脉瘤患者应该及时治疗。

蛛网膜下腔出血，即使经治疗，死亡率仍然很高。近几十年来，死亡率已经下降到入院人数的5%~10%。再出血可发生在动脉瘤闭塞之前，据报道再出血的死亡率高达70%~90%。与蛛网膜下腔出血相关的其他主要死亡原因是血管痉挛、脑积水等神经外科并发症，低钠血症，以及全身并发症，包括神经源性肺水肿和神经源性休克心肌（应激性心肌病，以日语“Tako Tsubo”——章鱼壶命名，超声心动图显示的左室心尖球样扩张与章鱼罐子特别相似）。随着治疗方案的改善，这些并发症的发生率正在下降。在SAH后观察到的心电图变化包括心律失常、ST段改变和压低，或“神经源性”T波。这些可能是SAH后下丘脑受损伤，导致循环系统内儿茶酚胺过量，影响了心电图的复极阶段。在严重的情况下，也会发生一定程度的心内膜下缺血，这可以通过检测心肌酶来确定。

动脉瘤破裂后，神经功能缺失是常见的。出血、血管痉挛引起的缺血性神经功能缺损和脑积水都可能损伤神经功能。在发病后6周，脑梗死发生率高达26%。血管痉挛是导致神经系统迟发性损伤的主要原因。大约1/3的幸存者遗留中度到重度残疾，尽管大多数存活患者的格拉斯哥（Glasgow）预后评分为4分或5分，但2/3动脉瘤成功夹闭的患者不能恢复到发病前的生活状态。在那些神经功能恢复良好的患者中，只有1/4的患者在一年后重返工作岗位。

不良预后的预测因素包括临床因素、患者自身因素和放射学因素。入院时世界神经外科联合会（WFNS）分级和Hunt-Hess分级（见**第49章**）越高的患者，死亡率和神经功能障碍越高。同样的，在CT上Fisher分级越高，脑血管痉挛的发病率越高，相应增加并发症的发生率。年龄是患者预后不良的独立危险因素，年龄超过70岁，死亡率及不良结局显著增加。

争议——癫痫的预防和处理

SAH后癫痫非常常见，常发生于发病后第一天。急性SAH后癫痫发作的风险约为3%。据报道，总体长期癫痫发病率在5%~27%，ISAT研究人员指出，5年内癫痫发病率为5%~10%。危险因素包括年轻患者、大脑中动脉瘤破裂、脑内血肿、硬膜下血肿，临床分级或放射分级差。另外，开颅手术治疗与介入手术相比，癫痫的发生率更高。

癫痫发病机制包括SAH后急性颅内压增高、血管痉挛、皮质功能障碍、早期扩散性皮质去极化，以及颞叶皮质损伤。癫痫发作对大脑的不利影响有继发性急性颅内压升高、血流动力学和气道不稳定。大脑对氧气的利用减少，代谢紊乱如酸中毒。在破裂动脉瘤未治愈的情况下癫痫发作可能会导致毁灭性的后果，如再出血。所有这些后续副作用都与不良结局有关，所以在癫痫发作发生时要积极治疗，要提高癫痫预防措施。

由于SAH后癫痫发作率相对较低，使用抗癫痫药（antiepileptic drug，AEDs）预防SAH后癫痫发作存在争议，对其使用尚无共识。苯妥英钠等抗癫痫药物可能会产生明显的副作用，并且副作用可能会超过它们的益处。左乙拉西坦等药物具有良好的抗惊厥作用，且不良反应较少，如需要预防癫痫发作，应考虑使用它们。应该在术后一周内预防性使用抗癫痫药物。其他减少癫痫发作风险的策略包括预防血管痉挛及皮质缺血，维持正常的生理代谢参数。

癫痫的治疗包括血液循环和气道支持，以及终止持续性癫痫发作的药物治疗。尽管SAH后癫痫的发生风险相对较低，但是一旦出现癫痫发作，应该应用AED。与预防应用一样，药物的选择应考虑其疗效和副作用。

延伸阅读、参考文献、EBRAIN的相关链接

扫描书末二维码获取。

第 49 章 蛛网膜下腔出血的治疗

Roberto Rodriguez Rubio・Brian P. Walcott・Michael T. Lawton 著
刘方军 译，伊志强 审校

蛛网膜下腔出血的治疗

脑动脉瘤破裂导致的蛛网膜下腔出血（subarachnoid haemorrhage，SAH）需要进行先进的医学处理，最大限度地提高患者的预后。在急性期，处理的重点是快速诊断，通过开颅夹闭或者介入栓塞将动脉瘤隔离于循环系统之外，防止再出血。在接下来的几天到几周，重点转向保证脑灌注，防止延迟性缺血。虽然对各种治疗方式和处理方案有争议，但是外科手术、血管介入技术、对血管痉挛处理的进步，进一步降低了这一挑战性疾病的致残率和致死率。

术前

蛛网膜下腔出血的临床表现

蛛网膜下腔出血（SAH）或蛛网膜下腔周围的脑表面出血，可由外伤性和非外伤性病因引起。总的来说，创伤是最常见的蛛网膜下腔出血的病因。非创伤性（自发性）蛛网膜下腔出血最常见的病因是脑动脉瘤破裂，其他原因包括 Call-Fleming 综合征、硬脑膜动静脉瘘、动静脉畸形和软脑膜转移瘤等。本章将重点讨论动脉瘤破裂引起的蛛网膜下腔出血的处理，着重于预防动脉瘤再出血的治疗技术及并发症的防治。

动脉瘤性蛛网膜下腔出血是非常严重的，在脑动脉瘤破裂前，往往不知道它的存在（或无症状）。据估计，动脉瘤破裂后，1/3 的患者会在入院前去世，即使幸存下来，致残率和死亡率都很高（van Gijn and Rinkel，2001）。因此，了解蛛网膜下腔出血的临床表现和快速诊断是预防或减轻继发性损伤的关键。

动脉瘤破裂最常见的表现是突发剧烈的头痛，患者通常称之为“一生中最严重的头痛”。偶尔，头痛可能没那么强烈，或者很快消失，患者可能不会迅速就医。其他体征和症状包括恶心、呕吐、脑膜刺激征、畏光，甚至意识水平降低（Suarez et al.，2006）。偶尔，也会出现巨大动脉瘤局部压迫导致的局灶性神经功能障碍、脑实质出血、硬膜下血肿或局限性蛛网膜下腔大血肿。此外，由于动脉瘤压迫动眼神经或颅内压增高，会导致第 3 和第 6 脑神经麻痹。动脉瘤性蛛网膜下腔出血也可引起癫痫（Rhoney et al.，2000）。评估动脉瘤性蛛网膜下腔出血患者临床状态的标准是 Hunt-Hess 分级表，这是很具有历史意义的评分表。这个量表是应用最广泛的一种，它将蛛网膜下腔出血的临床表现分为 5 个等级。1 级：患者完全无症状或有轻微临床表现，如轻微头痛或颈部僵硬。2 级：患者有中度症状，除脑神经功能障碍外无其他神经功能缺失。3 级：患者有轻度意识丧失伴有局灶神经功能障碍。4 级：患者中度意识丧失，（如昏迷），严重的局灶神经功能缺陷，或自主神经功能障碍的早期阶段。5 级：患者深昏迷或去脑强直（资料来自 Hunt & Hess，1968）。另一个流行的分级标准是更现代的世界神经外科医生联合会评分量表（**表 49.1**），可用于评估风险和预后（Rosen and MacDonald，2005）。当出现急性脑积水建议行脑室

表 49.1 世界神经外科医生联合会蛛网膜下腔出血评分量表

级别	GCS	运动功能障碍
Ⅰ	15	−
Ⅱ	14~13	−
Ⅲ	14~13	+
Ⅳ	12~7	±
Ⅴ	6~3	±

GCS，Glasgow 昏迷评分

造瘘术。

检查

对疑似动脉瘤性蛛网膜下腔出血患者的诊断中，无论是否进行脑脊液分析，最开始要集中于各种影像学检查。临床病史对确认是否存在蛛网膜下腔出血很重要。尽管脑脊液（通过腰椎穿刺获得）化验历来是第一步检查，但头部计算机断层平扫（CT）的有效性和便捷性已经改变了这种模式。

蛛网膜下腔的急性出血表现为基底池、脑沟或脑室的高密度病灶，在最初 24 小时内通过 CT 扫描检测蛛网膜下腔出血的灵敏度超过 95%（**图** 49.1）。头颅 CT 平扫也有助于判断是否存在由于出血破坏脑脊液吸收功能导致的急性脑积水，以及排除导致腰椎穿刺风险的颅内占位性病变。CT 显示的出血方式，可以帮助引导我们在随后的脑血管成像过程中关注特定解剖区域（**图** 49.2）。

对于有典型动脉瘤性蛛网膜下腔出血症状的患者，如果 CT 平扫未发现出血，可进一步行脑脊液化验，以最大限度地提高诊断敏感性。在患者出现症状几天后才进行医学检查的情况下，脑脊液化验特别有用。在这些情况下，CT 扫描的敏感性降低（48 小时后为 70%，7 天后为 50%），脑脊液颜色变黄提示近期出过血。脑脊液黄染可以通过肉眼观察，理想情况下用分光光度法（测量血红蛋白和胆红素在光谱中的吸收率）进行评估，蛛网膜下腔出血后 6 小时至 3 周内都能检测到脑脊液黄染的存在。影响脑脊液化验特异性因素是高胆红素水平、高蛋白水平和腰椎穿刺中的创伤。

如果证实了蛛网膜下腔出血，下一步的检查是确定出血是来自破裂的脑动脉瘤还是其他疾病。不同的医疗机构有不同的检查模式，但是通常通过 CT 血管造影或导管血管造影获得脑血管成像。三维（3D）重建 CT 血管成像速度快，在检测直径≥2 mm 的动脉瘤时，其灵敏度和特异性超过 95%。血管造影术，也称为数字减影血管造影术（digital subtraction angiography，DSA），仍然是检测颅内动脉瘤的金标准，具有比 CT 血管造影更高的敏感性和特异性。DSA 能分辨小动脉瘤，也能清楚显示周围正常血管。DSA 的局限性在于普及性低，血管痉挛影响造影剂的显示，手术操作相关的小风险及并发症，如脑缺血和腹股沟血肿。

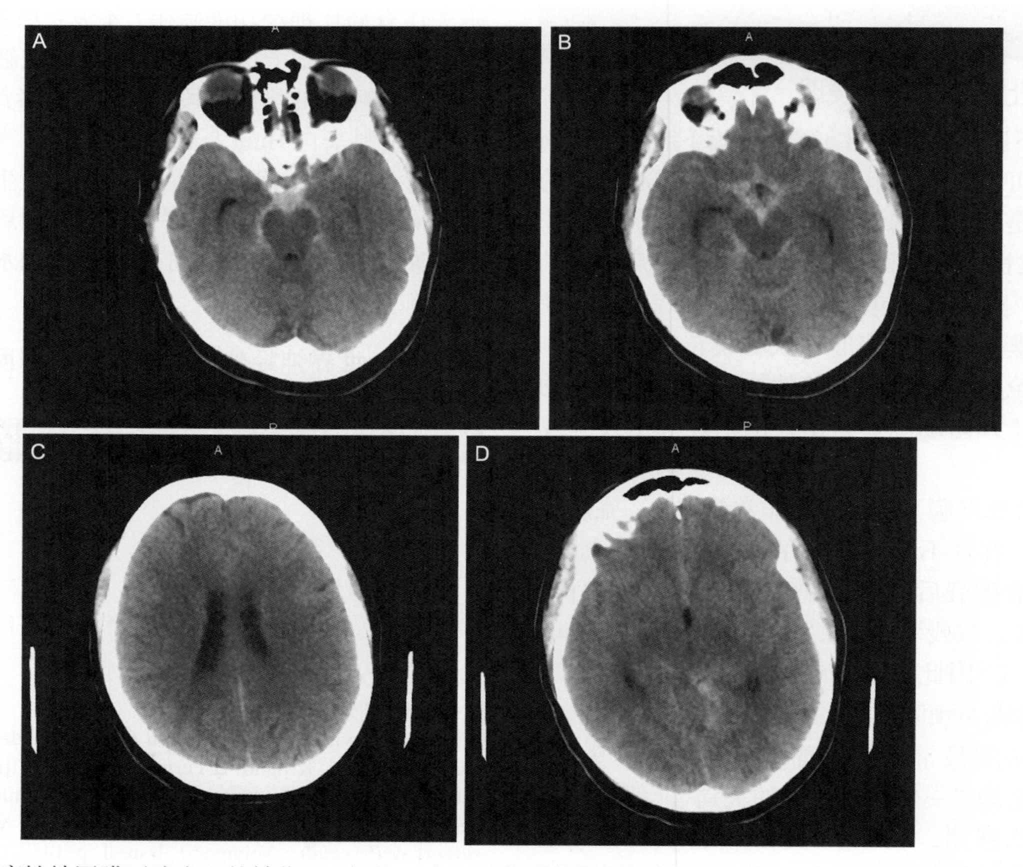

图 49.1 动脉瘤性蛛网膜下腔出血的轴位 CT 扫描，出血延伸到外侧裂和纵裂，A 到 D 是从下向上的代表图像

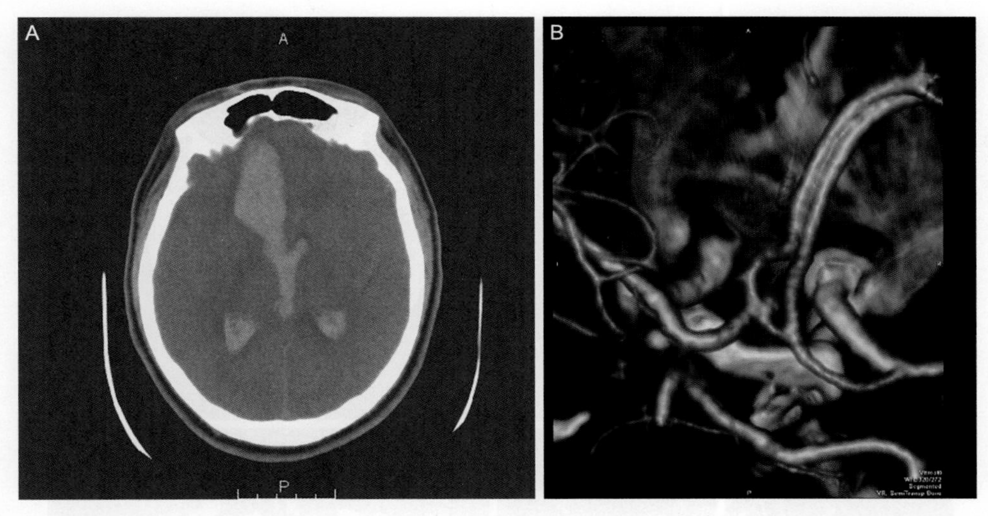

图 49.2　昏迷患者的动脉瘤夹闭术及血肿清除术。一名 35 岁男性患者在办公室工作的时候出现昏迷，发现有脑积水、脑室内出血、轻度蛛网膜下腔出血以及额叶血肿，这是前交通动脉瘤出血的特有模式。CTA 显示一个 5 mm 的囊袋状前交通动脉瘤，指向前方和下方。急诊手术给予血肿清除和动脉瘤夹闭术

磁共振成像是对大型或巨大动脉瘤的一种额外的、补充性的成像技术。它可以提供动脉瘤与相邻结构的信息及关系，如视神经或脑干，以及动脉瘤内的血栓情况。

术前处理

动脉瘤性蛛网膜下腔出血的患者应在专门的医疗中心进行治疗。由擅长脑血管疾病的神经外科医生、神经介入放射科医师、神经重症医师和神经内科医师组成的多学科团队提供治疗，这样才能得到较好的结果（Bardach et al.，2002）。破裂脑动脉瘤的最终治疗方法是将动脉瘤与循环系统隔离，以防再出血。在此之前，我们在重症监护室管理患者，以便立即采取措施防止动脉瘤再破裂，同时保证脑灌注。

许多急性中枢神经系统疾病抢救的核心是维持气道通畅、呼吸和循环。处于昏迷状态的患者需要气管插管以预防误吸，确保氧合，并优化气体交换以控制潜在的颅内高压。我们建议患者进行持续的全身血压监测（通常通过桡动脉插管），将收缩压维持在 140 mmHg 以下，以防止动脉瘤再出血（Connolly et al.，2012）。除了可以通过静输药物来降低血压，通过非药物干预疼痛和焦虑也能起到降压的作用。如果出现急性脑积水，应通过脑室穿刺术引流脑脊液以降低颅内压。

一旦确诊为动脉瘤性蛛网膜下腔出血，应通过心电图和超声心动图对心功能进行进一步评估。而大多数心脏病是自限性的，在制订手术和血管痉挛治疗方案之前，认识到任何潜在的心脏损害是很重要的。心功能异常常见于蛛网膜下腔出血后 48 小时，心电图改变包括高峰值 T 波或脑 T 波、ST 段压低和 QT 段延长。心肌酶轻度升高和心律失常很常见，但通常是良性的。也能见到急性神经心源性损伤性心肌病，表现为显著的左心室收缩功能障碍，由交感神经末梢过度释放儿茶酚胺引起心肌缺血导致（van der Bilt et al.，2014）。

在蛛网膜下腔出血后的最初几个小时内优先考虑的其他处理措施包括选择性给予抗癫痫药物预防癫痫发作和给予钙通道阻滞剂尼莫地平预防血管痉挛（Barke and Ogilvy，1996）。在特殊情况下，如果确诊了动脉瘤，但是几天内没有可用的治愈手段，可以进行抗纤溶治疗。

非动脉瘤性中脑周围蛛网膜下腔出血

当自发性 SAH 不是动脉瘤导致时，出血的模式可以分为两种。第一种，中脑周围型（**图** 49.3），血液主要局限于中脑周围的基底池并且受 Liliequist 膜限制，但可包括近端侧裂池的一部分。第二种，弥漫型，血液扩散进入远端侧裂池或纵裂池。

虽然非动脉瘤性出血有着典型的良性过程，但最近的证据表明，脑积水、血管痉挛和卒中都可能发生，特别是弥漫性出血模式（Walcott et al.，2015）。虽然全脑动脉造影检测出血病因方面具有极好的灵敏度，但它肯定不是 100% 敏感。第一次导管血管造影阴性的血管病变，间隔 1~6 周后可再次行血管造影检查，能提高检测的灵敏度（Grannan et

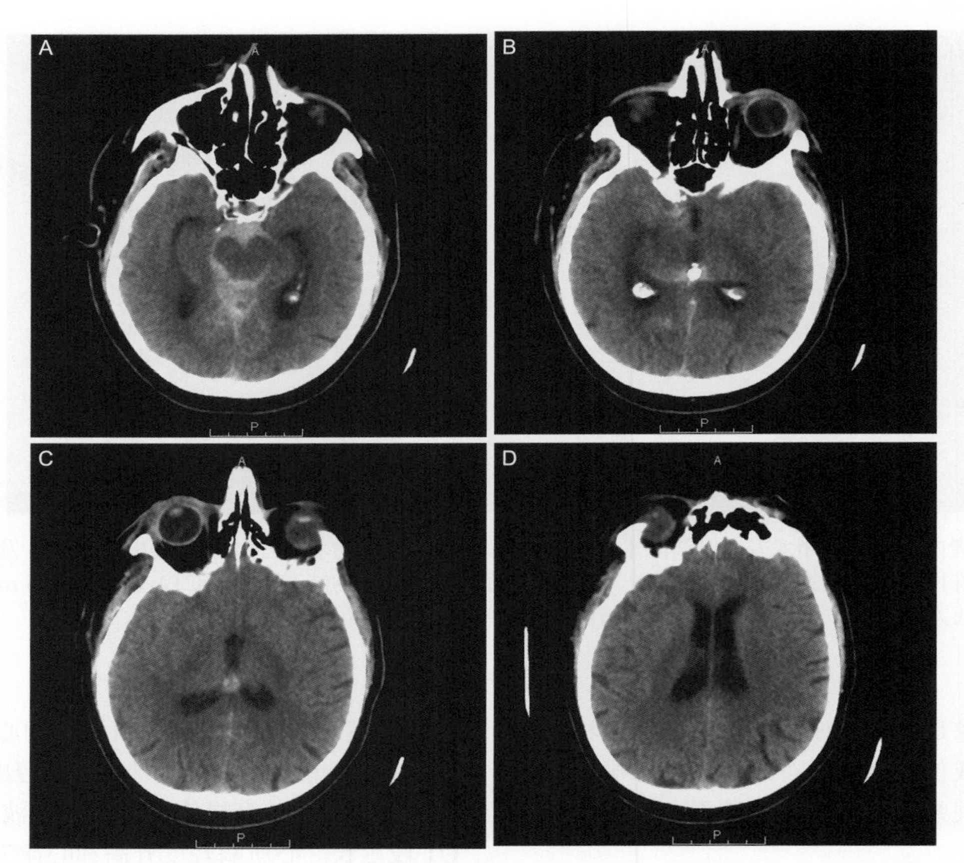

图 49.3 中脑周围出血型。非动脉瘤性 SAH 患者轴位头部平扫 CT，出血主要局限于中脑周围的基底池。典型的图片如 A~D，位置依次从下往上

al., 2014），尤其是临床上高度怀疑血管病变时。重复神经血管成像检查的确切时间和方式未得到前瞻性试验支持，建议主要基于大数据中心的经验。未检出的动脉瘤可能会产生毁灭性的后果，在对这些患者进行检查期间必须保持警惕。

动脉瘤的治疗

动脉瘤的血管内治疗

血管内弹簧圈栓塞是一种相对现代的动脉瘤闭塞方法。在 20 世纪 90 年代早期，第一次使用弹簧圈栓塞技术治疗脑动脉瘤患者（Guglielmi et al., 1992）。与显微外科夹闭相比，累积经验少，长期随访少。然而，这两种方法都已被证明是有效的治疗动脉瘤的方法，以安全地消除流入动脉瘤的血流为最终目标（Molyneux et al., 2015）。一个最近的对美国所有动脉瘤患者手术方式的分析，有力地证实了这两种技术的普及性，目前有一半以上的动脉瘤采用血管内栓塞治疗。某些辅助设备可以帮助栓塞，如腔内支架装置和球囊辅助。使用血流导向装置的血管内治疗，有或没有辅助性的栓塞，也是一种新兴的治疗选择。有了这些方法，许多以前“无法栓塞”甚至“无法治疗”的动脉瘤现在可以接受血管内治疗。

弹簧圈栓塞术

适应证

大多数动脉瘤既可以用显微外科技术夹闭也可以用弹簧圈栓塞术治疗。治疗建议通常是在全面评估不同治疗方法对同一动脉瘤患者的预期风险和益处后提出。这些因素通常与动脉瘤本身结构有关。一般来说，颈体比（长宽比）为 2∶1 的动脉瘤是可以用弹簧圈栓塞的。其他因素包括颈部尺寸（<5 mm，有利）和与邻近动脉的密切关系（不利）。通常有利于血管内治疗的其他因素包括动脉瘤位置（椎基底动脉系统）和患者年龄（高龄）。这些需要个性化分析，必须考虑到单个患者和动脉瘤的所有具体特点。由能够进行栓塞和夹闭的手术者结合临床条件和动脉瘤结构进行评估是最理想的。

技术

患者仰卧位，然后全身麻醉，或者，如果患者在透视过程中能够屏住呼吸并保持不动，也可以在清醒的情况下进行。双侧腹股沟部位都以无菌方式准备，穿刺股动脉（通常是右侧）。接下来，用 Seldinger 技术引入鞘管，由肝素化盐水组成的冲洗系统连接鞘管，以防止血栓栓塞并发症。引导导管，通过 0.35° 或 0.38° 弯曲或 j 形导丝引导，也连接到一个连续的肝素冲洗系统，在透视引导下从腹股沟到主动脉弓，根据动脉瘤的位置，再进入颈内动脉或椎动脉。

三维血管造影（旋转血管造影）通常可以更好地描述动脉瘤的大小、形态和邻近的神经血管结构。根据所想要的硬度或形态选择微导管，然后用导引导管将微导管引到动脉瘤处。通过动脉瘤的形状和测量值决定第一个弹簧圈的尺寸和形状。通常第一个弹簧圈被用来建立一个适合动脉瘤的框架，可以与随后的弹簧圈一起填充。间断的在放置弹簧圈前后行超选择性血管造影，可以确认弹簧圈在动脉瘤腔内的位置，并显示动脉瘤的残腔。当弹簧圈放置满意位置后，术者可以解脱弹簧圈，然后决定是否进行下一个弹簧圈的放置。

弹簧圈展开时的视觉触觉生物反馈、小弹簧圈不能展开、动脉瘤的填充密度以及动脉瘤填充后的残余空腔，是判断停止置入弹簧圈的一些指标。栓塞完成后，调整微导管并进行最后的血管造影（**图 49.4**）。撤掉所有导管，股动脉穿刺处可以用手工压迫止血，或血管压迫止血器压迫止血。

球囊辅助栓塞技术

适应证

宽颈动脉瘤，术中破裂风险较高的小动脉瘤，分叉部动脉瘤，动脉瘤颈上有分支血管发出，单纯栓塞是很有难度的。利用球囊辅助技术，通过重塑动脉瘤颈部、保护载瘤动脉及（或）分支，降低栓塞难度。球囊辅助技术也有助于保持微导管在动脉瘤腔内，减少弹簧圈置入过程中的“踢管”，可以使栓塞更加致密。

技术

与未破裂动脉瘤相比，不能对蛛网膜下腔出血的患者实施肝素化。将一个或两个弹簧圈置入动脉瘤腔内后，就可以使用肝素化。将球囊导管与微导管（通过侧孔）一起置入导引导管的近端。当弹簧圈接近动脉瘤时，用 100% 的造影剂将球囊填充至适当

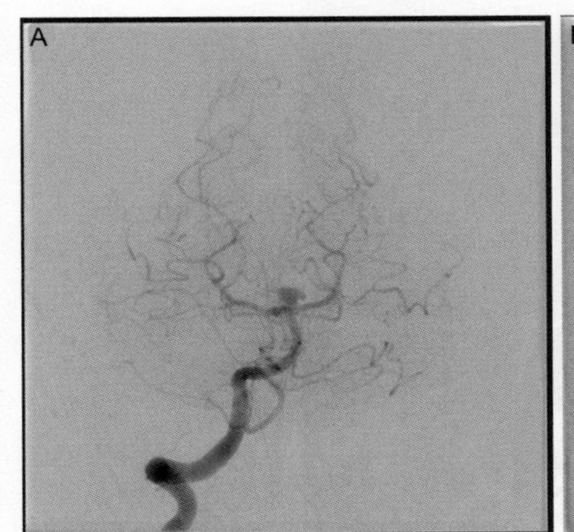

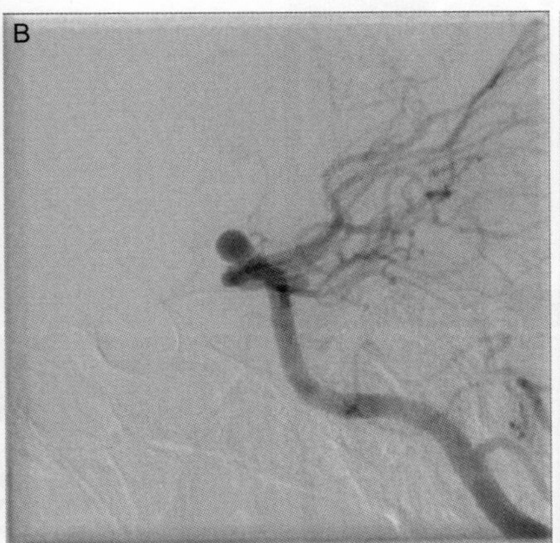

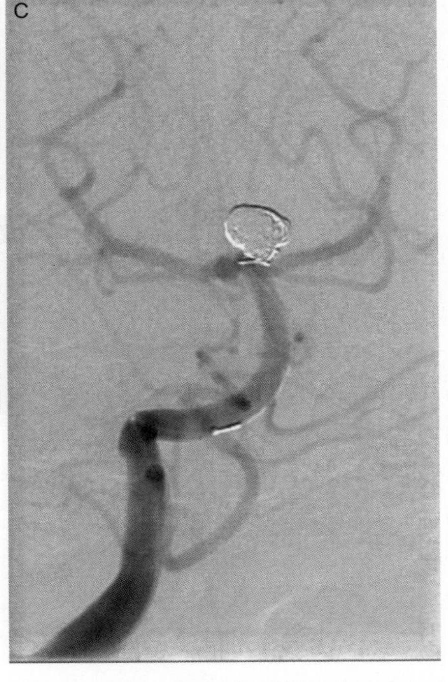

图 49.4 介入栓塞治疗基底动脉顶端动脉瘤。60 岁女性患者，表现为“一生中最严重的头痛”和弥漫性蛛网膜下腔出血。造影发现 7 mm 的基底动脉顶端动脉瘤（A、B）和较小的小脑上动脉和大脑中动脉动脉瘤。根据出血的弥散方式判断最大的不规则动脉瘤是责任病变。用弹簧圈填塞基底顶端动脉瘤（C），患者完全康复

的大小。随后可以继续置入弹簧圈，注意球囊充盈后远端血管的缺血时间。

体感诱发电位和运动诱发电位是一种有用的监测技术，特别是在麻醉患者中。当它们发生变化时，应该松瘪球囊。当弹簧圈成团后，松瘪球囊，评估弹簧圈的稳定性，如果弹簧圈没有从动脉瘤中脱出，从导引导管中撤出微导管。

双微导管技术

适应证

宽颈动脉瘤可采用支架辅助技术或球囊辅助技术栓塞及塑形，这些方法会导致一些血管栓塞的并发症。支架辅助栓塞，患者需要长期抗血小板治疗，这在处理破裂动脉瘤时中可能会产生一些问题。在这种情况下，可以采用双微导管技术，有助于实现更安全、更密集的弹簧圈栓塞，而无须抗血小板治疗。

技术

两根微导管通过导引导管进入动脉瘤腔内。由于单个微导管置入弹簧圈后，弹簧圈会通过宽颈向后脱出并进入载瘤动脉，因此第二个微导管也放置在动脉瘤腔中，在第一个成篮弹簧圈解脱之前，放置额外的弹簧圈。通过这种方式，将弹簧圈顺序置入，它们可以彼此“锁定”；或将弹簧圈同时置入，它们可以彼此“交织”。然后解脱其中一个弹簧圈。释放随后置入的弹簧圈，其中一根弹簧圈连接到推送丝，起到支撑作用。通过可用的导管继续栓塞，直到完成闭塞动脉瘤。这项技术大大提高了弹簧圈的稳定性，可以在不放置支架的情况下对一些宽颈动脉瘤进行弹簧圈栓塞治疗。

血管内弹簧圈栓塞的主要并发症

破裂动脉瘤的血管内弹簧圈栓塞并发症发生率低，常见于栓塞导致的卒中（4%~5%）、术中动脉瘤破裂（7%）（图 49.5）、弹簧圈移位、动脉瘤栓塞不全、动脉瘤复发（20%）、栓塞后动脉瘤再出血、造影剂肾病、腹股沟血肿（Owen et al.，2015；Molyneux et al.，2015；Spetzler et al.，2015；Stapleton et al.，2015a）。

虽然弹簧圈栓塞是治疗破裂动脉瘤的一线方法，

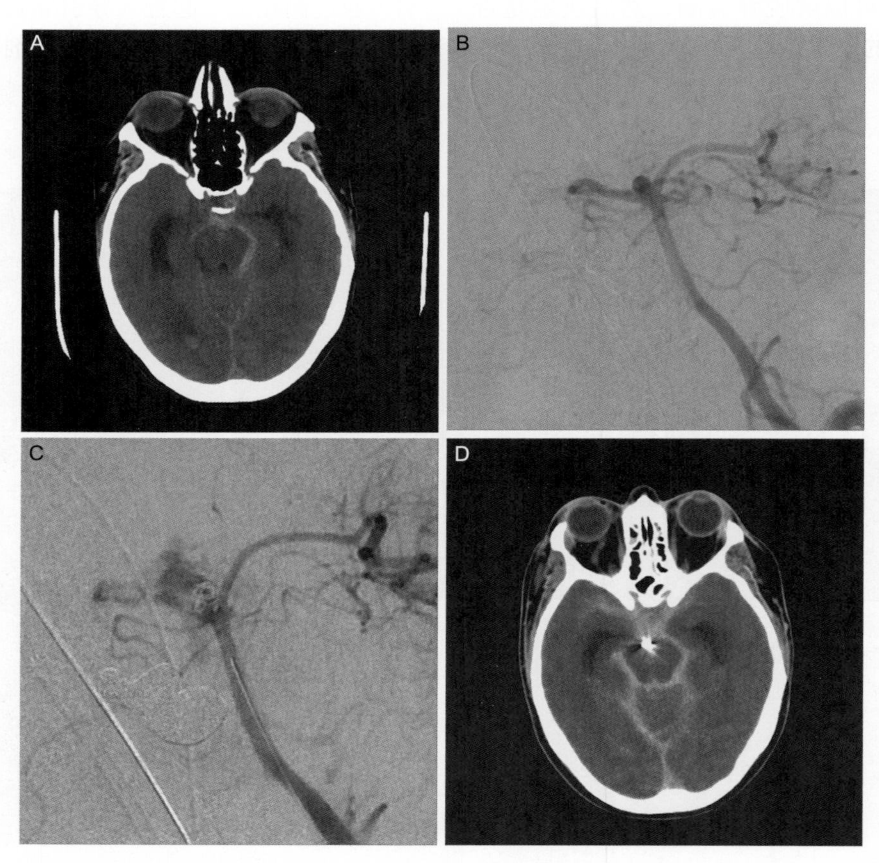

图 49.5 基底动脉尖动脉瘤栓塞术中破裂。（A）轴位 CT 显示破裂的基底动脉尖动脉瘤所致蛛网膜下腔出血。（B 和 C）右前斜位造影显示破裂的基底动脉尖动脉瘤（B）和活动性造影剂外渗（C），发生于弹簧圈栓塞术中破裂。（D）轴位 CT 显示基底动脉尖动脉瘤术中破裂后蛛网膜下腔出血增多和造影剂积聚

尚需考虑复发动脉瘤的后期再治疗（血管内治疗和可能的手术治疗）。栓塞术后复发的因素包括动脉瘤大小、长宽比、绝对宽颈、动脉瘤内血栓、吸烟、随访时间、家族倾向、填塞 / 堵塞的弹簧圈的质量、出血形式。治疗适应证尚未确定，要考虑复发的程度和比率、年龄、再出血以及临床医生 / 患者的选择。

显微外科手术夹闭动脉瘤

时间最长的治疗脑动脉瘤的标准方法是动脉瘤夹闭术。Dandy 于 1937 年完成了首例动脉瘤夹闭术，随着 Yasargil 引入显微技术，动脉瘤夹闭术已经发展成为并发症发生率低、效果好、精细精致的手术。器械和技术的进步水平代表着血管内治疗的最新进展，显微外科也不例外。新技术和术中影像的发展降低了开放性动脉瘤手术创伤，对患者更有吸引力，并逐渐降低了手术风险。动脉瘤夹闭术对于形状不规则的复杂的动脉瘤或血管内治疗失败的动脉瘤尤其有效（Davies and Lawton，2014）。

动脉瘤的手术入路主要取决于动脉瘤的位置。大多数位于前循环的动脉瘤（前交通动脉瘤、后交通动脉瘤、大脑中动脉分叉动脉瘤）可以通过翼点入路，根据动脉瘤的解剖结构有细微的变化。起源于大脑前动脉远端（A2 段及以上）的动脉瘤，通常采用双额叶开颅和半球间入路。对于上基底干动脉瘤（基底动脉顶端动脉瘤、小脑上动脉瘤），翼点开颅加眶颧部切除，充分分离侧裂，可以缩短安全到达这些病变所需的手术路径。其他后循环动脉瘤，如小脑后下动脉瘤，一般通过远外侧开颅手术入路，而椎基底动脉交界处的动脉瘤可通过乙状窦后开颅手术入路。显微外科手术的全部手术路径包括颞下、乙状窦前、经岩骨、枕下、眶上、经眼睑及其组合或演变。选择开颅术式是为了既要充分显示动脉瘤，又要尽可能地减少对脑组织的牵拉。

翼点开颅经外侧裂入路

额颞蝶骨开颅术，又称翼点开颅术，是动脉瘤外科医生最常见的开颅术式，因为大多数动脉瘤发生在前循环。它能够显露额顶岛盖，分离外侧裂进入 Willis 环。简言之，患者颅骨固定，头部向动脉瘤对侧旋转 15°~20°，头部后仰约 20°，使得颧弓成为手术区域的最高点。然后给予保护性体位，将头部抬离心脏水平面。弧形皮肤切口于耳屏前 1 cm 从颧弓处，弧形延伸至中线，终止于中线发际后。牵开皮瓣显露颧骨根部后下方和关键孔前方。因为面神经的额支位于颞浅筋膜的表层脂肪层，所以不要进入这层，防止损伤面神经额支。从颧弓沿皮肤切口切开颞肌至颞上线，沿颞上线下 1 cm 至关键孔。颞肌向翻，沿颞上线留一筋膜和肌肉条，用于在关颅时缝合肌肉，改善美容。接下来，在颞上线后方钻孔，并使用高速钻进行额颞开颅术。游离骨瓣后，用磨钻磨除翼点和蝶骨小翼，一直到眶上裂。当显露了连接前颅窝和中颅窝之间眼眶的脂肪时，就说明骨质磨除充分了。半圆形切开硬脑膜并向前翻转，多处用丝线牵开硬膜。显露完成后，应直接显示侧裂两侧的额叶和颞叶，视线从硬膜到颈动脉池应该完全无遮挡。

双额开颅前纵裂入路

双额开颅术是一种标准化的技术，用于纵裂入路治疗大脑前动脉远端动脉瘤，如胼周动脉瘤。这些动脉瘤通常位于中线，但深至大脑镰。因此，只需显露一侧就可以。双额开颅的特点（骨瓣只有一小部分越过对侧）允许用缝线牵拉上矢状窦，从而可以直视动脉瘤。患者仰卧位，头部居中，对于更远端的动脉瘤，头部可以偏向一侧，与地面呈 45° 倾斜。对于右侧入路，因为开颅偏于右侧，切口开始于右侧颧骨，结束于对侧颞上线。然后将皮瓣向前翻，显露从同侧颞上线到对侧眉间的眶上额骨。颞肌应不受干扰。铣下稍过中线的矩形骨瓣，2/3 位于冠状缝前。从颅骨内面剥离硬脑膜时要小心防止静脉窦损伤。半圆形剪开硬脑膜，其基底处为上矢状窦。可见纵裂，沿蛛网膜下腔向下分离就能显示动脉瘤。

额眶颧开颅经外侧裂入路

额眶颧入路大大提高了标准翼点开颅术的显露程度，最大限度地减少了牵拉，提高了对大的、巨大的或复杂的前循环动脉瘤以及上基底干动脉瘤的可操作性。也给深部搭桥旁路手术提供了操作空间。彻底去除眶壁，硬膜瓣翻向下方，去除颧弓，神经外科医师手术可达范围包括眶上、侧裂、颞前、颞下等区域。手术路径可以根据动脉瘤的确切位置进行调整。改良的额眶颧入路在不需要增加显露的情况下可以不断颧弓，保留颧弓的完整性。

远外侧开颅术脑桥延髓前入路

远外侧开颅术为大多数小脑后下动脉瘤提供了良好的通路。患者采用坐位或病变侧朝上的 3/4 俯卧位。上方的手臂用软垫吊带托住挂在手术床的末端。然后从三个方位来固定头位：①头屈曲，直到下颌与胸骨相距一个手指的间距；②头向病变对侧旋转

45°（使鼻子向下朝向地板）；③身体向地板侧向弯曲 30°。这些动作使斜坡垂直于地面，使神经外科医生可以向下观察椎动脉的轴线。同侧乳突位于最高点。用布带将患者的同侧肩部牵开，以打开颈枕下角。虽然存在变化，但经典的"曲棍球棒"切口如下：首先从颈部中线开始，下方起于 C4 棘突，上方至于枕骨粗隆，沿上颈线向外侧延伸至乳突，向下至乳突尖。下一步，去除 C1 后弓到双侧椎动脉沟。其次，去除从下方枕骨大孔到上方单侧横窦水平的枕骨，尽量向外，然后再回到枕骨大孔。开颅后，用咬骨钳和高速磨钻更大范围地打开枕骨大孔，去除部分对侧枕骨。最后，磨除枕髁的后内侧 2/3。髁突磨除的前界到髁导静脉或硬膜开始向内侧弯曲时，可以沿硬膜切线平面进行观察。磨除髁突可以使硬脑膜瓣完全平坦地反折到髁突上，这类似于翼点开颅术中将蝶骨嵴磨平。

弧形硬膜切口从颈部中线开始，穿过环窦，达骨窗外侧缘。切开硬膜后，显露椎动脉颅内段及延髓外侧和小脑下方夹角处的手术操作空间（Rodríguez-Hernández and Lawton，2011）。

颅内手术技术

夹闭动脉瘤的过程比开颅手术要复杂得多，不是简单将动脉瘤夹夹到动脉瘤颈。有许多的手术细节，如蛛网膜下腔分离技术和突发情况处理，这些都对患者的预后产生影响（Lawton，2011）。

在动脉瘤手术中，重点在于仔细、广泛地分离蛛网膜下腔。通过在高倍镜下打开蛛网膜下腔，不损伤脑组织的情况下显露到动脉系统的手术通路。这项技术包括三种基本操作：显微剪刀剪开、双极镊扩张和略微弯曲的钝头剥离子（如 Rhoton #6）剥离。通过开放这些天然的脑池，分开额叶和颞叶，引流脑脊液，无需过度操作或牵开脑组织就可以接近动脉瘤。以前交通动脉瘤为例，首先解剖外侧裂，然后从颈动脉到视交叉再到终板池。

外科医生要按照动脉瘤近心端、动脉瘤远心端、动脉瘤颈的顺序进行显露，但是由于动脉瘤体和穿通动脉的阻挡，常使得操作复杂困难。在此期间，可以选择性临时阻断，加强手术医生的信心，使动脉瘤体变软，更好地显示穿支动脉。巴比妥类药物能抑制脑电图（EEG）并提高全身血压，有助于防止缺血，但最重要的是提高手术效率和选择性使用临时阻断。当一切都准备好后，始终在完全直视的情况下进行永久夹闭。各种类型的夹闭已经定形：简单夹闭、多个交叉夹闭、堆叠夹闭、重叠夹闭以及这些类型的组合。串联夹闭，用开窗夹夹闭动脉瘤颈的远端，然后用较短动脉瘤夹夹闭未被开窗动脉瘤夹覆盖的瘤颈近端，也是一种非常有效的技术。串联夹闭利用了一个物理特性，即开窗夹的力量在夹的远端最大。这样可以使夹持力均匀分布在整个动脉瘤颈部，防止血流再通。

无法控制的动脉瘤术中出血是神经外科最可怕的并发症之一，如何处理，决定了患者的生死。对术中动脉瘤破裂的处理应以平静有序的方式进行：填塞、吸引、用临时阻断夹近端控制、永久性动脉瘤夹夹闭。可以用小的棉片压迫在破裂处，吸引器吸除术区的血液。近端控制减缓出血，通常能够完成分离及夹闭。用永久动脉瘤夹夹闭后，无论是否出现术中破裂或其他情况，术者必须花时间检查一下，检查动脉瘤是否闭塞，载瘤动脉及远心端是否通畅，穿通动脉是否通畅，以及是否有动脉瘤颈残留。尽管有些中心继续使用术中导管血管造影，我们常规使用术中吲哚菁绿血管造影进行检查（Raabe et al.，2005）。

动脉瘤的特殊注意事项和位置

前交通动脉瘤是最具有挑战性的。A1 和 A2 构成"H"形，术中要分清这些结构，确保不会误夹分支。在分离过程中，手术路径要保证动脉瘤相关血管的安全。对于向前突出的动脉瘤，分离过程如下：同侧 A1 和同侧 A2 的外缘，然后是对侧 A1 和 A2。相反，对于向下突出的动脉瘤，因为对侧 A1 被动脉瘤底遮挡，顺序变为同侧 A1 和 A2，对侧 A2 和被动脉瘤体遮挡的对侧 A1。如果动脉瘤和视交叉粘连，不适当地牵拉额叶，容易导致动脉瘤过早破裂（解剖学细节详见**第 46 章**）。

对于向上突起的动脉瘤，先分离同侧及对侧 A1，这样能够实现近端控制，然后分离双侧 A2。这种动脉瘤可能是最难夹闭的，通常需要跨过同侧 A2 的开窗动脉瘤夹，避免动脉瘤颈有残留。有时，尽管有可能导致相关穿支动脉的损伤，但有些前交通动脉瘤需要夹闭整个前交通动脉。

对于颈内动脉瘤（后交通动脉瘤和脉络膜前动脉瘤），术中头部旋转的程度取决于动脉瘤基底的体表投影。对于动脉瘤向后突出的，需要更大程度的头部旋转才能从颈内动脉后面显露动脉瘤的颈部。对于侧向突出的动脉瘤，必须注意颞叶的牵拉，因为颞叶可能附着在动脉瘤上，并且有过早破裂的危险。脉络膜前动脉分支有可能双干，与动脉瘤颈关系密切，识别和保存所有这些分支非常重要。胚胎性大脑后动脉非常重要，但是常与动脉瘤的形成有关。对于颈内动脉分叉动脉瘤，需要仔细识别和解剖内侧和外侧豆纹动脉，以避免被动脉瘤夹夹闭。在这个位置的动脉瘤夹特别容易扭曲载瘤动脉。

大脑中动脉（middle cerebral artery, MCA）动脉瘤夹闭需要对整个动脉瘤进行充分的解剖显露，因为M2分支数目经常变化。这些动脉瘤可能需要“动脉瘤夹重建”（即使用多个动脉瘤夹在不损害远端分支的情况下，将整个动脉瘤颈部夹闭）。

胼胝体周围动脉瘤是一个挑战，因为在识别和控制载瘤动脉之前会遇到动脉瘤的阻挡。然而，通过胼胝体周围动脉的血流明显低于Willis环底部的大动脉，术中破裂更容易控制。影像导航是一个有用的辅助手段，便与设计开颅及计划手术路径。

治疗复杂动脉瘤的先进技术

对于什么是难治性动脉瘤没有标准的定义，尽管可以认为不能直接夹闭或栓塞治疗的动脉瘤是复杂的。复杂动脉瘤也被描述为最大直径超过10 mm，或有腔内血栓形成，之前栓塞过，严重钙化，或有梭形或血泡样动脉瘤（**图**49.6）。治疗这些病变往往需要先进的技术或辅助设备。

先进的血管内技术

颅内支架辅助栓塞

对于某些宽颈动脉瘤，需要使用支架支撑将弹簧圈放置到动脉瘤腔中。支架丝可以“囚禁”动脉瘤内的弹簧圈，防止弹簧圈脱出进入载瘤动脉（**图**49.7）。由于支架等腔内装置容易发生血栓栓塞并发症，患者通常接受为期数月的双联抗血小板治疗，至少给予长期的某种形式的抗血小板治疗。新一代的支架现在有“低轮廓”配置（使用编织设计），有更好的顺应性，能顺应载瘤动脉的形态，比以前的血管支架更可靠和更均匀贴壁。“婴儿”支架用于远端颅内循环动脉瘤的栓塞正在评估中。

腔内血流导向

血流导向支架是一种相对较新的脑动脉瘤治疗方法，其腔内血流被重新导向载瘤动脉远心端，而不是动脉瘤内。这是通过使用一个低孔隙率网状编织支架来实现的。有时也会在动脉瘤内放置辅助弹簧圈，以立即关闭动脉瘤，防止“球阀”血流动力学效应引起的迟发性出血，这种假设效应可能在小比例治疗后患者中发生。已经报道了转流支架治疗颈内动脉海绵状段和床旁段动脉瘤的一些良好的初步结果（Brinjikji et al.，2013）。但载瘤动脉血流的重新定向会导致穿支动脉缺血，限制了该方法在其他血管领域广泛应用。

囊内扰流装置

另一个相对较新的血管内治疗模式是囊内分流，在动脉瘤囊内放置一个装置（编织血管内桥“WEB”装置），提供一个穿过动脉瘤宽颈的血流屏障，最终重建载瘤动脉并诱发动脉瘤腔内血栓形成和闭塞。该装置主要用于宽颈分叉动脉瘤，如颈动脉末端、基底动脉尖和大脑中动脉分叉处的动脉瘤，具有良好的初步结果（Lubicz et al.，2013）。然而，这种装置的临床经验仍然有限，在许多国家，如美国，它仍

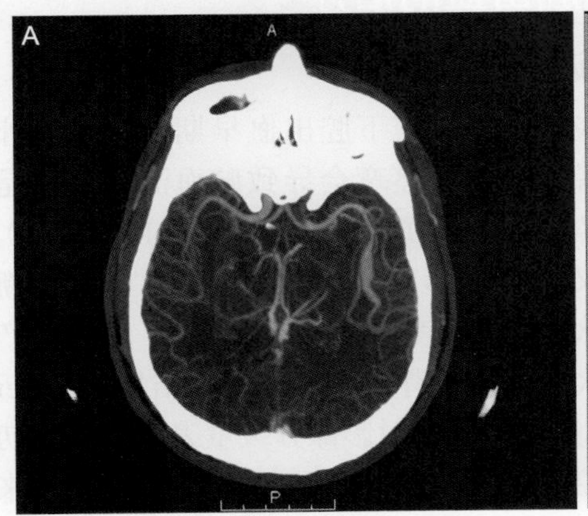

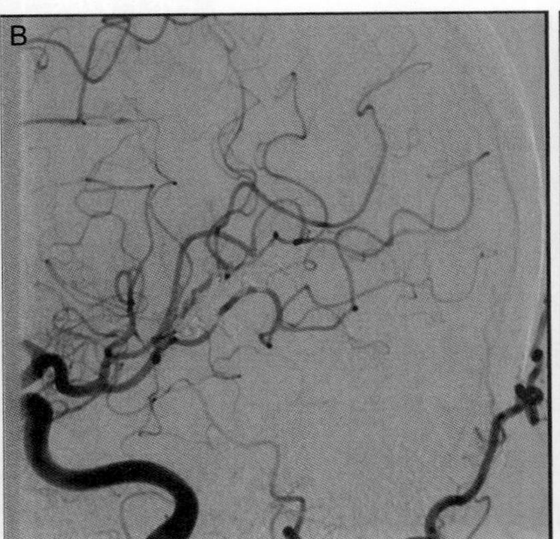

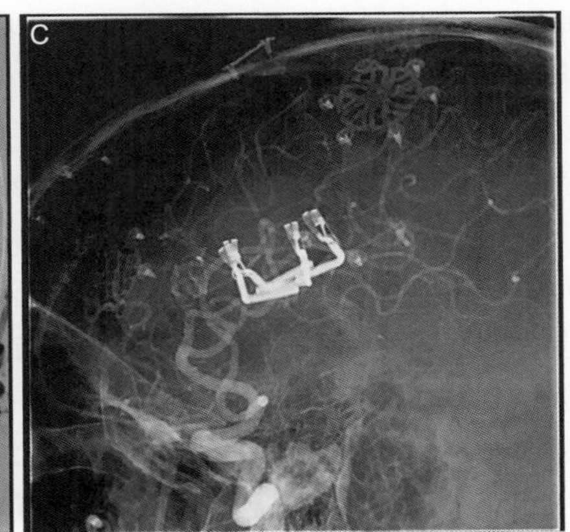

图49.6　梭形夹层动脉瘤的复杂血管重建。一名37岁的男性以“一生中最严重的头痛”为症状出现在急诊室。左侧大脑中动脉梭形动脉瘤破裂导致蛛网膜下腔出血。（A）在手术室用颅外-颅内搭桥技术进行血管重建。成功用开窗、直角动脉瘤夹重建血管壁。患者术后完全康复。随访两年的血管造影显示（B、C）重建的M2段没有残余动脉瘤

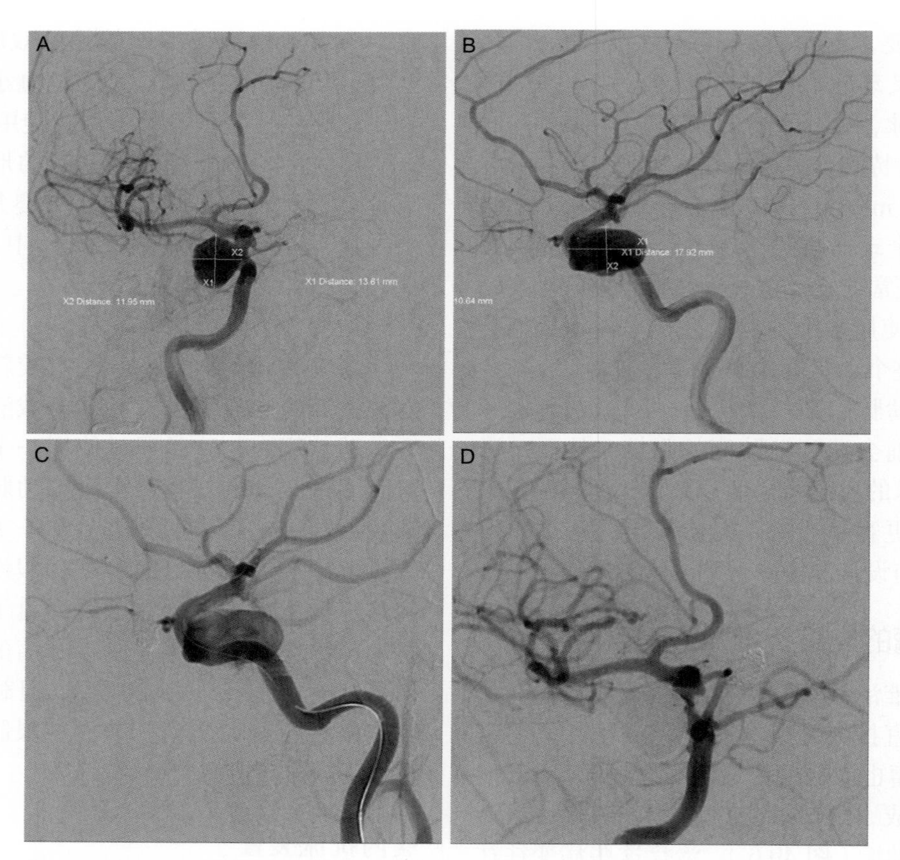

图 49.7 支架辅助颈内动脉瘤栓塞。术前血管造影成像（A 和 B）显示囊性宽颈海绵状段动脉瘤，单独栓塞难以治疗。（C）成功的置入颅内血管支架，并随后进行了栓塞。术后即刻造影（D）显示动脉瘤闭塞。另外一个床突上动脉瘤也被栓塞

在研究中。

高流量旁路手术

对于某些动脉瘤，直接夹闭动脉瘤，重建载瘤动脉是不可能的。虽然这种情况的例子相对少见，但可以看到累及多个 MCA 分支的巨大梭形 MCA 动脉瘤，血泡状或夹层动脉瘤，巨大床突旁 ICA 段延伸到海绵状段的动脉瘤等。对于这些病变，有必要将动脉瘤从循环中排除，同时也要保留通向远端分支的重要血流。这可以通过动脉瘤孤立和脑血管搭桥来实现。通过将动脉瘤远端的血管与供体动脉吻合，可以替代自然循环模式的血流。从历史上看，供体动脉血流是从颈外动脉（如颞浅动脉或经插入移植血管的颈外动脉）获得的，并与颅内循环进行吻合。最近，颅内 - 颅内旁路已成为许多情况下可行的治疗选择，不需要中间移植血管，缩短了旁路长度（Sanai et al.，2009；Abla and Lawton，2014；Davies and Lawton，2014）（**图 49.8**）。随着技术的发展和血管内器械的扩展，旁路手术的适应证有望减少，但不会消失。例如，许多巨大的颈内动脉床突旁动脉瘤现在正接受转流支架治疗。随着血管内技术治疗不太复杂病变的增加，以及先前血管内治疗后复发动脉瘤的增加，需要越来越复杂的外科解决方案，因此，应保持和提高旁路术的熟练程度（Owen et al.，2015）。

蛛网膜下腔出血的治疗

血管痉挛 / 迟发性脑缺血

对于那些度过蛛网膜下腔出血早期并接受治疗的动脉瘤患者，脑血管痉挛会导致脑血流受损，是迟发缺血和卒中的主要原因（Kassell et al.，1985）。血管痉挛定义为在造影或 CT 血管造影上显现的新发的颅内动脉狭窄（轻度、中度或重度），是血液产物与颅内动脉的血管平滑肌相互作用的结果。Fisher 表（**表 49.2**）是经典的放射影像分级量表，它根据初始蛛网膜下腔血液形态和动脉瘤破裂后的出血量来预测血管痉挛的发展。虽然许多患者出现血管痉挛，但只有不到一半的患者会出现症状，在没有其他解释的情况下，出现与放射或超声显示的血管痉挛区

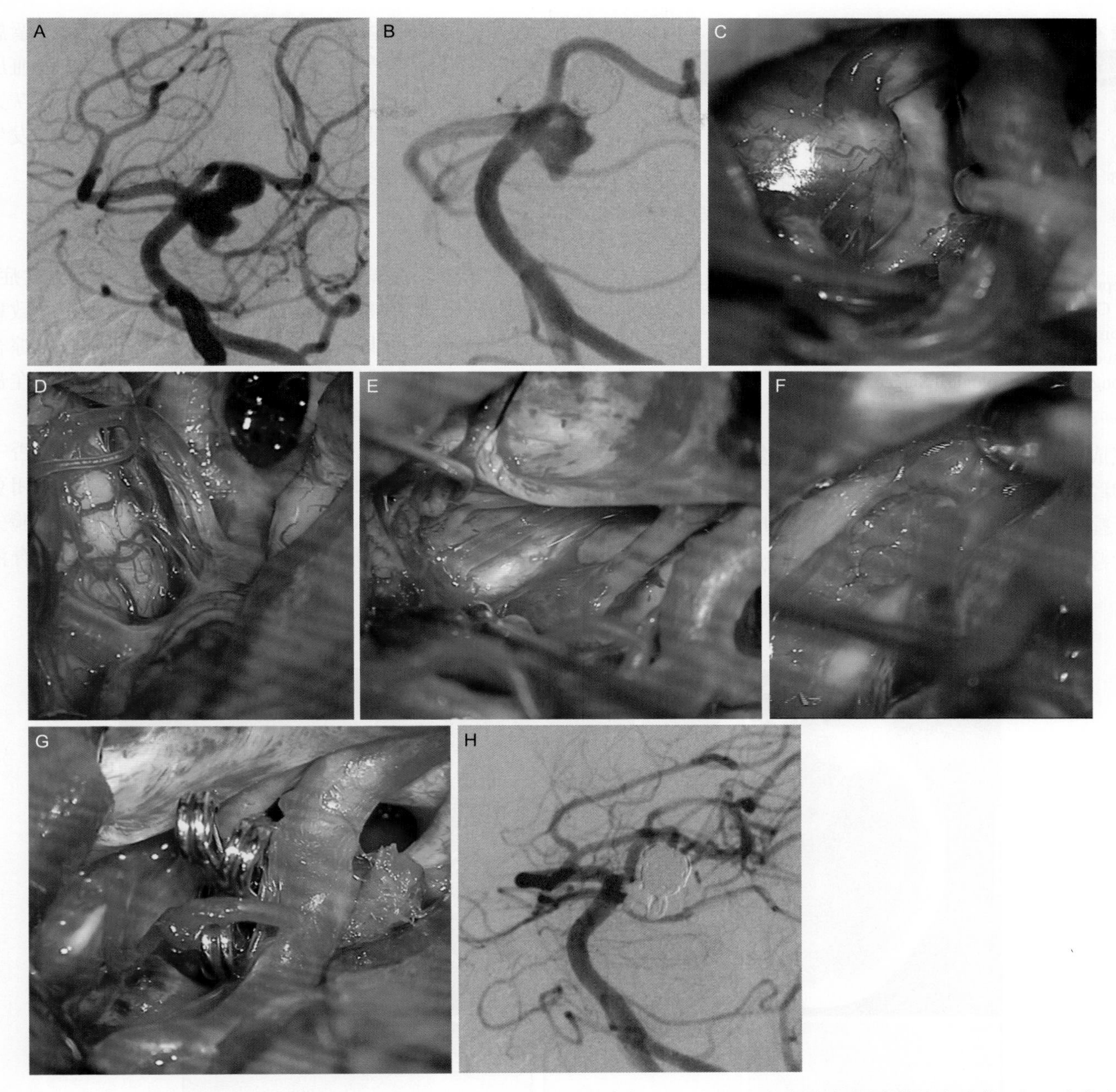

图 49.8 显微外科夹闭颅内转流治疗未完全栓塞的复杂小脑上动脉瘤。（A）无法完全栓塞的破裂的多叶状 SCA 动瘤（右椎动脉造影，前斜位）（B）然后考虑夹闭。（C）弹簧圈占位效应和粘连的动眼神经使动脉瘤不能夹闭，因此采用旁路/孤立术。（D）以大脑中动脉 M1 的颞前动脉（ATA）为供体动脉至 SCA 的 s2 段，（E）通过天幕边缘的切口暴露。（F）通过端侧吻合创建了 ATA-SCA 旁路（G）成功夹闭瘤颈并部分闭塞 SCA 起源。（H）术后血管造影显示动脉瘤完全闭塞，通过 SCA 的血流保留。注意由于来自前循环的血流通过旁路与 SCA 血流汇合，冲刷效应导致 SCA 的 S2 段造影剂的对比度降低

域有关的神经症状。唯一广泛应用的预防血管痉挛的药物是口服尼莫地平，通常服用 21 天（Barker and Ogilvy，1996）。

目前可用的血管痉挛检测手段除了依靠超声或计算机断层血管造影（CTA）的无创成像外，还依赖于一系列的临床检查。灌注成像可用来检测有临床意义的脑血流变化。此外，全脑动脉造影可用于诊断血管痉挛。血管痉挛的任何影像学监测的目的都是在神经系统恶化之前识别血管直径或血流的变化。了解这些变化后可以迅速给予治疗，包括升高血压和动脉内血管扩张治疗（**图** 49.9），如果患者继续出现症状应预防永久性损伤（Athar and Levine，2012）。

虽然实现形式各不相同，血管痉挛的监测可以通过每日经颅多普勒超声和重复的神经系统检查来

表 49.2 Fisher 量表

级别	CT 表现
1	无出血表现
2	蛛网膜下腔出血厚度小于 1mm
3	蛛网膜下腔出血厚度 1 mm 以上
4	任何厚度的蛛网膜下腔出血伴脑室或脑实质内出血

Reproduced with permission from Fisher, C.M.; Kistler, J.P., Relation of Cerebral Vasospasm to Subarachnoid Hemorrhage Visualized by Computerized Tomographic Scanning, *Neurosurgery*, Volume 6, Issue 1, pp. 1–9, Copyright © 1980 Oxford University Press and the Congress of Neurological Surgeons (CNS).

完成。对于由血管痉挛导致的经颅多普勒超声或改变神经状态改变的患者，应给与 CTA 检查。对 CTA 血管痉挛患者或 CTA 阴性或无 CTA 但临床高度怀疑血管痉挛的患者，应进行有或无药物或机械性动脉内血管扩张的导管内血管造影检查。所有血管痉挛患者应在开始血管内介入治疗前接受系统性升高血压治疗。对于昏迷患者，我们常规在出血后第 4~7 天行血管造影监测，因为他们的临床体征对即将发生的缺血不太敏感。

脑积水

脑积水是蛛网膜下腔出血相对常见的并发症，总发病率为 20%~30%。在急性期，脑积水可导致昏迷、脑灌注减少，甚至危及生命的中央脑干疝综合征。紧急脑室穿刺外引流可以纠正这种情况，在最初的神经评估期间要将消除脑积水作为一个因素。

最终，脑脊液外引流的患者需要确定其是否一直依赖外引流，即刻夹闭外引流系统比逐渐夹闭更好一些（Klopfenstein et al.，2004）。对于夹闭试验失败的患者，脑室腹腔分流术是最常见的重建脑脊液

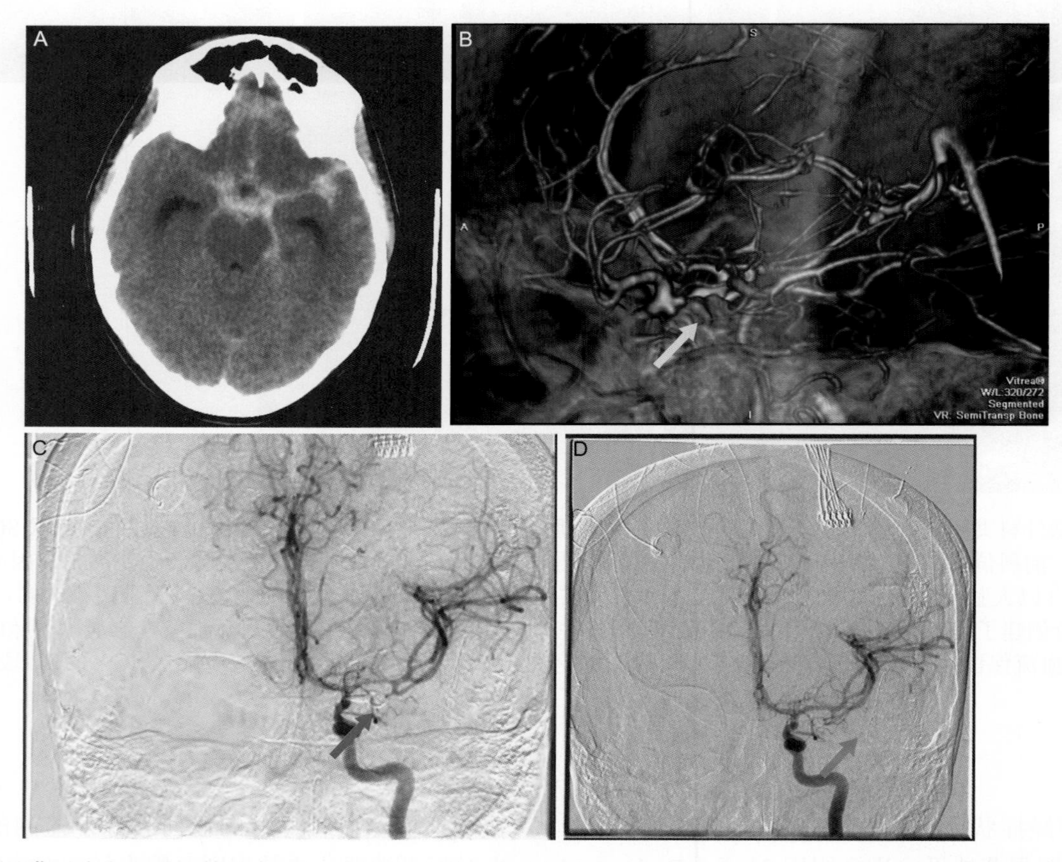

图 49.9 蛛网膜下腔出血和血管痉挛。（A）头部计算机非强化轴位普通断层扫描显示弥漫性蛛网膜下腔出血，（B）三维重建的计算机断层扫描血管造影，显示颈内动脉瘤（灰色箭头）导致蛛网膜下腔出血。（C）4 天后，患者出现右上肢运动无力和找词困难。数字减影血管造影显示严重血管痉挛（红色箭头），左侧大脑中动脉 M1 段狭窄。（D）患者接受了动脉内尼卡地平治疗，影像学显示血管痉挛消失（蓝色箭头）。替代药物包括动脉内维拉帕米。虽然球囊血管成形术具有更持久的治疗效果，但是有更高的手术并发症风险，因此仅限用于局灶性、近端和动脉内药物难以治疗的血管痉挛。治疗后这个患者所有的神经症状都消失了。如果在梗死发生前就开始血管痉挛的治疗是有效的，如果出现新的神经功能缺损，患者应该紧急接受治疗

动力学的方法（15%~20% 的 SAH 患者）。

所有的患者，不管初次住院期间是否需要脑室外引流，都应该在蛛网膜下腔出血后的几周内监测进行性脑积水的临床症状。影响分流率的因素包括蛛网膜下腔出血的程度、术中终板的开放程度和脑室外引流术后的脑室炎。

血清钠和容量平衡

低钠血症是动脉瘤性蛛网膜下腔出血的常见电解质紊乱（Sherlock et al.，2006）。有时，这可归因于抗利尿激素分泌不当综合征（syndrome of inappropriate antidiuretic hormone secretion，SIADH）。SIADH 导致水排泄受损。任何中枢神经系统疾病，如蛛网膜下腔出血，都可以增强抗利尿激素的释放（见**第 25 章**）。水的滞留和低钠血症的发生会对动脉瘤性出血患者的临床进程产生深远的影响。低钠血症可导致脑水肿及随后的颅内压升高和持续性脑缺血。

动脉瘤破裂后低钠血症的另一个不太常见的原因是脑耗盐，它常常预示着脑血管痉挛的发生。在这种情况下，利钠肽被释放，导致盐排泄过多，严重的相对低血容量。在重症监护环境中，正确的诊断和严格控制血清钠水平和容量状态是良好预后的必要条件。

蛛网膜下腔出血导致的这两种情况的治疗包括高渗盐水、肠内补充盐和盐皮质激素。在危重、有症状的患者中，由于担心加重低血容量和增加脑缺血的风险，通常不用限液的方法使血清钠正常化。

蛛网膜下腔出血的预后

动脉瘤破裂引起的原发性脑损伤可能很严重，并决定了整个临床过程（Stapleton et al.，2015b）（**图 49.10**）。无论采取何种干预措施防止动脉瘤再破裂，老年、血肿多或深昏迷患者预后都很差。另一方面，发病时临床分级良好的患者可能会出现血管痉挛，并出现严重的迟发性脑缺血。包括从未到医院或神经外科医生就诊的患者，蛛网膜下腔出血的死亡率约为 35%。总的来说，大多数在初次出血中幸存

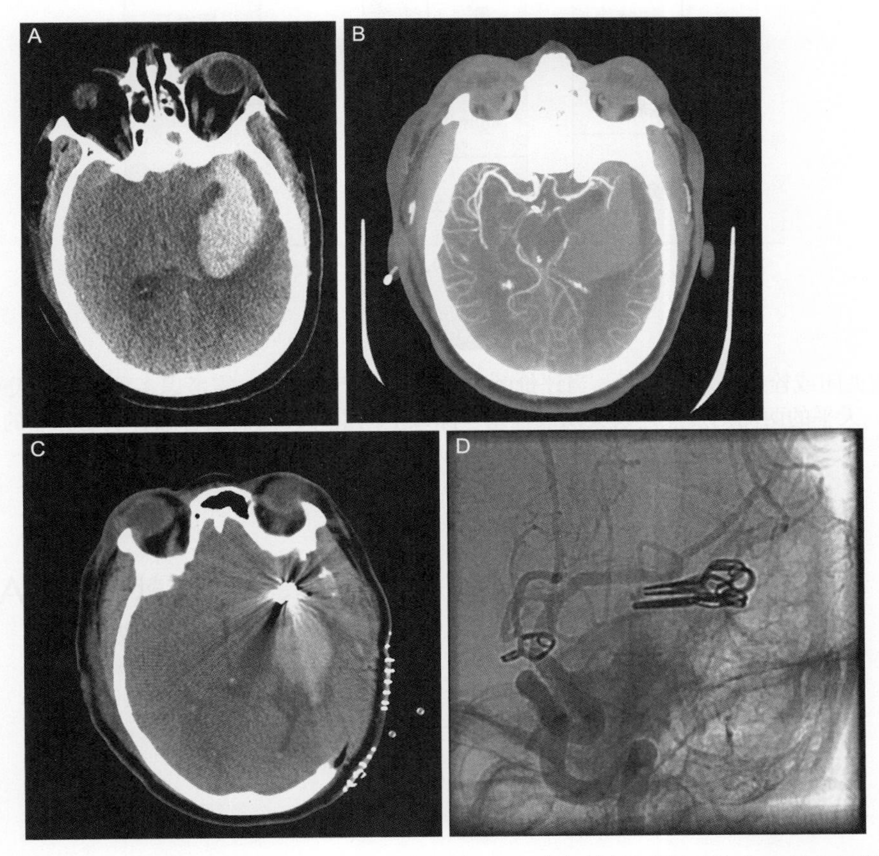

图 49.10　脑动脉瘤破裂伴大量外侧裂血肿。（A）头部 CT 平扫表现为急性蛛网膜下腔出血伴左侧额颞部及外侧裂大量血肿。（B）头部 CT 血管成像最大信号投影（MIP）显示左侧大脑中动脉（MCA）分叉动脉瘤。（C）术后头颅 CT 显示动脉瘤夹伪影，部分血肿清除术和去骨瓣减压术降低颅内压。（D）左颈内动脉数字减影血管造影显示显微外科术后完全夹闭大脑中动脉瘤。手术中同时夹闭了意外发现的前交通动脉瘤

下来的患者，接受治疗后会有良好的预后（约 2/3）（Hop et al.，1997；Vergouwen et al.，2011）。尽管如此，许多患者仍会表现出轻微的认知缺陷（约 1/2）和情绪问题，影响他们的日常生活（约 1/2 对生活不满意），并使他们不能重返工作岗位（只有 1/3 的人重返以前的工作岗位）。尽管蛛网膜下腔出血仅占出血性卒中的 5%，但与缺血性卒中和脑内出血一样缩短患者的寿命。为高危患者制订出血前检测动脉瘤的筛查方案，改进治疗技术，改善血管痉挛的管理，这些努力将继续不断的改善未来的预后。

争议

在破裂动脉瘤的治疗中，持续时间最长的争论是选择夹闭还是栓塞？两个主要的试验已经解决了这个问题，国际蛛网膜下腔出血动脉瘤试验（ISAT）（Molyneux et al.，2015）和 Barrow 破裂动脉瘤试验（BRAT）（Spetzler et al.，2015）。ISAT 组的最终长期随访显示，尽管神经外科手术组的死亡率更高，夹闭组和栓塞组之间的依赖性概率没有差异。但是，三项随机试验（包括 ISAT）的 meta 分析无法显示血管内治疗和神经外科夹闭治疗之间的死亡率的显著差异（Lanzino et al.，2013）。

BRAT 试验虽然只提供了 6 年的随访，对于前循环动脉瘤，两种治疗方式差别不大，对于椎基底动脉循环动脉瘤，栓塞术比夹闭术具有显著优势。选择偏差、术者的技术和熟练程度、外部效度以及治疗组之间的交叉使这些结果的解释复杂化。

“夹闭或栓塞”是动脉瘤治疗计划的重点（**图 49.11**）。患者最好由多学科协作治疗团队来服务，该团队可以根据动脉瘤的特征、临床情况、最佳可用证据和术者的技术水平来权衡治疗的风险和益处。

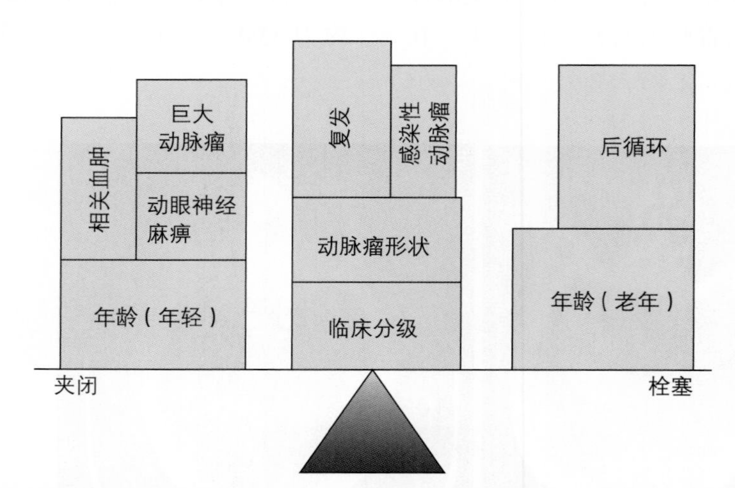

图 49.11 影响动脉瘤夹闭或栓塞决定的因素。当评价颅内动脉瘤治疗方案时，需考虑多种因素。天平的中间是影响动脉瘤栓塞或夹闭的因素。天平的两侧则强烈建议夹闭或栓塞。除以上因素外，尚需结合患者及动脉瘤的具体情况做决定

延伸阅读、参考文献、EBRAIN 的相关链接

扫描书末二维码获取。

第 50 章　脑动静脉畸形和硬脑膜动静脉瘘

Michael Morgan 著
杨希孟 译，陆军 审校

脑动静脉畸形的病理生理学、分类、流行病学、遗传学和自然史

病理生理学

脑动静脉畸形（brain arteriovenous malformations of the brain，bAVM）是脑实质内动脉和静脉异常连接形成的血管团，它们之间缺乏毛细血管。该异常血管团与正常的动脉及静脉系统相连接。这就造成了血流在正常动脉和静脉系统之间的 bAVM 内快速通过，因为该血管床内血流阻力较正常情况下有所降低（以前也被称为“分流”）。大多数 bAVM 引起的临床和病理结果均与这种动静脉分流相关。bAVM 在中枢神经系统无特殊好发部位，与脑叶大小成比例分布。

动静脉分流对颅内的生理影响可以通过该血管系统上的压力分布情况得到最好地说明（图 50.1）。由于血流阻力下降，向 bAVM 直接供血的动脉内的压力低于相应的正常动脉内的压力，类似的，bAVM 引流静脉内的压力则高于相应的正常静脉内的压力。此外，这些供血动脉与引流静脉上的分支血管也会受到这些压力分布的影响。考虑到颅内侧支循环不断适应剪应力的变化，血管系统的病理改变与这些生理性改变相适应。血管的扩张和血管壁不成比例的变薄，或者称为退变，与正常剪应力的增加、较低的局部动脉内压、较高的局部静脉内压和搏动减弱相关。这些均归结于 bAVM 引起的循环阻力降低。这些改变通过内皮型一氧化氮合酶（eNOS）的上调和内皮素的下调伴血管发生因子（如血管内皮生长因子，VEGF）的重塑来介导。因为这些随之而来的从正常血管向异常血管的转变，bAVM 通常没有可以明确辨认的开始或结束的边界，而用过渡区来反映 bAVM 引起的生理性变化造成的病理改变。病变被称为 bAVM 通常要以异常中心血管团（被称为“巢”）为基础。事实上，外科医生、病理学家或放射学家均能指出什么是异常或哪些是正常。但是，bAVM 中反映生理性异常的过渡区通常被忽视，因为通过直接肉眼观察来评估它们是非常困难的。

bAVM 的持续存在引起的许多病理生理学改变会导致临床症状的出现。包括如下几个方面：

1. 高流量的磨损导致 bAVM 血管的完整性破坏、破裂出血进入脑实质或蛛网膜下腔。由于剪应力和后续的血管壁退化：动脉瘤可能发生在 bAVM 间隙（巢内动脉瘤），或者在近端动脉上[相关近端颅内动脉瘤（associated proximal intracranial aneurysms，APIA）]；静脉系统可发生静脉扩张或静脉网。这些脆弱的血管可能在某个时间点破裂。静脉出口狭窄的加重或者静脉内血栓形成导致 bAVM 内压力的突然增加，后者会加速畸形的破裂。
2. 较低的供血动脉内压（相对于邻近脑实质动脉内正常压力）和较高的引流静脉内压（相对于相应静脉血管内正常压力）（窃血）可能造成神经功能缺损和癫痫。
3. 血红蛋白的溢出可造成铁沉积，进而可能形成致痫灶。
4. 因供血动脉管腔的变化和（或）缺血导致的扩散抑制可能造成复杂性偏头痛的发生。
5. 大静脉的牵拉、静脉内血栓形成引起的静脉壁的拉长、颅内压的升高、出血或并发偏头痛都可能导致头痛的发生
6. 静脉窦压力升高有时会导致颅内高压和视盘水肿
7. 在新生儿和婴儿中，肺动脉高压伴心力衰竭可能会发生。

流行病学

至少有些 bAVM 存在先天性起源，因为有报道发现 bAVM 在某些胚胎发育相关的特定组织体节性受累疾病中发现（Bonnet-Dechaume Blanc 综合征或 Wyburn-Mason 综合征）（Morgan，1985）。尽管 bAVM 经常被认为是先天性的，但支持此观点的证

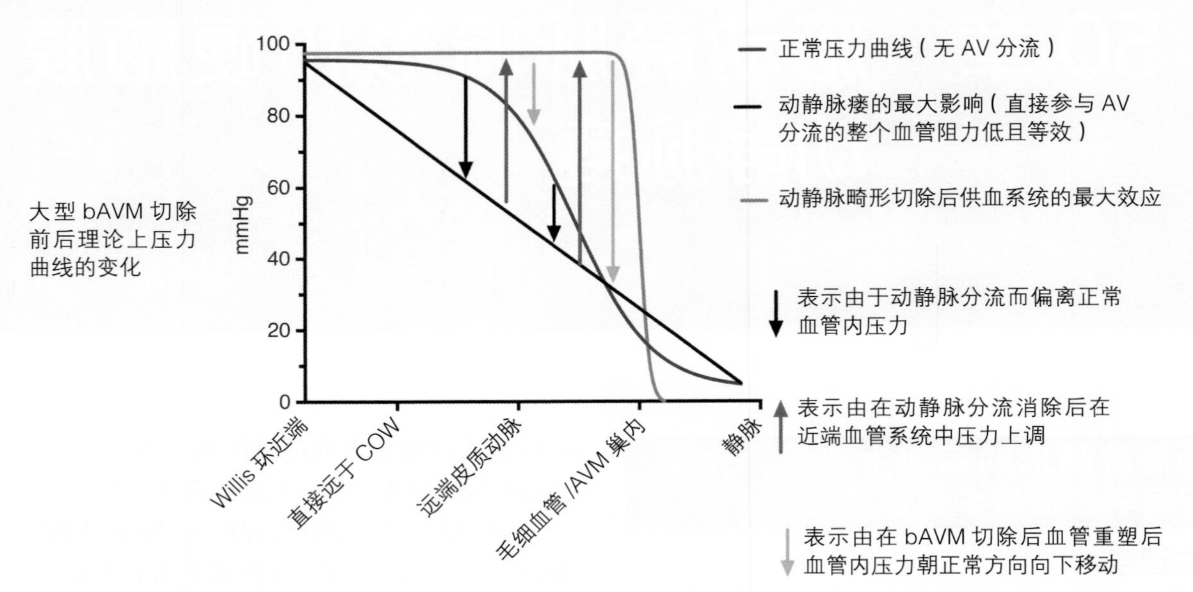

图 50.1 沿着大脑脉管系统的假想压力分布图，从 Willis 环近端的动脉到静脉流出，其中包含 bAVM。蓝色代表正常状态，表明在较小的动脉和小动脉中大多数阻力。当通过动静脉分流存在降低阻力时，压力曲线向黑线移动。这导致动脉压力降低和静脉压力升高。突然切除动静脉分流，当脉管系统明显扩张时，由于重塑前存在的较大的动脉和静脉而产生的阻力较小，因此压力超过正常压力（绿线）。动脉和静脉重塑后，压力分布恢复正常

据受到了各种挑战。有关 bAVM 可以在以后生涯中发生的报道证实了 bAVM 出现具有一定的年龄范围。但是，多数 bAVM 可能从幼儿时期开始出现。bAVM 是可恢复的病变，尽管有报道称部分 bAVM 可自发消失，但这种情况并不常见。对于大多 bAVM，从早期即发生，一生中持续存在，除非有意去除掉。bAVM 年发病率为 0.9~1.5/10 万人，成人中患病率为 10~100/10 万人。

遗传学

bAVM 通常是散发的（除非是遗传性出血性毛细血管扩张症或毛细血管畸形）。有三个 bAVM 发育相关模型曾被提出：发育过程中原始动静脉连接退化失败；小静脉的扩张或原发障碍；Notch4 诱导的来源于毛细血管的动静脉分流形成（Murphy et al., 2014）。

就像 bAVM 的病理学表现是其对动静脉分流的生理学反应，bAVM 疾病本身可能并非一种疾病，而是具有共同表型的多种基因型。这与遗传性出血性毛细血管扩张症（hereditary haemorrhagic telangiectasia，HHT）一致，HHT 是一种常染色体显性遗传病，具有和 bAVM 相似的表型（累及皮肤、黏膜表面、肺、肝和中枢神经系统的动静脉分流和毛细血管扩张）。目前有两个基因的多个突变被确定与 HHT 相关，这些基因在血管新生方面起到重要作用，包括染色体 12（HHT2），影响激活素受体样激酶（affecting activin receptor-like kinase-1，ALK1）；染色体 9（HHT1，最常见类型），前者的受体，内皮因子。

更加密切相关的家族性疾病是常染色体显性遗传毛细血管畸形，表现为皮肤毛细血管畸形和脑、四肢或面部的动静脉畸形（无腹部或胸腔内器官受累），已被描述为具有 RASA1 突变（Eerola et al., 2003）。

自然史和临床表现

临床表现为出血起病占到大约 50%（Stapf et al., 2003；Wedderburn et al., 2008；Gross and Du，2013；Korja et al., 2014），且没有性别或年龄倾向。未破裂的 bAVM 年出血风险为 1%~3%，近期破裂的 bAVM 年出血风险为 4%~6%（Gross and Du，2013；Kim et al., 2014；Mohr et al., 2014）。bAVM 特异因素也影响远期破裂风险。证据支持最多的两个增加出血的因素为颅内动脉瘤（Brown et al., 1988；Redekop et al., 1998；Stapf et al., 2002；Da Costa et al., 2009）和深静脉引流（或仅有深静脉引流）入大脑大静脉系统（Gross and Du，2013）。未破裂的 bAVM 中存在相关的动脉瘤会增加破裂风险，接近于破裂 bAVM 的出血风险（Brown et al., 1988；Redekop et al., 1998；Stapf et al., 2002；Da Costa et al., 2009）。但是，由于存在动脉瘤或仅有深静脉引流的比例大大低于所有未破裂 bAVM 的半数，同时 bAVM 并不常见，因此，应当谨慎使用更准确的破裂风险评估方案。

尽管报道的破裂结局差异很大，但可以合理地估计40%的病例会出现严重残疾或死亡。文献报道中低至10%、高至89%的风险不一致性可以主要通过以下原因来解释：病例的选择，是否在单次出血后进行短期随访，或者是否多次出血后进行长期随访（Drake，1979；Fults and Kelly，1984；Crawford et al.，1986；Brown et al.，1988；Ondra et al.，1990；Laakso et al.，2008；Da Costa et al.，2009；Van Beijnum et al.，2009；Kano et al.，2014）。

非出血性临床表现包括癫痫（25%）、头痛（16%）、非出血引起的神经功能缺损（8%）、颅内高压（1%）和高输出量心力衰竭（<1%且限于婴儿）（Hayashi et al.，1996；Galletti et al.，2011；Gross and Du，2013；Bervini et al.，2014）。这些临床表现及其出现的原因在上文已作解释。

大约25%的未经历出血的患者在10年内功能会下降（Brown et al.，1988）。这可能限于大型bAVM或由于癫痫发作或进行性神经功能缺损所致。

诊断、分级和检查

诊断

确定性诊断可通过数字减影血管造影（digital subtraction angiography，DSA）进行。DSA可以在解剖学上辨认参与的血管结构，也可确认快速的动静脉分流（**图50.2**）。非破裂bAVM在平扫CT上的表现可以是稍高密度占位，边界清晰，被周围正常脑组织环绕。可能有少量钙化灶。非破裂bAVM在平扫MRI T1和T2加权像上表现为血管流空影，通常可以识别出扩张的动脉和静脉。破裂bAVM在平扫CT或MRI上可能被血肿掩盖。MR和CT血管成像均可以辨认解剖学外观，同时动态序列可发现动脉期静脉造影剂充盈，证实存在动静脉分流。但是，如果考虑治疗，那DSA是必要的，因为它可以清楚地显示出完整的供血动脉（这可能包括颈外动脉供血）、引流静脉和血管结构特征如弥漫性、动脉瘤的存在和静脉狭窄。这些结构特征可能会影响到预期的自然病程和治疗风险。

弥漫性bAVM需要与增殖性血管病鉴别，这些病变是对梗死或颅内出血（尤其在年轻人中）的反应，虽然与bAVM相似，但它们缺乏bAVM中静脉引流早显模式。它们不是bAVM，不具有相同的出血风险。

评分

有用的评分系统包括Spetzler-Martin评分系统（Spetzler and Martin，1986）、Lawton-Young评分系统和Pollock-Flickinger评分。前两个预测手术的风险，而第三个用来预测聚焦照射后不伴有神经缺损的闭塞可能性（**表50.1**）。5分的Spetzler-Martin评分可以分别合并为Spetzler-Martin 1和2，Spetzler-Martin 3以及Spetzler-Martin 4和5，对应Spetzler-Ponce A、B和C类（Spetzler and Ponce，2011）。

检查

检查受人口学资料、bAVM相关因素和临床表现所影响。检查可限于诊断性的MRI或CTA，因为预期不会有进一步的干预（例如老年未破裂bAVM），

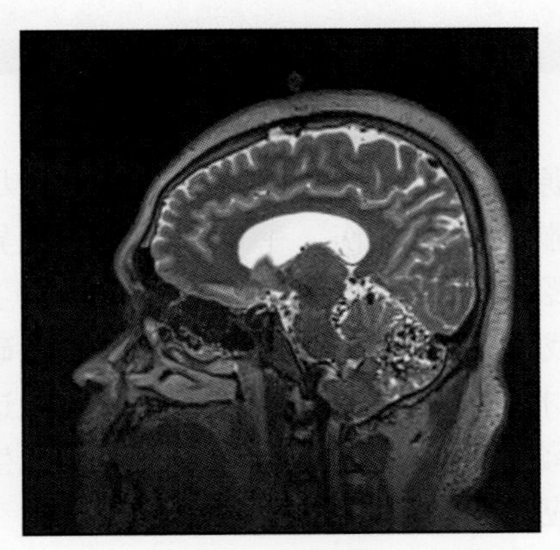

T2 MRI显示小脑bAVM中典型的血管流空

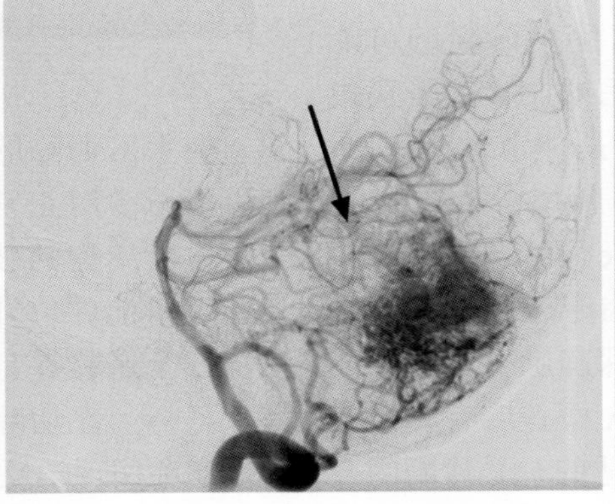

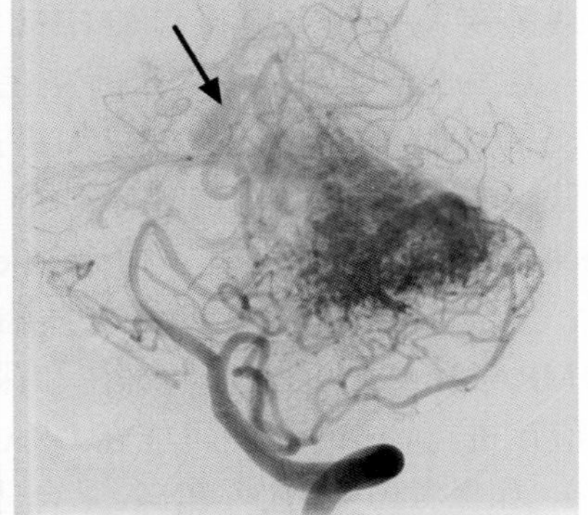

DSA动脉早期表现为bAVM的典型显影伴有引流静脉早显（箭头）。左椎动脉注射（左侧在侧位相，右侧有前后位）

图50.2　bAVM在MRI（T2）和DSA上的典型外观。引流静脉早显是bAVM的特征（箭头）

表 50.1 脑动静脉畸形分级系统

分级（参考）		基本分数	额外分数	分数范围	含义
Spetzler-Martin 分级（Spetzler and Martin，1986）	手术风险序数分类	1 = 大小 * <3 cm；2 = 大小 3~6 cm；3 = 大小 > 6 cm	1 代表深层静脉引流 **，1 代表功能区 ***	1~5	含义见下文
Lawton-Young 分级（Lawton et al.，2010）	手术风险序数分类	年龄小于 20 岁的 Spetzler-Martin 分级 + 1；+2 分（年龄 20~40 岁）；+3 分（> 40 岁）	1 表示非出血性表现，1 表示弥漫性 bAVM	2~10	Lawton-Young 得分分别为 4、5、6、7 和 8 的不利结局风险为 10%、20%、25%、40% 和 65%
Spetzler-Ponce 分级（Spetzler and Ponce，2011）	手术风险序数分类	简化 Spetzler-Martin 分级（SMG）： A = SMG 1 或 2 B = SMG 3 C = SMG 4 或 5		A、B 或 C	SPC A 的不良结局发生率低于 10%，SPC B 低于 20%，SPC C 低于 30%（46）。在某些研究中，SPC A 类的长期不良结局风险不大于 4%（5、7、49、50、51）
Pollock-Flickinger 评分（Pollock and Flickinger，2008）	预测放射外科闭塞同时无神经功能缺损	= 0.1 × 体积 ****（ml）+ 0.02 × 年龄（岁）	如果位于基底神经节，丘脑或脑干，则为 0.5	连续得分从 <1 到 > 2	≤1 时，无闭塞或不良后果的风险为 10%；分数 > 1 且 ≤1.5 时，风险 30%；分数 > 1.5 时，风险 > 40%

* 大小为最大直径，单位为厘米

** 深静脉引流包括与 Galenic 系统连通的引流

*** 功能区指 bAVM 位于原发性运动或感觉皮质、语言皮质、内囊、中脑、脑干、小脑脚。

**** 体积可以通过将三个正交最大直径（cm）除以 2 来近似得出。

a: Source data from Spetzler RF, Martin NA: A proposed grading system for arteriovenous malformations. *J Neurosurg* 65:476–483, 1986.

b: Reproduced with permission from Lawton, Michael T.; Kim, Helen, A Supplementary Grading Scale for Selecting Patients with Brain Arteriovenous Malformations for Surgery, *Neurosurgery*, Volume 66, Issue 4, pp. 702–13, Copyright © 2010 Oxford University Press and the Congress of Neurological Surgeons (CNS).

c: Source data from Spetzler RF, Ponce FA: A 3-tier classification of cerebral arteriovenous malformations. *J Neurosurg*. 2011; 114:842–849.

d: Reproduced with permission from Pollock, Bruce E.; Flickinger, John C, Modification of the Radiosurgery-Based Arteriovenous Malformation Grading System, *Neurosurgery*, Volume 63, Issue 2, pp. 239–43, Copyright © 2008 Oxford University Press and the Congress of Neurological Surgeons (CNS).

或者必须进行急诊干预（如危及生命的脑出血）。但是，当这样明确的干预措施并不明显，那就需要做进一步的检查。病史上来说，HHT、脑出血、脑脓肿或肺疾病家族史应该增加 HHT 鉴别诊断的可能性。复发性鼻出血、黏膜和手指毛细血管扩张病史更支持 HHT 的诊断。此外，如果是体节性 bAVM，皮肤或视网膜检查可能显示动静脉瘘（如 Bonnet-Dechaume Blanc 综合征）（Morgan et al.，1985）。但是，大部分 bAVM 不会出现这些临床表现。从 CTA 和 MRA，bAVM 的大小、部位和深静脉引流的可能性应该进行评估（虽然可能在 DSA 检查后有轻微改变）。如果考虑要治疗，DSA 是合适的，是诊断的金标准（注意肾功能）。

如果 bAVM 较小且弥漫（HHT 的特征），需要进行肺部 CT 检查来看是否存在肺动静脉瘘。HHT 患者若存在肺动静脉瘘，则提示其存在最大风险，因为动静脉瘘与脑脓肿相关（包括其他感染性栓子）。

治疗

手术

手术切除的原则是切除所有的动静脉分流，尽可能减少对正常脑功能的损伤，手术过程中避免异常血管结构的破裂出血（Hernesniemi et al.，2010）。通过术前评估计划切除区域周围的正常脑组织来确定安全区，并且术中尽可能在安全区操作来实现这一目标。在切除动静脉分流的过程中，应该考虑生理学和病理学反应。应采用如下的原则：

1. 最大限度地减少附带的脑损伤：
   a. 麻醉旨在控制平均动脉压和搏动压，促进脑组织松弛并防止缺血；
   b. 患者体位摆放以确保最佳的脑组织松弛，可最大程度地减少牵拉，并防止颅骨切开边缘的脑疝；

c. 颅骨切开的位置和大小适合 bAVM 和近端动脉暴露（包括穿过中线），并在发生灾难时允许采用其他方法；

d. 由于分流诱发的局部缺血并伴有与麻醉有关的低血压，脑组织牵拉应降低（尽管在 bAVM 上牵拉是合理的，前提是不存在相关的静脉流出损害）；

e. 如果高速动脉血流从供血动脉一直流向正常大脑，则必须检查从正常转变为异常，然后再恢复为正常的动脉血管。

2. 所有的供血动脉必须在静脉引流受到干扰之前加以控制：

a. 早期控制浅表供血动脉（包括使用临时阻断夹，直到确定最终的分区位置）；

b. 在手术早期沿着非常有限的边缘，在肿瘤切除术中通常采用的螺旋状环切术之前，通过脑沟分离和皮质切开术控制深部供血动脉；

应该记住，虽然豆状动脉和脉络膜动脉在解剖学上被认为是深动脉，但浅表系统也提供深部供血。这是因为高剪应力导致动脉和静脉之间的流动角变宽。这导致一些浅表动脉潜入离 bAVM 一定距离的脑沟深处，在较深的位置进入 bAVM。

c. 为了防止损伤主要的引流静脉，直接位于该静脉深处的动脉（通常的解剖结构不仅存在于 bAVM 中，而且在全身动脉和静脉并存的地方也可以观察到）应该被最后分离和控制，通常在 bAVM 的静脉脐部切除后。

d. 当存在穿硬膜动脉供血时，通过在离 bAVM 一定距离处切开硬脑膜，在 bAVM 上形成一个硬脑膜岛来控制硬膜外动脉供应，以防止这些动脉受到张力。

硬脑膜应在硬脑膜与 bAVM 之间的血管连接点一定距离处切开。当大脑镰受累时，最好从受累硬脑膜的对侧接近。

e. 为了尽量减少掀开骨瓣时的出血，当存在经颅骨供血的情况下，可以在许多狭窄的条带中进行颅骨开放，使出血在每一步都得到控制。

3. 静脉必须留下，直到所有的动脉都得到控制。重要的考虑是：

a. 与白质内 bAVM 相连的动脉化小血管通常为静脉；

这些静脉离开并返回到 bAVM 的血管簇，这是由于血管重塑，其目的在于使由高于正常的剪应力和角动量引起的血流动力学功最小化。这些血管绝大多数不需要结扎，但应该用双极和吸引器扫回 bAVM 边缘。由于血管周围空间仅在小动脉（而不是静脉）周围较大，这些血管周围缺乏脑脊液（CSF）可能是区分动脉和静脉的线索。由于 bAVM 内的静脉是浅表的，分离这些血管的累积效应将损害 bAVM 深鼻锥的静脉引流，使深鼻锥紧张，容易出现问题性出血。通过早期排除深部动脉供应，保留进出白质的静脉来尽量减少边缘静脉引流的损失，bAVM 的深部部分将更容易切除。

b. 最后一条主静脉应在 bAVM 的团块通过其静脉脐后分开，以确保所有的供血动脉都已分离出来。

4. 结扎畸形团的血管通常更困难，因为相比类似大小的血管，畸形团的血管壁更薄。结扎技术因其是在脑沟内还是作为皮质切开术的一部分而有所不同：

a. 用高质量的双极或微血管夹分离脑沟内的小血管；

i. 双极应该是高质量的，有绝对干净的镜面点和低设置（以确保血栓阻止血管内流动前血管壁不会爆裂）。透热闭塞的长度通常需要比处理其他疾病时考虑的更长。

Ii. 微血管夹是一种有用的对双极电凝的辅助，能够在非常薄壁的血管阻止血流，而双极电凝的效应热可能导致出血，而不是血栓形成（Sundt and Kees，1986）。此外，在具有多个分支终止于 bAVM 的一段较长的重要脑动脉上，在这些终接分支的起始处放置微血管夹可能比电凝对动脉造成更少的内皮损伤。

b. 皮质切开术中的小血管分离是通过更宽的、绝缘的双极电凝来实现的，双极利用邻近的组织来帮助强化要包括在热效应靶中的壁。

5. 吸引器应该高质量的（例如 #3 或 #4），利用最低的抽吸来清除脑脊液和血液。这减少了切除过程中细薄壁血管的意外破裂。如果出现问题性出血，应立即使用带有较大吸引器的单独吸引器系统。

6. 关颅前 bAVM 床应无出血。由于与 bAVM 相关的薄壁动脉，在大多数与其他病理相关的切除床上相比，通常会出现最小的血管收缩。因此，所有出血点都需要止住，任何出血点都不能被材料覆盖。后者可能导致灾难性的脑实质内出血。如果出血点不能很容易地用双极或微血管夹堵住，则需要将出血源追踪到大脑中，以达到血管可以被止血的点。这可以通过外科医生使用两个细吸引器来实现，一个用于吸吮出血点，另一个用于围绕出血点进行解剖。与特定位置的bAVM相关的血管解剖细节见第46章。

放射治疗

使用伽玛刀，一种直线加速器或质子束放射治疗，其将产生的辐射聚焦到覆盖bAVM的焦点上，在1~4年的时间内使血管发生反应，导致bAVM血栓形成。在bAVM病灶周围，18 Gy或更高的边缘剂量很有可能消除所有分流（Flickinger et al.，2002）。这是一种有效的治疗方法，随着时间的推移可实现闭塞，治疗风险低，闭塞率取决于边际剂量（取决于bAVM体积和位置）和患者年龄。由于闭塞的时间延迟可能是相当大的，因此需要考虑在这个潜伏期内bAVM的自然出血风险。bAVM照射的体积越小，照射到周围大脑的剂量相对于距离的下降就越大。这一点很重要，因为超过12 Gy的剂量可能会对某些脑组织（如视神经）产生不利影响。在制订放射治疗方案时，需要根据放射评估精确计算体积。但是，可以将三个正交最大直径（单位：cm）相乘并除以2得到近似值。无事故有效治疗的可能性可根据Pollock-Flickinger评分（PFS）得出，如下所示（总结见**表50.2**）：

= [0.1 × 体积（ml）]+[0.02 × 年龄（岁）]+[0.5 × 部位]

部位 = 0 表浅（半球/胼胝体/小脑）

部位 = 1 深部（基底节/丘脑/脑干）

消除的时间框架类似于S形曲线。SPC A和B类bAVM在报道中提供的数据尤其符合S形曲线（并将S形曲线的生成纳入以下假设，即在放疗后的头6个月中没有闭塞，超过5年以后也无进一步的闭塞），产生的闭塞率如**图50.3**所示（Flickinger et al.，2002；Kano et al.，2014）。较小的bAVM的达到50%累积闭塞率约为2年9个月，较大的bAVM为3年至3年6个月。在潜伏期（治疗结束到完全闭塞之间），出血率与未经治疗的自然病史相似。通过将未来出血的自然史纳入闭塞率曲线，可以生成出血率预测曲线（**图50.4**）。因此，推荐大型bAVM进行放射治疗是不合理的。然而，对于这些较大的bAVM，可以进行计划的分阶段减少容积策略，通过放射外科手术、质子束或分批放疗等（Karlsson et al.，2005；Huang et al.，2012；Kano et al.，2012a；Ding et al.，2014；Hattangadi-Gluth et al.，2014）。尽管采取了这样的策略，但支持这种策略的证据很少。一项关于此类治疗策略的前瞻性、意向性队列研究表明，治愈的病例少于死于出血的病例（Kano et al.，2012a）。因此，对于不太可能对单一治疗产生反应的病例，很难支持放射治疗策略。

表50.2 由Pollock-Flickinger得分得出的放射治疗的预期结局（Pollock and Flickinger.，2008）

=[0.1 × 体积（ml）] × [0.02 × 年龄（岁）]+0.5（如果是基底神经节、丘脑或脑干）

Pollock-Flickinger得分	70个月无事故有效治疗	神经系统功能的mRS下降（95%置信区间范围）
≤1	90%	0~10%
>1且≤1.5	70%	10%~20%
>1.5且≤2	60%	15%~30%
>2	<50%	25%~50%

栓塞

通过选择性插管和血管内栓塞bAVM通常作为：尝试减少术中出血风险来辅助手术；减小bAVM目标体积来辅助放射治疗；消除bAVM或近端血管结构上出血高风险的区域（如动脉瘤）来辅助放射治疗或保守治疗；或者作为单一和确切的消除治疗。bAVM通常通过前向性的动脉选择性插管进行评估（尽管经过静脉逆向性到位也有可能性）（Kessler，2011；Perreira，2013）。目前，栓塞最常用的材料为乙烯-乙烯醇聚合物栓塞剂（EVACE）。相比于之前的胶栓塞剂，EVACE具有易于控制释放的优点，这得益于它的非黏合性。

与消除病灶通常作为手术和放射治疗唯一目标不同的是，定义血管内栓塞在bAVM中的作用特别困难，因为其有各种各样的策略。有关首选栓塞治疗bAVM实现完全栓塞的数据有限。这是因为以栓塞开始合并其他治疗的可能性有很多种（完全栓塞，为放射治疗准备或为手术治疗准备）。治疗目的的转变使得结果分析变得困难。我们所获得的在EVACE之前的栓塞材料相关数据显示，永久残废率为8%，死亡率为1%，治愈率为5%（Frizzel and Fisher，1995）。对于EVACE，致残、致死和紧急手术发生率为6.6%，动静脉分流的完全消除率为27%（Morgan et al.，2013）。在一个前瞻性、多中心研究中，致残率被报道为5.1%，致死率为4.3%，完全栓塞率为

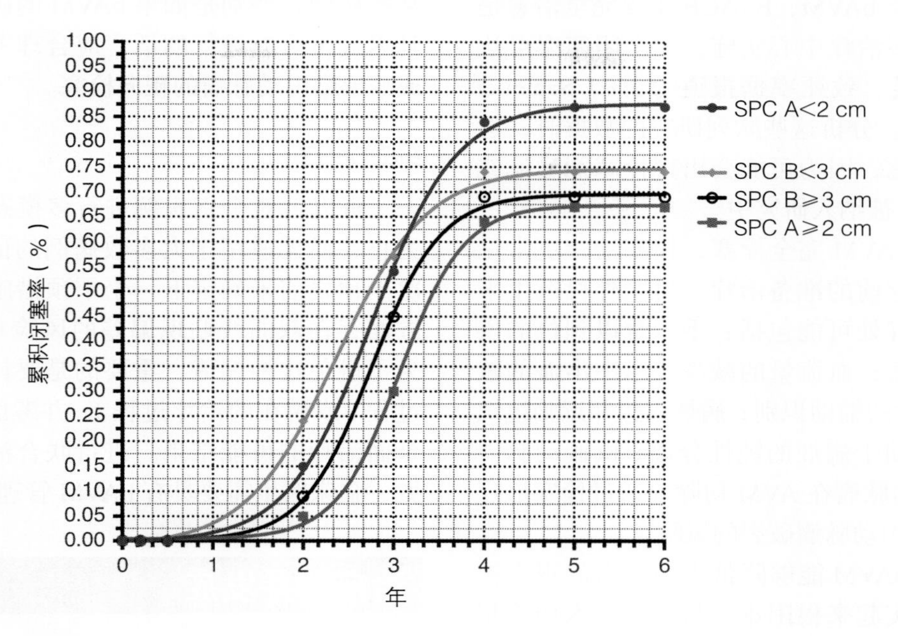

假设：
1. 头 6 个月内没有闭塞率。
2. 超过 5 年没有再闭塞。
3. 闭塞率最好用 S 形曲线拟合来表示。
数据推导：
Kano 2012（SPC A）和 Kano 2014（SPC B）。

图 50.3　由 Kano 及其同事的报道推算出，通过放射外科手术治疗的 SPC A 和 SPC B bAVM 的预期闭塞率。他们还发现，小直径的 bAVM 在这两组中更容易消失

Data from Kano H, Flickinger JC, Yang H-C, et al., Stereotactic radiosurgery for Spetzler-Martin Grade III arteriovenous malformations, *Journal of Neurosurgery*, Volume 120, Issue 4, pp. 973–81, 2014; and Kano H, Lunsford LD, Flickinger JC, et al., Stereotactic radiosurgery for arteriovenous malformations, Part 1:management of Spetzler-Martin Grade I and II arteriovenous malformations, *Journal of Neurosurgery*, Volume 116, Issue 1, pp. 11–20, 2012.

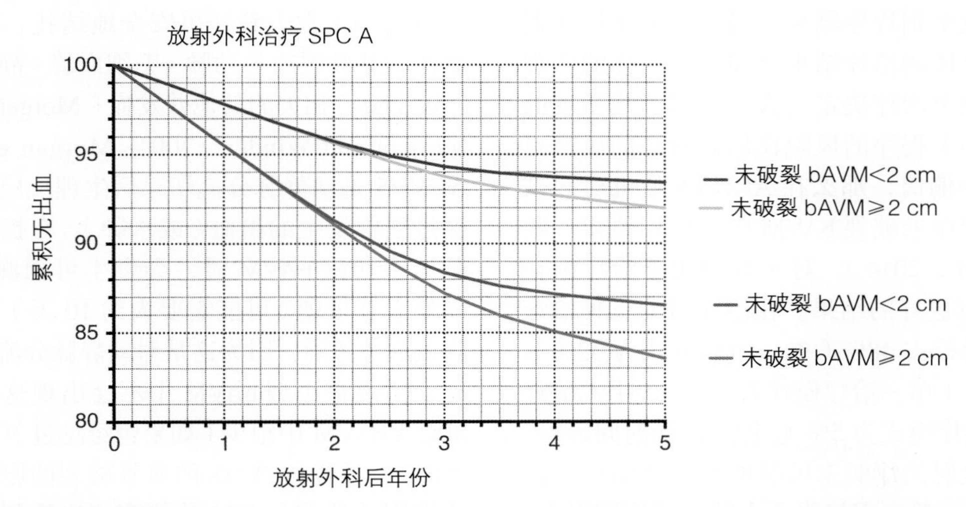

图 50.4　由 Kano 及其同事的报道得出，SPC A bAVM 接受放射外科手术后累积免于出血的比例曲线；根据 meta 分析得出，从诊断后自然出血史与未闭塞的比例相结合得出的

Data from Gross B, Du R, Natural history of cerebral arteriovenous malformations: a meta-analysis, *Journal of Neurosurgery*, Volume 118, Issue 2, pp. 437–43, 2013; and Kano H, Lunsford LD, Flickinger JC, et al., Stereotactic radiosurgery for arteriovenous malformations, Part 1:management of Spetzler-Martin Grade I and II arteriovenous malformations, *Journal of Neurosurgery*, Volume 116, Issue 1, pp. 11–20, 2012.

23.5%（Pierot et al.，2013）。据我们获得的资料显示，对于 SPC A 类 bAVM，EVACE 实现完全治愈是可能的，并在许多治疗中心实施，完全闭塞率可达 98%，同时，致残、致死率据报道为 3%（Saatci et al.，2011）。但是，分析这些队列研究的数据时，选择性偏倚需要考虑，因为可能会出现栓塞剂反流或难以到位的患者未被纳入研究中。

相比于实现 bAVM 完全栓塞，栓塞治疗更常见于手术或放射治疗前的准备治疗。对于外科医生来说，栓塞治疗的好处可能包括：手术难以到位的供血动脉的靶向闭塞；血流量的减少；术中出血的减少；术中供血动脉的辅助识别；病灶周边邻近脑组织有限的梗死带有助于病灶的钝性分离；供血动脉内压力增加导致的动脉瘤在 AVM 切除前通过栓塞治疗（减少了手术过程中动脉瘤破裂的风险）。

手术前栓塞 bAVM 能够降低术中出血的观点被广泛接受，但证实起来很困难。与单纯手术切除相关，术前栓塞联合手术的总体致残率、致死率和成功率可能未被改善（Morgan et al.，2013；Bervini et al.，2014；Korja et al.，2014）。与不联合术前栓塞直接进行放射治疗相比，栓塞治疗后进行放射治疗不太可能闭塞同等的残余 bAVM 体积（Andrade-Souza et al.，2007）。

手术和血管内技术的无数细微变化，加上各种不同复杂性病变的操作依赖性因素，使得在不了解机构结果并将其置于正确背景下的情况下，无法量化栓塞对 bAVM 治疗的贡献。因此，为了规划管理路径，需要了解负责治疗 bAVM 患者的机构的整体管理结果以及个别程序结果。当进行液体栓塞剂进行治疗并且个体的治疗结果已知，但整体的管理结果未知时，做出治疗决定的人存在双曲线贴现的风险，因为第一个程序的风险比后续程序的风险更大。理解了这种偏倚，那么在 ARUBA 随机对照试验里，栓塞治疗在未破裂 bAVM 中的作用值得一些反思（Mohr et al.，2014）。对照组相比于治疗组在 33 个月随访时有更好的结果。在治疗组的三种治疗模式中，放射治疗占 48%（单一治疗方式为 32%），栓塞治疗占 44%（单一治疗模式为 31%），手术治疗占 18%（单一治疗模式为 5%）。因为随访时间较短，人们不会认为放射治疗对未破裂的 bAVM 治疗的低效性有显著影响。鉴于仅接受手术的病例比例很小，这确实表明在进一步治疗之前栓塞治疗或单独栓塞的治疗策略最有可能归因于劣等治疗。因此，栓塞术在大多数未破裂 bAVM 的管理中可能是不合适的。

在破裂 bAVM 的治疗中，有时很明显出血的来源来自相关的近端颅内动脉瘤或畸形巢内动脉瘤。在某些病例，特别是如果 bAVM 的确定性切除手术将延迟或不可能进行的话，应合理考虑进行供血动脉或畸形巢内动脉瘤的靶向栓塞。

综合治疗

可以针对个别病例进行多模态治疗，但到目前为止，尚无适用于大多数病例的证据。如果在下一次干预之前未确定下一个干预措施，则在评估风险方面存在双曲线贴现偏差的风险（参见上文栓塞）。为了避免这种偏倚，重要的是要计划好后续的治疗过程（或潜在的治疗过程），并考虑并发症的发生和全面治疗的可能结果。进行联合治疗的决定非常细微，临床医生需要具有 bAVM 管理经验和专业知识。

治疗的并发症

开颅手术引起的手术并发症，如感染、硬膜下出血和周围血栓形成，都可在手术切除 bAVM 时发生（Morgan et al.，1993）。这些并发症的发生率与寻求的强度有关，尽管很严重并且带来管理上的挑战，但它们不会影响最终的改良 Rankin 量表评分（mRS）。bAVM 的显微外科手术具有特定的并发症，涉及功能区脑切除和因动静脉分流的消除而引起的血流动力学扰动。这些可能是互相作用的并且依赖动静脉分流的大小、位置和等级而定。为了减少切除术缘包含功能区脑组织对大脑造成直接损害的可能性，外科医生需要判断供血动脉的部位，从最后一个分支到正常大脑，可安全地结扎，而不发生近端供血动脉破裂或与动脉 - 毛细血管 - 静脉高压综合征（ACVHS）相关的其他并发症（Morgan et al.，1999；Morgan and Winder，2001；Morgan et al.，2003）。ACVHS 是动静脉分流切除后生理反应引起的或在切除过程中发生的出血（或水肿）。在扩张的动脉和静脉床中切除 bAVM 时，会发生可预测的生理反应，需要血管重塑（可能需要大约 10 天）或血栓形成以降低这种风险。因为这是对动静脉分流程度的生理反应，所以在小型 bAVM 中不会出现这种并发症。在 SPC A bAVM 中很少（如果曾经见过）（Morgan et al.，2003）。导致 ACVHS 的血管破裂的原因可能来自无法识别的残留 bAVM 并伴有流出道闭塞（如果没有流出道则可能没有流入，所以 DSA 不能总是将其识别出来），静脉闭塞（“闭塞性充血”）（Al-Rodhan et al.，1993），微循环自动调节功能不佳（正常灌注压力突破）（Spetzler et al.，1978；Sekhon et al.，1997），或近端薄壁小扩张小动脉壁破裂（Drake，1979；Sekhon et al.，1997）。统一的破坏力是向远端投射到先前低压区域的近端动脉压（见**图 50.1**）。当近端脉管明显扩张且无法通过血管收缩反应时，这一点尤其明显，通常应在剪切应力显著降低（抑制 eNOS 表达）并增加搏动性（增加内皮素 -1 的释放）后进行（Faraci et al.，1995；Mazzuca and Khalil，2012）。由于这些血管的半径大小，扩张的近端脉管系统中的阻力非常低，因此也有助于扩大压力。预计的压力会传递到闭塞点，因此，许多近端血管区域可能会因这种突然升高的压力而容易受到影响，直到动脉重构消除这种威胁为止。这符合 Poiseuillie 等式：

$$\text{血流量} = \frac{\text{压力梯度} \times \text{半径}^4}{\text{管腔长度}}$$

如果流量等于零，则动脉与流出道之间的压力梯度必须等于零。

SPC A 类 bAVM 发生 ACVHS 风险很小，除非在相当大的大脑表面上有大量多余的静脉引流（易导致蔓延性静脉阻塞和静脉梗死或闭塞性充血的风险）。在这种情况下，当 bAVM 床术后出血的风险降至最低时，可以考虑谨慎使用抗凝或抗血小板治疗。对于更复杂的 bAVM，此抗血小板或抗凝治疗方案是不合适的。预防和处理 ACVHS 的基石是血压控制。对于小于 4 cm 的 SPC A 和 SPC B 类 bAVM，预防高血压是必不可少的（例如，预防收缩压升高到 140 mmHg 以上）。但是，对于大型 SPC B 或 SPC C 类 bAVM，降低血压可能是希望达到的。维持脑灌注压至少为 50 mmHg，平均血压（在脑水平）小于 70 mmHg 对于降低灾难性 ACVHS 的风险似乎是成功的（Morgan et al.，2003）。通过降低血压，抑制收缩期峰值，降低脉搏波的上冲频率以及减少心输出量（如有必要）等综合措施，可以将 ACVHS 的风险最小化（**表** 50.3）。但是，至关重要的一点是，在任何时候正常脑部均不能因为治疗导致局部缺血。

保留正常功能的脑组织对于避免并发症至关重要。这就要求：保留向正常功能脑组织的供血，以及引流正常功能脑组织的静脉；最大限度地减少对功能区脑组织的损伤（例如谨慎地使用牵拉和分离，以最大限度地保护大脑）；避免止血海绵或其他止血材料掩盖不断发展的血肿（最好让出血直接进入腔内）；避免因头部位置不当导致静脉梗死和脑挫伤，从而导致颅骨切开术边缘的脑疝。

放射外科的主要并发症是在治疗后 4~40 个月发生不良放射反应（adverse radiation effects，ARE），原因是对放疗的炎症反应，7%~10％的病例发生（Boothe et al.，2013；Kano et al.，2014）。这种并发症的风险与 bAVM 的大小和复杂性有关，而对于 SPC A 类 bAVM 则要少得多（Kano et al.，2012b）。ARE 与接收 12 Gy 的脑体积有关。ARE 导致水肿和神经系统疾病，通常可以解决。但是，ARE 可能会危及生命，并永久性地致残。该病的治疗药物包括

表 50.3　治疗方案和动脉 - 毛细血管 - 静脉高压综合征（ACVHS）的预防

策略	方法	可能的药物	使用限制	潜在不良影响的改善
避免血压突然升高	预防癫痫发作和疼痛，以减少血压升高的瞬时发作		诱发便秘可能会加剧 GIT 问题	
降低平均血压	对血压进行实时滴定，以确保平均压力 <70 mmHg 的脑部安全灌注压（例如，脑部灌注压力 > 50 mmHg）	用于连续滴定控制的硝普钠和其他基线药物（例如 ACE 抑制剂和 β- 受体阻滞剂）	累积高剂量有毒；拉直自动调节曲线，使正常人的大脑在较低的血压下易受伤害	加入其他降压药以减少所需的实时降低血压的剂量
降低收缩压上升率	由于扩张的近端冗余血管中的脉动较大，因此应适当降低收缩期的上升	β- 受体阻滞剂	降低脉搏频率会增加卒中体积，可能适得其反	轻度（但安全）减少心输出量可能有利
心输出量减少	轻度减少心输出量以减少卒中体积	巴比妥类	需要确保足够的终末器官灌注和诱发的昏迷，增加了治疗的复杂性，包括监测颅内压（ICP）并防止免疫抑制。长时间使用会在脂肪存储中积聚大量巴比妥类药物，从而导致需要相当长的呼吸机支持时间	液体潴留可能需要加利尿作用； ICU 管理； 警惕评估感染状况； 改变许多药物的代谢

皮质类固醇、维生素E磷酸二酯酶抑制剂和VEGF抑制剂（Boothe et al.，2013）。此外，在需要手术干预的情况下，2%病例，最长至术后18年，可发生晚期囊肿形成（Kano et al.，2014）。放射外科治疗后的合并发病率和死亡率（包括潜伏期破裂的自然史）在图50.4中给出。

栓塞的主要并发症包括出血（由于过早阻塞了流出静脉和微导丝穿破动脉壁）以及阻塞了供应关键脑组织的动脉。有时会发生与动脉通路相关问题（股动脉闭塞、夹层、假性动脉瘤形成）、栓塞并发症（来自股动脉、髂动脉、主动脉和颈部动脉插管）和动脉解剖相关的并发症。发生这种情况的风险将取决于对每个患者执行的栓塞程序的复杂性和数量。因此，各机构之间的风险差异会很大，因为各个中心在手术、放射外科手术和栓塞的分工有所不同。采用EVACE进行治疗的较大病例数研究显示，其目标可能是积极进行栓塞，主要发病率和死亡率的风险平均为7%（范围从1%到大于10%）（Morgan et al.，2013）。

表 50.4 bAVM 治疗比较（括号内为来源参考）

治疗方法	修改因素	治疗引起不良结局导致永久性神经功能缺损（mRS>1）	年度破裂风险（参考文献）	预计的5年累积破裂率	达到50%病灶消除的时间	后期研究中5年后消除率，%（参考文献）
未经处理	出血起病	不适用	3.7%~5.9%（Gross and Du，2013；Kim et al.，2014）	20%	不适用	不适用
	未破裂	不适用	1%~2.7%（Gross and Du，2013；Kim et al.，2014）	10%	不适用	不适用
	未破裂，伴有动脉瘤	不适用	类似于破裂的（Gross and Du，2013；Brown et al.，1990）	>10%；<20%	不适用	不适用
放射外科	未破裂的SPC A或B <2 cm	<3%	不变，直到消失	7%	2.5~3.0年	85%（Kano et al.，2014；Kano et al.，2012b）
	破裂的SPC A或B> 2 cm	<3%	不变，直到消失	8%	3.0~3.5年	70%（Kano et al.，2014；Kano et al.，2012b）
	破裂的SPC A或B<2 cm	<3%	不变，直到消失	14%	2.5~3.0年	85%（Kano et al.，2014；Kano et al.，2012b）
	破裂的SPC A或B>2 cm	<3%	不变，直到消失	16%	3.0~3.5年	70%（Kano et al.，2014；Kano et al.，2012b）
外科手术	SPC A	6%~10%（34）；可能<3 %（Korja et al.，2014；Spetzler and Ponce，2011）	<1%	<1%	不适用	>99%
	SPC B：<20岁以下；20~40岁的年龄、破裂或致密（并非两者兼有）	10%~24%（Spetzler and Ponce，2011）；可能接近20 %（Korja et al.，2014；Kim et al.，2015）	<1%	<1%	不适用	97%
	其他SPC B（Lawton-Young评分＞6）	>39%（Kim et al.，2015）	<1%	<1%	不适用	97%
	SPC C	>50%（Korja et al.，2014）	<1%	<1%	不适用	96%

结果 / 预后

有关各种治疗途径结果的总结，请参见**表** 50.4。SPC A 类 bAVM 的手术风险据报道为 6%~10%，也有报道低于 3%（Gross and Du，2013；Korja et al.，2014）。这种风险可能会作为一个整体推广到所有 SPC A 类 bAVM（Korja et al.，2014）。对于年龄较大的、未破裂的和弥散性的 SPC B 类 bAVM，手术的风险显著增加（Kim et al.，2015）。Lawton-Young 分组允许围绕这些因素对 SPC B 类 bAVM 的风险进行分层（**表** 50.4）（Kim et al.，2015）。因为存在风险，在 20 岁及 20 岁以上的 SPC C 类 bAVM 人群中很少必须进行手术治疗。除非有非常微妙的原因，通常不建议在 20 岁以下 SPC C 类 bAVM 患者中进行手术治疗。据报道，SPC C 类 bAVM 病例的合并残废率和死亡率大于 20%（Korja et al.，2014）。但是，由于这些病例来自高度选择的病例，他们并不能代表这些病例的普遍风险，因此有理由推断 SPC C 类 bAVM 进行手术的风险至少为 50%（一半的不良结果会导致 mRS> 2）。

放射外科手术的结果取决于 bAVM 接收到的放射剂量和大脑接收到的放射剂量（同上）。

将手术的风险与自然史和放射手术的风险相叠加（包括在治疗和闭塞之间的潜伏期中预期的出血风险）可以比较治疗方案（**图** 50.5）。看来如果考虑 10 年的时间跨度，与 SPC A 类 bAVM 的自然病史相比，手术和放射外科手术似乎是更好的选择。对于破裂的 SPC A 类 bAVM，手术相对于放射外科手术的优势是显而易见的。未破裂的 SPC B 类 bAVM 最好通过放射外科手术治疗，因为其闭塞畸形团的预期很高。为了使外科手术适合于 SPC B 类 bAVM，需要考虑远超过 10 年的时间范围。尽管治疗方式的选择

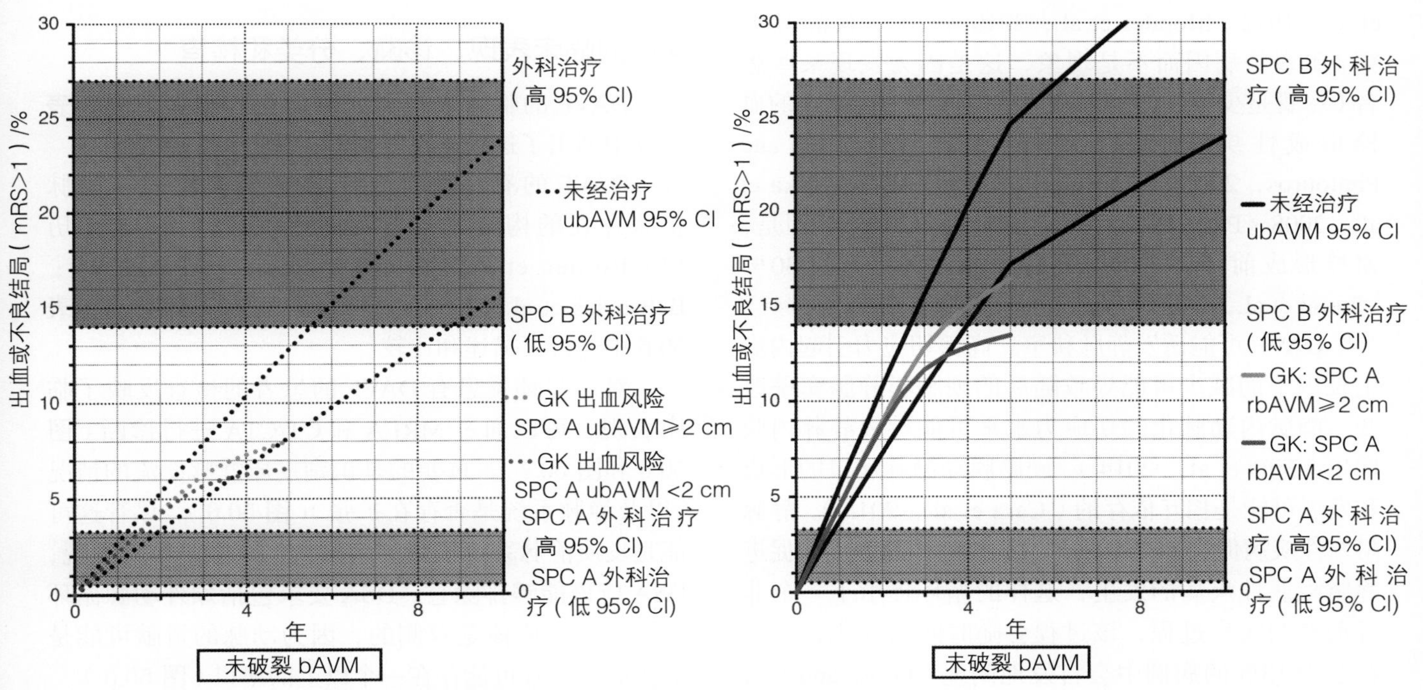

图 50.5　并发症风险展示图，手术并发症导致永久性 mRS 大于 1（蓝色条带代表 SPC A 手术的 95%置信区间范围，灰色条带代表在 SPC B 上手术的 95%置信区间）（来自未经治疗的出血随时间变化的结果数据，黑线）（来自放射外科手术之后的数据，深绿色 <2 cm 直径；浅绿色 > 2 cm）（见**图** 50.4）

Data from Korja M, Bervini D, Assaad N, Morgan MK, The role of surgery in the management of brain arteriovenous malformations: A prospective cohort study, *Stroke*, Volume 45, Issue 12, pp. 3549–55, 2014; and Gross B, Du R, Natural history of cerebral arteriovenous malformations: a meta-analysis, *Journal of Neurosurgery*, Volume 118, Issue 2, pp. 437–43, 2013; and Kano H, Flickinger JC, Yang H-C, et al., Stereotactic radiosurgery for Spetzler-Martin Grade III arteriovenous malformations, *Journal of Neurosurgery*, Volume 120, Issue 4, pp. 973–81, 2014; and Kano H, Lunsford LD, Flickinger JC, et al., Stereotactic radiosurgery for arteriovenous malformations, Part 1: management of Spetzler-Martin Grade I and II arteriovenous malformations, *Journal of Neurosurgery*, Volume 116, Issue 1, pp. 11–20, 2012.

最好由随机对照试验回答，并且已经完成一项（Mohr et al.，2014），但外部有效性受到质疑，限制了其推广（栓塞术同上）（Korja et al.，2014）。

硬脑膜动静脉瘘

AVF 的病理生理、分类和自然史

硬脑膜动静脉瘘（dural arteriovenous fistulae，DAVF）具有 bAVM（同上）中的部分动静脉异常。bAVM 在桥静脉之前的静脉系统内具有瘘口，而 DAVF 的瘘口定位在该点之外。DAVF 包含一个或多个瘘口，其中心在桥静脉（软膜静脉和硬脑膜静脉窦之间的桥接）以及硬脑膜内静脉壁内的瘘口（包括硬脑膜静脉窦）。它们通常是后天获得的，但可能是先天性的（例如，某些类型的大脑大静脉血管瘤；请参阅 Johnston et al.，1987）。DAVF 的检出率是 bAVM 的 1/3（Satomi and Satoh，2008）。

DAVF 的病因很可能是静脉血栓形成（Houser et al.，1972；Morales et al.，2010）。硬脑膜静脉狭窄 / 闭塞是病因而不是现象，这是因为发现某些患者（尽管是少数）已被识别为获得性或遗传确定的血栓形成性疾病（Kraus et al.，2002；Wenderoth and Phatouros，2003；Saito et al.，2008；Wysokinska et al.，2008；Pasi et al.，2014；Hwang，2015）。但是，血栓形成前状态占 DAVF 病例的比例不超过 30%（Izumi et al.，2007；Wysokinska et al.，2008）。

DAVF 可能诱发静脉狭窄。高剪切应力引起内皮生长因子的减少可能导致随后的硬脑膜静脉窦壁改变。静脉内动脉化的切应力水平可能导致静脉内膜增生（Fitts et al.，2014）。硬脑膜动静脉瘘口的形成和发展可能是相互依存的（Casa et al.，2015）。静脉阻塞性疾病促进 DAVF 的形成，DAVF 的形成又促进静脉阻塞性疾病的发生，这样的循环提示了一个非常动态的疾病过程，该过程会随时间而变化，并且在至少 13% 的病例中会自发地闭塞（Gross and Du，2012）。

DAVF 最令人担心的后果是脑实质内（或偶发的自发性急性硬脑膜下）出血（Duffau et al.，1999）。仅在有皮质静脉引流的情况下才发生出血，并且每年出血的风险为 4%~11%（Davies et al.，1997a；Davies et al.，1997b）。此外，当存在单一皮质静脉引流或具有张力的皮质静脉引流（扩张或广泛的皮质静脉分支）时，发生出血的风险明显增高（Baltsavias et al.，2015）。如果皮质静脉引流且扩张，则年风险至少为 10%，并且可能接近 50%（Butlers et al.，2012；Gross and Du，2012）。出血后再出血的时间间隔非常短，因此必须紧急进行明确的治疗（Butlers et al.，2012）。据报告，出血死亡率为 40%（Gross and Du，2012）。静脉引流的方式可能会随着时间推移而变化，对那些被认为具有较低出血风险的人应确保监测。DAVF 的部位中更容易出现单一软脑膜静脉反流的，通常位于较深的中线或旁中线位，如前颅底的筛骨区域、小脑幕缘、前直窦和岩窦。相比之下，海绵状和横窦乙状窦位置的可能性较小（尽管可能仍有）软脑膜静脉反流。

非出血性静脉高压综合征可以是由于软脑膜静脉高压而引起的局灶性或全身性静脉高压脑病，广泛性静脉窦高压综合征（导致颅内高压）和局灶性静脉窦高压综合征（最引人注目的是海绵窦综合征，对眼睛健康构成威胁）。有时，深静脉曲张发展可能导致导水管阻塞而引起脑积水。神经功能缺损的发生率在比例上与出血相似，并且发生在静脉引流模式相似的患者中（Gross and Du，2012）。

AVF 的临床表现、诊断、分类和检查

DAVF 的临床表现方式可能会有很大差异。**表 50.5** 中列出了这些表现及其潜在原因。

DAVF 的有用分类基于静脉引流模式与静脉扩张存在的构架关系，因此反映了它们的自然历史（Borden et al.，1995；Cognard et al.，1995；Baltsavias et al.，2015）。三种有用的分类系统在**表 50.6** 中进行了描述和比较。

对那些怀疑患有 DAVF 的患者的检查反映了临床表现。可以通过 MRI/A 和 CT/CTA 进行诊断（**图 50.6** 和**图 50.7**）。重要的是识别皮质静脉反流的情况（以及静脉系统是否存在扩张）（**图 50.6**）。尽管这可能是皮质静脉系统扩张的结果，但可能不容易发现，DSA 应该能够排除它。DSA 要求包括颈外动脉循环造影，并且应该是双侧的，因为动脉的贡献可能是双侧的，并且可能存在一个以上的瘘口（**图 50.6**）。

除了建立动静脉瘘的血管构筑外，还应评估血栓形成的易感性（如果有的话）。对于非常年轻的患者，还应评估动静脉瘘对心脏的影响（请参阅儿科部分）。

治疗

通常仅存在皮质静脉反流（因为这些患者有出血风险）、静脉窦高压（导致颅内高压）或海绵窦综合征（对眼睛健康造成威胁）的情况下才建议治疗。但是，偶尔进行治疗的目的是减轻症状（例如可听见

表 50.5 DAVF 的临床表现

临床表现	临床细微差别	解释
颅内杂音	通常位于横窦乙状窦的患侧。然而，它可能在闭塞乙状窦的瘘对侧耳朵上。杂音可能很大，使患者在夜间保持清醒。安静时，靠近患者的人甚至可以听到。杂音峰值在心脏收缩期，但通常持续到舒张期。用听诊器可以听到，并且压迫同侧颈内静脉可能会减轻杂音	由乙状窦内的湍流或高流量引起
可触及的肿物	在乳头后枕动脉路径中触诊	扩张的供血动脉（例如枕动脉）
头疼	需要考虑某些因素	1. 脑膜血管的募集和扩张 2. 硬脑膜静脉窦内血栓形成 3. 上颌静脉扩张导致三叉神经痛 4. 颅内高压（见下文） 5. 巧合的
神经功能缺损	1. 大脑局灶性神经功能缺损 2. 全面认知功能缺损 3. 脐静脉高压性脑病或脑积水导致的行走困难 4. 海绵窦综合征或脑神经缺损（部分或全部）	1. 局灶性静脉高压性脑病。这可能导致转瞬即逝、起伏不定或进行性局灶性神经功能缺损。这是由于皮质静脉高压导致缺血 2. 广泛性静脉高压性脑病。这会导致全脑广泛认知能力下降和昏迷。DAVF 的深静脉反流到大脑内部静脉或双侧皮质静脉中，这是上矢状窦引流阻碍的常见原因。在这种情况下，通常会有颅内静脉流出严重受阻，例如双侧横窦狭窄 3. 脑神经受压或缺血。这是海绵窦 DAVF 的一种常见表现形式。这可能与海绵窦血栓形成（全部或部分）与海绵窦内静脉高压的相互作用有关。另外，蛛网膜下腔内扩张的引流静脉可能导致颅神经受压，并可能导致面肌痉挛 4. 从静脉曲张梗阻到中脑导水管梗阻所致的脑积水 5. 从颅内 DAVF 主要向脊髓引流引起的静脉高压性脊髓病（这可能是典型的脊髓 DAVF 累及圆锥引起的）
出血	通常是实质性的，但可能是急性自发性硬膜下出血	请看自然史
癫痫发作	局灶的或全身的	仅在幕上软脑膜静脉反流的情况下发生
颅内高压，伴乳头水肿和头痛	大型 DAVF 可能会发生	由于静脉窦内压力增加而发生。因为蛛网膜下腔的压力 - 静脉窦压力梯度出现变化，这个梯度驱动了脑脊液的吸收
婴儿高输出心力衰竭	瘘口大的婴儿	在没有静脉流出障碍的情况下，直接分流到桥静脉中，可在婴儿和新生儿中产生很大比例的心输出量。当存在于新生儿中时，它们可能是主要的心脏问题，因为流向颅内瘘口的高流量可能出现肺动脉高压合并充血性心力衰竭的典型表现

的杂音）。应该记住的是，可能有其他缓解症状方法（例如，在背景白噪声的情况下入睡）。并且随着时间的流逝，DAVF 可能会自发形成血栓。在减轻杂音时，请务必牢记，可能无需治疗即可缓解症状，并且至关重要的是，良性动静脉瘘不会通过改变静脉引流而转化为危险的 DAVF。

外科手术

外科手术通常考虑两种通用方法。第一种是从 DAVF 上断开反向皮质静脉反流，使 DAVF 完好无损，但没有任何皮质静脉回流。这消除了出血的危险。第二种方法是切除 DAVF 本身。在此过程中，至关重要的是，静脉窦切除术不要干扰正常的皮质静脉引流。

1. **离断皮质静脉引流**。可以将其应用于所有位置，

表 50.6 围绕与颅内出血、静脉高压性脑病的风险相关的 DAVF 有用分类

病理	Borden-Wu-Shucart 分类（Borden et al.，1995）	Cognard 等对 Djindjian 和 Merland 分类的修改（Cognard et al.，1995）	DES 系统（直接软脑膜静脉引流；单一软脑膜静脉引流；软脑膜静脉应变 *n* =not/no（Baltsavias et al.，2015）	表现	性别和两个最常见的部位	出血或神经功能缺损（不包括脑神经缺损）的人群百分比）（Baltsavias 4）	预后（Gross and Du，2012）
直接进入硬脑膜静脉窦或脑膜静脉，顺向或正向静脉血流，无反向皮质静脉引流	Ⅰ	Ⅰ	nD、nE、nS	杂音	女性多见；横窦乙状窦或海绵窦	0	不太可能出血
直接进入硬脑膜静脉窦或脑膜静脉，反向硬脑膜静脉流出，无反向皮质静脉引流	Ⅰ	Ⅱa	nD、nE、nS	杂音	女性多见；横窦乙状窦或海绵窦	0	不太可能出血
直接进入硬脑膜静脉窦或脑膜静脉，同时静脉窦反向流出和反向引流进入皮质静脉，不伴有皮质静脉扩张	Ⅱ	Ⅱa 和Ⅱb	nD、nE、nS	杂音，静脉高压性脑病，出血，颅内高压	女性多见；横窦乙状窦或海绵窦	0	6%的年度风险
直接进入硬脑膜静脉窦或脑膜静脉，同时静脉窦反向流出和反向引流进入皮质静脉，伴有皮质静脉扩张	Ⅱ	Ⅱa 和Ⅱb	nD、nE、S	杂音，静脉高压性脑病，出血，颅内高压	女性多见；横窦乙状窦或海绵窦	66%	6%的年度风险
直接进入硬脑膜静脉窦或脑膜静脉，仅反向引流至不显示扩张的皮质静脉	Ⅱ	Ⅱb	nD、E、nS	杂音，静脉高压性脑病，出血，颅内高压	女性多见；横窦乙状窦或海绵窦	15%	6%（95% 置信区间，0.1% ~19%）的年度风险
直接进入硬脑膜静脉窦或脑膜静脉，仅反向引流至表现出水肿的皮质静脉	Ⅱ	Ⅱb	nD，E，S	杂音，静脉高压性脑病，出血，颅内高压	女性多见；横窦乙状窦或海绵窦	90%	6%（95% 置信区间，0.1%~19%）的年度风险
直接进入桥静脉，同时皮层静脉反向引流和静脉窦逆行引流	没有定义	没有定义	D、nE、nS	静脉高压脑病，出血，颅内高压			
直接进入桥静脉，仅皮质静脉反向引流，无静脉扩张	Ⅲ	Ⅲ	D、E、nS	静脉高血压性脑病，出血，	男性多见；小脑幕和岩骨	75%	10%（95% 置信区间，4%~20%）的年度风险；
直接进入桥静脉，仅皮质静脉反向引流并伴有皮质静脉扩张	Ⅲ	Ⅳ	D、E、S	静脉高压性脑病，出血	男性多见；小脑幕和岩骨	>90%	21%（95% 置信区间，4%~66%）的年度风险
髓周静脉引流（脊髓）		Ⅴ					

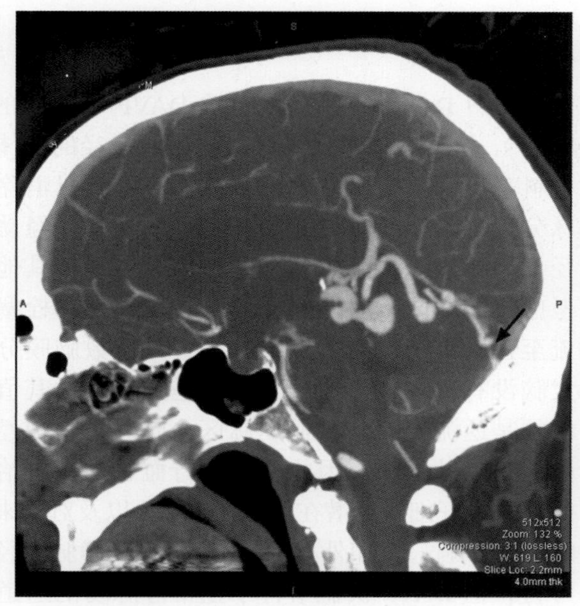

CTA 矢状面显示 DAVF 位于直窦内天幕边缘，Borden Ⅲ型表现为全面认知障碍，且无直窦充盈。

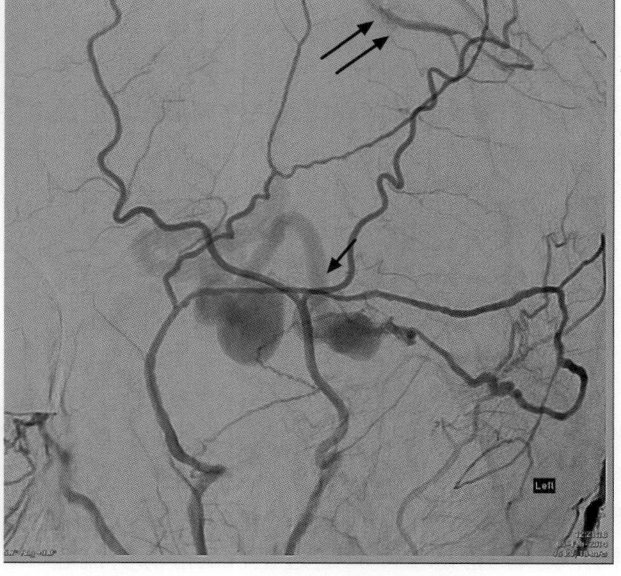

颈外动脉 DSA 显示逆行实质性静脉引流（箭头）。识别出第二个瘘，与镰相关（双箭头）。

图 50.6　CTA 和颈外 DSA 证实了 DAVF 伴有反向软脑膜静脉引流的特征。这位 60 岁的成年男性患者表现出全面性（全脑）认知能力下降。还有第二个小的 DAVF，其与镰相关，与上矢状窦相通

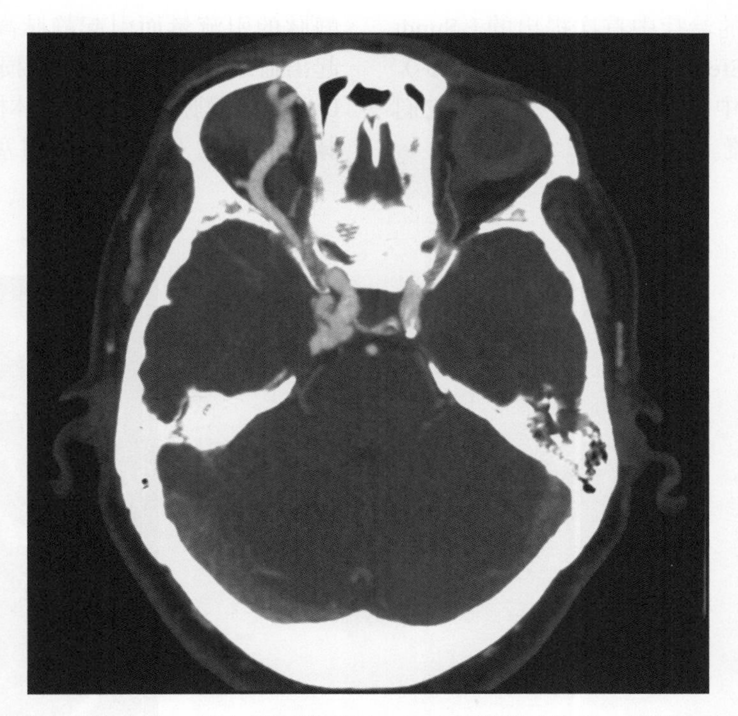

图 50.7　CTA 上动脉期可见眼上静脉充盈，是右侧海绵窦区 DAVF 的证据（注意：横窦充盈不足，因此可以认为眼上静脉是提前充盈）

只要存在皮质静脉反流，并且在大多数情况下是最佳治疗方法。脊膜 AVF 和脑膜 AVF 类似。尽可能最小的方法，在靠近硬脑膜的静脉入口处应用血管夹，将消除出血的风险。但是，在执行此操作时会遇到一些困难：

a. 因为动脉化静脉的支流可能靠近硬脑膜的出口，所以血管夹的位置必须足够靠近硬膜，以防止继续分流。

b. 在此时关闭夹子时，重要的是不要撕裂从硬膜流出的引流静脉（由于相对硬的硬膜中的静脉固定而使之成为可能）。因此，缓慢闭合血管夹对于使紧张的静脉在血管夹片内滑动以避免过多的张力是重要的。

c. 粗大而紧张的动脉化静脉可能会极大阻塞血管夹目标点的入路。在规划手术时，需要考虑这种进入障碍。举例来说，当以进入岩上静脉为目标时，可以通过幕上颞下的方法，将天幕从内侧向外侧分开，以从上方暴露岩上静脉，而避免静脉本身阻碍入路，这可能更容易实现。

2. **切除 DAVF 累及的静脉窦**。由于引入了液体栓塞剂和经静脉途径静脉窦内球囊临时保护静脉窦腔，因此几乎不需要这种方法。但是，为了完整起见，如果所累及的静脉窦不再通过正常的静脉引流起作用（即已形成血栓，或者所累及的部分不包含来自大脑的重要支流并且存在侧支静脉引流），则可以切除 DAVF 包括静脉窦 。尽管在进行血管内或简单的分离手术的情况下很少进行手术，但在治疗中仍可能会偶尔出现。这种方法是由 Sundt 医师在横窦乙状窦 DAVF 的治疗中首次提出的（Sundt and Piepgras，1983；Efekhar and Morgan，2013）。必须仔细考虑切除段中包含的静脉，以确保它们不存在正常的前向血流。

栓塞

治愈 DAVF 的关键是消除 DAVF 中包含的“静脉足”。这可以通过经动脉或经静脉途径的液体栓塞材料来实现。可以采用许多方法来栓塞以消除动静脉分流，包括经动脉途径和经静脉途径。经动脉途径类似于栓塞 bAVM 的途径。但是，还有其他需要考虑的问题。其中最主要的是头皮缺血和栓塞剂反流至正常大脑供血的侧支。尽管大多数脑膜分支对大脑没有贡献，但情况并非总是如此，尤其值得关注的是返流到到脑供血动脉区。此外，脑神经可能由脑膜动脉供应。因此，在进行血管内介入治疗之前，需要仔细考虑潜在的侧支供血（以及对未来治疗的潜在影响，例如外科手术入路）。经静脉途径尽管可行，但 DAVF 供血平行于正常静脉窦的通道可能会使治疗变得复杂。这可能会使静脉窦闭塞后仍无法治愈 DAVF。在栓塞过程中，静脉窦支架成形（将供血的动脉钉入窦中）或球囊扩张可以保护静脉窦的功能。进行经静脉治疗时的重要考虑因素是避免在手术过程中未减少动脉血流量的情况下增加皮层静脉的引流量而引起静脉高压性脑病。这可能会引起出血或加剧神经功能缺损（例如，**图 50.8**）。当对 DAVF 的静脉分支进行液体栓塞剂栓塞时，在存在静脉窦的情况下，存在窦闭塞的风险。这可以通过在

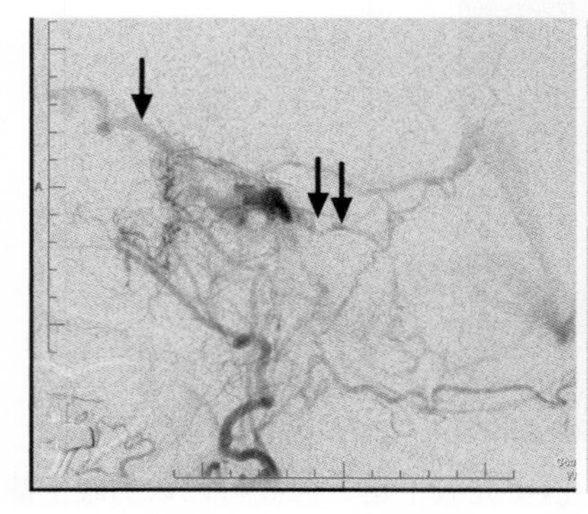

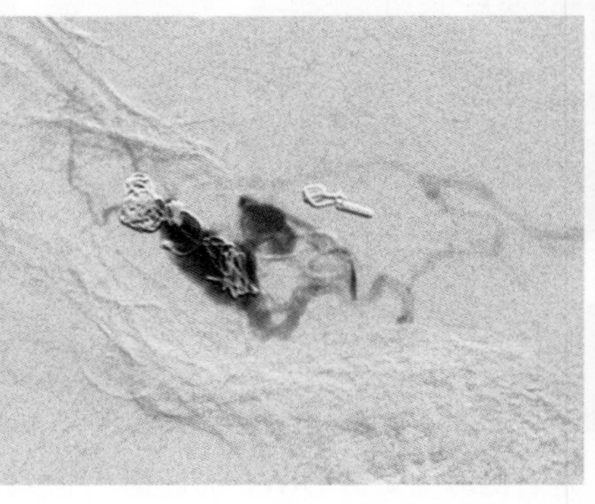

左颈外动脉注射（左）显示海绵窦 DAVF 伴眼上静脉充盈（箭头）和脑实质静脉逆流进入颅后窝（双箭头）。经岩静脉入路的手术期间（右），眼上静脉早期闭塞，随后 DAVF 完全逆行进入颅后窝皮质静脉（在最后闭塞流出道之前）。动脉瘤夹在伴发颈内动脉瘤上

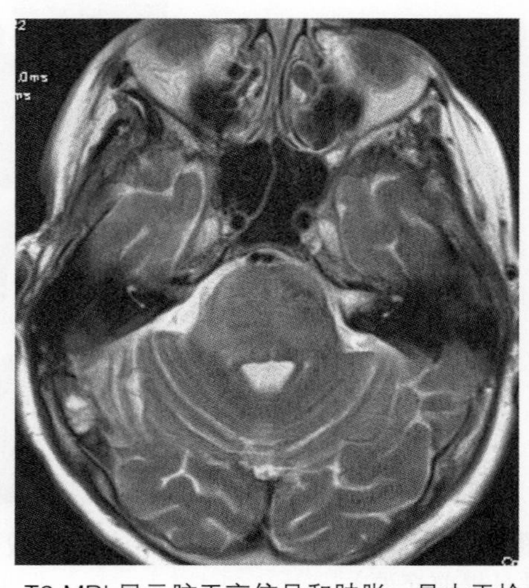

T2 MRI 显示脑干高信号和肿胀，是由于栓塞时血流重新导向并流入颅后窝皮质静脉引起的静脉高压性脑病，患者意识丧失的时间延长，醒来后伴有偏瘫

图 50.8 左海绵窦的 DAVF 表现为眼眶充血和危险的继发性青光眼。颈外动脉注射（左）显示出眼上静脉的特征性增大（箭头），从岩下窦到脑桥前静脉有危险的静脉流出（双箭头）。通过经静脉导管插入术和海绵状窦的线圈闭塞治疗，最初在眼上静脉附近向前方堆积。逆行流入脑桥静脉系统，直到最终被阻塞（中间图像）。患者缓慢苏醒并最终醒来，但合并偏瘫，通过 MRI（右图）可以看出，严重的静脉高压导致了临床和放射学特征（T2 上的高信号和脑桥肿胀）

液体栓塞剂注射期间静脉窦内球囊辅助来防止。但是，在球囊充盈期间，可能会阻碍正常的静脉引流，当目标是治愈动静脉瘘而非减轻症状的较小目标时，应将使用球囊留给更具侵略性的 DAVF。

聚集放射

尽管尚未通过 DAVF 治疗的验证，但在一些横窦乙状窦 DAVF 的病例中，放射治疗与栓塞术相结合已被证明是成功的（Loumiotis et al.，2011）。当没有逆行软脑膜静脉回流（因此没有立即的出血威胁）时，这可能是治疗严重症状性杂音的重要组成部分。一些横窦乙状窦 DAVF 患者，经动脉栓塞后进行放射治疗在减少杂音方面风险非常低，是一种有希望的治疗方式（Loumiotis et al.，2011）。

关于 DAVF 治疗的总结可以在**图 50.9** 所示的决策算法中看到。

并发症管理

外科和血管内治疗共同常见的并发症是：

1. **治疗时出血**。
   a. 在静脉高压的情况下，牵拉可能会引起出血。当存在静脉高压性脑病时，在消除逆行皮质静脉引流之前，必须非常小心地处理脑组织。开颅手术时，由于静脉高压而难以放松。但是，额外的牵拉引起的静脉阻塞可能导致静脉曲张和出血。尤其是在窦汇区手术中，俯卧体位会加剧问题，坐位可能在颅骨切开术时导致脑疝。当静脉高压明显时，应将牵拉保持在最低水平。
   b. 关于与血管内修复相关的出血风险，最有可能发生在静脉闭塞时，即在完全闭塞之前，逆行皮质静脉流出的压力（例如 Labbe 静脉分布）会暂时升高而实现。
2. **静脉梗死**。这是由于无意的闭塞或由于延伸的静脉血栓形成而导致的静脉正常前向血流的丧失而引起的。至关重要的是，只有逆向引流的静脉才能安全断开。
3. **静脉高压性脑病**。这与出血发生的基础相同。可以在**图 50.7** 中看到一个示例。
4. **蔓延式静脉窦血栓形成**（尤其是在静脉狭窄点）。随着流量的减少，可能发生进行性静脉窦阻塞。具有多处狭窄的静脉窦特别脆弱。如果其蔓延至下一个正常分支流入口，但不超出此范围，则不会发生临床后果。但是，如果这种蔓延超出了这

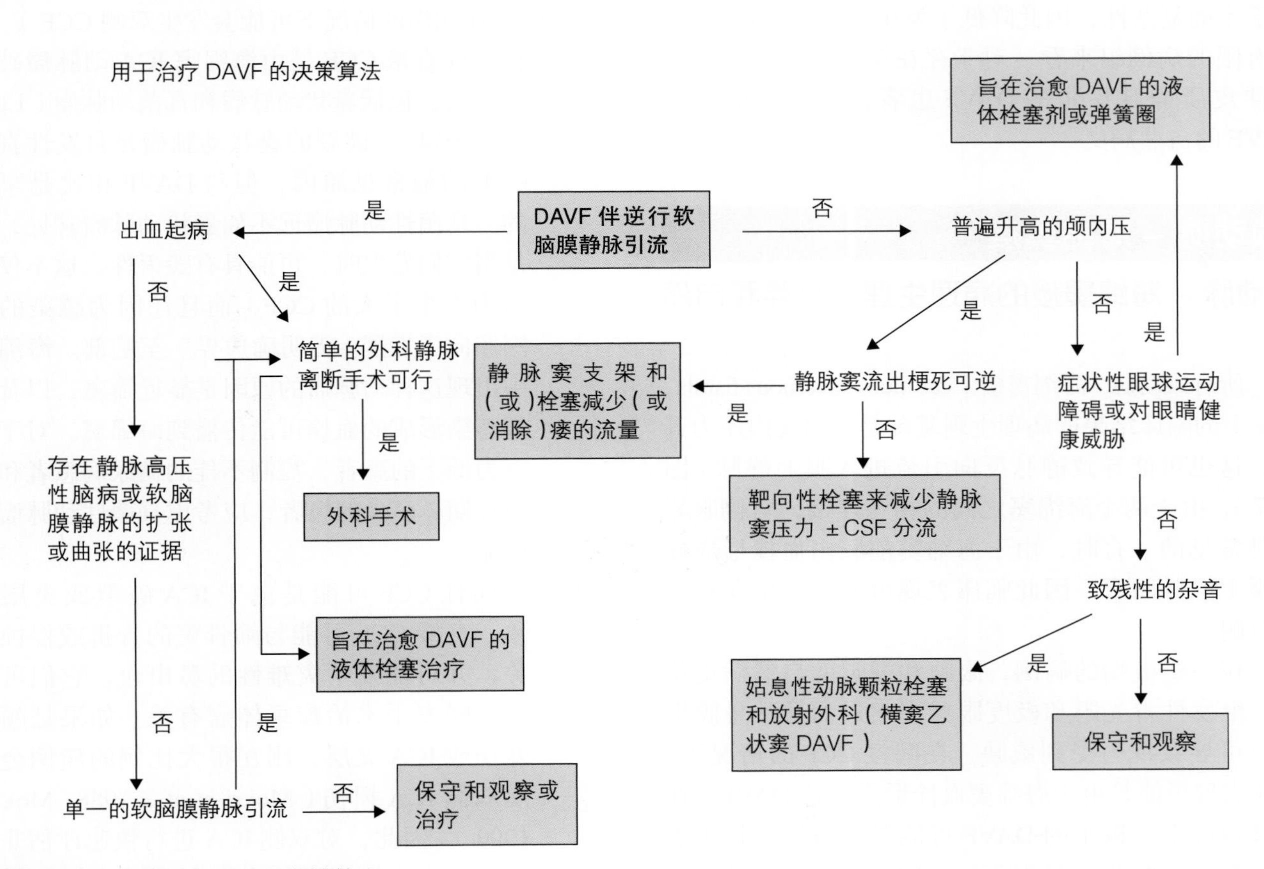

图 50.9 用于治疗 DAVF 的决策算法

一点（例如，穿过窦汇，则可能会导致灾难性后果）。在通过有或没有造影剂的CT扫描监测治疗后的血栓形成将有助于评估这种风险。此外，预防静脉血栓形成是非常重要的，尤其是因为可能存在血栓形成状态（参见上文）。

5. **深静脉血栓形成**。由于某些DAVF患者倾向于出现血栓形成状态，因此预防和警惕深静脉血栓形成（DVT）是合适的。

此外，手术还存在以下风险：

6. **假性脑膜膨出形成**。这是由于表浅静脉窦（上矢状窦和横乙状窦）的切除以及随后的硬脑膜闭合而发生的。除非存在相关的CSF循环障碍，否则通常可以在数周（数月）内解决。
7. **伤口愈合不良**。如果在手术前进行头皮动脉栓塞术，可能会出现伤口愈合问题。可以通过栓塞时仅在脑膜血管上进行来避免这种情况。

结果

外科手术和血管内治疗均具有较高的成功率且风险较低（例如Eftekhar and Morgan，2013）。由于方法的多样性和大型研究的数量有限，因此难以量化风险。在旨在仅从DAVF中消除皮质静脉引流的手术的情况下，动脉化静脉夹闭的方法有限，降低了手术的复杂性，因此降低了发生并发症的可能性。从有限的病例组来看，对于存在反向的皮质静脉引流伴皮质静脉扩张的DAVF患者，治疗可能优于DAVF的自然病史。

颈动脉–海绵窦瘘

颈动脉–海绵窦瘘的病理生理、分类和自然史

所有颈动脉-海绵窦瘘（carotico- cavernous fistula，CCF）的临床结果的病理生理基础是海绵窦内压力升高。这也可能导致静脉反向引流进入眼上静脉（**图50.7**）。由于两个海绵窦之间的相互连接，对侧眼累及是常见的。有时，由于海绵窦前腔内血栓形成导致眼上静脉闭塞，因此临床表现可能仅发生在CCF的对侧。

在一些极端的病例，眼睛和视觉的自然病史很差。继发性青光眼和极度眼球突出进而导致角膜损害，可导致视力受到威胁。在间接CCF的情况下，临床表现可能是由于海绵窦血栓形成合并DAVF。在这种情况下，极小的DAVF可能导致极端的临床表现。在直接CCF的情况下，可能会发生眼部动脉反向血流，从而导致视网膜缺血，当与高静脉压共同作用时，可能导致即时永久性视力丧失。

可能会发生除眼睛以外的问题。可能出现反向皮质静脉引流（大脑中静脉或脑桥静脉分支至岩下窦）。如果存在，则需要考虑与DAVF相关的注意事项（请参见前面）。

CCF可以是直接的，也可以是间接的。一些作者使用Barrow分类，将CCF分为四种类型（A-直接型；B-间接型，颈内动脉供血；C-间接型，颈外动脉供血；D-间接型，颈内和颈外动脉供血）（Barrow et al.，1982）。

1. 间接CCF是DAVF，与上述讨论一致。DAVF占CCF的绝大多数。它们位于海绵窦壁中，并可能（有时）与反向皮质静脉引流有关（Davies et al.，1997a；Davies et al.，1997b）。
2. 直接CCF可能是散发性或创伤性的。这些瘘通常起病突然且严重，这是因为潜在的非常高的流量，可能包括颈内动脉（ICA）（正向和反向）眼动脉以及通过后交通动脉参与贡献的后循环。因此，取决于血流的大小和Willis环的完整性，缺血可能威胁到各个大脑区域以及视力。由于它们的大小以及海绵窦之间的相互连接，两只眼睛都可以被累及，这使责任动脉的侧别识别变得困难（也要记住，在创伤的情况下可能会发生双侧CCF）。
   a. 自发性直接CCF是由海绵窦ICA动脉瘤破裂引起的，包括囊状动脉瘤和真菌动脉瘤（Lu et al.，2014）。破裂的囊状动脉瘤是自发性直接CCF的最常见原因，但与DAVF相比是罕见的。真菌性动脉瘤远不如囊状动脉瘤常见，但是当它们发生时，可能具有毁灭性，这不仅是因为发生了大的CCF，而且还因为感染的范围倾向于发展（无明确边界）至脑部。海绵窦中出现这种动脉瘤的原因是靠近筛窦，以及面部感染形成的血栓可能传播到海绵窦。对于免疫力低下的患者，控制不佳的糖尿病患者和疑似长期鼻窦炎的患者，应考虑真菌性动脉瘤的可能。
   b. 创伤性CCF可能是由于ICA破裂或夹层所致。直接CCF可能与筛骨窦的骨折或侵蚀有关，并可能发生灾难性的鼻出血。它们可以与经蝶窦手术治疗垂体瘤有关。如果是颅脑外伤或ICA夹层，则在很大比例的病例会出现双侧ICA损伤（Mokri et al.，1988；Mokri，1990）。因此，对双侧ICA进行快速评估非常重要。临床线索可能会有所帮助，例如霍纳

（Horner）综合征。然而，在存在对侧海绵窦综合征的情况下诊断霍纳综合征极具挑战性，但一旦做出诊断，应立即引起人们的担忧，因为临床情况可能非常不稳定。

CCF 的临床表现、诊断和检查

静脉高压过高可能会因静脉充血、继发性青光眼而导致红眼肿胀，并可能导致视力下降、眼球突出和限制性眼球运动。在直接 CCF 的情况下，起病突然，并且临床表现是极端的。但是，当海绵窦动脉瘤破裂导致直接 CCF 时，可能是第六脑神经麻痹和疼痛之后出现了明显的海绵窦综合征（对于浆果动脉瘤）或窦内血栓形成所致的海绵窦综合征（在真菌性动脉瘤的情况下）。对于间接 CCF，起病可能是渐进的，可能会变得极端，但通常在起病时是缓和的。此外，进行性海绵窦血栓形成可能临床上无症状。如果静脉窦血栓已知形成而症状无法改善，可能预示着 DAVF 的存在。CCF 可以在临床上得到确诊，因为闭眼后在额部放着听诊器可以听见杂音。

临床情况可能使诊断变得困难。对于头部受伤的患者，与 ICA 走行相邻的骨折，应接受 CTA。头部外伤后延迟出现的实发性结膜水肿和眼球突出应立即引起对直接 CCF 的怀疑。

可以通过 CT 或 MRI 确认眼上静脉的扩张来诊断（**图** 50.8）。与非增强检查相比，增强检查更有帮助，不仅可以更容易地识别出扩张眼上静脉，而且可以评估海绵窦内是否存在血栓形成和反向皮质静脉引流。

对于怀疑为间接 CCF 的患者，应从眼睛的健康状况中了解是否急于进行治疗，因为 CCF 可以自发消退的可能性大于 10%（Gross and Du，2012）。检查必须包括眼科医生对视力状态、眼压和眼睛保护的充分性进行评估。如果清楚地看到视力或眼睛受到威胁或逐渐恶化，或者有证据表明皮质静脉存在反流，则进行 DSA 检查并考虑治疗是适当的。

DSA 能明确诊断。在直接 CCF 的情况下，需要紧急进行 DSA 检查，并有可能介入治疗。颈内和颈外血管都需要检查以评估其供血。对于直接 CCF 中 ICA 远端没有逆行动脉血流的情况下，应为 ICA 提供足够侧支供血。这可以通过海绵窦 ICA 破裂远端的 ICA 逆行来证明。当存在前向的远端 ICA 血流时，应考虑在 DSA 检查时进行球囊闭塞试验，该试验可以安全进行。间接 CCF 可能仅在颈外血管造影上可见，并且可能见于现症状的眼睛的对侧。因此，对于间接 CCF（海绵窦 DAVF）（**图** 50.7），应进行双侧颈内外动脉 DSA 检查，以确保准确诊断。对于直接 CCF，如果考虑旁路手术，则需评估颞浅动脉是否合适。

治疗

间接 CCF 治疗

间接 CCF 的治疗需要与眼科专家协调。除非对视力或眼睛的威胁迫在眉睫，否则保守的方法是合理的（前提是不存在具有扩张性的反向皮质引流静脉），因为自发消退的可能性大于 10%。但是，当两只眼睛都累及时，应及早考虑治疗。

当做出干预的决定时，首选血管内治疗。打开海绵窦并填充促进血栓形成的材料的手术选择仅是历史上感兴趣的。在流出物仅流入大脑中静脉的情况下，可以考虑手术断开进入海绵窦时动脉化的静脉。鉴于在大多数情况下，只有眼睛处于危险之中，不宜通过旁路手术干预。

血管内治疗通常是经静脉的，要么通过眼上静脉（通过上眼睑）进入海绵窦，要么通过岩下窦进入。目的是阻塞静脉窦，以阻止血流反向流入眼上静脉，对侧海绵窦，通过大脑中静脉进入皮质静脉或通过岩下窦进入脑桥静脉。由于海绵窦内局部血栓形成，到达治疗部位可能困难，单一入路被证明可能是不充分的。

直接 CCF 治疗

可以通过重建（血管内方法）或闭塞（血管内或手术）ICA 来治疗直接 CCF。在重建的情况下，可以采用血流导向支架、覆膜支架、可脱球囊或支架辅助弹簧圈栓塞瘘口（Lu et al.，2014）。由于流量较大，与 DAVF 相比，静脉途径治疗直接 CCF 的问题更大。但是，如果经动脉途径未能完全闭合瘘口，则可在 ICA 支架置入后使用静脉途径（Lin et al.，2015）。治疗的选择取决于动脉壁的健康状况。将弹簧圈放入假性动脉瘤中可能会有问题，除非预计动脉的愈合可能会阻塞 ICA，而这可能是适宜的治疗选择。当进行了血管重建后，重要的是要进行后期检查排除假性动脉瘤的发生。

当确定建立了充分的侧支供血时，闭塞可以作为直接 CCF 的治疗。如果评估现有侧支供血不足，则应在闭塞动脉之前考虑高流量或低流量旁路手术。这也可能影响闭塞技术。如果认为不需要旁路手术，则在 DSA 时可通过血管内手段轻松实现闭塞。至关重要的是将动脉破裂点包括在被闭塞的区域中。近端闭塞可能导致眼动脉或 ICA 反向血流加重并导致局部缺血。在需要旁路手术的情况下，如果确认需要最少的额外流量，则 STA-MCA 低流量旁路是合理的。这种情况的一个例子是，在球囊闭塞试验过程中没有出现临床症状，但 DSA 上相比对侧，目标半球的毛细血管或静脉充血明显延迟（横流延迟）。如果由于临床指标、球囊阻塞试验或 DSA 检查认为需要维持 ICA 血流，则适合采用大流量旁路手术。为了提供最低 150 ml/min 的流速以替代 ICA 流量并防止梗死，可以使用隐静脉、桡动脉作为旁路血管。高流量旁路比 STA-MCA 旁路具有更高的手术风险，但在第一周后具有相似的长期通畅性（Sia et al.，2011）。

并发症管理

眼科监测和管理对于评估和管理继发性青光眼和角膜保护至关重要。

间接 CCF 并发症管理

对于经静脉途径治疗的海绵窦 DAVF，前面部分关于 DAVF 的并发症是相通的。最典型的与海绵窦综合征（导致眼眶和脑叶静脉功能不足，直到形成侧支）和在完全闭塞之前的过程中大脑的静脉高压有关，可能导致静脉高压性脑病（通常为脑桥）或同一大脑区域内的出血（图 50.7）。

直接 CCF 并发症管理

对于直接的 CCF，要在保留 ICA 的基础上进行治疗，则需要考虑并避免一些并发症。其中最担心的是：

1. **栓塞**。由于这些病变的稀有性，没有大型病例研究能显示出栓塞的并发症。但是，从动脉瘤的治疗推断是合适的。在动脉瘤的血管内治疗之后，无症状栓塞是一种相对普遍的现象，并且据报道，在复杂的动脉瘤治疗例如支架辅助栓塞的情况下，多达一半的病例在脑部 MRI 扫描中显示出明显的栓塞现象（Hahnemann et al.，2014）。然而，这些事件中很少有会导致不良的临床结果，并且在使用血流导向支架后，发生率可能为 1% ~5%（Saatci et al.，2012；McDonald et al.，2015）。这可能会在支架或弹簧圈放置时或不久之后。预先使用抗血小板药物并持续使用长达 6 个月是预防栓子的适当方法。但是，即使采取了这种预防措施，手术者也必须准备检查栓子并取回或溶解它。在大约 25% 的病例中，对最初推荐的氯吡格雷处理的反应不充分（Oran et al.，2015）。因此，注意患者对治疗的个体化反应可能会降低栓塞率。
2. **动脉瘤的复发（或假性动脉瘤）**。由于这些病变的稀有性，没有大型病例研究可以显示复发率。但是，从动脉瘤的治疗推断是合适的。对于动脉瘤的治疗，在血流导向装置治疗的动脉瘤中，有 10% ~40% 可能发生动脉瘤栓塞不全或复发（McAuliffe et al.，2012；Saatci et al.，2012；Toma et al.，2013；Fischer et al.，2014）。
3. **ICA 闭塞**。尽管闭塞可能是对这些病变的有效治疗，但如果不适当，计划外或已确定不能耐受闭塞，则可能会导致灾难性后果。如果尽早进行，可以进行紧急血运重建，并且可以预防灾难性卒中（请参阅卒中部分）。由于可能会预先使用氯吡格雷和阿司匹林，因此与血管内解决方案相比，采用高流量旁路进行外科血运重建术的需求较小。至于血管内治疗，时间是决定性因素，如果在闭塞后 6 小时内无法实现血运重建，尝试进行血运重建可能弊大于利。
4. **远端出血**。已经报道了在血流导向支架展开后远端出血的记录。其机制可能是栓塞的结果，也可能是由于动脉壁张力的改变，从而未能在 Willis 环中减弱动脉压力波。

对于通过闭塞治疗的直接 CCF。通过 DSA 检查的证据（例如，无神经功能缺损的 ICA 反向血流）或球囊闭塞试验，确定 ICA 可以被牺牲而没有血流动力学诱发的卒中的危险时，可以进行 ICA 闭塞。但是，应考虑以下并发症：

1. **栓塞**。从闭塞点开始的血栓形成将继续发展到下一个最重要的分支点。这通常是眼动脉。但是，如果眼动脉的持续供应导致远端 ICA 没有足够的血流所致的剪应力，则血栓蔓延可能会穿过眼动脉并继续发展。该过程可能继续累及临床上重要的动脉，包括脉络膜前动脉和末端 ICA。在向 ICA 供血的侧支血流进入 ICA（即后交通动脉）或 ICA 终止（即大脑前动脉）并向远端脉管系统提供正常正向血流的位置，血栓 - 血流界面可提供栓子的来源。要防止这种情况，需要使用抗血小板药物并至少维持正常的血压。栓塞，即使很小，也可以通过抗凝治疗，但如果存在近端闭塞，则不易通过取栓来治疗。在经验丰富的术者，如果手术时间较短，则导管可通过前交通动脉或后交通动脉进入栓塞部位（在相当长的时间内不损害侧支血流）可使血栓溶解。
2. **瘘再通**。当出现视觉症状复发或未能改善时应怀疑闭塞不完全或再通。CT 扫描显示眼上静脉持续增大则支持这一考虑。当怀疑再通时，行 DSA 检查来确诊和计划治疗是必要的。

3. **血流动力学性缺血**。尽管球囊闭塞试验是可靠的，但可能会被错误解释（由于技术问题或临床阈值错误），患者不能耐受后续的闭塞。如果尝试逆转阻塞时间超过一个短时间段，不建议去除闭塞材料，因为可能出现血栓栓塞。血流动力学诱发的缺血应迅速识别，并在紧急情况下升高血压。如果不能迅速逆转局部缺血，则应立即进行巴比妥诱导昏迷（始终保持正常至高血压）和颞浅至大脑中动脉搭桥的血运重建。在这种情况下，高流量旁路有潜在的危险，原因是重新血管化所需时间，以及充血和卒中后的出血性转化风险（Sia et al.，2011）。
4. **闭塞后晚期动脉瘤形成**。ICA 闭塞可能与对侧 ICA、同侧 PCA（后交通和前交通）动脉瘤有关，因为剪切应力增加（Roski et al.，1981）。这种重要的并发症虽然不常见，但对于那些未经旁路而进行闭塞治疗的患者，应该进行长期监测。

对于旁路手术治疗的直接 CCF，颞浅至大脑中动脉旁路和高流量旁路（以桡动脉或隐静脉作为颅外循环和 ICA 之间的通路）之间的手术复杂性存在很大差异。高流量旁路手术的并发症发生率为 5% ~13%，而颞浅至大脑中动脉旁路的并发症发生率为 0.5% ~5%（Sia et al.，2011）。处理这些并发症非常复杂，通常涉及快速识别和紧急外科手术，因此，治疗应在具有相当专业知识的脑血管外科领域中心进行。

结果

间接 CCF 结果

在大多数情况下，对眼睛的临床评估是评估动静脉瘘是否治愈的准确方法。例外是，当眼睛好转但瘘持续存在合并反向皮质静脉引流或岩部引流，反之，由于同时发生眼下静脉阻塞，眼睛仍有症状。但是，侧支静脉容量通常会随着时间的推移而改善，随后眼部问题也会逐渐改善。大多数患者迅速好转，复发很少见。

直接 CCF 结果

直接 CCF 有许多要考虑的结果。其中包括眼睛，局部动脉部位，ICA 远端供血，直接或间接对侧动脉系统以及创伤或感染（包括脑神经和脑脊液漏出的可能性）造成的结构性损伤。当 ICA 被保留时，动脉的愈合需要被视为已经发生。对于创伤或任何假性动脉瘤，很难预测出健康的动脉愈合的机会。当通过闭塞治疗直接 CCF 时，对局部部位愈合的关注较少，但对于远端缺血的可能性则存在更大的关注。由于流量增加和切应力，存在后交通动脉或前交通动脉中形成动脉瘤的可能，但风险很小。直接或间接 CCF 消除需要考虑的因素是，眼睛的症状和体征可能开始迅速好转，但随后却无法继续消退。有时可以通过海绵窦血栓形成来解释。海绵窦血栓形成引起的静脉功能不全可能需要一段时间才能恢复，随后眼睛才能恢复。

用 ICA 闭塞和搭桥治疗直接 CCF 患者除眼睛结局外，还具有与搭桥相关的结局。高流量旁路产生不良后果的最常见原因是旁路的急性闭塞（发生在大约 7% 的病例中）。鉴于这些病例要么没有通过球囊闭塞试验而失败，要么有临床或放射学证据表明不能耐受 ICA 闭塞，所以这将导致明显的致残率就不足为奇了。经验丰富的医生所做的颞浅至大脑中动脉旁路手术的通畅率预计为 98%（Sia et al.，2011）。在第一周中幸存下来之后，长期通畅率对于高流量旁路和颞浅动脉旁路而言都是极好的，并且这些通畅是相似的（Sia et al.，2011）。

延伸阅读、参考文献、EBRAIN 的相关链接

扫描书末二维码获取。

第 51 章 颈动脉疾病和脑缺血

Kieron Sweeney · A. O'Hare · Mohsen Javadpour 著
刘二腾 译，陆军 审校

引言

由于颈动脉疾病和脑缺血的发病率较高，需要准确、及时的诊断和治疗才能降低与这些疾病相关的发病率和死亡率。在这里，我们讨论这些疾病的流行病学、病理生理学、临床表现、检查和治疗，并进一步讨论内科、介入和外科治疗方案的现有证据。

脑缺血和脑卒中 / 梗死

病因学

脑缺血和脑卒中涉及多种病理过程。这些病理过程可以影响大血管或小血管，并分为血栓性、栓塞性或闭塞性原因。血栓性缺血最常见病因是动脉粥样硬化（下文讨论）。栓塞性缺血最常见病因是心房颤动所致的心源性，其次是主动脉或颈动脉粥样硬化。这两个原因都可以影响大血管和小血管。闭塞性疾病，如纤维素样坏死或脂性透明变性，主要影响小血管，由于中膜的增厚而导致腔隙性卒中或白质病。由于动脉粥样硬化原发血管的斑块脱落闭塞了小血管导致腔隙性卒中。

这些过程都有着共同的危险因素。常见危险因素包括年龄、性别、种族、家族史和遗传学。常见的可变危险因素包括高血压、吸烟、糖尿病、血脂异常和饮食。

血栓性脑卒中的罕见原因包括脑静脉窦血栓形成（Ferro and Canhao，2014）和高凝状态（遗传和获得性），血管夹层引起的创伤性闭塞，创伤所致占位性病变导致占位效应，从而引起大脑镰下疝，导致大脑前动脉（anterior cerebral artery，ACA）梗死，或小脑幕缘疝导致大脑后动脉（posterior cerebral artery，PCA）梗死，偏头痛或血管痉挛引起的痉挛性闭塞、炎性血管炎和其他闭塞性疾病，如辐射的延迟效应、Moya 纤维肌发育不良、脑淀粉样血管病和 CADASIL（Caplan，2015）。

发生率

缺血性脑卒中约占所有脑血管意外（cerebrovascular accidents，CVA）的 87%。在全球范围内，缺血性脑卒中的发生率存在很大差异，因为年龄、吸烟和饮食等危险因素有很大的差异性。全球疾病负担工作组发表了关于缺血性脑卒中的报告。这一系统的综述比较了全球各国报告的发病率，并根据收入对其进行了分类（Bennett et al.，2014）。从 1990 年到 2010 年，高收入国家的缺血性脑卒中发病率有所下降，而中低收入国家的发病率一直居高不下。西欧的发病率为 127.65/10 万，2010 年降至 102.39/10 万。1990 年撒哈拉以南中部非洲的发病率为 136.36/10 万，在 2010 年增加到 166.69/10 万。这是由于吸烟和预期寿命延长。

脑缺血和脑卒中的病理生理学

大脑是人体代谢最活跃的器官之一。它只占总体重的 2%，但需要 15%~20% 的心输出量和 20% 的总耗氧量。与其他器官不同，大脑的能量储备有限，完全依赖于血液供应（Clarke and Sokoloff，1999）。大脑的功能单位是神经元。神经元代谢严重依赖于有氧线粒体代谢，为离子泵系统消耗大量能量，以维持膜电位和参与动作电位。神经元有氧代谢的底物是葡萄糖、乳酸和酮体，神经元活动的最终产物则被挤压到细胞外环境中，它们是 K^+ 和谷氨酸等。星形胶质细胞充当神经元（↑ K^+、↑谷氨酸、↓葡萄糖、↓乳酸）的代谢传感器，继而与微血管内皮细胞偶联，从而改变与局部神经元活动有关的局部血流［脑血流（CBF）调节在其他地方讨论］。大脑的代谢需求在存在区域差异，灰质和皮质的代谢比白质束更活跃。白质的平均 CBF 约为 50 ml/100 g，灰质约为 20 ml/100 g 和 70 ml/100 g。

脑缺血是血流量的减少导致供给脑组织的氧气

和葡萄糖的减少。梗死是脑组织不可逆转的死亡。当CBF降至30 ml/（100 g · min）时，可能会出现神经系统症状。CBF进一步降至15~20 ml/（100 g · min）将导致可逆性伤害或“电衰竭”。这种状态仅能耐受几个小时。CBF降至10~15 ml/（100 g · min）会导致不可逆的神经元损害，2分钟内ATP含量将耗尽，随后发生Na/K ATP泵的故障。这会阻止正常的膜电位恢复，并且细胞会因Ca的流入而去极化。这种去极化作用会扩散，导致缺血级联反应释放出谷氨酸盐。细胞凋亡触发神经元死亡。

缺血半暗带模型是应用最广泛的模型。该模型由灌注动脉或小动脉组成，其核心是不可逆损伤的脑组织（神经元、星形胶质细胞/少突胶质细胞），周围有一个可逆的低灌注组织区域。影响半暗带组织体积的主要因素是侧支循环的质量和再灌注的时间（Jung et al.，2013）。侧支循环包括Willis环、相邻动脉区域之间的软脑膜连接以及颈外动脉和颈内动脉循环之间的吻合。

椎基底动脉和颈动脉缺血综合征的临床表现

缺血性脑卒中是指突然出现的神经系统症状，造成永久性缺陷，可以根据病因和临床症状（TOAST—Trial of Org 10172 in Acute Stroke Treatment）或血管区域和表现症状[牛津社区脑卒中计划分类（Oxford Community Stroke Project classification，OCSP）]进行分类。症状和体征与受影响的血管相对应的大脑区域有关。

前循环体征和症状

大脑前动脉（ACA）卒中症状

大脑前动脉区梗死并不常见，仅占脑卒中的1.3%（Arboix et al.，2009）。ACA分为三个部分。A1发出内侧豆纹动脉，偶尔还发出Heubner返动脉。由于存在前交通动脉的交叉血流，A1节段闭塞往往没有远端闭塞严重，并且可能导致五种腔隙性卒中综合征中的任何一种：纯运动、纯感觉、混合运动-感觉、共济失调性偏瘫和构音障碍手笨拙综合征。ACA远段供应胼胝体前叶、额叶内侧和顶叶，A2有时发出Heubner返动脉。因此，A2远段闭塞可导致腔隙性卒中综合征、失联综合征、尿失禁、对侧下肢瘫、对侧下肢感觉丧失，以及失用。

大脑中动脉（MCA）卒中症状

大脑中动脉区梗死是迄今为止最常见的脑卒中类型。大脑中动脉分为四个部分，提供大脑凸面皮质和额叶、顶叶和颞叶的皮质下白质的大部分，基底节和前后内囊的大部分。M1发出外侧豆纹动脉，这些血管的闭塞可导致腔隙性脑卒中综合征（见上文）。M2分为上干和下干。下干闭塞可导致视野缺损，如对侧同向偏盲或上象限偏盲。在优势半球，它导致感觉性失语；在非优势半球，它导致结构性失用。上干闭塞导致对侧偏瘫，手臂和面部比腿部受到更大的影响，优势侧半球出现偏身感觉丧失和运动性失语，非优势侧半球则出现偏身忽略。向优势半球下顶叶供血的上干的M4段分支如果闭塞，可导致格斯特曼（Gerstmann）综合征，即失写、失算、左右混淆和手指失认。

M1段主干闭塞可导致恶性MCA综合征，其梗死组织肿胀超过2~5天，导致占位效应逐渐加重，大脑廉下疝和颞叶沟回疝，这将造成中脑受压，并可能损害ACA和PCA区域的血供，进一步加重脑疝。如不治疗，其死亡率达80%。该情况下去骨瓣减压手术的作用将在后面讨论。

后循环体征和症状

大脑后动脉（PCA）卒中症状

大脑后动脉闭塞占所有缺血性脑卒中的5%~10%。PCA可分为四个部分。P1段：旁正中穿支的闭塞导致丘脑和中脑梗死，其特征为嗜睡、认知障碍和垂直性动眼神经麻痹。当存在单一优势丘脑穿支（一种罕见的变异）时，该动脉被称为Percheron动脉，其闭塞导致双侧内侧丘脑梗死。当大脑脚的血液供应来自P1段的穿支时，梗死导致严重偏瘫或轻偏瘫。P2段：丘脑膝状体动脉的闭塞导致严重的对侧偏身感觉过敏和共济失调。如果梗死导致偏身感觉丧失和偏身疼痛，该综合征被称为丘脑疼痛综合征或Dejerine-Roussy综合征。中脑腹内侧梗死累及动眼神经束和（或）核团，沿大脑脚分布[皮质脊髓束和（或）皮质球束]，可引起同侧动眼神经和对侧肢体偏瘫，即韦伯（Weber）综合征。当梗死涉及中脑背侧被盖（包括动眼神经核、红核、臂结膜）或小脑上脚纤维交叉，导致动眼神经麻痹和对侧小脑共济失调时，称为Benedikts综合征。如中脑被盖内的梗死范围也累及大脑脚，可导致动眼神经、对侧肢体偏瘫和对侧小脑性共济失调，则被称为Claude综合征。由于累及黑质，可表现为帕金森病的症状

（Ruchalski and Hathout，2012）。脉络膜后动脉闭塞累及外侧膝状体，可导致扇形盲，即一种楔形或扇形的视野缺损。P3段和P4段提供枕叶皮质（距状沟）、顶叶（楔前叶）、部分颞叶（钩状回、前梭状回、颞下回）和胼胝体压部。这些血管的阻塞可因视野丧失而产生一系列视觉症状，如伴有或不伴有黄斑保留的同向偏盲（大脑中动脉的侧支代偿）、视觉失认症、面容失认症和伴有或不伴有失写的失读症。Anton（-Babinski）综合征是一种视觉失认症（伴有虚构的皮质盲），患者否认自己因双侧大脑后动脉梗死而失明。Balint综合征涉及视觉共济失调，双侧顶枕叶同时梗死导致丧失自主性但存在反射性眼活动（Cereda and Carrera，2012；Ruchalski and Hathout，2012）。

椎基底动脉脑卒中症状（头侧至尾侧）

基底动脉头端（顶端）发出P1s。因此，基底动脉顶端闭塞可引起中脑、丘脑、颞叶和枕叶的缺血，并可产生一系列体征，被称为基底动脉尖综合征。这些体征包括意识障碍、嗜睡和垂直性凝视瘫痪，可伴四肢瘫痪但并不常见（Caplan，1980）。

小脑上动脉（superior cerebellar artery，SCA）可分为四段（桥前段、脑池段、四叠体段和皮质段）。近段SCA向脑桥、中脑和下丘供血，因此其近段闭塞可导致脑干顶端缺血表现，如同侧Horner综合征，对侧痛、温觉丧失和对侧滑车神经麻痹（脑桥上外侧被盖），以及小脑体征，如同侧肢体测距不准、构音障碍和共济失调。

小脑前下动脉（anterior inferior cerebellar artery，AICA）起源于基底动脉的中部至尾部1/3，供应脑桥下外侧被盖（三叉神经、面神经、前庭神经、耳蜗核和脊髓丘脑束）、小脑中脚和小叶。闭塞可导致眩晕、呕吐、耳鸣、构音障碍、面瘫、听力损失、Horner综合征、疼痛和体温损失、同侧共轭凝视麻痹（由于小叶）和测距不准。当所有这些症状和体征同时出现时，该综合征被称为脑桥外侧综合征或Marie-Foix综合征。

基底动脉由椎动脉汇合而成，终止于P1s的分叉处。它发出脑桥内侧穿支，供应脑桥基底内侧（皮质脊髓束）；旁正中穿支供应脑桥被盖内侧（包括第四脑室底、外展核、内侧纵束和脑桥旁正中网状结构；脑桥短旋支，供应脑桥基底和被盖的外侧；最后是长旋支，供应脑桥基底和被盖的最外侧部分。基底动脉的其他分支，小脑上动脉和小脑前下动脉在前面已经讨论过了。穿支闭塞可导致共济失调偏瘫，其特征为对侧无力和对侧共济失调。旁正中动脉和短旋支闭塞可导致对侧偏瘫、同侧面部无力和同侧侧视麻痹，这被称为桥下内侧综合征或Foville综合征（Kataoka et al.，1997）。如果没有合并面部症状，被称为脑桥腹侧综合征/Raymond综合征。如果凝视麻痹是由展神经麻痹"引起的"，为脑桥腹侧综合征/Millard–Gubler综合征。闭锁综合征是由于双侧脑桥基底部损伤，但脑桥被盖良好，导致皮质脊髓束和皮质球束受损，同时核上眼球运动通路和网状结构完好，使垂直眼球运动、眨眼和意识完好无损。

颅内椎动脉或V4段产生两组主要分支。中间分支包括脊髓前动脉（供应延髓内侧）和盲孔分支（位于延髓桥连接处，供应远至被盖和第四脑室底部）。外侧分支包括小脑后下动脉（posterior inferior cerebellar artery，PICA）、小脑下脚环形分支、延髓外侧和橄榄结构（Akar et al.，1994）。小脑后下动脉分为四段，分布于延髓外侧、小脑后下半球和下蚓部。脊髓前动脉闭塞可导致对侧偏瘫、对侧感觉缺失和同侧伸舌无力，也称为内侧髓质综合征或Dejerien综合征。闭塞小脑下动脉可导致一系列与延髓外侧有关的体征和症状，包括三叉神经尾侧核、前庭核、疑核、脊髓丘脑束、下行交感神经和小脑（网状体）。症状包括同侧面部疼痛和体温下降、共济失调、眼球震颤、眩晕、声音嘶哑、吞咽困难、Horner综合征和对侧半感觉丧失，称为延髓外侧综合征或Wallenberg综合征。

脑缺血和脑卒中的检查

急性卒中患者的评估可分为两个阶段。紧急评估包括使用诸如NIHS量表（见**表**51.1）等临床评分系统，以及影像学检查。影像学检查方法由实际情况决定，例如血管内介入治疗和快速的影像检查。非紧急评估包括"代谢综合征"的检查。

标准的成像方式是非增强CT（见**图**51.1）。这是一种筛查工具，用于排除缺血性卒中的类似情况，如出血性卒中或占位性病变。CT平扫可发现大脑中动脉早期缺血，可以计算Alberta卒中计划早期CT评分（ASPECTS）（参见**表**51.2；**图**51.2），明显低密度区及其体积，高密度动脉征。在神经血管介入的中心，CT血管成像（CTA）可以提供有关闭塞位置、侧支供应质量和血管狭窄的信息（见**图**51.3和**图**51.4）。如果CTA包含主动脉弓和颈部血管，则可以获得关于脑卒中病因和干预技术难度的重要信息。CTA被用于四个重要的血管内治疗临床试验：

表 51.1 NIHS 量表

指示	规模定义	指示	规模定义
1a：意识水平（LOC）	0= 反应灵敏 1= 不灵敏，但在轻微刺激下可唤醒 2= 不灵敏；需要反复强烈的刺激 3= 无反应	6：运动腿 6a：左 6b：右	0= 无下落 1= 能抬起，不能维持 2= 能对抗部分重力 3= 不能对抗重力 4= 没有任何运动 UN/X= 截肢或关节融合
1b：LOC 问题 - 两个定向问题	0= 两项均正确 1= 一项正确 2= 均不正确	7：肢体共济失调	0= 无共济失调 1= 在一个肢体中存在 2= 在两个肢体中存在 UN/X= 无法测试
1c：LOC 命令 - 两项命令	0= 均正确执行 1= 一项正确执行 2= 两项均不正确	8：感官	0= 正常 1= 轻度至中度损失 2= 重度到完全的感觉丧失
2：凝视	0= 正常 1= 部分凝视麻痹 2= 强迫凝视	9：语言	0= 正常 1= 轻度至中度失语 2= 重度失语 3= 不能说话或完全失语
3：视野	0= 视觉损失 1= 局部偏盲 2= 完全性偏盲 3= 双侧偏盲	10：构音障碍	0= 正常 1= 轻度至中度构音障碍 2= 重度构音障碍 UN/X= 不可测
4：面瘫	0= 正常 1= 轻微轻瘫 2= 严重轻瘫 3= 完全瘫痪	11：忽视和注意力不集中	0= 正常 1= 视觉、触觉、听觉、空间或个人注意力不集中 2= 严重的忽视或一种以上的偏侧忽视
5：上肢运动 5a：左 5b：右	0= 无下落 1= 能抬起，不能维持 2= 能对抗部分重力 3= 不能对抗重力 4= 没有任何运动 UN/X= 截肢或关节融合		

Reproduced with permission from T Brott, HP Adams, CP Olinger, JR Marler, WG Barsan, J Biller, J Spilker, R Holleran, R Eberle, V Hertzberg, Measurements of acute cerebral infarction: a clinical examination scale, *Stroke*, Volume 20, Issue 7, pp. 864–70. Copyright © 1989 Wolters Kluwer Health, Inc.

ESCAPE、MR CLEAN、EXTEND-IA 和 SWIFT。CT 灌注通过脑血流量或脑血容量评估梗死核心的体积，通过 MTT 或 Tmax 评估可挽救的半暗带的体积，以及通过不匹配比系数来评估半暗带与核心梗死灶的比率。MRA、DWI 和 MR 灌注等 MR 成像提供了与 CTA 和 CT 灌注相似的信息。但是，在急性卒中使用 MRI 检查存在很多逻辑上的问题，例如非工作时间的使用、扫描时间和病情不稳定的患者的监测（Menon et al.，2015；Na et al.，2015）。

脑缺血和脑卒中的内科治疗

治疗的目标是将闭塞血管再通，迅速恢复血液供应，以挽救半暗带，并通过纠正低血压、高体温和严格的血糖控制等一系列措施保障半暗带的灌注。对于需要再灌注治疗的高血压患者，使用拉贝洛尔、尼卡地平或硝普钠可将收缩压降至 185 mmHg 以下或舒张压降至 110 mmHg 以下，并在治疗后将收缩压维持在 180 mmHg 以下或舒张压维持在 105 mmHg 以下（Jauch et al.，2013）。在再灌注治疗后，患者还应进行体格检查和病因治疗。

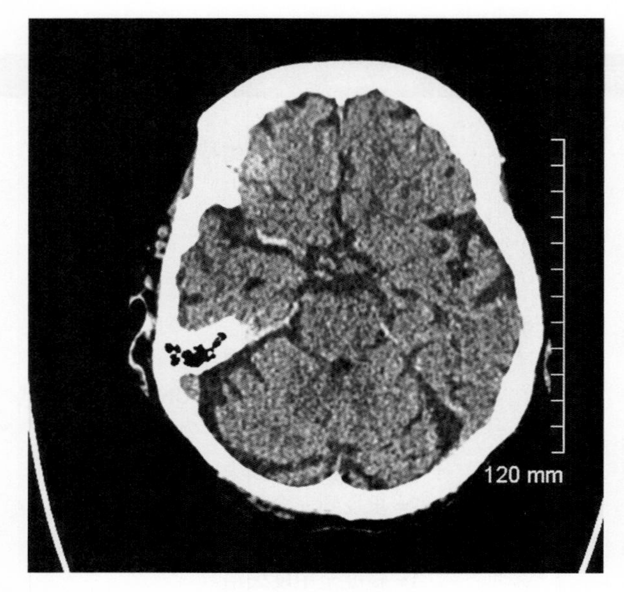

图 51.1 平扫 CT 脑显示右脑高密度中动脉（MCA）

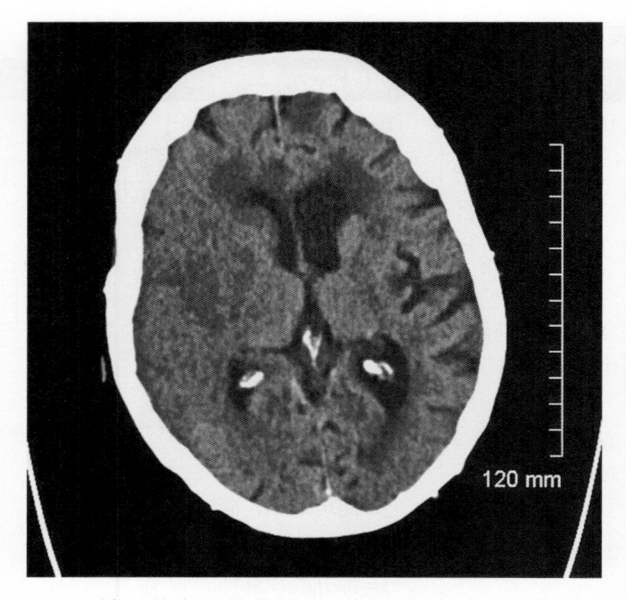

图 51.2 神经节水平的平扫 CT 脑显示 ASPECTS 评分为 7

表 51.2 ASPECTS 评分用于评估大脑中动脉梗死的严重程度。在基底节和基底节上方的区域内，两个标准轴位 CT 上，初始分数为 10，每累及一结构或者区域，扣 1 分，得分≤7 表示结果差

CT 级别	
基底节层面	尾状核、壳核、内囊、岛叶皮质、M1（额盖 / 前 MCA 皮质）、M2（颞前极 / 岛叶皮质外侧 带）、M3（颞后极 / 后 MCA 皮质）
基底节上方层面	M4（靠近 M1 上方的 MCA 前区）、M5（高于 M2 的 MCA 中段）、M6（紧靠 M3 上方的 MCA 后区）

Reprinted from *The Lancet*, Volume 355, Issue 9216, Philip A Barber, Andrew M Demchuk, Jinjin Zhang, Alastair M Buchan, Validity and reliability of a quantitative computed tomography score in predicting outcome of hyperacute stroke before thrombolytic therapy, pp. 1670–74, Copyright (2000), with permission from Elsevier.

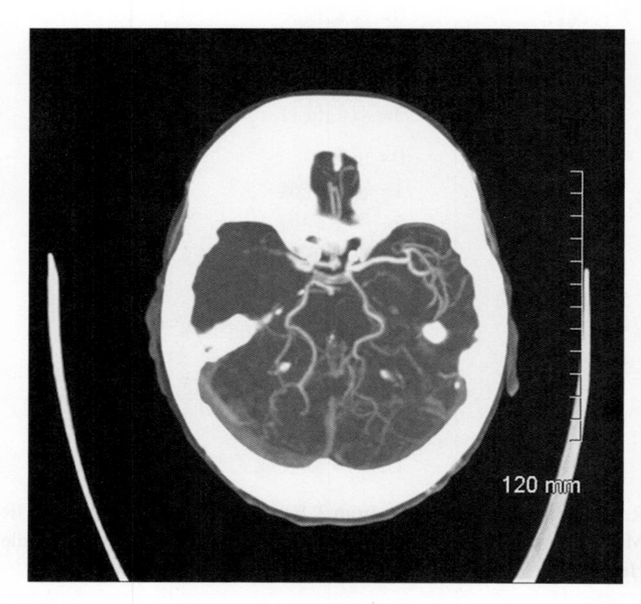

图 51.3 CT 血管造影显示右侧 MCA 有充盈缺损（最大密度投影 5 mm）

溶栓

重组组织型纤溶酶原激活剂（recombinant tissue plasminogen activator，rt-PA）静脉溶栓的应用是由 1995 年 NIND 发表的标志性文章确立的。这项试验随机将 600 名患者分为治疗组和安慰剂组。发病后 3 h 内单次给予 rt-PA 0.9 mg/kg（最大剂量 90 mg）。治疗组在所有预后指标，NIHSS 评分、Barthel 指数、GOS 和 mRS 评分方面均显示出改善的结果，并且脑出血的风险是可接受的。最近的 ECASS-Ⅲ试验将时间窗口增加到 4.5 h（有关Ⅳ rt-PA 患者选择的纳入和排除标准，请参见**表** 51.3）。随着使用灌注成像技术来选择筛查发病患者，溶栓的时间窗可能进一步推后（Burton et al.，2015）。但超过 4.5 h 进行静脉溶栓，会有较高的 SICH 风险。大血管闭塞如颈内动脉（ICA）和大脑中动脉（MCA）近端的 IV rt-PA 再通率也会降低。

手术及介入管理

动脉内溶栓（IA）是一种直接将溶栓剂输送到闭塞部位的神经血管介入治疗方法。到目前为止，只发表了一项试验，即 PROACT II 试验。证明了脑卒中后 6 小时内应用重组尿激酶原治疗有效，但 SICH

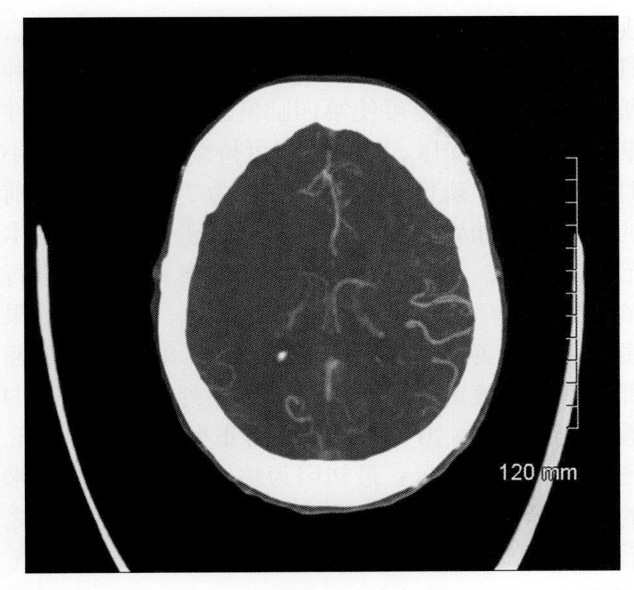

图 51.4　颅内血管 CT 血管造影显示右侧 MCA 区远端充盈减少且不对称

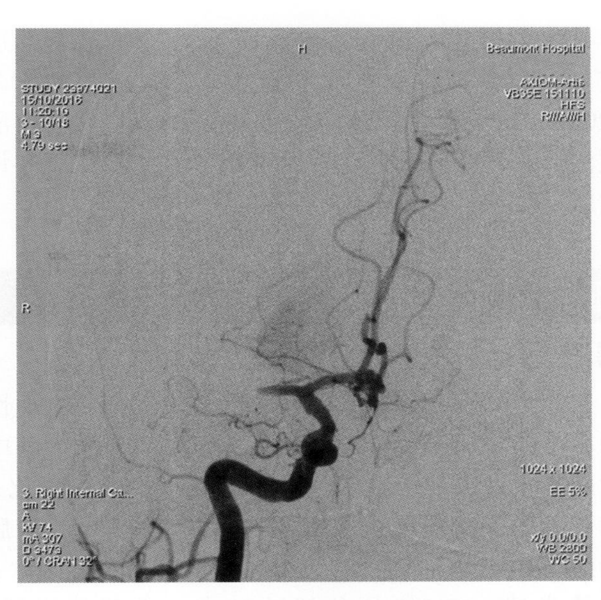

图 51.5　右侧颈内动脉的注射数字减影血管造影显示右侧 MCA 有充盈缺损

发生率会增加。该药物尚未获得食品和药品管理局（FDA）的批准。

随着各种设备的发展，血栓清除术得到了长足的发展，线圈型取栓器，例如 MERCI，与取栓支架，例如 Stryker 公司的 TREVO® 和 Covidien 公司的 Solitaire FR™。取栓支架已被证明优于线圈型取栓器。最近的几项随机临床试验表明，与静脉溶栓相比，血栓清除术的时间窗可达 6 小时。这些随机试验包括 MR CLEAN、ESCAPE、SWIFT PRIME、EXTEND-IA、REV ASCT 和 THRACE（Ding，2015）。这些试验均提示血栓清除术 90 天 mRS（0~2）有显著改善，治疗大动脉闭塞的疗效优于使用或者不使用静脉 rt-PA 的最佳药物治疗，因此被提前终止。目前的建议是：大动脉闭塞的患者，使用取栓支架进行血栓清除术（6 小时内）应该作为静脉溶栓（4.5 小时内）的辅助手段。如果静脉溶栓有禁忌证，推荐单独进行血栓清除术治疗大动脉栓塞（见**图** 51.5）。

表 51.3　r-tPA 治疗的适应证、相对禁忌证和绝对禁忌证

适应证	相对禁忌证	绝对禁忌证
年龄：>18 岁	最近 14 天内有过大手术或严重外伤	颅内出血证据
诊断为缺血性脑血管事件		颅内出血史
发病时间 3~4.5 h	血糖 <2.7 mm/L 或 >22.2 mm/L	椎管内手术、严重头创伤或过去 3 个月内脑卒中
	血小板计数 <10 万	临床表现提示蛛网膜下腔出血，即使 CT 正常
	凝血功能障碍：INR>1.7；aPTT>40 s	活动性内出血或急性创伤，如骨折
	最近 3 周内有过胃肠道（GI）或泌尿生殖系统（GU）出血	过去 7 天内在不可压迫的部位进行过动脉穿刺
	最近 3 个月内心肌梗死（MI）	已知的脑动静脉畸形（arteriovenous malformation，AVM）、肿瘤或动脉瘤
		收缩压 >185 mmHg，舒张 >110 mmHg
		癫痫急性发作

Data from Demaerschalk, B.M., et al., Scientific Rationale for the Inclusion and Exclusion Criteria for Intravenous Alteplase in Acute Ischemic Stroke: A Statement for Healthcare Professionals from the American Heart Association/American Stroke Association. *Stroke*, volume 47, Issue 2, pp. 581–641. 2016.

如果患者不符合溶栓治疗或血栓清除术的适应证，应立即接受抗血小板治疗。包括收缩压>220 mmHg或舒张压>120 mmHg的患者。接受再灌注治疗的患者至少应等待24小时，在CT或MRI评估后再接受抗血小板治疗。

脑卒中减压开颅术

幕上

恶性大脑中动脉综合征（前面讨论过）占缺血性脑卒中的5%~10%，死亡率高达80%。恶性大脑中动脉卒中遵循三个临床过程：① 96 h内迅速恶化；②数天内逐渐恶化；③最初恶化，随后平稳，最后得到改善。出现恶性大脑中动脉综合征的预测因素：优势半球、NIHSS评分超过20分，非优势半球、NIHSS评分超过15分；白细胞升高；血清标志物如血清S100B或MMP-9升高；早期（48 h内）累及超过50%的大脑中动脉区域，松果体移位超过4 mm，或96 h内前间隔移位7.5 mm，6 h内磁共振DWI梗死体积超过80 cm^3，或14 h内超过145 cm^3，出现颅内压升高症状，如恶心和呕吐（Staykov and Gupta，2011；Wijdicks et al.，2014）。目前已经发表了7个随机对照试验（Hatefi et al.，2014）。恶性大脑中动脉综合征的减压手术明确降低了死亡率，但在增加预后良好（mRS 1~3分）患者数量的同时，也增加了预后差（mRS>3分）的患者的数量，其对存活患者的功能结局存在争议。到目前为止大多数研究中的功能结局的评估方法是基础的mRS评分，其忽略了以患者为中心的因素，如神经心理结果、生活质量和经济负担。是否进行减压手术治疗应是多学科团队与患者家属共同做出的决定。

手术过程

手术采用标准问号型或者T型切口。额颞顶去骨瓣手术切口前后径至少应达到12 cm。在冠状位上，开颅手术应向上到达瞳孔中线上方，向下到达前、中颅窝底部，距离最少为10 cm。广泛切开硬脑膜，可以用移植物扩大硬脑膜。

幕下

不同于幕上脑卒中的去骨瓣减压术，目前还没有针对幕下脑卒中减压术的随机对照试验，需要基于病例、进一步观察性和回顾性研究。现有报道提示去骨减压术使死亡率显著降低和并获得良好的功能结局。后循环卒中的体征和症状前文已经叙述，出现脑卒中症状时，进行神经检查，以确定缺血区域，具体是小脑、脑干还是小脑。梗死小脑的细胞水肿所产生的占位效应可使第四脑室消失，导致梗阻性脑积水或脑干受压。这一过程可持续1~7天，72小时达到高峰。病情恶化的可能性为7%~32%。目前的观点是：如果水肿导致了病情的恶化，符合手术治疗适应证。现有两种手术治疗方案：①首先进行脑室外引流（external ventricular drain，EVD），如果患者无法改善，则进行枕下减压术；②术前右侧额部脑室外引流或术中顶叶后部脑室外引流术。EVD通常设置在15~20 cmH_2O，以防止小脑扁桃体上疝。已发表的研究显示：最初因为临床恶化并有脑积水的影像学证据而进行EVD的患者中，20%~30%之后还需要进行枕下减压手术治疗（Amar，2012；Wijdicks et al.，2014）。

手术过程

手术采用标准的正中切口，暴露枕外隆突至第一颈椎C1，骨瓣尽可能大，去除C1后弓，Y形切开硬膜，进行硬膜成形术。有些学者建议切除梗死组织。

内科学和麻醉学的神经保护措施

与创伤性脑损伤（traumatic brain injury，TBI）的治疗方案相似，见**第41章**。

短暂性脑缺血发作和颈动脉内膜切除术

手术前

动脉粥样硬化

动脉粥样硬化是动脉内膜的慢性疾病。它主要由三个相互作用的机制驱动，即炎症、氧化应激和肾素血管紧张素系统功能障碍。脂质、纤连蛋白和钙在内膜下积聚，产生动脉粥样斑块，导致血管逐渐狭窄。随着斑块进展，上面的内皮可能会溃疡，导致血小板活化和凝血级联反应，从而形成血栓。斑块部位的闭塞或分离，从而导致远端血管发生血栓栓塞（Tousoulis et al.，2011；Husain et al.，2015）。

导致动脉粥样硬化相关的危险因素包括代谢综合征或X综合征。代谢综合征有不同的定义，但它们都有相同的过程，如①胰岛素抵抗引起的高血糖、葡萄糖耐受减退或2型糖尿病；②体重，如BMI增加、向心性肥胖或种族和性别腰围测量；③血脂异常，甘油三酯升高，高密度脂蛋白降低；

④血压超过 140/90 mmHg（或国际糖尿病联合会为 130/85 mmHg）。其他标准包括微量白蛋白血症、尿酸代谢紊乱和血清炎症标志物（ESR、CRP）。代谢综合征的核心是血糖调节障碍（van Rooy and Pretorius，2015）。

短暂性脑缺血发作（transient ischaemic attacks，TIA）表现为一过性神经功能缺损，之后完全消失，没有梗死的证据。这些不同动脉区域的体征和症状之前讨论过，由于侧支循环供血到缺血区域，其可以完全消失。大多数 TIA 持续时间不到 5 分钟，患者在检查时可能已经康复。患者主诉症状可能有手臂、腿部或面部无力、不稳、恶心、眩晕或头晕、神志不清或健忘等症状（Markus et al.，2013）。TIA 后 90 天内发生缺血性卒中的风险约为 17%，大部分发生在 48 小时内，因此，TIA 需急诊诊断和治疗（Giles and Rothwell，2007；Gupta et al.，2014）。ABCD² 等评分常用于预测后续脑卒中的风险（参见**表 51.4**：≥4 高风险，≤3 低风险）。

TIA 的诊断通常用平扫 CT，这有助于排除 TIA 类似疾病。24 小时内进行磁共振弥散加权成像（DWI）有助于确定其表现是由于脑缺血，97% 的扩散受限病灶对应有脑梗死（Souillard-Scemama et al.，2015）。血管成像应包括主动脉弓和颈部血管以及颅内血管，以评估动脉粥样硬化狭窄或闭塞的证据。MRA、CTA、超声（US）、导管造影在检测颈动脉病变及评估狭窄程度方面具有较高的敏感性和特异性。MRA 可能提供关于斑块特征信息，可用于预测未来事件的风险（Mono et al.，2012；Zhao et al.，2013）。心电图和心脏超声可用于评估心源性栓子的病因。其他的检查用于筛查代谢综合征，包括空腹血糖、糖耐量试验、糖化血红蛋白、血压测量、体重测量和血脂变化。

表 51.4 ABCD

危险因素	得分
年龄	
≥60 岁	1
血压	
收缩压≥140 mmHg 或舒张压≥90 mmHg	1
TIA 的临床特点	
单侧无力伴或不伴言语障碍	2
言语障碍无单侧无力	1
时间	
TIA 持续时间≥60 分钟	2
TIA 持续时间 10~59 分钟	1
糖尿病	1

Reprinted from *The Lancet*, Volume 366, Issue 9479, PM Rothwell, MF Giles, E Flossmann, CE Lovelock, JNE Redgrave, CP Warlow, Z Mehta, A simple score (ABCD) to identify individuals at high early risk of stroke after transient ischaemic attack, pp. 29–36, Copyright (2005), with permission from Elsevier.

根据病因以及危险因素选择治疗方案。如果病因是心源性房颤（持续性或阵发性），则开始长期抗凝，或者抗血小板治疗，如双嘧达莫和阿司匹林。糖尿病患者的目标血压≤140/90 mmHg 或 130/85 mmHg。血脂异常用他汀类类药物，目标低密度脂蛋白低于 2.59 mmol/L。高血糖可以通过调整饮食或口服降糖药来治疗。鼓励戒烟和运动。目前对颈动脉血运重建的指征：出现症状且血管狭窄超过 50% 或无症状性血管狭窄超过 70%。是否进行颈动脉内膜切除术（carotid endarterectomy，CEA）或颈动脉血管成形术和支架置入术（carotid angioplasty and stenting，CAS）取决于血管和斑块解剖以及患者的并发症等因素。

手术

颈动脉内膜切除术

颈动脉内膜切除术（carotid endarterectomy，CEA）的证据来自几项设计良好的、针对有症状和无症状的颈动脉疾病的、国际性随机对照试验。北美症状性颈动脉内膜切除试验（NASCET 1991 和 1998）和欧洲颈动脉外科试验（ECST 2003）分别招募了 659 名和 1807 名患者。每项试验不仅确定了 CEA 在缺血性事件二级预防中优于最佳内科治疗（抗血小板治疗和降低危险因素），对其进行的 meta 分析更是帮助制订了当前的治疗方案。对于有症状的患者（短暂性脑缺血发作、一过性失明或非致残性卒中），同侧颈动脉狭窄超过 70% 的患者应在 2 周内进行 CEA 治疗。对于狭窄率为 50%~69% 的患者，仅推荐在并发症发生率低于 6% 的大容量中心接受 CEA 治疗。狭窄小于 50% 的，不建议进行 CEA。对于同侧狭窄超过 70% 且对侧颈动脉接近完全或完全闭塞的患者，尽管手术致残的风险较高，仍建议在同侧进行颈动脉内膜切除术。

无症状颈动脉研究（1995 年）和无症状颈动脉手术试验（2004 年）比较了无症状颈动脉疾病患者的最佳药物治疗（抗血小板治疗和降低危险因素）与最佳药物治疗和 CEA 的疗效。从 CEA 中获益不明显，狭窄程度的影响也较小。与有症状的患者相比，无症状患者 5 年风险降低需要治疗的病例数明显增加，围术期残疾和死亡的影响也更加明显。因此，应当基于患者的并发症和手术中心的并发症发生率来选择无症状患者进行 CEA 治疗（Brott et al.，2011）。

手术技术

手术可以在局部麻醉（LA）或全身麻醉（GA）下进行（Link et al.，2014）。在术中，可以使用转流管来维持脑血流。有些监测方法（局麻清醒状态下手术、EEG、SSEP、TCD 或残端压）可以用于颈动脉夹闭期间的监测，如果有低灌注的迹象，可以选择应用转流管。

体位：仰卧，同侧肩卷，颈部伸展，头部转向对侧。

切口：在胸锁乳突骨前缘后方呈曲线状，从乳突尖下方 1 cm 至下颌角（避开腮腺）下方 1 cm 至胸锁关节上方 1 cm。

入路：分离颈阔肌，显露颈筋膜、颈外静脉和耳大神经，使其离开胸锁乳突肌外侧缘，供应耳垂的感觉。

胸锁乳突肌（SCM）向外移动，暴露出颈动脉鞘，然后进入颈动脉鞘。面总静脉可以作为颈动脉分叉处的标志物，对其结扎。找到迷走神经和舌下神经并对其进行保护。找到舌下神经的颈袢，必要时可牺牲颈袢。

动脉内膜切除术：静脉注射肝素。小心暴露颈总动脉和颈内动脉（见图 51.6）。依次保护甲状腺上动脉、颈内动脉和颈总动脉。如果 EEG、SSEP 或 TCD 出现同侧改变，应采用转流。在颈总动脉的中部切开动脉，并用 Potts 剪刀继续向头端延续。从颈总动脉到颈内动脉找到正常的动脉内膜。将斑块从内膜上轻柔剥离，一直到颈内动脉远端。颈外动脉（ECA）外翻后可以剥离其中的斑块。清除松散的碎片后，用肝素盐水冲洗。内膜瓣用 7-0 prolene 线由内向外缝合固定。用 5-0 prolene 线单纯缝合或者采用补片（自体静脉、聚四氟乙烯或涤纶编织）缝合动脉切口。缝合之前进行顺行和逆行回血冲洗清除碎屑。先松开颈内动脉阻断使其回血，排出残存的空气或者碎渣，然后重新夹闭颈内动脉，再松开颈内动脉和颈总动脉的阻断，使碎渣进入颈外动脉。

缝合：术中多普勒可以评估血管的通畅程度。可放置伤口引流管。然后逐层缝合关闭伤口。

颈动脉疾病的血管内治疗

血管内治疗的选择包括栓子保护装置辅助的 CAS。颈动脉内膜切除术高危患者进行脑保护装置辅助的支架置入血管成形术试验（SAPPHIRE）将有症状和无症状的手术高危患者随机纳入 CEA 组和 CAS 组。根据并发症和手术解剖因素，将存在以下一种或多种情况的患者定义为手术高危患者：NYHA Ⅲ或Ⅳ型心衰竭；COPD；对侧狭窄超过 50%；对侧喉返神经麻痹；既往进行过颈动脉血运重建；既往进行过颈部根治性手术或放疗；以及既往胆囊癌（CABG）。在该研究中，对于无症状的手术高危患者，CAS 组

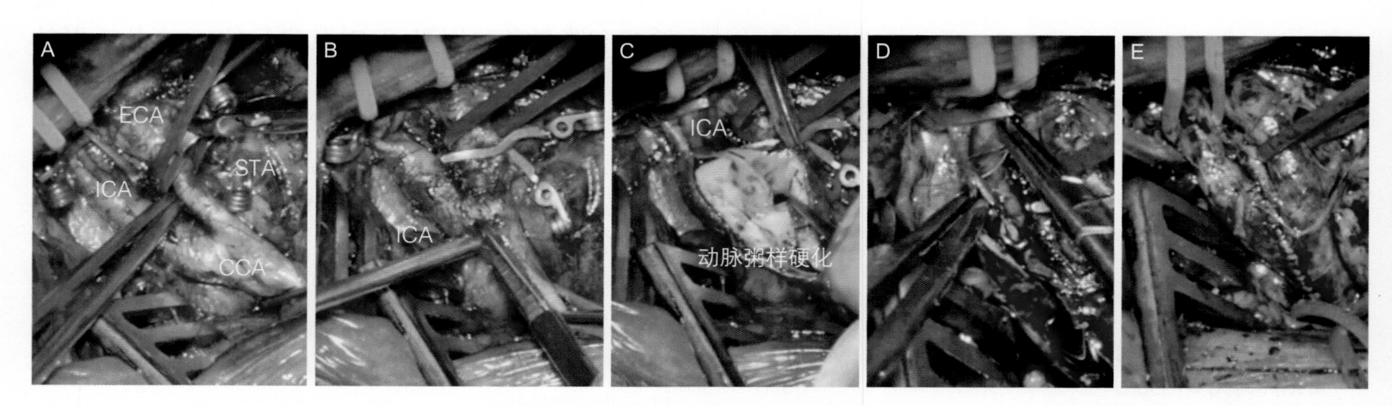

图 51.6 颈动脉内膜切除术。术中的图片说明了颈动脉内膜切除术的步骤。颈动脉分叉处充分暴露，吊索放置在颈内动脉（internal carotid artery，ICA）、颈外动脉（external carotid artery，ECA）和颈总动脉（common carotid artery，CCA）周围。静脉注射肝素后，血管夹夹闭 ICA、CCA、ECA 和第一个 ECA 分支：甲状腺上动脉（superior thyroid artery，STA）上。（B）用刀将颈动脉球上方的 ICA 中点切入 CCA，充分暴露动脉粥样斑块的范围。（C）解剖器用于定位动脉粥样斑块与血管介质之间的平面。将动脉粥样硬化从 ICA 和 CCA 周围剥离，残端随后进入 ECA 并被切除。任何内膜皮瓣（特别是 ICA 远端）都要用细线缝合。（D）血管从远端至近端用连续的缝线缝合，确保血管口径无扭曲或变窄。（E）结扎最后的缝线之前，松开支架将血液流回到内膜切除部位并排除空气。血管夹以特定的顺序打开，以避免栓子进入颅内循环：ECA、CCA、ICA

Courtesy of Dr Kirkpatrick, Department of Neurosurgery, Addenbrookes's NHS Trust, Cambridge, UK

的预后比 CEA 组更好。在其他所有的基于症状和风险的患者中，还没有证据表明 CAS 优于 CEA（Ooi and Gonzalez，2015）。随着血管内技术的改进，上述情况可能会有所改变。

并发症管理

术后控制血压对于预防高灌注损伤至关重要。任何新出现的术后神经系统障碍都需要紧急进行卒中检查，以排除 ICA 急性闭塞或栓塞现象。最后，出现颈部血肿是急症，需要立即保持气道通畅和清除凝血块。如果气管插管失败，应立即通知耳鼻喉科医生，进行气管切开术。

争议

去骨瓣减压术治疗大脑中动脉供血区恶性梗死

减压术明显降低大脑中动脉供血区恶性梗死（malignant MCA infarction，MMCAI）的死亡率。随着死亡率的下降，患者预后良好（mRS 1~3）和预后差（mRS>3）的数量均有所增多。接下来我们对年龄和功能预后方面的争议进行探讨。

年龄和生存

已经证实，去骨瓣减压术能够提高 60 岁以下患者的生存率。近期经 DESTINY Ⅱ证实，61~80 岁的患者也存在这一趋势。

年龄和功能预后

功能预后似乎是去骨瓣减压术治疗大脑中动脉供血区恶性梗死具有争议的问题。使用非特定的宽泛度量标准如改良 Rankin 量表（Modified Rankin Scale，mRS）进行评估备受诟病，原因有以下两点：首先，mRS 是一个 7 个分值的量表，衡量的是运动功能和幸存者照顾自身需求的能力。它忽略了神经心理学、生活质量、照顾者的负担和医疗保健系统等其他因素；其次，此量表中什么是好的结局或坏的结局是一个重要问题，因为所有主要和次要结局衡量标准在这一点上都只有二分类。研究表明，如果设定 mRS 为 0~4 为良好结局，mRS 为 5~6 为不良结局，DHC 可以增加良好结局比例，如果将 mRS 0~3 作为良好结局，治疗组和对照组之间将无明显差异。这是由于手术组中（mRS 为 4）患有严重残疾的幸存者增加所致（Yang et al.，2015）。mRS 为 4 的定义为没有外界帮助无法满足自己的身体需要或行走。

最近的 meta 分析和随机对照试验显示，年龄与患有严重残疾的幸存者之间可能存在直接联系，因此，单纯使用年龄而忽视患者的生物学因素和并发症，可能与使用 mRS 一样存在争议（Juttler et al.，2014）。

延伸阅读、参考文献、EBRAIN 的相关链接

扫描书末二维码获取。

第 52 章　颅内外搭桥手术治疗脑缺血

Mathew R. Guilfoyle・Peter J. Kirkpatrick 著
黄亚波 译，伊志强 审校

引言

症状性颈部（C1 段）颈内动脉（internal carotid artery，ICA）狭窄或闭塞最好通过直接动脉内膜剥脱术或血栓切除术来解决。对于更远端的病变，这一策略通常是不可行的，恢复脑灌注需要通过各种间接和直接的旁路技术将血液从颅外循环转移到颅内循环。然而，尽管经历了 50 年的实践和技术的改进，颅外 - 颅内（extracranial-intracranial，EC-IC）搭桥术治疗脑缺血仍然存在争议，关于如何最佳地选择患者进行手术，以及是否有临床益处，存在相互矛盾的证据和观点。

EC–IC 搭桥术的类型

直接旁路

与闭塞颈内动脉（或椎动脉）后采用高流量搭桥手术治疗复杂动脉瘤或切除肿瘤不同的是，脑缺血的血运重建是为了补充血流而不是替代原有血流。30~50 ml/min 的流速足以增加缺血阈值以上的灌注量并达到脑血管自动调节范围。到目前为止，最常见的“低流量”EC-IC 搭桥术包括将颞浅动脉（superficial temporal artery，STA）的后（顶）或前（额）支与同侧大脑中动脉（middle cerebral artery，MCA）的皮质支（M3 或 M4）吻合。手术技术将在稍后详细介绍。在椎基底动脉供血不足的情况下，可以使用颞浅动脉或枕动脉直接搭桥进入后循环，但是临床上很少应用。

间接旁路

目前已经提出了几种相关的技术，这些技术可以促进颅外向颅内循环供血的侧支循环的建立。缺血性脑组织强烈表达血管生成生长因子（Lanfranconi et al.，2011），间接搭桥的目的是消除物理障碍，以促进连接颅外和颅内循环的新生血管形成。这些手术最常应用于儿童，或因供体和受体血管太细而无法行直接搭桥术的成人。

软脑膜血管成形术指将颞浅动脉的一个或两个分支解剖出几厘米，然后将动脉的外膜袖套缝合到软脑膜上，使其与皮质表面直接接触。或者可以将颞浅动脉缝合到剪开的硬脑膜的游离边缘，并将其铺设在脑表面[脑 - 硬脑膜 - 动脉血管形成术（encephaloduroarteriosynangiosis，EDAS）]，或者将富含血管的颞肌从其血管蒂上分开，并覆盖至皮质表面[脑 - 颞肌血管形成术（encephalomyosynangiosis，EMS）]；这些选择通常合并称为脑 - 颞肌 - 动脉血管成形术（encephalomyoarteriosynangiosis，EMAS）。为了促进更大范围的皮质（包括大脑后部和前部区域）的侧支循环的建立，钻多个骨孔并打开硬脑膜可能是一种简单但有效的手术步骤。

间接搭桥手术的最大益处在术后一年内可能不明显，因此有相对急性症状或进行性症状加重的患者不适合进行单纯间接血运重建手术。许多外科医生都主张采用 STA-MCA 吻合术和某种间接搭桥术相结合的方法。

适应证和患者选择

在大多数患者中，颈内动脉远端或其末端分支的狭窄或闭塞，要么是动脉粥样硬化的结果，要么是烟雾病（moyamoya disease，MMD）的结果；较罕见的病因包括慢性夹层、穿透伤或医源性损伤。

确定是否进行 EC-IC 搭桥手术的关键是需要了解潜在疾病的自然病史以及估计未来卒中的风险。不管病因如何，偶然发现血管改变但实际无症状的患者发生缺血性事件的风险较低，通常不建议进行预防性手术。该组患者应该处理血管危险因素，并监测其症状的发展，在某一时点可能有必要进行干预。与此形成鲜明对比的是，出现累及整个血管区域、处于危险中的大面积脑梗死的患者也不适合进行血运重建。

动脉粥样硬化性狭窄性或闭塞性疾病

在20世纪60年代末Yasargil首次引入STA-MCA搭桥术之后（Y asargil et al.，1970），这项技术在治疗严重ICA或MCA动脉粥样硬化性狭窄或闭塞的高危卒中风险的患者中迅速获得广泛普及。由数百名患者组成的一系列研究表明，这种手术远期疗效好且安全：据报道，5年吻合血管通畅率超过95%，围术期死亡或严重残疾的发生率低于5%（Chater，1983；Sundt et al.，1985）。

为了研究血运重建术组与单纯药物治疗组相比是否能降低未来卒中风险的问题，EC-IC搭桥研究小组进行了一项涉及北美、欧洲和日本的71个医疗中心的多中心随机对照试验（Group，1985）。符合条件的患者有颈内动脉远端或大脑中动脉M1段的闭塞或严重狭窄，并有临床证据表明在前三个月内有短暂性脑缺血发作（包括黑曚）或轻度卒中。总共招募了1377名患者，所有患者都接受了阿司匹林和积极的高血压控制，663名患者被随机分配接受STA-MCA搭桥手术。在方法上来说，这项研究进行得很好，并且手术在技术上非常成功，无论是在高容量单位还是低容量单位，吻合血管通畅率都达到了96%左右。试验的主要发现令人震惊：与单纯接受药物治疗的患者相比，接受搭桥手术的患者卒中发生率明显更高。平均而言，累积风险估计为14%，尽管大多数缺血事件发生在手术后的早期，随机分组后五年的累积卒中次数在两组之间是相似的。多个亚组分析未能确定任何具有特定临床特征的患者在血运重建术后获益。尽管这项试验的批评者质疑这项研究在更广泛的人群中的普适性，因为参与研究中心的大量患者在研究之外接受治疗，但在1985年发表该研究后，EC-IC搭桥手术的数量急剧下降。

作为对EC-IC搭桥试验的反思，人们通过使用单光子发射计算机断层扫描、正电子发射断层扫描（PET）、磁共振灌注、氙气CT和增强CT灌注等技术来量化脑血管储备及反应性，从而重新聚焦如何改进对于手术患者的选择（Schmiedek et al.，1994；Grubb et al.，1998a；Patel et al.，2010）。本质上，所有这些方法都包括首先测量基础脑血流灌注，然后应用血管扩张刺激药物（如高碳酸血症或静脉注射乙酰唑胺）后的重复测量。对于严重狭窄的患者，由于血管最大限度地扩张以扩大脑血容量、保持血流并维持组织氧合时，远端血管床的自动调节能力在基线时已经耗尽。对血管扩张刺激的反应，与周围区域的充血形成对比，受影响区域的相对血流量减少，因为它无法进一步扩张血管，或者进入邻近大脑的流量增加引起局部缺血区域的“盗血”效应，血液流速和通过时间进一步恶化（图52.1）。使用PET测量组织的氧提取分数（oxygen extraction fraction，OEF）也可以量化，并且随着这一分数的增加，意味着越来越严重的盗血效应和局部缺血。已经提出了一个定义宽松的分级系统，从Ⅰ级发展到Ⅲ级，在Ⅰ级中有血管舒张能力的丧失，但没有明显的盗血；在“严重”的Ⅰ级和Ⅱ级中有显著的盗血效应和（或）OEF增加；在Ⅲ级中有明显的缺血，不能通过OEF的增加来补偿（Grubb et al.，1998a）。

灌注成像研究的集体分析表明，对于有证据表明对血管扩张刺激有明显盗血效应的患者，每年卒中的风险在10%~20%（Grubb et al.，1998b；Garrett et al.，2009）。此外，STA-MCA搭桥手术可显著改善脑血管储备和反应性，并将卒中风险降低了约2/3（Garrett et al.，2009）。

这些有希望的研究表明，可以筛选出可能受益于血运重建手术的亚组患者。颈动脉闭塞手术研究（Carotid Occlusion Surgery Study，COSS）是一项随机对照试验，入组标准为术前120天内发生缺血性事件以及使用乙酰唑胺后同侧大脑半球OEF增加（PET成像显示）的动脉粥样硬化性颈内动脉闭塞患者，分别进行STA-MCA搭桥术和单纯最佳药物治疗后，比较两组的疗效（Powers et al.，2011）。在随机选择的194名患者中，有97人被分配接受搭桥手术，最终有93人接受了手术。COSS由于搭桥手术无效而提前终止，其结果与早期的EC-IC搭桥试验的结果非常一致，再次表明，尽管吻合血管通畅率极高（>96%），但手术组在术后30天内患同侧卒中的风险显著增加（14.4% *vs*. 2.0%）；两组患者术后两年的累积卒中风险没有差异（21.0% *vs*. 22.7%）（Powers et al.，2011；Grubb et al.，2013）。

日本EC-IC搭桥试验（JET）的研究方法与COSS相似，随机选择196名狭窄性或闭塞性疾病且对最佳药物治疗效果不佳的患者（不管是否进行EC-IC搭桥手术）。在一项中期分析中，有迹象表明接受搭桥手术的98名患者的进一步卒中发生率略有下降，但该试验的全部结果和细节从未公布（JET Study Group，2002）。

值得注意的是，与最初的EC-IC搭桥试验相似的血管内支架植入术治疗（即血管造影显示的颅内动脉狭窄并在过去120天内发生缺血性发作）的随机试验也没有显示出介入治疗比最佳药物治疗更有益处

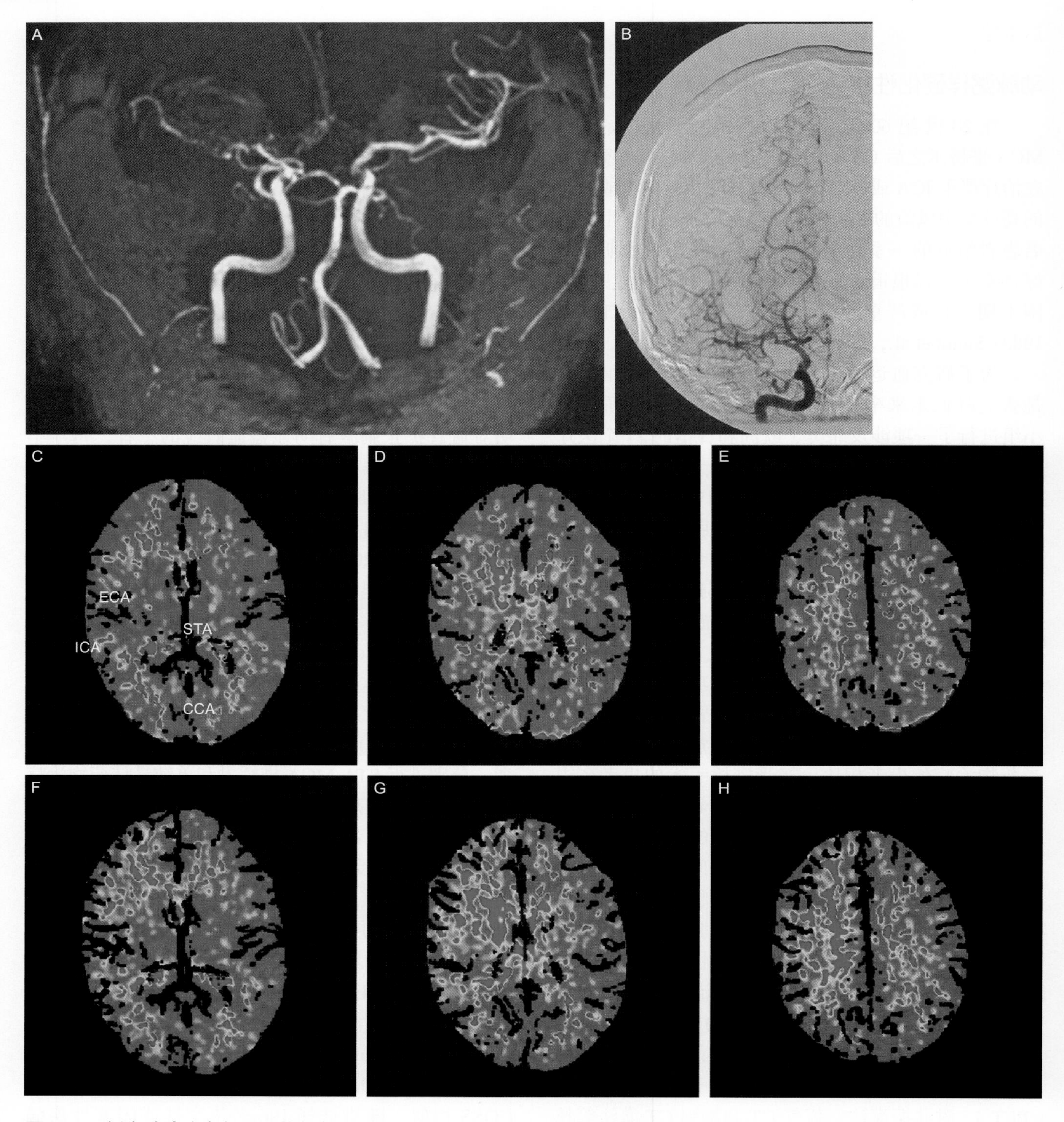

图 52.1 颅内动脉狭窄与脑血管储备影像学检查。（A 和 B）MRA 和 DSA 显示右侧 MCA M1 段狭窄（白箭头）。（C~E）增强 CT 灌注成像的基线平均通过时间（mean transit time，MTT）参数图；右侧 MCA 供血区域灌注轻度延迟。（F~H）在注射乙酰唑胺后，相应的 MTT 图显示出右侧 MCA 供血区域的延迟灌注现象恶化，表明脑血管储备耗尽和盗血现象

（Chimowitz et al.，2011）。在总共 451 名患者中，接受支架治疗的患者 30 天内卒中的风险为 14.7%，而未接受支架治疗的患者 30 天内卒中的风险为 5.8%。

总而言之，这些试验清楚地表明大多数动脉粥样硬化性颅内动脉狭窄患者适合接受最佳的内科治疗。然而，仍有少数患者没有形成足够的侧支代偿，继续发生短暂性缺血事件，或者尽管有最佳的药物治疗，但由于脑灌注不足，仍有躯体残疾和认知障碍的症状。这一组患者应该仔细评估行 EC-IC 搭桥手术的潜在可能性，以防止进一步的卒中并使症状

得到缓解。

烟雾病

出现缺血性事件的 MMD 患者在 12 个月内再次卒中的风险为 15%~50%；以出血为表现的患者的临床病程更具危害性。因此，对于有症状的 MMD 患者，目前的观点倾向于手术干预，以降低进一步卒中或出血的风险。目前还没有随机对照试验比较直接或间接 EC-IC 搭桥术对 MMD 患者进一步缺血事件的影响，而且首选的血运重建技术仍不清楚。间接搭桥手术被认为是更安全的选择，但已发表的病例系列研究表明，直接和间接技术发生缺血性或出血性卒中的总体风险相当，约为 5.5%；围术期死亡率低于 1%（Kazumata et al.，2014）。相比之下，就血管造影结果（通过血管造影结果评估 MCA 区域血运重建的范围）而言，STA-MCA 吻合手术效果优于间接搭桥手术，并且更有效地降低中期卒中复发的风险（3.5% vs. 11.2%）（Kazumata et al.，2014）。

最近的一项小型随机对照试验研究了直接 EC-IC 搭桥术预防 MMD 患者再次出血事件的效果（Miyamoto et al.，2014）。术前一年内发生出血的 80 名患者被随机分配到内科治疗组或双侧 STA-MCA 搭桥手术组。与更大的前瞻性随访研究结果相比，手术组的每年再次发生出血的风险较低（2.7% *vs*. 7.6%）（Jiang et al.，2014；Miyamoto et al.，2014）。

STA-MCA 搭桥手术

术前检查

所有患者都应该由神经内科或神经外科医生进行全面评估，以明确诊断，并确保治疗得到优化。需要 CT 或 MRI 来确定脑梗死范围，并结合灌注成像和乙酰唑胺激发试验来确认动态的血管盗血现象。全脑血管造影用于定位狭窄 / 闭塞的位置，或 MMD 的严重程度。在进行血运重建之前，明确是否伴发动脉瘤和其他血管畸形是非常必要的。必须进行选择性地颈外动脉造影，以评估现有侧支循环对颅内循环的代偿程度，以及 STA 的通畅度和直径，通常要求最小直径为 1 mm。术前血管造影提示供体动脉和受体动脉的匹配性，将决定选择直接搭桥手术还是间接搭桥手术，尽管通常要等到术中直接探查血管时才能最终做出决定。一般建议患者在围术期继续进行抗血小板治疗，以降低早期吻合血管闭塞的风险。

手术步骤

在全身麻醉诱导期间，应持续进行动脉压监测，以确保维持正常血压；即使是轻微的低血压也可能导致这些脆弱的患者出现严重的脑缺血。

患者仰卧在手术台上，头部放在马蹄形头枕上；也可以使用三钉头架固定，但不是必需的。应触诊或用多普勒探头确定 STA 分支的走行，以设计皮肤切口。可以采用从耳屏前开始的直线型切口，切口位于 STA 主干的前缘，但我们更倾向于采用 Y 形切口，“Y”的每条分支都沿着 STA 及其终末分支的大致走行路径（**图 52.2A**）。一定要避免肾上腺素渗入设计好的切口，因为这会收缩供体血管；普通的局部麻醉药物应当采用谨慎的皮下注射。

切开皮肤，显露出帽状腱膜下层，STA 走行其中。该血管的近端主干在颧骨位置的皮肤上最为表浅，但通常最好首先识别出更远端一个分支。一旦识别出动脉，就将其近端解剖剥离，在其表面保留一束结缔组织袖套，并在距血管几毫米的地方沿着血管将分支剥离出来（**图 52.2B**）。根据可用血管的直径和长度选择额支或顶支作为供体血管，然后将另一分支尽可能向远侧剥离开，以使得 STA 能够被移动，向一侧缩回并得到保护。在吻合手术完成之前，供体血管需保持连续性通畅。

切开颞肌且翻转，然后在远端外侧裂上进行小骨瓣开颅手术。在手术显微镜下，检查皮质血管并选择合适的受体血管，通常是分支最少的最大直径的血管，其具有足够的长度以允许使用临时阻断夹。用显微剪刀切开蛛网膜，并将目标受体血管的分支电凝后剪断，从而获取一段约 15 mm 的受体血管。

将一张对比鲜明的卡片从皮质血管下方通过并垫在其下方，以便于缝合（**图 52.2C**）。静脉注射肝素（5000 IU），然后切断供体血管 STA 分支。确认其血流通畅，将动脉包括其末端“骨骼化”（从末端开始约几毫米），然后将其末端带至受体血管，同时要确保供体动脉能够充分活动以避免受到牵拉。临时阻断夹阻断 STA，受体血管上的吻合位点两端的血管壁被微血管夹夹住（**图 52.2D**）。使用显微剪刀将受体动脉吻合位点切开一个小口，使其接近 STA 的口径。然后用 10-0 尼龙缝线进行间断端侧吻合，首先将受体动脉切口的两端分别与供体血管末端的两端加以缝合以固定血管，然后依次用 3~5 针完成两侧吻合（**图 52.2E~H**）。用钝性探头间断确认受体血管的通畅性。也可以使用连续缝合，但间断缝合提供了更高的精确度，必要时更容易修正，并且更适

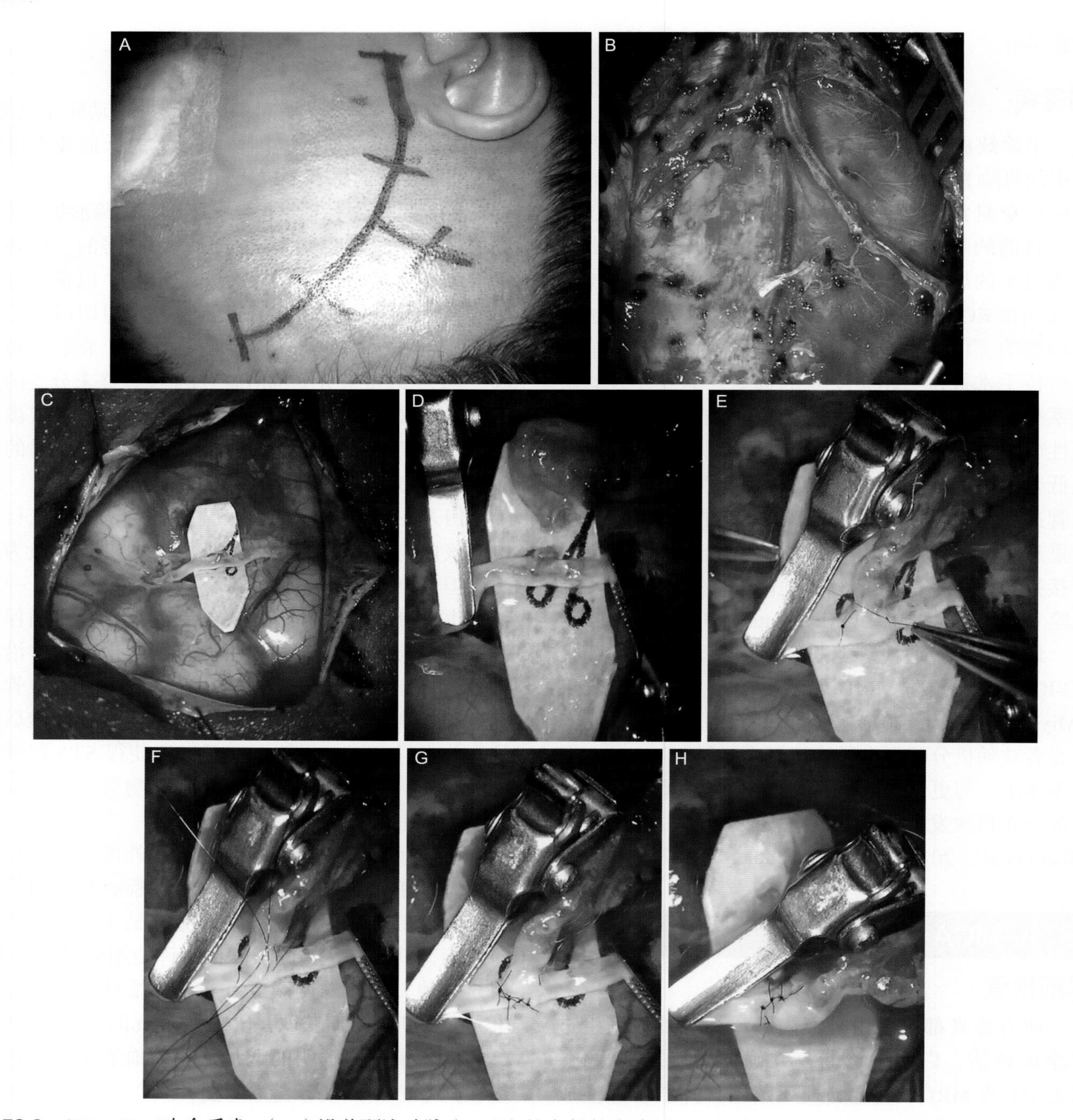

图 52.2 STA-MCA 吻合手术。（A）沿着颞浅动脉（STA）的走行行皮肤切口。（B）解剖 STA 分支，标记后（顶）分支。（C）开颅手术后，解剖并准备受体血管。（D）STA 末端的“骨骼化”与皮质动脉靠拢，并用夹子夹住。动脉切开处用虚线标记。（E）吻合口两端用 10-0 尼龙缝线固定缝合。（F~G）沿一侧间断缝合，然后打结。（H）在吻合的后壁重复相同的操作步骤

合于调整供体和受体血管口径的不匹配程度。

一旦吻合完成，就从皮质血管和 STA 上依次取下临时阻断夹，并检查吻合口情况。少量出血可以用止血剂和轻柔的压迫来控制，如果需要，也可以用 10-0 缝线补救缝合。使用多普勒探头和术中吲哚菁绿血管造影术可确认吻合血管通畅和血流方向。在 EC-IC 旁路建立的同时，静脉滴注 200 ml 20% 甘露醇以改善血流，并在关颅前监测 10~15 分钟。如果担心供 / 受体血管或吻合口闭塞，可以使用未使用的 STA 分支作为出口，以评估来自 STA 的顺行血流和来自皮质血管的逆行血流。

缝合硬脑膜，骨瓣复位时应该确保 STA 在穿过骨窗边缘时不会受到压迫。颞肌筋膜、皮肤和帽状腱膜按常规方式逐层缝合。

术后护理

建议在手术后的12~24小时内密切监测和控制液体平衡和血压，以避免术后低血压和脑缺血，并尽量降低出血和脑肿胀的风险。可以用多普勒超声定期检查吻合血管的通畅性。出院医嘱还应包括严格避免对供体血管施加任何压力，例如弹性面罩。

结论

大多数动脉粥样硬化性颅内动脉狭窄的患者在医学上都能得到最佳内科保守治疗，但对于某些难治性症状、影像学可证实灌注不足的患者，通过直接EC-IC搭桥手术进行血运重建仍是一个重要的治疗选择。对于有症状的MMD患者，直接或间接搭桥手术可显著降低缺血性发作和出血再次发作的风险。动脉粥样硬化或MMD导致的无症状狭窄的患者则不需要手术。

参考文献

扫描书末二维码获取。

第 53 章　颅内巨大动脉瘤和搭桥手术

Mario Teo · Omar Choudhri · Michael Lawton 著
黄亚波 译，伊志强 审校

引言

根据颅内动脉瘤和蛛网膜下腔出血的联合研究，巨大颅内动脉瘤被定义为最大直径在 2.5 cm 或更大的病变，占所有颅内动脉瘤的 2%~5%（Locksley，1966；Sughrue et al.，2011）。它们仍然是最难治疗的脑血管病变之一。

巨大动脉瘤的自然病史普遍较差。Drake 报告说，在他保守治疗的一系列巨大动脉瘤中，2 年的死亡率为 68%，5 年的死亡率为 80%（Drake，1979）。因此，保守治疗的策略在大多数情况下是不合适的，尤其是在较年轻的人群中。在较早的一系列研究中，直接手术夹闭或塑型重建术分别适用于 30% 的后循环和 50% 的前循环巨大动脉瘤患者。随着颅底入路、显微外科技术和神经麻醉技术的进步，当代一系列研究表明，多达 2/3 的巨大动脉瘤可以直接夹闭或塑型重建（Darsaut et al.，2011；Sughrue et al.，2011）。此外，血管内技术的稳步发展使得巨大动脉瘤的血管内治疗成为可能，无论是否使用支架或球囊辅助等辅助技术，以及最近的分流装置。

尽管取得了显著的进展，但目前关于治疗巨大动脉瘤的安全性和完全闭塞率的最佳数据和报道结果仍然来自外科手术系列报道（**表** 53.1，Sughrue et al.，2011）。

病理学和病理生理学

囊状动脉瘤是巨大动脉瘤最常见的亚型，约 60%~70% 位于前循环在颈内动脉（internal carotid artery，ICA）的海绵窦段、床突旁区和颈动脉分叉区，大脑中动脉（middle cerebral artery，MCA）近端，大脑前动脉（anterior cerebral artery，ACA）/ 前交通动脉（anterior communicating artery，ACoA），出现的概率逐渐减少）。后循环动脉瘤位于基底动脉尖、基底动脉中段、椎动脉、椎基底动脉交界处，很少位于小脑后下动脉（posterior inferior cerebellar artery，PICA）和小脑前下动脉（anterior inferior cerebellar artery，AICA）。其他类型的巨大动脉瘤包括梭形或蛇形动脉瘤亚型（以夹层为假定病因）和感染性亚型。梭形动脉瘤的破裂率被认为很低，而且血管造影显示疾病的进展性是不可预测的。

颅内动脉瘤形成的病理基础尚不清楚，在其他地方也有报道。在巨大动脉瘤形成后，动脉瘤内搏动且不规则的血流向瘤壁施加压力，导致动脉瘤囊性扩张、变薄和生长。在试图修复动脉瘤的过程中，血管内腔内皮细胞表面会发生血栓形成和重塑。然而，持续的慢性、不规则、搏动性血流会损害愈合过程，并导致胶原蛋白沉积紊乱、管壁动脉粥样硬化变性、不同阶段血栓形成和营养不良性钙化。因此，巨大动脉瘤是一种伴随着血栓形成和溶解的周期性循环的动态损伤。

临床表现

与小型动脉瘤不同，巨大动脉瘤患者经常（60%~80%）出现血栓栓塞事件或由占位效应引起的与神经血管压迫有关的症状，尤其是占据小容积颅后窝的后循环动脉瘤。动脉瘤破裂引起蛛网膜下腔或实质内出血的可能性较低（20%~30% 病例），其结果比占位效应更差（Hamburger et al.，1992）。动脉瘤的快速生长（通常由急性血栓形成引起）可以出现类似急性出血的严重头痛。其他很少出现的症状包括癫痫发作（通常由大脑中动脉动脉瘤引起）和偏瘫。

表 53.2 占位效应症状与巨大动脉瘤的位置相关联。

术前检查

曾经采用普通颅骨 X 线摄片诊断钙化的巨大动

表 53.1　已发表的巨大动脉瘤的外科和血管内治疗经验

		患者	完全闭塞		搭桥手术	良好	差	死亡率	发病率	随访	再次治疗	再出血
作者	年份	*n*	*n*	%	*n*	%	%	%	%	（年）	%	%
血管内弹簧圈												
Higashida[39]	1990	39	24%	62	0/39	NA	NA	NA	NA	0.5	NA	NA
Gobin[1]	1966	9	5/9	56	0/9	100	0	0	11	0.5	33	0
Tateshima[45]	1999	28	17/28	61	0/28	73			18	3.3	82	4
Hallacq[46]	2002	5	1/5	20	0/5	60	20	20	20	1.0	0	0
Sluzewski[44]	2003	29	5/29	17	0/29	75	4	21	10	3.1	55	7
Henkes[38]	2004	47	10/47	21	0/47	NA	NA	NA	NA	NA	NA	NA
Kolasa[20]	2004	7	4/7	57	0/7	85	14	0	NA	NA	NA	NA
Murayama[48]	2006	33	19/77	25	0/33	NA	NA	NA	NA	NA	NA	NA
Jahromi[40]	2008	39	14/39	36	0/39	63	8	29	20	1.3	54	5
Shi[43]	2009	9	9/9	100	6/9	78	11	11	11	1.0	0	0
Lylyk[41]	2009	8	4/6	67	0/8	NA	NA	NA	0	0.5	0	0
显微血管夹												
Peerless，Drake[47]	1990	118	97/118	82	0/118	58	26	14	NA	NA	NA	NA
Kodama, Suzuki[48]	1982	49	NA	NA	NA	61	16	22	NA	NA	NA	NA
Yasargil[37]	1984	30	26/30	87	6/30	67	23	10	NA	NA	0	0
Hosobuchi[49]	1985	82	80/82	98	15/82	84	9	7	38	10.0	0	0
Heros[50]	1986	25	25/25	100	NA	72	12	16	NA	NA	NA	NA
Sundt[51]	1990	315	310/315	98	81/315	80	6	15	NA	NA	NA	NA
Ausman[31]	1990	62	62/62	100	23/62	84	11	5	NA	NA	NA	NA
Tamaki[29]	1991	4	4/4	100	0/4	100	0	0	0	NA	NA	NA
Lawton, Spetzler[6]	1995	136	132/136	97	40/136	85	9	6	11	2.2	1	0
Shibuya, Sugita[36]	1996	29	NA	NA	NA	84	7	8	NA	NA	NA	NA
Kattner[19]	1998	29	29/29	100	1/29	87	10	3	20	7.0	0	0
Samson[26]	1999	44	NA	94	NA	NA	NA	NA	NA	0.5	0	0
Lawton[22]	2002	28	28/28	100	1/28	75	11	14	5	1.6	0	0
Jafar[18]	2002	29	29/29	100	29/29	93	3	3	10	5.0	0	0
Lozier[23]	2004	19	6/16	38	2/19	36	47	16	89	7.4	0	0
Gonzales[32]	2004	8	8/8	100	1/8	63	38	0	50	1.0	0	0
Kolasa[20]	2004	13	13/13	100	0/13	76	23	0	NA	NA	NA	NA
Krisht[21]	2007	11	11/11	10	0/11	88	12	2	27	0.5	0	0
Hauck[17]	2008	62	56/62	90	9/62	68	32	15	42	1.0	0	3
Sharma[28]	2008	181	106/118	90	11/181	86	5	9	12	NA	0	0
Cantore[15]	2008	99	99/99	10	41/99	89	3	8	3	8.5	1	1
Xu[30]	2009	51	51/51	100	0/51	84	14	2	NA	0.5	NA	NA
Sano[27]	2010	109	109/109	100	0/109	63	16	22	4	NA	0	0
Sughrue（当前研究）	2010	140	118/140	84	52/140	80	7	13	10	1.9	1	1

（续表）

		患者	完全闭塞		搭桥手术	良好	差	死亡率	发病率	随访	再次治疗	再出血
作者	年份	*n*	*n*	%	*n*	%	%	%	%	(年)	%	%
血管内 – 手术联合治疗												
Hacein-Bey[16]	1998	5	4/5	80	1/5	80	20	0	0	1.9	0	0
Arnautovic[14]	1998	8	8/8	10	0/8	87	13	0	13	2.0	0	0
Ponce[25]	2004	8	NA	NA	5/8	76	0	25	38	1.5	0	0

NA，不可用

Reproduced with permission from Sughrue, Michael E.; Saloner, David, Rayz, Vitaliy L.; Lawton, Michael T. Giant Intracranial Aneurysms: Evolution of Management in a Contemporary Surgical Series, *Neurosurgery*, Volume 69, Issue 6, pp. 1261– 70, Copyright © 2011 Oxford University Press and the Congress of Neurological Surgeons (CNS).

脉瘤（20% 的病例），并且可以重建包括鞍区在内的颅底影像（Pia and Zierski，1982）。CT 和 CTA 可以测量动脉瘤大小，载瘤血管直径，评估其与颅底的解剖关系，以及显示血栓和钙化的动脉瘤内容物。

另一方面，MRI 可以观察到巨大动脉瘤及其与脑实质的关系，以及由动脉瘤快速生长或急性血栓形成引起的病灶周围水肿。在巨大血栓性动脉瘤中，可以发现层状含铁血黄素和高铁血红蛋白形成的“洋葱圈”特征。

六血管造影（DSA）是获得载瘤血管解剖、动脉瘤形态、相关的穿支血管、血管闭塞可能性、搭桥方案的评估、颅内 - 颅内和颅外 - 颅内侧支血管等解剖信息的金标准。为了评估血管储备，可以根据需要行球囊闭塞试验（balloon test occlusion，BTO），包括 Allcock 试验（椎动脉造影时压迫同侧颈动脉）和低血压刺激。降压刺激包括用硝普钠静脉滴注将平均动脉压降低 20 mmHg，或平均动脉压的 25%（以较大者为准）。

考虑到所有这些信息丰富的放射学研究，包括患者的神经系统状况、并发症 、预测的治疗风险、当地经验以及患者家庭的选择偏好，最佳治疗策略可以基于个人情况与多学科合作团队而制订，该团队包括血管外科医生、介入神经放射科医生和神经血管专家。

手术策略

对于不适宜直接夹闭动脉瘤颈的患者，有必要采用其他技术治疗动脉瘤。一个好的策略是夹闭动脉瘤近端或远端的病变血管，同时采用旁路搭桥术来重建远端区域的血运，导致血流逆转（**图 53.1 和图 53.2**）。一般来说，高流量搭桥术适用于 BTO 失败的患者，低流量搭桥术适用于低血压刺激后 BTO 失败的患者。原位搭桥手术策略用于特定位置的动脉瘤，不需要从颅外循环重新引导血流。据报道，这种技术在成对的 ACA 和 PICA，以及颞动脉至 M2 原位旁路血管中用于治疗相应位置的巨大动脉瘤（Bederson and Spetzler，1992；Sanai et al.，2009）。

在深低温停循环下行巨大基底动脉尖和大脑中动脉动脉瘤夹闭等手术是高风险的，并已被更安全的替代方法所取代，如腺苷阻滞（短暂房室传导阻滞）、快速心室起搏和通过旁路血管行近端阻断（Sughrue et al.，2011）。腺苷和快速心室起搏都会引起一过性低血压，从而降低动脉瘤的张力，从而实现安全的操作和夹闭。

颅内外搭桥术

选择搭桥的类型

一般而言，当考虑到可能需要闭塞主要的载瘤血管时，诸如颞浅动脉（STA）或枕动脉（OA）这样的“低流量”血管（通常提供 25~30 ml/min 的流量）不足以重建整个半球的血运。在这种情况下，需要“高流量”血管，如桡动脉（50~150 ml/min）或大隐静脉（100~200 ml/min）。除了血流量要求以外，供体血管的选择还取决于供体血管的可用性、受体血管的大小和手术团队的习惯。

桡动脉供体移植血管容易出现严重的血管痉挛，这个问题可以通过合理升高血压扩张血管和罂粟碱浸泡来克服（Mohit et al.，2007）。桡动脉供体移植血管的优点包括供体和受体血管之间的直径匹配度较高，因此在吻合技术上更容易操作，并且在吻合部位引起的湍流较少（Houkin et al.，1999；Mohit et al.，2007；Kocaeli et al.，2008）。

表 53.2　动脉瘤位置和占位效应引起的症状

动脉瘤位置	占位效应相关的症状和体征
前循环	视力障碍
颈内动脉海绵窦段	眶后区头痛
	复视
	面部感觉缺失
	垂体功能低下（偶尔）
	鼻衄（少见）
颈内动脉眼动脉段或床突旁段	单侧眶后区头痛
	视力下降
	不对称性视野缺损
颈内动脉分叉	视野缺损（同向性偏盲）
	偏瘫
	抽搐
	垂体功能低下（少见）
大脑中动脉	抽搐
	偏瘫
大脑前动脉 - 前交通动脉	视野缺损（双颞侧偏盲）
	视力下降
	激素水平改变（下丘脑受压）
	个性改变
基底动脉干	复视
椎 - 基底动脉汇合处	面部感觉缺失
小脑后下动脉	言语、吞咽困难
	后组颅神经功能缺失
	步态不稳
	小脑症状
	长束征

Source data from Kalani MYS, Spetzler RF. Giant Aneurysm. In: Spetzler RF, Kalani MYS, Nakaji P. 2015. Neurovascular Surgery. 2nd Edn. Thieme Publishers.

另一方面，大隐静脉移植（saphenous vein graft，SVG）更容易获取，提供更大的血流量，并且不容易出现明显的血管痉挛。然而，直径不匹配和脆弱的内皮细胞可能会导致供体移植血管远端吻合手术更加困难。将静脉瓣膜系统破坏的静脉受体血管逆转的方法可以减轻直径不匹配，但是有继发于血管内皮细胞破坏的血栓形成风险。

供体血管的选择

通常，在高流量搭桥手术中颈动脉分叉处远端的颈外动脉（external carotid artery，ECA）是首选供体血管。避免累及颈内动脉是很重要的，因为在吻合过程中夹闭颈内动脉可能导致脑缺血，特别是在BTO已经失败，不能耐受颈内动脉闭塞的患者中。如果由于解剖变异或无法获取而不能使用ECA，则可能需要与颈总动脉进行吻合术，以便在吻合过程中允许ECA到ICA之间的侧支循环。

在低流量搭桥术中，根据受体血管与供体血管的距离，选择包括（颞浅动脉额支或顶支）、枕动脉和耳后动脉（posterior auricular artery，PAA）。

高流量颅外 – 颅内搭桥术在前循环动脉瘤中的应用

低流量搭桥术的技术方面在本书其他章节中已经介绍，因此我们将在本节重点讨论高流量搭桥术，并通过一个病例来阐述手术步骤（**图 53.3**）。

手术是在全身麻醉下进行，同时行神经监测、亚低温（33~34 ℃）、导尿、中心静脉压和动脉压监测（以确保最佳体液管理）。

患者仰卧位，头部固定在Mayfield头架上，同侧肩部垫高，头部旋转至对侧，以确保颅骨手术区域与地面平行。

开颅术

翼点开颅术采用头皮弧形发际线内切口，取肌皮瓣翻向颅底，磨平蝶骨嵴，然后根据磨除蝶骨翼的范围悬吊硬脑膜后剪开。在显微镜下广泛分离外侧裂，显露大脑中动脉的M2各分支，通常不使用M1分支作为受体血管，这样最大限度地减少对豆纹穿通动脉的损伤。选择直径匹配的M2段作为受体血管，剪开蛛网膜从而剥离血管。将一块对比度明显的血管垫片放置在受体血管下方。我们通常在血管垫片下方放置抽吸微管，以保持冲洗和渗血下手术区域的视野清晰（**图 53.3A**）。

显露颈部

可以选择在舌骨水平沿皮纹走行，做颈部皮肤横切口，显露颈动脉分叉部。另一种方法是沿胸锁乳突肌前缘作纵向切口，尤其是在颈动脉分叉部难以显露的情况下采用。在胸锁乳突肌内侧，打开颈深筋膜和颈动脉鞘，显露颈总动脉，并暴露颈动脉分叉部以上长达2 cm的颈外动脉，为颈外动脉作为供体血管行端侧吻合术做准备。这样可以留出足够的空间在应用临时阻断夹后进行搭桥手术。

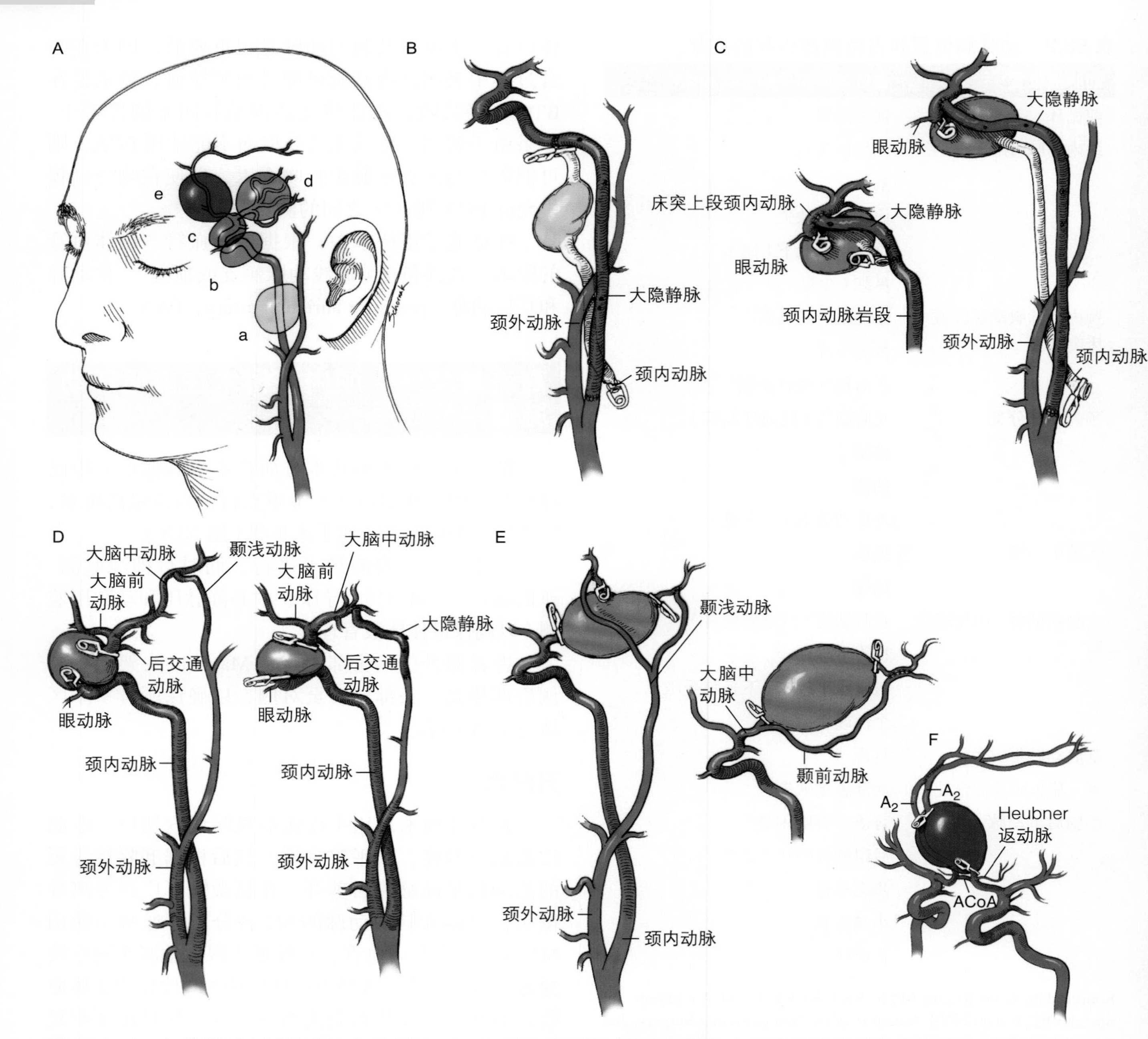

图 53.1 （A）前循环血运重建技术示意图。（B）可以通过使用大隐静脉作为移植血管的颈内动脉颈段 - 岩骨段搭桥手术，来实现位于颅底的颈内动脉（ICA，internal carotid artery）动脉瘤的孤立和血运重建。（C）ICA 海绵窦段动脉瘤可以使用大隐静脉移植血管，采用 ICA 岩骨段 - 床突上段（C3~C5）搭桥手术，或颈段 - 床突上段搭桥手术。（D）ICA 床突上段动脉瘤可以通过颞浅动脉 - 大脑中动脉（STA-MCA）搭桥手术后进行孤立。另一种策略是以大隐静脉为移植血管的 STA-MCA 搭桥手术。（E）大脑中动脉瘤可以采用 STA-MCA 双支血管搭桥术进行孤立术和血管重建术。或者颞前动脉至 MCA 的原位搭桥手术可以用于特定动脉瘤。（F）采用 A2-A2 原位搭桥手术可以孤立 ACA 动脉瘤并进行血运重建术

供体移植血管的获取

在获取 SVG 时，我们常规检查患者是否有静脉曲张或以前的手术史是否损伤过大隐静脉。手术获取从踝关节（内踝）到膝部的静脉长度达 20~25 cm。亦可在腹股沟区识别股动脉，股静脉位于其内侧，大隐静脉依据股静脉的位置而得到定位。然后向膝部远端进行分离，获取一长段移植血管。在分离过程中，结扎后剪断所有侧支，以确保管腔不会狭窄或受损。充分显露头颈部切口，结扎止血彻底后剥离出 SVG，并用肝素化生理盐水冲洗管腔，清除其内的血凝块，同时对结扎的侧支行压力测试，防止漏

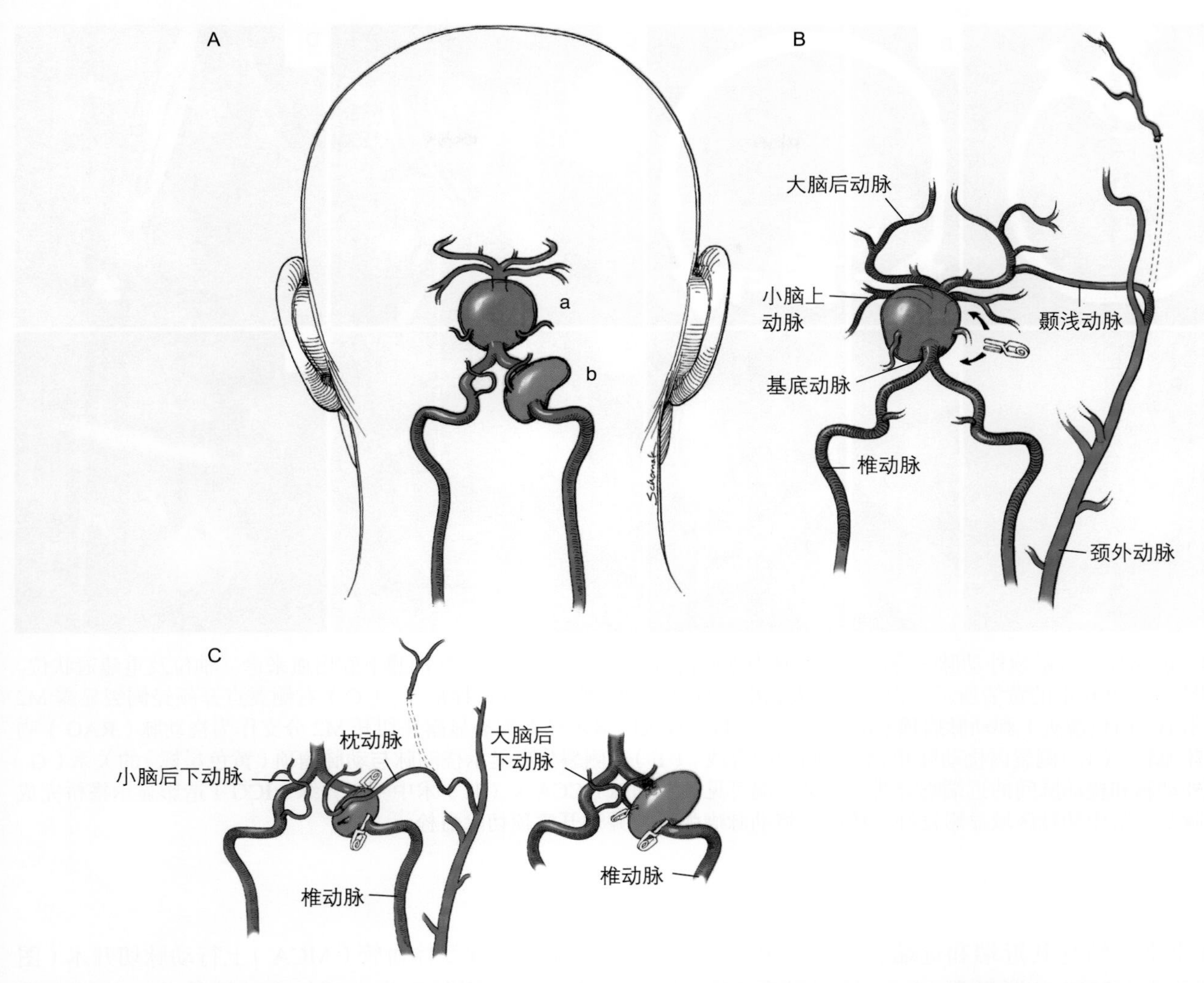

图 53.2 （A）后循环血运重建技术示意图。（B）基底动脉中段动脉瘤可以在动脉瘤的近端或远端夹闭，并通过 STA-PCA 搭桥手术或 STA-SCA 搭桥手术进行血运重建。我们倾向于在 SCA 下方的无穿支血管区域夹闭基底动脉。在某些病例中，可以使用双支 STA 作为 PCA 和 SCA 的供体血管进行双血管搭桥手术，可以应用于脑干血运重建。（C）可以永久夹闭 VA 近端和 PICA 的起始处来孤立椎动脉动脉瘤，血管内弹簧圈栓塞 VA 的远端。PICA-PICA 原位搭桥手术用于远端区域的血运重建，或者可以采用 OA-PICA 搭桥手术

Courtesy of Barrow Neurological Institute, reprinted with permission.

血的发生。剥除 SVG 的两端 1~2 cm 的外膜和结缔组织，以便于吻合。SVG 的静脉瓣膜可以采用椎间盘剥离器来破除之，而 SVG 的通畅性可通过肝素化的生理盐水双向冲洗来确认。也可以采用颠倒移植血管的方向（其踝端或膝端用于颈部近端吻合），以确保血流沿瓣膜方向流动，从而避免使用瓣膜切开术，因为瓣膜切开术可能会损坏内膜，并导致血栓形成。

桡动脉的获取

桡动脉移植血管（radial artery graft，RAG）是一种很好的移植血管选择，其直径与供受体血管匹配良好。虽然我们已经介绍了内镜技术，但是我们更倾向于开放手术。在获取 RAG 之前，一个重要的先决条件是完成改良 Allen 实验，以评估手的尺侧侧支循环。在腕部皮肤折痕以近 1 cm 处和肘部皮肤折痕以远 1 cm 处，设计曲线型皮肤切口，通过触诊或手持式多普勒超声检查使切口走行在桡动脉搏动路径上的中线处。肱桡肌和桡侧腕屈肌及其筋膜构成桡动脉的间隙。切开筋膜，显露疏松蜂窝组织中的桡动脉。一旦进入桡动脉筋膜层面后，从近端至远端进行剥离。动脉与其伴行静脉一起作为血管蒂被剥离。将浸泡在罂粟碱中的明胶海绵铺在未被处理的桡动脉上。桡动脉近端取自桡返动脉的起始点下方，远端掌浅动脉的起始点近端。侧支采用 Weck 血管夹夹闭或电灼法进行处理，将对桡动脉的损伤降至最低。移植血管用蓝色墨水标记近端和远端。桡动脉一旦

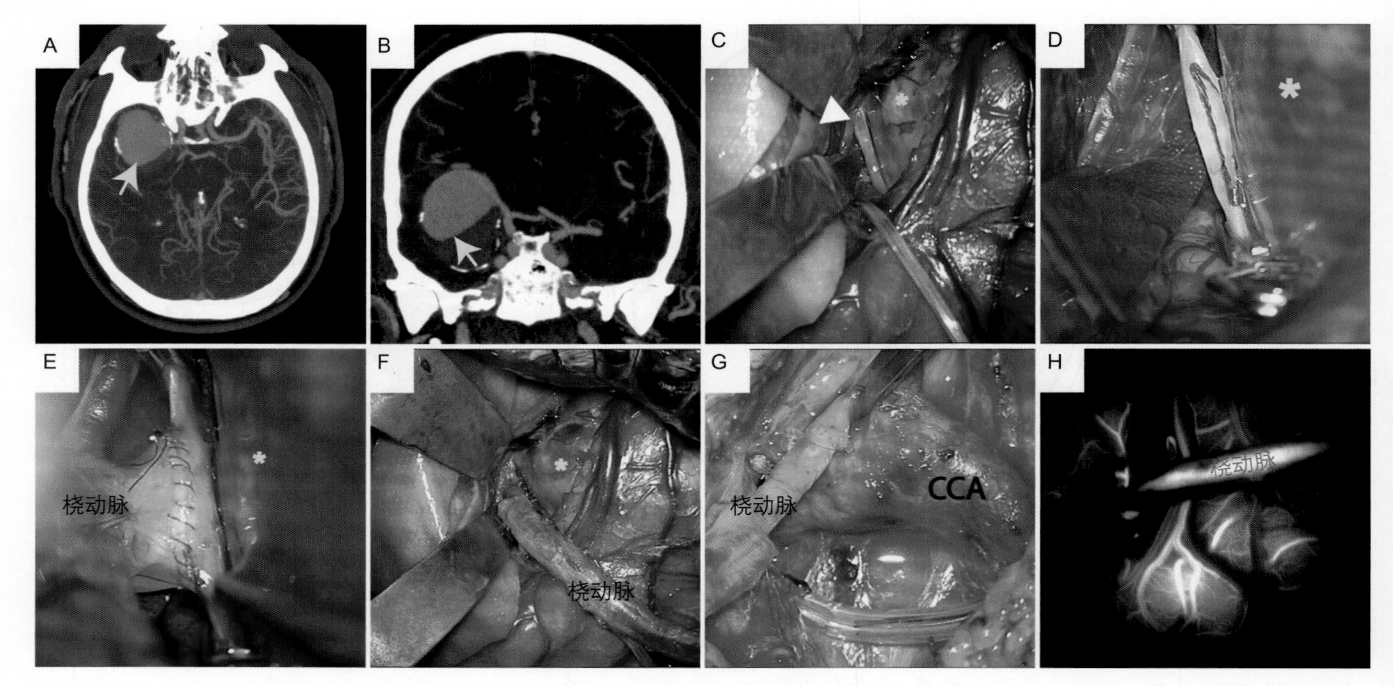

图 53.3 前循环高流量颈外动脉—桡动脉—大脑中动脉搭桥。36 岁女性患者，蛛网膜下腔出血来诊。轴位及重建冠状位。CTA（图 A 及图 B 中的黄箭所示）提示右侧大脑中动脉巨大动脉瘤伴部分血栓形成。（C）右侧翼点开颅经侧裂显露 M2 分支流出道（白色箭头）和动脉瘤顶（黄色星标）。（D）放大图显示经右侧裂显露并切开 M2 分支作为桡动脉（RAG）吻合的受体血管。（E）侧裂内桡动脉和 M2 之间的吻合线。（F）经侧裂分离显示桡动脉与动脉瘤顶（黄色星标）的关系（G）颈部颈外动脉和桡动脉间的近端吻合线。分叉近端可见颈总动脉（CCA）。（H）术中吲哚菁绿（ICG）造影显示搭桥完成后桡动脉及大脑中动脉区域显影良好。然后，将动脉瘤弧点，并切开瘤顶切除血栓

被分离出来，结扎其近端和远端，然后切开。用肝素生理盐水（2500 U 肝素和 60 mg 罂粟碱在 250 ml 生理盐水中配制的溶液）冲洗桡动脉近端，同时行压力测试。

耳前或耳后皮下隧道

在获取移植血管前建立皮下隧道，从耳前或耳后的皮下通过，在皮下隧道中放置一对 Roberts 钳，待皮下渗血稳定后，采用一把 Kelly 钳夹住一根胸管，使其从开颅手术的切口穿过皮下隧道到达颈部切口。然后将移植血管从胸管内穿过，防止移植血管拉伸或扭曲。一旦移植血管通过，移除胸管。需要进行足够的皮下分离，以避免移植血管受压后闭塞。移植血管完成颅内吻合后，移除临时阻断夹，使得移植血管的管腔充盈，血管保持足够的张力，确保移植血管不会打结或扭曲。

血管吻合术

在临时阻断之前将平均动脉压（MAP）升高至 90 mmHg（以增加侧支循环中的血流量），保持 33~34 °C 的低体温，静脉滴注丙泊酚以防止动脉瘤突然破裂。在受体血管（MCA）上行动脉切开术（**图 53.3B**），并用肝素化生理盐水冲洗管腔。移植血管和受体血管用靛红或无菌标记笔染色，以便在显微吻合过程中更好地观察这些动脉。用 10-0 或 9-0 缝合线来缝合吻合口的两端，侧壁采用连续或间断的方式缝合（**图** 53.3C）。我们更喜欢采用连续缝合的技术，便于改进对吻合部位对位和直径匹配的校正。

缝线应该从移植血管外壁穿入受体血管内壁，或者从受体血管外壁穿入移植血管内壁，然后结打在吻合口的外面。缝合时必须非常小心，不要缝住血管后壁。临时阻断时间应尽可能短。一旦吻合完成，就要松开受体血管上的临时阻断夹，吻合口周围可能会有少量渗血。

移植血管中的反流血很重要，可以通过血流灌注移植血管的内皮细胞，以最大限度地减少缺血的影响。在此之后，将肝素化的生理盐水注入移植血管的游离端并进行冲洗，同时在 MCA 吻合口附近应用动脉瘤临时阻断夹阻断移植血管。

然后，移植血管与颈外动脉（ECA）段使用 9-0 Prolene 线施行连续或间断端侧吻合术（**图 53.3D**）。由于血管的深度增加吻合手术的难度，可以使用动

脉悬吊丝带将ECA更好地呈现在手术视野中。在ECA近端和远端应用临时阻断夹后，在动脉上切一个椭圆形的切口。将SVG剪切成一定长度（以最大限度地减少血管打折和迂曲），游离端呈鱼嘴样张开，然后按照颅内阶段的描述进行吻合手术。

在完成搭桥后，松开移植血管远端的临时阻断夹以重新确认血液回流，随后移除ECA的阻断夹以建立移植血管内的顺行血流。术中采用血管造影术、吲哚菁绿荧光血管造影术、Charbel Transonics血流探头或超声多普勒血流测量方法来监测载瘤血管的通畅性（**图** 53.3E）。

关颅与术后护理

关闭颅骨和颈部手术切口的多层伤口时都需要注意仔细止血，并且在骨瓣复位、颞肌对位和最终皮肤缝合过程中要监测移血管的通畅性。术后应避免弹力头套对移植血管的外部压迫，患者在ICU严格维持正常血压和正常血容量。用手持式多普勒仪定期监测移植血管。

然后用血管造影术证实患者搭桥血管通畅，可以即刻或者延迟几天后，在全身麻醉下采用血管内治疗闭塞同侧载瘤动脉。对搭桥血管和潜在巨大动脉瘤的长期监测应遵循当地治疗指南。

后循环高流量颅外－颅内搭桥手术

鉴于后循环巨大动脉瘤的手术入路困难，因此手术特别具有挑战性。尽管夹闭塑型术可以用于某些特定的巨大后循环动脉瘤，但是还是经常需要进行颅外-颅内搭桥手术和动脉瘤孤立术（Patel and Kirkpatrick，2009）。大脑后动脉（posterior cerebral artery，PCA），小脑上动脉（superior cerebellar artery，SCA）和小脑后下动脉是常见的受体血管，并且颞浅动脉或枕动脉被用作许多此类搭桥手术的供体血管。虽然枕动脉是一条强大的供体血管，但它可能没有足够的血流量来供应整个后循环。此外，枕动脉提供的长度可能不足以到达颅后窝的深度。Pisapia等回顾当代关于后循环搭桥手术的文献，发现34例高流量搭桥术治疗后循环复杂动脉瘤的病例。这些病例中有12例是使用桡动脉完成的，其余22例是使用大隐静脉完成的（Pisapia et al.，2011）。椎动脉V3段和颈外动脉是最常见的供体血管，据报道移植血管的长期通畅率为95%。对于一些巨大的冗长扩张性后循环动脉瘤，采用EC-IC和IC-IC搭桥手术进行血流逆转或降低其流量的治疗可能是最佳的治疗方法，使用RAG进行的MCA-PCA搭桥手术是重建基底动脉远端血运的首选技术（Lawton et al.，2016）（**图** 53.4）。

外科治疗的结果

依据外科手术治疗颅内巨大动脉瘤的一系列最新的文献报道，证实外科手术可以明显改善患者的预后（**表** 53.1），越来越多的医生采用搭桥技术联合间接巨大动脉瘤闭塞术。根据资深作者自己的经验，在13年的时间里，140例患者共141个巨大动脉瘤接受手术治疗。100个动脉瘤（71%）位于前循环，41个位于后循环。46%的动脉瘤采用直接夹闭治疗，51%采用载瘤动脉闭塞的间接手术治疗，38%采用搭桥手术治疗。108个动脉瘤（77%）完全闭塞，14个（10%）动脉瘤有微小残留，16个（11%）动脉瘤因其血流逆转或血流量降低而不完全闭塞。手术死亡率为13%，永久性神经系统功能障碍的发生率为9%。与搭桥相关的并发症包括移植血管闭塞（7例）、由于动脉瘤不完全闭塞所致动脉瘤出血（4例）及动脉瘤血栓形成伴穿支或分支动脉闭塞（4例）。总体而言，平均随访2年，114例（81%）取得良好的预后，109例（78%）经过治疗后症状得到改善或没有加重（Sughrue et al.，2011）。

搭桥术治疗的结果

如**表** 53.3所示，高流量EC-IC搭桥手术是安全、有效的手术方式，同时闭塞复杂巨大颅内动脉瘤患者的载瘤血管，大多数患者可以获得良好的预后和闭塞动脉瘤。搭桥手术的通畅率为90%或者更高，据文献报道手术并发症发生率为5%～20%，包括术后缺血性卒中或出血、移植血管闭塞或感染性并发症。在较早的文献报道中术后30天内的死亡率较高，但是在现代的文献报道中术后30天内的死亡率保持在1%或更低的水平。最大宗的搭桥手术回顾性研究中，报道搭桥手术治疗93例颅内巨大动脉瘤（ICA占46%，MCA占32%，后循环占18%），其血管通畅率为96%，平均随访3年，94%的患者长期预后良好（Shi et al.，2015）。

血管内治疗的结果

宽颈巨大动脉瘤，并且伴有腔内血栓形成，载瘤动脉及其分支血管扭曲，此类巨大动脉瘤并不适合血管内治疗（**表** 53.1）。这些解剖因素不利于使用

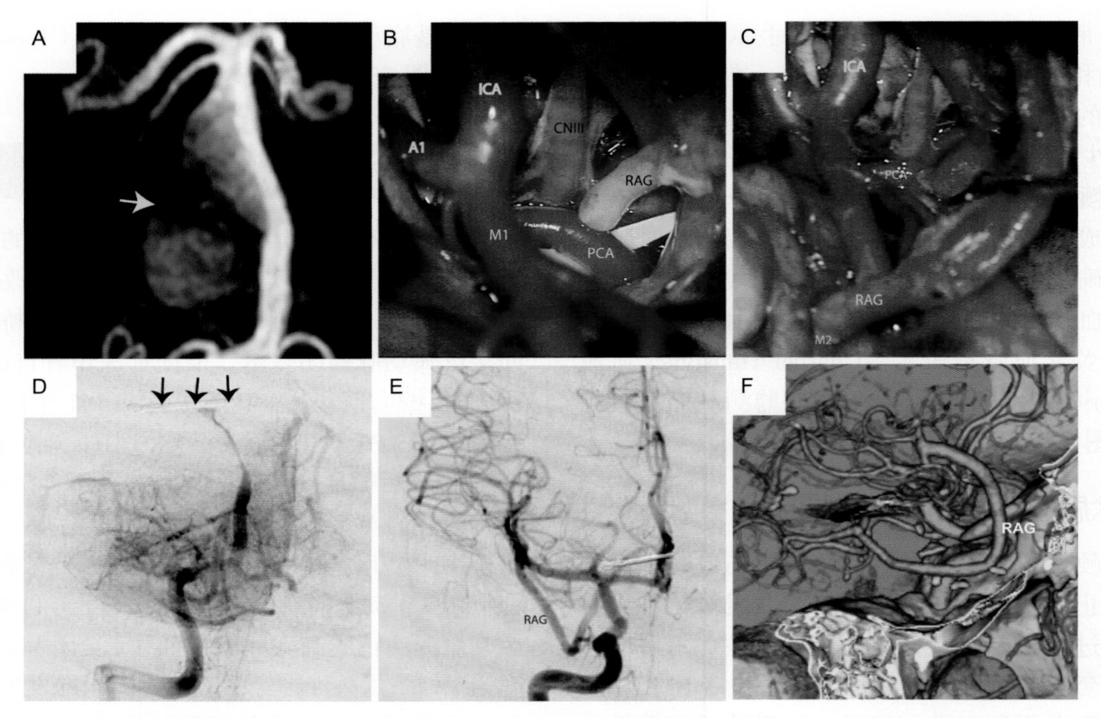

图 53.4 后循环高流量大脑中动脉—桡动脉—大脑后动脉搭桥。44 岁男性患者，巨大基底动脉干动脉瘤（图 A 箭头所示），伴部分血栓形成。经右侧眶颧入路，用桡动脉作移植血液，行大脑中动脉—大脑后动脉搭桥术，在小脑上动脉起点近端闭塞动脉瘤流出道。（B）右侧经侧裂显露扩展颈动脉动眼神经三角，完成大脑后动脉—桡动脉吻合。周边结构如颈内动脉，A1、M1 和动眼神经（CN Ⅲ）可显露。（C）另一经侧裂视角显示桡动脉和 M2 及大脑后动脉吻合口。（D）术后右侧椎动脉正位造影显示椎基底动脉近端显影，夹闭动脉瘤流出道后，远端血流改道。动脉瘤内血栓形成，动脉瘤未显影。（E）右侧颈内动脉前后位造影显示大脑中动脉—桡动脉—大脑后动脉血流通畅，前循环血流经桡动脉灌注后循环。（F）术后 3D 重建 CTA 斜侧位显示桡动脉充盈良好，巨大动脉瘤已闭塞

弹簧圈完全闭塞动脉瘤。此外，动脉瘤复发的可能性非常高，需要多次治疗，偶尔还会出现再次出血，以及动脉瘤进行性增大引起的神经功能障碍加重。像支架或球囊辅助这样的技术经常被用于治疗巨大动脉瘤，增加术中风险（Lylyk et al.，2009）。Jahromi 等（2008）报道 39 个巨大动脉瘤的血管内治疗经验（其样本量为最大之一），结果显示完全闭塞率为 36%，支架辅助率为 66%，平均每个动脉瘤治疗两次。累积治疗复发率为 32%（12 例），治疗死亡率为 16%（6 例）。总体而言，11 名患者在随访后期死亡（29%）。尽管血管内技术有所进步，但是同一作者在 2007 年至 2012 年发表其后续研究结果，在最后一次随访中显示 31% 的手术相关死亡率和 46% 的永久性神经功能障碍或死亡（Dumont et al.，2014）。

血流导向装置最近已经获得批准用于治疗 ICA 近端动脉瘤（从岩部到垂体上段）（Lylyk et al.，2009；Nelson et al.，2011；Fischer et al.，2012）。它们可以使血流转向正常方向，随着时间的推移，病变血管会发生新生内皮化并隔绝动脉瘤，从而导致动脉瘤内的血栓形成。在某些情况下，血流导向装置被证实可以保留被覆盖的穿支血管的血流，但是包括支架内晚期血栓形成、延迟性出血和动脉瘤周围水肿在内的并发症并不少见（Alderazi et al.，2014）。用于颅内动脉瘤治疗的支架（Pipeline for Intracranial Treatment of Aneurysms，PITA）和用于动脉瘤无法栓塞或栓塞失败的支架（Pipeline for Uncoilable or Failed Aneurysms，PUFS）在治疗前循环近端动脉瘤中的试验结果是有前景的（Nelson et al.，2011）。然而，在后循环中应用的试验结果不太理想（Siddiqui et al.，2012）。这对于巨大的基底动脉梭形扩张性动脉瘤来说尤其如此，这些动脉瘤内有层状血栓，使用多个重叠的短血流导向装置，导致穿支动脉闭塞和迟发性破裂的发生率很高。此外由于使用血流导向装置需要服用双联抗血小板药物，在蛛网膜下腔出血的情况下其附加风险导致疗效不太理想。

然而目前批准的血流导向装置并不适用于动脉分叉，也不适用于带有穿支血管的大脑中动脉和基底动脉（basilar artery，BA）的梭形动脉瘤，这可能

表 53.3 已发表的颅内巨大动脉瘤搭桥手术经验总结

						手术并发症			最后随访时患者预后	
研究	研究期间	患者数量	适应证	搭桥手术类型	桥血管通畅率 (%)	死亡率 (%)	并发症 (%)	平均随访时间（年）	非常好 / 良好 (%)	一般 / 差 (%)
Hacein–Bey et al. (1997)	1992—1997	9	ICA GIA	高流量 ECA-SVG-M2 STA-M2	89		11	1.8	100	
Houkin et al. (1999)	1989—1998	43	ICA GIA	高流量 ECA-RAG-M2	95		4	7.2	N/A	
Jafar et al. (2002)	1990—1999	30	ICA GIA	高流量 ECA/ CCA-SVG-MCA ECA/ CCA-SVG-ICA	93	3	6	5.2	N/A	
Van Doormaal et al. (2006)	1999—2004	34	ICA GIA	高流量 ECA-SVG-ICA	100 （17% 返修率））	6	12	4.4	79	
Cantore et al. (2008)	1990—2004	41	ICA GIA PC GIA	高流量 ECA/ ICA-SVG-M2	93	10	5	8.5	85.4	
Patel et al. (2010)	2005—2007	9	ICA GIA ICA 分离	高流量 ECA-SVG-M2	88 （22% 返修率）	0	22	N/A	100	0
Kalani et al. (2013)	1983—2011	16	MCA GIA	高流量和低流量 STA-MCA (13) ECA-SVG/ RAG-MCA (3)	94	0	19	4.9	94	6
Ishishita et al. (2014)	1996—2011	38	ICA GIA	高流量 ECA-RAG/ SVG-M2	95	0	5	3.9	100	0
Shi et al. (2015)	2004—2013	93	ICA GIA MCA GIA PC GIA	高流量和低流量 ECA/IMA-RAG/ SVG-MCA/PCA STA-MCA OA-PICA/AICA	96	1	5	3.0	94	5

ACA，大脑前动脉；ACoA，前交通动脉；AICA，小脑前下动脉；BA，基底动脉；CCA，颈总动脉；ECA，颈外动脉；GIA，颅内巨大动脉瘤；ICA，颈内动脉；MCA，大脑中动脉；OA，枕动脉；PC，后循环；PCA，大脑后动脉；PCoA，后交通动脉；PICA，小脑后下动脉；RAG，桡动脉移植血管；STA，颞浅动脉；SVG，大隐静脉移植血管；VA，椎动脉；N/A, 不详

会导致穿支闭塞而造成灾难性后果。

结论

巨大动脉瘤是一种不常见但是极具挑战性的病变，且自然病史较差，因此将并发症发生率和死亡率降至最低是治疗的关键。一部分巨大动脉瘤可以通过夹闭术、夹闭塑型术或弹簧圈栓塞治疗。然而一些病例的治疗仍然需要应用复杂的血运重建术和血流逆转技术。随着血管内技术的不断发展，未来可能会有越来越多的此类病变不需要开放手术就能成功治疗。与此同时，血管内重建术或栓塞术治疗后复发动脉瘤以及在颈内动脉海绵窦段和床突旁段以外使用血流导向装置的不确定结果等问题持续存在，使外科治疗成为此类巨大动脉瘤患者的首选治疗方法。

延伸阅读、参考文献

扫描书末二维码获取。

第 54 章　自发性颅内血肿

Berk Orakcioglu · Andreas W. Unterberg 著
殷祥栋 译，伊志强 审校

自发性颅内血肿的病理生理学、流行病学、发病率和危险因素

流行病学 / 发病率

自发性颅内血肿（intracerebral haematoma，ICH）占所有卒中的 20%，男性略占优势。发病率随着年龄和抗凝 / 抗血栓治疗的增加而升高。由于人口结构的变化，到 2050 年，发病率可能会增加 35%（Stein et al.，2012）。这与种族起源有关：在白种人中，发病率为 20/10 万，而在日本为 60/10 万。发作后第一周和第一年的死亡率分别为 31%~34% 和 53%~59%（Flaherty et al.，2006）。

分类

ICH 可以通过多种方式进行分类：出血来源、血肿的解剖位置、其他室腔（比如脑室）是否存在血肿。按描述性解剖分类可将出血部位分为脑叶、基底节、丘脑、脑干或小脑，以及是否破入蛛网膜下腔或脑室。ICH 会累及脑实质，不管出血部位典型或者不典型，可诊断为颅内血肿。在较年轻的患者中，典型的 ICH 可见于基底节或丘脑。一般推测可能是豆纹动脉或丘脑小动脉破裂引起出血，且与急性或慢性高血压的发作密切相关。在老年患者中，脑叶血肿被称为非典型血肿，通常与淀粉样血管病变有关。在年轻患者中，非典型部位的血肿应怀疑由血管畸形或肿瘤引起，需行进一步血管检查。

危险因素

ICH 的主要危险因素是基底节出血区的动脉高压和老年人中伴有皮质出血的淀粉样血管病变。5%~10% 的 ICH 发生在肝素或维生素 K 拮抗剂（华法林最为常见）用药期间。使用维生素 K 拮抗剂抗凝与每年 0.5%~1% 的脑出血风险相关，在这些患者中只有一半存在药物过量。口服抗凝药物（oral anticoagulant，OAC）治疗的患者发生自发性脑出血的风险更高，如果不逆转 OAC 药物治疗，死亡率更高（Kuramatsu et al.，2015）。

其他已知的危险因素包括心脏病、血液系统相关疾病、凝血功能障碍（血友病、血管性血友病综合征）、血小板减少症、白血病和弥散性血管内凝血病。

与缺血性卒中不同，糖尿病、高胆固醇血症和吸烟并不是 ICH 的危险因素，而低胆固醇水平可使脑出血的风险增加一倍。脑静脉血栓形成可在不同部位诱发 ICH。

病理生理学

ICH 最重要的特征之一是血肿大小或水肿早期进展（**图 54.1**）可导致继发性神经功能恶化。

血肿增大可能发生在脑出血后的 24 小时内，而炎症过程在脑出血后很快开始，水肿可在脑出血后持续数周（**图 54.2**）（Xue and Del Bigio，2000）。

对 ICH 患者的连续 CTA 分析发现，早期“斑点征”（6小时内）是不良结局的强有力预测因素（Mayer et al.，2009；Demchuk et al.，2012）。“斑点征”是指起病早期血肿内的造影剂外渗。理论上，随着血肿体积的增加，颅内压（intracranial pressure，ICP）升高的风险增加，随之 CBF 和 $P_{br}O_2$ 降低，导致局部或整体缺血。细胞毒性和（或）血管源性水肿是否在周围性出血的病理生理学中起关键作用仍然是一个有争议的问题（Butcher et al.，2004）。这些继发性脑组织改变可能是影响患者预后的最重要因素。病理生理因素在初期几个小时内的作用尚不清楚（Kirkman and Smith，2013）。

血肿降解产物和凝血因子引发的继发性神经元损伤级联反应主要是基于凝血酶和铁毒性。炎症过程和血脑屏障的紊乱促进出血周围组织的水肿形成（Nakamura et al.，2006；Xi et al.，2006）。

和血管源性水肿的促进因素一样，代谢作用也被认为是晚期加重的原因。血肿对周围血管的压迫被认为是引起缺血伴细胞毒性水肿的原因。然而，大

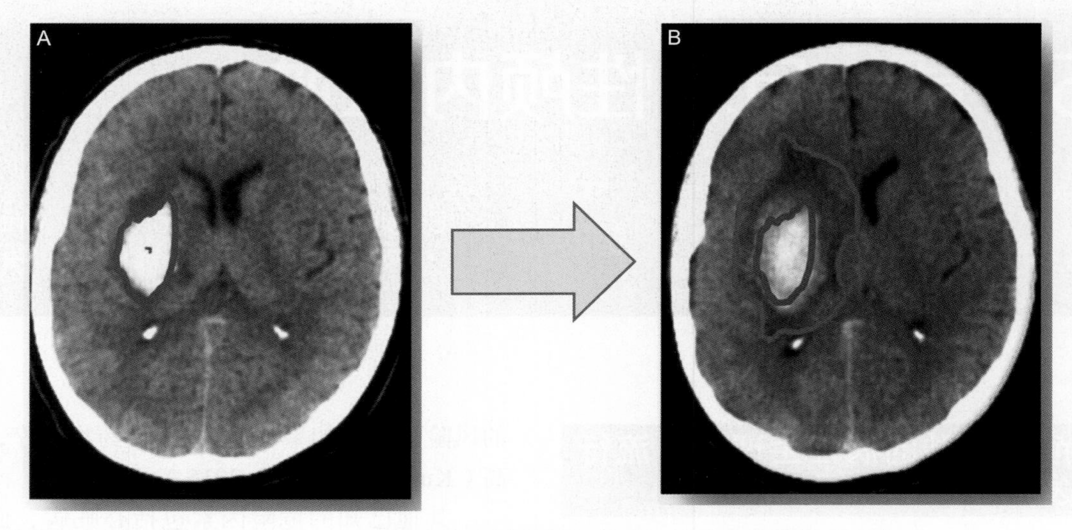

图 54.1　壳核出血伴轻度占位效应（A）；随后原发病灶周围出现水肿，导致中线结构受压（B）

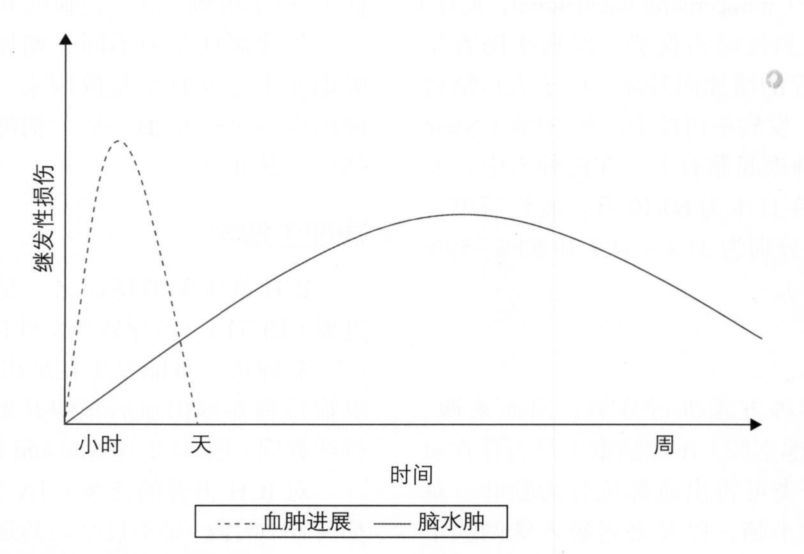

图 54.2　原发性 ICH 后血肿和水肿进展的时间轴

多数学者发现虽然灌注减少，但出血周围却没有明显的缺血。线粒体功能障碍似乎起了一定作用，但其起源尚不清楚（Kim-Han et al.，2006）。新的实验数据表明，线粒体功能障碍引起的缺血更有可能出现在较大的血肿中（Orakcioglu et al.，2015）。

ICH 的另一个主要原因（15%，由于人口结构的变化有增加的趋势）是脑淀粉样血管病（cerebral amyloid angiopathy，CAA）。在这些患者中，淀粉样蛋白可在大脑动脉皮质的内、外膜中发现。随着年龄的增长，这些变化易导致脑叶血肿和淀粉样蛋白沉积增加。

波士顿（Boston）标准总结了 CAA 的诊断标准。为了明确诊断，必须做组织病理学检查。然而，波士顿标准有助于在没有组织学关联的情况下对脑叶血肿进行临床分类（见**专栏** 54.1）。

临床表现和检查

根据血肿的位置、大小和动态变化，患者有不同的临床表现。**专栏** 54.2 总结了某些部位出现的症状。然而，随着血肿大小的增加，有可能出现临床表现的加重。患者应在发作后的早期阶段收入卒中病房或神经重症监护病房。

一般来说，ICH 应被视为一种严重威胁生命的事件。即使发病时症状轻微，出血进展也可能导致快速的神经功能恶化。ICH 急救的重点是：①确定并治疗出血的根本原因（如 AVM）；②一般重症监护，确保重要功能；③有针对性的神经重症措施控制颅

专栏 54.1　脑淀粉样血管病变（CAA）波士顿标准

确诊的 CAA

尸检组织学发现：
- 脑叶、皮质或皮质下血肿
- 严重 CAA 伴相关血管病变
- 未发现其他原因

有病理支持的 CAA

临床资料和病理发现：
- 脑叶、皮质或皮质下血肿
- 组织学上有一定程度的 CAA 表现
- 未发现其他原因

较为可能的 CAA

临床和影像学表现为：
- 多处血肿，主要为脑叶、皮质或皮质下（包括小脑）
- 年龄≥55 岁
- 未发现其他原因

有可能的 CAA

临床和影像学表现为：
- 单发大叶、皮质或皮质下血肿
- 年龄≥55 岁
- 未发现其他原因

内压升高；④限制血肿进展的特殊治疗；⑤评估是否存在手术治疗方案（如 EVD，手术清除巨大血肿）。

检查

因为计算机断层扫描（CT）广泛的应用，低廉的价格，并且可在入院时迅速执行，CT 仍然是 ICH 影像学诊断的金标准。检测有临床意义的 ICH，其敏感性和特异性接近 100%。一旦发现 ICH，加做增强序列（CT 血管造影、CT 静脉造影）可能对其潜在病因提供有价值的信息。对于年轻患者的非典型血肿，这些附加的方法对于排除潜在的血管异常（如动脉瘤）是必要的。如果出现蛛网膜下腔出血（动脉瘤性 SAH）或脑室周围血肿破入脑室（AVM），则将血肿归类为不典型血肿。不同阶段的潜在钙化和血凝块成分（海绵状血管瘤）也应怀疑为非典型血肿，需要进一步检查。

在诊断脑出血的敏感性和特异性方面，梯度回波和 T2 加权磁共振成像（MRI）与 CT 相当（Masdeu et al.，2006）。包括 MR 血管成像在内的 MRI 也可用于早期 ICH 的检测。然而，MRI 的实用性较低，技术复杂性较高，成本较高，检查时间也较长。镇静插管的患者应由神经重症监护室和 MRI 室的医生照看。MRI 的一个优点是其对提示 CAA 诊断的微出血的敏感性。

一旦发现 ICH，就应确定出血量来判断预后。一个很好的估计 ICH 出血量的方法是公式 a*b*c/2（Kothari，1996）。出血量 30 ml 或以下可能与可接受的功能预后相关，而出血量大于 60 ml 则往往与功能预后差和生活不能自理相关。

最近的报告强调了“斑点征”的重要性。在早期

专栏 54.2　ICH 的典型症状与部位的关系

壳核
- 对侧偏瘫
- 病变侧共轭凝视偏斜
- 同侧偏盲
- 如果 ICH 位于优势侧，则为失语

丘脑
- 对侧感觉症状
- 最初的意识减退进展为昏迷
- 偏瘫
- 偏身共济失调（高达 20%）
- 中脑受压引起的动眼肌症状（如 Parinaud 综合征）
- 神经心理障碍

尾状核
- 偏瘫
- 常累及脑室合并脑膜炎

脑桥
- 最初意识状态下降，逐渐发展为昏迷
- 四肢瘫痪
- 异常屈曲或伸展
- 内侧病变中双侧颅神经功能障碍
- 被盖定位：核间眼肌麻痹、瞳孔扩张和对侧偏瘫

中脑
- 最初意识减退进展为昏迷
- Parinaud 综合征

小脑
- 最初意识状态下降，逐渐发展为昏迷
- 共济失调
- 头晕
- 凝视性麻痹
- 颅内压增高的征象

CTA 显示斑点征阳性的患者可能出现血肿增大，进而预后更差。然而，在 CAA 患者的脑叶血肿中，很少有斑点征阳性。该征的存在是否会影响治疗分层仍然存在争议（Evans et al.，2010）。

典型的高血压血肿不常规进行 CT 增强检查。然而，如果临床上充分怀疑有非典型血肿，提倡至少行 CTA 来排除真正的血管病变，如动脉瘤或动静脉畸形。

在非典型病例中，CT 或 MR 均未显示出血来源时，可采用数字减影血管造影（digital subtraction angiography，DSA）。如果怀疑有血管炎或有潜在的动静脉畸形时也可以使用 DSA，在这些情况下其优于非侵入性血管造影。

内科治疗

保守治疗方案的关键目标是维持重要功能，保证脑灌注和氧合，以及控制随后引起血肿进展的主要危险因素。对于较大的血肿，可能需要采取 ICP 监控措施来达到这些目标。

血压管理

关于自发性颅内血肿后血压升高的预后价值，尚未有研究得出明确的结果。大多数研究表明，血压显著升高与不良临床预后相关。大多数急性脑出血患者存在高血压，并且很大比例有高血压病史。即使患者没有高血压病史，作为颅内压升高的一种生理反应，血压仍会升高。从理论上讲，血压升高可能导致血肿增大和水肿的进行性进展，从而导致更差的结果。因此，在脑出血的紧急处理中应采取针对性的、积极的降压措施。INTERACT Ⅱ研究的结果证实，将收缩压降到低于 140 mmHg 的目标是安全的。尽管该研究作者可以证明血肿进展能显著降低，但并未观察到对预后的相关影响（Anderson et al.，2013）。考虑到这些发现，欧洲卒中组织（ESO）新的脑出血管理指南推荐在急性情况下维持正常至轻度升高收缩压水平（Steiner et al.，2014）。

癫痫治疗

癫痫发作的发生率为 7.5%，在 ICH 中比在其他卒中亚型中更常见（Passero et al.，2002），而 ICH 中的癫痫发作预示着预后不佳。在大多数病例中，癫痫发作发生在起病 3 天内，并伴有脑叶出血，这可能是主要的临床症状。重要的是，非惊厥性发作是脑出血患者病情恶化的原因之一。如果怀疑癫痫发作，应立即行脑电图或连续脑电图监测。此外，迟发性癫痫发作与脑叶血肿、微出血和酒精滥用引发有关（Rossi et al.，2013；Madžar et al.，2014）。

在癫痫发作的急性治疗中，苯二氮䓬类药物是首选，在后续治疗中，苯妥英钠、左乙拉西坦和丙戊酸是常用的抗癫痫药物。

专栏 54.3 信息专栏

纠正抗凝和积极控制血压是 ICH 重症监护或手术治疗的基础。

手术治疗

选择合适手术的患者，其关键因素是血肿大小、患者年龄、基础病、位置（脑叶还是深部）和患者的临床病程。

外科治疗的基本原理

如前所述，ICH 是一种和出血量相关的原发性占位性病变。随着毒性和代谢过程的发生，出血性水肿很可能发生在血肿和脑实质之间的边界处（Butcher et al.，2004）。实验数据表明，血肿的局部力学效应会限制出血周围灌注，从而促进继发性神经元损伤（Orakcioglu et al.，2014）。这些继发性变化和伴随的组织肿胀可能持续数天，往往导致神经功能恶化。一旦发生继发性功能恶化，晚期血肿清除的手术可能会错过获得更好预后的治疗窗口。在 STICH Ⅱ试验中，最初保守治疗的患者中有 21% 出现水肿相关的神经功能恶化而转为手术治疗。与最初接受手术的患者相比，这个亚组的最终结果更差。STICH Ⅱ的亚组分析提示 GCS 为 9~12 且无脑疝临床症状的患者应考虑手术治疗。

这里提出的关于出血和病理生理机制的理论考虑，建议早期手术清除颅内血肿。尽管术后影像学的结果良好，但两项大型随机对照多中心研究（STICH Ⅰ和Ⅱ）并没有提供证据说明早期血肿清除的策略在临床上是有益的（Mendelow et al.，2005；Mendelow et al.，2013）。

因为现代手术微创技术仍然是一个有前景的治疗选择，STICH Ⅰ和Ⅱ都没有个体化的手术治疗的相关研究。在随机对照 MISTIE Ⅱ研究中，有证据表明，立体定向放置导管到血块中，同时通过连续的 rt-PA 促进血凝块的减少，可显著减轻出血周围水肿（Mould et al.，2013）。MISTIE Ⅲ将内镜下凝块减少和溶解与“标准内科治疗”进行比较，也未发现对结果有显著的有益影响（Hanley et al.，2019）。

其他的微创手术包括使用导航钻孔入路的内镜治疗。最近，有经验的亚洲中心报道了一项回顾性研究，发现微创内镜下血肿清除可降低早期死亡率，从而使中等大小血肿患者的功能得到改善。这可能主要归因于精细的外科手

专栏 54.3 （续）

术方法，包括神经导航和现代内镜设备。需要前瞻性随机对照临床试验来比较这种治疗方式与传统开颅血肿清除术以及单独保守治疗对长期死亡率和功能预后的影响。

在比较保守治疗和手术治疗的随机对照研究中，尚未对颅后窝脑出血进行研究。只有一项研究比较了幕下血肿清除的两种手术技术，表明小骨瓣开颅术比更大的减压手术更有益（Tamaki et al., 2004）。从回顾性病例系列中可以明显看出，其病理生理学与幕上脑出血不同，由于颅后窝的空间有限，手术更可能用于巨大血肿。手术指征为第四脑室闭塞（不论临床症状或ICH大小），GCS评分小于14，血肿直径大于30 mm且不小于7 mm（Da Pian et al., 1984；Mathew et al., 1995；Kirollos et al., 2001）。然而，2014年的ESO指南得出结论，RCT没有足够的证据来明确建议如何、何时以及对哪些幕下ICH患者进行手术治疗。

争议部分

ICH患者应尽可能转移到专门的神经重症监护室或卒中病房。必须仔细评估患者的具体特征（即年龄、危险因素、血肿位置和大小等）、神经系统和病前状况、凝血障碍以及包括血管检查在内的诊断检查，以决定最佳的个体化治疗方案。是否进行手术不仅取决于这些因素，还取决于能否应用特定技术，如内镜和其他微创手术。经过仔细讨论后，一旦倾向于手术清除血肿，就应该使用神经导航或立体定向方法来降低手术相关的并发症，从而有助于改善结果。治疗脑出血患者的手术措施如下：

- 怀疑颅内压升高或脑室内受累者行脑室造瘘及外引流术；
- 导航/立体定向钻孔和沿血肿长轴留置导管并连续重复rt-PA溶栓治疗和抽吸（MISTIE操作）；
- 导航/立体定向钻孔和沿长轴的内镜下血肿清除术；
- 导航辅助小骨瓣开颅及显微神经外科血肿清除术；
- 部分病例采用去骨瓣减压术（即窦静脉血栓形成的脑出血）。

大多数争议存在于基底节深部有较大血肿的年轻患者。由于仍然缺乏评估继发性神经功能恶化的有价值的指标，是否应该进行手术仍然是个不确定的问题。如果第一时间不赞成手术，继发性脑肿胀和水肿可能会进展，推迟手术可能成为唯一的选择。在STICH Ⅱ中，21%的保守治疗患者接受了延迟手术，其中大多数出现了继发性恶化。理想情况下，这些患者可以在神经功能和影像学进展之前接受手术，但选择标准尚不明确。

专栏 54.4 病例介绍

一名35岁的亚洲女性突发性头痛，右侧偏瘫和面瘫。CT显示继发于严重高血压的巨大基底节血肿。初始GCS评分为14，但GCS在早期进展为8，血肿进展明显，提示可采用内镜下血肿清除术。术后患者迅速恢复为中度偏瘫，早期GCS为15分。术后第3天的MRI（图54.3B）显示术后早期血肿清除，水肿进展得到控制，且颅内压正常。

专栏 54.4的案例说明了神经重症医生、神经内科医生和神经外科医生之间进行跨学科决策的必要性。即使最初由于患者的早期良好临床状况而优先选择最佳药物治疗，但起始的GCS为14可能增加了随后恶化的可能性。因此，即使患者的临床状况发生轻微变化，也应重新评估上述手术方案。

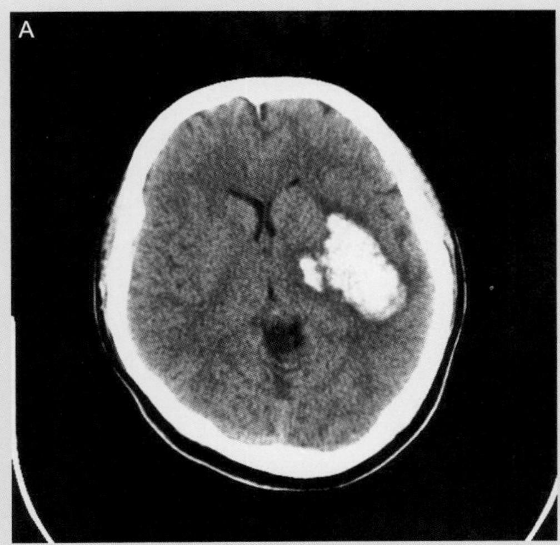

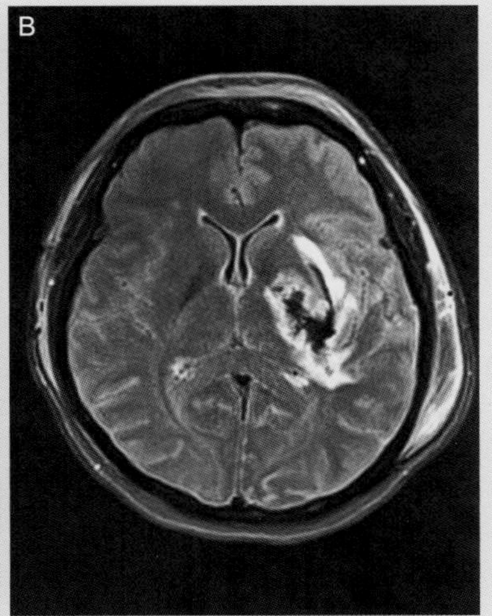

图 54.3 （A）CT显示继发于重度高血压的巨大基底节血肿。（B）术后MRI显示血肿清除，水肿程度局限，术后早期ICP正常

抗凝、抗血小板治疗和凝血功能障碍的治疗

在所有 ICH 患者中，近 40% 在 24 小时内出现进行性血肿增大（专栏 54.3）。为了限制继发性神经功能恶化，有必要采取上述医疗措施（即降低血压）来减轻血肿扩大。为了快速评估凝血疾病，抗血小板药物的有效程度，并帮助加速凝血管理，即时诊断已得到广泛应用（Beynon et al.，2013；Beynon et al.，2014）。如果证实有溶栓功能障碍，则应考虑使用氨甲环酸、去氨加压素或新鲜冷冻血浆，尽管尚无证据支持这一实用的治疗建议（Campbell et al.，2010；Sprigg et al.，2014）。

根据创伤性颅脑损伤的指导方针，最新数据显示 OAC 或 NOAC（新型口服抗凝剂）相关的 ICH 应通过停止抗凝，给予维生素 K，并考虑特异性逆转（如凝血酶原复合物浓缩物，PCC）来限制血肿扩大（Le Roux et al.，2014）。4 小时内 INR 的逆转小于 1.3 和 4 小时收缩压小于 160 mmHg 与较低的血肿增大率和较好的预后相关，恢复 OAC 治疗与较低的缺血事件风险相关（Kuramatsu et al.，2015）。

延伸阅读、参考文献、EBRAIN 的相关链接

扫描书末二维码获取。

第 55 章　海绵状血管瘤和血管造影隐匿性病变

Janneke van Beijnum · Hiren Patel 著
李春伟 译，伊志强 审校

引言

脑海绵状畸形（cerebral cavernous malformations，CCMs），也称为海绵状血管瘤，是由异常扩大的毛细血管腔组成的血管畸形，没有介入实质（见本章毛细血管扩张症一节），没有供血动脉及引流静脉（见**第 50 章**动静脉畸形）。10%~20% 的 CCMs 与发育性静脉畸形（developmental venous anomaly，DVA，正常静脉解剖学的极端变异，见本章后文）有关，CCMs 的发生可能是潜在的遗传性疾病的结果，对于有阳性家族史或多发性病变的患者，建议进行基因分析。对于无症状的 CCMs，在绝大多数病例中采用保守治疗似乎是合理的，只有当患者出现症状时才需要进行后续的影像学检查。CCMs 手术治疗的适应证是病灶反复出血、具有占位效应而引起相关症状，以及确定病灶为致痫灶的难治性癫痫患者。在手术风险极高的特殊情况下，可考虑立体定向放射治疗。

病理学

组织学描述

在显微镜下，CCMs 表现为桑葚状畸形，大小可从几毫米到几厘米不等。CCM 内不同阶段出血的证据可通过周围脑组织的含铁血黄素染色来判断。在显微镜下，它们由紧密堆积的单层内皮细胞组成不同的腔隙。腔壁由结缔组织组成，缺乏组织胶原蛋白和明显的肌肉层，这在正常血管和动静脉畸形中是存在的。此外，腔隙内壁内皮细胞之间缺乏紧密连接，这可能有助于 CCMs 反复发生小的出血，这是典型的 CCMs 特点。CCMs 基底层存在特征性的含铁血黄素沉积，但没有累及其中的神经组织，这使 CMMs 与毛细血管扩张症相区别（Wong et al.，2000；Haasdijk et al.，2012）。

发病机制、遗传学和家族性综合征学说

通过研究与家族性 CCMs 相关的基因，解开了部分 CCMs 的发病机制。据报道，近 20% 的患者有家族性 CCMs 发生，尽管一些散发病例也可能表现为常染色体显性遗传，但其表现形式不一，且为不完全显性遗传。在墨西哥血统的西班牙裔美国患者中，由于 KRIT1（k-rev 相互作用捕获蛋白 1）基因（Q455X）的共同突变，家族遗传病例的比例可能高达 50%（Haasdijk et al.，2012）。

表 55.1 概述了三种已知基因的突变与 CCMs 有关。由于这些 CCM 基因编码的蛋白质与血管内皮细胞之间的连接形成有关，因此，丧失功能的突变可能导致内皮亚单位之间存在间隙的异常血管的形成。

虽然 CCMs 是血管性病变，但原位杂交研究表

表 55.1　CCMs 的遗传因素

	染色体	可能的功能
CCM1 KRIT1	7q11.2-21	细胞黏附（ICAPα）、细胞扩散（malcavernin）、内皮细胞迁移方向（HEG1）、肿瘤抑制基因（RAP1a）
CCM2 MGC4607 malcavernin	7p13	管腔形成（PDCD10）、血管通透性（Rac1）、迁移（p38 MAPK 信号传递激酶）
CCM3 PDCD10	3q26.1	细胞凋亡（malcavernin），内皮细胞迁移方向（SSTK24）
不明基因	3q26.3-27.2	

HEG1，玻璃心受体 1；ICAP1α，β1 整合素调节因子整合素胞质衔接蛋白 1 的 α 亚型；KRIT1，k-rev 相互作用捕获蛋白 1；PDCD10，程序性细胞死亡 10；STK24/25，丝氨酸 / 苏氨酸蛋白激酶

Adapted with permission from Remco A Haasdijk, Caroline Cheng, Anneke J Maat-Kievit, Henricus J Duckers, Cerebral cavernous malformations: from molecular pathogenesis to genetic counselling and clinical management, *European Journal of Human Genetics*, Volume 20, Issue 2, pp. 134–40, Copyright © 2011 Springer Nature.

明，KRIT-1、MGC4607 和 PDCD10 在星形胶质细胞、神经元和各种上皮细胞中均有表达。因此，CCMs 也可能是内皮细胞和神经细胞之间信号传递错误的结果，那么，又提出了一个问题，即 CCMs 的主要缺陷是源于血管还是神经元（Haasdijk et al.，2012）。

此外，家族性 CCMs 与散发性 CCMs 相比，与 DVA 相关的可能性较小，散发性 CCMs 几乎有一半的病例与 DVA 相关。这表明，CCM 的发展存在潜在不同的致病机制（Petersen et al.，2010）。

与 CCM1 相关的突变最为常见，其次是 CCM2，CCM3 则较为罕见。几乎所有至少有一个受影响亲属的 CCM 患者都会有一个 CCM 基因的突变，而在 60%~80% 有多个病变但没有受影响亲属的患者中，情况也是如此（Denier et al.，2006；Haasdijk et al.，2012）。虽然 CCM3 家族中受影响的亲属数量一般较少，但与 CCM1 和 CCM2 表型相比，临床病程似乎更加凶险，在家族性和散发性病例中，病变数量更多，出血更频繁，并且在儿童期即表现出（Denier et al.，2006；Shenkar et al.，2015）。

建议

- 对有 CCM 家族史或多发病变的患者进行基因分析。

临床表现和放射学检查

临床表现

CCMs 的发生率在每年每 10 万人中 0.17~0.56（Brown et al.，1996；Al-Shahi et al.，2003）。在之后一项以人口为基础的前瞻性研究中，一半以上的 CCMs 是尸检（11%）或影像学检查（46%；见 Al-Shahi et al.，2003）时偶然发现的。然而 1965—1992 年进行的一项回顾性研究具有较低的发病率（Brown et al.，1996），因此可以推测 CCMs 发病率的增加是 20 世纪 80 年代以来 MRI 扫描日益普及的直接结果。

CCMs 最常出现在 40~50 岁，女性可能略高（58%）。大约一半的 CCMs 患者无症状，而约 1/4 的患者出现单次或反复癫痫发作。首次发作的患者极有可能发展为长期癫痫，因为只有 6% 的患者会被治愈。几乎有一半的 CCM 患者在诊断为癫痫后随访的 5 年内两年无发作（Josephson et al.，2011）。此外，患者可表现为出血（约 12%）或局灶性神经功能缺损（约 15%）（Al-Shahi Salman et al.，2012）。

放射学检查

CCMs 在血管造影中不显影，因此可称为血管造影隐匿性病变，或隐匿性血管畸形。虽然 CCM 可凭借脑出血或钙化在 CT 扫描上诊断，但通常在 MRI 影像上进行诊断（见**图** 55.1~ **图** 55.5）。CCMs 在 MR 扫描上可有特征性表现，经典的表现为“爆米花”样病变，周围有低信号边缘，这是由于反复微出血后含铁血黄素沉积所致（在 T2* 加权序列上，见**图** 55.1~ **图** 55.3）。放射学上，CCMs 可分为四种类型（**表** 55.2），梯度回波序列（gradient-echo sequence，GRE）（分别见**图** 55.4 和**图** 55.5 与**图** 55.2 和**图** 55.3 相比）显示 CCMs 远优于 T2，原因是血红素造成了磁敏感性伪影（Zabramski et al.，1994；Lanzino and Spetzler，2007）。

CCMs 最常见的发生位置是脑叶（67%），其次是幕下（脑干 14%，小脑 13%）。位于深部的病变相对罕见（6%）（Al-Shahi Salman et al.，2012）。

建议

- 血红素敏感的 MRI 序列，如 GRE 或敏感性加权序列应用于检测多发 CCMs。

表 55.2 CCMs 的放射学分类

种类		T1	T2
Ⅰ	（亚）急性出血并伴有放射线外延伸的征兆	超强度出血焦点	*IA* 型 CCMs 的出血灶过强或过弱，通过过弱的边缘延伸，而 *IB* 型 CCMs 的出血灶没有延伸
Ⅱ	亚急性大出血	网状混合芯材	网状混合核心，边缘低密度（典型的”爆米花”病变）
Ⅲ	慢性溶血性出血 通常见于家族性 CCMs	等强度或低强度病变	标准 T2 低密度病变，边缘低密度 *GRE*：与 T2 相比，放大率更高
Ⅳ	典型的见于家族性发生的 CCMs	通常不可见	标准 T2 通常不可见 *GRE*：小点状低密度病变

Source data from Zabramski JM, Wascher TM, Spetzler RF, Johnson B, Golfinos J, Drayer BP, Brown B, Rigamonti D, Brown G. The natural history of familial cavernous malformations: results of an ongoing study. *J Neurosurg* 1994; 80:422–32.

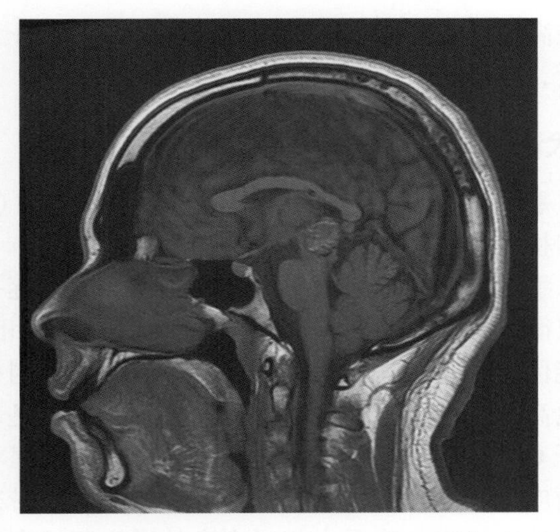

图 55.1　中脑海绵状血管瘤的矢状 T1 MR 图像

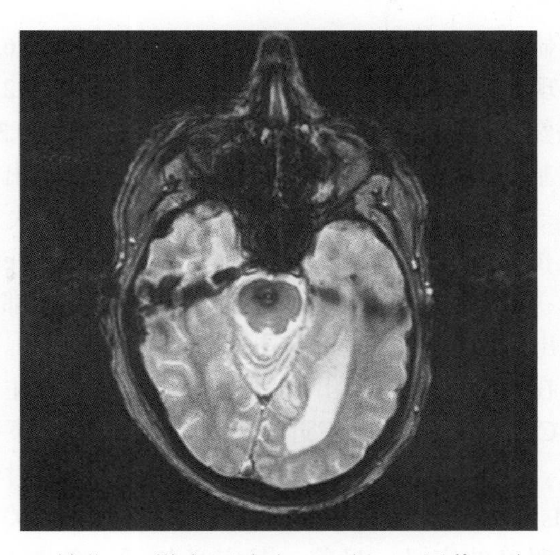

图 55.4　轴位 T2 梯度回波（GRE）MR 图像，由于其敏感性，较好地显示了脑桥海绵状血管瘤

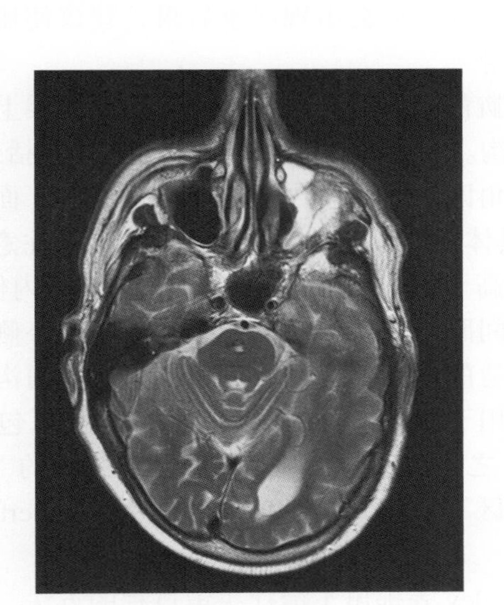

图 55.2　脑桥海绵状血管瘤的轴位 T2 快速自旋回波（FSE）MR 图像

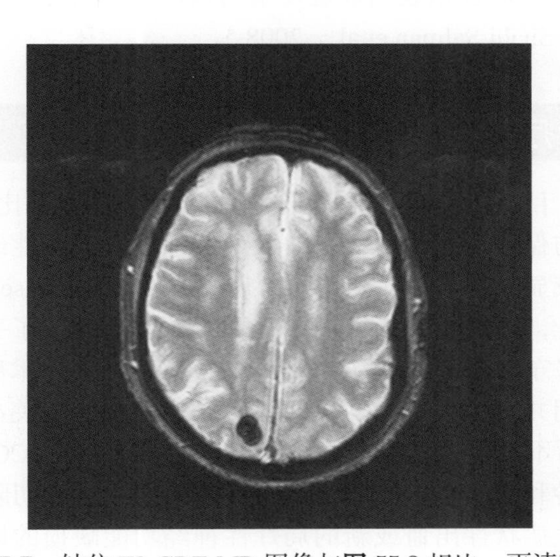

图 55.5　轴位 T2 GRE MR 图像与**图** 55.3 相比，更清晰地显示了海绵状血管瘤

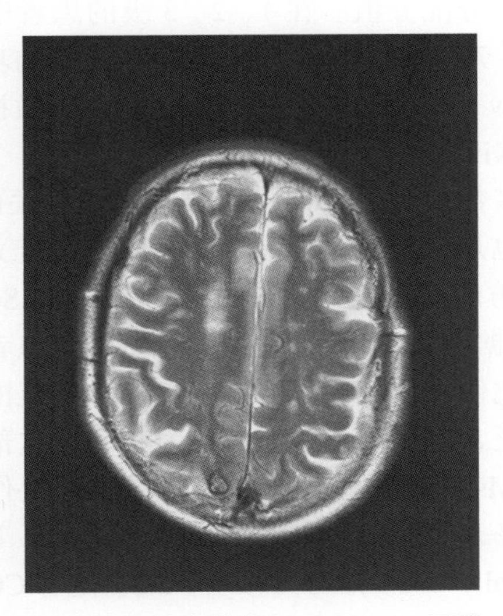

图 55.3　小海绵状血管瘤轴位 T2 FSE MR 图像

CCMs 的自然史

与动静脉畸形一样，关于 CCMs 自然史的可靠数据很少。大多数自然史研究都有偏向性，因为它们描述的是因某种原因没有接受治疗的选定患者，以及对接受治疗的患者进行的短期未治疗的跟踪。此外，这些研究绝大多数是以医院为基础的，并没有对一般人群进行观察。

一般认为，首次发生 CCM 相关出血的年风险率较低（每年 0.4%~0.6%），而后续出血的风险要高得多（每年 3.8%~23%），但这种风险会随着时间的推移而降低（Al-Shahi Salman et al.，2012；Flemming et al.，2012）。一项以医院为基础的大型回顾性研究数据显示，在出现出血的患者中，年出血率为6.2%，在出现非出血相关症状的患者中，年出血率为2.2%，在偶然发现的CCM的患者中，年出血率为0.33%。一项基于人群的前瞻性研究显示，最初出现出血的患者5年累计再出血风险接近30%，而首次出现出血的5年风险仅为2.4%（Al-Shahi Salman et al.，2012）。出现过大出血、男性性别和多发病灶都会增加大出血的风险（Flemming et al.，2012）。

在解读CCMs和出血率的数据时，需要注意的是，CCMs可以在没有近期明显出血的情况下引起症状。此外，CCMs有微出血倾向，导致放射学上CCMs典型的MR表现。这就需要对CCM相关出血进行明确的定义。目前，其定义如下：急性/亚急性症状发作的临床事件，并有放射学、病理学、手术或CSF证据表明最近发生的病灶外或病灶内出血（Al-Shahi Salman et al.，2008）。

治疗策略和预后

目前还没有随机对照试验将治疗方式相互比较，或与保守治疗进行比较。此外，也没有观察性研究比较显微手术切除和放射治疗的效果（Samarasekera et al.，2012）。一项基于人群的队列研究比较了手术和保守治疗，得出的结论是，由于CCM切除术后的早期并发症，手术与较差的短期功能预后相关。手术后不良预后的其他预测因素包括脑干部位的CCM、高龄和男性性别。此外，与保守治疗相比，切除后发生症状性出血或新的局灶性神经功能缺损的风险更高，而死亡率相当，手术组有1名患者（4.0%）在癫痫发作后死亡，而保守组有4名患者（3.7%）发生CCM相关死亡（Moultrie et al.，2014）。

保守治疗的管理

对于所有患者，在考虑任何干预措施之前，必须仔细评估风险和收益之间的平衡。最近的研究表明，CCM治疗的风险不容忽视，与保守治疗相比，CCM切除可能与短期预后不佳有关（Moultrie et al.，2014；Poorthuis et al.，2014）。一项系统性回顾显示，切除或立体定向放射手术（stereotactic radiosurgery，SRS）后，死亡、出血或新的/恶化的永久性神经功能障碍的总体发生率约为6例/每100人每年。如果患者出现出血或病变位于脑干外，手术风险较低（Poorthuis et al.，2014）。这表明，对于偶然发现的CCMs应强烈考虑保守治疗，除非随访期间出现临床出血或症状性生长。此外，对于有症状的CCMs且存在高治疗风险的患者，例如在功能区（如脑干）的患者，应考虑保守治疗。

手术切除

手术切除的适应证一般是既往出血病史和（或）伴有相关症状和体征的病变生长。

手术风险应根据每个患者的自然病史，逐一进行权衡。一般来说，与非功能区的CCMs患者相比，功能区或手术无法到达的CCMs患者的切除门槛应该更高。手术经验是这一决策的关键，尤其是对于脑干CCMs。当考虑切除脑干CCMs时，海绵状血管瘤应达到软膜或室管膜表面，以减少手术带来的神经功能损害。脑干中相对安全的进入区域在下文中进行了总结（Giliberto et al.，2010）。然而，如果重要结构损伤后会出现严重后果，建议使用术中电生理监测。

中脑背侧的安全进入区位于四叠体层上下和中脑外侧沟。在第四脑室底，安全进入区包括正中沟、面上三角区（面丘的上方）、面下三角区（面丘的下方）。具体而言，对于内侧沟入路，必须注意在面丘水平或高于面丘水平，因为可能会遇到内侧纵束，导致核间眼肌麻痹。在这种情况下，前外侧入路是比较合适的。在髓内，后正中裂、后中间沟和后外侧沟可用于相对安全的入路。腹侧入路区包括SCA和PCA之间的区域、Ⅴ和Ⅶ脑神经之间的“三叉神经周围区”、橄榄后沟和前外侧沟（Giliberto et al.，2010）。

Kivelev等提出了治疗决策过程的方法，并根据他们小组制订的分级量表报告了结果。在该量表中，根据位置（幕上1分；如果是幕下、基底节或脊柱，则为2分）和先前存在的神经功能缺陷（如果存在则为1分）分配分值。在1、2、3级的患者中，分别有87%、79%和46%的患者获得了良好的功能预后（Glasgow结果评分5分：正常活动、轻微神经功能缺损）（Kivelev et al.，2011）。

大多数探讨手术切除与癫痫发作相关的CCMs的研究也是有限的，缺乏对癫痫的严格定义，以及预后随访的衡量标准（von der Brelie and Schramm，2011）。据称，药物难治性癫痫的CCM患者的无癫痫发作比例可达到约88%。手术切除的范围可能需要更广泛，以更好地控制癫痫发作。在这部分患者中，CCMs导致的慢性癫痫患者无癫痫发作的比例能到80%，而散发的癫痫患者能达到91%（von der Brelie et al.，2013）。手术步骤无疑会随着CCM位置和手术入路的不同而有所不同。

术前咨询是极其重要的，以便让患者了解疾病的自然史、手术的获益（预防未来的大出血及相关的发病率和死亡率）和风险（包括术后大出血、感染、局灶性神经功能缺损、CSF 漏、癫痫和生命危险）。脑干 CCMs 切除后的病程可能与术后一定程度的暂时性神经功能恶化、长期接受重症监护有关，甚至有可能进行气管切开术和（或）经皮内镜胃造瘘术（percutaneous endoscopic gastrostomy，PEG）以及随后的康复需求。

在一项汇总分析中，术后并发症（30 天内死亡的复合、症状性出血、新发或恶化的局灶性神经功能障碍）的风险在幕上优势半球约为 7.7%（95% CI，5.2~11），脑干约为 50%（95% CI，37~64）（Moultrie et al.，2014）。

在选择合适的手术方式时，术前三个切面的 MRI 影像会有所帮助。CCM 手术入路选择的一个关键原则是找到最短的路径，将神经损伤降至最低（尤其是脊髓或脑干的 CCMs），并避开手术路径上的“盲点”。两点法可帮助手术入路的选择，利用一条延伸至颅骨的线，该线包括 CCM 中心的一个点和 CCM 累及软膜表面的第二个点（或者，能够安全进入大脑 / 脊髓的点）。

虽然手术过程中手术标志物（如黄荧光）可以引导外科医生从软膜或室管膜下进入点到识别出 CCM，但是无框架导航可以带来更大的获益。术中监测也可能有用，尤其是在功能区切除 CCM 时（Lanzino and Spetzler，2007；Nader et al.，2014）。

对于非功能区的 CCM，常用的手术方式是解剖病灶四周脑胶质面，先进行减瘤以简化手术切除，从而滚动着将病变从胶质面完整切除。理想情况下，为了把不完全切除的风险降到最低，应尝试将周边胶质连同病变一同切除。

切除功能区的 CCMs 则是另一种完全不同的手术方式。基本上采取“由内向外”的切除方式，即通过进入并切除 CCM，使其周边脑组织自行塌陷，之后再仔细处理 CCM 与周边被挤压以及功能区脑组织的界面，以减少周围脑组织伤害。

如果 CCM 与 DVA 相关，在切除时应保留后者，因为它代表正常静脉系统的一部分。只有 DVA 的小分支可以烧灼，如果主干牺牲了，则可能会导致静脉性脑梗死，造成潜在的灾难性后果（Lanzino and Spetzler，2007；Nader et al.，2014）。

立体定向放射外科

CCMs 进行 SRS 的目的是通过诱导海绵状血管瘤中形成血栓 - 闭塞，从而预防出血。由于 CCMs 是血管造影隐匿性病变，SRS 的效果不能像 AVMs 那样通过影像学评估，而完全依赖于随访期间出血的发生情况（Nagy and Kemeny，2013）。由于复发性颅内出血的风险随着时间的推移而降低（Al-Shahi Salman et al.，2012；Flemming et al.，2012），一些研究所描述的 SRS 后出血风险降低是否可以归因于这种治疗是值得怀疑的。因此，SRS 应仅限于重要功能区或手术无法到达的区域，如基底节和脑干（其中海绵状血管瘤不存在于表面）。

SRS 相关的发病率包括治疗后出血和放射性损伤。约有 7% 的患者因 SRS 后出血导致持续神经功能减退。治疗剂量在 12~15 Gy，并将 CMS 靶点定义在含铁血黄素素环内，辐射相关并发症一般在 1%~7%。一些 SRS 治疗 CCM 合并药物难治性癫痫患者的研究报道，40%~50% 的患者在随访时无发作（Nagy and Kemeny，2013）。另一项研究，对 CCMs 导致癫痫发生的患者进行对照分析显示，87% 的患者在手术后无癫痫发作，而 SRS 后为 64%（Hsu et al.，2007）。

建议

- 鉴于在 CCM 的治疗在循证医学方面的证据存在较大的局限性，只能提出有限的建议。
- 关于 CCMs 患者的治疗决策应该基于个体化（Samarasekera et al.，2012）。
- 在绝大多数情况下，对无症状的 CCMs 采取保守的方法似乎是合理的。
- 只有当患者出现症状时，才需要进行后续的影像学检查。
- 对于 CCM 患者，如果出现反复的出血，或是 CCMs 引起占位效应或神经系统体征和症状，或是引发难治性癫痫，则可以考虑手术切除病灶。对于难治性癫痫患者，应进行术前评估，以确定致痫灶。
- 对于功能区的 CCMs，鉴于发病率和死亡率相当高，手术的门槛被提高，但在反复病灶外出血和神经功能下降后可考虑。
- 在特殊情况下可以考虑 SRS，例如脑干海绵状血管瘤的反复出血，这些病灶没有累及软膜表面，因此具有很高的手术风险。

其他血管造影隐性畸形

发育性静脉畸形

DVA是正常静脉系统的极端变异。它们通常没有症状，尽管DVAs可能会因为流入量增加、静脉流出受阻或小的动静脉瘘导致静脉压力增加而出现症状。DVA如果发生出血，通常是由于合并的CCM所致（Osborn，1994；Pereira et al.，2008）。DVAs被认为是对胚胎发育过程中的代偿性反应，从而再通和扩张先前存在的经髓静脉（Pereira et al.，2008）。

DVAs在CT和MRI上均可被诊断，表现为弯曲状强化信号影或流空，并伴有扩张的增强髓静脉（"水母头征"）。其检出率约为每年每10万例患者中0.43（0.31~0.61），其中至少1/5的病例中合并CCM（AlShahi et al.，2003；Meng et al.，2014）。此外，同一MRI切面有三条或更多髓静脉的DVA、幕下病变以及多发DVAs则更可能与CCM相关（Meng et al.，2014）。血管造影的静脉期显示经髓静脉的水母头样静脉引流至回流静脉，进而又引流至浅静脉或深静脉系统（Osborn，1994）。

建议

- 在大多数患者中，DVA是正常变异，不需要治疗。如果在诊治脑内出血（intracerebral haemorrhage，ICH）时诊断为DVA，应排除相关CCM。

毛细血管扩张症

毛细血管扩张症由扩张的毛细血管巢组成，毛细血管壁上无平滑肌或弹性纤维。中间脑实质的存在可区分毛细血管扩张症和CCM。最常见的位置是脑桥。

毛细血管扩张症常常多发，大多在MR检查或尸检时偶然发现。通常它们可与CCMs同时发现。与CCMs相似，毛细血管扩张症在血管造影上一般不显影，但葡萄状病变可表现为淡淡的腮红样显影，在MRI上可表现为弧形的增强区。在T2或GRE序列上可表现为多个低密度病灶。

值得注意的是，脑毛细血管扩张症并不属于遗传性出血性血管扩张症（hereditary haemorrhagic telangiectasia，HHT）。HHT是一种常染色体显性遗传的神经皮肤疾病，其特征为皮肤黏膜毛细血管扩张以及肺、肝、脑和脊髓的动静脉畸形和瘘（Osborn，1994）。

争议

SRS在CCMs诊治中的作用尚有争议。文献多限于单一中心的病例分析，专家的意见也大相径庭。

一些人认为SRS对CCMs的治疗效果与对AVMs的效果相同，而另一些人则认为它仅作为挽救性治疗，甚至根本不作为挽救性治疗（Lanzino and Spetzler，2007；Lunsford and Sheehan，2009；Nagy and Kemeny，2013；Lu et al.，2014；Nader et al.，2014；Mouchtouris et al.，2015）。由于SRS对CCM的影响只能通过比较出血的发生率来评估，因此目前的文献仅限于比较SRS前后的出血率（Samarasekera et al.，2012）。一项纳入5个三级回顾性研究的meta分析显示，其中4项脑干CCMs在SRS后出血率降低，但有一项研究的出血率变化不显著，反而略有增加。12%的患者在SRS后出现新的神经功能障碍，2.2.%的患者在CCM出血后死亡。遗憾的是，没有尝试评估可能存在的偏差（Lu et al.，2014）。

此外，由于CCMs颅内再出血的风险随着时间的推移而降低（Al-Shahi Salman et al.，2012；Flemming et al.，2012），一些研究中看到的SRS后出血风险的降低是否可以归因于SRS，或者可能仅仅只是CCMs的自然史。

在一本关于颅内立体定向放射外科的手册中，提出了一个结论，即SRS后出血风险的降低是有限的，而并发症的风险却很高。因此，在一级随机对照试验提供相反的证据之前，应限制对CCMs采取SRS（Lunsford and Sheehan，2009）。

延伸阅读、参考文献、EBRAIN的相关链接

扫描书末二维码获取。

第十二篇　脊柱外科原则

第56章　脊柱外科的手术原则

Simon Thomson · Chris Derham · Senthil Selvanathan 著
吴超 译，于涛 审校

术前注意事项

患者选择

在许多脊柱疾病中，手术和非手术治疗的结果是相似的，理解背部和颈部疼痛的多因素性质是至关重要的。外科手术在处理一些软组织来源的疼痛诱导因素方面是有效的，但对于继发因素导致的疼痛无明显效果，手术往往会使病情变得更糟。由于手术通常只是患者众多治疗选择中的一种，在决定手术是否是患者的最好治疗手段之前，应充分考虑以下因素：患者的并发症、未决诉求、人格类型等。但是在一些患者中，比如患者有进展性脊髓病伴椎管狭窄，那么即使患者合并某些严重的并发症，也应考虑优先手术治疗。

一些患者有明确的手术指征，但是可能选择不做手术，这是法律赋予患者的权利，医生必须尊重患者的选择。然而，有些患者可能会在几乎没有任何手术指征的情况下要求手术，医生需拒绝手术，在这种情况下，外科医生没有义务进行手术，但通常应该提供给患者其他的治疗意见。有些情况下，通过评估脊柱疾病患者手术的风险与获益，决定是否进行手术是存在困难，且非常具有挑战性的。选择合适的患者进行合适的手术，需要外科医生具有相当丰富的临床经验。

知情同意和术前宣教

至少在英国，知情同意通常被认为是一个纯粹的法律程序，但它不应该仅仅被简化为讨论手术风险、利益和替代方案。患者需要获得许多其他信息，包括住院时间、手术后的活动以及何时回归正常工作。患者对手术预期的理解是很重要的，例如，希望通过颈前路椎间盘切除术缓解颈部疼痛的患者很可能会感到失望，希望术后在医院住院5天的患者也不愿意尽早活动。然而，值得注意的是，尽管对进行髋关节和膝关节手术的患者进行了广泛的告知和宣教，有些令人惊讶的是，它并没有显示出可以改善患者术后焦虑或提高手术效果（McDonald et al., 2014）。

抗凝药物的使用

在脊柱手术过程中，大多数药物的使用都比较一致，但抗凝和抗血小板治疗需要特别关注。

应该停用华法林，逆转它的抗凝作用通常需要5天的时间。根据华法林治疗的适应证，可以考虑采用大剂量低分子肝素的桥接治疗。手术前高剂量低分子肝素也需要停用，它的抗凝作用在24小时后逆转。利伐沙班是一种新的Xa因子抑制剂，用于代替华法林。对于外科医生来说，有一点需要特别注意，与华法林不同，利伐沙班的抗凝血作用不是立即可逆的，在大约2天内就会很快消失。关于抗凝药物在第5章中深入讨论。

择期脊柱手术前是否停用抗血小板药物存在争议。抗血小板药物包括阿司匹林、磷酸二酯酶抑制剂双嘧达莫、二磷酸腺苷（ADP）受体抑制剂氯吡格雷（不可逆）和替格瑞洛（可逆）。非甾体类抗炎药也能抑制血小板，但与阿司匹林不同的是，这种作用只有在它们还在血液循环中时才会产生，因此当药物停止使用时，其抗血小板活性会迅速消失。

阿司匹林通过不可逆地阻断环加氧酶起作用。血小板没有细胞核，不能代替酶的作用。血小板平均存活10天，因此如果停止服用阿司匹林，整个血小板群需要10天才能恢复。然而，正常的止血过程仅需要20%的正常血小板就可以维持，且研究表明逆转阿司匹林的作用只需2~4天。此外，现在有越来越多的证据表明，当阿司匹林停止后，会发生血小板反弹现象，增加血栓形成的风险（Gerstein et al., 2012）。

在2011年发表的一项大型研究中，研究对象为行择期非心脏手术的患者，这些患者术前因存在某种疾病需继续口服阿司匹林，研究对象被随机分为两组，其中一组手术前10天持续口服安慰剂，而另外一组口服阿司匹林，研究结果显示两组患者在重大血栓或出血事件方面没有差异（Mantz et al.，2011）。在脊柱手术方面，2015年发表了一项非随机研究，研究对象为接受脊柱手术的心脏支架患者，患者分为持续服用阿司匹林组与术前至少5天停用阿司匹林组，对比显示，两组出血相关并发症无差异（Cuellar et al.，2015）。

一些置入心脏支架患者，特别是药物洗脱支架，如果在支架置入一年内停用抗血小板药物是高危的。针对这种患者，建议在停止使用抗血小板药物前与心脏病专家进行讨论。相反，如果发生出血概率很高，硬膜下手术的操作将面临产生严重不良事件的很高风险，在这种情况下，通常需要停止抗血小板药物。

手术注意事项

患者体位摆放

脊柱手术常常采用俯卧位、仰卧位、侧卧位，偶尔采用截石位，正确的手术体位至关重要。

所有脊柱后入路手术均采用俯卧位，当对后颈椎进行手术时，常常用头钉将患者的头部固定在头架（Mayfield头架或Sugita头架）上，并且屈曲下颌，头端上抬，以最大化肩部后侧和枕骨之间的操作空间。但需要注意的是，要确保下颌不要紧贴手术台，并且头架要保持清洁。手术中通常保持头位于高位，手臂置于患者身旁。抬高患者头部可改善静脉回流，从而有助于减少术中出血。

腰椎或胸椎手术采用俯卧位时，可将患者置于可弯曲腰部、形成腰桥的支撑架或者手术台上。重要的是要保证支架的宽度正确——如果支撑架太窄，腹部会受到挤压，进而增加术中的静脉压力；支撑架太宽，会导致患者躯体支撑不足。另外，一些外科医生采用肘膝位，这种体位确实能有效降低静脉压，但要注意避免神经受压导致的神经麻痹。

行俯卧位时，确保颈部不要过度牵拉伸展，特别是在肘膝位时。腋窝要避免受压，肩膀需处于舒适的位置，男性外生殖器也不能受压。眼睛是最危险的器官，应该保护角膜，避免受压；消毒皮肤时从项部绕向前方。眼睛受压会导致失明，在任何情况下都应该非常小心地检查眼睛。

仰卧位常用于颈椎前路手术。头部通常用环形或马蹄形头圈固定，在肩膀后面垫一块卷起来的毛巾或其他支持物有助于使颈部得到适当的伸展。有些外科医生会选择使用牵引，但对于有较大颈椎间盘脱垂的患者应该特别小心，因为颈部伸展和牵引可能会导致脊髓损伤，眼睛应该用纱布或其辅料进行保护，以减少意外损伤的风险。

侧卧位用于极外侧椎间融合手术（extreme lateral interbody fusion，XLIF）。准确的体位摆放是进行安全有效手术最基本的要求之一。一旦患者摆完体位并固定良好，使用X线透视获得真实的侧位片和前后位片，可最大限度地降低定位错误的风险，并可减少椎间融合器位置放置不正的风险。根据术前定位，手术台面有时会被“断开”使得腰椎侧弯，从而打开椎间盘空间，特别是在L4/5水平。手术操作面垂直于矢状面，这样进入腹膜腔时，腹腔内脏器官向前移动，以减少腹腔脏器受损的风险。XLIF入路时存在损伤腰丛的风险，推荐XLIF入路进行神经监测评估，特别是经腰肌入路行L4/5椎间盘手术时。XLIF入路的禁忌证包括血管解剖异常、双侧腹膜瘢痕及Ⅱ级以上的椎体滑脱。

相比XLIF，前路腰椎椎间融合术（anterior lumbar interbody fusion technique，ALIF）避免了髂嵴的阻挡，可以提供更好到达L5/S1椎间盘节段的通路。与XLIF入路相比，ALIF入路的体位更为简洁，术者可在髋和膝关节适度外展的普通仰卧位上进行，术者可从侧位患者的一侧或者双下肢之间进行手术操作。由于血管解剖结构的影响，相比L4/5节段，ALIF更常应用于L5/S1节段。ALIF入路过程中可能出现相关的并发症，除了明显的血管损伤外，还包括内脏损伤、逆行性射精和交感神经功能障碍。

X线的使用和脊柱节段定位

X线广泛应用于脊柱手术中，以评估骨位置、螺钉轨迹和确定脊柱节段。X线是电离辐射，使用时必须严格控制，以确保环境安全和和工作人员安全。不恰当的使用X射线是存在风险的。

当使用X射线时，存在视差的风险。当标记针离骨组织太远，而X线机覆盖的范围与病变范围不一致时，可导致视差的发生。将标记针靠近标记的骨结构，并确保X线机的正确位置，可以将视差的发生降至最低。通常可以通过观察终板或前后位（AP）下的椎弓根结构来检查图像的质量。

手术节段错误始终是脊柱手术的一个风险。术者需谨慎避免各种陷阱如腰椎骶化、骶椎腰化、颈椎klippel-feil畸形、先天性C2-C3融合以及椎体数量异常。最容易出现节段错误的部位是胸椎。有多种方法可用于检查手术的脊柱节段水平，包括在前后位平片上从骶骨向上计数，从C2向下计数及以T12为标志计数。建议计数由两个人独立完成，以减少发生错误的风险。术前有人使用皮肤标记，但这种方法并不十分准确，如果采用这种方法，患者应该在与手术台上相同的位置接受X线检查。术前注射亚甲蓝染料也被成功地用于标记脊柱节段水平。

当手术到达病变时，术中X线将有助于确认脊柱节段。在对肥胖患者实施手术时，即使经验非常丰富的术者，在做手术切口时，也常常会向上或向下偏离一个节段。

手术显微镜和影像导航

手术显微镜在现在的神经外科手术室里随处可见。这些仪器的照明和放大功能使得伤口更小，手术更精确。

由于影像导航适用于颅脑手术，所以其在神经外科中得到广泛应用。当脊柱手术运用影像导航，可以减少手术中X线的使用，降低了患者和手术室工作人员的辐射剂量。并且影像导航技术可以实现在任何平面上的可视化，当术中解剖结构不典型时具有很大指导价值。

影像导航的注册配准依赖于被锚定到相邻椎体的参考点，然后从棘突和椎板上的多个点或通过X线片对感兴趣的椎体进行记录。最后可以根据术前CT扫描图像评估螺钉的轨迹。

术中神经电生理监测在脊柱外科手术中应用

体感诱发电位（somatosensory evoked potentials，SSEP）是通过头皮获取并经皮测量大脑感觉皮质的信号。通常使用双极电刺激周围神经，如手腕处的正中神经或脚踝处的胫后神经，电信号通过脊髓背柱传递至大脑皮质。

单个刺激的信号太小，无法被检测到，并且信号会在脑电活动的背景中丢失。信号平均技术可以对100~1000个信号进行平均，这样可以得到更好的信噪比。然而，平均这些信号数需要几分钟，因此SSEP不能即刻反馈脊髓功能。

运动诱发电位（motor-evoked potentials，MEP）是在给予运动皮质刺激后从肌肉中测量出来。MEP不需要信号平均，但患者收到刺激后可能肌肉会发生“跳动”，所以当应用刺激时，手术应短暂停止，因此MEP不能像SSEP那样连续运行。运动信号在皮质脊髓束中传递，皮质脊髓束在脊髓的腹侧。使用运动诱发电位时，麻醉师不应该使用肌松药，且通常需要全静脉麻醉。因此，SSEP和MEP是互补测试，经常一起使用。

在SSEP监测中，潜伏期比基线增加10%，或振幅减少50%提示脊髓背侧损伤，这可用于防止手术中脊髓进一步损伤。MEP的反应情况和SSEP则有所不同，波形的任何形态学及振幅改变或波形消失都表明前皮质-脊髓束的病理破坏，一些神经生理学家可能认为这是一种“全或无”的反应（即当这种反应被记录下来时，脊髓发生了不可逆转的损伤）。重要的是要认识到，尽管上述变化是敏感的，它们不是特定的脊髓损伤，假阳性也很常见。其他因素如温度、血压的变化、使用挥发性麻醉剂和肌肉松弛剂也会影响读数。

神经生理学监测目前常规应用于脊柱侧凸手术，作为“唤醒测试”的替代方法。它在脊柱外科的其他领域，特别是在髓内肿瘤手术中得到了广泛的应用。在一些国家，神经生理监测是进行所有脊柱手术的常规部分，但这并不是世界各地的标准做法。

脊柱手术中的骨融合

如果骨融合失败，所有的金属内固定最终也会失败。恶性病变导致的脊髓压迫患者的融合节段必须要长于创伤性脊髓损伤的患者，因为前者发生融合失败的概率大，而后者的融合率要高。

在前路颈椎间盘切除术中，颈椎融合率超过90%，但腰椎融合率相对较低（Fraser and Härtl，2007）。虽然融合失败可以发生在脊柱的任何一个节段，但在腰椎更常见。融合失败最常见的表现是脊柱疼痛，尤其是在运动时疼痛加剧。融合失败最好是用动态X线或CT扫描来证实。

在手术过程中，可以通过去皮质骨、植入自体骨（通常取自体髂骨）或使用几种不同的内植物促进融合，常用的包括异体松质骨或皮质骨、脱钙骨基质或合成磷酸钙基骨移植物替代品。所有这些都提供了一个支架，成骨细胞可以沿着这个支架迁移（**图56.1**）。

重组骨形态发生蛋白-2（recombinant bone morphogenetic protein 2，rhBMP-2）可促进成骨细胞分化，并能有效促进脊柱融合。最近的数据提出了对BMP-2的重大安全问题，包括危及生命的不良事件。并发症包括植入物移位、沉降、感染、泌尿生殖系统不良反应、逆行射精、神经根炎、异位骨形成、骨溶解和整体预后较差等（Garragge et al.，2011）。

一项关于非甾体抗炎药物是否抑制骨融合的综述得出结论，在服用非甾体抗炎药的患者中，骨不愈合的合并优势比为3.0，但如果只使用高质量的研

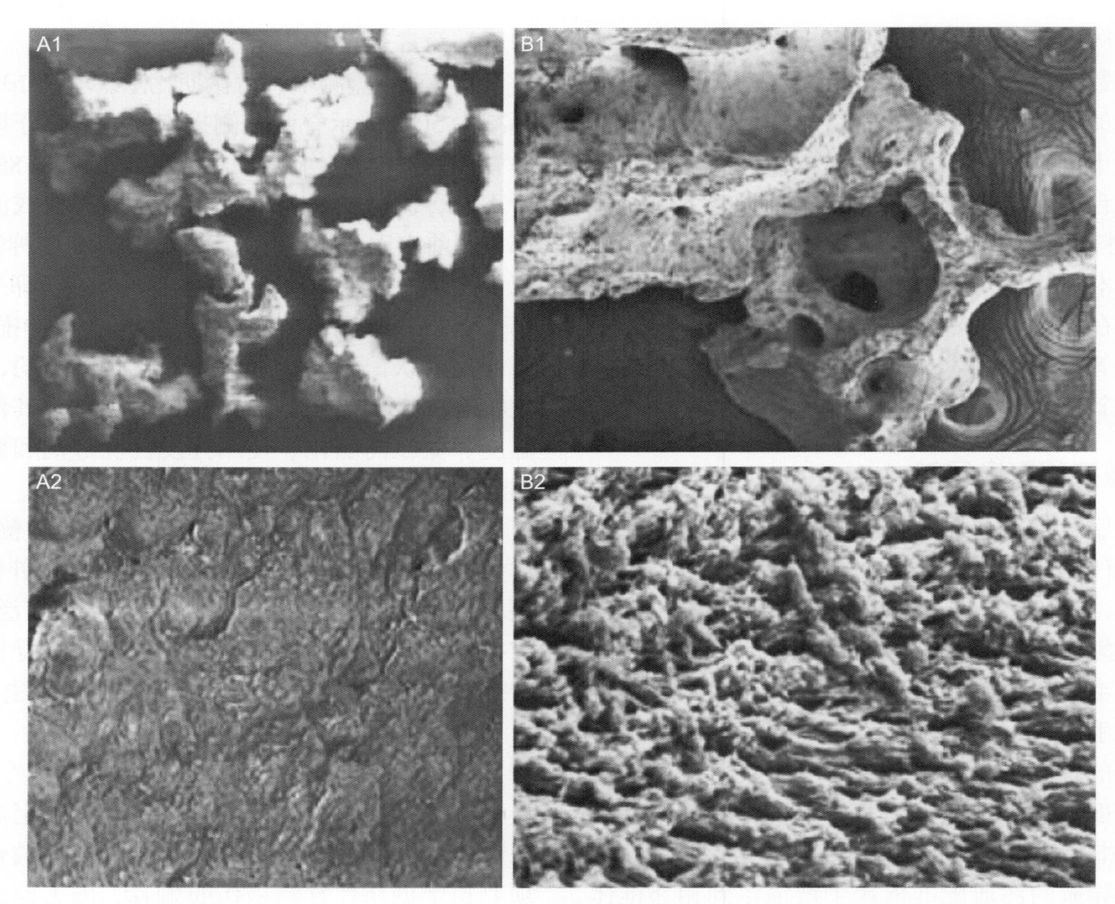

图 56.1 合成骨替代品 NanoBone®（A1、A2）的扫描电子显微镜图像，而 B1 和 B2 显示了异种材料 Bio-Oss® 的特征（上排：×25，比例尺 =1 mm；下排：×2000，比例尺 =20 μm）（见 Ghanaati et al.，2013）

究，这一优势比就不显著了（Bydon et al.，2010）。另外，吸烟也会抑制脊柱融合（Bydon et al.，2014）。

脊柱外科手术内植物

脊柱的内固定手术出现在四肢的内固定手术之后。这些内固定物可用于矫正脊柱畸形（侧凸和后凸）并维持脊柱稳定（骨折、脱位、恶性肿瘤、感染和退行性病变手术）。在过去的几十年里，人们使用了各种形式的内植物，包括挂钩和钢丝棒，但这些都依赖于椎板的完整性，现在很少使用。脊柱内固定的革命性进展是钉 - 棒固定系统的产生。钉 - 棒系统利用椎弓根和侧块作为固定点，这些结构是脊柱的强固定点。此外，钉 - 棒系统可完成骶骨内固定，并可与椎板切除术结合使用。现在的钉 - 棒系统的材质是非铁金属，可允许 MRI 扫描。

螺钉由两部分组成（钉体部分和钉帽部分，钉帽内可放置金属棒）。螺钉的不同类型取决于钉帽的类型、钉帽和钉体连接处的类型、螺钉是全螺纹还是部分螺纹，以及钉体是否中空。

钉帽和钉体连接处的类型是螺钉设计的要点之一。连接处决定了钉帽和钉体的活动度，目前有两种类型：单向螺钉和多向螺钉。

单轴螺钉（图 56.2）的钉帽和钉体连接处是无活动度的，适用于脊柱畸形矫正手术，但会导致金属棒的塑形存在困难。另外，多向螺钉的钉帽和钉体连接处为一球形接头，接头密闭在钉帽内部，球形接头使得顶帽可以围绕钉体转动。多向螺钉的优势在于为螺钉与棒连接提供了一定的灵活性。多向螺钉的薄弱处位于钉帽和钉体的接合处，而不是在钉体和金属棒，很少出现断钉和断棒，具有一定的安全性优势。

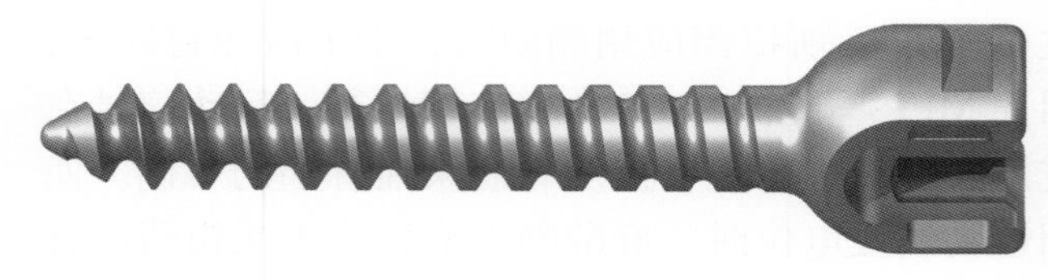

图 56.2 单轴固定头螺钉

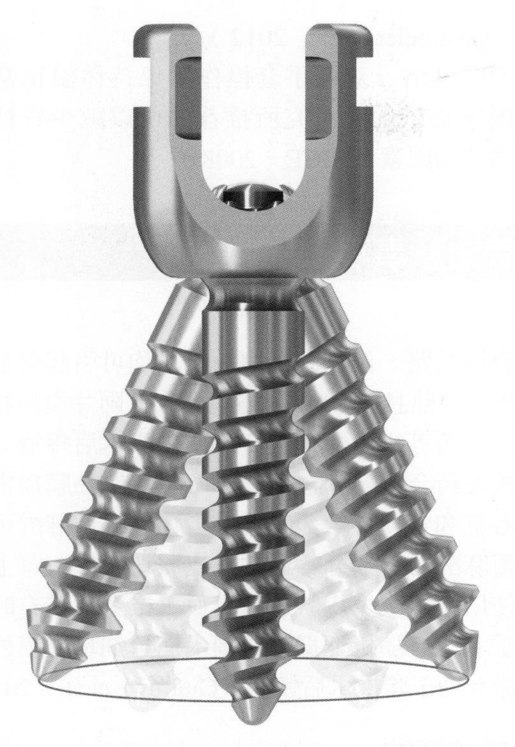

图 56.3　多轴螺钉显示头部和体部之间可以在多个方向移动

多轴螺钉（**图** 56.3）又可分为单平面和多平面两种。单平面或单轴螺钉只允许在头 / 尾平面运动。这在脊柱侧凸病例中是有用的，因为多轴元素有助于棒的位置，而内侧 / 外侧运动的缺失使椎体旋转。

多平面多轴螺钉可以是无偏置的，也可以有偏置的或有偏好的角度。非偏置角度多轴螺钉可提供每个平面的 30° 的角度（即可以完成 60° 锥形运动）。带偏角的多轴螺钉钉头的偏移角，可提供在一个方向上多达 55° 的角度。这种高度的成角使螺钉能够放置在最佳解剖位置，同时避免了金属棒的困难塑形。

螺钉钉体也有多种设计类型，有全螺纹或光滑螺钉。光滑螺钉有一个 10 mm 的无螺纹段，用于 C1 侧块，光滑区的设计是为了防止螺纹刺激 C2 神经根。另一种光滑螺钉是拉力螺钉，它也有一个无螺纹段，并且远端有一半是螺纹。这用于齿突骨折，其中螺纹区位于齿状突内和无螺纹区位于 C2 椎体内，拧紧螺钉后使得齿状突和 C2 椎体压缩对位，从而加强骨融合。拉力螺钉与光滑螺钉的主要区别在于拉力螺钉完全拧入后的螺钉头与椎前筋膜平齐，而光滑螺钉拧入 C2 后的螺钉的钉帽位于椎体外并可以容纳金属棒。

有些螺钉钉体是中空的，这使得克氏针能够引导螺钉的放置或通过螺钉将骨水泥注入椎体。

螺钉的螺距是螺钉旋转 360° 所走过的距离。小螺距螺钉在一圈内移动的距离较短，用于皮质骨，通常具有较高的抗拉力强度，而长螺距螺钉每一圈移动的距离较远，用于松质骨，所需的攻入力较小。外径（或公称直径）和芯径也是两个常用的参数。螺钉的长度是从钉帽的基部到尖端间的距离。在螺钉持力差的地方，可以使用补救螺钉——它通常比它所取代的常规螺钉有更宽的直径和更粗的螺距。

有的螺钉尖端是圆钝的，需要先钻一个导向孔和在骨皮质上开洞，然后将螺钉攻入骨质内。另一种类型的螺纹尖端是自攻类型的，它有切割凹槽在尖端，但仍然需要先开一个引导孔。最后，自钻螺钉是尖锐的，不需要提前开一个先导孔。

前路椎体结构经常使用钢板固定，所使用的是锁定或非锁定 / 动态钢板。在锁定刚板中，螺钉被锁定在板中，以便固定螺钉与板的角度。相反，当骨折处于“稳定”时，允许使用动态板保持一定运动。大多数钉板系统都具有阻止术后远期螺钉从钢板内拔出的方法。需要注意的是，钉 / 板系统和钉 / 棒系统的结构主要抵抗分散力，而椎间融合器主要抵抗压缩力，因此结合这两个系统可能会获得最佳的稳定性。

人工椎间盘置换术于 1966 年首次尝试（Fenstrom），后来在颈椎中被放弃。随后，特别是近 20 年来，它在腰椎和颈椎都得到了进一步发展。目前有 10 年的腰椎间盘置换术随访数据显示 Oswestry 残疾指数（ODI）有所改善（Le et al.，2004）。几种不同的椎间盘设计可用金属、聚氨酯或超高分子量聚乙烯（UHMWPE）制成（**图** 56.4）。脊椎在人一生中要弯曲大约 1 亿次，这对人工椎间盘置换提出了很高的要求，手术精确地将它们置于中线是很重要的。人工椎间盘植入术会面临包括植入物移位、关节融合、吞咽困难（颈椎间盘）和植入物骨折等并发症。

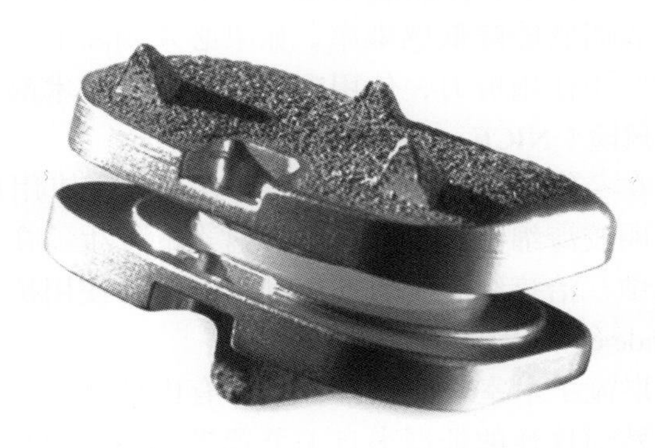

图 56.4　用钴铬钼和高分子聚乙烯制成的可活动的人工颈椎间盘

微创脊柱外科手术

脊柱手术常常切口较大且需要广泛地肌肉剥离，因此常常发生术后疼痛、感染和伤口愈合不良等问题。微创入路手术利用多种先进技术，在减少切口和肌肉损伤的情况下，可使得外科医生进行相同的减压和（或）融合手术。具体的技术在其他章节详细介绍，此处仅描述其基本原则。

脊柱微创开放手术要求精准定位手术切口，并使用适当的牵开器和长柄器械完成。手术显微镜是必不可少的，不仅因为它的光学放大性，也因为它可以提供与视线平行的照明。已经开发出可以提供手术路径的通道，内部可插入一系列扩张器。手术通道可以为诸如腰椎间盘切除术、椎板切除术和颈椎椎间孔切开术等减压手术提供良好的通路。通过 2 cm 切口完成极外侧椎体间融合技术便是一个很好的例子。

内固定器械的植入也可以使用微创切口入路，首先通过穿刺道植入椎弓根螺钉，然后将一棒向下旋转进入螺钉头。这种方法的主要弊端是难以促进骨融合，因此该技术可能最适合恶性脊髓压迫病例。

微创手术的优点在于术后疼痛程度轻，可减少镇痛药物的使用，且住院时间更短。也存在一些缺点：微创手术的操作相对传统开放式手术更困难，存在操作通道放置错误的风险、更多 X 线暴露的风险、骨融合不良的风险，并且微创手术的设备通常比较昂贵。

预防感染措施

神经外科手术围术期感染的预防，包括全身抗生素的使用，在**第 95 章**中有介绍。这里只考虑脊柱手术特有的因素。

在脊柱中，皮肤脱毛通常是不必要的，也没有证据表明它能降低感染率。如果必须剃除毛发，发现相对于使用剪刀，使用剃须刀会增加手术部位感染的风险（NICE，2008）。

在一项大型非随机的研究中，术中使用庆大霉素明胶海绵可减少术后椎间盘炎的发生。在这项研究中，治疗组和安慰剂组都没有全身使用抗生素（Rohde et al.，1998）。

层流手术室一直被推荐用于有内植物的骨科手术，然而这样的证据来自关节置换手术，没有脊柱手术相关的随机研究。并且最近的一项研究表明，层流甚至可能是导致手术部位感染的危险因素，这和层流手术室患者体温过低及手术室人员站位不佳有关（Gastmeier et al.，2012）。

术前淋浴、双层手套操作和保持体温正常也是英国国家临床优化研究所推荐的可以减少脊柱手术相关感染的因素（NICE，2008）。

术后注意事项

镇痛

脊柱后路、经胸和经腹的手术均可引起明显的术后疼痛。扑热息痛（对乙酰氨基酚）、阿片类药物和非甾体抗炎药等止痛药物被广泛使用于术后疼痛。但非甾体抗炎药会影响骨融合，并可引起胃黏膜损害、哮喘、心脏和肾损害等药物反应。伤口局部麻醉可以作为均衡麻醉的一部分，通常在皮肤切开前与肾上腺素一起使用，以减少皮肤边缘出血。椎旁阻滞有时用于经胸手术，有随机证据表明围术期单剂量硬膜外芬太尼阻滞有助于腰椎术后镇痛（Guilfoyle et al.，2012）。

静脉血栓预防

术后早期活动、合理饮食、穿戴弹力袜和（或）弹力靴是术后减少静脉血栓栓塞风险的标准做法。

低分子肝素被广泛使用于静脉血栓的预防，但对于是否应在术前使用或术后多长时间使用，目前尚未达成一致（Bono et al.，2009）。脊柱手术中深静脉血栓的发生率为 0.29%~31%，并且非常依赖于所使用的筛选方法。有证据表明，低分子肝素可降低脊柱手术中 VTE 的风险；但也有证据表明，由于担心术后硬膜外血肿形成，低分子肝素未得到充分利用，尽管术后硬膜外血肿的报道发生率仅在 0~1%（Hamidi and Riazi，2015）。

理疗

理疗广泛应用于脊柱术后康复，主要包含以下五个方面：动员患者自主活动、脊柱活动度练习、稳定性练习、神经运动练习以及为患者提供建议和宣教。

在最近的一篇综述中，有一些低质量的证据表明理疗可以改善术后患者的预后（Gillmore et al.，2015）。然而，理疗中哪一项内容最重要、术前理疗的作用以及应该在门诊还是住院进行理疗尚不清楚。推荐门诊进行理疗的程度及进行何种程度的理疗干预，目前存在较大的分歧。

延伸阅读、参考文献、EBRAIN 的相关链接

扫描书末二维码获取。

第 57 章 脊柱稳定性

Peter R. Loughenbury · Richard M. Hall 著
吴超 译，于涛 审校

脊柱的解剖

脊柱是连接头颅和骨盆的一系列骨性结构，人类的脊柱已经高度进化，以适应直立行走和两足步态，这样脊柱就像一个垂直杆，由韧带和肌肉保持位置。脊柱内部有独特的机械构造和力学结构，脊柱与颅骨和骨盆之间有复杂的生物力学关系。从头端到尾端，脊柱椎体的体积逐渐增加，以承受施加于从头端到尾端逐渐增加的负荷和压力。在颅颈交界处，因头颅的大部分重量通过椎体进行分散，故此处椎体后肌群不发达，肌肉附着面积较小。然而，增加的重量转移到骨盆导致骶骨间的广泛融合，以便更有效地将压力转移到下肢。

脊柱由 24 个活动椎体（7 个颈椎，12 个胸椎，5 个腰椎），4~5 个融合在一起的骶椎和 4 个融合的尾椎组成。骶椎以上的可活动椎体之间的运动受到椎间盘、后方成对的滑膜关节突关节、椎间韧带和椎旁肌肉的限制，这些不同结构的相互作用对于维持正常的脊柱生物力学和功能是必不可少的。成人脊柱的长度为 72~75 cm，其中椎间盘的高度占 1/4。脊柱的长度约占人体总身高的 40%，脊柱的长度相对固定，身高的差异一般和四肢的长度相关，而和脊柱的长度关系小。此外，曾有报道指出，脊柱的高度在一日内可有约 2 cm 的差异，另有报道指出，由于椎间盘的脱水，随着年龄的增长，脊柱的高度会产生明显的高度损失。

脊柱的主要作用是保护脊髓，维持人体运动时的稳定性和灵活性，并可控制上下肢的协调运动。脊柱包含复杂的关节并且可以运动，可以在每个脊柱节段上提供局部稳定和整体的稳定，以适应及执行这些上述功能。在矢状面上，腰椎和颈椎存在向前的生理弯曲（脊柱前凸），胸椎和骶骨存在向后的生理弯曲（脊柱后凸）。这种生理弯曲是人类在开始行走的早期发育阶段形成的。由于骶椎之间是融合，所以骶椎的生理弯曲是永久性的，但其他部位的生理弯曲可发生不同程度的改变，以保持人体的不同姿势。在直立状态下，前柱（由椎体和中间的椎间盘组成）负责承担大部分负荷，脊柱后方结构保护椎管，这些结构也包括小关节突关节，它们可以限制脊柱的过度旋转、屈伸、侧凸和平移。在骶椎以上的椎体，典型的两个相邻的椎体间（不包括 C1 和 C2 之间）的关节包括两个后方的小关节（由上下关节面构成）和椎体之间的椎间盘，这样，每个椎体之间的三个关节形成了一个三角结构。

椎体解剖特点及不同节段椎体的差异

虽然椎体的解剖结构存在局部差异，但椎体的宽度、前后径和高度从头端到尾端均有增加的趋势，这种趋势与椎体抗压强度的增加相关，尾端的椎体往往承受更大的轴向载荷。椎体由松质骨和皮质骨外壳组成，松质骨的微结构是适应应力的，使小梁沿着施加负荷的线定向分布，以抵抗动态载荷。

C1（寰椎）的构造（**图** 57.1A）不同于其他椎体，因为它没有椎体结构。寰椎包含一个前弓，前弓的后方与枢椎齿突紧密相接，寰椎同时包含一个后弓，后弓在中线上形成后结节。关节突朝向内侧，允许屈 / 伸和旋转运动。C2（枢椎）（**图** 57.1A）是非常典型的颈椎椎体，包括齿突结构，齿突作为枢椎椎体的延续，位于 C1 前弓的后方，枢椎同时拥有脊柱中最大的棘突结构。C3 到 C7 的颈椎椎体形态比较一致（**图** 57.1B），通常称为（枢椎）下颈椎。C3 到 C7 的椎体前外侧上的钩突与上面椎体的相应关节相连，这个关节（钩椎关节）是颈椎的旋转关节。胸椎的各个椎体形态也比较一致（**图** 57.1C 和**图** 57.1D），具有较长且向下方生长的棘突和垂直方向的小关节突。从 T1 到 T12 有肋椎体关节，在椎体和相应的肋骨之间提供关节。从 T1 到 T10 的横突上也有肋 - 横突关节，肋骨、胸骨和肋间结构为脊柱提供了额外的稳定性。腰椎（**图** 57.1E 和**图** 57.1F）的椎体粗壮，呈肾形，腰椎椎

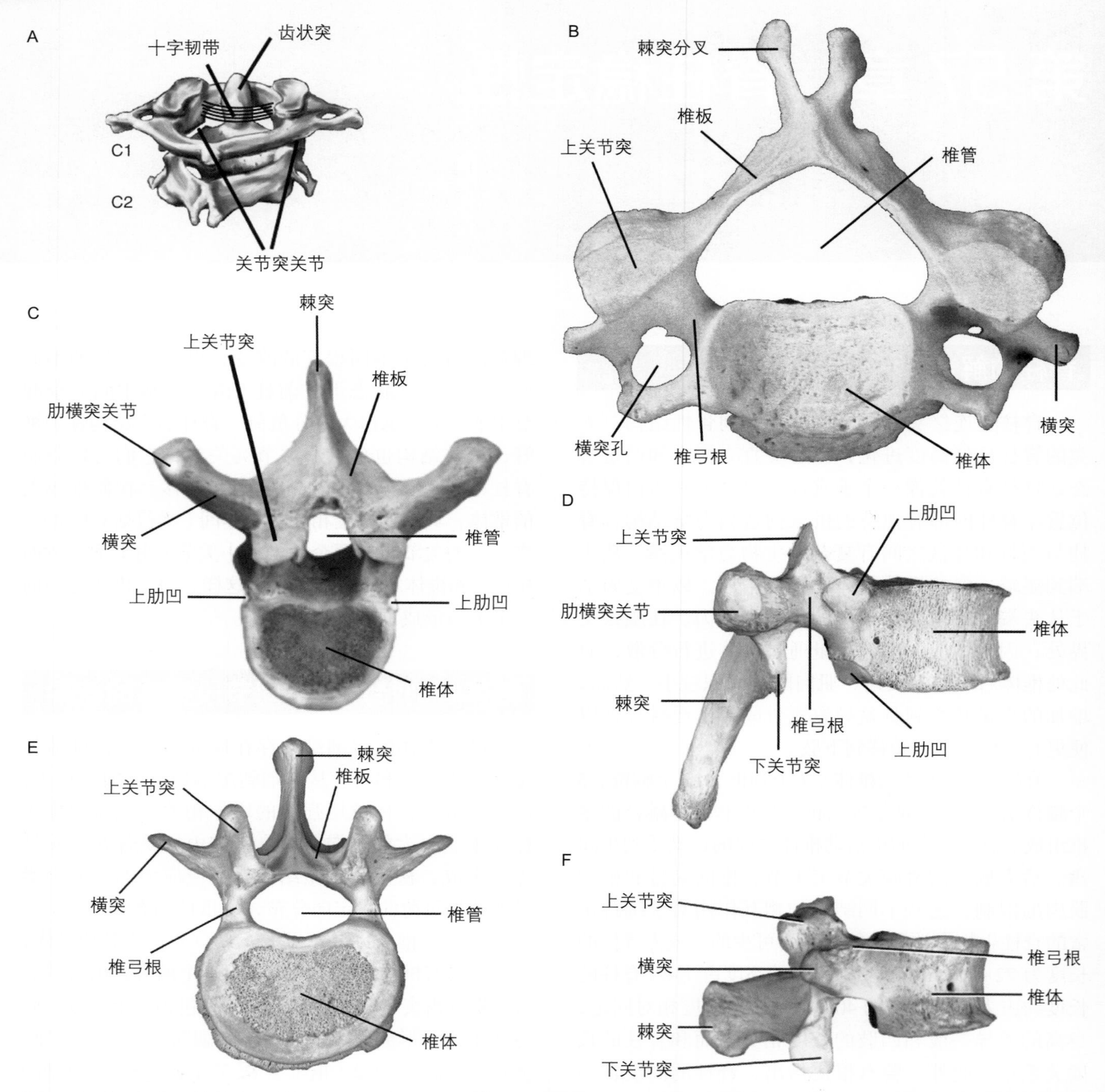

图 57.1 （A）寰枢椎关节的解剖；（B）典型颈椎椎体的轴位观；（C）典型胸椎体的轴位观；（D）典型胸椎椎体的侧位观；（E）典型腰椎椎体的轴位观；（F）典型腰椎椎体的侧位观

体的棘突垂直生长，关节突关节面呈矢状面。

椎间盘

椎间盘位于上位椎体的下终板和下位椎体的上终板之间，它是一个复合结构，中央髓核被多层纤维环包围（**图** 57.2）。椎间盘的作用是传递负载，提供椎体间的活动并维持脊柱稳定。脊柱轴向载荷被有效地传递，依赖于椎间盘的特殊构造。椎间盘的髓核主要由水（80%~90%）、2 型胶原蛋白和多种亲水蛋白聚糖组成。纤维环与这些蛋白多糖的相互作用形成了独特的流体静力学结构，当髓核受压时，水分会渗出，椎间盘的高度会降低，但由于髓核的膨胀，力可以传递到纤维环内多层（薄片）的斜形纤维上。胶原纤维（1 型胶原）与垂直方向呈 60°~70° 的角度，胶原纤维在每一个层次上交错分布。纤维尚可连接到椎体的软骨终板和椎体壁的皮质骨上（Sharpey 纤

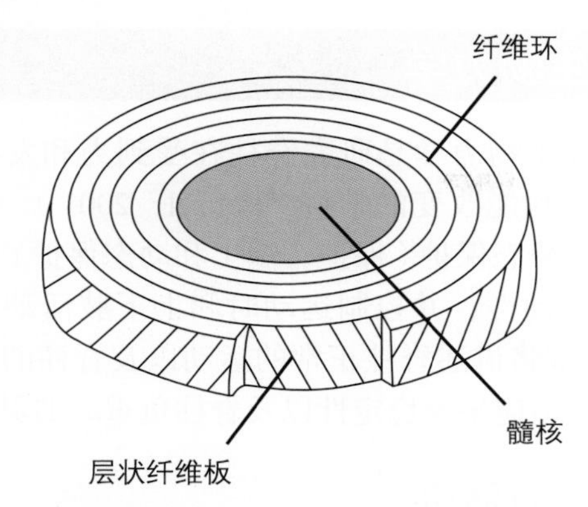

图 57.2 椎间盘结构

维）。当纤维复合体受到负荷时，纤维处于张力之下，纤维环的构造可允许拉力向多个方向分布，以预防纤维环破裂，如果纤维环破裂，髓核可通过裂口疝出。椎间盘缺乏神经支配，仅由感觉（主要是伤害性的）和神经节后交感（血管舒缩）神经纤维支配。

椎间盘抗轴向压缩的能力随着年龄的增长而降低，随着年龄的变化髓核的蛋白多糖含量会发生变化，水分含量会减少。终板的硬化会阻碍椎间盘的营养供给，导致椎间盘高度的丢失以及髓核化学成分的变化。纤维环纤维的走向能抵抗拉力，也能有效抵抗旋转力，然而它们不能抵抗直接的压迫，因此椎间盘突出经常出现在脊柱生理或病理弯曲的凹侧。弯曲脊柱椎间盘的不对称负荷也可导致髓核向凸侧移动，在正常的腰椎前凸中，屈曲会导致腰椎环的前压迫和髓核的后向移位。椎间盘膨出是由于椎间盘纤维环受压所致，经常在脊柱磁共振图像上看到。椎间盘膨出不应与椎间盘突出相混淆，椎间盘突出是指髓核通过纤维环上的裂口从其正常解剖位置移位到椎管内。

脊柱的后方结构

椎体后方结构包括椎板、棘突和双侧小关节突。椎板构成椎体后方的骨性弓状结构，可以保护椎管内的神经结构。棘突在中线位置上为韧带和肌腱提供了广泛的附着点，附着在椎体后方结构上的椎旁肌肉和韧带维持脊柱的运动，并为脊柱提供整体稳定性。棘突尖端通常朝向尾侧，在颈椎和上胸椎角度有所增加，胸腰椎和腰椎部位的棘突向尾侧成角较少，C3~C6 的棘突为典型的分叉结构。

小关节突（关节突或关节突关节）是两个相邻椎骨上、下关节突之间构成的滑膜平面关节。脊柱不同节段的小关节方向不同，对相应节段生物力学有重要影响。在颈椎中，小关节突关节位于冠状面，这增加了颈椎屈伸、侧弯和旋转的范围；在腰椎区方向是矢状面，因此可阻止过度的旋转，但对屈伸及侧弯运动影响小；胸椎的小关节为中间方向，使得胸椎椎体间各方的运动均受到阻力；腰骶关节（L5/S1），关节突关节有更明显的冠状位，这是该水平椎体前脱位发生率较低的一个因素，在关节突关节完整的情况下，尽管 L5/S1 椎间盘间隙垂直，但 L4/5 椎体退行性滑脱更常见。在脊柱伸展运动期间，有更大的压缩负荷向小关节突关节转移。

椎管的直径在脊柱的不同位置是不同的，胸椎管最窄，在大多数解剖研究中 T7 节段显示椎管横断面积最小，腰椎和颈椎节段的椎管更宽。由于病理过程或正常退变，椎管可能会变得狭窄，由于颈椎和腰椎的活动范围大，故发生椎管狭窄也更常见。椎间盘脱水引起的纤维环膨出，骨关节炎引起的小关节增生，椎间盘高度丧失引发的黄韧带增厚，均可导致腰椎管狭窄。这些原因导致的腰椎管狭窄，椎管横截面上往往呈现出典型的“三叶草状”。

脊柱的前方骨结构和后方结构通过椎弓根相连。脊柱的不同节段，椎弓根的大小和方向存在差异，了解这种差异对理解经椎弓根内固定过程至关重要，其中 T4 的椎弓根最小。在脊柱椎体的外侧，横突起自在椎弓根和椎板的交界处，它们为椎旁肌提供附着点，因此有助于运动和稳定性的控制。尽管横突在很大程度上与关节突关节的方向一致，但是它在脊柱上的投射角度仍存在变化。横突孔位于颈椎的横突上，C1 至 C6 的横突孔中有椎动脉和静脉走行。C7 的横突上也存在横突孔，但椎动脉走行于 C7 的横突孔外。

脊柱韧带和肌肉组织

有大量的韧带维持着脊柱的稳定性，这些韧带包括棘间韧带、前纵韧带、后纵韧带、黄韧带、横突间韧带和关节囊韧带。棘间韧带通过每一节的棘突之间，由于它们与旋转轴的距离，提供了显著的屈曲阻力。前纵韧带（anterior longitudinal ligament，ALL）是从颅底延伸到椎体前部骶骨的大韧带。它与椎体的附着较强，但与椎间盘的附着较弱。它位于旋转轴的前方，因此抵抗伸展。后纵韧带（posterior longitudinal ligament，PLL）要小得多，从斜坡延伸至尾骨。它明显弱于前纵韧带，对屈曲的阻力有限。通常认为 PLL 包括两个不同的层次（浅层和深层），与前纵韧带相比，它在椎间盘水平有较强的增宽附着，与椎体的附着较松。盖膜是后纵韧带向颅方向的延伸。后纵韧带可起到抑制髓核突出的作用。

黄韧带从 C2 延伸到 S1。它靠近旋转轴，虽然有明显的抗拉强度，但对脊柱屈曲的阻力相对较弱。它因其呈黄色而得名，这种黄色是因为富含弹性蛋白，富含弹性蛋白可以防止韧带在伸展和弯曲时变得松弛进而缩小椎管直径。两侧黄韧带在中线汇合处留下一窄长纵行间隙，通过此间隙进入椎管，可更安全地实施后路中线减压手术。关节囊韧带在维持脊柱稳定性方面也起着重要的作用，特别是在颈椎。硬脊膜通过几个硬膜外韧带固定在整个脊柱周围的结构上，这些韧带或可以为椎管内的神经结构提供了稳定性（Hoffman 韧带）（Wadhwani et al.，2004）。

除前纵韧带和后纵韧带外，枢椎和颅底间还由几根韧带加强连接。十字韧带分横部和直部两部分，直部由 C2 到颅底的小束纤维构成，横部为 C1 侧块的内侧面之间的横形纤维，横部更为明显。韧带走行于齿突的后方，可有效预防寰枢椎半脱位。齿突尖韧带为细小薄弱的韧带，连接齿突尖与枕骨大孔前正中边缘。通常认为齿突尖韧带没有实际功能，但可能含有脊索残余。翼状韧带起于齿突尖外侧，斜向外上，止于颅底两侧枕髁内侧面，有限制头及寰椎在枢椎上过度旋转的作用。后方寰枕筋膜从 C1 延伸至颅底，寰枢筋膜从 C1 延伸至 C2。这些筋膜取代了枢椎部位的黄韧带。

脊柱解剖中的先天性变异

先天性脊柱畸形或由椎体形成失败或分节失败所致（McMaster and Ohtsuka，1982）。这些畸形常与泌尿生殖系统、心脏或神经根管闭合异常一起出现，并可随着脊柱的生长脊柱畸形逐渐进展。由此产生的畸形可以是三维的，导致椎体侧方偏移和旋转畸形（脊柱侧凸），矢状面异常，导致后凸过度或前凸过度。在生长过程中，畸形可以在没有先天性异常的情况下发生，而且往往没有明确的原因（特发性脊柱畸形）。脊柱畸形将在后面的章节中详细介绍。

颈椎多节段融合畸形可视为 Klippel-Feil 综合征。这可能是由于在妊娠 3~8 周时颈椎椎体的形成失败或分节失败所致。患者可能表现为典型的临床三征：后发际线低、短蹼颈、颈部活动范围受限（Kim，2013）。有的患者还可能合并相关的肾病、先天性心脏病、脑干异常、先天性颈椎狭窄和颈椎侧凸，在 30% 的 Klippel-Feil 综合征患者中可见 Sprengel 氏畸形（一种隐发的肩胛骨常伴有肩胛骨翼化、发育不全和肩胛脊柱连接）。缓解颈部不适的保守治疗是主要的治疗方法，当出现脊柱不稳或神经系统恶化，则需选择手术治疗。Klippel-Feil 患者需要避免碰撞运动，成年后经常出现颈椎退行性疾病。

脊柱生物力学

脊柱生物力学是研究脊柱在受到力和发生位移后结构和功能改变的学科（Benzel，2001）。脊柱的功能包括静态保护（保护脊髓）和动态保护（提供稳定性和活动性，并控制运动时和上下肢活动的协调性）。本节将讲述脊柱正常的运动以及脊柱的解剖结构是如何适应平衡稳定性以及脊柱负重时的灵活性。

正常的脊柱活动

脊柱的屈伸活动主要发生在下颈椎和腰椎。在 C0/C1 处允许有大约 15°、C1/2 处允许有 10°、上颈椎每节段间允许有 7°，下颈椎允许有 20° 的屈伸活动范围。腰椎的节段间屈伸活动度向尾侧递增，L5/S1 的屈伸活动度为 20° 左右。胸椎由于肋骨的固定作用，屈伸运动受限。颈椎和腰椎屈伸活动度的增加是这些区域退行性疾病发生率较高的原因。脊柱的旋转运动主要发生在颈椎，C1/2 处活动度为 45°，从 C2/3 到 T8/9，每个水平段的旋转活动度在 7° 到 10° 之间。C0/1 处没有旋转，下胸和腰椎区域很少发生旋转运动。脊柱侧屈运动活动度在每个节段类似，每节段活动度约为 5°，而 C1/2 是一个例外，这个水平上没有侧屈运动。

脊柱内在稳定性

脊柱内部解剖结构的相互作用提供了内在的稳定性，因此，尽管脊柱是多节段结构，但脊柱是相对稳定的，仅用少量的肌肉活动就可以保持直立。椎间盘不允许椎体在水平方向上产生大量的运动，无论是否负载都是如此，因为髓核的亲水性对纤维环提供了持续张力的“预负载”效应，椎间盘高度的增加也会使纵向韧带处于紧张状态。髓核的可移动性使其成为一个动态系统，不对称的负载使髓核从负载侧向椎间盘凸面移动。这些负荷也可被脊柱后方的结构分散平衡，特别是在屈伸运动中。基于脊柱这种固有的稳定性，脊柱关节最基本的力学模型是一级杠杆；力学围绕一个支点达到平衡状态，而不增加机械损伤。杠杆可以看做是一个简单的刚性杆，支点是杠杆围绕其旋转的点。在这个模型中，支点是小关节，可平衡富有弹性结构的后方韧带结构和椎间盘。

功能性脊柱单元

功能脊柱单元（functional spinal unit，FSU）或运动节段包括两个相邻的椎体以及之间椎间盘和相关的韧带（图 57.3）。它被认为是具有整个脊柱生物力学特征的最小的解剖脊柱节段（White and Panjabi，1990）。通过对脊椎的生物力学测试，我们可以了解单个 FSU 以及整个脊柱节段在正常活动和病理过程中的负荷和运动。正常行走时，腰椎间盘承受 1~2.5 倍体重的负荷（Huang et al.，2005）。直立姿势时，大约 80% 的体重通过脊柱前方结构转移，其余的通过椎体后方结构转移。前屈时脊柱前方受到的负荷会增加，后伸时脊柱后方受到的负荷会增加。在站立和脊柱负重过程中，由于腰椎小关节的垂直方向，脊柱前方结构受压，后方结构提供前后平移稳定性。当不平衡的力量作用于前屈肌，产生屈伸、侧向弯曲和旋转等基本运动时，脊柱运动就发生了。

瞬时轴向旋转

当外力作用在 FSU 上时，就会产生一个弯矩，并导致其绕轴旋转或有绕轴旋转的趋势，这被称为瞬时（螺旋）旋转轴（instantaneous axis of rotation，IAR），并可定义为空间中椎体围绕其旋转的点，它的位置是可变的，取决于椎体水平和脊柱的运动。它通常位于中线后，上终板下方。可运用带有三个轴的标准笛卡尔坐标系——x 轴、y 轴和 z 轴（图 57.3），来描述围绕 IAR 的运动。为了从解剖学角度理解这个坐标系统，我们将这三个轴确定为颅 / 尾方向、前 / 后方向（神经结构的腹 / 背）和左 / 右方向。脊柱的平移和旋转都可以发生在这些轴上，这产生了关于 IAR 的 12 个可能的运动，或 6 个可能的成对运动，即“6 个自由度”。在脊柱运动过程中，每个脊柱节段的 IAR 的运动方式类似于髓核的运动—当前弯曲力矩应用于 FSU 时，IAR 向后方向运动。

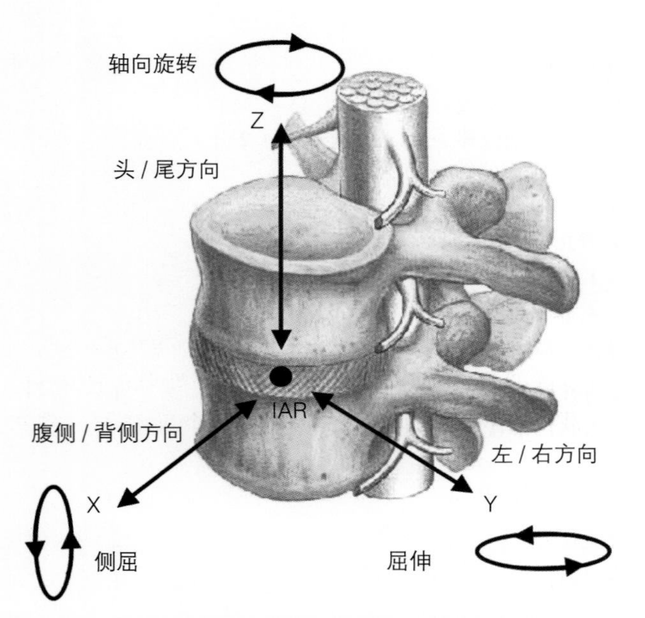

图 57.3　功能脊柱单元显示了瞬时旋转轴和用于描述 6 个自由度运动的笛卡尔坐标系

荷载 / 变形关系

前面概述的力学模型中假定固体结构是刚性的，而在现实中没有一个固体结构是真正刚性的，对于生物组织来说更是如此。Hooke 定律中指出，对于较小的位移，变形的大小与所施加的力成正比，这种关系发生在材料变形的弹性阶段，当应力（施加在一个区域上的力）被移除时，应变（长度的变化）完全恢复。对于较大的位移，达到材料的弹性极限（阈值点），超过这一点，线性关系就不复存在，这被称为塑性变形区，导致材料结构的永久变化，因此当应力消除时，应变不会完全恢复。如图 57.4 所示的应力 - 应变曲线所示，测试结构到破坏点将揭示极限强度，曲线下的面积与破坏前吸收的能量成正比。

骨、韧带和肌腱都表现出与图 57.4 相似的应力 - 应变关系。然而，它们也是黏弹性材料，所以这种关系同时与速率和时间相关。在较低的荷载下，恒定荷载的应用导致随着时间推移的渐进变形的黏性行为，而在较高的荷载下，弹性行为是可见的，渐进变形不发生，黏弹性在材料的蠕变特性（施加恒定荷载时随时间的渐进变形）和应力松弛特性（施加恒定应变时应力的渐进减小）中表现得很明显。此外，重复加载可能导致不同的应力 - 应变曲线与净能量损失（热），这一特性称为滞后现象。

耦合运动

脊柱的运动通常是耦合的，因此沿着一个轴的

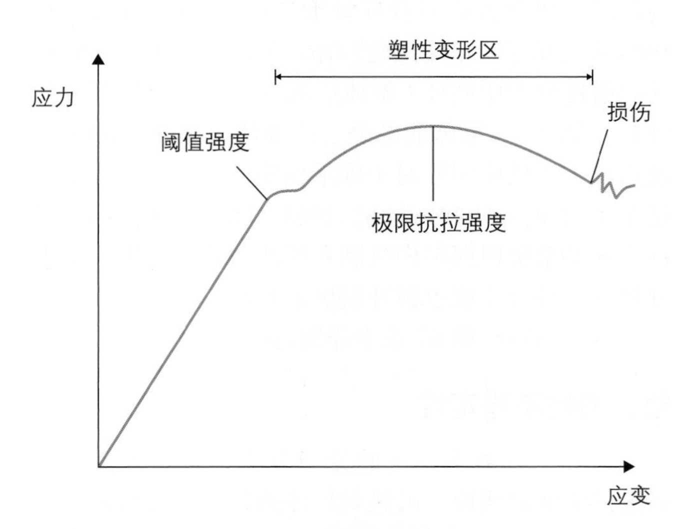

图 57.4　生物组织典型应力 - 应变曲线

运动与围绕另一个轴的运动是相连的。这主要是由于关节突关节的朝向，在颈椎中很明显，侧凸导致棘突旋转，远离弯曲的凹面。腰椎则相反，侧凸使棘突向凹陷处旋转。这是理解脊柱运动时需要考虑的一个重要概念，也是生长性或退行性脊柱侧凸畸形发展的关键。此处，侧位偏移导致椎体的强制旋转，可形成临床所见的三维畸形。

脊柱稳定

脊柱的临床稳定性被 White 和 Panjabi（1990）定义为“在生理负载下脊柱限制位移发生的能力，各结构能够维持其相互间的正常位置关系，以免引起脊髓或者脊神经根的压迫和损害”。将这一定义应用于临床实践，可能会引起重大争论，在实际情况中，不同程度的稳定性取决于力学或临床情况。Panjabi（1992）还引入了个体 FSU 的“中性区”概念，即椎间运动范围的初始部分，在此期间有最小的内阻，在这个范围内，运动不受该椎体水平固有稳定性的限制。当运动超出这个范围时，固有稳定性导致刚度增加，运动受到限制。作为临床医生，我们更关心的不稳定的定义，可以帮助我们判断哪些情况需要临床干预，以改善患者的预后。

柱理论

传统上，在临床环境下识别急性稳定性，是将脊柱视为一系列柱体。1963 年，Holdsworth 提出了一种描述脊柱骨折的“两柱模型”：前柱（椎体、椎间盘、ALL 和 PLL）支持压缩负荷，后柱（脊柱后方结构）抵抗张力。基于这种理论，累及后柱意味着脊柱的不稳定，可能需要进行干预维持稳定。在此之前，已经从损伤机制方面对脊柱骨折进行了描述。Denis 在 1983 年提出了“三柱理论”的概念，将 Holdsworth 描述的前柱分为中间柱（椎体后部分、纤维环后部分和 PLL）和前柱（椎体前部分、纤维环前部分和 ALL），他指出，评估中间柱对于确定损伤机制和评估稳定性是最有用的（Holdsworth，1963；Denis，1983）。最近的分类系统根据损伤机制和所涉及的结构进一步细分骨折，评分系统也被开发出来判断识别不稳定的部位，这些问题在**第 67 章**中详细讨论。

急、慢性不稳定性

另外一种对不稳定的分类方法，是要考虑到不稳定发生的时间段。虽然对具体的时间没有精确的定义，但大多数情况下，将不稳定性分为急性不稳定或慢性不稳定。急性不稳定常见于创伤后，也可见于退行性疾病的晚期阶段、肿瘤或感染性疾病。急性不稳定可进一步分为两种情况，一种是脊柱所有柱的完整性丧失，另一种是前柱或后柱的完整性丧失。White 和 Panjabi（1990）设计了一种评分系统（**表 57.1**~**表 57.3**），以用于评估颈椎、胸椎和腰椎急性临床不稳定性的程度。评分包括放射学完整性的丧失和临床疼痛或神经损伤的证据，5 分以上表示临床不稳定。该评分系统比较全面，但相对复杂，很少用于临床实践。在临床实践中，我们会经常发现，当肌肉痉挛发生时，脊柱存在延迟性急性不稳定的风险。在急性不稳定期，肌肉对稳定性的维持起到积极的作用，但当外伤后的 10~14 天，肌肉痉挛消失后，脊柱可能会出现不稳定。在颈椎椎板切除术患者的长期随访中发现，这些患者存在发生不稳定的高风险（10%~45%），明显体现了这一点。几乎所有颈椎损伤的患者都必须进行至少 6 周的动态影像学随访，以确保脊柱保持稳定。

慢性不稳定比较难以定义，通常涉及畸形的渐进性进展，在生理负荷条件下即可导致过度疼痛或神经刺激，这个缓慢的过程可以被描述为“冰川不稳定”，并逐渐发展为整体畸形。当单一水平过度变性

表 57.1 急性颈椎不稳评分系统

评价要素	分值
前方结构受到破坏或无功能	2
后方结构受到破坏或无功能	2
拉伸测试阳性	2
放射学标准 A. 屈 / 伸位 X 线 1. 矢状面位移 >3.5 mm 或 20%（2 分） 2. 矢状面旋转 >20°（2 分） 或 B. 静止位 X 线 1. 矢状面位移 >3.5 mm 或 20%（2 分） 2. 相对矢状面成角 >11°（2 分）	4
异常的椎间盘变小	1
发育性椎管狭窄 1. 矢状位椎管直径 <13 mm 或 2.Pavlov 比 <0.8a	1
脊髓损伤	2
神经根损伤	1
超过预期负荷的风险	1

[a] 椎管前后径和椎体前后宽度的比值。

表 57.2　急性胸椎及胸腰段不稳评分系统

评价要素	分值
前方结构受到破坏或无功能	2
后方结构受到破坏或无功能	2
肋椎关节断裂	1
放射学标准 1. 矢状面位移 >2.5 mm（2 分） 2. 相对矢状面成角 >5°（分点）（2 分）	4
脊髓或马尾神经损伤	2
超过预期负荷的风险	1

Source data from Panjabi, M., White, A., Basic Biomechanics of the Spine, *Neurosurgery*, Vol 7, No.1, (July 1980), pages 76–93.

表 57.3　急性腰椎不稳评分系统

评价要素	分值
前方结构受到破坏或无功能	2
后方结构受到破坏或无功能	2
放射学标准 A. 屈 / 伸位 X 线 1. 矢状面位移 >4.5 mm 或 15%（2 分） 2. 矢状面旋转 >5°（L1-2、L2-3、L3-4）； > 20°（L4-5）；> 25°（L5-S1）（各 2 分） 或 B. 静止位 X 线 1. 矢状面位移 >4.5 mm 或 15%（2 分） 2. 相对矢状面成角 >22°（2 分）	4
马尾神经损伤	3
超过预期负荷的风险	1

Source data from Panjabi, M., White, A., Basic Biomechanics of the Spine, *Neurosurgery*, Vol 7, No.1, (July 1980), pages 76–93.

（由于退变、肿瘤或感染）时，受影响的水平可视为“功能失调性运动节段”，从而导致慢性不稳定。

脊柱的整体序列

每个运动节段的固有稳定性维持脊柱的整体稳定，并允许头部在骨盆上方以最小的肌肉活动保持平衡。Debousset（1994）提出了一种“经济圆锥”的概念，描述矢状面平衡在维持姿势和躯体稳定性中的作用，躯干在一个狭窄的姿势范围内，能在不需要外力支持的情况下保持直立和平衡，在这个范围之外，需要增加肌肉活动来保持直立的姿势，这可能会导致站立和运动期间肌肉疲劳和不适。人体为了能在最省力的状态（最经济的能量消耗状态）下保持直立姿势，重心应该落在两脚之间，同时保持双眼平视，这种状态下可能是冠状面或矢状面失平衡的状况，在过去的二十年里，学者们对这些概念的兴趣与日俱增。

可用矢状轴（sagittal vertical axis，SVA）评估脊柱的整体矢状位平衡，矢状轴是经 C7 椎体中心所作的铅垂线与 S1 后上缘的水平距离（Jackson and McManus，1994），矢状面轴向距离一般在 5 cm 内。铅垂线位于 S1 后上缘的前方时 SVA 为正值，位于 S1 后上缘的后方时为负值。SVA 提供了一个简单和快速的测量脊柱整体矢状位平衡的方法，但对姿势的变化高度敏感，也没有将骨盆的位置考虑在内。通过测量 C7 铅垂线在冠状面上平分骶骨的偏移量，同样可以评估冠状面不平衡。其他的矢状面平衡指标（脊柱 - 骶骨角、T1- 骨盆角、T1 和 T9 脊柱 - 骨盆倾斜度）和矢状面失衡与脊柱融合术后临床预后较差有关（Bess et al.，2016）。

脊柱与骨盆的关系较难描述，而且个体之间的骨盆形态有相当大的差异。当尝试矢状面平衡的手术矫正时，理解这种关系是至关重要的。骨盆入射角决定了骶骨相对于骨盆的相对方位，是成人中的恒定参数（Duval-Beaupere et al.，1992）。它与骨盆倾斜度和骶骨倾斜度密切相关（**图** 57.5），公式如下：

骨盆入射角（PI）= 骨盆倾斜度（PT）+ 骶骨倾斜度（SS）。

由于 PI 在成人中是恒定的，由于整体矢状面失衡引起的 SS 的变化可以通过改变 PT 来补偿，但这影响了下肢的生物力学，会使站立时产生不适。无症状成人的平均 PI 为 52°+/-10°，平均 PT 为 13°+/-6°，平均 SS 为 41°+/-8°（Vialle et al.，2005）。骨盆应被认为是脊柱和下肢之间的关键连接，纠正矢状面失衡时应尽可能评估这些参数，并尝试恢复脊柱和骨盆的正常关系。

骨骼疾病对脊柱稳定性的影响

骨质疏松症是一种骨骼疾病，其特征是单位体

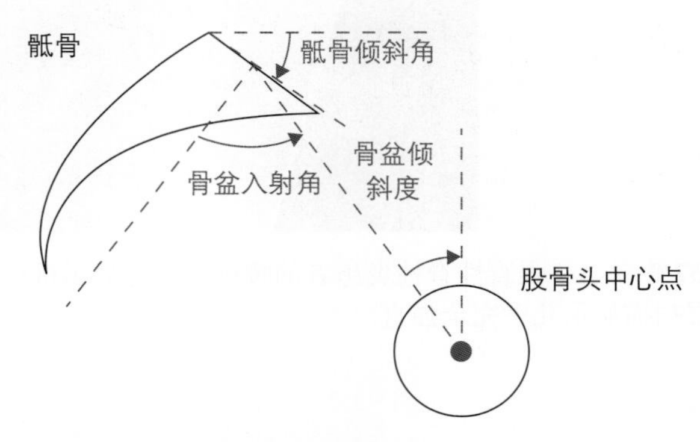

图 57.5　骨盆参数影响脊柱序列

积骨量低，骨组织微结构推变，导致骨骼脆性增强，骨折风险增加（Consensus Development Conference，1993）。骨质疏松的诊断通过双能X线吸收法骨密度仪（DEXA）扫描估计骨密度（bone mineral density，BMD）进行判断，预估密度与健康人群的平均值相比，正常骨密度在这个平均值的一个标准差内。低于平均值1~2.5个标准差被认为骨质减少，低于平均值2.5个标准差为骨质疏松。通常骨密度报告会给出两个值，“T值”（受检者骨密度与同性别、同种族的健康青年群体骨密度的比较值）和“Z分数”（被检者的骨密度与同性别、同年龄、同种族人群的骨密度的比较值）。

患骨质疏松症的危险因素包括生活方式因素（吸烟、过量饮酒、低体力活动和低体重）、家族史、某些遗传多态性、低钙摄入量、低维生素D水平和一些内科疾病（皮质类固醇使用、甲状腺疾病、吸收不良综合征、慢性疾病、例如类风湿关节炎、慢性肝和肾病、结节病、1型糖尿病和慢性阻塞性肺疾病）。治疗骨质疏松首先应该从改变生活方式做起，以减少这些危险因素，并重点预防脆性骨折，这可导致严重的并发症和提高患者的死亡率。应该进行钙和维生素D水平的检测，以确定是否需要补充这些物质，也有一些药物已被证明可以增加骨密度和降低脆性骨折的风险，包括双磷酸盐、结合雌激素-黄体酮激素替代（HRT）、雌激素替代和特立帕肽。

为了帮助指导患者合理服用补充剂和药物，位于谢菲尔德大学的世界卫生组织代谢病合作中心开发了一种FRAX工具（骨折风险评估工具），内容包括临床骨质疏松危险因素和股骨颈骨密度（kani et al.，2009）。该评分可在线获得，可用于评估患者发生衰竭性骨折的风险。建议对合并以下情况的50岁以上的绝经后妇女和男性需进行骨质疏松的治疗：

- 髋关节或椎体骨折
- T值在-1.0和-2.5+之间
  - 10年髋关节骨折的风险为3%或更高
  - 10年发生严重骨质疏松骨折的风险为20%或以上
- T值低于-2.5

强直性脊柱炎

强直性脊柱炎是一种以HLA-B27阳性和类风湿因子滴度阴性为特征的脊椎关节病。男性患者更常见，男女患病比例为4∶1，通常在30多岁出现临床症状。强直性脊柱炎存在遗传易感性，但遗传模式尚不清楚。本病早期出现的主要特征是背痛，随着临床病程的进展，脊柱屈曲畸形表现为特征性的X线变化（椎体呈方形，垂直韧带骨赘）（图57.6）。脊柱强直由下往上发展，最终整个脊柱变得僵硬。颈椎晚期畸形可导致该区域出现“下巴贴近前胸”的外观，此处发生骨折时，神经损伤和死亡率的发生率高于普通人。

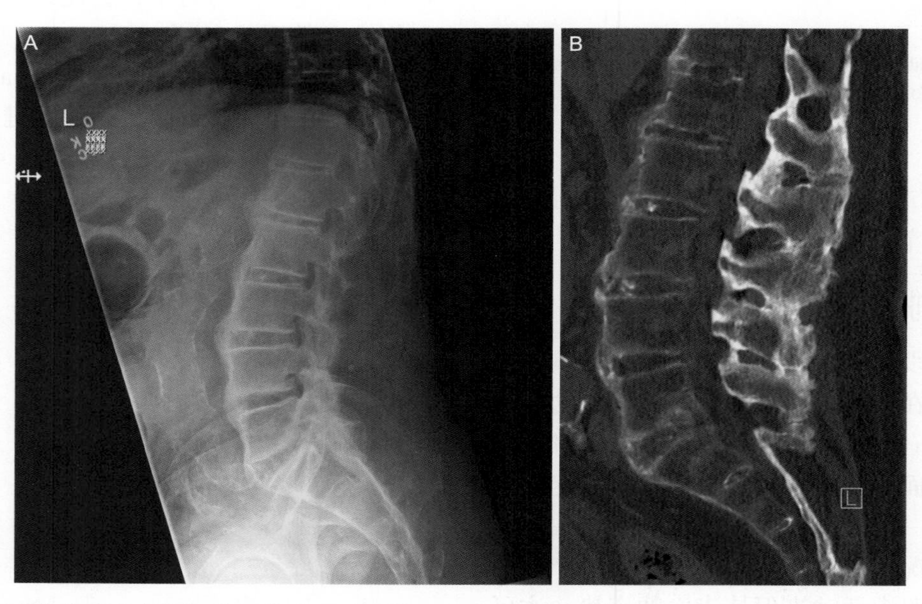

图57.6 （A）强直性脊柱炎患者的腰椎侧位片显示椎体呈方形和垂直韧带骨赘，（B）同一患者三年后的中矢状位计算机断层扫描显示几乎完全强直

延伸阅读、参考文献、EBRAIN的相关链接

扫描书末二维码获取。

第 58 章　脊柱生理

Sadaquate Khan・Kevin Tsang・Lamia Nayeb 著
司雨 译，于涛 审校

脊髓解剖

总览

脊髓从枕骨大孔延伸到腰部上段，是一个宽圆柱形结构。由高度组织化的中枢神经细胞和相关神经胶质细胞组成，周围被椎管保护。负责上肢和下肢运动功能的灰质在颈髓和腰髓区域形成颈膨大和腰膨大。脊髓的长度在男性中大约为 45 cm，在女性中大约为 43 cm。虽然存在个体差异，但是脊髓末端圆锥状髓质通常在成人的第一腰椎和第二腰椎之间终止（Saifuddin et al.，1998）。在发育过程中，椎管生长超过脊髓生长，因此在 10 岁时，脊髓圆锥从新生儿的 L3-4 左右上升到成人位置（Patten，1996）。终丝是一条从脊髓圆锥的末端延伸出的变细的条状纤维带，终丝附着于尾骨，使脊髓稳定。脊髓硬膜是颅脑硬脑膜层的延续，覆盖脊髓和马尾神经。每个椎骨水平两侧均有齿状韧带，可以进一步稳定脊髓。从功能上讲，脊髓节段可分为 31 段，每段发出双侧成对的脊神经。

血管通过三个动脉向脊髓供血。源自两个椎动脉的脊髓前动脉供应脊髓前部，并在其延伸过程中，从前方的节段性髓动脉接收额外的血液输入。两根脊髓后动脉为脊髓后部提供血液供应，通常由椎动脉在水平段上发出，但偶尔由小脑后下动脉发出。它们也从节段性髓动脉获得额外的血液供应。Adamkiewicz 动脉是最大的节段性动脉，通常从第九胸椎至第十二胸椎水平的左侧产生。**第 64 章**将更详细地介绍脊髓血管解剖。

横截面结构

与脑神经组织不同，脊髓的灰质位于中央，而白质形成一个外部纵向层（**图 58.1**）。在任何水平的横截面中，灰质都类似于 H 形或蝴蝶形区域，由中央灰质联合在中线桥接，中央管位于它的中心。该区域可分为三个“灰质柱”：前柱、后柱和外侧柱。灰质也可被细分为 10 个在细胞学上不同的层组成的系统，称为 Rexed 分层，从后到前分别为Ⅰ层到Ⅻ层。特异的Ⅹ层（灰质连合和中央胶质）对应于沿脊髓全长延伸的灰质中心管（Patestas and Gartner，2016）。

灰质的前部称为前角，传达运动信息。它由支配梭外肌的大型 α 运动神经元神经纤维（即 Rexed 分层的Ⅸ层）、支配梭内肌纤维的较小的 γ 神经元和少数小神经元（Rexed 分层的Ⅷ层）组成。在 Rexed 分层的Ⅸ层，支配伸肌的神经元比支配屈肌的神经元更靠前。

灰质后部（即后角）接收感觉相关信息，并细分为接收特定感觉信息的多个 Rexed 分层（Ⅰ至Ⅵ）。最重要的是分层Ⅱ（Rolando 的明胶质），它是脊髓丘脑束第一级和第二级神经元之间突触的部位。分层Ⅴ处理来自皮肤、肌肉、关节和内脏伤害感受器的信息，而分层Ⅵ参与简单的脊髓反射。这些分层的神经元（Ⅳ、Ⅴ和Ⅵ）共同构成了脊髓丘脑束。

外侧柱是仅在 T1 和 L2 水平之间存在的前灰质柱的后外侧投影，与节前交感神经活动有关。在 S2 和 S4 段之间也存在灰质外侧柱，传递节前副交感神经活动。

脊髓传导束

这些是脊髓白质内的上行和下行纤维束。主要包括感觉性的脊髓丘脑束和背侧束以及运动性的皮质脊髓前束和外束。

脊髓丘脑束

来自皮肤的关于疼痛和温度的信息通过脊髓周围传入神经元的一级感觉神经元轴突进行传达，进入后根。这些轴突通过后根入髓区附近 Lissauer 通道进入脊髓，在脊髓内部它们上行一到两个节段，与 Rolando 胶质（Rexed 分层Ⅱ）中的第二级神经元形成突触。在之前的一两个脊髓节段内，通过前连合到

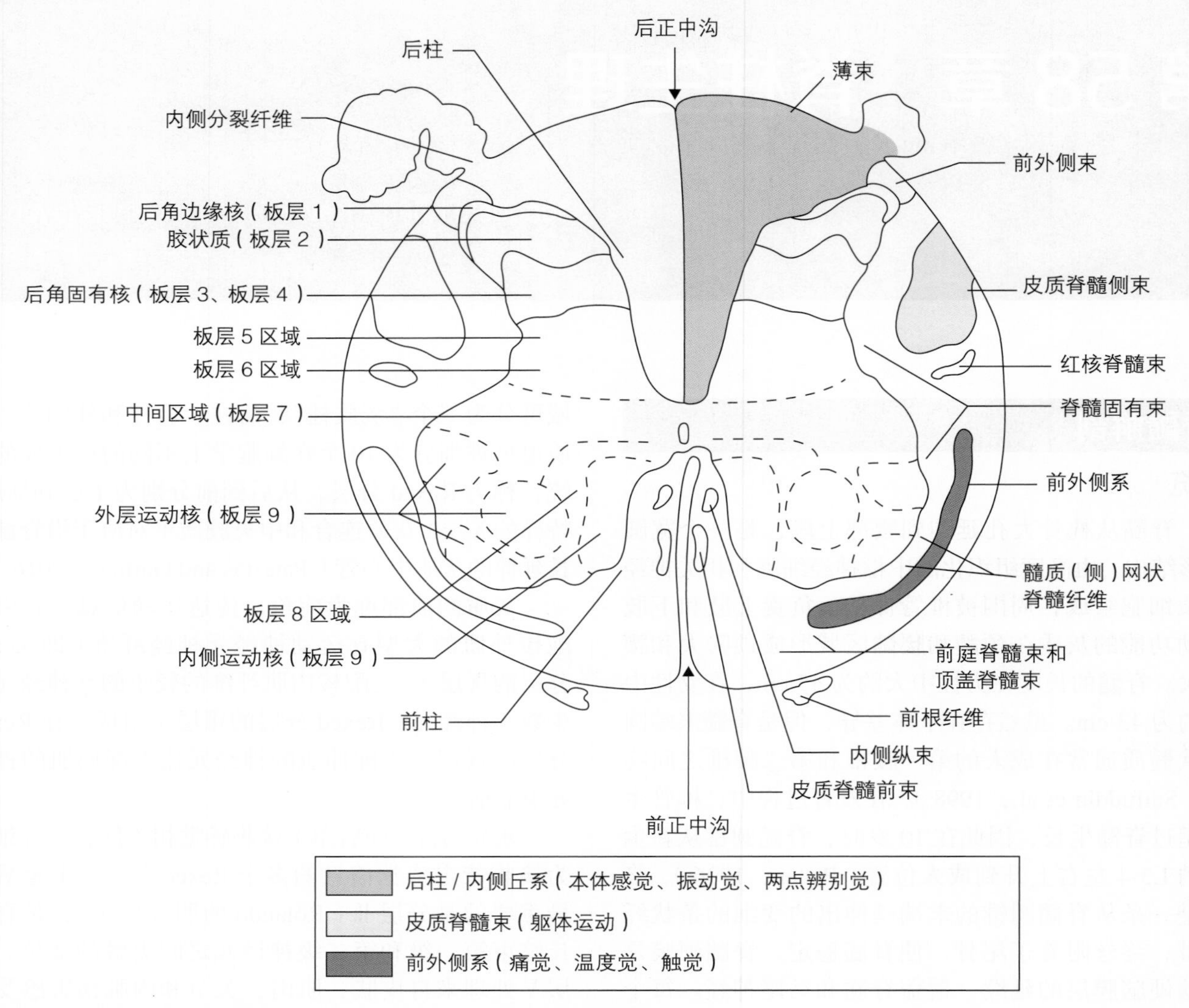

图 58.1 胸椎脊髓横截面显示 Rex 板层结构、上行和下行纤维束

This image comes from: Figure 5.2, page 86, Haines DE, *Neuroanatomy: An Atlas of Structures, Sections and Systems*, 6th Edition, Lippincott Williams & Wilkins.

对侧脊髓的前外侧区域，并通过延髓腹侧作为脊髓丘脑侧束上升。它们依次与丘脑腹后外侧核（ventral posterolateral nucleus，VPL）中的三级神经元突触突触，这些神经元将信息主要传递到中央后回的感觉皮质。

相邻的纤维，即脊髓丘脑前束，传达有关粗触觉和压力的信息。该途径的第二级纤维也通过前部交界处进入对侧脊髓的前部区域。

面部的疼痛感和温度感通过脑神经传递至上颈髓内的三叉神经束，与 Lissauer 束连续。二级神经元形成三叉神经丘脑束，至丘脑腹后核（ventral posteromedial nucleus，VPM），然后与三级神经元形成突触，从而将信息传递到感觉皮质。

在与三叉神经核相连的脊髓丘脑束胶质内，由于二级传入感觉神经元与其他传入神经元、中间神经元和下行神经元之间发生的许多相互作用，疼痛的感觉被进一步调节。通过激活胶质中的抑制性中间神经元，激活传递非伤害性感觉（轻触、振动和压力）的较粗传入神经可阻止疼痛刺激通过伤害性传入神经（delta 和较小的无髓鞘纤维）传递（McCance and Huether，2009）。这种相互作用构成了疼痛门控理论的基础，该理论被提出来解释为什么按摩疼痛区域可以缓解疼痛，并且该原理被经皮神经电神经刺激（transcutaneous electrical nerve stimulation，TENS）装置所利用。脊髓丘脑束纤维通过脊髓中脑束将信息传递到中脑的导水管周围灰质（periaqueductal grey，PAG），该束将释放脑啡肽的神经元投射到中脑的中缝大核（nucleus raphe magnus，NRM）。从

NRM 释放的血清素神经递质激活明胶质内的抑制性中间神经元，导致内源性阿片类药物（脑啡肽或强啡肽）的释放；它们与伤害性 delta 和 C 传入神经元的 mu-阿片受体结合。占用 mu-阿片受体会减少 P 物质的释放，从而抑制疼痛传递（Patestas and Gartner，2016）。

背侧（内侧丘系）束

精细触觉、振动和本体感觉是通过外周传入神经元的第一级轴突从皮肤、肌肉和关节传递的。这些神经元的轴突在同侧的背侧脊髓中不间断地上升为两个束，外侧的楔束（来自上肢的感觉信息）和内侧的薄束（来自躯干和下肢的感觉信息），到下延髓。它们分别与楔核和薄核的二级感觉神经元的轴突形成突触。这些轴突在髓质中作为内部弓状纤维交叉，形成内侧丘系，将信息传递到丘脑的 VPL 核。它们依次与投射到中央后回的躯体感觉皮质的三级轴突突触。

皮质脊髓束（锥体束）

上运动神经元（upper motor neurons，UMN）主要从运动皮质（中央前回）不间断地下降到脊髓。大多数（80%~90%）交叉发生在 C1 椎体上部水平的下延髓，然后继续延伸，成为皮质脊髓束。皮质脊髓侧束纤维主要支配肢体肌肉组织。

那些没有退化的纤维形成皮质脊髓前束，并在其功能水平或以上水平穿过前连合。该束仅存在于上索中，并在中胸段完全消失。皮质脊髓前束带有纤维，可支配近端躯干肌肉。

这两个束的纤维支配对侧腹角的下运动神经元（lower motor neurons，LMN），通常称为前角细胞，其产生轴突，支配躯干、上肢和下肢的肌肉。

上行的背侧和腹侧脊髓小脑束通过来自肌梭、高尔基腱器官、触觉和压力感受器的感觉信息进一步微调运动功能。这些通过终止于背角的初级传入神经元传递信息，与二级神经元突触直接传递信息到小脑。脊髓小脑背侧束初级神经元的起源在 T1 至 L3-4 水平被称为 Clarke 柱（或背核，Rexed 分层Ⅶ）；从这里，二级神经元通过小脑下脚在同侧上行到小脑，而腹侧脊髓小脑束的神经元交叉两次通过小脑上脚到达同侧小脑。脊髓小脑背侧束处理来自下肢的信息。类似的楔小脑束由 Clarke 柱头端的轴突组成，通过小脑下脚到达髓质中的楔核，传递来自上肢的信息（Latash，2008）。

锥体外束

中脑和脑干产生的其他下行运动束受大脑皮质、基底神经节和小脑调节。

来自中脑头端红核的轴突在腹侧被盖交叉处交叉，并在外侧索中作为红核脊髓束下降，在皮质脊髓侧束的腹外侧，终止于颈椎。它通过红核和大脑运动皮质接收来自小脑的传入信号，以调节肌肉运动和张力。刺激它会导致肢体的屈曲和肢体伸展的抑制（Snell，2010）。

内侧和外侧网状脊髓束分别出现在脑桥和髓质的网状结构中，并影响所有脊柱水平的反射和运动功能。网状结构接受来自红核、前庭核和基底核的输入纤维，而这些核又受小脑的影响。前束在同侧下降，与 α 和 γ 运动神经元形成突触，促进随意运动和增加肌肉张力。后束在双侧下降以达到相反的效果，抑制运动并降低肌肉张力。

内侧前庭脊髓束接收来自同侧内侧前庭核的输入，并作为内侧纵束的延伸下降到颈髓和上胸段，影响头部的运动和姿势。它还刺激脊髓副神经的下运动神经元。最终，它有助于响应姿势和平衡的变化而做出适当的转向。主要在小脑控制下，外侧前庭脊髓束接收来自外侧前庭（Deiter）核的纤维并在同侧下降以终止所有脊髓水平的 α 和 γ 神经元，进而调节伸肌运动功能，此外通过刺激有助于维持姿势下肢伸肌和屈肌抑制（Sengul and Watson，2012）。

顶盖脊髓束被认为会通过影响姿势来响应对中脑上丘的视觉刺激。其轴突从上丘突出，在背侧被盖交叉处交叉，下行终止于颈脊髓（Rexed 分层Ⅵ、Ⅶ、Ⅷ）。

脊髓自主功能

脊髓自主神经功能分为从 T1-L3 发出的交感神经和从 S2-S4 节段发出的副交感神经（图 58.2）。脑神经中的副交感神经传入和传出通路将不在本节中讨论。脊髓自主神经对于维持正常的内脏功能以及体内平衡至关重要，包括肠道、膀胱和性功能（图 58.3 和图 58.4）。

交感神经系统

交感神经节前纤维从 T1 到 L3 离开脊髓到达交感神经链的水平或通过交感神经链支配椎前神经节和肾上腺髓质。

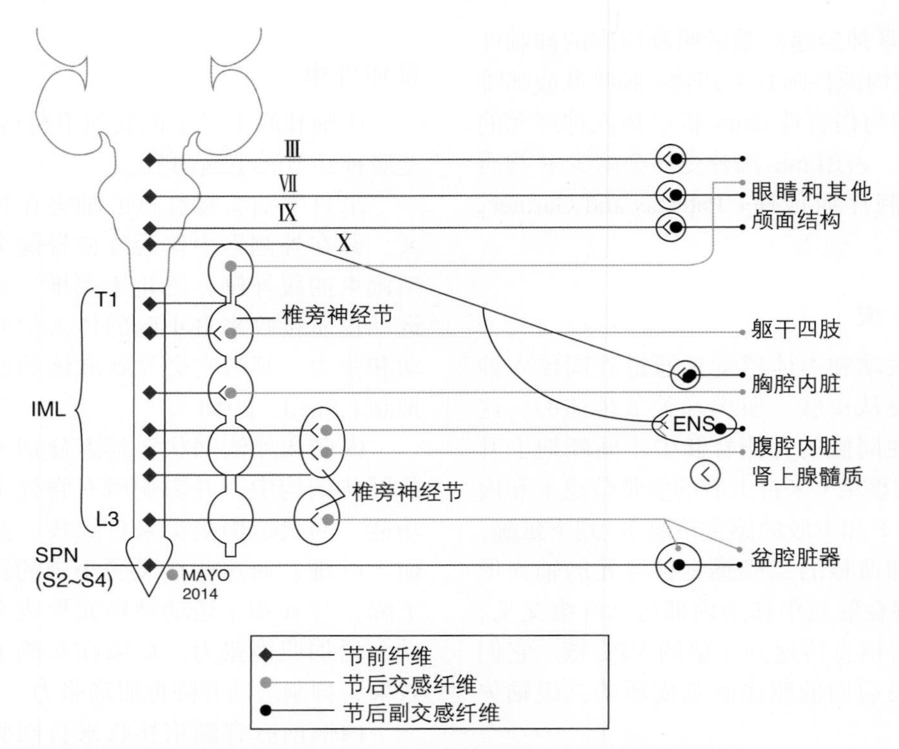

图 58.2 自主神经系统。IML，中间外侧核；SPN，骶副交感神经核；ENS，肠神经系统

Adapted from Benarroch EE. *Basic Neurosciences with Clinical Applications*. Philadelphia [PA]: Butterworth Heinemann/Elsevier; 2006. Chapter 20, Peripheral autonomic control of visceral organs; pp. 679–720. Used by permission of Mayo Foundation for Medical Education and Research.

椎旁交感神经节后传出神经支配面部、躯干、四肢和胸腔内脏。椎前神经节后交感神经传出神经支配腹部和盆腔内脏。节前交感神经是胆碱能，除了支配汗腺的节后交感神经，其他均是肾上腺素能神经。

副交感神经系统

脊髓副交感神经起源于骶副交感神经核（sacral parasympathetic nucleus，SPN），位于 S2 至 S4 水平之间，支配膀胱、直肠和性器官。节前和节后副交感神经是胆碱能神经元（Benarroch，2006）。

膀胱功能的脊髓控制

膀胱功能的正常控制需要脑桥排尿中枢的支配，而脑桥排尿中枢又受到来自多个幕上区域（主要是额叶）的输入的调节。这包括前扣带回、视前下丘脑、杏仁核、床核、终纹和中隔核。脑桥排尿中枢通过副交感神经、交感神经和躯体传入和传出神经元协调正常的尿液储存功能。任何这些通路的中断都会导致膀胱功能紊乱（图 58.3）。

膀胱副交感神经

源自 S2-S4 根的传出节前副交感神经纤维在下腹神经丛中形成突触，节后纤维起源于此处并继续支配逼尿肌和内括约肌。节后副交感神经在排尿开始时释放大量乙酰胆碱，导致逼尿肌松弛和内括约肌收缩。

传入的副交感神经纤维通过阴部神经传递膀胱壁和内括约肌的扩张。这是在脊髓中间外侧柱中的有髓 纤维中传播的。

膀胱交感神经

膀胱的传出节前神经支配起源于 T9 至 L2，经骨盆神经、腹下丛和腹下神经到达下腹下神经节。节后纤维支配逼尿肌和内括约肌，其中去甲肾上腺素的释放导致在排尿储存阶段逼尿肌松弛和内括约肌收缩。

走行在下腹神经中的交感传入神经也有部分参与，它也传达膀胱扩张的感觉。

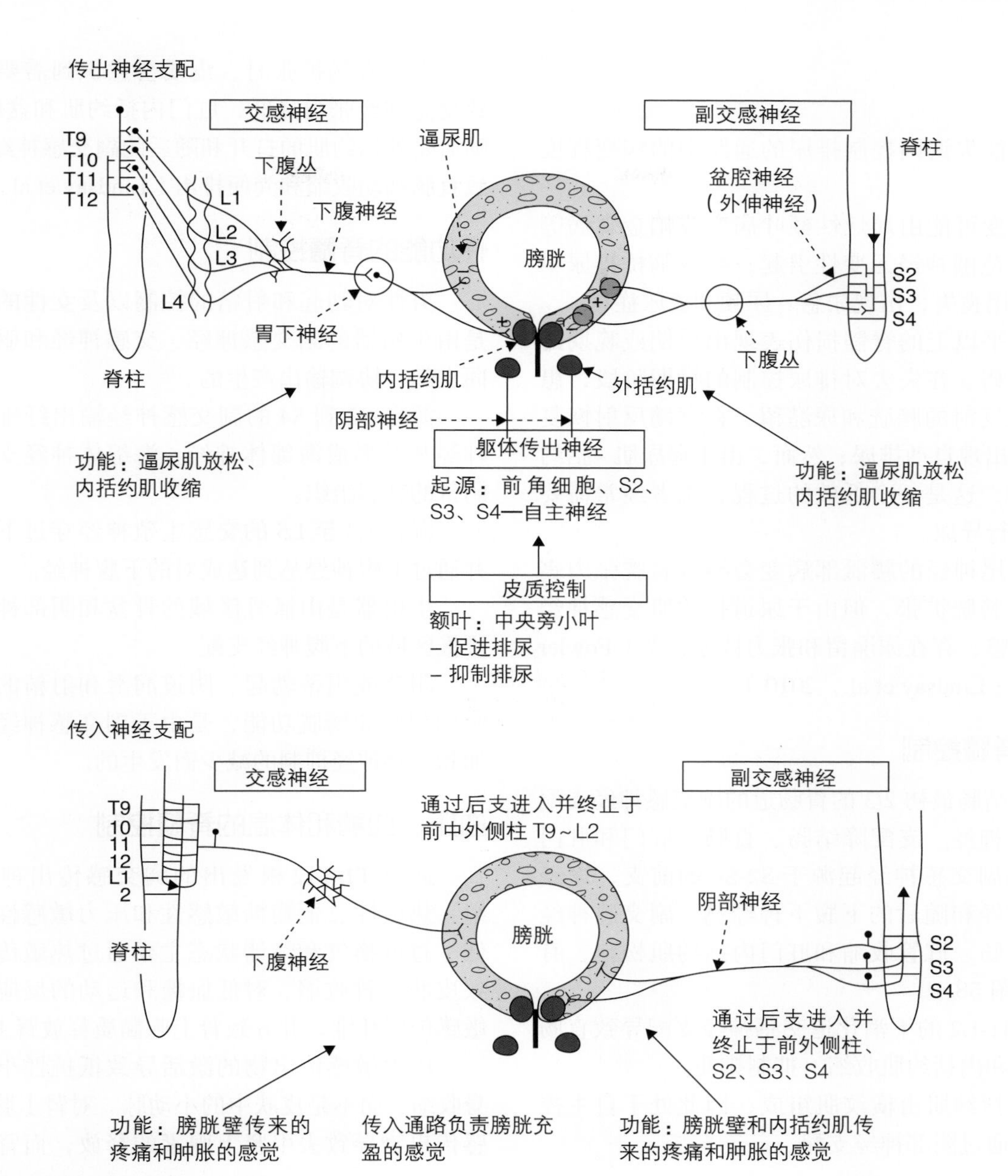

图 58.3　膀胱的自主神经支配

膀胱的体神经

外括约肌或尿道括约肌由横纹肌组成，接收源自 S2-S4 前角细胞的纤维，运动神经元位于 Onuf 核（也包含副交感神经核）并通过阴部神经传递。

自主排尿的协调

排尿的储存阶段通过交感神经支配，有意识地抑制排尿。此时外括约肌收缩，逼尿肌放松和内括约肌收缩。

自主排尿的开始涉及脑桥排尿中枢、骶脊髓、逼尿肌以及内外括约肌之间活动的协调。排尿之前是外括约肌横纹肌松弛，通过阴部神经和内括约肌松弛，通过下腹神经丛的副交感神经流出。来自下腹神经丛的副交感神经支配也引起逼尿肌收缩和膀胱排空。

自主抑制和开始排尿由额叶中央旁小叶控制，并通过脑桥排尿中枢协调括约肌松弛和逼尿肌收缩（Fowler et al.，2008）。

排尿障碍

排尿功能失调因控制排尿的通路中的病变程度而异。

桥上病变可能由局灶性额叶病变或帕金森病等疾病中的大范围神经元变性引起，导致脑桥排尿中枢的抑制作用丧失，出现尿急、尿频和夜尿症状。

腰骶水平以上的脊髓损伤表现出早期或晚期的泌尿功能障碍。在失去对排尿控制的早期阶段，患者会出现无反射的膀胱和尿潴留。在脊髓反射恢复的后期，会出现自动排尿；然而，由于逼尿肌 - 括约肌协同失调，这是一个低效的过程，患者经常需要间歇性地自行导尿。

影响马尾神经的腰骶部病变会导致膀胱张力丧失和无痛性膀胱扩张，但由于尿道括约肌交感神经输出纤维完整，存在尿潴留和张力性尿失禁（Fowler et al.，2008；Lindsay et al.，2010）。

肠功能的脊髓控制

包括横结肠最初 2/3 的胃肠道的副交感神经支配是通过迷走神经。支配降结肠、直肠、肛门和肛门内括约肌的副交感神经起源于 S2-S4 的前支，途经骨盆内脏神经和随后的下腹下神经丛。副交感神经传出引起直肠、肛管收缩和肛门内括约肌松弛，有助于排便（**图** 58.4）。

来自 T11-L2 的下消化道交感神经支配导致直肠和肛管松弛和内括约肌收缩，抑制排便。

肛门外括约肌由横纹肌组成，因此处于自主控制之下。它通过阴部神经支配。

大便直肠扩张时，皮质会意识到需要排便，导致交感神经张力降低，肛门内括约肌和盆底肌松弛。随后是外括约肌的打开和随后的副交感神经活动，导致直肠蠕动收缩和粪便排出（Lindsay et al.，2010）。

性功能的脊髓控制

男性对勃起和射精的控制以及女性的唤醒反应是由生殖器的副交感神经、交感神经和躯体神经共同支配、协调输出产生的。

源自 S2 到 S4 的副交感神经输出纤维通过盆腔神经丛并形成海绵体神经。海绵体神经支配阴茎和阴蒂的勃起组织。

源自 L3 至 L5 的交感生殖神经穿过下腹神经丛并通过下腹神经丛到达成对的下腹神经。

生殖器是由骶骨区域的骨盆和阴部神经以及胸腰椎区域的下腹神经支配。

阴茎或阴蒂勃起、阴道润滑和射精的过程，同时抑制肠和膀胱功能，是由于副交感神经的协调增加和交感神经抑制的减少而发生的。

血压、血糖和体温的脊髓控制

通过 T1-T12 根发出的胸交感传出神经分为三组：热敏性、葡萄糖敏感性和压力敏感性。体温过低、过度换气和情绪状态主要通过热敏传出纤维导致皮肤血管收缩。对低血糖和运动的反应会激活糖敏感传出纤维，并导致肾上腺髓质释放肾上腺素。

压力敏感传出物的激活导致抵抗性小动脉的全身收缩，而不是皮肤中的小动脉。对肾上腺的压力敏感传出物导致去甲肾上腺素的释放，而肾传出物导

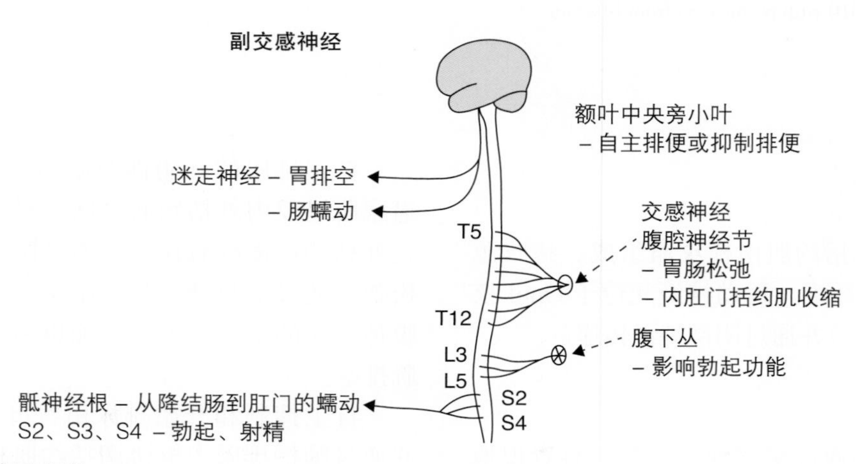

图 58.4 肠的自主神经支配

Reprinted from Kenneth W. Lindsay, Ian Bone, Geraint Fuller, *Neurology and Neurosurgery Illustrated*, Fifth Edition, pp. 429–87. Churchill Livingstone, Copyright © 2010 with permission from Elsevier.

致肾素分泌增加，肾钠吸收和血流量增加（Guyenet，2006）。

脊髓损伤类型

脊髓损伤（Spinal cord injruy，SCI）与几乎一半的脊柱创伤相关，可分为完全性或不完全性（Teufack et al.，2012）。不完全性损伤根据脊髓受累的情况进一步细分。因此，临床医生了解脊髓的解剖学和生理学对于准确诊断和正确决策非常重要（Wheeler and Fok，2003；Krishna et al.，2014）。**表 58.1** 概述了各类型的经典特征。

完全脊髓损伤

这意味着由于完全脊髓横断、严重挫伤或脊髓出血（Wheeler and Fok，2003），脊髓损伤水平以下的脊髓功能完全丧失（即 ASIA A）。这种损伤后感觉和运动功能的丧失并不总是直接对应于脊柱创伤的程度。

由于所有上行和下行神经束的功能丧失，在损伤水平存在完全的运动和感觉丧失。如下所述，自主神经系统也可能受到影响。然而，由于部分的上行性水肿，患者也可能表现出比实际损伤水平高出两到三个水平的功能降低（例如，C6/7 脱位的患者可能在 C6 以下完全丧失功能，肩部无力和上臂感觉改变）。在损伤水平以上看到的缺陷通常会随着时间的推移而改善，这与损伤平面下的功能完全丧失不同。由于骶骨传出神经的丧失，会阴和肛周感觉完全丧失以及肛门张力丧失。患者，如果是男性，在入院时也可能出现阴茎异常勃起。这是自主神经功能障碍的征兆（S2-S4 副交感神经输出海绵状神经），是预后极差的预测因素。自主神经功能障碍也可能表现为神经源性休克或自主神经反射障碍。前者表现为由于血管舒缩张力丧失引起的心动过缓和低血压。这与胸部交感神经（压力敏感）输出纤维的损伤有关。因此，它见于 T1 水平以上的损伤（尽管 T6 是主要的传出神经，因此 T1 和 T6 之间的中断也可能导致神经源性休克）。自主神经反射异常最常发生在患者排尿或排便时，导致无法控制的高血压。其处理和意义在其他章节中描述。

表 58.1　脊髓损伤的类型

损伤类型	受影响的脊髓束	临床表现
完全	全部	完全丧失运动和感觉功能，包括括约肌功能，低于伤害水平
前索	皮质脊髓束 脊髓丘脑束	伤害水平以下瘫痪合并疼痛和温度觉丧失
中央索	皮质脊髓束	肢体无力，手臂比腿部受影响更大
后索	后柱	去轻触，振动和关节位置感
半切	皮质脊髓束 脊髓丘脑束 后柱	同侧运动功能、轻触觉、振动以及位置觉丧失 对侧痛温觉损伤

部分脊髓损伤

这意味着在损伤水平以下某些功能可以维持（即 ASIA B~D）（Krishna et al.，2014）。这种功能的减少可能没有特定的模式。

前索综合征

这很可能是由于脊髓前动脉受损导致脊髓缺血和梗死。脊髓前动脉是单根血管，起源于两个椎动脉，在脊髓腹侧下降至终丝水平，供应皮质脊髓束的前部和外侧束以及脊髓丘脑前束和外侧束。它由来自主动脉的多根神经根动脉汇入和加强，最明显的是从 T9 和 T12 之间的左侧进入的 Adamkiewicz 动脉。动脉或附属血管的破坏会导致腹侧脊髓缺血和梗死。

X 板层中的皮质脊髓束和运动核受累最严重，患者表现为痉挛性截瘫。脊髓丘脑束也受累，尽管后柱没有受到影响，这可能导致分离性感觉丧失（即疼痛和温度丧失，但保留轻触、振动感和本体感觉）。预后很差，只有 10%~20% 的患者功能恢复。

中央索综合征

这往往发生在患有颈椎管狭窄的老年患者中，并遭受过伸损伤。据推测，这可能是由于脊髓挫伤或出血所致。无论哪种方式，脊髓中央区域都会受到破坏，主要影响皮质脊髓束，但也会影响脊髓丘脑束和后柱，具体取决于损伤程度。

皮质脊髓束排列有顺序，近端纤维（上肢）位于内侧，远端纤维（下肢）位于外侧。这导致手臂的典型运动功能丧失比腿部更严重。然而，背侧的下肢感觉纤维在内侧（薄束）而上肢感觉纤维在外侧（楔束）排列，因此感觉丧失可能与运动功能障碍不同。

后索综合征

这种情况非常罕见，在文献中只有案例研究，为了完整性而将其包括在内。脊髓后动脉有两条，分别起自各自的椎动脉（偶见小脑后下动脉），有良好的节段性动脉侧支，因此不常见单纯的脊髓后部损伤和梗死。仅后柱（薄束和楔束）受到影响，患者表现为失去轻触觉、振动觉和本体感觉，但保留疼痛和温度觉。

脊髓半切综合征

脊髓半切最有可能是不完全脊柱损伤的结果。受影响的三个主要束是皮质脊髓束、脊髓丘脑束和后柱。

皮质脊髓束和背柱在下降前都在髓质中交叉，因此患者会失去同侧的运动能力、轻触觉、振动感和本体感觉。然而，脊髓丘脑束不是水平交叉的，而是跨越多个水平。这意味着特定水平的损伤会影响尾部两到三个水平的交叉纤维，但也会影响损伤水平的非交叉纤维。

延伸阅读、参考文献、EBRAIN 的相关链接

扫描书末二维码获取。

第 59 章　脊髓病理学

Chris McGuigan · Karen O'Connell · Eavan McGovern · Iain McGurgan 著
司雨 译，于涛 审校

引言

脊髓的病理改变可以以急性、亚急性或慢性方式出现，通常与神经外科术后表现相似。在医生或神经科医生治疗之前可能会寻求神经外科意见，因此神经外科医生必须了解可能影响脊髓的常见医学状况并识别可能有助于诊断的一些检查结果。从而避免不必要的检查或干预。

本章将讨论模仿脊柱外科病理改变的常见症状表现，包括急性痉挛性截瘫和急性弛缓性麻痹。本章还涵盖了前角细胞、神经根、外周神经、神经肌肉接头和肌肉的内科疾病，这些疾病可能与具有局灶性表现的神经外科疾病相混淆。

第 1 节：急性痉挛性截瘫 / 四肢轻瘫

具有病因的急性痉挛性四肢瘫痪 / 下肢轻瘫最常由脊髓炎症引起，通常称为横贯性脊髓炎（transverse myelitis，TM），该术语由 Suchett-Kaye 于 1948 年首次使用（Suchett-Kaye，1948）以描述感染后脊髓炎一例。它的临床特征是急性或亚急性运动、感觉或自主脊髓功能障碍。横贯性脊髓炎通常继发于其他原发性神经或全身性疾病，包括多发性硬化症或神经结节病。在儿童中，最常见的原因是感染后或接种疫苗后的自身免疫现象。在 15%~30% 的病例中，横贯性脊髓炎可能是特发性的。

估计的发病率为每百万人 1.3~8 例（Bhat et al.，2010），当包括多发性硬化症等脱髓鞘疾病时，发病率更高。预后差异很大，通常取决于发病原因，大部分在前三个月恢复，但症状可能会在最初出现后持续改善长达一年。脊髓休克的迹象（严重无力、张力减退和无反射）可能在发病时出现，而不是通常的上运动神经元体征，并且与较差的结果相关。

临床表现

横贯性脊髓炎是一个包罗万象的术语，因此临床症状和严重程度可能会有所不同，具体取决于病变的大小和位置。典型症状包括无力、麻木或感觉改变、疼痛、共济失调和膀胱或肠道功能障碍。仔细询问病史通常会发现，症状通常会在数小时到数天后发展，而不是在发病时达到最严重的程度。在急性期，临床上通常无法将其与其他急性脊髓病原因（包括压迫性病变）区别开来，因此需要立即进行紧急影像学检查和评估。

症状通常是双侧的，但并不总是对称的；例如，在伴有半脊髓损伤的经典 Brown-Séquard 综合征中，患者有同侧运动无力和对侧感觉障碍。这种无力通常与反射亢进有关。然而，临床医生应注意，在疾病的早期阶段，可能会出现弛缓性麻痹和深部腱反射减弱，类似于格林 - 巴利综合征等周围神经系统疾病。明确的感觉平面很常见，可以帮助区分脊髓或脑部病变。临床上感觉平面通常位于实际脊柱病变下方的许多节段，在进行后续成像研究时需要考虑这一点，例如感觉病变 T5 可能是颈髓炎的结果，因此应考虑在感觉水平以上对整个脊髓进行影像学检查。这有助于排除马尾神经综合征的膀胱功能障碍患者。神经性疼痛可表现为胸部或腹部周围的“带状”或紧绷感，进一步提示病因是脊髓起源。

诊断和检查

当有脊柱感觉运动或自主神经功能障碍的急性或亚急性发作的患者，临床病史已排除压迫性病变时，应怀疑该诊断。需要在磁共振成像（MRI）（**图 59.1**）或腰椎穿刺（总是在成像后进行）中发现潜在炎症的证据，这使得 MRI 和腰椎穿刺对于确定诊断至关重要。特发性急性横贯性脊髓炎的诊断标准炎已被提出并在**表** 59.1 中进行了概述。其他测试是针对确定根本原因的。

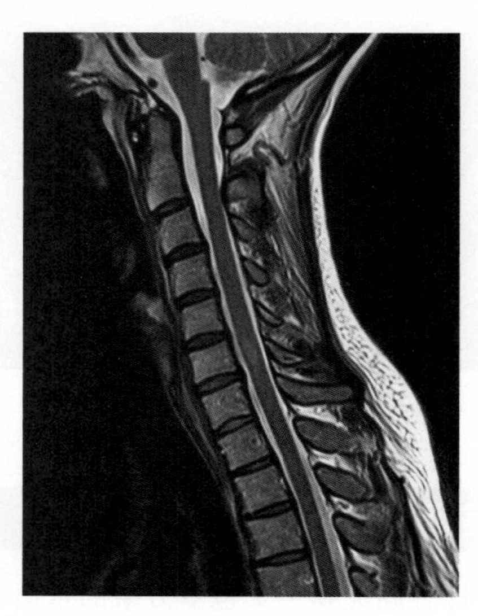

图 59.1 颈椎磁共振 T2 加权像显示高信号病变，提示脱髓鞘

表 59.1 特发性急性横贯性脊髓炎的标准

入选标准	排除标准
脊髓的感觉、运动或自主神经功能障碍逐步发展	过去 10 年内存在脊柱辐射的病史
双侧体征和（或）症状（尽管不一定是对称的）	清楚的动脉分布，临床缺陷与脊髓前动脉血栓形成一致
明确定义的损伤水平	脊柱动静脉畸形表面异常血流
通过神经影像学检查（MRI 或脊髓造影，不采用脊柱 CT）排除轴外压缩性病因	结缔组织疾病的血清学或临床证据（结节病、白塞病、干燥综合征、SLE、混合性结缔组织疾病等）
脊髓内的炎症表现为 CSF 胞吞，IgG 指数升高或钆增强。如果症状发作时未达到任何炎症标准，则在症状发作后 2~7 天重复 MRI 和腰穿评估	梅毒、莱姆病、HIV、HTLV-1、支原体、其他病毒感染的中枢神经系统表现（例如 HSV-1、HSV-2、VZV、EBV、CMV、HHV-6、肠病毒）*
症状发作后 4 h 至 21 d 恶化至最低点（如果患者醒来时出现症状，从醒来时症状必须变得更加明显）	脑部 MRI 异常提示 MS
	临床上明显的视神经炎的病史

*不排除与疾病相关的急性横贯性脊髓炎。

横贯性脊髓炎的病因

横贯性脊髓炎可能与自身免疫性、感染性、副肿瘤性、全身性炎症或多灶性神经系统疾病有关。下文概述了常见的与之相关疾病的一些关键特征。

多发性硬化症

横贯性脊髓炎可能随时发生在诊断为多发性硬化症（multiple sclerosis，MS）或首次出现神经系统事件（临床孤立综合征）的患者中，如**专栏** 59.1 中所述。L'hermitte 征，其特征是沿脊柱或四肢放射的电击感，通常由颈部屈曲（背柱病变的延伸）引起，被认为是脱髓鞘疾病的临床标志之一，应该怀疑 MS 或视神经脊髓炎谱系障碍（见下文）。在 MS 中，MRI 上看到的脊柱病变通常很短，跨越一个椎骨节段或更少（**图** 59.1）。它们往往位于偏心、背侧或侧向位置，通常涉及不到一半的脊髓。MRI 脑部脱髓鞘证据（**图** 59.2）和脑脊液分析阳性寡克隆带也可以支持该诊断。

视神经脊髓炎谱系障碍

视神经脊髓炎（neuromyelitis optica，NMO）是一种影响中枢神经系统的炎症性疾病，不同于 MS。它通常涉及视神经和脊髓，表现为视神经炎和脊髓炎的反复发作。它与血清水通道蛋白 -4 免疫球蛋白抗体有关。与 MS 相比，病变通常纵向扩展，跨越三个以上的节段，并且位于脊髓的中心。在急性期也可能有水肿的迹象。预后通常不如多发性硬化症，更有可能导致永久性残疾，50% 的患者在诊断后至少一只眼睛失明和需要帮助行走（Wingerchuk and Weinshenker，2003）。

专栏 59.1 案例 1

一名没有既往病史的 23 岁女孩，来急诊就诊。在过去的四天里，她的双腿逐渐无力，双腿一直延伸到胸部有麻木感。她还存在排尿困难。在检查中，她双腿的力量降低（4/5 级），右侧比左侧更明显，双侧深腱反射活跃，足底伸肌反应阳性。她的针刺感也降低到 T6 平面。在她的脖子弯曲时，她描述了“电击感从双臂和背部放射”。脊髓 MRI 显示 C6 处有强化病变。随后的 MRI 脑部显示许多非强化病变，呈典型的脱髓鞘分布。腰椎穿刺显示阳性的寡克隆带。这些发现支持临床孤立综合征的诊断，可能是多发性硬化症的首发事件。

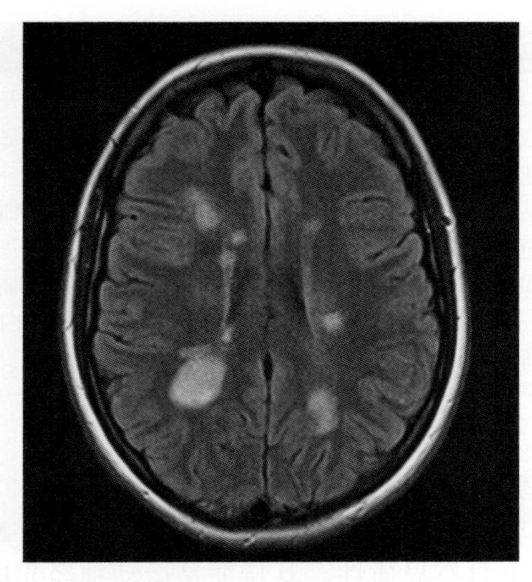

图 59.2 脑的 T2 轴突显示多发性脑室病变与脱髓鞘相一致，这是多发性硬化症的典型特征

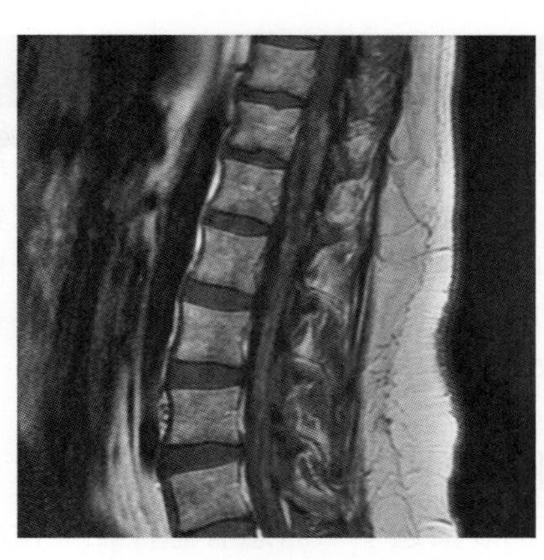

图 59.3 静脉注射钆造影剂后矢状腰椎 MRI T1 显示结节病导致的延髓和马尾弥漫性、结节性、软脑膜增强

一部分出现视神经或脊髓炎症反复发作的患者具有与神经脊髓炎一致的临床表型，但水通道蛋白 -4 IgG 呈阴性。神经脊髓炎谱系疾病（neuromyelitis spectrum disorders，NMOSD）一词已发展为涵盖那些有和没有水通道蛋白 -4 IgG 抗体但具有一致临床表型的患者（Wingerchuk et al.，2015）。髓鞘少突胶质细胞糖蛋白（MOG）抗体的检测约占 NMO 水通道蛋白 -4 抗体阴性 NMOSD 病例的 20%，并且往往具有更有利的临床过程，在脊髓 MRI 上以短节段脊髓下段病变占优势（Sato et al., 2014）。

神经结节病

结节病是一种免疫介导的多系统疾病，其特征是存在非干酪样肉芽肿。在大约 10% 的病例中，它会影响神经系统。患者通常有系统性结节病病史，或在随后的调查中发现系统性受累的证据。孤立的神经结节病很少见。最常见的表现是脑神经病变，但脊髓受累并不少见，并且因脊髓萎缩和残疾导致较差结果（Sohn et al., 2014）。最常见的部位是颈胸椎，大多数髓内病变延伸超过三个节段。在 50% 中，还可以看到软脑膜增强（**图** 59.3）。**专栏** 59.2 概述了一种不太常见的涉及马尾和脊髓圆锥的表现。与 NMO 发病相比，神经结节病通常更为缓慢，患者可能并存神经根病或脑神经病，提示更多弥漫性中枢神经系统（central nervous system，CNS）受累。明确诊断依赖于 CNS 组织活检，但考虑到相关发病率，如果有神经外受累的病理证据，并伴有相容的神经系统综合征，则可能是该疾病。

专栏 59.2 案例 2

一名 39 岁的女士存在 6 个月的行走困难的病史，需要拐杖活动以及反复尿路感染和便秘。她 5 年前被确诊患有肺结节病，因此她不需要任何治疗。检查时，她有双侧下肢无力的证据，近侧更为明显（4/5 级），双侧下肢的针刺感降低至 L2 水平。反射减少，巴氏征阴性。她有一个紧急的脊柱 MRI 检查（**图** 59.3），该检查显示马尾神经足和延髓的广泛的软脑膜增强与神经结节病保持一致。根据先前关于肺结节病的病理学证据以及她的临床和放射学发现，对她做出了神经结节病可能的诊断。

结缔组织疾病

系统性红斑狼疮（systemic lupus erythematous，SLE）和干燥综合征也可能出现横贯性脊髓炎，应包括在鉴别诊断中。与 NMO 相似，病变通常延伸到多个节段。筛查包括 ANA、抗 Ro 和抗 La 在内的自身抗体，可能有助于诊断。

副肿瘤疾病

这些是炎症性脊髓炎极为罕见的原因。通常会出现弥漫性中枢神经系统受累，并伴有脑炎、运动障碍或癫痫发作的证据。单独的脊髓炎很少见，与横贯性脊髓炎的其他原因相比，通常具有更隐匿的病程。有许多可以筛查的神经元抗体，它们的神经系统表现通常早于潜在肿瘤的诊断。

治疗

如果患者感觉患有炎症性脊髓病，可以用大剂量皮质类固醇进行经验性治疗。进一步的治疗是针对具体病因来选择的。

第 2 节：急性弛缓性麻痹

导致急性弛缓性麻痹的症状可能与马尾综合征和脊髓休克的原因相混淆。在评估急性发作的肢体无力患者时，仔细询问病史和检查有助于区分内科和外科原因，通常通过解剖学方法定位损伤水平来确定可能的原因。

基于解剖位置的鉴别诊断

专栏 59.3 描述了一名患有急性弛缓性麻痹、腱反射消失和既往腹泻病史的女性。这种表现最常见的医学原因是格林 - 巴利综合征（Guillain-Barré syndrome，GBS）（Marx et al.，2000）。弛缓性麻痹的内科原因的鉴别诊断范围很广，可以通过解剖位置来考虑（**表** 59.2）。

专栏 59.3 案例 3

一名 42 岁的女性在食用未煮熟的鸡肉后 10 天因对称性双侧肢体无力和短暂的腹泻入院。检查显示窦性心动过速（110 bpm）、弛缓性无力和下肢反射消失。脑神经评估显示双侧面部无力。值得注意的是，在针刺感觉的检查中不存在感觉水平。最初的血液检查是正常的。大脑和脊柱的 MRI 是正常的。进行了腰椎穿刺，脑脊液（CSF）分析显示细胞计数和葡萄糖水平正常，蛋白质浓度升高。

全部脊髓或脊髓前柱

如前所述，急性完全性横贯性脊髓炎最初可能表现为“脊髓休克”。在此期间，自相矛盾的运动体征表现为弛缓性麻痹和缺乏深腱反射。

如果弛缓性麻痹发作突然且疼痛，考虑脊髓前柱梗死是很重要的。这种表现的原因包括分支血管（Adamkiewicz 动脉）的动脉粥样硬化、主动脉夹层和主动脉手术。较少见的可能是脊髓前动脉血栓形成、血管炎和感染性心内膜炎。

前角细胞

某些病毒偏爱脊髓前角细胞，并可能导致弛缓性麻痹。它们包括肠道病毒（脊髓灰质炎病毒、肠道病毒 71、B 组柯萨奇病毒）、黄病毒（西尼罗河病毒、日本脑炎）和弹状病毒（狂犬病病毒）（Berger，2012）。肠道病毒很容易通过呼吸道和胃肠道分泌物传播。西尼罗河病毒是最有可能引起弛缓性麻痹的病毒。它通过蚊子叮咬传播，在美国非常流行（Davis et al., 2006）。狂犬病病毒通过蝙蝠、小动物和狗传播。1/3 的感染患者出现“麻痹性狂犬病”和急性弛缓性麻痹的临床表现（Yousaf et al., 2012）。

运动神经元疾病（motor neurone disease，MND）在临床上具有异质性，其特征是运动神经元进行性退化。典型的临床表现是进行性运动综合征，具有上下运动神经元体征的临床证据（Turner and Talbot，2013）。然而，它可以呈现为下运动神经元为主的表现。偏爱前角细胞的 MND 亚型包括进行性肌肉萎缩和连枷腿综合征（Ludolph et al., 2015）。临床上，运动神经元疾病可表现为足下垂或局灶性无力，因此应完成彻底的临床检查，寻找上下运动神经元混合体征和延髓功能障碍的证据。同一患者的压迫性脊髓型颈椎病和偶发的周围神经病可能会模仿上下运动神经元混合体征，因此颈椎成像通常用于 MND 的诊断工作。

周围神经

如上述病例所述，格林 - 巴利综合征是弛缓性麻痹最常见的医学表现。如果 8 周后临床症状继续恶化，则应考虑慢性炎症性脱髓鞘性多发性神经病。莱姆病由硬蜱传播，在北美、欧洲和亚洲流行（Solomon and Shapiro，2014）临床上，它可引起多发性神经根病，也可能涉及面神经的下运动部。

某些病毒直接侵入脊神经根和周围神经（HIV、CMV、VZV、EBV）。卟啉症虽然罕见，但可能表现为弛缓性麻痹，但往往是不对称的。这种情况通常先于腹部和精神症状。

表 59.2 急性弛缓性麻痹的鉴别诊断

脊髓全部 / 脊髓前柱	前角细胞	周围神经	神经肌肉接头	肌肉
横向脊髓（HSV、EBV、VZV、肺炎支原体）	肠病毒（小儿麻痹症病毒、肠道病毒 71）	莱姆病、壁虱瘫痪	肉毒杆菌	急性肌炎
血管性（脊髓前动脉综合征）	弹状病毒（狂犬病病毒）	病毒（HIV、CMV、EBV、HSV）	重症肌无力	周期性瘫痪（急性低钾性周期性瘫痪）
	疱疹病毒（HSV2）	卟啉症	重症监护	

神经肌肉接头

重症肌无力和肉毒杆菌中毒等神经肌肉疾病可能会出现弛缓性无力。然而，诸如易疲劳性无力、脑神经受累和瞳孔受累等相关特征有助于排除神经肌肉疾病作为潜在诊断。

肌肉

急性肌炎可能出现在最近的病毒性疾病之后。临床上，无力与受累肌肉疼痛有关，并可能伴有发热。急性低钾性周期性麻痹表现为劳累和富含碳水化合物的膳食后无力。经常有阳性家族史；2/3 的病例是常染色体显性遗传（Maurya et al.，2010）。

基于病史的鉴别诊断

评估这种临床情况的一个重要的初始步骤是详细的临床病史。记录病史时要考虑的问题包括：最近的旅行史（脊髓灰质炎流行地区，到美国旅行），既往感染（上呼吸道或胃肠道感染症状），昆虫或动物咬伤（蜱虫或狗咬伤），最近接种疫苗（H1N1 流感疫苗接种），血管危险因素（既往卒中 /TIA）和家族史（家族性低钾性周期性麻痹）。在这种情况下，患者患有前驱腹泻疾病，随后检测出空肠弯曲杆菌感染呈阳性。空肠弯曲杆菌是最常见的 GBS 感染，在 30% 的病例中观察到，通常在 10 天后出现神经系统症状（Poropatich et al., 2010）。

在考虑鉴别诊断时考虑症状的演变也很重要。无力，即在发病时最大，没有进一步的演变，很可能是血管性的（脊髓前动脉闭塞）。然而，在数天到数周内逐渐发展的无力更可能是由于炎症、免疫介导或感染过程。一个更缓慢的进展过程，在数月内发展，应提示考虑神经退行性疾病，如 MND。

根据检查结果进行鉴别诊断

检查结果可以提供有用的线索，帮助进一步缩小鉴别诊断的范围。生命体征异常（体温升高、低血压）有助于识别弛缓性麻痹的潜在感染性原因。

如上述案例所述，自主神经不稳定经常出现在 GBS 中。出现完全性横贯性脊髓炎的患者在病变水平以下会出现自主神经功能障碍。在早期病例中检查时没有感觉水平是可能的。如果存在，可能会考虑横贯性脊髓炎。后者也可观察到膀胱受累。检查皮疹并从临床病史中询问先前皮疹的证据很重要。游走性红斑是莱姆病最常见的临床表现（Solomon and Shapiro，2014）。它通常在一到两周后出现在原始蜱叮咬的部位。它可能类似于牛眼，中心区域有红斑，周围有光晕。颊黏膜和手足上的水泡性皮疹提示肠道病毒 71，而皮疹分布的皮疹提示带状疱疹。

在这种情况下，另一个有用的发现是双侧面部无力。双侧面部无力和对称性弛缓性麻痹的存在使得诊断 GBS 的可能性很高。面神经受累也可见于莱姆病。值得注意的是，尽管弛缓性麻痹已被纳入 GBS 的诊断标准，但仍有 10% 的患者存在反射保留或增强（Fokke et al., 2014）。

基于调查性检查的鉴别诊断

一项重要的初步调查是脊柱 MRI，以排除炎症、缺血或结构性原因，以解释临床表现。GBS 可能在钆 MRI 上表现为近端神经根强化。腰椎穿刺可以帮助进一步缩小差异。如本例所示，人们会预期 GBS 中的白蛋白细胞学分离（高蛋白，正常白细胞计数）。同时，病毒性病因表现为淋巴细胞增多、高蛋白浓度和正常葡萄糖水平。

在疑似感染病例中，诊断通常通过脑脊液（CSF）或血清（HSV2、VZV、肠病毒、伯氏疏螺旋体）中的病原体特异性血清学或抗原来确认。在考虑 MND 时，诊断是临床的，但神经生理学测试可以为去神经支配的存在提供支持。

第 3 节：模仿外科手术病理的医学疾病的重点报道

区域性疼痛

疼痛是包括脊髓压迫在内的几种神经外科常见的早期症状，它通常会导致神经障碍和神经根病。急性或慢性神经源性疼痛也是许多内科疾病的特征，可能与手术表现相混淆。中枢性卒中后疼痛是一种常见的中枢神经性疼痛综合征，可产生慢性半身疼痛，尤其是在丘脑和外侧髓质梗死的情况下，因此应考虑既往卒中史是否存在弥漫性疼痛综合征。

局限于单肢的感觉障碍和（或）无力的疼痛表明周围神经系统存在疾病，通常需要检查神经根受压。

复杂区域性疼痛综合征（complex regional pain syndrome，CRPS；以前称为反射性交感神经营养不良、灼痛或 Sudeck 萎缩）在其早期阶段会在身体区域（通常是肢体）产生灼痛或跳动的疼痛。它具有强烈的女性优势，并且可能在发作之前发生诸如创伤、手术、心肌缺血、脑血管事件或情绪障碍等刺激性事件（Veldman et al., 1993）。疾病后期的体征，如软组织水肿、肌肉萎缩、皮肤增厚、挛缩和骨质疏松，有助于区分CRPS与包括神经根病和周围神经病在内的鉴别诊断，尽管这种区分在症状上可能更具挑战性。可帮助诊断CRPS的检查结果包括与神经根、周围神经或神经丛干不相符的疼痛或感觉障碍分布。此外，受影响区域和对侧之间的温度或肤色差异是一个有用的迹象。临床诊断；然而，偶尔会采用包括自主神经测试和骨闪烁扫描在内的检查。

带状疱疹是由背根神经节中潜伏的水痘 - 带状疱疹病毒感染的再激活引起的。受影响的皮区（通常是胸部和腰部）的灼痛或刺痛是最常见的临床特征，并且在经典水疱性皮疹发展之前作为前驱症状出现。在某些情况下，还可能发生相关的脊髓病（Frohman and Wingerchuk，2010）。原因不确定的诊断实验室测试包括病毒培养或聚合酶链反应（polymerase chain reaction, PCR）。皮疹消退后疼痛持续超过一个月被定义为带状疱疹后神经痛，并被认为代表病毒损伤引起的背角神经元过敏。与异常性疼痛和麻醉相关的受影响皮区的单侧神经性疼痛可能被误解为神经根病，因此在所有区域性疼痛病例中，引出皮疹既往史的重要性。

影响周围神经丛的情况也可以引起一些脊髓损伤。更常见的非创伤性臂丛神经炎之一是臂神经炎，也称为神经痛性肌萎缩或Parsonage-Turner综合征。这种以男性为主的特发性病症通常表现为急性发作的严重单侧肩痛。多达1/3的病例可能会出现双侧疼痛，但这种疼痛在出现时是不对称的（van Alfen and van Engelen，2006）。通常在发病后几周内，通常由上躯干支配的肌肉（例如前锯肌、三角肌、冈上肌、冈下肌）出现无力。大多数情况下还会出现感觉症状，在与供应最薄弱肌肉的神经分布相对应的分布中发现麻木或感觉迟钝，并且反射可能减弱或消失。大约一半的患者报告了先前的疾病或事件，例如病毒或细菌感染、创伤、手术、结缔组织疾病、疫苗接种或怀孕。还存在一种遗传性（常染色体显性遗传）形式，其特征是从儿童期或成年早期开始反复发作疼痛并伴有附加性无力。诊断主要在临床上进行，但磁共振（magentic resonance，MR）成像可用于排除臂丛神经的压迫或浸润，神经传导和肌电图（electromyographic，EMG）研究可用于排除单神经病 / 神经根病并确认去神经支配。治疗以保守为主。

感觉障碍

与前面讨论的感觉障碍的普遍原因不同，仅限于肢体部分的感觉丧失强烈表明外周过程，所有感觉模式（触摸、温度、疼痛、振动和本体感觉）的参与也是如此。

对称性感觉丧失

区分对称性感觉丧失的中枢（即脊髓病）和外周（即多发性神经病）原因有时具有挑战性。彻底的神经系统检查应有助于区分，随着张力的增加，上运动神经元模式的无力（上肢伸肌和下肢屈肌较弱）、反射亢进、缺乏肌束震颤和严重萎缩，提示中枢原因。双侧感觉障碍患者的本体感觉和振动觉不成比例丧失提示脊髓后柱受到影响，例如维生素B12缺乏（脊髓亚急性联合变性）、三期神经梅毒（脊髓痨），更罕见的是获得性铜缺乏，但也是脱髓鞘性多发性神经病的一个特征（如下所述）。

术语“多发性神经病”是指多根周围神经的疾病，通常是对称的，并且对远端神经的影响最为显著。患者通常表现为对称的远端感觉（灼痛或麻木）或运动（无力）症状。根据病因，表现可能是逐渐发作并遵循慢性临床过程，或者症状可能急性发展并自行产生限制。多发性神经病通常分为轴突性或脱髓鞘性，这代表了潜在医学病理学方面的有用区分，尽管存在相当大的重叠。

轴索病通常首先累及下肢（即它们与长度有关），逐渐发展为感觉丧失和感觉障碍，最明显的是足部灼痛感，随后累及上肢（称为手套和袜子样分布）和运动症状。检查结果包括远端感觉和反射丧失。这些通常是由代谢和毒性疾病引起的；然而，感染性或血管疾病可导致不对称性轴索性多发性神经病。

脱髓鞘性多发性神经病倾向于优先影响运动纤维，无力代表早期临床表现，后期发展为感觉迟钝和本体感觉减退。检查时可能会出现全身无力，在远端肌肉中更明显，与弥漫性反射减退 / 反射消失和主要是大纤维（有髓鞘）感觉障碍（本体感觉和振动感受损）有关。存在几种遗传性周围神经病，其病理学可以是轴突性或脱髓鞘性。尽管已经描述了广泛的范围，包括许多作为更广泛的全身性疾病的一部分发生的遗传性运动和感觉神经病（HMSN，也称为Charcot-Marie-Tooth病）是此类遗传性神经病中最常见的家族。迄今为止，已描述了7类HMSN，其中30多种构成疾病已被识别，并且髓磷脂基因的致病突变正在不断被发现（Klein et al.，2013）。HMSN 1型和2型通常都是显性遗传的，共同占大多数病例。HMSN 1是一种脱髓鞘形式，其特点是神经粗大肥大和神经传导速度缓慢。HMSN 2主要位于轴突，与临界缓慢 / 正常神经传导速度相关。如果没有明确的家族史（例如，迟发或未在亲属中诊断出的轻度疾病），病史和检查的某些特征指向遗传性周围神经病的诊断。这些包括儿童反复跌倒史、踝关节扭伤或骨折、长期缓慢进展的病史、腿部畸形如弓形足或倒置的香槟瓶外观（由于腿部肌肉萎缩）以及感觉丧失没有明确的感觉症状。诊断基于临床怀疑、电生理研究和基因检测，可以避免神经活检的侵入性检查。尚未开发出针对 HSMN 的特定治疗方法，管理主要是支持性的，重点是物理治疗。

非对称型感觉丧失

仅限于肢体部分的感觉丧失提示周围神经或神经根的疾病。单神经病和神经根病分别由个体周围神经或神经根的疾病引起。在某些情况下，区分对应于单个神经分布或神经根分布（即皮节 / 肌节）的临床症状可能很困难，可能需要进行神经传导研究和 EMG。单神经病和神经根病的非压迫性原因包括感染（特别是带状疱疹和莱姆病）、糖尿病、伴有神经 / 神经根缺血的血管炎、肿瘤浸润、肉芽肿病或淀粉样变性以及脱髓鞘。

多发性单神经炎的特征是对至少两条独立的神经造成孤立性损伤，导致不对称的感觉和运动周围神经病变。常见的相关疾病包括糖尿病、血管炎、结缔组织疾病和淀粉样变性，其中炎症引起的血管闭塞导致周围神经缺血。疼痛通常在发作时出现，脚下垂是常见的表现。除了评估相关疾病和神经传导研究 /EMG 的血液检查外，外周神经（特别是容易触及和经常累及的腓肠神经）活检有助于在开始治疗前确定诊断（Bennett et al.，2008）。

背根神经节水平的病理学也可导致不对称的感觉丧失。感觉神经元病是相对罕见的疾病，其特征是背根神经节中感觉神经元的退化，导致几乎纯感觉丧失的非长度依赖性分布（Camdessanché et al.，2009）。它们可能是副肿瘤性的，也可能是与干燥综合征、HIV 感染和顺铂毒性有关。除了检测上述相关疾病外，诊断还基于电生理学研究，最近皮肤活检已被用于确认小纤维变性的非长度依赖性。

无力

局部肌肉无力是压迫性脊髓病的常见表现；然而，在鉴别诊断中必须考虑一系列内科疾病。

如前所述，例如，表现为双侧足下垂或握力下降的远端对称性无力通常与多发性神经病有关。近端对称性肌肉无力，例如难以上楼梯、从坐姿站起或梳理头发，通常是肌病而非神经病的指征，例如多发性肌炎、皮肌炎或包涵体肌炎。代谢疾病，如甲状腺功能减退、甲状旁腺功能减退和药物性肌炎（例如用他汀类药物治疗降低胆固醇）都应考虑在内。其他提示肌病过程的特征包括孤立的肌肉无力（没有感觉症状和保留的反射）和迟发性肌肉萎缩，这通常在神经病变的早期发生。EMG 有助于排除主要的神经源性过程，是一种有用的诊断辅助手段，而肌肉活检和 MR 扫描经常被采用。

延伸阅读、参考文献、EBRAIN 的相关链接

扫描书末二维码获取。

第十三篇　脊柱外科

第60章　颈椎病

Navin Furtado · Georgios Tsermoulas · Adikarige Haritha Dulanka Silva 著
许菲璠 译，伊志强 审校

退行性颈椎病的病理学

退行性颈椎病是一个广义上的定义，包括若干导致关节结构（如椎间盘、小关节突、钩椎关节）改变的病理过程，从而可能引起神经组织受压、畸形、疼痛和残疾。充分理解脊柱生物力学和相关病理机制有助于症状性患者的处理与治疗。

骨骼肌组织的退变从生物学角度上来说是难以避免的，但是其退变速度与身体负重及使用强度呈正相关。其他危险因素也可以加快脊柱退变过程，包括：吸烟、遗传、局部创伤和感染。

在颈椎部分，椎间盘承受头部和颈部的负重。颈椎的轴向负荷通过椎间盘髓核转化为作用在纤维环和椎体终板上的环向应力。这种持续的机械负重改变了髓核的细胞成分，使得亲水性蛋白聚糖减少，胶原蛋白增多（Ⅱ、Ⅲ、Ⅵ、Ⅸ型）（Urban et al.，2000）。继而，椎间盘的力学结构开始发生改变，椎间隙高度降低，最终纤维环及椎体终板破裂导致髓核疝出。颈椎所受压力继而转移至小关节，导致局部活动度增大，在退变过程中骨赘增多可以适当改善脊柱稳定性（Galbusera et al.，2014）。在增生韧带中可见的组织学改变包括：非纤维性软骨增生、化生及毛细血管增生（Inamasu et al.，2006）。

最常见的病变层面为C6-7、5-6节段。55岁以下患者，软性椎间盘突出包括突出髓核侵犯椎管或椎间孔，导致脊髓和（或）神经根受压，从而分别引起临床脊髓和（或）神经根损伤症状。对于老年患者，神经压迫更多来自于骨性增生及硬化增厚的椎间盘。多节段退行性改变可能影响正常颈椎曲度，导致颈椎变直或反弓、过度前凸或侧弯改变。

当颈椎管横截面积减少30%以上时，颈椎退变可以导致颈椎管狭窄和脊髓受压改变（Yu et al.，1986）。正常颈椎管前后径约为18 mm，正常脊髓直径为10 mm。

脊髓型颈椎病所导致的脊髓损伤有多种病理生理学机制参与。椎管狭窄引起的静态压迫导致脊髓直接损伤，而广泛颈椎不稳（>3.5 mm）引起的动态压迫会导致慢性脊髓缺血。神经炎症反应触发级联细胞事件，引起皮质脊髓束脱髓鞘、中央灰质变性和中间神经元的丧失，以及前角细胞萎缩和胶质细胞增生（Kalsi-Ryan et al.，2013）。

临床表现与检查

患者临床表现因病情严重程度及进展速度可能存在差异性。脊髓损伤往往涉及双侧运动和感觉传导束。常见症状包括：双侧脊髓受损平面以下乏力（四肢瘫痪、麻痹）、感觉异常、麻木、刺痛、分离性感觉障碍等。临床体征主要包括：肌张力增高、腱反射异常、病理征阳性（霍夫曼征和巴宾斯基征）。部分患者可能出现括约肌功能障碍。早期症状可能不明显，手部活动异常特别是精细动作障碍可能逐渐出现，随之进展为动作笨拙、步态不稳和反复摔倒。

退行性颈椎病临床上常表现出神经根性病变特点。由神经根受压引起的神经根病变可以导致运动及感觉功能障碍，伴随受损神经根分布范围的深肌腱反射减弱。沿颈部向上肢远端放射的根性疼痛是最主要的颈椎病症状，同时合并颈椎活动度减小。感觉症状特别是沿神经根分布的针刺感常见。神经根压迫试验可以诱发阳性疼痛出现。

磁共振是确诊颈椎病的主要手段。低头仰头位X线平片用于判断颈椎稳定性以便于制订手术策略。颈椎CT和双斜位X线片有助于评估骨质增生程度和椎间孔狭窄情况。脊髓造影能够很好评估脊髓受压程度，但是很难看清极外侧神经根孔狭窄。

治疗

应选择个体化治疗方案，充分考虑压迫位置、矢状位曲度、是否存在神经根性损伤、轴性疼痛、年龄、并发症以及对手术技术的熟练程度等。

对于大多数脊髓型颈椎病患者应考虑手术减压，因为 80% 患者会随时间逐渐加重而非自发性改善。对于颈髓受压损伤的轻症或无症状患者，手术时机的选择尚存争议。但医生应提醒颈椎退变患者颈部外伤可能突然加重脊髓损伤的风险。

对于症状性脊髓型颈椎病患者，早期积极治疗通常能获得满意预后。慢性神经功能障碍不容易改善。术前应与患者充分沟通手术风险与获益。

对于神经根型颈椎病，随机研究显示：相比保守治疗（如物理治疗），手术可以立即改善症状，但是远期效果两者基本相同。因此，推荐保守治疗作为一线治疗选择。如果症状持续不缓解或加重，则推荐手术治疗。

对于退行性脊髓型颈椎病患者，手术减压的首要目的是阻止疾病进展。手术后，60%~70% 脊髓型患者症状得到改善，30% 病情不再进展，10% 继续发展。而对于神经根型颈椎病，90% 患者上肢症状可以获得改善。

后纵韧带骨化和黄韧带骨化

后纵韧带骨化（ossification of posterior longitudinal ligament，OPLL）在日本的发病率（2%~4%）高于西方国家（0.1%~1.7%）。地域差异造成的遗传影响尚不明确。非胰岛素依赖型糖尿病、糖耐量受损、肥胖、低甲状旁腺素血症和佝偻病均可能与 OPLL 有关。韧带内出现异位骨化，OPLL 和 OLF 的组织学特点包括：骨化、韧带增生、细胞增殖和血管增生。

OPLL 分为四种类型：①连续型（骨化韧带覆盖连续多个节段）；②节段型（骨化韧带位于不连续椎体后方）；③混合型（连续型与节段型同时存在）；④局灶型（骨化韧带仅位于椎间盘水平）。

由于生物力学改变及正常韧带组织缺失，OPLL 患者的手术治疗需要个体化设计。OPLL 增加了颈椎前路手术的难度及术中硬脊膜损伤风险。当骨化物跨过椎间隙，局部颈椎活动度减小，后纵韧带与硬脊膜囊粘连融合。颈后路手术更为常用，但如果选择颈前路手术，通常需要进行更为广泛的椎体切除减压。

黄韧带骨化（ossification of ligamentum flavum，OLF）在日本发病率同样较高，女性多于男性，50 岁以上人群发病为主。骨化物位于黄韧带内，与上下椎板相连。

类风湿性关节炎

类风湿性关节炎（rheumatoid arthritis，RA）是一种可以影响颈椎的全身性自发免疫性疾病（在欧洲和美国成人占 1%）。抗风湿药和相关生物制剂的发展减少了 RA 所致颈椎病数量（Kaito et al.，2013）。早期使用现代药物治疗可以防止出现关节病理性破坏损伤，但如果已经存在损伤，则无法阻止其进一步加重。

RA 的病理生理学机制为滑膜细胞产生的异常抗原导致持续性细胞激活与免疫复合体产生（类风湿因子 IgM）。细胞因子（IL-1、IL-6、TNF-α）介导慢性炎症启动，导致滑膜内颗粒组织沉积（类风湿性关节翳），从而产生蛋白水解酶破坏相邻软骨、韧带、肌腱和骨组织（Reiter and Boden，1998）。

破坏性滑膜炎导致韧带松弛及骨侵蚀，伴颈椎椎体不稳及半脱位。颈椎不稳或关节翳增生可以引起神经间接或直接压迫。位于寰枕和 C1~2 的上颈椎关节受损最常见，这主要是由于提供核心牵拉力和稳定性的环绕枕骨 - 寰枢椎区域的正常韧带结构在病情进展过程中受到损伤。RA 在颈椎最常见的病理改变包括：C1~2 不稳（65%）、颅底凹陷（20%）以及下颈椎半脱位（15%）（Kim et al.，2015）。

下颈椎半脱位源于小关节面和钩椎关节存在不稳。可以出现沿颈椎矢状位和冠状位的椎体平移运动（伴或不伴旋转运动）。异常颈椎序列包括：椎体滑脱、后凸畸形、侧弯畸形或“楼梯”畸形。手术减压及固定融合适用于颈椎不稳与颈椎管狭窄伴脊髓受压、神经功能障碍的患者。

枕颈部发育异常

寰枢椎半脱位

横韧带、齿状突韧带及翼状韧带损伤可以导致 C1-2 不稳。可见于类风湿性关节翳、强直性脊柱炎、软骨发育不全、唐氏综合征、莫基奥（Morquio）综合征及外伤等。非激素类药物使得治疗类风湿性关节炎的激素用量明显减少，从而降低了寰枢椎半脱位发病率。

寰枢椎半脱位在动力位颈椎 X 线片或动力位 MRI 上可以看到 C1 脊椎相对于 C2 脊椎的过度活动。从寰椎前弓后缘至齿状突前缘的寰齿间距正常值应小于 3 mm（儿童小于 5 mm）。对于寰齿间距大于 8 mm 的无症状患者或存在脊髓病变的所有患者，建议行手术固定治疗。颈部疼痛是这类患者存在颈椎不稳的一个特征表现。术前尚无脊髓损伤时，手术预后较满意，因此建议早期行 C1~2 椎间融合手术。然而，有些 RA 患者虽然存在明显 C1~2 半脱位，但没有脊髓损伤症状，寰齿间距与神经功能预后无明显相关性。寰齿后间距是指齿状突后缘至寰椎椎弓前缘，正常值大于 14 mm，与神经功能预后相关性更好。

旋转型寰枢椎半脱位

寰枢椎旋转型半脱位最常见于儿童，详见**第 85 章**。

颅底凹陷

颅底凹陷是由于寰枕关节和 C1~2 间关节（如齿状突）发育不良并向枕大孔内下陷的病理改变，可合并脑积水、脊髓空洞或进行性脊髓病变。影像学上有许多参数可以用来诊断颅底凹陷（**图 60.1**）。Chamberlain 线是指由硬腭向枕骨大孔后缘所作连线，正常情况下齿状突尖不应超过该线 3 mm。针对无法确认枕骨大孔后缘的情况，McGregor 提出了改良方法。McGregor 线是指硬腭与枕骨鳞部最低点之间连线，正常人齿状突尖不应超过该线 4.5 mm。McRae 线是最简单的参考线，指枕骨大孔前后缘之间连线，正常情况齿状突尖低于该线 5 mm，若超过则为颅底凹陷。McRae 线同时还是诊断 I 型小脑扁桃体下疝畸形的参考线，正常小脑扁桃体应高于该线，而成年患者小脑扁桃体下缘低于该线超过 5 mm，儿童大于 3 mm。由于骨性破坏及增生，有时候很难判断齿状突。此时可以测量 C1 前弓与 C2 椎体间的位置关系。当颈1前弓接近C2椎体下1/3时，提示严重颅底凹陷。

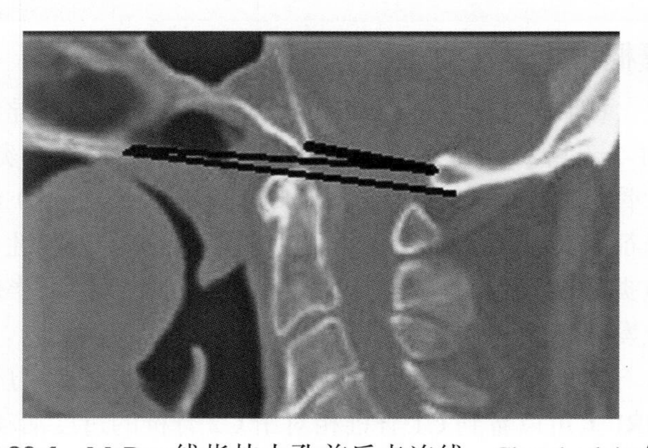

图 60.1 McRae 线指枕大孔前后点连线。Chamberlain 线指从硬腭后缘至枕大孔后缘连线。McGregor 线指硬腭后缘至枕骨最低点连线。正常齿状突尖应不超过 Chamberlain 线 3 mm，不超过 McGregor 线 4.5 mm，位于 McRae 线下方 5 mm

有些学者将由于颅底骨质软化引起的类似影像学改变称为“颅底压迹”。这是由于颅底 - 枕骨以及枕髁的骨质异常导致枕骨大孔内折，引起上颈椎脱位移向枕大孔方向并导致脑干受压。而颅底凹陷是由于韧带松动导致齿状突向上移位进入枕大孔。

颅底凹陷最常见的病因是类风湿关节炎，其他病因还包括：Klippel-Feil 综合征、成骨不全、软骨发育不全、小脑扁桃体下疝畸形、颅锁骨发育不全、Schwartz-Jampel 综合征、Morquio 综合征、甲状旁腺功能亢进、软骨病、佝偻病和 Paget 病。

颅底凹陷的治疗方法多样，包括局部治疗或联合牵引、前路减压、伴 / 不伴枕大孔减压的颅颈融合手术等，但所谓最佳方法尚未达成共识。应充分考虑椎动脉的解剖变异。如果存在腹侧组织压迫，应选择经颈椎前方入路。当不存在脑神经麻痹时，颈椎后路融合是治疗关键，术前颈部牵引有助于预测术中是否能够获得充分神经减压。当存在脑神经麻痹或颈椎牵引存在风险时，应考虑经鼻或经口腔切除齿状突。多数专家推荐先进行颈前路减压然后再做后路融合，但也有少数专家建议“先后再前”。

扁平颅底

扁平颅底是指颅底骨质变平，除非合并其他异常，否则一般无明显临床异常表现。颅底角是由鼻根与垂体窝中心连线以及枕大孔前缘与垂体窝中心连线所组成的夹角。扁平颅底指该角度大于 143°，颅底后凸是指该角度小于 125°。扁平颅底常合并颅底凹陷、软骨发育不全、唐氏综合征、寰枕畸形、锁骨颅骨发育不全、颅面畸形、成骨不全、Paget 病、软骨病、佝偻病、骨纤维结构发育不良或甲状旁腺功能减退。

血清反应阴性的脊柱性关节病

该类疾病包括一系列病因不明但相互关联的慢性炎症情况，如：强直性脊柱炎、Reiter 综合征、银屑病关节炎、炎症性肠病关节炎和难以鉴别的脊柱性关节炎。

强直性脊柱炎最为常见，80%~98% 患者携带 HLA-B27 基因型。全身性炎症反应导致肌腱与韧带和骨骼衔接处发生炎症，同时合并继发性关节间骨桥（骨刺）形成。颈椎问题表现为由于关节及韧带骨化导致的典型颈部僵直以及严重时出现颈椎后凸畸形。使用立位全脊柱 X 线片和（或）临床照片测量颏额垂线角可以评估整体脊柱畸形和平衡。对颈椎畸形的手术矫形应仅限于排除合并有胸腰椎畸形和髋/膝关节畸形的情况。骨量减少是病情变化的特点之一，会影响包括脊柱固定在内的整体手术方案。

弥漫性特发性骨骼肥大

该病也称为Forestier病，总发病率为6%~12%，常见于50岁以上患者。主要特点为连续3个节段的非边缘化韧带骨赘形成（包含4节椎体），影像学上显示为连续的前纵韧带骨化，但保留椎间隙高度。该病发展与强直性脊柱炎不同，不存在关节面僵硬、骶髂关节侵蚀、硬化或关节内骨融合，也没有骨质疏松。

临床表现包括僵直和疼痛。相关椎间盘退行性改变和骨质增生会导致脊髓神经根病。强直性脊柱炎和弥漫性特发性骨骼肥大容易导致僵直的颈椎在轻中度外伤作用下发生骨折。多数颈椎管狭窄导致症状性脊髓神经根病的患者会选择积极手术治疗。合并巨大颈椎前方骨质增生、吞咽困难、喘鸣和声音嘶哑的患者也有少部分具有手术指征。

颈椎前路手术

自20世纪50年代（Cloward，1958），颈椎前路手术逐渐开始被用于脊髓和神经根减压。

前路减压技术包括椎间盘切除和椎体次全切除。神经减压后有两种选择，一是做椎间融合，二是做保留椎体间活动度的非融合手术。对于椎间融合患者，可以使用自体骨、异体骨或人工椎间融合器。

颈椎前路手术指征

来自脊髓或神经根前方的压迫应当选择前路手术。对于颈椎后凸畸形也可以用于纠正颈椎曲度。禁忌证包括压迫来自脊髓或神经根后方以及广泛的后纵韧带骨化。既往有颈部手术史和（或）颈部放疗伴或不伴随声带功能障碍应视为相对禁忌证。颈椎前路手术后常出现无症状的喉返神经麻痹，除非喉镜检查证实双侧声带正常，否则二次手术时应选择从首次手术侧进行。声乐工作者（如歌手）行该类手术时应慎重考虑声带损伤的风险。

技术问题

椎体后缘跨椎间隙广泛骨赘形成，特别是合并后纵韧带骨化时需要做椎体次全切除以获得充分减压。

单节段椎间盘切除的椎体融合率为100%，随着切除节段增多而逐渐降低。如果需要切除多节段椎间盘，颈前路钛板塑形固定可以有效增强颈椎融合稳定性。吸烟与非甾体类抗炎药则不利于椎体融合。

超过一个节段的椎体次全切除患者其椎间植入物松动率和手术失败率均会升高。因此，许多医生喜欢采用多节段椎间盘切除或联合使用颈后路固定融合技术，以增加力学稳定性及融合效果。

有证据表明单一节段椎间盘切除患者，单纯减压和减压后椎间隙填充植入物两者间预后没有显著差异。不使用植入物可以减少治疗费用及手术时间，并避免植入物相关并发症，如取材部位疼痛。与其他技术相比，自体骨移植一直被视为经典的标准术式。但是，随着现代人工融合器（碳纤维、钛合金、聚醚醚酮等材料）的出现，有效避免了供体局部并发症，如疼痛、伤口感染、血肿、外周神经损伤或刺激。

颈椎前路钛板固定增加了颈椎弯曲时的稳定性，通过外科手段提供了强有力的颈前方固定，有助于纠正后凸畸形，但是也有证据表明钛板会增加吞咽困难的发生率。

不同钉板系统组合可分为三类：动态、固定或半固定系统。动态或半固定系统允许相邻椎体与植入物间自然融合，增加钛板与植入物之间的承重均衡以改善融合效果。

总结

从长期预后来看，颈前路椎间盘单纯切除或自体骨移植相较颈前路椎间盘切除植骨融合术或椎体次全切除植骨融合术而言没有明显优势。每种技术都有自己的优缺点。获得最佳手术效果的优选方案应主要取决于患者自身病理特点及主刀外科医生的临床经验（见**专栏** 60.1 和**图** 60.2）

颈椎前路椎间盘切除术

患者仰卧位，头部枕于头圈上，肩部下方垫肩垫，保持轻度仰头姿势。轻度头高位有助于静脉回流但也会减小椎间隙高度。

皮肤切口参考病变层面，根据体表解剖标记和影像学资料进行定位。C3/4大致位于舌骨尾侧，C4/5位于甲状软骨水平，C5/6位于环甲膜水平，C6/7位于环状软骨水平。

手术切口多为直切口，选择在颈部自然皮纹内可以减少术后瘢痕，或偶尔选择沿胸锁乳突肌前缘

专栏 60.1 病例 1：颈前路多节段固定融合

这位 54 岁男性患者主诉为颈部疼痛，尿急和平衡功能障碍。MRI 提示颈椎 C4-5，C5-6，C6-7 节段退行性改变（椎间隙变窄、骨质增生），其中 C6-7 最严重，合并该节段脊髓信号改变。该患者接受了 3 个节段的 ACDF 手术（**图 60.2A~C**）。

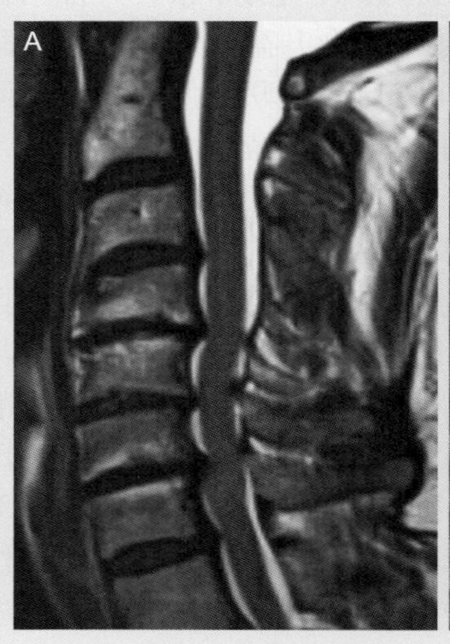

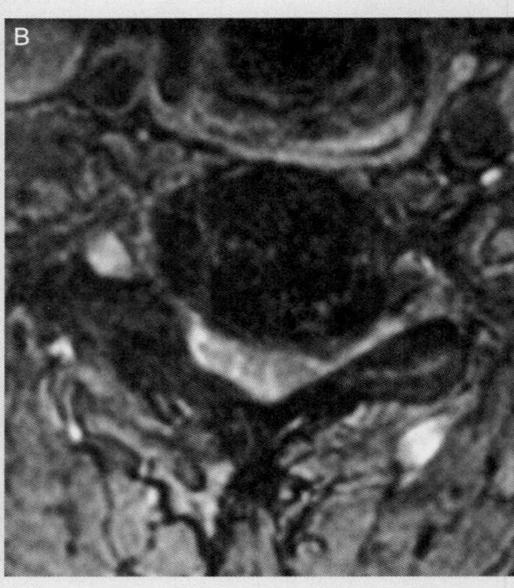

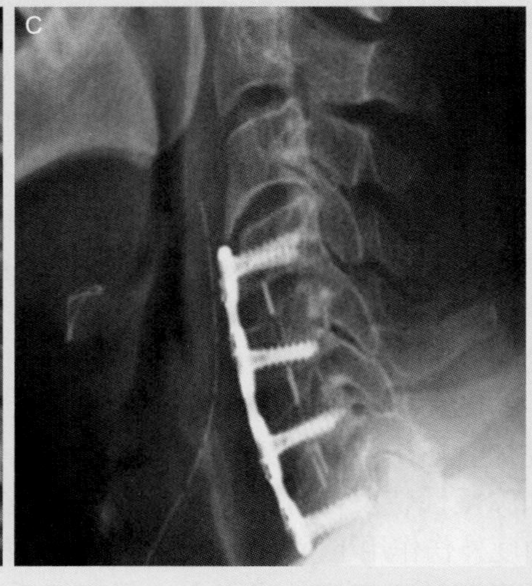

图 60.2 （A）术前矢状位 T2W MRI 可见来自颈前方的以 C6-7 节段为主的多节段脊髓压迫，C6-7 节段脊髓可见轻度脊髓信号改变。（B）术前轴位 T2W MRI：C6-7 节段椎间盘突出及骨质增生导致该节段颈椎管狭窄伴脊髓压迫。（C）术后 1 天。X 线片显示椎间融合器和螺钉位置满意

做斜切口。颈部左、右侧均可选择。喉返神经在右侧解剖路径偶有变异，术中容易损伤，而左侧胸导管在低位切口入路时更容易损伤，特别是近颈胸交界处。多数右利手医生习惯选择在颈部右侧手术，反之亦然。

颈阔肌水平离断或沿上下纵向分离。打开颈筋膜浅层，经胸锁乳突肌和颈动脉鞘内侧与气管食管外侧间隙的无血供区域游离至椎前筋膜。钝性分离通常足以获得充分显露，游离过程中要格外注意鉴别和保护颈动脉鞘结构。

切开椎前筋膜显露椎体、椎间盘和颈长肌。沿颈长肌内缘向两侧适当剥离，将牵开器拉钩置于颈长肌下方以防止损伤距离颈长肌内缘侧方约 1 cm 的交感神经链。将细针头插入病变椎间盘，C 形臂下再次确认手术节段。

切除椎间盘的范围以钩椎关节为两侧边界（**图 60.3**）。使用 caspar 牵开器或颅骨牵引打开病变椎间隙。咬除椎体前缘骨赘，使用刮勺、椎板咬骨钳和磨钻切除椎间盘。注意避免过多切除骨性终板，否则易引起植入物沉降。

从头端向尾侧走行的纤维束提示为后纵韧带，切除后深方为硬脊膜囊。对于脊髓型颈椎病患者，要彻底切除椎体后方的骨质增生。对于神经根型颈椎病，要注意椎间孔区走行神经根的充分减压。

切除间盘后，植入融合器。如果使用前路钛板，应注意避免损伤相邻节段椎体。使用可吸收线关闭伤口，多数医生会留置伤口引流管。

颈椎前路椎体次全切除术

对于单节段椎体次全切除，手术切口方法与椎间盘切除术相同。椎体次全切除是指切除上下椎间盘之间的椎体中央骨质。对于多数患者，15~18 mm 的减压宽度较为适宜。

使用填充满骨屑的钛笼重建并恢复颈椎曲度，椎体前方固定钛板。**表 60.1** 显示颈前路手术的相关并发症。

颈椎非融合手术

颈椎非融合手术被视为颈椎间盘切除 + 固定融合术的替代方案。其原理是保留颈椎局部活动度。关于人工椎间盘在体内的长期有效性及是否能减轻邻椎病等问题尚存争论（见争论部分）。

非融合手术适用于主要为软性椎间盘突出的年轻患者。禁忌证包括：关节炎（强直性脊柱炎、类风湿性关节炎）、感染性关节病、后纵韧带骨化、血清阴性的脊柱性关节病、严重骨质增生以及颈椎不稳

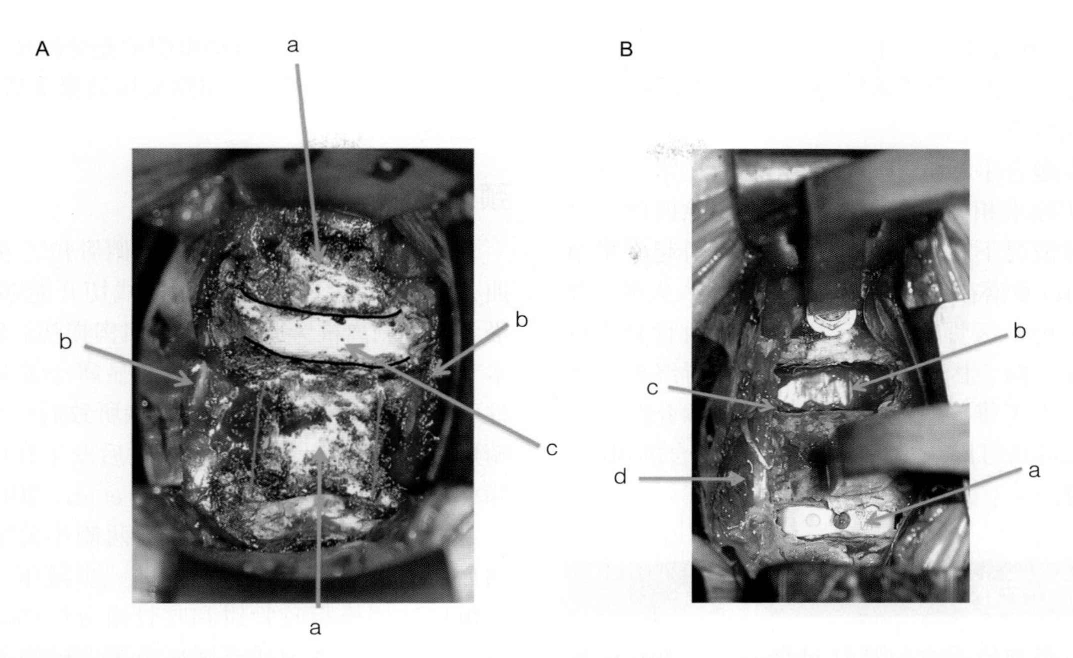

图 60.3　（A）显露颈前路 C5-6 椎间隙。a，C5（上）和 C6（下）椎体。b，两侧颈长肌。c，C5-6 椎间盘。黑实线显示 C5 下终板和 C6 上终板，以及两侧钩椎关节（提示向两侧减压范围）。蓝实线显示对 C6 椎体做椎体次全切除时两侧的磨除边界。（B）C5-6 和 C6-7 ACDF 手术。a，C6-7 椎间盘切除植骨融合。b，C5-6 椎间盘切除后可见深方脊髓。c，骨性斜面提示 C6 上终板钩椎关节的起点。d，右侧颈长肌。置入 C5 和 C6 椎体内撑开钉以打开椎间隙

表 60.1　颈前路手术相关并发症

并发症	发生率	评价
声音沙哑	4%	常继发于喉返神经麻痹，双侧麻痹可能引起完全气道闭塞。由于喉返神经走行于气管食管沟内，故神经压迫可能发生于牵开器与气管插管气囊之间。在安置好牵开器后从新对气囊放气充气可能减少该并发症
吞咽困难	10%	危险因素包括：多节段手术、高龄、厚钛板、下颈段手术。要小心植入物移位
出血	2%~3%	危险因素包括：未做术后伤口引流、止血不充分（尤其是显露过程中）。出血可以引起气道梗阻及术后软组织水肿
硬膜撕裂	0.5%	常见于合并 OPLL 的患者（最高达 25%） 术中需要修补硬脊膜（可使用缝线、夹子、纤维蛋白胶）
食管损伤	<1%	危险因素包括：既往手术瘢痕 可能引起致命损伤。需要耳鼻喉科或胸外科医生参与修补
四肢乏力加重	0.5%~5%	小心摆放体位，避免颈部过度后仰 避免对椎间隙过度牵拉或在硬膜囊表面过多操作 术后及早行核磁排除血肿可能
Horner 综合征	<1%	由于向两侧过多牵拉颈长肌引起 多数患者可以自行缓解
感染	1%	危险因素包括：全身性免疫抑制（如糖尿病）、食管穿孔的抗感染治疗。植入物不一定非要取出
临椎病	2.9% 每年	融合术后每年约有 2.9% 的患者会出现临床症状
其他少见并发症		融合器移位 血管损伤（椎动脉、颈动脉、颈静脉） 胸导管损伤 死亡（0.1%）

（滑脱≥3.5 mm 或成角≥11°）。

所有考虑行非融合手术的患者都应术前做 CT 和动力位 X 线检查。

颈椎非融合手术的术野显露和减压技术与颈前路椎间盘切除术相同，但应避免过度切除两侧钩椎关节。特殊情况下，钩椎关节不稳可能引起手术节段过度活动以及潜在不稳和人工椎间盘植入失败。要格外注意避免术区骨屑残留，以减少术后骨刺形成或异位钙化风险。因此，不使用磨钻进行终板准备而直接安置人工椎间盘是最好的。有文章介绍使用非甾体类抗炎药可以减少术后早期椎间融合的风险，见**专栏** 60.2。

颈椎后路手术

颈椎后路减压手术包括针对脊髓型颈椎病的椎板切除或椎板成形术以及针对神经根型颈椎病的椎间孔扩大成形或颈后路椎间盘切除术。颈后路手术适应证包括：黄韧带肥厚及关节面增生、3 个节段以上的椎间盘突出、后纵韧带骨化、先天性多节段颈椎管狭窄、椎间孔狭窄。

颈后路手术更适合于老年患者，因为多节段病变更为常见且术后颈椎稳定性相较年轻人可以适当忽略。颈后路手术可以避免出现声音嘶哑、吞咽困难及邻椎病。如果存在不稳或后凸畸形，可以考虑进行后路固定融合。

手术目的是获得神经组织的充分减压。回顾性研究显示颈后路减压与颈前路减压效果大致相当（Luo et al., 2015）。

颈椎板切除术

颈椎板切除术患者体位为俯卧位，头部轻度屈曲，头架固定。沿颈后正中白线切开能够减少出血。沿骨膜下剥离椎旁肌可以减少肌肉损伤。X 线定位手术节段。避免过度肌肉剥离及显露小关节以防止脊柱不稳和进行性畸形（椎板切除所致后凸畸形和鹅颈畸形）。大宗文献报道椎板切除后发生脊柱不稳的发病率约为 6%~46%（McAllister et al.，2012）。

椎板切除可以使用磨钻沿两侧小关节面内侧开槽后完整取下。切除黄韧带进一步减压。替代方法也可以使用椎板咬骨钳和咬骨钳分块切除。应将两侧小关节内缘视为适当减压范围。硬膜外静脉丛出血可能会影响术野，应充分止血，见**专栏** 60.3。

改良颈后路手术

颈椎板切除术的改良术式可以减少肌肉分离并保留颈椎后方张力带结构以减轻术后出现颈椎不稳的风险（**表** 60.2）。

颈后路椎间孔扩大成形术

小关节骨质增生、钩椎关节增生和椎间孔区椎间盘突出可以引起神经根受压及无脊髓症状的根性

专栏 60.2 病例 2：两个节段的人工椎间盘置换术

这位 41 岁女患者主诉为颈部僵硬伴上臂沿 C5 和 C6 神经根分布范围的放射性疼痛。左侧肢体肌力 4 级，Lhermitte 征阳性。影像学提示 C4-5、C5-6 节段椎间盘退行性改变。随后为该患者进行了两个节段的人工椎间盘置换术（**图** 60.4A~C）。

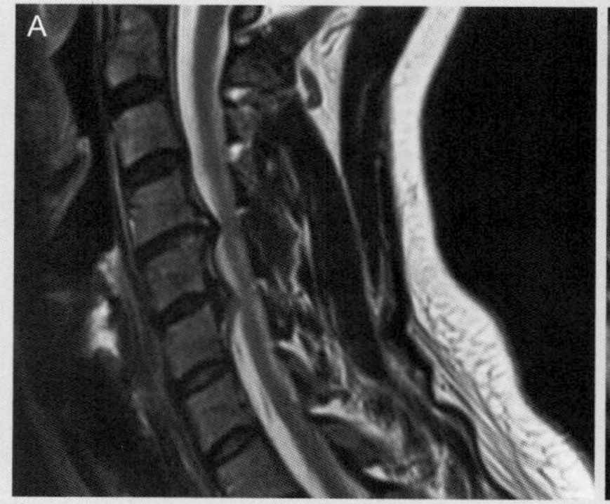

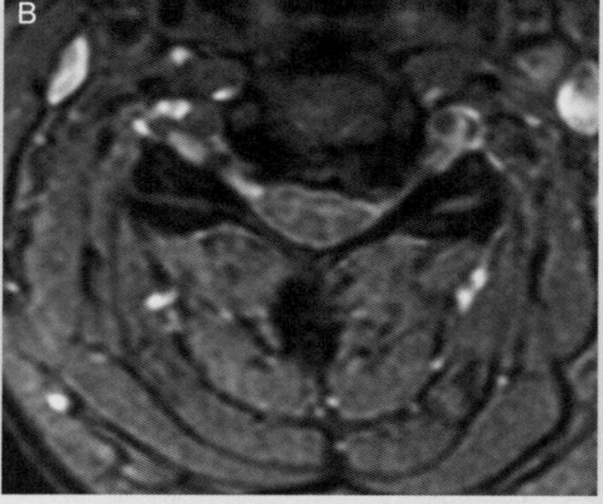

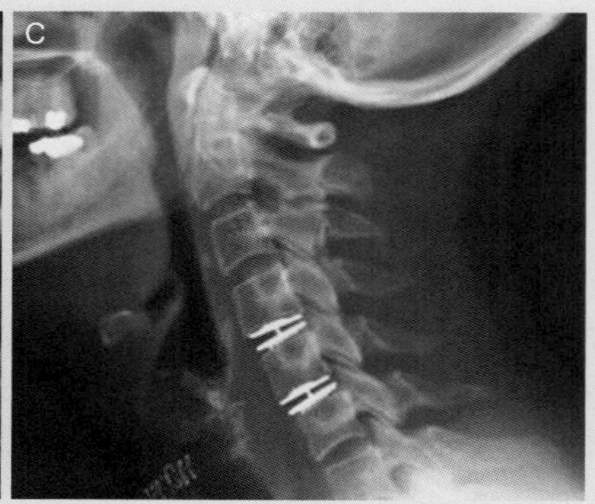

图 60.4 （A）术前矢状位 T2W MRI。C4-5、C5-6 椎间盘左侧旁中央型突出引发左侧压迫。（B）术前轴位 T2W MRI。C4-5 左侧旁中央型椎间盘突出导致颈椎管及椎间孔狭窄，C5 神经根受压。（C）术后 1 天颈椎 X 线显示椎间盘位置满意

专栏 60.3　病例 3：颈椎板切除 + 侧块螺钉固定融合

这位 74 岁患者表现为脊髓型颈椎病特点。影像学发现严重的颈椎管狭窄和脊髓压迫，伴 C3-4 水平髓内信号改变。由于颈动脉粥样硬化和颈椎曲度丧失，故为该患者选择了颈后路固定融合手术（**图** 60.5A~C）。

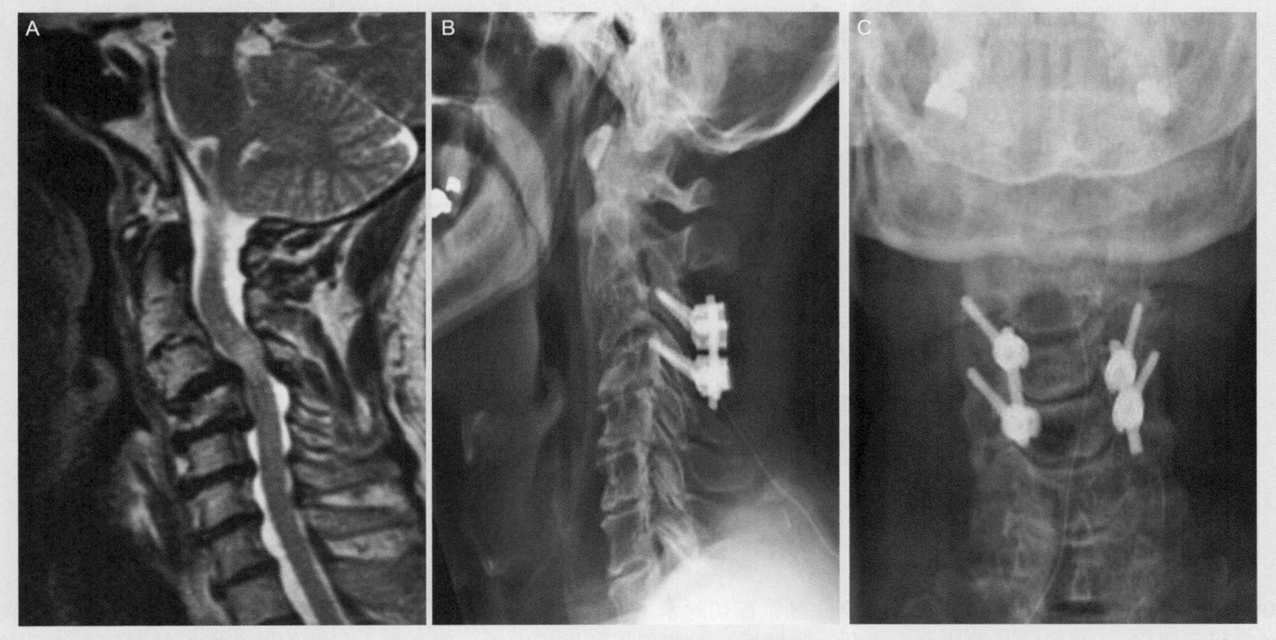

图 60.5　（A）术前颈椎矢状位 T2W MRI。C3-4 脊髓受压，合并因颈椎前凸消失和后凸畸形导致的髓内信号改变。（B）X 线侧位片显示 C3-4 椎板切除减压术后 C3 和 C4 的侧块螺钉位置。（C）冠状位 X 线可见侧块螺钉固定钉道

表 60.2　改良颈后路手术

	评论
跳跃式颈椎板切除术	2002 年由 Shiraishi 等提出，跳跃式切除椎板可以部分保留中线结构。见**图** 60.6A
颈椎板成形术	颈椎管容积通过敞开椎板及切除黄韧带得到扩大。两种常见方式分别为单开门（**图** 60.6B，Hirabayashi et al.，1983）和双开门手术（**图** 60.6C，Kurokawa et al.，1982）

疼痛。椎间孔扩大成形术可以在不显露中线结构的基础上实现神经根减压。

患者体位与颈椎板切除术相同。手术显露可以仅做病变同侧肌肉剥离（开放手术）或经肌间隙入路（微创通道技术或神经内镜）。显露病变头尾端椎板及走行神经根表面的小关节面。术中 X 线定位病变节段，使用高速磨钻、小号椎板咬骨钳或超声骨刀切除头尾端部分椎板，在关节面内缘下方咬除部分骨质以减压走行神经根（**图** 60.6D）。关节面破坏应小于一半，否则容易影响局部稳定性（Raynor et al.，1985）。

个别情况下，突向椎间孔区的软性椎间盘可以通过增大椎间孔扩大成形的下边界及部分切除下关节突的方法实现切除。将钝钩置于神经根下方，松动并切除游离髓核，见**专栏** 60.4。

颈后路手术并发症包括：持续性颈痛和后凸畸形。小心筛选适合手术患者可以有效降低并发症。如果存在脊柱不稳，可以考虑做固定融合。术后神经功能障碍时有报道，其中 C5 神经根麻痹最常见。对于脊髓受压患者，在摆放体位时要格外小心避免颈椎过度屈曲及牵拉（Nassr et al.，2012）。总体来说，颈后路减压手术是适应证广、安全、有效的操作。

寰枢椎半脱位手术

通过手术方法对不稳定的寰枢椎复合体（**图** 60.8）进行加固曾经主要是通过颈后路椎板下钛缆固定和椎板间加固实现，但现在除了作为补充选择，这些方法已经较少使用（**表** 60.3）。Magerl C1-2 经椎弓根螺钉固定或后路 C1 侧块螺钉联合 C2 椎弓根螺钉 Harms-Goel 技术是目前最常用的两类手术方式（后文会进一步讨论）。螺钉固定技术从生物力学角度看优于钛缆加固技术，因为它直接限制了 C1-2 关节面

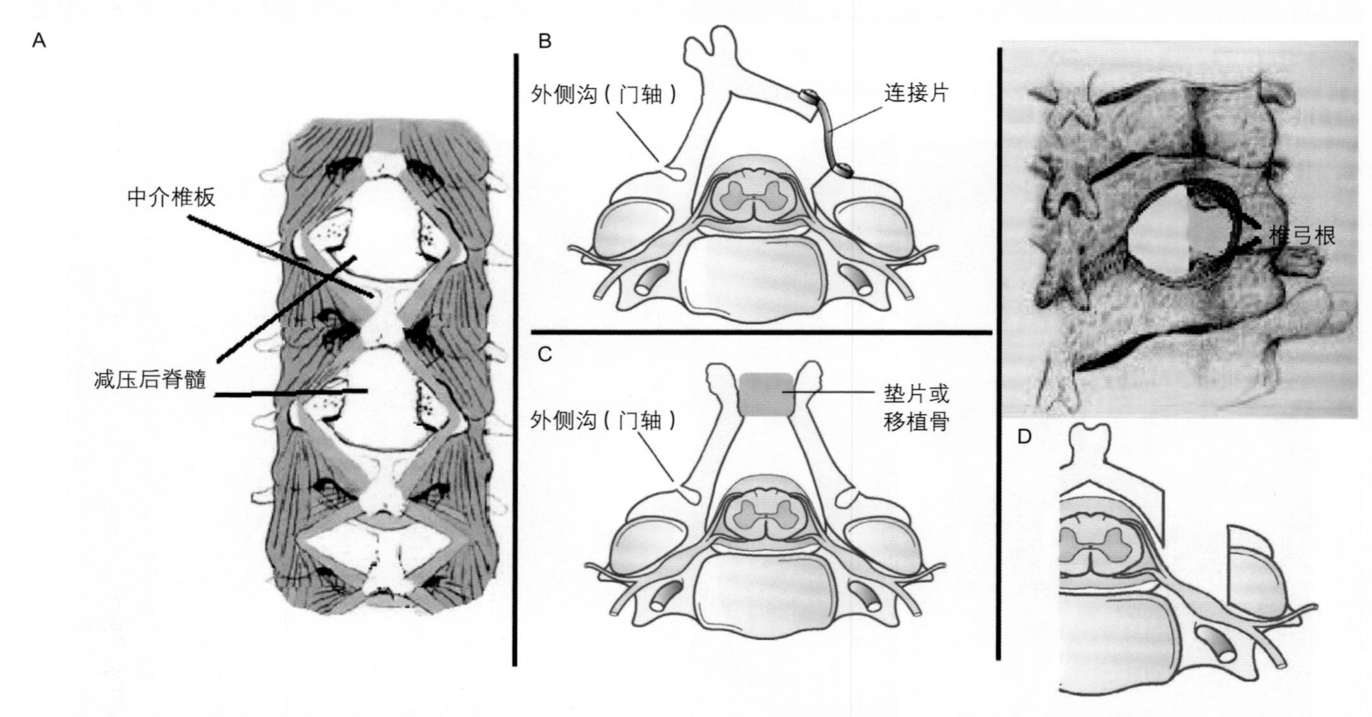

图 60.6 微创颈后路减压手术。（A）跳跃式颈椎板切除术。交替切除椎板和黄韧带，保留间隔椎板和结构。不用剥离相邻棘突附着肌肉。（B）单开门技术。磨开一侧椎板，对侧仅保留椎板内板，以该侧为门轴侧敞开椎板棘突复合体，并用内固定板维持椎管开放状态。（C）双开门技术。沿中线切开棘突，在两侧椎板外侧开槽（准备门轴）后向两侧敞开椎板，切除黄韧带。在两侧椎板间植入骨块以保持椎管扩大效果。（D）椎间孔切开术。通过切除叠瓦状骨质及黄韧带来对相邻椎弓根间的走行神经根进行减压。使用探针来确认减压效果

专栏 60.4 病例 4：微创颈后路椎间孔切开术

这位 41 岁患者曾做过 C5-6 ACDF 手术，主诉为右上肢 C7 神经根分布范围疼痛。MRI 提示 C6-7 椎间盘向右侧后方突出压迫 C7 神经根。本患者采用了颈后路微创 C6-7 椎间孔切开术（图 60.7A–C）。

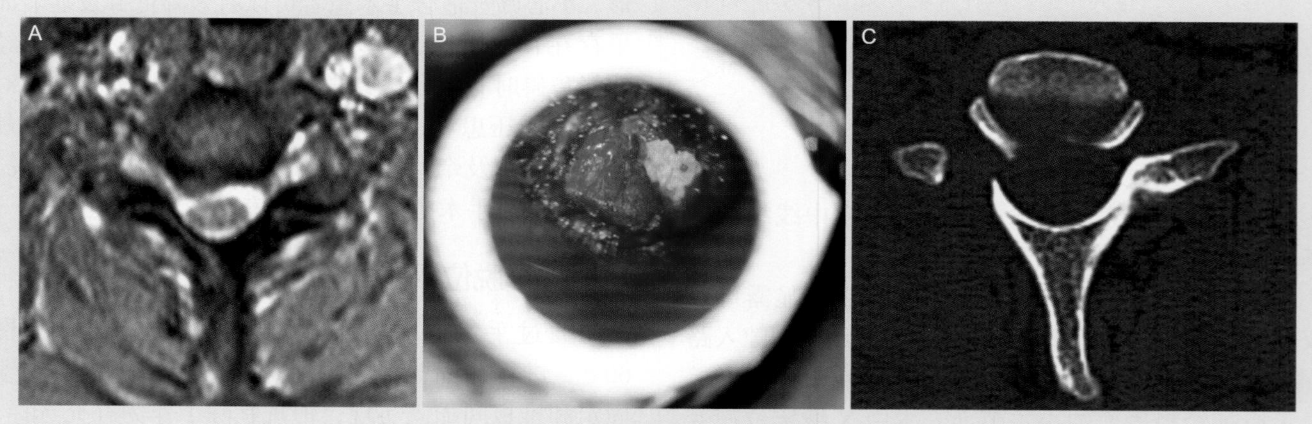

图 60.7 （A）术前 T2W MRI 轴位像。C6-7 椎间盘向右侧后方突出压迫 C7 神经根引起根性疼痛。（B）术中显微镜下微创切开右侧 C6-7 椎间孔，深部可见减压后的 C7 神经根。（C）术后 CT 轴位像显示右侧 C6-7 椎间孔切开及神经根减压

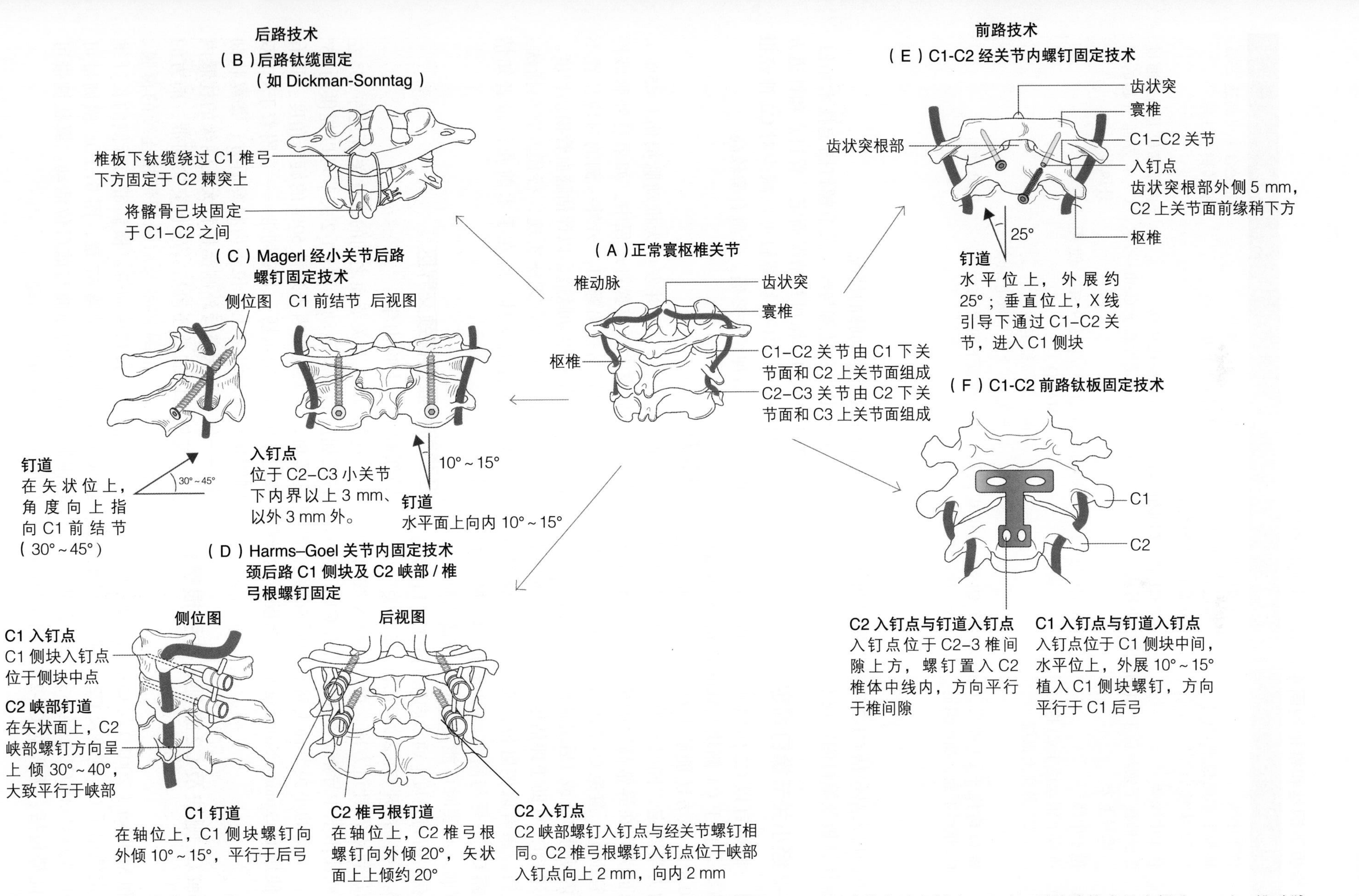

图 60.8 维持寰枢椎稳定的外科技术。（A）正常 C1-C2（寰枢椎）关节的解剖后视图（含椎动脉位置）。颈后路技术见左侧（B~D），颈前路技术见右侧（E~F）；椎动脉位置已表明。（B）颈后路钛缆固定技术：椎板下钢丝及 C1-C2 椎板间植骨。（C）Magerl 经小关节后路螺钉固定技术：入钉点已标注，两侧钉道如图显示（矢状面 - 由下向上；轴位 - 由两侧向中央）。（D）Harms-Goel 关节内固定技术：C1 侧块螺钉联合 C2 峡部或椎弓根螺钉固定。注意入钉点根据 C2 峡部或椎弓根需作出调整。（E）前路 C1-C2 经关节固定术：入钉点位于 C2 上关节突下方，齿状突根部中线旁 5 mm，针道如图显示。（F）前路 C1-C2 钛板固定技术：如图显示 C1 和 C2 入钉点。前路手术相对后路手术较少使用

表 60.3 以椎板下钢丝和椎板钩固定技术为基础的外科原则演变

技术	原则	植骨块	优势	劣势
Gallie（1939）	位于中线 椎板下钢丝位于 C1 下方包裹 C2 棘突	单独植骨块支撑 靠近 C1 椎弓 覆盖于 C2 棘突上	避免椎板下钢丝 通过 C2 下方	非融合率可高达 25% 旋转稳定性差
Brook and Jenkins（1978）	位于中线旁 2 根椎板下钢丝位于 C1 和 C2 椎弓下方	在 C1 和 C2 间植入两块骨块	融合率高达 93% 旋转稳定性高于 Gallie 技术	由于椎板下钢丝通过 C2 下方而引起的额外风险
Dickman et al.,（1991）（图 60.8）	位于中线 椎板下钢丝位于C1椎弓下方，于 C2 棘突上盘绕	在 C1 和 C2 椎板间植入一块骨块	融合率高达 97%（使用 HALO） 改善旋转稳定性 避免 C2 下方椎板下钢丝	
椎板钩技术	椎板钩位于 C1 椎弓上面及 C2 椎弓下面，加压固定	在 C1 和 C2 椎板间植入一块骨块	避免椎板下钢丝通过	移动骨瓣

的活动。前方经口入路包括 C1-2 经关节螺钉和从 C1 侧块至 C2 椎体钛板及螺钉固定技术。

Magerl C1–2 经小关节螺钉固定

各使用一根螺钉以 C2 两侧峡部为进针点，经 C1-2 小关节突，止于 C1 侧块（Magerl and Seeman, 1986；**图 60.8**）。该方法能够为 C1-2 小关节提供最稳定的生物力学固定，同时有效防止旋转。该术式的主要禁忌证为存在异常高跨的椎动脉。操作上要格外小心血管损伤，避免 C1 侧块前方穿孔，从而导致咽部、颈内动脉和（或）后组脑神经的损伤。

术前头颈 CTA 有助于评估椎动脉走行，术中 X 线引导下置钉。患者取俯卧位，头架固定，颈部适当屈曲。显露 C1 后弓与侧块、C2 椎板、C2 峡部和 C2-3 小关节面。必要时可能需要向尾侧适当延长后正中切口以获得置钉角度（通常向尾侧至 C7-T1 棘突旁 1~2 cm）。可以打开 C1-2 关节囊以显露关节面。**图 60.8** 显示进钉点及针道方向。可以选择 X 线引导下钻孔置钉或使用术中导航。钻孔后置入 C1-2 经小关节螺钉。在暴露的小关节面上进行植骨有助于骨融合。通常使用 Dickmann-Sonntag 后路椎板下钢丝来强化固定。

Harms–Goel C1 侧块及 C2 峡部 / 椎弓根螺钉固定

Harms 和 Melcher（2001）与 Goel 等（2002）针对关节间固定使用了 C1 侧块及 C2 峡部 / 椎弓根螺钉固定（**图 60.8**）以取代 C1-2 经小关节螺钉固定。

其主要优势包括：无需对 C1-2 进行解剖复位，且适用于高跨椎动脉的情况。

手术定位和显露与经小关节螺钉固定技术相似。对 C2 神经根的保留可视情况而定。置钉点和针道方向详见**图 60.8**。C1 侧块螺钉可以减少对 C2 神经根的刺激及术后神经性疼痛。骨融合率较高。

并发症

两种术式的主要并发症为椎动脉损伤（<5%），常发生于显露术野或置钉过程中。如果意外刺破椎动脉，不要轻易拔出螺钉。另外一侧的对应位置不再置钉，尽早行椎动脉造影以评估脑血管损伤程度。

如果 C1-2 内固定无法实现，替代方案包括枕 - 颈固定或外骨骼支具。应在手术前获得患者知情同意。

经颈前路显露枕颈交界区

局部解剖与生物力学

枕髁与 C1 上关节面之间的寰枕关节允许 15° 左右的屈曲和伸展运动，而 C1-2 关节可以提供约 45° 旋转角，这大致相当于颈椎 50% 的旋转角度。具有稳定作用的结构包括：①横韧带——它附着于 C1 双侧侧块内面的结节上，位于齿状突后方；②翼状韧带——位于齿状突背外侧至枕骨大孔前缘的枕髁内侧。其他辅助韧带还包括：齿状突尖韧带、前方的寰枕筋膜、与前纵韧带及后纵韧带相连续的覆膜、后方的寰枕筋膜和黄韧带。横韧带与背侧的长纤维组成了十字韧带（见**第 57 章**，**图 57.1**）。横韧带可以限制寰枢关节的屈曲与前后位活动。翼状韧带可以限制寰枕关节旋转运动。

开放性颈前入路

前方经口及经鼻入路C1-2固定术主要适用于需要前方减压并切除齿状突的患者。可以选择开放手术或神经内镜。该类术式已极少用于类风湿性疾病，类风湿性关节炎主要通过单纯后路固定融合治疗。口咽部感染是该类手术的禁忌证。

患者呈仰卧位，头颈部两侧预留好摆放C形臂的空间。根据主刀医生的手术习惯，选择开刀手术或内镜手术。有两种固定技术可供选择：C1-2经关节螺钉固定或C1侧块及C2椎体T型板螺钉固定（**图60.8**）。

C1-2经关节螺钉固定术一般选择咽部黏膜直切口，而T型板技术则选择U形切开黏膜。保持在沿C2椎体中线外侧12 mm内操作可以避免损伤椎动脉。如果需要扩大显露，一般选择经口咽下颌骨劈开扩大入路。

绝大多数颈前入路手术都是在专科医疗中心进行。手术并发症包括内脏损伤，如食管、气管、咽部、舌头。还包括颈内动脉、颈内静脉及第9~12对脑神经。

值得注意的是，手术相关并发症与以下有关：咽部黏膜瓣的愈合不良、腭咽闭合功能不全合并食道反流、因软腭切开导致的言语障碍以及经面或经颞下颌入路骨切除所导致的牙齿咬合不齐。

经鼻神经内镜扩大入路

经鼻齿状突切除适用于颅底凹陷的病例。鼻腭线用来评估该入路可及最低范围。颅底凹陷患者上抬的齿状突可以使用神经内镜经齿状突基底部进行磨除。如果需要向下方进一步扩大，可以采用经口入路神经内镜辅助治疗。

沿中线经鼻咽后壁做直切口或黏膜瓣可以用来显露斜坡下部、枕骨大孔前缘以及寰椎前弓。该术式可以避免切开上颚。使用高速磨钻切除寰椎前弓，由浅入深在C2椎体上磨断齿状突基底部，直至见到深方的横韧带和硬脊膜。将游离齿状突从枕大孔小心拉下来。为了锐性切开齿状突尖韧带和翼状韧带，可能需要适当扩大切除枕骨大孔前缘。完整取出游离的齿状突，解除对硬膜囊压迫（**图60.9**）。切口边

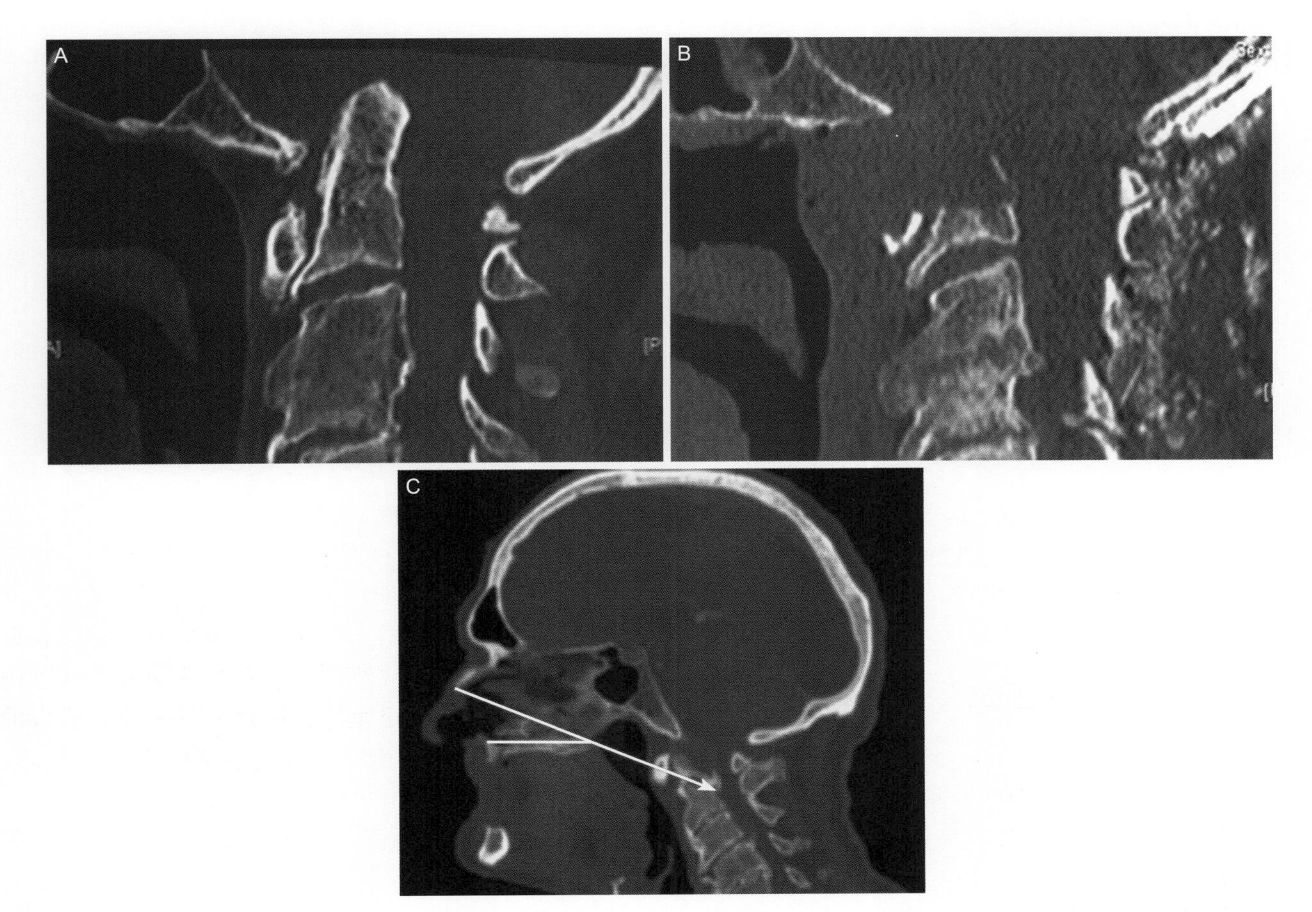

图60.9 经鼻内镜齿状突切除及颅颈交界区减压术前CT重建矢状位显示颅底凹陷。（B）术后CT重建矢状位显示内镜下切除齿状突。（C）Kassam鼻腭线标记的是经鼻内镜入路的下限范围

缘距离很近，所以不必须缝合，除非出现脑脊液漏。由于该术式会引起C1-2不稳，后续需要进行局部固定。

有关颈椎退行性疾病治疗的争论

只有极少量临床研究能够提供高级别证据以指导退行性颈椎病的治疗。常见争论包括：手术适应证及时机、微创与开放手术、前路与后路手术。目前尚没有Ⅰ级或Ⅱ级证据比较前路与后路手术效果，现有研究证实两者效果大致相当（Fehlings et al.，2013；Lawrence et al.，2013）。

邻椎病是颈前路椎间盘切除术患者难以回避的问题之一。Hilibrand 等（1999）发现症状性邻椎病发病率大约为2.9%每年。相关争论集中于邻椎病是否由关节融合导致还是由疾病自然病史所引发。有关研究发现颈椎固定融合后相邻节段生物应力（椎间隙压力）和活动度增加。

前瞻性试验研究了颈椎间盘置换术的脊柱生物力学效应，并比较了人工椎间盘置换和固定融合的预后。对于单节段椎间盘切除手术，颈椎间盘置换与固定融合效果类似（Buchowski，2009），但对于多节段病变，人工椎间盘置换患者需要二次手术的概率有所下降。椎间盘置换手术费用较高。临床数据显示更倾向于椎间盘置换手术（Ren et al.，2014）。尽管对于颈前路椎间盘切除患者更推荐椎间盘置换术，但仍需腰更有力的长期随访数据支持。

延伸阅读、参考文献、EBRAIN 的相关链接

扫描书末二维码获取。

第 61 章　胸椎病

Kieron Sweeney · Catherine Moran · Ciaran Bolger 著
许菲璠 译，伊志强 审校

引言

胸椎在解剖学、生物力学、病理学和手术学方面具有一定的特殊性。颈椎自然曲度前凸、胸椎后凸与腰椎前凸三者共同维持了整个脊柱的矢状位平衡。胸椎及其胸肋关节使胸椎稳定性最大化、活动度最小化，因此胸椎间盘脱出率较低。

发病率

胸椎病发病率为每年百万分之一（McInerney and Ball，2000）。在诊治其他脊柱疾病时偶然发现胸椎间盘突出的概率高达 11%（Awwad et al.，1991）。0.2%~4.0% 的症状性椎间盘突出位于胸椎部位，胸椎间盘突出占所有症状性椎间盘突出手术的 0.2%~1.8%。男 / 女发病率约为 1∶1，与颈 / 腰椎间盘突出类似，胸椎病同样好发于 30~60 岁年龄段（McInerney and Ball，2000）。由于胸廓对上胸椎的稳定作用，胸椎间盘突出常见于胸 7 水平以下，尤其是胸 11-12 水平范围。多数椎间盘突出为中央型或中央偏外侧型。退行性改变是胸椎间盘突出的首要病因，仅有 25% 源于脊柱外伤。创伤性椎间盘突出通常见于年轻患者。30%~70% 椎间盘存在钙化，且多数钙化椎间盘位于硬膜下（图 61.1）。

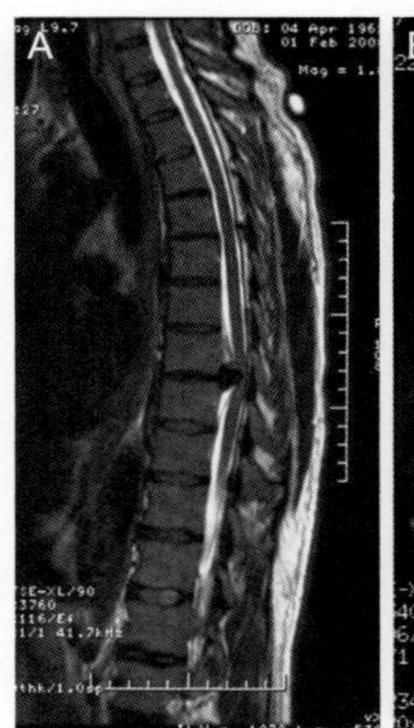

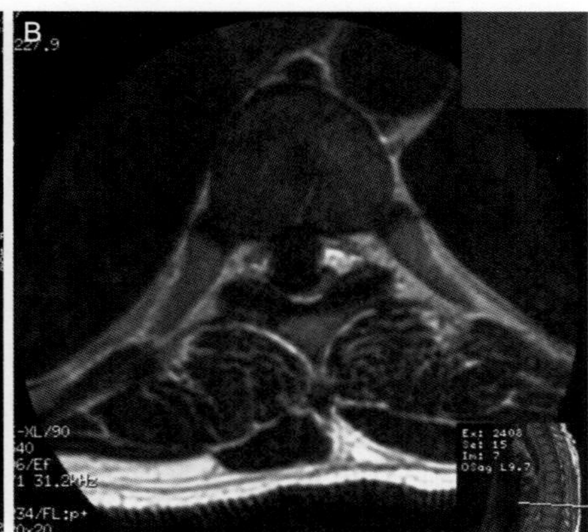

图 61.1　巨大胸椎间盘。在 T2 像上可见明显脊髓受压

临床表现

脊髓病变的常见临床特点及主诉包括：痉挛性瘫痪、感觉障碍、括约肌功能障碍、疼痛、背部轴性疼痛及向胸阔前方放射的根性疼痛（Stillerman et al.，1998）。但是，不同胸椎间盘突出患者之间的主诉症状和体征可能存在较大不同，这取决于突出椎间盘所在脊柱水平、位置、大小、压迫时间、神经血管的代偿能力以及致病原因。大多数文献认为疼痛是发病时最主要症状。疼痛可以是单侧或双侧，其放射区域取决于突出层面。胸 1-2 椎间盘突出可表现为上肢根性痛及手部肌肉乏力。胸椎中部椎间盘突出所引发疼痛可以沿胸廓放射，而下胸段椎间盘突出可以引起腰腹部疼痛。临床表现依时间顺序逐渐发展。由于退变引起的椎间盘突出最先表现出疼痛（胸腰部或放射性疼痛），其次为感觉障碍、运动障碍、括约肌功能障碍（Arce and Dohrmann，1985）。对于创伤性椎间盘突出，疼痛后短期即可出现脊髓损伤表现（Arseni and Nash，1960）。然而，最多 25% 的患者可能没有疼痛，而是主诉轻度神经功能障碍或步态异常，容易影响早期诊断。

发病机制

神经功能症状和体征是由于神经受压和血供不足引起的。由于胸 4-9 节段的脊髓血供较差，该范围的突出压迫可以导致严重的脊髓损伤。

治疗

保守方法

对于无症状性胸椎间盘突出的自然病史鲜有文献报道。无症状胸椎间盘突出的发病率为 15%~37%（Wood et al.，1995）。作者回顾了 90 例无症状患者的胸椎 MRI 以评估解剖异常，在平均 26 个月的 MRI 随访中发现突出椎间盘仍然没有引起症状，但是小的突出间盘倾向于不变或增大，而突出明显的间盘反而容易缩小（Wood et al.，1997）。

手术

手术指征包括：顽固性疼痛、脊髓损伤表现、括约肌功能障碍等。主要手术适应证为脊髓损伤导致的神经功能障碍。作者自身的临床经验是：尽管由于诊断不及时可能使患者长期存在神经功能障碍，但是手术减压仍然有助于神经功能的显著恢复。对于仅表现为神经根性疼痛的患者，一旦通过神经阻滞确认病变节段，则可以使用相对微创的手术方式进行受压神经根减压。然而对于多数患者，外科干预通常是指开放手术。手术策略主要取决于：椎间盘突出层面、病变椎间盘与神经组织的相对位置关系、病变椎间盘的成分（软性或钙化）以及突出椎间盘是否位于硬脊膜下（Arts and Bartels，2014）。在以上这些因素中，突出椎间盘的层面和其与神经组织的相对位置关系对手术方式的决策最为重要（**表 61.1**）。

在外科干预前，所有患者均需进行：①全脊柱MRI 检查以确认病变水平；②突出间盘位置的 CT 检查以判断病变间盘是否存在钙化成分。

胸椎间盘突出的手术入路

当选择手术入路时，术前最应该考虑的核心问题包括：突出位置、突出方向（中央型、中央偏外或侧方突出）、突出物大小、任何相关或可能出现需要固定的脊柱畸形、任何突出间盘存在钙化的证据。椎板切除术曾被作为治疗胸椎间盘突出的手术方式，但其并发症率高达 60%（Fessler and Sturgill，1998），因此目前已不再使用。

建议术前标记手术位置。术中应再次使用 C 形臂或术中 CT 二次核实。术中神经监测可根据实际情况酌情使用，但根据作者经验，更核心的问题是手术入路设计既要能够清楚显露突出椎间盘结构，又不能影响受压脊髓。

准确定位病变节段非常重要。应使用前后位及侧位 X 线片进行核对，可以从骶骨往上或从颈 2 往下计数椎体节段。包含突出椎间盘的全脊柱 MRI 至关重要，可以参考颈 2 和骶骨进行病变节段的定位。

表 61.1　中央型椎间盘突出

节段	入路
胸 1-4	经胸骨
胸 2-6	经右侧胸廓
胸 6-12	经左（或右）侧胸廓

前路经胸骨手术

该术式适用于胸 1-4 节段、中央型、钙化、突出于硬膜下的椎间盘病变。

技术要点如下。患者仰卧位，两侧肩胛骨下方垫高以保持颈肩部轻度伸展。下胃管以便于术中触诊判断食道位置。

手术切口沿胸锁乳突肌内侧缘向内下至胸骨角。有些学者推荐经左侧胸锁乳突肌切口手术，因为左侧喉返神经在气管食管沟内更容易辨认。沿肌纤维走行方向分离颈阔肌，于骨膜下游离肩带肌、胸锁乳突肌、胸舌骨肌在胸骨和锁骨的附着处，以保留以上肌肉术后收缩功能。用手指在胸骨下方游离出深达上纵隔的界面。将胸腺推向一侧。使用摆锯离断胸骨，放置胸骨牵开器，向两侧分开胸膜。

类似颈前入路手术，沿内侧的气管食管与外侧的颈动脉鞘之间可以钝性分离出一层无血管间隙。左侧的头臂静脉和动脉向下外方牵拉。向深部继续沿食道和椎前筋膜间分离无血管间隙可见两侧颈长肌（该处可放置牵开器；Zengming et al.，2010）。关闭伤口时应逐步逐层进行，留置胸腔引流管，术后常规复查胸片。

主要手术并发症包括：血管损伤、胸部淋巴管损伤、气管损伤、食道损伤以及胸膜损伤 / 气胸。

前路经胸廓手术

该术式能够最大限度从前方显露脊髓和突出椎间盘，尤其适用于中央突出型椎间盘，是外科医生治疗此类疾病需要掌握的核心技术。作者推荐该术式用于治疗所有钙化及所谓的“巨大”椎间盘突出。所谓“巨大”椎间盘突出是指术前影像学提示占位效应大于椎管横截面积 40% 的情况（Hott et al.，2005）。

手术适应证包括：胸 2-12 节段突出、中央型、钙化、硬膜下椎间盘突出。

手术技术如下（**图 61.2~ 图 61.6**）：患者取侧卧位，腋下放置腋垫，双下肢屈曲，膝盖间夹枕头。对于高节段椎间隙（胸 2-6），皮肤准备应包括肩部和肩胛骨区。经右侧入路适合于高节段病变，便于更好地显露脊柱结构，因为主动脉弓和降主动脉紧邻椎体左侧。经左侧入路便于显露胸 8 及以下节段，因为肝和膈肌可能阻挡右侧路径。此外，左侧入路可以使胸导管损伤的风险降至最低。麻醉时常使用双腔气管导管。

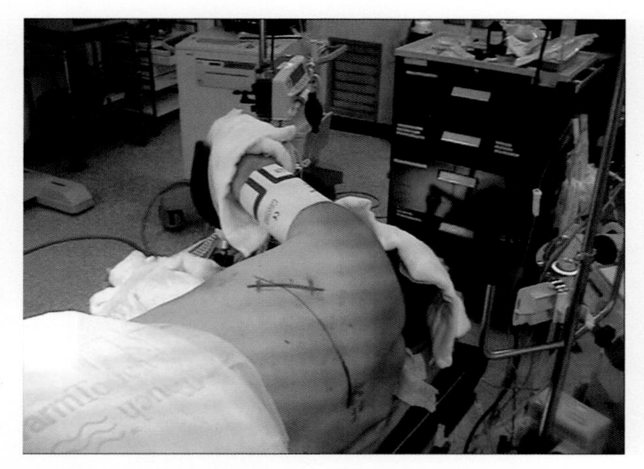

图 61.2 患者右侧卧位，切口线位于左侧腋中线，以前后位及侧位 X 线片定位的椎间隙水平为中心

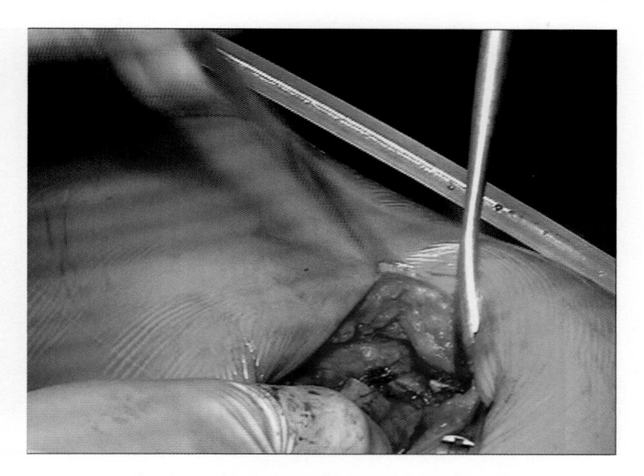

图 61.4 切断肋骨并从下方取出，以显露胸膜

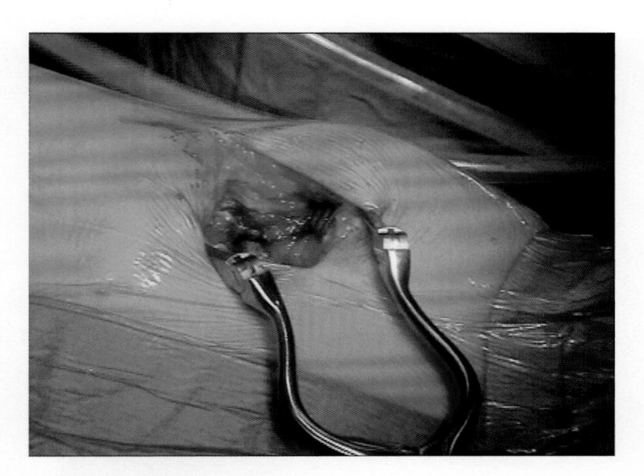

图 61.3 切口线位于对应肋骨上

术中定位椎间隙节段及肋间水平后标记切口线。对于高位节段病变的开放手术入路，切口线从胸 1 棘突开始，平行于肩胛骨内侧缘，向下至肩胛骨下角，再向外侧至第七肋骨肋缘。对于低节段病变，切口线位于准备切除的肋骨水平。不管是选择全开放还是微创开放手术，手术切口的中点都应位于病变椎间盘所对应的腋中线水平。

对于胸椎高节段病变，手术需要辨别、分离背部如斜方肌、背阔肌、斜方肌、前锯肌等有助于回缩肩胛骨以显露胸廓的肩带肌。对于低节段病变手术，应辨别、分离背阔肌和前锯肌以显露肋骨。剥离肋间肌并使用骨膜剥离子剥净肋骨下缘，沿肋骨向前向后尽可能分离肌肉。

切断肋骨（后部尽可能接近肋骨头/肋横突关节，前方尽量接近胸肋关节）。对于微创开放入路，不需要向前切开肋骨，但需要安置一个撑开器使医生可以经胸腔或于胸膜腔后操作。如果选择胸膜腔后操作，应使肺部膨胀以便于游离胸膜并减少胸膜撕裂。如果选择经胸腔操作，则肺部应排气，将病变间盘节段表面的胸膜壁层切开并使胸膜瓣基底部居中。

应仔细辨别奇静脉、左侧主动脉、交感神经丛、肋间血管神经束及肋骨头。在肋间动静脉起始部（至少远离椎间孔 1 cm）结扎离断，以减小血管损伤风险。切除肋骨头显露椎间隙。切除病变椎间盘及上下部分椎体结构。骨性切除范围取决于椎间盘突出的上下范围。为了延长轴完整显露突出椎间盘，对于巨大突出间盘，必要时可以切除部分椎弓根的上下缘。目的在于在脊髓前方开放足够空间，以便于从前方解除突出椎间盘对脊髓的压迫。

闭合伤口时应逐步分层进行，包括修补任何可能的硬脊膜漏口。经胸腔手术时应留置引流管一根。如果存在硬脊膜破损，应留置腰大池外引流。

手术并发症包括：血管损伤、右侧胸淋巴管损伤、食管损伤、胸膜损伤/气胸、交感神经丛损伤。

后外侧入路：肋横突切除术

该术式的适应证为侧方软性椎间盘突出。

手术技术如下：患者呈俯卧位，以病变层面为中心做后中“T”形切口、旁正中直切口或曲线切口。

辨别并离断在横突附近的斜方肌或背阔肌。使用骨膜剥离子剥离肋骨表面的残余肌肉及肋骨下方。清除横突及椎板处的所有肌肉。在肋横关节处离断肋骨头，保护好肋骨下方神经血管束后，将整根肋骨从前方离断取出。切开横突显露椎弓根。推开胸膜壁层以切除椎弓根。标准肋骨切除术可能受空间所限而无法有效推开胸膜，腹侧甚至侧方显露可能仍旧受限。

手术并发症包括：血管损伤、右侧胸部淋巴管

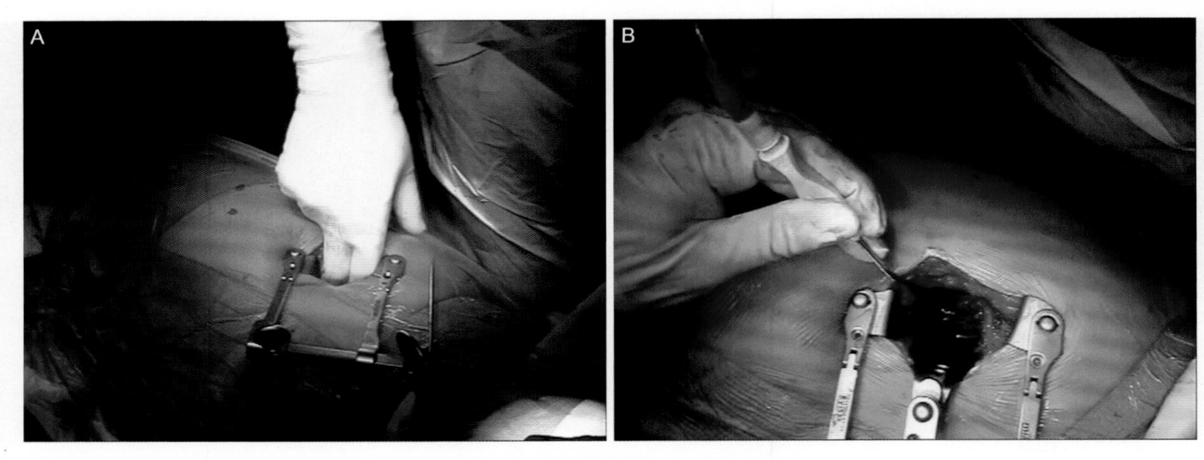

图 61.5 钝性剥离胸壁内胸膜。将深部牵开器插入至椎体表面

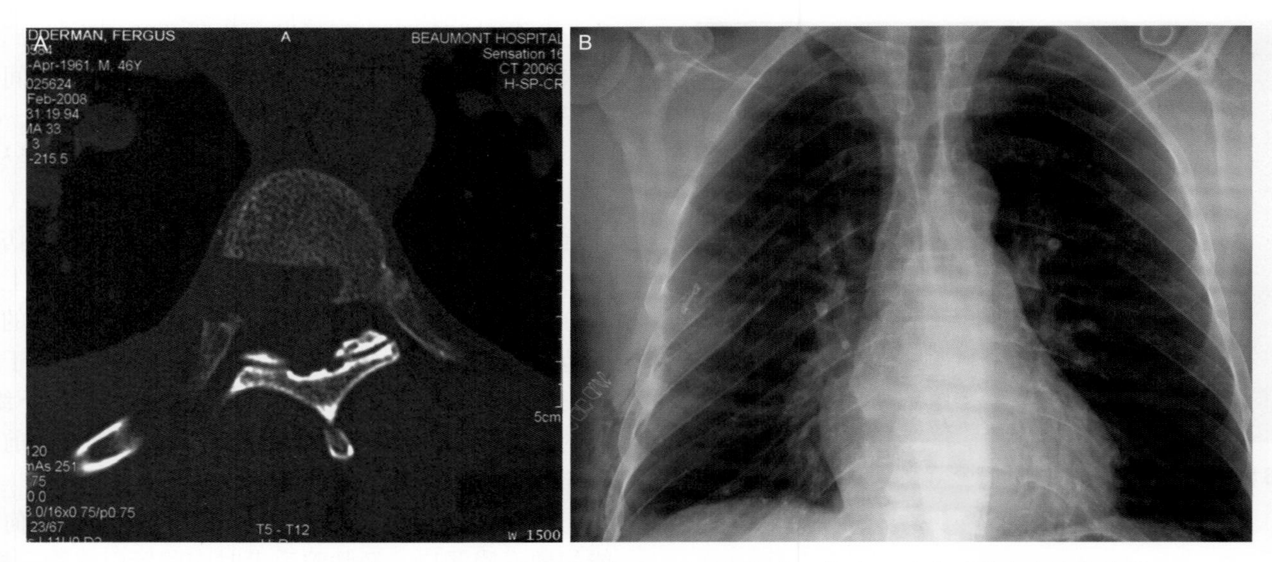

图 61.6 （A）术后 CT 显示骨切除范围及完整切除突出椎间盘。（B）术后 X 线片显示微型钛片连接的肋骨

损伤、食管损伤、胸膜损伤 / 气胸及交感神经丛损伤。

后外侧入路：外侧腔外入路

该术式的适应证为侧方软性椎间盘突出。

手术技术如下：患者呈俯卧位，手术切口取决于突出层面，或者沿棘突做中线直切口，或者做曲线切口（直线部分位于棘突上，沿肩胛骨下角做曲线）。在横突附近离断斜方肌或背阔肌。将竖脊肌的外缘向中线翻转。使用骨膜剥离子剥离肋骨表面的残余肌肉及肋骨下方。清除横突及椎板处的所有肌肉。

在肋横关节处离断肋骨头，在侧方 12 cm 以外处切断肋骨。保护好肋骨下方神经血管束后，将整根肋骨从前方游离取出。切开横突显露椎弓根。推开胸膜壁层以切除椎弓根。必须考虑突出间盘所在脊柱水平。当位于胸 4 以上时，由于肩胛骨遮挡，手术更为困难。需要离断菱形肌和斜方肌，因此很容易造成运动功能损伤。

手术并发症包括：血管损伤、右侧胸部淋巴管损伤、食管损伤、胸膜损伤 / 气胸、交感神经丛损伤、硬脊膜撕裂、脑脊液漏、胸廓造瘘可能、神经根损伤和感染等。据某些文献报道，并发症发生率可高达 53%（Lubelski et al.，2012）。该术式中离断肌肉可能导致失血量增多、术后疼痛及住院日延长。

后外侧入路：经椎弓根入路（单侧或双侧）

该术式适应证为侧方软性椎间盘突出。双侧入路可以对中央型椎间盘突出进行减压，但也会更容易导致脊柱不稳。

手术技术如下：患者呈俯卧位，沿棘突做后中线直切口。沿棘突和椎板做骨膜下肌肉剥离至两侧小关节突。使用小号枪状咬骨钳切开椎板，显露神经根及硬脊膜囊。切除上位椎体的下关节面和下位椎体的上关节面以及横突上缘以显露椎弓根。先于椎弓根皮质骨内磨除松质骨，然后切除上下方皮质骨。向侧方切除临近椎管的皮质骨后，进一步向外侧切除部分椎板。磨除部分上下关节面。切开侧方椎间盘纤维环，使用刮勺和髓核钳小心清除椎间隙内髓核碎片。

术后脊柱不稳较少见，因此一般不需要做脊柱固定。手术并发症包括：神经根和脊髓损伤。

后外侧入路：经关节突保留椎弓根入路

该术式的适应证为侧方软性椎间盘突出。

手术技术如下：患者呈俯卧位，沿棘突做后中线直切口。沿棘突和椎板做骨膜下肌肉剥离至两侧小关节突。使用小号枪状咬骨钳切开椎板，切除上位椎体的下关节突内侧缘以显露神经根及硬脊膜囊。关闭切口时应分层逐步缝合。手术并发症包括神经根和脊髓损伤。

微创手术

微创手术技术在神经外科中越来越受到重视。尽管这些技术可以通过减少手术部位组织损伤来降低并发症发生率，但是其学习过程有一定难度，因此也可能会因为技术不成熟而引起显著的并发症（Elhadi et al.，2015）。微创手术包括：小切口手术、视频辅助胸腔镜和内镜技术。Eihadi 等发表的系统性文献综述比较了微创手术和传统开放手术的预后效果，发现局限于单个节段的软性胸椎间盘突出很适合于微创技术，但是伴有钙化且与硬膜囊粘连的椎间盘更适合于开放手术。可惜的是，该综述并不包括小切口手术。

胸腔镜下椎间盘切除术

患者呈侧卧位，麻醉使用双腔气管插管，在准备好切口通道后，嘱麻醉师换对侧单肺通气。手术通道直径约 15 mm，分三个通道插入手术器械，另单独开放一个直径约 1 cm 的胸腔镜通道。将胸膜从脊柱表面分离。胸廓切开术由于广泛分离肌肉和牵拉肋骨易引起术后严重神经痛，而胸腔镜手术可以有效减少该并发症发病率。类似开放胸腔切开术，首先磨除肋骨头和椎弓根，清楚显露脊髓，在邻近突出椎间盘的椎体上磨出一个骨槽，继而间盘碎片会随之缓慢进入该骨槽内。

小切口技术

作者之前发表过介绍小切口胸膜腔后入路手术的文章。先在腋中线做一个 4 cm 长切口，然后切除一根肋骨，使用钝性花生米剥离器将胸膜从胸腔内壁剥开，插入一个长牵开器有助于持续同侧肺通气并免除使用术后胸部引流管。切除突出椎间盘的方法如前所述，继而将肋骨复位固定。对于巨大中央型椎间盘突出，作者习惯经左侧入路，因为强韧的主动脉使术中操作更安全容易。许多作者都报道过小切口手术的成功案例（Moran et al.，2012；Snyder et al.，2014）。其他需要考虑的因素包括：外科医生的手术经验（Falavigna and Piccoli Conzatti，2013）。

预后

对于需要手术治疗的情况，神经功能恢复和疼痛管理是多数患者需要考虑的问题（Moran et al.，2012）。既往文献报道，术后神经功能恶化及麻痹等手术并发症发生率较高，椎板切除术的相关并发症发生率为 18%~75%（Arseni and Nash，1960；Fessler and Sturgill，1998）。

自从弃用了椎板切除术而更多采用腹侧入路（如经胸廓或背外侧入路）后，手术效果得到了显著改善。然而，开胸术后疼痛综合征会在多达 50% 的术后患者中发生，其中 30% 患者可能长期存留该症状（Karmakar and Ho，2004）。

骨质疏松症和椎体压缩性骨折

骨质疏松症是一种骨质异常，可能增加骨折风险。骨折风险与骨强度成反比，骨强度反映的是骨密度、骨微结构和重塑等功能（NIH Consensus Development Panel，2001）。骨密度是通过双能 X 线骨密度仪测量。影响骨密度的因素包括：年龄相关的骨质流失和激素状态。最新研究显示，松质骨丢失可能最早出现于 30 岁的男性和女性。但是，直到中年皮质骨才会开始出现丢失。年龄相关性骨流失被认为与肾羟化维生素 D 成为其活性成分的能力降低有关，导致血钙浓度降低及继发性甲状旁腺功能亢进。

激素相关性骨质疏松对于女性影响大于男性。从绝经期开始，血浆雌二醇和雌酮水平下降导致骨生成与溶解失平衡从而引起进行性骨含量下降。净骨溶解引发细胞外钙浓度升高，继而激活代偿机制以阻止高钙血症引起全身钙含量负平衡。

相对而言，性激素突然下降不会发生在男性身上。但是，由于性激素结合蛋白增多，男性睾酮和雌二醇会出现一个缓慢下降的过程（Drake et al.，2015）。

有关雌激素的药物替代方面，选择性雌激素受体调节剂已经获批用于治疗绝经期后骨质疏松症。双磷酸盐是一种无机焦磷酸盐，对羟磷灰石具有高亲和性。它可以在破骨细胞和Howship腔隙间形成一道非降解性屏障。破骨细胞吞噬双磷酸盐导致细胞凋亡。

由于急性或慢性疼痛，骨质疏松可以显著增加椎体压缩性骨折的发病率。进行性后凸畸形会引起脊柱不稳，从而增加摔倒风险或呼吸功能障碍。因此，建议65岁以上女性定期筛查骨质疏松。对于小于65岁的女性或65岁以上男性，个体化危险因素分析有助于预测骨质疏松的发生。相关高危因素包括：女性、白人或亚洲裔、低体重/体重指数、家族史、早停经、长期久坐、酗酒、低钙或低维生素D饮食、缺少日晒、服用药物（糖皮质激素或抗癫痫药）、类风湿性关节炎以及多数全身性炎症疾病。实验室检查包括：血沉、空腹血糖、血钙、果糖、碱性磷酸酶、肌酐和24小时尿钙。双能X线吸收测定法是排查骨质疏松的影像学金标准，因为其能够预测骨折风险。MRI反转恢复时间序列则有助于鉴别新、旧损伤。

骨质疏松的治疗分为非药物和药物治疗。非药物治疗包括：锻炼和饮食。身体锻炼可以降低年龄相关性骨质丢失。奶制品饮食和鱼类可以增加维生素D的摄入量。药物治疗包括：双磷酸盐（剂量依赖性药物，有助于减少骨转换和骨折风险）、激素替代治疗、选择性雌激素受体调节剂。

椎体成形术和椎体后凸成形术

椎体成形术适用于因骨质疏松引起的、对保守治疗效果不佳的急性症状性压缩性骨折。患者可以在局麻强化或全麻下手术。患者呈俯卧位，在C形臂或术中CT引导下做单侧或双侧穿刺。使用11~13号穿刺针经椎弓根或椎弓根旁（椎弓根与椎体连接处）穿刺至压缩椎体前1/3或1/4位置。将聚甲基丙烯酸甲酯水泥沿穿刺针缓慢注射到椎体内，直到水泥填充至椎体后缘为止。如果发现有骨水泥渗出椎体，则应当立即停止注射。相关并发症包括：脂肪或骨水泥引起的肺栓塞、神经根性疼痛以及相邻椎体骨折。

椎体后凸成形术同样适用于因骨质疏松引起的、对保守治疗效果不佳的症状性压缩性骨折，并有助于恢复脊椎矢状位平衡。操作方法类似椎体成形术，区别在于穿刺针经终板下方置于椎体中央位置，借助各种工具制作出一个工作通道以便可扩张球囊通过。在术中X线引导下扩张球囊，同时监测其容积和压力。当椎体高度恢复或达到球囊最大容积/压力，或球囊接近皮质骨表面1 mm以内时停止充气。取出球囊，将聚甲基丙烯酸甲酯水泥缓慢注射入椎体腔内。并发症包括：脂肪或骨水泥引起的肺栓塞、根性疼痛、神经并发症及相邻椎体骨折。

用于评估以上这些操作的短期和长期典型指标包括：疼痛评分（VAS）、伤残评分（ODI）、并发症（骨水泥渗漏、神经功能损伤）、椎体前方高度、脊柱后凸角度、相邻节段椎体骨折和住院日。与保守治疗相比，两种手术方式在预后方面都是安全有效的。在相邻椎体骨折发病率上，后凸成形术与椎体成形术之间没有发现明显差异。而与保守治疗相比，两种手术均能降低相邻椎体骨折发病率。相较椎体成形术而言，后凸成形术可能在恢复椎体前方高度及后凸角度方面稍有一些优势（Ma et al.，2012）。

关于椎体成形术和后凸成形术的手术时机目前尚存争论。椎体成形术的主要手术指征是控制疼痛，因此其最佳手术时机很难确定，有些专家建议伤后2~12个月内进行椎体成形术都是安全有效的（Nieuwenhuijse et al.，2012）。由于后凸成形术的手术指征是恢复脊柱矢状位平衡及缓解疼痛，因此手术时机似乎更为重要。恢复椎体高度在急性或亚急性椎体骨折时最为有效，因此手术治疗的精准时机选择非常必要（Crandall et al.，2004）。

争议

为骨质疏松性骨折患者行常规MRI检查

MRI可以用于鉴别急性或慢性骨折。在急性骨折愈合期，可以发现出血。此外，正常脂肪骨髓提示显著骨髓水肿，并在3个月内逐渐减少（Brinckman et al.，2015；Piazzolla et al.，2015）。这种现象可以在T2加权序列上看到高信号或者在T1压脂相上鉴别。最新研究指出，急性骨折的特定T1和T2相特点有助于预测骨折不愈合（Tsujio et al.，2011；Takahashi et al.，2016）。其他在骨质疏松性骨折时使用MRI的适应证还包括是否可能存在由于肿瘤骨转移导致的病理性骨折，可以通过增强MRI及弥散加权序列予以求证（Pozzi et al.，2012）。

延伸阅读、参考文献、EBRAIN的相关链接

扫描书末二维码获取。

第 62 章　腰椎疾病

Christopher G. Kellett・Matthew J. Crocker 著
郭胜利 译，佟怀宇 审校

引言

有关腰椎退变的观察可以追溯到希波克拉底（Hippocrates）和盖伦（Galen）。但是直到上世纪，腰椎退行性椎间盘病变才被公认。近年来，影像学和手术技术的进步带来了新的治疗方法，使这个领域的发展方兴未艾。腰椎疾病普遍存在，对这一具有挑战性的领域有一个合理的认识是神经外科医生的明智之举。

腰椎退行性病变

关键概念

本节将讨论三个关键概念：脊柱功能、运动节段和脊柱骨盆平衡。

脊柱功能

脊柱有三个主要的生物力学作用，即承重、活动和保护神经系统。

作用在椎间盘上的力是身体各部分和支撑物重量总和的数倍。无论健康椎间盘的负荷模式和它的静力学特性如何，负荷被平均分配到椎体终板。经椎间盘造影证实，与其他关节一样，异常的负荷会导致腰椎间盘局灶性退行性变和疼痛（McNally et al., 1996）。

脊柱的肌肉组织具有机械优势，肌肉长度的微小变化会导致运动范围的大幅增加，使脊柱承受巨大的压力。脊柱韧带具有张力和拉伸的特性，脊柱的稳定性与韧带的张力和刚性密切相关。没有确凿证据表明超出正常运动范围的平移或侧屈运动与疼痛有关，但据传腰椎滑脱表明节段性不稳定会导致疼痛。

因退化引起完整的支撑结构的丧失通常会导致神经组织的机械和化学损伤，例如椎间盘突出、腰椎管狭窄和脊椎滑脱。

运动节段

Schmorl 和 Junghanns（1971）首次描述了“运动节段”，该运动节段由两个椎体、椎间盘和相关的小关节突组成。节段性韧带包括纵韧带、黄韧带和棘突间韧带。固有的节段性肌肉（夹肌、竖脊肌等）提供拮抗作用和稳定性。“三关节复合体”由 Kirkaldy-Willis 等率先提出（1978），强调椎间盘和小关节突之间密不可分的关系。一种成分的变性会导致整个节段的变性，从而导致疼痛、畸形和神经受损。Panjabi（1992a，1992b）将脊柱描述为具有三个平衡子系统（被动的、主动的和神经反馈系统）的动态神经肌肉系统。

脊柱骨盆平衡

理想的矢状面对线能够使脊柱以最小的能量消耗支撑身体的重量，脊柱的不平衡会导致肌肉疲劳、畸形、疼痛和侧弯及轴位失衡的社会心理影响。治疗脊柱疾病时，骨盆、脊柱和整体矢状面平衡之间的关系至关重要。神经外科医生将遇到许多平背综合征患者。利用患者的全脊柱站立正位及侧位 X 线片可以用于测量脊柱骨盆的几何形状，从而揭示矢状失衡的程度以及恢复平衡所需的矫正程度。脊柱骨盆参数在**第 57 章**和**第 66 章**涉及。

病因学和病理生理学

80％的人一生中经历过下腰背部疼痛，其中10％的人发展为慢性疼痛。在英国，每年有 830 万个工作日因骨骼肌肉问题而损失，病假两年后，患者重返工作岗位的可能性不大。腰痛的自然病史是良性的，在大多数情况下，疼痛会在 2~4 周内消失，超过 90％的疼痛会在 12 个月时消失。随着 65 岁以上老年人在未来 25 年内翻番，腰背疼痛将对社会经济产生更大的影响。

传统上，退行性疾病与职业性重复负荷有关，此外，还涉及年龄、男性性别及吸烟等因素。另外，越来越多的证据表明遗传起着重要的作用。家族性退行性椎间盘病已经被认识到，候选的基因包括编码胶原蛋白的 Sox9、维生素 D 受体金属蛋白酶 -3 和白介素 -1 等。

退行性变的级联

退化过程具有三个不同的阶段（Kirkaldy-Willis et al.，1978）。当退变超过了维持稳定结构的临界值时，脊柱就会出现不稳定的现象。

首先，以轻度创伤或反复劳损为特征的功能障碍会导致继发于节段性肌肉疲劳、痉挛和发炎的轴向背部疼痛。椎间盘退变表现为纤维环撕裂和核基质改变，然后出现小关节滑膜炎和软骨退变。其次，不稳定以椎间盘内部破裂和吸收、小平面囊松弛和半脱位为特征。最后，稳定的特征是骨赘形成和关节僵硬运动减少，黄色韧带增厚以及周围神经被侵犯致神经元损伤。

腰椎病

“腰椎病”包括与运动节段退变有关的系列疼痛及临床症状，主要表现为轴向下背部疼痛，神经功能受损和神经根痛可能并存。

大多数腰椎病患者表现为非特异性腰痛。一小部分患者（10% ~15%）表现为与椎间盘或小平面变性和不稳定相关的疼痛。在无症状患者的 MRI 发现退行性表现很常见，但是在年轻患者中很少有伴有 Modic 改变和明显的小面变性的椎间盘疾病。某些临床体征会特异性的指向疼痛产生的根源和适当的治疗方法。

腰椎管狭窄

1961 年，Friedman 首次描述了腰椎管狭窄症（lumbar canal stenosis，LCS）及其临床表现。在过去的 30 年中，大约 1% 的患者因此接受手术，这个数量增加了 8 倍，主要是在 65 岁以上的年龄组。LCS 即椎管或神经孔狭窄，可分为先天性（特发性或软骨发育不全）和后天性（退行性、腰椎峡部裂、创伤性或代谢性）。

先天性腰椎管狭窄比较罕见的，大多数发生在 30~40 岁。退行性腰椎管狭窄较常见，主要发生在 60 岁以上。其主要症状是神经源性跛行，主要是在站立和行走中发生根性腿痛、腿脚沉重、麻木和感觉异常。影像学受压程度与临床症状严重程度相关性较差。应该注意外周血管疾病存在的危险因素，详细询问病史有助于鉴别血管性跛行和神经源性跛行。

临床特征包括背部疼痛，行走时伴有腿脚沉重和麻木的臀部放射痛，休息及弯腰时可缓解症状。马尾综合征罕见，但患者可能表现为慢性疾病合并或不合并急性椎间盘突出。运动可能会使检查结果变得更精准。矢状位平衡的评估发现，通过膝关节屈曲和髋关节过伸以补偿腰椎曲度的增加。

韧带增厚导致椎管中央受侵犯，由于椎间盘高度的丧失和变形而导致脊柱缩短会引起肥厚的黄韧带屈曲膨胀，这种情况在腰椎伸展时会加重，可能同时存在的腰椎滑脱会进一步使椎管直径缩小，加重神经损伤。

跛行发生的机制可能是继发于机械压迫和血管功能不全，马尾的长期压迫会导致脑脊液（CSF）分泌减少、微血管改变和炎症。静脉充血会妨碍新陈代谢，并且在运动时，神经根的小动脉会因失去血管舒张功能而无法适应代谢需求的增加。

大多数患者的症状会进展，但一小部分患者会通过保守治疗得到改善。

当存在严重的并发症、影像学与临床症状缺乏一致性以及症状较轻微或呈间歇性发作时，保守治疗是合理的。治疗方法包括使用非甾体类抗炎药、肌肉松弛剂、理疗、纠正姿势和硬膜外类固醇浸润。

由于缺乏 1 级证据和患者的异质性，直接对接受手术和保守治疗的 LCS 患者进行比较具有误导性。尽管缺乏相关证据，但普遍认为对于中度至重度症状的患者手术效果优于非手术治疗。

尽管很少见，但进行性神经功能缺损和括约肌功能受损是手术的绝对指征。手术方案取决于脊髓受压程度、中央或侧面受压程度以及是否并存畸形。手术方法包括椎板切除术、选择性减压、椎板成形术、棘突间牵引、单独减压或减压并融合。见**图 62.1**。

椎板切除术与选择性减压并椎板成形术

椎板切除术可治疗中央压迫引起的椎管狭窄，这对存在严重狭窄、畸形和需要广泛的侧方减压的情况下是有利的。最大程度的压迫来自椎板下增厚的黄韧带。在中度压迫的情况下，可通过单侧入路切除黄韧带（保留中线韧带和对侧肌肉）。椎板切开术和“over-the-top”技术可对对侧椎管进行减压。中度侧隐窝和椎间孔狭窄可以用选择性减压技术处理，例如椎板切开术、内侧小关节切除术和椎间孔外肌肉间入路。

腰椎椎板成形术与颈椎椎板成形术相同，但是，

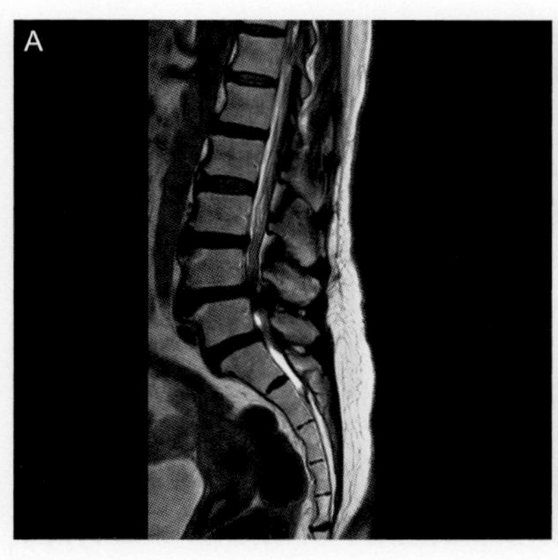

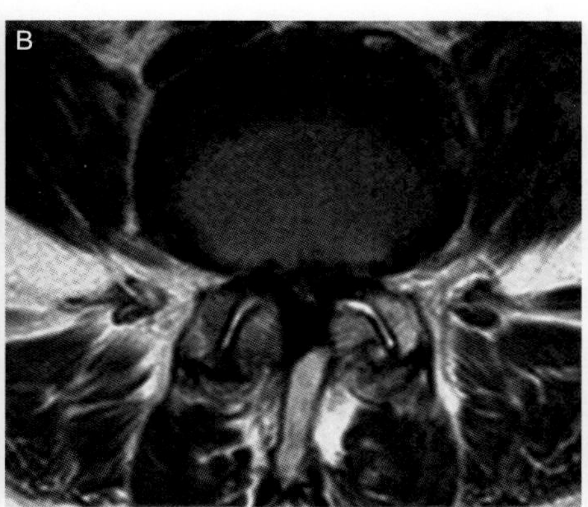

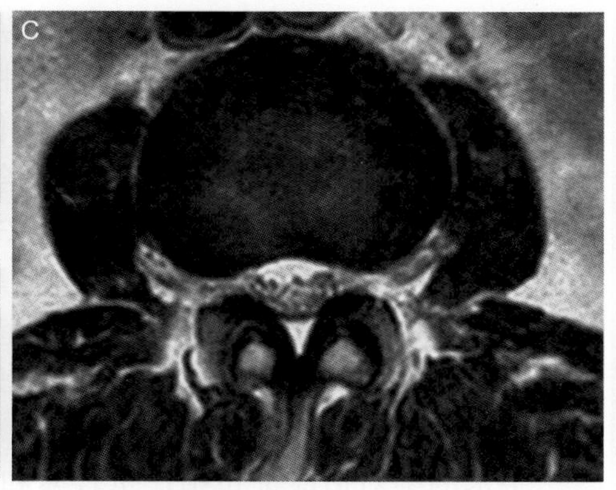

图 62.1 T2 MRI。（A）矢状位：L4/5 腰椎管狭窄症和退行性腰椎滑脱；（B）轴位：继发于椎间盘突出、小关节增生和黄韧带增生的马尾神经受压；（C）轴位：非狭窄平面的比较

由于手术时间长，椎板成形术在 LCS 的治疗中并不常用，也没有证据表明其优于其他方法。

棘突间牵引装置

棘突间牵引装置（interspinous distraction devices, ISD）需要通过棘突间韧带插入垫片，以保留棘上韧带。牵引降低了椎间盘内压力，牵开了关节面和神经孔，使黄韧带伸直，并减少了异常节段运动。它们可以在多个节段使用，L4/5 最常见，由于 S1 棘突小，所以无法在 L5/S1 使用。禁忌证包括脊椎滑脱、肿瘤、外伤、不稳定或高度退行性椎体滑脱和骨质疏松。

根据目前的证据和 2010 年 NICE 指南，ISD 对合适的患者在短期和中期内是有效的，虽然可能出现失败并需进一步手术，但没有重大的安全问题。因此，在临床管理和知情同意充分的情况下可以使用这种治疗方案。

减压融合（器械与非器械）

当有节段性不稳定的证据时，建议联合减压和融合。很难在影像上找到融合的确切证据。一般认为，在存在畸形、中重度腰痛、复发性和交界性狭窄的情况下，或当需要进行大于 50% 的双侧小关节切除减压时，应考虑融合。

有限的证据表明，与单纯减压相比，退行性腰椎滑脱患者的减压加非器械融合可显著改善背部和腿部疼痛。没有证据表明器械融合术在临床结果方面优于非器械融合术，然而，器械融合术确实有更高的融合率。没有证据表明椎间融合（ALIF、PLIF、TLIF 和 XLIF）能改善整体预后。

腰椎间盘突出症与马尾综合征

腰椎间盘突出症（lumbar disc herniation，LDH）是椎间盘在相邻椎体边缘以外的局灶性移位。腰椎间盘突出症和神经根病是脊柱手术最常见的适应证。有症状的腰椎间盘突出症的患病率约为 3%，最常见于 30~50 岁年龄组。腰椎间盘突出症与年龄相关的椎间盘改变有关，创伤性椎间盘突出症并不常见。职业因素（频繁的举重、扭动和振动）和遗传易感性易患腰椎间盘突出症。它通常是良性的，大多数患者在术后 1 个月内恢复。破裂的椎间盘碎片由于被巨噬细胞吞噬，可能在 6 个月内被完全分解。

椎间盘突出的位置决定了哪根神经根受累（即突出物是中央的、侧隐窝的、孔内的还是孔外的）。根据突出椎间盘的形态以及是否突破后纵韧带，腰椎间盘突出症可分为以下几类：突出的椎间盘引起了纤维环变形，但未突破纤维环；突出的椎间盘虽然突破了纤维环但是连续的；突出的椎间盘呈一个独立的碎块。

神经根性疼痛可能是继发于机械和化学刺激。研究表明，单纯的神经根压迫会导致麻木，但不会导致疼痛。压迫导致缺血、水肿和炎症。脑脊液和血流量的减少会导致营养供应减少和清除有害化学物质的能力减弱。

急性腰痛可能先于神经根症状，足下垂和神经系统不协调的病例应考虑周围神经损伤的可能性。

临床特征包括皮肤痛、感觉异常和坐姿、站立和 Valsalva 动作增加的麻木感；肌肉无力、反射减退、活动范围缩小；止痛步态、脊柱受压疼痛；Lasegue 征阳性、Lasegue 征逆转（上腰椎受压）或交叉 Lasegue 征（大盘）。

MRI 是标准的检查方法，而高分辨率计算机断层扫描（CT）或脊髓造影可用于 MRI 检查的替代方法。神经生理学有助于排除周围神经损伤。

保守治疗通常应用在没有马尾综合征或急性足下垂的情况。保证短时间的卧床休息（3 天）是关键，最佳的镇痛包括消炎药和理疗。大多数症状会在 3 个月内消失。持续的严重坐骨神经痛伴感觉运动障碍需要早期行手术治疗，硬膜外和口服皮质类固醇激素可作为辅助治疗。

手术的绝对适应证包括严重轻瘫和马尾综合征。相对适应证包括非反应性严重的坐骨神经痛和最佳保守治疗后持续症状超过 6 周。

手术技术

鉴于无症状椎间盘突出症的发生率高，患者的选择至关重要，临床症状与影像学结果一致且对保守治疗至少 6 周无效的患者，应考虑进行手术。Ⅰ级证据表明与保守治疗相比，手术能改善短期结果，但手术的效果随着时间的推移而下降。标准的手术方式是椎板间入路和显微腰椎间盘切除术。经皮穿刺技术包括内镜椎间盘摘除术、化学髓核溶解术和自动经皮腰椎间盘摘除术。

椎板间入路和显微椎间盘切除术

椎板间入路采用正中切口和双侧或单侧骨膜下剥离肌肉进入椎板间隙。显微椎间盘切除入路与椎板间入路相同。患者取俯卧或侧卧位，患侧在上方。所使用的标准技术类似于 Yasargil、Caspar 和 Williams（**专栏 62.1**）所描述的技术。

专栏 62.1 腰椎间盘切除术

- 在椎间盘平面确定后，在与椎间盘间隙相对应的棘突外侧切开 1.5~2.5 cm 的切口
- 切开棘上韧带旁的腰背筋膜
- 骨膜下剥离椎板上的肌肉
- 置入 Williams 或 McCullough 牵引器
- 显微镜下暴露椎板下极
- 4~5 mm 的高速磨钻用来使磨除椎板，并行内侧小关节切开术
- 可以用刮勺将黄韧带从椎板下分离出来，也可以用 15 号刀片将黄韧带从椎板表面切开，并用 Watson-Cheyne 切开后纵韧带
- 然后可以用 2~3 mm 的 Kerrison 咬骨钳去除黄韧带，露出覆盖在神经根上的硬膜外脂肪。为了帮助识别神经根，可以用 Watson-Cheyne 解剖探查椎弓根
- 神经根显露后，用神经根牵引器将神经根肩部牵开，以显露椎间盘间隙
- 硬膜外间隙中游离的碎片可以用微型垂体咬骨钳清除
- 硬膜外静脉出血可用低功率双极点烧止血
- 下面的后纵韧带和纤维环可用 15 号刀片切开
- 进行充分的椎间盘切除以对神经根充分减压
- 手术是通过切开椎间孔完成的（切除韧带并切开小关节的上关节突）
- 手术前进行充分的止血

并发症

- 椎间盘突出复发（5%）
- 脑脊液漏
- 神经根损伤
- 椎间盘炎

马尾综合征

马尾综合征（cauda equina syndrome，CES）是一种罕见病，年发病率在 1 / 33000~1 / 10 万，是神经外科临床实践中的主要争议。其特点是中央或较大的中央旁椎间盘突出，最常见于腰 4-5，撞击马尾神经，特别是中央性的骶神经根。较小的椎间盘突出可能导致椎管先天性狭窄的患者发生马尾综合征。在腰椎管狭窄的情况下，症状可能是超过几个小时的急性发作，也可能是慢性发生。

根据膀胱和肛门感觉运动受累的程度区分完全性和不完全性病变很重要。假说认为骶神经节前和感觉神经的直径越小越容易受到机械压迫和炎症的损害。

临床特征包括严重的下腰痛，双侧神经根性腿痛（较低的 L5/S1 椎间盘碎片移位疼痛可能消失），排尿功能障碍（尿感改变和尿流不良），肌肉无力，会阴部和生殖器感觉障碍。

完全性病变预后不佳，以神经源性膀胱为特征（继发于低张力的感觉迟钝和扩张，以及括约肌无法协调和收缩导致尿潴留和溢出性尿失禁）。肛门括约肌张力丧失导致大便失禁和生殖器麻木，并伴有三角区感觉丧失和性功能障碍，通常是晚期的症状。

手术时机具有极大的争议，在没有Ⅰ级证据的情况下，临床医生必须务实并以患者的最佳利益行事。顺理成章的是，马尾神经越早减压，恢复的机会就越大。Ahn 等对 322 名患者的 meta 分析（2000）表明了在症状出现后 48 小时内进行减压可得到最佳结果。在症状出现后 24 小时内尽快减压，这似乎是理所当然的，也是被普遍接受的。

标准的手术方式是双侧椎板切除术。对有经验的外科医生，切除大的椎间盘碎片可以通过半椎板切除和内侧小关节切除，或椎板切开和开窗，其优

点是保留了中线结构，较少发生肌肉萎缩，并可减少因椎板切除导致的后背部疼痛。参见图 62.2。

腰痛

80% 的人在一生中会经历过一次背部疼痛。大多数人会经历非特异性腰痛（non-specific back pain，NSBP），在影像上会有一些退行性改变。非特异性腰痛是一种排除性诊断，无神经根压迫或严重潜在病理的特征。疼痛通常是弥漫性的，可能会辐射到大腿。非特异性腰痛是一种良性的自限性疾病，应排除的特异性腰痛的原因，包括肿瘤、炎性疾病、感染、创伤、退行性疾病和畸形。

健康管理包括排除严重的病理和通过一个整体的方法来解决患者的健康信念、期望、回避行为、就业问题和潜在的二次获益。

严格的保守治疗是最重要的：到 12 周，90% 的人将不再痛苦。治疗包括多学科的合作，包括优化止痛、疼痛专家的治疗、定期锻炼、物理治疗、工作调理计划以及适当的心理评估。

椎间盘、小关节和腰椎不稳定可能是特异性腰背部疼痛产生因素，可能对干预有反应

腰椎间盘疾病

腰椎间盘支撑大部分脊柱负荷，充当高效的“减震器”，承受巨大的平移和旋转力。随着年龄的增长，椎间盘会发生机械失效，会发生一些相关的化学和形态学变化，包括椎间盘中的核 / 环区分丧失，1 型和 2 型胶原的比例和分布发生变化，胶原交联断裂，从而增加了纤维环对机械应力的敏感性。纤维环破裂和变形造成了矢状位 / 冠状位椎间盘高度的丧失、核基质蛋白多糖碎裂和椎间盘脱水。软骨细胞数量减少，角蛋白 / 硫酸软骨素比增加，P 物质由于神经纤维新生血管和新神经产生增多，促炎细胞因子，乳酸水平升高和 pH 降低，这些都是有害的。

在椎体终板中，异常的机械负荷导致炎症和 Modic 改变，终板钙化伴随着血供和营养供给减少。对机械应力的敏感性增加，这可能是 Schmorl 结节和椎体边缘增生钙化的原因。

椎间盘疾病的临床特征包括深部中枢性疼痛、大腿前部或腹股沟疼痛，以及在屈曲和长时间坐位时椎间盘负荷加重。

MRI 是腰椎间盘疾病检查的金标准。1988 年，Modic 根据 MRI 信号特征对终板改变进行了分型（**专栏 62.2**）。

随着感染成为下腰痛的潜在致病因素，人们对 Modic 1 型改变重新产生了兴趣。Albert 等（2013）在一项双盲随机对照试验中，介绍了应用复方阿莫西林治疗腰痛和椎间盘 Modic 1 型改变的患者，疗程为 100 天。研究结果令人鼓舞，与安慰剂组相比，抗生素组的致残指数在统计上有显著改善。参见图 62.3。

平片和 CT 在显示椎间盘高度降低、硬化、骨赘

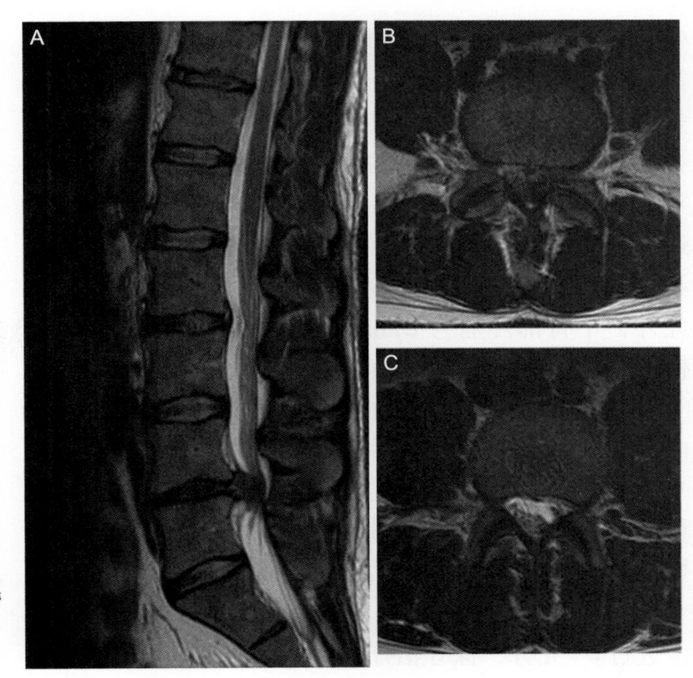

图 62.2 （A）T2 矢状位：巨大的 L4/5 椎间盘突出和马尾神经受压；（B）T2 轴位：硬脊膜受压，完全无脑脊液信号；（C）T2 轴位：腰椎管正常横断面对比

专栏 62.2 Modic 分型

1 型（脊髓炎症和水肿）
- T1 呈低信号，T2 呈高信号

2 型（脂肪脊髓交界型）
- T1 和 T2 均呈高信号

3 型（软骨下骨硬化型）
- T1 和 T2 均呈低信号

Data from Modic MT, Steinberg PM, Ross JS, et al., Degenerative disk disease: assessment of changes in vertebral body marrow with MR imaging, *Radiology*, Volume 166, Issue 1, pp. 193–9, 1988 Radiological Society of North America.

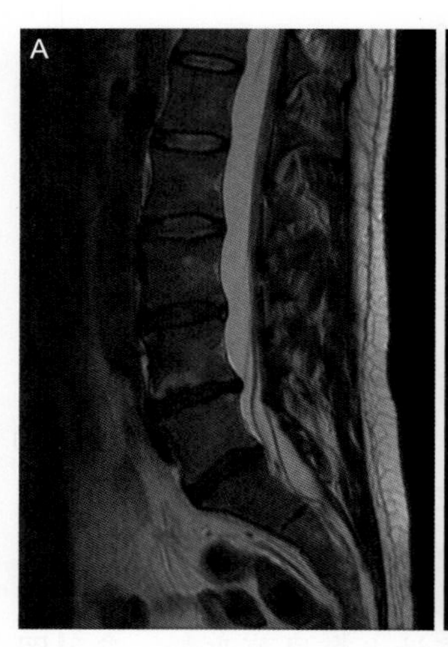

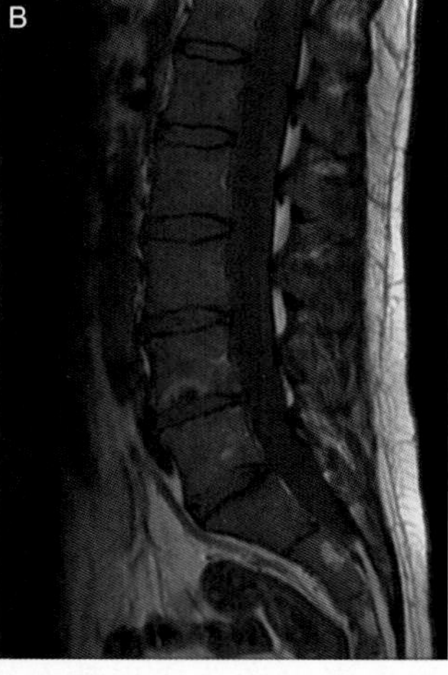

图 62.3 （A）T2 矢状位和（B）T1 矢状位：Modic2 型改变伴有 L4 下终板 Schmorl 结节

生和真空现象上也有一定的价值。腰椎间盘造影可作为选择合适患者进行融合手术的辅助手段。被认为是引起疼痛的椎间盘在 MRI 上被识别并注射，同时，必须对一个 MRI 上正常的椎间盘进行注射，以作为对照，从而确保有效性。单独来讲，症状与椎间盘造影之间的相关性较差，但是，在严重的 Modic1 型和 2 型改变的情况下，症状与椎间盘造影是一致的。此外，下背部疼痛与 Dallas 椎间盘图分级所描述的椎间盘破裂严重程度之间存在相关性。这与 McNally 等（1996）的结论是一致的，他认为椎间盘有明显的内部破裂后仅仅将负荷转移到纤维环是令人痛苦的。

非手术治疗方案包括严格的镇痛、转诊给疼痛科专家、理疗、减肥、定期运动（核心强化活动）和抗生素治疗试验。心理评估和咨询也是需要的。

手术干预在充分的保守治疗被认为是失败后应该进行。“充分”保守治疗的时间是仁者见仁、智者见智的，如果认为手术是患者的最佳选择，则应尽早手术干预。

腰椎间盘疾病的手术治疗可包括：非器械融合、器械融合、椎间盘置换术、动态稳定、椎间盘电热治疗、生物制剂的椎间盘内给药和干细胞植入。

腰椎间盘疾病的手术治疗

非器械融合术

目前很少单独使用非器械融合术，建议将骨性的后外侧融合术与椎弓根螺钉（器械）固定相结合。在临床实践中，目前因继发的相关术后疼痛，很少行髂骨嵴取骨术。后路取骨及使用人工骨替代物是目前比较常用的方法。后外侧融合术因其较高的融合率和令人满意的临床结果而成为与其他非融合术相比较的金标准手术（**专栏** 62.3），这项技术最早于 1911 年用于治疗结核病。

后路椎间盘切除和椎间融合也可以与后外侧融合术结合进行，使融合率提高到近 90%，但神经损伤的风险更大。没有证据表明前路融合优于后路融合术，并有逆行射精和血管损伤的风险。

器械融合术

椎弓根固定技术

椎弓根内固定术始于 20 世纪 70 年代，由于其生物力学稳定性优于经椎板螺钉或椎板钩，迅速成为首选固定器械（**专栏** 62.4）。

这项技术使外科医生能够通过椎弓根进入脊柱的前柱、中柱和后柱，椎弓根是脊柱中最坚固的骨性结构。椎弓根螺钉植入的学习曲线比较陡峭，但对经验丰富的外科医生，椎弓根螺钉的并发症发生率较低，与非器械融合相比能够提供更好的融合率。椎弓根螺钉允许外科医生在需要时广泛减压，而不存在术后不稳定的风险。

专栏 62.3 后外侧融合术：手术要点

- 俯卧位，腰椎处于中间位置
- 中线入路和骨膜下分离肌肉暴露小关节和横突，应用术中透视确定腰椎节段
- 必要时进行减压
- 使用高速磨钻去除后方骨皮质作为融合床
- 髂后上嵴具有良好的成骨性、骨传导性和骨诱导性，仍然是植骨的首选，也可使用减压时收集的自体骨碎片作为植骨替代物

专栏 62.4　椎弓根螺钉：Magerl 技术

- 术前影像学和椎弓根解剖应详细研究。椎体异常可能妨碍螺钉的植入（例如腰椎发育不良和椎弓根发育不良）
- 与 Roy-Camille 技术相比，该技术允许更长的螺钉长度，因此具有更好的生物力学强度
- 患者取俯卧位，腰椎中立，中线入路，骨膜下剥离肌肉。旁正中劈开肌肉入路的创伤更小，不易引起肌肉萎缩，且疼痛更少
- 充分暴露横突和椎弓根，注意保留不融合节段的小关节
- 进钉点位于冠状面横突平分线与矢状面上关节突下外侧的交点处
- 该进钉点可以靠近终板的中间轨迹
- 建议构造的上螺钉（横向过程中的第一个）和更多的超级形式轨迹略低的入口点（横向过程中的较低）和更多的超级形式轨迹被推动在不涉及融合的尾部椎骨的下铰接方面上
- 为避免撞击未参与融合的椎骨的下关节面，建议对上位螺钉采用略低的进钉点（横突下 1/3）和更偏向上内侧的钉道
- 从 L1 到 S1 内倾角从 15° 增加到 30°，术中应使用正位和侧位透视
- 椎板切开术可在螺钉进钉时使用球探在椎管内侧裂口处探查
- 非器械融合术中的磨除皮质的横突可为自体或替代骨移植提供了一个骨融合床
- 根据脊柱前凸的长度和轮廓裁剪的钛棒用螺帽固定并拧紧。万向头螺钉使得无论角度如何都能被容易放置
- 应注意不要将肌肉夹在钉棒结构中导致坏死和疼痛

并发症

- 复位丢失、椎弓根断裂和螺钉断裂
- 螺钉移位
- 神经损伤
- 硬膜撕裂
- 邻椎病
- 血管损伤

椎弓根螺钉固定可以通过椎间融合器来强化。最常见椎间融合器是聚醚醚酮（polyetheretherketone，PEEK）或肽笼，通常在椎间盘切除和终板制备后植入。自体髂骨嵴移植和同种异体股骨头环移植也有报道。椎间融合可通过后路、后外侧（经椎间孔）、外侧（极外侧）或前方入路实现。椎间融合的优点是通过恢复椎间隙高度、椎间盘切除和终板骨赘切除来提高融合率、恢复对线和椎间孔减压（见**图** 62.4）。

经椎间孔入路（TLIF）切除小关节面，单侧入路直接对神经根进行减压，减少对神经根的牵拉和出血。极外侧入路（XLIF）是一种经腰肌入路的微创手术，患者取俯卧位，植入椎间融合器和侧板。优点是手术时间短，出血少。这种手术方式可同时纠正退行性脊柱侧凸，从而成为老年患者的更好的选择。术中电生理监测可尽量避免腰丛损伤。L5/S1 间隙因髂骨阻塞而无法实施这种术式。前路手术（ALIF）的优点是保留了后路结构，充分的减压，且损伤神经结构的风险最小。并发症包括血管损伤和交感神经链损伤，后者导致逆行射精的风险增加。

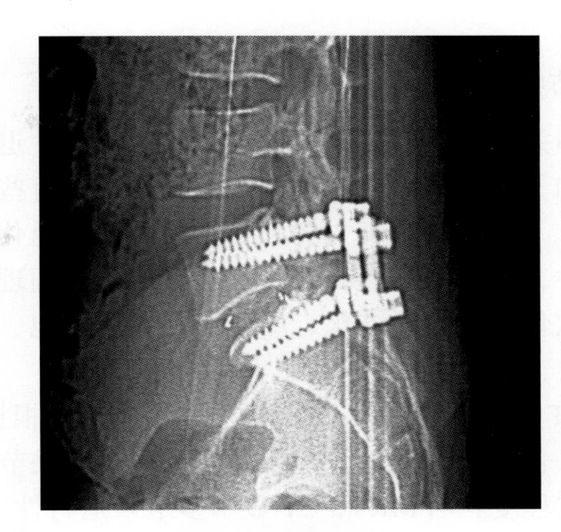

图 62.4　后路腰椎融合术后复查 X 线

椎间盘关节成形术

Fernstrom 于 20 世纪 50 年代首次使用 Fernstrom 球进行腰椎关节成形术。20 世纪 80 年代出现了以 SB Charité 和 ProDisc-L 植入物为标志的现代椎间盘置换术。这种替代品是基于金属板插入一个塑料球和插座形状的装置。该入路为腹膜后入路，与 ALIF 相关的并发症相似。禁忌证包括肥胖症、外伤、医源性因素导致的后路不稳、1 级以上腰椎滑脱、骨质疏松症和外伤。严重的关节突关节病是相对的禁忌证。来自 FDA 的 Ⅰ 级证据表明 Charité 和 ProDisc-L 植入物（Blumenthal et al.，2005；Zigler et al.，2007）与融合相比，在中短期内显示出相似的临床疗效，并且在某些方面更具优越性。David（2007）报道长期临床结果与融合相当，但并发症发生率更低，邻椎病的发生率也更低。腰椎间盘关节成形术已被 NICE 批准，临床医生应发表他们的经验，目前这些植入物的长期效果和有效时间尚不清楚。

动态稳定性

动态稳定是在保持运动范围和减少相邻节段疾病的基础上，同时减少运动节段的负荷。临床数据仍然有限，到目前为止还没有长期随访。

小关节病

小关节支持着 20% 的脊柱负荷。节段性退行性变增加了小关节的负荷和关节病的发生。有些证据表明，下腰椎的垂直方向和各方向的加速退化与不稳定性，畸形和疼痛有关。关节突退变的病理改变包括软骨变薄和纤维化、渗出、关节囊松弛、关节半脱位、骨赘生成和滑膜肥大伴囊肿形成。

CT 诊断小关节病效果最好，Weishaupt 根据 CT 和 MR 表现设计了一个分级系统来描述小关节病变的严重程度。当 MR 和 CT 显示多节段退行性变时，SPECT 可能有助于定位活动性疾病。MRI 上的小关节积液与 SPECT 显示的活动性病变相关。

临床特征包括随活动改善的晨僵，疼痛会随着伸展和扭转运动加剧。位于腹股沟、臀部或大腿后部的疼痛，并可能有局限性椎旁压痛。

保守治疗（包括疼痛专家进行的脊柱注射）是主要治疗方法。“内侧支阻滞（medial branch blockade，MBB）”优于关节内注射。注射疗法应在不同的时机进行，以提高诊断的有效性。有证据表明，MBB 阳性反应预示着射频消融可能有良好的反应。有限的数据表明，射频消融术可以在短期及长期缓解小关节病变导致的疼痛。

不稳定性

“不稳定”仍然是一个神秘的概念；腰椎活动范围正常或无症状的活动度异常是最具争议的疼痛综合征。异常运动更可能会导致纤维环和椎体终板（疼痛发生器）的负荷异常，这增加了脊柱肌肉组织和腱附件的负荷，导致疲劳和疼痛。

临床特征包括背部“屈曲”，疼痛突然随着的轻微运动而增加，背部在运动时“锁定”和“僵硬”并伴有肌肉痉挛。

有报道称腰痛与不稳定有关，表现为动态 X 线片上异常的平移和角度。治疗的重点是提高核心力量，动态稳定装置已被证明可以改变负载模式，这可以解释其在短期内与融合效果相似。

注射治疗

硬膜外注射

硬膜外皮质类固醇注射是一种有效的辅助手段，短期内可缓解腰椎和神经根疼痛。注射类固醇和短效局部麻醉剂的组合，解决根性疼痛的炎症成分，没有证据表明长期有效。腰段硬膜外注射可以通过椎板间（位于关注水平以上）入路进行，也可以通过骶裂孔尾端进行。

腰段硬膜外注射的适应证包括腰椎管狭窄、多节段受累、非特异性疼痛、伴有急性纤维环撕裂的腰痛和无手术适应证。并发症包括脓肿、蛛网膜炎、硬膜外血肿、脑脊液瘘和副神经麻痹。

选择性神经根阻滞

选择性神经根阻滞是一种有效的诊断和治疗方法，用于在影像学与临床症状缺乏一致性时确定或排除手术节段。此外，它们可用于没有神经功能缺损的急性神经根病的短期疼痛缓解。手术时的影像（作者研究使用 CT）对于进入椎弓根下方和神经根上外侧的“安全三角”至关重要。并发症包括疼痛增加、神经根损伤、永久性神经缺损、脑脊液漏和脓肿。

脊椎滑脱

希腊语“olisthanein”的意思是滑倒，Killian 在 1854 年创造了“脊椎滑脱”一词。脊椎滑脱是指关节间的缺陷，可能导致脊椎滑脱。脊椎下垂是指椎体严重滑脱和完全错位。1782 年比利时产科医生 Herbunux 首次描述了这种疾病，1976 年 Wiltse、Newman 和 MacNab 提出了被广泛接受的病因分类（**专栏 62.5**）。

1932 年 Meyerding 分类描述了滑脱的程度，其中 1 级为 1%~25%，2 级为 26%~50%，3 级为 51%~75%，4 级为 76%~100%，5 级为脊椎下垂。

峡部裂型脊椎滑脱

峡部通过椎弓根连接椎弓和椎体，如果峡部断裂，椎体和棘突有可能偏离相应的下关节突和下一椎体的上关节面。令人惊讶的是，虽然施加在峡部的压力巨大，它却是脊柱中最薄弱的骨结构之一。

峡部缺失在儿童晚期出现，在青少年或成年早期成形，其最常见于 L5/S1 节段。其出现的病因是重复的机械应力导致峡部下内侧皮质与上外侧疲劳性骨折。峡部疲劳骨折在运动员中最常见，通常可通过保守治疗治愈。不愈合导致的 A 型骨折处可见纤维组织。重塑、延伸和再愈合形成了 B 型。不到 20% 的腰椎滑脱患者会出现临床症状。峡部型比退行性变更容易出现滑脱。一些学者认为，滑移角（由 S1 上终板和 L5 下终板上端板上的两条线的交点定义的角度）可预测疾病进展。推荐进行临床观察和站立侧位 X 线检查。

临床特征包括运动导致滑脱水平加剧而引起的

专栏 62.5 脊椎滑脱

- 峡部裂最常见于 L5/S1
  - A 型 - 峡部缺失
  - B 型 - 缺损愈合伴部分延长
  - C 型 - 急性双侧骨折
- 退行性变最常见于 L4/5
  - 椎间盘和小关节退变
- 发育不良
  - L5/S1 交界处发育不良
    - L5 楔形发育
    - 穹隆状 S1 上椎体缘
    - L5/S1 关节面水平方向
    - 拟峡型
- 外伤
  - Aihara 分类
- 病理
  - 代谢性骨病
  - 结缔组织病
  - 感染
  - 肿瘤

Reproduced with permission from Leon Wiltse, P. Newman, and Ian MacNab, Classification of Spondylosis and Spondylolisthesis, *Clinical Orthopaedics and Related Research*, Volume 117, pp. 23–9, Copyright © 1976 Wolters Kluwer Health, Inc.

隐匿性中央腰痛、滑脱水平的骨性台阶改变、腰椎前凸增加、扁平臀、蹒跚步态、大腿后部疼痛、腘绳肌痉挛、神经根性疼痛（继发于峡部纤维软骨块压迫最常见于 L5），但中枢性压迫、神经源性症状和马尾综合征少见。年轻患者的 Phalen-Dixon 征表现为坐骨神经危象、腘绳肌痉挛、步态和姿势异常，但是拇长伸肌无力或踝关节背屈是罕见的。

治疗方法

治疗方案包括保守治疗，如严格的疼痛管理及转诊给疼痛专家，限制体力活动，固定和物理治疗。手术治疗的适应证包括：即使充分的保守治疗但疼痛仍然剧烈、进行性神经功能缺损、进行性滑脱和高滑脱角。

手术方法包括直接用椎弓根螺钉修复椎弓根缺损，自体骨移植到缺损部位，神经根彻底减压，后外侧（器械固定或非器械固定）或椎体间融合，或横突线缆捆绑，非器械固定自体骨移植融合。

在有明显的神经根压迫症状的情况下，Gill 所描述的减压，包括切除疏松的后方组织、肥大的纤维软骨和全关节面切除术。建议在行峡部滑脱减压术后行融合术。Caragee（1997）报道单纯减压后假关节发生率较高，且预后较差。器械固定合并植骨融合是否会改善预后以及术后是否需要支撑仍存在争议。

在没有神经根症状的情况下，不需要减压，可以通过中线入路或使用 Wiltse 技术进行融合：在中线切开皮肤和筋膜后，在内侧多裂肌和外侧最长肌形成的凹槽上切开双侧椎旁筋膜。充分利用锐性切开筋膜及钝性分离肌肉间隙，这个平面可充分显露峡部、横突和对小关节进行固定和融合。

器械固定融合可通过椎弓根螺钉固定或椎体间融合实现。这两种技术在效果上是相似的，并不能降低假关节的发生率。一些学者认为融合可以改善继发于不稳定和神经根刺激导致的神经根症状。椎弓根螺钉固定还有另外一个优点，可以减少腰椎滑脱。据称，复位可提高融合率，但引起神经根损伤的概率会增高，见图 62.5。

退行性腰椎滑脱

退行性腰椎滑脱常见于中老年人，通常继发于退行性椎间盘疾病对小关节产生的额外压力。在女性和非裔患者中更为常见，最常发生在 L4/5，这可能与 L4/5 小关节呈矢状方向有关，而 L5/S1 小关节的冠状方向不易发生前移。表现类似为腰椎管狭窄和根性疼痛，这些疼痛是由于 L5 神经根被滑脱的下关节突、肥大的小关节和疝出的椎间盘压迫所致。马尾综合征较少见，但可能发生在亚急性椎间盘突出时。自然史表明，这是一种相对良性的疾病，进展率低至 25%，滑脱很少进展到 Meyerding 分级一级以上。

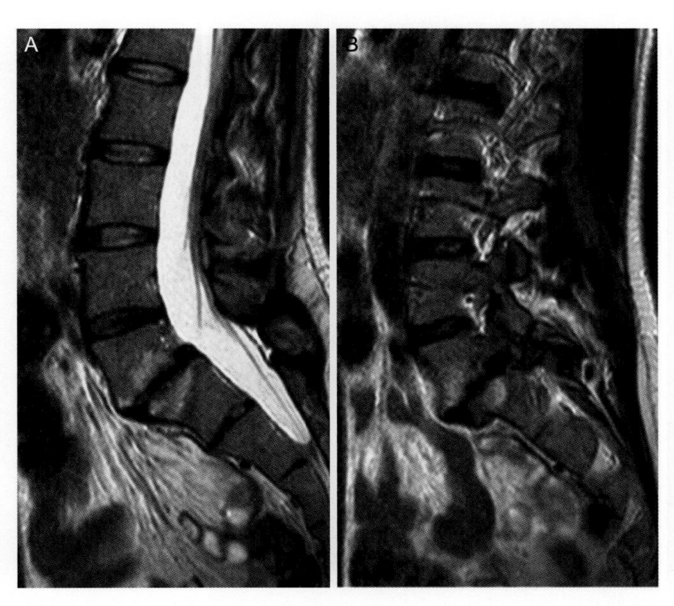

图 62.5 A、B 图示矢状位 T2 像。（A）示 L5 发育不良和 1 级峡部滑脱。（B）示 L5 峡部溶解

非手术治疗包括有效的疼痛管理和物理治疗，当有神经根症状时，可使用硬膜外或神经周围阻滞治疗。在采用充分的保守治疗后仍然有症状的患者应采用手术治疗。几项研究表明，手术治疗与药物治疗相比，在功能和疼痛方面效果更好，见**图** 62.6。

对于退行性腰椎滑脱，单独减压或减压并融合仍有争议，治疗应基于个体因素，如年龄、并发病、骨质量、继发于不稳定的腰痛、动态 X 线片、滑脱程度和术中发现的节段不稳定。

脊柱滑膜囊肿

这些相对罕见的囊肿与脊椎病有关，通常是偶然发现的，最常见于 L4/5，也可见于颈胸段。据称，最常见于异常运动导致的黏液样变性和滑膜肥大。

组织学上，囊肿壁可能有或没有滑膜（神经节囊肿），但是这仅仅是一种学术观点。临床表现通常为神经根性疼痛，其由于小囊肿导致的关节下间隙受压导致。偶尔会有继发于囊肿出血的急性恶化，很少有马尾综合征，通常会自行缓解。

这些囊肿通常可以根据 MR 特征和位置与其他病变相鉴别。鉴别诊断包括神经鞘瘤、突出的椎间盘碎片或硬膜内椎间盘碎片、脊膜囊肿、蛛网膜突出、神经周围囊肿或转移性沉积。

尤其重要的是要认识到这些囊肿，因为它们可能在手术过程中被不经意地引流，并被错误地认为是椎间盘突出碎片。根据囊肿的组成和是否有出血，MR 特征可能有所不同。囊肿壁钙化在 T1 和 T2 呈低信号，出血在 T1 呈高信号。可见囊肿清楚地与小关节间隙沟通，从而区别于神经来源的囊肿。注射造影剂后，囊肿可出现囊肿壁强化。

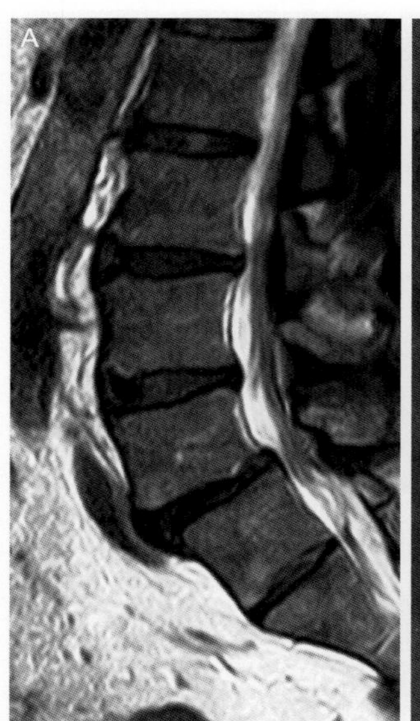

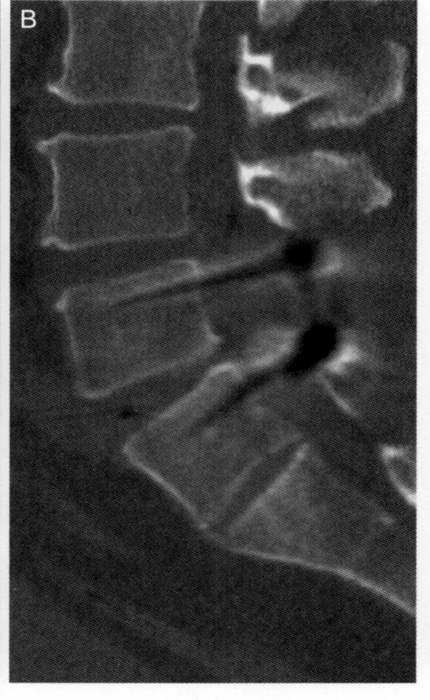

图 62.6 （A）T2 矢状位 MR 显示 1 级腰椎滑脱。（B）同一患者术后 CT 显示后路椎间融合后滑脱复位

治疗方法

现有的文献均由少数病例系列组成，经过适当的保守治疗（包括严格的镇痛、关节突和靶向神经根周围注射）后考虑采用手术治疗。标准的方法是开放性囊肿摘除和椎间孔切开 + 融合。单纯减压的复发率约为 2%。融合的复发率较低，对于有节段性不稳定的临床或放射学证据的患者应考虑融合。微创切除和抽吸也有报道，但复发率较高。见**图** 62.7。

脊膜囊肿

这些罕见的含有脑脊液的薄壁囊肿可能由蛛网膜憩室、硬脑膜憩室或腰椎内神经根鞘形成，通常是 MRI 偶然发现的。可根据 Nabor 分类（见**专栏** 62.6）。

Tarlov 囊肿（Nabor 2 型）

患病率为 5%~9%，大多数囊肿是偶然发现的，最常见于 S2 和 S3 神经根，骶骨常有变形，其病因不明，但可能是由于神经周围间隙不完全闭塞和脑脊液搏动所致。它们出现在神经根和背根神经节交界处的神经内膜和神经束膜之间，包裹或涉及神经根，受压的神经纤维形成囊壁的一部分。与脑膜憩室相比，脑膜憩室与蛛网膜下腔有潜在的联系，Tarlov 囊肿发生在背根神经节附近，与蛛网膜下腔自由沟通。

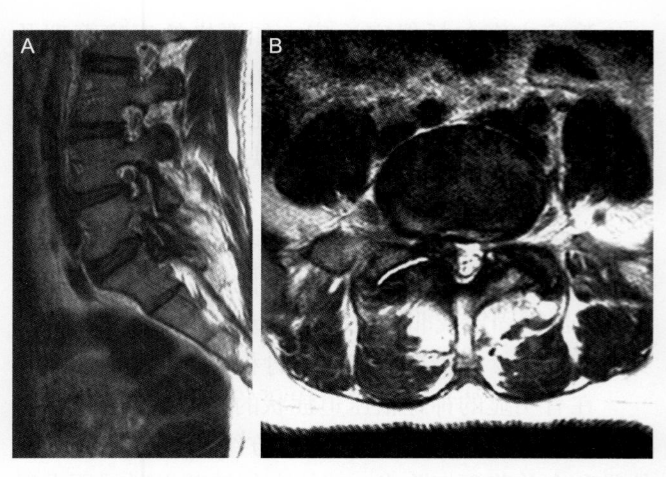

图 62.7 T2 MRI 矢状位（A）和轴位（B）图像显示右侧 L5/S1

专栏 62.6 脊膜囊肿

- 1 型 - 无神经组织的硬膜外脊膜膜囊肿
  - 1a 型 - 硬膜外蛛网膜囊肿
  - 1b 型 - 骶骨脊膜膨出
- 2 型 - 含神经组织的硬膜外脊膜囊肿（轴位神经 /Tarlov 囊肿）
- 3 型 - 硬膜内蛛网膜囊肿

Source data from Nabors MW, Pait TG, Byrd EB et-al. Updated assessment and current classification of spinal meningeal cysts. *J. Neurosurg*. 1988;68 (3): 366-77.

CT 脊髓造影检查晚期或无充盈，而其他脑膜囊肿则是早期充盈。

囊肿很少会产生占位效应，并伴有 Valsalva 手法会加重的疼痛。骶骨不全骨折通常继发于扇形骶骨。

该囊肿通常无症状，其常见的临床特征可包括进行性骶神经根痛、麻木和感觉异常、骶骨、会阴或直肠疼痛以及肠、膀胱和性功能障碍。

非手术治疗包括充分的疼痛管理，据报道脑脊液引流可以暂时缓解症状，很少出现经过严格疼痛治疗后仍出现进行性症状加重，以至于需要进行手术的患者。有病例报告显示，可通过 CT 引导下注射纤维蛋白封闭腰 - 腹腔或膀胱 - 蛛网膜下腔效果良好。确切的治疗方法包括骶板切除术、囊肿开窗 / 切除术和骶棘肌皮瓣闭合术，建议在电生理监测下进行手术。

骶髂关节病

骶髂关节是髂骨和骶骨之间的一个滑膜和纤维关节，它将重量从轴骨转移到阑尾骨，其可进行轻微的旋转和滑动。韧带松弛通常会导致怀孕期间骶髂关节疼痛。骶髂关节炎是一系列疾病的表现，可能与腰椎病理相似。常见的症状包括腰部、臀部和大腿疼痛，久坐会加剧疼痛。New York 标准提出了一种基于 X 线平片上硬化和强直程度的分级系统。疾病的确诊应该基于病史和临床检查。可通过骨盆挤压分离试验和 X 线片上的病理变化确诊。临床表现提供了潜在病因的线索（对称和双侧，不对称和双侧，或单侧）。鉴别诊断包括炎症性关节炎、感染和肿瘤。

治疗包括治疗潜在的病因，严格的疼痛管理，骶髂关节注射和物理治疗。关节融合术是患者在接受充分的保守治疗后仍出现进行性和失能性疼痛的选择。

尾骨痛

尾骨痛是指尾骨周围的疼痛，久坐和从久坐后站立会加重症状。确切的发病率未知，但危险因素可能是肥胖和女性。该疾病在男性中相当罕见，值得进一步研究潜在的病理，体检时有明显的压痛。直肠检查可见尾骨移动范围增大或减少。

病因包括骨关节炎、局部创伤、过度活动、感染、盆腔炎性疾病 / 慢性感染和肿瘤（原发性局部骨肿瘤、神经鞘瘤、盆腔肿瘤或转移性肿瘤的直接播散）。90% 的病例可通过保守治疗痊愈。包括非甾体抗炎药（NSAIDs），腰围固定，鼓励腰椎前凸和使用特别设计的垫子以减少对该区域的压力。手法复位可能会发现脱臼的尾骨并有治疗作用。

其他选择包括皮质类固醇局部注射、尾侧硬膜外皮质类固醇注射、交感神经阻滞或尾骨切除术（有效率各不相同，只有在保守措施用尽后才应考虑）。

术后症状缓解不满意和术后并发症的处理

“failed back syndrome”是指脊柱手术后未能达到满意程度的患者群体。这一术语并不意味着治疗失误，更多的是指患者出现超出预期的持续疼痛，这可能会导致工作能力的丧失并妨碍重返工作岗位。当手术效果不佳时，应回答三个问题：一、手术方式的选择正确吗？例如：对退行性腰椎滑脱患者行单独减压术患者术后腰痛加重。二、诊断正确吗？例如在髋关节和膝关节存在病变的情况下进行腰椎手术，或在肩关节或尺神经或正中神经病变并存的情况下进行颈椎手术。糖尿病、血管炎和营养缺乏等导致神经功能障碍的疾病应始终牢记。三、对这个患者来说是正确的治疗方法吗？例如：对患者的动机、期望水平和心理健康的评估很重要，并充分意识到潜在的次生利益和可能的诉讼。

这种思考方式有助于反思性实践，然而，有时会出现超出临床医生控制的不好的结果。复发性或持续性轴性和根性疼痛可能由以下情况引起：残留的椎间盘和骨赘压迫、复发性椎间盘突出、邻近节段疾病、硬膜外瘢痕形成和纤维化、术后椎间盘炎（感染性和无菌性）、假性脑膜膨出形成、硬膜外血肿、蛛网膜炎、永久性神经根损伤、牵拉或切开硬膜时的损伤、连体神经根（在与手术相邻的节段压迫），进行性脊椎病和不稳定、未能认识到矢状位失衡导致的肌肉疲劳和畸形、肌筋膜综合征和复杂的局部疼痛综合征并存。

确定疼痛的性质是很重要的。烧灼痛是继发于神经损伤的神经病理性疼痛的特征，包括复杂的局部疼痛综合征。这种类型的疼痛最好用神经营养药物治疗，并转诊给疼痛专家，也可考虑脊髓电刺激等神经调节。

矢状面失衡可通过背部伸肌的收缩纠正，骨盆倾角增大会导致疼痛和疲劳。疼痛会导致失能，而畸形会导致不良的自我形象和水平凝视障碍，从而产生社会心理影响。畸形的矫正可通过积极的外科手术实现，如 Smith–Peterson 截骨术和椎弓根截骨术。

硬膜损伤和假性脊膜膨出

硬膜不慎损伤的的发生率约为 15%，在翻修手术中发生率更高。就其本身而言，它很少导致损伤，但可能会出现一些并发症，包括神经根或马尾神经损伤（挫伤或撕裂伤）、持续性脑脊液漏（假性脑脊膜膨出或脑脊液瘘）、脑膜炎、蛛网膜炎和慢性头痛。

在翻修手术中，由于瘢痕组织的形成和可辨认的组织平面的丢失，这种情况更为常见。在有慢性椎管狭窄的老年人中，硬膜可能非常薄。潜在的病理变化可能导致硬膜或神经根套位于不正常的位置。器械不慎滑动和 Kerrison 不慎卡住硬膜造成的损伤最为常见。外科医生应该小心地将骨刺磨圆，因为这可能导致迟发性脑脊液漏。

治疗方法包括显微镜下破损修复，如果硬膜切口很小，神经根疝出会使硬膜很难缝合，应该注意防止术中缝线刮伤或扎住神经根。在这种情况下，硬膜切口应该延长，并在缝合过程中使用棉片保护神经根。如果硬膜破口在腹侧面，可以从背侧切开硬膜后进行硬膜内修补。如果神经根套受累或有硬膜缺损较大，这时强行缝合硬膜可能卡压马尾神经，在这种情况下，可使用患者的血液、脂肪或肌肉移植修补硬膜。作者倾向于使用分层的组织、粉碎的肌肉组织和凝固的血液或者纤维蛋白封闭剂，如 Tisseel。

术后的恢复通常需要 3~5 天的平卧位休息，如果硬膜开口很小，蛛网膜保持完整，没有脑脊液漏，那么在硬膜缝合后可不进行严格的平卧位。切口和腰椎引流管的使用是有争议的，是否采用基本取决于外科医生的偏好。对于卧床休息的患者，预防下肢深静脉血栓是很重要的。

含有脑脊液的硬膜疝出称为假性脊膜膨出。肌肉张力过高可引起创伤、脑脊液瘘和感染。症状包括低压性头痛、腰痛和神经根症状。磁共振检查是必要的，为鉴别血肿和感染，可抽吸后进行相应的实验室检查，β-2 转铁蛋白生物标志物可以区分脑脊液和血肿。对于有症状的假性脊膜膨出，可尝试进行腰椎引流，最终修复需要按照前面所述进行开放性修复。在修复失败或硬脊膜破口难以确定时可使用 MR（脂肪抑制序列）、MR、CT 和数字减影脊髓造影。在复发病例中，建议联合整形科考虑皮瓣重建。

术后椎间盘炎

术后椎间盘炎罕有发生，发生率约为 1%，80% 的病例一般在术后第一个月内出现。危险因素包括老年人、糖尿病、免疫抑制和伴随的全身感染。

临床特征包括中至重度腰痛和痉挛、发热、活动范围受限和压痛，但神经根症状罕见，很少有患者会出现伤口感染。

手术后无菌或化学性椎间盘炎的发生均有报道。临床医生除了应进行积极的影像学检查，还应关注感染性血液指标，如白细胞计数（中性粒细胞）、CRP 和血沉（erythrocyte sedimentation rate，ESR）。提示感染的 MR 表现包括椎前和硬膜外增强，伴有椎间盘强化和终板水肿。

若怀疑出现术后椎间盘炎，应进行细菌培养。在大约 40% 的病例中，椎间盘穿刺活检提供了阳性微生物学指标。表皮葡萄球菌、金黄色葡萄球菌、革兰阴性菌和链球菌最常见。厌氧菌、结核菌和真菌不常见。每周应观察感染指标，直至稳定或正常。

可进行积极的心理引导治疗（某些情况下可在社区进行）至少持续 6 周静脉注射抗真菌作用的抗生素。如果感染对口服药物（如氟氯嘧啶和梭酸）有反应，则可在微生物学的指导下进行长时间的观察。在治疗结束前，可进行增强 MRI 扫描以进行对比。在耐药的病例中，可考虑通过开放或微创的方法进行椎间盘切除和冲洗。

文献报道的结果不一，大约 80% 的患者腰痛明显改善，这与腰椎间盘术后的结果相似。

蛛网膜炎性粘连

蛛网膜炎会累及硬脊膜的三层，炎症会导致神经根粘连，有学者认为，粘连过程除了机械损伤性拴系，还引起了流向神经根的血液和脑脊液减少。MR 增强提示处于急性期，应进一步密切关注和监测，特别是在潜在病因不确定的情况下。

MRI 上可观察到三种类型，即中央型粘连、中央索发育和神经根与鞘膜粘连型，所形成的空腔中脑脊液被炎性组织所取代（CT 血管造影上被阻塞或呈“蜡滴征”)。

蛛网膜炎性粘连偶尔与退行性疾病有关，通常是偶然发现的。继发于外伤的蛛网膜炎性粘连通常与脊髓空洞的形成有关。发展为蛛网膜炎的危险因素包括意外的硬膜损伤、脑脊液漏、鞘内出血、感染、创伤、脊柱麻醉、曾做过脊髓碘油造影和肿瘤形成。

与蛛网膜炎相关的神经根性疼痛预后较差，治疗的目的是通过完善的疼痛管理，理疗和心理支持达到症状缓解。手术的效果不能令人满意，手术方式包括切除狭窄的硬膜外瘢痕组织和椎间孔。

复发性腰椎间盘突出症的治疗

复发性腰椎间盘突出症的严格定义是在最少6小时的无痛期后在先前手术节段的同侧或对侧再次出现疼痛，复发率在5%~12%。鉴别诊断包括进行性神经周围纤维化和蛛网膜炎。

腰椎MR增强成像提供有价值的诊断信息，与突出的髓核相比，神经周围疤痕增强，如神经鞘膜和神经根向病变处收缩提示纤维化；相反，神经鞘膜移位提示复发性突出碎片。没有证据表明保守的死骨切除术或环切术与更积极的椎间盘切除术相比会影响复发率。

应仔细记录病史，明确疼痛的性质，弥漫性烧灼性疼痛提示神经性疼痛，对手术无反应。有假说提出神经周围纤维化可能导致神经根收缩、慢性缺血和神经损伤。

硬脊膜切开后再手术会增加20%的神经损伤的风险。因此，一些作者主张采用更积极的方法，包括从外侧切除椎间盘突出平面的同侧小关节，并使用该通道对突出椎间盘和神经根受压迫区的内侧减压。这种方法要求器械融合合并或不合并椎间融合，据称这也降低了再次复发的风险。

Dower等(2016)的meta分析指出，没有证据表明常规融合治疗复发性腰椎间盘突出症可改善预后。因此，推荐针对不同患者采用实用的和个性化的治疗，如果有临床或影像学上表明节段性不稳定，那么应施行融合术。同样，如果术中行小关节切除术时发现广泛的纤维化，应准备实施融合术。

脊柱内镜和微创手术的经验随着内镜下经椎间孔腰椎间盘切除术、微创经椎间孔腰椎间融合术和经皮椎弓根螺钉固定术的发展而不断发展。在未来，对这些技术进行长期的随访是有趣的。

伴有神经根症状的退行性腰椎滑脱：单纯减压与减压并融合(器械与非器械)

据报道，单纯减压术后腰椎滑脱并再次出现症状的发生率高达50%。术前动力位(侧位)腰椎X线片不能预测腰椎不稳，但有时可发现异常平移(大于4mm时)。Mardjetko(1994)的meta分析证实了减压融合(器械和非器械)与单纯减压的临床效果。Gibson和Waddell(2005)进行的meta分析和系统评价证实了内固定与非内固定融合相比融合率更高、临床疗效更好，同时并发症发生率更高。脊柱患者结果研究试验(SPORT)发现，在比较各种不同的融合技术时，结果没有显著差异。

延伸阅读、参考文献、EBRAIN的相关链接

扫描书末二维码获取。

第 63 章　脊柱肿瘤

John Brecknell・Boon Leong Quah 著
范存刚、汤韫钰 译，范存刚 审校

多样性

对脊柱神经外科医生而言，脊柱肿瘤的病变类型、临床表现及其治疗所必备的手术操作技术均十分复杂：就病变类型而言，既可以是长达十余年的观察中保持不变的良性病变，也可以是数小时内进展为截瘫的恶性病变；在手术操作技术方面，既包括最精细的显微手术，也包括对多个脊柱节段进行内固定的手术操作。本章涉及的内容很宽泛，但未包括脊柱的非肿瘤性占位的治疗，也未包括儿童脊柱肿瘤的特殊治疗方法。

将复杂的脊柱肿瘤分为两大类（起源于硬膜囊内的肿瘤和起源于硬膜外的肿瘤）有助于使其简化，同时位于这两个腔室的肿瘤很少见。起源于硬膜内的肿瘤主要是位于枕骨大孔以下的各类肿瘤，其病理类型主要为良性肿瘤；起源于硬膜外的肿瘤以转移性恶性肿瘤为主，也包括源于脊柱结缔组织和血液系统的肿瘤。

常见的基本临床表现

虽然脊柱肿瘤的类型各不相同，但仍有一些共同之处，特别是在临床表现和检查方面。在脊柱肿瘤患者得以诊断之前，用于阐明每例患者上述特征的临床方法也有共同之处。

疼痛

疼痛是脊柱肿瘤患者最常见的症状。当患者的疼痛位于局部时，通常为肿瘤作用于脊柱内的痛觉感受器所致，有直接应力变形、静脉充血和椎骨的病理性骨折等多种机制参与。这种疼痛通常为持续性，呈进行性加重，表明肿瘤在增长。夜间和卧位时疼痛加剧，这种现象通常为平躺时硬膜外静脉丛扩张导致静脉充血加重所致。在转为直立位以及运动时疼痛突然加剧提示可能发生了病理性骨折。

疼痛也可发生在肿瘤的远隔部位，这类疼痛多为脊柱的神经结构受压所致。由肿瘤或变形的脊柱结构使一条或多条神经根受压是引起放射痛的较为常见的原因，马尾神经受压可导致神经源性跛行。脊髓损伤可引起伴有烧灼样感觉异常的中枢性神经痛。虽然这类疼痛可能最常见于脊髓本身的肿瘤，但也可由外部压迫（如转移瘤）致脊髓损伤引起 。

80%~90% 的转移瘤所致脊髓压迫症患者的首发症状是疼痛，95% 的患者在就诊时已有疼痛（Cole and Patchell，2008）。3/4 以上的脊柱原发性骨肿瘤以疼痛就诊，约半数没有其他症状。一项报道了 438 名患者的大宗病例的作者认为，这种局部疼痛通常为骨内肿瘤扩张所致，但病理性骨折和神经根压迫也可引起局部疼痛（Dang et al.，2015）。仅稍过半数的硬膜内肿瘤患者会出现疼痛（Wu et al.，2014）；但位于脊髓圆锥以下的肿瘤大部分可引起疼痛，其比例升至 80% 以上。

神经功能缺损

脊柱肿瘤的另一类重要症候群为受累的脊柱神经结构功能障碍所致，其中以脊髓受累最为重要。虽然作用于脊髓的压力可直接造成轴突损伤并引起脱髓鞘，但血管机制可能是造成脊髓损伤的主要原因——初期为静脉受压引起脊髓充血和水肿，后期为动脉功能不全引起脊髓缺血和梗死（Baptiste and Fehlings，2006）。

虽然转移瘤所致脊髓压迫症作为一种临床综合征以神经功能缺损为特征，但所有以脊柱肿瘤就诊的患者中，无论其肿瘤类型如何，约半数会出现神经功能缺损。神经功能缺损按发生率依次为无力、感觉障碍、平衡障碍和尿失禁。

其他表现

脊柱畸形可能为转移瘤或原发性骨肿瘤引起的肌肉骨骼破坏所致，但作为主要特征或唯一的就诊表现者罕见。以脊柱侧凸就诊的髓内肿瘤罕见，但也可见于儿童。

值得注意的是，脊柱肿瘤也可偶然发现。在磁共振时代，脊柱专业的所有医务人员都会遇到常见的椎体血管瘤。在磁共振时代以前，一项基于病理学或放射学平片的研究估算这类良性血管肿瘤的患病率约为10%（Fox and Onofrio，1993），而最近伊朗的一项因其他原因行MR检查的研究估算该病的患病率高达27%（Barzin and Maleki，2009）。原发性骨肿瘤（4%，Dang et al，2015）和硬膜内髓外肿瘤（4/18，Marchetti et al，2013）的病例系列也报告了一些占比较低的偶发案例。然而，偶然发现的脊髓本身的肿瘤却极为罕见（0/89，Li et al，2014）。转移性脊柱肿瘤通常是在原发灶诊断后为进行肿瘤分期检查时发现，即使并非完全偶然，通常也是无症状的病灶。

鉴别诊断

脊柱疼痛是“几乎普遍存在的人类疾病”（Hall，2014）。例如，约1/4美国成人在过去3个月里至少有一天背痛。腰背痛的终生患病率可能高达80%，其中绝大多数并无明确异常发现（Srinivas et al.，2012）。由于脊柱肿瘤较为少见，其发生率较腰背痛低几个数量级，因此很容易被忽视。也许正是基于上述缘由，良性硬膜内肿瘤患者从症状出现到诊断的中位时间通常可长达25个月（Manzano et al，2008），甚至在没有先前确诊原发灶的情况下，脊柱转移瘤患者从症状出现到诊断的时间也可长达200天（Quraishi et al，2014）。

累及脊柱并表现为疼痛和神经功能障碍的病变范围十分广泛。感染性病变可引起脊柱破坏并危及脊髓，也可浸润至硬膜外腔。虽然继发于骨质疏松的不全性骨折很少引起神经功能缺损，但可能难以与继发于肿瘤的骨折相鉴别。退行性脊柱疾病以轴向脊柱痛和脊髓病就诊，与硬膜外肿瘤相似，或表现为类似于硬膜内髓外肿瘤的根性疼痛。疼痛表现缺如有助于鉴别脊髓病的许多神经源性病因与肿瘤。

影像学

自20世纪90年代广泛应用以来，磁共振成像（magnetic resonance imaging，MRI）已成为检查脊柱疼痛和神经功能缺损的首选成像方式。虽然基于医疗保健经济学或避免对正常人过度医疗应适当限制MRI在脊柱疼痛这类常见主诉患者中的应用（Srinivas et al.，2012），但对于有危险信号或6周内新发疼痛的患者，MRI可作为一种非侵袭性检查方法；如果不进行MRI检查，则难以对可能存在的严重脊柱肿瘤做出诊断。

MRI平扫或钆增强扫描是疑诊脊柱肿瘤患者的首选检查方法。MRI提供了对脊柱各腔室极高的分辨率，能提供充足的信息以区分血液与囊液、增强的实性肿瘤与脊髓。尤其重要的是，根据现有的影像资料，通过分析肿瘤与脊髓和硬膜的关系可确定肿瘤位于脊柱的哪个腔室（**图63.1**）。如疑为转移瘤所致脊髓压迫症，在24小时内进行全脊柱MRI是金标准。

如有MRI检查禁忌，可使用计算机断层扫描（computed tomography，CT）脊髓造影术（**图63.2**）。脊柱CT可作为MRI的补充检查手段，为评估骨性结构的首选影像学检查，在肿瘤侵犯或破坏脊柱骨性结构的成像和显示病理性骨折方面具有重要价值。脊柱CT也可用于压缩骨折和脊柱不稳定患者进行器械固定的手术计划。胸部、腹部和骨盆CT可广泛用于寻找其他部位转移灶和原发灶，核素骨扫描也有助于筛查其他部位的骨转移灶。CT是引导脊柱肿瘤经皮穿刺活检的主要影像学检查，但肿瘤活检很少用于硬膜内病变。

单纯X线平片检查对脊柱肿瘤的诊断不敏感，仅用于术中确定脊柱节段和器械固定术后成像。对于富血管肿瘤，如血管母细胞瘤、脊椎血管瘤和肾转移癌，数字减影血管造影（digital subtraction angiography，DSA）可作为确定供血血管的脊柱节段和进行异常血管成像的重要手段。此外，还可在DSA检查过程中进行栓塞治疗，以减少术中出血。超声检查仅限于儿童患者和术中定位。

治疗方式

脊柱肿瘤患者的即刻处理措施包括镇痛、预防血栓栓塞以及对必要部位进行制动。肿瘤性脊柱破坏的不稳定很少像创伤性脊柱破坏那样严重，通常卧床休息即可。地塞米松是一种合成的糖皮质激素，具有抗炎作用，有助于镇痛和改善神经功能。对某些血液系统肿瘤而言，地塞米松还具有抗肿瘤功效，能迅速缓解脊髓受压。快速使用地塞米松也可以改善转移瘤所致脊髓压迫症患者的运动功能转归（Sorensen et al.，1994），且广泛用于脊柱肿瘤手术治疗前，以通过神经保护效应改善神经功能转归。

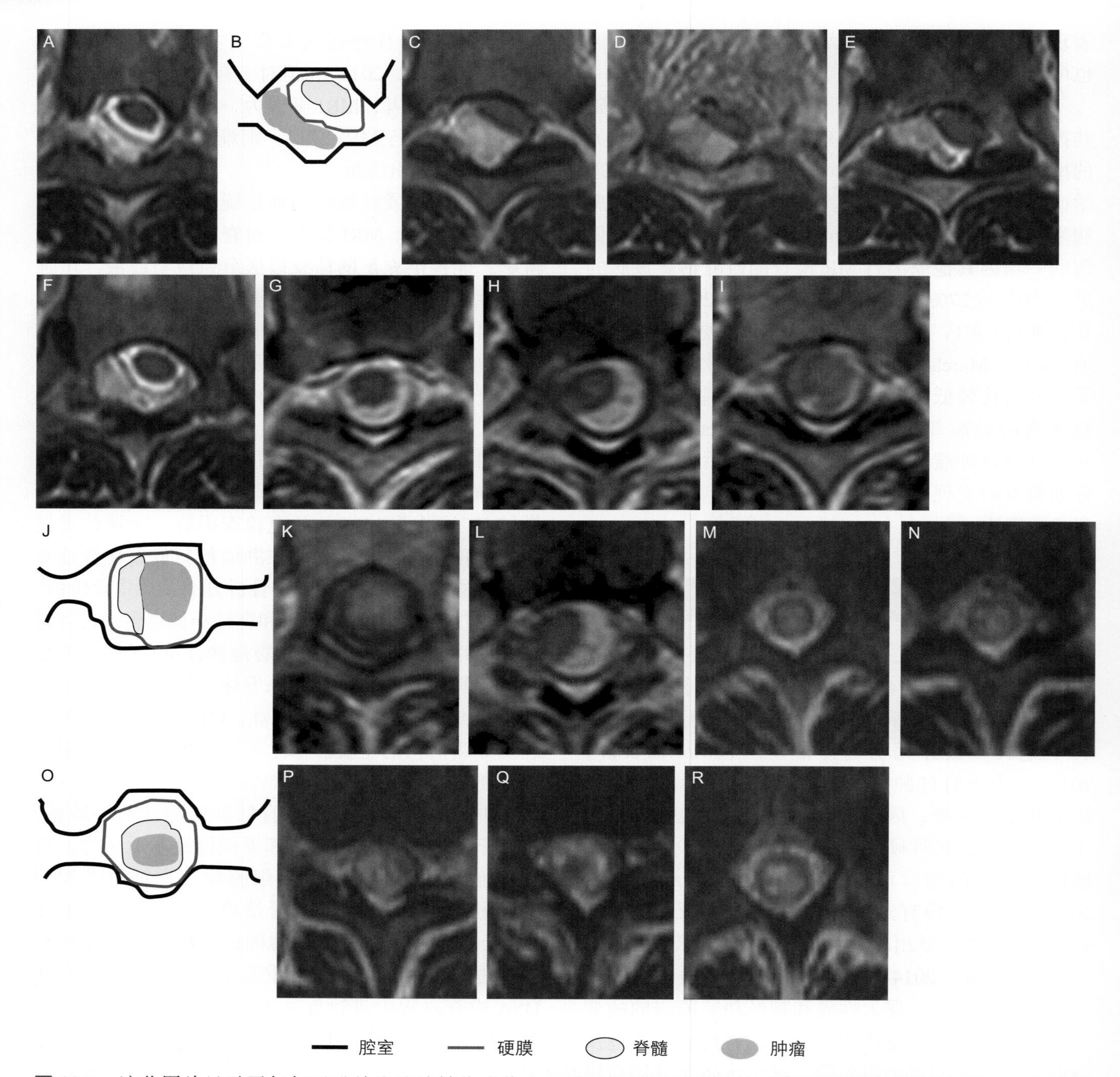

图 63.1 这些图片显示了如何通过关注连续轴位成像中肿瘤与脊髓和硬膜的关系确定脊髓肿瘤所处的腔室：硬膜外（A~F）、硬膜内髓外（G~L）或髓内（M~R）

手术

大部分脊柱肿瘤患者应向脊柱外科咨询，以明确手术干预在诊断、缓解症状、改善预后甚或治愈肿瘤方面的作用。对于某些患者而言，特别恶性肿瘤广泛播散、预后很差的患者，手术治疗可能价值不大；但对于大部分硬膜内肿瘤患者，手术为治疗方案的核心环节。

以骶骨为参考点进行肿瘤的矢状位成像是骶骨、腰椎和胸椎肿瘤手术计划所必需的。枕骨可作为颈椎和上胸椎肿瘤的参考点。这些术前影像有助于术中通过影像增强器进行肿瘤定位并合理地设计手术切口。摆放体位时应特别注意预防皮肤、周围神经和面部受压引起损伤。麻醉诱导期使用单剂抗生素（如头孢呋辛 750 mg）预防感染是合理的。如果术前已使用低分子肝素预防因活动减少导致静脉血栓栓塞（venous thromboembolism，VTE），可在术前 24 小时停用，术后不再使用，以降低术中出血和术后

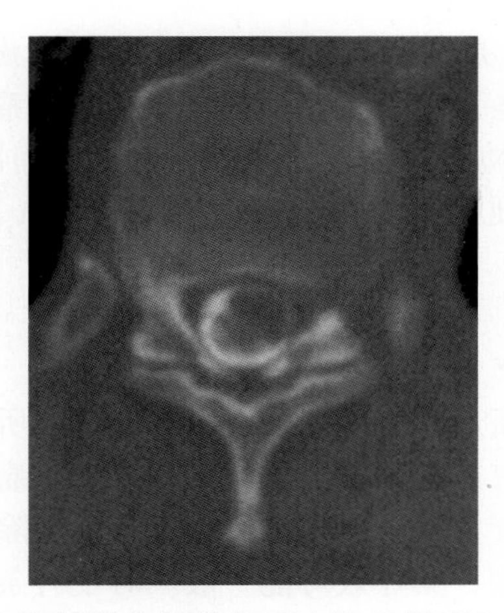

图 63.2　胸椎硬膜内髓外肿瘤（神经鞘瘤）的 CT 脊髓造影

血肿的风险。术中常使用分级加压弹力袜和间歇性小腿加压。

椎管内入路

椎板切除术是切除椎管内肿瘤的标准手术入路。虽然该入路能为处理硬膜内和硬膜外的椎管病变提供良好显露，但仍有术后疼痛和椎板切除术后脊柱后凸等困扰，在儿童患者中尤为明显。为此，有人开始探索替代的手术入路，包括椎板成形术、半椎板切除术（**图** 63.3）和微创的脊柱手术技术。半椎板切除术也可用于转移瘤所致的脊髓压迫症（metastatic spinal cord compression，MSCC）的脊髓减压，不会使脊柱不稳定加重，可作为更大范围器械固定手术的替代方法，如下文所述（**图** 63.3；另见 Millward et al.，2015）。

向侧方扩展的体积较大的肿瘤可能需要切除小关节和椎弓根，以充分显露肿瘤并实现全切。虽然腹侧入路手术已用于切除脊柱肿瘤，但硬膜外和硬膜内肿瘤的腹侧部分均可从背侧和背外侧进行切除，无需过度牵拉脊髓。

硬膜内入路

如备有术中超声，建议在打开硬膜前进行超声检查以了解是否充分显露了肿瘤的上极和下极。通常纵向切开硬膜，然后打开蛛网膜、探查肿瘤。可以将齿状韧带切断，以处理起源于脊髓腹侧的肿瘤。髓外的实性肿瘤可通过超声吸引器进行囊内减压，囊性肿瘤可先吸除囊液，然后在显微镜下将瘤壁从周围结构上分离。源于一条神经根的神经鞘瘤可以在肿瘤上极和下极切断神经根，将肿瘤完全切除，通常不会引起神经功能障碍。然而，如肿瘤累及多条神经根或一条特别粗大的运动根，手术医生可以尝试从神经根上剥离肿瘤，或将每条未受损的神经根上的小块肿瘤残留。虽然多数硬膜下髓外肿瘤与周围结构之间的界面清晰，可行根治性切除；但也有一些肿瘤可能粘连紧密，如黏液乳头状型室管膜瘤尤为明显。

髓内入路

在显露脊髓后，于显微镜下辨认正常结构有助于肿瘤定位。体积较大的肿瘤或肿胀的脊髓常使正常解剖结构扭曲变形，此时标志背侧中线脊髓切开术的背侧正中静脉和后正中沟、标志背根进入区的背根和后外侧沟的辨认可能十分困难。显露肿瘤后，用超声吸引器进行肿瘤内减压，将活检组织送冰冻切片检查。术中及早辨认肿瘤与脊髓之间的界面可

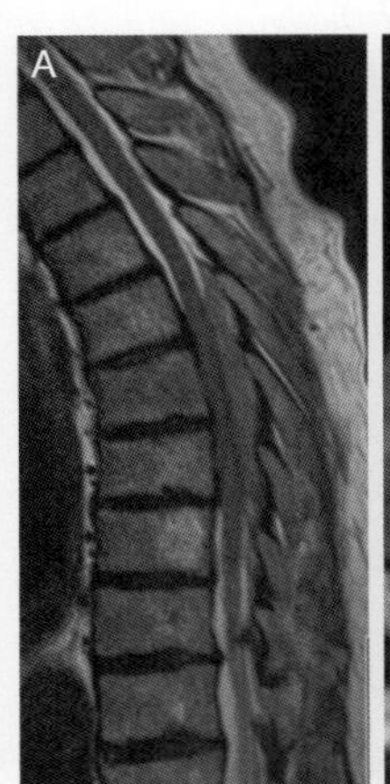

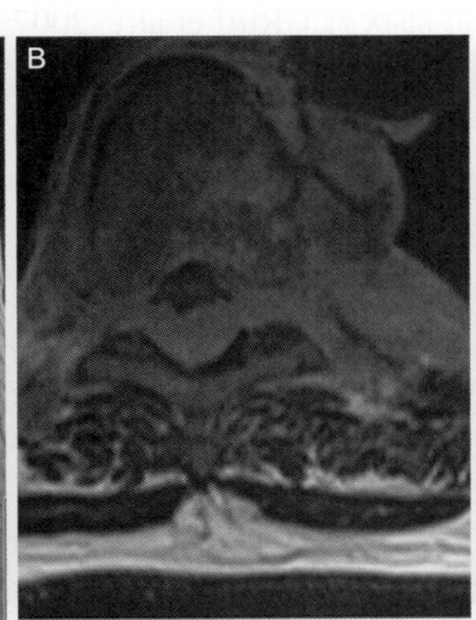

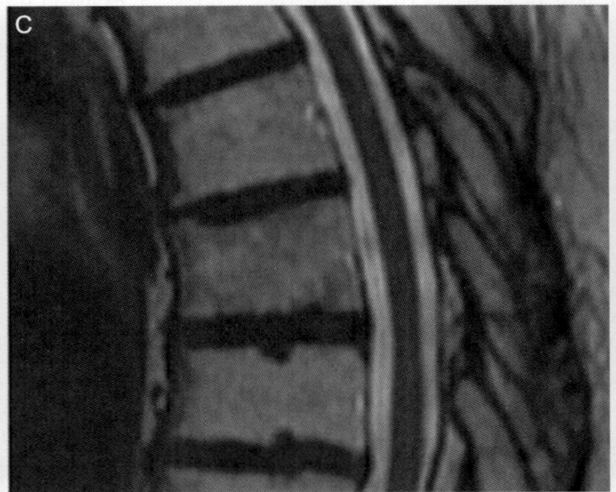

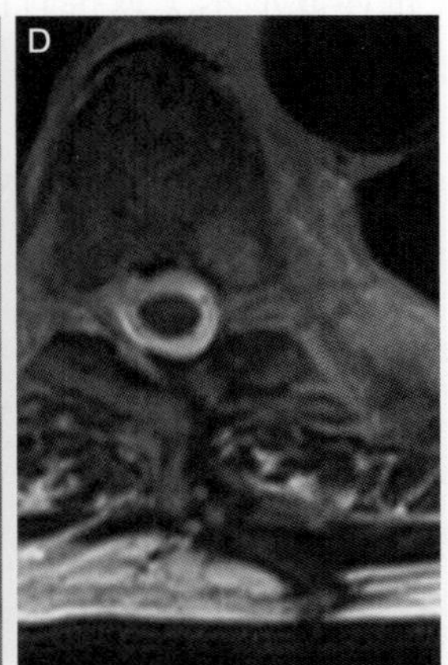

图 63.3　胸椎淋巴瘤。一名 74 岁男性患者以进行性截瘫及下肢疼痛就诊。正中矢状面 T2 加权（A）和轴位钆增强 T1 加权（B）MRI 扫描显示位于硬膜外有强化的占位性病变。患者接受半椎板切除以进行活检和减压。术后矢状位（C）和轴位（D）MRI 成像如图所示

指导手术切除范围，也可以根据术中病理结果和术中电生理监测确定手术切除范围。虽然室管膜瘤通常可以实现全切（**图** 63.4），但星形细胞瘤常与脊髓的边界不清。

器械固定

脊柱骨性结构来源的肿瘤可通过多种入路进行切除，入路的选择以便于处理病变为宜。颈椎前路手术早已为神经外科所熟知，但经体腔和体腔外入路在胸腰椎病变的广泛应用改变了位于椎体内的肿瘤的手术入路（Young et al.，1980；参考 Patchell et al.，2005）。不仅具有破坏性的肿瘤本身会影响脊柱的力学完整性，用于治疗这类肿瘤的切除术亦是如此。从事脊柱肿瘤治疗的手术医生应掌握各种前路和后路器械固定技术，以恢复脊柱的稳定性。

近年来，对转移性脊柱肿瘤和原发性骨肿瘤的治疗倾向于采用后路手术。现代基于椎弓根螺钉的器械固定无需在前方植入承重装置即可实现跨越病变节段的脊柱稳定。微创脊柱手术已用于肿瘤累及脊柱节段的减压和固定（Ziari et al.，2012），同样也可通过单纯背侧入路完成。用于放疗和化疗耐药的孤立性转移瘤（如肾细胞癌、脊索瘤和其他骨肿瘤）的全椎体切除术或整块椎体切除术也可以通过单纯背侧手术入路完成。

脊柱肿瘤的手术风险很高。**表** 63.1 重点列出了主要的潜在并发症，但并不详尽。这些风险应在患者咨询病情时明确地强调，尽可能予以避免，并在与患者讨论病情时予以清晰地解释。

经皮椎体成形术

经皮经椎弓根将骨水泥直接注射至椎体骨髓腔（椎体成形术）或椎骨内球囊扩张后形成的间隙（后凸成形术）是治疗骨质疏松性椎体压缩后疼痛的有效方法。这类手术对脊椎痛性骨转移和骨髓瘤患者也很有效。椎体成形术可有效且安全地治疗痛性骨转移，即使对有硬膜外软组织转移灶者亦有效（Sun et al.，2014）。

肿瘤学治疗

虽然新近有证据支持手术对转移瘤所致脊髓压迫的治疗有效，但放疗仍是多数此类肿瘤急诊患者的主要治疗方式。放疗也可用于难以切除和复发的硬膜内肿瘤，其疗效可能一般。对于有条件的脊索瘤和软骨肉瘤患者，质子束治疗能使患者获益。

通过立体定向放射外科进行聚焦放疗应用于颅内肿瘤的治疗已有 60 余载，目前也用于脊柱肿瘤的治疗。放射外科作为不断增大的硬膜内髓外肿瘤的一种治疗方法，可以实现影像学稳定、神经功能保护甚至改善，发生脊髓放射性坏死的风险很低（Marchetti et al.，2013）。在脊柱转移瘤的治疗中，放射外科的疗效可能较常规放疗更持久，对放疗不敏感的病变以及常规放疗后复发的病变也能奏效（Gerszten et al.，2009）。化疗对脊柱肿瘤的治疗价值有限，但对血液系统恶性肿瘤（特别是淋巴瘤）累及脊柱者可能发挥治愈作用。

康复

在治疗过程中，脊柱肿瘤患者通常情绪十分低落，如疼痛未经适当治疗得以缓解，患者可能会出现抑郁、焦虑和乏力等心理和精神障碍（Jones et al.，2003）。脊柱神经康复是治疗过程必不可少的一个组成部分，在专业化的中心尽早制订个体化治疗计划能使患者最大获益。已有研究证实，康复治疗能改善患者的抑郁状态（Ruff et al.，2007）。

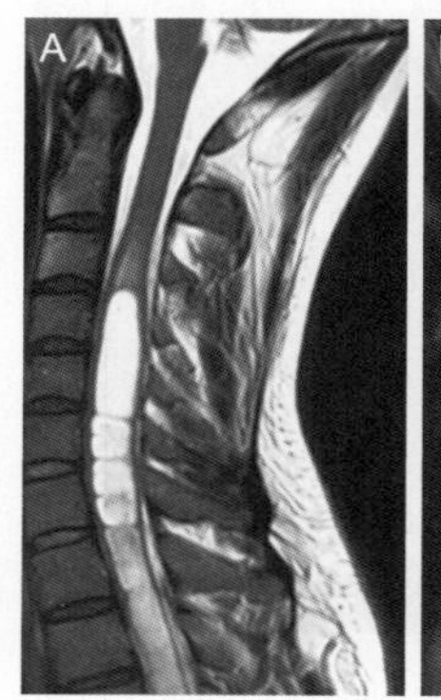

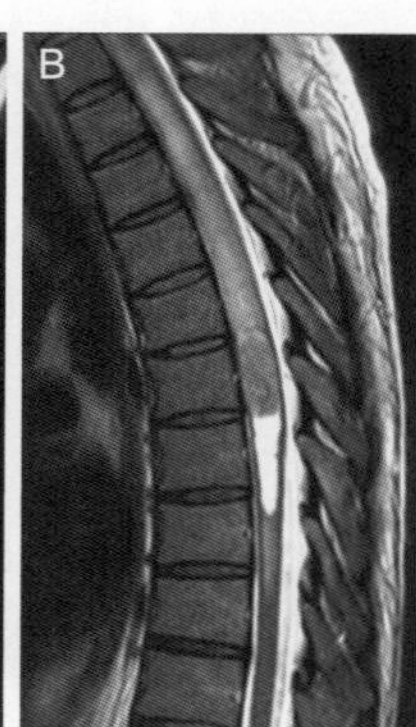

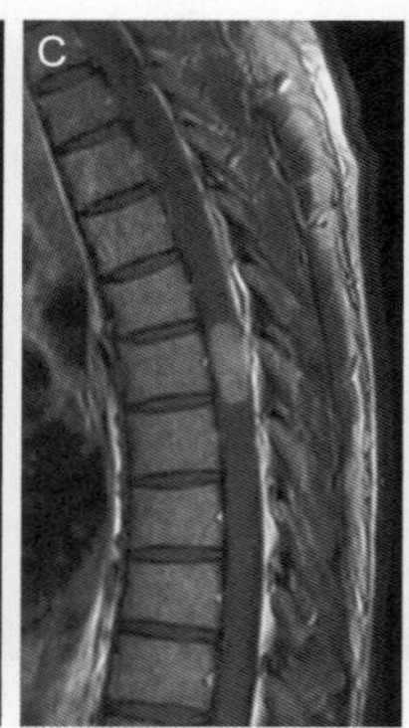

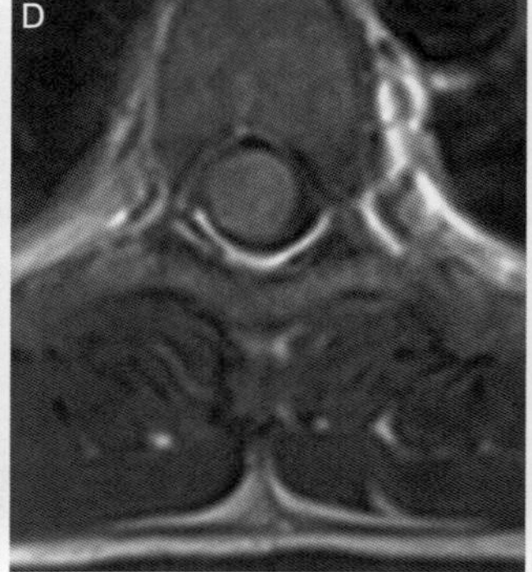

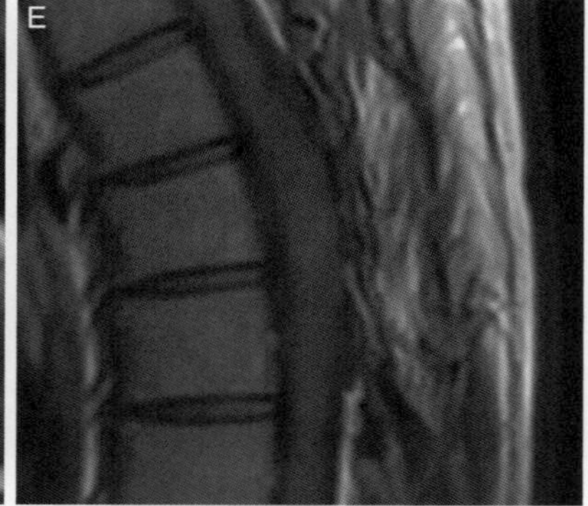

图 63.4 一名表现为进行性瘫痪的 30 岁男性患者，其诊断为室管膜瘤（WHO Ⅱ级）。注意在空洞尾端附近有增强的肿瘤（A~D）；（E）为肿瘤切除术后 4 年 MRI。患者神经功能恢复良好

表 63.1 脊柱肿瘤手术相关并发症

并发症		
概述	良性肿瘤	恶性肿瘤
出血	DSA+ 栓塞对某些肿瘤（如血管母细胞瘤、转移性肾细胞癌）是有用的。总体而言，恶性肿瘤手术的术中失血风险增加	
感染	同时使用类固醇激素、年龄过大或过小、糖尿病等共患病均增加感染风险	
脑脊液瘘 +/- 假性脊膜膨出	只有在出现临床症状时才需干预，手术治疗方法包括腰椎引流、手术修复	
脊髓拴系	缝合软膜可降低拴系风险，但硬膜成形术却未显示出保护作用	
脊髓空洞症	手术部位发生脊髓拴系者脊髓空洞风险增加 切除肿瘤并重建脑脊液流通常会使术前空洞缩小乃至消失	
血管损害	术前 DSA+/- 栓塞治疗会增加血管损害风险	
永久性神经功能恶化，包括四肢瘫和截瘫	约 20% 患者会出现永久性运动、感觉、括约肌（或上述不同组合）功能障碍；迟发性术后脊髓病的风险 <4%。几乎所有的髓内肿瘤患者都会出现脊髓背柱功能障碍。脊髓监测等实用技术能为外科医生提供额外信息，有助于降低上述风险	
肿瘤复发	完全切除者复发率很低。然而，未全切的黏液乳头状室管膜瘤是一个例外	恶性肿瘤几乎总会复发
肿瘤种植	非常罕见	在活检部位发生种植，尤其是肉瘤。在进行确切的肉瘤切除手术时，应将活检针道周围的组织一并切除
脊柱畸形	在儿童病例中脊柱畸形的问题更为突出，常因肿瘤所致神经功能障碍引起或在术后出现	

肿瘤分组的具体情况

脊髓髓内肿瘤

脊髓髓内肿瘤（intramedullary spinal cord tumours，IMSCT）较为罕见，占中枢神经系统肿瘤的4%以下，占硬膜内脊髓肿瘤的30%。最常见的肿瘤类型是室管膜瘤和星形细胞瘤。在多数病例系列中，室管膜瘤较星形细胞瘤多见；星形细胞瘤在年轻组患者中占优势，随着年龄的增长，室管膜瘤更常见（Manzano et al.，2008）。血管母细胞瘤的发生率较低，其他各种发育性肿瘤和囊肿也较少见，如脂肪瘤、皮样囊肿、表皮样囊肿和神经肠源性囊肿。**表** 63.2 列出了较为常见的 IMSCT 特征。

值得注意的是，虽然髓内肿瘤切除与良好的肿瘤预后和患者长期活动能力具有相关性，但脊髓切开术本身并非没有并发症。最近一项报道的 278 例患者中，61% 的患者术后神经功能状态加重，约 20% 的患者永久性加重（Klekamp，2013）。

脊髓硬膜内髓外肿瘤

脊髓硬膜内髓外肿瘤（intradural extramedullary spinal tumours，IDEM）发病率为 IMSCT 的两倍以上，但仍不常见。此类肿瘤约占硬膜内肿瘤发病率的 70%，人群发病率为 0.8~1.3/10 万人·年。神经鞘肿瘤为最常见的 IDEM（**图** 63.5），其次是脊膜瘤和黏液乳头状室管膜瘤（Traul et al.，2007）。IDEM 多为良性、单发肿瘤；其他特征见**表** 63.3。发生在髓外硬膜内的肿瘤类型十分广泛，包括转移性肿瘤、副神经节瘤、表皮样和皮样囊肿、脂肪瘤和畸胎瘤。

手术主要适用于进行性增大的、引起症状的肿瘤。某些神经鞘瘤、脊膜瘤和发育性病变不会进展，仅予以定期监测即可，从而避免了手术的潜在风险。然而，黏液乳头状室管膜瘤的生物学表现有所不同，值得特别注意。

黏液乳头状室管膜瘤

黏液乳头状室管膜瘤几乎仅发生于腰椎节段，通常为孤立性病变。由于其独特的发生部位，患者症状多表现为圆锥或马尾神经功能障碍。这类肿瘤可能会充满整个腰骶管（**图** 63.6）。尽管黏液乳头状室管膜瘤的分类属“良性”（WHO 分类 1 级的肿瘤），但其行为学具有侵袭性，有复发和沿脑脊液播散的倾向，患者在一生中可能需多次手术治疗（Boström et al.，2011）。黏液乳头状室管膜瘤可侵蚀骨质使之呈扇状花边样改变，也可侵透硬膜并与马尾神经根紧密粘连。黏液乳头状室管膜瘤的首选治疗方案是

表 63.2 室管膜瘤、星形细胞瘤和血管母细胞瘤的特征

		肿瘤类型		
		室管膜瘤	星形细胞瘤	血管母细胞瘤
MRI 特征	T1WI	可变	低信号	等信号至低信号
	T2WI	低信号	高信号	等信号至高信号（可见增粗的供血和引流血管）
	位置	脊髓中央	偏心生长	通常较表浅
	增强	均匀强化	不均匀强化（LGG 无强化；毛细胞型星形细胞瘤和 HGG 明显强化）	明显增强
	边界	通常较清晰	不清	边界清晰的结节
	脊髓空洞 / 囊肿	常伴发	不太常见（毛细胞型星形细胞瘤可伴囊变）	常伴有囊肿
GTR 的可能性		可能	不太可能	可能
组织学	亚型（最常见者以粗体表示） WHO 分级	室管膜下瘤（罕见） 1 室管膜瘤 2 间变性室管膜瘤 3	毛细胞型星形细胞瘤（罕见） 1 低级别星形细胞瘤 2 间变性星形细胞瘤 3 胶质母细胞瘤 4	血管母细胞瘤 1
	最常见亚型的显微镜下特征	由均匀一致的细胞形成的细胞层，细胞核呈卵圆形，有纤细的胞质突起 血管周围假菊形团 有丝分裂罕见 / 无	微囊性变的肿瘤基质内可见分化良好的肿瘤性星形细胞 （无坏死或微血管增生） 有丝分裂：Ki-67/MIB-1<4%	两种主要成分：内皮细胞和周细胞；内含脂质的大空泡基质细胞 囊肿壁和空洞壁含 Rosenthal 纤维 一般无有丝分裂（MIB-1: 0~2%）
	免疫组化	GFAP、S-100 蛋白、波形蛋白	GFAP 波形蛋白（肿瘤级别越高，阳性可能性也越高）	基质细胞不表达内皮细胞标志物（在 RCC 中呈阴性），但表达 D2-40 Ab 和抑制素 -A（在 RCC 中呈阳性）、波形蛋白、VEGF
症状学关联		NF2（染色体 22q12）	NF1（染色体 17q11） TP53 基因突变 /Li-Fraumeni 综合征 Ollier 病	VHL（染色体 3p25）

缩写：T1WI，T1 加权成像；T2WI，T2 加权成像；LGG，低级别胶质瘤；HGG，高级别胶质瘤；NF1，1 型神经纤维瘤病；NF2，2 型神经纤维瘤病；VHL，von Hippel-Lindau 综合征；GTR，全切除术；免疫组化，免疫组织化学；VEGF，血管内皮生长因子；GFAP，胶质纤维酸性蛋白；RCC，肾细胞癌；Ab，抗体；Ollier 病，也称遗传性多发性内生软骨瘤 1 型

手术全切肿瘤，偶然发现的体积小的无症状肿瘤可以早期手术治疗，此时全切肿瘤和治愈的机会较高，也可降低病变播散和进展为难以手术切除的肿瘤的风险。实际上，由于肿瘤囊壁较薄且质地柔软，整块切除肿瘤有时很难实现。在手术过程中应尽早辨认终丝，通过神经刺激器和插入肛门外括约肌的肌电图电极有助于辨认终丝。

脊柱原发性骨肿瘤

脊柱原发性骨肿瘤同样罕见，而脊椎转移瘤要常见得多。脊柱原发性骨肿瘤的病理类型广泛，具有双峰状的年龄分布特征，主要累及青年和老年。这类肿瘤起源于结缔组织成分的细胞，分类上属于肉瘤组，可分为恶性肿瘤（**表 63.4**）和良性肿瘤（**表 63.5**）两大类。这类肿瘤的治疗属于跨区域的专业单元范畴。

恶性骨肿瘤

脊索瘤（**图 63.8 和图 63.9**）是最常见的成人原发性恶性脊柱骨肿瘤，通常为中线肿瘤，多见于枢椎和腰骶部。肿瘤生长缓慢，但为破坏性病变，分

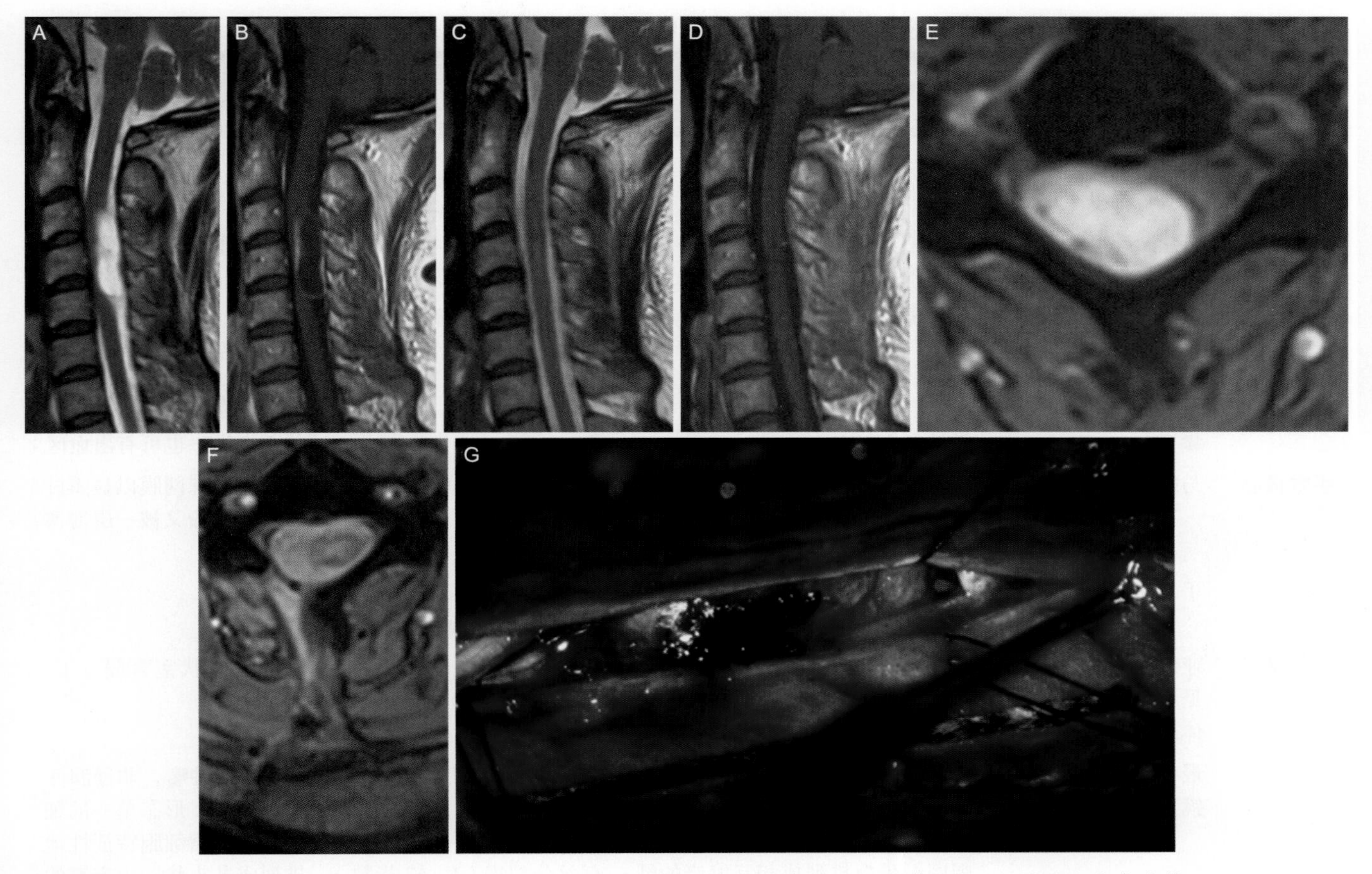

图 63.5　单侧旁矢状面入路和半椎板切除术（A~F）切除颈椎神经鞘瘤的 MR 图像。（G）所示为术中成像

块切除后复发率很高。研究显示，沿肿瘤未侵犯边界进行完整的根治性整块切除能显著降低复发率并改善患者生存期（Fuchs et al.，2005）。

骨肉瘤是最常见的原发性脊柱肉瘤，预后极差（Sansur et al.，2007）。骨肉瘤发生的危险因素包括 Paget 病和放射治疗。遗憾的是，很难实现整块切除。尽管有多种治疗方案可选，但原发性脊柱骨肉瘤的治疗仍属姑息性治疗。

软骨肉瘤（图 63.10）有特征性的影像学表现，虫蚀样溶骨区和肿瘤基质内“环状和弧形”钙化灶在 CT 上最易于观察。骨外和硬膜外扩展常见，MR 是证实该特征的首选检查。幸运的是，多数软骨肉瘤为低级别肿瘤。与分块切除相比，广泛的整块切除与患者生存期和无复发间期延长具有相关性（Quiriny and Gebhart，2008）。

多发性骨髓瘤和浆细胞瘤

多发性骨髓瘤（multiple myeloma，MM）是一种以单克隆浆细胞增殖为特征的全身性血液系统恶性肿瘤（图 63.11），世界范围内约占全部癌症的 1%，发病率约为 5.5/10 万（Ferlay et al.，2013），好发于老年人，首诊中位年龄为 70 岁。浆细胞瘤是组织学上与 MM 相同但无全身表现的、隐袭起病的孤立性病变。

脊柱是最常见的骨骼受累部位。MM 引起的症状性脊髓压迫症的治疗仍是尚有争议的领域。因软组织造成脊髓压迫者以紧急局部放疗为首选，手术一般用于有骨性或结构性相关的脊髓压迫表现的 MM 患者，且仍需放疗以巩固疗效。然而，Rao et al.（2006）在对一组临床和影像学均不稳定的颈椎 MM 患者进行回顾分析后建议，单纯放疗是一种有效的姑息治疗方式，无需进行手术治疗。MM 患者的骨密度很低，会影响器械固定的使用。

血管瘤

脊椎血管瘤是一种良性肿瘤，也是最常见的原发性脊柱肿瘤（图 63.12 和图 63.13）。这类病变通常为影像学上偶然发现，MRI 特征地表现为 T1 和 T2 加权成像均呈高信号，根据这些表现无需活检即可得出诊断。椎体血管瘤很少出现症状，但这类肿瘤中的小部分可引起骨骼扩张并导致病理性骨折，亦可延伸至硬膜外腔并压迫神经结构。较大的病变在

表 63.3 神经鞘肿瘤、脊膜瘤和黏液乳头状室管膜瘤的特征

<table>
<tr><th colspan="3" rowspan="2"></th><th colspan="6">肿瘤类型</th></tr>
<tr><th colspan="2">神经鞘瘤</th><th colspan="2">脊膜瘤</th><th colspan="2">黏液乳头状型室管膜瘤</th></tr>
<tr><td rowspan="7">MRI 特征</td><td colspan="2">T1WI</td><td colspan="2">高信号</td><td colspan="2">等信号</td><td colspan="2">低信号</td></tr>
<tr><td colspan="2">T2WI</td><td colspan="2">高信号</td><td colspan="2">等信号至高信号</td><td colspan="2">高信号</td></tr>
<tr><td colspan="2">部位</td><td colspan="2">累及感觉神经根
在椎管内均匀分布</td><td colspan="2">以硬膜为基底；后侧 / 后外侧；胸段常见</td><td colspan="2">几乎仅累及终丝</td></tr>
<tr><td colspan="2">增强</td><td colspan="2">不均匀</td><td colspan="2">均匀；“硬膜尾征”</td><td colspan="2">均匀</td></tr>
<tr><td colspan="2">边界</td><td colspan="2">清晰</td><td colspan="2">清晰</td><td colspan="2">清晰</td></tr>
<tr><td colspan="2">水肿</td><td colspan="2">无</td><td colspan="2">不确定</td><td colspan="2">常伴水肿</td></tr>
<tr><td colspan="2">囊变</td><td colspan="2">常见</td><td colspan="2">无</td><td colspan="2">并不少见，也可有出血区</td></tr>
<tr><td rowspan="2">手术核心</td><td colspan="2">与蛛网膜的关系</td><td colspan="2">两层蛛网膜（类似于颅内神经鞘瘤）均需打开</td><td colspan="2">肿瘤和脊髓之间有清晰的蛛网膜界面</td><td colspan="2">需要打开蛛网膜以显露肿瘤，而肿瘤又被一层薄薄的囊包裹</td></tr>
<tr><td colspan="2">手术切除</td><td colspan="2">分块切除，可牺牲受累的感觉神经根</td><td colspan="2">分块或整块切除，电凝或切除其下方的硬膜</td><td colspan="2">整块全切</td></tr>
<tr><td rowspan="3">组织学</td><td>亚型（常见者以黑体表示）</td><td>WHO 分级</td><td>神经鞘瘤
神经纤维瘤</td><td>1
1</td><td>良性
非典型（罕见）
恶性（罕见）</td><td>1
2
3</td><td>黏液乳头状室管膜瘤</td><td>1</td></tr>
<tr><td colspan="2">最常见亚型的显微镜下特征</td><td colspan="2">由两种完全不同的肿瘤性施万细胞组成：Antoni A 型（细胞密集；纺锤形细胞，致密的细胞周围网织蛋白排列成相互缠绕的纤维束；特征性的 Verocay 小体），Antoni B 型（细胞稀疏；细胞松散排列于黏液样基质中，周围网织蛋白很少）</td><td colspan="2">因亚型和分级不同而异。
常见亚型：脑膜上皮型，砂砾体型
有丝分裂率（Ki 67 指数）通常 <4%
网织蛋白很少像神经鞘瘤那样密集</td><td colspan="2">有囊壁的肿瘤，非浸润性含有圆形、形态单一的细胞核的肿瘤细胞特征性地排列成乳头状，由丰富的黏蛋白 / 黏液样间质核心包裹
有丝分裂和坏死罕见</td></tr>
<tr><td colspan="2">免疫组化</td><td colspan="2">S-100：高表达，弥漫性表达
GFAP：局灶性表达，少见着色
Ⅳ型胶原和层粘连蛋白阳性：见于所有神经鞘瘤的基底膜表面</td><td colspan="2">EMA、波形蛋白：阳性
S-100：不确定
细胞角蛋白：局灶性
GFAP 阴性</td><td colspan="2">GFAP、S-100、波形蛋白：阳性
细胞角蛋白：无</td></tr>
<tr><td>症状学关联</td><td colspan="2"></td><td colspan="2">NF2（染色体 22q12）
Carney 综合征（17q23-q24）（黑色素性神经鞘瘤）</td><td colspan="2">NF2（染色体 22q12）
既往放疗
Castleman 综合征（脊索瘤型）</td><td colspan="2">NF2（染色体 22q12）</td></tr>
</table>

缩写：T1WI，T1 加权成像；T2WI，T2 加权成像；NF1，神经纤维瘤病 1 型；NF2，神经纤维瘤病 2 型；GTR，大体全切除；GFAP，胶质纤维酸性蛋白；EMA，上皮膜抗原；免疫组化，免疫组织化学

矢状和冠状位 CT 上表现为特征性的“蜂窝状”改变或“灯芯绒征”，即增粗的骨小梁形成明显的垂直条纹。引起症状的椎体血管瘤的治疗方法包括手术切除、椎体成形术、血管内栓塞和放射治疗。

脊柱转移瘤

在本章描述的各类重要的临床病变中，脊柱转移性恶性肿瘤是最常见的。癌症的骨骼转移性种植以脊柱最为常见，约 40% 死于癌症的患者尸检时有脊柱转移灶。随着更有效的癌症治疗方法的涌现，癌症患者的生存期不断延长，脊柱转移瘤的发病率也不可避免地随之升高（Sciubba et al.，2010）。脊柱转移瘤最常见的来源是肺癌、乳腺癌（**图 63.14**）和前列腺癌，但肾细胞癌、胃肠道恶性肿瘤和黑色素瘤也很常见。骨髓瘤种植的确可能是转移性的，但本章在原发性骨肿瘤中加以讨论。

当不断增大的肿瘤侵及硬膜外腔或引起椎体病理性骨折时，会引起脊髓压迫；一旦神经功能障碍

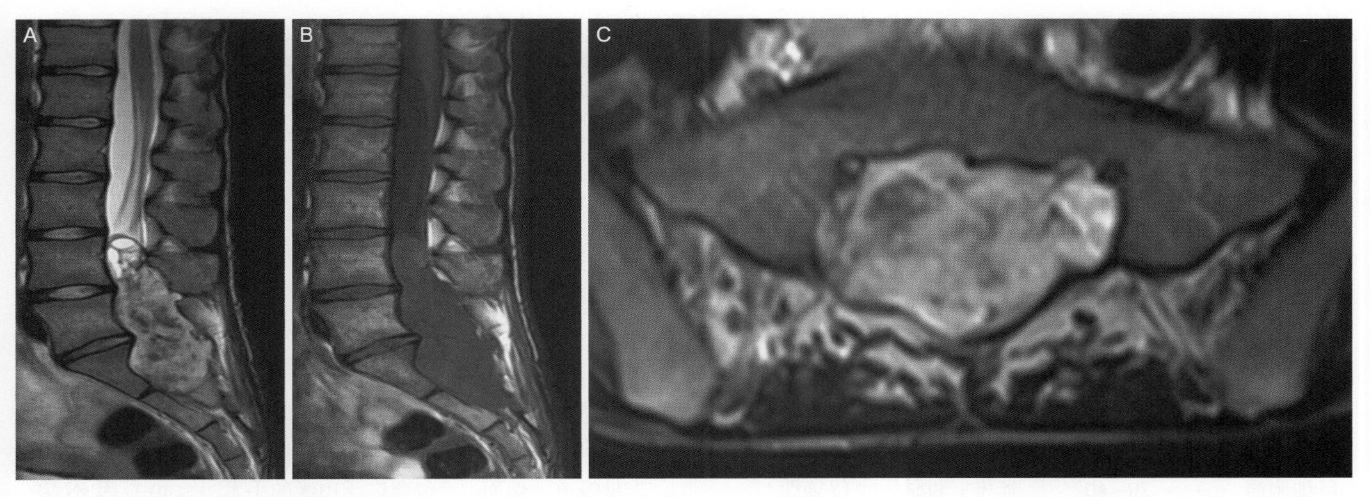

图 63.6　黏液乳头状室管膜瘤晚期表现为后部结构破坏和骶骨体受侵蚀边缘呈扇形（A、B）。肿瘤侵犯尾侧神经根和硬膜，影响手术切除。由于无法直接缝合硬膜，因此在直接放置脊柱引流管后缝合伤口（C）

Courtesy of Dr Allinson, Department of Pathology, Addenbrooke's Hospital, Cambridge.

表 63.4　恶性原发性脊柱骨肿瘤

肿瘤类型	年龄（岁）	脊柱位置	起源	临床表现	中位生存期（月）	5 年生存率（%）	转移	治疗
脊索瘤	60 岁	骶骨（如位于颈椎则好发于 C2）	脊索残留物	疼痛、畸形、神经功能缺损	74	50~85	不常见	包括广泛边缘的整块切除，放射治疗（对化疗不敏感）
骨肉瘤	两个峰值：10~30 岁和 50 岁	骶骨，后部结构	骨		11	18~41	肺转移很常见 Paget 病以及放射治疗后的恶性变	包括广泛边缘的整块切除 切除、化疗、放疗（通常为单纯姑息治疗）
软骨肉瘤	50 岁	胸椎，后部结构	软骨		26	40	不常见 骨软骨瘤的恶性变	手术切除（对放、化疗不敏感）
尤因肉瘤	10~30 岁（青少年）	骶骨，后部结构	小圆形蓝色细胞肿瘤		37	55~73	常转移至肺和骨 很少位于硬膜外	手术、化疗、放疗

进展，MSCC 就会表现为肿瘤急症。突发的功能障碍可能为脊髓梗死所致，较渐进性起病者预后更差。多数脊柱转移瘤患者已确诊为恶性肿瘤，但仍有高达 20% 的脊柱转移为患者首诊时的表现（Cahill, 1996）。此类患者的检查应包括骨髓瘤筛查、男性前列腺特异性抗原化验、女性乳腺检查和胸腹盆腔 CT 筛查。

脊柱外科医生常应邀会诊，对 MSCC 手术治疗的可行性做出判断。无论先行手术抑或放疗，均应及时决定、快速治疗，同时尽可能咨询熟悉患者病情的肿瘤学家并进行磁共振成像检查。治疗方案的确定需要考虑许多因素，这些因素可分为四组（**图 63.15**）。肿瘤因素包括恶性肿瘤对放疗和化疗敏感性以及患者的分期和预后。神经系统因素包括神经系统压迫的症状和功能障碍，以及可解释这些表现的影像学所见的压迫性病变。持续时间超过 24 小时的全脊髓病变在减压后获得改善的可能性极低。生物力学因素主要是肿瘤对脊柱结构的影响。机械性疼痛和畸形可作为手术固定的指征，但需要相邻脊柱节段完好才能行器械固定。加做 CT 扫描有助于明确上

表 63.5 良性原发性脊柱骨肿瘤

类型	年龄（岁）	部位	临床表现	恶性变	治疗	复发率（%）
血管瘤	任何年龄	胸椎；椎体	意外发现	无	引起症状的病变可行外科切除和（或）放射治疗	（低）
骨样骨瘤	10~20	腰椎；椎体	夜间疼痛可由水杨酸盐缓解，NSAIDs<2 cm	无	手术切除	<4.5
成骨细胞瘤	10~30	腰椎；椎体	非特异性疼痛；>2 cm	有	手术切除	<15
动脉瘤样骨囊肿（见图 63.7）	<20	胸腰椎；后部结构	疼痛、畸形、神经功能缺损	无	完全刮除和切除。不完全切除复发率高	<30
巨细胞瘤	20~40	骶椎；椎体	侵袭性 复发率高	未见报道。然而，术后放疗诱发肉瘤的风险为 10%	包含广泛边缘的手术切除 放疗与预后改善无关	<40（因不完全切除及病灶内边缘而增加）
（骨）软骨瘤	30~40	C2；后部元件	神经功能缺损罕见脊柱侧凸	有（软骨肉瘤）	手术全切	缺乏数据
软骨母细胞瘤	青春期	因罕见而不适用	疼痛，神经功能缺损	未见报道	手术全切 未全切者复发率高	24~100

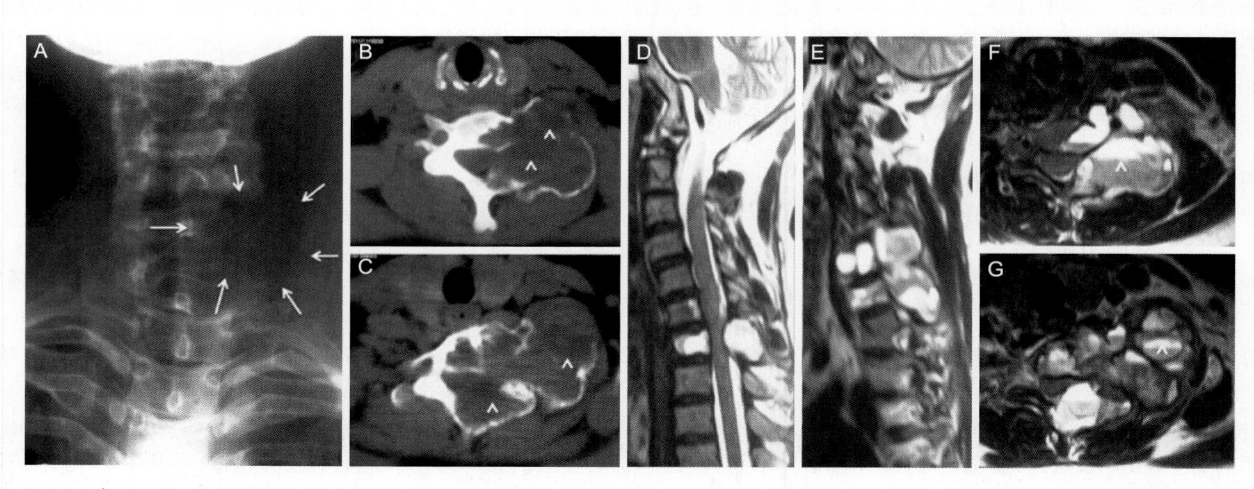

图 63.7 一名 47 岁女性颈痛患者，其病理诊断为动脉瘤样骨囊肿。（A）前后位 X 线显示 C6~C7 椎骨左侧溶骨性破坏性病变（箭头）。（B、C）显示累及锥体和后部结构的多房扩张性病变的液 - 液平（箭头）。同一名患者的磁共振成像，矢状位（D、E）和轴位（F、G）T2 加权成像显示多个液 - 液平（箭头），表明不同时期的出血成分

述信息，但脊柱长节段受累的患者不太适合手术固定。患者因素是最重要的，包括功能状态、共患病、年龄（Chi et al.，2009）以及患者意愿。

诸如 Tokuhashi et al.（2005）多位作者已将上述某些因素纳入各种评分系统，这些基于精算生存表的评分系统为患者预后提供指导，并有助于决策制定。然而，不应盲目使用这些数字，也不能替代肿瘤医生和患者进行充分讨论。Sciubba et al.（2010）建议对脊髓受压、神经功能障碍进展迅速、脊柱不稳定、放疗不敏感以及放疗后复发的肿瘤患者进行手术减压和内固定。

争议

毫无疑问，2005 年 Patchell 发表的具有里程碑意义的研究改变了手术治疗 MSCC 的临床实践。此前一项对比椎板切除术联合放疗与单纯放疗治疗 MSCC 的随机对照试验发现，两组之间的神经功能转归没

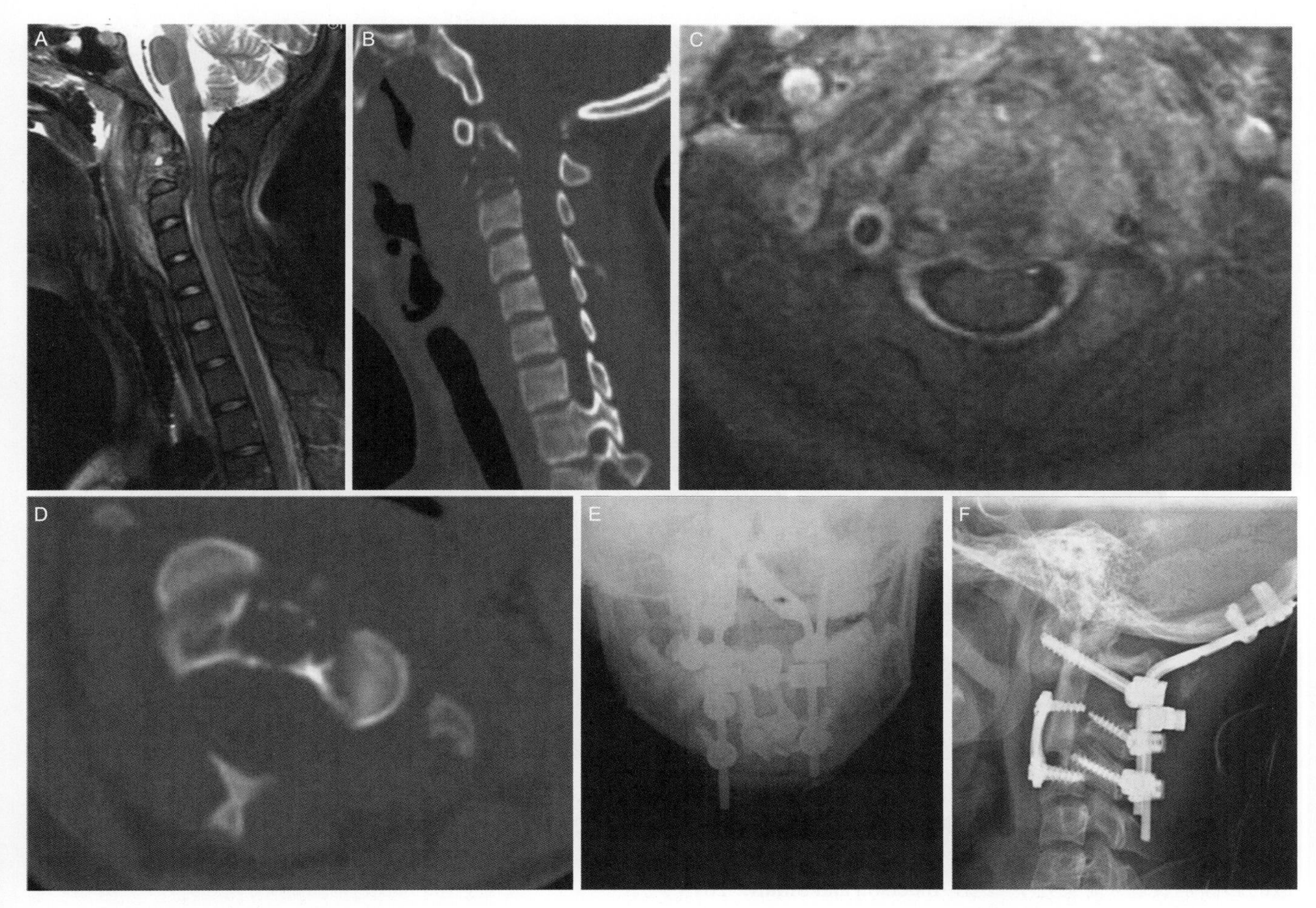

图 63.8　脊索瘤。术前矢状位 T2 加权 MRI（A）显示 C2 椎体广泛破坏，病变自斜坡于椎体前方延伸至 C5（箭头）。术前矢状位 CT 重建（B）显示扩张性病变累及 C2 椎体（箭头）。术前轴位 T2 加权 MRI（C）和钆对比剂增强扫描显示 C2 椎体广泛浸润，椎动脉周围可见肿瘤（箭头）。术前 CT 轴位像（D）显示 C2 椎体骨质受累（箭头）。根治性扩大经口 - 经下颌切除术，随后切除后部结构并行器械固定和融合。C2 全切除、器械固定和融合术后的正位（E）和侧位（F）X 线片（参见 Walcott et al.，2012）

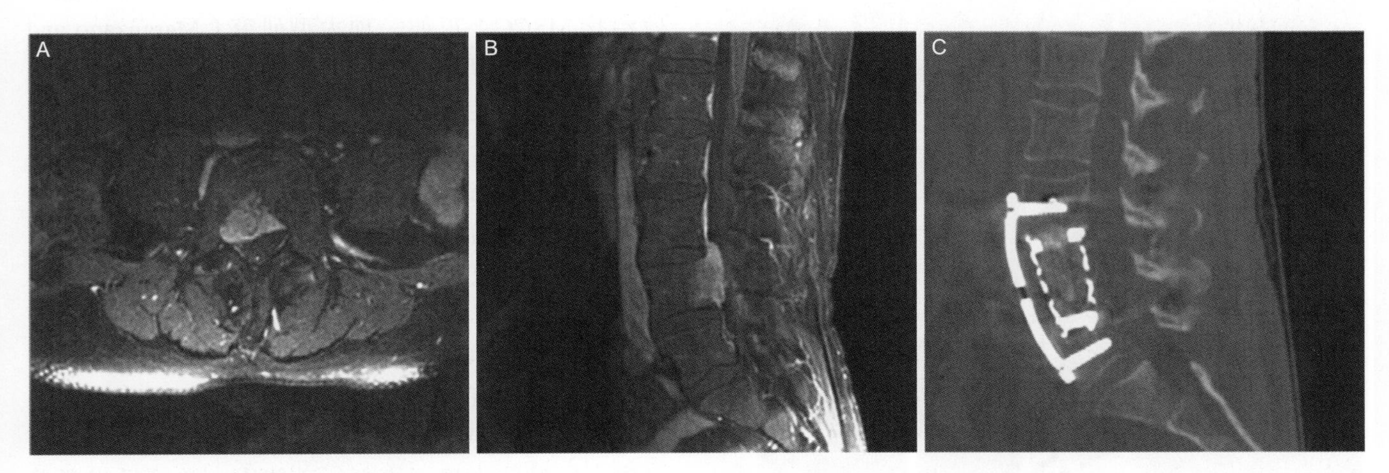

图 63.9　腰椎脊索瘤的 CT 和术前磁共振轴位像（A）；腰椎脊索瘤术前磁共振矢状位成像（B）；术后侧位 X 线片（C）（参见 Ozaki et al.，2002）

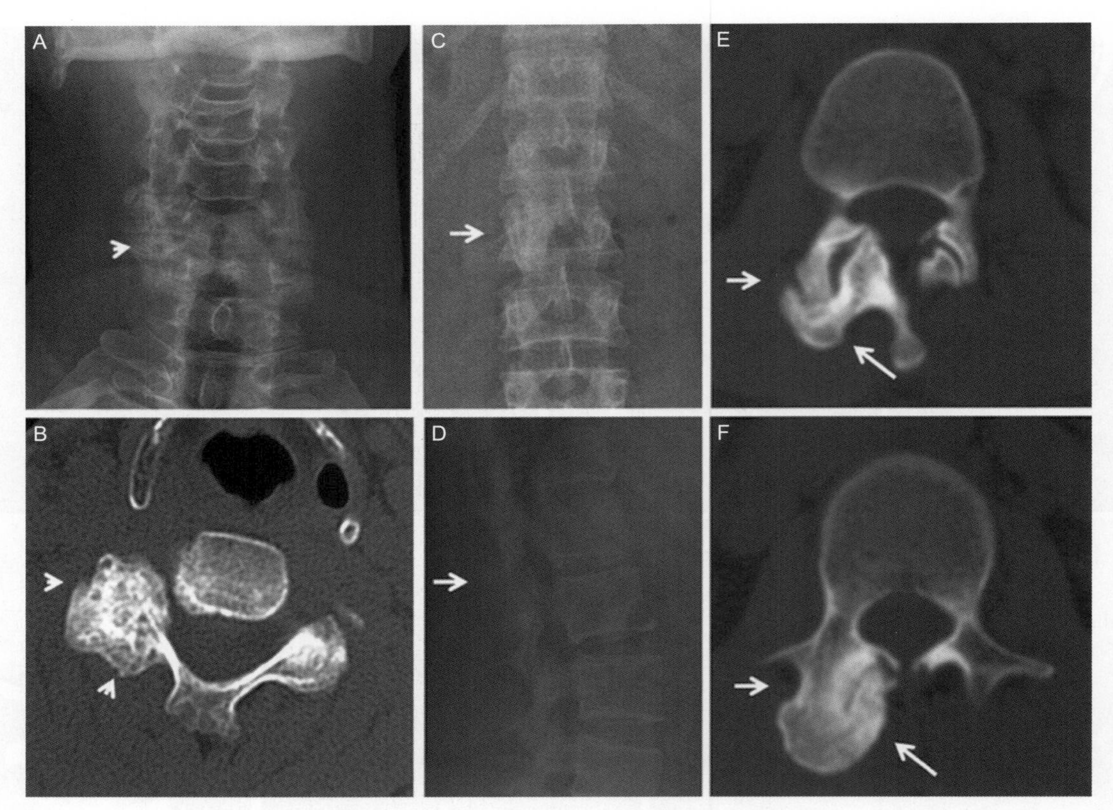

图 63.10 两位不同的脊柱骨软骨瘤患者。第一位患者为 45 岁男性，起源于右侧 C5~C6 小关节的骨软骨瘤。（A）颈椎前后位 X 线片；（B）轴位计算机断层扫描（computed tomography，CT）显示一个轮廓清晰的分叶状成骨肿瘤（箭头）。第二位患者是以背痛就诊的 36 岁女性。（C、D）前后位和侧位 X 线片；（E、F）轴位 CT 扫描显示 L2 椎体右上关节突有类似的影像学表现（箭头处）（参见 Anderson and Smith，2013）

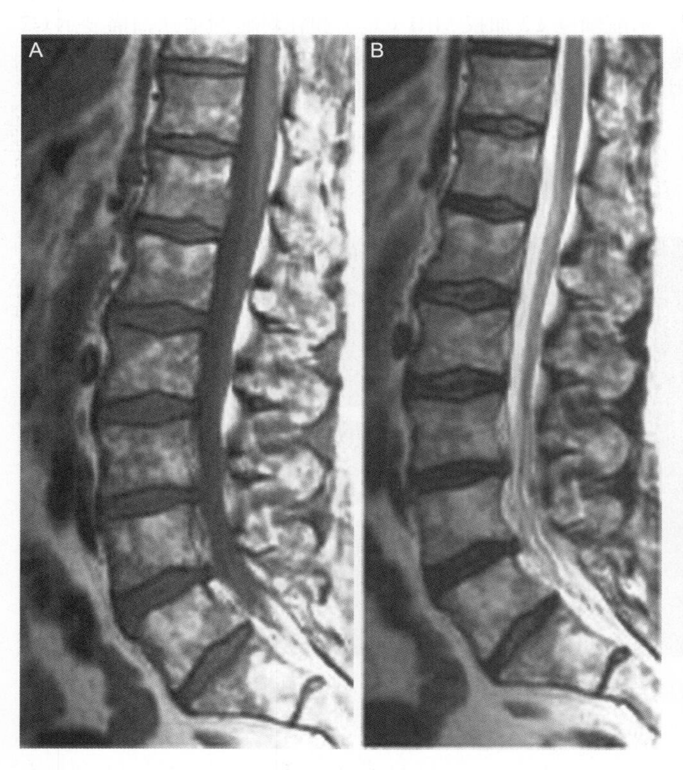

图 63.11 多发性骨髓瘤。腰椎矢状位（A）T1 和（B）T2 加权成像显示从下胸椎到腰椎的骨髓中均有相似的混杂异常信号区域

有差异（Young et al.，1980）。当时估算椎板切除术的并发症发生率为 10%，加之椎板切除术对椎体压缩引起脊髓腹侧压迫者无效，使手术治疗 MSCC 的方式逐渐遭到废弃，转而采用单纯放疗。放疗能有效治疗 MSCC，正如一项大型研究（Maranzano and Latini，1995）所示：109 名尚能行走的患者中除 2 人外均保留了行走能力，82 名已丧失行走能力、尚有一定肌力的患者中 60% 恢复了活动能力。

Patchell et al.（2005）报道了一项纳入 101 名 MSCC 患者的随机对照试验，其中 50 名患者随机接受手术和术后放疗，另 51 名患者仅行放疗，中期分析后提前终止了该项试验停止。该试验的主要终点是行动能力，手术治疗组在治疗后有 84% 能行走，而单纯放疗组仅有 57% 能行走。该项研究还表明，手术治疗在维持患者能行动能力的持续时间、使术前已失去行动能力患者恢复行动能力、治疗后患者的尿便控制功能以及生存期方面有显著优势。虽然有压倒性的证据支持手术治疗较单纯放疗能使 MSCC 患者有更多获益，但在文献中并非没有相反的证据，一项较大宗、但为回顾性的病例配对分析显示与单

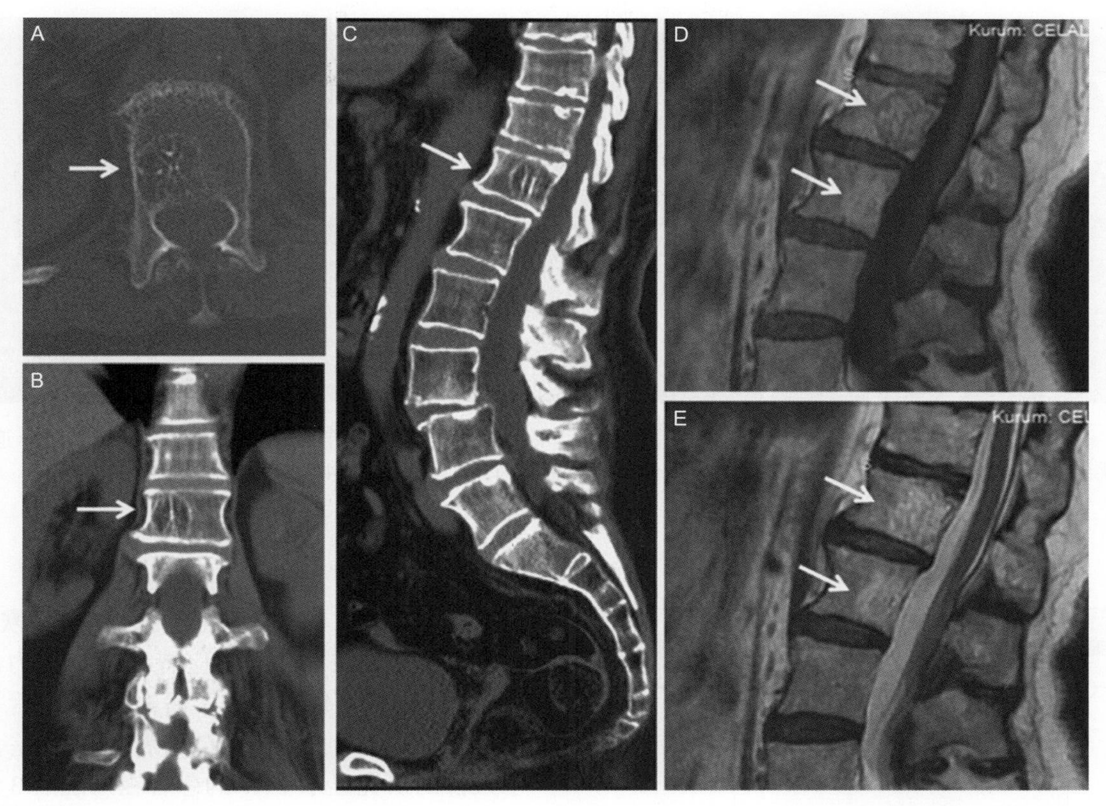

图 63.12　血管瘤。（A）轴位 CT 显示多发点状硬化区，形成白色波点征。（B）冠状位和矢状位重建 CT 成像显示 T12 椎体明显的垂直小梁形似蜂窝状，构成“灯芯绒”征。（D）矢状位 T1 和（E）T2 加权磁共振成像显示 T12 和 L1 椎体有两个高信号的血管瘤（箭头）

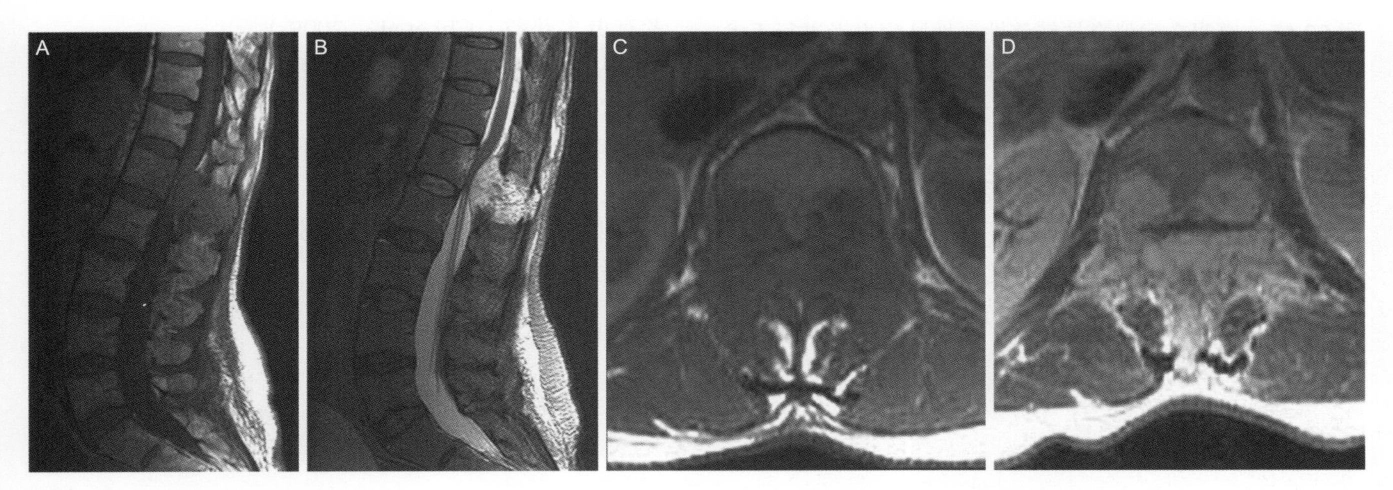

图 63.13　血管瘤。T1（A）和 T2（B）矢状位 MRI（箭头）显示累及椎体后部和后部结构的外生型占位性病变。注射造影前（C）后（D）的轴位 MR 显示血管瘤有强化，硬膜囊受压（箭头）

纯放疗相比，手术并未使患者有显著获益（Rades et al.，2010）。

如果我们接受手术的确较单纯放疗有潜在获益，也并不意味所有 MSCC 患者均应接受手术治疗。在 INDEX 研究（Patchell et al.，2005）中，历经 10 年从 7 个神经肿瘤中心招募了 101 名患者。对于发病率为 5~8/100 000 的疾病而言，该研究令人惊讶（Lobalaw et al.，2003），提示存在选择偏倚，因此该治疗可能仅适用于 MSCC 患者的一个小亚组。挪威某地区在 18 个月内有 903 名经急诊转诊接受 MSCC 治疗的患者，其中仅 58 名（6.4%）接受了手术治疗（Zaikova et al.，2011）。

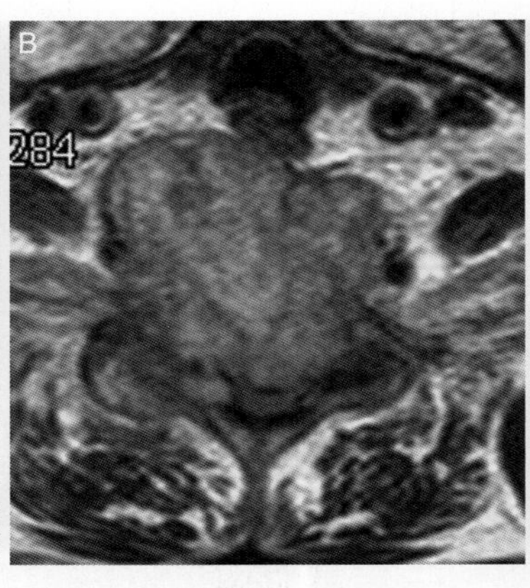

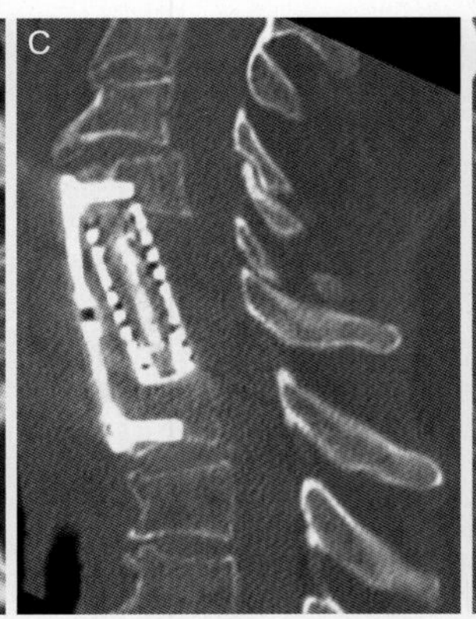

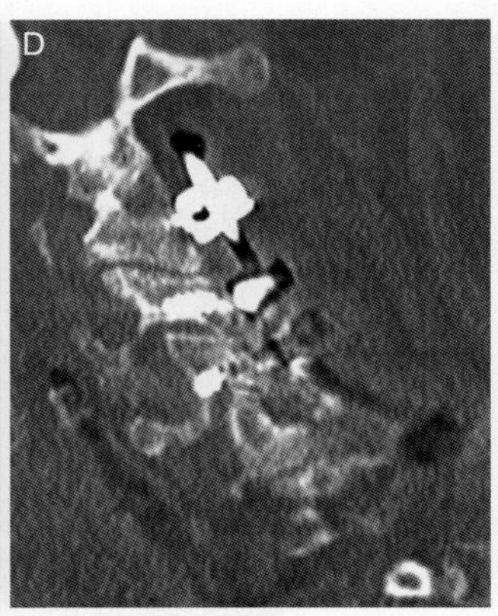

图 63.14 一名以数日内进行性加重的行走困难就诊的患者。磁共振成像显示一个破坏性的颈椎病变伴脊髓压迫，在本次首发症状就诊时患者诊断为乳腺癌转移，接受了两个节段椎体切除术，随后行 C4 至 T1 的后路器械固定

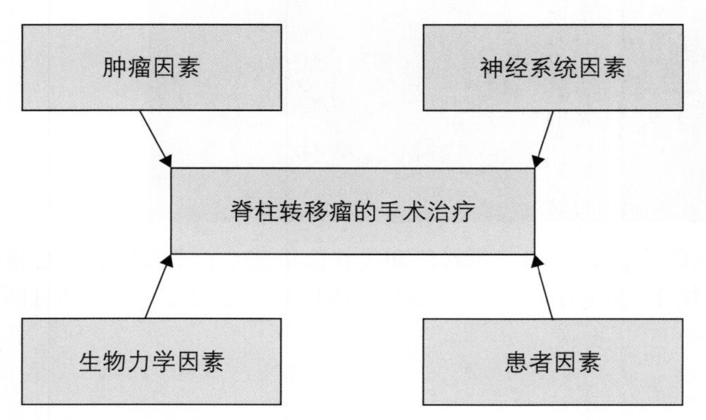

图 63.15 说明在建议脊柱转移性恶性肿瘤患者进行手术治疗时需要考虑的多重因素

因此，手术治疗研究的患者很可能仅能代表 MSCC 的一个小亚组，以前路胸腰椎减压术和重建是主要术式，报道显示该术式的并发症发生率高达 52%，死亡率高达 13%（Dunning et al.，2012），可能不适合晚期患者。脊柱前路手术的术后恢复期长达 3 个月，建议在 6 个月内应持续限制体力活动，症状改善的时间可能发生在术后 18 个月以后（RNOH，2018）。总体而言，MSCC 患者预后较差，一项基于人群的研究显示 74% 的患者在入院后 3 月内死亡（McLinton and Hutchison，2006）。对于生存期达到或接近术后康复期的患者而言，手术很难使患者获益。值得注意的是，Patchell 研究的一个亚组分析表明，65 岁以上患者中手术与单纯放疗相比不能使患者有更多获益（Chi et al.，2009）。

从事 MSCC 手术治疗的医务人员应明确该治疗可能为患者带来的潜在获益，但同时也应明确手术仅适用于一小部分 MSCC 患者。

延伸阅读、参考文献、EBRAIN 的相关链接

扫描书末二维码获取。

第64章 脊髓的血管病变

Daniel Walsh 著
卞立松 译，伊志强 审校

脊髓正常血管解剖

动脉供应

脊髓由单支腹侧动脉，即脊髓前动脉（anterior spinal artery，ASA）和两支背动脉，即脊髓后动脉（posterior spinal arteries，PSA）形成的穿支动脉供血。根动脉的分支沿着背根和腹根到达脊髓。前轴位于脊髓腹中间沟内唇，由一系列神经根髓动脉形成，而后轴由神经根软膜血管形成。

胚胎发生

这些腹侧轴和背侧轴本身在子宫内形成成对的节段动脉。从子宫内的第6周到第4月，前节段动脉对发生融合，最终形成ASA。同时一些节段动脉发生退化。62条节段血管（31条背侧和31条腹侧）中，4~8条保留在腹侧，10~20条保留在背侧（Lasjaunias et al.，2001）。

脊髓前轴最早形成，后轴在胎儿发育15~20周时成熟。融合失败是ASA偶尔能见到开窗的原因。

前节段动脉退化的程度有很大的变异性，但有两个相对恒定的残留动脉。

腰膨大动脉（也称为Adamkiewicz动脉或根髓大动脉）通常起源于左侧。75%的人发生在T9和T12之间。当它在该区域外出现时，通常有第二大的保留的节段动脉，出现在其头侧或尾侧。

颈膨大动脉起源于甲状颈干和肋颈干，恒定地在C5/6水平进入椎管。同样，该处也常有变异，有直接起源自锁骨下动脉的报道（Miller，1993）。

根动脉

脊髓内的供血来源于根动脉。根动脉发出根髓动脉和根脑膜动脉，在各个节段，根髓动脉分为前后支伴随神经根进入椎管为脊髓供血。

这种外部动脉供应有相对良好的侧支循环，特别是在颈部。肋颈干的闭塞相对不太会导致脊髓前部梗死，因为颈深动脉和颈升动脉会形成侧支循环向脊髓动脉前轴提供代偿供血。

根脑膜动脉供应神经根的硬膜鞘和内容物，但不到达脊髓。硬脊膜动静脉瘘就是由这些动脉供血的。脊髓分支负责脊髓的内部供血，脊髓动静脉畸形和髓周动静脉瘘的供血动脉来自脊髓分支。

到达脊髓后，每个神经根脊髓动脉分别通过根软膜动脉或根髓动脉进入后轴和（或）前轴参与脊髓供血（**图64.1**）。

根软膜动脉

根动脉的终末支伴随脊神经根到达脊髓表面，形成PSA。这些到达脊髓的分支被称为根软膜动脉，它们从脊髓表面进入脊髓，向脊髓的周边部分供血，并在白质和灰质交界处形成分水岭。根软膜动脉和根髓动脉的小分支走行于软膜表面并环绕脊髓。被称为冠状血管。它们发出穿支血管进入脊髓浅表白质，并与前循环形成浅表吻合。

根髓动脉

前轴通过根髓动脉的放射状分支灌注前部灰质的大部分，同时也灌注白质柱的前侧、外侧、后侧的部分。每支根髓动脉都分出上升支和下降支，形成脊髓前动脉轴。沟联合动脉经腹侧前正中沟穿入脊髓，形成放射状穿支血管，灌注脊髓。

动脉吻合和“圆锥篮状吻合”

冠状血管与径向穿支血管沿脊髓形成纵向的和节段的吻合。根软膜系统和根髓系统在脊髓不同节段供血范围也不同。在颈髓二者供血基本持平，而在胸髓根软膜血管供血占比更高，但不可靠，这与众所周知的胸髓易受到缺血损伤有关，当然胸髓静脉引流也可能是原因之一，下面会提到。腰骶段供血主要依赖于中央根髓血管系统（Hassler，1966）。

脊髓前后轴的供血在圆锥部位形成很好的吻合

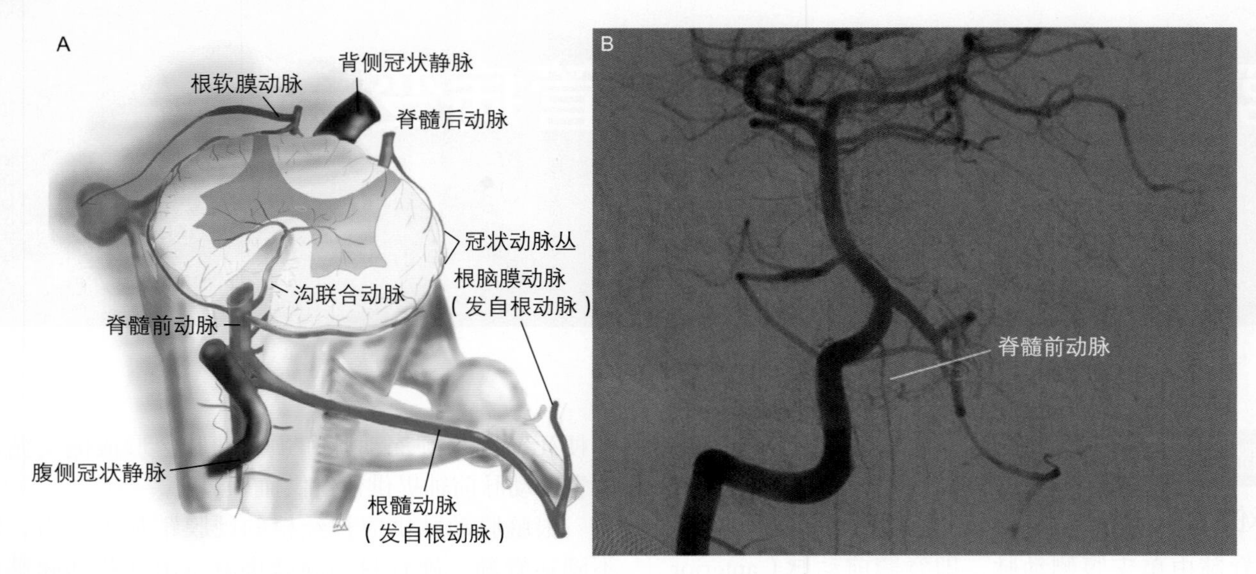

图 64.1 （A）脊髓前后动脉轴示意图；（B）脊髓血管造影（右椎动脉注射）

网，被称为圆锥篮状吻合（Lasjaunias et al.，2001）。ASA 沿圆锥前表面向下逐渐变细，分出 1~2 个分支与 PSA 连接（Martirosyan et al.，2015）。终丝动脉是前轴在圆锥以下的终末延续。

静脉引流

脊髓血液主要通过背侧和腹侧的冠状静脉丛引流沿脊髓纵轴分布的静脉毛细血管网。Thron 特别描述了横贯胸髓的大静脉，其增加了腹侧和背侧静脉血之间的沟通，但同时也导致胸髓的静脉引流能力相对过剩，可能导致胸髓易充血受损伤（Thron，1988）。

脊髓血管造影

导管内脊髓血管造影仍然是评估脊髓结构性血管病的金标准。需要对脊髓的每一节段的动脉按顺序定位，同时检查 Willis 环和骶内侧动脉。通常由股动脉进入，但如果存在严重的腹主动脉和髂动脉疾病，通过肱动脉入路也可以方便地检查胸髓和颈髓血管情况。

因此，对脊髓进行完整的血管造影检查是一个时间相对较长的过程，可能需要分期进行或全麻操作，以确保患者能够在整个过程中保持舒适和平静。生理运动（如呼吸和胃肠蠕动）可能会降低成像质量，这在全身麻醉下则更容易控制。分期检查还能做到分次辐射暴露和分次造影剂清除。

我们专门采用磁共振血管成像或 CT 血管成像做脊髓血管横断面成像帮助探查病变节段，从而进一步做介入血管内造影（Zampakis et al.，2006；Amarouche et al.，2015）。

脊髓血管造影的神经系统并发症在经验丰富的术者手中非常罕见，但其技术要求很高，故比脑血管造影的应用频率要低得多（Chen and Gailloud，2011）。非神经系统并发症包括血管损伤、腹膜后血肿、肺水肿和造影剂过敏。

脊髓的固有血管在血管造影上通常较直。脊髓静脉是典型的窦状，位于中心，比动脉更直，根髓血管以典型的“发卡”样形态终止。

自发性脊髓出血

自发性硬膜外脊髓出血

自发性脊髓硬膜外出血（spontaneous spinal epidural haemorrhages，SESH）通常是抗凝药使用的结果，与结构性血管病变无关。这种出血占非创伤性脊髓损伤原因的 11.8%（Citterio et al.，2004）。目前尚不清楚新型口服抗凝血剂（novel oral anticoagulants，NOACs）的引入将如何影响其发病率。

在对 553 例自发性中枢神经系统（central nervous system，CNS）出血患者的系统回顾中，SESH 患者明显更年轻。在一个小队列研究中，约 88% 的患者接受了手术减压，死亡和良好的预后各占结果的 21%。同样的作者进行了一项尸检研究，没有发现与创伤性脊髓损伤有任何不同的细胞炎症反应，因此建议从创伤中获得的脊髓保护经验可以有效地用于

SESH（Furlan et al.，2012）。

脊髓动脉瘤和脊髓蛛网膜下腔出血

0.6%~1% 的颅内蛛网膜下腔出血可能是由脊髓病变引起，这些病例中大多数病因是脊髓血管畸形或海绵状瘤。脊髓动脉的孤立性囊状动脉瘤是导致蛛网膜下腔出血的异常罕见的原因（Handa et al.，1992；Massand et al.，2005）。

脊髓后动脉的动脉瘤似乎更罕见，更有可能是特发性的。据报道，脊髓前动脉动脉瘤与真菌性感染、类风湿性关节炎、纤维性肌肉发育不良和白塞病有关。据报道大多数动脉瘤都是通过手术治疗成功的。一例白塞病患者通过预期治疗痊愈（Geibprasert et al.，2010）。

有病例报道显示，脊髓蛛网膜下腔出血与各种硬膜内肿瘤相关，最常见的是神经鞘瘤、室管膜瘤和血管母细胞瘤。

缺血性脊髓病

脊髓梗死比较罕见，通常是主动脉手术或严重的动脉粥样硬化性主动脉疾病的并发症。保持脊髓血流量大于 10 ml/（100 g · min）（Gharagozloo et al.，1998）可显著降低主动脉夹闭时的脊髓缺血，可通过控制鞘内脑脊液压力以增加脊髓灌注压（spinal cord perfusion pressure，SCPP）。动物实验显示，夹闭主动脉前行脑脊液引流可显著改善 SCPP（McCullough et al.，1988），有些胸腹部主动脉瘤修复时会采用这种方法。

慢性缺血性脊髓病最常见的病因是动静脉瘘。脊髓引流静脉的动脉化被认为会大大削弱脊髓的气体传输，从而导致细胞损伤并最终死亡。硬脊膜动静脉瘘是常见的病因，但不同结构的脊髓血管畸形也可引起缺血。

缺血性脊髓病的体征和症状

症状的出现往往是隐匿的，故诊断延误常见。在作者关于硬脊膜动静脉瘘（spinal dural arteriovenous fistula，SDAVF）系列的个人研究中，在诊断前，症状的中位持续时间是 18 个月。患者多为男性（比例为 1：1.5），年龄在 60~70 岁。

运动症状和感觉症状往往同时出现。患者描述感觉改变，常有东西在皮肤下爬行的感觉。后期出现感觉平面。感觉改变通常从远端开始，并上升到躯干。疼痛可能会出现类似腰椎神经根病的症状，而且通常会随着用力而加重（Jellema et al.，2003）。据报道步态障碍发生率为在 20%~69%（Atkinson et al.，2001）。典型表现是混合型上、下运动神经元症状以及本体感觉受损。括约肌和性功能常受影响，该类症状在治疗成功后恢复的可能性最小。

临床高度怀疑时应及时检查和治疗。动静脉分流引起的颈髓的缺血相对少见，根据我们的经验，更可能是由 Cognard V 型硬脑膜动静脉瘘引起的。因此在这种情况下，对 Willis 环和颈外动脉循环进行全面的血管造影检查是必要的。

检查

单独出现的脊髓缺血有非常多的鉴别诊断。若确认没有血管结构异常，则需要筛查潜在的神经炎症和肿瘤，但这方面内容超出了本章的范围。

MR 通常出现脊髓肿胀，表现为体积明显增大。提示缺血诊断。中、下胸段最常受影响，多数病例可见脊髓圆锥水肿（Muralidharan et al.，2013）。T2 相显示中央高信号，外周相对低信号环，反映了脊髓毛细血管脱氧血（Gilbertson et al.，1976）。当存在相关的动静脉分流时，可在脊髓上看到扩张的冠状静脉丛，形成多个小的血管流空影。当 MR 的这些表现突出时，提示病理性硬脊膜动静脉瘘（图 64.2A）。软膜分流可以有相似表现，但靠近脊髓表面的动脉血管密集团的存在可能会提示软膜分流。

MR 和 CT 血管成像都被用来显示硬脊膜动静脉瘘的结构。我们使用时间分辨成像对比动力学 MR 血管成像来评估瘘所在的水平，并在该水平和紧邻的节段进行定向导管血管造影，以确认瘘的存在，并确定附近是否有明显的节段动脉。对于多发瘘或实质内动静脉畸形，该检查不能提供特别有用的信息（Amarouche et al.，2015），还是要首选导管内血管造影。

二维血管断层成像对结构复杂的病灶制订手术计划有一定的帮助。微导管造影可得到横断面图像，并可分辨畸形的动脉和静脉相。如图 64.3B 所示，其中脊髓血管畸形与圆锥的关系比轴向 MR 或常规血管造影能更好地显示。这有助于在这例脊柱侧弯解剖复杂的示例病例中更好的规划手术入路。

脊髓血管畸形

在本节中，我们将更详细地研究结构性血管畸形（spinal vescular malformation，SVM），涉及其血管结构、分类和临床的关系。了解脊髓血管畸形的

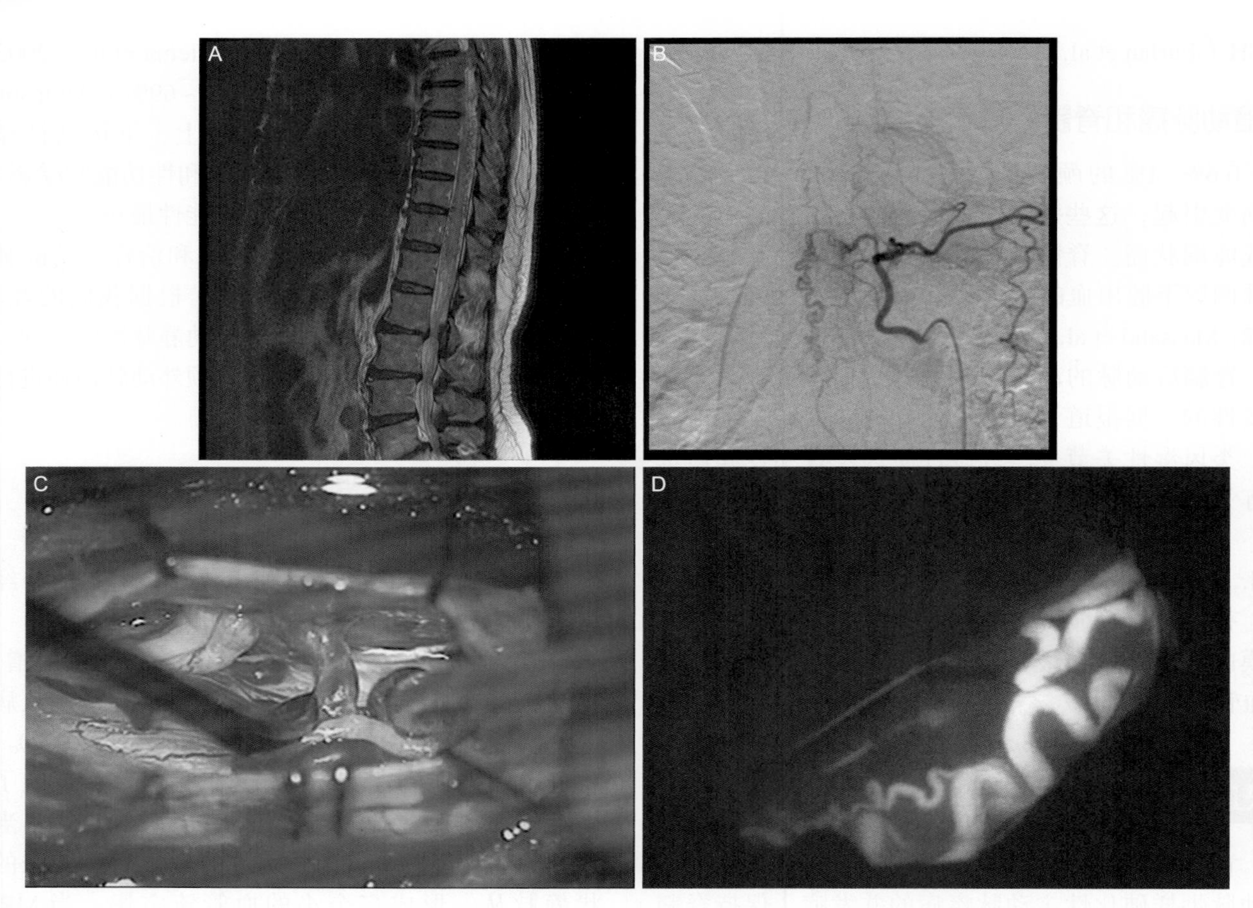

图 64.2 （A）硬脊膜动静脉瘘（SDAVF）患者的 MRI 表现；（B）SDAVF 的血管造影表现；（C）瘘口从硬脑膜引流至脊髓冠状静脉丛；（D）ICG- 造影显示背侧冠状静脉动脉化

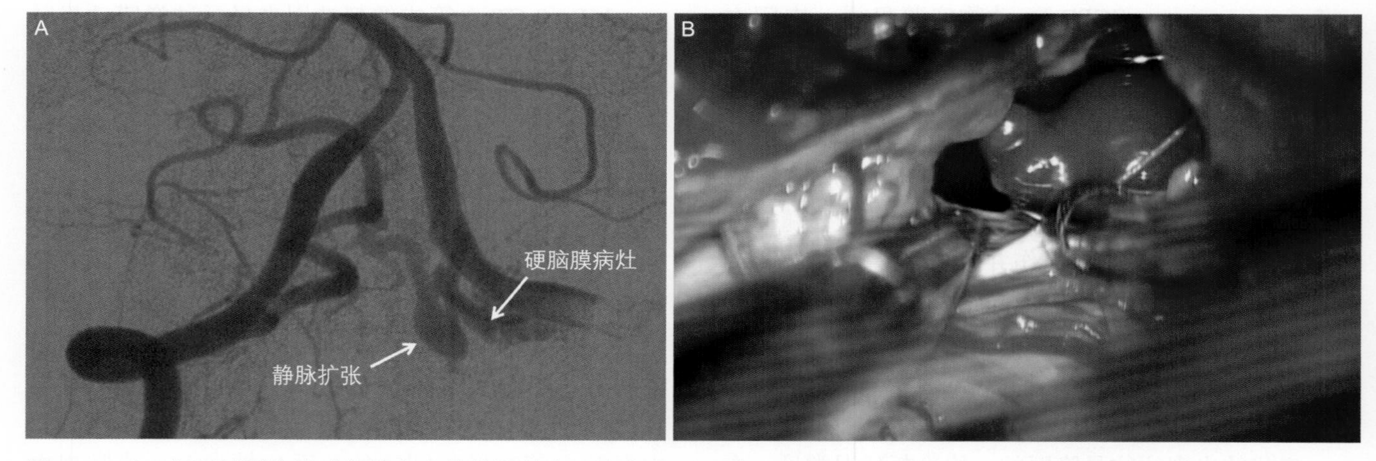

图 64.3 （A）颈髓硬脑膜动静脉瘘合并静脉扩张。患者出现网膜下腔出血发现此病变。（B）通过远侧入路显示静脉呈瘤样扩张

结构是治疗它的重要步骤。

分类系统

多年来，关于脊髓血管畸形的分类系统激增，这个主题在第一次接触时就令人生畏。事实上，仍然没有一个被普遍接受的分类系统。外科医生倾向于基于解剖学的分类系统，

而放射科医生则倾向于动静脉分流的血流动力学和病因学分类。本质上，分类系统需要回答以下三个问题：

1. 动静脉分流发生在哪里？
2. 如何达到病变？
3. 有合并的其他病变吗？

2002 年，Bicêtre 医院提出了一种具有吸引力的简洁的系统，将脊髓畸形大致分为动静脉畸形和动静脉瘘（Rodesch et al.，2002）。他们建议根据发病机制将动静脉瘘（arteriovenous fistula，AVF）和动静脉畸形（arteriovenous malformation，AVM）归为三种类型之一：

第 1 组：基因遗传性病变（例如，与遗传性出血性毛细血管扩张症相关）。

第 2 组：有体节联系的基因非遗传性病变。迄今为止，在一个脊髓节段内累及多种组织的血管畸形被称为幼稚型或体节性动静脉畸形。在一个脊髓节段内的所有组织都受累，被称为 Cobbs 综合征。这可能是 CLOVES 综合征中脊髓病变的一个相对常见的原因（Alomari et al.，2011）。将颅面血管畸形归类为脑面体节性动静脉综合征（CAMS 1~3），可以根据受累的体节进行描述，而不是依赖于命名者描述，如 Wyburn-Mason 综合征或 Bonnet-Dechaume-Blanc 综合征。同样的系统可以应用于脊髓体节病，根据受累节段不同，描述 SAM 1~31 型病变。也存在多体节受累的变异情况（Bhattacharya et al.，2001）。

第 3 组：孤立性病变。这一组的病变可能代表了第 1 组和第 2 组病变的表达不完全，但它也可能包括获得性病变，这意味着可以将绝大多数的脊髓血管畸形归于这一组。对这一组进行亚组分类是有用的，以前称为幼稚型或体节性动静脉畸形Ⅲ病变属于 Bicêtre 第 2 组，并且将会有Ⅳ型病变属于第 1 组或第 2 组的情况（例如，被描述为毛细血管畸形 -AVM 综合征的 Ras 病；Eerola et al.，2003；Tiex et al.，2010）。

这样的命名系统是有用的，因为它提示人们考虑不常见的结构畸形或涉及一种以上组织类型的潜在相关病变。例如，识别第 1 组病变应及时进行基因学咨询，与患者沟通可能存在遗传性出血性毛细血管扩张症（hereditary haemorrhagic telangectasia，HHT）潜在的肺部和中枢神经系统并发症。正如最初所写的那样，椎旁和硬膜的畸形被排除在外，使该系统的实际应用有限，并招致了批评（Rodesch et al.，2002）。我们发现将这些病变纳入第 3 组是切实可行的。许多椎旁动静脉畸形可能被认为是节段病变的不完全表达。有获得性髓周瘘和硬脊膜瘘的例子，它们归在第 3 组。

一个将 SVM 分类为Ⅰ~Ⅳ组的系统已经存在了多年，由来自法国、英国和美国的一大批临床科学家不断发展完善。出于这个原因，一些作者在描述它时会提到其与美 - 英 - 法的联系（Black，2006）。

Merland 提出了一个关于髓周瘘有用的细分（Gueguen et al.，1987），该细分是由 Djindjian 首先描述的（Djindjian et al.，1977）。Heros 建议将髓周瘘视为离散型Ⅳ型病变（Heros et al.，1986），而其他人则将其描述为瘘型动静脉畸形（瘘型脊髓动静脉畸形 SCAVM），因为它们通常主要由髓根动脉供应，其被认为是脊髓血供的一部分。

最好不要拘泥于一种命名法。现在出现了进一步的细分，相对于从前的理解，曾经被认为不同的一些病变被发现其实有更多的共同点。本章的其余部分采用了前面描述的 Bicêtre 系统的改良版（**专栏 64.1**）。**表** 64.1 总结了美英法体系。对血管结构的理解比命名更重要。

硬膜外（椎旁）血管畸形

这些病变罕见，仅向硬膜外静脉丛引流。可自发出现（Willinsky，1993），或作为外伤后的并发

专栏 64.1　改良的脊髓血管畸形 Bicêtre 分类

第 1 组

基因遗传性病变（例如：与遗传性出血性毛细血管扩张症相关）

第 2 组

有体节联系的基因非遗传性病变 - 脊髓动静脉体节综合征（SAMS）

第 3 组

获得性或第 1 组或第 2 组表现不完全的孤立性病变

椎旁血管畸形

硬脊膜动静脉瘘

　a）孤立性瘘

　b）多发瘘

髓内动静脉畸形

髓周瘘

　a）孤立性简单瘘，有小的静脉扩张

　b）1~2 条供血动脉，中度静脉扩张 +/- 瘘管部位的静脉囊袋

　c）巨大的多瘘口病变

表 64.1　美英法脊柱血管畸形分类

Ⅰ类	脊髓硬脑膜动静脉瘘 • 孤立性瘘 • 多发性瘘
Ⅱ类	髓内 AVM
Ⅲ型	幼年或偏角动静脉畸形（SAMS）
Ⅳ类	髓外瘘 • 单纯瘘，微小静脉扩张 • 1~2 条供血动脉，中度静脉扩大 +/- 瘘管部位的静脉袋 • 巨大多瘘病变

症出现（Johnson et al.，1990）或出现在神经纤维瘤病一型患者中（Deans et al.，1982; Benndorf et al.，2000）。也可以是 Bicêtre 所建议的那样，是一种基因非遗传性畸形的不完全表达（见前面描述）。

无症状的椎旁畸形在断面影像上会偶然遇到。根据静脉充血的程度不同，当压迫硬膜囊或神经根时会出现症状。**图** 64.4 展示了一例表现为严重腰椎放射痛的椎旁动静脉瘘病例。瘘被栓塞后，腰痛快速且完全消失。可逆性的脊髓病也有报道（Willinsky，1993）。

这些病也可表现为自发性硬膜外血肿，尤其是在儿童中（Lonjon et al.，1997; Sivakumaran et al.，2016）。3%~18% 的血肿被认为是由血管畸形引起的（Kubo et al.，1984; Graziani et al.，1994）。

治疗包括血管内介入治疗及外科手术治疗，基于已发表病例，对于有症状的病变结果通常是良好的。

硬脊膜动静脉瘘

SDAVF 占临床上脊髓血管畸形的 70%~85%（Merland et al.，1980；Symon et al.，1984），男性发病率是女性的五倍，通常在 50 岁左右起病。这不同于其他类型的脊髓血管畸形，后者通常在 30~40 岁起病（Djindjian et al.，1977; Rosenblum et al.，1987）。SDAVF 被认为是获得性病变，其发病机制尚不清楚。

SDAVF 最常见于胸椎。在我们病例中，胸椎占 68.5%。颈椎和骶椎各占不到 5%，腰椎占 21%。多发瘘的发病率约为 2%（Krings et al.，2004）。

瘘发生在靠近脊神经根出口处的硬膜上。静脉在此处引流向神经鞘及其内容物供血的根脊膜动脉的血液。动脉化的静脉在神经根下方穿行硬膜，容易识别。静脉通常直接从椎弓根下方进入。在静脉穿过硬膜处仔细观察，可以发现供应瘘口的明显的动脉。在此处切断静脉会闭塞动静脉分流。不需要切除硬脊膜来治疗瘘。

动脉化的静脉直接连接冠状静脉丛，造成脊髓充血，这在缺血性脊髓病的章节中已有描述。硬脊膜动静脉瘘引起的蛛网膜下腔出血极为罕见，常与颈髓瘘有关。腰髓瘘和胸髓瘘出血的病例也有过报道（Koch et al.，2004）。静脉瘤和静脉扩张在这种情况下很常见。

显微外科治疗

通常通过（半）椎板切除术或椎板切开术在硬膜内暴露瘘口。管状牵开系统和光纤照明的应用使得可以通过微创入路进行手术。术中找到静脉穿行硬膜处，电凝切断，并电凝其周围的硬膜。仅电凝切断供血动脉可能会导致短暂的症状改善，但必然会出现其他硬脑膜动脉供血继而出现瘘的复发。

当背侧冠状静脉丛动脉化时，静脉充盈，略呈粉色。当闭塞动静脉分流时，则静脉塌陷，其被覆

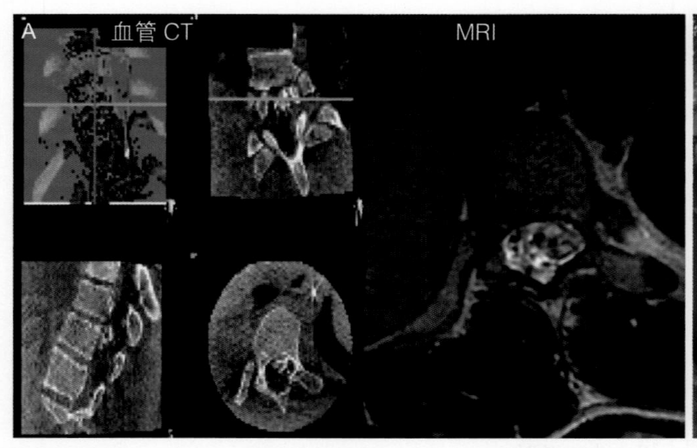

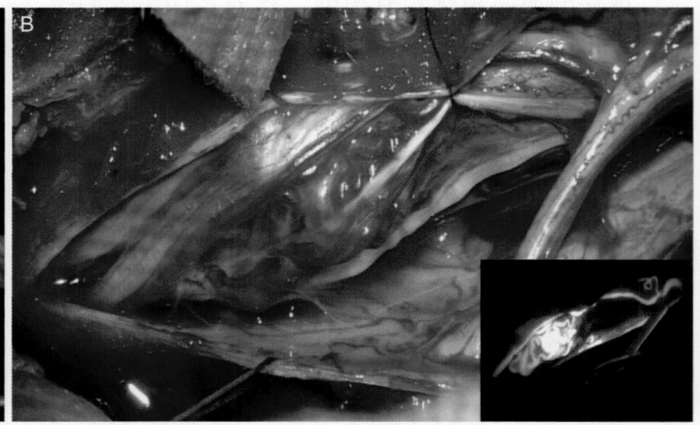

图 64.4　（A）二维（2D）血管断层摄影显示圆锥腹外侧表面有致密的髓内动静脉畸形；（B）肋骨横突切除后显示手术野

的蛛网膜出现小圆齿状改变。但在相对低的动静脉分流中，肉眼变化并不总是很明显。微多普勒检查（Iacopino et al.，2001）或吲哚菁绿血管造影（ICG-VA）可用于确认静脉血流的正常化。ICG-VA 也有助于发现异常动脉并将其与动脉化的静脉区分开（Walsh et al.，2013）。**图** 64.2A~D 显示了在 ICG-VA 上观察到的血流变化。

目前硬脊膜动静脉瘘的标准治疗是显微外科手术切断瘘口。最近的一项对 2004 年以来的英语文献的 meta 分析，包括了 35 项涉及 1112 名患者的研究。其中外科手术闭塞率为 96.6%（94.8%~97.8% 95%CI）。氰基丙烯酸正丁酯（NBCA）或 Onyx 血管内治疗闭塞率为 72.2%（95%CI，68.1%~75.9%）。血管内治疗明显更有可能出现瘘的晚期复发（Bakker et al.，2015）。

手术并发症发生率也比较有利。在 Steinmetz 及其同事进行的 meta 分析中，手术和血管内治疗的并发症比例分别为 1.9% 和 3.7%。这两种治疗方法都是相对安全的，而且大多数并发症很轻。术中将瘘行点状断开意味着冠状静脉本身的风险很小。

外科手术治疗的一个重大风险是脊髓节段定位错误。可在术中通过仔细透视来降低这种风险。血管内置入的弹簧圈（Britz et al.，2004）或注入的 Onyx（Timo Krings et al.，2010）有助于术中识别相应脊髓节段。

血管内治疗

为了达到有效的治疗效果，栓剂必须达到引流静脉穿过硬脊膜后的近端，重复前面描述过的动静脉分流的"点"断开。单独用颗粒和弹簧圈栓塞供血动脉，不能产生持久效果。液体栓塞剂如 Onyx 或 NCBA 经动脉输送时能有效地穿透硬膜至引流静脉端。如果术中造影发现，栓塞剂未能到达引流静脉，则需要进一步治疗。而且进一步治疗不宜延迟，若引流静脉通畅，不能寄希望于瘘口自发形成血栓而闭塞。若不及时治疗，这些病例会出现进一步的临床恶化（Andres et al.，2008）。

栓塞治疗的治愈率明显低于手术切断瘘口。一些作者主张在诊断性血管造影术时尝试栓塞。采用该方案应告知患者冠状静脉逆行血栓形成的小风险，后者可导致神经功能恶化。

SDAVF 的治疗结果

只要闭塞了动静脉分流，血管内治疗和手术治疗 SDAVF 的结果是相似的。Aminof 和 Logue（1974）对患者步态及排尿控制障碍进行了分级（**表** 64.2），该系统仍用于评价治疗结果。

在一项 154 例手术治疗患者的研究中，45% 的患者在出院时下肢力量有所改善。约 12% 的患者感觉改善，15% 的患者括约肌功能改善，而 17% 的患者括约肌功能恶化。大多数患者在治疗后短期内症状没有变化。利用 Aminof-Logue 步态和排尿联合评分作为功能障碍的综合评价指标，发现 45% 的患者在平均随访 31 个月时有所改善，而 34% 的患者保持在术前基线（Bakker et al.，2015）。括约肌功能障碍的预后不良。Steinmetz 发现，在括约肌功能有任何改善的 33% 的患者中，经过更长时间的随访，其中 11% 的患者出现恶化，89% 的患者改善或稳定（Steinmetz et al.，2004）。

髓内动静脉畸形

脊髓动静脉畸形（spinal cord arteriovenous malformations，SCAVM）是由脊髓固有的动脉到静脉引流的分流形成的。有人将血管球（或血管巢）的变异类型与瘘型 AVM 区分开。血管球（血管巢）型动静脉畸形有一个位于软脊膜深部的离散病灶，在结构上与脑动静脉畸形相同。可以将它们描述为紧密型、弥散型或混合型。我们将瘘状病变作为单独的一个疾病类型——髓周瘘（perimedullary fistula，PMAVF）。在文献中这一区别是令人困惑的，这也显示了有时

表 64.2 Aminoff-Logue 分级系统

等级	定义
步态	
0	正常
1	腿部无力、步态异常或活动不受限制的站立
2	活动受限
3	需要一根棍子或类似的支撑物
4	需要拄着拐杖或两根拐杖才能走路
5	不能站立、卧床或坐轮椅
排尿	
0	正常
1	尿等待、尿频或尿急
2	偶尔尿失禁或尿潴留
3	永久性尿失禁或尿潴留

当有各种静脉 - 静脉或其他生理血管吻合充血时，评价血管巢的困难。

这些病变也可细分为高、低流量病变。高流量病变的特点是血管重塑：动脉扩张，发生动脉瘤和静脉囊袋。多见于儿童和 HHT 患者。在对 155 名患者的回顾研究中，Rodesch 等观察到 31.6% 的动脉瘤发生率（Rodesch et al.，2002）。

这种血管压力与髓内或蛛网膜下腔出血的增加有关。也可能表现为缺血性脊髓病，或血管扩张引起的神经压迫症状。据报道，约 30% 的患者有神经性疼痛。

偶然发现的病变的自然病史尚不清楚。一项对包含超过 3 例病例的研究进行的汇总分析表明，每年的出血率为 4%，大约一半的这些病变首发症状表现为出血。同样的数据显示，部分治疗在一定程度上降低了出血风险，在所有类型病变中部分治疗后出血复发率为 2%~3%（Gross and Du，2013a）。

血管内治疗

血管内治疗在这些病变的治疗中占有重要地位，尤其是那些主要来自脊髓前动脉供血的病变。治疗目标可能与脑动静脉畸形略有不同，有证据表明，部分治疗不仅可以减轻缺血症状及占位效应，而且可能有利于影响出血风险。Onyx 或 NCBA 胶是目前最常用的液体栓塞剂，可穿透到达血管巢内。弹簧圈可用于治疗静脉囊袋、扩张和动脉瘤

由于治疗的血管结构存在相当大的差异，治疗结果也不尽相同。所以，术者必须仔细判断每个步骤，以免栓塞材料误栓塞导致缺血损伤。

在包含 104 例患者的 16 项研究中，33% 的液体栓塞剂治疗导致分流完全闭塞（Gross and Du，2013a）。与手术相比，10 年的 Aminof-Logue 步态和排尿功能评分结果相似。随访期间无再出血记录。与 Onyx 或 NCBA 胶（0~11%）相比，聚乙烯醇（PVA）颗粒栓塞（17%）明显更容易发生再通。

显微手术

在某些选定的病例中，手术切除是一种有效的治疗方法，其并发症发生率主要取决于畸形的位置和达到病变的难度。Spetzler 建议将圆锥致密动静脉畸形作为一种亚型，特别适合手术治疗（Spetzler et al.，2002）。

手术切除的原则类似于颅内同类病变，但技术方面的某些细微差别值得注意。首先，作为相对低流量的病变，有利于先处理静脉端，而不用担心像颅内病变一样出现脊髓出血或充血肿胀。其次，要避免过度剥离软膜，尽量在“原位”离断瘘，不要试图完全切除畸形的所有组成部分。当血管内栓塞后进行手术时，无需切除完全栓塞的畸形部分，以免进一步干扰神经组织。

大多数病变可通过后方或后外侧入路进行手术。我们再次发现，二维血管断层扫描有助于计划手术入路，术中常规使用神经电生理监测，特别是通过 Delta 波和运动诱发电位来监测前方运动束的改变（**图 64.4A**）。

在 Gross 的分析中，78% 的病例得到根治性切除。93% 的患者长期 Aminof-Logue 步态评分得到改善或维持稳定，94% 的患者排尿评分相同或更好。很多患者术前都有明显的功能障碍，因为出现症状而寻求治疗（Gross and Du，2013a）。

放射外科

脊髓动静脉畸形的体积对放射外科治疗具有吸引力。其面临的挑战也是颅内同类疾病所没有的。应用现代图像引导系统有助于消除呼吸运动的影响，将高度适形的放射线聚焦特定靶区，进而消除病变。

Sinclair 等报道了他们使用射波刀（CyberKnife™）平台治疗 15 例硬膜内 AVM 的经验。为避免脊髓放射损伤，分为 2~5 次治疗。在平均 27.9 个月的随访中，只有 1 例畸形被根治。对这些病变的短时间随访限制了对其疗效的总结（Sinclair et al.，2006）。Hida 等报道了 10 名患者使用 LINAC 的 10 年经验。未观察到任何一例患者病变完全闭塞，但在 49 个月的中位随访中，未观察到随后的出血或任何的放射毒性（Hida et al.，2003）。

脊髓对辐射的耐受性仍在研究之中。目前认为，病变完全闭塞的机会似乎很低，但考虑到部分治疗可以改善其他并发症的预后，这些病变的放射治疗值得进一步研究。

髓周瘘

髓周动静脉瘘（perimedullary arteriovenous fistulae，PMAVF）是脊髓表面固有动脉与引流静脉之间的直接交通。通常起源于前动脉轴，偶尔也会遇到根软膜瘘。根据供血动脉的数量、流量和大小对瘘进行再分类（见**专栏** 64.1 和**表** 64.1）。在文献中，它们有时被称为软膜动静脉瘘或瘘型脊髓动静脉畸形（SCAVM）。

大多数 PMAVF 表现为缺血性脊髓病，但约 32% 的患者发生出血，其临床病程与 SDAVF 不同（Gross

and Du，2013b）。它们可能作为孤立的病变发生，也可能与遗传疾病相关，例如HHT（髓周大瘘）或CM-AVM Ras病。

此外，由于这些不常见病变大多是在有症状时才发现的，因此缺乏可靠的自然史数据。虽然已发表的结果令人鼓舞：A型病灶的闭塞率为93%，C型病灶的闭塞率为71%。但关于治疗的数据仅限于相对较小的病例。显微手术和血管内治疗是主要的治疗手段。C型病变特别适合血管内治疗，因为增生的供血动脉便于导管导入。A型和B型病变可通过血管内治疗、外科治疗或联合处理。我们中心常发现不适合手术治疗的PMAVF，适合血管内治疗（Amarouche et al.，2015）。

文献中关于放射外科的经验很少。有一例报道使用射波刀治疗，但没有任何结果数据。有可能斯坦福的一些病例（射波刀）是瘘型AVM，但没有提供所有结构的详细信息。我们用射波刀治疗了1例中胸段的A型PMAVF，随访18个月没有任何效果。

脊髓海绵状血管瘤

可以合理地认为，海绵状血管瘤不属于脊髓血管病变的讨论范畴。除非与深静脉异常（deep venous anomaly，DVA）相关，否则它们是低压力、血管造影隐匿性病变。对所有海绵状血管瘤的自然史了解甚少，尤其是罕见的脊髓海绵状血管瘤。

海绵状血管瘤文献多为手术病例。当病变出现症状时，建议进行治疗。对于血液成分缓慢渗出到周围组织为特点的病变，其出血的定义是有疑问的。相比症状性微出血，明显的出血是否该作为导致功能障碍的预测因素？

髓内海绵状血管瘤

最近的一项meta分析包含40项符合分析标准的研究，涵盖632例患者（Badhiwala et al.，2014）。约376例患者报告了预后数据。胸髓是最常见的病变部位，占55.2%，其次是颈髓（38%）、颈胸段（2.4%）、腰髓（2.1%）、圆锥（1.7%）和胸腰段（0.6%）。年出血率为2.1%。其中，脑海绵状血管瘤与多发性海绵状血管瘤并存的病例约占50%。

作者的结论是，症状性病变的手术干预是有数据支持的。有急性症状的患者的治疗结局优于慢性症状患者。超过80%的接受手术的患者在最终随访时症状改善或稳定，尽管术后早期恶化是常见的（27%）。虽然干预与良好结局相关，但应该注意的是，在这些研究中只有10%的患者接受了保守治疗。

硬膜外海绵状血管瘤

硬膜外海绵状血管瘤很少见，偶尔需要外科治疗。单纯的骨内病变可能是最常见的，但很少有症状。硬膜外病变可因其大小和位置而产生神经根性疼痛和（或）脊髓病。92%的患者手术切除可获得良好的结果（Mühmer et al.，2014）。

放射外科和脊髓海绵状血管瘤

当需要干预时，手术切除仍然是标准治疗方法。有报道描述了一例椎旁海绵状血管瘤因出血而放弃手术后，行放疗取得明显成功（Sohn et al.，2009）。报道过一例中胸段髓内海绵状血管瘤的放射治疗，但仅以随访6个月作为疗效的证据（Martin et al.，2012）。几乎没有证据支持这种应用。

关键参考文献、参考文献、EBRAIN的相关链接

扫描书末二维码获取。

第 65 章　椎管脑脊液动力学

Graham Flint 著

范存刚、汤韫钰 译，范存刚 审校

病理生理学

颅后窝和椎管内脑脊液柱在每分钟约 70 次动脉压力波影响下产生“往复”运动，同时也受静脉压力波的影响。静脉压力波频率较低，时间不规则，但波幅较大，任何 Valsalva 样动作均可引起静脉波幅变化。静脉波造成颅内和椎管内的腔室之间大量的液体流动。任何 Valsalva 样动作均可引起由椎管硬膜囊至颅内的脑脊液净流量，Valsalva 动作结束时脑脊液液体返回椎管，伴随椎管硬膜外静脉塌陷使硬膜囊再次扩张。

颅椎交界处的脑脊液流动部分受阻时，脑脊液的流体动力学也会发生某些变化。在咳嗽、用力等情况下，液体仍会自由流入颅内，但不会轻易反流。此时，多余的脑脊液暂时滞留在颅内，在由蛛网膜颗粒吸收前会有一段持续数秒的颅内压增高。这种压力分离性头痛病史的准确描述为头痛并非发生在咳嗽或用力时，而是在咳嗽或用力后立即出现。类似的，患者由弯腰状态站起后也会发生头痛。

如果脑脊液沿椎管的自由运动受阻，动脉压力波也可能会产生不良影响。在解剖结构正常的情况下，脑脊液的收缩压力波分散于整个椎管。如果椎管内脑脊液的部分通道受阻，同样的能量不能很容易地扩散，转而作用于脊髓外表面。类似的，当疝出的小脑扁桃体反复“撞击”脑脊液柱而后者被有效地滞留椎管内时，脑脊液收缩压力波则难以自由地反冲至颅内。

因此，我们可以设想一种正常的解剖状态，小脑扁桃体、脑干和脊髓在连续的脑脊液柱内呈节律性振荡，脑脊液柱随心动周期同步上下摆动。在 Valsalva 动作期间，脑脊液进入颅内时后脑结构会向上抬起，直至用力消失后才返回。椎管任何部位的脑脊液运动受阻均可引起上述正常脑脊液流动模式严重紊乱，正常压力波变形，产生明显的症状，某些情况下还可引起进行性加重的解剖学改变。

临床检查

磁共振成像（magnetic resonance imaging，MRI）是疑似椎管脑脊液运动障碍疾病的主要检查方法。理想的成像应包括整个神经轴，这是因为椎管脑脊液病变可能与颅内的解剖异常有关，抑或表现为颅内信号改变。T2 序列能清晰显示正常的脑脊液通道，也能显示异常的液体积聚。此外，明亮的白色信号表明脑脊液流动停滞，而灰色的“漩涡”提示脑脊液湍流。有时，可能难以区分脊髓的空洞前水肿与明显的空洞，此时 T1 成像可辅助诊断。动静脉瘘引起的水肿可能会误诊为空洞前水肿。标准 T2 成像难以显示蛛网膜网，但重加权 T2 成像则可以显示蛛网膜网。还需要进行增强扫描以排除相关的肿瘤性病变。

心脏门控相位对比流动研究显示脑脊液在收缩期和舒张期进行“往复”运动，有助于评估解剖学上处于临界值的扁桃体下降。如果脑脊液运动有明显障碍，则可根据脑脊液流量（减少）和流速（增加）进行定量测量。

直立位 MRI 可以显示从水平到直立位变化的细微解剖运动。这些发现有助于诊断解剖学上小脑扁桃体下降程度处于临界值的脑脊液运动梗阻。

超声影像可用于术中定位椎管内异常积聚的脑脊液，也可以用于确定硬膜外减压是否有效地缓解了颅椎交界处脑脊液运动障碍。

电生理检查可作为辅助的诊断手段。即使出现的症状与影像学表现不符，在临床体检中也未发现支持诊断的体征，体感诱发电位（somatosensory evoked potentials，SSEPs）也可能出现异常。运动诱发电位和 SSEPs 也可用于辅助术中决策——是否需要将打开硬膜作为颅椎体减压术的一部分。

脊髓空洞症

脊髓空洞症是脊髓内出现充满脑脊液的空洞，

可有多种不同的表现（图 65.1）。一些权威学者认为脊髓积水和脊髓空洞症有区别：前者本质上是胚胎性脊髓中央管扩张，由室管膜衬覆；后者是沿脊髓中央管逐渐形成的，以胶质组织衬覆。无论是脊髓积水抑或脊髓空洞症，其解释所面临的挑战均为空洞形成原因如何，以及何种因素决定空洞会增至多大。多数空洞无论其大小如何，很可能与椎管的某个部位脑脊液正常流动的梗阻有关（专栏 65.1）。这种梗阻不一定很明显，但多次序列成像可揭示空洞发展的方向。空洞通常向远离梗阻部位的方向发展，这意味着空洞“保持固定”的一端位于脑脊液流动梗阻部位。

脊髓空洞症的流行病学数据并不准确，有明显的地域和种族差异，其估计值也随时间变化而异，这可能反映了所研究的人群构成的变化。据研究工作估计，人群年发病率为 $0.5\sim1.0/10^5$ 人，患病率为 $5\sim10/10^5$ 人。随着磁共振成像的广泛应用，检出了更多处于疾病演变早期阶段的病例，这些患者很少出现神经功能障碍。目前检出更多的 Chiari 畸形病例，其中至少半数没有伴发脊髓空洞症。

临床表现

脊髓空洞症的平均发病年龄为 30~40 岁，但其年龄范围很广，可以从儿童到退休人群。临床特征可分为基础病变所致的表现和空洞本身引起的症状（专栏 65.2）。

典型的临床表现为斗篷状分布的分离性感觉丧失、爪形手和手部肌肉萎缩，其表面有烫伤瘢痕，以及上肢和腹部反射消失伴下肢腱放射亢进，这些表现目前在临床上仍可见到，仅是偶尔遇见而已。目前更多患者表现为脊柱或四肢疼痛或躯体感觉障碍，如动作笨拙和失衡感觉。疲劳是一种常见但不够特异的主诉。这些症状可能误诊为纤维肌痛所致，在最终确诊时可能会引发患者不满。

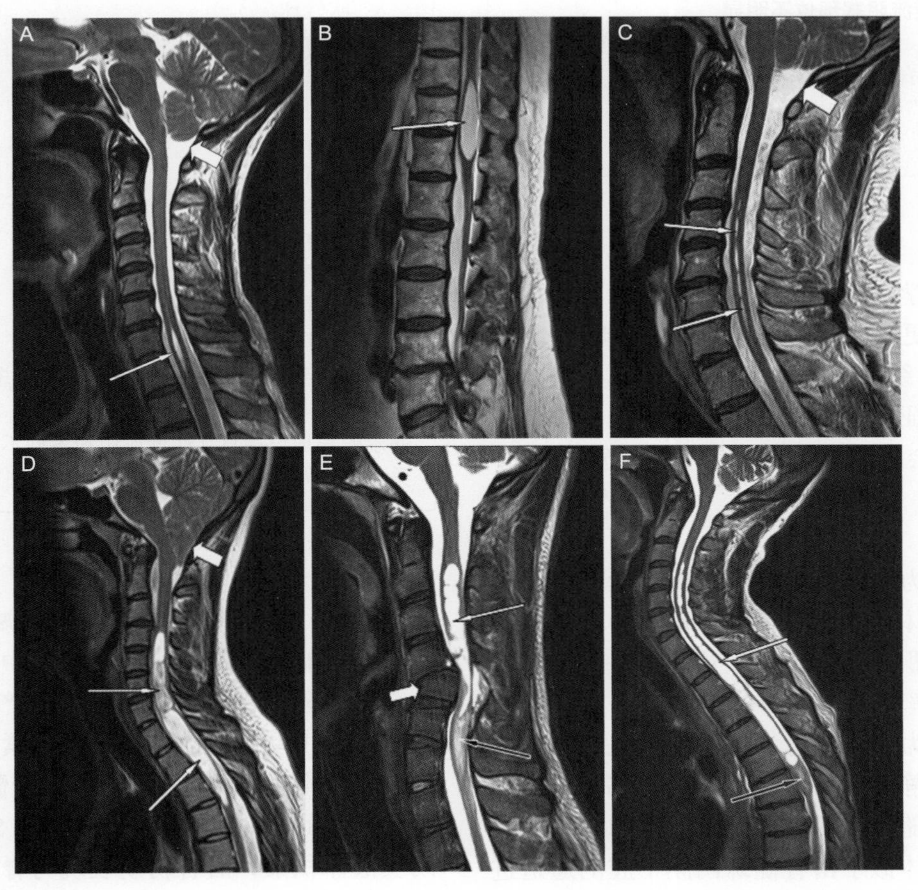

图 65.1 脊髓空洞症的形态学变异。T2 加权 MR 成像显示：（A）纺锤形空洞，两端尖（长箭头）。脑脊液在椎管内流动未受阻。小脑扁桃体位置相对较低，但未通过枕骨大孔下降，枕大池开放（短箭头）；有些人将其称为 0 型 Chiari 畸形。（B）由脑脊液充盈的短小、有张力的空洞，两端呈圆形（箭头所示），有时称为胶质室管膜囊肿。（C）异常明显的中央管（长箭头）和宽开口的枕大池（短箭头）。（D）由 1 型 Chiari 畸形（短箭头）引起的大且有张力的空洞（长箭头）。（E）紧邻 C5 椎体损伤（短箭头）处上方的创伤后空洞（长、白色箭头）。下方，脊髓形成空洞前水肿（长的黑箭头）。（F）广泛的空洞（白色箭头），可见明显的囊袋形成，后者是由其下方的髓内肿瘤向上扩展形成的（黑色箭头）

专栏 65.1 脊髓空洞症的分类和病因

后脑相关病变
- 1 型 Chiari 畸形
  - 先天性颅后窝狭小
  - 颅缝早闭（如 Crouzon 综合征）
  - 小脑占位引起的慢性压力锥
  - 椎管脑脊液漏 / 腰大池 - 腹腔分流
  - 良性颅内压增高
- 1.5 型 Chiari 畸形 ± 脊髓栓系
- 2 型 Chiari 畸形 + 开放性脊柱裂
- 颅底蛛网膜纤维化（出血后 / 炎症性）
- 颅骨增厚或软化疾病 ± 颅底凹陷（如 Paget 病、佝偻病）

原发性脊柱病变
- 脊髓损伤 *
- 感染——化脓性或结核性 *
- 蛛网膜下腔出血——颅脑或脊髓 *
- 蛛网膜囊肿或蛛网膜网
- 髓内肿瘤

* 炎症后蛛网膜纤维化是常见因素

特发性——脑脊液流阻塞部位不明显
- O 型 Chiari 畸形
- 明显的中央管（脊髓积水）
- 孤立的"纺锤形"空洞
- 胶质室管膜囊肿

专栏 65.2 后脑相关脊髓空洞症的临床特征

局部压力
- 颅底硬膜
  - 枕部头痛
- 神经结构
  - 延髓 / 后组脑神经
    - 复视 / 斜视 / 眼球震颤
    - 眩晕 / 共济失调
    - 耳鸣
    - 面部疼痛 / 麻木
    - 构音障碍 / 发声障碍 / 吞咽困难
    - 睡眠呼吸暂停
    - 晕厥
  - 长传导束
    - 躯体感觉障碍
    - 主观无力 / 疲劳

脑脊液流梗阻
- 压力分离性头痛
  - 咳嗽 / 打喷嚏
  - 用力
  - 向前屈身
  - 吹气球
- 空洞形成
  - 中央灰质
    - 肌肉萎缩
    - 爪形手
    - 霍纳综合征
    - 脊柱侧凸
  - 长束
    - 脊髓丘脑感觉丧失
    - 中枢神经性疼痛
    - 下肢痉挛
    - 自主神经紊乱（膀胱、肠道、多汗症）

偶尔的表现包括直立性低血压和各种不自主的肢体运动，类似锥体外系综合征

真正的解剖学上的延髓空洞症罕见，延髓或后组脑神经的特征更可能是由潜在的 Chiari 畸形所致。偶尔可通过发际线较低发现伴发的骨骼异常，如 Klippel-Feil 综合征。青少年脊柱侧凸也是一种常见表现。幼童可能会出现呼吸困难，并由此危及生命。

充盈机制

有人可能认为，脑脊液在椎管内的运动受阻可引起脊髓外的液体压迫。这种情形确实会发生，但脊髓内的脑脊液积聚更为常见，这究竟是如何发生的尚未得到充分解释。

早期理论认为，当枕骨大孔发生梗阻时，脑脊液在动脉搏动或静脉压力波驱动下经闩部进入脊髓中央管。然而，随着使用水溶性造影剂的脊髓造影术问世，显示液体似乎由脊髓蛛网膜下腔的通道进入空洞。脊髓空洞症动物模型的实验研究支持上述解释。为了使脑脊液进入一个自身处于张力状态的空洞，必须有某种形式的瓣膜机制。当椎管脑脊液通道发生梗阻时，收缩压力波不能自由扩散，从而形成跨脊髓实质的透壁压，迫使脑脊液沿血管周围间隙流动，而这些间隙可能发挥了瓣膜作用。

也可能也有其他机制参与其中。在脑脊液流发生部分梗阻的部位以下，可能会产生 Venturi 效应，后者也是由动脉压力波动所致。紧邻梗阻部位下方的脑脊液流速增加，在髓外产生较髓内更低的压力，由此改变了作用在毛细血管床上的 Starling 力，引起间质液体积聚，后者初期表现为脊髓水肿，此后汇合成充满液体的腔。

因此，动脉能量似乎是引起空洞形成和充盈的可能性最大的驱动力。静脉压力波具有较大的振幅和较长的持续时间，可能通过液压"挤压"效应导致此后的空洞进展。

后脑相关脊髓空洞症

Chiari 1 型畸形是脊髓空洞症最常见的病因（**图 65.2A**）。Chiari 1 型畸形是一组表现各异的疾患（**专栏 65.1**），但通常认为是中胚层发育异常所致，即颅后窝容积过小、难以容纳小脑。该病可能有遗传基础，正如某些品系的狗 Chiari 样畸形发病率很高所证实。家族性聚集偶尔也可见于人类。颅后窝容积可能是主要遗传特征，扁桃体疝为继发性发育所致。患者通常在骨骼发育完成多年后才出现症状，表明颅内压等其他因素可能发挥作用；实际上，约 1/5 的显性良性颅内压增高患者在 MRI 扫描中可见扁桃体下移。

Chiari 2 型畸形由脊柱闭合不全引起。神经管尾端闭合失败导致脑脊液渗漏至羊膜囊，阻碍颅后窝结构正常发育（**图 65.2B**）。

有时可见介于 1 型和 2 型之间的 MRI 表现，延髓和闩部以及小脑扁桃体均下移，但没有脊柱闭合不全或后脑整体下降（**图 65.2C**）。

所有这些类型的 Chiari 畸形均可伴发脊髓空洞症，但形成脊髓空洞的决定因素尚不清楚。脊髓空洞症也可见于没有明显后脑疝者，而减压手术也能使空洞萎陷，此类谓之 Chiari 0 型畸形，推测为脑脊液在颅椎交界处的运动受阻所致，可能为薄层蛛网膜网或枕大池过于拥挤所致。一般而言，MRI 上所见的解剖学下降程度与患者症状的严重程度之间的相关性较差。因此，影像学上测量的扁桃体下降的绝对值对评估具体患者的价值有限。

后脑疝的临床特征可以从局部结构受压和脑脊液运动梗阻两方面考虑。神经痛和面部不自主运动可能酷似血管压迫所致的脑神经根病。睡眠呼吸暂停会使某些 Chiari 畸形患者就诊于耳鼻喉科。猝倒发作是一个值得特别关注的问题。一旦排除了心脏和癫痫等病因，即应考虑延髓压迫和非器质性病因。明显由类似 Valsava 样动作引起的暂时失去知觉当然需要考虑手术治疗，但对晕厥发作的病因尚不明确者不宜推荐手术治疗。

后脑疝的典型症状是压力分离性头痛，由任何类似 Valsalva 的活动引起，如咳嗽、打喷嚏、大笑、喊叫、紧张、吹气球或向前弯腰等。

脊髓病变所致的脊髓空洞症

多种病变可引起枕骨大孔以下的椎管脑脊液通路梗阻（**专栏 65.1**），其中最常见的是瘢痕形成，多由既往感染或出血后的蛛网膜炎引起。出血可以发生在颅内，也可以直接进入椎管，其中脊髓损伤（spinal cord injury，SCI）是最常见的椎管内出血病因。

创伤后脊髓空洞症的形成可能会进一步加重 SCI 患者已有的负担。虽然脊髓空洞症在人群中相对罕见，但在 SCI 患者中相当常见，每 20 名 SCI 患者就有 1 名甚至多名会出现脊髓空洞症。患者在临床上多表现为疼痛加剧或膀胱控制能力改变。其他症状包括多汗、肌肉痉挛加剧、运动力量丧失以及感觉平面上升。从初始损伤到出现症状之间的潜伏期从数月至数年不等。与 Chiari 畸形类似，尚不清楚何

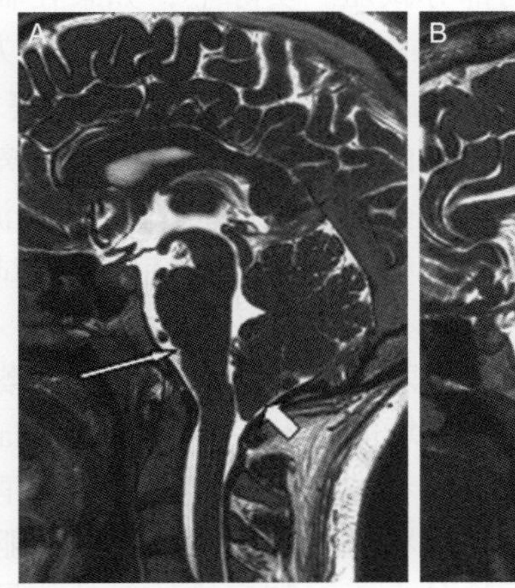

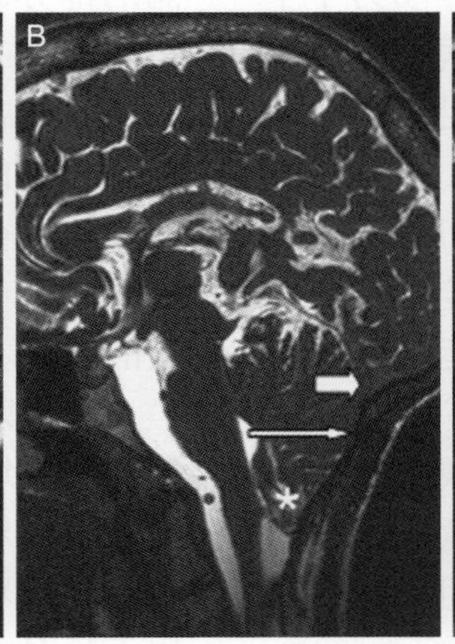

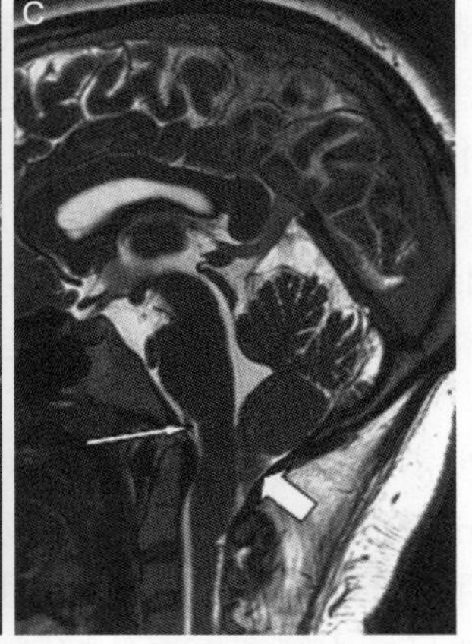

图 65.2 后脑疝。显示各种 Chiari 畸形的 MR 图像。（A）1 型，小脑扁桃体自枕骨大孔突出，占据枕大池（短箭头）。脑桥 - 延髓交界处的位置正常（长箭头）。（B）2 型，由于腰骶部椎管闭合不全，延髓和较明显的部分小脑（星号）由扩大的枕大孔疝出并进入上颈椎管。颅后窝发育不良，窦汇（短箭头）邻近枕大孔后缘（长箭头）。（C）1.5 型，其特征与 1 型相似，但脑桥 - 延髓交界处位置较低（长箭头），小脑扁桃体通过枕骨大孔下降。小脑扁桃体疝的形态与 Chiari 1 型相似（短箭头）

种因素决定哪些 SCI 患者会形成脊髓空洞症。针对 SCI 患者年龄、受伤机制、受累脊髓节段、神经功能缺损程度、初始治疗为手术抑或保守治疗等可能预测因素的研究均未得出一致的答案。

特发性脊髓空洞症

对几乎所有神经系统症状持续时间较长的患者进行 MRI 扫描时，会检出较以往更多的脊髓空洞症患者。这其中也包括某些没有明显潜在病因的脊髓空洞症，特别是未找到脑脊液流梗阻部位者。其中一些所谓的“病变”仅为持续存在的脊髓中央管，实则为胚胎残余所致。婴儿的脊髓中央管一直保持通畅；随年龄增长，特别是在青少年时期，中央管的容积减小，但仍有约 1% 在脊柱磁共振扫描上可见到脊髓中央管。

其他更明显的脊髓空洞（**图 65.1C**）也面临三个问题：①为什么会出现空洞；②空洞是否为患者症状的病因所在；③应该如何治疗？目前第一个问题尚无明确答案。患者症状通常包括躯体感觉障碍和不适，其特征为中枢神经源性疼痛。不存在手术治疗的问题，其所产生神经功能缺损的可能远超过任何潜在获益。使用神经营养药物、TENS、针灸和理疗的标准疼痛治疗方案可能会有所帮助。如未能奏效，腰椎穿刺和脑脊液引流可能会使患者获益，但该治疗相应的生理机制尚不清楚。

脊髓空洞症的治疗

大部分 Chiari 畸形患者无需手术治疗。许多作者主张，如伴发脊髓空洞则应进行手术，但该做法的价值类似于无论患者是否有症状均对脑积水进行分流术。许多脊髓空洞症患者已达到液体动力学平衡状态，此类患者仅需随访观察即可。病情加重通常是逐渐的，但患者会有明显感知。有足够的时间进行影像学随访并仔细考虑手术的必要性。突然加重并不常见，通常发生在一连串的体力活动后。然而，没有必要因为 Valsava 样动作可能会引起空洞扩张而禁止体育锻炼。相反，只需提醒患者在运动过程中避免屏气即可。

本病患者很少需要急诊手术，至少成人无需急诊手术，但 Chiari 畸形患儿偶尔因发生危险状况需进行手术治疗。手术治疗的主要目标为阻止运动功能障碍加重，次要目标为缓解疼痛、控制感觉障碍、减少出汗和痉挛、恢复已丧失的功能。手术方案包括开放梗阻的脑脊液通道、直接引流空洞以及降低整个脑脊液通路的总压力。

颅椎减压术为开放梗阻的脑脊液通道的最好例证。如果脑脊液通道充分开放，手术医生可以预期至少 3/4 患者的脊髓空洞会萎陷。这种情况并非立即发生，需要六个月才能做出有意义的评估。颅椎减压术的并发症包括化学性脑膜炎、脑脊液漏、细菌性脑膜炎、脑积水，以及偶尔发生的急性脑肿胀。孤立性第四脑室和脑下垂是非常难处理的并发症；实际上脑下垂可能是由上方的高颅压所致，而非下方缺乏支撑引起。手术牵开器对枕大神经的损伤会产生令人不适的感觉障碍，这种感觉障碍在术后会持续一段时间。

另一个人工建立脑脊液流动通路的例证是通过椎板切除术和硬膜内蛛网膜粘连松解术治疗外伤后脊髓空洞症。与颅椎交界处相比，椎管腔更狭小，术后可能会再次粘连并反复造成脑脊液循环梗阻。椎管脊髓空洞症的手术成功率不及颅椎交界部位。一般而言，任何手术使空洞永久性萎陷的可能性均与硬膜内蛛网膜粘连程度成反比。

对于蛛网膜粘连过于广泛（如化脓性或结核后脑膜炎）的患者，直接进行空洞腔引流可能更合适。其缺点包括需要切开脊髓，会造成一定程度的背柱功能丧失。该引流管与其他脑脊液分流系统一样，随时间推移也有发生堵塞的趋势，超过半数的患者不太可能有长期疗效获益。患者易于形成新空洞，其原因在于引起空洞充盈的机制尚未解除。空洞液引流的部位包括胸膜腔、腹腔或脊膜囊本身。一种特殊形式的直接引流是将脊髓横断，仅适用于完全截瘫且其他引流措施失败的患者。

此外，还可以通过降低整个硬脊膜囊的压力以降低椎管脑脊液柱的动脉脉搏的振幅，从而实现空洞的部分减压。实际上，如果在临床就诊时即有脑积水表现，上述方案可作为首选方法。脑室 - 腹腔分流术甚或显微镜下第三脑室造瘘术可以降低 Chiari 畸形患者的颅内压，缓解压力分离性头痛，甚至可使伴随的空洞萎陷。脊髓 - 腹腔分流术可能对其他类型的脊髓空洞症有效，特别是尝试建立人工通路失败的患者。

即使术后脊髓空洞的空腔已萎陷，并非患者的所有症状均能在术后缓解。对 Chiari 畸形患者而言，大部分患者的压力分离性头痛会消失或减轻，眼部和运动症状也得以改善。然而，躯体疼痛和感觉障碍无论是由于小脑扁桃体对长传导束的压力抑或空洞引起，往往会在高达半数的患者中持续存在。实际上，神经病理性疼痛仍然是脊髓空洞症治疗的主要挑战，通常严重影响患者的生活。

轴外脑脊液积聚

除脊髓内脑脊液异常积聚外，我们还可能遇到椎管中其他腔室内的脑脊液病理性积聚。这类脑脊液积聚可能位于硬膜外或硬膜内，其囊壁内可能有神经成分或没有神经成分。这类脑脊液积聚本质上为囊性病变，提示存在某种瓣膜机制，造成囊内充盈容易但排空困难。由此产生的压力可能刺激邻近脊膜，产生脊柱局部疼痛；如累及神经根，可能还会出现神经根体征。胸椎管或颈椎管的积液可能会引起“水压性脊髓病”，引起不同程度的运动、感觉和自主神经紊乱。

这些病变的病因尚不清楚，已提出的假设包括创伤、炎症和先天性缺陷。已有一些家族聚集性病历的报道，并发现与多种胶原蛋白疾病有关。

椎管硬膜外囊肿

硬膜外积液于下胸椎最常见，多位于背侧（图 65.3）。这类病变提示有潜在的硬膜缺损，其缺损部位可能毗邻神经根。如果疼痛难忍或脊髓病征象突出，手术治疗较为合理。较小的囊肿可以直接切除，但对于较大的囊性积液行多节段椎板切除欠合理。如能在术前对硬膜缺损进行影像学定位，则可通过更小范围的显露封堵硬膜缺损。否则，可能需要选择分流至腹膜腔、胸膜腔或脊膜囊。

蛛网膜囊肿和蛛网膜网

椎管脑脊液通道可由蛛网膜组织的薄层隔膜阻塞，这类隔膜在影像学检查上难以发现。在矢状位或轴位成像上，脊髓移位可作为蛛网膜隔膜的线索（图 65.4）。重要的是明确造成梗阻的隔膜并非源自更广泛的硬膜内囊肿的顶部结构，这类囊肿通常位于脊髓背侧。

如患者无外伤、脑膜炎、椎管内出血或既往手术史，通常认为此类病变为特发性。患者的主要表现包括神经性疼痛和运动性脊髓病。高位病变可能会引起头痛，这可能与脊膜囊的顺应性较正常情况有所降低有关。

运动功能障碍进行性加重为手术治疗指征。对于孤立的蛛网膜网或较小的蛛网膜囊肿可行手术切除，对于广泛的囊肿行开窗术可能更为有效。遗憾的是，虽然从解剖学角度手术获得成功，但患者的神经病理性疼痛可能仍会持续存在。

腰椎穿刺能暂时降低囊肿外的充盈压力，可作为一项有用的测试，明确患者的症状是否为病变引起，也可直接进行囊肿抽吸。

Tarlov 囊肿

这类神经周围囊肿常在磁共振扫描时偶然发现，多位于骶管，但也并非仅位于骶管内，往往呈多发。在组织学上，囊壁中有神经成分，可能引起脊柱、会阴或下肢疼痛。使用止痛方法进行保守治疗是首选治疗策略。如因囊肿的液压作用于低位骶神经根，引起明显括约肌控制或性功能问题，则有手术治疗指征。由于囊肿壁非薄，并且与重要结构粘连紧密，常难以剥离。目前有多种手术技术用于该病的治疗，

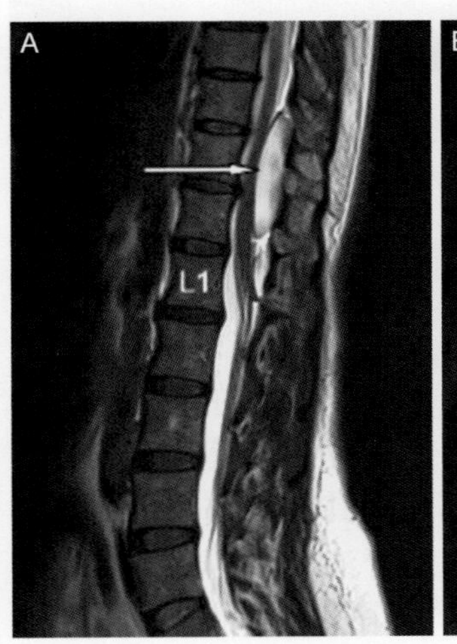

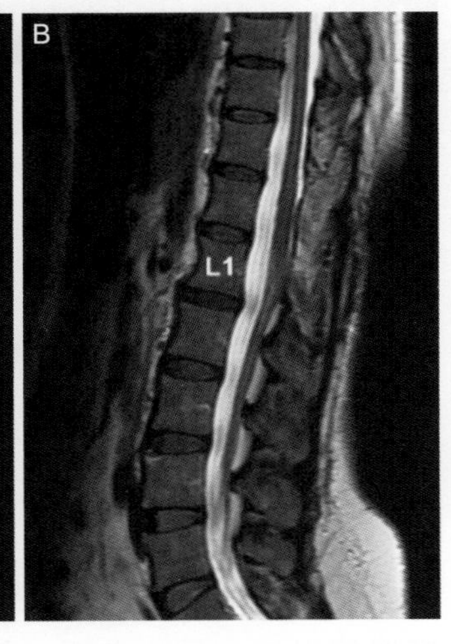

图 65.3　硬脊膜外囊肿。（A）T2 矢状位 MRI 显示硬脊膜外由脑脊液充盈的囊肿（箭头）。（B）两年后的术后表现

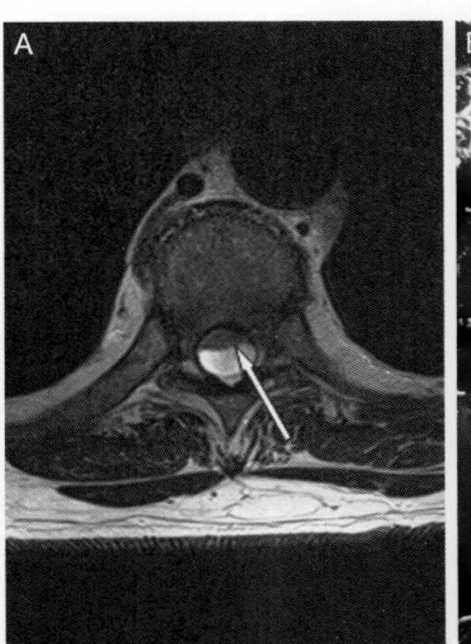

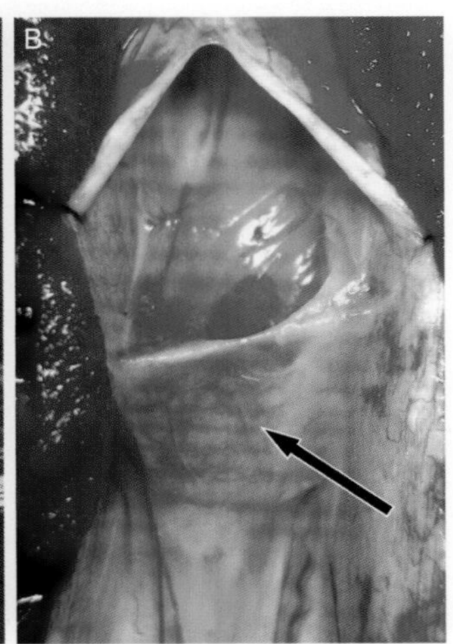

图 65.4　蛛网膜网。（A）胸椎轴位 T2 MRI 成像，显示由脊髓蛛网膜网上方的静水压引起的脊髓向前移位和受压（箭头）。（B）术中见硬膜内蛛网膜网（箭头所示）形成横贯硬膜囊、位于脊髓背侧和外侧的隔膜

包括开窗术、囊壁折叠术和分流管置入术，此外也可注胶。在计划开放性手术治疗前，可先行试验性抽吸。

自发性低颅压综合征

低颅压性头痛是腰椎穿刺术后常见的后遗症，其特点是直立位加重，平卧位可缓解。在没有植入任何脑脊液分流装置的情况下，自发出现的低颅压性头痛常提示脑脊液在椎管的某个部位有自发性渗漏，其病因包括先前创伤、胶原蛋白功能疾患或硬膜憩室（**图** 65.5A），但许多病例似乎是特发性的。

除了直立性头痛外，患者还可能出现听力改变、复视和脊柱疼痛等症状，然而脊柱疼痛部位并不足以定位脑脊液渗漏部位。不太常见的表现包括锥体外系运动障碍和意识状态改变。一个有趣的症状是溢乳，由“逆 Monro-Kellie”效应引起：颅内脑脊液容量减少引起包括垂体在内的颅腔内容物血流灌注增加，从而导致泌乳素分泌增加。

血流增加也是头颅增强 MRI 扫描中广泛脑膜强化的特征性表现的原因所在（**图** 65.5B）。此外，还可见脑组织下陷和小脑扁桃体疝，偶尔可见硬膜下血肿，更细微的征象包括横窦扩张和视神经鞘塌陷。

椎管中渗漏部位的定位常较为困难。同位素脑池造影和计算机断层扫描（computed tomography, CT）脊髓造影可用于定位，但需要接受大量电离辐射。使用鞘内钆造影剂进行 MR 脊髓造影可作为备选检查方法，但 T2MR 成像也可生成类似常规脊髓造影的影像。腰椎穿刺可能显示较低的初压，如与灌注成像相结合还可能出现较低的平台压。

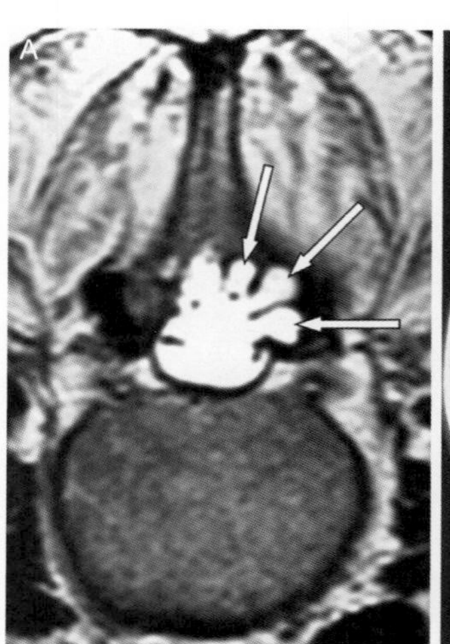

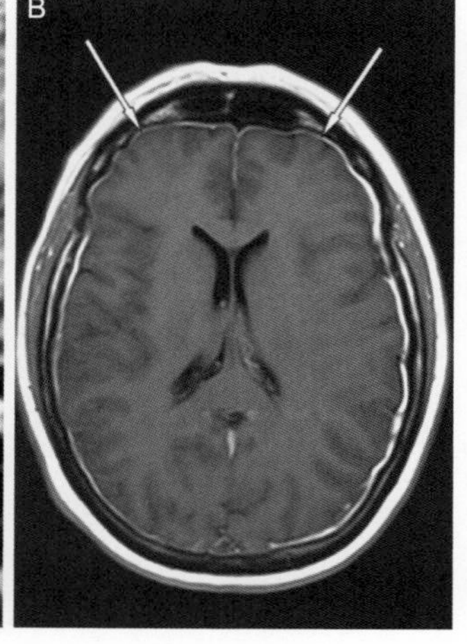

图 65.5 自发性低颅压。（A）脊柱轴位 T2 MRI 显示硬膜憩室（箭头），可能为脑脊液渗漏的部位。（B）头颅轴位 T1 对比 MRI 显示椎管内脑脊液渗漏引起的弥漫性脑膜强化（箭头）

自发性低颅压治疗初期可行保守治疗，包括卧床休息、足量补液和简单镇痛，如同腰椎穿刺后头痛的处理，其目标是渗漏处可自行愈合。如症状持续存在，可用硬膜外血液补片治疗。如可以找到渗漏部位则针对该部位进行治疗，但通常是“盲”操作，必要时可重复治疗。手术修补适用于某些特例，且仅在渗漏部位已经明确（例如需要结扎硬膜憩室）时才可采用。

脊髓疝

脊髓前疝虽然并非椎管脑脊液循环障碍类疾患，但其 MRI 表现与蛛网膜网形成类似，如脊髓向前移位和背侧脑脊液容积增大。如果误判了病变的真实性质，可能会进行不适当的手术。相位增强 MRI 或 CT 脊髓造影可用于确诊脊髓疝，并将其与椎管蛛网膜囊肿相鉴别。

因此，临床评估至关重要。该病以中年患者多见，表现为前脊髓综合征，初期多累及一侧脊髓。随着脊髓前柱自硬膜囊前方缺损（最常见于胸椎）逐渐脱出，其症状发展会持续一段时间，往往是渐进性发展。患者可能表现为一侧下肢的脊髓丘脑感觉丧失，另一侧下肢的上运动神经元功能障碍。脊髓背柱功能往往未受累，但如果未治疗，患者可能会进展为更完全的脊髓病。

仔细的显微手术可减缓脊髓疝，在脊髓和硬脊膜之间插入一片人工合成的隔膜有助于防止复发。

争议

在 Chiari 畸形和脊髓空洞症手术领域，争论的一个主要方面是进行颅椎体减压的最佳手术方法。在所使用的各种方法中，唯一的共同之处是均需切除骨质。此外，手术医生操作的解剖范围也有很大差异（**专栏** 65.3）。

有一个很好的理由可以解释为何许多外科医生控制其操作范围，这是因为开放蛛网膜下腔通道不可避免地引起化学性脑膜炎，其程度或轻或重。因此会给患者带来不适，使脑脊液压力增加，有时还会引起脑脊液漏；此时如能除外脑积水，最好行腰穿置管引流。另一方面，部分切开硬膜甚至完全不切开硬膜则难以实现伴发的脊髓空洞萎陷。一些外

专栏 65.3　颅椎减压技术

- 仅行骨性减压
- 部分硬膜松解
- 打开硬膜
- 打开蛛网膜 *
- 小脑扁桃体减容
- 硬膜成形术
- 丙烯酸树脂颅骨修复

* 通常不可避免地需打开硬膜

科医生提倡先不打开硬膜，如无效可再进一步手术。然而，这会使患者需要进行另一个较大的、令人不适的脑部手术。

小脑扁桃体减容的额外操作有引起小脑肿胀的风险，这可能导致第四脑室梗阻并引起脑积水。然而，该操作确实能去除向脊膜囊内孤立的脑脊液柱施压的“活塞”。虽然单纯的外部减压可以打开脑脊液通道，但随后放置的硬膜补片会在补片、小脑扁桃体和颈髓 - 延髓交界处形成粘连。此时，椎管脑脊液动力学障碍会较术前严重得多。在这种情况下，与初次手术相比，再次手术非常困难，危险更大，成功的可能性更低。损伤背柱并引起浅触觉和关节位置觉丧失是一个特殊的手术风险。

因此，作者倾向于打开硬膜和蛛网膜，减容小脑扁桃体，从而形成一个人工枕大池，第四脑室可向该池自由开放，该池也可与基底池和椎管脑脊液通路自由交通。没有必要使用硬膜移植物，因为这类硬膜修补很难做到水密缝合。脑脊液会漏到周围，并将补片挤压至其下方的神经结构上，从而引起脑脊液循环障碍。

延伸阅读、EBRAIN 的相关链接

扫描书末二维码获取。

第 66 章　脊柱侧凸和脊柱畸形

Nigel Gummerson 著
张一博 译，佟怀宇 审校

引言

脊柱畸形是指由于疾病、外伤或发育异常导致的脊柱失去了正常的形态。

在讨论脊柱畸形之前，我们必须首先知道何为正常脊柱。从前面及后面观，脊椎是直线形；在冠状面上没有明显的曲线（在正常范围内可有轻微的横向曲线）。从侧面观，矢状面轮廓是脊柱的形状。矢状面轮廓随着生长和年龄的增长而变化。

在出生时，脊椎全长是平缓的 C 形曲线。当孩子开始控制头部并开始爬行时，颈椎出现正常的前凸；腰椎前凸则在行走时开始出现。在整个生长过程中，脊柱矢状轮廓都在不断发展，直到达到正常的成人形态。脊柱的矢状面的轮廓永远不会固定，会随着脊椎年龄的增长而不断变化，年龄越大，脊柱越后凸。

正常脊柱轮廓可达到在冠状面上使头部和胸廓位于骨盆中心轴上的效果。在矢状面上，重心落在骶骨和股骨头之间。正常的身体表面轮廓是由头部、肩部、胸廓、骨盆之间的相对位置构成。

传统上，我们将脊柱畸形分为脊柱侧凸（影响冠状面）和脊柱后凸（影响矢状面）。实际上，脊柱是一个复杂的系统，冠状面的变化会导致矢状面的变化，而矢状面的变化伴随着旋转（在轴向平面）。因此，脊柱畸形是一个三维问题。对于发育和老化的脊椎，都会随着时间的推移而退变；存在第四维度。

在过去的 30 年里，人们对腰椎和骨盆之间的关系有了越来越多的了解。患者会倾斜骨盆以代偿脊柱畸形，而这种代偿是有限度的。从正常位置向前或向后旋转骨盆会影响髋关节功能。因此，在考虑脊柱正常与否时，必须要考虑到骨盆的情况。

脊柱形态的临床评估

辨别轻度到中度的脊柱畸形比较困难。我们大多数人醒着的大部分时间都是衣着整齐，处于不断运动之中。运动和衣着掩盖了脊柱畸形可能导致的体表形状的细微变化。

临床上评估患者脊柱形态，必须完整暴露患者，要求他们脱下衣服，只穿内裤，并且保持静止的直立状态。我们可以观察到腰部皱纹、躯干移位和肩部高度的任何差异。脊柱旋转异常可能表现为后胸壁不对称或腰部不对称。让患者身体前倾，腰部弯曲，通常会使这些不对称（由于旋转）更加明显。这是 Adam 前弯试验。在这种姿势下，脊柱旋转（相对于水平面）可以用脊柱侧凸测量仪测量。

检查患者是否在髋关节和膝盖完全伸展的情况下直立站立；矢状面畸形的患者直立站立时会弯曲臀部和膝盖，这样可以向后倾斜骨盆，补偿脊柱畸形。

有几种影像技术可用于描绘后面观的脊柱形态图形（例如，英国牛津的 ISIS 2- 集成形状成像系统）。这可以量化后胸廓的不对称，在不使用电离辐射的情况下监测脊柱侧凸的进展，其在评估手术结果方面有帮助。

脊柱形态的 X 线（放射学）评估

脊柱形态的 X 线评估是通过 AP 和全脊柱侧位 X 线片来实现的。这些都应该在患者站在标准体位的情况下进行。脊柱在站立时会发生变形，因为脊柱是负重的，所以仰卧拍片（和仰卧位 MRI 扫描）的价值是有限的。其他因素，如手臂的位置或支撑，会改变重心，从而改变脊柱在 X 线片上的外观。理想的 X 线片应该包括 C7、整个肋骨、骨盆和两侧股骨头。

矢状面和骨盆的 X 线评估

正常脊柱在前后位 X 线片上是笔直的，在矢状面上有四个弯曲。骶椎后凸是固定的，骶骨融合。通过测量 T12 上终板与 S1 终板之间的夹角（正常范围为 40°~60°），可测量腰椎前凸度。按照惯例，椎后凸是从 T5 的上终板测量到 T12 的下终板（肩部通常遮挡高位的胸椎）。T5~T12 脊柱后凸的正常范围为 10°~40°。大部分腰椎前凸发生在最下面的腰椎间盘；上腰椎相对直，下胸椎也是如此。因此，从 T10 到 L2 的节段相对较直（正常为后凸 0°~20°）。病理改变（如 Scheuermann 后凸畸形）会破坏矢状面轮廓。见图 66.1。

将骨盆包括在 X 线片上是一种很好的做法，因为骨盆的解剖和位置对脊柱有根本性的影响，它是腰椎曲线的基础。上半身的重心应该在骶骨和股骨头之间。有一种观点认为，脊柱在骨盆上方的一个潜在的“圆锥”内是“平衡的”。在这个圆锥内，保持站立所需的肌肉力量最小。当脊柱或重心移出这个圆锥时，脊柱就会变得“不平衡”，保持站立所需的肌肉力量就会增加（Jean Dubousset，经济圆锥）。

直接测量重心并不容易，所以我们用 C7 椎体中心和 S1 终板后缘的相对位置代替。从 C7 椎体下落的垂直线应落在整个脊柱侧位 X 线片上 S1 终板后缘 2.5 cm 的范围内。这是矢状垂直轴。

全脊柱平衡在这个范围之外的患者据说会有失代偿的矢状位脊柱畸形，该组患者的生活质量评分较低。

通常测量的三个影像学脊柱骨盆参数：

- 骶骨倾斜角（SS），S1 终板相对于水平面的角度（正常值 39° ± 8°）。
- 骨盆倾斜角（PT），股骨头至 S1 终板中点相对于垂直平面的夹角（正常值 13° ± 6°）。PT<25° 是脊柱畸形手术后的理想结果之一。参见图 66.2。
- 骨盆入射角（PI），垂直于 S1 终板绘制的线与连接 S1 终板中点与股骨头的线之间形成的角度。PI 随骨盆的生长而变化。一旦骨骼生长完成，PI 就固定了，只能通过骨盆或骶骨骨折或截骨术来改变。PI 等于骶骨倾斜角与骨盆倾斜角之和（正常值55° ± 10.6°）。高PI的患者的腰椎前凸往往较大。

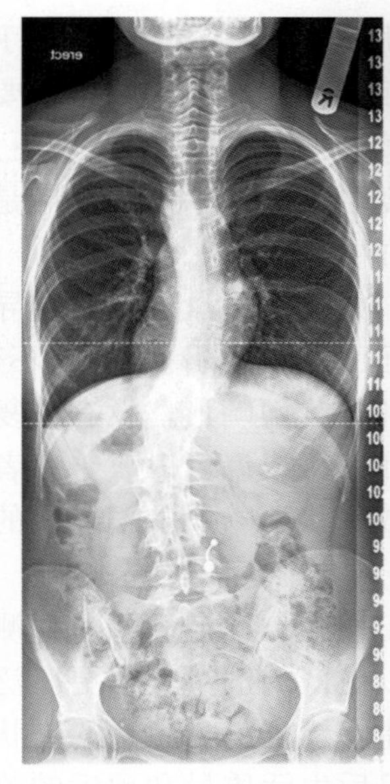

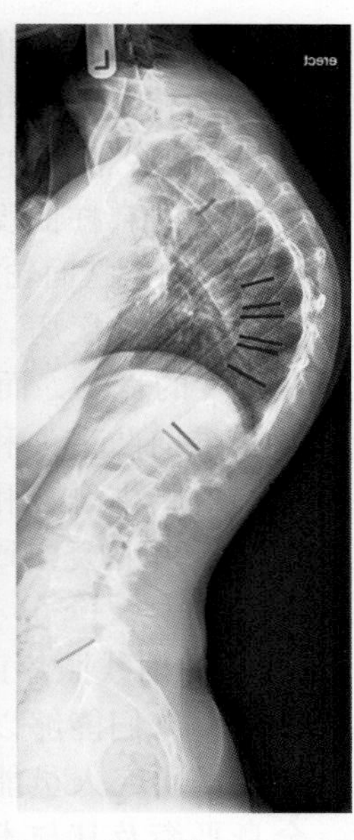

图 66.1 Scheuermann 后凸畸形。侧位 X 线片上可见胸椎后凸增大，连续三个节段楔入至少 5°（终板标为绿色）。AP 片显示一个小的脊柱侧凸，这在 Scheuermann 中很常见，在这种情况下，腰椎前凸（黄色）（L1-S1）为 75°（正常范围 40°~60°），胸椎后凸（橙色）（T5-T12）为 96°（正常范围为 10°~40°）

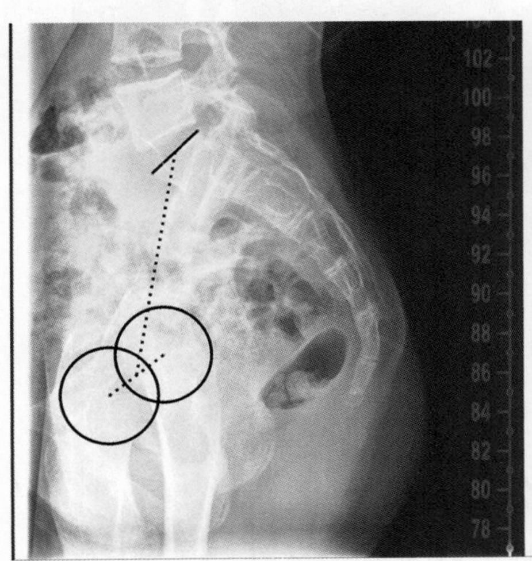
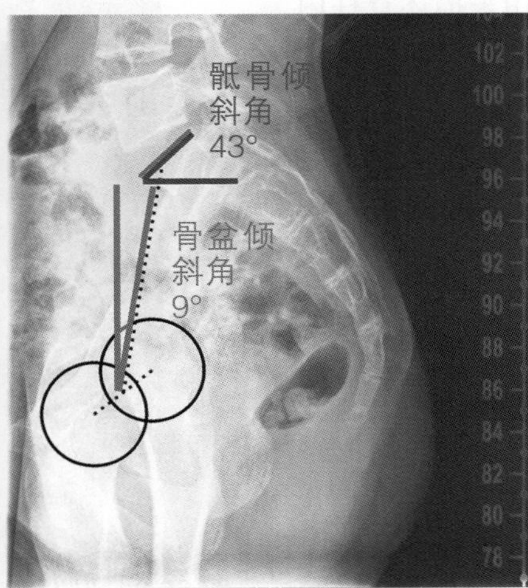

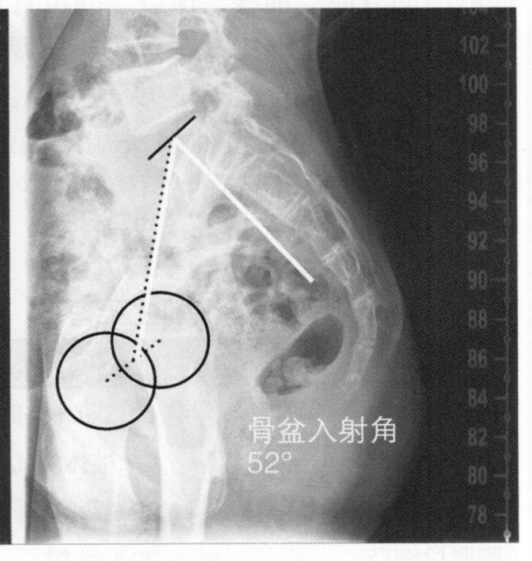

图 66.2 骨盆参数。股骨头轮廓可以用于确定其中点。S1 终板也标记出来。从 S1 中点到股骨头中点画一条线。建立水平和垂直线可以测量骶骨倾斜角（SS）和骨盆倾斜角（PT）。通过以 S1 终板中点向下画一条垂直线测量骨盆入射角（PI）。这些角度之间有固定的几何关系，例如 PI = SS + PT

PT＜25° 和 PI＜9° 的腰椎前凸，与脊柱畸形手术后的阳性结果有统计学相关性。然而，同样重要的是要认识到，一些患者的脊柱天生“S 形”程度更大，而另一些患者的脊柱曲度更平坦：手术的目标是恢复其原本和谐的矢状面轮廓。

常见的退行性疾病，如腰椎间盘疾病，会导致脊柱前柱高度的丧失，而后柱部分的高度保持不变。这会导致腰椎前凸丢失和矢状面畸形。没有恢复正常腰椎前凸的腰椎融合和减压或许可以改善患者的根性腿痛，但可能会导致矢状面畸形和不理想的手术结果。

“全身式”射线照片正变得越来越普遍，探测器技术的进步使人们能够以更低的剂量获得更广泛的成像。这使得研究人员能够检查整个患者的矢状面平衡。全身平衡及其与术后生活质量和预后的关系是一个不断发展的课题。

脊柱侧凸的 X 线评估

脊柱侧凸的基本特征是脊柱冠状面弯曲超过 10°。

脊柱侧凸可以是结构性的，也可以是非结构性的。非结构性弯曲是可完全校正的弯曲。非结构性曲线可能是由于姿势、疼痛、瘫痪或骨盆倾斜造成的（例如，如果是腿长不均导致的弯曲，那么当患者坐着时，脊柱弯曲将会变直）。结构弯曲具有固定组成，并且不会完全拉直（即它们不会校正为零度）。随着时间的推移，非结构弯曲可能会形成结构性的弯曲。

脊柱侧凸曲线通常通过曲线的位置、方向和程度来描述。曲线可以描述为具有凸面（曲线的“外部”）和凹面（曲线的“内部”）。凸面的方面描述了脊柱侧凸的方向。曲线“顶点”的位置用来描述脊柱内的位置。顶端是离中线最远的椎间盘或椎体（即从中央脊柱垂直轴移位最多）。见**表** 66.1。

弯曲程度是通过曲线头端最倾斜的椎体的上终板到曲线尾端最倾斜的椎体的下终板之间的夹角来测量的。这个角度就是 Cobb 角。

表 66.1 从顶点位置识别主要弯曲

曲度类型	顶点位置
颈椎侧凸	C1 到 C6/7 间盘
颈胸段侧凸	C7 椎体到 T1 椎体
胸椎侧凸	T1/2 间盘到 T11/T12 间盘
胸腰段侧凸	T12 到 L1
腰椎侧凸	L1/2 间盘到 L5

脊柱侧凸研究学会定义

Cobb 角度测量仅仅是 3D 曲线的二维（2D）近似。为了完整地描述一条曲线，我们需要记录弯曲的脊柱节段数、旋转畸形和矢状面畸形。Cobb 角为描述脊柱弯曲提供了一种有用的速记方法，也是我们目前了解最多的一种测量方法。见**图** 66.3。

脊柱侧凸

脊柱侧凸是一种常见的、发展相对缓慢的疾病。除了一些神经肌肉疾病外，年轻患者的脊柱侧凸往往是活动的和有弹性的。儿童脊柱侧凸倾向于表现为美容问题，而成人脊柱侧凸倾向于表现为轴性脊柱疼痛和神经根性症状。

儿童脊柱侧凸的分类

儿童脊柱侧凸可按发病年龄、病因或两者一起进行分类。

特发性脊柱侧凸传统上分为“婴幼儿”（0~3 岁）、“幼年”（4~9 岁）和“青少年”（10~18 岁）。我们现在使用术语“早发性脊柱侧凸”（0~9 岁）和“迟发性脊柱侧凸”（10~18 岁）。这里的重要因素是肺部发育。早发性脊柱侧凸可导致胸廓发育不良综合征。

胸廓发育不良综合征是肺生长受限，胸廓无法支持正常呼吸的结果。脊柱侧凸可能会限制胸椎的

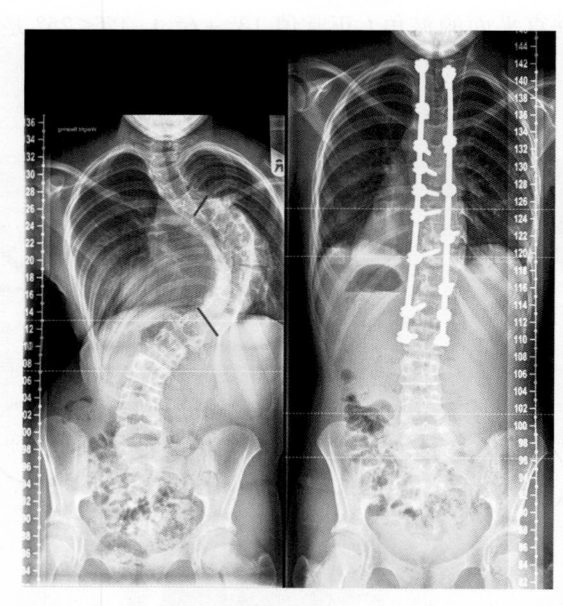

图 66.3 迟发性特发性脊柱侧凸（术前、术后前后位片）。Cobb 角的测量如图所示。在曲线顶部最倾斜的椎体的上终板上画一条线，在曲线底部最倾斜的椎体的下终板上画一条线。在本例中，胸廓曲线的 Cobb 角为 108°

高度（正常肺功能需要 18~22 cm 的 T1 到 T12 高度），或者因为侧凸的顶端旋转到胸部，侵占了可供肺部使用的空间，从而限制了肺的生长。天性脊柱侧凸中的肋骨异常也可能导致这一问题。

胸部和肺部生长的细节是复杂的，对于不同年龄的早发和晚发之间的界限也有争论。在 10 岁时，胸部体积是其最终大小的 50%。迟发性脊柱侧凸不太可能引起肺功能的任何改变，除非曲度变得非常大（>90°）。

在先天性（15%）或神经肌肉（10%）病例中，脊柱弯曲的病因可能很明显。在大多数情况下，很难查到明确的病因（特发性）。最常见的，有 70% 的儿童脊柱侧凸是特发性的。一小部分脊柱畸形患者有潜在的综合征。

先天性脊柱侧凸和脊柱后凸

第 85 章描述了脊柱的胚胎发育。先天性脊柱侧凸的分类是描述性的。先天性畸形可分为分节缺陷、发育缺陷、混合性缺陷和一小部分难以描述的复杂畸形。这种分类来自于 McMaster 和 Ohtsuka（1982）的工作，该工作主要基于普通的 X 线。Kawakami 等建议对该系统进行更新，分析畸形的 3D-CT 表现。CT 可显示 50% 的患者在平片上所见的额外异常。

三维 CT 分析可以更好地了解异常的相对（3D）位置，并提供更多关于节段间融合和异常后方解剖的信息。

先天性脊柱侧凸的一个重要方面是要考虑到相关的肋骨异常。Jarcho-Levin 综合征（脊柱胸椎骨质疏松症）可见多根肋骨融合。这种情况会导致胸部生长明显减慢，并导致胸部功能不全综合征的早期死亡。另一种较轻的形式，脊柱肋骨发育不良，导致的肋骨问题不太严重，对预期寿命没有明显影响。孤立性肋骨异常可见于没有这些症状的病例，反映肋骨和椎体的共同胚胎起源是体细胞的硬核组，非综合征性肋骨异常最常见于未分段。

先天性脊柱侧凸畸形进展的自然病史是多种多样的。大约 50% 的先天性脊柱侧凸患者会有明显的进展，25% 没有进展，其余的只有轻微进展或根本没有进展。进展的机会取决于异常的位置和类型。进展是不对称生长的结果。

先天性脊柱畸形最良性的形式是阻滞椎体。这是双侧分节失败的结果。阻滞椎体不会导致渐进性弯曲，但当存在多个阻滞椎体时，可能会导致躯干缩短。

嵌顿或未分节的半椎体进展的可能性很小。楔形椎体每年只会导致 1°~2° 的进展。单个半分节或完全分节的椎体将以每年 1°~3.5° 的速度进展，胸腰椎交界处的进展更快。多发性半椎体的进展会更快。腰骶半椎体会导致代偿性的腰椎和胸椎弯曲，随着时间的推移，这些曲线会变得僵硬（和结构性）。早期手术正是为了防止这一结果。

未分段的肋骨每年会导致 2°~9° 的进展。同样，胸腰椎交界处的情况更糟。

最麻烦的组合是未分段的肋骨与对侧完全分节的半椎体的混合缺陷。胸腰椎交界处是发生这种畸形最糟糕的部位，在此节段它可能以每年超过 10° 的速度进展，当发现时需要及早（预防性）手术治疗。

先天性脊柱后凸比脊柱侧凸少见。脊柱后凸可能以每年 2°~7° 的速度进展。大多数后凸畸形位于下胸段或胸腰椎区域。如果不进行治疗，一些先天性后凸畸形患者可能会变成截瘫。

先天性畸形有继续观察和手术治疗两种选择。支撑和理疗都不能改变这些畸形的自然病程。渐进性弯曲需要手术治疗。进展的可能性可以通过 CT 和 MRI 检查来确定。手术前应积极寻找相关因素，并考虑潜在综合征的可能性。手术介入前对肺功能的评估，作为基线，将有助于指导治疗并告知预后。

手术选择范围从半骨骺阻滞术（短节段前向生长停滞超过曲线凸度）到更复杂的截骨术，如椎弓根减压截骨术（pedicle subtraction osteotomy，PSO）、半椎体切除或椎体切除。参见**图** 66.4。

治疗的选择将取决于畸形的性质和发病时的年龄。半骨骺阻滞术等技术依赖于弯曲凹面的显著生长潜力，对老年患者用处不大。

在进展性畸形的情况下等待“保持增长”不会有什么好处。在这些病例中，通常需要合并前后路融合。在可能的情况下，应该保留“正常”水平，但可能需要对整个曲线进行内固定，以恢复正常的脊柱平衡。

每一种先天性弯曲都必须根据其自身的特点进行评估，但一般来说，对于有多于一个半椎体、单侧肋骨或混合缺陷的曲度，应该考虑早期手术治疗，因为这些脊柱弯曲往往会进展。

神经肌肉性脊柱侧凸

大脑、脊髓、神经或肌肉的疾病可能导致无法维持正常的脊柱平衡，从而导致脊柱侧凸。例如脑瘫、迪谢内（Duchenne）肌营养不良、弗里德赖希（Friedreich）共济失调和创伤后瘫痪。

这些弯曲的发生频率和严重程度在不能走路

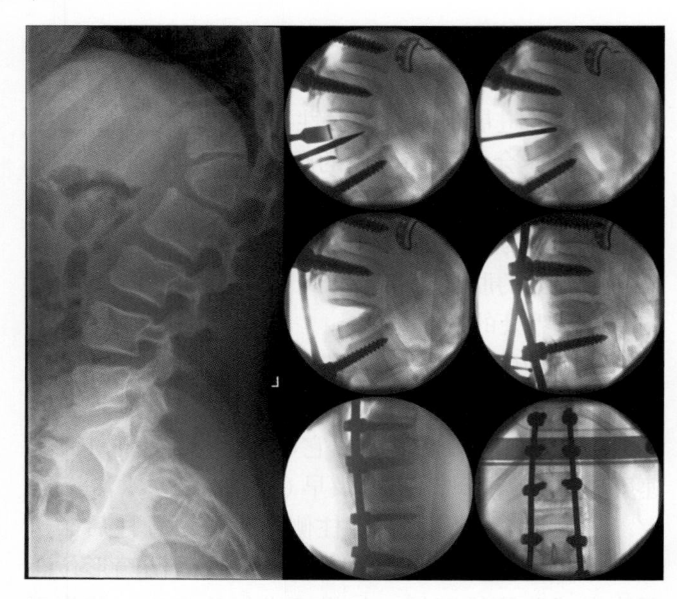

图 66.4　椎弓根减压截骨术治疗先天性脊柱后凸。在畸形矫正中可能需要脊柱截骨术。在这种情况下，一块楔形的骨（后方结构、椎弓根和躯干）被切除，使得脊柱在神经结构周围变短。这会产生角度校正，其旋转轴位于椎体的前面。这种截骨术通常会产生 25°~30° 的矫正

的儿童中更严重。仍在行走的儿童通常能保持脊柱平衡。

神经肌肉弯曲一般无痛，但确实会引起坐姿和卫生问题。不良的坐姿平衡可能意味着孩子不得不使用手臂来帮助平衡，剥夺了他们使用该手臂的权利。

早发性神经肌肉弯曲可能导致胸廓发育不良综合征。神经肌肉疾病的患者需要一个多学科团队的照顾。对于许多神经肌肉脊柱弯曲的患者来说，非手术治疗是合适的。所有人都应理疗以及坐姿矫正。

保守治疗失败是手术治疗（通常是后路内固定脊柱融合术）的指征。这样做的目的是防止弯曲进展，恢复坐姿平衡。

综合征性脊柱侧凸

有很多可能导致脊柱侧凸的综合征。例如神经纤维瘤病、马方氏综合征、埃勒斯 - 当洛斯（Ehlers-Danlos）综合征、成骨不全等。对这些罕见情况的详细讨论超出了本文的范围，但非常仔细地检查患者的临床体征是有用的，其可能暗示潜在的综合征。如果怀疑有潜在的综合征，则需要考虑临床遗传学者的观点。

重要的是要意识到综合征性脊柱侧凸的一些常见陷阱，这些陷阱很多，而且随着症状的不同而有所不同。本组患者手术并发症发生率高于特发性脊柱侧凸。

特发性脊柱侧凸

特发性脊柱侧凸是一种没有任何其他潜在问题的结构性脊柱畸形。根据定义，畸形是天生的，尽管有许多关于病因学的理论，其根本原因尚未确定。

早发性特发性脊柱侧凸（EOIS）

早发性特发性脊柱侧凸（early onset idiopathic scoliosis，EOIS）很少见（美国为 1%，欧洲约为 5%）。它通常向左侧弯曲，在出生后发展，但在出生时不存在。这在男孩中更为常见（男：女 =3：2）。EOIS 与其他疾病密切相关，如马蹄内翻足、发育性髋关节发育不良、斜颈和腹股沟疝。EOIS 的分类是描述性的，有用的区分特征是弯曲程度大小、肋骨 - 椎体角度差（顶端）和肋骨头部的外观。

90% 的 EOIS 的患者会自愈。有趣而又令人费解的是，脊柱右侧弯曲的女孩比脊柱左侧弯曲的女孩预后要差得多。进行性 EOIS 与胸廓发育不良综合征和随之而来的预期寿命缩短有关。

历史上对这组患者的描述很可能包括许多有脊柱侧凸潜在原因的患者。曲度小于 20° 的假定 EOIS 患者中约有 22% 有潜在的神经轴异常（即他们不是真正的特发性）。在一个系列中，8/10 的神经轴异常患者需要神经外科手术治疗。

为了预测预后，根据肋骨 - 椎体角度差（RVAD）来区分曲线是帮助的。参见**图** 66.5。这个测量是由 Mehta（1972）定义的，是从肋骨长轴和曲线顶端垂直于椎体终板的线测量的左右两侧的角度大小之差。Mehta 表明，如果角度的差异小于 20°，那么曲线自然缓解的可能性为 85%~90%。她接着描述了第二个特征：肋骨头部在顶点的凸面上的相位。“一期”肋骨头部不与椎体重叠，在 84%~98% 的病例中与分辨率有关。“二期”肋骨头部确实与椎体重叠，并与 84%~97% 的病例进展有关。双曲线比单曲线更有可能进展。

有人认为 EOIS 是宫内塑型的结果；与此相反的是，EOIS 在出生时很少见到。其他人则认为这是从孩子的位置“塑造身体”的结果。如果婴儿处于侧卧位，则会形成一条曲线；这一点得到了该组斜头畸形的观察结果的支持。

大多数脊柱外科医生一致认为，对于进展性 EOIS，连续塑形是一种合理的非手术治疗选择。由于儿童的生长速度很快，刚性支架几乎没有什么用处，但可以模制连续石膏管型，如 Cotrel 推广的、Mehta 使用的效果良好的石膏管型（伸长 - 反旋 - 屈

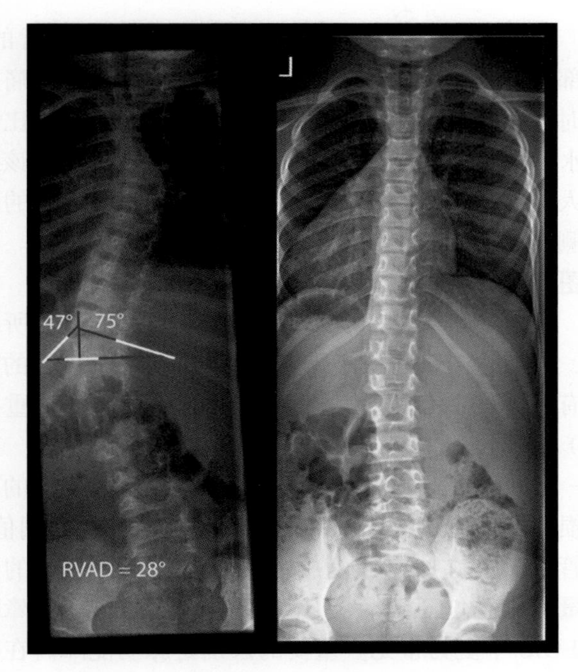

图 66.5 肋骨-脊椎-角度差（RVAD）。在这个病例中，首发时（9个月大）的RVAD为28°，这是一个可能进展的标志。曲线是渐进式的，并用连续石膏管型（EDF管型）治疗。这条曲线在6岁的时候几乎已经矫正

曲管型或EDF管型），以控制细小的进展性弯曲。

大弧度（大于约50°Cobb角）最好手术治疗。处于两难境地是，早期脊柱融合将阻止胸部生长，而这反过来将导致胸廓发育不良综合征、呼吸衰竭和预期寿命缩短。因此，手术治疗的目标是在保持生长的同时控制曲线。目前已经尝试了许多技术。

通常推荐的技术是双棒生长系统。在这里，曲线是在近端和远端（通常两端各有两个水平）测量的，但曲线的中心不受干扰。两边各有一根杆子用来连接近端和远端的内固定装置。传统的棒状物必须每4~6个月加长一次才能生长，这就需要重复多次的外科手术。所有这些病例最终都会遇到伤口感染或棒折断等并发症，这是由于器械反复穿过同一疤痕而造成的。一种带有可伸缩的内置磁电机的杆子最近已进入临床使用，在门诊中可以使用外部磁铁重复延长，从而消除了重复手术的需要。

另一种可能的解决方案是选择性地抑制曲线凸度上的生长。这项技术在一定程度上还是试验性的，没有被广泛采用。

迟发性特发性脊柱侧凸（LOIS）

迟发性特发性脊柱侧凸（late onset idiopathic scoliosis，LOIS）是一种比较常见的情况。小曲度比大曲度更常见。曲度 >10° 的患病率为2%，曲度 >30° 的患病率为0.2%~0.3%。总体而言，每10000名儿童中只有6名需要治疗LOIS。

曲度为10°时，性别比接近1：1，而曲度大于20°时，男女之比为1：5。临床上不存在小曲度。关于小曲度的数据来自学校筛查计划（Glassman et al., 2005）。学校筛查计划基本上已经被放弃，因为没有可靠的治疗方法可以提供给有小曲度的儿童，这可能会改变曲线的自然历史。

迟发曲线的形成是一个潜在的过程。家长们没有注意到小曲度改变也就不足为奇了。

迟发性发性脊柱侧凸的分类

对于这个多维问题，我们还没有找到理想的分类系统。目前，使用最广泛的分类是Lenke等的分类（2001）。这为我们提供了一个有用的工具，它对LOIS曲线进行可重复的描述，可以指导治疗，并促进研究。Lenke分类基于静态直立和仰卧弯曲X线片。包括三个部分：曲线型、腰椎矫形器和矢状胸矫形器。

这种分类是二维的，既涉及矢状面也涉及冠状面。旋转畸形未分类。工作仍在继续以寻找真正的3D分类。这些分类系统没有解决患者抱怨的问题——容貌问题。

迟发性特发性脊柱侧凸的病因学

特发性——自发性或由不明或未知的原因引起

关于LOIS的病因学有很多理论，但仍有许多不清楚之处。内分泌、神经、肌肉和骨骼原因都已被假定。这在身材修长（外形型）的女性中更为常见。该畸形为前凸合并脊柱侧凸。脊柱变形时曲线的旋转可能会在标准侧位X线片上显示出后凸的外观，但去旋转的视图会给出更准确的评估。有一种理论认为，相对于后部生长，脊柱前部过度生长会降低胸椎后凸的稳定性，然后胸椎后凸会发生弯曲，从而产生脊柱侧凸。

有8%~20%的LOIS患者，其一级亲属与之相关。寻找相关基因的工作仍在继续。脊柱侧凸很可能是多个基因之间复杂相互作用的结果。

迟发性特发柱侧凸的自然病史

迟发性曲线进展的主要驱动力是增长。剩余增长指标有助于预测曲线进程。这些剩余生长的指标可能是按时间顺序的、内分泌的或骨骼的成熟标志。

年龄本身就是预测剩余生长潜力的粗略指标。

月经初潮年龄增加了更多信息。女孩在月经初潮前18个月和月经初潮后18个月生长迅速。使用手部和手腕的X射线对骨龄进行正式评估也很有用。Risser分级是在正位X线片上看到的髂骨隆起的融合程度。0级时，凸起尚未出现。到了五年级，它就完全融合了。1~4级代表从外侧向内侧逐渐融合到髂骨隆起。年龄、青春期和骨龄可以帮助预测进展的风险（**表66.2**）。

即使有显著的剩余生长，小曲度的弯曲也不太可能取得进展。5°~19°曲线的数据显示，如果儿童的Risser分级为0~1，则有22%的进展，而如果儿童的Risser分级为2~4，则仅有1.6%的进展［请注意，5°的曲线低于目前可接受的脊柱侧凸诊断阈值（10°）］。

表66.2 曲度进展的风险预测

影响因素	进展风险（>5°）
年龄<10	88%
年龄>15	29%
初潮前	53%
初潮后	11%
Risser 0级	68%
Risser 3~4级	18%

Data from Lonstein JE, Carlson JM., The prediction of curve progression in untreated idiopathic scoliosis during growth, *The Journal of Bone and Joint Surgery Am*, Volume 66, Issue 7, pp. 1061–71, 1984.

从长远来看，LOIS患者的预期寿命是正常的。背部疼痛的发生率并不高于普通人群，但当疼痛发作时，可能会稍微严重一些，持续的时间也会比平均水平稍长一些。这一组原因不明的背部疼痛应该促使人们寻找其他可能的原因，特别是导致疼痛的脊柱侧凸的病理因素，如骨样骨瘤或椎弓峡部裂。参见**图66.6**。

在这个群体中，人们对身体形象的认识有所提高，当然，畸形也有心理上的影响。患有LOIS的女孩有更高的饮食失调发生率和更低的BMI（体重指数）。

除非曲度非常大，否则LOIS不会引起明显的心肺损害。曲度为90°经常被引用为这种折中的阈值，尽管事实上在所有曲度中都可以看到某种程度的可测量的肺功能障碍。相比之下，严重的肺功能障碍在EOIS中更为常见。重要的区别是肺功能障碍在何种情况下变得临床显著。曲度大于50°的患者可出现劳力性呼吸困难症状。

有长期数据表明，即使在骨骼成熟之后，所有曲度都会略有进展。年均进展0.5°。曲度越大（>50°），进展越快。

许多LOIS患者将再次以成人的身份出现在脊柱外科医生面前，曲线上有进展和退化，有疼痛的症状，可能还有神经根受压。

迟发性特发性脊柱侧凸的治疗

理疗对那些背部疼痛的孩子很有帮助。没有很好的证据表明物理疗法可以改变潜在的曲线。

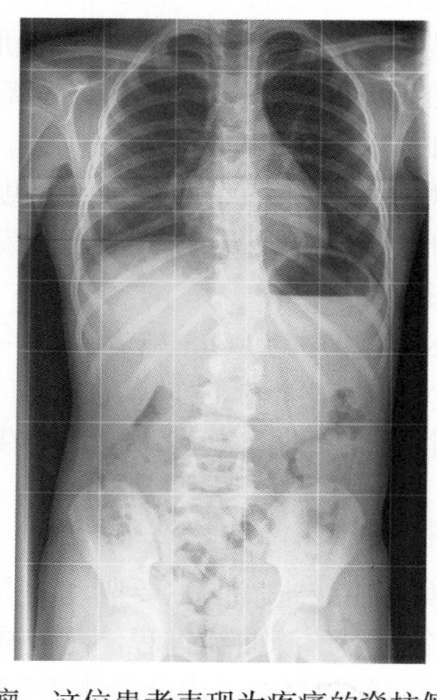

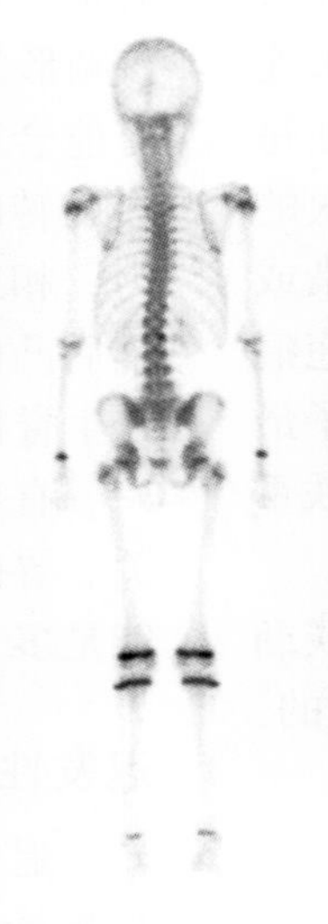

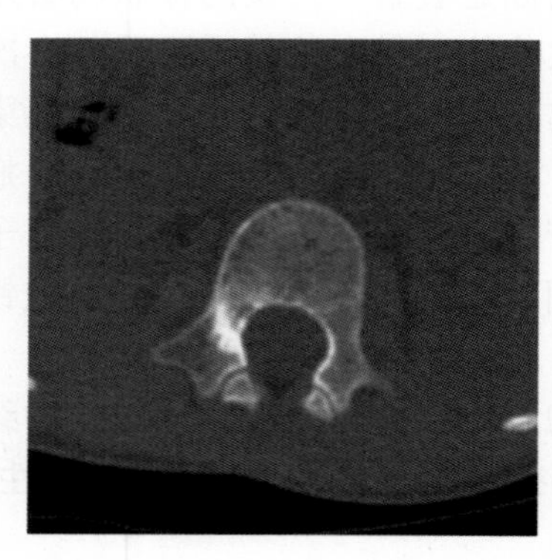

图66.6 骨样骨瘤。这位患者表现为疼痛的脊柱侧凸，并通过放射性核素骨扫描进行了进一步的研究。骨扫描可见L2椎弓根摄取增加。轴位CT扫描显示周围有一个硬化灶

支撑可能在治疗小曲度时起作用，其目的是防止曲度进展，而不是纠正曲度。支撑需要一天 17 个小时或更长时间才能成功。支具有潜在的严重的生理和心理障碍。理想情况下，支撑需要在快速增长之前开始，并且需要患者和医护人员做出重大承诺。动态（弹性）支撑已经开发出来，并仍在评估中。

手术可以改变潜在的脊柱形状和美容外观。小于 40° 的曲度不太可能因美容原因而需要手术治疗。脊柱侧凸手术的目的是防止恶化，留下一个稳定和平衡的脊柱，并最大限度地安全地进行美容矫正，保留尽可能多的运动节段。整容矫正相当于使肩部水平，躯干居中，腰部褶皱平衡，矫正脊柱轴向旋转，以减少肋骨或腰部突出。

要确定融合程度，大多数情况下遵循的简单规则是确定终椎（即终板从水平面倾斜最大的椎体，并融合从上端椎体到下端椎体的所有结构曲线）。应该选择最高的水平，以确保肩部变平或保持水平，在从融合到非融合的交界处应该有一个正常的矢状面轮廓。最低节段的选择应基于站立片上的中间和稳定的椎体，以及检查弯曲的椎间盘间隙所获得的矫正度。

灵活的弯曲使矫正相对简单。刚性曲线需要一些松解才能实现最佳矫正。所有小关节都被松解，作为实现融合的一种手段。小关节和黄韧带可以去掉，椎间盘也可以去掉，从而增加灵活性。僵硬的弯曲需要更广泛的截骨或完全切除脊柱。

需要就采取的方法和融合哪些节段做出决定。大多数脊柱侧凸手术是通过后路手术进行的。前路手术可能适用于更大、更僵硬的曲度，通常与后路固定相结合。关于融合的精确程度的选择将由方法的选择和矫正的程度决定。

脊柱畸形手术干系重大，具有很大的风险。这些风险可以通过系统化的方法来管理和降低。这涉及许多方案，包括术前计划、患者血液管理（氨甲环酸和细胞回收）以及使用体感诱发电位和运动诱发电位进行脊髓监测（见**第 56 章**）。如果电生理学显示持续性异常，则可提示进行“唤醒”测试。

Scheuermann 后凸畸形

这种情况有很多名称，但通常被称为舒尔曼（Scheuermann）病或舒尔曼后凸畸形。Scheuermann 首先将这种情况描述为青少年痛苦的固定脊柱后凸的发展。X 线片显示椎体楔形，椎体前缘受压。

Sorensen 完善了诊断标准，要求至少三个有异常后凸的相邻椎体前方楔入超过 5°。

据报道，发病率在 0.9%~30%，但 1% 到 6% 的数字更合理。一些研究发现，这种情况在男孩中更常见，另一些研究发现没有性别差异。

尽管有很多理论，原因尚不清楚。在这些理论中，有人认为椎体前部可能有异常的血液供应，或者在椎体终板下可能有异常的骨化。

理疗和伸展运动对这些患者有帮助。支撑对弯曲度小于 65° 的患者也有作用，可能会帮助减轻患者背部疼痛。

手术适用于不能接受的美容情况（曲度 >70°），如果保守治疗失败，可致残或加重疼痛。手术的目的是将后凸矫正到正常范围的上限。过度矫正可能会导致相邻水平连接问题。矫正是通过缩短后柱，多节段截骨术来实现的。

成人脊柱畸形

大多数成年脊柱畸形患者表现为新生退行性脊柱侧凸。脊柱内都会发生退行性改变，但不利的退行性改变，如狭窄、腰椎滑脱、侧滑和腰椎前凸丧失等可能会导致症状。值得考虑的是，在这组患者中是否存在潜在的代谢性骨骼疾病，如骨质疏松症。骨质疏松症可能是曲度进展的一个因素，患者是否应该接受手术治疗将是一个考虑因素。

少数成年脊柱畸形患者在青少年特发性曲度内出现退行性改变和曲度进展。

与儿童患者不同的是，成人患者会出现疼痛和神经根性症状。冠状面畸形相对不重要。对临床影响最大的是矢状面和骨盆参数。局灶性半脱位、腰椎前凸丧失和整体脊柱失衡与残疾相关。

随着人口老龄化，接受成人畸形手术的潜在患者越来越多。然而，对畸形矫正的热情必须被现实的目标和认识到在这类手术中潜在的重大并发症所冲淡。医学上的并存可能意味着一些患者的身体状况不够好，无法承受所需的大手术。

简单的减压（不矫正畸形）可能会缓解神经根性症状，但如果不解决失去前凸和整体脊柱平衡的问题，“小融合”可能会让患者处于更糟糕的状态。在许多情况下，需要选择是什么都不做或做一个小的减压手术，或者考虑做一个更大的手术和矫正畸形，后者通常需要截骨或多个椎间融合器。

如果要解决畸形，那么矫正的目标是恢复患者的矢状椎排列。

要提防成年畸形患者，他们在站立或行走时会出现畸形，但当他们躺下时就会消失。这可能是躯干前曲症（驼背），这是一种与帕金森症相关的轴性肌肉病。

脊柱后凸

破坏性病变，如创伤、肿瘤和感染，都可以产生局限性的脊柱后凸。在某些情况下，在未受累的相邻脊柱节段上有足够的灵活性，以维持正常的整体脊柱平衡。在其他情况下，局部破坏可能导致整体矢状位脊柱失衡，治疗患者时应考虑这一点。

创伤、肿瘤和感染的治疗在本书的其他地方有更详细的讨论（参见第10篇的相关章节）。

延伸阅读、参考文献、EBRAIN的相关链接

扫描书末二维码获取。

第十四篇　脊柱损伤

第 67 章　脊髓损伤的治疗

Saksith Smithason • Bryan S. Lee • Edward C. Benzel 著
王科大 译，苏亦兵 审校

引言

脊髓损伤(spinal cord injury，SCI)，指由各种创伤性或非创伤性原因导致的暂时性或者永久性脊髓功能损害。关于脊髓损伤的病理生理学研究已经取得了一些重大进展。目前关于脊髓损伤的原发和继发损伤机制研究都指向直接的且不可逆的细胞损害。及时、合理的治疗对于保护急性脊髓损伤患者一部分神经功能组织是非常有必要的。

脊髓损伤的治疗通常住院时间长，康复耗时久，且耗费高。脊髓损伤后神经功能的恢复很大程度上取决于损伤的严重程度。脊髓损伤的治疗、外科减压手术的方式及时机的确定仍然至关重要，但也存在争议。后期进一步的流行病学研究对于优化保健计划和成本控制是非常有必要的。

流行病学

发病率、患病率、性别和地理分布

全球脊髓损伤的年发病率为 15~40/100 万，发达国家为 11.5~53.4/100 万(Botterell et al.，1975)。在美国，每年有 12000 例因脊髓损伤而导致的截瘫或四肢瘫痪新发病例，其中 4000 例在到达医院前死亡，1000 例在住院期间死亡(Sances et al.，1984)。每年幸存且送达医院的脊髓损伤患者约在 50/100 万。然而，世界范围内急性脊髓损伤的患病率也各不相同。可能某项研究中某个国家的脊髓损伤发生率为 583/100 万，而另一项涉及多个国家的脊髓损伤的研究，这一数字可能为 130~1125/100 万(Griffin et al.，1985)。大多数国家脊髓损伤患者的年龄分布峰值在 20~30 岁。通常认为男性比女性更容易遭受创伤性脊髓损伤。脊髓损伤患者男女比为 3~4∶1，且 2/3 的脊髓损伤病例发生在 30 岁以下的年轻群体(Griffin et al.，1985)。然而，近来脊髓损伤患者的平均年龄和老年人比例呈现逐渐增加的趋势(Sekhon and Fehlings，2001)。在脊髓损伤地理分布方面，加拿大的一项研究证实农村居民的脊髓损伤发生率是城市居民的两倍(Dryden et al.，2003)。交通事故、高处坠落、体育运动和暴力伤害是脊髓损伤的主要原因。

经济影响

由于脊髓损伤通常需要长时间的住院和康复治疗，通常需要耗费巨大的经济成本。1990 年，美国脊髓损伤的治疗成本约为 40 亿美元(Stripling，1990)。1992 年的一项全国研究表明，脊髓损伤患者在受伤后的前两年平均住院时间为 171 天，初始的平均住院费用接近 10 万美元(Harvey et al.，1992)。现如今，脊髓损伤的治疗费用要更高。此外，医疗服务、医疗用品、医疗设备和康复的费用也很高昂(Harvey et al.，1992)。脊髓损伤的终生治疗费用从不完全脊髓损伤的 5 万美元到高颈段四肢瘫的 200 万美元不等(Harvey et al.，1992)。

病理生理学

原发性损伤和继发性损伤

急性脊髓损伤的原发损伤机制通常认为是不可逆的；一般由创伤性骨折或脱位导致正常保护结构移位而引起的快速、剧烈的脊髓受压和扭曲(Fehlings and Tator，1995)。继发性损伤指由原发损伤引发的一系列级联损伤反应，如缺血、缺氧反应、电解质紊乱和脂质过氧化反应等(Fehlings and Tator，1995)。在脊髓损伤发生的最初几分钟内，通过缺血、缺氧、离子转运、脂质过氧化、自由基形成、蛋白酶激活和前列腺素诱导的凋亡等一系列事件导致随后的细胞死亡(**图 67.1**)(Carlson et al.，1998)。继发损伤通常认为由于血管损伤导致最初存活的细胞坏死(Tator and Koyanagi，1997)。然而，从原子吸收光谱学分析，继发损伤只占整个脊髓损伤病理过

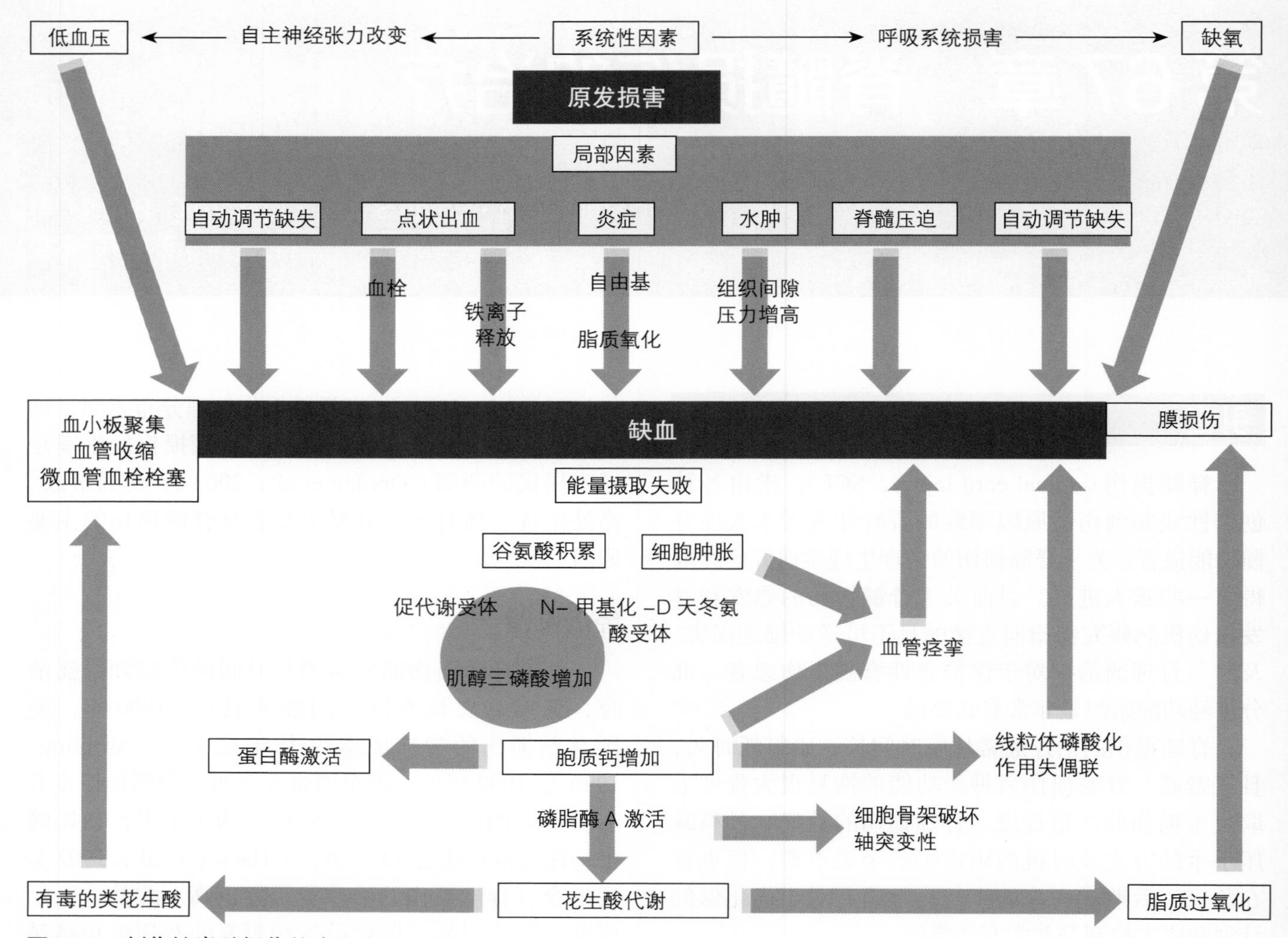

图 67.1 创伤性脊髓损伤的病理生理过程

程的百分之十（Young et al.，1982）。脊髓损伤的血管损伤机制包括脊髓血流量的改变，如在脊髓损伤动物模型中可以看到伤后至少 24 小时的脊髓持续缺血并恶化（Rivlin and Tator，1978）。虽然这种缺血的机制尚不清楚，但机械损伤引起的血管痉挛、血管内皮水肿、血栓形成导致的局灶性出血损伤以及兴奋性氨基酸等可能参与其中（Sekhon and Fehlings，2001）。

组织学发现

急性期（伤后 3~5 天）脊髓损伤标本的组织学主要表现为脊髓灰质的严重出血，这可能与前中央沟动脉损伤有关。周围白质也显示多发病变，包括脱髓鞘和轴突水肿（Tator and Koyanagi，1997）。虽然没有发现脊髓大动脉的完全闭塞，但是在变性的后索可见髓内静脉的闭塞。通常认为，早期机械性应力或继发性损伤导致的髓内静脉闭塞可能是引起白质病变的主要原因（Tator and Koyanagi，1997）。

脊髓损伤的治疗

院前阶段、初步检查和复苏

在创伤现场，应该通过高级创伤生命支持指南（advance trauma life support，ATLS）对患者进行处理（Kortbeek et al.，2008）。首先，脊髓损伤患者应小心地使用类似 kendrick 解脱装置进行固定，同时使用硬颈托，尤其是在救治交通事故导致的脊髓损伤患者。转运过程中，必须通过固定头部和躯干来维持颈椎稳定，同时建议使用血管升压药物来维持收缩压高于 100 mmHg（Gondim et al.，2004）。脊髓损伤的院前处理至关重要。大约 25% 的脊髓损伤患者存在因伤后处置不当而导致的损伤加重（Bernhard et al.，2005）。

医院阶段及二次检查

患者到达医院急诊后应立即取出硬板以防褥疮。同时，必须监测呼吸状态，因为 1/3 的脊髓损伤患者在伤后 24 小时内需要气管插管。高颈段损伤会导致膈肌和肋间肌麻痹，而下颈段损伤通常只影响肋间肌。在颈 5 水平以上脊髓损伤的患者中，我们经常可以看到伴随呼吸的腹部反常运动。因此，常常建议对肺活量小于 1 L 的脊髓损伤患者进行气管插管（Ball，2001）。二次检查时，需要对脊柱进行全面评估，因为当患者保持仰卧位时，许多损伤可能不明显。建议联合使用低分子肝素、旋转翻身床或气动压缩袜预防深静脉血栓形成。第一步是确定脊髓损伤是完全性还是不完全性。在宣布脊髓完全损伤之前必须评估膀胱直肠功能。为了准确和一致地评估脊髓损伤后的神经功能，美国脊髓损伤协会脊髓损伤量表（ASIA）由于其应用简单并与之前使用的 Frankel 量表类似而被广泛应用（**图 67.2**）（Kirshblum et al.，2011）。

甲基强的松龙（甲泼尼龙）琥珀酸钠（MPSS）已在五项人体脊髓损伤试验中得到广泛研究。美国关于急性脊髓损伤的三项多中心、随机、双盲研究（NASCIS）对脊柱创伤的处理有着重大的影响（Bracken et al.，1990）。在一项 NASCIS 研究的基础上，甲基强的松龙琥珀酸钠（MPSS）被认为对脊髓损伤患者具有神经保护作用。研究中还提出了各种剂量与给药建议。然而，在 NASCIS Ⅱ期和Ⅲ期研究中也发现了一些缺陷，据称该结论是基于非标准化的试验设计和人为统计得出的（Sayer et al.，2006）。尽管 MPSS 在脊髓损伤中应用存在研究数据的相互矛盾，且 MPSS 本身存在已知的并发症及缺乏有效性的证明，但其在美国急性脊髓损伤中仍被广泛使用，而且许多中心仍在坚持使用 MPSS 以避免任何可能的法律后果（Hurlbert，2000）。

影像检查

昏迷或不配合治疗的患者在被证实有脊髓损伤之前，应被认为存在脊髓损伤。经观察发现，99.3% 的颈椎、胸椎和腰椎骨折可以通过螺旋 CT 检查出来，而那些螺旋 CT 漏诊的损伤仅需要简单地治疗或者不需要治疗（Brown et al.，2005）。脊柱 MRI 可以清晰地显示神经结构、韧带和间盘。MRI 由于其检查耗时较长不常规用于多发创伤患者的评估。MRI 对于 CT 结果不能解释的神经系统状态的患者最实用，最常用于 CT 表现无异常的神经系统受损患者。MRI 可用于排除颈椎小关节半脱位或脱位患者复位操作前后是否合并椎间盘挤压。

颈椎牵引

Halo 牵引支架已被提倡用于多发创伤患者，它有利于脊髓损伤患者进一步必要的诊断评估和多发创伤患者相关脊髓损伤的紧急手术治疗。闭合颈椎复位和牵引的好处是有争议的。颈椎牵引成功率约为 80%，牵引后神经功能改善率在 80% 左右，但是因椎间盘突出引起的神经功能恶化也可能发生。需要强调的是，颈椎牵引不是普遍采用的治疗方法。

颈椎间隙

关于多发性创伤患者颈椎间隙的问题仍有争议。冠状位和矢状位重建 CT 扫描有助于骨损伤的显示。如果需要对软组织进行评估则需要 MRI 检查。MRI 可以明确是否存在损伤以及明确损伤范围。MRI 上显示的脊髓受压程度、肿胀情况以及脊髓实质出血等往往预示脊髓损伤不良的预后（Miyanji et al.，2007）。为明确钝性伤后脊柱的稳定性，必须对临床和影像学证据进行彻底和系统地评估。

死亡率

脊髓损伤的死亡率从 1970 年的 38% 已经下降到 1997—2000 年间的 15.8%（Bilello et al.，2003）。伤后死亡主要与高颈段脊髓损伤、心血管紊乱或者呼吸损伤有关。脊髓损伤当时和伤后数小时内死亡率最高。死亡率在入院后往往急剧下降（Evans et al.，2013）。创伤性脊髓损伤后早期死亡风险增高的因素如下：年龄大于 20 岁，男性，一种或多种伴随疾病，伴随全身损伤（损伤严重分级，ISS 大于 15 分），以及合并颅脑损伤（Varma et al.，2010）。

预后

入院 ASIA 损伤量表分级（AIS）可以预测伤后 1 年的神经功能恢复情况，因为脊髓损伤严重程度往往与预期恢复水平相关。10%~15% 的脊髓损伤患者可以从最初的 AIS A 级恢复到不完全损伤，仅 2% 的患者可以从 AIS A 级恢复至 AIS D 级（Tator et al.，1999）。对于 AIS C 级的脊髓损伤患者，伤后 1 年 ASIA 运动功能评分平均改善约 43 分，其中约 70% 可以恢复至 AIS D 级或者 AIS E 级（Kirshblum et al.，2011）。颈髓损伤患者的 ASIA 运动功能评分平均可以提高 9.6 分，而胸椎和腰椎脊髓完全损伤患者的 ASIA 运动功能评分仅提高 2.6 分（Kirshblum et al.，2011）。截瘫患者伤后 1 年可以行走的概率约为 5%，而四肢瘫的患者行走的概率为 0（Wilson et al.，

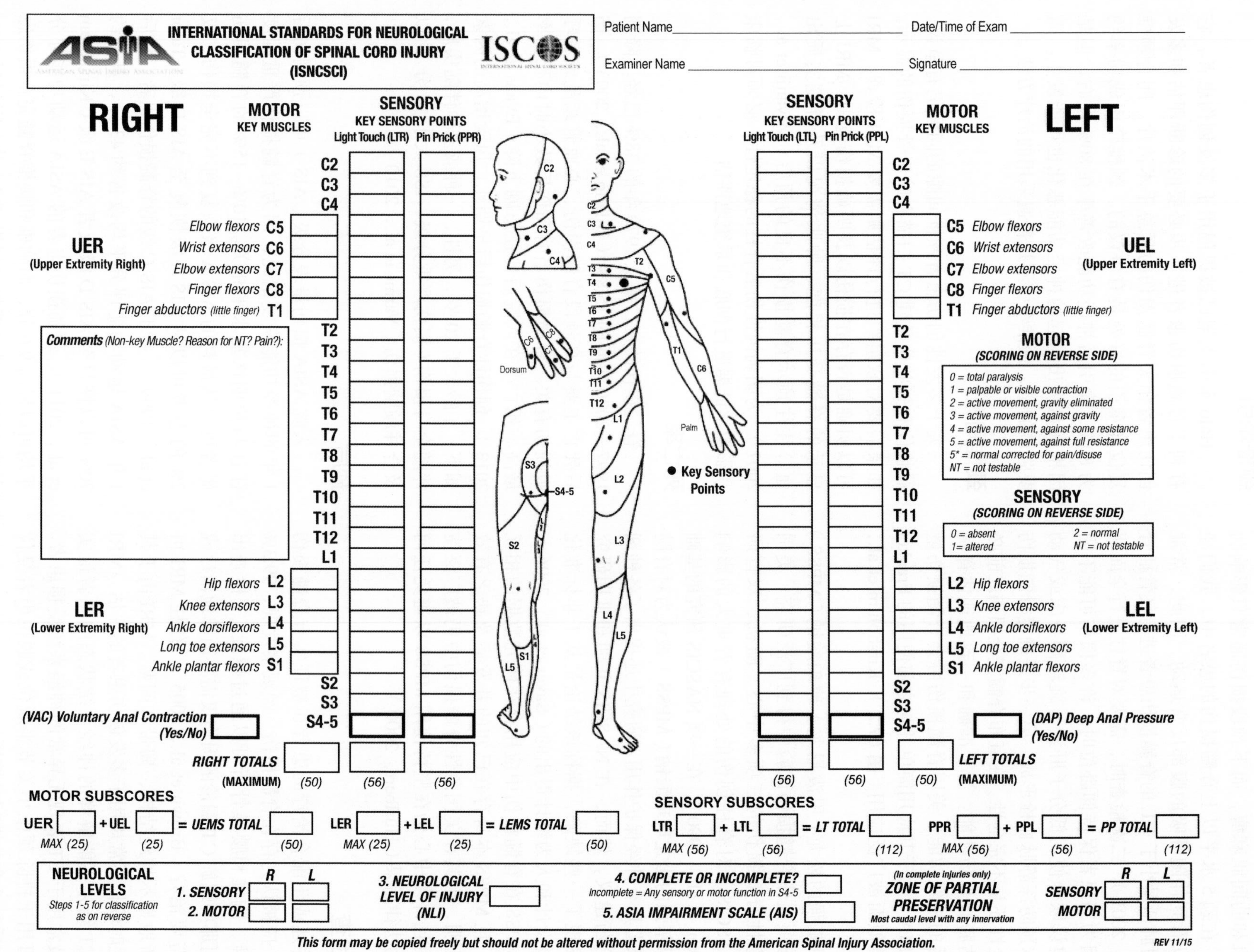

ASIA ISCOS

INTERNATIONAL STANDARDS FOR NEUROLOGICAL CLASSIFICATION OF SPINAL CORD INJURY (ISNCSCI)

Patient Name ______ Date/Time of Exam ______

Examiner Name ______ Signature ______

RIGHT

MOTOR KEY MUSCLES

SENSORY KEY SENSORY POINTS Light Touch (LTR) Pin Prick (PPR)

C2
C3
C4

UER (Upper Extremity Right)
Elbow flexors C5
Wrist extensors C6
Elbow extensors C7
Finger flexors C8
Finger abductors (little finger) T1

T2 T3 T4 T5 T6 T7 T8 T9 T10 T11 T12 L1

Comments (Non-key Muscle? Reason for NT? Pain?):

LER (Lower Extremity Right)
Hip flexors L2
Knee extensors L3
Ankle dorsiflexors L4
Long toe extensors L5
Ankle plantar flexors S1

S2
S3
S4-5

(VAC) Voluntary Anal Contraction (Yes/No)

RIGHT TOTALS (MAXIMUM) (50) (56) (56)

LEFT

SENSORY KEY SENSORY POINTS Light Touch (LTL) Pin Prick (PPL)

MOTOR KEY MUSCLES

C2
C3
C4

UEL (Upper Extremity Left)
C5 Elbow flexors
C6 Wrist extensors
C7 Elbow extensors
C8 Finger flexors
T1 Finger abductors (little finger)

T2 T3 T4 T5 T6 T7 T8 T9 T10 T11 T12 L1

MOTOR (SCORING ON REVERSE SIDE)
0 = total paralysis
1 = palpable or visible contraction
2 = active movement, gravity eliminated
3 = active movement, against gravity
4 = active movement, against some resistance
5 = active movement, against full resistance
5* = normal corrected for pain/disuse
NT = not testable

SENSORY (SCORING ON REVERSE SIDE)
0 = absent
1 = altered
2 = normal
NT = not testable

LEL (Lower Extremity Left)
L2 Hip flexors
L3 Knee extensors
L4 Ankle dorsiflexors
L5 Long toe extensors
S1 Ankle plantar flexors

S2
S3
S4-5

(DAP) Deep Anal Pressure (Yes/No)

LEFT TOTALS (MAXIMUM) (56) (56) (50)

MOTOR SUBSCORES

UER ___ + UEL ___ = UEMS TOTAL ___ MAX (25) (25) (50)

LER ___ + LEL ___ = LEMS TOTAL ___ MAX (25) (25) (50)

SENSORY SUBSCORES

LTR ___ + LTL ___ = LT TOTAL ___ MAX (56) (56) (112)

PPR ___ + PPL ___ = PP TOTAL ___ MAX (56) (56) (112)

NEUROLOGICAL LEVELS
Steps 1-5 for classification as on reverse

1. SENSORY R L
2. MOTOR R L

3. NEUROLOGICAL LEVEL OF INJURY (NLI)

4. COMPLETE OR INCOMPLETE?
Incomplete = Any sensory or motor function in S4-5

5. ASIA IMPAIRMENT SCALE (AIS)

(In complete injuries only)
ZONE OF PARTIAL PRESERVATION
Most caudal level with any innervation
SENSORY R L
MOTOR R L

REV 11/15

图 67.2 脊髓损伤神经功能分级标准

Muscle Function Grading

0 = total paralysis
1 = palpable or visible contraction
2 = active movement, full range of motion (ROM) with gravity eliminated
3 = active movement, full ROM against gravity
4 = active movement, full ROM against gravity and moderate resistance in a muscle specific position
5 = (normal) active movement, full ROM against gravity and full resistance in a functional muscle position expected from an otherwise unimpaired person
5* = (normal) active movement, full ROM against gravity and sufficient resistance to be considered normal if identified inhibiting factors (i.e. pain, disuse) were not present
NT = not testable (i.e. due to immobilization, severe pain such that the patient cannot be graded, amputation of limb, or contracture of > 50% of the normal ROM)

Sensory Grading

0 = Absent
1 = Altered, either decreased/impaired sensation or hypersensitivity
2 = Normal
NT = Not testable

When to Test Non-Key Muscles:

In a patient with an apparent AIS B classification, non-key muscle functions more than 3 levels below the motor level on each side should be tested to most accurately classify the injury (differentiate between AIS B and C).

Movement	Root level
Shoulder: Flexion, extension, abduction, adduction, internal and external rotation **Elbow:** Supination	C5
Elbow: Pronation **Wrist:** Flexion	C6
Finger: Flexion at proximal joint, extension. **Thumb:** Flexion, extension and abduction in plane of thumb	C7
Finger: Flexion at MCP joint **Thumb:** Opposition, adduction and abduction perpendicular to palm	C8
Finger: Abduction of the index finger	T1
Hip: Adduction	L2
Hip: External rotation	L3
Hip: Extension, abduction, internal rotation **Knee:** Flexion **Ankle:** Inversion and eversion **Toe:** MP and IP extension	L4
Hallux and Toe: DIP and PIP flexion and abduction	L5
Hallux: Adduction	S1

ASIA Impairment Scale (AIS)

A = Complete. No sensory or motor function is preserved in the sacral segments S4-5.

B = Sensory Incomplete. Sensory but not motor function is preserved below the neurological level and includes the sacral segments S4-5 (light touch or pin prick at S4-5 or deep anal pressure) AND no motor function is preserved more than three levels below the motor level on either side of the body.

C = Motor Incomplete. Motor function is preserved at the most caudal sacral segments for voluntary anal contraction (VAC) OR the patient meets the criteria for sensory incomplete status (sensory function preserved at the most caudal sacral segments (S4-S5) by LT, PP or DAP), and has some sparing of motor function more than three levels below the ipsilateral motor level on either side of the body.
(This includes key or non-key muscle functions to determine motor incomplete status.) For AIS C – less than half of key muscle functions below the single NLI have a muscle grade ≥ 3.

D = Motor Incomplete. Motor incomplete status as defined above, with at least half (half or more) of key muscle functions below the single NLI having a muscle grade ≥ 3.

E = Normal. If sensation and motor function as tested with the ISNCSCI are graded as normal in all segments, and the patient had prior deficits, then the AIS grade is E. Someone without an initial SCI does not receive an AIS grade.

Using ND: To document the sensory, motor and NLI levels, the ASIA Impairment Scale grade, and/or the zone of partial preservation (ZPP) when they are unable to be determined based on the examination results.

ASIA
AMERICAN SPINAL INJURY ASSOCIATION

INTERNATIONAL STANDARDS FOR NEUROLOGICAL CLASSIFICATION OF SPINAL CORD INJURY

ISCOS
INTERNATIONAL SPINAL CORD SOCIETY

Steps in Classification

The following order is recommended for determining the classification of individuals with SCI.

1. Determine sensory levels for right and left sides.
The sensory level is the most caudal, intact dermatome for both pin prick and light touch sensation.

2. Determine motor levels for right and left sides.
Defined by the lowest key muscle function that has a grade of at least 3 (on supine testing), providing the key muscle functions represented by segments above that level are judged to be intact (graded as a 5).
Note: in regions where there is no myotome to test, the motor level is presumed to be the same as the sensory level, if testable motor function above that level is also normal.

3. Determine the neurological level of injury (NLI)
This refers to the most caudal segment of the cord with intact sensation and antigravity (3 or more) muscle function strength, provided that there is normal (intact) sensory and motor function rostrally respectively.
The NLI is the most cephalad of the sensory and motor levels determined in steps 1 and 2.

4. Determine whether the injury is Complete or Incomplete.
(i.e. absence or presence of sacral sparing)
*If voluntary anal contraction = **No** AND all S4-5 sensory scores = **0** AND deep anal pressure = **No,** then injury is **Complete.***
*Otherwise, injury is **Incomplete.***

5. Determine ASIA Impairment Scale (AIS) Grade:

Is injury Complete? **If YES, AIS=A** and can record ZPP (lowest dermatome or myotome on each side with some preservation)

NO ↓

Is injury Motor Complete? **If YES, AIS=B**

NO ↓ (No=voluntary anal contraction OR motor function more than three levels below the motor level on a given side, if the patient has sensory incomplete classification)

Are at least half (half or more) of the key muscles below the neurological level of injury graded 3 or better?

NO ↓ **AIS=C**　　**YES** ↓ **AIS=D**

If sensation and motor function is normal in all segments, AIS=E
Note: AIS E is used in follow-up testing when an individual with a documented SCI has recovered normal function. If at initial testing no deficits are found, the individual is neurologically intact; the ASIA Impairment Scale does not apply.

图 67.2 （续）

2012；Wilson et al.，2013）。

完成的试验

GM1 神经节苷脂

目前脊髓损伤最大的前瞻性、随机临床试验是一项关于 GM1 神经节苷脂的临床研究，该研究入组了超过 750 名的脊髓损伤患者。Ⅲ级临床证据表明神经节苷脂通过优化脊髓灌注可以改善脊髓损伤患者预后（Hurlbert，2006）。然而，在脊髓损伤患者长期随访中其效果并不明确。因此，目前还未在临床使用。

甲状腺激素释放激素、加环利定、尼莫地平和强啡肽

一项甲状腺激素释放激素的 NASCIS 试验证实其能够使不完全脊髓损伤患者的 Sunnybrook 神经功能评分得到改善。然而，这项研究被指出存在统计学上的Ⅰ类错误（仅仅分析了 20 名患者）（Pitts et al.，1995）。加环利定试验虽然统计学效力不足，但在治疗组中显示出了益处，但这种益处在 1 年随访中并未持续（Hirbec et al.，2006）。尼莫地平试验比较了尼莫地平、甲基强的松龙琥珀酸钠和安慰剂（NASCIS Ⅱ方案）。两种药物都没有显示出对脊髓损伤改善有帮助（Hall，2011）。强啡肽 A，一种内源性阿片类药物，在 NASCIS Ⅱ试验中也没有显示出其对脊髓损伤有帮助（Bracken et al.，1990）。

进行中的试验

新的关于创伤性脊髓损伤模型的试验有两方面：①抑制继发性脊髓损伤的神经保护药物和②促进轴突修复和再生的神经再生药物（图 67.3）。

神经保护方面：脑脊液引流、电刺激、亚低温和利鲁唑

有证据表明，脊髓损伤患者型腰大池脑脊液引流可以降低截瘫的发生率（Coselli et al.，2002）。沿脊髓长轴方向建立磁场对于促进轴突生长也有改善（Shapiro et al.，2005）。将心脏停搏期间低温的保护作用应用于脊髓损伤动物模型结果呈现出多变性（Kwon et al.，2008）。最近的实验提示将全身体温降至 33° 可以使脊髓损伤患者获益。但是，目前的证据不足以将亚低温治疗作为脊髓损伤治疗的标准指南。利鲁唑，一种钠离子阻断和抗癫痫药物，与 MPSS 联合使用，即使在受伤 10 天的脊髓损伤动物模型中，也显示出对脊髓具有保护作用（Wang et al.，2004）。

神经再生能力

细胞替代治疗一直是人们关注的焦点。活化自体巨噬细胞移植在Ⅰ期试验中显示出了良好的结果，但由于资金问题，多中心Ⅱ期试验被暂停（Knoller

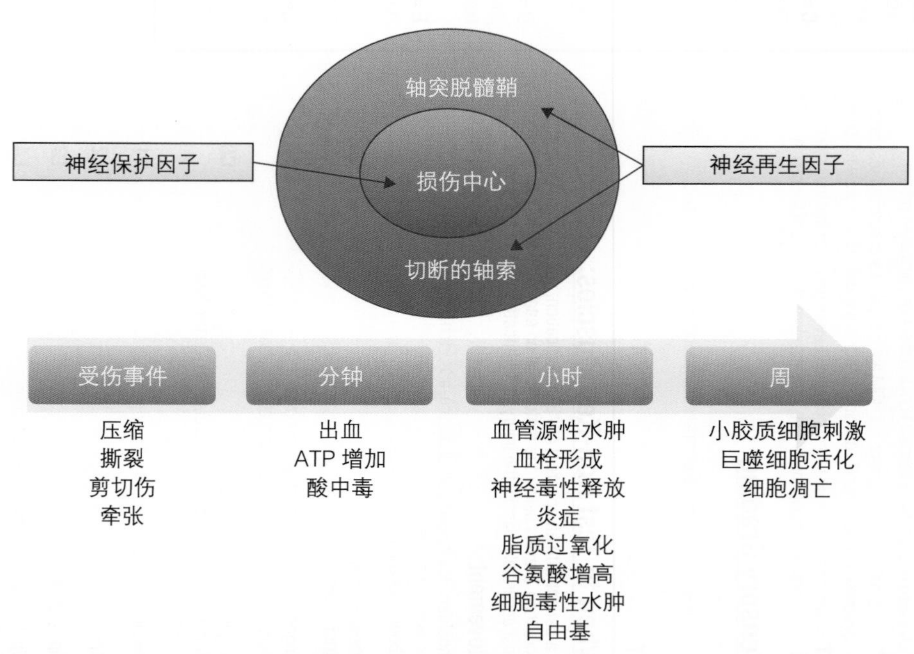

图 67.3 影响脊髓损伤严重程度的原发和继发损伤机制。原发损伤诱导继发损伤的病理级联反应，这一过程自伤后数秒持续至伤后数周

et al., 2005)。施万细胞在促进周围神经再生方面起着重要作用。嗅鞘细胞移植通过1年随访发现是安全可行的。然而，长期随访结果不确定(Lima et al., 2006)。一项人自体骨髓基质细胞联合粒细胞巨噬细胞集落刺激因子的试验显示，在急性脊髓损伤患者中可以获益，但在慢性脊髓损伤患者中没有获益(Park et al., 2005)。人胚胎干细胞移植在大鼠脊髓损伤模型中显示出良好的效果。然而，由于肿瘤发生的风险，FDA暂停了人体试验(Keirstead et al., 2005)。rho是一种轴突生长抑制蛋白，它会导致神经元生长停止，神经突回缩；在一项体外研究中，rho相关的激酶抑制剂和C3转移酶证明了皮质神经元的有效再生(Dergham et al., 2002)。局部注射活化的自体巨噬细胞可以使神经毒性肿瘤坏死因子的合成降低(TNF-α)，从而促进神经保护和神经再生(Bomstein et al., 2003)。

结论

脊髓损伤是一个全球性的问题，对经济、社会及个人都产生了巨大的影响。目前对原发性损伤的治疗证明是可行的。为了预防和减少脊髓损伤的发生，人们已经做出了努力并取得了一些成功。脊髓继发性损伤涉及多种病理生理过程。临床指南的建立旨在减少继发性损伤。目前正在研究新的药理和生物制剂来介导次生机制。从过去完成的试验中汲取经验教训，更有效的脊髓损伤管理显然需要多种治疗方式。脊髓损伤治疗的目标是尽量减少初始损伤，保留剩余功能，并加强康复。希望通过各专业科学家和临床医生的合作，在我们有生之年能够完成脊髓损伤后的神经修复。

争议

脊髓损伤早期减压手术

动物脊髓损伤模型已经证明早期减压对脊髓损伤有好处(Dimar et al., 1999)。然而，在人类，特别是在多发创伤患者中，早期减压是否获益仍不清楚。第一项关于手术时机的前瞻性随机研究发现，脊髓损伤患者伤后72小时内颈椎减压手术相比于伤后超过5天者无明显获益(Cadotte et al., 2010)。第一个外科手术治疗急性脊髓损伤的随机、前瞻性研究证实神经功能得到改善，认为在脊髓损伤24小时内进行减压手术的患者AIS至少有两个以上等级的改善(Fehlings et al., 2012)。

先前存在退变的脊柱(伴有椎管狭窄)的剧烈伸展性损伤可导致典型的脊髓中央性损伤。中央型脊髓损伤综合征早期减压预后也不佳(Schneider et al., 1954)。因此，对于脊髓中央管综合征患者不建议早期手术。但是，后来又有研究证实早期手术有效(Aito et al., 2007)。关于脊髓中央管综合征的治疗仍存在许多未知之处。因此，实践模式往往依赖于临床经验而不是科学证据。

关于损伤机制、损伤节段及减压时机对胸段脊髓损伤功能预后的报道较少。一项回顾性研究比较了三组患者的恢复和预后数据：对照组(n=93)，伤后72小时内早期手术组(n=156)和伤后超过72小时晚期手术组(n=49)。结果显示早期手术组在呼吸机依赖、ICU时间、住院时间、死亡率和肺衰竭等方面明显好于晚期手术组(Schinkel et al., 2006)。

延伸阅读、参考文献、EBRAIN的相关链接

扫描书末二维码获取。

第 68 章　颈椎损伤

Calan Mathieson・Chris Barrett・Likhith Alakandy 著
阎涛 译，苏亦兵 审校

引言

颈椎骨折的治疗是一个复杂而有趣的话题。在过去的许多年中已经发展出许多专业术语和分类，以能更好地理解并区分这一大类的患者。尽管如此，在这一类患者的治疗方法选择上很难达成共识。本章将主要讨论与颈椎骨折治疗有关的决策过程。

脊柱外科医生在治疗急性颈椎损伤患者的主要目标是预防继发性神经损伤以及脊柱畸形的发生，必要时通过重建脊柱稳定性来减轻患者的疼痛症状。评估如何实现这些目标可能非常具有挑战性。外科医生将会面临很多问题。什么样的患者应该接受手术治疗？哪种手术可以使脊柱获得最好的稳定性？哪些患者只需要用颈托或 Halo 支架予以治疗？治疗初期是否需要通过牵引减轻损伤？还有时机选择的问题，外科医生应该什么时间开始这些治疗？

颈椎骨折的发病率

颈椎骨折的年发病率估计在 9.2~12/100 000（Hu et al.，1996；Brolin and von Holst，2002）。以男性患者为主，存在两个发病年龄高峰，分别是在 15~45 岁年龄段和 65~80 岁年龄段。这两个年龄段组的患者损伤机制有所不同，老年人最常见的是摔倒后导致 C2 齿突骨折，而年轻人主要是因为高速损伤导致的颈椎损伤（Blizzard et al.，2016）。总体而言，有接近 10% 的颈椎骨折将合并有神经系统损伤。

颈椎损伤和头部损伤的关系密切。据报道，在头部损伤的患者中合并有颈椎损伤的发生率在 4%~14%（Nazir et al.，2012）。在那些中度至重度颅脑损伤的患者中发生颈椎损伤的风险极高。NICE 指南建议对任何符合头部 CT 诊断标准的颅脑损伤患者都应同时进行颈椎 CT 检查。

对潜在的颈椎损伤患者进行评估

评估潜在的颈椎损伤需要仔细询问病史，认真查体和影像学检查。当然，要获得完整的病史和全面的查体需要患者有清醒的意识可以很好地配合。对于意识清楚的患者，如果没有颈部的疼痛或压痛，神经功能正常，没有牵拉伤（和没有醉酒状态），即使没有影像学检查，也可以排除颈椎损伤的可能。NEXUS（National Emergency X Radiography Utilization Study）指出应用这些原则时，可以排除严重的颈椎损伤（Eyre, 2006）。

但是，对于那些意识不完全清楚或有牵拉伤，以及醉酒状态的患者，仍要求做全面的放射学检查。可以选择侧位、开口位和前后位（AP）X 线检查和颈椎 CT 检查。在急性期不建议做屈伸位的影像学检查。MRI 扫描有助于评估后方韧带复合体和椎间盘结构的损伤。MRI 扫描将提供有关椎管内内容物的一些重要信息。所以，在必要情况下，在做完 CT 检查后，还应该完善 MRI 检查。

对于那些符合头部 CT 检查标准的创伤患者也应该进行颈椎 CT 检查。中度或重度的颅脑外伤患者可能在几周内都无法进行神经学评估。在这种情况下，如果在薄层 CT 扫描没有发现骨质损伤而且不存在移位的情况下，作者建议可以去掉颈托。通过常规的 CT 检查漏诊韧带损伤的风险非常低，并且继发于佩戴颈托而在颈椎周围区域皮肤出现压疮的风险也并不十分明显（Eastern Association for the Surgery of Trauma，2015）。如果患者在随后的治疗过程中神经学症状有所改善，则应对颈椎再次进行评估。

在评估期间应尽一切努力保持脊柱对位，以最大限度地减少继发性损害的发生。对强直性脊柱炎的患者应特别提高注意。这些患者特别容易遭受颈椎骨折，经常遇到此类患者在低速的冲击力下即已发生颈椎骨折。当固定此类患者时应加倍小心，因为他们的颈椎形态决定了不太容易将这类患者放置到完全放平的位置。他们应当固定在损伤前的既有的屈曲位置，而不要求达到完全仰卧的姿势。还应该对那些具有危险（即高速损伤）机制的患者和老年患者提高警惕（Clinical Effectiveness Committee，2010）。

颈椎创伤的评估

诊断颈椎骨折后，应继续对患者进行适当的治疗，以减少继发性神经损伤的风险。应当对患者继续进行仔细的固定、导尿、留置鼻胃管、给予低分子肝素和质子泵抑制剂。然后，应寻找进一步的信息，使外科医生能够对骨折的明确处理做出适当的抉择。

在评估颈椎损伤时，必须考虑许多重要因素。这些可以通过详尽的病史、细致的查体和全面的检查而获得。我们不能单纯依靠放射学评估，就对如何最好地处理颈椎损伤做出十分明智的决定。

当询问病史时，必须考虑患者的年龄，是否存在强直性脊柱炎或骨质疏松等基础疾病，损伤发生的速度和机制（是屈曲型损伤还是过伸型损伤？）。受伤后肢体的疼痛和无力在病史的记录中非常重要，此外其他部位的损伤也应详细记录。

应该仔细检查患者以发现神经系统体征，有无压痛，有无棘突间距离增大，以及脊柱周围淤青和畸形。

影像学检查通常包括X线检查，CT检查，有时也包括MRI检查。

分类系统

许多临床医生和学者都使用分类系统来帮助进行沟通，理解和决策制订。多年来，已经有了许多不同的分类系统，以简化和细分颈椎损伤。对这些系统的批评大致可分为两类，即该系统要么过于复杂而无法被广泛采用，要么过于简单而对于颈椎损伤的患者难以细分。这些分类系统中的一些是有可取之处的，因为它们强调了在治疗过程中能够做出明智决策所需信息的关键要素。

分类系统使用前述的不同方面。较早的分类系统倾向关注于损伤的机制上，而较新的分类系统则更倾向于放射学和神经系统的方面。

Allen分类

1982年，Allen等发表了基于受伤机制的颈椎损伤分类系统。分类包括屈曲压缩、垂直压缩、屈曲牵张、伸展压缩、伸展牵张和侧方屈曲等6类。根据损伤的放射学严重程度进一步细分每个子类别。常用的词语，例如爆裂骨折，大致相当于中等程度的屈曲压缩骨折。后纵韧带复合体十分重要，严重的伸展损伤常常合并这一重要结构的完全破坏。作者证明，神经损伤的概率随着脊柱损伤的类型和严重程度的增加而增加。

可以在其他地方找到该分类系统的完整说明。尽管今天这些分类仍然有用，但这些子类别都是基于普通X射线来评判的。借助CT和MRI扫描的现代成像方法已促使开发出了更新的分类系统。

下颈椎损伤分类评分系统（SLIC）

C1和C2的解剖结构与颈椎中其余五个椎骨的解剖结构非常不同。（Vaccaro et al.，2007）。下颈椎可被视为C2椎体下边界以下的任何水平的颈椎。下颈椎损伤和分类评分系统从形态学，韧带和神经学方面得出评分。见**表68.1**。

在存在关节面错位、前椎间盘间隙异常变宽、运动段后凸畸形、STIR MRI序列上出现高信号的情况下，韧带复合体破裂被认为是可能的。

颈椎损伤严重程度评分（CSISS）

该系统可用于对不稳定性骨折进行分级（Anderson et al.，2007）。根据解剖部位将颈椎分为前柱、左侧柱、右侧柱和后柱四部分。该系统系统，根据颈椎四个柱的骨骼和韧带结构的损伤严重给予0~5分的评分。将分数相加，得出最终的CSISS分数。

表68.1　下颈椎损伤分类评分

骨损伤形态	间盘韧带复合体	神经功能状态
0 无异常	0 完整	0 完好
1 压缩	1 可疑损伤	1 神经根受累
2 爆裂	2 撕裂	2 完全型脊髓损伤
3 牵张分离		3 不完全脊髓损伤
4 移位或旋转		4 不完全脊髓损伤伴进行性脊髓压迫
		+1 在神经功能缺损的情况下

Reproduced with permission from Alexander Vaccaro, R Hulbert, Alpesh Patel, et al., The Subaxial Cervical Spine Injury Classification System: A Novel Approach to Recognize the Importance of Morphology, Neurology, and Integrity of the Disco-Ligamentous Complex, *Spine*, Volume 32, Issue 21, pp. 2365–74, Copyright © 2007 Wolters Kluwer Health, Inc.

使用该系统进行的评估已证明具有良好的观察者间系数，范围从0.75~0.98，平均为0.88。据称，根据这种分级系统可以预测是否需要手术。但是，这仅适用于得分大于7（均接受手术治疗）的患者，而得分低于7的20名患者中只有4名接受了手术治疗。

作者建议使用这些评分系统来熟悉它们。但是，在计算分数之前，应先考虑患者情况的各个方面，并确定其最佳治疗方法。这一评分系统只能作为一个指导，并不能被用于所有的患者。例如，对于那些不能耐受麻醉，不宜通过外科手术处理老年患者。其他的一些患者可能就是单纯拒绝手术。由于合并其他损伤，有些患者需要严格卧床休息一段时间。这可能意味着当上述评分提示手术治疗时，这些患者只能通过卧床休息保守治疗骨折。

常见的命名性颈椎骨折的治疗

Jefferson 骨折

这类骨折是C1的爆裂骨折。它最初是用于描述C1的四点骨折，其中有两个骨折影响前弓和两个骨折影响后弓。在C1也经常看到其他形式的骨折。示例见**图** 68.1。接近30%的C1骨折合并有C2骨折。

孤立的C1骨折很少引起神经系统损伤，因为骨折部分倾向于向外移动，远离神经组织。典型的C1骨折损伤机制是轴向受力。评估横韧带的损伤非常重要，通常可以通过在CT扫描中测量寰齿间隔来间接评估横韧带的损伤。成人通常小于3 mm，儿童小于5 mm。有时在轴向CT扫描中可以看到韧带撕脱的C1侧块内侧的小骨块。当横韧带破裂时，C1的侧块向外移动。在经口PEG位像或冠状CT重建像上，可以测量C1的侧边缘和C2的侧边缘之间的距离。Spence规则规定，如果两侧的总和超过7 mm，则横韧带就会存在破裂。只有极少数的C1骨折仅需要手术干预。如果横韧带受损，患者通常需要运用Halo支架固定；如果横韧带完好，则患者只需要佩戴颈托加以保护。

Hangman 骨折

Hangman骨折是一种枢椎外伤性滑脱。见**图** 68.2。尽管从历史上看，这些骨折是在司法绞刑后被注意到的，但这种骨折最常见的损害机制是道路交通事故。

Hangman骨折有其特定的分类系统。由Levine和Edwards修改的Effendi分类系统已在12篇评估这些损伤治疗的论文中使用（Li et al.，2006），见**表** 68.2。

最近的一项meta分析（Li et al.，2006）指出，

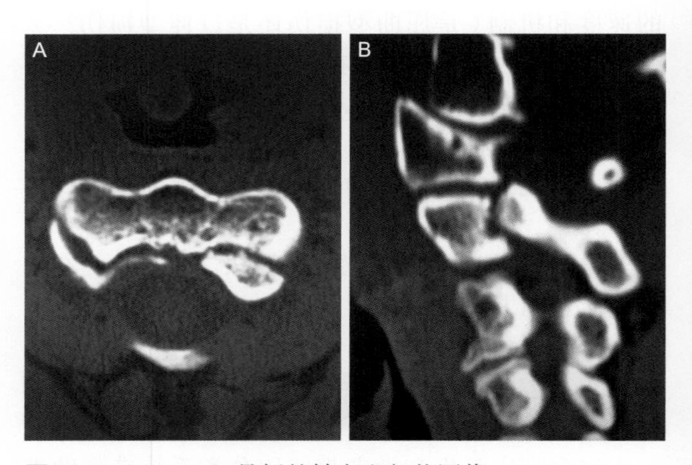

图 68.2 Hangman骨折的轴向和矢状图像

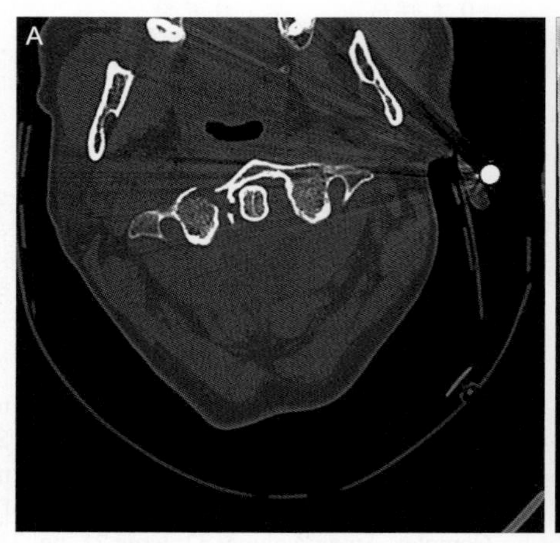

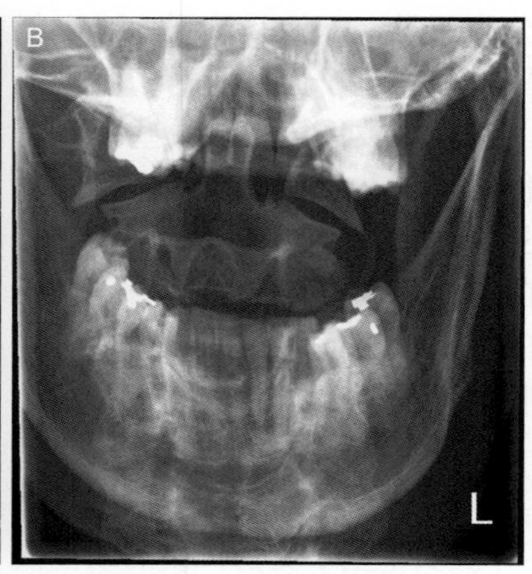

图 68.1 （A）寰椎前弓骨折。（B）侧块移位伴C1环骨折、横韧带破裂

表 68.2　Levine 和 Edwards 分类（Orthopaedics-One, 2012）

Ⅰ型	骨折移位<3 mm，无 C2–C3 成角，稳定
Ⅱ型	明显 C2–C3 成角，骨折移位>3 mm，C2–C3 椎间盘破裂，不稳定
Ⅱa 型	比Ⅱ型更明显的成角，没有骨折移位，由于屈曲 - 分离暴力骨折不稳定
Ⅲ型	严重的 C2–C3 成角和骨折移位，有时有单侧或双侧的 C2–C3 前脱位，不稳定

Reproduced with permission from A Levine and C Edwards, The management of traumatic spondylolisthesis of the axis, *Journal of Bone & Joint Surgery*, Volume 67, Issue 2, pp. 217–26, Copyright © 1985 Wolters Kluwer Health, Inc.

有 62.5%的文章主张对 Hangman 骨折的主要治疗方法应是保守治疗。meta 分析的结果表明，在大多数Ⅰ型、EffendiⅡ型和 Levine-EdwardsⅡ型骨折，无需进行手术干预。Levine-Edwards Ⅱa 和Ⅲ型骨折的患者应考虑进行手术治疗。

因为这些骨折可能同时存在 C2/3 椎间盘的损伤，因此，如果不进行手术融合，则导致骨折很难愈合。保守治疗通常是佩戴 Halo 支架。

前路和后路方法都可以治疗 Hangman 骨折。作者更喜欢采用 C2/3 颈椎间盘切除术和融合的前入路手术方式。可以通过刻下切口到达合适的脊椎水平。

齿状突骨折

齿状突骨折（**图 68.3**）在跌倒后的老年患者中最常见，但在颈椎过度屈伸或过度伸展损伤后的年轻患者中也可能发生。该损伤占所有颈椎骨折的 10% ~15%。据 Anderson 和 D'Alonzo 所述，骨折有三种类型（**表 68.3**）。

表 68.3　Anderson 和 D'Alonzo 分类

Ⅰ型	韧带撕脱引起横韧带上方的齿状突尖端断裂
Ⅱ型	在横韧带下方的齿突底部骨折
Ⅲ型	C2 椎体骨折，使齿状突与其余椎体分离

Reproduced with permission from Lewis Anderson and Richard D'Alonzo, Fractures of the Odontoid Process of the Axis, *Journal of Bone & Joint Surgery*, Volume 56, Issue 8, pp. 1663–74, Copyright © 1974 Wolters Kluwer Health, Inc.

这类骨折重点需要和游离齿突小骨相鉴别，这是一种良性的、慢性的、发育过程中齿突骨化中心发育不良造成的陈旧性骨折而导致长期的骨不连。

Ⅰ型骨折非常少见，但除镇痛外无需其他任何治疗。Ⅲ型骨折通常运用 Halo 支架保守治疗就可能达成融合（对于无法忍受 Halo 支架的老年患者则应佩戴颈托）。

治疗Ⅱ型骨折仍然存在很大争议。与Ⅰ型和Ⅲ型骨折相比，它们的不愈合率更高（20% ~30%）。有些患者，尤其是老年人，患有Ⅱ型齿状突骨折，但没有横韧带破坏，会发展成纤维性骨不连，也没有任何症状。但是，在其他情况下，患者可能会出现疼痛，僵硬，脊髓病和慢性不稳定。使用颈托或 Halo 背心进行非手术治疗无法达到固定的效果，并且与手术技术相比，其骨不连的风险更高。尤其是老年患者，对 Halo 背心的耐受性很差，在这些患者中，颈托可能是唯一的选择。

治疗齿状突骨折的常用外科手术技术是前路齿状突钉固定或后路使用经关节面螺钉或 Harms 技术进行 C1/C2 融合。

前路手术具有可以保持活动的优势，因此应被视为Ⅱ型骨折的首选手术治疗方法（Apfelbaum et al.,

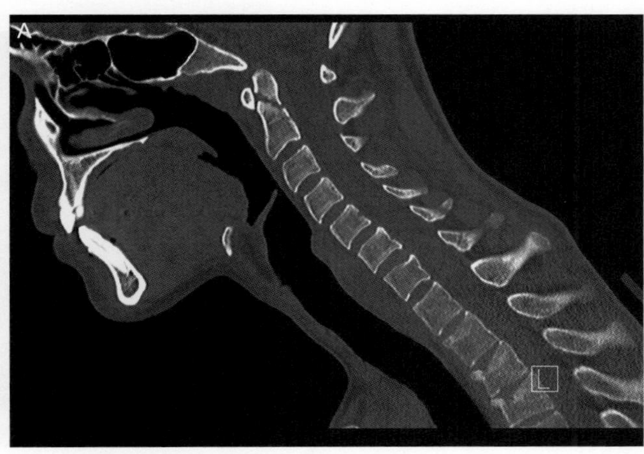

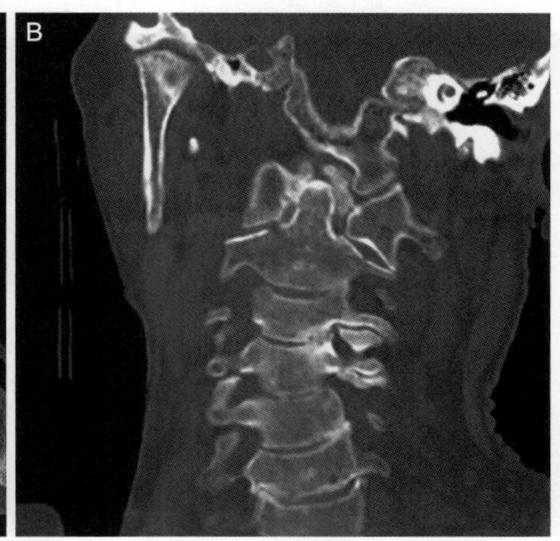

图 68.3　（A）Ⅱ型齿状突骨折。（B）Ⅲ型齿状突骨折

2000）。但是，并非所有的患者都适合于骨折的直接前路固定。应通过 CT 和 MRI 扫描仔细评估患者的寰椎横韧带的完整性，对于横韧带破裂的患者，应采用 C1/C2 后路固定治疗。骨折的形态也是重要的考虑因素。粉碎性骨折或骨折线不适合放置螺钉的情况也应该采取后路方法。同样，如果将脊柱平缓伸展，不能轻易将骨折复位到满意的位置也不适合采用前路方法。对于体型较大的患者或有桶状胸腔的患者可能难以获得最佳的螺钉轨迹。骨质较差是相对手术禁忌，因为螺钉经过远端骨折会形成“奶酪接线”。在非急性骨折中，骨折愈合的机会明显较低，在这种情况下，如果骨折不稳定，则应考虑采用 C1/C2 后路固定。单螺钉前齿状突的固定有较低的并发症发生率和较高的融合率，应成为首选（(Subach et al.，1999；Lee et al.，2004）。

小关节骨折脱位

单侧（**图 68.4**）或双侧（**图 68.5**）的小关节骨折脱位是下颈椎段最常见的严重损伤类型。它们通常是体育运动或车辆事故后因为屈曲和分离损伤而发生的。当通常原本位于下方小关节面后面的上方的小关节面“跳”到下方小关节面的前方时，会发生单面骨折脱位。

这会产生旋转错位，当从侧面 X 射线观察时，旋转错位表现为上方椎体的前半脱位 25%。脊髓很少受到影响，但在该水平存在的神经根可能受到损害，并可能发生神经根病。可能会发生没有骨折的脱位，有时还会看到部分脱位或高位小关节面。C7/T1 的水平可能会受到影响，因此，当 X 射线应当能显示 T1 的顶部才算足够。

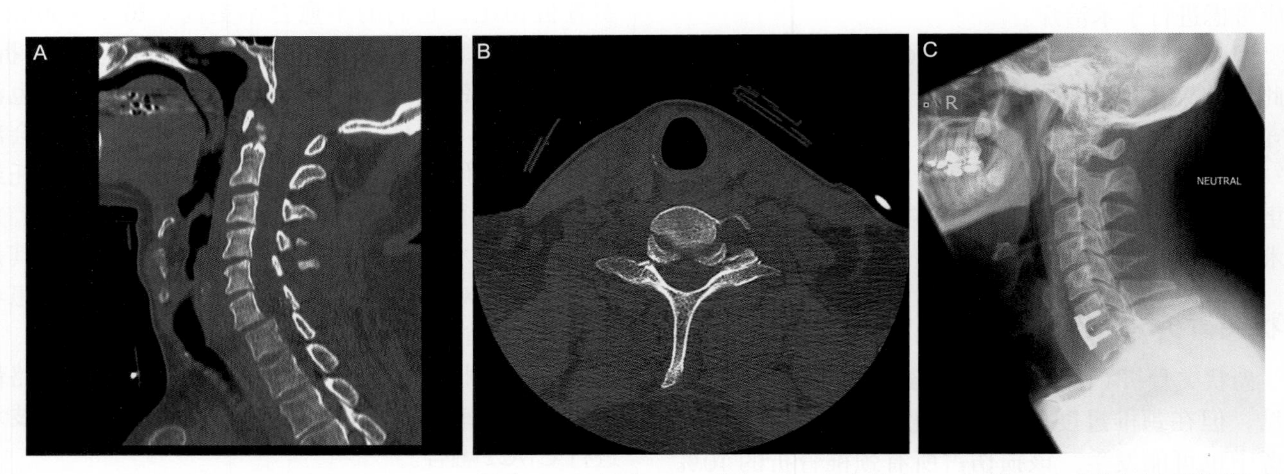

图 68.4 C6/7 处的单关节面脱位。（A）在矢状位 CT 扫描中 25%脱位。（B）在轴向 CT 扫描上显示的左侧“跳跃”的小关节面。（C）术后 X 线片显示复位，颈椎前路椎间盘切除术和融合术

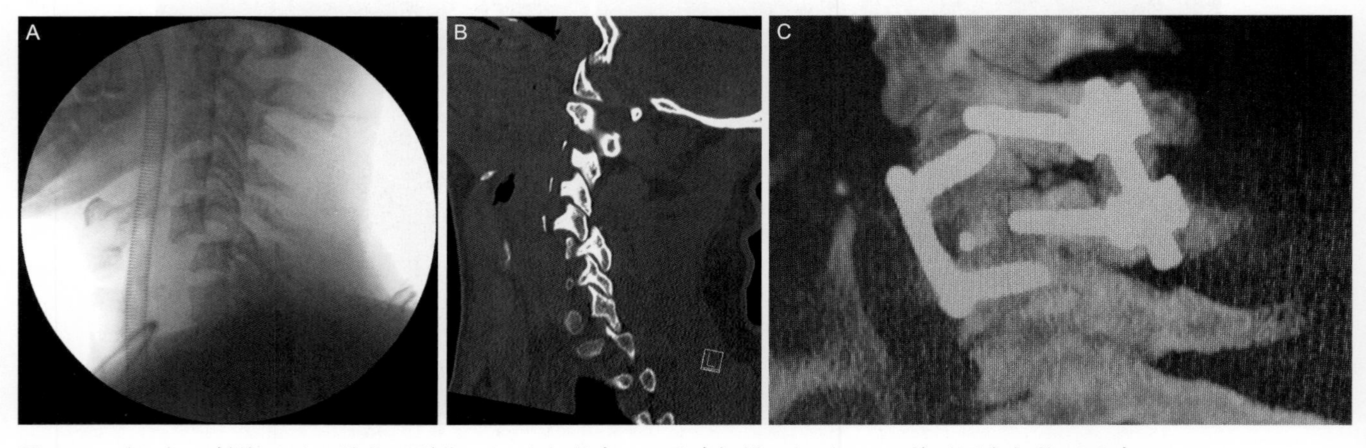

图 68.5 （A）X 射线显示双关节面脱位。（B）矢状旁 CT 重建扫描。（C）C4/5 前后固定矢状面重建 CT

双面关节面骨折脱位通常伴有脊髓损伤，以完全性脊髓损伤为常见。

这些损伤不是旋转损伤，是真正的前半脱位，X线平片显示有 50%或更多的半脱位。

这些骨折的治疗方法在本章的争议部分中介绍。

其他轴下骨折

患者可能出现椎板、关节间隙或棘突等未移位的颈椎骨折，例如铲土者骨折（棘突撕脱性骨折，最常见为 C7）见**图 68.6**。对于大部分这类骨折的治疗通常只需要佩戴颈托等非手术方式，但也需要仔细观察，因为有一小部分患者会有进一步进展。对于影响关节间隙的骨折尤其如此，有些作者建议尽早进行手术干预或固定 Halo 支架。

过度伸展引起的泪滴撕脱骨折是椎体下部、前部的骨折，很容易被忽略（见**图 68.7**）。当见到泪滴骨折，并且 MRI 确认椎间盘和（或）韧带损伤时，手术是最确定的治疗方法。因为是韧带损伤，它们往往不容易愈合，大多数作者建议进行手术融合。

颈椎骨折的治疗选择

颈托

合适的硬质颈托是限制颈椎运动的有效方法，特别是屈曲和侧屈。在外科手术方面，颈托通常用于在愈合过程中使相对稳定的损伤脊椎不动，并经常在外科手术固定后为脊柱提供额外的支撑。在急诊过程中也会经常使用颈托作为辅助，以防止继发性脊髓损伤。不常见的是，它们也可用于减轻软组织损伤后的不适症状。在较低的颈椎和胸椎水平骨折，颈托的固定有效性会有所下降，在这种情况下可能需要颈胸支具或 Halo 支架才能获得有效的固定。

安装说明

各种制造商提供了一系列硬性颈托。典型的设计是两件式硬壳，由皮带固定，并衬有可移动的软垫。除了将与压力有关的并发症的风险降至最低，舒适且合身的颈托还可以增加患者的依从性。在脊椎不稳定的患者中应用颈托时，必须在整个过程中保持头部和颈部正确对位。首先将颈托的后部小心翼翼地滑到脖子下面，然后将前部紧紧贴在患者的脖子上，并用绑带固定。在骨折相对稳定的情况下，可以让患者在站立时佩戴颈托。一旦颈托就位，重要的是要确保支撑物从下颌骨延伸到胸骨切迹，并且压力点要适当填充。气管开口和中线孔应在中线。

并发症

颈托相关的最主要的并发症是压疮。这种与颈托相关的皮肤问题的风险包括从轻微的红斑到严重的溃疡，并且随着使用时间的延长，多达 10%的患者会出现这些并发症。

颈椎牵引

颈椎骨折和创伤性半脱位 / 脱位通常通过考虑复位、减压和稳定的原则进行治疗。目的是实现骨折复位，并在可能的情况下实现脊髓减压。显然，仅靠牵引是无法实现稳定的。

颈椎牵引是闭合复位的一种形式，可以在闭合复位之前使用或偶尔使用。在这种情况下，如果可以实现良好的重新对位，并且如果因为患者无法尽早进行手术以稳定脊柱，则可以用于将患者暂时或最终外固定（Halo 支架或 Minerva 支架）。

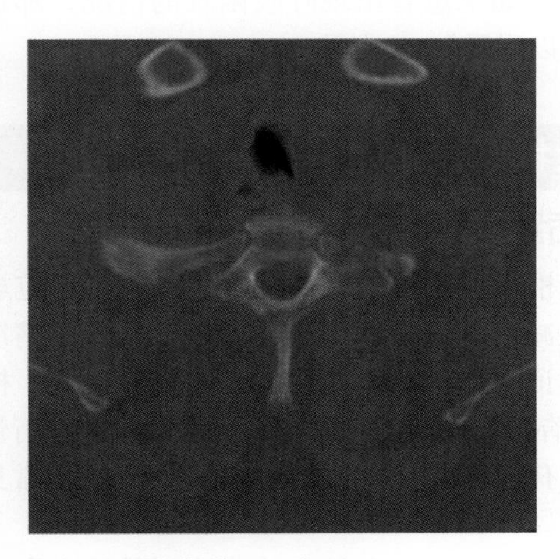

图 68.6　铲土者骨折轴位 CT 表现

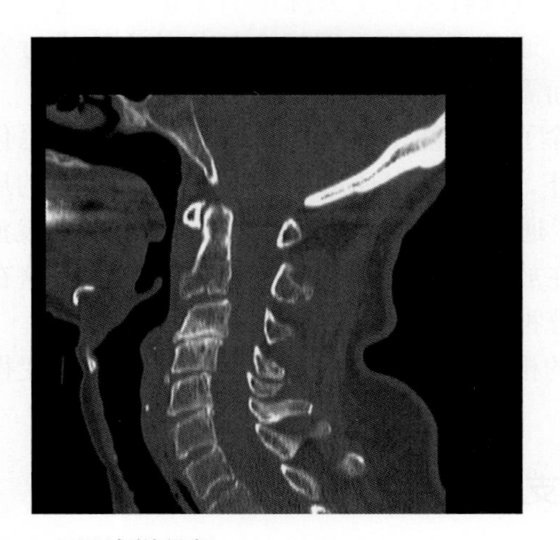

图 68.7　C2 泪滴样骨折

施加牵引力最有效的方法是使用直接固定在头骨上的钳子或 Halo 环。应该避免使用吊索或皮带的系统，因为极有可能会导致下巴上的压疮，并且这样在精确的方向上施加力会更加困难。然后，通过穿过滑轮的绳索将圆环连接到垂直放置的配重上，从而最大限度地减少摩擦，并确保力的水平分量直接作用在头骨上。

Gardner-Wells 钳仅依靠两个销钉固定。它们相对容易操作，特别是如果临床医生在数小时内不能得到更多的援助。销钉上有可见的指示，可有效提示何时将颅骨销钉拧紧至正确的扭矩。

Halo 环（通常但不总是不完整的环或 C 形）至少需要四点颅骨固定。它比钳式固定更难操作，并且通常使患者更不舒服，特别是对于后部或顶针部位可能难以实现足够的局部麻醉时。但是，显著的优势是，一旦实现了足够的复位，便可以更轻松地安装临时或永久的 Halo 支架。

一旦将钳子或 Halo 环放置于头骨，则将绳索连接并穿过滑轮。通过调节皮带轮的角度，可以沿所需方向施加力。重要的是，不要过度屈曲以减少骨折，因为据报道这样做会导致呼吸情况恶化（Harrop et al.，2001）。应该逐渐增加牵引的重量，这需要有良好的护理，通常需要仔细镇痛并偶尔使用苯二氮䓬类药物。定期进行侧位 X 射线检查，并仔细观察患者是否出现新的或恶化的神经系统症状，这是十分必要的。

关于合适的牵引重量，存在各种经验法则，通常取决于所涉及的颈椎水平。从枕骨远端开始计数，每节段增加 2 磅的重量（即 C5 损伤，则需要 10 磅的初始重量）。需要强调的是，通常需要更大的重量才能完成复位，但应该在仔细的临床和放射学观察下，循序渐进地增加牵引重量。如果出现神经功能恶化，应减轻或完全去除牵引重量，并进行 X 射线检查。通常不可能采用闭合复位的方法进行完全复位，而需要在全身麻醉进行切开复位。

除了有可能出现神经系统和呼吸系统恶化的情况之外，颈椎牵引还可能出现 Halo 环销钉的局部并发症。通常大小的牵引力不足以引起此类并发症的发生。在放置牵引之前，应进行 MRI 检查。这在完全或部分神经功能缺损的情况下尤其显得重要。例如，较大的椎间盘碎片或血肿可能使闭合复位变得十分危险。

Halo 支具固定

Halo 支具是固定颈椎的一种更牢固且有创的固定方式。它是由一个可以用固定针固定在颅骨外表面的圆环组成，通过可调节的金属杆连接到带有衬里的硬质背心或外套（Lind et al.，1988）。这使患者可以活动，同时提供比颈托更好的固定度。可调节杆可精确控制需要固定颈椎的位置。Halo 冠和背心的固定也可用于在术前转移过程中以及在某些情况下补充手术固定以提供稳定性。

在使用 Halo 支具固定时，至关重要的是在整个过程中必须使头部和颈部保持正确对位。Halo 环通常通过四个销钉固定在颅骨上，两个销钉位于额骨区域，距眶缘上方一厘米，两个销钉位于耳后部，位于顶壁后部。在局麻下将销钉插入，在额部钉钉时应该闭上眼睛。使用扭矩扳手来防止拧得太紧。然后，把背心的前部组件和后部组件放置到合适位置并用绑带固定。金属杆固定在背心上并连接到 Halo 环上。这些多功能杆可在调整脊椎位置时提供更多灵活性。固定所有连接杆后，用 X 射线确认颈椎的位置。应定期检查该装置，在此期间重新拧紧硬件并检查针脚是否松动或感染。脊柱的位置也应进行放射线检查。Halo 支架固定治疗的持续时间取决于个体，但是对于大多数骨折，持续三个月的时间就足够了。

大多数患者可以良好耐受 Halo 支架，但有一部分患者在开始佩戴时会不适应、活动困难以及难以入睡等问题。针脚松动通常以疼痛为特征，并且明显可见（Vertullo et al.，1997）。定期检查针脚的位置可以避免发生这样的情况，特别是在开始阶段。针脚感染发生在 10%~20% 的患者当中，这种感染常常是比较表浅的感染。这种情况可能需要抗生素治疗以及更换针脚的位置。更严重的感染如颅骨骨髓炎和继发于颅骨的颅内脓肿也有报道，但是相当少见（Rizzolo et al.，1993；Van Middendorp et al.，2009）。Halo 环或背心的直接压迫可能导致压疮或局部的皮肤破溃。如果患者出现呼吸困难的情况，那这类患者就难以耐受 Halo 支具。

手术技术

颈椎后路内固定（C3~C7）

颈椎后路固定术应用于已经存在不稳定或可能因外科减压手术后即刻或迟发的不稳定的情况。具体适应证包括外伤引起的骨或韧带不稳定，椎间盘炎 / 骨脊髓炎引起的不稳定和后凸畸形，退行性脊柱疾病伴有后凸畸形以及需要减压的地方（最常见于脊髓病）。

非常重要的一点是，除非达到骨性融合或理想的骨折愈合，否则无论采用何种专业技术，任何固定方法最终都会失败。因此，在进行固定和减压后，外科医生应该行脊柱融合术。这涉及去皮移植受者部位的标准方法，然后进行局部或远距离采购的自体骨移植（例如，在椎板切除术后取骨或取髂骨植骨）。

存在许多可能的技术，并且这些年来已经逐渐发展。颈椎后路钢丝和经关节面螺钉最好是在其他方法无法实现或失败的情况下进行的。

文献报道了颈椎椎弓根螺钉的一系列病例。下部颈椎（C6 和 C7）的椎弓根可能具有足够的位置防止椎弓根螺钉，而颈椎中段则较少。尽管如此，作者们认为从 C6 向上的椎间孔中存在椎动脉会带来一种特殊的额外并发症，使得侧块螺钉的放置仍然是后路颈椎固定的金标准技术（Yoshihara et al.，2013）。

术前检查应包括一般性因素，例如在俯卧数小时的情况下是否适合麻醉。特殊考虑的因素包括骨质疏松症的可能性。虽然这不是手术的绝对禁忌证，但如果骨骼质量极差，需要小心，否则螺钉可能无法获得足够的固定力。在这种情况下，如果没有在术后使用 Halo 支具外固定，则可能无法实现侧块融合。

标准的术前检查可能包括 CT 和 MRI 以及动态影像学检查，包括 X 线平片或 CT。重建 CT 扫描通常是最有用的检查，因为可以估计螺钉的大小和轨迹，并发现常见的凹坑。这些将包括极小的侧块，通常在 C3 处，使得螺钉置入困难或椎动脉走行异常。如果外科医生对椎动脉的走向有特殊的担忧，则需要进行颈部血管的 CT 血管造影。

在全身麻醉下，患者 Trendelenburg 俯卧位，放在合适的床垫和手术台上。作者大力提倡使用头架（例如 Mayfield 钳），而不要使用泡沫头枕或枕头。这样可以根据需要进行术中调整，从而实现更精确的定位。它还可以避免对脸部或眼睛施加任何压力，并始终为麻醉师提供良好的通道。

一旦患者就位，应行颈椎侧位片以确定手术切口范围和颈椎形态。轻度的屈曲位有利于更好的手术暴露，但也应当避免过度屈曲。

正中切口切开，然后沿中线切开至棘突水平，分离棘突旁两侧肌肉，以充分暴露椎板和侧块。

需要进一步的侧位 X 线片以确认要椎体水平。通常可以直接看到脱位并从后方将脱位复位，有时可能需要钻掉下方小关节才能进行复位。应注意避免损伤神经根。

外科医生应仔细确认每个侧块的外侧、上侧和下侧边缘：侧块的内侧边缘位于向下扫掠的椎板、末端且轮廓明显变化的点。

侧块呈现出正方形。进入点实际上在该正方形的中点，或者在下象限的边缘处（**图 68.8**）。高速钻头磨开骨皮质。

此时有两个主要考虑因素是：将磨钻应向侧方偏向足够位置，以避开椎间孔中的椎动脉；并尽可能向上方，以避开损伤椎间孔中的神经根（**图 68.9**）。几种不同的螺钉角度都有过应用。一般而言，轴向和矢状面的角度都应约为 20°。放置在相邻小关节上的器械可以很好地指示矢状面内的螺钉轨迹，无论如何应通过 X 射线照相检查或图像引导对其进行确认和指导。

钻孔完成后，使用球形探针仔细检查通道是否可能存在裂口。放置 3.5 mm 直径的所需长度的螺钉（如果计划进行单皮质固定，通常在 14~16 mm 左右；如果使用双皮质固定，则稍长一些），一旦所有螺钉都以同样的方式放置就位，将直径为 3 mm 的棒材切割并定型为所需的长度和形状，并将其放置在两侧的多轴螺钉头内。经过合适地拧紧后，将进行最终的 X 射线检查。然后以标准方式进行冲洗，融合和伤口闭合。

后路 C1/C2 融合

第 58 章已介绍此技术。

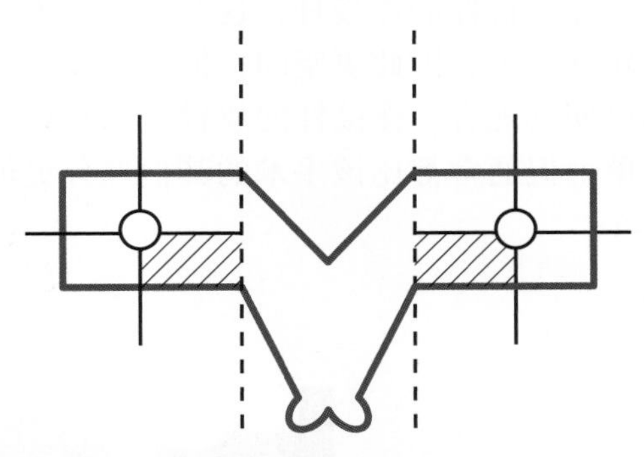

图 68.8 外科医生视角下暴露的侧块。螺钉进入点通常在正方形的中点或下象限内（阴影）

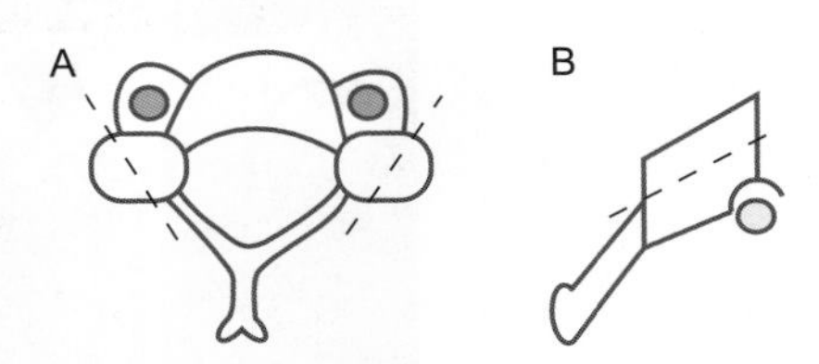

图 68.9 示意图，显示了轴向（A）和矢状（B）平面上的适当螺钉轨迹。在轴向平面上，外科医生必须足够侧向地避开椎动脉（红色），而在矢状平面上必须充分地避开神经根（黄色）

颅颈固定

如果存在枕颈脱位或严重不稳定的 C1 骨折，将会使用颅颈固定。从枕骨固定到 C2 或下颈椎椎骨会使枕骨和寰枢关节完全无法活动。此种手术方法仅应在其他方法无法满足要求的情况下使用（即在严重不稳定的情况下，请参阅 Bhatia et al.，2013）。

仔细的术中定位以确保尽可能的“解剖”位置至关重要：过度屈曲的姿势可能会使吞咽困难，过度伸展的姿势使走路变得困难。

一旦患者适当地定位，就从下枕骨突出部做一切口（切口的下端以计划固定的节段下极为准）。剥离肌肉以暴露枕骨以及椎板和侧块。C1、C2 和下颈椎螺钉置入的技术将在其他地方描述。在所有情况下，至关重要的是详细的术前检查（包括 CT 扫描 +/– 对比），尤其要注意任何会妨碍螺钉安全放置的静脉异常。

中线枕骨髁在接近枕骨大孔时逐渐变薄。双皮质固定应优先考虑。内外板必须钻孔并攻丝以允许螺钉放置。如果硬膜破裂、出血或脑脊液漏发生，通常将螺丝插入孔中即可将其塞住。通常需要对骨板进行轮廓处理和（或）使枕骨的凹凸不平变得光滑，以使板牢固地固定而不晃动。

一旦枕骨板和颈椎装置就位后，必须放置杆以将两者连接。外科医生可以塑形使直杆轮廓更合适或使用预先弯折好的连接杆，这些杆可能不需要进一步的轮廓加工，因此更坚固，但几乎总是需要修整两端以使其配合。连接杆的放置，从直观上看似乎很简单，但通常都比该手术的其他部分更加困难和耗时。

如果患者因为外伤而需要行枕颈固定手术，对所有可见的骨质去除皮质、与骨移植材料一起包装和（或）合成骨替代品是至关重要的。从长远来看，如果不能骨质融合，并且头部相对于颈椎具有较大的机械杠杆臂，则所有金属固定物都将失效。通常有必要在术后数周内进行外部固定，直到确信融合正在发生。

颈胸融合

使用前面介绍的技术和胸椎椎弓根螺钉（参见**第 67 章**），可以治疗需要将颈椎结构延伸到胸椎上部的不稳定的交界骨折。颅颈胸固定术可能是一种对患者极端痛苦的治疗方法，如果有可能应该尽量避免这种方法（Tanouchi et al.，2014）。

前齿状突螺钉固定

在全身麻醉下，患者仰卧位，颈部轻度过伸位。应拍摄前后位和侧位 X 线片，并获得开口位图像。放射状的开口器使嘴在术中始终保持张口位，气管插管放置在一侧，以确保充分显露齿状突（**图 68.10A**）。

通过使用侧位 X 射线将预期的螺钉轨迹投射在表面上来标记皮肤切口，通常在 C5/6 椎间盘水平。应用标准的颈前路方法，沿着颈动脉鞘与气管和咽之间的间隙向下分离到椎前间隙。横向自固定式牵开器放置在部分分开的长直肌下方。然后，在侧位 X 射线引导下，使用一个带角度的牵开器牵开到 C2/3 椎间盘间隙，同时保留在椎前间隙内。将一根克氏针插入 C2 椎体的下唇中，然后在前后位和侧位 X 线引导下将克氏针部分钻入 C2 椎体中。将外部导管上的

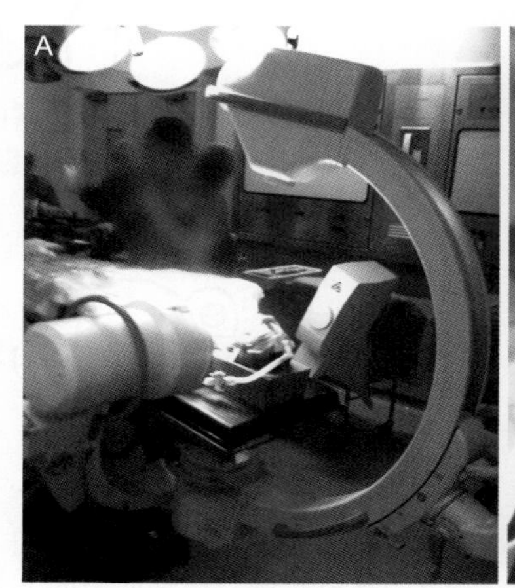

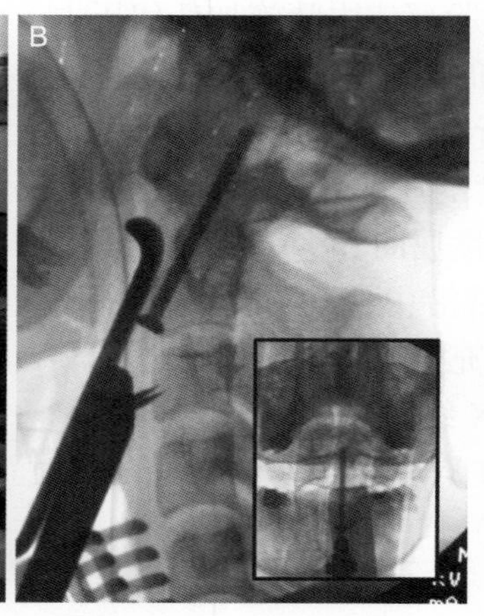

图 68.10 （A）设置了两个图像增强器，以在两个平面和颈椎的伸展位同时获得齿状突的图像。（B）术中侧位和 AP 位 X 线片，显示牵开器，导引螺钉和单个方头螺钉的位置

尖刺固定到C3上，然后进入内部导管。导管穿过克氏针，以用作钻头的导向器。使用更宽的空心钻头在C2/3椎间盘和C2皮质的环上边缘钻出一个空间以放置螺钉头。一旦将外套管牢固地固定到位，就可以取下克氏针。使用3 mm钻头的电钻，以外套管作为导向，沿着克氏针标记的轨迹钻出一个导向孔。如有必要，可以调整患者的头部或C2椎体位置，使远端碎片复位以达到合适的解剖位置。然后将钻头推进到远端碎片中，使其刚好穿过齿状突的外皮质进入根尖韧带。然后用一个4 mm的丝锥扩大此孔，使其穿过外套管。在此步骤结束时，可以使用丝锥上的标记来测量螺钉的长度。考虑到骨折端最终将被固定在一起，螺钉应选择小于骨折端间距的型号。使用前后位和侧位X片引导下将半螺纹的4.0 mm钛合金方头螺钉插入导向孔中并拧紧，以确保骨折碎片被充分压缩，并且螺钉头沉入沉孔中（**图68.10B**）。

有证据表明，早期手术干预可导致较低的不愈合率（Apfelbaum et al.，2000；Rao and Apfelbaum，2005）。老年患者和骨质疏松症患者发生螺钉固定失败的风险明显更高。可能发生松动和螺钉退回的情况，如果骨接合处失败，则会在骨折部位产生持续的应力。据报道，老年患者吞咽困难的发生率增加，因为食道纤维化程度更高，因此对回缩的耐受性较差（Vasudevan et al.，2014）。这种情况下喉上神经受到损伤的可能性会增加，喉上神经供应环甲肌并向喉黏膜提供感觉神经支配，它在大约C3/4的水平刺甲状腺舌膜。

颈椎前路融合术

颈椎前路椎间盘切除术和融合术或颈前路椎体切除术都是处理颈椎损伤的常用方法。这些方法将以非常高的融合率提供两柱的稳定性。移除受影响的椎间盘后，外科医生将放置自体骨移植物或装有骨碎片的融合器，然后放置前颈椎板。许多外科医生认为，在仅以稳定为目的的创伤病例中，无需切开后纵韧带。有关这些技术的说明，请参见**第58章**。

取下椎间盘后，可通过使用椎体中的销钉在一个椎骨上旋转另一个椎骨，同时施加牵引力，对单侧骨折脱位进行复位。但是，如果在受伤后将手术延迟了2~3周以上，则关节面可能会部分融合，并且从前方复位的难度会更大。

争议：单侧和双侧关节面骨折

在颈椎手术的患者中，通常诊断是明确的。困难往往存在于治疗方案的选择：保守或是手术；前路还是后路，或是前后路联合；两个、三个或是更多节段。

此类决定最终取决于临床判断。一般而言，有些原则至少可以用来指导治疗。需要进行更广泛手术的指征包括明显移位，多节段受累，双侧受累，MRI上存在韧带断裂和脊髓损伤的证据。

使用这些原则，可以考虑单关节面骨折的情况。尽管此类患者可能有神经根病和根性损害（通常为单侧），但大多数患有此类损伤的患者并没有严重的脊髓损伤。对侧小关节可能是完好的，损伤仅限于单个水平，没有证据表明MRI上的韧带完全破裂。在这种情况下，可能根本不需要任何手术，如果能够实现合理的复位，则可以应用Halo支架和背心来维持正确的位置，固定充分的时间以达到骨折的愈合。

如果位置有丢失或患者倾向手术，可选择手术治疗，但不一定需要同时做前路和后路的手术。如果对位良好，单做前路或后路手术可以取得满意的复位、良好的融合和稳定性。这可避免长时间手术甚至是实际上的第二个手术。然而，一些医生倾向于做360°融合，以保证额外安全性。

相反，双髋臼骨折/脱位是一种非常不同的损伤。这些患者通常有完全的神经损伤，MRI可见韧带断裂。就其本质而言损伤是双侧的，且涉及严重的移位。

考虑到这种损伤的不稳定性，许多外科医生会考虑使用前路和后路固定以恢复稳定性，促进融合和神经系统康复。然而，另外有一些外科医生会认为仅通过前路或后路融合手术也可以治疗这类损伤。作者认为，最佳的手术方式通常是后路复位固定术，然后进行前路融合术，除非神经系统给功能不全且有较大的椎间盘脱出。在这种情况下，后路复位作为首选治疗方法可能会使情况变得更糟。其他外科医生通常会先进行前路手术，然后再进行后路手术。如果不能从前方进行复位，则甚至可以采用前-后-前的方式。对于哪种技术最好，人们几乎还没有达成共识。

延伸阅读、参考文献、EBRAIN的相关链接

扫描书末二维码获取。

第 69 章　胸腰椎损伤

Bedansh Roy Chaudhary・Shiong Wen Low 著
史良 译，苏亦兵 审校

引言

胸腰椎创伤可以使用 Magerl 评分或胸腰椎损伤和严重程度评分（TLICS）进行分类。治疗方法可以是保守疗法，包括药物镇痛和支具固定，也可以是经后路、经胸腔或环脊柱融合固定的手术治疗。

这一章将着重讨论胸腰椎损伤的分类和外科治疗，着重介绍椎弓根螺钉置入技术及微创技术的进展。

骨折分类

成人的胸腰椎创伤分类系统包括：Holdswort 分类，其主要根据损害机制进行分类；Whitesides 分类，其基于建筑起重机原理定义了脊柱两柱概念进行分类；Punjabi 和 White 发展了稳定性评分系统；Denis 建立了一种基于脊柱三柱稳定性的力学分类。

1994 年 Magerl 及其同事基于超过 1400 例经其治疗的胸腰椎骨折患者进行连续回顾并设计了一种形态学分类系统（Magerl et al.，1994），其是当时最完善的骨折形态学分类。此分类将胸腰椎损伤分为 3 类，即压迫、牵张及旋转损伤，相应的标记为 A，B，C 类骨折，A~C 损伤逐级加重，各组别还将进一步细分。

Magerl 分类较为复杂，其 55 种不同胸腰椎骨折的亚型分类，对专业的医师来说使用都有困难，因此日常临床较少使用。此外，孤立的横向或棘突骨折也未包含在 Magerl AO 分类中。

为了解决这些问题，AO 脊柱分类小组致力于更新 AO 胸腰脊柱损伤分类共识，努力为全球提供一个可靠、敏感、简单而强大的临床和学术工具，并尽可能完善胸腰椎损伤分类的系统，最终于 2005 年达成目标，出版了 TLICS（Vaccaro et al.，2005）。

2013 年 Vaccaro 等发表了 AO 脊柱胸腰段损伤分类系统（图 69.1），其中包含了一些临床修正（Vaccaro et al.，2013）。此版 AO 脊柱胸腰椎伤害分类体系是建立在三个基本参数之上：骨折形态、神经损伤和临床修正参数 。

形态学分型 A 型为压缩性损伤，一般为最轻微的损伤类型——压迫性损伤，只影响椎体不影响韧带组织。椎板的纵向骨折可能存在，但不构成韧带张力。分为 5 种亚型，即 A0~A4。A0 是无结构性骨折，包括横突或棘突的骨折，其不危及脊柱的结构完整性。A1 为单纯边缘楔型压缩性骨折，未累及椎体的后路。A2 骨折为劈裂或双终板骨折，未累及椎体后路。A3 为累及后壁的不完全性爆裂性骨折，但只有一个终板骨折。A4 骨折是完全爆裂性骨折，并累及后壁和两端终板。

B 型是牵张型伴张力带损伤，可能是后张力带、前纵韧带或骨组件损伤。包括 3 个亚型 B1~B3。B1 亚型是单纯跨越骨性结构破坏伴张力带断裂或 chance 骨折，属于单节段骨折。B2 型是后张力带断裂伴或不伴韧带性结构破坏，通常表现为 A 型骨折。B3 是一个过伸性损伤，累及椎间盘或椎体，特别是在椎体后壁的前纵韧带破裂，导致脊柱过度伸展时发生。

C 型损伤是移位 / 分离损伤。C 型损伤的特点是脊柱骨折节段头尾端在任何平面上的移位超出了正常的生理范围，所以没有亚型，A 型骨折也可能存在 C 类损伤。

入院时的神经系统状态评分按照以下方案：N0，神经完整；N1，短暂性神经缺陷，很快恢复；N2，存在放射状神经根损伤的症状或体征；N3，不完全的脊髓或马尾神经损伤；N4，完全性脊髓损伤；NX，用来表示一些特殊情况，如颅脑损伤或镇静而无法完成神经系统检查。

有两个明确的临床修正参数可以使用。M1 修正参数用于针对骨折伴有影像学检查（如 MRI）发现的不确定的张力带损伤情况。该修正参数对骨结构稳定而韧带功能不全的患者是否需要选择手术治疗有指导意义。M2 参数表示患者特异的并发症或伴随性疾

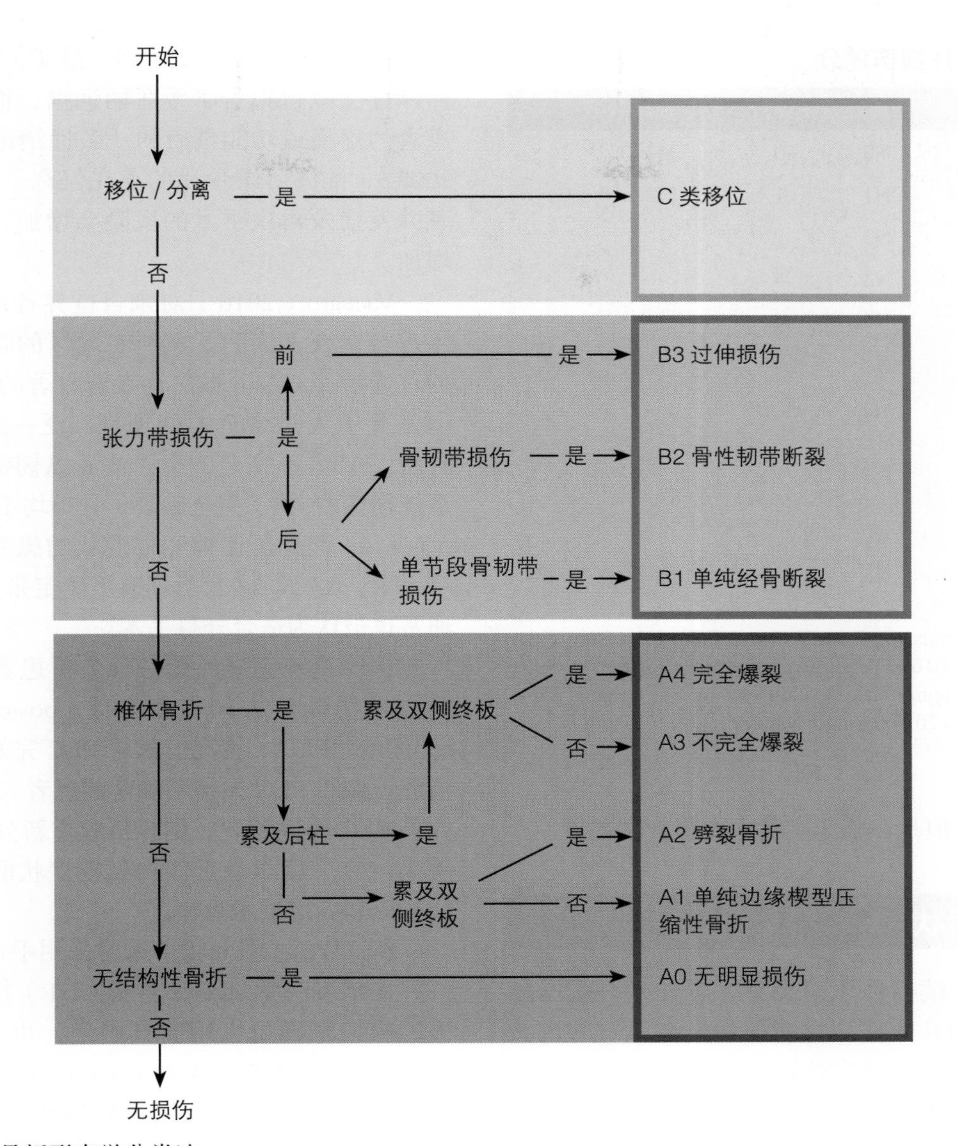

图 69.1 胸腰椎骨折形态学分类法

病，这些并发症会对患者的手术决策造成影响，例如强直性脊柱炎或受伤脊椎周围的皮肤烧伤。

Kepler（Kepler et al.，2015）发表了 AO 脊柱损伤评分系统，以损伤特征作计算分数，通过统计总分来决定保守治疗或手术治疗（**表** 69.1）。

胸腰椎骨折的外科治疗

对于脊柱损伤的患者，应按照高级创伤生命支持指南（**第 65 章**）原则进行治疗。而脊髓损伤患者也应该遵从该指南。本章中只讨论特殊的胸腰椎骨折相关手术指征和手术技术。

X 线虽然广泛用于评估骨质疏松相关的粉碎性骨折患者，但其在急性脊柱损伤时评估作用有限。所有的患者都需要全脊柱 CT 三维重建检查，其可显示三个平面维度图像。CT 扫描可观察骨折形态、软组织肿胀及脊柱或身体附近的其他部位损伤。同时，CT 扫描还能提供与手术计划相关的信息，如椎弓根的大小，也可用于图像导航系统。然而，CT 扫描并不排除韧带受伤。

有持续神经系统症状的所有患者或者 CT 上有明显脊柱损伤的患者都应该行 MRI 扫描。MRI 应包括 T1、T2 和 STIR 序列。T1 和 T2 图像可显示出脊髓或神经根的压迫，而 STIR 序列对于骨折、椎间盘和韧带损伤更为有效。

手术的目的是实现神经减压，生物力学稳定和

表 69.1 AO 脊柱损伤评分

骨折类型		神经系统评分		临床参数	
A0	0	N0	0	M1	1
A1	1	N1	1	M2	0
A2	2	N2	2		
A3	3	N3	4		
A4	5	N4	4		
B1	5	NX	3		
B2	6				
B3	7				
C	8				
评分 0~3		保守治疗			
评分 4~5		保守治疗 / 外科治疗			
评分 6~13		外科治疗			

Reproduced with permission from Vaccaro, A.R., Schroeder, G.D., Kepler, C.K. et al (2016) The surgical algorithm for the AOSpine thoracolumbar spine injury classification system. Eur Spine J, 25(4), 1087–94. Copyright © 2016 Springer Nature.

骨性结构重建，但是在临床实践中有很大的差异。

神经系统症状

对大多数持续神经压迫患者，脊柱外科减压融合手术是首选治疗方法。脊髓损伤是在原发的机械性损伤基础上，引发继发连锁反应，包括出血、血管痉挛、缺血、水肿、兴奋毒性介质释放、炎症和进一步的神经元凋亡。

因此，手术的 2 个目标为：首先是减压和去除损伤病变，而通过恢复脊髓的正常灌注，防止继发性神经细胞凋亡；其次是防止可能在运动时发生神经细胞的进一步损伤，并允许早期康复运动。

患者只要有神经根受压症状，就应进行手术评估，评估应基于生物力学稳定性而不仅仅是神经损伤的症状。

骨折的稳定性

当存在神经损伤时，不稳定的骨折、危险移位和晚期神经损伤都应该进行手术固定。外科医生面临的挑战是确定哪些骨折是稳定的，可以进行保守治疗，而哪些骨折需要固定。

多年来，没有任何一处骨折如神经系统完整的胸腰椎爆裂骨折的治疗引起了如此大的争议（Anderson et al.，1991；Miyanji et al.，2006；Aleem and Nassr，2016；Vaccaro et al.，2016）。最近 Cochrane 的一篇回顾性文献也报告了矛盾的证据，而没有任何关于患者的疼痛或功能预后的一致性结论（Koller et al.，2008）。椎体后缘骨片的存在仅有一定的临床意义，其并发症及再次手术的风险会增加，手术费用也会增加。

Vaccaro（2016）对来自世界各地 483 名外科医生进行调查，询问了其所在地区的临床病例及他们的首选治疗方法。虽然存在着显著的区域实践差异，但是关于 A 型骨折的处理是广泛一致的。A1 或 A2 骨折，A3（不完全破裂）或后纵韧带完好、无神经系统损伤的 A4（完全破裂）骨折均不适合手术治疗。A3 或 A4 型骨折伴神经根症状的患者通常被认为适合手术，A3 或 A4 骨折伴有不确定张力带损伤（M1）通常也被认为适合外科手术。

神经系统完好的爆裂性骨折患者应该进行 MRI 检查后明确后方韧带复合体（posterior ligamentous complex，PLC）情况。如果 PLC 完好，建议非手术治疗。对于 PLC 损伤不确定的患者，可以考虑手术。如果 PLC 明显断裂，则骨折应重新分类为 B2，建议手术治疗。爆裂骨折伴神经根症状的患者可考虑进行减压和固定手术治疗。

B 型骨折（**图 69.2**）通常采用手术治疗，但是有一些文献表明骨 chance 骨折（B1）排列整齐，有适当的骨接触面可以用支具固定，也可以愈合（Kim and Lenke，2005；Lakshmanan et al.，2009；Wood et al.，2015）。但应注意患者后凸畸形小于 10°，没有神经损伤，而且有能力遵守密切随访的前提。

C 型损伤，也就是移位性或旋转性损伤，生物力学上被定义为不稳定的类型。它们通常是手术复位固定（**图 69.3**）。

骨折的节段也可以预测稳定性。高胸段或中胸段骨折由于胸腔和胸骨支撑较为稳定，而颈胸或胸腰段骨折则相对不稳定。在相同的放射学特性下，高速损伤比低速损伤更容易不稳定。强直性脊柱炎常伴有骨质疏松症，chance 骨折更为常见。由长阶段融合后的骨折稳定性大大低于正常个体 chance 骨折。这些情况下，多节段的手术干预应该执行。而骨质疏松症和其他并发症则是手术的相对禁忌证。

在过去的十年里，脊柱的矢状面稳定在预测手术和预后中作用越来越显著。虽然这一准则在畸形手术中得到了深入的研究，但它在创伤中的作用却没有明确的定义，并更有争议。

Koller 等研究了创伤后畸形在胸腰椎爆裂骨折患者长期预后中的作用。他们随访了 21 例接受保守

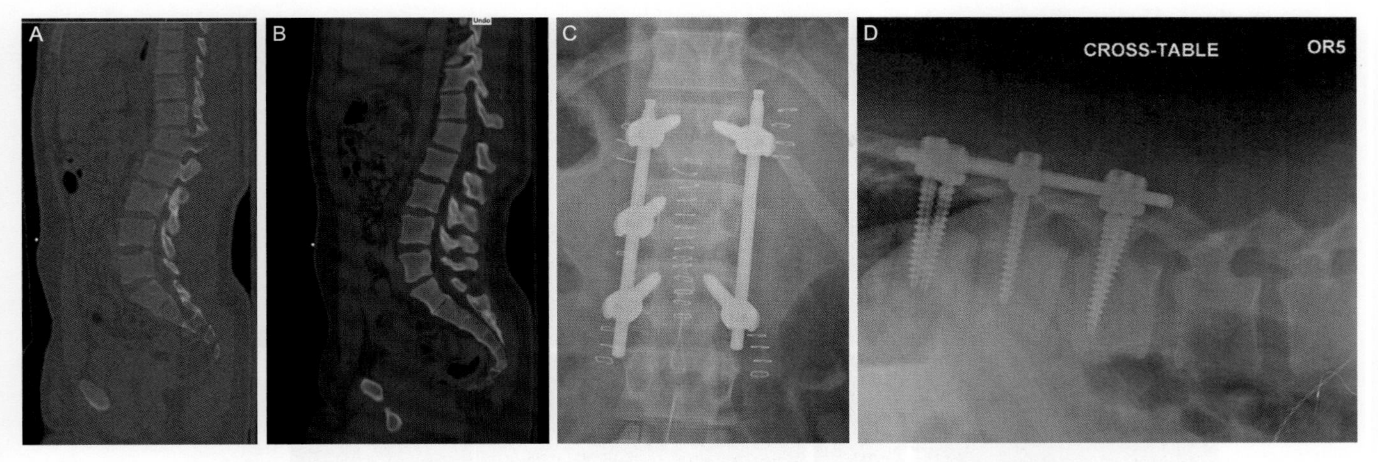

图 69.2　一名 23 岁的男性，在一场高速单车交通事故中有系安全带。他出现了这种孤立的损伤。他的神经完好无损。有明显的后凸，棘间和棘上韧带断裂，棘间韧带明显可见扩宽，以及对侧关节突断裂。进行了受伤节段上下各一个节段的经皮固定，以及有限的开放棘间融合。椎弓根螺钉置入为损伤的右侧椎弓根

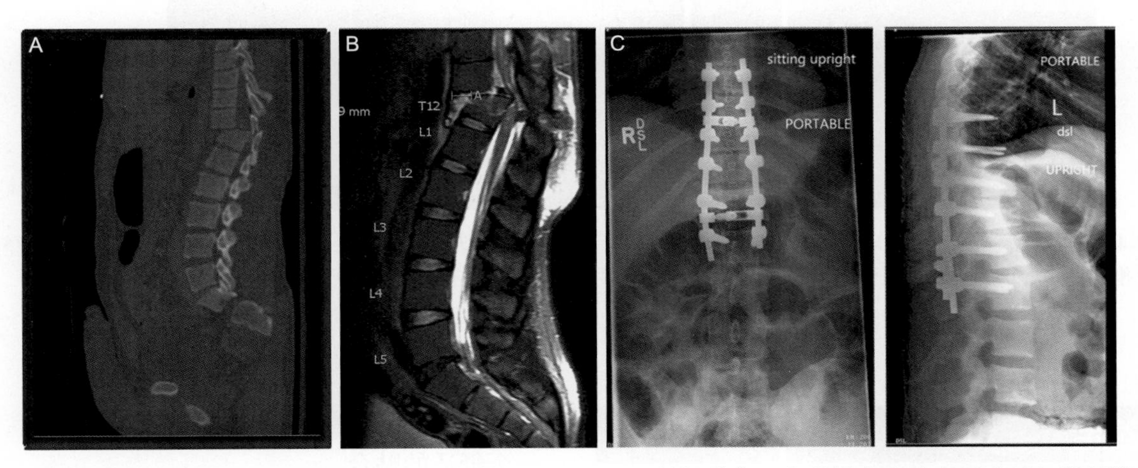

图 69.3　一名建筑工人在楼梯上被重物砸伤。CT 扫描显示 T11-T12 骨折脱位。患者是在事故现场进行气管插管，没有临床检查，因此磁共振成像评估神经功能。此种 C 类损伤采用切开复位、后路内固定融合术以及脊髓减压术治疗。术后，患者恢复了部分骶神经功能和部分大小便自主控制功能

治疗的患者，平均 9.5 年。他们根据 SF-36 及 Visual Analogue Scale-spine scores 发现后凸畸形和腰椎前凸的丢失是患者预后不佳的主要因素（Koller et al., 2008）。他们得出结论，对较严重的爆裂骨折患者，进行后凸畸形的矫正应被考虑。

外科医生面临的挑战是单独的后路内固定治疗并不能有效预防脊柱后凸。Lakshaman 等（2009）已经证明，在爆裂骨折中，即使后凸畸形最初通过正确的后路固定加以矫形，但往往有一个“摆动”的问题，患者在长期随访中往往恢复到其基线畸形状态。他们最终的结论：爆裂骨折后路手术治疗，如没有其他强适应证，如不稳定或神经功能障碍，单纯的为适度纠正脊柱后凸，其手术价值尚不明确（Vaccaro et al., 2016）。

Wood 等对 47 例胸腰椎爆裂骨折但稳定患者进行了前瞻性随机对照研究，在最终的随访期内（从 16~22 年），在仅后路固定手术治疗组和非手术组之间，脊柱后凸角度无明显差异（Miyanji et al., 2006）。而 Pekmezci 等在他们的论文中则提出一种微创的开放椎体切除并经皮后路椎体截骨固定技术，其用于治疗单节段外伤性腰椎爆裂骨折。他们随访 12 个患者，平均 38 个月。他们能够有效地维持纠正的角度，并且患者预后良好（**图** 69.4）。

因此，作者结论是胸腰段爆裂性骨折后严重的后凸畸形可能被认为是合适的手术指征，特别是对于腰椎前凸与骨盆位置明显不匹配的患者。为了维持矫正效果，除后路常规固定外，也常常需要前路固定。

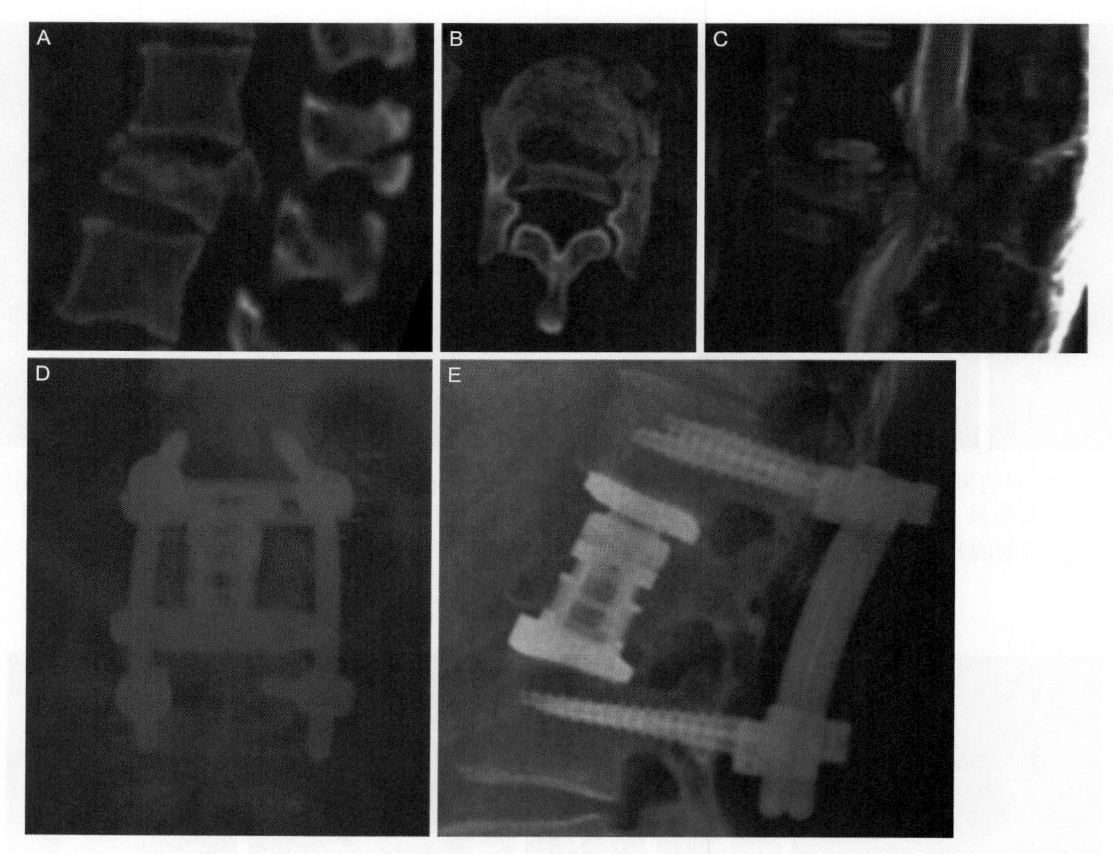

图 69.4 48 岁男性患者从 4.57 米（15 英尺）高处坠落后发生 L1 爆裂性骨折（A~C），无神经功能障碍。行经皮置入后路短节段椎弓根螺钉，前路减压稳定骨折。在术后 12 个月的随访中没有显示出矫正异常的迹象（D~E）

支具固定

胸腰骶段矫形器（thoracolumbosacral orthoses，TLSO）是一种硬质脊柱外固定支具，其可跨越胸、腰、骶段脊柱以便限制脊柱活动、矫正畸形，或改善某些节段的功能。TLSO 支具可限制运动、稳定损伤结构、减少疼痛、增强稳定性、促进愈合、防止畸形发展。在保守治疗、手术后或手术不能完全确保安全的患者应该使用这些矫正支具。

Jewett 过伸矫形器可减少下胸段和腰段的屈曲。它通过胸骨前部和耻骨上施加压力，产生胸腰椎向后的定向压力以达到稳定的作用。其主要用于下胸段和胸腰段骨折。Jewett 矫形支具的禁忌证为不稳定或爆裂骨折。

一种定制的 TLSO，有时称为折叠式矫形器，可为胸、腰椎提供坚固的外部支撑，有效范围可达 T3 到 L4。它是用聚丙烯或塑料塑形以适合患者的需要。其前面覆盖了从胸骨切迹到耻骨联合的区域，背侧覆盖了从肩胛骨到尾骨的区域。模具与身体之间有柔软的填充物，并用尼龙搭扣带调节松紧，以提供一个舒适的贴合。

TLSO 支具在所有的运动平面提供了最大程度的外部固定。TLSO 通常用于非手术治疗的 T3-L4 骨折患者，包括爆裂性骨折、压缩性骨折和 chance 性骨折。而术后 TLSO 的使用是为了限制活动能力和增加骨质融合率。

TLSO 支具可提供各种尺寸定制版。其优势是可方便快捷的使用。然而，如果安装有问题可能会导致脊柱不稳定或者不舒适。病态肥胖，需要增加侧向稳定性，存在胸管，结肠造口术，或被支撑区域内有较大伤口时 TLSO 支具受到限制。最常见的并发症是支撑物与身体接触点的皮肤和软组织压疮。

腰围是用尼龙搭扣带包裹腹部，并结合后部钢板支撑。腰围提供前、外侧躯干包裹。这有助于提升腹内压。后部的钢板可限制腰椎的屈伸。这与其他矫形器相比稳定性较弱。它往往使用在由腰椎间盘突出、腰肌痉挛或稳定的单柱压缩型腰椎骨折引起的腰疼。

后路胸腰椎融合固定技术

通常有三种不同的椎弓根钉置入方法。第一种方法是徒手操作，在 X 射线引导下，寻找解剖标志，以得到穿刺起点和路径。第二种是术中经皮穿刺法，使用数字透视引导椎弓根钉置入。最后一种是在计算机辅助导航下完成的。

在所有病例中，外科医生术前都需要进行 CT 扫描，注意患者椎弓根的大小、穿刺通道及解剖结构变异。应制订详细的操作计划。

徒手置入椎弓根螺钉最重要的部分是选择合适穿刺点的能力。不同水平的胸椎的解剖标志也不同。一般来说，我们使用 Kim 和 Lenke（2005）所描述的解剖方法。为便于记忆，我们将胸段椎体分为三组，见**图** 69.5。

徒手螺钉置入

使用可透视放射线的手术台。为了防止交界性脊柱后凸，应小心剥离肌肉以确保上、下节段的关节突囊、棘上和棘内韧带完整。显露脊柱后确定解剖

胸椎	
T1～T3 水平以上，椎弓根起始点位于横突中点，与关节突外侧交汇点	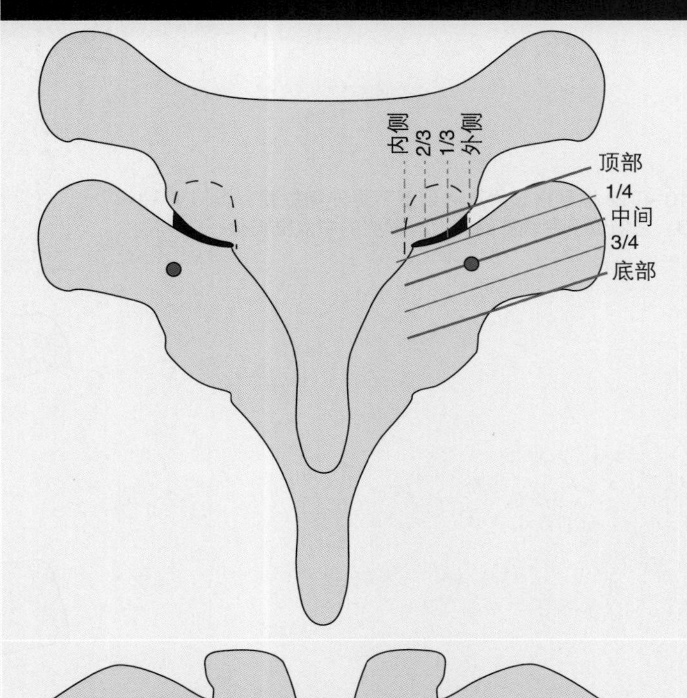
T4～T6，椎弓根起始点位于关节突侧方 1/3，距离横突上边缘 1 / 4 的地方交汇点	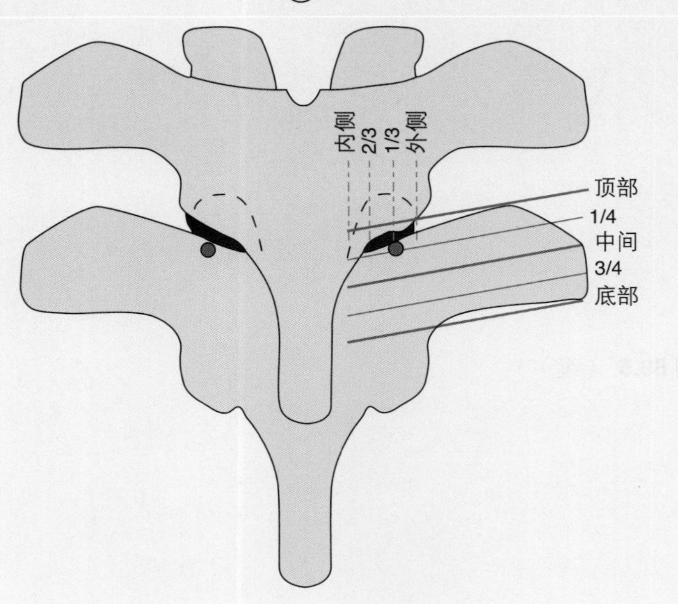

图 69.5 胸椎

胸椎	
T7～T9 椎弓根起始点是所有胸段的最近端和内侧位置，其位于小关节突的外侧 1/3 与横突的上缘交汇点	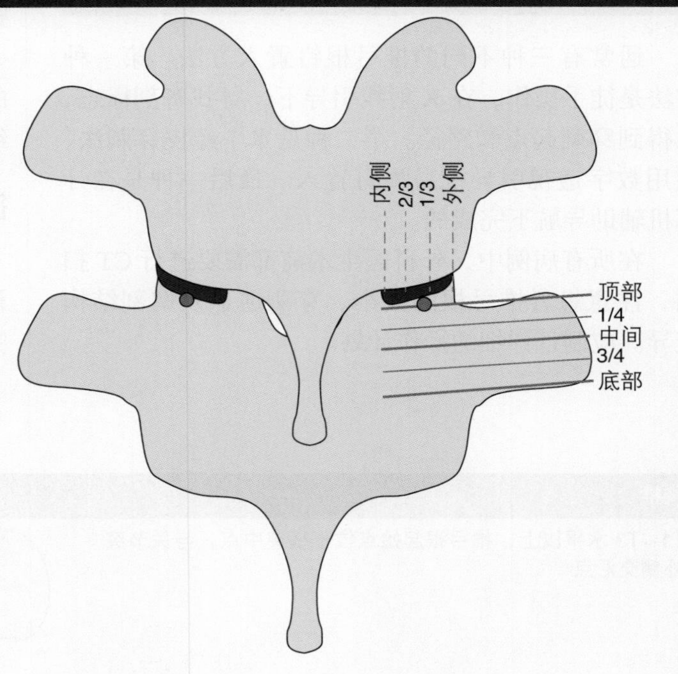
T10～T12 椎弓根起始点回到更下更外侧位置，类似于 T1–T3。它们位于在峡部的侧面与横突的中点交汇处	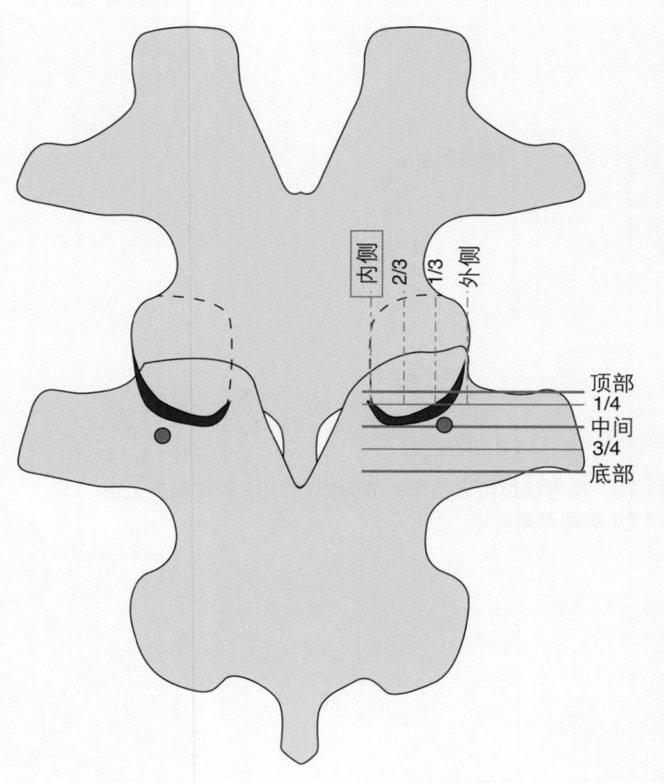

图 69.5 （续）

胸椎

腰椎椎弓根起始点均位于横突和峡部的侧面正中交叉点

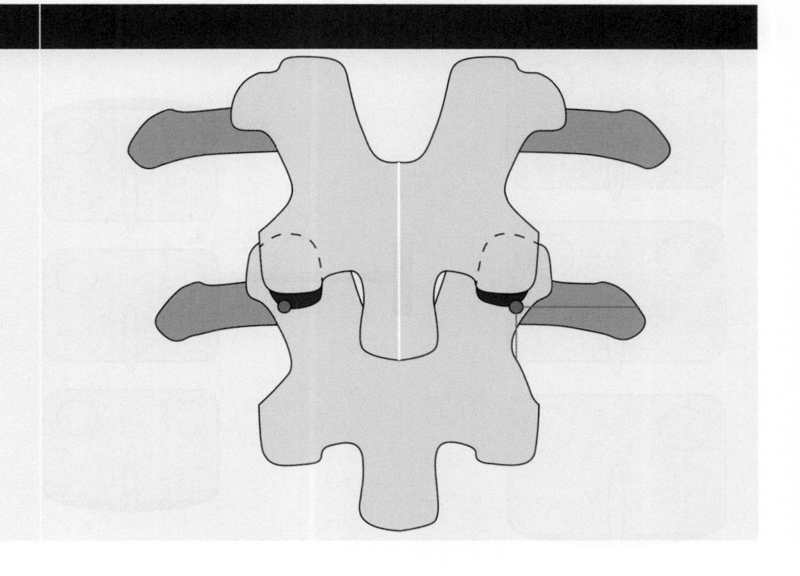

图 69.5 （续）

标志，确定关节突、横突和峡部来引用穿刺点，通过 X 线可以用来识别椎弓根，并确定上述结构。一旦确定了穿刺点，可用锥子或高速毛刺打磨穿透外层骨质。这可以防止使用时椎弓根探针打滑。横突的内侧部分需要去除，以使椎弓根钉头在胸椎的正确位置。在腰椎，部分关节突可能需要去除，然后使用弯曲的椎弓根探针插入椎弓根。AP 和侧位 X 线的结合可以用于监测探查的过程，探针不应穿过椎弓根内侧壁，直到椎弓根探针进入椎体。弧形椎弓根探针最常使用，其第一次使用时弯曲方向应远离椎管 20 mm。一旦到达预计深度，它就会旋转 180°，再次探查。边拧边施加恒定的压力前进，然后用声音来触诊四周和椎弓根的质地。在椎弓根预期深度处，如果没有感觉到阻力，预示其置入太深了。使用与椎弓根钉尺寸类似的小于 1 mm 的螺锥扩开椎弓根通道。拔出螺锥时，再次确认椎弓根的声音以确保这个新通道没有打穿骨皮质。再次感觉通道四周和底部，然后在 X 射线引导下，小心地按照之前的通道插入螺钉。

放射线透视下通道技术

本章介绍的第二种椎弓根螺钉置入方法是术中 X 线下通道椎弓根钉系统。技术的关键在于获得每个需融合的椎体的影像学资料。

为了正确置入椎弓根螺钉，一个正确的 X 线透视位置应该是 C 型臂的横梁平行于椎体的终板，棘突位于在椎弓根之间椎体的中间。椎弓根钉置入点应该位于右侧椎弓根 3 点钟位置，左椎弓根 9 点钟位置。参见**图** 69.6。

然后插入套筒，用槌缓慢推进套筒到达椎弓根内侧壁。为了避免内侧壁裂开，重要的是要在 AP 位 X 线片上观察到椎弓根内侧壁穿过之前，在侧方 X 线片上进行确认套筒已经进入椎体。参见**图** 69.6B。

然后再次拍摄侧位 X 线片，以证明套筒在穿过内侧壁之前已经进入了椎体。注意随着安全地进一步推进，正位 X 线片套筒将显示有内侧壁的突破。参见**图** 69.6C。

然后取出套筒的内芯，置入一根导丝，探查椎体的底部。注意，因为椎体的前壁不平，在侧位脊柱的 X 片上显示到达顶点之前导丝可能会碰到前壁。然后移除套筒，确保导丝保持在正确的位置。然后沿导丝插入松质骨螺杆。拍摄侧位 X 线片以确保钢丝没有打折，或无意中向前移动突破椎体前壁。最后，将松质骨螺杆沿导丝置入，再次拍摄侧位 X 线片确保导丝未缠绕，如果导丝缠绕，可能会发生丝锥或螺丝位置无法与导线对齐的情况。

图像导航下椎弓根螺钉置入

除了应用 X 线外，椎弓根螺钉可以在其他图像导航下置入，椎弓根螺钉可以通过通道（经皮穿刺）或开放手术等非通道技术置入。

神经导航系统参考必须安全连接到椎体的棘突上，并用椎板背面解剖学的标记或由微创病例的 X 线系统进行注册。

图像导航技术可以减少 X 射线暴露，同时允许三维重建，对解剖结构异常的患者有很大帮助。它

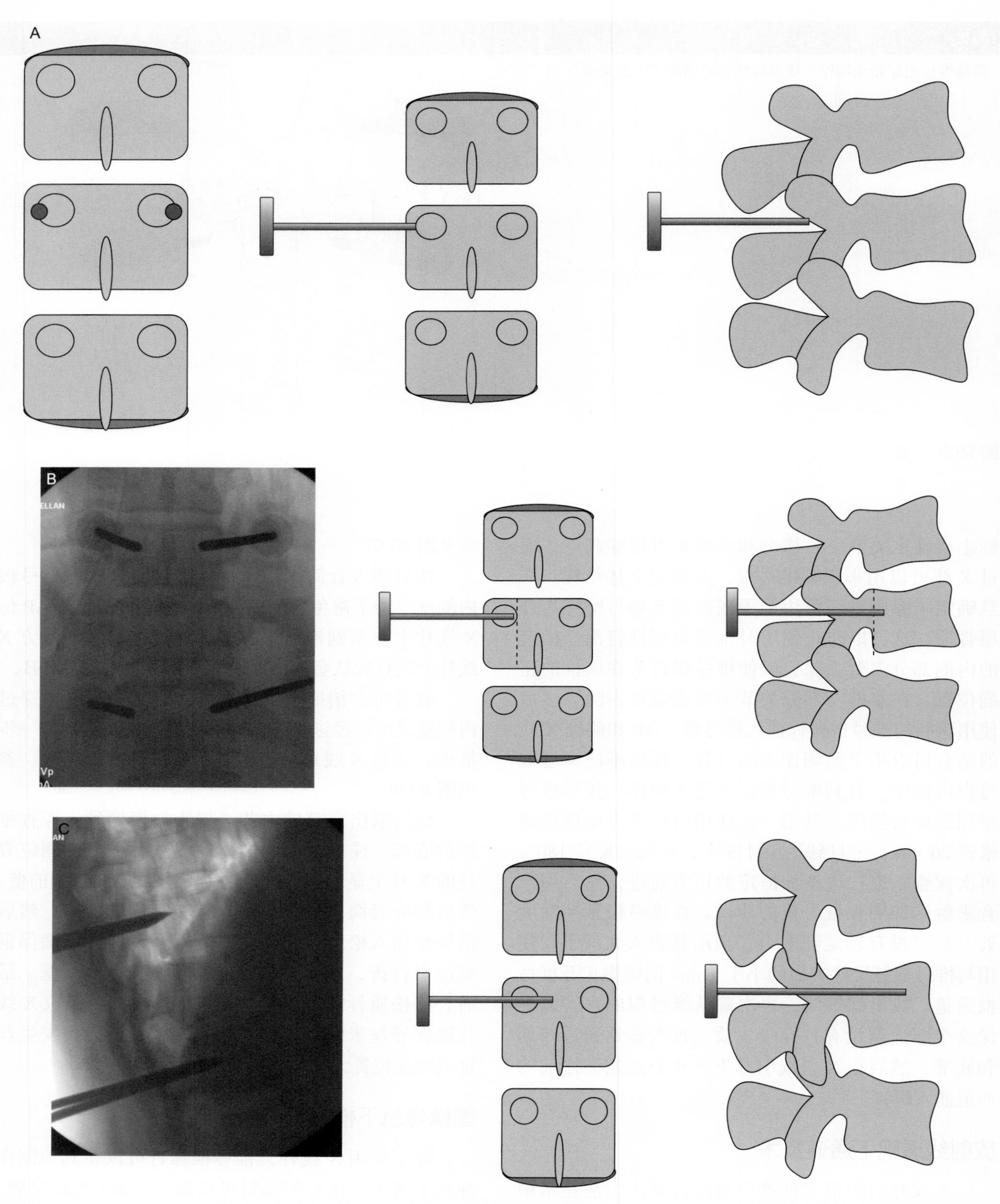

图 69.6 椎弓根螺钉置入技术。终板必须是位于棘突在中间（A）。前后位（B）和侧位（C）视图允许外科医生在椎弓根中定位螺钉。在前后位视图中，螺钉不应该穿过内侧壁，直到螺钉尖端可见已进入椎体

至少较其他技术更为精确。

椎弓根螺钉置入的并发症包括椎弓根壁的破坏，其可达 20%，但其不到一半患者会有症状而需要再次处理。破坏可能位于内侧，导致脊髓或马尾受压，也看位于外侧，多累及可能受损的部位或下方血管及神经根。而术后神经根疼痛最常见由螺钉破坏椎弓根壁压迫所致。在插入螺丝之前，通过椎弓根探子探查椎弓根周边骨质，或通过神经生理监测，X 线片仔细解读和定位，应用神经导航，或者用探查椎弓根破裂阻抗设备等方法可减少椎弓根破坏的情况。

当螺钉直径过大时，椎弓根钉在置入过程中可发生椎弓根骨折。通过选择正确的螺钉尺寸及缓慢置入螺钉以便椎弓根有适应过程，可以避免这种并发症。

如果椎体融合失败，螺钉可能松动、脱落或断裂。与所有内固定技术一样，如果骨质不能融合，金属结构就会失效。必须鼓励患者戒烟及应避免使用非甾体类抗炎药，同时术中去除骨外皮质并植骨，均可有助于促进融合。

预后与随访

无论手术治疗还是保守治疗患者均需要物理和康复治疗。一些外科医生需要通过 CT 评估螺钉和骨折位置，但这不是强制性的。每隔 3~6 个月应拍 X 光片直到发生骨质融合，以监测进行性脊柱后凸或其他不稳定情况。

延伸阅读、参考文献、EBRAIN 的相关链接

扫描书末二维码获取。

第 70 章　脊髓损伤的康复治疗

Fahim Anwar · Wail Ahmed · Tamara Tajsic · Damiano G. Barone · Harry Mee 著
刘龙奇 译，苏亦兵 审校

急性期脊髓损伤的康复

脊髓损伤修复的重要性

康复实际上是针对残障人群的教育过程，使他们能够达到并维持最佳的身体、智力、心理和社会功能水平（World Health Organization，2011）。脊髓损伤（spinal cord injury，SCI）康复的重要性源于以下事实：专业的 SCI 康复单元可使四肢瘫痪者的预期寿命从大约一个月提高到了几乎正常的预期寿命。

急性期脊髓损伤的诊断和病理生理变化

康复的先决条件是通过采集病史、全面的常规和神经系统检查以及回顾相关检查（例如放射影像）了解诊断。更重要的是，结合病史、体格检查和影像学检查有助于确定脊髓损伤的类型，例如完全脊髓损伤、脊髓前柱损伤或马尾综合征。此外，明确复合创伤中的相关损伤及其对其他功能障碍和康复需求的影响，对于指导康复的过程和方向至关重要。例如，据报道 5% ~15% 的严重颅脑损伤患者发生急性脊髓损伤（Michael et al.，1989）。因此，在这些病例中，对颅脑损伤的严重程度评估和康复优先于脊髓损伤的康复。

理解与急性脊髓损伤相关的常见病理生理变化，例如神经源性休克、脊髓休克和体位性自主神经功能紊乱，对于康复团队采取必要的相关干预措施非常重要。在 SCI 后脊髓休克的急性期，膀胱和肠道的神经功能障碍类型主要是反射消失（和无力）而不是反射性（和痉挛性）功能障碍，后者为慢性期的主要特征。因此，两者的护理和照料是不同的。又如在体位性自主神经功能紊乱患者中，除药物治疗外，物理治疗将集中在使用倾斜台使患者的自主反应逐步适应其新生理状态。

确定神经损伤水平以及 SCI 分级

重大创伤和脊髓损伤康复服务的标准做法是使用国际脊髓损伤神经分类标准（ISNCSCI，2015）记录检查结果。这是一张国际范围内广泛应用的表格，该表由美国脊髓损伤协会（ASIA）和国际脊髓学会（ISCoS）设计，并自 1992 年结盟以来定期审查（Kirshblum et al.，2011；Kirshblum and Waring，2014）。

在 SCI 患者中进行神经系统检查的主要目的是确定是否存在感觉或运动功能缺损平面，从而确定神经损伤平面（neurological level of injury，NLI）。感觉平面定义为具有完整针刺觉和轻触觉的最末端皮节。运动平面的定义为关键肌肌力至少 3 级以上（仰卧位），且在该节段以上关键肌肌力为完整的 5 级肌力水平。神经功能损伤平面是感觉和运动损伤平面中的最高平面（Kirshblum et al.，2011；Kirshblum and Waring，2014；ISNCSCI，2015）。如果患者四肢肌力下降但没有感觉平面（即所有皮节针刺和轻触感完整），则损伤可能发生在脊柱上而不是 SCI。

另一个目的是使用 ASIA 损伤量表（AIS）确定 SCI 的分级。根据定义，如果 S4 和 S5 节段无任何感觉或运动功能，则损伤为完全 SCI（AIS A）。如果 S4 或 S5 存在任何感觉或运动功能，则损伤为不完全 SCI（AIS B、C 或 D）。AIS B 定义为感觉不完全，在神经功能损伤平面以下，包括 S4 和 S5 节段，保留感觉功能而非运动功能（轻触、针刺或肛门深压），并且身体任意一侧的损伤平面以下肌力不超过 3 级。AIS C 定义为运动不完全，在骶尾节段保留了运动功能以进行肛门自主收缩，或者患者符合感觉不完全的标准，并且身体任意一侧的运动功能保留了同侧运动水平以下的 3 级以上，包括非关键肌肉。AIS C 为损伤平面以下不到一半的关键肌肌力大于等于 3 级。AIS D 为运动不完全（如 AIS C 中所定义），损伤平面以下至少一半（或更多）关键肌肌力大于等于 3 级。确定 NLI 和 AIS 的重要性在于建立 SCI 诊断并预测长期可能的功能结局。

卧床康复与主动运动

与晚期减压或完全不进行手术相比，SCI 早期减压是否在神经功能预后方面获益还存在争议。目前尚无相关的随机临床试验，但是一些病例对照研究发现手术不能改善神经系统的预后。早期手术可以使患者早期运动，从而降低肺部并发症（如肺炎或肺不张）的发生率，并有效地减少住院时间和总体住院费用（Donovan，1994；Fehlings and Perrin，2006）。

自主神经系统和心血管系统干预

严重急性 SCI 的患者面临发生危及生命的循环不稳定和呼吸功能不全的风险。原发性脊髓损伤诱发若干涉及血管损伤的继发性损伤机制，从而导致血流减少、自主调节功能失调、微循环受阻、血管痉挛、血栓形成以及大出血。急性 SCI 还会引起全身性血管改变，例如心动过缓（颈髓损伤中常见）、心律不齐、平均动脉压降低、外周血管阻力降低以及心输出量减少。全身性低血压并伴随自主调节功能失调，可减少脊髓灌注并加重缺血。受伤后 7~10 天可能再次发生危及生命的循环不稳定。在一系列以积极的方式进行治疗（关注血压、氧合和血流动力学表现）的急性 SCI 患者的临床病例中，未报告有害作用，并提示神经系统预后得到改善（Hawryluk et al.，2015）。美国神经外科医师协会指南和神经外科医师代表大会的建议（AANS and CNS，2002）见表 70.1。

胸部和通气干预

脊髓损伤后常见呼吸功能不全和肺功能不全，尤其是颈髓水平发生损伤时（Reines and Harris，1987；Como et al.，2005；Berlly and Shem，2007）。呼吸和肺功能不全最有可能发生在受伤后 7~10 天

表 70.1 AANS 和 CNS SCI 管理指南摘要

1	在重症监护病房或具有类似监测环境的护理单元管理急性 SCI 患者，在该护理单元中可以监测心脏、血流动力学和呼吸，从而发现循环功能障碍和呼吸功能不全。
2	避免全身性低血压（定义为收缩压＜90 mmHg）并尽快纠正低血压。
3	急性脊髓损伤后的前 7 天，维持平均动脉血压在 85~90 mmHg，以改善脊髓灌注。

Reproduced with permission, Guidelines for Management of Acute Cervical Spinal Injuries, *Neurosurgery*, Volume 50, Issue suppl 3, p. S1, Copyright © 2002 Oxford University Press on behalf of the Congress of Neurological Surgeons.

（Berney et al.，2010a；Berney et al.，2010b）。AANS 和 CNS（AANS and CNS，2002）指南建议，应立即对所有颈椎高位（C4 或更高）损伤的患者进行插管，对脊髓低位损伤的患者根据具体情况进行评估。然而，在急性情况下，T11 以上任何节段的脊髓病变都会破坏呼吸力学。

危重机械通气患者由于无效咳嗽和分泌动员能力受损而发生气道间隙受损（Hassid et al.，2008）。对 C5 以上节段病变的患者进行早期气管切开术可能会减少使用呼吸机的天数和呼吸机相关性肺炎的发生率（Como et al.，2005）。在特定患者中横膈起搏器可能是有用的。咳嗽增强技术可提高咳嗽效率，包括无创面罩式咳痰机（mechanical insufflation-exsufflation，MI-E）、人工辅助咳嗽和肺复张（AANS and CNS，2002）。

胃肠系统干预

严重急性 SCI 通常伴有麻痹性肠梗阻，如果长时间如此，则引起的腹胀会导致板状膈肌，进而影响通气，在四肢瘫痪患者中更甚。应在受伤后 48 小时内采取静脉输液，并置入鼻胃管。所有急性脊髓损伤的患者都将获益于接受药物预防应激性溃疡。治疗的持续时间尚不确定，但应持续治疗至不存在危险因素为止（Anwar et al.，2013）。

肠道管理干预

神经源性肠道功能障碍是由源自脊髓的外在神经支配的损失引起，包括骨盆内脏（S2~S4；副交感神经）、肠系膜上下（T9~T12；交感神经）、下腹部（L1~L3；交感神经）和阴部（S2~S4；躯体）神经支配。

通常，神经源性肠道可归因于骶髓上脊髓损伤导致的上运动神经元或反射性肠道与骶段和（或）马尾部完全损伤而引起的下运动神经元或无反射性肠道。

肠道护理的目的是定期、有计划地完全排空肠内容物（no authors listed，1998）。在制订肠道护理方案之前，必须采集病史，并进行常规和神经系统检查，包括评估骶段（S4~S5）的感觉、运动和反射功能。

膀胱管理干预

在脊髓休克早期，产生的神经源性膀胱松弛且反射消失，导致尿潴留并伴有尿失禁。在此阶段进行膀胱治疗的目的是使膀胱减压，以防止膀胱输尿

管反流和尿路感染。该治疗通过留置导尿管完成。使用封闭的引流系统、适当固定导管并定期更换导管有利于避免导管相关感染（Consortium for Spinal Cord Medicine，2006）。

压疮的预防

压疮是一项继发于SCI的严重并发症。引起压疮的主要原因是在骨隆突处长时间接受外部压力，如骶骨和坐骨结节。这导致上覆软组织的局部缺血，最终可能引起坏死。肌肉对由压力引起的局部缺血更为敏感，其次为皮肤和软组织。压疮可引起凶险的败血症，因此可能是致命的。根据组织损伤的程度对压疮进行分级。美国国家压疮咨询委员会（NPUAP）分级系统被广泛用于压疮的分级（Haesler，2004）。

压疮的预防在SCI患者中至关重要，受伤后尽快在急诊处置中开始，并持续至慢性恢复期，对大部分SCI患者而言需终生预防压疮。减压措施包括改变受压部位或改变体位、机械倾斜和倾斜台。根据所使用的技术，应每15~30 min进行一次最佳的减压方式，持续30~120 s。在慢性期，前倾体位、左右倾斜、使轮椅向后倾斜65°或更大角度或进行适当时长（即2 min）的减压是最有效的减压方式。

营养干预

急性、重症脊髓损伤后，患者常为蛋白质分解代谢。肌肉萎缩引起的体质变化导致大量氮流失、长期负氮平衡和快速体重减轻，前两周尤甚。然而，SCI后由于神经支配的肌肉松弛，SCI患者的高代谢亢进反应变得迟钝。推荐在急性期和慢性期使用间接量热法评估能量消耗（AANS and CNS，2002）。SCI患者的营养支持应满足热量和氮的需求，而不是达到氮的平衡，这样的营养支持是安全的，并且可以减少急性脊髓损伤后发生的分解代谢和氮消耗过程的有害影响（AANS and CNS，2002）。早期肠内营养（在72小时内启动）似乎是安全的，但尚未显示出对急性SCI患者的神经功能状态、住院时长或并发症的发生率产生影响（Rowan et al.，2004）。目前尚无报道评估SCI患者营养补充剂的组合或构成。有关颅脑损伤患者营养支持的文献支持从高氮肠内或肠外溶液开始的方案，在该方案中至少15%的蛋白质热量、不超过15%的葡萄糖或右旋糖、总能量的至少4%应为必需脂肪酸，以及添加维生素、必需元素和微量矿物质（AANS and CNS，2002）。

多学科康复团队干预

多学科康复团队（由一名接受过康复和脊髓治疗培训的顾问医师领衔）的早期介入，对于改善功能、预防并发症和避免进一步恶化至关重要。团队应在脊髓损伤急性期完成初步评估以制订个体化的康复计划。物理治疗应关注维持所有关节的最大活动范围、帮助床上运动、提高体能，预防继发性并发症，如应用夹板支具预防肌肉挛缩。患者可以耐受坐姿后应立即安排坐位和姿态康复计划。使用倾斜台可以帮助改善急性期的自控能力、疲劳和运动耐受性。急性期肺部干预包括胸部物理治疗、体位引流、呼吸运动和使用咳嗽辅助装置。

职业理疗师可以帮助改善上肢伸展和支具使用、轮椅坐姿及水肿的管理。早期开始言语和语言治疗有助于增强沟通，使用辅助技术促进独立吞咽功能恢复并评估。

心理干预

接受由脊髓损伤引起的残疾是一个终生的过程。脊髓损伤的急性期普遍出现急性应激反应，如果不及时治疗可能会导致创伤后应激障碍。因此，在急性期开始早期心理干预至关重要，以减少这些心理状况的影响并改善生活质量。心理干预可能是有帮助的，包括提供情绪支持、促进适应过程、及早识别和管理焦虑和抑郁，以及鼓励自我护理、独立性和心理健康。

预后和家庭支持

脊髓损伤对患者及其家属而言是灾难性的。他们通常在伤后不久就咨询预后情况。神经功能恢复可发生在低于损伤节段的正常节段。ASI损伤量表（AIS）分级为C或D级的患者中更常见神经功能恢复。分级为ASI C（年龄<50岁）和ASI D的患者预期可在康复出院后行走（有或没有辅助装置）（Burns et al.，1997）。带领康复团队的顾问在患者SCI的急性期解释预后和支持家人方面发挥着至关重要的作用。

慢性期脊髓损伤的康复

并发症的医疗管理

自主神经反射异常

自主神经反射异常是SCI的潜在危重临床综合征，可导致急性难治性高血压，进而引发癫痫发作、视网膜出血、肺水肿、肾衰竭、心肌梗死、脑出血和死亡。它的发生是由于自主神经系统过度活跃，导致T6及以上节段神经系统损伤的SCI患者突然出现过高的血压（Krassioukov et al.，2009）。T6及以上节段脊髓损伤的SCI患者中，有48%~90%会出现自主神经反射异常，完全性SCI的可能性高于不完全性SCI。

源自损伤节段以下的完整周围神经的任何有害或非有害刺激都会导致交感神经产生强烈的交感神经活动。这会导致血管收缩及高血压。大脑通过下调抑制信号来关闭交感神经系统来对此作出反应。但这些信号无法通过受损伤的T6及以上节段。同时，大脑通过完整的迷走神经激活副交感神经系统并产生心动过缓。刺激消除后，反射性交感神经活动随即消失，见**表**70.2。

早期识别对于预防危重并发症至关重要。管理原则（Acute Management of Autonomic Dysreflexia，2001；Krassioukov et al. 2009），见**图**70.1。

静脉血栓栓塞

血栓栓塞性疾病常见于颈椎脊髓损伤的患者，具有显著的发病率（AANS and CNS，2002）。推荐低分子肝素联合气动加压袜或电刺激作为静脉血栓栓塞（venous thromboembolism，VTE）的预防性治疗方案。已有许多关于脊髓损伤后预防性治疗VTE 6~12周可获益的报道（AANS and CNS，2002）。推荐重症颈椎SCI患者进行持续3个月的深静脉血栓和肺栓塞的预防性治疗。不建议腔静脉滤器作为常规预防措施，但推荐将其用于抗凝失败的患者或不适合抗凝和机械装置治疗的患者（AANS and CNS，2002）。

痉挛的管理

痉挛被定义为一种运动障碍，其特征为快速的紧张性牵张反射的增加（肌张力），伴腱反射亢进，进而导致牵张反射过度兴奋，它是上运动神经元综合征的组成成分（Feldman et al.，1980）。痉挛影响70%的脊髓损伤患者（Johnson et al.，1998；Noreau et al.，2000）。

脊髓损伤中痉挛的病理生理是多因素的。病理生理学的主要解释为由于缺乏下调抑制信号而引起α运动神经元相对过度兴奋。对于脊髓损伤患者，这种过度兴奋主要是由于抑制性冲动无法到达α运动神经元。然而，最新文献记载，肌梭敏感性增加以及脊髓运动神经元内在性质的变化引起脊髓运动神经元的传入信号增加，这导致运动神经元的过度兴奋，引起在牵张反应中自持放电（Nielsen et al.，2007）。同样，肌肉的内在性质也出现变化，导致肌肉纤维和肌腱顺应性产生生理变化，从而引起痉挛（Friden and Lieber，2003）。

痉挛并不总是有害的，在某些情况下，脊髓损伤的患者可以利用它来移动、动员或进行日常生活。对于下肢而言，痉挛有助于促进血液循环、预防水肿并降低深静脉血栓形成的风险（Ashworth，1964）。痉挛的有害影响包括功能恶化、日常生活和卫生保健中的困难、姿势异常、挛缩、压疮和疼痛。

对痉挛进行全面的多学科临床评估对于计划任何治疗都是至关重要的。目前已有若干临床量表

表70.2　自主神经反射异常的原因、体征和症状

自主神经反射异常的触发原因示例	自主神经反射异常的症状	自主神经反射异常的体征
• 膀胱膨胀或刺激；尿路感染、结石、附睾炎或阴囊压迫 • 由于粪便梗死导致的肠管扩张 • 肠道内器械：结肠镜检查 • 痔疮 • 肛裂 • 胆结石 • 压疮 • 骨折 • 深静脉血栓形成 / 肺栓塞 • 烧伤 • 脚趾甲增长 • 妊娠，尤其分娩 • 月经 • 性交	• 双侧头痛 • 视力模糊 • 鼻腔充血 • 不安 • 焦虑 • 受伤节段以上皮肤潮红	• 高血压 • 心动过缓 • 瞳孔散大 • 受伤节段以下鸡皮疙瘩 • 受伤节段以上多汗 • 受伤节段以下皮肤干燥 • 心律失常、房颤

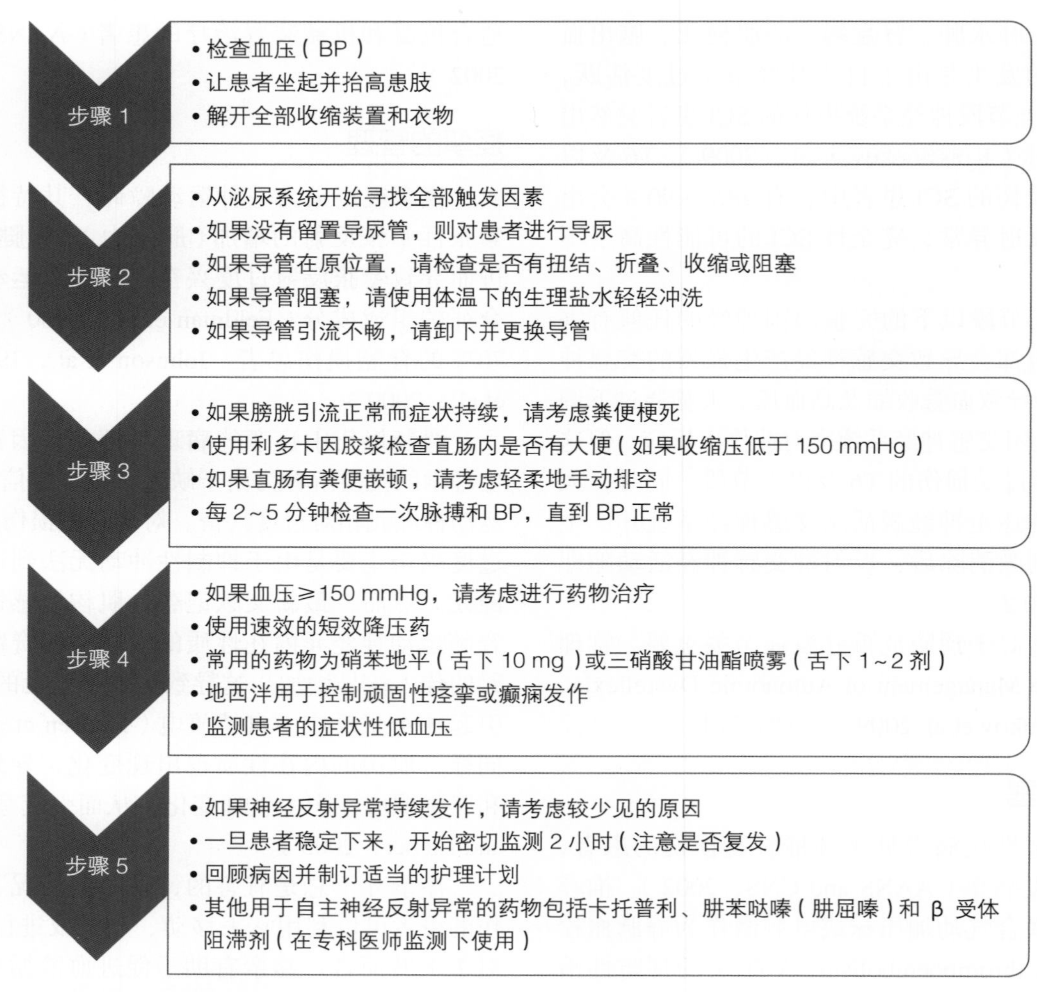

图 70.1 自主神经反射异常的管理原则

可以量化痉挛。临床实践中应用最广泛的量表是 Ashworth 量表和改良的 Ashworth 量表。

多种因素可加重痉挛，例如感染、压疮、月经疼痛、脚趾甲持续生长和肾结石。因此，治疗痉挛之前必须寻找并治疗这些恶化因素。痉挛可以是局部的、多灶性的、区域性的或全身性的。物理疗法是痉挛的一线治疗方法。在关节的正常运动范围内，持续被动拉伸肌肉有助于减少痉挛。应该定期进行该“活动度”运动，以防止痉挛发展。在轮椅上保持良好的姿势以及在床上保持体位有利于持久拉伸痉挛肌肉。可以在床上和轮椅上使用各种矫形器和装置，以帮助保持正确的体位。

口服药物可用于多灶性、区域性和全身性痉挛。最常用的口服药物是巴氯芬。它是一种 γ- 氨基丁酸（GABA）类似物，可通过抑制单突触和多突触脊髓反射来减少痉挛。最大剂量为每天 100 mg，分为 3~4 次服用。常见的副作用是恶心和镇静。突然停用巴氯芬可能导致戒断症状，如癫痫发作和精神病。

如果巴氯芬不能耐受或无效，可使用替扎尼定。它是一种中枢 α2 肾上腺素能激动剂，通过减少在脊髓中间神经元水平上的兴奋性神经递质的释放来减少痉挛。它耐受性良好；最大剂量为每天 36 mg，分 4~5 次服用。替扎尼定有可能引起可逆性肝损害，因此在使用过程中需要严格监测肝功能。

丹曲林是一种骨骼肌松弛剂，通过抑制肌质网释放钙而减少痉挛。最大剂量为每天 400 mg，分 3 次服用。与替扎尼定相似，丹曲林也影响肝，因此需监测肝功能。由于它是一种外周作用的药物，因此会产生镇静作用。

因为与 GABA 受体结合，苯二氮䓬类药物（地西泮和氯硝西泮）也用于治疗痉挛和疼痛性痉挛。长时间使用苯二氮䓬类药物会导致镇静和认知障碍，因此不推荐使用。

加巴喷丁也可用于控制痉挛或与其他口服药物联合用。它还有助于缓解肌痉挛痛。常见的副作用是镇静和体重增加。同样的，可乐定可用于减少痉挛，但是由于其副作用，它在临床实践中的使用受到限制。

靶点注射肉毒杆菌毒素对于局部痉挛可能非常有效。它通过抑制乙酰胆碱从突触前神经末梢释放来削弱肌肉能力。肉毒杆菌毒素的作用持续3~6个月，需要重复注射。在肌电图（EMG）或超声引导下定位肌肉注射，可以增强效果。苯酚神经和运动点阻滞是注射肉毒杆菌毒素的有效替代方法。苯酚是一种神经溶解剂，以浓度为3%~7%的水溶液使用。需要针电刺激来定位神经和运动点。苯酚的作用持续6个月以上，可以根据需要重复进行。苯酚的副作用包括淤伤、肿胀、出血和神经性疼痛。也可联合注射苯酚和肉毒杆菌毒素治疗多灶性或区域性痉挛。

鞘内泵入巴氯芬可成功治疗脊髓损伤患者的全身性痉挛。植入泵之前，患者应对鞘内测试剂量的巴氯芬有所反应。使用手持遥控装置可调整巴氯芬的剂量，该装置可以设定特定的给药间隔。需定期向泵内加药。输液泵故障或导管问题可能导致巴氯芬停药症状。对于顽固性下肢痉挛，可选择鞘内注射苯酚。然而，该方法应仅用于没有膀胱、肠道或性功能，且已制订了有效的膀胱和肠道管理计划的患者。由于治疗窗窄以及依赖性风险，不推荐将大麻产品用于治疗痉挛（Karst et al.，2010）。

明确的肠道管理

慢性期肠道管理的目的是确保遵守常规的肠道护理方案并处理并发症。发生脊髓休克后，如果神经功能恢复，SCI患者可能具有完全或不完全的反射性肠道功能、完全或不完全的无反射肠道功能、混合性肠道功能（圆锥病变）或正常肠道功能。神经源性肠道功能障碍的严重程度取决于SCI的节段和完整性。SCI节段和AIS分级越高，功能障碍越严重。

为保持可预测的粪便稠度，应定期服用泻药（膨胀剂、渗透剂、软化剂），而刺激性导泻剂（如番泻叶）应仅在计划排便前服用，因为此类药物会增加肠道蠕动，从而导致粪便进入乙状结肠和直肠导致排便。

其他更具侵入性的神经源性肠道管理包括经肛门冲洗、顺行性大肠灌肠、结肠造口术（和经皮内镜结肠造口术）、骶前神经根刺激器（SARS）和骶神经刺激器。

图70.2概述了神经源性肠道管理（no authors listed，1998；Multidisciplinary Association of Spinal Cord Injured Professionals，2012）。

明确的膀胱管理

脊髓休克阶段（数周至数月）后，神经源性膀胱功能障碍的程度取决于SCI的水平（脊髓*vs.*圆锥*vs.*马尾病变）和程度（完全与不完全）。因此，临床病史（包括使用频率/容积图）、一般检查和神经系统检查（包括骶骨节段的运动、感觉和反射功能）在神经源性膀胱的管理中起着重要作用。脊髓病变通常会导致反射性神经源性膀胱[神经源性逼尿肌过度活跃（neurogenic detrusor overactivity，NDO）]，从而引起膀胱痉挛，表现为尿管或耻骨上膀胱造瘘管周围漏尿或间歇性自导管插入之间漏尿。有时，由脊髓梗死（例如，从T6到圆锥）引起的脊髓损伤（骶髓节段以上）可能会导致无反射性膀胱，类似于圆锥或马尾损伤，表现为尿潴留伴充溢性尿失禁。

脊髓损伤导致的骶上病变中断了“脑桥排尿中心”和“骶髓排尿中心”之间的神经通路（Blaivas et al.，2008）。这通常会导致逼尿肌外括约肌协同失调症（detrusor external sphincter dyssynergia，DESD），其特征是在非自愿逼尿肌收缩期间尿道括约肌自发收缩（Blaivas et al.，2008）。

神经源性膀胱管理通常从间断夹闭导尿管开始，以训练膀胱。可以通过导管与尿袋之间的阀门实现夹闭导管。夹闭导尿管通常联合口服抗胆碱能药物进行，以松弛脊髓完全损伤（AIS A）或感觉不完全损伤（AIS B）患者的膀胱。1~2周后，通常通过增加导管闭合时间至每天3~4个小时，或者直至患者有排空膀胱的冲动，来进行膀胱训练。膀胱训练过程中出现膀胱充盈感（或排空冲动）的患者可能经过锻炼后在无尿管情况下成功自主地排空膀胱。重复性超声检查以测定排尿后残余尿量，通常认为小于100 ml是正常的。无法排空膀胱或排空膀胱不完全（排尿后残余尿量大）的患者应进行导尿，以维持安全的泌尿系统低压。对于手部功能良好的患者（截瘫患者和一些低水平四肢瘫痪患者），膀胱管理的理想方法是学习每隔4~5小时进行一次清洁的间断自我导尿（clean intermittent self-catheterization，CISC），具体取决于口服摄入量。对于手部功能受损的患者，相较于尿道插管更适合长期耻骨上膀胱造瘘，以避免生殖器并发症（溃疡、尿道撕裂、尿道下裂）和反复感染。

视频尿动力学研究在测定膀胱内压力、诊断膀胱输尿管反流以及检查DESD的严重性方面十分有用。但这些研究不是为特定患者确定最佳膀胱治疗方案的方法。

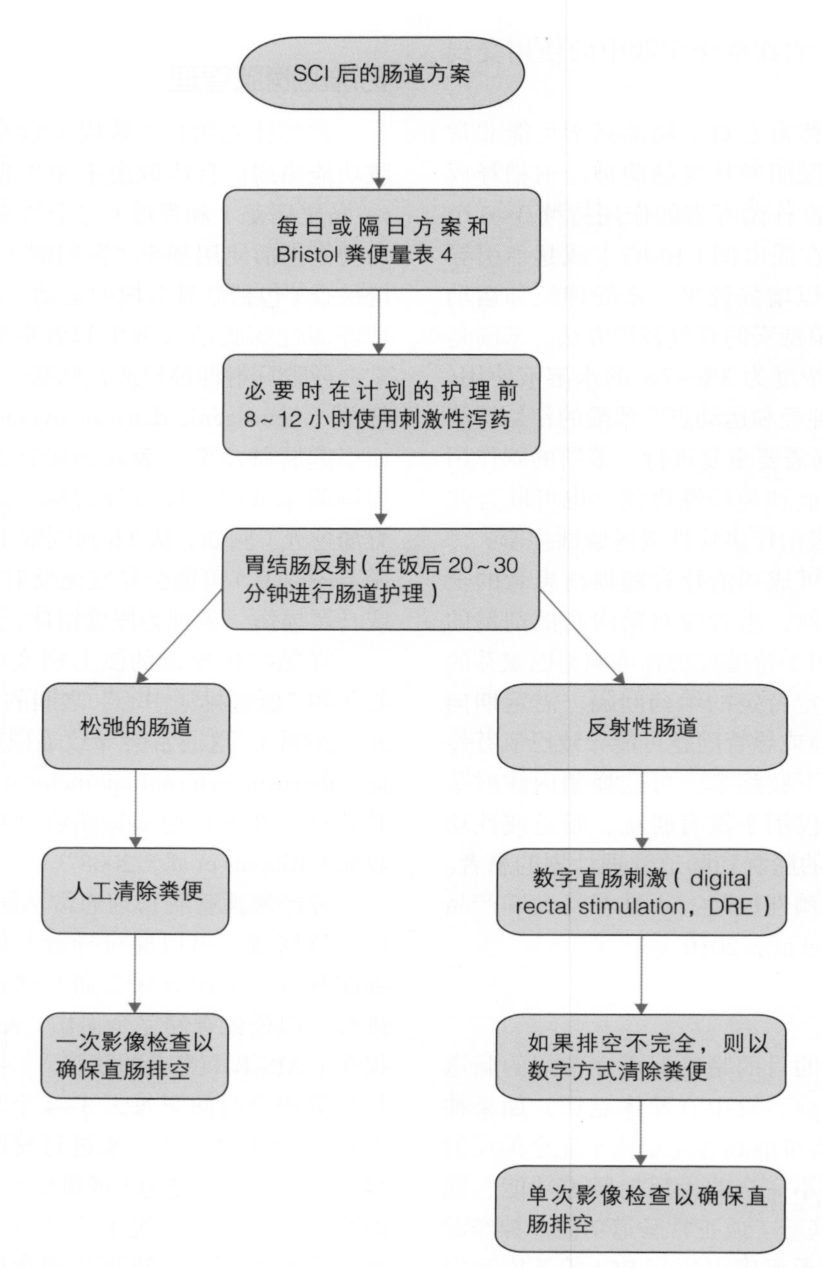

图 70.2 神经源性肠道管理

Data from https://www.mascip.co.uk/wp-content/uploads/2015/02/CV653N-Neurogenic-Guidelines-Sept-2012.pdf; also Neurogenic Bowel Management in Adults with Spinal Cord Injury, *Journal of Spinal Cord Medicine*, volume 21, issue 3, pp. 248–93. © 1998 Taylor and Francis.

在严重 DESD 患者中，膀胱内注射肉毒杆菌毒素可有效治疗痉挛性尿失禁的 NDO 症状。其他方法包括外科膀胱扩张术、神经调节、神经刺激和骶前神经根刺激（sacral anterior root stimulation，SARS）。

性功能管理

脊髓损伤后常见性功能障碍，且以非常不同的方式影响男性和女性。脊髓损伤的女性可能会发生会阴部感觉改变、性高潮延迟，并需要更多刺激才能达到性高潮。同样的，由于缺乏阴道润滑，导致性交时阴道刺激。使用水基润滑剂有助于防止这种情况。对于女性而言，身体形象可能是性功能障碍的重要因素，接受这些缺损可使得性关系幸福而令人满意。急性期，女性会出现月经周期紊乱，但受伤后的 3~6 个月内可自然恢复。一旦月经周期恢复规律，生育能力通常不会受到影响。多学科的专业人员团队可共同管理脊髓损伤后患者的妊娠。

在男性中，T11 及以上完全损伤将导致心因性勃起功能丧失，但患者仍可实现反射性勃起。这类患者中不到 10％可以射精（Subbarao and Garrison，

2016）。相反，T12及以下完全损伤将导致反射性勃起丧失，而可能保留心因性勃起，但通常不能射精（Subbarao and Garrison，2016）。脊髓损伤后常出现男性生育问题，这主要与射精不足有关。可以通过电刺激射精、宫内人工授精或体外受精来解决。

异位骨化

异位骨化（heterotropnic ossification，HO）是异位部位（如软组织）形成骨组织。20%～30%的脊髓损伤患者发生异位骨化（Snoecx et al.，1995）。异位骨化的病因和发病机制尚不清楚。在脊髓损伤中，肌肉外伤（撕裂、断裂、出血）被认为会引起异位骨化（van Kuijk et al.，2002）。HO最常见部位是髋部（Sullivan et al.，2013）（图70.3），但也可发生在肘部、肩部、手和膝关节周围。

急性期碱性磷酸酶升高可能提示怀疑HO。同位素骨扫描和MRI扫描对急性期的HO诊断具有高敏感性。由于早期钙沉积不足，X射线不会显示HO。

非甾体抗炎药（NSAIDs）可治疗HO。然而，由于其副作用以及在骨折后抑制骨愈合的作用，非甾体抗炎药的使用受到限制（Johnson and Lanig，1996）。治疗已形成的HO旨在终止HO过程，维持受损关节的运动范围并防止疼痛。目前尝试治疗HO的药物十分有限。研究主要集中在吲哚美辛和依替膦酸的使用上，这些药物作为预防措施在早期给予时最为有效。依替膦酸已显示可防止继发性HO的形成，但治疗时长尚待明确，并且存在骨质软化的风险。

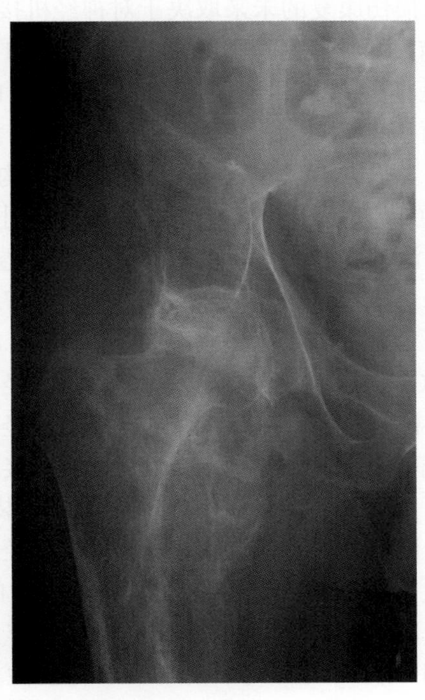

图70.3 髋关节周围的异位骨化

当HO影响生活质量或导致继发性并发症时应考虑手术治疗。应在HO稳定期行手术治疗，因为在急性期手术存在大出血风险。术后给予依替膦酸、非甾体抗炎药、放射治疗等可以降低复发风险。

神经病理性疼痛的治疗

脊髓损伤后的疼痛可能对积极的康复治疗产生影响，并且也对生活质量和日常生活活动产生负面影响。脊髓损伤后疼痛的发病原因尚不清楚。脊髓损伤后有两种不同类型的疼痛：神经病理性疼痛（继发于脊髓损伤）和骨骼肌肉性疼痛（是一种脊髓损伤的结果）。临床上神经病理性疼痛可以分为三类（Cardenas et al.，2002）：脊髓损伤疼痛（在病变水平以下）、过渡区疼痛（在病变水平双侧）、神经根痛和内脏痛。详细的病史纪录、体格检查及随后的重点检查，有助于做出诊断并区分诸如脊髓空洞症等病症。

脊髓损伤后的慢性疼痛治疗是艰难的，知晓这一点十分重要。治疗的目的是控制疼痛并改善生活质量。应探索并适当治疗影响痛觉的心理因素，以改善治疗效果。可通过多种治疗方式来控制疼痛，例如物理疗法、认知行为疗法、自我管理策略、生物反馈、针灸、经皮神经电刺激、正念疗法和药物干预。系统性的疼痛治疗计划可包含以上所述方法。

非甾体抗炎药（NSAIDs）和对乙酰氨基酚用作脊髓损伤患者疼痛的一线治疗，其效果不一。长期使用非甾体抗炎药与胃溃疡和急性肾损伤的风险有关。

抗抑郁药和抗惊厥药用于治疗神经病理性疼痛。三环抗抑郁药（阿米替林、去甲替林和丙咪嗪）可有效治疗神经性疼痛，但抗胆碱能副作用可能会限制其使用。但是一项随机对照研究显示这些药物未能在脊髓损伤人群中缓解神经病理性疼痛和伤害性疼痛（Cardenas et al.，2002）。

抗惊厥药（加巴喷丁、普瑞巴林、拉莫三嗪）是钙通道调节剂，已在脊髓损伤患者中进行了研究。加巴喷丁（每天300～3600 mg）因可引起嗜睡和体重增加而限制了它的使用，但其可有效缓解截瘫患者的神经病理性疼痛（Levendoglu et al.，2004）。普瑞巴林（每天50～600 mg）较加巴喷丁耐受性更好，且副作用更具优势。在完全和不完全脊髓损伤的患者中，普瑞巴林可有效减轻疼痛和改善睡眠（Siddall et al.，2006）。在一项随机对照试验中，拉莫三嗪在整个样本中均未显示具有统计学意义的效果，但在不完全损伤患者中，拉莫三嗪可显著减轻损伤水平及以下的疼痛（Finnerup et al.，2002）。尚未进行 5- 羟色胺去甲肾上腺素再摄取抑制剂（例如度洛西汀和文拉法辛）在脊髓损伤性疼痛中的研究，但这类药物通常在神经性疼痛中非常有效。

阿片类药物已被用于治疗 SCI 后的疼痛，疗效各异，只有曲马多对疼痛有积极作用。长期使用阿片类药物可能会导致严重的副作用，尤其是嗜睡、便秘、呼吸抑制、内分泌异常、耐受性、成瘾以及阿片类药物引起的痛觉过敏。仅在无法耐受口服或口服无效的顽固性疼痛情况下，才考虑鞘内给药。一项临床试验联合使用吗啡和可乐定，并显示效果良好（Siddall et al.，2000）。尚未对脊髓刺激、深部脑刺激和背根进入区病变的长期疗效和安全性进行临床评估。

肌腱移植手术的作用

在不完全颈髓损伤患者中，肌腱移植手术可以通过恢复手部的某些有用功能来帮助患者实现自理。然而，这类手术十分复杂，需要丰富的经验，并且直到神经系统检查稳定且患者已接受大量的康复治疗后才可实施。

计划肌腱移植手术需全面的临床评估。肌腱移植手术的目的是恢复肘部弯曲或伸展、腕部弯曲或伸展或改善抓握能力。

术后大量的上肢康复有助于改善手术效果。必须注意的是，在康复阶段由于肌腱移植的愈合，患者可能会失去使用肢体或手的能力达 12 周。

脊髓损伤后的骨骼肌干预

一旦患者病情稳定并且能够耐受治疗，即可开始 SCI 后的骨骼肌干预。骨骼肌干预结果可能因 SCI 的类型和位置而有所不同。干预的三个主要原则是增加力量、预防和治疗挛缩以及改善运动表现。力量训练对脊髓损伤患者有效。上肢的力量训练目的是帮助 SCI 患者自己实现有效和安全从地板转移到轮椅，并参与功能性任务。下肢的力量训练可能有助于借助辅助装置行走或站立移动。

被动运动对于预防挛缩至关重要，伸展运动可用于治疗挛缩。尚不清楚被动运动和伸展运动的最佳运动量和持续时间，应根据 SCI 水平以及患者的需求进行调整。基于运动学习的原则，重复练习以改善 SCI 患者的运动任务。最近的一项临床试验表明，即使在受伤 3 年后，强化理疗仍可改善 AIS C 和 D 病变患者的力量和步态（Jones et al.，2014）。

在不久的将来，骨骼系统的最新进展可能会改变 SCI 后肌肉骨骼干预的前景。

干细胞移植

SCI 的干细胞疗法是一个主要的研究热点，并且已在动物 SCI 模型中试验了若干干细胞。这些细胞包括从脂肪、骨髓、脐带、鼻腔黏膜和牙髓中获取的胚胎干细胞（多能）和间充质细胞（多能）。尽管胚胎干细胞具有多能性，移植后可分化成任意组织，但由于伦理问题以及患者需要免疫抑制的事实，其使用受到限制。另一方面，间充质干细胞是多能干细胞，且不需要免疫抑制。然而，近期的研究并未深入了解其分化和修复神经细胞的能力。最近已经开发了诱导的多能干细胞。这些是经过基因处理成为神经细胞的成熟细胞。这些细胞取自患者组织，因此不需要免疫抑制。由于基因处理需要较长时间，这类细胞在脊髓损伤的急性期使用受限（Doulames and Plant，2016）。理论上，经基因处理也存在随机突变的风险。

由于新植入的细胞可能在脊髓中引起占位效应，而引发严重的风险，因此限制了干细胞疗法的使用。仍需进行大型随机对照试验，以确保 SCI 中干细胞治疗的安全性和有效性。在美国和欧洲，正在进行几项使用神经干细胞、间充质干细胞和胚胎干细胞的临床试验（Scope，2018）。

SCI 中的神经机接口

脊髓损伤康复的未来取决于对神经机接口（也称为脑电脑接口、BCI 或脑机接口 BMI）的研究。神经接口是神经系统和读取 / 刺激电极之间的直接连接，继而连接到外部硬件。电极可以置于深部也可以在表面。前者可以放置在大脑深部的结构中（几厘米），也可以放置在大型神经的实质中，例如帕金森病使用的深部脑刺激器。也可使用皮质穿透装置（微米到毫米），这可以提供更大的神经元分辨率。另一方面，可以将浅表电极放置在大脑皮质（皮质脑电图，ECoG）或头皮（脑电图，EEG）。神经接口电极可以植入神经系统（大脑、脊柱、周围神经）和肌电器官（肌肉）的任意位置，从而有可能直接连通系统的任意两个部分（或与任何外部神经修复装置）。通过刺激和记录运动、感觉和（或）自主神经系统并完全绕过受伤部位，BCI 可用于恢复 SCI 后的受损功能。一个著名的例子是 Utah array，已在非人类灵长类动物和 I 期人类研究中使用，以将慢性 SCI 患者的运动和感觉皮质连接到肌肉或外部神经修复装置。

功能恢复的优先级取决于多种因素，包括SCI水平、ASI分级和个人意愿（Anderson，2004；Snoek et al.，2004）。对于四肢瘫痪患者，优先考虑的是手臂和手的某些功能恢复，而任何水平的SCI患者均需恢复膀胱和肠道功能。步行和站立能力是SCI人群生活质量的巨大改善（Collinger et al.，2013a）。

神经机器接口的最基本形式是功能性电刺激（functional electric stimulation，FES），它有助于在SCI后刺激无力的肌肉。FES可以通过表面电极或深部装置得以应用。表面电极倾向于刺激肌肉本身，而植入装置可以靶向刺激肌肉或支配特定肌群神经。理论上，FES有助于改善SCI后上肢功能、站立和行走能力。若干外部FES系统正在临床试验中应用，以改善SCI患者的抓握能力（Collinger et al.，2013b）。植入式FES系统需要一定的技术水平以及大量手术干预，然后才能产生作用。

硬膜外和椎管内刺激脊髓可以改善不完全SCI患者的行走能力是基于以下事实：脊髓中存在中枢模式发生器，能够在不需要任何感觉反馈的情况下提供腿部的节律运动（Collinger et al.，2013b）。一些临床试验正在研究硬膜外脊髓刺激改善不完全SCI患者的步行能力（Herman et al. 2002；Huang et al.，2006）。

神经机接口也用于改善SCI后的膀胱控制。通过植入起搏器刺激骶前神经根，可以帮助实现控尿和改善生活质量。对于保守治疗逼尿肌过度活跃失败的完全SCI患者，可获益于该刺激。市售刺激系统由外部部分和植入装置组成。外部刺激器放置在植入装置内，以实现对骶前神经根的一般刺激。通常联合刺激与脊神经背根切断术，以防止反射性膀胱和括约肌收缩。SARS联合脊神经背根切断术也有助于治疗自主神经反射异常和DESD（Martens and Heesakkers，2011）。然而，脊神经背根切断术限制了SARS在不完全SCI患者中的应用，因为它会导致其他盆腔感觉丧失（Martens and Heesakkers，2011）。近期，阴部传入神经刺激迅猛发展，以替代SARS和脊神经背根神经切断术。该方法对于膀胱控制的反射通路完整的患者具有作用。该方法的过程相对简单，且无需联合脊神经背根神经切断术。正在进行进一步的研究以针对膀胱的传入和传出通路建立闭环系统并提供半独立系统（Chew et al.，2013）。

目前还有其他项目正在进行临床前试验，包括皮质内微刺激以恢复感觉、基于脑电图（EEG）的脑机接口、脑机接口（解码神经信号以操作装置并向用户提供脑部活动的反馈）、基于ECoG活动的脑机接口（通过硬膜下或硬膜外电极记录以进行精确功能定位）。未来计算机技术的进步将转化为易于使用的植入物和装置，不出现重大并发症，且更具美观。

延伸阅读、参考文献、EBRAIN的相关链接

扫描书末二维码获取。

第十五篇　周围神经外科

第 71 章　电生理诊断学

Alan Forster・Robert Morris 著
伊骏飞 译，李良 审校

引言

临床神经生理学在神经外科手术中提供了宝贵信息，可鉴别中枢和周围神经系统损伤的类型及量化损伤的严重程度，监测手术范围内及邻近区域组织的安全性，辨别神经结构。总之，它可协助确定解剖结构（如，找到脊髓脂肪瘤内的神经根或丘脑内的神经核团），评估功能的完整性（如，从皮质到任何相关的肌肉的运动通路），监测手术操作涉及区域的神经的功能（如，在三叉神经微血管减压术中或在脊柱侧凸手术中监测面神经），在功能性手术过程中提供指导（如，选择性脊神经背根切断术）。

术中监测在临床应用已久，近年来技术和设备的进步极大地扩展了其在协助神经外科医师和保护患者方面的作用。1950 年定位致痫灶和定位语言皮质技术的发展，革新了癫痫手术技术（Penfield and Jasper，1954）。1960 年多伦多的塔斯克（Tasker）和爱丁堡的吉林汉姆（Gillingham）从放置在人类丘脑的微电极中记录信号，指导运动障碍的手术。诸如 Møller 之类的先驱更是早就扩展了神经电生理监测在颅底手术中的应用（Møller et al.，1981；Møller et al.，1982；Møller and Jannetta，1983）。

本章介绍神经生理学在定位与监测的功能和在不同手术中的应用。

正常神经生理学的基本原理

神经元由胞体、树突和轴突组成。树突和胞体处理来自其他神经元的信息，轴突接收信息并产生电信号（动作电位），引起突触处释放神经递质。突触是两个神经元在非常近的距离内传递信息时的连接点。正常神经元生理学模式图如**图 71.1** 所示。

动作电位 / 膜电位

当细胞膜去极化至阈值时会产生动作电位。细胞内外存在离子浓度差，因此细胞膜的静息电位约为 –60~70 mV。细胞外部的刺激会改变细胞膜对特定离子的通透性，引起膜电位的变化。这些细胞外部的刺激包括跨膜电位的传导或细胞外液中神经递质的激活。这些刺激将打开特定离子通道，增加细胞膜对该离子的通透性，驱使膜电位趋近于该离子的平衡电位。

神经递质增加细胞膜对钠离子或钙离子的通透性时会引起去极化（膜电位趋近 0 mV），而增加钾离子或氯离子的通透性则会引起超极化（膜电位向负值增大的方向移动）。动作电位产生的阈值为 –60~ –50 mV。到达此阈值时，电压门控性钠通道开放，细胞膜对钠离子通透性迅速增加，钠离子快速、大量的内流导致膜电位迅速变化，在有髓轴突中引起动作电位，以高达 100 m/s 的速度沿膜传播。在细胞外予电刺激，也会产生动作电位。自发产生或外部诱导的神经冲动均可应用于临床监测。

突触功能

突触间隙约为 20 nm。动作电位到达突触前膜时，神经递质被释放到突触间隙中并与突触后膜上的受体结合，开放突触后膜的离子通道，引起膜电压的变化。通过这种方式，突触前膜的电位可传递到突触后膜。γ- 氨基丁酸（GABA）是最常见的抑制性神经递质。GABA 与突触后膜 GABA-A 受体结合，开放氯离子通道，从而引起突触后膜超极化；或与 GABA-B 受体结合，通过 G 蛋白与钾离子通道连接使突触后膜超极化。谷氨酸盐是一种兴奋性神经递质，可与 N- 甲基 -D- 天冬氨酸（NMDA）受体、AMPA 受体和 kainite 受体结合。这些受体激活阳离子通道，钠、钾或钙离子进入突触后神经元，引起细胞膜去极化。神经元由此被其他神经元的树突激活或抑制。

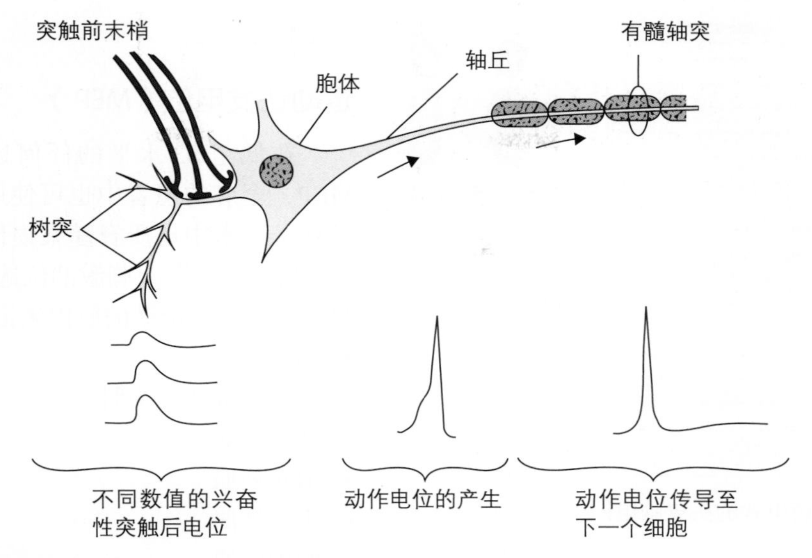

图 71.1　兴奋性突触后电位（EPSPs）产生神经元电活动，以动作电位的形式传递

神经纤维分类

根据神经直径、传导速度和髓鞘形式可对周围神经纤维分类。A 纤维是直径较大的有髓纤维，传导速度快（10~100 m/s），可进一步分为：

A-α 纤维：肌梭和腱器官。

A-β 纤维：皮肤的机械感受器和肌梭的第二受体。

A-γ 纤维：支配肌梭活动的运动神经。

A-Δ 纤维：自由神经末梢的快痛觉传导纤维。

B 纤维是直径稍小的有髓纤维，为自主神经，传导速度可达 15 m/s。C 纤维是直径最小的有髓纤维，传导速度减低，最高为 2 m/s，传导慢痛觉信号和温度觉。

与神经外科有关的神经生理学原理

脑电图

脑电图（EEG）记录来自头部不同区域的电活动，分为头皮脑电图、皮质脑电图（ECoG）(使用硬膜下带状或栅格状等电极记录）和使用深部电极记录的立体定向脑电图（SEEG）。脑电图是复合电位，主要来自突触后电位。通过测量两点之间的电位差来确定电场，EEG 的每个通道代表两个特定位置之间的电位差。这些电位差可以平均到单个公共参考点，也可以在 EEG 各电极之间测量。常规使用“10–20”系统放置电极，但该系统并不能完全覆盖前颞叶区域，如有必要则需用额外的电极进行补充。

图 71.2 为一位成年癫痫患者的头皮脑电图。使用的标准“10-20”系统放置电极位。奇数代表左侧，偶数代表右侧。F= 额叶，Fp= 额极，P= 顶叶，O= 枕骨，T= 颞叶，X1-X2 为备用导联，此处用以记录心电图（ECG）。部分导联可见正常的 α 节律，如通道 16（T5-O1）。通道 9、10 和 11 中的慢波活动是该区域潜在的神经胶质瘤造成损害的结果。右上方为在图中绿线位置处分析的“压缩谱阵密度”，定位了出现慢波活动的区域，但头皮脑电图上的这种频谱分析有时会有误差。

头皮脑电图主要记录来自大脑皮质的信号，无法提供如海马和基底神经节等脑深部结构的详细信息。但是部分慢波活动可以透过肿瘤（**图 71.2**），例如额叶的慢波活动可以反映中线深部损伤。头皮脑电图可以提示异常功能区的位置，例如癫痫灶或占位性病变，或显示功能异常的程度。与功能成像相比，头皮脑电图的空间分辨率低，且异常改变常缺乏特异性，但其具有更好的实时性。头皮脑电图还可以反映麻醉深度，应用于重症监护。头外伤的患者可能会出现亚临床的癫痫发作。在一项研究中，监测 144 名头外伤的儿童，在 30% 的患者中发现癫痫发作与 ITU 住院时间相关（O’Neill et al.，2015）。

脑电图监测还可以应用于一些血管手术，如动脉瘤手术和颈动脉内膜剥脱术。持续脑电图监测可迅速发现由缺血引起的双侧不对称的改变，虽然体感诱发电位（SSEP）可能更敏感，但 SSEP 应用的平均叠加技术需要一定时间才能记录到有警报意义的改

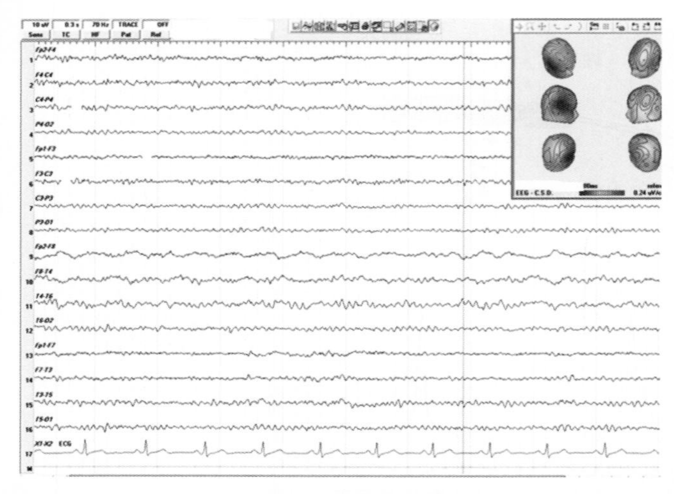

图 71.2 一位成年癫痫患者的头皮脑电图

变。原始的实时脑电图或经过后期处理的脑功能监护仪（CFAM）发现脑电活动的迅速下降，是颈动脉剥脱术中提示可能需要放置转流管的敏感指标。CFAM可连续显示经过处理的两秒前的EEG，几乎可以实时反映动态变化。在使用巴比妥类药物减少大脑活动时，脑电图或脑功能监测可协助诱发较为理想的爆发 - 抑制状态。

皮质脑电图（ECoG）和立体定向脑电图（SEEG）用于在癫痫手术前和手术中定位致痫灶。在视频遥测过程中记录的癫痫发作和传导可协助制订手术计划，有时还可用于指导确定切除范围。除了通过此类电极记录外，还可以通过给予刺激束定位皮质功能或诱发癫痫发作（Cossu et al.，2012）。单脉冲电刺激（SPES）作为一种主动诱发技术可以定位兴奋性皮质（Valentín et al.，2002）。上述技术可用于指导复杂的癫痫手术。

诱发电位（EP）

与诸如EEG和肌电图（EMG）等自发电位不同，诱发电位（evoked potentials，EP）是外部刺激产生的一种电信号。诱发电位可以检测许多传导通路，包括运动诱发电位（motor evoked potentials，MEP）、体感诱发电位（somatosensory evoked potentials，SEP），视觉诱发电位（visual evoked potentials，VEP）、脑干听觉诱发电位（brain stem auditory evoked potentials，BSAEP）和视网膜电图（electroretinography，ERG）。大部分的诱发电位会被麻醉剂所减弱或完全阻断，因此应用异丙酚和瑞芬太尼的全静脉麻醉方案可取得最好的监测效果。虽然肌松药会阻断MEP和EMG，但在插管过程中应用的肌松药在需要监测时通常已完全代谢。

运动诱发电位（MEP）

在低至S3水平的任何远端肌肉上均可记录到MEP，全麻的患者中也可使用MEP以降低颅脑（和脊柱）手术中皮质脊髓束损伤的风险（**图 71.3**）。根据“皮质小人”上刺激部位选择对侧记录点，首选有最大的皮质支配区的肌肉来记录。常用的肌肉包括：

- 颏肌
- 三角肌或肱二头肌
- 伸指总肌
- 拇短展肌
- 小指展肌
- 股内侧肌
- 胫骨前肌
- 拇展肌

通常用一对针电极记录相关通路上的肌肉的信号，或刺激运动皮质后，用放置在蛛网膜下腔或硬膜外的电极直接在脊髓上记录在运动传导通路远端产生的信号——称为D波（直接波）。在麻醉的患者中通过单次经颅骨刺激通常可引起D波，D波是在脊柱外科手术中监测皮质脊髓束损伤最可靠的指标，但是电极移位时会造成假阳性（Ulkatan et al.，2006）。

MEP刺激方式包括经颅骨的电刺激或磁刺激、皮质刺激、皮质下刺激、皮质脊髓束（包括髓内）和周围神经刺激。在手术前可使用磁刺激定位运动区和言语区。在术中麻醉状态下，通常采用成串的电刺激，以“5个刺激串”最为常用，它由脉冲间隔为2~4 ms的五个脉冲组成。Taniguchi使用单极探头以高频（300~500 Hz）脉冲刺激初级运动皮质，以定位运动皮质和在麻醉下状态下监测皮质脊髓束的功能，通常用硬膜下带状电极紧贴大脑皮质记录（Taniguchi et al.，1993）。在唤醒手术中，负极最好放置于头皮的麻醉区域（例如头顶）。麻醉下岛叶胶质瘤切除术中也可以监测运动通路，先用硬膜下条带状电极通过SEP皮质翻转定位运动区，然后用与运动皮质接触的点（作为正极，头皮电极为负极）刺激运动皮质。在切除过程中监测所诱发出的运动反应，如果在手术期间MEP恶化，则可以及时采取治疗措施（休息，冲水，应用罂粟碱）（Neuloh et al.，2007a）。用探头刺激面丘并在面部肌肉和舌肌上记录反应，当发生转变时提示进入第四脑室底，这种技术可用于确定中线位置，判断脑干肿瘤的安全手术入口（Sala et al.，2007）。在脊柱外科手术中，皮质脊髓束受刺激

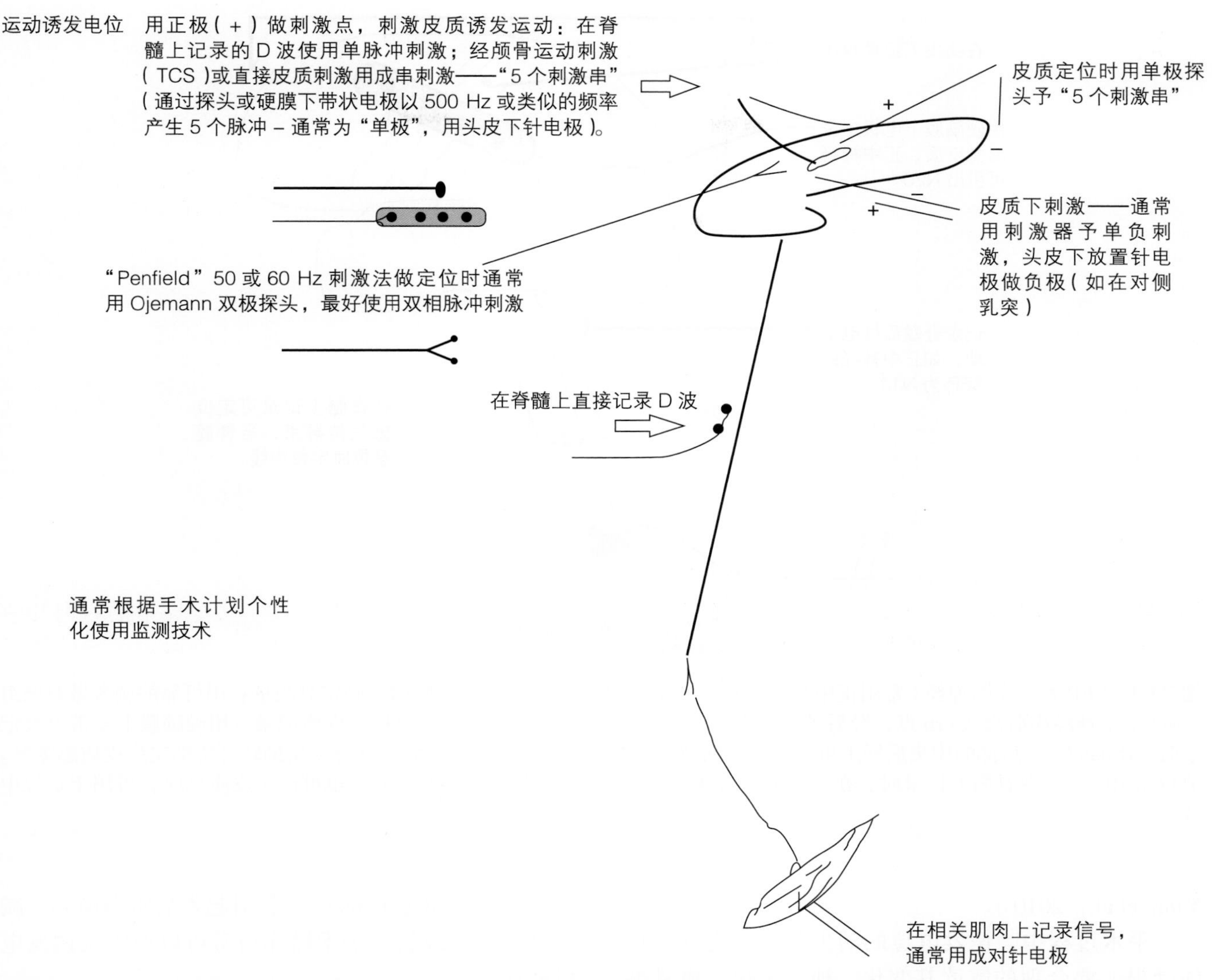

图71.3　动作诱发电位可经颅骨刺激：术前定位通常采用磁刺激，术中用“5个刺激串”经颅骨电刺激以监测整个通路。条件允许时，可通过硬脑膜下带状电极或探针直接刺激皮质：探针刺激可在皮质和皮质下水平定位运动区。远端记录点常选择肌肉（MEP）或脊髓（D波）：对于脊髓手术，在手术平面以上的肌肉做记录可作为参照

后引起的运动反应可能提示内侧椎弓根断裂，在髓内肿瘤手术中则提示手术操作靠近的皮质脊髓束。

体感诱发电位（SEP）

在周围神经上刺激时，神经系统的近端可记录到刺激所引起的反应（**图71.4**）。例如，对正中神经和胫后神经的刺激可在神经根、脊髓、脑干和感觉皮质中记录到。正中神经的体感反应（SEP）是在手腕处予电刺激（约200刺激强度），通过平均技术在Erb点、颈椎和皮质记录刺激所引起的反应。潜伏期延长和波幅下降提示手腕至皮质的体感通路上的任意水平可能发生损伤。

与EEG类似，在感觉皮质记录到的潜伏期为20 ms的负向波（N20）能够定位感觉皮质，并反映皮质功能。血管痉挛引起的局部缺血可导致N20消失（例如，在动脉瘤或岛叶手术中）。在ITU中，如果正中神经SSEP的皮质反应消失，而皮质下反应（例如颈椎的N13）存在，则提示皮质功能受损，预后欠佳。在脚踝处刺激胫后神经引起的皮质反应为P40。胫后神经的信号沿薄束上行，在左右脚踝刺激并在脊髓上记录相应反应，可指导定位后正中沟，当髓内肿瘤使原有的解剖结构易位时可协助寻找安全的手术入口。体感诱发电位主要用于在脊髓手术中监测背柱而非运动功能。在脊髓后部刺激在脚踝处和头皮处记录感觉反应（在下肢肌肉记录运动）可作为一种替代技术（Quinones-Hinojosa et al.，2002；

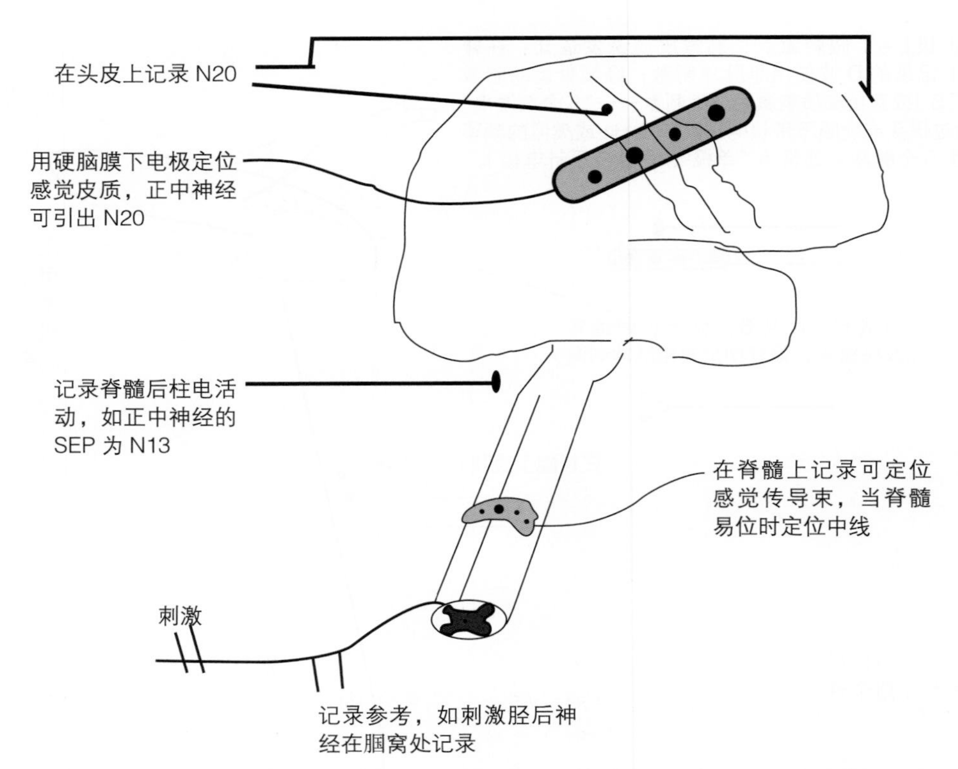

图 71.4　SEP 刺激周围神经（常用正中神经或胫后神经），以引出可见的肌肉收缩来确定刺激量：用可靠的刺激做对照组（例如正中神经用肘窝或 erb 点，胫后神经用腘窝）：可在脊髓、脑干、可放置电极的皮质记录。用硬脑膜下条带电极记录时，Rolandic 沟后部的中央后回上可记录到负向波，同时在运动区出现正向波，这种皮质翻转可协助定位皮质感觉区。值得指出的是，在脊髓上记录时：在脊髓上刺激既可以在双侧脚踝处诱发感觉反应，也可产生皮质反应，可用于定位中线

Yanni et al.，2010）。

手术过程中，诱发电位的消失并不一定预示功能受损，要合理的解读其变化。神经牵拉、血管事件、刺激或记录电极的移位均有可能对诱发电位产生影响。固定位置不佳时肢体受压导致的神经丛麻痹也会引起反应消失，这种变化在调整体位后可逆转。

在手术部位的近端和远端同时记录有助于解读信号变化。在 SEP 中，多个神经根同时被刺激，因此可能无法检测到单支神经根损伤。在臂丛手术中可能会同时出现两个水平的损伤。如果刺激近端神经残端可以引起皮质 SEP，则一定存在尚完整的神经根，提示并非所有神经根均被撕脱。

脑干听觉诱发电位（BSAEP）

通过插入式耳机在术中予咔哒音刺激，在乳突和头顶放置记录电极，收集约 1000 次 EEG 信号加以平均得到脑干听觉诱发电位。正常的短程听觉诱发电位有五个波形，其中Ⅲ波和Ⅴ波通常最清晰。对听神经有潜在的损伤性的操作或牵拉会使Ⅲ波和Ⅴ波的潜伏期延长。Ⅴ波潜伏期延长 0.9 ms 以上可以使听力图发生可测量的变化：Ⅴ波的波幅降低 50％或潜伏期延长超过 1 ms 可能会引起术后听力障碍。减少神经牵拉或暂缓手术操作通常可以使听觉诱发电位恢复。

BAEP 主要应用于桥小脑角手术中，例如三叉神经痛、听神经瘤和面肌痉挛。术中通过记录对 500 Hz 的音频信号的直接反应可以定位听神经瘤内的听神经（Butler et al.，1995），用放置在神经上的电极记录咔哒音刺激也可以定位和评估神经功能。

在颅脑损伤中，听觉诱发电位的潜伏期延长是预后良好的指标（Fischer et al.，2008）。

神经传导速度（NCS）

测量周围神经传导速度（nerve conduction studies，NCS）可以检测运动、感觉和反射通路，应始终结合临床解读 NCS 结果。

检查内容包括：

1. 运动成分（M 波）　刺激周围神经并在该神经支配的肌肉中记录（例如，正中神经和对应的拇短展肌）。测量内容包括潜伏期（从刺激到记录到反应之间的时程）和波幅，测量结果受前角细胞、轴索、髓鞘、神经肌肉接头或神经病变本身的影响。

2. 感觉成分 在被刺激的神经上的另一点，而非肌肉上记录。感觉神经波幅小于运动振幅。
3. F 波是动作电位沿运动轴索逆行传到脊髓，激活前角细胞后引起肌肉的延迟反应。F 波的潜伏期反映肢体和脊髓之间的传导功能，而非肢体内节段性的传导功能，其传入和传出均为运动轴索。
4. H 反射是另一种延迟反应，可以有效地评估腱反射。例如，在腘窝刺激胫神经并在腓肠 - 比目鱼肌群记录，可用于鉴别 L5（H 反射存在）和 S1（H 反射消失）神经根病。

顺行记录的感觉神经动作电位（sensory nerve action potential，SNAP）的波幅反映了有功能的感觉神经轴索的数量。因此，尺神经 SNAP 减低的病因不仅有肘管综合征，还可能是其他 C8 神经根节后损伤（例如，糖尿病性神经病或胸廓出口综合征）。对检查结果的判读必须结合临床。在臂丛神经损伤中，感觉神经的波幅是评估损伤严重程度、判断神经根损伤水平以及鉴别节前或节后损伤的依据。值得注意的是，断裂的神经在发生沃勒变性前，其远端在约 1 周内仍保留功能。因此损伤当天的电生理检查具有误导性。颈椎病通常损伤神经节近端，因此尽管患者有手麻症状，感觉传导仍可能为正常。

神经受压时会出现传导阻滞（如尺骨或腓骨神经病变）。压力的增加早期会导致传导阻滞，随后出现局灶性传导减慢：轴突的凋亡导致波幅下降，其中感觉轴索损伤先于运动。

运动神经传导速度检查（**图 71.5**）记录肌肉的反应（复合肌肉动作电位 -CMAPs），其波幅反映了激活的轴索 / 肌纤维的数量。轴索丢失和肌肉萎缩时动作电位较小，局部脱髓鞘时远端刺激点的潜伏期延长（例如腕管综合征、吉兰 - 巴雷综合征和断裂神经的再生）。

重复神经刺激重点在检测神经肌肉接头功能，可用于诊断肌无力和相关疾病（Kimura，2001）。

NCS 可协助诊断诸如腕管综合征（CTS）之类的卡压性神经病。神经的局部卡压通常会导致局部的传导减慢（见**图 71.5**）。CTS 的临床症状可能存在误导，其临床诊断的准确率约为 50%，在进行手术前应进行神经传导检查。疾病的严重程度取决于正中神经传导速度在跨手腕前后减慢的程度（与尺神经传导速度相比）（**图 71.5**）。感觉神经传导速度减慢是最敏感的指标，运动潜伏期延长仅在运动功能严重损伤时才出现（Bland，2016）。

肘关节附近尺神经运动传导速度减慢和波幅下降（波幅下降 50% = 传导阻滞）能够定位尺神经卡压部位，“寸进法”也可在术前确定压迫部位（Kimura，2013）。术中使用后种技术可以显示局灶性减慢的部位，并改善预后（Kim et al.，2003）。

肌电图（EMG）

肌电图（EMG）用表面电极或针电极测量肌膜的电活动。兴奋性良好的运动单位在肌肉收缩时的募集电位呈“干扰相”（**图 71.6A**）。如果神经有轴突缺失，大力收缩时运动单位募集异常，仅有少量甚至是单个运动单位以高频放电（**图 71.6B**）。

在神经损伤中，存在单个放电的运动单位证实至少有一个轴突与肌肉相连。这在评估神经丛损伤或作为神经再生的证据方面有重要意义。失神经支配持续约三周后，肌膜会出现“去神经增敏”现象，肌电图表现为自发电位，如纤颤电位和正尖波（**图 71.6C**）。自发电位也见于肌强直和肌炎等疾病。运动单位中不同肌纤维放电的变异性可用“Jitter”衡量，在运动终板不稳定时“Jitter”增加（例如重症肌无力或再生神经中不稳定的末端轴突）。结合临床和神经传导速度检查，肌电图异常的肌肉的分布情况可以协助疾病的定位和定性，如神经根病、卡压性周围神经病、周围神经病、运动神经元病和多灶性神经传导阻滞。

术中肌电图在提示支配可记录肌肉的运动神经的损伤风险中有重要作用。自由 EMG 可以通过视觉和听觉两种形式在神经被刺激时提示外科医生。例如，听神经瘤手术中，刺激面神经时，放置在面部肌肉中的一对针电极会记录到肌肉放电。肌电反应是非线性的，因此最初刺激产生的放电可能很短暂，但进一步的神经激惹可能会引起长达数分钟的持续放电。前庭神经鞘瘤切除术中，放电的形式与刺激面神经的严重程度相关，其中 A-train（有高度同源性、高频放电形式）是预测术后面神经损伤的可靠指标（Prell et al.，2007）。

术中监测

单一脑神经的术中监测

CN Ⅱ

在枕叶皮质记录闪光刺激所诱发视觉反应可用于监测视神经和视觉传导通路（Sasaki et al.，2010）。麻醉患者可在视束上记录视觉反应。在清醒患者中，刺激视束会引起光幻视，在相关皮质内刺激视觉通路则会诱发以往的回忆。

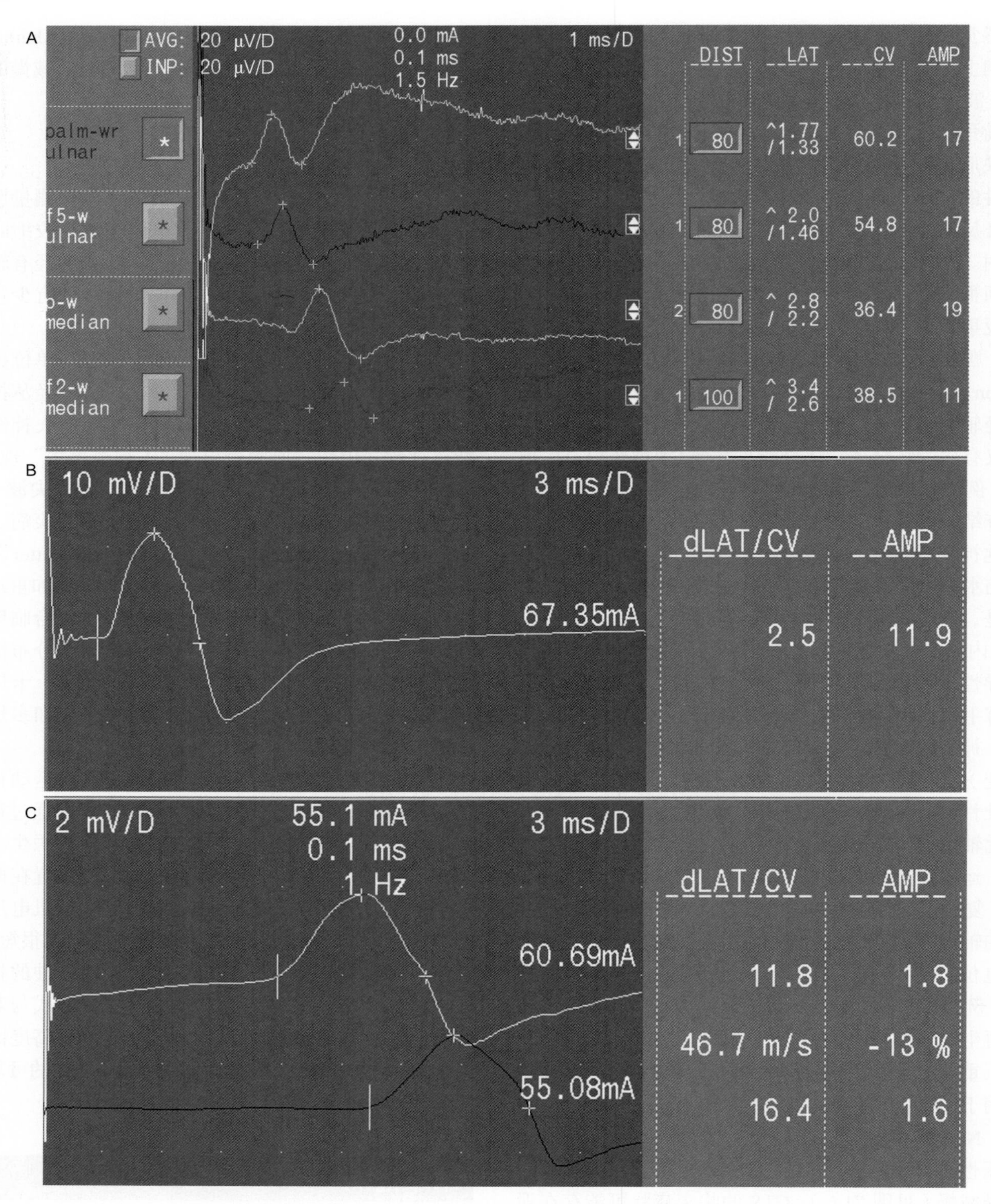

图 71.5 （A）正中神经在手掌到手腕之间传导速度为 36.4 m/s，明显低于同部位的尺神经速度 60.2 m/s，手指到腕关节处正中神经的速度为 38.5 m/s，也显著慢于尺神经的 54.8 m/s。（B）正中神经运动远端潜伏期正常（手腕到拇短展肌），这是一例轻度腕管综合征。（C）该名患者，在手腕处刺激正中神经时，其运动反应延迟了 11.8 ms（较严重的腕管综合征）。第二条线为在肘部刺激，检查肘部到腕部的正中运动传导（注意，其他受检神经反应需正常，即异常并非系统系疾病的局部表现）

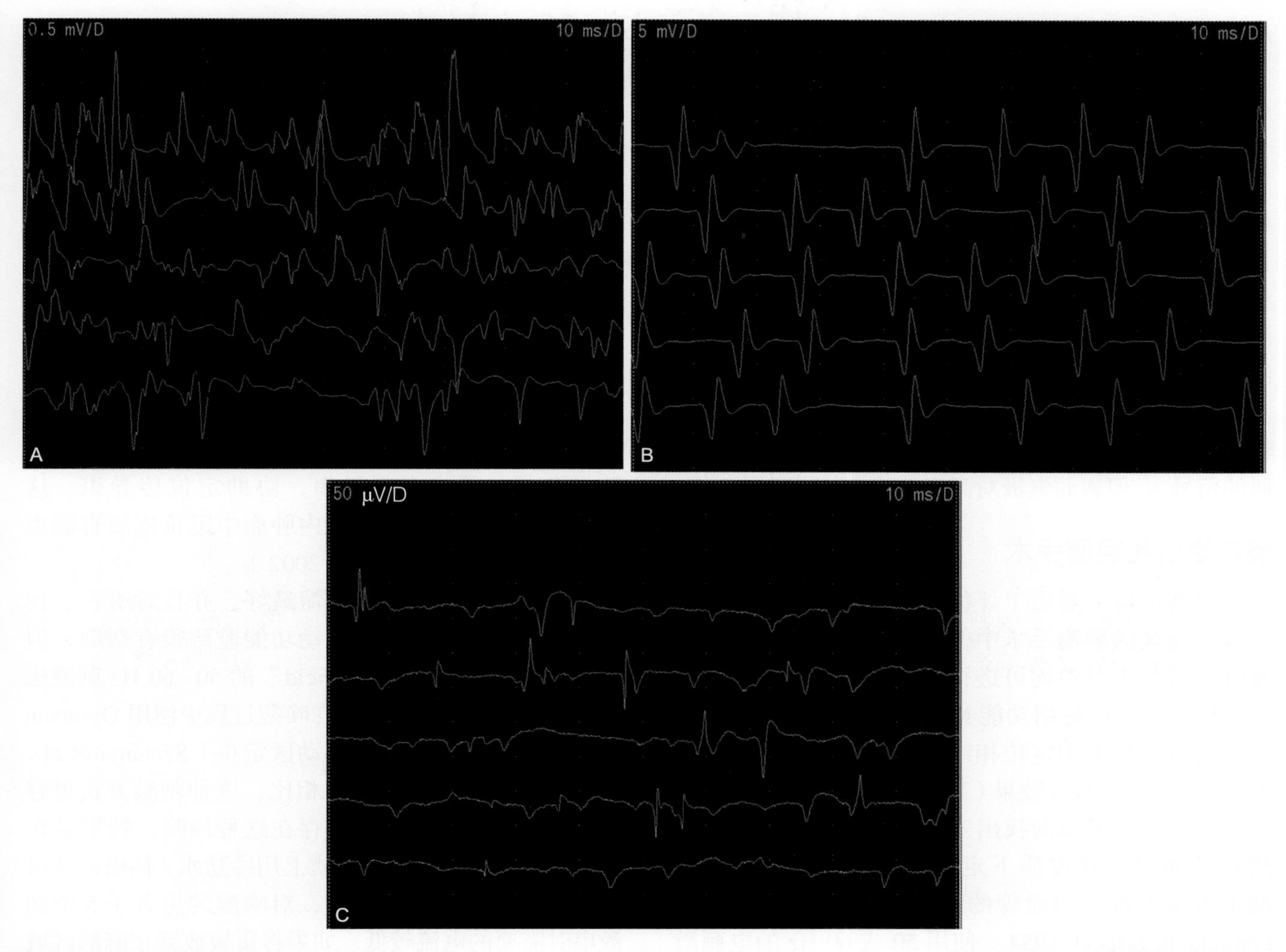

图 71.6 （A）肱二头肌正常的干扰相肌电图。（B）严重减少至离散电位的干扰相。（C）严重失神经支配的拇短展肌中出现的纤颤波和正锐波，提示 C8/T1 神经节后病变

CNⅢ、Ⅳ、Ⅴ、Ⅵ、Ⅶ、Ⅸ、Ⅹ、Ⅺ

应用自由肌电图和使用单极或双极探针刺激的诱发肌电图可以监测上述脑神经。监测第三、第四和第六对脑神经时需将针电极插入眼外肌中。

记录三叉神经的肌电图通常选择咬肌，但是自由肌电图和诱发肌电图只能评估下颌支的运动成分。瞬目反射可以测试感觉通路——在清醒患者中予单一刺激，术中则予成串刺激。在海绵窦中，术中可用探针刺激、在面部肌肉中记录，以检测 V1 和 V2（Al Masri et al.，2014），使用成串刺激最容易诱发出瞬目反射的 R1 波。

前庭神经鞘瘤手术中，使用刺激可定位尚未显露的面神经。但是，如果神经已被切断，损伤远端仍会对刺激产生反应。此外，刺激量过大时电流会扩散（“电流跳跃”），可能会引起误判，或者相反，术腔中的盐水可能会使刺激电流分流，导致刺激失败。

在治疗三叉神经痛的三叉神经微血管减压中，存在听神经损伤的风险（主要是由于牵拉），因此，听觉诱发电位是主要的监测项目。

在面肌痉挛中，导致痉挛的病因引起一种类似 F 波的反应“侧方扩散”（例如，在垫开责任血管前，刺激面部颧支时在下颌支支配的肌肉中可引起反应）。解除责任血管对第七对脑神经的压迫后，侧方扩散波会出现变化，通常会消失。这种变化通常提示预后良好。在三叉神经痛手术中，牵拉第八对脑神经的会影响听力，因此通常需要监测 BAEP。

在微小的听神经瘤中可用 BSAEP 监测第八对脑神经：在听觉纤维上直接记录信号是可行的。当患侧听力受损时，通常无法记录到反应信号。如果肿瘤较大，则可通过另一侧耳朵的 BSAEP 监测脑干，通

过 SEP 监测传导束。

通过颅骨的运动刺激并在脑神经支配肌肉记录产生的反应，验证脑神经的完整性：刺激伪迹是一个问题——相比于直接反应，喉部肌肉（如环甲肌、声带肌、舌肌和上颚）长潜伏期的反应更容易记录，可能会反映部分语言通路，甚至吞咽功能。常使用相同强度的单个刺激作为对照，因为高电流可能会激活周围神经的远端部分（即，刺激不经颅骨直接激活神经远端）。对于某些肌肉（例如声带肌），特殊的细“钩状”电极更为适合，在长时间的手术中不易脱落。表面肌电图记录有特殊用途（例如，通过气管插管表面放置喉部电极，可记录迷走神经支配的咽喉肌的信号），但表面电极对高频的放电信号显示不佳。

皮质定位和唤醒手术

皮质定位主要用于评估运动和语言功能。靠近语言功能区的肿瘤手术中，定位和监测运动功能在麻醉或清醒患者中均可进行，但语言功能仅能在唤醒下评估。术前应用功能 MRI 和磁刺激定位运动区和语言区，与术中定位相结合，能达到在语言皮质上 / 附近手术的最佳效果（Bello et al.，2008）。

定位技术可协助找出安全的手术入口，持续监测运动通路，在皮质下定位皮质脊髓束，对于辅助手术和发现受损血管的痉挛都具有重要的价值。Penfield 和 Jasper（1954）使用 50 或 60 Hz 的电刺激（双极或单极刺激均可）来确定主要的运动区，但现在大多数人更倾向于 Tanaguchi 和 Schramm 在 1993 年提出的“5 个刺激串”的方法。

通常使用五个 500 Hz 的正极脉冲刺激运动皮质，用 2 mm 的单球刺激器放置皮质上作为正极，插入前额或头顶的独立针电极作负极（如图 71.3）。与 50 Hz 的方法相比，这种短程、高频的刺激串所需要的刺激量更小，且更不易诱发癫痫。用成对的针电极插入对侧运动投射区的肌肉中记录其对刺激的反应，在具有最大的皮质运动投射区的肌肉中通常能观察到最佳反应，如拇短展肌、小指展肌（或第一骨间肌）。通常还使用以下肌肉，包括颏肌、三角肌或肱二头肌、伸指总肌、股内侧肌、胫前肌和拇展肌。在皮质下（包括脊柱）手术时，刺激器为负极刺激、其他电极作为正极，直接刺激皮质脊髓束。

有一种简单、可靠的技术可以显示麻醉或唤醒患者的主要运动区。通过 SEP 能找到 Rolandic 沟（皮质翻转，通常刺激对侧正中神经），从而定位运动皮质，通过直接刺激可确认运动区。SEP 中，Rolandic 沟后的中央后回在 20 ms 处出现负向波，而中央前回则为正向波，从而可定位运动皮质。因此，使用横跨 Rolandic 沟的四触点（或更长的六触点或八触点）带状电极来定位运动皮质和感觉皮质。在适当的情况下，可以用探针刺激以进一步的定位。将条带固定放置在该区域，使用运动皮质上的一个接触点重复刺激以监测运动通路。在岛叶肿瘤切除术中，血管痉挛很可能损害运动通路，而这种由 Neuloh 等发现（2007b）的方法在该手术中效果显著。他的研究中，约有 44% 的患者出现 MEP 的恶化。通过休息，冲水和应用罂粟碱，29% 的患者恢复，无法恢复的患者术后出现了神经功能缺损症状。

切除运动区下肿瘤时，在皮质下可用单极探针做负极，予 5 个刺激串，协助定位传导束。这种负极刺激还可用于在髓内肿瘤中定位皮质脊髓束（Quinones-Hinojosa et al.，2002）。

患者对唤醒手术的反馈最好，并且对语言、视觉、更高级的功能以及运动功能监测很有帮助，但并不适合所有患者。“Penfield”的 50~60 Hz 刺激法可诱发运动反应，通常是在唤醒过程中使用 Ojemann 双极刺激器进行语言和运动区定位（Szelényi et al.，2011）。与“5 个刺激串”相比，这种刺激方式更容易诱发癫痫，虽然两者都存在这种风险，特别是在过度刺激的情况下。在皮质上用冷盐水 / 林格冲洗可终止癫痫发作。如前所述，对唤醒的患者予 5 个刺激串时需要的电流较低。如果将负极放置在麻醉区域（例如头顶）中，这种刺激通常不会引起疼痛。目前有几篇研究表明，当肿瘤位于语言区时，唤醒手术肿瘤全切率更高，术后功能障碍更少，效果改善显著（Sacko et al.，2011）。较大的刺激会产生肌肉可见的收缩，针电极更容易记录较小刺激诱发的反应。在寻找阳性反应时，应使用阈值刺激量来排除反应为阴性的刺激点。如果可能，应评估脑电图以监测迟放电并尽早发现癫痫发作。在定位中使用过高的电流会增加癫痫风险，同时电流的扩散可能会导致术者过度谨慎和肿瘤切除的不彻底。总体而言，癫痫发作风险为 4.9%（Serletis and Bernstein，2007），可用在发作的皮质上冲冷盐水治疗。麻醉师应用过多的化学药物控制癫痫发作会使清醒的患者昏睡，无法配合唤醒。

在麻醉患者中，通过“5 个刺激串”在环甲肌诱发的长潜伏期反应可监测某些语言通路（Deletis et al.，2011），在上颚和舌头中也可以看到类似的反应。

辅助运动区损害引起的显著力弱通常在几天或几周内会自发缓解。该区域损伤时，患者无法完成特定运动指令（Nakajima et al.，2015），例如，无法活动某些手指：同侧和对侧手均可能受影响。理论上，如果能直接从对侧肌肉记录到完整的皮质刺激诱发的运动反应，而主动运动逐渐消失，则表明正在切除辅助运动皮质。运动功能在约一个月内会恢复。运动前区手术可留下永久性的损伤，对唤醒的患者通过皮质和皮质下刺激可最大程度减少损伤（Rech et al.，2017）。

在清醒的患者中可通过闪光、颜色或视野变换等刺激定位视觉通路。脑深部电刺激手术期间，在麻醉患者中可以用闪光刺激诱发患者视觉通路的反应，通过微电极记录来自苍白球下视束的信号。

与语言相关的区域存在巨大的个体差异（Ojemann，1979），最简单的测试是通过 50 Hz 刺激诱发延后表达，图像识别和动词生成检测了其他重要的语言功能（Rofes et al.，2017）。

5 个刺激串更少引起癫痫发作，并且在大多数情况下更有效。

功能性手术的神经生理学和微电极记录

脑深部电刺激（deep brain stimulation，DBS）现已发展为神经外科的重要领域。DBS 的作用机制尚不明确，对不同的靶点的不同刺激方式会产生不同作用。刺激调节了相邻细胞或纤维的活动。McIntyre 等认为去极化的阻断、突触失活、突触抑制和刺激诱导的神经网络活动的调节是 DBS 作用机制的 4 种主要假说（McIntyre et al.，2004）。

植入电极通常有四个触点，触点间的不同组合可组成多种刺激模式，通过电流刺激来影响靶点区域的功能。改变刺激频率和刺激量能够调整治疗效果。

目前，运动障碍手术的主要靶点是丘脑（主要用于震颤）、苍白球（主要用于肌张力障碍或帕金森病）、丘脑底核（用于帕金森病）和近期出现的脚桥核（也用于帕金森病）。对于神经性疼痛，靶点包括丘脑的 VPL 和脑室周围灰质（PVG）。刺激 PVG 可以在相应区域产生温暖的感觉，而刺激 VPL 则发生感觉异常。运动皮质电刺激治疗疼痛的靶点是运动皮质和前扣带回（Boccard et al.，2014）。还有许多其他靶点，包括治疗强迫症的伏隔核和治疗进食障碍的下丘脑。

神经生理学可用于精准定位靶点和正确放置电极。术中通常唤醒患者做功能测试。通过电刺激定位靶点、确定治疗窗、明确与邻近结构的距离，并避免刺激引起的副作用（例如靠近内囊会引起肌肉收缩）。此外，可以考虑使用阻抗测量或微电极记录来分辨电极植入路径中穿过的结构。

目标电极的最终位置至关重要，微电极可提供靶点附近的电活动信息，还需要良好的成像技术和使用微电极或阻抗测试的定位技术。细胞外微电极主要用于在 DBS 手术中记录相邻神经元的动作电位。白质仅有偶发的棘波，而灰质则显示出更持续的电活动，不同位置的神经元放电模式不同。这种技术在靶点的精准定位中非常有用，如在帕金森病手术中确定丘脑下核（STN）（图 71.7）。通常情况下，STN 自发放电的频率约为 40 Hz，在帕金森病中其放电频率增加，而亨廷顿舞蹈症中则减少。STN 兴奋性谷氨酸能神经元放电频率的增加导致 GPi 抑制性 GABA 能神经元放电增加，抑制丘脑或脑干靶细胞，

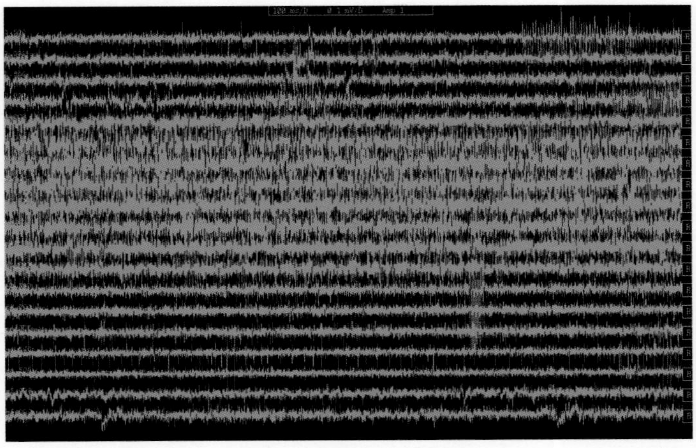

图 71.7　微电极通过丘脑底核（STN）过程中记录的多细胞电活动。放置电极过程中，每个通道按顺序记录，因此顶部的通道信号起源于 STN 深处，一些规则的细胞放电（右上角）可能起源于黑质；STN 细胞快放电引起电活动增加（中间），通过扩音器产生如“撕扯尼龙搭扣”的声音。脑深部电刺激电极应跨越这个区域放置

从而引起帕金森病患者运动减少的症状。对于肌张力障碍患者，剧烈运动会带来技术操作上的困难，因此经常在麻醉下测试苍白球。肌张力障碍患者中，GPi 记录显示其自发放电减少，由强直性放电转变为位相性放电。这种改变进而导致对丘脑的抑制减少，运动区和运动前区活动因此增加。电极在壳核、GPe 和 GPi 中的位置发生变化时，其记录到的放电模式也随之改变。闪光在视觉通路诱发的反应，可以用微电极在苍白球下方的视束中记录下来。从丘脑的 Vim 中可能记录到与震颤有关的节律性爆发放电。

当影像技术无法清楚地显示靶点时，神经生理技术对于靶点定位必不可少。影像技术的进步使得 DBS 电极在没有神经生理信息时也能成功植入，但这种方法仍存在争议（Ashkan，2008）。

脊柱手术中的运动和感觉监测

对于脊柱外科手术，“多模式”监测是最佳方案（Kothbauer et al.，1997）。通常结合使用运动、体感和 EMG 技术。自 1970 年代以来，SEP 被用于脊柱侧凸手术（Nash et al.，1977），但其不能可靠地预测运动通路的损伤。“多模态监测”包括从周围肌肉或从脊髓背侧（D 波）记录的运动诱发电位、SEP、自由肌电和诱发肌电图。这些技术对髓内肿瘤意义重大，也可应用于髓外肿瘤、甚至简单的减压手术（Ney et al.，2015）。

在脊柱和圆锥手术中，可能会损伤外周神经。目前外科医生可用的主要信息是神经受刺激时其所支配肌肉收缩引起的肌电活动和神经对电刺激的反应，经颅骨刺激也可用于确认结构的完整性和监测脊髓功能。

圆锥肿瘤和马尾手术可能很复杂。在复杂性脊柱脂肪瘤手术中，神经生理监测是“必要的”（Pang，2015）。诱发肌电图建议使用同心刺激器，刺激速度为 10/s，刺激神经根的电流为 0.3~3 mA，刺激脊髓的电流最高为 2 mA。此外，应记录腓神经和胫后神经 SEP，包括括约肌在内的多块肌肉的肌电图和 MEP，括约肌也可用于球海绵体反射的监测（Skinner and Vodušek，2014）。

置入椎弓根螺钉时可能会破坏椎弓根壁。如果螺钉植入路径靠近神经根，沿该路径刺激或对螺钉刺激时，受到刺激的神经根所支配的肌肉可能会收缩。如果在靠中线处断裂且脊髓受到刺激时，在较低节段也能记录到刺激的反应。监测依赖于可靠的刺激和肌肉记录，须选择被检测神经支配的肌肉做记录点，且神经和肌肉必须功能良好。在肥胖患者中，如果成对的针电极无法准确插入肌肉中，信号记录可能会不准确。这个问题在胸椎手术中尤其突出。

参考文献、EBRAIN 的相关链接

扫描书末二维码获取。

第 72 章　卡压综合征

Grainne Bourke・Mobin Syed 著
伊骏飞 译，李良 审校

引言

周围神经卡压综合征很常见（**表 72.1**）。在上肢中，腕管综合征（carpal tunnel syndrome，CTS）约占卡压性神经病的 90%。在欧洲人口中，其年发病率为 0.1% ~0.35%，患病率为 1% ~7%（Bongers et al.，2007；Dang and Rodner，2009），远高于尺神经综合征（0.03%）、桡神经综合征（0.003%）或感觉神经痛（4.3/1 万人·年）（Nordstrom et al.，1998；van Slobbe et al.，2004；Latinovic et al.，2006）。由于 CTS 在工作年龄人口中高发，因此其对经济有显著的影响（Foley et al.，2007）。

病生理机制

周围神经通过特定的行径到达其外周的靶器官。这些由骨骼、韧带、纤维管、肌肉腱膜和筋膜所组成的通路，可能阻碍有效的神经滑动，或成为神经受压的潜在病因。例如，在肘关节屈伸过程中，肘管的"滑轮系统"（内侧肌间隔、Struthers 弓、内上髁沟和尺侧腕屈肌肌腱）使尺神经在肘部周围可滑动偏移 9.8 mm，在前臂为 14.5 mm（Wilgis and Murphy，1986）。我们也是通过分离这些结构以缓解神经压迫。

表 72.1　上肢卡压性神经病和卡压点

神经	部位：卡压综合征	卡压解剖结构
正中神经	手腕：腕管	腕横韧带下
	前臂近端：旋前圆肌综合征	卡压在旋前圆肌的两个头之间或指浅屈肌的纤维弓
骨间前神经	前臂近端：骨间前神经	卡压在旋前圆肌的两个头之间或指浅屈肌的纤维弓
尺神经	手腕	Guyon 管
	上臂 / 肘：肘管	尺侧腕屈肌的两个头之间，Osborne 韧带，Struthers 弓形组织
桡神经	前臂 / 肘：骨间后神经卡压	旋后肌两个头之间的 Froshe 弓

实验已证实，神经压迫可引起继发于压力的解剖畸形和神经外血流量改变。改变程度取决于压迫的大小和持续时间。早期改变为神经内水肿，影响神经内转运。神经内压升高会引起微循环障碍，导致神经间断缺血。临床上，这些微观解剖的变化与间歇性感觉异常和感觉阈值升高相关（Ochoa et al.，1972；Rempel et al.，1999；Mackinnon，2002）。

进行性压迫会导致局部脱髓鞘，引起持续的感觉异常、麻木和活动灵活性改变。压力持续增高将引起弥漫性脱髓鞘和轴突变性，临床上表现为肌萎缩、不可逆性的感觉异常和疼痛（Rempel et al.，1999）。

神经穿过关节时神经内部和包绕在神经周围的结缔组织会增加。这种变化也可能会导致压迫，因为周围神经袖的血流改变会引其纤维化和增厚，从而加重神经压迫症状并干扰正常的神经内外滑动机制（Rempel et al.，1999；Mackinnon，2002）。

双重卡压

Upton 和 McComas 于 1973 年首先提出双重卡压的概念：神经全长上的一处压迫虽然不足以引起症状，但会使神经更易受第二个压迫部位的影响。这两个水平上的压迫共同产生症状。减轻其中一个部位的神经压迫可能足以缓解症状，传统上认为应首先解决远端的问题（Upton and McComas，1973）。

腕管综合征

病因学

大多数 CTS 是特发性的。从组织学上看，这些患者表现为神经水肿增加，非炎症性的纤维化。在腕横纹以远 1 cm 处的压力最大，对应腕横韧带的最厚点（Ikeda et al.，2006）。有研究认为，其他一些局灶性病因也可能会增加腕管内压力：脂肪瘤、神经节、血管瘤和解剖变异，如蚓状肌起源过高，掌短肌或永存正中动脉。

糖尿病、类风湿性关节炎、甲状腺功能减退、肢端肥大症和慢性肾衰竭等全身性疾病会增加腕管综合征的易感性。在儿童中需注意除外黏多糖贮积症。怀孕是暂时性的危险因素，高达 45% 的妊娠晚期女性会出现症状。

腕管的解剖

腕管是一个以腕骨和腕横韧带为边界的骨纤维管道，其中腕横韧带为致密的筋膜结构，尺侧附于钩骨和三角骨，桡侧附于大多角骨结节和舟骨结节。正中神经与指深、浅屈肌腱和拇长屈肌腱共同穿行其中，由前臂走行至手掌。了解正中神经的解剖变异在神经松解术中非常重要。据报道，正中神经运动支和手掌感觉支的解剖变异很大，可能有 3 种形式穿过腕横韧带，以韧带外最常见（46%~90 %），其次是韧带下（31%）和韧带内穿出（23）%。

临床症状

CTS 的诊断主要根据临床症状、客观体征和诱发诊断试验（**表** 72.2）。典型症状包括夜间麻木，严重时患者可从睡眠中痛醒，正中神经支配区的刺痛感和鱼际肌无力。改变腕管压力 / 容积比的动作（例如在驾驶时握住方向盘或在阅读时握着书）也会诱发出类似的症状。2006 年，Graham 等（Graham et al.，2006）（**专栏** 72.1）验证了临床诊断标准的专家共识。

最常用的诱发性试验可能是 Tinel-Hoffmann 征——在叩击时出现神经支配区域的麻木不适感。这种检查的敏感性较差，但特异性较高（即，如果患者的 Tinel 体征阳性又有 CTS 病史，则很可能患有 CTS），但是 Tinel 征阴性并不能排除该诊断（Davis and Chung，2004）。其他诱发诊断试验包括 Phalen 试验，反向 Phalen 试验和 Durkan 试验（**表** 72.2）。测试感觉阈值的 Semmes-Weinstein 单细试验和评估两点辨识觉也是有用的检查感觉的方法（Gelberman et al.，1983）。这些检查可能会显示手掌区域感觉无异常，因为支配手掌感觉的掌皮支不穿过腕管。

检查

建立研究模型时应排除其他疾病（如颈神经根

表 72.2 常见的诱发性试验

神经	卡压点	诱发性试验和阳性表现
正中神经	腕管综合征	• Tinel-Hoffmann 征：在腕管区叩击时出现正中神经支配区域的感觉症状（circa 1915） • Phalen 征：前臂直立位时屈曲手腕，在 1 分钟内出现症状（1966） • 反 Phalen 征：伸直手腕，症状在 1 分钟内缓解 • Durkan 征：直接压迫腕管，30 秒内出现桡侧手指症状。使用校准器时敏感度为 89%，特异度为 96%（1994）
	前臂近端	• 旋前肌征：症状在肘伸直前臂抗阻抗旋前时出现 • 肱二头肌腱膜纤维化：症状在抗阻抗屈肘时出现 • 指浅屈肌腱弓：症状在中指抗阻抗屈曲时出现
尺神经	Guyon 管	• 压迫 Guyon 管近端 • 反 Phalen 征：伸直手腕，症状在 1 分钟内缓解
	肘管	• Tinel 征：敲击肘管在尺神经支配的手指中产生感觉症状 • 屈肘 • 压迫肘管近端

专栏 72.1 无加权的临床诊断标准清单

正中神经支配区的麻木和刺痛感
夜间麻木
鱼际肌的无力和（或）萎缩
Tinel 征
Phalen 试验
两点辨别觉消失
改善 / 加剧因素 *
夹具和（或）类固醇注射后改善
驾驶和手部用力等活动后加重
共病情况 *
妊娠
糖尿病
甲状腺功能减退

* 这些因素在 logistic 回归模型中无显著性。
Reprinted from *The Journal of Hand Surgery*, Volume 31, issue 6, Brent Graham, Glenn Regehr, Gary Naglie, James G. Wright, Development and Validation of Diagnostic Criteria for Carpal Tunnel Syndrome, pp. 919.e1–7, Copyright (2006), with permission from Elsevier.

病、周围神经病变），并评估易感疾病（如甲状腺功能减退、糖尿病和炎性关节炎）。检查项目包括血液检查、电生理检查和影像学。

电生理检查可协助临床诊断。然而，该检查只有在患者存在脱髓鞘或轴突丢失时才呈阳性。在间歇性缺血和可逆性传导阻滞中，神经传导速度并无异常。而在糖尿病患者中，神经传导速度的结果常更为异常。

目前已有通过电生理对CTS分级的研究。神经传导速度的结果与临床症状评分有相关性。疾病严重程度与较高年龄组之间的相关性已被证实，同时轻型疾病在年轻女性中更为常见（Padua et al.，1997；Bland，2000）。

在临床中，神经传导速度检查可应用于既往病史和临床评估提示CTS但无法定论时，也可在CTS中确认诊断。

超声作为一种无创检查方式，在腕管综合征中的应用已被认可。通过超声可测量横截面积、神经弹性，观察局部组织运动情况，用多普勒可测定神经周围血流特征。该检查的灵敏度已达到97.9%，不亚于神经传导速度（85%）（McDonagh et al.，2015）。

MRI可用于评价异常的正中神经或腕管解剖，包括神经内外肿瘤和血管异常。磁共振弥散张量成像的作用尚在评估中，暂无定论。

治疗

非手术治疗

对基础疾病（如炎症性关节炎）的非手术治疗可以缓解某些患者的症状。与肢端肥大症相关的CTS，当原发病治愈后，大多数CTS症状在6周内可缓解。

腕关节支具固定等非手术治疗可有效地缓解症状，在怀孕女性和症状早期的青年女性中效果良好。但是，夜间支具固定与其他治疗方式相比的获益尚缺乏足够证据支持（Page et al.，2012）。

有研究表明甲强龙注射液可在注射后10周内缓解症状，但在一项随机安慰剂对照研究中，75%的患者在类固醇注射后1年内仍进行了手术减压（Atroshi et al.，2013）。

还有某些其他非手术疗法在临床试用中，包括激光疗法、离子导入疗法、电疗法、热疗法、利尿剂和非甾体抗炎药；然而，这些治疗尚没有足够的证据支持。

注射治疗

这是一项无菌操作。正中神经靠近腕横纹，位于桡侧腕屈肌和掌长肌之间深部。掌皮支在桡侧从正中神经分出，靠近神经走行，但不进入腕管（**图72.1**）。

使用1 ml类固醇和1 ml局部麻醉剂。最常使用10 mg/ml的曲安奈德。在腕横纹水平，用细针以30°角从掌长肌腱尺侧进入。回吸以确认针尖不在血管内。推注时应没有阻力。请患者告知是否感到刺痛或疼痛，出现上述症状表明针尖可能位于神经内，需及时撤回。注射并发症包括类固醇混合物误放于神经内和血管内，这两者均会导致严重的后遗症。

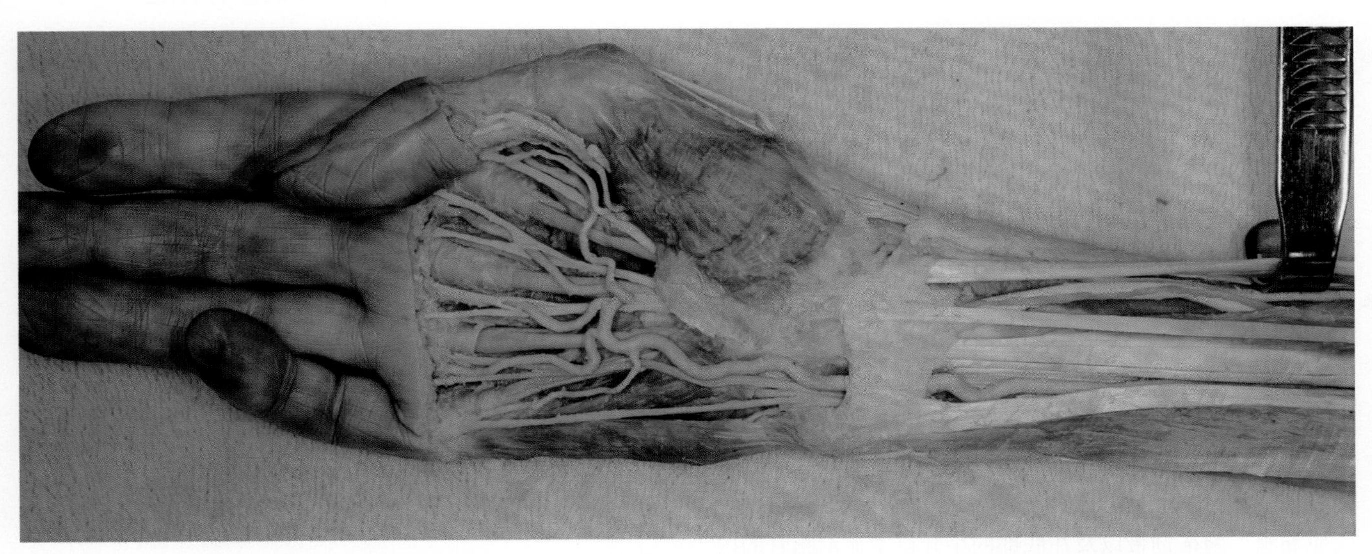

图72.1　正中神经（黄色）靠近腕横纹，位于桡侧腕屈肌和掌长肌之间深部。掌皮支（紫色）在桡侧从正中神经分出，不进入腕管

手术治疗

手术治疗长用于非手术治疗效果不佳或出现进展性神经压迫症状（即感觉丧失或运动障碍）时。手术涉及松解腕横韧带，可以通过开放手术或内镜行腕管减压术。

最常用的术式是开放的腕管减压术。在成人中，这是一种局部麻醉手术，在有无肾上腺素的情况下均可进行。在手术后期需要使用止血带，以确保术野中结构良好的可见性。

在腕横韧带上方做一个切口，该切口与环指屈曲时桡侧边界一致，平行于鱼际纹由近侧延伸至远端腕横纹。直视下分开腕横韧带时，使用自动拉钩牵开皮肤和软组织（**图 72.2**）。这种方式能够识别所有的解剖变异，并避免损伤运动支。用可吸收的缝线进行单层皮肤缝合。可使用简单的敷料以保留手部完整的活动度，但通常会在手术部位上局部施压，并建议患者在接下来的 48 小时内举起手。

1989 年，Chow 首次使用两个切口行内镜下腕管减压术。这种技术的获益立时可见：恢复快、疤痕小和术后疼痛轻（Chow，1989）。Agee 改良了手术技术，以单切口观察前屈肌腱滑膜和腕横韧带的 plane（Agee et al.，1994）。该手术可以在局部浸润麻醉下进行，但区域麻醉可能更常见。

腕管减压术：开放还是内镜

这两种技术都有广泛的应用，哪种方式更好仍存在争议。不同医疗机构在决定最合适的手术方式时要考虑的主要因素包括并发症、重返工作的时间、设备成本、手术时间和技术专长。

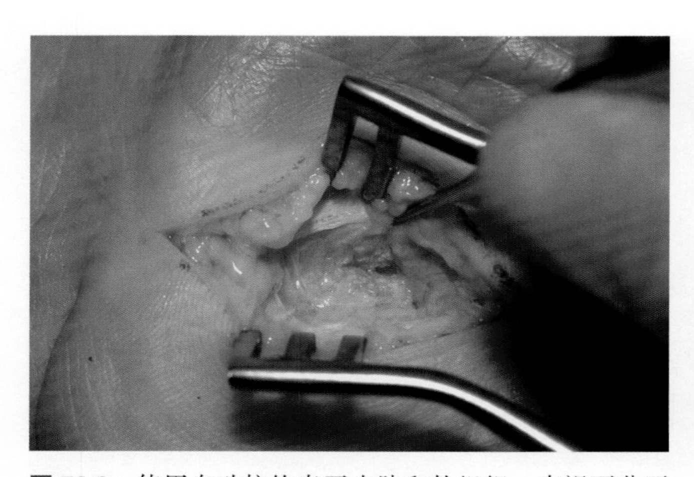

图 72.2 使用自动拉钩牵开皮肤和软组织，直视下分开腕横韧带。从表层到深部逐层分离：皮肤、皮下脂肪、掌长肌筋膜、腕横韧带以及在底部的小开口中显示腕管的内容物

既往研究认为，内镜下腕管减压术的神经血管并发症的发生率更高，学习曲线更陡峭。但近期的一个多中心系统研究和 meta 分析并不支持“并发症发生率更高”的结论（Vasiliadis et al.，2015）。内镜下腕管减压术的患者可以更早地恢复工作，疤痕触痛更少，术后握力更好。患者术后确实有更多的暂时性的神经系统症状，但两者在术后 6 个月的效果并无差异（Sayegh and Strauch，2015）。

如果不考虑内镜下腕管减压术中所使用的设备的成本，那么这两种手术的成本没有实质性的区别（Sayegh and Strauch，2015）。但是，在工作人群组中，两者复工的时间有统计学差异（内镜组早 8 天），这使内镜对行业确实具有成本优势（Saw et al.，2003）。如果有适当的设备和内镜专业人员，对有早复工需求的患者而言，应考虑使用内镜下腕管减压术。

预后和并发症

总体而言，75% 的外科减压术患者预后良好，8% 的患者病情恶化。接受类固醇注射的患者初始有效率为 70%，但随着时间延长会复发，再次注射类固醇可能同样有效（Bland，2007）。在超过 70 岁的人群中，减压并不能完全缓解症状或恢复功能，但患者主诉症状有显著缓解（Leit et al.，2004）。

开放性腕管减压术最常见的并发症是约有 25% 的患者诉瘢痕疼痛，其次是瘢痕僵硬和肿胀。其他有报告的并发症包括运动支、掌支或正中神经主干损伤和肌腱粘连。大约有 20% 的患者有复发。

肘管综合征

病因学

肘管综合征是继 CTS 之后第二大最常见的卡压性神经病。它是肘部最常见的嵌压性神经病，在男性中更为常见。发病率为 20.9/10 万人 · 年（Mondelli et al.，2005）。吸烟是一种危险因素，这可能与其对微循环的病生理影响有关，而不是吸烟时肘部活动的机械作用的结果（Bartels and Verbeek，2007）。在年轻的行政管理人员中较常见后上髁卡压，在体力劳动者中则为肱尺腱膜卡压（Omejec and Podnar，2016）。增加易感性的系统性疾病与 CTS 的状况类似。

解剖

最近端的卡压点的是 Struthers 弓形组织，它距肱骨内上髁近端约 8 cm，是由臂部深筋膜延伸至内侧肌间隔的增厚的筋膜。尺侧副韧带从尺侧腕屈肌（flexor carpi ulnaris，FCU）延伸至 Osborne 韧带底）构成肘管的后侧壁（即顶）。神经通道在 FCU 的两个头和屈肌 - 旋前肌深腱膜之间延续（**图** 72.3）。

临床表现

临床症状包括小指、环指尺侧和手背尺侧的刺痛或感觉异常。患者抱怨从睡眠中麻醒，屈肘时症状加重。晚期表现为尺神经支配区的手指感觉丧失和手内在肌萎缩。后者可用以鉴别卡压是源自近端的肘部或远端的手腕 Guyon 管。诊断依靠临床症状，通过诱发性试验证实（**表** 72.2）。

检查

排除潜在的系统性疾病的研究如前 CTS 中所述。有意义的影像检查包括 X 射线、超声和 MRI。这些检查不仅有助于确定神经的解剖结构，而且有助于排除骨骼畸形、肿瘤和其他引起压迫的软组织异常。

结合短节段神经传导速度检查与超声检查，可将卡压定位于内上髁后神经沟或肱尺弓内（Omejec and Podnar，2016）

治疗

非手术治疗

非手术治疗方法包括夹板固定、物理治疗和活动矫正。在没有肌萎缩或持续性麻木的情况下可选择以上治疗方法。有约一半接受治疗的患者症状会得到缓解（Dellon，1989）。

手术治疗

有肌无力、持续麻木或症状明显的患者，如采用非手术治疗无法改善症状，则应接受手术治疗。

手术在局部或区域麻醉下借助止血带进行。手术选择包括单纯减压术（开放或内镜下）、尺神经前置术（肌下或皮下）和内上髁切除术。

所有手术的共同点是重建神经解剖通道，以使其更容易滑动并消除潜在或实际卡压的因素。从近端到远端按照如下顺序依次松解神经：Struthers 韧带，Osborne 韧带、FCU 筋膜。在神经的解剖通道中沿其全长分离尺神经，从而确保了对 FCU 的分支和前臂内侧及后侧皮神经的保护。

关于手术技术以及原位减压 *vs*. 神经前置术，神经前置部位的选择（肌下、肌内或皮下）之间存在重大争议。研究表明，在适用神经前置术的情况下，原位减压也能取得相同的结果。如果减压后神经在肘屈曲时存在半脱位的倾向，则可考虑神经前置术，因为原位减压联合神经前置术的成功率超过 90%。

内镜下减压术

研究认为，内镜下肘管减压术切口小，其预后和并发症与开放手术类似，同时避免了较大的疤痕，并具有早复工作的好处。然而，目前尚无此方面更大的随机研究。

内上髁切除术

King 和 Morgan 最早报道应用此方法治疗创伤

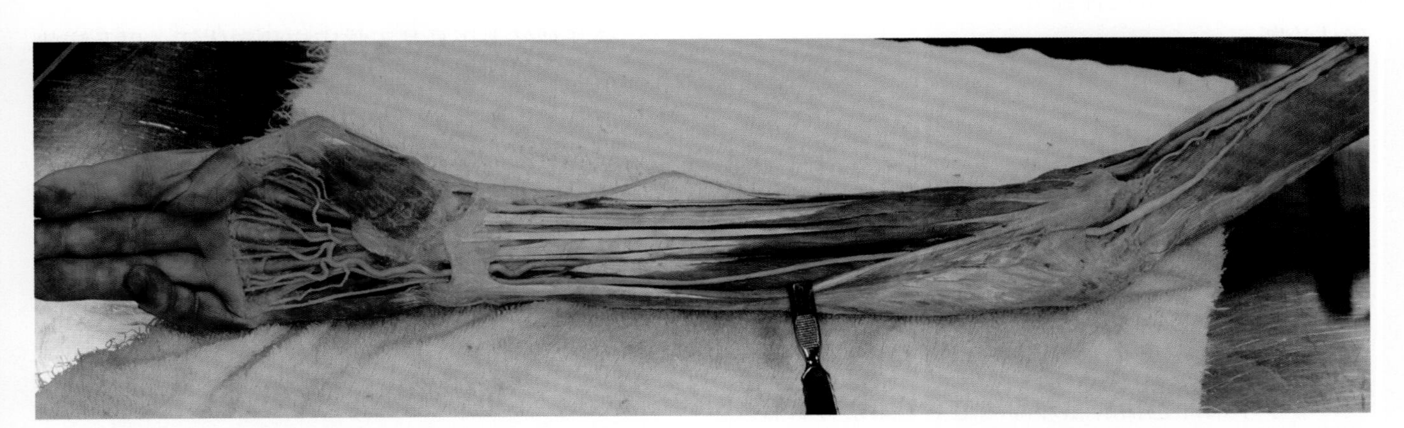

图 72.3 尺神经穿行于手臂的屈肌和伸肌间，穿过内上髁沟，内上髁沟顶部被移除以充分暴露。尺神经于尺侧腕屈肌两个头之间进入前臂

后尺神经炎，随后应用于治疗肘管综合征。这种方法背后的理念是，它可以允许一定程度的神经前置，同时避免会牵拉尺神经的明显切除。尸体研究显示，与单纯减压相比，内上髁骨切除术治疗后的尺神经张力明显降低（Hicks and Toby，2002）。过度切除特别是切除一部分内侧副韧带后，会导致内侧肘关节不稳定（Efstathopoulos et al.，2006）。手术包括在肘关管内松解尺神经，骨膜下暴露内上髁，以及切除根尖部分（20%），确认保留内侧副韧带的附着点。据报道，高达 45% 的患者在内上髁切除术后出现持续性肘部疼痛。

感觉异常性股痛

病因学

股外侧皮神经在经过骨盆走行至大腿外侧的过程中的卡压被称为麻痹性痛感，在男性和超重的人群中更常见。

神经穿过筋膜时解剖变异性大，因此在体位变化时易于受到压迫。见于脊柱外科手术俯卧位后以及从髂嵴和前骨盆取移植骨块的手术后。

临床表现

患者在大腿前外侧处出现疼痛、刺痛和感觉异常。外侧皮神经为纯感觉神经，因此仅有感觉症状和体征。衣服或皮带的外源性压力、髋关节过伸和长时间站立会加剧症状。

诱发性试验可再现刺痛和疼痛，例如 Tinel-Hoffmann 测试——在神经走行邻近髂前上棘时压迫神经。另一种有用的诊断性测试是将一些局部麻醉剂注入 Tinel-Hoffmann 测试阳性的部位。如果患者随后症状缓解并出现神经分布区的麻木感，则可以确认诊断。

检查

该病是临床诊断。然而，由于临床评估尚无定论，神经传导速度和超声检查目前是最有用的诊断工具。其他的影像学检查（如 MRI）有助于排除脊髓近端的神经压迫、神经内和神经外肿瘤的鉴别诊断。

非手术治疗

非手术治疗包括解除外部压迫（例如紧身衣服或皮带）、减肥和消炎药。

超声不仅可以用于诊断，还可以作为治疗手段。通过超声引导可直接或间接注射类固醇（Onat et al.，2016）。

手术治疗

非手术治疗失败且持续存在明显症状的患者可采用手术治疗。手术治疗也适用于盆腔手术后出现症状的患者。

手术在诊断和治疗中都起着重要作用。探查和神经松解是有效的。如果神经被束缚或包埋在瘢痕组织中，则应考虑植入可增加神经滑动潜力的正常组织。

既往研究认为，在某些情况下，神经切除术与神经松解术一样有效（de Ruiter and Kloet，2015）。

其他卡压性神经病

在临床中还可以看到其他卡压性神经病，包括桡神经卡压（桡管综合征、骨间背侧神经麻痹），肘部正中神经卡压和 Guyon 管处尺神经受压（Kumar and Bourke，2016）。在肩带附近肩胛上神经和胸长神经等近端神经也容易受压。由于没有皮肤感觉成分可协助评估，且患者表现为活动时加剧的肩部疼痛，因此这种卡压更隐匿。这些较不常见的卡压综合征不在本章内详细讨论。

总结

腕管综合征和肘管综合征等神经卡压综合征很常见，可出现所有年龄段中。该病影响工作人群，且需要在手术后请假以恢复和进行康复训练，因此有一定经济负担。

诊断神经卡压是基于临床症状和体征，以及症状和体征的延伸。超声可能是当前临床实践中最有用的影像手段，因为它可以在运动过程中动态评估。电生理检查也很有价值，但最好用作临床检查的辅助。

延伸阅读、参考文献

扫描书末二维码获取。

第 73 章 锁骨上臂丛神经和周围神经损伤

Jonathan Perera・Marco Sinisi 著
沈胜利 译，李良 审校

引言

锁骨上臂丛神经（supraclavicular brachial plexus，SBP）损伤非常罕见，通常与外伤相关。SBP 损伤（SBP injury，SBPi）不仅会导致严重的身体障碍，也会引发心理和羞耻感问题。

流行病学

由于全球差异、报道不足和对轻型损伤的认识缺乏，外伤性臂丛神经损伤（brachial plexus injury，BPi）发病率极难确定。Goldie 和 Coates（1992）曾报道英国每年约发生 500 例臂丛神经损伤，主要由道路交通事故导致。

Keep 在 2013 年指出，随着道路安全性整体提高，英国高能交通事故幸存者数量正逐步增加。1990—2012 年间，道路交通事故死亡人数减少了 66%，重伤人数减少了 62%。大多数 SBPi 由机动车碰撞导致，在大多数报道中该比例高达 60%（Allieu and Cenac，1988；Azze et al.，1994；Doi et al.，2000）。回顾现有数据，SBPi 主要是年轻男性由高能量多发伤摩托车事故所致，并与长骨骨折和头部损伤相关。在英国，摩托车手虽然只占道路通行总人数的 1%，却占道路死亡 / 重伤总人数的 20%，每年约 7000 人重伤（Clarke et al.，2003；Rhee et al.，2011；Keep and Rutherford，2013）。尽管这些事件数目很大，SBPi 却只占多发伤患者的 1%，Allieu 在 1988 年报道其年发生率为 0.3/100000~6.3/100000。

Narakas 的七法则

关于 BPi 有 7 个“70% 统计数据”，即 70% 的病例与道路交通事故有关，70% 的事故是摩托车手，70% 的患者是复合伤，70% 的病灶在锁骨上，70% 的病灶涉及至少一处神经根撕脱伤，70% 的撕脱伤发生在 C7、C8 或 T1 神经根，70% 的神经根撕脱伤患者会发展为慢性痛（Narakas，1985）。

损伤机制

与所有医学诊断一样，SBPi 的类型和严重程度可以通过准确的病史来诊断。理解受伤机制至关重要，其重点包括解剖、力的大小和力的矢量。神经拉伸超过 12% 或缺血超过 8 小时将导致严重的神经损伤。颈神经根撕裂仅需 200 N 大小的力。神经根发出时走行的角度非常重要，因为受到撞击时上半身处于不同位置会产生不同矢量的力，从而造成不同的损伤。一种典型的损伤是手臂和头 / 颈部之间被拉开，手臂被水平拉向下方将导致上神经丛损伤，而手臂被水平拉向上方则导致下神经丛损伤。

肩关节脱位是一种严重的损伤，是锁骨上或锁骨下臂丛神经（infraclavicular brachial plexus，ICBP）损伤的危险因素。损伤通常发生在上干，主要累及肩胛上神经和腋神经。许多复合伤患者中都存在一条连接胸小肌和胸壁的异常筋膜带，这使得 SBP 汇入 ICBP 的空间减小，进而导致这些患者更易受伤。以平均 70 kg 的男性为例，假设减速时间为 1 s 多，则很容易计算出产生上述大小力所需的起始速度。如果力正好施加在 SBP 上，要想撕裂神经根，仅需 2.24 m/s（5 mph）的起始速度。

解剖和损伤分类

臂丛神经由 C5~T1 共 5 条脊神经组成。神经根由脊髓发出，在颈后三角形成上干（C5~C6）、中干（C7）和下干（C8~T1），见图 73.1。有时 C4 或 T2 亦会参与其构成而分别被称为“前置型”或“后置型”。

SBP 位于锁骨上部，包括臂丛的根、干和股，但不包括束和支，后两者属于 ICBP。SBPi 也包括更近端的损伤，因此也根据损伤部位在背根神经节（dorsal root ganglion，DRG）的近端或远端而分为神经节前或节后损伤。

Birch 在 2011 年将节前损伤分为 5 类。A 型，过渡区（transitional zone，TZ）中心的撕脱伤；B1 型，TZ 远端的损伤；B2 型，有完整的硬膜套；B3 型，椎管内的神经根断裂，无 DRG 移位或硬膜破裂；B4 型，局限于背根或腹根的撕脱伤（**图 73.1**）。

神经撕脱伤患者的 DRG 并未受损，因此感觉神经不会发生沃勒变性，这类患者也不会出现 Tinel 征阳性（Tinel，1915）。直接和间接神经损伤可通过 Seddon 分类进一步细分（Seddon，1942），见**专栏 73.1**。该分类适用于轴突损伤，而非整条神经的损伤。Sunderland 分类（Sunderland，1951）将 Seddon 分类中的第Ⅲ类进一步细分为三级：保留神经束膜、保留神经外膜和神经完全横断，因此将神经损伤共分为 1~5 级。

Erb 氏点是指 C5 和 C6 神经根汇成臂丛神经上干的部位，位于胸锁乳突肌后缘中点，颈丛神经的皮支（枕小神经、耳大神经、颈横神经和锁骨上神经）均从此处向浅表走行。这在临床上非常重要，因为

专栏 73.1 神经损伤分类

Ⅰ类：神经失用，无解剖连续性中断、支持结构完整的神经传导功能障碍。
预后：数天或数周内快速、完全恢复正常。

Ⅱ类：轴索断裂，轴突及其髓鞘连续性破坏，神经内膜完整
预后：多变，一般良好，近端损伤和无法再植入肌肉的损伤预后较差。

Ⅲ类：神经断裂 - 神经全层的破坏。若不进行适当的手术干预则没有恢复的可能性。是整条神经的完全断裂或破坏。
预后：预后差，尤其是未进行干预时；通常不能完全恢复。

Reproduced with permission from H. J. Seddon, A Classification of Nerve Injuries, *The BMJ*, Volume 2, issue 237, Copyright © 1942 BMJ Publishing Group Ltd.

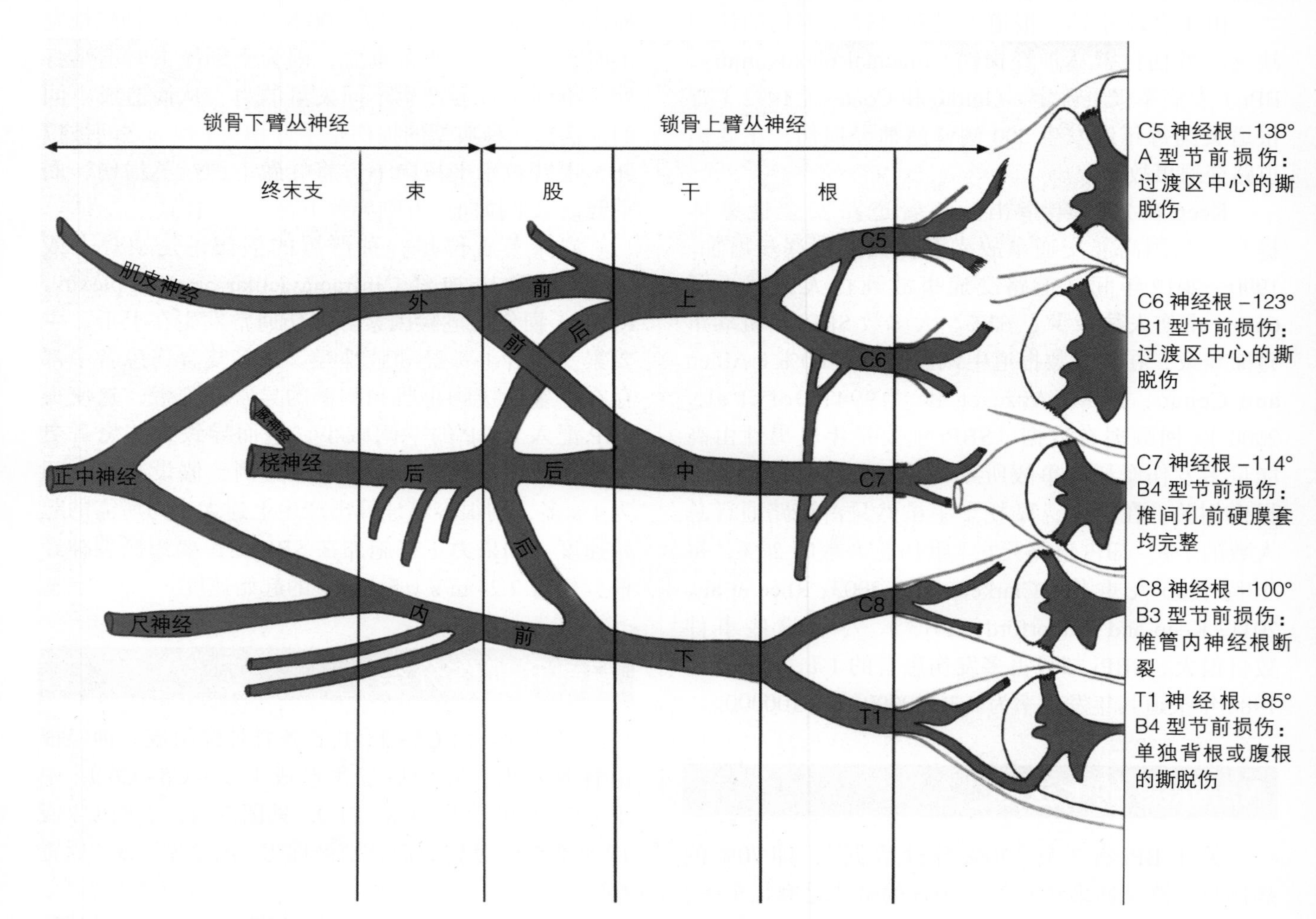

图 73.1 臂丛神经、神经根、神经根角度及不同类型节前神经撕脱伤示意图
Courtesy of Mr Jonathan R. Pereta.

施加在上半身和头颈部的力在此汇聚，常导致 SBPi。全神经丛损伤，尤其是累及下神经丛的 SBPi，通常与 Horner 综合征（上睑下垂、瞳孔缩小、无汗和眼球内陷）有关。这是由于节前损伤以及直接的脊髓、头部或血管损伤会同时导致交感干损伤，如 Rhee 在 2011 年所述。其他损伤有时会加重症状、混淆诊断或被遗漏，包括腋动脉损伤、锁骨下和椎动静脉损伤、骨折、脱位和上半身的肌肉损伤。

临床表现

SBPi 节前损伤、SBPi 节后损伤和 ICBPi 三种损伤类型可单独或联合出现。

节前损伤或撕脱伤的典型表现是在感觉障碍的手臂上出现挤压性的、持续的剧烈刺痛。疼痛通常沿着受损脊神经的皮节分布。Kato 在 2006 年曾报道，超过 50% 的撕脱伤患者在伤后 24 小时内出现明显疼痛，90% 的患者在伤后 6 周内出现明显疼痛。节前损伤的患者 Tinel 征阴性，其他体征包括神经根水平或周围神经分支（胸长神经、肩胛背神经和膈神经）受损以及相应肌肉的功能障碍。

与 SBPi 患者相反，神经节后损伤患者 Tinel 征阳性、无 Horner 综合征、无前锯肌、菱形肌和膈肌功能障碍，而且在神经传导试验中不产生感觉神经动作电位（sensory nerve action potentials，SNAPs）。Erb 氏麻痹或上臂丛神经病变（C5、C6）会出现一种被称为“服务员小费”的特征性姿势，即肩内收内旋、肘伸、前臂旋前。Klumpke 氏麻痹或下臂丛神经病变（C8、T1）则会出现肘屈、前臂旋后、手腕过伸和由于手部小肌群无力导致的爪形手。Erb 氏麻痹和 Klumpke 氏麻痹均分别被描述为源于肩部过压或过抬引起的产伤，但也可发生于成人，损伤机制类似。

检查

SBPi 的主要影像学检查包括磁共振成像（magnetic resonance imaging，MRI）、计算机断层扫描（computed tomography，CT）和脊髓造影术。

针对 SBP 和颈椎的磁共振成像对 SBPi 非常重要，但是传统 MRI 对 SBP 部分结果的解读仍有较大挑战。20 世纪 90 年代以来，有两项新的磁序列被研发并应用，即 Filler 等在 1993 年（Filler et al.，1993）提出的磁共振神经成像（magnetic resonance neurography，MRN）和 Ramsbacher 在 1997 年（Ramsbacher et al.，1997）提出的磁共振脊髓成像（magnetic resonance myelography，MRM）。这些序列可用来评估 SBPi 中的节前和节后神经。MRN 需要 3T 及以上的 MRI 机器，为周围神经非侵入性成像提供了一种极佳的方法。MRM 可用来检测节前 SBP，亦是非侵入性的，而且在检测神经损伤方面和传统的脊髓造影术效果相当。MRM 不需要向椎管内注入造影剂，也无辐射。综合应用这两种成像技术可革命性地改变 SBPi 的诊疗过程，特别是在非专科中心。

CT 和 CT 血管造影术也是非常重要的影像学检查手段，尤其是对于多发伤患者。大多数创伤单位都能在事故和急诊科附近快速、方便地进行这些扫描。一旦患者稳定下来，就可以安全地进行扫描以判断有无危及生命和肢体的损伤。血管损伤和（或）血肿在 SBPi 中很常见，这会导致 SBP 周围显著的纤维化反应，再加上原发损伤，如果不进行手术干预，将足以导致永久的神经传导障碍。

传统使用 X 线透视的脊髓造影术和 CT 脊髓造影术都需要硬膜内注射。脊髓造影术对评估神经根撕脱和寻找继发的脑脊膜膨出和假性脑脊膜膨出非常有用。由于下颈椎和上胸椎产生的伪影，SBP 的下神经根较难分辨。

X 线片

X 线片是一种快速简便的影像学技术，例如，胸部 X 片可以显示半膈抬高，进而表明膈神经损伤和胸部创伤。颈椎 X 片可显示横突骨折进而提示神经根撕脱伤。上半身 X 片可以显示肱骨、肩胛骨、锁骨骨折以及肩带损伤，这都和 SBPi 和 ICBPi 有关。

电诊断检查

对于 SBPi 来说，电诊断检查是系统的感觉运动功能检查和影像学检查的极佳辅助手段。与其他检查方法类似，电诊断也需要有经验的临床医生去进行检查并准确解读。主要的检查方法包括肌电图（electromyography，EMG）和神经传导检测（nerve conduction studies，NCS），见**表** 73.1。肌电图用于检测肌肉在静息和活动状态下的电活动。失神经支配肌肉的变化最早在损伤后 1 周即可观察到（Dumitru and Zwarts，2005），且这种变化可被检测到的速度与神经长度成反比。轴突越长，沃勒变性需要的时间就越长，因此近端肌肉很快就能出现 EMG 改变，而远端肌肉则需要 3~6 周才会出现失神经支配改变。当神经损伤较重时，可立即出现 EMG 改变，但只有经验丰富的神经生理学家才能检测出来。EMG 和 NCS 都能显示受损的神经节段，但无法显示轴突横断。SNAPs 和运动单位动作电位（motor unit action

表 73.1 神经损伤的 EMG 和 NCS 大致表现

	传导速度	MUAPs	CMAPs	SNAPs	注意
神经失用	正常	无	正常，近端稍弱	减弱	节间变薄导致永久性传导减慢
轴索断裂	降低	无	与轴突损失成比例减弱	减弱	正向尖波和纤颤
神经断裂	无	无	与轴突损失成比例减弱	无	

potentials，MUAPs）是判断节前和节后神经损伤的重要手段。损伤位于背根神经节近端时 SNAPs 得以保留，因此节前损伤时 SNAPs 正常而 MUAPs 异常（**表** 73.1）。

组胺试验

由于 BPi 影像和诊断技术的提高，该试验已不常规进行。正常情况下，皮内注射组胺会出现下述三联反应：由于直接的毛细血管扩张导致的红色反应，继而由于血管渗透性增加、液体渗出过多而出现风团，以及由于感觉神经分布区轴突反射介导的动脉扩张而引起的周围部位红色耀斑。

组胺试验可用于鉴别节前和节后损伤。节前损伤时传入轴突完整，因此会出现正常的伴有红色耀斑的三联反应。而节后损伤时感觉细胞体和轴突连接中断，传入轴突变性，因此只会出现前面的红色反应和风团，而没有红色耀斑。

治疗

开放性 SBPi 需要紧急处理，而闭合性 SBPi 患者手术时机尚有争议。早期干预的好处包括疼痛缓解和预后改善，尽管有时推迟手术时间有助于炎症消退（Kato et al.，2006；Birch，2011；Birch，2015；Hems，2015）。关于 SBPi 手术治疗一直存在两种主流思路，一种提倡早期手术，另一种提倡推迟手术直到所有急性期问题解决为止（Birch，2015；Hems，2015）。中间阶段受原发损伤炎症期的影响，往往会使预后变差（Hems，2015）。炎症期消退后的晚期修复则可改善预后（Hems，2015）。重建的主要目的是恢复最佳的上半身功能及缓解疼痛。Kato 等（2006）发现越早进行手术，患者的疼痛缓解越明显，部分原因是早期手术后功能恢复减轻了疼痛（**图** 73.2）。

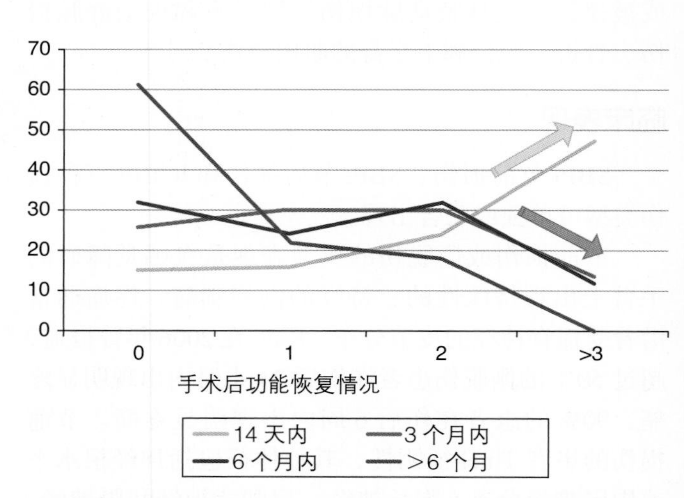

图 73.2 图示 SBPi 后 14 天内手术的患者与伤后 6 个月以上手术的患者结局有明显差异

Data from Birch R; 2011; Peripheral Nerve Injury Unit, Royal National Orthopaedic Hospital.

与开放性损伤一样，血管损伤也需紧急手术。出血、感染和血肿形成会导致严重的纤维化，严重者可导致正常组织层次消失，整个神经丛形成一堵瘢痕组织墙，导致无法手术。受伤病史非常重要，因为施加在 SBP 上的能量不同，损伤的严重程度以及可能的恢复程度也不同。所有的完全性损伤都需要手术探查，因为它们极不可能自行恢复。许多患者会出现疼痛，疼痛会使患者逐渐衰弱，影响他们后续的物理康复治疗及职业治疗。

采用工作或规律锻炼的注意力分散疗法能非常有效地缓解疼痛，而且日常生活越正常，效果越好（Birch，2015）。同等损伤程度下，越早回归工作的患者往往疼痛越轻、预后越好（Kato et al.，2016；Birch，2011）。疼痛的严重程度可以推断是否发生了撕脱伤（Parry，1980；Kato et al.，2006；Birch，2011）。

手术

体位和皮肤切口

患者采用公园长椅位，使用头圈，头略微伸展 5°～10°，并向对侧倾斜约 10°。为了使臂丛神经得到充分的暴露，头部位置的摆放非常重要，尤其是神经根水平，如果不伸展头部是无法达到的。通过倾斜分体式手术台将胸部抬高 30°，见**图** 73.3。为了在锁骨上区充分显露臂丛神经，我们认为行 Langer 氏

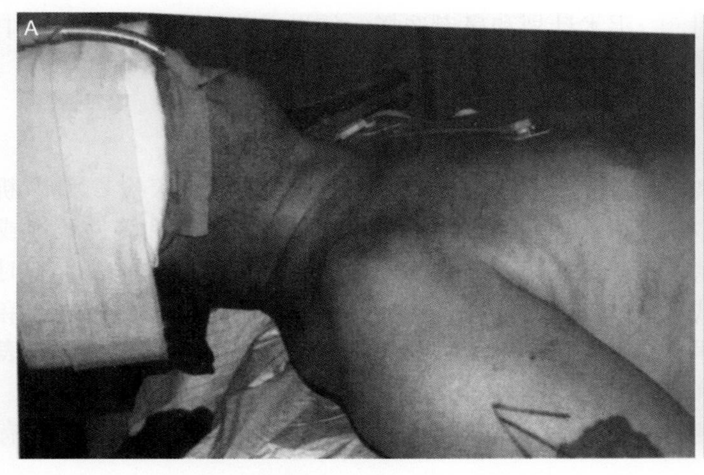

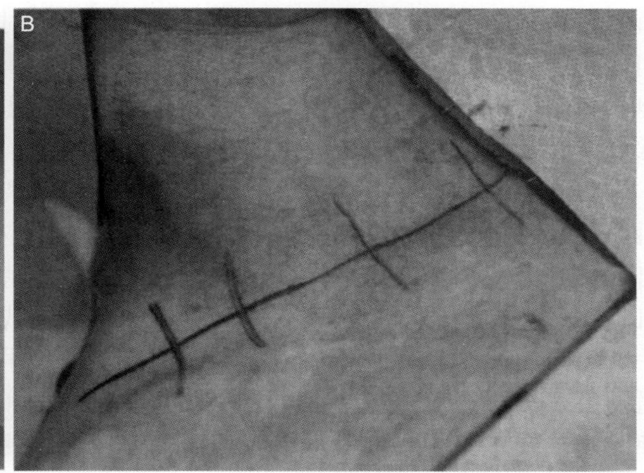

图 73.3　经锁骨上横入路显露臂丛神经患者体位摆放及标记切口线
Reproduced with permission of Medtronic, Inc.

线颈部切口即足够，即从锁骨内侧上方 1~2 cm 开始向后延伸 10~15 cm（Langer，1861）。这样可以避免沿胸锁乳突肌做切口，同时为从神经根水平到干及股水平分离神经丛提供了足够的空间。

从切开颈阔肌开始进行分离，并辨认出内侧的胸锁乳突肌前表面、颈丛的锁骨上分支、外侧的颈外静脉以及上方的耳大神经。分离结束后采用 Joll 氏甲状腺拉钩维持术野开放。

分离胸锁乳突肌和颈外静脉以游离静脉并向外牵拉静脉。有时需要游离、结扎和切断静脉。分离这些结构后，辨认其深方的肩胛舌骨肌，这是该区域唯一的横肌，需要将其从邻近结构上分离出来。随后将其用可吸收强力缝线缝合，以便在手术结束时将其修复。脂肪垫和颈横血管必须被切断并牵开。这些血管壁很薄，只能将其烫闭。有时这些血管会大得多，尤其是在淤血的情况下。

下一步是辨认膈神经，它位于前斜角肌的前表面。有时在臂丛外伤中，尤其是伤后数月时，该部位明显纤维化，很难分离。沿着膈神经游离可以找到 C5 神经根。

少数情况下，C6 也参与膈神经的组成。C5 神经根从椎间孔发出后，向后发出一分支支配菱形肌，即肩胛背神经，并在距起点 1~2 cm 的地方与 C6 汇合组成上干。在 C6 的下表面是胸长神经，它斜穿过中斜角肌，由 C5、C6、C7 以及偶尔还有 C8 的分支构成。

分离出 C5 和 C6 神经根后，在其后外侧可显示上干，正好位于肩胛上神经前后支前方，之后在其下方分离辨认中干和下干。肩胛背动脉在上干和中干之间横行走行，与神经丛相对。

中干和下干位于上干的下方和稍前方。为了在根部暴露这些神经干，需要分离部分前斜角肌。沿锁骨下动脉追踪非常关键，尤其是在严重外伤后有大量瘢痕组织时。锁骨下静脉在该水平位于前斜角肌前方、锁骨下动脉下方，所有横行穿过臂丛的静脉都起源于此。因此切勿过多牵拉这些静脉，否则它们可能会在汇入锁骨下静脉时损伤，甚至锁骨下静脉本身都可能受损。

分离出这三支主干后即可显露其前、后分股。上干和中干的前股共同组成前外侧束，下干的前股单独构成前内侧束，所有后股共同组成后束。

重建

SBPi 常用的重建技术包括直接修复、神经移位术和神经移植术，以恢复患者主要的上半身功能，其最终结果都是将可正常工作的神经或神经束转移到已丧失功能的神经上。神经移位术可有多种方式，但都受供体和受体神经位置的限制。神经移位术后患者有望获得至少 3 级的肌力（Medical Research Council，1976）。

常见的神经移位术包括将脊副神经转移至肩胛上或腋神经，桡神经束转移至腋神经、尺神经和（或）正中神经束转移至肌皮神经，以及将肋间神经转移至肌皮神经、腋神经、桡神经、正中神经或尺神经。常用的神经供体包括上臂和（或）前臂的内侧皮神经和腓肠神经。

神经根回植术应在伤后 4 周内完成。由于大部分损伤为外伤性撕脱，神经根本身已严重损伤，如不采用神经束移植，将无法进行直接修复。通常采用纤维蛋白胶或将神经与软膜缝合的方法来进行移植。伤后预期肌力弱于伤前，可能需要一年多的时间才能达到 MRC 分级肌力 3 级的水平。越远端的肌肉肌力越弱，但也存在腕部和手部功能几乎接近正常、结局极佳的案例（Htut et al.，2007）。

功能性游离肌肉移植术极少使用，它是将游离肌瓣连同其供血动脉、引流静脉及运动神经一起取出并移植到一个新的位置。常用的供体肌肉是股薄肌，在臂丛神经损伤中它被用来恢复肘关节屈曲或手指屈曲功能（即代替肱二头肌或指深屈肌）。手术通常由整形科医生进行，需要采用血管显微吻合和神经修复技术。考虑到手术风险，需要进行详细的手术计划和患者选择。如果成功的话，患者可从中获益并恢复 4 级的肌力（Doi et al.，1998）。

周围神经损伤

周围神经麻痹很常见，只要临床检查和诊断正确，治疗方法很简单。通常与急性和慢性压迫或者是外伤有关。正中神经和尺神经最常累及，有时也被称为远端臂丛神经损伤，桡神经和腓总神经麻痹亦同样重要。上述各神经的功能和表现总结于**表 73.2**。

一旦诊断明确，即可开始给予适当的治疗。有

表 73.2 上下肢重要神经压迫汇总表

神经	常见麻痹部位	受累肌肉	感觉	重点检查
正中神经（C5~T1）	胸三角筋膜 髁上突 +Struthers 韧带 腕管	蚓状肌 1 和 2 拇对掌肌 拇短展肌 拇短屈肌 大鱼际肌萎缩	桡侧为主，掌侧前三指	鱼际肌萎缩 Phalen 试验和 Durkin 试验
AIN（C5~T1）来自正中神经	Kiloh-Nevin FDS 浅弓 腱膜 旋前圆肌浅头	指深屈肌桡侧半 旋前方肌 拇长屈肌	n/a	无法做 OK 手势；内旋无力
尺神经（C8~T1）	肘管综合征（5 处） Guyon 管	蚓状肌 3 和 4 所有骨间肌 拇收肌 拇短屈肌深头 小鱼际肌萎缩	尺侧 / 第四指	Froments 征 小鱼际 + 第一 DIO 萎缩 Wartenberg 征和 Jeanne 征
桡神经（C5~T1）	副肩胛下 - 圆 - 阔肌 肩胛下动脉 三角间隙 外侧肌间隔	肱三头肌 肘肌 肱桡肌 桡侧腕长 / 短伸肌 旋后肌 整个后室、伸肌、拇长展肌	上臂外 / 后侧、肘部、手，主要是前三指的桡、背侧	典型的垂腕，取决于损伤平面
PIN 来自桡神经	桡管综合征	桡侧腕短伸肌（通常来自桡神经） 指总伸肌 小指伸肌 尺侧腕伸肌 旋后肌 拇长展肌 拇短伸肌 拇长伸肌 食指伸肌	支配腕囊背侧的感觉纤维，不累及皮肤	疼痛 手指掌伸无力 垂腕
腓总神经（L4~S2）	膝盖以上 腓骨颈 膝盖以下	深 前室：胫骨前肌、踇长伸肌、趾长伸肌、第三腓骨肌 浅 外侧室：腓骨短、长肌	腓肠外侧神经（L2~3）小腿 / 膝部外上部 腓浅神经（L4~S1）小腿和足背外侧缘 腓深神经（L4/5）仅累及第一趾	足下垂 TA、EHL 和趾长伸肌（extensor digitorum longus，EDL）不同程度的力弱

时候治疗方法相当简单，预后又好，但有些时候则不然。

通常需要进行手术治疗，尤其是在神经卡压部位出现非进展性的 Tinel 征阳性时。手术减压最为简便，操作得当时效果也最好，以腕管减压术效果最为明显。预后好的一大关键因素是需要配备一名优秀的健康专业人员（职业治疗师和理疗师），以帮助术后评估和康复锻炼。

修复术需要用细尼龙缝线和纤维蛋白胶在显微镜或手术放大镜下进行操作。可采用神经外膜修复术或神经束修复术。在有张力的情况下不能进行神经修复，因为会导致修复失败。这种情况下应进行神经移植术，通常采用腓肠神经或前臂皮神经，因为它们只是单纯的皮神经。在没有机会行直接修复或者距离过长的情况下，有不计其数的神经和肌腱可被用来转移以恢复肢体功能。

结论

SBPi 是一种严重的致残性疾病，通常累及年轻健康的成年患者。需要紧急转诊、评估和治疗才能获得最佳的预后。神经损伤在以前被认为是不可逆的，在现代快速干预的情况下已并非如此。因此，建议尽快将患者转诊至周围神经专家。

延伸阅读、参考文献

扫描书末二维码获取。

第 74 章　周围神经肿瘤

Rikin Trivedi · Vincent Nga 著
沈胜利 译，李良 审校

引言

周围神经鞘瘤（peripheral nerve sheath tumours，PNST）包含一组临床病理学分类明确的疾病，从良性肿瘤到高级别恶性周围神经鞘瘤（malignant peripheral nerve sheath tumours，MPNST）。虽然大多数 PNSTs 为散发，但仍有一些众所周知存在遗传倾向的肿瘤，如神经纤维瘤病 1 型（neurofibromatosis type 1，NF1）、神经纤维瘤病 2 型（neurofibromatosis type 2，NF2）、神经鞘瘤病和 Carney 综合征（Carney complex）（Rodriguez et al.，2012）。

神经外科医生在会诊中经常诊治累及四肢及躯干的周围神经肿瘤，大多数累及周围神经系统的肿瘤为神经鞘膜良性肿瘤。本章重点讨论良性及恶性周围神经鞘瘤的病理学、诊断、治疗及预后。

分类

PNSTs 可分为良性与恶性。目前已经发现了一些不同的良性亚型，包括施万细胞瘤（神经鞘瘤）、神经纤维瘤和神经束膜瘤。2016 年 WHO 对神经系统肿瘤分类进行了修订（**表 74.1**）（Louis et al.，2016）。这些修订包括将黑色素型神经鞘瘤单独分为一类，将混杂性神经鞘瘤合并，以及在 MPNST 中划分出 2 种亚型：上皮样 MPNST 及 MPNST 伴神经束膜分化。

表 74.1　2016 年 WHO 周围神经鞘瘤分类

良性周围神经鞘瘤	恶性周围神经鞘瘤
神经鞘瘤	上皮样 MPNST
细胞型神经鞘瘤	MPNST 伴神经束膜分化
丛状神经鞘瘤	
黑色素型神经鞘瘤	
神经纤维瘤	
非典型神经纤维瘤	
丛状神经纤维瘤	
神经束膜瘤	
混杂性神经鞘瘤	

Reprinted from *WHO Classification of Tumours of the Central Nervous System*, Revised. Fourth Edition, Edited by Louis DN, Ohgaki H, Wiestler OD, Cavenee WK, International Agency for Research on Cancer, France, Copyright (2016).

PNST 的病因未知。这些肿瘤可散发，也可能与遗传疾病相关，特别是 NF1 和 NF2。这两种疾病都呈常染色体显性遗传，其中 NF1 在 17 号染色体上有突变，NF2 在 22 号染色体上有突变。NF1 患者易患多发神经纤维瘤及 MPNST。NF2 患者则易出现脊髓及脑神经受累。

神经鞘瘤

神经鞘瘤是一种施万细胞起源的良性肿瘤。病理特征为包膜完整的梭形细胞肿瘤，有明确的 Antoni A 区（梭形细胞紧密排列）、Antoni B 区（细胞数目少、体积小）、玻璃样变性血管壁及栅栏样细胞核。与神经纤维瘤不同，神经鞘瘤起源于神经鞘膜内部并取代了束膜，而非包裹束膜。肿瘤细胞 S100 蛋白强阳性，细胞周围有丰富的Ⅳ型胶原蛋白。近期发现的神经鞘瘤经常出现的阳性标志物还包括平足蛋白（podoplanin）（Jokinen et al.，2008）、钙网膜蛋白（calretinin）（Fine et al.，2004）和 SOX10（Nonaka et al.，2008）。

神经鞘瘤的病理类型包括经典型、细胞型、丛状和黑色素型神经鞘瘤。细胞型神经鞘瘤虽然少见，却是一种需要辨别的重要变异型，因为它细胞数量大、呈束状生长、有丝分裂活跃、偶尔对局部有破坏性。诊断的重要线索包括有良好的包膜，其中有淋巴聚集，出现泡沫样组织细胞聚集，并且 S100 蛋白弥漫高表达，细胞周围Ⅳ型胶原表达。值得注意的是，S100 蛋白弥漫表达在梭形 MPNST 中极为罕见。细胞型神经鞘瘤可能有更高的局部复发率（5%~40%），但实际上没有恶性倾向、不会转移。丛状神经鞘瘤是一种独特的亚型，常出现在浅表部位，以神经内结节样生长为特点。比较麻烦的是一些解剖位置较深的罕见的丛状神经鞘瘤，它们的细胞数量更高，有丝分裂也更活跃。S100广泛表达及Ⅳ型胶原蛋白免疫阳性可确诊。黑色素型神经鞘瘤是一种罕见的独特的肿瘤，有恶性倾向，以上皮样细胞及显著黑色素沉着为特征。约半数的Carney综合征患者存在砂粒体（Carney，1990）。

对散发和NF2相关的神经鞘瘤进行比较基因组杂交技术（comparative genomic hybridization，CGH）分析显示，22号染色体长臂片段缺失是这两组患者之间的主要差异。NF2抑癌基因编码的神经鞘蛋白（schwannomin/merlin）是一种在细胞间信号通路发挥作用的细胞膜蛋白，帮助介导生长停滞。

神经纤维瘤

神经纤维瘤是良性的无包膜的肿瘤，由纤维黏液样基质中散在的梭形细胞组成。大体标本上呈黄白色，切面有光泽。神经纤维瘤与神经鞘瘤之间至关重要的组织学差异在于，神经纤维瘤在截面上可见神经束受累；所以术中正常神经纤维与肿瘤之间没有明确分界。它们的生长模式要么是在神经内部生长、界限分明，要么是在神经外软组织中弥漫浸润生长。神经纤维瘤相对常见，尤其在浅表皮肤部位，表现为局限、带蒂的生长。S100阳性细胞的比例差异较大。

临床病理亚型根据生长模式不同可分为局灶型、弥漫型和丛状神经纤维瘤。局灶型皮肤神经纤维瘤最常见，多数为散发病例。弥漫型神经纤维瘤以斑块样增大为特征，通常出现在头颈部，约10%的病例最终被证实与NF1相关。丛状神经纤维瘤是最少见的类型，而且几乎都与NF1相关。这一类型的特征是大量相邻神经束受累，显微镜下表现为类似于局灶型和弥漫型神经纤维瘤混杂排列的区域。它具有恶变倾向，被认为是NF1患者的MPNST前病变。NF1基因的突变位于17q11.2，编码神经纤维蛋白（neurofibromin），一种细胞内信号蛋白，可促进Ras-GTP信号级联反应失活，并上调环磷酸腺苷（cyclic adenosine monophosphate，cAMP）水平。当有功能的神经纤维蛋白缺乏时，细胞增殖和存活将会增加。

神经束膜瘤

神经束膜瘤是一种伴有神经束膜高度分化的良性肿瘤。有两种不同类型：神经内神经束膜瘤及软组织神经束膜瘤。神经内神经束膜瘤以孤立增大的周围神经为特征，这是由一个或多个神经束膜受累所致。组织学上表现为“假洋葱头”，它们由复杂的神经束细胞增殖组成，向神经内膜延伸，并呈同心圆包绕着一个个神经纤维及神经内毛细血管。软组织神经束膜瘤与之相反，基本没有相关联的神经，而且通常较局限，可能有包膜。典型的组织学表现为细长的细胞，伴有非常精致、相互重叠的拉长的细胞突起，组成松散的神经束。肿瘤细胞表达波形蛋白（vimentin）和上皮细胞膜抗原，但不表达S-100蛋白、结蛋白（desmin）、肌肉特异性肌动蛋白（muscle-specific actin）和CD34。

混杂性神经鞘瘤

混杂性神经鞘瘤（hybrid nerve sheath tumours，HNST）是2016年WHO分类中新划分出的一类周围神经肿瘤。这类肿瘤包括神经纤维瘤/神经束膜瘤、神经鞘瘤/神经束膜瘤、神经纤维瘤/神经鞘瘤混杂的肿瘤。在已报道的病例中，肿瘤位置基本都在手指、足趾及四肢。这类肿瘤通常为孤立性，且位于真皮和皮下组织。亦曾有非典型部位，如结肠等的报道（Lang et al.，2012）。

恶性周围神经鞘瘤

MPNST为恶性肿瘤，起源于周围神经，或起源于神经外软组织但表现为神经鞘膜分化。NF1患者中的恶性梭形肿瘤，在除外其他诊断之前需考虑为MPNST。MPNST也可能出现在放疗后。常见的组织学表现包括细胞形态变化，轮匝、栅栏或花环样排列，当肿瘤与某个神经相关时，向神经周围及神经内部扩散，以及其分布区域内的大面积坏死（Hruban et al.，1990）。

在这些肿瘤中，50%~70%表达S-100蛋白，绝大多数病例TP53阳性。虽然MPNST没有能用于诊断的独特细胞遗传学特征，但在适当的情况下可以通过检测分子遗传学变异来协助诊断，包括表皮生长因子受体（epidermal growth factor receptor，EGFR）扩增及NF1和CDKN2A的缺失。

上皮样MPNST是MPNST中一种独特而罕见的亚型，它的特征是肿瘤以巨大的上皮样细胞为主要成分。该肿瘤在浅表部位较为常见，与经典型MPNST

不同的是，该肿瘤中 S100 蛋白高表达，而且通常呈弥漫分布。在原有的神经鞘瘤内发生的 MPNST 中，绝大多数为上皮样 MPNST。

特别要注意的是，丛状神经纤维瘤是 NF1 患者发生 MPNST 前最主要的可识别的良性病变。相比之下，由神经鞘瘤恶变为 MPNST 的现象非常罕见，而且通常表现为上皮样改变、血管肉瘤，或由小细胞组成的肿瘤。罕见情况下，MPNST 也可能起源于节细胞神经瘤或节细胞神经母细胞瘤，起源于嗜铬细胞瘤则更为罕见。

CGH 数据显示，MPNST 中，17q 远端增多和 13q14-q21 缺失较为常见。其他经常报道的变异还有 5p、7q、8q 的增多和 9p 片段的缺失。

临床表现

任何年龄和性别都可能会患 PNST。散发的 MPNST 在 40~50 岁最为常见。而与 NF1 相关者确诊 MPNST 的时间可提前 10 年。MPNST 占所有软组织肉瘤的 5%~10%。尽管在一般人群中较为罕见，MPNST 在 NF1 患者中发生率为 5%~42%。

PNST 患者通常表现为可见或可触及的肿块、疼痛、无力、感觉改变，或是影像学检查偶然发现的肿块，但多数周围神经肿瘤最初发现时表现为无症状的肿块。触诊肿块时可有触痛或感觉异常。运动神经受累者可能有无力，或者是更为常见的精细运动功能的轻微受损。自主神经功能障碍可能表现为皮肤的质地、颜色和温度变化，以及产生汗液量的变化。应该特别检查患者有无 NF1 相关症状（牛奶咖啡斑，神经纤维瘤，Lisch 结节，视神经胶质瘤，腋窝、腹股沟雀斑，特征性骨骼异常及家族史）。

任何体积快速增长或症状快速进展的情况都应怀疑是否有囊肿形成、出血或是恶变，并且患者需要进行相应评估。

检查

以往周围神经肿瘤是通过病史、临床检查及电生理检查诊断的。虽然 CT 能够显示内部钙化和继发骨质改变，但 20 世纪 80 年代出现的 MRI 已成为周围神经肿瘤影像学诊断的金标准。MRI 使得软组织可以在高分辨率下清晰显示，能够发现肿块，显示受累神经的解剖，以及与周围重要结构（如血管等）的关系。高分辨率神经造影 MR（MRN）使得分辨率进一步提高，并且通过对比帮助显示周围神经肿瘤的明确位置、形状、大小及是否可切除。

MRI 也可提供肿瘤性质的线索，可以帮助区分良性和恶性病变。良性神经鞘瘤通常为 T1 像等信号或者稍高信号，T2 像高信号（**图 74.1**），不均匀增强。大多数神经纤维瘤及一部分神经鞘瘤表现为 T1 像中央高信号、周围低信号（称“靶征”），而 T2 像信号强度相反。相反，MPNST 通常呈不均匀强化，较为不连续，且更容易出现出血及坏死区域。在动态监测中，肿瘤迅速增大常提示恶变。

代谢显像采用 ^{18}氟代脱氧葡萄糖（^{18}fluorodeoxyglucose，^{18}FDG）正电子发射断层扫描技术（positron emission tomography，PET）可以提供肿瘤分级的重要信息。^{18}FDG PET/CT 是 NF1 患者检测 MPNST 最有效的影像学手段。最大标准摄取值（maximum standardized uptake value，SUV_{max}）比值大于 1.5 的阴性预测值为 98.8%，阳性预测值 61.5%。但是，从假阳性率上说，它对于 NF1 相关的 MPNST

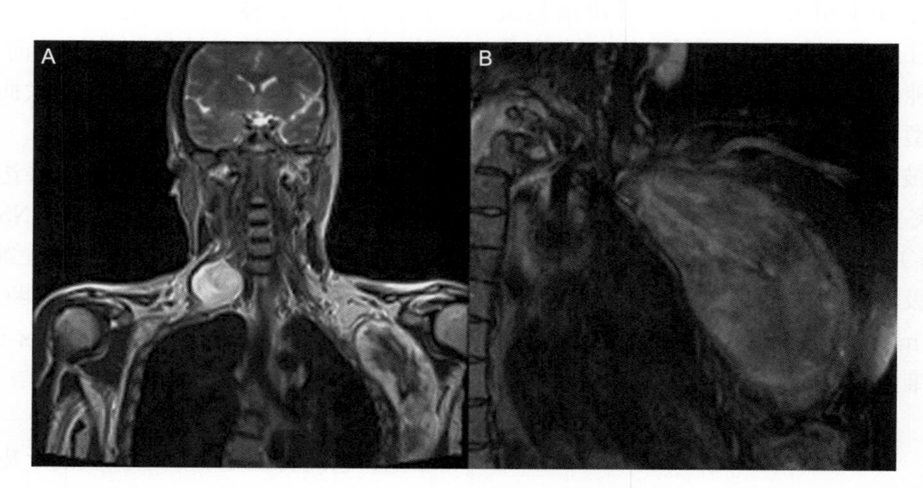

图 74.1 （A、B）一位 28 岁女性 NF1 患者的 MRI T2 加权像，显示左侧锁骨下神经丛神经鞘瘤及右侧锁骨上神经丛肿瘤

诊断特异性不够高（Combemale et al.，2014）。近期一项研究显示，26 例怀疑 MPNST 的 NF1 患者进行了立体定向 PET/CT（肿瘤 / 肝比值 SUV_{max} 大于 1.5）引导下穿刺活检术，结果显示诊断的准确率为 96%（Brahmi et al.，2015）。

一些电生理检查，如肌电图（electromyography，EMG）和神经传导检查（nerve conduction studies，NCS）经常用于周围神经肿瘤患者。EMG 和 NCS 检查可以帮助进行肿瘤定位、识别亚临床损害及记录基线功能以便将来对比。这些检查在累及四肢多条神经的神经丛水平的肿瘤中格外有用。

治疗

由于良性 PNST 通常生长缓慢，出现症状之前不需进行干预。手术切除指征包括疼痛、神经症状、恶性可能、改善外观和组织学诊断。丛状神经纤维瘤应密切监测其大小变化及症状进展。影像学提示为良性的 PNST 无需活检，除非临床表现不典型。

诊断不明确时应行组织学诊断。由于 NF1 患者中恶变风险高，当肿瘤生长迅速或疼痛快速进展时应放宽经皮活检的指征。组织标本可由细针抽吸或针芯活检取得。为了降低可疑病灶的假阴性率，可行 PET/CT 立体定向引导下活检。

PNST 切除手术可采用全身麻醉、区域阻滞或局部麻醉（**图 74.2**、**图 74.3** 和**图 73.4**）。应避免使用肌松药，因其会妨碍术中神经生理监测和刺激。摆放患者体位使病变周围神经得到最大暴露。皮肤切口位于神经上方，从肿瘤近端 2~4 cm 开始，向远端延伸 2~4 cm。分离皮下组织暴露病变部位，严密止血。从正常解剖部位开始显露神经，再逐渐深入肿瘤部位。辨别肿瘤近端和远端的正常边界非常重要。常用手术放大镜或显微镜来观察肿瘤，可能需要神经内松解术来辨认穿过肿瘤的神经束。

神经刺激器可用来协助判断无神经束通过的入点。将神经束从瘤囊上轻轻提起并分离，建立无神经束分离层面。使用超声吸引器进行瘤内切除有助于体积较大肿瘤的分离。术中进行 EMG 监测可提醒术者避免过度牵拉神经束。

进出神经鞘瘤的无功能性（通过刺激判断）神经束可能需要切断以切除肿瘤。大多数施万细胞瘤可以从包膜上剥离下来并完整切除。肿瘤包膜没必要切除因为与肿瘤复发无关。相反，神经纤维瘤中扩大的神经束通常仍有功能，切除肿瘤时不可避免地需要牺牲一根或多根神经束。有时当牺牲掉非常重要的神经束时应考虑神经移植，常用的神经供体是腓肠神经，还可选用前臂内侧皮神经和桡神经感觉支。巨大丛状神经纤维瘤的手术目的通常是减瘤以减轻神经压迫症状。应行冰冻切片以判断是否为恶性。然后逐层关闭伤口，注意避免将神经卡于狭小的腔隙中。

病灶局限、边界清晰的的 MPNST 可手术完全切除。这一点非常重要，甚至是对于巨大的、非肢体部位的恶性肿瘤来说——常见于 NF1 患者，即使扩大全切可能与严重的并发症相关。数据支持手术全切的独立预后重要性（Dunn et al.，2013）。对大多数大的（>5 cm）高级别肢体肉瘤，建议辅助放疗以减少局部复发风险，但是对 NF1 患者是否行辅助放疗需要与患者充分沟通，因为放射性肉瘤风险增加。尽管没有专门针对 MPNST 辅助化疗的随机对照试验，辅助化疗仍然是治疗积极患者的一种选择。近期报道的由肉瘤协作研究联盟（Sarcoma Alliance for Research，SARC）开展的 SARC006 Ⅱ期临床试验，评估了联合多柔比星、异环磷酰胺和依托泊苷化疗在 48 位局部晚期转移性 MPNST 患者中的疗效。结果显示，在大多数病灶局限的患者中，新辅助化疗产生的反应使后续局部治疗变得可行，最终获得了令人鼓舞的疾病稳定率（Widemann et al.，2013）。

臂丛神经肿瘤是一种不常见的疾病，涉及多数神经外科医生不熟悉的手术区域，因此在临床上具有一定的挑战性。针对这类肿瘤的治疗不仅需要对臂丛神经的复杂结构有所了解，还需要对可能遇到的各种肿瘤合适的手术入路有足够的认识。建议采用锁骨上前入路治疗大部分神经根和神经干的肿瘤，采用锁骨下入路治疗累及神经束和远端神经丛的病变。后入路用来治疗累及椎间孔水平的脊神经、C8-T1 神经根及下干的肿瘤，也推荐用于肿瘤有残留或复发或曾接受放疗的患者。

无论选择何种手术入路，大多数神经鞘瘤切除手术步骤都相似。简单来说，确定肿瘤的近、远端，并游离肿瘤与周围的神经血管结构。通过束间分离、术中电刺激辨别肿瘤近、远端受累及未受累的神经束。运用这些技术辨别出有功能和功能障碍的神经束，从而可以牺牲掉无功能性神经束。逐渐游离肿瘤及邻近但已移位的神经束，将肿瘤从残余神经上剥离开。最后，将包膜从剩余的神经束上锐性剪除（Das et al.，2007）。

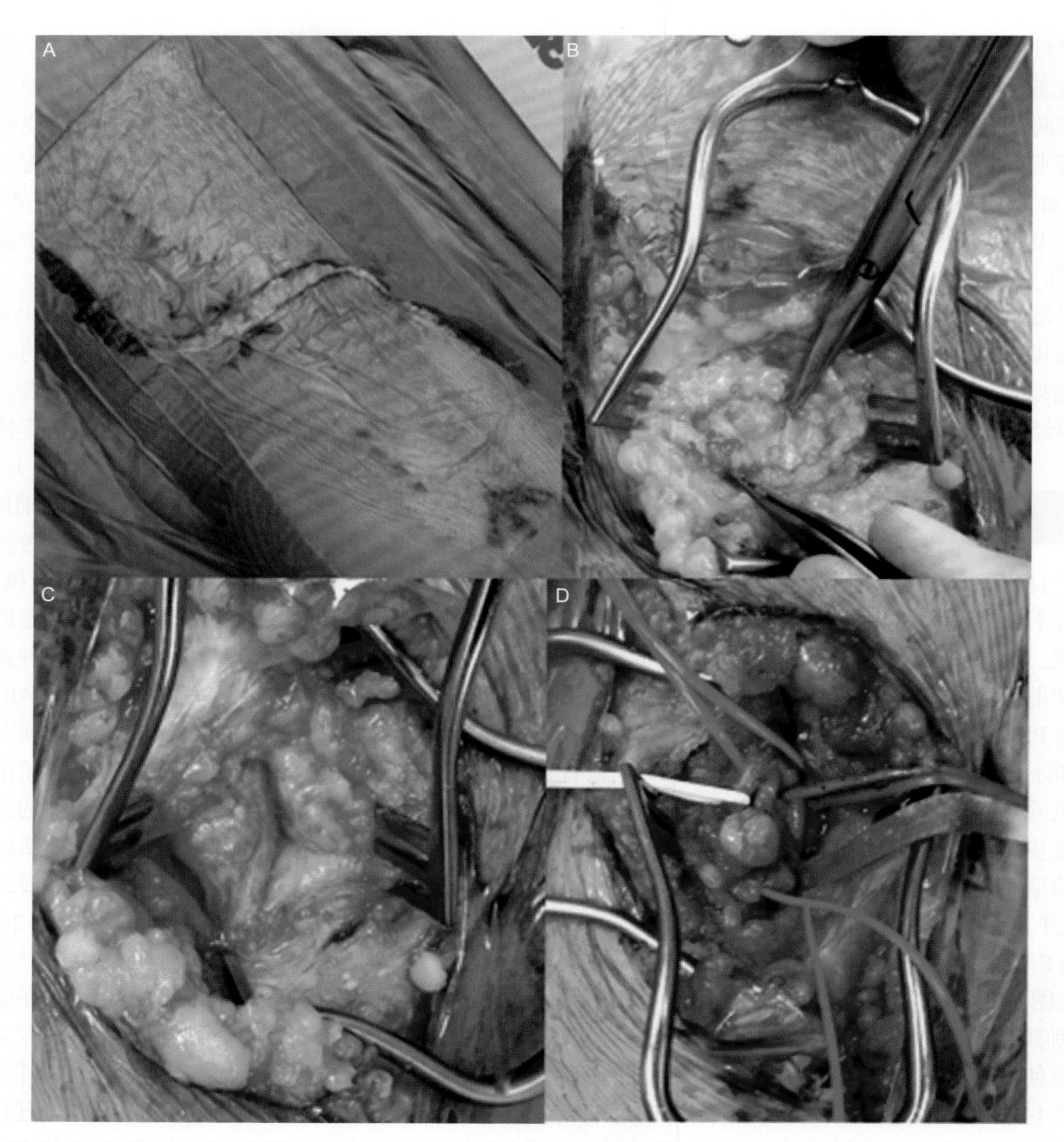

图 74.2 胫后神经鞘瘤。（A）左腘窝弧形切口。（B）锐性分离显露肿瘤。（C）分离伴行的神经束。（D）辨认肿瘤起源的神经束

结局

大多数良性 PNST 可完整切除，很少复发，除非肿瘤过大或既往做过手术，否则都能在不损伤或对载瘤神经损伤很小的情况下实现全切。

MPNST 转移风险高，预后差。不同报道的长期预后差异很大，5 年生存率 15%~50% 不等。肿瘤体积大（>5 cm）是不良预后的最稳定因素，其他因素还包括肿瘤分级、手术切缘情况、局部复发、躯干部位以及异质性横纹肌母细胞分化。尽管 p53 核表达、AKT 和 TOR 通路激活以及 MET 活化与不良预后有关，但目前为止还没有明确的或广泛可重复的分子预后因子（Farid et al.，2014）。

NF1 患者一生中出现 MPNST 的风险介于 8%~13%，是 NF1 患者死亡的最常见原因。一些大型研究报告显示，与散发性肿瘤相比，NF1 患者中出现 MPNST 者预后更差、对细胞毒药物化疗反应更差，最差的情况下 5 年生存率最高仅 50%。一项纳入了数项欧洲研究的 meta 分析显示，尽管 2000 年前 NF1 可能是不良预后因子，但鉴于 NF1 患者更好的整体监测、更早期的干预以及影像学和诊断技术的提高，该负向影响可能会消失（Kolberg et al.，2013）。

晚期或转移性 MPNST 患者的预后通常较差。在

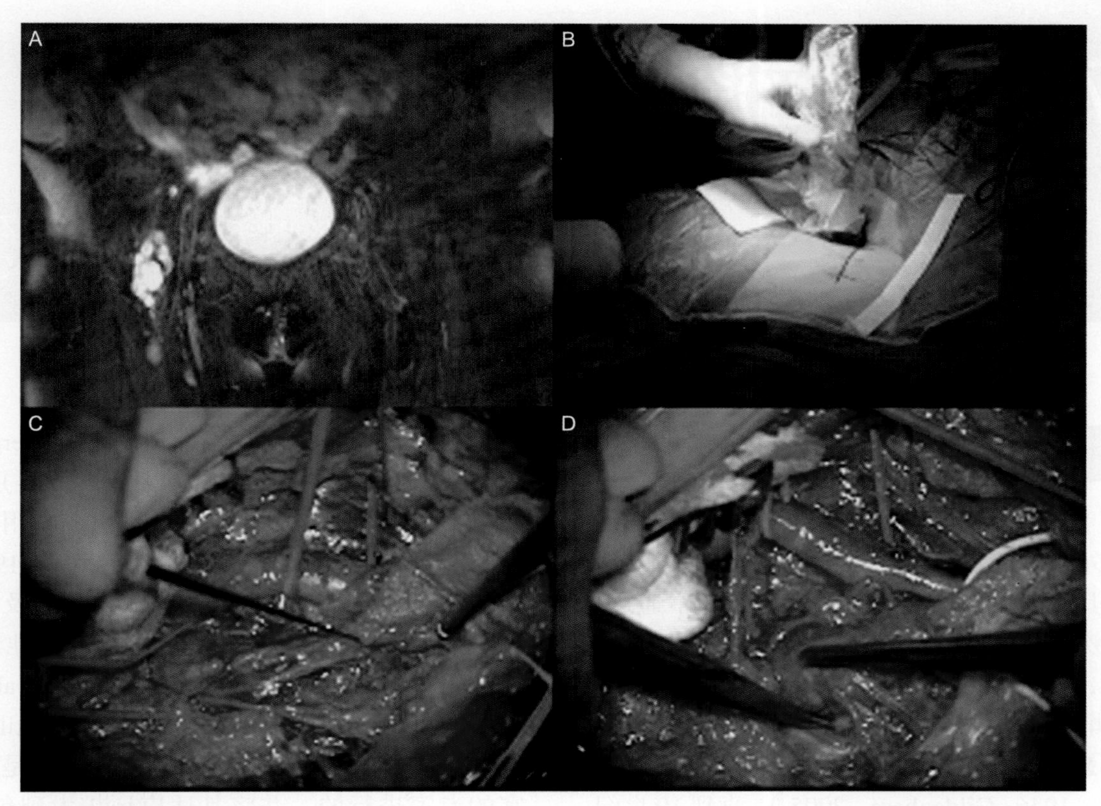

图 74.3　右生殖股神经鞘瘤。（A）MRI T1 加权像显示来源于右生殖股神经的对比增强、边界清楚的肿瘤。（B）术中超声确认肿瘤位置。（C）辨认股神经、股动脉和股静脉。应用神经刺激器辨认无神经束的层面。（D）使用锐性分离和显微外科技术切除肿瘤

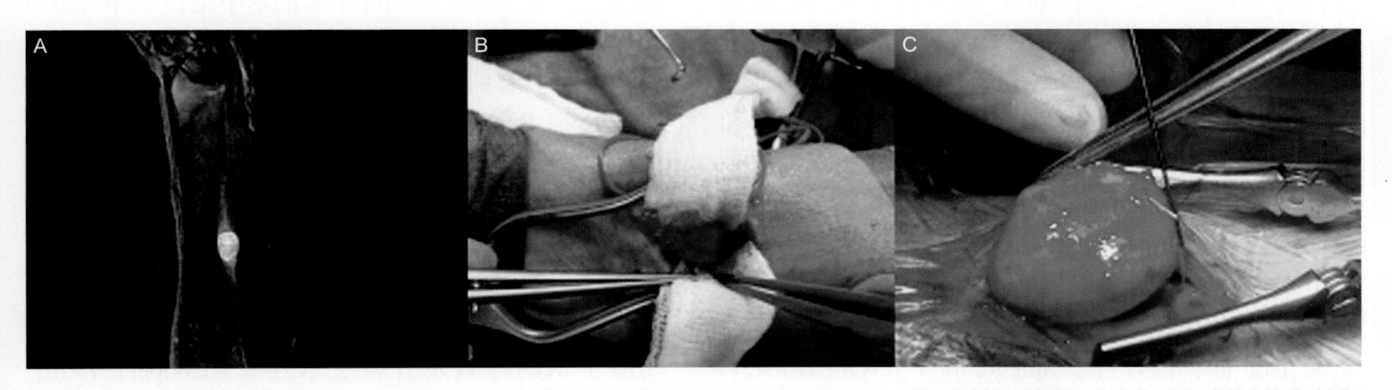

图 74.4　右正中神经鞘瘤。（A）MRI T1 加权像显示来源于右正中神经的对比增强的神经鞘瘤。（B）应用锐性分离游离肿瘤和正中神经。（C）切除肿瘤前应用神经刺激器辨认无神经束层面

一项多机构回顾性研究中，来自多个软组织肉瘤试验的 MPNST 患者实体瘤的疗效评价标准（Response Evaluation Criteria in Solid Tumours，RECIST）反应率为 21%（Kroep et al.，2011）。

延伸阅读、参考文献

扫描书末二维码获取。

第十六篇　功能性神经外科

第 75 章　脑深部电刺激原理

Erlick A.C. Pereira・Alexander L. Green・Tipu Z. Aziz 著
范世莹、刘冲、李仁鹏 译，孟凡刚、胡威、张建国 审校

引言

在 20 世纪早期 Victor Horsley 和 Harvey Cushing 建立神经外科以及 18 世纪末期 Benjamin Franklin 发现电流及其对肌肉的影响之前，就已经有了通过电刺激治疗疾病的理念。文献记载最早可以追溯到古罗马帝国，Tiberius 皇帝时期一位患有痛风的自由民踩在了电鳐上，电击大大缓解了他的痛风，所以当地医生 Scribonius 建议将其用来治疗痛风和头痛（Kellaway，1946；Gildenberg，2005）。直到 19 世纪，动物实验应用电刺激脑干和大脑皮质引起运动，电刺激才成为一项正式的科学研究（Flourens，1824；Fritsch and Hitzig，1870；Morgan，1982）。英国神经外科之父 Horsley，在 19 世纪 80 年代首次将电刺激直接用于人脑，利用这种技术识别功能皮质并指导肿瘤的切除（Vilensky and Gilman，2002）。

除了开拓性的神经刺激技术之外，Horsley 和 Clark 联合发明的立体定向装置，是促使脑深部电刺激（deep brain stimulation，DBS）技术成为可能的另一伟大进步（Horsley and Clarke，1908）。立体定向使用固定在头部的框架，通过外部坐标系，并参照大脑图谱定位脑结构，根据头骨或大脑的标志点来计算靶点坐标。1947 年，Spiegel 和 Wycis 将 Horsley-Clarke 立体定向装置用于人类的立体定向神经外科手术（Spiegel et al.，1947）。尽管化学注射或热凝这种不可逆性损伤手术已成为标准治疗方式，但许多先驱依然主张在术中使用可逆性的电刺激以确定靶点位置是否准确（Hassler et al.，1960；Spiegel，1982）。

DBS 作为一种临床治疗方式从一系列转化研究项目中脱颖而出。植入式神经刺激装置是由 Roger Avery 和 Thomas Mortimer 等工程师联合外科医生以及公司合作开发的（Sweet and Wepsic，1968；Mortimer et al.，1970）。术中刺激被用于描绘感觉丘脑和其他脑深部结构的功能图（Tasker et al.，1982）。动物研究和人类神经外科消融手术的经验观察增加了脑深部结构的功能解剖知识（Gildenberg，2005；Gildenberg，2006；Pereira and Aziz，2006）。20 世纪 50 年代和 60 年代间断性 DBS 首次成功用于治疗癌性疼痛（Heath and Mickle，1960；Gol，1967），随后，在 20 世纪 70 年代，丘脑、内囊以及导水管周围灰质 DBS 用于治疗三叉神经痛及其他慢性疼痛综合征（Adam et al.，1974；Hosobuchi et al.，1973；Hosobuchi et al.，1977；Richardson and Akil，1977）。在过去的四十年中，DBS 治疗疼痛一直是由经验丰富的专家进行的，并将其适应证扩大到包括卒中、截肢、多发性硬化、神经丛病和失败的背部手术综合征等（Pereira and Aziz，2014）。

尽管在 20 世纪 50 年代到 70 年代的整个时期，DBS 用于癫痫病灶和切除手术的术中定位（Spiegel et al.，1950），并在帕金森病震颤和运动障碍等运动障碍性疾病中起到作用（Hassler et al.，1960；Alberts et al.，1965；Bechtereva et al.，1975），但是，直到 20 世纪 80 年代末 DBS 才被推广到这些适应证。延缓其推广使用的关键因素包括：药物治疗这些疾病的成功——苯妥英钠、卡马西平和丙戊酸钠用于治疗癫痫，左旋多巴用于治疗帕金森病（Parkinson’s disease，PD）（Cotzias et al.，1967）；PD 及癫痫的消融和切除手术的疗效及外科手术经验（Cooper，1956；Svennilson et al.，1960；Jensen，1975）；以及与目前技术相比早期笨重的神经刺激器模型既不可靠，还存在更大的损伤和感染风险（Mullett，1987）。

在首次用于疼痛治疗的十多年后（Hosobuchi et al.，1973），丘脑 DBS 被用来治疗药物难治性 PD 震颤（Benabid et al.，1987）。基于灵长类动物的研究确定了丘脑底核（基底神经节结构）作为消融和 DBS 治疗的靶点（Bergman et al.，1990；Aziz et al.，1991）。随着丘脑和苍白球毁损手术的复苏（Narabayashi et al.，1984；Laitinen et al.，1992）、神经刺激技术小型化和可逆化的进步，灵长类动物研究中的科学发现促进了 PD 外科手术在 20 世纪 90 年

代的复兴，特别是在过去的十年中，DBS 作为治疗药物难治性帕金森病的首选疗法，其他运动障碍性疾病、疼痛和情感障碍也成为这一治疗方式的可能适应证。**表 75.1** 汇总了目前 DBS 的适应证及其解剖靶点。

立体定向手术

Horsley 和 Clarke 发明了立体定向手术，这种方法可以对脑部核团进行毁损。该方法需要精确定位，并且在一定程度上尽可能减少对其他结构的损害（Horsley and Clarke，1908）。相传，Clarke 在凝望着星空并思考自己在星空中的位置时，构想出一个装置，通过这一装置可以将颅内探查装置插入，这一装置通过横向放置的颅钉、与插入外耳道的耳塞相连的横杆以及靠在鼻子和眶缘的横杆固定在动物头部，并将其固定在笛卡尔坐标系中。希腊语“stereos”表示“solid”，“taxis”表示“arrangement”，他们据此创造了“stereotaxic”一词，通过这一方法，可以研究大脑的每一立方毫米并将其记录下来（Horsley and Clarke，1908；Pereira et al.，2008）。

立体定向手术有三个基本概念。首先，大脑在坐标系（通常是笛卡尔坐标系）中是一个几何体；其次，可以在这一几何体中定义合适的参考点（例如前后联合）来计算手术靶点；第三，在这一坐标系中，可以用合适的手术器械对这些靶点进行操作。

几何体和参考点

通过将头部固定在与给定参考原点相交的三个正交平面上，可以在空间中描述头部中的任意一点。

表 75.1　DBS 的适应证及其常用靶点

适应证	DBS 靶点
帕金森病	苍白球内侧部、丘脑底核
肌张力障碍	苍白球内侧部
震颤	丘脑腹中间核、未定带
抑郁症	膝下前扣带回、内囊前肢
强迫症	内囊前肢
抽动秽语综合征	丘脑腹内侧核、内囊前肢、苍白球内侧部
癫痫	丘脑前核、丘脑中央正中核
丛集性头痛	下丘脑后部
慢性疼痛	丘脑腹后核、脑室周围和导水管周围灰质

因此，原点的横向距离（X）、前方距离（Y）以及垂直上方距离（Z）可以用 mm 来量化。

当头部固定在立体定向框架（无框架系统）中时，可以用其与 X、Y 和 Z 三个方向上距零参考点的距离来描述大脑中的可视靶点。其中包括现代 MRI 成像中用于治疗 PD 的丘脑底核和苍白球内侧部。不可视靶点例如丘脑腹中间核，可以根据其与深部脑标志物（如前后联合中点）的已知距离，或使用立体定向图谱进行粗略定位。Jean Talairach 首次描述了使用前后联合（the anterior and posterior commissures，AC-PC）作为完全颅内参考框架的一部分（Talairach et al.，1957）。立体定向图谱是从多个平行于参考平面的切片的固定脑标本中编制的，对切片进行染色，以突出显示脑深部核团和传导纤维。Schaltenbrand 图谱是最常用的，它是根据大脑切片（正交或与 AC-PC 线平行的切线）编制的（Schaltenbrand and Wahren，1977）。将直接或间接靶点定位与术中患者清醒状态评估、多通道微电极或 DBS 宏电极电生理记录相结合以提高疗效，这可能对外科医生有帮助。

设备

大多数立体定向系统由坐标框架和定位装置组成，这个框架有一个刚性的金属“基环”平台固定在头骨上防止移位，它通常是由 4 颗钉子插入颅骨表面。常用的框架有 Cosman-Roberts-Wells（CRW）（**图 75.1**）和 Leksell 头架。CRW 头架的零点位于框架中心，而 Leksell 头架的零点位于其右后上方的角上，100 mm、100 mm、100 mm 位于其 X、Y、Z 的中心。可以在进行 CT 或 MRI 扫描之前在这一平台上安装一个定位系统，头部相对于框架的位置可以通过计算机软件计算（也可以用 Leksell 框架手动计算），从而将感兴趣的大脑结构转换到“立体定向空间”，即框架的坐标系中。定位装置上的“N”形杆可以计算 Z 值。

弧半径、极点和焦点坐标系可以用于立体定向设备。焦点坐标系统将患者的头部放到带框架的探头上，现在除放射外科外几乎很少使用。极坐标系仅用于第一代立体定向框架（如 Clarke 改良的 Horsley-Clarke 框架、Spiegel-Wycis 框架和欧洲仍然流行的 Riechert-Mundinger 框架），它是通过角度和深度确定探测路径的。在笛卡尔坐标系中定位靶点时，制订计划时选择的入颅点给出了探测装置相对于靶点的方位角和倾斜角。在靶点和入颅点确定的情况下，探针路径即为它们之间的直线，这一直线穿过立体

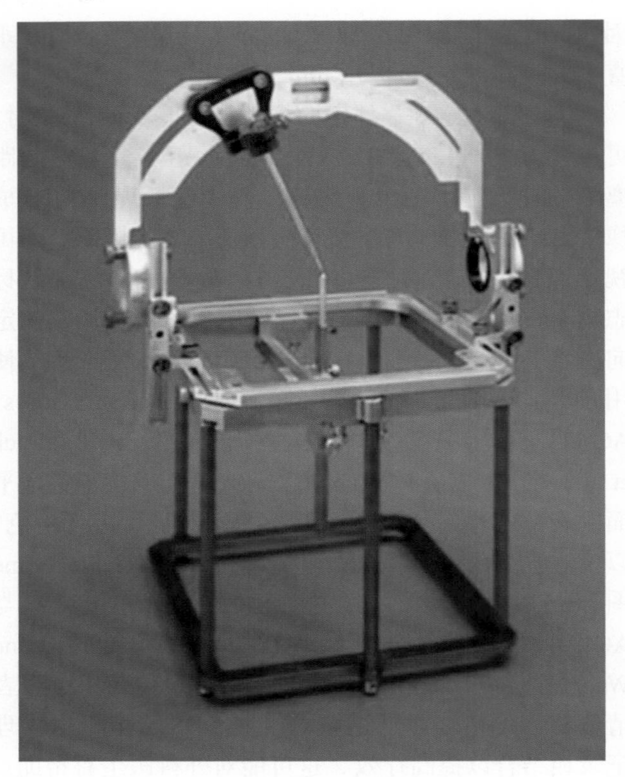

图 75.1 CRW 精度弧光系统检查其虚拟靶点坐标

定向弧弓到框架中某一固定深度。在现代常用的圆弧半径系统中，路径可以由两个角度（Arc 和 Ring）和一个线性长度（半径或深度）确定。在常用的圆弧半径框架（如 CRW 和 Leksell）中，固定半径的半圆弧可以在笛卡尔坐标系中自由移动，前后旋转 180°，探针架可以在正平面上沿圆弧平移。因此，只要靶点坐标和深度确定，就可以从任一路径上穿至靶点。

笛卡尔虚拟坐标系统（如 CRW）包括一个模拟靶点并提供安全检查的指针，以减少人为错误，并在将头架固定在头上且探针穿至颅内靶点之前确定头架能够准确定位靶点（**图** 75.1）。当立体定向框架使用极坐标时，这种模拟系统更为重要，因为它们提供了一种安全检查，检查探针携带框架和虚拟的笛卡尔靶点之间的相交角——两者同时出现错误的可能性是极小的。

许多 DBS 外科医生使用 CRW 框架，并通过算法将立体定向 CT 与术前 MRI 融合，以减少 MRI 中组织结构的空间漂移（**图** 75.2）。其他医生多使用 MRI 兼容的 CRW 和 Leksell 框架直接从立体定向 MRI 中定位靶点，在现代高分辨率的扫描设备中，空间漂移问题不大。一些医生继续单独使用 CT 或脑室造影进行 DBS，有些使用计算机化的无框架系统甚至是全程自动化的机器人。

DBS 硬件

目前最常用的电极是四触点电极，一根电极上有 4 个触点，每个触点长 1.5 mm，触点之间有 0.5 mm 的间隔区。DBS 有几种可以调节的刺激参数。通常情况下，刺激可以是单极刺激（远隔的脉冲发生器作为正极）或双极刺激，即每根电极四个触点的任意组合，每一个触点都可以作为正极或负极。电压通常可以从 0~10 V，频率从 2~300 Hz，方波脉冲的宽度从 60~500 μs。刺激可以是连续的，也可以在

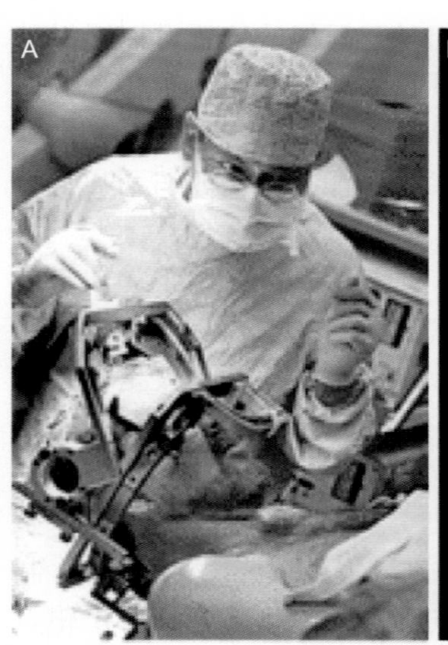

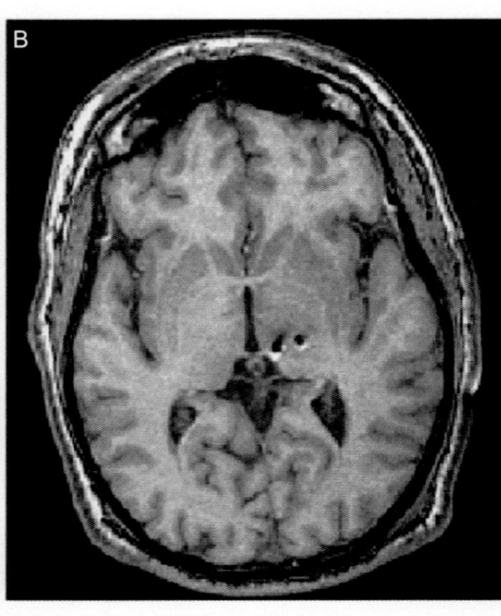

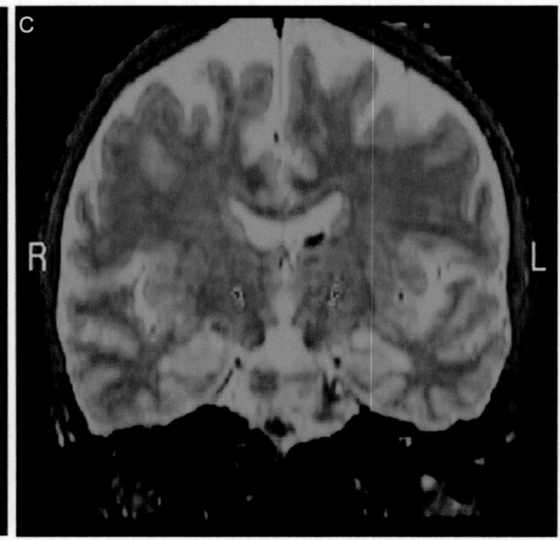

图 75.2 （A）术中清醒 DBS；（B）DBS 治疗疼痛的轴位 MRI；（C）冠状位 MRI 和 CT 融合显示 DBS 治疗帕金森病中的丘脑底核

开关状态之间循环，每个状态的持续时间应不少于0.1 s。

DBS电极固定在颅骨上，通过皮下隧道的导线连接到植入到胸部或腹部皮下的含有电源的脉冲发生器（起搏器）上（图75.3），有些起搏器可以经皮充电。

DBS机制

围绕DBS机制的主流观点是高频DBS抑制靶点结构内的神经元放电，而低频DBS激活神经元放电。高频“干扰”的证据主要来源于其与毁损手术的相似性，如苍白球切开术和丘脑切开术，它们的临床结果是相似的。低频驱动理论主要来源于观察到的低频DBS会加重某些PD的症状，并认为脚桥核低频DBS治疗冻结步态以及室周灰质低频DBS治疗慢性疼痛可分别激活运动和镇痛神经环路。然而，人类和非人灵长类动物的电生理实验表明，低频和高频DBS都能够激活靶点核团的传入和传出神经元的轴突以及纤维通路（McIntyre et al.，2004）。

DBS更基本的原理首先包括对神经元及其组成部分产生的电活动的影响；其次是这些影响如何通过相关的神经环路，例如基底核、丘脑和皮质回路；最后，DBS如何影响大脑中调节性的单胺类和其他神经递质。在这里，我们将重点放在DBS对神经元生理的直接电效应上，因为后面的突触神经递质释放和神经解剖回路调节原理可以认为是继发于这一效应的。

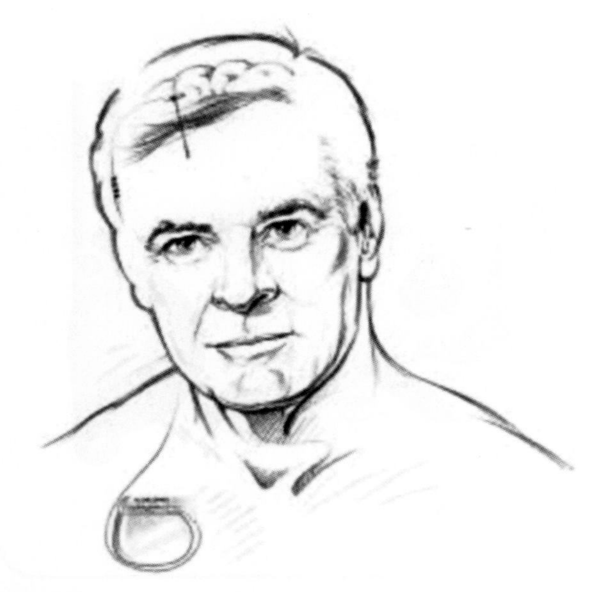

图75.3 DBS电极、皮下延长导线和植入的脉冲发生器

Reproduced with permission of Medtronic, Inc.

局部电效应

DBS通常激发周围神经元组织的动作电位（Kringelbach et al.，2007；Montgomery and Gale，2008）。有效的DBS有赖于在目标靶组织中激发足够的动作电位，同时限制电流的传播，以免激发不必要的相邻结构中的动作电位。增加电流强度或电压可以改善预后，但会增加不良副作用的发生。因此，为每位患者制订DBS电场的电生理策略是可取的。改变刺激参数（如电压和脉宽），也可以改变激活神经元的数量。轴突末梢阈值最低，其次是轴突、树突，最后是神经元胞体，较大的轴突对低脉宽的刺激反应更大。因此，在考虑DBS激活哪些神经元时，一般原则是：首先，远离电极的神经元不太可能受到刺激；其次，与神经元胞体相比，在低电压DBS刺激下，轴突会受到刺激产生动作电位；再次，较大的轴突比较小的轴突对低电压刺激更有反应；最后，有分支的轴突在较低的刺激电压下也会被激活。神经元相对于DBS电场的方向也与此有关，面向电压梯度方向的神经元比垂直于电压梯度方向的神经元更容易达到阈值。同样有趣的是，离DBS负极最近的神经元比靠近正极的神经元更容易被激活，因此在单极DBS中，通常指定脉冲发生器为正极。

未来发展

目前，大多数起搏器都是以固定的频率持续发出刺激，这是一种相对简单但有效的治疗方式。然而，持续刺激会扩散到其他纤维束，或者扰乱病理性活动背景下的正常脑信号，从而引起不必要的副作用。例如，这些“正常”脑信号的改变可能会影响情绪和认知。通过专门针对异常振荡进行刺激，可能能够实现间歇性刺激，从而使正常信号得以恢复。事实上，有证据证明，间歇性刺激比持续性刺激更有利于控制症状（Little et al.，2016）。其他发展前景包括具有遥测功能的起搏器，它可以帮助识别多种疾病的病理标志。对姿势有反应的起搏器也可以减少副作用，比如在脊髓电刺激的情况下，仰卧位比直立位需要更低水平的刺激。这种起搏器是用方向加速器确定运动和位置的。

良好的临床效果有时会受到触点与靶点附近结构的距离的限制。例如，可以在丘脑底核放置电极，但如果电极太靠近内囊，治疗窗内的刺激就会引起副作用。为了克服这一问题，科技公司已经生产出新的电极结构，例如将环形触点分成两个到三个，甚至将32个触点排列成一个类似鱼鳞的阵列（**图75.4**）。试验证明，后者在灵长类动物中具有方向性（Martens et al.，2011），在临床病例序列中，也可以记录多个触点的局部场电位，以便更好地定位（Bour et al.，2015）。

目前结构MRI通常用于电极定位。虽然还没有充分评估，但弥散张量成像定位效果可能更佳，它能够定位与其他区域或可能的网络部分相连的核团的特定区域，而不仅仅是核团本身。正如在肿瘤手术中所证明的，弥散张量成像可以用来识别纤维束，纤维束如果受到刺激就会引起副作用，因此可以避免这些副作用。也有可能通过躯体学方法确定同质结构（如丘脑）内的最佳电极位置（Hyam et al.，2012）。

在分子和细胞治疗领域，有许多正在进行的转化研究，但很少有治疗方法能证明具有与DBS相当的安全性和有效性。神经营养因子、干细胞、胎儿细胞移植的临床试验都收效甚微（Astradsson and Aziz，2016）。然而，单侧DBS的确为对侧生物治疗植入提供了一种很好的潜在控制性手术（Rowland et al.，2015）。

毁损手术

由于DBS具有更高的安全性和可逆性，使用射频消融的毁损手术已基本被DBS取代，但在某些情况下，苍白球切开术、丘脑切开术甚至丘脑底部切开术仍然是有效的替代治疗方式，尤其是在资源有限、DBS经济条件不允许、临床随访可能有挑战性的情况下（Pereira and Aziz，2013）。其他特定的适应证包括DBS术后并发的慢性感染、金属过敏、跌倒或强迫性头部撞击对植入的DBS硬件的风险，或寿命有限的姑息性治疗，如癌症疼痛的扣带回切开术或严重晚期帕金森病的苍白球切开术（Bulluss et al.，2013；Viswanathan et al.，2013）。用电损伤发生器射频热凝脑组织是最常用的毁损手术，但通常需要进行颅骨钻孔，且需要用刚性探针穿经脑组织到达要毁损的靶点。另一种非侵入性的毁损方式是伽玛刀放射外科手术，其缺点是需数月才能起效，而磁共振引导的高频聚焦超声有良好的初步临床证据（Elias et al.，2013；Witjas et al.，2015）。

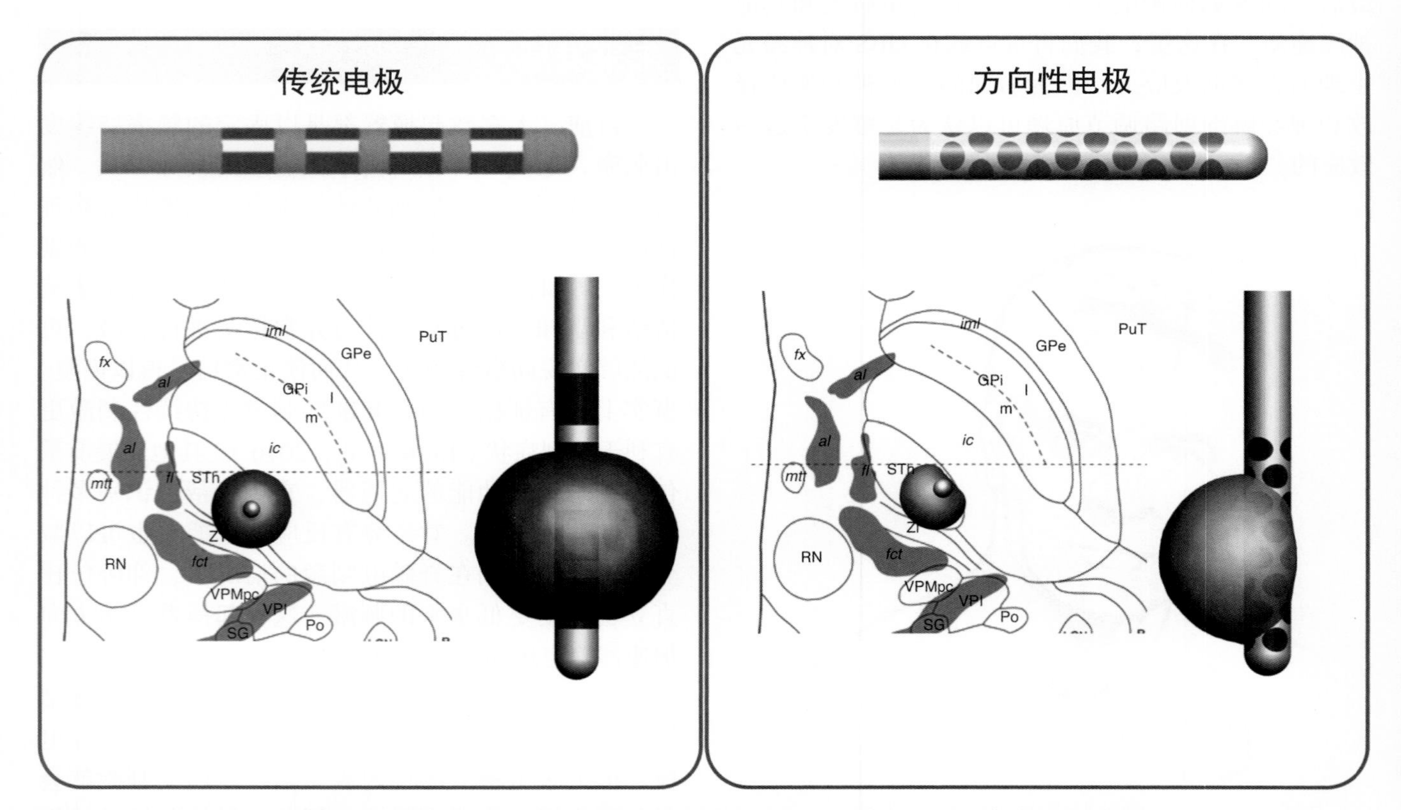

图75.4 方向性电极的多触点阵列优化DBS刺激脑神经核团。STN，丘脑底核（帕金森病DBS常用靶点）；ic，内囊

Reproduced with permission of Medtronic, Inc.

结论

DBS 需要准确地植入电极，尽管存在无框架和机器人替代方案，通常使用固定在头部的立体定向框架。对于所有的 DBS 靶点，局部相互作用和更广泛的功能性神经解剖学回路，孰轻孰重还没有完全阐明。然而，一般的原理是，从植入的电池中通过的脉冲电流产生一个局部场电位，进而导致周围的神经元达到产生动作电位的阈值或发生超极化。这类神经元可能从突触释放神经递质，并改变控制运动、癫痫发作或其他行为（如痛觉减退或抽搐）的脑深部神经回路功能。DBS 的替代方法包括射频热凝、伽玛刀放射外科或聚焦超声。未来的发展包括成像方面的进展，如弥散张量 MRI、方向性电极驱动的电场、分段电极、智能闭环 DBS 以及利用立体定向神经外科进行分子和细胞治疗，如基因治疗、神经营养因子药物输送、胎儿和干细胞移植。

延伸阅读、参考文献

扫描书末二维码获取。

第 76 章 运动障碍性疾病

Keyoumars Ashkan・Ismail Ughratdar 著
王乔、刘冲、张墨轩 译，孟凡刚、季玉陈、冯涛 审校

引言

运动障碍性疾病包括多种神经系统疾病，这些疾病主要影响运动的速度、流畅性、自由度和动作的质量。运动障碍大致上可以分为自发运动过多型（运动过度）和目的性运动能力缺失型（运动减少）（**表** 76.1）。异常运动可能是节律性的（如特发性震颤），也可能是缓慢而持续的（如帕金森病）。在大多数情况下，这些异常的动作无法被有意识地控制或抑制。

对典型和重叠表现的不同诊断会影响治疗方式和手术效果，因此必须谨慎地进行临床评估和相关研究。详细的病史和特定的检查可以对大多数患者进行确诊，必要时可以通过电生理诊断和结构影像增加诊断准确率。

本章将从临床评估、发病机制和临床治疗等方面对常见运动障碍性疾病进行回顾，另外对外科治疗及其效果、相关争论进行简短的介绍。

表 76.1 运动障碍的分类

运动减少	
帕金森病 / 帕金森综合征	• 特发性、继发性（药物、中毒、感染、外伤、血管病变） • 运动迟缓、震颤、僵直和姿势不稳
进行性核上性麻痹	• 垂直凝视障碍、锥体外系症状、额叶功能障碍
多系统萎缩	• 帕金森综合征、小脑和自主神经功能障碍 • 进展迅速
僵人综合征	• 进行性躯干肌肉强直、僵硬并伴有肌痉挛
运动过多	
不宁腿综合征	• 继发于不适感的难以遏制的想要活动四肢的冲动
特发性震颤	• 动作性震颤 / 姿势性震颤 • 相关常染色体显性遗传
抽动秽语综合征	• 突然的、重复性的无节律的动作和话语，涉及离散肌群
肌张力障碍	• 持续的肌肉收缩导致肢体扭曲和重复性动作，或者异常的姿势
面肌痉挛	• 一侧面部的不自主运动
亨廷顿舞蹈症	• 认知、运动及精神障碍
斜颈	• 肌张力障碍导致的头颈部非对称性姿势
眼睑痉挛	• 双侧眼睑异常收缩
书写痉挛	• 特定任务下（如书写）出现的手部肌张力障碍

帕金森病

帕金森病（Parkinson’s disease，PD）是一种逐渐进展的慢性神经退行性疾病，主要表现为运动迟缓、肌强直、静止性震颤和姿势不稳。该病通常为单侧、隐袭起病，并伴有抑郁、疲劳以及睡眠障碍等非运动症状。

分类

帕金森综合征包括上文提到的运动症状，并且根据病因学分为以下 4 类：

a. 原发性 / 特发性 / 帕金森病（最常见）
b. 继发性 / 获得性（感染、药物、外伤、血管性因素）
c. 遗传性帕金森综合征（罕见）
d. 帕金森叠加综合征——有类似帕金森样临床表现的一类原发性神经系统退行性病变（如多系统萎缩）

流行病学

PD 是仅次于阿尔茨海默病的第二常见的神经退行性疾病。在英国，PD 发病率为（8~18）/100 000 人年，患病率为（108~164）/100 000。发病率与患病率都随年龄增长显著升高。50 岁之前较少发病，但在 60 岁之后近 1% 的人出现 PD。随着人口老龄化

PD 患者不断增加，预计到 2030 年全球 PD 患者数量将增加至 870 万~930 万人（Dorsey et al.，2007）。

研究表明男性比女性更易患 PD（1.3∶1，患病率和发病率）。尽管存在一定的确认偏倚，但是粗略的研究显示，欧洲和北美洲的高加索人更易患 PD，而非洲人患病率最低。有研究称吸烟和饮用含咖啡因的饮料可以预防 PD，但机制不明（Goetz and Pal，2014）。

发病机制

PD 发生发展的基本机制是黑质致密部（substantia nigra pars compacta，SNc）多巴胺能神经元的退行性变导致多巴胺缺失（Dauer and Przedborski，2003）。PD 有下列 3 个病理特征：

- 路易小体——这种嗜酸性神经元内包涵体被认为是神经元变性的标志。
- SNc 多巴胺能神经元死亡，并导致神经黑色素的丢失和该结构的褪色。
- 小胶质细胞清除死亡细胞中的神经黑色素。

要明确这种相对选择性的多巴胺缺失是如何导致 PD 的，需要对基底神经节的功能解剖和神经环路有详细的认识。大体上这条神经通路从前运动皮质途经纹状体，然后再回到辅助运动皮质。该神经环路的活动是由作为“油门”的 SNc 和作为“刹车”的丘脑底核（subthalamic nucleus，STN）调节的。帕金森病患者 SNc 功能缺失，导致运动缓慢，失去运动控制能力。

显然，该模型对 PD 的病理生理学进行了粗略的简化。从更复杂的层面讲，STN 和 SNc 的功能受到直接和间接通路调节（**图 76.1**）。直接通路来源于一组单突触投射到苍白球内侧部（GPi）和 SNr 的神经元，而间接通路来源于另一组投射到 GPe 且与 STN 有双向联系的神经元。PD 患者多巴胺缺乏导致纹状体苍白球 GABA 能神经纤维活性增加，抑制苍白球外侧部（GPe）神经元对 STN 的作用。从 STN 投射到 GPi 的谷氨酰胺能神经元受到刺激，进而增加对丘脑的激活（Calabresi et al.，2014）。

然而，上述模型并不能对所有实验室或临床研究结果做出解释。因此在过去的十年中，对于 PD 病理生理学理论的关注点已经从放电频率变成了放电模式，而现在人们更加关注神经元集群间的过度同步化活动。当大脑被唤醒并积极参与精神活动时会产生 β 波。已证实基底节神经元在 20 Hz 的 β 频段的过度同步化与 PD 有关（Little et al.，2012）。治疗性脑深部电刺激（deep brain stimulation，DBS）的宏电极可以检测到这种局部场电位的波动。

诊断

PD 的诊断通常以临床表现为依据。根据英国帕金森病协会脑库标准（Hughes et al.，1992）（**专栏 76.1**），诊断可能的帕金森病时，需要有运动迟缓及其他一项主要症状（强直、静止性震颤、姿势不稳）。此外，对多巴胺治疗反应良好是诊断的一个重要标准。其他帕金森综合征患者对多巴胺治疗的反应较 PD 患者差。

在评估疑似 PD 时，神经影像学往往不能提供准确诊断，但为了排除某些结构异常和其他疾病，需要对大脑进行磁共振成像（magnetic resonance imaging，MRI）。尽管临床应用仍存在争议，正电子发射断层扫描可显示早期 PD 患者壳核中后部示踪剂摄取减少。

使用单光子发射计算机断层扫描（single photon emission computed tomography，SPECT）对 PD 患者多巴胺转运体（dopamine transporter，DAT）进行成像，可以显示壳核放射性示踪剂摄取不对称减少，而尾状核对示踪剂摄取的减少程度较轻微（**图 76.2**）。而健康对照者、特发性震颤患者和药物引起的帕金森综合征患者的放射性示踪剂摄取是正常的。纹状体 DAT SPECT 可区分临床上可能的 PD 和特发性震颤，灵敏度为 79%~100%，特异度为 80%~100%（Vlaar et al.，2007）。然而，它不能区分 PD 和大多数帕金森综合征。

临床评估

详细的病史和神经科查体（**图 76.3**）对于准确诊断和随后的治疗至关重要。应该对其他疾病（如特发性震颤），以及共存的和可逆性的继发性帕金森综合征致病因素（如药物因素）进行仔细鉴别，最好由运动障碍疾病专业的神经病学家对患者进行检查。若感觉系统查体正常，但是考虑到 PD 有增加黑色素瘤的风险，可能建议进行皮肤检查（Bertoni et al.，2010）。通常体检可以发现许多基本症状，因此应该进行彻底的评估。此外，还应关注非运动症状（Chaudhuri et al.，2006）。

一些临床评定量表可以用于评估 PD 的严重程度、进展情况和对治疗的反应。这些量表的具体内容不在本书讨论范围之内，其中几个功能神经外科医生常用的量表列举如下：

- UPDRS（Unified Parkinson’s Disease Rating Scale，统一帕金森病评定量表）是最常用的 PD 临床评估

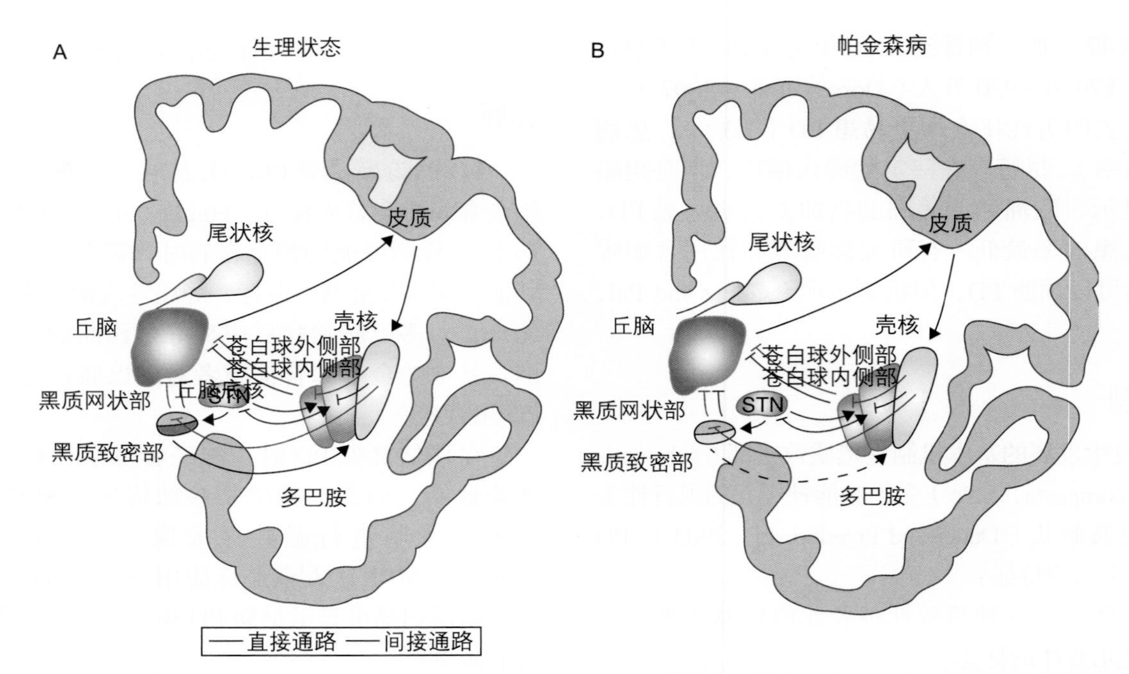

图 76.1 （A）在生理条件下，SNc 产生的多巴胺（dopamine，DA）可以激活直接通路（红线）中纹状体 MSN 的 D1 受体，抑制间接通路（蓝线）中纹状体神经元的 D2 受体。输出核团 GPi 和 SNr 投射到丘脑，然后再通过传出神经构成皮质 - 基底节 - 丘脑 - 皮质环路。（B）在帕金森病中，黑质神经元的退行性变减少了纹状体 MSN 上多巴胺受体的激活。直接途径和间接途径的不平衡导致输出核团的异常激活以及向皮质投射的丘脑神经元的过度抑制

量表，常用于跟踪随访患者的病程进展。它由 6 部分组成，通过访谈和临床观察相结合的方式进行评估。UPDRS-Ⅲ是一项由临床医生评分的运动状况评估。最近运动障碍协会对 UPDRS 进行了修订，新出版的 MDS-UPDRS 强调了对非运动症状的评估。
- 改良后的 Hoehn-Yahr 分期用于描述患者症状的进展情况及疾病分期。

药物治疗

可用于治疗 PD 的药物种类很多，具体用药取决于患者的病情差异（如病程分期、残疾程度）。大多数治疗方法本质上是对症治疗，并不能延缓或逆转疾病的自然进程。一些潜在的神经保护剂已经在动物和（或）早期临床研究中展现出一定的前景，进一步的研究正在进行之中（Stocchi and Olanow，2003）。包括教育、支持、锻炼、物理治疗、职业治疗、语言治疗和营养在内的非药物管理，也有助于提供整体的护理关怀。

是否对 PD 患者进行药物治疗取决于症状对患者日常生活的影响程度或者对工作的干扰程度。目前治疗 PD 运动症状的主要药物有：
- **左旋多巴**（L-dopa）是治疗 PD 的首选药物，尤其对运动迟缓疗效显著。左旋多巴也可以改善震颤和僵直症状，但是对姿势不稳疗效较差。左旋多巴与外周脱羧酶抑制剂（卡比多巴、苄丝肼）联合，可以阻止其在透过血脑屏障之前在外周循环中转化为多巴胺。

有相当一部分患者经过左旋多巴治疗后会出现左旋多巴诱发的并发症，比如运动波动、异动症和肌张力障碍。至少 50% 的患者经过 5～10 年的治疗后会出现这些症状（Schrag and Quinn，2000）。
- **多巴胺受体激动剂**（如普拉克索、罗匹尼罗、罗替戈汀和阿扑吗啡注射液）可单独用于治疗早期 PD，也可以与其他药物联合用于治疗晚期 PD。多巴胺受体激动剂可延迟需要进行左旋多巴治疗的时间点，但是也可能导致冲动控制障碍（性欲亢进、病理性赌博）（Weintraub et al.，2006）。鉴于与左旋多巴相比多巴胺受体激动剂可更少地引起运动症状波动，并且有证据表明早发型 PD 更容易出现左旋多巴诱导的异动症，因此建议对较年轻的 PD 患者（年龄＜65 岁）起始治疗时使用左旋多

专栏 76.1　英国帕金森病协会脑库诊断 PD 标准

核心诊断标准

行动迟缓（随意运动起始缓慢、重复动作的速度和幅度逐渐减小），并且存在下列至少一项：

- 肌强直
- 4~6 Hz 静止性震颤
- 非视觉、前庭、小脑或本体感受功能障碍引起的姿势不稳。

排除标准

- 反复卒中伴阶梯样进展的帕金森病症状、反复头痛或者明确的脑炎病史
- 动眼危象
- 症状初期的神经抑制剂治疗
- 1 个以上的亲属受累
- 症状持续缓解
- 发病 3 年后仍为严格的单侧症状或对称发病
- 核上性凝视麻痹
- 小脑体征
- 早期严重的自主神经受累
- 早期严重的痴呆，出现记忆、语言和行为障碍
- 巴宾斯基征
- 影像学检查示脑瘤或交通性脑积水
- 排除吸收障碍情况下对大剂量左旋多巴为阴性反应
- MPTP 接触史

支持诊断标准

3 项及以上并结合核心诊断标准方可确诊 PD

- 单侧发病
- 静止性震颤
- 呈进展性
- 持续的非对称性受累（先发病侧重）
- 对左旋多巴反应好（70%~100%）
- 严重的左旋多巴诱发的舞蹈症
- 左旋多巴反应在 5 年以上
- 临床病程在 10 年以上

巴受体激动剂。

- **单胺氧化酶 B（MAO–B）抑制剂**（如司来吉兰、雷沙吉兰）对 PD 症状有一定的改善，但是单药治疗对许多患者疗效并不显著。目前尚无足够的临床研究对 MAO-B 抑制剂与其他抗帕金森病药物进行比较，因此其相对风险与收益并不明确。不良反应包括恶心、头痛、失眠和精神错乱，特别是在老年患者中可出现（Riederer and Laux，2011）。
- **抗胆碱能药物**。PD 患者多巴胺缺失会导致胆碱能递质系统相对亢进，因此胆碱能药物会加剧 PD 症状而抗胆碱能药物可以缓解 PD 症状。单一用药时对有严重震颤而无明显僵直或步态障碍的 70 岁以下患者最为有效。该类药物对经左旋多巴或多巴胺受体激动剂治疗后仍存在持续性震颤的进展期患者也有效。不提倡对存在精神症状而无明显震颤的老年患者使用该药。
- **金刚烷胺**是一种抗病毒药物，具有相对较弱的抗帕金森作用，毒性较低，用于治疗早期或轻中度的年轻 PD 患者，以及异动症严重的晚期患者。副作用包括皮肤网状青斑、踝关节水肿、精神障碍、幻觉、梦魇、肝功能异常以及认知改变。
- **儿茶酚氧位甲基转移酶（COMT）抑制剂**（如恩他卡朋）作为左旋多巴的增效剂可以延长左旋多巴的效果，但单独使用时无明显疗效。该药主要用于存在剂末现象、症状波动的患者。

特发性震颤

震颤是一种不自主的运动，其特征为身体某一部分围绕一固定点进行有节奏的振荡样运动。特发性震颤（essential tremor，ET）以前被称为良性特发性震颤，是姿势性或动作性震颤最常见的神经系统病因，常累及上肢，也可累及头部和声带等其他部位。尽管症状存在差异，ET 仍可能被误诊为 PD。

流行病学

人群中 ET 的患病率为 0.4%~4%，男性和女性患病率无明显差别（Benito-Leon and Louis，2006）。头部震颤在女性患者中可能更为常见，而姿势性手部震颤在男性中可能更为严重。约 50% 的 ET 患者为常染色体显性遗传的家族性病例。

ET 的发病率随年龄增长而增加，有两个发病高峰——第一个是在青春期后期至成年早期，第二个是在老年期。目前来看，ET 发病平均年龄在 35 岁至 45 岁之间，也常见 65 岁甚至 70 岁发病者。震颤的幅度也会随着病程缓慢增加，震颤的频率却随着病程增加而降低。8~12 Hz 的震颤常见于年轻人，6~8 Hz 的震颤常见于老年人。虽然 ET 是进展性的，但没有证据表明发病年龄与疾病严重程度之间存在关联。新生儿和婴儿中曾有罕见 ET 病例的报道。

发病机制

ET 的确切病理生理学仍是一个谜。来自尸检和

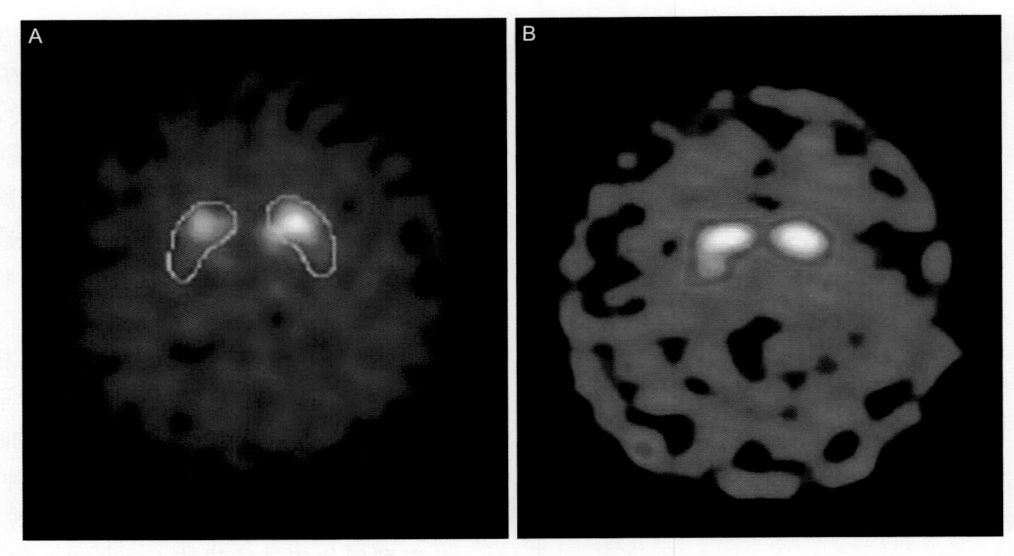

图 76.2 DAT 扫描显示正常人的对称信号（A）与帕金森病患者的不对称信号（B）

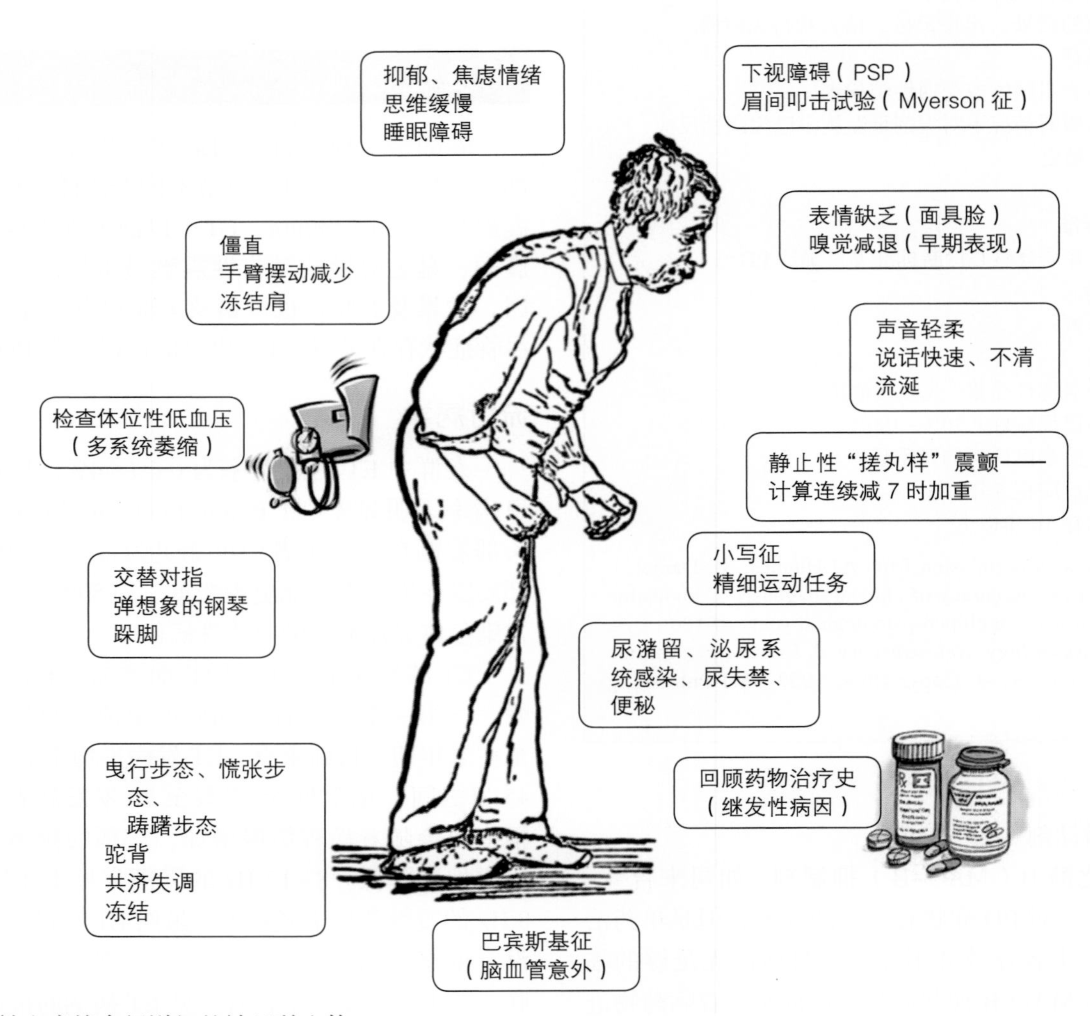

图 76.3 帕金森综合征详细的神经科查体

Reprinted from *A Manual of Diseases of the Nervous System*, W.R. Gowers, 1886, London J.& A. Churchill.

影像学研究的各种假说指出，ET 的发病机制可能为小脑 - 脑干 - 丘脑 - 皮质环路功能障碍，也可能是位于脑干附近的格 - 莫三角（Guillain Mollaret triangle）的中枢振荡器和下橄榄核的功能异常（Helmich et al.，2013）。

遗传学

ET 具有家族遗传性，在至少 50%~70% 的确诊病例中表现为外显不全的常染色体显性遗传，一些更精确的研究认为 17%~100% 的病例是家族性的。由于测量偏倚等问题，家族性发病的真实数据可能很难确定（Deng et al.，2007）。部分散发病例病因不明。

临床表现

ET 表现为颤抖的运动或感觉，典型的症状为上肢远端对称的 8~10 Hz 姿势性震颤，通常为低振幅快频率。疾病初期震颤的持续时间较短，但随着病情发展可变为持续性震颤。预测进展的因素包括发病之初的不对称震颤和单侧震颤。颈部肌肉可能受累，导致头部震颤（约 30%），嗓音、面部和下颌肌肉也可能受累。震颤的频率趋向于稳定，但振幅受情绪和生理状态影响变化很大。患者在睡眠时不会出现震颤，大部分研究称摄入酒精后症状会有所改善。ET 有时很难与严重的生理性震颤（由甲状腺功能亢进、发热或药物引起）鉴别，因此在诊断时应认真考虑上述情况。

随着时间的推移，这种震颤会影响患者的生活能力，造成进食、穿衣和个人卫生等方面的困扰，从而导致抑郁、焦虑状态、社交障碍或酗酒。少部分患者可能发展为严重的残疾，影响他们的就业和社会活动（Lorenz et al.，2011）。

诊断

像大多数运动障碍疾病一样，诊断主要依靠临床症状（**专栏 76.2**）。生化检查（甲状腺功能、血浆铜蓝蛋白）和影像学检查（MRI）是有效的替代筛查方式。SPECT 显像有助于帕金森病的诊断，从而减少 ET 的误诊。其他 PD 和 ET 震颤的鉴别要点如**表 76.2** 所示。

专栏 76.2　运动障碍学会震颤诊断标准

典型特发性震颤（ET）核心诊断标准

- 双手及前臂明显且持续的对称性姿势性和（或）动作性震颤
- 可单独或合并出现头部震颤，但不伴有姿势异常

典型 ET 的排除标准

- 其他异常体征，如肌张力障碍
- 存在加剧生理性震颤的因素，包括正在或近期服用致震颤的药物和药物戒断状态等
- 心因性震颤的病史或临床表现
- 明确的突然起病或进行性恶化
- 原发性直立性震颤
- 孤立性声音震颤
- 孤立性位置特异性或任务特异性震颤，包括职业性震颤和原发性书写震颤
- 孤立性舌或下颚震颤
- 孤立性下肢震颤

Reproduced with permission from Kailash P. Bhatia, Peter Bain, Nin Bajaj, et al., Consensus Statement on the classification of tremors. from the task force on tremor of the International Parkinson and Movement Disorder Society, *Movement Disorders*, Volume 33, Issue 1, pp. 75–87, Copyright © 2017 John Wiley and Sons.

表 76.2　PD 和 ET 震颤的其他鉴别要点

临床特征	帕金森病震颤	特发性震颤
发病年龄	>50 岁	20 岁和 60 岁两个高峰
性别	男性≥女性	男性 = 女性
家族史	<10%	>50%
对称性	单侧起病	双侧对称
震颤频率	4~6 Hz	4~10 Hz
特征	静止性震颤，偶见动作性震颤	姿势性、动作性震颤
部位	双手、前臂、下颌、舌	头、双手、嗓音
关联症状	运动迟缓、僵直、走路困难、姿势不稳	无
对下列药物反应：		
– 酒精	无	改善
– 左旋多巴	有	无
– 扑米酮 / 普萘洛尔	无	有

药物治疗

如果能够耐受，β 受体阻滞剂特别是普萘洛尔（60~320 mg/d）是治疗 ET 最常用的药物。一项临床试验中有 12%~66% 的患者出现了晕厥、头晕、乏力、阳痿和心动过缓等副作用（Zesiewicz et al.，2005）。存在心传导阻滞、哮喘或 1 型糖尿病的患者禁用普萘洛尔。

与普萘洛尔相同，**抗惊厥药物**扑米酮对ET同样有效。在治疗开始时扑米酮的副作用通常更为严重，包括镇静、嗜睡、乏力、恶心、呕吐、共济失调、萎靡不振、头晕、失稳、神志不清、眩晕和急性中毒反应。如果能够忍受副作用，联合应用β受体阻滞剂和扑米酮可以取得较好的疗效。其他抗惊厥药物如加巴喷丁和托吡酯也可以减轻震颤。

人们很早就知道**酒精**可以缓解ET。ET患者餐前或参加社交活动前可少量饮酒。然而长期饮酒会导致耐受，从而需要越来越多的酒精来达到同样的效果。一旦停止饮酒，戒断性震颤的出现会使得病情更加复杂，且饮酒会增加肝病风险。ET患者是否存在更高的酒精成瘾风险尚存争议。

苯二氮䓬类药物仅作为ET晚期的选择，因为该类药物效果有限，且存在药物滥用及停药导致戒断症状和震颤加重的可能。

肉毒杆菌毒素（botulinum toxin，BTX）注射治疗ET作用有限。对上肢震颤的轻度改善主要与剂量依赖的双手无力有关，而就嗓音震颤而言，该药可能导致呼吸困难、声音嘶哑和吞咽困难等副作用。

肌张力障碍

肌张力障碍是一种以肌肉持续不自主收缩产生扭转和重复性动作或异常姿势为特征的临床综合征。Herman Oppenheim在1911年首次描述了该病（Klein and Fahn，2013）。它是一种异质性的疾病，有多种表现形式和病因，可影响运动、言语、姿势、视觉等多种功能。通常而言，异常的姿势不是固定的，可以出现缓慢的扭转动作（手足徐动）。患者常十分痛苦且虚弱。

分类

肌张力障碍的分类方法较为复杂。早期的分类方法将肌张力障碍分为原发性肌张力障碍和继发性肌张力障碍（如脑瘫）。该分类经历了多次改进，目前已达成共识，将肌张力障碍按照临床表现和病因两类别进行分类（**专栏76.3**），不再使用原发性和继发性肌张力障碍等容易混淆的术语（Albanese et al.，2013）。

流行病学

据估计，英国大约有70 000成人和儿童患有肌张力障碍，发病率为1/900。虽然很难准确量化，但根据最低患病率估计，原发性肌张力障碍是继ET和

专栏76.3 肌张力障碍的分类

类别1，临床特征

发病年龄
- 婴儿时起病（出生~2岁）
- 儿童时起病（3~12岁）
- 青少年时起病（13~20岁）
- 成年早期起病（21~40岁）
- 成年晚期起病（>40岁）

累及部位
- 局灶性（如书写痉挛、睑痉挛）
- 节段性（2个及以上相邻部位肌群受累、头颈部肌张力障碍）
- 多灶性（2个及以上不相邻部位肌群受累）
- 全身型（+/- 腿部受累）
- 偏身型

时间模式
- 病程
- 稳定型
- 进展型
- 变异性
- 持续型
- 活动特异型
- 日间波动型
- 发作型

关联特征
- 孤立性肌张力障碍
- 混合性肌张力障碍
- 合并神经系统或其他系统受累表现

类别2，病因学
- 神经系统病理
- 有神经系统退行性变证据
- 有结构病变证据
- 无神经系统退行性变或结构病变
- 遗传性或获得性
- 遗传性
- 常染色体显性
- 常染色体隐性
- X染色体连锁隐性
- 线粒体缺陷

获得性
- 围产期脑损伤
- 感染
- 药物
- 中毒
- 血管性
- 肿瘤性
- 脑损伤
- 精神性

原发性
- 散发性
- 家族性

帕金森病之后的第三常见的运动障碍疾病。

遗传学

遗传形式对于肌张力障碍的临床鉴别十分重要，同时也可以在众多疾病类型中提供有价值的病因学信息。遗传性肌张力障碍可根据已知致病基因名或已有20多个并在不断增加的肌张力障碍基因位点进行分类。DYT基因位点系统是按照医学文献中出现相关报告的时间顺序进行分配命名的，理论上一旦明确了潜在的遗传原因，就应该移除该基因座命名。然而，实际上并没有发生这种情况，因此常同时使用肌张力障碍基因位点和基因名（如DYT1/TOR1A）（Charlesworth et al.，2013）。

DYT1/TOR1A是早发型肌张力障碍的致病原因，并以低外显率的常染色体显性方式遗传。已知有TOR1A突变的患病个体或无症状个体的后代有50%的遗传致病突变风险，30%~40%出现临床症状的风险。

发病机制

肌张力障碍的发病机制尚不清楚。有趣的是，大多数研究报告显示DYT1肌张力障碍中没有明显的神经退行性变或细胞减少。一项研究描述了脑干中的泛素和torsin-A阳性包涵体。功能MRI研究表明脚桥核参与肌张力障碍的“代谢网络”。

尽管一些研究指出继发型肌张力障碍小脑传出存在问题，通常认为其病理改变与基底神经节有关。虽然该病的病理生理学研究已经取得了许多进展，但仍需大量工作来完善这些假说。

诊断

因为肌张力障碍临床表现及病因多种多样，且常与其他运动障碍疾病叠加存在，其诊断存在一定的困难。肌张力障碍主要依靠临床诊断，因此最好由运动障碍专业的神经科专家进行评估。家族遗传史十分重要，多达44%的患者有类似的运动障碍的亲属。仔细询问用药史以排除继发性原因也很重要。

血液检查包括肝功能、血浆铜蓝蛋白等。神经影像学检查有助于排除结构性病变，并可用于研究潜在的深部脑电刺激的解剖学原理。对DYT和其他突变的遗传筛查和遗传咨询对于早发型原发性肌张力障碍患者及其亲属至关重要。

通常使用下列量表对肌张力障碍进行评估：

- Burke-Fahn-Marsden肌张力障碍量表（Burke-Fahn-Marsden Dystonia Rating Scale，BFM-DRS）用于对身体9部位进行肌张力障碍严重程度的测验，满分120分。该量表能够反映肌张力障碍活动的严重程度与频率。分数越高症状越严重。
- 痉挛性斜颈程度简况（Cervical Dystonia Impact Profile，CDIP-58）包括58项共8个量表，分数越高代表疾病越严重。
- 多伦多西部痉挛性斜颈评分量表（Toronto Western Spasmodic Torticollis Rating Scale，TWSTRS）也是痉挛性斜颈的常用评估量表。该量表包括3部分：严重程度（0~30分）、残障程度（0~30分）、疼痛（0~40分）。

药物治疗

根据症状的严重程度，采用多学科联合治疗肌张力障碍，包括药物治疗、联合医疗保健（物理治疗、心理治疗、语言治疗和职业治疗）以及必要时的手术治疗。

物理康复疗法治疗局灶性肌张力障碍十分有效，目的是尽可能地恢复和维持自理能力。认知行为疗法、自律训练法在肌张力障碍相关的抑郁症和焦虑症的管理中发挥着重要作用。肌肉痉挛和姿势异常可引起明显疼痛，可能需要进一步的疼痛治疗。如有言语困难，则需要进行语言治疗。

药物治疗通常用于缓解症状。目前没有一种特效药，通常需要多种药物联合才能有效治疗。

- 左旋多巴——在原发型肌张力障碍中，左旋多巴是长期治疗多巴反应性肌张力障碍的关键药物。
- 苯海索——通常作为治疗肌张力障碍的一线药物，但需注意监测其抗胆碱能副作用。
- 巴氯芬——有一定的疗效，但会引起嗜睡、流涎、肌无力等。
- 苯二氮䓬类药物——因呼吸抑制和成瘾被限制使用。
- 可乐定——可引起困倦。
- 加巴喷丁——可能对稳定情绪和提高睡眠质量有帮助。
- 肉毒毒素A注射——特别适用于局部肌张力障碍（如睑痉挛、书写痉挛）。可以在EMG或超声引导下进行注射。超适应证用于儿童特定肌群疼痛和痉挛的治疗。
- 巴氯芬鞘内注射——对局部和全身性肌张力障碍有效，并且与口服巴氯芬相比引起睡眠障碍风险更小。

也可考虑饮食支持、职业治疗、遗传咨询和社会支持等其他疗法。

手术治疗

对于药物难治性运动障碍疾病，则须考虑手术治疗。手术干预有可能避免运动障碍疾病的长期并发症（例如肌张力障碍患者的畸形和挛缩），因此手术被越来越多地用于这类疾病的早期治疗。当代功能性神经外科技术的起源可以追溯到 Irving Cooper 医生，他无意中结扎了一位 PD 患者的脉络膜前动脉，结果意外地改善了其震颤和强直症状（Cooper，1953）。该方法基本上被行之有效的特定区域毁损技术所取代。然而，鉴于毁损疗法尤其是双侧毁损术的不可逆性和并发症，使得高频 DBS 成为运动障碍的金标准手术方法。

毁损术

该手术首先要获取立体定向影像，然后通过深入到基底神经节核团的绝缘射频电极，使目标核团内的一小块区域凝固，疗效往往立竿见影。考虑到其不可逆转性，该技术在很大程度上已被 DBS 所取代。几十年来，它的应用逐渐减少；然而，对于功能神经外科医生而言，这种毁损手术仍然是一种有用的方法。其具备价格低廉、感染率低、相对安全等优势，并且能够避免因调整刺激参数或更换电池而反复就诊。

最近开展的高强度超声聚焦（high-intensity focused ultrasound，HIFU）技术，可以在实时 MRI 测温的引导下对靶点核团进行无切口的微创毁损，并进一步提高毁损手术的安全性。

脑深部电刺激

DBS 是指利用高分辨率成像（特别是 MRI）识别基底节区靶点核团，并使用立体定向技术植入永久电极的治疗技术。该过程通常在局部麻醉下进行，以便于利用神经生理学和临床表现确定电极的最佳放置位置。随后，电极通过延长导线在皮下走行与植入胸壁或腹壁的可植入式脉冲发生器（implantable pulse generator，IPG）相连。IPG 作为电池和编程设备，接受外部调整参数，改变电极输出信号。

植入手术

PD 的移植和修复疗法历史悠久，可追溯到 20 世纪 70 年代，但目前仍仅在部分临床试验中使用。一项随机研究对 40 名严重 PD 患者进行人类胚胎多巴胺神经元移植或对照假手术治疗，结果显示移植细胞可存活，对年轻患者有一定疗效，但对老年患者则无明显效果。此外，在移植后 4 年内移植物能够保持活性并持续带来临床收益，影像学变化与临床结果可靠相关。与此相反，在另一项前瞻性 24 个月的双盲安慰剂对照试验中，对 34 例晚期 PD 患者进行胚胎黑质移植，发现对病情较轻的患者有轻微的治疗效果。但是约 56% 的接受移植治疗的患者发展为关期肌张力障碍（Olanow et al.，2003）。其他团队也描述了这种异动症，并认为可持续长达 11 年。目前，神经移植仍是一种实验性疗法。需要进一步的研究来证实其客观疗效，明确适应证，确定最佳的移植细胞和植入部位。

手术治疗效果

帕金森病

有充足的证据表明，DBS 可以有效改善晚期 PD 患者的运动症状，对震颤、强直和运动迟缓有显著的长期疗效。一般来说，DBS 有望改善 UPDRS-Ⅲ衡量的运动症状达 50%，缩短关期时间达 70%，延长良好运动能力状态约 20%（Alamri et al.，2015）。总的来说，震颤和强直长期改善率比运动迟缓高。左旋多巴治疗有效的轴性症状通常也会得到改善。此外，经 STN-DBS 治疗，药物相关并发症如运动波动和异动症可减少 60%~70%。尽管疗效显著，但 DBS 治疗并没有改变 PD 的自然神经退行进程，因此从长期来看，轴性症状和运动不能会不断加重，认知功能同样会随着疾病进展而下降。报道称 STN-DBS 后 5~10 年运动症状持续显著改善，尤其是震颤、强直、运动波动和异动症等。帕金森病患者每日服用的左旋多巴等效剂量可以减少 40%~60%，并可保持长达 5 年。

最近有研究表明 STN-DBS 的运动改善效果并不局限于晚期 PD 患者。前瞻性随机多中心 EARLYSTIM 研究中神经刺激组疗效明显[鉴于以上结果，DBS 更多地被提出用于 PD 致残性运动波动早期的治疗]。但是仍需等待该队列研究的长期结果（Schuepbach et al.，2013）。

非运动症状（non-motor symptoms，NMS）是 PD 的常见症状，严重影响患者的生活质量。虽然 DBS 相关文献主要关注运动症状，但也有证据表明 STN-DBS 可以改善特定患者的 NMS（Witt et al.，2008）。

特发性震颤

DBS的短期和长期疗效已经被反复证实，90%的患者上肢震颤显著缓解。几项研究比较了 DBS 和丘脑毁损术治疗 ET 的临床结果和并发症。60%~90% 的患者经过上述中的一种治疗后对侧上肢震颤几乎完全消失（Zhang et al.，2010）。尽管两种疗法都有显著的长期疗效，但随着时间的推移，一些患者的疗效可能会降低。与 DBS 相比，丘脑毁损术出现严重神经系统并发症的风险更高。目前，丘脑毁损术仅用于某些特定的药物难治性的严重震颤患者，这些患者因不符合 DBS 适应证、无法耐受 DBS 硬件、需要反复进行 MRI 扫描、无法按时接受 DBS 术后程控或经济条件不允许等原因而不适合接受 DBS 治疗。少数 ET 患者可能因其他健康状况手术风险过高，不能耐受 DBS 或丘脑毁损术。在这种情况下，可以考虑丘脑放射外科治疗。

肌张力障碍

丘脑和 GPi 的立体定向毁损手术已用于肌张力障碍的治疗。由于纳入标准、评估手段和手术技术的标准化欠缺，疗效难以评估。研究显示，丘脑毁损术可使 10/20 的原发性肌张力障碍患者症状改善 25%~100%，29 例继发性肌张力障碍患者中 68% 有 25%~100% 的改善。但是严重的副作用（15% 的偏瘫和高达 56% 的构音障碍或发音困难）限制了该疗法的应用。Buzaco 认为苍白球毁损术效果与丘脑毁损术效果相同，但副作用更少，证实了苍白球毁损术在减轻原发性或继发性肌张力障碍患者症状方面的有效性。这些报告中没有提及任何长期并发症（Speelman et al.，2010）。

虽然丘脑和丘脑底核电刺激也被用于治疗肌张力障碍，但 GPi 是目前 DBS 手术治疗肌张力障碍的首选靶点。据报道，在原发性全身性肌张力障碍中，BFMRS 的运动和残疾评分有显著改善（40%~80%）。类似的结果也出现在节段性肌张力障碍患者中。经过长达 10 年的随访，苍白球 DBS 治疗效果稳定。继发性肌张力障碍较为特殊，一般认为其对 DBS 治疗反应差，但有报告显示许多继发性肌张力障碍的临床结果令人满意，如迟发性肌张力障碍。对该患者群体 DBS 疗效的评估，更倾向于使用生活质量量表或患者报告进行评估，而不是已得到验证的运动障碍量表。

争议

近三十年来，DBS 已成为运动障碍疾病的有效干预手段，因此争议主要集中在手术技术的差异，而不是其疗效：

- 全身麻醉与局部麻醉。良好的 DBS 疗效依赖于准确将电极植入一个非常小且深入脑内的靶点。可以在术中利用 DBS 电极对清醒患者进行宏刺激，以确定缓解症状的最佳位置并避免副作用，并可以立即更换电极位置至更有效的靶点。但是一个术中清醒的患者需要在“关期”保持完好的认知功能来执行智力任务、进行配合并长时间保持不动。这些问题可以通过全身麻醉避免，但是只能依靠影像定位法和术中微电极记录进行电极定位。目前还没有比较两种方法效果的随机对照试验。
- 微电极记录（microelectrode recordings，MER）是一种电生理学技术，通过插入非常细小尖利的电极记录信号，并根据靶点核团放电模式和特征信号来验证其边界。但是 MER 需要专业知识、额外的花销和更长的手术时间。也有证据表明 MER 会增加颅内出血的风险。随着外科技术的进步，精确的影像引导下可以“直接”对靶点进行定位，一些外科医生开始质疑 MER 的常规应用。
- STN 与 GPi。因相关研究结论不一，一直存在关于采用 GPi 还是 STN 作为 DBS 治疗 PD 靶点的争论。过去 10 年中，总体观点倾向于对大多数患者选择 STN 靶点，而对以肌张力障碍为主或存在神经精神障碍风险的老年患者进行 GPi 刺激。最近的研究表明这两种方法的疗效相当。
- 复合左旋多巴 / 卡比多巴肠用凝胶和 DBS。口服左旋多由于胃排空而无法维持稳定的血药浓度，导致运动症状波动。因为可靠的药理学特征和便携式运载系统，复合左旋多巴 / 卡比多巴肠用凝胶（Duodopa）已成为运动波动患者的一种治疗选择。比较 Duodopa 和 DBS 的研究有限，一项研究表明，与 Duodopa 相比，DBS 在异动症持续时间和残疾方面改善更为显著（Merola et al.，2011）。虽然 Duodopa 有望成为 PD 患者尤其是 DBS 禁忌证患者的替代治疗方案，但必须注意 PEG 管置入相关的高并发症率。Duodopa 比 DBS 昂贵得多，因此成本问题也应注意。

延伸阅读、参考文献、EBRAIN 的相关链接

扫描书末二维码获取。

第77章 痉挛状态

John Goodden・Catherine Hernon・Brian Scott 著
李志保、王乔、韩春雷 译，孟凡刚、崔志强 审校

引言

本章回顾了成人及儿童痉挛状态的病因与治疗。由于这一人群复杂多样且年龄跨度大，本章中所提及的许多治疗仅适于其中部分患者群体。

痉挛状态是指一种导致运动抵抗增加的不自主、速度依赖的肌张力增高状态。痉挛状态主要由上运动神经元损伤（upper motor neurone lesions，UMNL）所引起，该损伤导致α和γ运动神经元下行抑制作用丧失或减弱，主要表现为反射弧内的改变，抑制性输入丧失导致反射亢进。根据上运动神经元损伤的病因，痉挛状态的影响可见于上肢或下肢。

痉挛状态既往多采用偏瘫、双侧瘫痪和四肢瘫痪这些术语来描述痉挛症状的分布及四肢的受累情况。然而，神经康复专家不建议使用这些术语，因为这些术语错误地暗示了其他肢体没有受到影响，而实际上这些肢体可能受到了轻微的影响。因此痉挛状态的描述既要说明主要受累的肢体，又要体现痉挛状态（例如，“主要影响双下肢的痉挛状态”而不是“双侧瘫痪”）。

痉挛状态的病理生理学基础

导致痉挛状态的脑或脊髓的病理生理改变尚不明确。然而，目前认为痉挛状态主要由网状脊髓束和皮质脊髓束或锥体束和脊髓中间神经元损伤所引起。这种损伤引起脊髓运动环路抑制性输入减少，从而导致反射弧过度活跃。神经电生理检查中H-M比例和F波幅值增高证明了运动神经元兴奋性的增强。

在脊髓内，可看到运动神经元、中间神经元和反射弧通路兴奋性的变化。在健康人中，1a抑制性中间神经元调节反射弧，其一部分功能是接受从皮质脊髓通路传入的下行神经元。当中间神经元受损和下行传入减少时，痉挛状态就会出现。

随着时间的发展，受影响的肌肉会逐渐挛缩，但是肌梭的敏感性通常不会改变。

病因

痉挛状态的病因包括先天性因素（脑瘫、脊髓栓系/脊髓闭合不全）和后天性因素（卒中、外伤、肿瘤、脱髓鞘病变、进行性神经退行性病变、感染、脑积水和脊髓空洞症）。因为痉挛状态是上运动神经元损伤导致的，所以不可能由脊髓圆锥以下的脊髓损伤引起。如果患者出现急性上运动神经元损伤，最初肌张力通常较低，表现为弛缓性瘫痪，随后会逐渐演变成痉挛状态。

脑瘫是儿童痉挛状态最常见的病因，而多发性硬化（multiple sclerosis，MS）是成人痉挛状态最常见的病因。

脑瘫在新生儿中的发病率为1/500。它是一种非进展性疾病，临床表现多样，包括痉挛状态、肌张力障碍、运动障碍和共济失调。虽然脑损害处于静态，但由于肌肉生长慢于邻近的骨骼，且关节受力不平衡，故脑瘫对肌肉骨骼系统的影响通常是进展的。这对发育中的骨骼和关节的形态是有害的。

多发性硬化是一种免疫介导的进展性退行性疾病，病程变化多样，可表现为复发-缓解和逐渐/快速进展。多发于北欧地区，发病高峰在30岁左右，男女比例为1∶3。英国的发病率最近估计为9.46/10万人，英格兰和威尔士的发病率为100~140/10万人，北爱尔兰为170/10万人，苏格兰为190/10万人，设得兰为295/10万人，奥克尼为402/10万人。

辅助检查、评估和诊断

痉挛状态患者应转诊给高年资医师进行全面评估。包括详细的病史记录和检查，做基本的血液检查（包括全血细胞检查/血尿素电解质检查）和血

液或尿液培养以寻找感染。在考虑神经退行性疾病时，家族史对儿童尤为重要。专科检查包括脑脊液（cerebrospinal fluid，CSF）检查、MRI 和 EMG/EEG。

当患者症状突然加重时，临床医生需要再次进行详细的病史记录和体格检查、血液检查和尿培养。引起病情恶化的常见因素包括感染（尤其是尿道或耳部感染）、更换药物、疼痛、褥疮、便秘、隐匿性骨折、足部矫形相关问题、深静脉血栓形成、心理压力高、疲劳，甚至是寒冷的天气。

痉挛状态的评估需要专业的多学科综合治疗团队（multidisciplinary team，MDT），包括评估哪些肌肉过度活跃，以及痉挛状态如何影响患者的日常生活（包括自我护理、活动、睡眠和工作）。一些开发的评分系统可以记录痉挛状态和功能限制的程度。改良 Ashworth 评分是最常用的评估痉挛状态严重程度的量表（Platz et al.，2005）（**表 77.1**），但也使用其他量表，如 Tardieu 评分。此外，还需要记录运动范围、肌力、生活质量、功能和步态（如果有关联）（Haley et al.，1992；Steinbok，2001；Platz et al.，2005；Haugh et al.，2006；O'Brien and Park，2006；Engsberg et al.，200；Harvey et al.，2007；Khan，2007；Delhaas et al.，2008；Gorton et al.，2009；Akerstedt et al.，2010；Gilmore et al.，2010；Ou et al.，2010；Dasenbrock et al.，2011；Reynolds et al.，2011；Tedroff et al.，2014）。这些评估应在治疗前进行，以便评估治疗的效果。

对于脑瘫儿童，粗大运动功能分级系统（Gross Motor Function Classification System，GMFCS）和粗大运动功能评估量表（Gross Motor Function Measure，GMFM）的测试是记录和总结儿童运动功能能力的有用工具。GMFCS 的分级是从 1 级（独立行走）到 5 级（坐轮椅）（**图 77.1** 和**表 77.2**）。GMFM 是标准化的观测工具，用于测量儿童粗大运动功能随时间的变化，将其汇总为单个分数，然后进行比较并跟踪疾病进度。

表 77.1　改良 Ashworth 评分

评分	描述	检查
0	无肌张力增高	可以任何速度自由活动
1	肌张力轻微增高	仅在抓住、释放或活动末出现最小的阻力
1+	肌张力轻度增高	在抓住、释放和活动剩余部分均出现最小阻力
2	肌张力较明显增高	整个活动都有中等阻力，但关节可自由活动
3	肌张力严重增高	肌张力高，并且关节难以活动
4	僵直	受累关节僵直不能屈曲或伸展

痉挛状态的治疗（包括康复、物理治疗及专业治疗）

治疗痉挛状态的多学科综合治疗团队应该由一名康复医师、物理治疗师、专科医师和多个外科医师（神经外科、整形外科、骨科）组成（Park and Albright，2006；Steinbok，2006；Abbott，2007；Ronan and Gold，2007）。谨慎地掌握疗效与副作用之间的平衡尤为重要。痉挛状态对患者的生活既有积极影响也有消极影响。比如，患者虽然存在腿部痉挛性僵直，但在这种状态下患者可以行走，解除这种痉挛状态后，患者肢体无力可能导致无法行走。

可以通过通讯辅助工具、夹板、定制的步行架和轮椅为患者提供帮助。其总体目的是保护功能，避免或减少痉挛状态和残疾的有害影响。常规的物理治疗是核心，以保持患者灵活性和避免肌肉 / 肌腱挛缩形成的进展。职业疗法和矫形检查对于保护皮肤、优化夹板和支撑、实现功能最大化和防止褥疮的发展是必要的。最后，良好的膀胱护理对预防复发感染（泌尿道感染是痉挛状态恶化的常见原因）也至关重要。

采用多种药物治疗有助于降低痉挛状态的有害影响。这些治疗的主要目的是改善肌张力、缓解痉挛状态、维持胃肠道正常功能和膀胱功能。

常见的抗痉挛状态药物有巴氯芬、丹曲林、替托尼定和地西泮（Papavasiliou，2009；Quality Standards of the American Academy of Neurology et al.，2010；Novak et al.，2013）。这些药物的副作用多种多样，包括嗜睡、虚弱、疲劳、镇静和记忆障碍。患者 / 护理人员在服用之前阅读了相关资料后，这些药物并不容易被患者接受。

巴氯芬是治疗痉挛状态的主要药物，特别是对脑瘫和脊髓损伤的患者。主要作用于突触前、后的 $GABA_B$ 受体，减少 α 运动神经元的兴奋性传递并减少痛觉。胃肠道（gastrointestinal，GI）吸收良好，但血脑屏障的通过性较差。因此，在临床疗效显现之前需要大剂量给药，但这有增加副作用

6~12 岁 GMFCS E & R：描述与插图

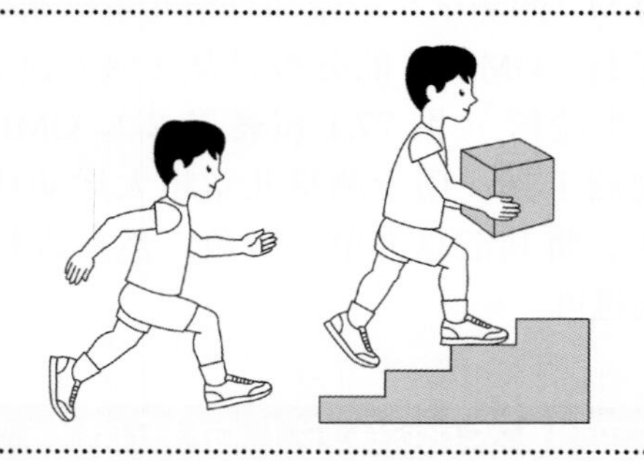

GMFCS 1 级

儿童可在家里、学校、户外和社区行走。可不扶栏杆爬楼梯。可做粗大动作，如跑步和跳跃，但说话、平衡和协调能力受限。

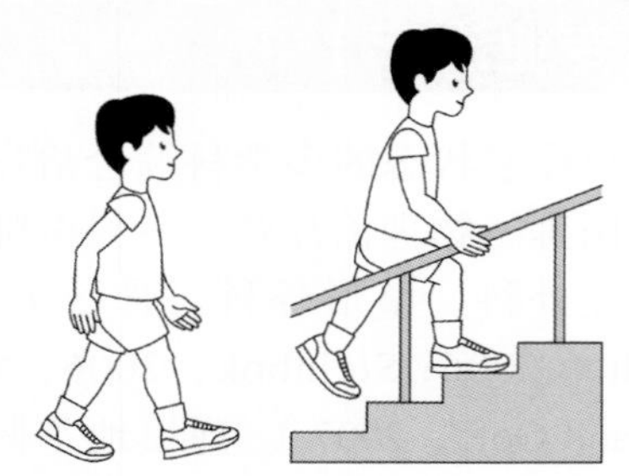

GMFCS 2 级

儿童可在大多数场景下走路，爬楼梯时需扶着栏杆。在不平坦的地形、斜坡、拥挤的区域或狭窄的空间中可能难以长距离行走和保持平衡。儿童可以在物理辅助、手动运动辅助设备或使用轮椅的情况下长距离行走。儿童只有很少的能力来执行粗大的运动功能，如跑步和跳跃。

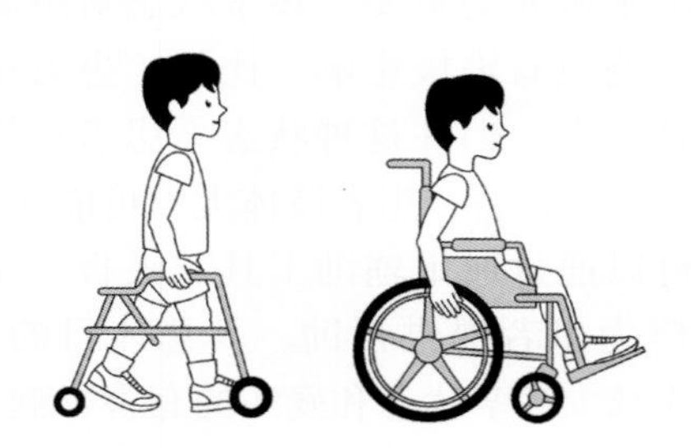

GMFCS 3 级

在大多数室内环境中，孩子们用手驱动辅助设备以便能够行走。在监督或帮助下，他们可以扶着栏杆爬楼梯。儿童在长途旅行时使用轮式设备，在较短距离内活动可以自行行走。

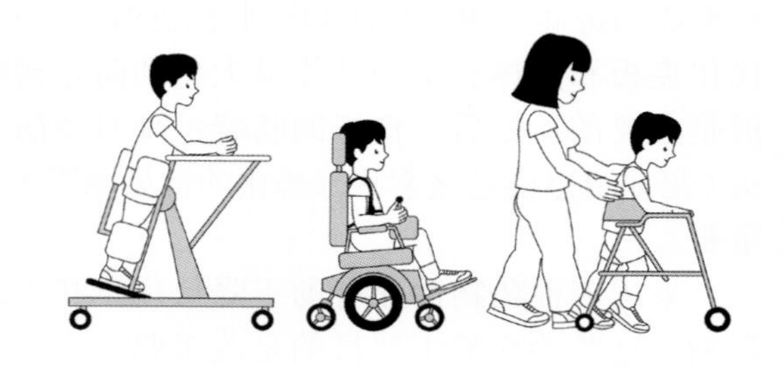

GMFCS 4 级

在大多数情况下，儿童使用物理辅助或动力驱动的移动方式。可以在家里在物理辅助或使用动力驱动的方式进行短距离行走，或定站立时需要身体支撑步行器。在学校、户外和社区中，儿童乘坐手动轮椅或使用电动移动工具。

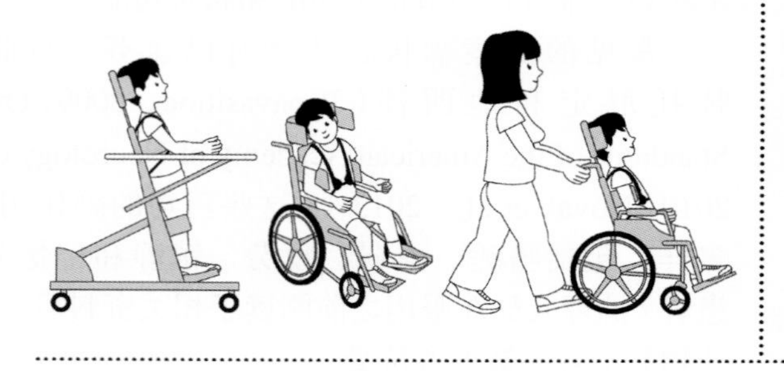

GMFCS 5 级

儿童在任何情况下都用手动轮椅活动。儿童在维持头部和躯干的反重力姿势以及控制腿部和手臂运动的能力方面受到限制。

图 77.1 粗大运动功能分级系统

表 77.2　粗大运动功能分级系统

GMFCS 分级	一般描述
1	步行不受限
2	步行受限
3	在手动运动辅助设备辅助下行走
4	自我移动受限，需要动力驱动设备辅助
5	借助手动轮椅活动

Reproduced with permission from Robert Palisano, Peter Rosenbaum, Stephen Walter, et al., Development and reliability of a system to classify gross motor function in children with cerebral palsy, *Developmental Medicine & Child Neurology*, Volume 39, Issue 4, pp. 214–23. Copyright © 2008 John Wiley and Sons.

（镇静、行为改变、意识障碍、共济失调、尿频和失眠）的风险。巴氯芬开始时小剂量给药，然后逐渐增加，直到获得最大疗效或产生副作用为止。如果停药，必须逐渐减少，以避免有癫痫发作、痉挛状态反弹或幻觉的风险。

丹曲林用于治疗上运动神经元损伤导致的痉挛状态、抽筋和痉挛。主要作用是减少去极化诱导的钙流入横纹肌浆网。其胃肠道吸收不充分，缓慢但稳定。副作用包括肌无力（使移动更困难）、镇静状态和肝损害。

替托尼定是一种中枢 α_2- 肾上腺素能受体激动剂。通常用于治疗多发性硬化、卒中和脊髓损伤导致的痉挛状态。作用时间较短，给药后 1~2 小时达到峰效应；3~6 小时后逐渐消失。因此，它通常用于特定的活动和最需缓解痉挛的时候。其药代动力学在不同的制剂中有所不同，并且在进食与否的情况下服用时也有所不同，在禁食条件下服用（进食后 >3 小时）更好。与其他药物一样，这种药物的剂量可以在几天内逐渐增加，停药也应该是渐进过程。

地西泮作用于 $GABA_A$ 受体，通过增加运动神经元的突触后抑制达到治疗痉挛状态和肌肉痉挛的作用。是完全性脊髓损伤患者的首选药。剂量增加或减少要逐渐进行。用药超过一周后可能会出现药物依赖性问题。药物副作用包括无力、镇静和体力下降。突然停药可能会导致抑郁、癫痫发作和急性戒断综合征。

肉毒素 A（Criswell et al.，2006；Steinbok，2006；Love et al.，2010；Quality Standards Subcommittee of the American Academy of Neurology et al.，2010；Williams et al.，2012；Novak et al.，2013；Cusick et al.，2015）是一种神经毒素，可永久性结合在神经肌肉接头处的突触前端抑制乙酰胆碱释放，使治疗的肌肉去神经功能。通常在超声引导下直接注射给药，以提高准确度和疗效的持久性。起效在 3~7 天内并维持 16 周，随着新的神经肌肉接头从芽生的神经根中长出，解痉作用逐渐消失。如果频繁使用肉毒素 A，会因抗体形成而使疗效下降。给药时一定要谨慎，肉毒素用量过少，可能疗效有限，但过量可能会导致全身反应和广泛的肌肉麻痹。目前已批准用于治疗成人上肢痉挛状态、不稳定膀胱、膀胱过度活动症以及颈部肌张力障碍。肉毒素 A 广泛用于儿童上下肢痉挛状态，但未得到许可。最好与拉伸、石膏矫正、肌肉锻炼、矫形调整结合使用。

痉挛状态的外科治疗

有几种手术策略用来缓解痉挛状态的不利影响。这涉及几个不同的学科。神经外科技术包括巴氯芬鞘内注射（intrathecal baclofen，ITB）、选择性脊神经后根部分切断术（selective dorsal rhizotomy，SDR）、经皮射频神经根切断术和脊髓切断术。除此之外，整形外科医生还可以实施选择性外周神经切断术（selective peripheral neurotomy，SPN）。骨科手术也很重要，因为痉挛状态可导致复杂的骨和关节畸形。由于篇幅的限制，我们重点介绍 ITB、SDR、SPN，并对骨科手术治疗该疾病进行概述。

巴氯芬鞘内注射

巴氯芬鞘内注射疗法是治疗成人及儿童痉挛状态和肌张力障碍的一种疗效确切的方法。1958 年由 Penn 和 Kroin 首次报道（Penn and Kroin，1985）。他们假定并证明了将巴氯芬直接注射入脑脊液内可达到和口服一样的疗效，而且所用剂量更小、副作用更少。这是因为脊髓中的 $GABA_B$ 受体位于表层，巴氯芬可直接起作用。然而，大脑中的 $GABA_B$ 受体位于深层，这意味着中枢不良反应会更少。

在考虑使用 ITB 疗法时，通常先从试验剂量开始（Albright and Ferson，2006；Delhaas et al.，2008；Phillips et al.，2015）。在全麻或局部麻醉下通过腰椎穿刺直接注射 50~100μg 巴氯芬，或通过腰穿置管进行连续试验剂量注射或试验灌注。进行试验剂量注射的目的是评估疗效及检测可能的副作用。然而，试验剂量对肌张力障碍患者的疗效可能不明显，而长期灌注的持续作用疗效会更好。

ITB 可通过外部可调控泵系统给药，该系统包含药物贮存器（10~40 ml）、电池和药物输送装置。手术时，患者左侧卧位。将泵植入到右前腹壁的皮下囊袋里。避免在左侧植入 ITB 装置，因为胃造瘘术通常在这一侧进行。泵囊既可以位于皮下（直肌筋膜浅部），也可以位于筋膜下（腹直肌和腹外斜肌筋膜深部）。筋膜下囊袋特别适用于瘦小的儿童（Vender et al.，2006；Motta et al.，2007；Fjelstad et al.，2009；Ammar et al.，2012；Motta and Antonello，2014）。囊袋成型后，在腰椎区域做一个小切口，然后用 Toohey 针通过腰椎穿刺插入鞘内导管。文献报道中对导管尖端的位置存在争议，即在上肢痉挛状态或肌张力障碍的患者中是否需要将导管尖端位置放得更高（Grabb et al.，1999；Albright and Ferson，2006；Dziurzynski et al.，2006；McCall and MacDonald，2006；Motta et al.，2007；Brennan and Whittle，2008；Sivakumar et al.，2010；Ughratdar et al.，2012；Varhabhatla and Zuo，2012）。一些研究表明，胸椎和腰椎的脑脊液脉冲式流动较少，因此将导管放置在此部位会导致巴氯芬扩散减少（Bernards，2006；Heetla et al.，2014）。术中导管尖端定位可通过 X 线引导完成。在某些情况下可将导管插入脑室内，以进行脑室内巴氯芬注射（Albright，2011；Rocque and Albright，2011；Bollo et al.，2012；Turner et al.，2012）。一旦导管植入到合适的位置后，就将导管通过皮下隧道穿到腹部囊袋并固定到输液泵上完成植入（**图** 77.2）。

植入后激活输液泵，系统就可以立即开始释放巴氯芬。剂量逐渐向上滴定，通常每 1~2 周递增 10%。ITB 剂量可以通过灵活的剂量程控来调节，在一天的不同时间提供不同量的巴氯芬。根据滴速和药物浓度的不同，药物储存器需要每 2~6 个月排空和重新注满一次。当电池寿命接近尾声时，还需要手术来更换药物泵。

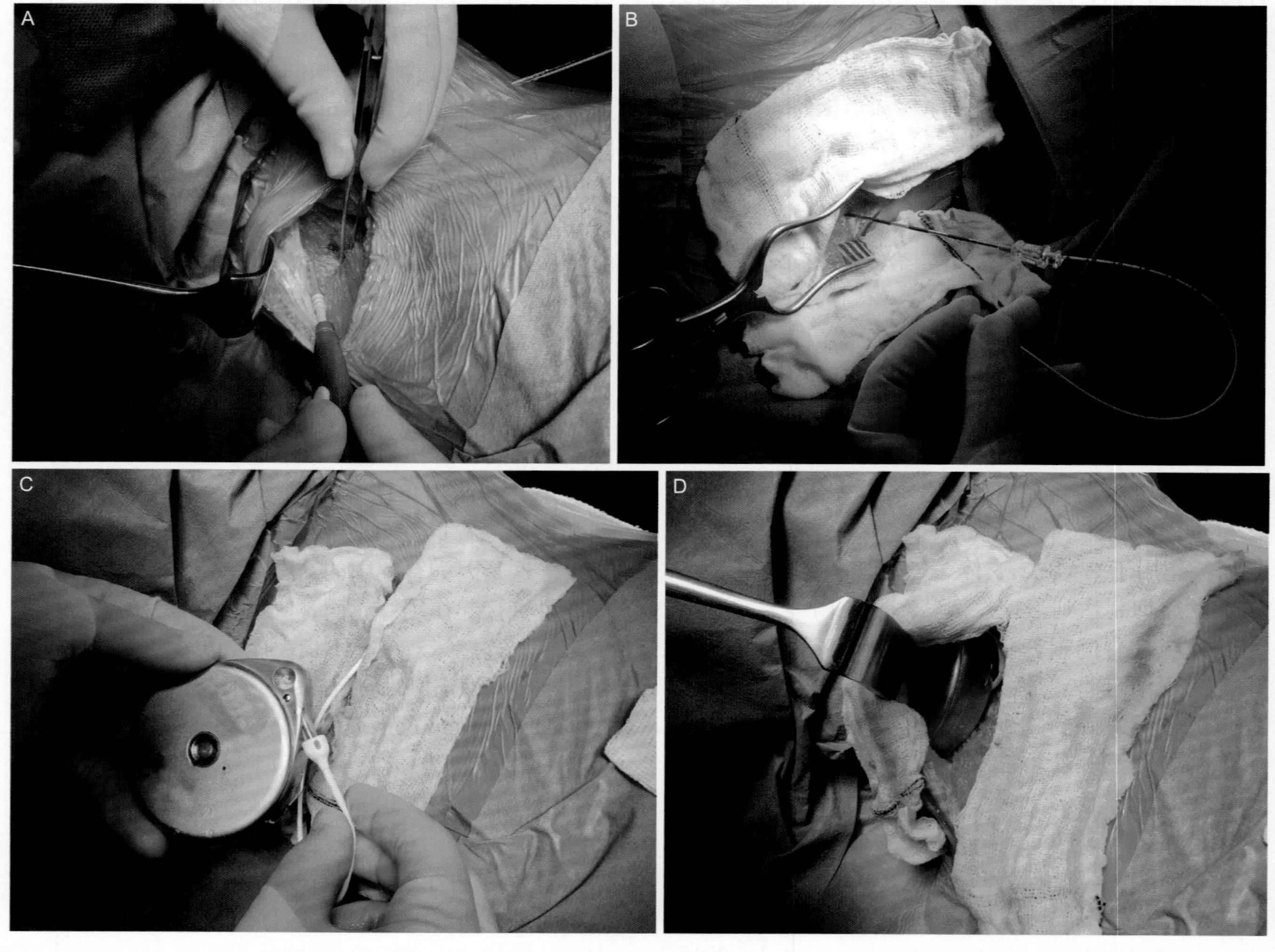

图 77.2 鞘内注射巴氯芬泵植入的术中照片。（A）经右上腹切口形成筋膜下囊袋。（B）通过中部腰椎穿刺插入腰椎导管。（C）导管与泵连接。（D）将导管盘绕在泵后面并植入体内

ITB 疗法的风险和不良反应包括手术本身的风险以及与药物泵系统障碍和药物加注过程相关的风险（Albright and Ferson，2006；Vender et al.，2006；Motta et al.，2007；Protopapas et al.，2007；Brennan and Whittle，2008；Fjelstad et al.，2009；Heetla et al.，2014；Motta and Antonello，2014）。

- **药物剂量不足或急性戒断**：如同任何机械设备一样，ITB 泵可能会出故障，导致急性的巴氯芬戒断综合征（一种危及生命的情况，可导致严重的痉挛加重、横纹肌溶解、肾衰竭，甚至死亡）。如果在加注药物的时候使用了错误的药物浓度，也会出现这种情况。
- **药物过量**可见于程控错误或加注药物时。给泵加药时关键是要确保针插入到泵内，而不是泵的旁边，使药物加到泵内，而不是泵的皮下囊袋中（囊式加注）。囊式加注会危及生命安全，需要立即从囊袋中吸出药物，并需要重症监护病房（intensive care unit，ICU）的支持性通气，直到巴氯芬作用消失。

选择性脊神经后根部分切断术（SDR）

SDR 是一种能永久降低或消除腿部肌张力增高的手术。主要适用于儿童，但不适用于成人。手术包括解剖和切断部分腰椎感觉神经根，以破坏异常反射弧。此技术较适于脑损伤稳定且没有进展的脑瘫。对于进展的神经退行性病变，SDR 的获益较为短暂。当痉挛状态是唯一表现时，则最好行 SDR；但当存在肌张力障碍时，SDR 往往会加重症状。

1898 年，Sherrington 在一只猫的脑瘫模型上进行了试验，首次报道了脊神经被根切断术（Sherrington，1898）。后来，Foerster 在 1913 年首次报道在人身上进行的 SDR（Foerster，1913）。然而，这两个报道都进行了腰椎感觉神经根完全切断，导致躯体感觉麻木和本体感觉障碍，从而增加了活动困难。后来 Gros（Gros et al.，1967）和 Fasano（Fasano et al.，1978）也进行了进一步研究，直到 Peacock（Peacock and Eastman，1981；Peacock and Arens，1982）最终报道了现代选择性脊神经后根部分切断术，该技术先利用神经电生理技术找到最异常的神经根，然后切断。此后的主要进展是明确了患者选择标准（Peacock et al.，1987），并将手术改进为 2 个节段椎板切除术（Park et al.，1993），后来又改进为单节段 L1 椎板切除术（Park and Johnston，2006）。

在考虑 SDR 时，需要仔细进行 MDT 评估。行 SDR 的典型患者是确诊为脑瘫，且动态性痉挛状态主要影响腿部从而限制活动的儿童。GMFCS 分级通常在 2~3 级，在辅助下可以活动，但需要足够的核心肌肉和腿部肌肉力量支持。

对于肌张力障碍和明显累及上肢的患者，SDR

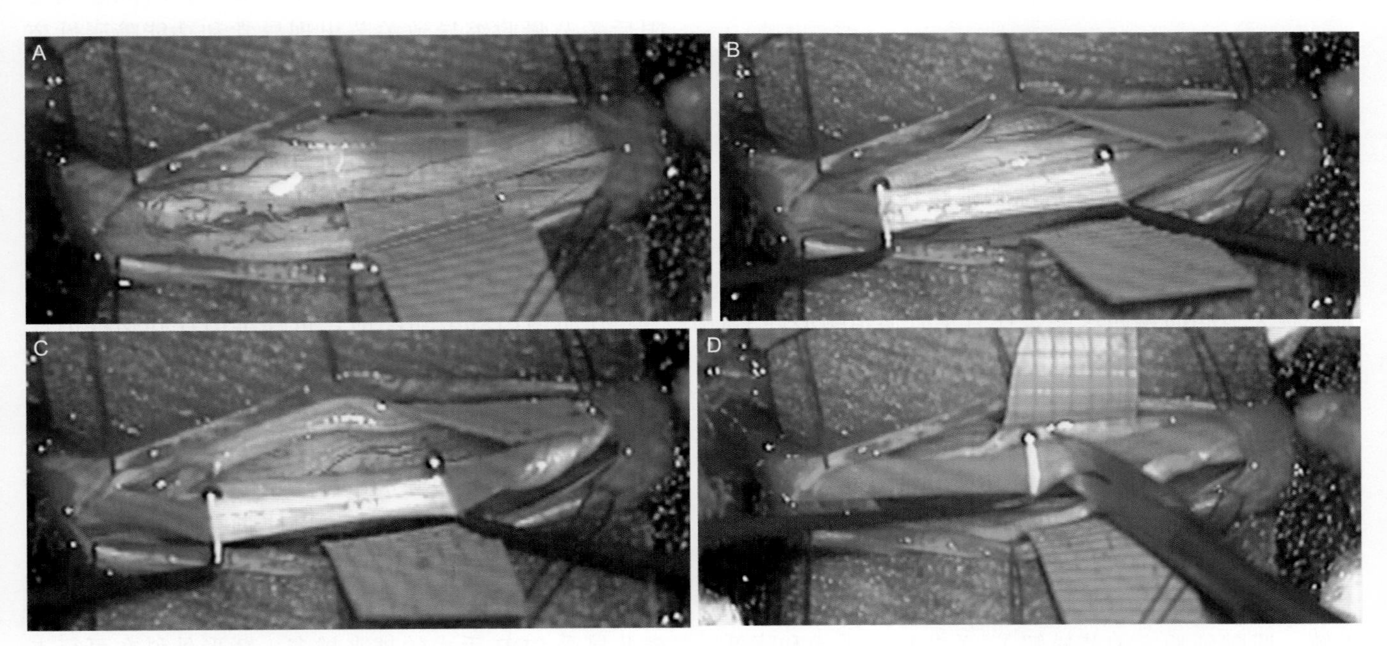

图 77.3 术中照片显示通过圆锥上单椎板切除术进行选择性脊神经背根切断术。（A）L2~S1 右侧背根与腹根分离，并使用绿色硅橡胶条隔离。（B）通过定制的神经钩进行双极刺激测试 L2 的第一分支。（C）测试 L2 的第二分支。（D）将反应最异常的分支切断

并不适用。对 GMFCS 4~5 级的患者疗效不确切。

手术通过切开圆锥上的 L1 椎板进行。从运动根分出 L1~S1 背根（感觉）。每个神经根再分成三个小根，术中进行神经生理学检查，找出异常活跃最显著的小根，然后再将三个小根中的两个小根切断（**图 77.3**）。因此，L1~S1 每条感觉根的大约 2/3 被切断。为了降低尿失禁的风险，通常要进行肛门括约肌监测。

一旦通过 SDR 消除或减轻了痉挛状态，随后会出现肌无力。这需要加强物理治疗来增强力量。SDR 后，患者在出院前需要接受 3 周的强化理疗。在此之后，需要进行定期的社区理疗，并鼓励患者坚持活动。

SDR 的风险与副作用包括任何神经外科脊髓硬膜内手术的常见风险（包括瘫痪、麻木和尿失禁）。然而，术中神经电生理监测能将这种风险降到最低（Hays et al.，1998；Mittal et al.，2001；Steinbok et al.，2009；Turner，2009；Fukuhara et al.，2011）。

SDR 的疗效已经在文献中得到了广泛的研究和报道，证实了该手术在控制痉挛状态和减少骨科手术方面的具有长期获益（Bolster et al.，2013；Dudley et al.，2013；Hurvitz et al.，2013；Langerak et al.，2013；Steinbok，2013；Tedroff et al.，2014；Josenby et al.，2015；Steinbok，2015；Vermeulen and Becher，2015）。痉挛状态控制程度与 SDR 手术中切断的细小神经根百分比有关，小于 50% 的切断比例会增加痉挛状态的复发。

上肢痉挛状态和选择性周围神经切断术（SPN）

上肢痉挛状态以痉挛性和弛缓性瘫痪相结合为特征。典型的表现是屈肌旋前肌痉挛和伸肌旋后肌的肌无力，导致肩内收、内旋，肘关节屈曲，前臂旋前，腕关节屈曲偏向尺侧，伴有掌心拇指畸形握拳。除非在睡眠或麻醉状态下，屈肌旋前肌张力随着被动拉伸而增加，并且保持恒定不变。使用拮抗剂时张力亢进的肌肉协同收缩，影响抓放能力。

MDT 管理的目的是维持功能和活动程度。在考虑手术治疗之前，应充分利用物理治疗、夹板固定、降低肌张力的药物和肉毒素注射等非手术措施。手术治疗包括再平衡（肌腱转移）、挛缩松解（肌筋膜松解、肌腱延长、关节松解）、关节稳定手术和降低肌张力的手术，此外还有 SPN 手术或选择性神经切断术（Zancolli，2003）。SPN 仅用于肌张力过高影响肢体功能的情况。

肉毒杆菌毒素治疗效果类似于 SPN，在考虑 SPN 前应首先选择肉毒素治疗。门诊局部麻醉阻滞也可用于评估相关神经切断术的疗效。

SPN 可单独使用或与肌腱转移、松解和关节稳定手术联合使用。手术包括在神经肌肉连接处切断牵张反射的传入和传出神经。切断相关肌肉本体感觉传入通路和传出通路导致痉挛的肌肉瘫痪。其目的是在不抑制有用的肌张力或损害剩余运动和感觉功能的情况下，以降低肌张力。由感觉和运动神经纤维组成的混合神经干不应被切断，因为这可能会导致传入神经阻滞性疼痛。术中神经电刺激与手术显微镜联合应用，分离出相应的运动支。将分离的运动支的大部分（50%~80%）切断并烧灼以防止纤维再生。切断的范围取决于神经对电刺激的反应（Sindou et al.，2007）。

术前准确地识别肌张力高的肌肉，并精确地对这些肌肉进行部分神经切断，是 SPN 术后疗效的关键。当切断量不足时可导致痉挛状态复发，但可再次手术。

矫形手术

痉挛性脑瘫是儿童矫形外科最常见的疾病之一。

起初，肌肉因痉挛或挛缩而表现为功能性缩短，但随着时间的推移，肌肉 / 肌腱单位因挛缩而出现结构性缩短。这种情况也发生在关节，长时间运动受限后关节囊收缩导致关节出现异常和功能障碍性姿势，如固定的膝关节屈曲。关节不稳定导致的脱臼在痉挛性脑瘫患儿中比较常见，例如严重内旋（扁平）足及髋关节半脱位和完全脱位（Ounpuu et al.，2002；Pirpiris et al.，2003；Soo et al.，2006；Ross and Engsberg，2007；Robin et al.，2009；Shore et al.，2012；Silva et al.，2012）。

在肌肉出现挛缩之前，抗痉挛治疗和物理治疗是公认的治疗方法，但如果挛缩形成后就需要恢复正常的解剖结构和功能。痉挛性脑瘫患儿临床表现主要有两类：能行走的和不能行走的。前者的治疗目的是维持或恢复站立和行走功能。后一类的治疗集中于预防髋关节脱位，可以使脚在鞋内维持舒适的位置，并保持舒适的坐姿。

目前在英国，GMFCS 评分为 2~3 级的可行走患儿接受 SDR 手术的越来越多，矫形外科在可行走患儿中的作用也在发生改变。以前的多节段软组织松解术（multilevel soft tissue release，MLSTR）是可行走患儿的主要治疗方法，但当患儿身高和体重逐渐增加后，该手术的疗效就会下降或不明显（Gough et al.，2004；Graham et al.，2005；Khan，2007；Gorton et al.，2009；Akerstedt et al.，2010；Harvey et al.，2012）。矫形手术对收缩和挛缩都适用。典型的是患儿会出现蹲伏或跳跃步态（臀部内收、臀部和膝盖弯曲、马蹄足），这是一种耗能的站立和行走方式。

7~13岁的患儿可接受矫形手术，但治疗应具有高度个性化。通常是一次性延长髋屈肌（缝匠肌和腰大肌）、膝屈肌（股薄肌、半腱肌、内侧半膜肌，或股二头肌外侧）和踝跖屈肌（腓肠肌或跟腱）。使用小夹板固定（通常于膝下用轻便的石膏固定4周），并进行早期强化康复。

如果患儿先接受了SDR手术，是否需要矫形手术，应在多学科合作下对患儿进行评估。通常情况下，某些部位的紧缩程度会有所改善，因此很少需要进一步矫形外科手术。分期骨科手术的最佳时机尚未确定，如果说需要进一步手术，最好在SDR手术后的几个月内进行，以促进康复。

尽管文献报道很少，但选择性的经皮肌筋膜延长术（"percs"）是美国最流行的MLSTR方法，该方法具有皮肤切口小、康复速度快以及肌肉瘢痕形成少的优点。

争议

目前，关于痉挛状态的治疗争议主要聚焦于SDR手术对痉挛状态儿童的术后疗效。之所以产生这种担忧主要是该手术的结果是不可逆的并且可能会使神经功能恶化。因此，严格的患者选择是关键。

当前，尽管大多数研究者接受了SDR手术对中等残疾（GMFCS评分2~3级）儿童的术后疗效，因为该手术可改善患儿的粗大功能和活动性，但对中等残疾患儿的SDR手术仍然存在争议。对SDR文献的主要批评是，研究通常是单中心、小样本和无病例对照的。SDR手术量小，专业性强，因此做大样本的病例对照研究具有挑战性。尽管有越来越多的最长达26年的随访报告，但一些研究者还引用了缺乏长期结果的数据（Langerak et al.，2011；Bolster et al.，2013；Dudley et al.，2013；Hurvitz et al.，2013；Langerak et al.，2013；Steinbok，2013；Tedroff et al.，2014；Josenby et al.，2015；Steinbok，2015；Vermeulen and Becher，2015）。另一些研究者则认为瘫痪或尿失禁的风险很高，但在文献报道中尚未得到证实。

然而，一些人也主张为残疾程度较重的儿童甚至使用轮椅的儿童（GMFCS 4~5级）行SDR手术，以替代ITB疗法（Gump et al.，2013；Ailon et al.，2015；Steinbok，2015；Vermeulen and Becher，2015）。对于这一部分患儿来说，治疗的适应证和目标是不同的，因为这部分患儿往往无法实现独立行走。他们也更可能存在痉挛状态合并肌张力障碍，这会使疗效不太确切。一些研究主张为GMFCS 4~5级儿童行SDR手术而不是ITB，以帮助他们保持个人卫生和行动方便，因为接受SDR手术意味着他们随后无需定期到医院复查，但ITB泵需要在随后数年里不断进行加药或更换。然而，这种情况尚未被研究证实，这无疑是未来临床试验研究的一个领域。对于这部分患者（GMFCS 4~5级），SDR手术可以消除或降低他们的支持移动能力，并对生活质量产生相对的负面影响。

此外，SDR手术治疗遗传疾病（Kai et al.，2014）、后天损伤（如脊柱创伤或感染后）（Langerak et al.，2014；Reynolds et al.，2014）以及偏瘫患者（Oki et al.，2010；Gump et al.，2013）也见有报道。

结论

痉挛状态需要详细计划多学科的评估和治疗。治疗策略应根据患者的功能和身体需求，联合康复科、药剂科和外科进行个体化治疗。患者需要定期复查，以确保适合患者的个体化治疗。治疗目标包括改善肌张力、减轻痉挛、控制胃肠道反应和维持膀胱功能，目的是保护功能并尽量降低痉挛状态及其不良影响。

延伸阅读、参考文献、EBRAIN的相关链接

扫描书末二维码获取。

第 78 章　疼痛病理生理学和外科治疗

Richard Mannion・Rokas Tamosauskas 著
赵学敏、王宁、高佳宁、陈希恒 译，王林、孟凡刚、罗芳 审校

疼痛传导通路——解剖及生理学

外界的感觉信息在传入大脑的通路中首先由初级感觉神经元（一级神经元）进行转导和传输，此类神经元在解剖及功能上具有异质性，它们的胞体位于脊髓背根及三叉神经节，其突触向两个方向进行投射传递：其一是向外周投射至所支配区域，二是向中央投射至脊髓（图 78.1）。

初级感觉神经元可分为以下几类：①大的有髓 Aβ 传入神经纤维，负责传递低阈值的机械感觉和振动觉；②细的有髓 Aδ 传入神经纤维，其胞体较小，负责传递快速疼痛（如针刺觉）；③小的无髓 C 纤维传入神经纤维，负责疼痛和温度觉的传递。这些神经元的外周终末分支作为“游离神经末梢”广泛分布在它们所支配的组织中，通过高度成熟、复杂的过程感受和转导经过严格管理的外周刺激。伤害性感受器在解剖、功能及神经化学上有所不同，它们通过特定的受体介导机制对特定刺激作出反应（Woolf and Ma，2007）。这种机制在初级感觉神经元中产生了可预测的刺激 - 反应效应，允许大脑对外界的感觉刺激进行可靠的、可重复性的编码。然而，值得注意的是，这些关系并不是“固定的”，它们在生理状态下保持不变，但在疾病状态下可以发生改变，初级感觉神经元可以改变表型，从而改变对外周刺激的编码功能，即转导和传输。事实上，它们甚至可以在没有外周刺激的情况下开始自发放电，这也是公认的自发性（即非刺激性）神经病理性疼痛的机制之一（Costigan et al.，2009）。

疼痛的转导和传输

在生理状态下，身体产生痛感是由于检测到潜在或实际已引起组织损伤的外周刺激而产生的，这就是伤害感受性疼痛。伤害性感受器，即能够检测伤害性刺激（如热、化学、机械）的初级感觉神经元，具有小的无髓传入纤维，胞体位于背根神经节，支配皮肤、肌肉和内脏等周围结构（Woller et al.，2017）。它们的中央轴突通过脊髓背根进入到背根入髓区，进而汇入脊髓背外侧的白质束状带 Lissauer 束。

除了谷氨酸等常见的神经递质外，伤害性感受器还优先选择在神经化学传递中起作用的几种肽类，如 P 物质和降钙素基因相关肽（calcitonin gene-related peptide，CGRP）。由于肽类递质的作用相对复杂，在这些神经递质被发现之后，早期并没有意识到其可能为疼痛治疗提供新的治疗靶点，但它们确实在感觉神经传递中发挥重要作用，通过与谷氨酸等递质协同，对背角的突触后神经元有显著的、更持久的作用。这些肽类递质能够存在于痛觉感受器的外周终端，同时从细胞体到细胞终端产生顺行性动作电位导致肽类释放，引起血管扩张、血浆外渗和免疫细胞募集，产生神经源性炎症。

这类神经元大多数是多模态的（即它们可以检测到不止一种类型的刺激）。通常情况下，它们检测机械刺激的激活阈值比 Aβ 神经元高（尽管这个伤害性阈值可能因组织不同而有所变异，例如角膜和皮肤）。已有研究发现，大量机械敏感蛋白包括机械门控离子通道具有不同功能和种类（Delmas et al.，2011；Delmas and Coste，2013）。

热敏性被认为是通过一个称为 TRPs 的受体蛋白家族（瞬时受体蛋白；Mickle et al.，2015）介导的。大约 40% 的初级感觉神经元表达 TRPV1 受体，其中有大量包含有小的无髓 C 纤维的神经元，离子通道以温度敏感的方式开放。TRPV1 被认为与热感知有关，有趣的是，在不同的疾病模型中，感觉神经元 TRPV1 的表达有所不同。在正常和疾病状态下，还有其他几种相关蛋白与冷感知、无害的热感知和有害的热感知有关（图 78.2）。

不同的电压门控离子通道由痛觉感受器优先表达而非痛觉初级感觉神经元，其中 Na^+ 离子通道最为典型（1.7、1.8、1.9）。这些通道对伤害性感受器

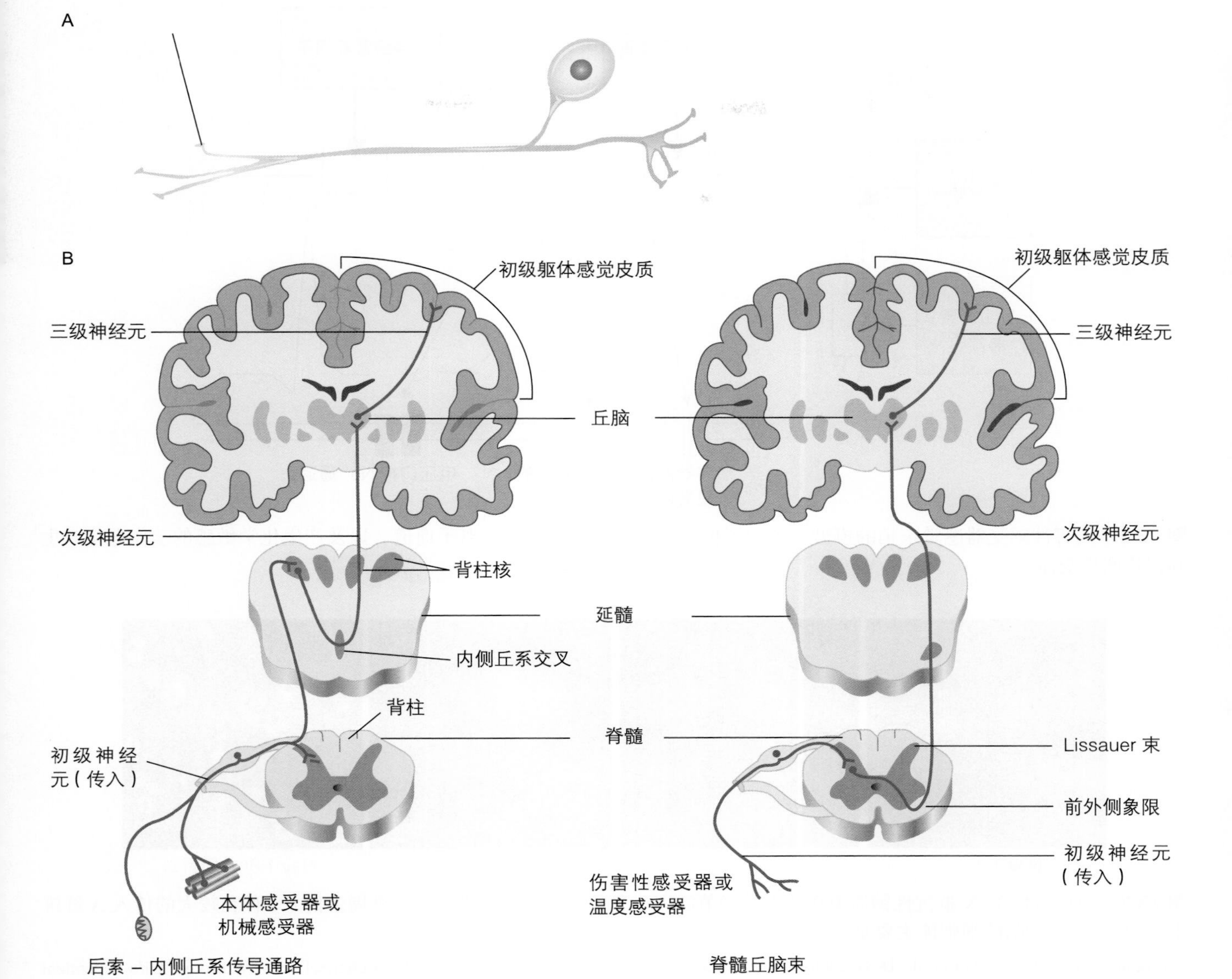

图 78.1 （A）初级感觉神经元只有一个离开细胞体的轴突，分成一个较长的外周轴突和一个较短的向中央突出的轴突。（B）主要感觉传导通路示意图

的正常感觉转导和传输至关重要。已有证据表明，编码这些通道的某些基因如果发生突变会导致遗传性慢性疼痛（Cummins et al.，2007）。值得注意的是，在诸如炎症和神经损伤后的慢性疼痛状态下，钠通道功能发生改变，从而使受体变得敏感（Liu and Wood，2011）。其他与伤害感受有关的离子通道还有酸敏感离子通道，也优先由痛觉神经元表达（Dubé et al.，2009），这些离子通道在低 pH 值环境下开放，这是由于在炎性组织中伤害性感受器更敏感、激活阈值降低的缘故（**图** 78.3）。

有一类伤害性感受器亚群在生理状态下保持沉默，对任何外周刺激（甚至有害刺激）都没有反应，但它们在组织或神经损伤后被激活，对机械或热刺激做出反应。这些神经元可能与炎症等疾病状态下的疼痛反应改变有关（见**图** 78.4）。

初级中继站——脊髓背角

一旦伤害性感受器被激活，动作电位就会沿着轴突通过背根神经节（或三叉神经节）进入脊髓。在脊髓水平，这些纤维穿过背根到达背根入髓区（dorsal root entry zone，DREZ）。在这里可以看到大的有髓 A 纤维轴突和小的无髓 C 纤维在解剖上相互分离。A 型纤维中央轴突进入同侧背柱向上传导。当它们从 DREZ 进入脊髓白质时，它们分出一个轴突侧支，进入脊髓背角的灰质。这个轴突在感觉门控中起着关键作用。

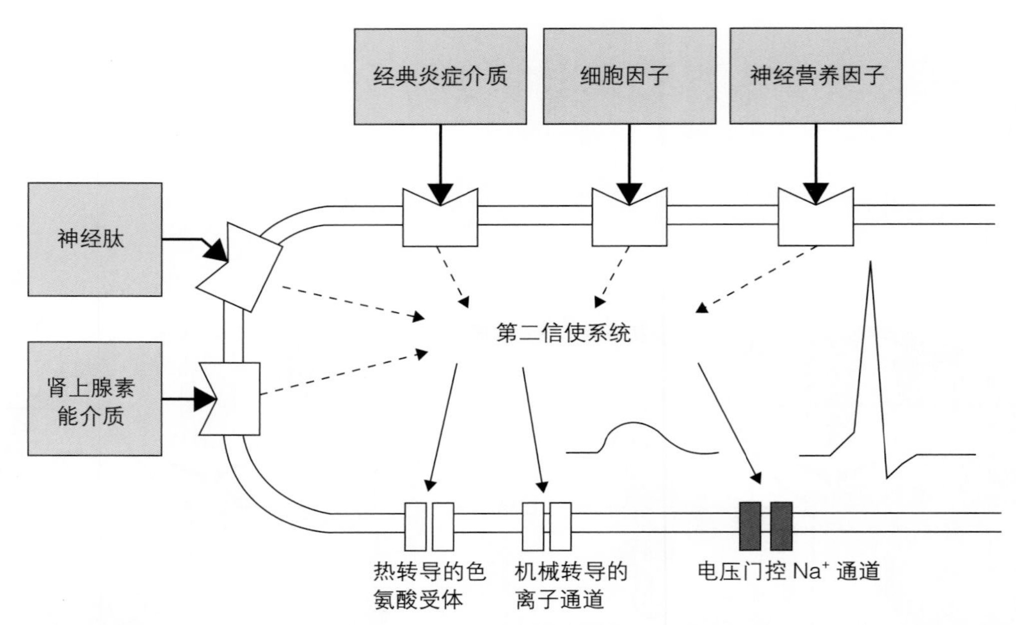

图 78.2 伤害性感受器感觉末梢的模型，展示了传递热刺激和机械刺激的离子通道，以及产生化学敏感的动作电位产生和促代谢性受体

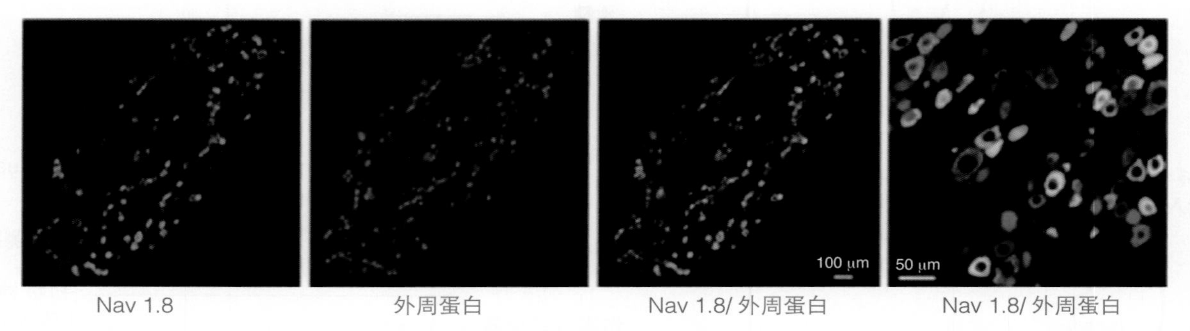

图 78.3 免疫组化 TTX 抵抗性钠通道在背根神经节的表达，免疫组织化学染色显示外周蛋白（一种在较大的传入 A 纤维中发现的蛋白）。阳性细胞体主要是小的伤害性感受器神经元

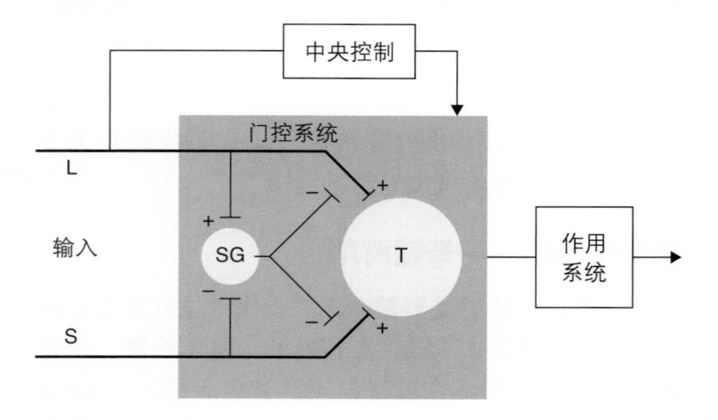

图 78.4 最初的模型是由 Melzack 和 Wall（1965）提出的。L- 大 /S- 小感觉神经元。T- 传递神经元。兴奋胶状质（SG）神经元，通过兴奋和抑制机制对投射神经元的感觉输入进行突触前调制，并从下行通路进一步控制

C 纤维进入 DREZ 后，可以直接进入背角，也可以在 Lissauer 束内向下或向上延伸几个节段后再进入并终止于背角。现已证实这些纤维进入并终止于背角的浅层，也称为胶状质。在这里，C 纤维与位于背角内的神经元细胞体树突产生突触连接，神经元的结构包括细胞体、轴突、树突、髓鞘等。其中大多数神经元是参与局部顺行和逆行中继的中间神经元，可以是兴奋性神经元，也可以是抑制性神经元。因此，后角的浅层含有广泛的兴奋性和抑制性神经递质和神经肽递质，它们构成了一个复杂的门控系统，控制着环境（内部和外部）信息传递到大脑。此外，还有一些神经元的胞体位于背角浅层或深层，它们的轴突在中央管前方的脊髓丘脑束（spinothalamic tract，STT）中节段性地穿过脊髓（见**专栏 78.1**）。

广动力范围神经元

广动力范围（wide dynamic range，WDR）神经元的胞体位于脊髓的后角，主要存在于较深的板层，接受来自 Aβ 纤维、A δ 纤维和 C 纤维的输入并作出反应。它们可以对无害和有害的刺激做出分级反应。这类神经元也有很大的感受野，而浅层神经元的感受野要小得多。因此，也有学者认为伤害性刺激可能是由神经元群体或神经网络编码的。

虽然存在复杂的神经元排列，通过顺行投射和逆行反馈实现兴奋性和抑制性传输的平衡，但在基础生理状态下，特定的外周刺激通常会产生可预测的反应。然而，当我们受到有害刺激时，我们对疼痛的体验可能会有很大的不同。早在我们理解疼痛解剖学和生理学之前很久就已经认识到，我们对疼痛的体验在很大程度上依赖于环境（即疼痛感知是与周围环境相关的）。1956 年 Henry Beecher 发现，在战场上遭受严重伤害的士兵几乎不需要止痛药，而平民伤亡中类似的伤害会产生更多的痛苦（Beecher，1956）。现在已知大部分的调节发生在第一个感觉中继，即脊髓的背角。

C 纤维输入的脊髓门控调节

通过背角的单突触和多突触传导通路，初级感觉传入汇聚到投射神经元。不同的信息传入可以调节其他传入信息的传递。因此，非伤害性信息传入可以抑制伤害性信息传入和对疼痛的感知；例如，抚摸受伤的部位可以减轻疼痛感。为了解释这种现象，梅尔扎克（Melzack）和沃尔（Wall）在 1965 年发表了门控理论（见**专栏 78.1**）。

脊髓内有几种不同的信息传递机制，可以增加或减少传输到大脑的感觉信息。涉及局部兴奋性和抑制性中间神经元，以及来自大脑的下行通路。直接电刺激中脑导水管周围灰质（periaqueductal gray matter，PAG）可产生一种阿片介导的深层次镇痛作用。PAG 投射到延髓腹侧（rostroventral medulla，RVM），包括延髓中缝核（富含 5- 羟色胺）。接着，这个区域投射到脊髓的背角，在那里它们也影响初级感觉神经元到中枢神经系统的传输。这些脊髓 - 延髓腹侧 - 脊髓通路被认为在初级中继的感觉处理中形成了一个“调节增益”的关键环路。有人认为，针灸镇痛的机制可能是通过激活下行通路，这种现象被称为弥漫性伤害性抑制控制（diffuse noxious inhibitory control，DNIC）。此外，这些调节机制并不是一成不变的，神经或组织损伤会使感觉信息传递到大脑的相互作用和影响发生改变（D’Mello and Dickenson，2008）。

专栏 78.1　闸门学说

1965 年，Melzack 和 Wall 在 *Science* 杂志上发表的 *The Gate Theory of Pain* 提出了一种机制，解释了在脊髓背角的第一次感觉中继时，伤害性输入是如何由感觉系统编码的。它主要关注在最近发现的来自大小感觉神经元的突触前控制的机制，根据这些输入之间的平衡来“控制”传入信息［参见 Mendell（2014）的全面综述］。它还结合了其他机制，如来自大脑的下行控制通路，以及伤害性和非伤害性信息传入汇聚到脊髓中相同的神经元，参与向大脑的传递。虽然后来发现并不是所有的预测都是准确的，但闸门学说推动了新兴的疼痛神经生物学领域进一步研究。它有助于改变人们对疼痛机制的既往认识，从固定的“标记线”疼痛路径转向适应性和非适应性过程调节生理性和病理性疼痛。参见**图 78.4**。

上行通路

背角投射神经元负责将感觉信息从痛觉感受器传递到大脑。这可通过多种途径予以实现，有些负责投射到丘脑，然后是新皮质，这是对有害刺激产生有意识反应的关键。其他途径产生更复杂的行为，如回避（远离有害刺激）、自主反应（如交感神经激活）和情绪方面（如恐惧、愤怒、悲伤）。因此，当感觉信息从初级感觉神经元传递到高级中枢时，不同的信息输入分别进入不同的靶点，这使得感觉系统的组织更加复杂，导致我们对每个结构（相对于另一个结构）的意义的理解更加困难，也给科学地研究这一过程增加难度。有趣的是，下面描述的“疼痛通路”中没有一条是针对有害输入的，它们都包含低阈值输入、有害输入和“广动力范围”的神经元。

脊髓丘脑束（STT）

这一纤维束被命名为脊髓的上行“疼痛传导通路”，但这过于简单化。STT 位于腹侧和腹外侧白质束内。它有两个部分，外侧部和腹侧部（前部）。外侧 STT 更多地参与到疼痛和体温感觉，而腹侧 STT 则参与到触觉和压力感觉。STT 的投射具有躯体拓扑关系，在颈髓中，颈纤维多位于内侧，腰骶纤维位于外侧。STT 的主要的投射目标是丘脑的腹后外侧核（ventroposterolateral，VPL），这是丘脑皮质感觉处理系统的一部分。

脊髓网状束（SRT）

这条通路还包括从Ⅴ板层的背角投射神经元发出的轴突，延伸到腹角（Ⅶ，Ⅷ）和内侧灰质（Ⅹ）的更深的板层。和STT一样，SRT也位于脊髓白质腹侧部，邻近外侧STT，并投射到多个目标区域，包括网状结构（位于中脑、脑桥和延髓）、丘脑（外侧和背侧网状核）、巨细胞网状核以及其他部位。

脊髓中脑束

这条通路位于外侧STT的腹侧，投射神经元胞体位于浅层（Ⅰ）、深层背角（Ⅳ、Ⅴ）及腹角（Ⅶ、Ⅷ）。它投射到臂旁核和PAG，这一区域已经成为脑深部电刺激治疗慢性疼痛的靶点（见下文）。臂旁区域位于中脑和脑桥的交界处，是外侧网状结构的一部分，向杏仁核、丘脑和下丘脑投射，与伤害性刺激的情绪反应有关。臂旁区被 认为包含一个与喜欢特定刺激有关的“享乐”区域，除了疼痛之外，还接受从孤立核输入的与嗅觉有关的信号传导，并与味觉有关。

疼痛通路——病理生理学

在生理状态下，伤害感受器检测到有害刺激的存在，并引起我们的警觉。虽然疼痛通常是一种不愉快的体验，但它是我们生存本能的重要组成部分，保护我们免受有害刺激（例如，手接触热板会快速撤离），或者降低损害的程度（肿胀的脚踝可以迫使我们减轻负重，有助于恢复）。缺乏伤害感受能力不可避免地会导致严重的或潜在的危及生命的损伤，少数人先天对生理疼痛不敏感，生活中会出现反复损伤，甚至过早死亡。其他例子还有糖尿病患者的沙尔科（Charcot）关节病，以及已知的面神经和三叉神经功能障碍患者出现的眼睛并发症。

需要注意的是，初级和次级感觉投射神经元、脊髓、脑干和丘脑的中间神经元以及它们接受支配的下行神经在内，在感觉通路中的功能是不固定的，就像电灯开关一样，处在一个预先设定好的、硬性连接的系统中。任一神经元的表型及其功能都是由局部化学和电环境决定的。因此，导致神经元局部环境改变的过程都可能会导致神经元表型的改变，从而对整个感觉系统产生功能上的影响（Woolf and Salter，2000）。

比较一下炎症和神经损伤（例如，创伤、压迫、肿瘤侵犯）这两种因素对机体的影响，可使我们对此有更清晰的认识。

炎症

组织发生炎症反应后，通常非疼痛的刺激（例如，轻压）也会引起疼痛（痛觉超敏）。如上所述，这种痛觉敏感性增加或异常通常是有利的，通过保护受伤区域免受进一步伤害并促进愈合。然而，在许多病理状态下产生的炎症反应往往对机体没有任何益处（例如类风湿关节），在这种情况下，慢性疼痛就成了疾病。现在人们更多地认识到神经系统和免疫系统之间的相互作用，在生理和病理状态下都能相互调节（McMahon et al.，2015）。

无论是组织损伤还是自身免疫触发，炎症都是由血管扩张、血浆外渗、组织肿胀、免疫细胞募集和炎性介质的释放所介导的。伤害性感受器的热敏感性和化学敏感性是指局部环境的改变，炎性细胞因子的增加（如白介素-1、白介素-6、肿瘤坏死因子α）、局部温度升高和pH降低会导致活动模式改变，引起疼痛加剧。这不仅仅是刺激增加导致反应增强，炎性细胞因子可以通过对表面受体和细胞内信号蛋白的翻译后修饰，以及伤害性感受器细胞体内的转录变化，改变感觉从外周组织到脊髓的传递过程。这些蛋白质表达和表型特性的变化导致功能的改变，因此相同的刺激会导致反应增强和更多动作电位的激活。任意部位的初级感觉神经元（外周终末、轴索膜、细胞体或脊髓的中央终末）都会因炎症发生功能的改变，主要是由化学环境改变或活动依赖的机制引起的蛋白质修饰介导的。

现已证明，外周组织中炎性细胞因子的存在与疼痛程度的增加和刺激与反应之间关系的改变有关。这会引起痛觉过敏（伤害性刺激引起的疼痛增加）和痛觉超敏（无害刺激引起的疼痛）等现象。此外，这些变化可能是长期存在的，了解这些变化可以让我们深入地了解慢性疼痛状态（这些特征通常表现为异常的疼痛行为［不像“生理的（伤害性的）疼痛”）］的一些特征的相关调节机制。

神经损伤

除了创伤或压迫（例如椎间盘突出）外，还有许多其他原因可导致周围神经损伤，包括引起多发性神经病的系统性疾病、肿瘤侵袭和炎症本身。现在的观念认为腰椎病或神经根型颈椎病不仅仅是一种压迫性神经病，可能存在机械压迫和相关的炎症反应之间复杂的相互作用。神经病理性疼痛模型和临床研究中已经明确了一些炎症标志物，这可能为药物治疗提供新的靶点，并重新评估外科手术在这些疾病中的作用。

当然，对于一些脊髓或神经根受压的患者，尤其是肠道或膀胱损伤或进行性神经功能障碍的患者，减压手术仍然是一种重要的具有循证依据的治疗方法。

然而，大多数神经病理性疼痛患者并没有神经压迫，也无从谈起进行减压手术治疗，对这些患者进行疼痛控制可能极具挑战性，可以说是临床中最棘手的问题之一。此外，这也是一个巨大的社会问题，这些患者通常有负性症状（感觉减退或丧失）和正性症状（痛觉过敏、超敏、感觉异常/感觉障碍、自发性疼痛、过度兴奋症）。周围神经损伤对初级感觉神经元有广泛的影响（Costigan et al.，2009），关键是不局限于损伤的神经元，还涉及相邻的未损伤的细胞和纤维。**表 78.1** 详细描述了周围神经损伤后发生的一些病理生理变化及其可能的临床表现。

慢性疼痛的脊髓机制——敏化作用和去抑制

外周炎症和神经损伤对初级感觉神经元功能的影响可导致中枢神经系统感觉处理的改变（D'Mello and Dickenson，2008）。潜在原因是多样性的，包括活动依赖机制以及蛋白质功能异常（转录和翻译后修饰），导致细胞活动和行为的变化。这些变化可能是永久的，并可能导致突触后活动改变、蛋白质表达异常，甚至背角神经元死亡。脊髓的变化表现为敏化作用和去抑制。

在神经损伤和炎症之后，慢性疼痛通常在空间上延伸到受损皮肤区域之外，产生继发性痛觉过敏区域，这与最初的损伤无关。这些症状不能用周围神经系统的变化来解释，而是反映了脊髓和脊髓上神经网络的变化。只有生理性的高阈值刺激才能引起疼痛伤害性机制的改变，从而导致病理性的低阈值疼痛过敏症。

导致这一变化的一个重要机制是中枢敏化（Latremoliere and Woolf，2009；见**专栏 78.2**）。神经损伤的其他长期后果包括基因转录和膜蛋白翻译后修饰改变引起的神经元表型改变，以及背角 GABA 能和甘氨酸能神经元活性下降。这种“去抑制”的机制包括减少下行抑制控制、细胞死亡导致 GABA 能或甘氨酸能中间神经元丢失，GABA 或 GABA 合成酶（如谷氨酸脱羧酶）降低，GABA 受体、甘氨酸能受体和阳离子 - 氯化物共转运体的性质改变等。这些机制的改变进一步促进了中枢过度兴奋和痛觉通路活性的增加。

在疾病状态下，中枢神经系统内的小胶质细胞（巨噬细胞样）在感觉传递和疼痛处理中扮演着一个新的角色（McMahon and Malcangio，2009）。神经或组织损伤后，小胶质细胞的形态和功能会迅速改变，这对感觉加工有重要的影响（Calvo and Bennett,

表 78.1　病理状态下在初级感觉神经元或其中央终末观察到的病理生理变化以及推测的临床表现

病理生理变化	疾病状态	症状
外周敏化	炎症	疼痛过敏症（痛觉过敏、痛觉超敏）
沃勒变性/脱髓鞘/轴索死亡	周围神经损伤	麻木/感觉减退
假突触传递	周围神经损伤	扩散性疼痛（感受区域增加）
异位激活：C 纤维	炎症、神经损伤	自发性灼痛（非刺激性）
细胞死亡：初级感觉神经元	周围神经损伤	麻木/感觉减退
细胞死亡：背角中间神经元（抑制性）	周围神经损伤	自发性疼痛、扩散性疼痛（感受野增加）
中枢敏化	炎症、神经损伤	疼痛过敏症（痛觉过敏、痛觉超敏）

专栏 78.2　中枢敏化

在生理环境下，特定的刺激会产生可预测的反应。然而，在组织或神经损伤后，初级伤害性感受器的活动增加，这可能会导致中枢及外周对相同刺激的反应增加，这就是中枢敏化。国际疼痛研究协会将其定义为“中枢神经系统中的伤害性神经元对正常或阈下输入的反应性增强”。中枢敏化的活动依赖性机制包括同突触长时程增强（伴随伤害性反应的夸大）和异源性突触活化（募集低阈值 Aβ 纤维进入疼痛传导通路），这些机制可能是由受损神经的异位活动驱动和维持的。

中枢敏化是由神经递质谷氨酸和各种神经肽递质激活几种蛋白激酶，导致突触后受体[如 N- 甲基 -D- 天冬氨酸（NMDA）受体]的翻译和转录后发生改变而产生的。中枢敏化是神经病理性疼痛的主要驱动力，降低中枢兴奋性的药物对这类疾病的临床疗效支持了这一观点，这些药物包括加巴喷丁类（如加巴喷丁和普瑞巴林）、三环抗抑郁药（如阿米替林）、SNRI（如度洛西汀）和 NMDA 拮抗剂（如氯胺酮）。中枢敏化已成为新止痛药开发的一个重要焦点，也是超前镇痛（即阻止初级痛觉传入信号向中枢神经系统传递）的理论基础。

2012）。中枢神经系统内的这些神经免疫相互作用为开发新的慢性疼痛管理策略提供潜在靶点（Scholz and Woolf，2007）。

因此，初级感觉神经元、脊髓中间神经元、投射神经元以及非神经元细胞的表型和功能的改变可以导致功能性脊髓中继的极度改变，并建立远远超过初级组织损伤时期的慢性疼痛状态。

脊髓上机制

外周组织或神经损伤后感觉系统的病理生理变化并不局限于初级感觉神经元或脊髓。在慢性疼痛患者的大脑中也检测到其结构、兴奋性和抑制性递质以及功能连接的变化。如何将这些变化与认知、感觉和情感痛苦体验联系起来，了解其中的因果关系，以及这些变化是否可逆，仍然是当前面临的挑战。

慢性疼痛的外科治疗方法

毁损手术治疗慢性疼痛具有很长的历史（Loeser，2006），早于现代人们明确理解疼痛的神经生物学机制及可能引起慢性疼痛的潜在机制之前即已进行。当然，距我们完全了解这些机制并能够为每个患者做出明确判断，甚至提供基于循证医学证据的有效治疗还有很长一段路要走（von Hehn et al.，2012；Vardeh et al.，2016）。目前许多用于管理慢性疼痛患者的“治疗方法”都是基于经验，我们目前无法预测哪些患者会对不同的疼痛干预措施（如药理学、注射疗法、针灸、理疗、TENS 等）有反应，也无法解释为什么有些人有反应，而另一些人没有反应。了解感觉的病理生理学，认识初级感觉神经元、脊髓和高级中枢发生的内在变化后，会在许多方面重新审视手术治疗慢性疼痛的理论基础，特别是毁损 / 不可逆手术，其可能不仅不会减轻疼痛，还会给患者引发更多的不适感。也许这就解释了这样的手术只会对部分慢性疼痛患者有短暂的效果，而且只对其中的部分患者有效，并且也已经认识到此类手术会加剧神经性疼痛症状。近年来，大多数神经外科中心都不再开展破坏性手术，而仅给那些预后不佳的晚期癌症患者实施。同时，在评价任何外科手术的实用性和有效性时还要考虑到安慰剂效应，特别是当只进行了短期随访时（参见 Colagiuri et al.，2015）关于安慰剂效应和潜在机制的观点，在外科领域得到广泛认可。

部分患者在专业医学中心经过严格筛选后，仍可进行合适的手术治疗，且手术疗效确切（见综述 Sindou et al.，1990）。

DREZ 毁损

20 世纪 70 年代，Marc Sindou 在里昂首次尝试了 DREZ 毁损手术，之后开始推广。目前这种手术方式仍在应用，用于治疗中枢性或非传入性疼痛综合征，如臂丛损伤、幻肢痛、创伤性脊髓损伤、癌症痛以及痉挛等，但比以前少得多。不同直径的感觉神经轴突混合在背根中，但在它们到达脊髓前就已完成组织分类。神经根分为不同的小根，在进入 Lissauer 束之前，小纤维位于外侧，而较大的纤维位于内侧，即更靠近背柱。

手术通过椎板切除或半椎板切开完成。打开 DREZ 上方的软脊膜，使用电凝或射频消融方式进行微创损伤。其并发症包括皮质脊髓束或背柱损伤、大小便失禁以及神经病理性疼痛不缓解或加重。现在人们普遍认为，对于所有其他侵入性较小的治疗策略都失败的患者，这是最后的治疗手段。

脊髓丘脑外侧束切断术

脊髓丘脑外侧束传导来自对侧的疼痛、温度和触觉信号，因此破坏或切断该束会导致对侧的痛觉和温度觉丧失。1911 年首次报道了开放的脊髓切开术，但该手术可引起较高的发病率及死亡率。经皮穿刺技术的发展使得该手术的创伤性明显减低，而脊髓切断术是公认的治疗单侧肿瘤性疼痛的方法。计算机断层扫描（CT）引导下可以实现更精确的穿刺定位并进行切断操作。内镜下脊髓切开术也在不断探索之中。

脊髓丘脑外侧束切断术的治疗原理是什么?

脊髓丘脑外侧束由来自对侧脊髓的交叉纤维组成。在每节段脊髓水平，一个二级神经轴突在同侧脊髓上行 2 到 5 个节段后交叉到对侧前外侧，并汇入脊髓丘脑外侧束。在 C1-2 水平，脊髓丘脑外侧束有明显的躯体定位关系：前内侧部分包含来自上肢、肩部、前胸的纤维，而后外侧部分包含来自下肢、下背部和骨盆的纤维投递（**图 78.5**）。

本文介绍了几种经皮脊髓丘脑外侧束切断术的方法。在局部麻醉下，在透视（经典技术）或 CT 引导下，经 C1-2 椎间孔将射频套管插入脊髓前外侧部分。其目的是穿透硬脊膜，进入与矢状面垂直的前外侧脊髓，齿状韧带的前面。理论上，感觉刺激应在温度觉（热或冷）方面产生明显变化，并伴有对侧刺痛，但不一定与疼痛区域重叠。由于邻近皮质脊

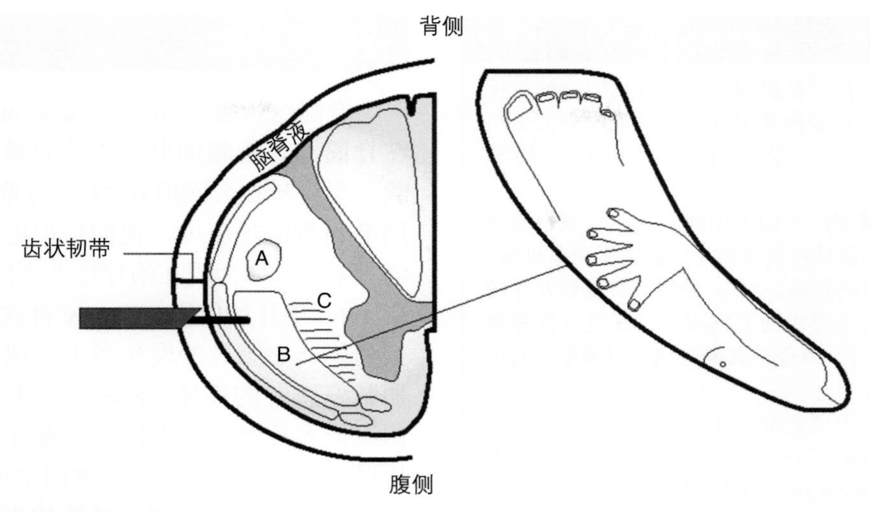

图 78.5 脊髓颈 2 节段的横断面示意图

Reproduced with permission from Alireza Feizerfan, and JHL Antrobus, Role of percutaneous cervical cordotomy in cancer pain management, *Continuing Education in Anaesthesia Critical Care & Pain*, Volume 14, Issue 1, pp. 23–6, Copyright © 2014.

髓束，运动刺激会产生同侧颈部和肩部肌肉的收缩。当对肢体对侧刺激时产生热感觉变化被认为是具有良好镇痛效果的可靠预测因子。然后，以递增的方式进行射频热凝，并持续监测同侧的运动功能。毁损完成后，两侧肢体对针刺的感觉应有明显差异。

本文介绍了 CT 引导下经椎间盘前路手术入路。部分学者主张使用侧向内镜技术进行激光毁损，以获得更高的精确度和准确度。

经皮脊髓丘脑外侧束切断术的适应证

对于 C5 以下由恶性肿瘤引起的单侧伤害性疼痛的患者，尽管有相应的姑息药物和介入治疗，但如果肺功能尚可，预期寿命 6 个月到 1 年，且能够配合完成经皮脊髓丘脑外侧束切断术，则可以考虑进行此手术操作。研究最多的患者群体是恶性间皮瘤、肺上沟瘤和转移性肺癌引起的疼痛患者。但也有一些低等级的证据表明，脊髓切断术对神经病理性疼痛无效。

手术疗效的佐证

大多数研究都是回顾性的，也有一些前瞻性的病例报道。最近的一篇系统回顾研究总结了经皮脊髓丘脑外侧束切断术治疗间皮瘤相关疼痛的情况。在 160 例患者中，94% 的患者在治疗后疼痛即刻完全或部分缓解。若患者寿命超过一年，疼痛复发也很常见。

并发症

经验丰富的医师通过严格挑选合适病例进行手术治疗，其并发症非常罕见（<1%）。术式相关的并发症包括同侧肢体（腿 > 臂）一过性或永久性运动无力、感觉障碍、同侧镜面疼痛、肋间 / 膈肌无力所致呼吸困难。其他并发症包括胸腔感染、立位低血压、尿潴留、大小便失禁、性功能障碍、意识模糊和死亡等。如果毁损影响附近脊髓小脑前束、网状脊髓束和皮质脊髓束可产生共济失调，或产生自主神经和运动控制障碍。

双侧脊髓丘脑外侧束切断术

只有极少数患者出现双侧癌痛或在单侧脊髓切断术后出现新的疼痛而进行治疗。目前关于疗效的资料很少，但已知双侧脊髓丘脑外侧束切断术的并发症发生率高，包括共济失调、运动无力、感觉障碍、大小便失禁、呼吸抑制和死亡。

实际问题

随着长期口服阿片类药物、经皮阿片类制剂（**专栏 78.3**）和鞘内给药系统的问世，采用脊髓丘脑外侧束切断术的患者数量一直在稳步下降。然而，恶性间皮瘤病例数量不断增加（预计在 2020 年左右达到峰值），若通过药物和介入治疗缓解疼痛效果不佳，手术对这些患者仍可能是一种有效的止痛方法。但随着手术量的减少和医生不愿意实施破坏性和不可逆转的治疗方法，这种手术方法可能会被逐步淘汰。

专栏 78.3 阿片类药物——止痛之王？

阿片受体是控制伤害性反应、享乐性反应、情绪反应、自主神经反应、神经内分泌反应和免疫反应的蛋白质。基因克隆只明确了三个受体基因，分别编码 μ、δ 和 κ 受体。

通过敲除相关基因产生的受体缺陷的小鼠表现出更强的疼痛敏感性。在急性疼痛模型中，μ 受体调节机械、化学和脊髓上控制的热痛觉，而 κ 受体调节脊髓介导的热痛觉和内脏痛。有高等级的证据表明，在炎症性和神经病理性疼痛的情况下，δ 受体在减轻痛觉过敏中起着重要作用。

内源性阿片肽。甲硫氨酸脑啡肽和亮氨酸脑啡肽作用于脊髓背角Ⅰ和Ⅱ层，三叉神经脊束核和中脑导水管周围灰质（periaqueductal grey，PAG）的阿片受体。它们也存在于胃肠道和肾上腺髓质。强啡肽对多个脊髓和脊髓上部位有作用，但被认为是弱止痛剂。β- 内啡肽的多种复杂作用一般仅存在于中枢神经系统。

阿片类药物在脊髓产生作用的部位位于在由脊髓背角初级传入神经元、投射神经元、星形胶质细胞和小胶质细胞的中央末端组成的四突触中。阿片类药物：

1. 通过关闭 Ca^{++} 通道和开放 K^{+} 通道使初级传入神经元细胞膜超极化，从而减少伤害性传入神经元的谷氨酸释放（突触前效应），减少来自外周的伤害性输入；
2. 减少突触后细胞内 Ca^{2+}，升高 K^{+}，从而阻断一些原本可能导致二级神经元过度兴奋的机制。

脊髓上部阿片类药物镇痛的位点

阿片类药物在脑内有多种机制和作用部位。阿片类药物与 5- 羟色胺（5-HT）、γ- 氨基丁酸能（GABA），以及可能的其他下行中枢调节系统相互作用。它们抑制自喙部中央内侧髓质（rostroventral medial medulla，RVM）输出的下行神经纤维传导。阿片类药物在调节疼痛体验方面也起着重要作用。

阿片类镇痛的外周作用。阿片受体也在背根神经节（dorsal root ganglion，DRG）合成，并沿着轴突运输到外周部位。在炎症模型中，在 DRG 处合成内源性阿片肽可能不受调节。

中脑束切断术

与丘脑切开术类似，这种手术也已经用于治疗卒中后疼痛和癌症疼痛，尽管数量不多，且有经验的外科医生较为稀少。中脑切开术适用于头部、颈部、肩部和手臂顽固性疼痛的患者，也被称为脊髓上的脊髓切开术。然而，手术疗效喜忧参半，而且像眼球运动功能障碍这样的并发症也很常见。这几年已很少使用这种手术方式，多首选其他侵入性较小的治疗方式。

脊髓电刺激

脊髓电刺激（spinal cord stimulation，SCS）是指在脊髓上直接施加电流以达到镇痛的目的。根据记载，至少早在公元前 63 年，古希腊人就已经尝试使用电刺激治疗痛风，他们使用电鳐作为治疗痛风的电流来源。作为现在治疗慢性疼痛的一种方法，SCS 自 1966 年开始使用，Shealy 首次将鞘内单极电极连接到体外心脏脉冲发生器上，成功地缓解了一名晚期肺癌患者的疼痛。Shealy 认为，直接电刺激大的初级传入神经元会“关闭”通过小的 A δ 和 C 纤维传播的伤害性信号（参见闸门学说**专栏 78.1**）。随着完全植入式脊髓电刺激系统的发展，SCS 已成为一种公认的慢性疼痛缓解方法（Song et al.，2014）。英国国家临床成果研究所（National Institute of Clinical Excellence，NICE）再次推荐 SCS 用于治疗慢性周围神经性疼痛，FDA 已批准 SCS 用于治疗躯干和四肢的慢性疼痛。

SCS 的作用原理

SCS 植入系统由两个主要部分组成：放置在硬膜外间隙的电极导线和位于皮下囊袋的植入式脉冲发生器（implantable pulse generator，IPG）（图 78.6）。电极可以选择性地设置为阴极、中性或阳极，从而产生直接影响周围脊髓结构的电流和电磁场。

阴极周围的神经元带的负电荷较少，会发生去极化，从而导致双向动作电位传播。当膜带更多

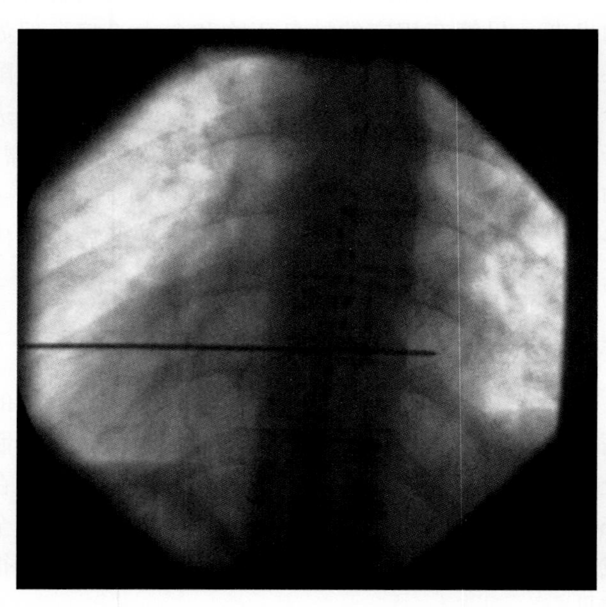

图 78.6 一例左下肢放射性疼痛和双侧腰痛患者，在下胸硬膜外间隙放置两根经皮圆柱形脊髓刺激（spinal cord stimulation，SCS）电极导线的前后观图像

负电荷时，阳极会产生局部轴突超极化。通过对电极触点设置不同的阴阳极组合，在相应的皮肤区域产生电场，从而改变感觉异常或达到镇痛的目的。Holshemer 用计算机模型解释了刺激效果是由以下几个因素决定的：负极相对于生理中线的位置；电极的极性设置；负极下的脑脊液（cerebrospinal fluid，CSF）深度；轴突直径和是否存在髓鞘；背柱、背根和背角内的轴突方向（各向异性）。近来刺激脉冲的参数设置不断优化，可以使用高频刺激、簇状放电刺激、高电流密度刺激和阈下刺激。其中一些新的刺激模式能达到显著的镇痛效果而不会产生感觉异常。

自 20 世纪 70 年代初以来，人们一直在研究以感觉过敏为基础的低频 SCS 的作用机制。有关 SCS 机制的研究主要来自动物，将临床前数据转化为临床实践是具有挑战性的。目前还没有一个确切的机制，主要考虑以下三个方面：首先，激活大直径的 Aβ 纤维（激活更多的 A-WDR 纤维可能与改善预后有关），抑制背角 WDR 神经元；其次，SCS 诱导神经递质的释放，其中一些是抑制性的，如 GABA，但也有 5-羟色胺（5-HT）、甘氨酸、腺苷和乙酰胆碱，在突触前和突触后都是如此；最后，刺激脊髓上通路可激活下行疼痛抑制系统，促进 WDR 神经元的突触释放 5-HT 和去甲肾上腺素。

一些临床证据已经证实了这些机制，我们都知道，低频 SCS 能缓解疼痛必须是患者体会到感觉异常（可能是由于 Aβ 纤维激活）与疼痛区域重叠。这也表明 Aβ 终末投射多会在脊髓背角的过度兴奋区域重新编排组合。此外，鞘内注射亚临床剂量的巴氯芬（一种 $GABA_B$ 激动剂）可以增强先前无效的低频 SCS 的效果，从而提示 GABA 在传统的基于感觉异常的 SCS 中起到了缓解疼痛的作用。

最近有研究表明， 10 kHz 高频 （10 kHz high frequency， HF10） 的无感觉异常 SCS 在缓解慢性顽固性腰腿痛方面优于传统的基于感觉异常的低频 SCS。与低频 SCS 相比，接受高频刺激的患者没有出现刺激相关性感觉异常，而且 Aβ 介导的感觉异常-疼痛重叠似乎与疼痛缓解无关。这表明 Aβ 纤维在高频 SCS 中可能并不重要，临床前研究表明 HF10 作用机制不同于传统低频 SCS。

适应证和禁忌证

SCS 对周围神经病理性疼痛非常有效，最常见的适应证是术后神经根性肢体疼痛。它在治疗中枢神经性疼痛方面的作用机制还不是很清楚。最近的研究表明，SCS 治疗腰痛的结果喜忧参半。随着高频刺激和多触点电极的引入，SCS 对某些类型的腰疼可能有良好的效果。

SCS 治疗的常见适应证如下：

- 椎板切除术后慢性神经病理性疼痛综合征；
- 复杂区域性疼痛综合征；
- 周围神经病变，包括创伤后和糖尿病性神经病变；
- 周围血管缺血性疾病引起的疼痛；
- 顽固性心绞痛；
- 骶骨刺激治疗骨盆疼痛。

SCS 治疗的禁忌证包括：①无法进行电刺激操作；②拟刺激部位存在心脏起搏器 / 植入式心脏复律除颤器 / 鞘内泵治疗设备；③局部或全身感染；④免疫抑制；⑤凝血障碍。相对禁忌证是病理学上不适宜手术的情况（神经根或脊髓压迫、脊柱不稳、椎管狭窄），即便是这样也面临着许多挑战，例如复发性椎间盘突出，再次手术产生并发症的概率更高。

SCS 的临床证据

North 等在 2005 年发表了第一篇关于 SCS 与腰背术后疼痛综合征（failed back pain syndrome，FBSS）患者再次手术的有利的 RCT 研究。2007 年，一项前瞻性的多中心随机对照试验（PROCESS）对 100 例 FBSS 患者进行了 SCS 治疗和常规药物治疗（conventional medical management，CMM）的临床疗效比较，6 个月后，SCS 组有 48% 的患者疼痛缓解 50% 以上，CMM 组为 9%（意向治疗分析），12 个月时两组疼痛缓解 50% 以上的比率分别为 34% 和 7%，24 个月时分别为 37% 和 2%（$P=0.003$）。而且，Oswestry 残疾指数和 EQ-5-D 问卷评估结果显示，SCS 组患者具有更好的功能改善和更高的生活质量（$P<0.0001$）（Kumar et al.，2007）。最近，一项前瞻性的多中心非劣效性随机对照试验比较了传统的辅助性 SCS 和高频刺激（10 kHz 频率的低电压刺激）在顽固性腰腿痛患者中的治疗作用。198 名患者被随机分为常规刺激和高频刺激两组，在治疗 12 个月后，高频刺激治疗腿痛（78% *vs*. 51%）和腰痛（78% *vs*. 51%）有效率均高于传统 SCS（Kapura et al.，2015）。

SCS 治疗的实际问题

1. **SCS 转诊的多学科评估**。在推荐患者进行 SCS 试验之前，需对患者进行综合评估。严格筛选适合手术的患者，才能使 SCS 成为一种经济有效的治疗方案。对于患者来说，要对 SCS 治疗有一个现实的期望值，了解 SCS 治疗的局限性，要知道 SCS 不会治愈他们的疾病或消除他们的疼痛，这也是 SCS 成功与否的先决条件。SCS 术前评估和教育也是手术成功的另一个重要因素。

2. **电极的选择**。电极根据放置的方式分为两种：经皮（圆柱）电极和开放（片状）电极。前者通过改良的 14G Tuohy 针在透视辅助下置入硬膜外间隙，既可以用于术中测试，在手术结束后取出，也可以通过打通隧道将其锚定在背筋膜上，转换为持久的试验性电极，进行 1~4 周的测试。圆柱形电极的优点包括易于植入和相对非侵入性。在撰写本文时，圆柱形电极的标准电极阵列为 8 个触点，其中一家制造商提供 16 个触点的经皮电极。圆柱形电极的缺点是容易移位，从而达不到治疗效果，刺激非预期靶点（如黄韧带）而导致电流扩散不佳，以及较高的电流需求。随着电极固定技术的不断提高，电极移位已很少见。可充电的 IPG 技术也缓解了电量过早耗尽的问题。

片状电极有一个有效面，可容纳多达排成三列的 16 个电极触点。它们必须通过在靶水平以下 1~2 个椎板间隙处行一个小的椎板切开术进行插入。电极上更宽的触点分布可能会增加刺激治疗有效的可能性，并降低刺激无效的可能。片状电极移位很少发生。它们也需要较少的电流来刺激前方的靶点，因为背面是绝缘的。但是片状电极的放置是一种创伤更大的手术，并发症可能会更多。片状电极占据了更多的硬膜外间隙，有脊髓受压的风险，特别是在颈椎水平。

在选择电极时需要考虑 MRI 的兼容性。截至撰写本文时，大多数电极和 IPG 已被认证为“限制条件性兼容头和四肢 MRI”，允许患者接受 1.5T 的头部 MRI 检查。一家 SCS 系统供应商已经开发出兼容 1.5T 全身 MRI 检查的电极和 IPG。

3. **IPG 的选择**。目前 SCS 市场所有的制造商除了提供不可充电的 IPG，也都可以提供可充电的 IPG。可充电 IPG 的寿命取决于充电循环的次数，而充电循环的次数又取决于刺激参数。对于大多数 SCS 设备，IPG 电池可以使用 5~10 年。IPG 的寿命是决定 SCS 治疗成本效益的重要变量之一，不可充电的 SCS 系统成本效益最低，高频刺激最高（McMahon and Malcangio，2009）。

并发症

据报道，并发症发生率高达 34%，但大多数症状轻微，且能恢复。这些症状包括电刺激时无镇痛疗效、刺激丧失、感觉异常或感觉障碍。原因包括电极移位、硬膜外纤维化或对刺激产生耐受性，这种耐受性可能是由脊髓的可塑性引起的。使用现在的电极固定技术，发生移位的情况很少，但可能需要重新放置或更换为片状电极。通过对患者进行教育、“开 - 关”循环设置和 IPG 参数调整，可重新达到刺激效果。一些研究数据表明，簇状放电刺激模式可能会降低耐受性。IPG 埋置部位的不适感很常见，有可能需要调整放置部位。极少患者会发生皮肤破溃。其他与设备相关的并发症包括导线断裂、IPG 故障和电池耗尽。

来自大型前瞻性试验的数据显示感染率低至 2%~3%，与其他外科假体植入的感染率一致。经皮体外测试、BMI>30 和二次手术是感染的危险因素。最常见的病原体是对甲氧西林敏感的金黄色葡萄球菌。即使是表浅部位的感染也令人担忧，应该及早积极治疗，以防止发生神经系统感染或装置取出。因此手术操作必须严谨，应适当应用抗生素，术区敷料保持无菌。

SCS 治疗的神经系统并发症非常少见。最常见的是在导线放置过程中不慎刺穿硬脑膜。脊髓损伤引起的偏瘫、四肢瘫痪均有报道。因此建议手术前通过 MRI 来评估硬膜外间隙，并预测电极置入过程中的潜在风险。

脑深部电刺激术

背景

脑深部电刺激术（deep brain stimulation，DBS）自 1954 年开始用于治疗复杂慢性疼痛（参见综述 Boccard et al.，2015）。DBS 是一种对多个脑内靶点进行电刺激的方法，这些靶点被认为是大脑中“疼痛神经基质”的一部分。DBS 镇痛效应的假说早在动物试验及精神分裂症研究的“疼痛闸门”理论发表前至少十年就出现了。Heath 是第一个采用间歇性隔核刺激成功治疗癌症晚期疼痛患者数周的人。

理论上，在众多脑内核团、神经束和神经束组成的网络中，DBS 有多个治疗靶点，又被称为“疼痛神经传导网络”。历史上，内侧隔核是最早刺激靶点。从 1973 年损毁的早期数据中发现：丘脑的腹后内侧核（ventroposteromedial，VPM）和腹后外侧核（ventroposterolateral，VPL）是另一个重要的刺激靶点。中脑导水管周围灰质和脑室周围灰质（periaqueductal grey and periventricular grey，PAG/PVG）也是啮齿类动物镇痛的重要靶点，DBS 刺激该区域可产生镇痛作用。最近，人们对前扣带回皮质的分离痛觉及其情感成分产生极大的兴趣。对中枢性卒中后伴发全身或偏身疼痛的患者可能产生更好的效果。

作用机制

DBS 的镇痛机制知之甚少。对疼痛神经传导网络中多个部分之间复杂的相互作用的理解仍不清楚，神经传导网络的层次关系尚未完全阐明。目前研究认为，中枢性疼痛状态最终会导致与疼痛感知和疼痛传递相关的神经细胞异常放电。关于持续的伤害性信号传入究竟如何改变神经细胞电生理学尚无定论。部分学者认为它提高了神经元放电频率的同步化。然而，也有部分学者提出了一种不同的机制，即细胞自发放电减弱。DBS 既可以同步化并“减缓”PAG/PVM 和 VPM/VPL 的异常放电，也可以增强上述结构中被抑制的神经活动。有趣的是，PAG 的 DBS 似乎确实影响内源性阿片类递质的释放，已有研究表明 PAG 可能对丘脑感觉核起上行调制作用。

DBS 的适应证

理论上，DBS 治疗对任何慢性神经病理性疼痛都应该有效。然而，目前大多数工作都是在患有中枢性神经病理性疼痛的患者身上进行的，且这些患者对其他多种治疗方式均没有明显疗效（**专栏 78.4**）。到目前为止，已发表的研究表明非典型面部疼痛、中枢性卒中后疼痛、臂丛撕脱痛和截肢后疼痛 / 幻肢痛患者效果最好。已有 DBS 治疗脊髓疼痛 /FBSS 的病例报道。

DBS 疗效

DBS 在疼痛治疗方面已进行了两项多中心研究。这两项研究都存在研究设计和数据收集的重要缺陷，以及患者的异质性和高流失率的问题。当随访时间超过 12 个月时，两项研究都没有达到 FDA 设定的主要结果，即 50% 以上的受试者疼痛缓解超过 50%。因此，在美国 FDA 没有批准 DBS 治疗慢性疼痛。此后有了更多的研究，包括一项随机的安慰剂对照试验。英国 NICE 已经批准使用 DBS 治疗经过严格筛选的其他治疗无效的难治性慢性疼痛患者。

并发症

DBS 的临床并发症主要包括手术并发症、硬件相关并发症和刺激相关并发症。DBS 手术的并发症包括颅内出血（4%）、感染（12%）、电极位置不准和罕见的死亡。硬件相关的并发症包括电极断裂、电极侵蚀和感染。刺激相关并发症是靶点周围神经

专栏 78.4　伤害性与神经性疼痛的药物治疗

尽管我们对慢性疼痛的多种发病机制有了更好的理解，在临床实践中其治疗仍然存在极大的挑战性。伤害性信息传入和抑制下行输出的平衡已向前者倾斜，外周和中枢敏化通常是神经病理性疼痛的主要驱动因素，下行抑制机制不能抑制躯体感觉系统的过度活动。大脑中疼痛神经传导网络的激活改变了疼痛体验，与大脑控制情感、压力和情绪的区域建立了联系。疼痛不再是生理上的伤害性反应，而已经成为一种复杂的生物 - 心理 - 社会现象。

慢性疼痛的药物治疗主要包括：

1. 减少外周伤害性输入和外周敏化；
2. 减少脊髓的中枢性敏化，防止躯体感觉神经系统产生可塑性改变；
3. 加强下行疼痛抑制；
4. 改变疼痛体验。

慢性疼痛治疗药物的选择取决于疼痛发生机制。在伤害性疼痛中，最重要的治疗策略是减少伤害性输入。非甾体抗炎药（NSAIDs）和阿片类药物是最有效的药物选择。NSAIDs 通过抑制 COX-1 和 COX-2 酶从而减少组织损伤部位前列腺素的合成来减轻炎症，这样就降低了外周敏感度。阿片类药物作用于外周神经系统（peripheral nervous system，PNS）和中枢神经系统（CNS）中的多个靶点，减少背角外周伤害性输入。它们还减少了通过二级神经元的信号传递，并增强了 RVM 的下行疼痛抑制，而且还会改变疼痛体验。

一旦躯体感觉系统发生改变，要考虑其他治疗策略（如突触前 TPVR1 和 2 上调，电压门控 Na+ 通道，钙通道 α2δ 亚单位上调，背角 WDRs 激活，AMPA 和 NMDA 受体激活，胶质细胞和星形胶质细胞激活，突触后 GABA 受体活性降低，二级神经元敏化，5- 羟色胺和去甲肾上腺素能下行疼痛抑制系统减弱，疼痛神经传导网络激活）。

外周脱敏可尝试辣椒素乳膏或贴剂（作用于突触前的香草素受体 TPVR1 和 2）、局部麻醉药物（如 LA 乳膏、利多卡因膏）、全身性 Na+ 通道抑制剂（如 TGN 中的卡马西平）、加巴喷丁类（如加巴喷丁和普瑞巴林）。

中枢脱敏可用加巴喷丁类（作用于大脑中钙通道的 α2δ 亚单位，从而增强去甲肾上腺素能下行通路）、5- 羟色胺和去甲肾上腺素再摄取抑制剂（三环类抗抑郁药、文拉法辛、度洛西汀、曲马多）、选择性去甲肾上腺素再摄取抑制剂他戊二醇、非选择性 NMDA 拮抗剂（氯胺酮、美沙酮）、α2- 激动剂可乐定来尝试。阿片类激动剂在治疗中枢敏化和神经病理性疼痛方面效果不佳，因此不应作为神经病理性疼痛治疗的主要药物。过度依赖阿片类药物可能导致对阿片类药物的耐受和（或）心理依赖（成瘾），这将导致用药剂量增加，并可能导致严重的医源性并发症（便秘、呼吸抑制、阿片类药物诱导的背角痛觉敏感、垂体肾上腺轴抑制、免疫抑制、认知下降）。

结构受到不必要的刺激引起的。

运动皮质电刺激（motor cortex stimulation，MCS）治疗难治性中枢性和周围性去传入疼痛综合征最早出现于20世纪90年代，并在一些小的研究中取得了一定的成功。MCS潜在的作用机制尚不清楚，尽管人们推测它可能通过激活躯体运动和感觉皮质之间的通路而导致感觉抑制，或者可能通过激活边缘系统发挥作用。有人对其长期疗效持怀疑态度，经颅磁刺激可能会成为患者选择的一种非侵入性筛查工具。

结论

慢性疼痛仍然是医学上跨越不同学科的一个巨大难题。过去25年的疼痛研究重新定义了我们对感觉生理学和疼痛生物学的理解。疼痛和伤害感受不再被认为是通过硬连接的、固定的，可以通过手术“重新连接”的环路来调节，许多治疗慢性疼痛的旧式外科技术已经很少应用。对疼痛神经生物学和不良适应感觉可塑性理解的增加，为有效的循证干预带来了新的机会（Yekkirala et al.，2017）。从外科的角度来看，最近基于电刺激的技术产生了振奋人心的结果，这一领域将继续快速发展。毁损性手术仍可通过有经验的外科医生在经过严格筛选的部分患者中进行，但手术无效的可能性及手术的不可逆转性，使得它们在当前的医学环境下难以推广。

参考文献、EBRAIN 的相关链接

扫描书末二维码获取。

第 79 章 脑神经血管压迫综合征

Marc Sindou · George Georgoulis
王宁、郭宇鹏 译，孟凡刚、陈国强 审校

引言

在过去几十年中，众多所谓的“特发性”（或原发性）高兴奋性脑神经（cranial nerve，CN）疾病是由血管压迫神经（neurovascular conflict，NVC）引发的，这一理念得到越来越多学者的认可。因此，显微血管减压术（microsurgical vascular decompression，MVD）成为治疗这些功能性脑神经疾病的首选方法。

高兴奋性脑神经疾病可发生于人体的第Ⅲ至第Ⅻ对脑神经。

- 三叉神经痛（trigeminal neuralgia，TN）是目前最常见的脑神经疾病。当今对三叉神经痛的发病原因有一个普遍的共识，即第Ⅴ脑神经感觉根存在着 NVC，而 NVC 往往位于三叉神经根部入脑干区（root entry zone，REZ），也可位于神经根的其他部位，而三叉神经的运动根则很少受累。
- 面肌痉挛（hemifacial spasm，HFS）绝大多数患者的病因也是由于颅内动脉血管压迫第Ⅶ对脑神经，而且压迫部位几乎总是在 REZ。
- 迷走 - 舌咽神经痛（vago-glossopharyngeal neuralgia，VGPN）在疼痛特征和治疗方案方面与 TN 非常相似，也是由 NVC 引起，但 NVC 部位是在第Ⅸ和（或）第Ⅹ对脑神经上。发病率为 TN 的 1%。
- 第Ⅷ对脑神经从脑干到内听道均有中枢髓鞘成分包裹，是所有脑神经中具有最长中枢髓鞘成分覆盖的神经纤维组织。其病变可能是耳鸣（耳蜗神经）和眩晕（前庭神经）的发病原因。这两种疾病的发病率很高而且病理生理学特征变化多样。不论何种类型的损伤均可导致神经纤维发生病理性改变，产生中枢突触重组效应，从而导致听力损害，这种发病机制与许多类型的神经性疼痛相类似。而部分患者的发病原因可能与 NVC 有关，其诊断有时较为困难。
- 除面神经外，运动性脑神经高兴奋性疾病较为少见。与眼球运动相关的脑神经（第Ⅲ对、第Ⅳ对、第Ⅵ对）功能障碍所导致的运动异常多数与其他病变有关而非 NVC。
- 文献报道，与咬肌有关的肌肉痉挛多是由于第Ⅴ脑神经的运动根发生功能障碍。虽然有部分学者认为痉挛性斜颈是由于第Ⅺ对脑神经存在 NVC 引起的，但在疾病分类中，应该将此类疾病归类为肌张力障碍或异动症，因为其疾病的起源可能是脑干或基底神经节功能异常，而不是由于副神经受压迫所致。关于舌下神经，目前有文献报道存在于第Ⅻ对脑神经根部的 NVC 可导致半侧舌痉挛。
- 部分假说认为血管压迫延髓腹外侧和第Ⅸ对至第Ⅹ对脑神经 REZ 的腹侧可能是神经源性特发性高血压的病因之一。
- 最后，少数情况下，同一个体中可同时存在多组脑神经受累而出现脑神经高兴奋性功能异常症状。

相关神经生理学机制的假说见**专栏** 79.1。

面肌痉挛

面肌痉挛的名称是根据临床症状进行定义：面神经支配的同侧面部肌肉出现慢性、不自主运动，部分患者可表现为痉挛性抽搐和眼口联动。原发性面肌痉挛的诊断必须满足以下三个标准：①除外面神经麻痹产生的后遗症；②症状为慢性进展性并局限于单侧面神经支配区域；③除了第Ⅶ对脑神经上存在血管压迫，且绝大部分位于 REZ 外，常规影像学检查无明显异常。

病理生理学

目前，有足够的证据表明原发性面肌痉挛与面神经 REZ 区受搏动性压迫导致支配面部运动的神经核出现功能改变（过度兴奋）有关（Gardner，1962；Gardner and Sava，1962；Møller and Jannetta，1984；Sindou，2005）。中枢神经元的过度兴奋会产生运动

专栏 79.1　神经生理机制假说

公认的有关血管压迫神经（NVC）导致高兴奋性脑神经（CN）疾病的机制有数个，而且各个机制之间有很好的互补性。

对神经根的慢性搏动性压迫会产生异位刺激，并通过局部脱髓鞘病变传导到邻近神经纤维通路。这些脱髓鞘区就像是新突触，由此产生假突触传递，换句话说，就是神经纤维间由于“短路”而发生“串扰”现象的中心（Gardner，1962）。这可以解释扳机点和产生放射状传播的临床表现。通常，NVC 多位于所谓的神经根 REZ 区（神经根进入 / 出脊髓区）。据我们所知，REZ 并没有权威的定义。然而，通常认为 REZ 相当于中央型髓鞘与施万细胞形成的髓鞘之间的移行区域，即过渡区（transitional zone，TZ）（图 79.1），脑神经中枢端和 TZ 被认为是“更容易兴奋”的结构。事实上，并不是所有的 NVC 都位于 REZ 区，有些则位于神经远心端区域。对于后一种 NVC，在手术显微镜下经常可观察到一个由于压迫而出现的灰色凹槽，这种表现多为搏动性动脉，或也有（非搏动的）静脉长期压迫导致的局灶性脱髓鞘病变。

机械搏动和局灶性脱髓鞘可能不是诱发疾病的唯一来源。通过逆行刺激激活相应的 CN 核（即通过“点火”现象），局部产生的异常神经信号传导会导致神经核细胞的过度兴奋和过度活跃。中枢神经系统产生的这种高兴奋性与许多 CN 高兴奋性疾病的癫痫样临床表现相一致，所以抗癫痫药物对该类疾病有独特疗效。

此外，也可能还有其他机制尚未被人们所认知，如遗传、免疫、内分泌和心理因素，可能在这些复杂的神经系统疾病的发病机制中也发挥作用。

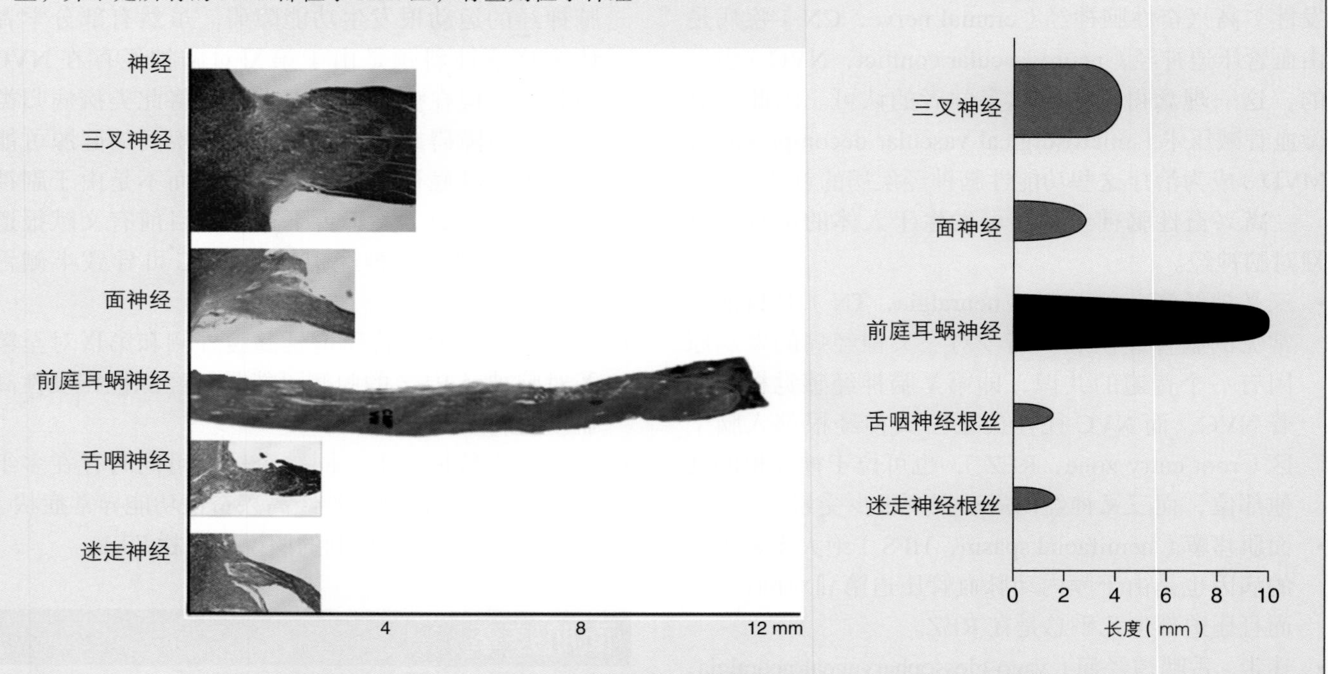

图 79.1　（A）用 Luxol 固蓝染色法对三叉神经、面神经、前庭耳蜗神经、舌咽神经和迷走神经根部进行染色，纵行切片后在同一评估标准下进行显微照片比较。中央髓鞘部分和施万髓鞘部分之间的过渡区（TZ）已进行画线分隔。（B）中央髓鞘部分长度的对比图，数据来源于相应神经根长度（附带直径）的平均值

放电，这种放电可能是由各种外周刺激以及通过脑干网状结构传递的情感事件引起。这种假说的机制与痉挛的临床症状和电生理特征相一致，也与医学影像资料和术中所见在面神经的 REZ 区存在血管神经压迫的事实相一致。在过去的三十年中，MVD 已被证实对治愈这种疾病具有很高价值（Barker et al.，1995）。关于与该疾病有关的发现、手术技术和治疗结果已有大量文献予以描述，相关信息可参阅已发表的文献（Huang et al.，1992；Sindou et al.，1997；Sauvain et al.，2001；Sindou and Keravel，2009b；Li et al.，2016）。

诊断

本病的患病率是 1/100 000（美国）。左侧与右侧的比例大约为 2∶1，女性与男性的比例大约为 2∶1。

在典型的原发性面肌痉挛患者中，痉挛通常起始于一侧眼轮匝肌的轻微、间歇性抽搐；继而出现低位面部肌肉抽搐。

肌电图（electromyography，EMG）记录显示为一个典型的电生理信号：阵发性面部肌肉收缩，联带

运动，侧方扩散反应阳性。

影像学检查有助于明确原发性 HFS 是由于神经受血管压迫所致。压迫血管通常为动脉：小脑前下动脉（anterior inferior cerebellar artery，AICA）、小脑后下动脉（posterior inferior cerebellar artery，PICA）和（或）椎基底动脉（vertebrobasilar artery，VBA），高分辨率 MRI 结合磁共振血管成像（MR-angio，MRA）可以清晰显示上述压迫血管。三维 MRI-T2 序列可清晰显示面神经的轮廓。值得注意的是，影像学检查可能有假阳性表现，即无症状人群的影像学检查中也可见血管神经接触现象。责任动脉一般位于脑干腹侧面神经 REZ。

外科治疗

本病口服药物治疗效果差，药物治疗首选方法是进行肉毒杆菌毒素注射，但当此治疗方式无明显疗效后，MVD 是唯一的治疗方法。

MVD 手术是由 Gardner（Gardner，1962）率先提出，随后由 Jannetta 总结并推广开来（Jannetta et al.，1977）。在同一患者可能存在一支或多支动脉压迫。在我们的 280 例患者中，责任血管为 PICA、AICA 和（或）VBA 的概率分别为 61%、56% 和 27%，其中多达 40% 的患者存在多支血管压迫现象（Marneffe et al.，2003）。手术探查不彻底，尤其是脑干部位血管遗漏可能是外科手术失败的主要原因。

大多数中心都是选择侧卧位进行此类手术。手术入路为乳突后锁孔开颅，骨窗直径在 1.5~2 cm，位于乳突顶端的后方，这样可从侧下方越过小脑绒球，并从下方到达面神经（**图 79.2**）。选择此入路有两方面需要特殊注意。首先，NVC 通常位于脑干的腹尾侧。其次，小脑半球从外侧向内侧牵拉会对第Ⅷ对神经产生拉伸作用，从而对患者的听力造成影响。当术中 BEAP 记录峰值Ⅲ和Ⅴ潜伏期延长时需特殊注意（Grundy et al.，1982；Møller and Møller，1989；Sindou et al.，1992；Polo et al.，2004）。

在处理压迫的动脉时，需小心不要撕脱穿支动脉，明确迷路动脉后再对 AICA 进行操作。机械性血管痉挛可能导致耳蜗缺血，尤其是 BEAP 记录的峰值Ⅰ振幅减小时更需提高警惕（Sindou et al.，1992；Polo et al.，2004）。应用医用材料将责任血管袢推离开神经根部，我们中心采用的是 Teflon 垫棉（材料为聚四氟乙烯，从整个完整垫片中抽离成细丝后制作成束状或球状。Edwards Outfow Tract Knitted 是将聚四氟乙烯制作成隔离血管神经的垫片，质地偏硬，而 Sauvage Knitted Polyester 法制作的隔离垫片则较柔软，其生产厂商信息为：Bard Peripheral Vascular，Inc. 1625 West 3rd Street，Tempe，AZ 85281 USA，https://www.crbard.com）。术中操作需注意不要在面神经和（或）前庭耳蜗神经上造成任何新的压迫，避免动脉扭转、打折。应用滴有少量 10% 浓度罂粟碱的生理盐水定期冲洗术区可以减轻血管的收缩反应，考虑罂粟碱的碱性较强，冲洗溶液浓度不宜过高，否则会产生毒性作用。

在 HFS 患者中，当刺激面神经的一个分支时，会在另一分支支配的面部肌肉中产生重复和扩散的肌电反应。Møller 和 Jannetta 提倡在 MVD 手术过程中进行侧方扩散反应（lateral spread responses，LSR）的肌电图记录，以确保减压过程充分、彻底（Møller and Jannetta，1987；Mooij et al.，2001）。然而，在我们报道的一组患者中，当 MVD 结束时 LSR 仍然存在，但术后症状却获得长期改善，因此，LSR 监测的可靠性仍需进一步验证（Hatem et al.，2001）。

结果

据不同作者报道，手术的长期治愈率为 85%~95%。术后临床症状完全缓解可能会有所延迟，时间大概为几个月到一年（Goto et al.，2002；Sindou and Keravel，2009a；Zhong et al.，2015）。在我们纳入有 280 例患者的研究中，术后 7 年进行随访时的治愈率为 87%，其中 12% 的患者术后出现延迟治愈，多为几个月。由于这个概率的存在，因此我们不建议早期就进行再次手术，观察时间最好持续至术后一年。已获治愈的患者，症状再次复发的概率很小，此项研究结果显示复发率为 1%~2%。

延迟治愈现象的存在充分说明 HFS 的病因不仅仅是由于动脉血管对面神经 REZ 的搏动性机械压迫所致。慢性血管压迫引起的面神经核脱髓鞘病变和运动神经元过度兴奋可能在疾病的发生过程中起到一定作用。考虑到可能是由于神经核团的病变导致临床症状，神经纤维的可塑性导致电生理变化的逆转往往需要一定时间，这些推测均可以解释延迟治愈现象（Møller and Møller，1989；Sindou，2005）。

MVD 很少有严重的手术并发症。文献回顾显示 MVD 并发症风险可概括如下：死亡率小于 1%，小脑梗死或出血并发症为 0.50% ± 0.30%。所有脑神经中，第Ⅷ对和第Ⅶ对脑神经出现并发症的概率较高，后组脑神经出现并发症的概率极小。MVD 术后出现残留部分有效听力和完全性的永久性听力障碍的概率分别为 2.45%~15.90% 和 1.18%~2.60%。一系列数据显示，患者术后出现永久性面神经麻痹

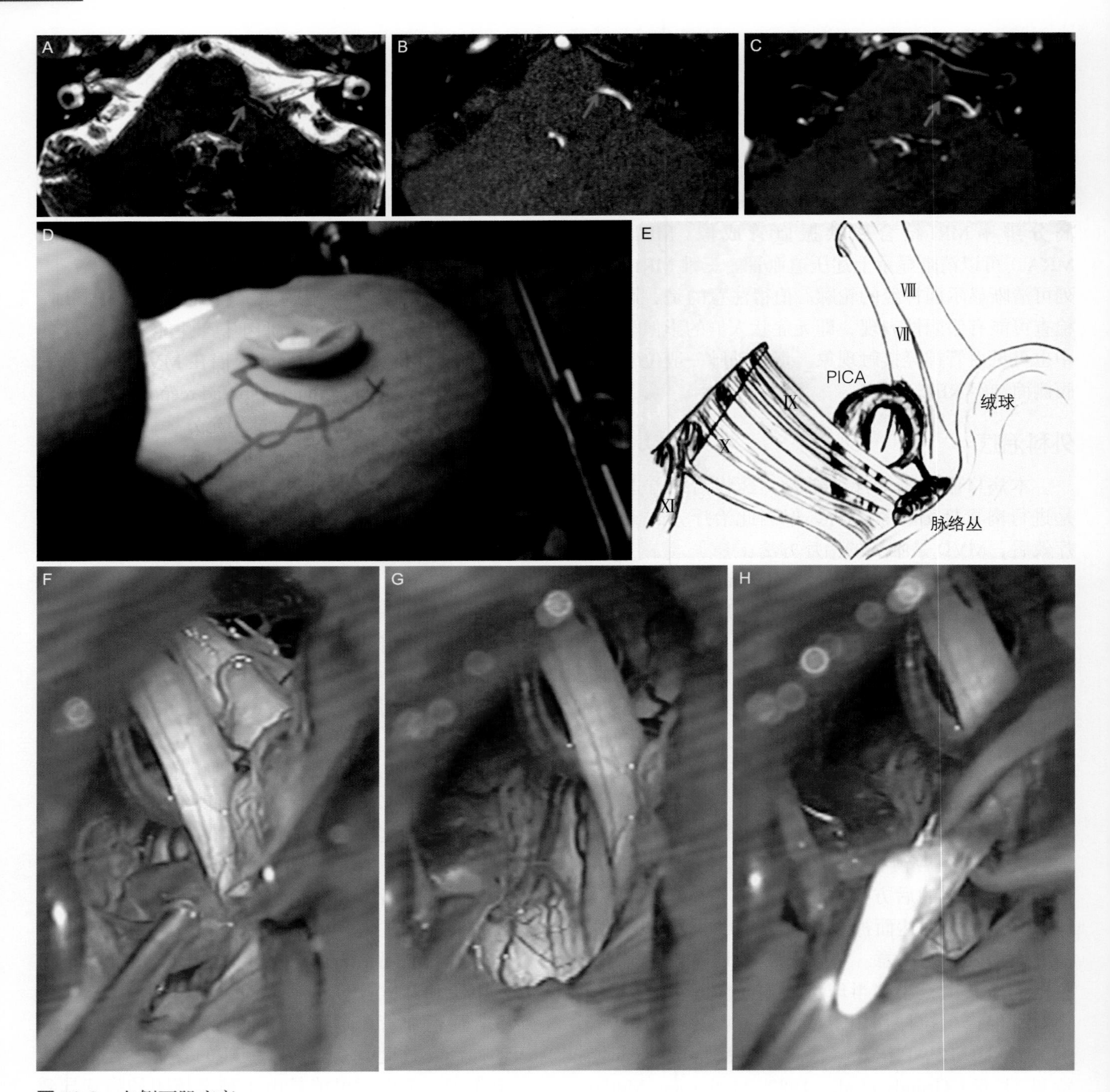

图 79.2 左侧面肌痉挛

磁共振影像所见：左侧面神经根部 REZ 区可见 PICA 环嵌入脑干，在 MRI T2 序列（A）、TOF 血管成像序列（B）和 MRI T1 强化序列（C）清晰可见。

外科手术入路：通过暴露乳突后方至乳突最高顶点范围进行颅骨切开术（D），从下方区域进入面神经 REZ 区，即沿着后组脑神经（第Ⅺ、第Ⅹ、第Ⅸ对脑神经）和经小脑延髓裂的上部 Luschka 孔出现的脉络丛处进入。NVC 多位于面神经 REZ 区和脑干结合处的腹尾侧（E）。

显微手术步骤：PICA 环压迫面神经 REZ 区，后者由于被前庭蜗神经遮挡而不可见（F）；PICA 血管环被推移离开面神经 REZ（第Ⅷ脑神经腹侧视角），呈灰色（G）；用一块长 1 cm，宽 0.5 cm 的半刚性 teflon 垫棉将血管环推移远离面神经 REZ 区（H）

（包含新发或持续存在且病变程度不限）的概率为0.8%~5.0%。据文献资料显示，迟发性面神经麻痹的发生率高达7.30%，且通常发生在术后第一周的末尾。但几乎所有患者的症状均可在几周到几个月内都恢复正常，其机制尚不清楚。后组脑神经出现功能障碍的概率为0.44%~2.18%，主要表现为声音嘶哑、饮水呛咳、吞咽困难。与脑脊液漏有关的并发症包括：脑脊液耳漏、假性脑膜膨出、脑脊液鼻漏，最终均可导致脑膜炎。但术中通过对硬膜进行水密缝合后，其发生率已明显降低。

三叉神经痛

三叉神经痛（TN）的定义也是来源于临床症状。根据国际头痛学会分类委员会的分类标准，典型TN表现为患者一侧面部三叉神经的一支或多支分布的范围内反复发作的短暂的电击样疼痛，突发突止，并且轻微刺激即可诱发（Headache Classification Committee，2013）。部分患者可表现为持续性面部疼痛，这种类型往往被称为非典型三叉神经痛。无论其临床表现是典型的还是非典型的（原发性），或者继发于神经系统疾病或其他疾病导致的（继发性）。当TN的发病除了神经血管压迫以外没有其他原因时，被称为经典型三叉神经痛，当其发病原因未明时，被称为特发性三叉神经痛。

诊断

- 患病率为7/10 000，年新发病率为5/100 000。
- 对TN的诊断主要靠临床检查。刺激依赖（即触发性疼痛）是TN的必要诊断标准。虽然部分TN患者可表现为轻微的面部感觉异常，特别是患病时间较长者，但绝大部分患者多不存在感觉障碍，对于疾病的正确诊断极为重要。值得注意的是，对于长期存在疼痛的经典型TN因长期合并有面部疼痛（即非典型形式），其阵发性发作的特点可消失或被其他治疗措施所掩盖。一些作者将TN的疼痛类型分为1型疼痛（如刀割样疼痛）和2型疼痛［如持续性疼痛或灼痛（=Burchiel分类）］。这两种疼痛类型可以发生于同一患者身上。但也需排除其他面部疼痛综合征，特别是既往进行治疗后效果不佳或考虑再治疗的患者，如其他治疗后出现的去三叉神经支配型疼痛和SUNCT综合征（伴有结膜充血及流泪的单侧短暂持续性神经痛样头痛）。
- 对抗癫痫药物主要是卡马西平或奥卡西平的反应，是明确诊断的一个重要指标，特别是发病的早期。
- 必要时进行多学科会诊也至关重要，包括口腔科、耳鼻喉科、颌面外科、眼科和神经内科，以排除继发性TN，如有必要将采取针对原发性疾病的专科治疗。事实上，部分继发性TN因其临床表现类似经典型TN而导致误诊的情况在临床上时有发生，特别是一些神经系统疾病，如多发性硬化症或桥小脑角肿瘤更易发生上述情况。
- 三叉神经根部影像学检查是选择治疗方法前必要的检查项目。需要扫描下面三个磁共振高分辨率序列：3D T2加权高分辨率、三维时间飞越法磁共振血流成像（TOF-MRA）、T1增强扫描，由于三者之间良好的互补性，使得采用1.5T的设备即对NVC检查的灵敏度达96.7%，特异度达100%（**图**79.3A~C和**图**79.4A~C）（Leal et al.，2010）。

3D-T2序列可获得三叉神经根部的精细图像。此序列就像进行脑池造影一样可显示不同的组织结构信息，脑脊液显示高信号，桥小脑角的其他结构显示低信号，缺点是血管和神经之间没有信号差别。3D-TOF-MRA序列如果只进行一个预饱和扫描，则只能看到高流量血管（主要是动脉血管）。3D-T1增强扫描序列则可以显示动脉和静脉，因为两者都被造影剂增强。因此同时进行3D-TOF-MRA序列和3D-T1增强扫描序列就可区分静脉和动脉。

如何明确错综复杂的动-静脉血管压迫也至关重要（Matsushima et al.，1983; Dumot and Sindou，2015）。在我们的一组病例中，静脉压迫占比约39%，其中单纯静脉血管压迫约占1/4，合并延长的小脑动脉血管共同压迫的有近3/4（Dumot and Sindou，2015）。压迫静脉可能来源于岩上静脉系统的脑池段（60%），也可能来源于三叉神经根在Meckel腔出口处的脑桥横静脉（40%）。

这种MRI检查方案也可以帮助我们预测血管压迫的程度：单纯接触（Ⅰ级），神经根部轻微变形（Ⅱ级），神经根部明显压痕（Ⅲ级）。在我们的患者中，其准确率可达84.6%（$P<0.01$）（Leal et al.，2010）。

应用3.0T磁共振设备，图像更精细，灵敏度更高：在我们的研究中，其灵敏度可达97.4%，这可用于检测小静脉所导致的NVC（Leal et al.，2011）。

高分辨率磁共振成像还可以准确显示三叉神经根的形态学异常，即整体萎缩、Meckel腔上方岩骨脊成角以及颅后窝的形态异常，如颅底扁平症、Arnold-Chiari畸形、脑池容量小等。

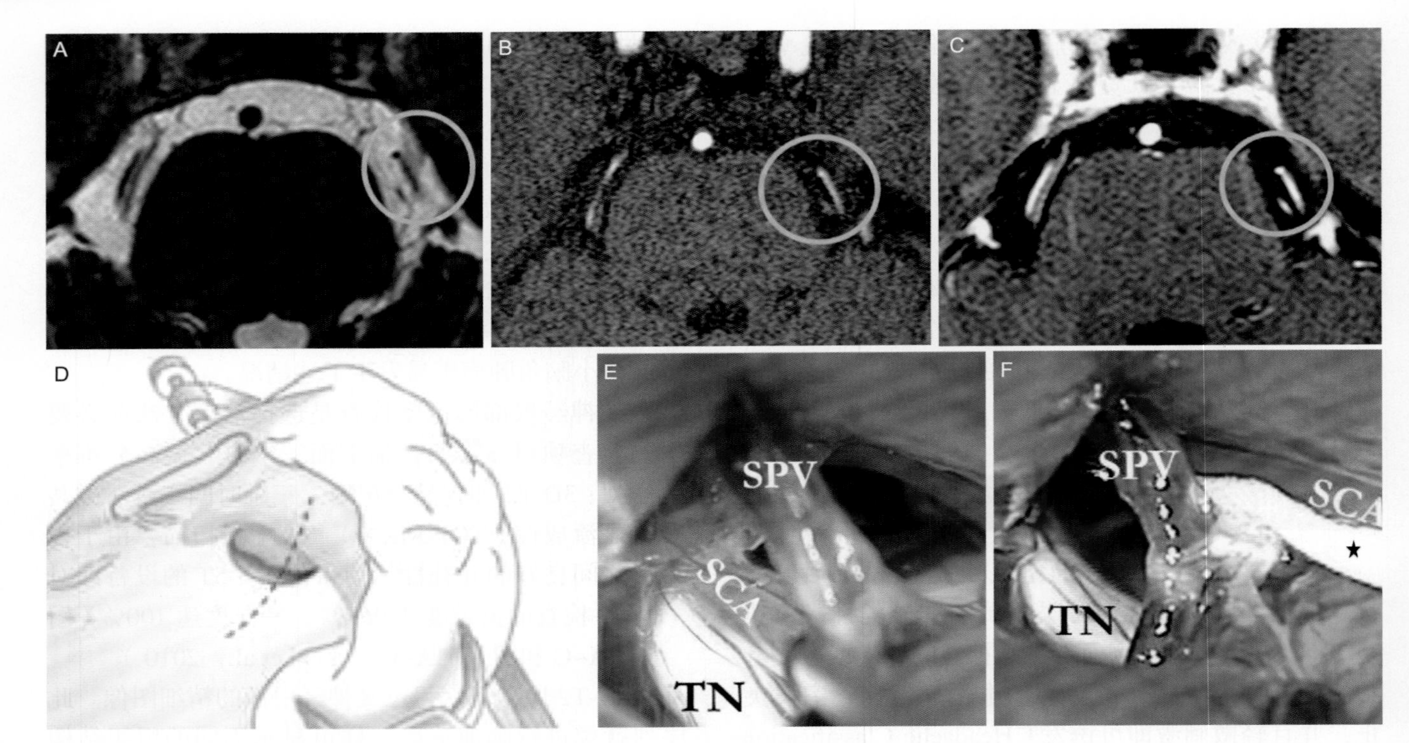

图 79.3 小脑上动脉（SCA）导致的血管压迫（左侧 TN）。（A~C）单纯 SCA 对三叉神经根产生压迫的影像学显示。（A）3D-T2 高分辨率序列显示神经根与压迫血管的走行关系；（B）三维时间飞越法磁共振血流成像（TOF-MRA）；（C）3D-T1 增强扫描。需要注意的是，T2 加权序列中看到的责任血管，在 3D-T1 增强扫描和 TOF-MRA 序列中也均可见，从而得出责任血管是高流量血管（如本例中显示的动脉血管，也即 SCA）的结论。（D~F）经幕下小脑上入路的显微外科入路（左侧）。SCA 粘在了三叉神经根上面（压迫程度二级）（E）；将动脉分离并推移离开神经根部后，用一小块 teflon 垫棉（★）将 SCA 和神经根部隔离出一定距离（F）。TN，三叉神经；SCA，小脑上动脉；SPV，上岩静脉。需注意的是，SPV 及其分支保留完整。还需要注意的是，teflon 垫棉（被 SPV 支撑）不要接触三叉神经根（“无新生压迫”）

解剖学发现及其功能结果

根据文献描述，在大多数原发性 TN 其神经走行区可见 NVC。既往研究显示，NVC 存在率为 76.3%~100%，平均 90.5%。我们根据手术中的所见初步研究显示，97% 的患者在三叉神经根处（TR）存在血管压迫现象（Sindou et al.，2002）。其中 90.70% 的患者为动脉压迫，其余 9.30% 的患者仅有静脉压迫。迂曲延长的责任动脉血管中，SCA 占 88%，AICA 占 25.1%，VBA 占 37.8%。其中，37.8%的患者存在不止一根血管压迫。术中未能识别或处理所有的 NVC，是手术失败或复发的主要原因。

与其他单中心团队研究结果一样（Sindou et al.，2002；Sindou et al.，2007；Dumot and Sindou，2015），仅 50% 的 NVC 位于传统描述的 REZ 区，40%的 NVC 位于神经根部在脑池段走行部分，10% 的患者其 NVC 位于三叉神经的远端即 Meckel 腔区域（图 79.5）。在最后这种类型其责任血管通常是脑桥横静脉，在神经根处有明显的凹陷，呈灰白色，是典型的局灶性脱髓鞘表现。此类患者手术过程中需完全探查整个神经根部即从脑干到 Meckel 腔出口整个区域，方可避免责任血管遗漏。

最近一项对于静脉与三叉神经关系的研究发现，38.7% 的患者存在明确的静脉压迫，有 1/4 的患者为单纯静脉压迫，3/4 的患者常合并有动脉和静脉血管共同压迫（Dumot and Sindou，2015）。

术前高分辨率成像上明确神经血管压迫程度非常重要，它对手术预后起着至关重要的作用。在我们的 Kaplan-Meier 法（KM）生存分析研究中，分别有 49.2% 和 33.2% 的患者显示为Ⅲ级或Ⅱ级血管压迫，术后 15 年的随访结果显示其治愈率仍分别高达 88% 和 79%。相反，17.2% 的患者术前影像显示为Ⅰ级程度压迫，术后其治愈率仅为 65%（Sindou et al.，2007）。血管压迫程度术前可以被可靠预测（在血管压迫程度高的患者中 $P<0.01$），并在进行手术决策时提供参考（Leal et al.，2010）。

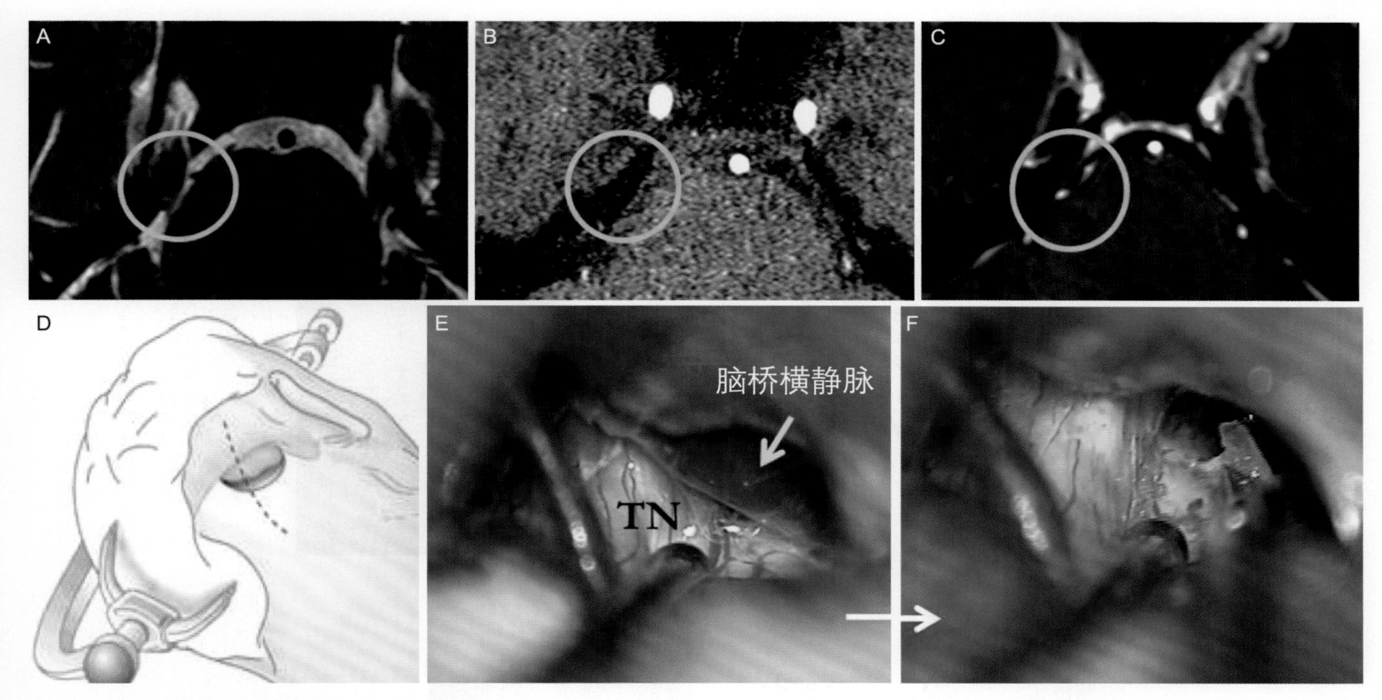

图 79.4　单纯静脉（脑桥横静脉）压迫所引起的 NVC（右侧 TN）。（A~C）神经根自脑桥发出后至 Meckel 腔出口段单纯静脉即横（桥）静脉压迫的影像学显示。高分辨率 T2 轴位视图显示神经根与周围血管交叉（A）。TOF-MRA 序列上不能显示在 T2 序列上所显示的压迫血管，但 T1 增强成像上又可见上述压迫血管，这说明为单纯静脉血管压迫。注意此例患者桥小脑角池的容积较小。（D~F）手术操作经幕下 - 小脑上入路进行（D）。横（桥）静脉（箭头所示）在 Meckel 腔出口处压迫三叉神经根的下侧面（E）。TN，三叉神经。电凝切断压迫静脉和推移垫开压迫静脉方可解除对三叉神经根压迫，达到治愈疗效（F）

三叉神经根或颅后窝解剖结构异常与血管压迫密切相关（Sindou et al.，2002；Sindou et al.，2007；Parise et al.，2010；Parise et al.，2013）。根据我们的观察，42% 的患者 TR 处有明显不同程度的萎缩，即神经轴位横断面直径缩小 1/3~2/3，而不再是圆柱形，这也可证明 TN 可能与神经退行性病变并存。有 18.2% 的 TN 患者表现为蛛网膜增厚，且与三叉神经根部粘连紧密。12.6% 的患者其神经根在穿过岩骨嵴时发生明显的成角现象，尤其是存在小脑萎缩患者，与所谓的三叉神经下垂现象相吻合（Gardner et al.，1956）。3.9% 的患者由于颅后窝狭小，神经根在脑桥和岩骨之间，即“理论上”桥小脑角池内存在 NVC。这些解剖异常情况在术前制订手术入路和术中采取手术决策时应充分考虑。

手术方法及临床疗效

神经外科手术适应证的标准基本包括，第一，排除继发性三叉神经痛，因此类手术需要特殊治疗措施；第二，TN 患者口服药物临床症状不改善或副作用大不能耐受，如全身乏力。

根据患者的具体情况，可以提供多种外科治疗选择，如通过经皮神经毁损术或放射外科技术，也可采用非破坏性的显微血管减压术。

显微血管减压术

1934 年，Dandy 首先观察到 TR 处经常有迂曲延长的动脉血管压迫的现象并将这一发现予以发表，他也是脑桥旁神经根切断术治疗 TN 的先驱者（Dandy，1934）。令人惊讶的是，首位将血管神经分离进行减压操作的人并不是他。Gardner 于 1959 年第一次进行了此项手术（Gardner and Miklos，1959）。其后，Jannetta 于 1967 年通过其发表的相关论文成功对此手术方法进行了推广（Jannetta，1967）。但在其论文中采用的是经颞下小脑幕入路来显露 TR。是 Hardy 首先将这种更容易、更安全的乳突后入路应用于临床（Provost and Hardy，1970）。显微血管减压术（microvascular decompression，MVD）方法随后由 Jannetta 通过发表大量学术论文的方式在世界范围内广泛推广开来（Jannetta，1976）。

MVD 的操作步骤如图 79.6 所示。

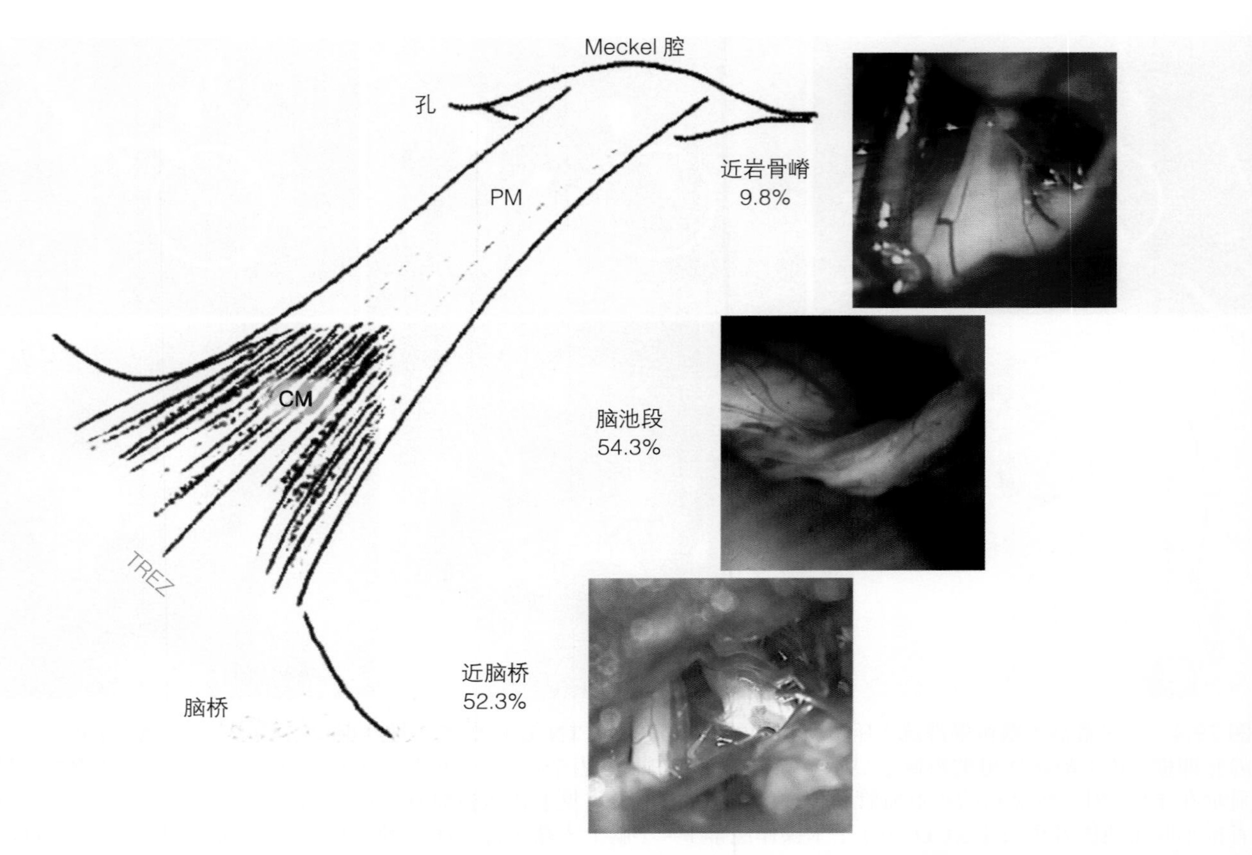

图 79.5 根据三叉神经根 REZ、三叉神经中段（脑池中段）和三叉神经 Meckel 腔出口段（近岩骨嵴）的不同情况，对三叉神经痛患者进行微血管减压术时血管压迫神经（NVC）的情况进行再分类。在 37.8% 的患者中，NVC 可不止一个。CM，中枢髓鞘；PM，外周髓鞘。手术过程中 NVC 视图展示。近脑桥：右侧 NVC 位于三叉神经根入髓区（TREZ）下侧，责任血管为 AICA 血管袢（用显微吸引器向外侧回拉分离），压迫程度Ⅲ级（明显的压痕，呈灰白色局灶脱髓鞘样病变）。脑池段：右侧 NVC 位于三叉神经的中上部，责任血管为 SCA 并向下挤压神经（压迫程度Ⅱ级）。近岩骨嵴：右 NVC 位于 Meckel 腔入口处下方，压迫血管来源于脑桥横静脉，压迫程度Ⅲ级。注意标记的灰色区域为局灶性脱髓鞘病变

在同一患者中，责任血管可能不止一根，这类患者占所有 TN 患者的 1/3（Sindou et al.，2002）。为避免责任血管遗漏，必须探查从脑干的 REZ 到 Meckel 腔之间的全部神经走行区域，并游离所有蛛网膜粘连。插入的 Teflon 垫棉主要是为了保持血管神经不再产生压迫，而需要将血管推移远离神经根部，但也要避免产生“新的压迫”损伤（**图** 79.3D~F 和图 79.4D~F）（Sindou et al.，2008）。

文献结果总结于**表** 79.1 中。一系列术后平均随访时间不少于 5 年的研究结果和 KM 生存分析均显示 MVD 手术可达到很高的疼痛缓解率（Tatli et al.，2008）。在 Jannetta 对 1185 名患者施行的 MVD 手术中，术后 10 年仍有 70% 的患者可获得优秀的疗效（Barker et al.，1996）。在我们的一组纳入 1800 名患者的研究中，且对前 362 名患者进行了 KM 生存分析，治愈率为 74%（即术后 15 年随访时仍无疼痛且无药物辅助治疗）；值得注意的是，非典型病例和典型病例术后其临床疗效均同样令人满意（Sindou et al.，2006）。

手术中发现明确的责任血管压迫（Ⅱ级或Ⅲ级）与术后治愈率有明确的相关性，在其术后 15 年时随访发现二者治愈率分别为 79% 和 88%。相反，当血管神经处于简单接触状态（Ⅰ级）时，长期缓解率仅为 65%（P=0.001）（Sindou et al.，2007）。更为重要的是，术前可以通过高可靠性的影像学检查来预测血管神经压迫程度（P<0.01）（Leal et al.，2010）。

MVD 的优势是它对神经功能保留的特性以及在发现明确有 NVC 存在时术后长期缓解率高。缺点是开颅手术的相应风险。

图 79.7 展示了对 TN 患者提供的治疗建议。

三叉神经射频热凝术

经皮三叉神经射频热凝术（radiofrequency thermorhizotomy，RF-ThRh）（**图** 79.8）是由 Sweet 详

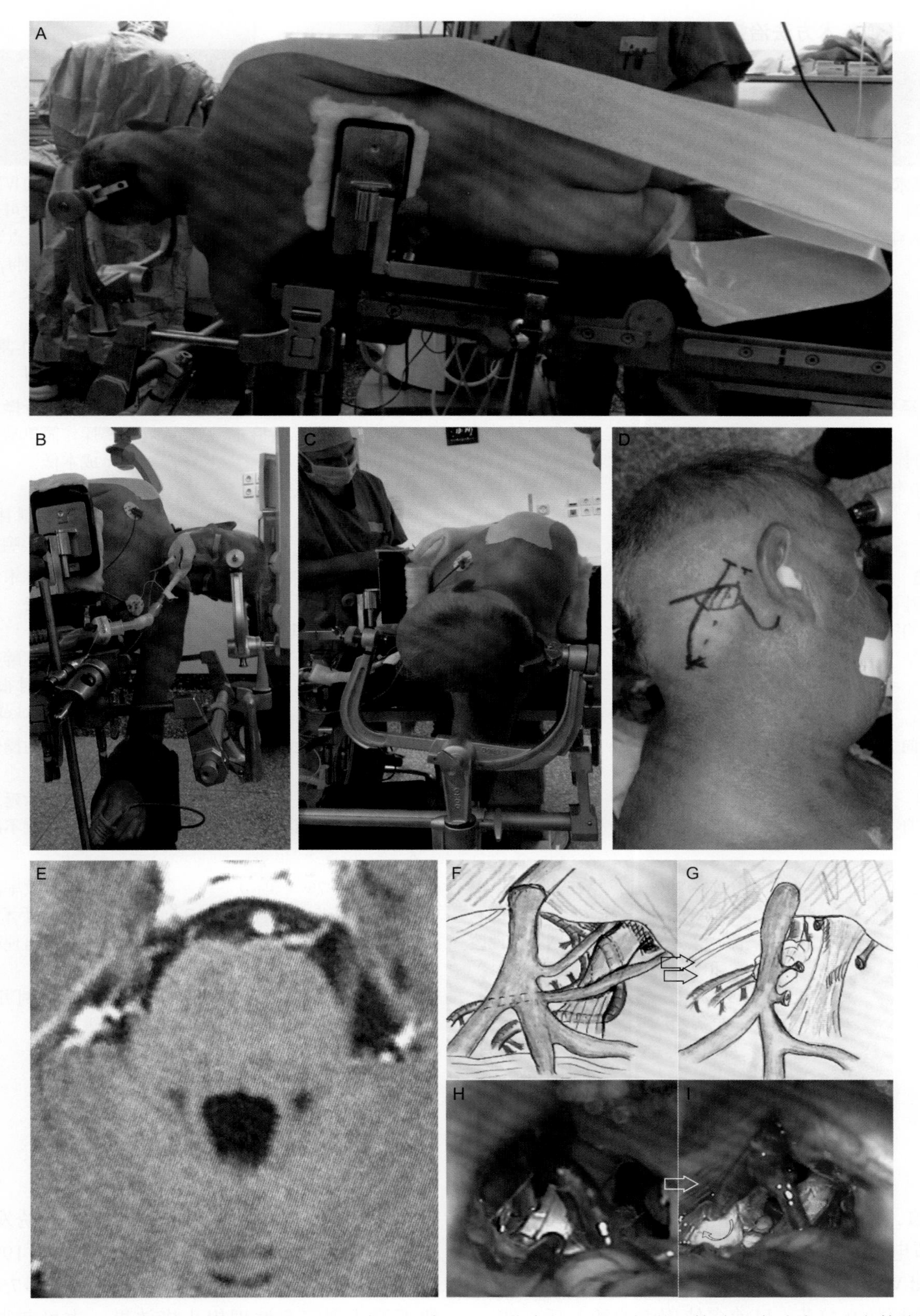

图 79.6　患者为右侧三叉神经痛，动脉（SCA）合并静脉（SPV 分支）压迫而行微血管减压术治疗。患者体位、手术入路和外科操作展示。（A）侧卧位，肩部适度牵引。手术床呈轻微头高脚低位，以降低头部静脉压。（B~D）注意颈部 / 头部向对侧偏转 15°（B），头部向对侧旋转 15°（C），枕骨嵴 / 横窦下方和乳突后部 / 乙状窦外侧为颅骨切开范围标志（阴影区）（D）。皮肤切口位于项线和乳突后部形成的角平分线内侧 1 cm 处。（E~I）磁共振 T1 增强序列显示 SCA 血管袢压迫于三叉神经腹内侧和来自于 SPV 系统的静脉分支压迫于三叉神经背外侧。插图（F、G）和手术照片（H、I）显示微血管减压术前后的三叉神经根。星号，SCA 血管袢；V，责任静脉为 SPV 的分支

表 79.1 各种手术方法治疗三叉神经痛的结果汇总（文献数据）

	即刻疼痛缓解：范围（平均值）	长期疼痛缓解：范围（平均值）	手术失败和神经痛复发率；死亡率	副作用 / 并发症范围（均值） T= 暂时性，P= 永久性	优势与劣势
射频热凝术 *n*=7483 例 FU: 3~26 年 （9 年）	81%~99% （94%） 取决于射频热凝强度和术后感觉障碍程度	20%~93% （60.4%）	39.6% （+）：颈动脉损伤，0.1%	• 麻木（P）：5%~98% • 咬肌功能障碍（T）：4%~24% • 角膜感觉减退（P）：5%~18%（12%） • 角膜炎：1%~8%（5%） • 滑车神经麻痹（T）：1%~2%（1%） • 感觉缺失（P）：0.8%~7%（3%）	• 短暂性的Ⅳ级麻醉 • 治疗部位可选择 • 若“扳机点”出现感觉减退则疗效持续时间较长 *vs*. • 手术操作复杂，需专业练习
甘油神经毁损 *n*=1310 例 FU: 1~10 年 （6.5 年）	42%~84% （68%）	18%~59% （38.5%）	61.5% （+）：无死亡报告	• 带状疱疹暴发：50% • 脑膜反应：经常性麻木 ± 感觉减退（P）：30% • 角膜感觉减退（P）：15% • 角膜炎：5%	• 局麻进行操作 • 操作简单易行 • 成本低 *vs*. • 不能控制甘油弥散区域，影响疗效
球囊压迫 *n*=1404 例 FU: 1~6 年 （4 年）	82~100% （96%）	54.5%~91.3% （67%）	33% （+）：颈动脉损伤，0.2%	• 面部麻木（±T）：39% • 咬肌功能障碍（±T）：66% • 翼腭窝血肿：偶尔可见	• 无严重麻木 • 无角膜炎 *vs*. • 需全身麻醉 • 球囊有时很难精准植入 Meckel 腔
立体定向放射外科 *n*=310 例 FU: 2~7 年 （5 年）		21.8%~88.9% （54%）（仍口服药物的患者人数）	46% （+）：无死亡报告	• 三叉神经分布区感觉减退 0~54%（32%） • 角膜感觉缺失：无 • 三叉神经支配区运动功能障碍：无	• 无侵入性操作 *vs*. • 疗效显示延迟 • 长期疗效不确定
微血管减压术 *n*=5122 例 FU: 5~15 年 （7 年）	80%~98% （91.8%）	62%~89% （76.5%） 高等级压迫（Ⅱ～Ⅲ级）：90%， 低等级压迫（Ⅰ级）：65%	23.4%［手术探查引起的蛛网膜炎性改变（*P*=0.04）］ （+）：死亡率为 0~1.2%（0.3%）源自小脑梗死	• 麻木：2%~7%（3%） • 听力障碍 / 步态障碍（P）：2.5% • 面神经麻痹（P）：0~2%（1%） • 滑车神经麻痹（T）：0~5%（1%） • 感觉缺失（P）：1%~3%（1.5%） • 小脑梗死：1% • 脑脊液漏（T）：2%~17%（4%）	• 长期有效率高 • “锁孔”手术 • 副作用出现率低 *vs*. • 部分病例可出现严重并发症

细阐述的，它是 Kirschner 在 1933 年首创的三叉神经半月节电凝术的一种改良形式（Kirschner，1933；Sweet and Wepsic，1974）。当进行射频治疗时需要在推注短效静脉麻醉药（目前多使用丙泊酚）后完成，必要时可重复使用。电极针在透视下采用 Hartel 路径穿过卵圆孔，到达三叉神经半月节后半部分，即三角丛，在这里走行着对应不同三叉神经分支的躯体感觉纤维。在 X 线和神经电生理学指导下，电极末端裸露部分（5 mm ± 2 mm）应放置在对应于不同疼痛区域的纤维中，后者是基于电刺激诱发的感觉异常和产生的肌肉反应明确的（Sindou，1999；Tatli and Sindou，2008）。射频热凝温度在 65~75 ℃，即便不能达到完全性理想止痛效果，也可获得较优秀的临床疗效。射频热凝毁损位置不要直接位于神经节本身，而应位于三角丛水平的远侧即三叉神经半月节后半部分，这样可以降低直接破坏半月节的 T 细胞而发生营养性溃疡的风险（Sindou and Keravel，1979）。患者术后要获得明显的感觉减退而又不丧失

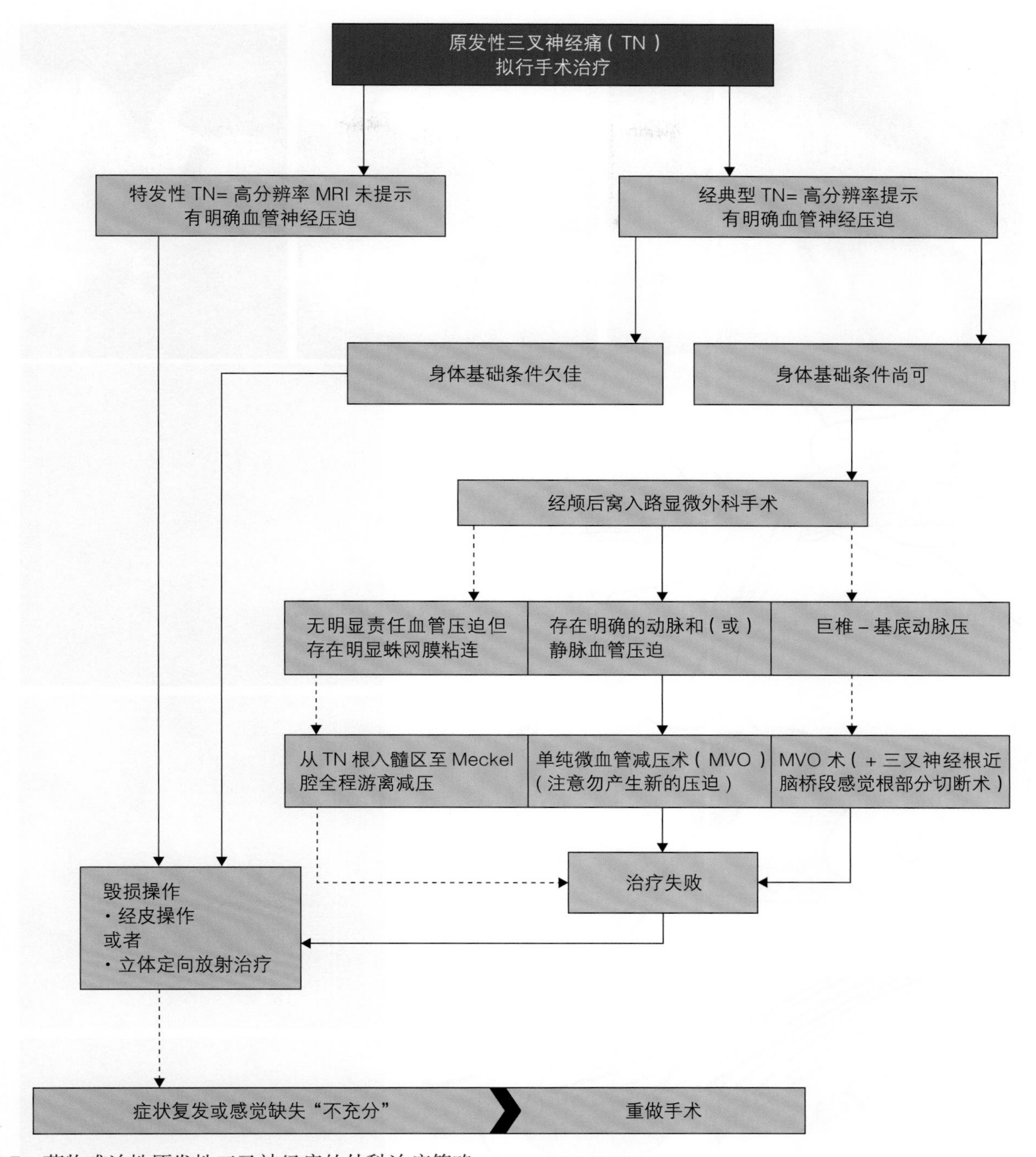

图 79.7　药物难治性原发性三叉神经痛的外科治疗策略

所支配区域重要的触觉，术中就需要精确地放置电极位置并进行逐渐毁损，虽费时费力但至关重要。

相关文献结果总结于**表** 79.1 中。在所有已刊发的报道研究中，临床疗效的持续时间与术中诱发的感觉减退的程度成正比（Sindou and Keravel，1979）。在我们的研究中，术后随访 5~25 年的复发率为 7%，缺点是 95% 的患者在原有疼痛区域存在明显的感觉减退。然而，约 98% 的患者对由此产生的麻木都有良好的耐受性，剩余 2% 的患者患有失能性感觉障碍（Sindou and Tatli，2009）。

RF-ThRh 的优势是可以根据患者的疼痛范围而选择治疗部位。缺点是难以精确做到目标神经纤维并达到最佳的感觉减退程度。如果热凝毁损过度，可能会加重原有非典型 TN 的疼痛程度，也可能会产生角膜炎。

RF-ThRh 特别适用于一般情况不佳的典型 TN 患者或继发于多发性硬化症 TN 患者（Kanpolat et al.，2001）。也可适用于发作性和（或）异常疼痛类型为

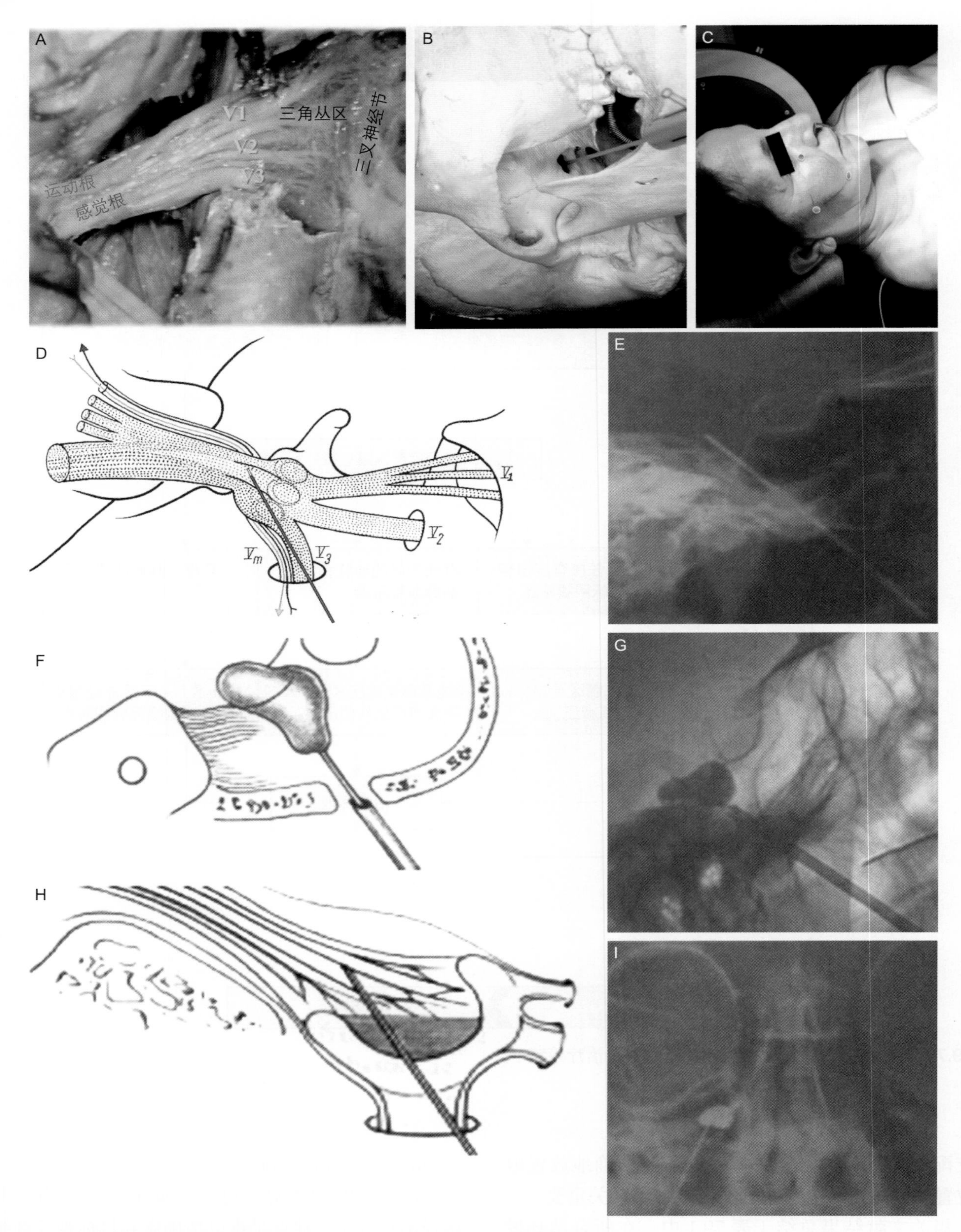

图 79.8 经皮穿刺技术治疗三叉神经痛（A~C）采用 Hartel 路径穿刺卵圆孔到达三叉神经半月节的颅骨标志和穿刺路径（右侧 TN）。电极针的入点位于口角旁 30 mm 处或双侧口角连线中点旁 60 mm 处。卵圆孔的定位标准是（i）侧位：在外耳道前壁（耳屏）的前方 35 mm；（ii）前后位：瞳孔的内侧边缘；（iii）通过 X 射线透视将电极针的深度导送至三角丛区（Tatli et al., 2008）。为获得准确的卵圆孔位置（如斜坡线和上岩嵴的交点），手术应在透视下进行（Tatli et al., 2008）。错误的（危险的）穿刺路径是（由后向前）：颈静脉孔、岩骨下颈动脉、破裂孔处颈动脉、通过眶下裂到达眶尖，或者通过眶上裂到达颈动脉旁组织

主要表现的继发性 TN 患者。

三叉神经半月节球囊压迫术

Mullan 在 20 世纪 80 年代引入经皮球囊压迫术（**图 79.8**）（Mullan and Lichtor，1983）。手术是在全身麻醉下进行，气管插管和 X 线引导下将 4 号 Fogarty 导管穿入卵圆孔。球囊处于 Meckel 腔壁内，并用甲泛葡胺充气的梨形球囊形状验证其位置的准确性。根据不同操作者经验，压迫时间维持约 5 分钟 ±2 分钟。压迫过程中可能会发生心动过缓。

文献结果分析见**表** 79.1。这种手术方法副作用很少，但咀嚼功能障碍（通常是短暂）发生率比较高。感觉减退特别是角膜感觉减退通常较轻微（Keravel et al.，2009）。

缺点是不能根据患者的疼痛部位进行精准治疗和相对较高的复发率。由于角膜炎的发病率低，此治疗方式主要适用于各种类型，特别是累及 V1 支的 TN 患者。

三叉神经半月节甘油注射阻滞术

经皮三叉神经半月节甘油注射毁损术（**图** 79.8），由 Håkanson 于 20 世纪 80 年代首先进行描述并推广开来，包括在 Meckel 腔三叉神经池内的脑脊液中注射甘油（Håkanson，1981）。手术在局部麻醉下进行，并在甲泛葡胺透视辅助下以便准确放置到神经池中。该技术操作简单，但需控制注射的甘油在三叉神经池内，若甘油外漏扩散则会产生严重并发症。

有关经皮三叉神经半月节甘油注射毁损术的文献结果见**表** 79.1。常见的副作用是带状疱疹、感觉异常和角膜炎（Tatli et al.，2008）。

由于其成本低廉，该方法在世界各地得到广泛应用。它的缺点是除了因其神经毒性而产生的潜在并发症外，疼痛控制范围和长期疗效方面缺乏可预测性。

立体定向放射外科治疗

Leksell 早在 20 世纪 70 年代就提出了立体定向放射外科（SRS）治疗 TN 的概念（Leksell，1971）。但直到磁共振成像技术的发展使得目标的精确定位成为可能后，这种方法才在最近十年流行起来。单次辐照剂量为 70~90 Gy，可以覆盖等中心距离为 4 mm 的范围。根据 Régis 团队的建议，为减少脑干照射，辐照靶点应位于 TR 的半月神经节后脑池段，即从三叉神经出脑干处至 Meckel 腔方向 7.5 mm 处，而不是三叉神经根入髓区（TREZ）（Régis et al.，2009）（**图** 79.9）。

有关立体定向放射外科治疗文献结果见**表** 79.1。文献报告的结果差别很大，可能是由于放射治疗的靶点和剂量不同所致。此外，不同作者对疼痛缓解的评估标准也不尽相同，在一些文献中，尽管患者术后仍需继续服药，但仍被归类为满意组。文献结果显示，有 0~54% 的患者术后会出现感觉迟钝并伴有麻木和感觉异常。虽然有些学者对此抱有争议，

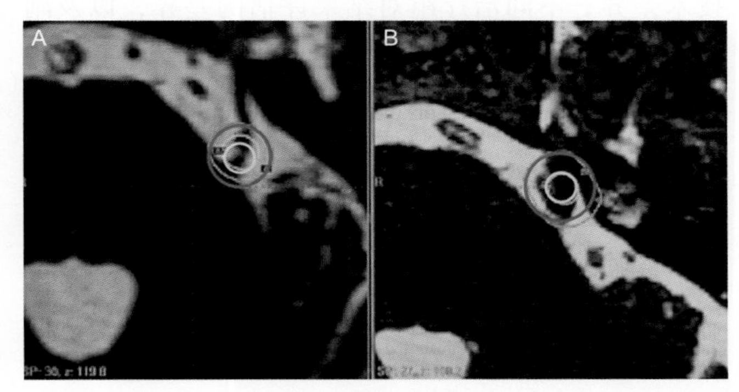

图 79.9 立体定向放射外科（SRS）靶点定位：该图显示了两个目前最常采用的在高分辨率 T2 序列上的治疗靶点。（A）治疗靶点为 TREZ；（B）治疗靶点为脑池段 TR。后者因治疗靶点远离脑干，故危险性较低，并发症发生率低。黄色圆圈代表 80 Gy 等剂量曲线；红色圆圈代表 30 Gy 等剂量曲线

图 79.8 （续）（D~E）射频热凝三叉神经毁损术的示意图和 X 线对照（侧位片）。注意三叉神经 V1 分支位于上内侧，V3 分支位于下外侧，而 V2 分支位于二者之间。电极的末端裸露部分应根据“扳机点”部位和疼痛区域而采取个体化定位。在患者清醒时，通过电刺激神经根引起感觉异常和（或）在相应的面部肌肉中触发三叉神经面部反射（尤其是眨眼反射），从而引导定位（Sindou 1999）。然后在短时全身麻醉提供镇痛（针刺测试）的前提下进行热凝治疗，此时，保持皮肤和黏膜的触觉尚未完全丧失和角膜反射未明显降低（棉棒接触测试）。（F~G）：三叉神经半月节和三叉神经丛的球囊压迫示意图和 X 线对照（侧位图）。注意膨胀起来的“梨”型球囊形状，这证明压迫部位为 Meckel 腔和三叉神经池，是理想的压迫部位。（H~I）：三叉神经池甘油注射示意图及 X 线对照（前后位）。手术过程中需要注意：碘造影剂应确保针头位于三叉神经池内；在患者清醒时注射甘油溶液

但却普遍认为疼痛能否缓解及持续时间取决于是否存在感觉减退及其程度（P=0.02）（Pollock，2006；Régis et al.，2016）。因此，Pollock 认为应当把 SRS 治疗 TN 技术归类为毁损效应组。

SRS 的优点是侵袭性小和并发症发生率低。缺点是疗效显现慢，一般多为术后几个月方可见疗效。然而，除那些难以忍受当下剧烈疼痛而积极救治的患者，大多数患者均能接受这种不足。

治疗策略

高分辨率 MRI 检查对于制订治疗策略具有极其重要的作用，因为它提供了必需的解剖学依据，从而能选择最合适的治疗方法。普遍的共识是，当患者情况良好时，MVD 可以作为首选治疗方法。经皮毁损技术或立体定向放射治疗技术对于影像上不能明确显示存在 NVC 的患者最有帮助，或者当患者身体状态一般时，它们也是有效的治疗手段。

鉴于已发表的一系列文献有着不同的侧重点，故难以明确各种神经外科方法治疗 TN 的优劣。原因是：不同团队对 TN 患者的选择标准不同；手术操作技术差异；不同治疗组对结果评估的差异，以及副作用和并发症的评估标准不同；较少有研究采用 KM 方法对患者长期疗效进行分析。

迷走－舌咽神经神经痛

舌咽神经痛更应该被称为迷走-舌咽神经痛（vagoglossopharyngeal neuralgia，VGPN），因为疼痛范围不仅覆盖于第Ⅸ对脑神经（CN Ⅸ）支配的感觉区域，而且还扩展到迷走神经（CN Ⅹ）支配的范围。VGPN 的发病率是 TN 的 1%。其定义也是来源于临床症状。VGPN 是指在咽后部、扁桃体窝、舌根、外耳道深部、下颌角下方发生的阵发性的、短暂的、剧烈的疼痛，通常持续几秒到几分钟，通常由吞咽、进食、咀嚼、咳嗽、打哈欠、说话等诱发（Headache Classification Committee，2013）。VGPN 有时也可能伴有心血管病症状，特别是晕厥（Chen and Sindou，2015）和特殊类型的消化系统症状（Anthérieu et al.，2016）。

病因学和病理生理学

VGPN 可以是继发性的，由于颅外或颅内肿瘤，或各种其他特定的病变。在过去的十年中，原发性 VGPN 和 TN 一样被命名为经典型 VGPN，最常见原因是 CN Ⅸ和Ⅹ受动脉血管压迫所致，但其压迫点并不总在 REZ。像 TN 一样，高分辨率 MRI 对压迫血管具有较高的灵敏度和特异性（Kawashima et al.，2010；Leal et al.，2010）。

诊断

VGPN 的诊断是基于疼痛的特征。临床检查并未发现任何明显的神经功能障碍。耳鼻喉科检查和 MRI 可排除颅外或颅内肿瘤、血管病变、Chiari 畸形等病变。在大多数典型 VGPN 患者中，高分辨率 MRI 显示压迫血管多为迂曲延长的动脉血管，一般为 PICA 和（或）VBA。

手术治疗

像 TN 患者一样，当以抗癫痫药物为基础的药物治疗症状改善不佳或不能耐受时，则应考虑手术治疗。在颈静脉孔进行经皮 RF-ThRh 不适用于原发性 VGPN，因为其造成 CN Ⅸ和Ⅹ运动功能受损的风险很高（Lazorthes and Verdie，1979；Tew et al.，1982）。需要指出的是，RF-ThRH 可应用于肿瘤源性疼痛患者。立体定向放射外科（SRS）最近取得的一些成果备受鼓舞（Dhople et al.，2009；Leveque et al.，2011）。对于经典的 VGPN，因为 MVD 的有效性和“功能保留”特征，应该作为首选治疗方法（Laha and Jannetta，1977；Chen and Sindou，2015）。

手术入路是在乳突尖后和髁突后的锁孔型开口颅骨切开术，沿着小脑扁桃体后 - 小脑绒球下方入路进入小脑延髓裂相关组织结构。这样的入路方式可以避免牵拉 CN Ⅷ及其相关并发症（**图** 79.10）。压迫血管，一般为 PICA 和（或）VBA，位于延髓和脑桥分界处 CN Ⅸ和Ⅹ REZ 的腹侧。此处蛛网膜常常增厚并黏附于神经根上，为了彻底有效减压，需将其广泛剪开并分离。

结果

文献结果已在其他论文资料中进行了回顾和详细分析（Chen and Sindou，2015）。简要地说，这篇综述包括了 28 篇文献，共 515 例患者，对数据资料进行统计显示 VGPN 行 MVD 术后的疼痛完全缓解率在 50%~100%，且副作用或并发症的发生率在可接受范围内。在我们组纳入的 36 例 VGPN 患者中，随访时间超过 2 年，94.4% 的患者疼痛获得完全缓解，无死亡病例、无一般并发症、无伤口感染报告。两例患者出现一定程度的神经功能障碍（永久性的），包括发音困难和吞咽困难。

最近的文献报告显示，MVD 是治疗原发性

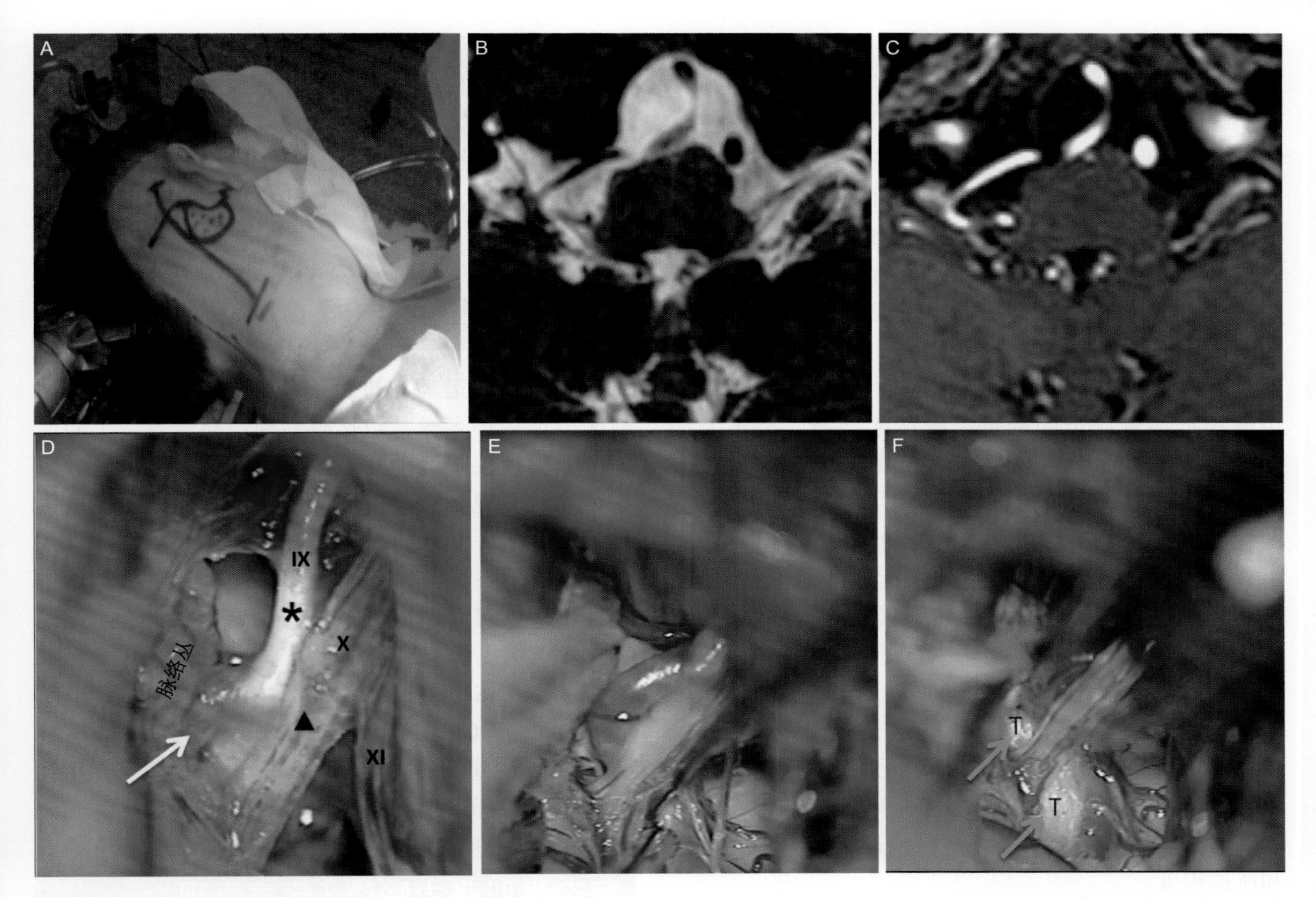

图 79.10　高分辨率 MRI-T2（B）和 T1 增强成像序列（C）显示，VGPN 患者（右侧）NVC 责任血管为右侧小脑后下动脉（PICA）。显微外科手术取右侧小脑绒球下入路，锁孔（乳突后、髁突后、乙状窦后）入路行迷走神经和舌咽神经微血管减压术的标志（A）。责任血管 PICA 位于 CN Ⅸ（＊）和 CN Ⅹ（▲）REZ 区腹侧。注意 CN Ⅸ和 CN Ⅹ的神经根存在萎缩和灰白色病变，表明为局灶性脱髓鞘改变（D）。当将粘连于神经血管周围的蛛网膜剪断并分离后，责任血管 PICA（黄色箭头）即可达到游离状态（E）。将 teflon 棉（T 标志）制作呈束状后放置于 CN Ⅸ和 CN Ⅹ的 REZ 与责任血管之间，避免二者再次接触

VGPN 的一种有效且相对安全的方法。SRS 有希望被纳入备选治疗方案，但仍需要更多的长期评估结果。经皮 RF-ThRh 可作为一项保留治疗方式，主要针对于已经有神经功能缺陷的肿瘤性疼痛患者的治疗。

耳鸣和眩晕

耳鸣

耳鸣是一种常见的症状，主要是由于内耳、外周或中枢神经系统损害后听觉传入障碍，导致中枢听觉结构的神经元过度活跃和（或）功能重塑（Møller，2007；Londero et al.，2009）。血管压迫起源的机制仍存有争议；在无症状患者中，小脑动脉血管袢与位于 CPA 池或内听道处的 CN Ⅷ关系密切也很常见。然而，在极特殊情况下，患有单侧耳鸣且不能耐受的患者，除了图像显示存在明确的 NVC 外，没有其他明确的原因，可考虑针对 CN Ⅷ行 MVD 术（De Ridder et al.，2012；Mathiesen and Brantberg，2015）。

治疗标准均是源于解剖学的依据：① MRI 图像上存在清晰的动脉血管袢压迫于 CN Ⅷ的 REZ 区、脑池段或内听道内处，导致神经走行出现扭曲变形；②神经电生理学脑干听觉诱发电位（BAEP）记录中峰值Ⅲ和Ⅴ的潜伏期增加。同侧前庭反射减弱也可以作为一个参考依据。

与此有关的文献报道很少，且结果一致性较差。尽管对患者的手术适应证已进行严格的筛选，但手术结果仍充满不确定性，特别是术前耳鸣症状已经持续较长时间的患者。

眩晕

在各种常见的前庭疾病中，要明确由 NVC 引起的阵发性前庭功能障碍性眩晕是相对困难的（Tilikete and Vighetto，2009）。根据 Hüfner 的统计资料显示，发病率约为 4%（Hüfner et al.，2008）。Jannetta 和 Møller 的研究认为，“致残性位置性眩晕”是该发病病因中最让人印象深刻的临床表现（Jannetta et al.，1984；Møller et al.，1986）。

当缺乏相关听觉症状和体征检查资料时，很难单纯根据血管压迫的证据准确诊断该病。事实上，在许多无症状患者中常可见到 CN Ⅷ与周围血管袢密切接触的现象。与听觉症状不同，前庭检查中发现的迷路内或迷路后病理形态异常资料既不具体也不可靠。在眼动记录中，眼震的快速成分无论是自发性的还是体位性的，均可指向受累侧或正常侧，分别代表前庭系统兴奋性过高或过低。此原理也同样适用于前庭功能检查的冷热水试验，试验中反应减弱或增强取决于受影响的前庭系统是低兴奋还是高兴奋。因此，在听觉检查中若缺乏明显的单侧检查异常，即 BEAP 记录中Ⅲ和Ⅴ的潜伏期增加，不能仅依靠前庭检查结果诊断该病，或确定 NVC 的部位和压迫程度。

无论进行何种的外科手术，其对象都应该是丧失生活能力的眩晕患者，即美国耳鼻喉头颈外科学会听力和平衡委员会颁布的功能量表上评分达到 5~6 级的患者（Committee on Hearing and Equilibrium guidelines for the diagnosis and evaluation of therapy in Menière's disease，1995）。当有足够的证据支持血管压迫时，考虑 MVD 具有功能保留的特性，仍被推荐为最好的治疗方法（Hüfner et al.，2008）。责任血管可能为 AICA 或 PICA，并在 REZ 处产生压迫，也可能为 AICA 的血管袢在 CN Ⅷ脑池段或邻近内听道处产生压迫。只有当纯音测听小于 50 dB，声音阈值低于 50% 时（美国耳鼻喉和头颈外科学会分类 C~D 级），且考虑保留听力功能对患者无明显意义时，方可考虑行损害性操作如前庭神经切断术（Møller et al.，1986；Committee on Hearing and Equilibrium guidelines for the diagnosis and evaluation of therapy in Menière's disease 1995；Lacombe，2009）。当然，在做手术前必须先明确对侧听觉功能。

在已发表的文献资料中，根据 Møller 和 Ryu 对一系列患者的临床资料统计显示，对眩晕患者的 CN Ⅷ进行 MVD 治疗后至少 3/4 有效（Møller et al.，1993；Ryu et al.，1998）。然而这些报告也有不足之处，即对此类患者与听觉和前庭功能有关的试验未进行系统地评估。此外，也缺乏相关功能测试。在这两组报告中，致残性并发症均罕有发生。在所有接受手术的患者中，报告显示只有 2% 的人会完全丧失听力。但是，大多数患者的听力都有一定程度的下降。

动眼神经综合征

神经源性运动亢进可引起眼外肌阵发性痉挛，临床表现多种多样，包括眼周神经肌强直、上斜肌阵挛、病理性眼运动联带运动、周期性痉挛等，且均可导致复视。病理生理学也各不相同，可能由多种疾病引起（Vighetto and Tilikete，2009）。其作用机制仍不清楚，常常涉及受累核团神经元活性的中枢性重建。然而，据文献报道，只有极少量明显的特发性病例显示与神经血管压迫有关（CN Ⅳ 3 例和 CNⅢ 1 例）（Samii et al.，1998；Mikami et al.，2005；Inoue et al.，2012；Fam et al.，2014）。

值得注意的是，其他几例报告为 NVC 并经 MVD 治疗的病例实际上是动脉瘤引起的神经麻痹。

复杂性肌张力障碍 / 疼痛表现

偶尔会有患者出现复杂的面部肌张力异常 / 疼痛表现，其发病机制不清，可能与心理机制调节异常有关。如术前影像数据中可明确存在 NVC，则可考虑行 MVD 治疗。我们组曾治疗过一位这样的病例：患者为女性，单侧咀嚼肌和面部肌肉的张力异常发作，表现极为痛苦，伴有不自主眼活动异常，时有跌倒。当给予患者进行 MVD 时将深嵌于脑桥延髓沟内的 AICA 血管袢推移离开后，患者症状完全缓解。

神经源性高血压

在所有假定的原发性高血压（hypertension，HT）的发病原因中，存在着这样一种机制：延髓腹外侧（VL）由于血管压迫而引起的神经源性功能障碍。虽然这种机制导致的 HT 患者数量巨大，但自从 Jannetta 及其团队在 20 世纪 70 年代末将这一假说应用于人类以来，无论是对狒狒动物试验或临床结果的研究均罕有报道（Jannetta and Gendell，1979；Jannetta et al.，1985；Geiger et al.，1998；Levy et al.，2001；Naraghi et al.，2001）。

外科手术数据

Jannetta 和 Gendell 在他们的第一份临床报告中观察到，TN 或 HFS 患者左侧延髓 VL 区存在着较高比例的神经血管压迫现象，且这些患者均存在高血压并发症（Jannetta and Gendell，1979）。值得注意的是，传递来自（左）心房压力感受器信号的舌咽神经和迷走神经复合体主要位于机体的左侧，而此类患者的血管压迫部位也多位于左侧延髓 VL 区，二者理论基本一致。

自此以后，仅有两项外科研究数据发表：一项是由 Jannetta 等对 53 例患者进行的回顾性研究，另一项是由 Geiger 等对 36 例患者进行的前瞻性研究（Jannetta et al.，1985; Geiger et al.，1998）。在这两组患者中，MVD 对药物控制不佳的 HT 患者的有效率分别为 84% 和 80%。

我们在此领域也进行了一项前瞻性研究，在 48 名合并有明显原发性高血压的 HFS 患者中，除了在面神经 REZ 区进行 MVD 外，在舌咽神经和迷走神经的 REZ 以及邻近的延髓 VL 区进行 MVD 手术，以期观察对患者血压（blood pressure，BP）的影响（Sindou et al.，2015）。在所有患者中，除 1 例患者外，所有入组患者的 HT 至少为 WHO Ⅰ级，其中 18 例尽管给予正规治疗仍为不稳定型，且在 MVD 手术中，CN Ⅸ和Ⅹ的 REZ 及邻近的延髓 VL 区均可观察到存在血管压迫现象。MVD 后进行末次随访时（2~16 年，平均 7 年），28 例患者 BP 恢复正常，其中 14 例患者无需任何降压治疗（$P<0.0001$）。同时，在 18 例 MVD 术前血压不稳定的患者中，在末次随访时只有 8 例患者仍存在血压不稳定（$P<0.02$）。这些研究结果间接证明了 MVD 治疗原发性难治性 HT 的有效性（**图 79.11**）。在侧别方面，30 例患者为左侧存在血管压迫，其中 17 例患者术后血压正常（11 例患者术后不需用药）；18 例患者为右侧存在血管压迫，其中 11 例患者术后血压正常（3 例患者不需要用药），但二者无统计学差异。

HT 的 MRI 表现

由于并非所有药物治疗无效的原发性 HT 患者在接受手术后均可获得良好的疗效，因此患者的选择应基于 MRI 检查结果，以此提供足够的可靠性依据。大多数文献报道显示，相较于正常血压组患者，MRI 影像上原发性 HT 患者在延髓 VL 区存在血管接触/压迫（vc/c）的概率明显增高（Sindou，2015）。左侧 vc/c 的发生率高于右侧 vc/c。然而，在上述前瞻性研究中未显示出有统计学差异（$P=0.178$），在回顾性研究中显示有统计学差异（$P=0.001$）。

但单纯依靠 MRI 影像信息很难区分延髓 VL 区和舌咽神经至迷走神经的 REZ 区存在动脉血管袢是血压升高的原因或是结果。通过对典型的原发性 HT 和继发性 HT 患者的 MRI 影像资料进行对比，后者（继发性 HT）在脑干处存在 NVC 比率低于原发性 HT 组，但二者无统计学意义。

讨论和结论

有观点认为在 CN Ⅸ至 CN Ⅹ的 REZ 水平及延髓 VL 区存在血管压迫，即可考虑将 MVD 作为可能来源于神经性 HT 的有效治疗方法，此观点似乎很有说服力，但仍需进一步验证（Sindou，2015）。尽管部分患者 MRI 影像显示存在巨大动脉血管压迫脑干的信息，仍需对患者做进一步筛查，而这一措施至关重要。对于那些尽管已经进行规律治疗，但血压仍然很高，且不稳定，而又有生命危险的患者，方可考虑进行减压手术。

全文总结——尾声

近几十年来，在众多的由血管压迫造成的脑神经疾病的鉴别和治疗方面取得了重要的进展，并明确其发病原因为兴奋性增高继而出现功能障碍。

在临床中必须严格把控微血管减压术（MVD）的指征，神经生理学检查和近来高速发展的高分辨率成像技术可为手术的成功施行提供很多有益的依据。

然而，并不是所有患者在接受手术后均可治愈。不可否认，在所有类型患者中，有部分患者的发病原因可能是由多因素机制引起的（如部分患者可能有或多或少的心理原因参与其中），其具体机制仍不清楚。为了更好地了解疾病相关机制，对患者的准确选择和提高手术的有效性和安全性，仍有大量工作要做。

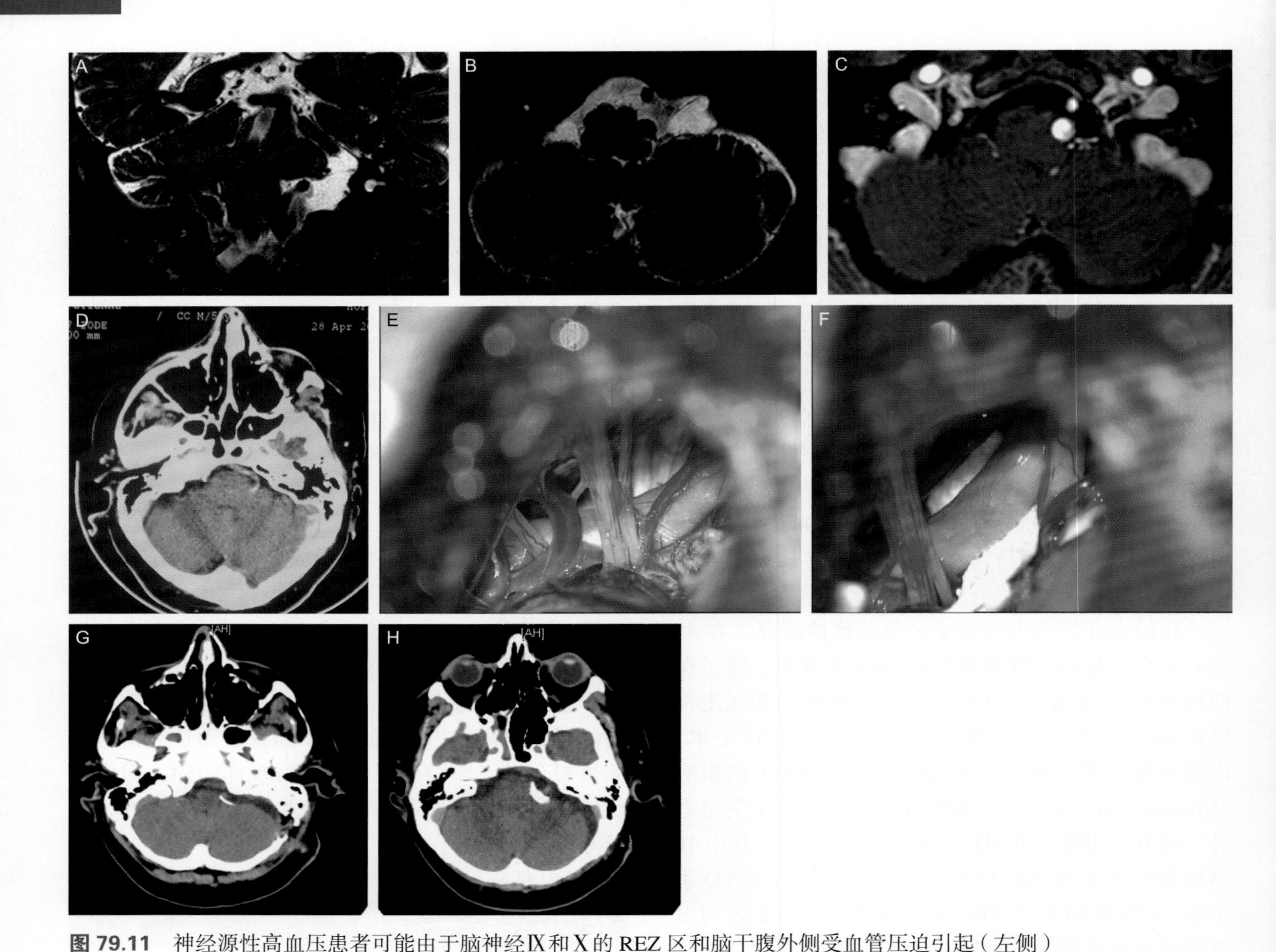

图 79.11 神经源性高血压患者可能由于脑神经Ⅸ和Ⅹ的 REZ 区和脑干腹外侧受血管压迫引起（左侧）
影像图片：左侧极度迂曲延长的椎基底动脉（VBA）压迫同侧延髓 VL 区，（A）MRI-T2 冠状位；（B）MRI-T2 轴状位；（C）MRI T1 增强成像，轴状位；（D）CT 轴状位成像显示极度迂曲延长的 VBA 位于脑干左侧。
手术视图：（E）左侧小脑延髓沟，VBA 压迫延髓 VL 区，CN Ⅸ和 CN Ⅹ的 REZ 及神经根也同时受到压迫。（F）在脑干和神经根之间置入一块中等偏硬的 teflon 垫棉后完成血管神经减压。（G、H）术后 CT 轴位扫描，注意 teflon 棉片（高密度影）的位置

延伸阅读、参考文献、EBRAIN 的相关链接

扫描书末二维码获取。

第 80 章　精神疾病的神经外科干预

Chris Bervoets・Bart Nuttin・Loes Gabriëls 著
任倩薇、范世莹、韩春雷 译，孟凡刚、崔志强 审校

引言

精神疾病是全世界最普遍的疾病之一，在普通人群中，有多达 1/3 人口患有焦虑症或抑郁症（Kessler et al.，2005a；Kessler et al.，2005b）。精神疾病的基本治疗方法包括药物治疗和心理治疗。此外，非药物、神经调控的治疗，包括电休克疗法、磁惊厥疗法、迷走神经电刺激、反复经颅磁刺激和脑深部电刺激等，也已经得到了研究。尽管这些治疗方式还处于临床开发的各个阶段，但它们代表了一个新的领域，它为精神疾病患者提供了更多的治疗选择，并有助于更好地理解这些疾病的神经生物学原理。关于神经生物学方面的理解，大多数精神疾病都有经过充分验证的动物模型，这一领域也取得了进一步的进展（van Kuyck et al.，2007）。同时，通过结合已发表的病例报告中的毁损术经验，以及神经影像学的信息，可以科学地进行靶点选择。此外，在使用 DBS 治疗其他疾病时进行的功能性神经影像学研究和生理学研究，可以促进对新靶点的研究。

关于精神疾病的神经外科治疗可以追溯到 1935 年，Egas Moniz 和 Almeida Lima 报道了一系列额叶白质切开术（后来由 Walter Freeman 和 James Watts 改名为“额叶切除术”），并首次使用“精神外科”一词（Feldman and Goodrich，2001）。Spiegel 和 Wycis 在 20 世纪 40 年代发展了立体定向技术，随后引入了计算机断层扫描和磁共振成像，这为更精准地处理大脑病变提供了机会。随着对特定脑区与不同行为之间联系的深入了解、精神病学标准化病因学系统的发展，以及越来越多地使用评估量表来评估治疗效果，使立体定向手术在精神疾病的治疗中取得了很大的发展（Larson，2008）。然而，为缓解严重的精神疾病症状而造成的不可逆的脑部损伤，使得人们很难接受毁损手术。20 世纪 90 年代，脑深部电刺激（deep brain stimulation，DBS）的发展重新引起人们对精神疾病的外科治疗的兴趣。DBS 是可逆的技术，且触点选择和刺激参数具有可调节性，不会损害治疗所涉及的神经回路，因此人们认为 DBS 比毁损术更具优势。此外，由于可以关闭刺激器，因此 DBS 可以在控制条件下进行更严格的临床试验，比如评估者不知道刺激器的开关状态。尽管尚需进行大规模的长期随访研究，但 DBS 为患有严重和无行为能力的精神疾病患者提供了治疗希望（Gabriëls，2010；Luyten et al.，2016）。在本章中，我们将（i）提供与神经外科手术相关的精神类疾病的病理生理基础；（ii）描述患者术前、术后管理以及手术操作；（iii）讨论阻碍该治疗技术在精神病学领域未来发展的问题。

患者的术前管理

患者选择

应仅考虑 18 岁以上且证明其他治疗方法无效，以及严重、慢性和致残性的精神疾病患者进行外科手术。平衡手术干预措施的潜在收益与风险（Gabriëls，2010）。强迫症、抽动秽语综合征和重度抑郁症可能受益于外科干预。在这些患者中，人格障碍史、活性物质（如毒品、麻药、酒精灯）滥用史或其他类 Ⅱ 症状（人格障碍和智能障碍）是手术的（相对）禁忌证。在患者选择中的关键问题仍然是对严重性、慢性、残疾及难治性标准的制订。使用经过验证的针对特定症状的临床研究评估量表评估其严重程度，例如强迫症（obsessive-compulsive disorder，OCD）的耶鲁 - 布朗强迫症量表（Yale-Brown Obsessive-Compulsive Scale，YBOCS）得分超过 30 分，严重抑郁症的蒙哥马利 - 艾森贝格抑郁量表（Montgomery-Åsbetg Depression Rating Scale，MADRS）超过 30 分。残疾则通常通过整体功能评估（Global Assessment of Function，GAF），评分小于 50 分进行判定。难治性需要由治疗该患者的精神科医生根据当前发布的指南中描述的所有治疗方法（指定剂量和治疗持续时

间）出具证明（Bandelow et al.，2008）。此外，精神科医生需要对患者和评估过程提供承诺，同意承担术后的（与 DBS 不相关的）管理责任。患者及其家庭也必须同意充分参与。同时建议由一名患者家庭成员或其他近亲参与评估过程。

术前筛查

初步选择适合手术的患者后，还需要另一位有经验的精神科医生的意见，在比利时进行强迫症外科治疗时，该名医生的评估意见也要添加到手术申请中。在比利时，由经验丰富的精神科医生、神经外科医生组成的多学科小组及伦理学家，对医疗记录进行彻底地审查，头颅 MRI 以及神经心理学测试也应添加到评估内容中。此外，必须满足知情同意的要求。

手术技术

损毁手术

扣带回前部毁损、尾状核下部神经束毁损、边缘叶脑白质毁损术和内囊前肢毁损术被认为是 4 种安全有效的治疗 OCD 的方法（Jenike，1998）。通常以上所有治疗方式都是双侧，并通过立体定向实施，以便精确损毁靶点区域脑组织。扣带回前部被认为是患有顽固性疼痛和并发混合性焦虑 - 抑郁状态患者进行外科手术的合适靶点（Fulton，1951）。目前，其手术适应证为难治性重度抑郁症、慢性焦虑症或强迫症。1964 年（Knight，1964；Knight，1969）引入了尾状核下神经束毁损术，首次限制了手术损毁区域的大小，并最大限度地减少标准额前叶毁损术所带来的副作用。手术目的是通过毁损尾状核头部下方的无名实性区域，以中断眶皮质与皮质下结构之间的白质联系。手术适应证包括重度抑郁症、强迫症和焦虑症。边缘叶白质毁损术（Kelley et al.，1973）包括尾状核下神经束毁损术和前扣带回毁损术。手术的目的是利用前者的毁损中断眶 - 额 - 丘脑环路，用后者中断 Papez 环路的重要部分。其手术适应证包括强迫症、焦虑症、抑郁症和其他各种精神类疾病。内囊前肢毁损术的目的（Talairach et al.，1949）是中断位于内囊前肢的额丘脑联系，它们在尾状核头和壳核之间通过。内囊前肢毁损术的临床指征包括抑郁症、慢性焦虑症和强迫症。

脑深部电刺激（DBS）

深部脑刺激可以对皮质下的深部靶点脑组织产生持久的电刺激。电极的放置取决于治疗的情况，并使用神经影像引导的立体定向神经外科技术，通过颅骨上的骨孔植入。每根电极由一个电极阵列组成，通常包含四个电极触点，跨度为 10~20 mm，具体则取决于电极类型。植入后，电极通过皮下延长线连接到一个或两个皮下植入的电池脉冲发生器（implanted battery-operated pulse generators，IPG）。IPG 通常植入到锁骨下或腹部。医生可通过操作程控仪非侵入式调控刺激参数（使用的触点、频率、脉宽和电压）。临床使用的参数包括刺激频率 60~130 Hz，脉宽 60~450 μs，电压 2~10 V，可以是单极刺激，也可以是双极刺激（Holtzheimer and Mayberg，2011）。尽管一般认为 DBS 比损毁治疗有优势，但仍然有颅内出血和感染的风险，以及与麻醉有关的并发症（Luyten et al.，2016）。此外，植入的电极或延长线断裂，延展性问题，以及由于电池寿命终止而需要频繁更换 IPG 也是 DBS 的不足之处（Nuttin et al.，2003；Visser-Vandewalle et al.，2003；Abelson et al.，2005；Houeto et al.，2005；Machado et al.，2005；Mayberg et al.，2005）。OCD 的第一个 DBS 靶点是内囊［其腹侧部分称为腹侧内囊（VC），包括纹状体末端的床核（BST）］和腹侧纹状体或 VS［有时包括伏隔核（NAcc）］。DBS 靶点的选择是基于 OCD 的立体定向毁损术（Jenike，1998；Lippitz et al.，1999；Dougherty et al.，2002；Greenberg et al.，2003；Sturm et al.，2003）。我们团队报道了在内囊前肢（Nuttin et al.，1999；Nuttin et al.，2003）和 BST（Luyten et al.，2016）应用 DBS 的情况。发现根据电极的几何形状和刺激参数设置，跨越该区域的 DBS 电极能够影响任何上述结构（Larson，2008）。在患有帕金森病和强迫症的患者中，偶然发现了通过刺激丘脑底核的特定亚区来缓解强迫症症状，此后，研究人员将注意力集中在皮质 - 纹状体 - 丘脑皮质回路中的这一节点上。此外，还有采用其他不同靶点［例如丘脑下脚和苍白球内侧部（GPi）］进行 DBS 治疗精神疾病的病例报道。

患者的术后管理

在患者的术后管理阶段，神经外科团队应与精神科团队密切沟通。由于神经外科手术被认为是患有慢性和严重精神病患者的最后治疗手段，因此患者和家属的术后心理和情感指导至关重要。通常情况下，患者的主要症状会出现早期和显著的变化，要在家庭或亲人中找到新的平衡通常需要一定的时间。

此外，优化刺激参数是一个复杂而漫长的过程，需要精神科医生和家人的支持。参数调整最好由同一位医生负责，以便个体化观察患者刺激相关的态度和行为变化。

未来的问题

通过基础研究，更好地理解情感的神经生物学原理，可能有利于更好地进行靶点选择以及更准确的电极植入。结合无创技术（例如经颅磁刺激、经颅直流电刺激）的进一步研究发现，神经调控方法的一个新研究领域目前正在扩展，即用于治疗难治性精神病患者。这些技术的优势在于可以进行双盲对照试验。这对于以前的具有不可逆性和侵袭性的毁损手术几乎是不可能的。当前使用的科学方法的进步，使得在研究中的关于神经外科手术治疗难治性精神病的安全性和有效性的循证声明成为可能。此外，侵入性手术的使用与高标准的伦理和临床审查委员会密切相关。

然而，我们应该对靶点的选择保持谨慎。首先，在DBS治疗中，对同一精神病适应证，有多种靶点可供选择，与此同时，其方法学的精确度不断提高，并且同一靶点可用于治疗不同的精神疾病。其次，刺激参数对患者的DBS疗效有影响。目前我们缺乏用于选择最佳参数的有效算法。Kuncel计算得出，在多个可能的解剖学靶点及在给定IPG的建议电荷密度限制内，可获得12 964个脉宽、频率和电压组合以及65个电极几何形状组合（Kuncel and Grill，2004）。当可以使用靶点的组织特征和网络连接图（由扩散张量成像建立）的数学模型来帮助临床医生选择，改善和优化单个患者的刺激参数时，也许可以在该领域取得进展（Astrom et al.，2009）。最后，随着诸如TMS等非侵入性神经调节研究的兴起，TMS的临床疗效探索应与DBS的结果进行比较，这将有助于在未来的治疗方法中同时提供有创和无创的神经调控。

参考文献

扫描书末二维码获取。

第十七篇　癫痫

第 81 章　癫痫和癫痫发作的分类

Andrew McEvoy · Tim Wehner · Victoria Wykes 著
亓蕾、李志保、王安妮 译，韩春雷、孟凡刚、任连坤 校

引言

癫痫发作是神经外科医生经常遇到的一种症状或一种颅内疾病的并发症。在接下来的章节中我们会探讨国际抗癫痫联盟（International League against Epilepsy，ILAE）在 2014 年提出的癫痫实用定义，概述癫痫发作的表现，回顾适合外科治疗的常见的两种癫痫病因：局灶性皮质发育不良和海马硬化，并对边缘系统的解剖进行概述。

癫痫发作是由于大脑神经元异常过度或同步化放电引起的一过性体征和（或）症状（Fisher et al.，2005）。不伴有任何临床事件的电发作称为“亚临床发作”。临床发作症状可分为明显的行为表现（“阳性症状”，如阵挛等非自主运动）、患者对自身及其周围环境的主观体验的改变（先兆）以及与患者基线相比的脑功能受损（“阴性症状”）。在特殊情况下，发作表现中的认知变化可能是轻微的，只有在对患者进行充分评估时才显现出来。癫痫发作首先是一种症状，可能提示存在急性的神经内科疾病（即存在诱因的发作）。传统意义上，癫痫是指无诱因的反复出现的发作。为了解释首次非诱发性癫痫发作后风险分级的流行病学数据，并纳入具有类似病理生理学的临床表现，ILAE 最近提出了一个实用性的癫痫定义（Fisher et al.，2014；另见**专栏 81.1**）。目前为止，第一种情况是神经外科最常见的。这一定义包括风险分级的一个要素。一定程度上来说，如果一个人在无任何诱因的情况下出现癫痫发作，10 年内若不接受任何治疗，那么存在 60% 的复发风险。

以下临床情况对诱发癫痫和癫痫的概念进行了叙述。

1. “婴幼儿热性惊厥”——在 5 岁以下的儿童中，多达 5% 的患儿在发热时会出现抽搐发作。这被认为是诱发的癫痫发作，但不构成癫痫（尽管再次发热时的复发风险为 40%）。

专栏 81.1　癫痫和癫痫发作的概念性定义和癫痫的实用性定义

癫痫发作是由于大脑中神经元的异常过度或同步化放电活动引起的一过性体征和（或）症状。癫痫是一种脑部疾病，出现下列任何一项即可确诊：

1 至少出现两次无诱因（或反射性）的发作，相隔 24 小时以上；

2 一次无诱因（或反射性）的发作，且在两次无诱因发作后，在 10 年内再次发作的可能性与一般复发风险（≥60%）相似；

3 癫痫综合征。

a) Reproduced with permission from Jerome Engel, Phillip Lee, Pierre Genton, et al., Epileptic Seizures and Epilepsy: Definitions Proposed by the International League Against Epilepsy (ILAE) and the International Bureau for Epilepsy (IBE), *Epilepsia*, Volume 46, Issue 4, pp. 470–2, Copyright © 2005 John Wiley and Sons.

b) Reproduced with permission from Samuel Wiebe, Masako Watanabe, Torbjörn Tomson, et al., ILAE Official Report: A practical clinical definition of epilepsy, *Epilepsia*, Volume 55, Issue 4, pp. 475–82, Copyright © 2014 John Wiley and Sons.

2. 急性中枢神经系统（central nervous system，CNS）病变（如脑膜炎或脑炎、硬膜下血肿、缺血性卒中、脑外伤等）的患者，在疾病早期即可出现癫痫发作（多于发病 7 天内）。上述情况下的癫痫发作多为诱发的癫痫发作。由于所有皮质病变都增加了癫痫的风险，这些患者可能有发生癫痫，然而，如果出现在疾病的急性期，则不能诊断为癫痫。如果急性中枢神经系统损害超过 1 周后出现无诱因的癫痫发作，那么再次发作的风险将超过 60%，因此即使是首次癫痫发作也可诊断为癫痫。
3. 如果患者有右额凸面脑膜瘤，出现左臂的局灶性运动发作，即使出现首次癫痫发作，也符合 ILAE 对癫痫的实际定义。这是因为脑膜瘤的存在增加了该患者再次出现癫痫发作的风险。

局灶性发作和全面性发作

全面性发作是指起源于双侧大脑半球网络内的某一节点，并在双侧大脑半球内迅速扩布（Berg et al.，2010）。

局灶性癫痫发作是指起源仅限于一侧大脑半球网络内的某一节点（Berg et al.，2010），它可局限于这一区域，或者局限于同侧大脑半球或双侧大脑半球内。因此，局灶性发作可发展为双侧肢体的发作（“继发的全面性发作”）。

传统意义上，癫痫发作可分为这两种类型。然而，发作症状学（即临床表现）可能不仅仅局限于某一种类型。例如，失张力发作、阵挛性发作、强直性发作和肌阵挛发作可能是全面性的或局灶性的（当仅影响一侧或单侧肢体时）。典型的失神发作（短暂的意识丧失，立即完全恢复）的临床表现可类似于局灶性发作（例如，起源于额叶）。相反，人们越来越认识到全面性强直阵挛发作可能具有局灶性发作的症状学特征。癫痫性痉挛是婴儿的一种常见发作类型，常见于结节性硬化症或其他脑部实质性病变，具有全面性和局灶性发作的特征，发作起始的脑电图即表现为双侧大脑半球受累，但在某些情况下可仅限于一侧大脑半球，此时可进行治愈性切除术（Chugani et al.，2015）。1998 年，Lüders 等提出的癫痫症状学分类，是专门针对癫痫发作的临床表现对癫痫发作进行的分类，并越来越多地被世界各地的癫痫外科中心使用。

神经外科医生遇到的绝大多数癫痫发作和癫痫（主要）是局灶性发作。传统上，这些发作被分为保留意识的发作（“简单部分发作”）和意识受损的发作（“复杂部分发作”）。虽然意识改变通常表明有发作（对驾驶、就业和休闲活动有影响），但不可能从患者的描述或行为表现可靠地推断癫痫发作期间意识是保留的还是受损的。

任何发作都可能导致这四个维度的改变：①自我和环境的主观性体验；②意识、认知和记忆的形成；③自主性的改变；④运动和行为表现。虽然后者通常是显而易见的，但前三个维度的记录取决于在癫痫发作期间和之后的评估方式。直接电刺激大脑的特定脑区可诱发发作的部分症状。这些症状包括初级视觉皮质的基本或复杂视觉幻觉或失明，以及初级感觉皮质的躯体感觉幻觉（刺痛感）。其他主观症状在边缘系统，特别在内侧颞叶杏仁 - 海马复合体的癫痫发作中非常典型。这些症状包括熟悉感（“似曾相识”）或陌生感（“似曾不相识”），上腹部和（或）胸部的上升感，以及（通常令人不快的）嗅觉和味觉幻觉，后者通常带有“金属”特征。在大脑皮质刺激过程中，可以诱发一些运动表现，具有可重复性。这些症状是中央前回的初级运动皮质支配的对侧面部和远端肢体的肌阵挛或紧张性收缩，额上回近端辅助感觉运动区支配的近端强直性收缩，和额眼区支配对侧头眼的偏斜。运动前区（通常位于初级运动皮质的正前方）的皮质电刺激可诱发所谓的负性运动现象（即运动或语言的中断或停止）。发作期间对这些症状和体征的观察表明，癫痫发作期间相应皮质区域在特定时间内受到影响。这些都是特别相关的症状和体征，因为单纯的主观症状（即癫痫先兆）或局灶性阵挛 / 强直性收缩发作往往无法通过头皮脑电图监测到。这是因为需要激活产生这些症状的皮质面积通常小于可以在头皮脑电图上记录到的发作模式所需的皮质面积。有面部、手臂或腿部局灶运动性发作的患者发作间期和发作期的头皮脑电可以完全正常。

另一方面，如咂嘴、咀嚼、摸索或抓握、蹬腿或踢腿以及全身旋转这些复杂的动作（自动症）一般不能通过皮质直接电刺激诱发，这表明这些症状为释放现象，并没有特定对应的皮质区域。更极端的症状包括，复杂的动作（术语“复杂”指的是动作的复杂性，而不是意识状态）可能表现为不合情境的“奇怪”行为（如跳跃、摇摆、殴打、喊叫、吹口哨或接吻）。

意识状态的改变是全面性和局灶性癫痫一个普遍存在和致残性的特征，几乎源于任何大脑区域。因此，意识的改变并不具有明确的定位和定侧价值。通常提到的“失神”是指短暂（通常 5~10 秒）的全面性发作，定义为意识丧失，伴或不伴轻微的动作症状，脑电图上出现广泛性的 3 Hz 棘慢复合波，且发作后意识立即恢复。因此，伴有意识丧失的局灶性发作并不是失神发作。

自主神经症状和体征常见于局灶性和全面性惊厥发作，通常反映交感神经兴奋（如心动过速和过度换气），但也可出现心动过缓和呼吸暂停。胃肠道症状包括发作性恶心、呕吐和排便。泌尿系症状是大小便失禁、发作期或发作期后的尿急和生殖器感觉。患者也可能主诉有发热感或面色发红。参与自主神经产生的大脑区域有内侧前额叶皮质、脑岛、杏仁核和扣带回。一般来说，发作性自主神经症状的定位和定侧意义不大。但颞叶内侧癫痫中见到的典型的胃气上升感是一个例外。

癫痫发作症状和体征定位的进一步证实，源于癫痫发作和发作后的特征与 MRI、发作期脑电图

（EEG）有关发作“病灶”的信息之间的相关性，以及最终癫痫灶切除术后癫痫发作停止。常见发作症状和体征的定位和定侧价值汇总见**表** 81.1 和**表** 81.2。

癫痫综合征

癫痫综合征是综合发作类型、发病年龄、并发症，有时还包括遗传因素在内的是一组临床特征的统称。尽管癫痫遗传学正在迅速发展，但癫痫外科很少涉及这一方面。局灶性癫痫综合征以往是根据致痫区域（即产生癫痫发作所必需且足够的区域）的解剖定位来划分的。值得注意的是“典型”发作并不完全与特定解剖位置相对应。其中一个原因是，癫痫的起始区（发作起始区）可能与首次出现癫痫症状的区域（症状产生区）不同。例如，胃气上升感（“腹部先兆”）是颞叶内侧癫痫的典型症状，但这一症状可由前岛皮质刺激引起，因此也见于岛叶癫痫。

颞叶内侧癫痫（mesial temporal lobe epilepsy，mTLE）是最常见的局灶性癫痫综合征。mTLE 的常见病理类型是海马硬化、海绵状血管瘤、低级别脑肿瘤、局灶性皮质发育不良、软化灶和错构瘤。然而，30%~40% 的患者 MR 异常不明显（Tatum，2012）。mTLE 患者常存在儿童期热性惊厥、中枢神经系统感染或急性中枢神经系统损伤的病史。在习惯性癫痫发作之前，通常有 5~20 年或更长时间的潜伏期。典型的先兆为胃气上升感，恶心或不自然的、通常令人不快的嗅觉或味觉幻觉，以及熟悉感（似曾相识感）或脱离现实感（陌生感），复杂的视觉或听觉幻觉，情感症状或恐惧感，但这些症状并没有定侧的价值（Ferrari-Marinho et al.，2012）。

在新皮质颞叶癫痫（neocortical temporal lobe epilepsy，nTLE）中，癫痫发作往往发生在成年早期。50%~75% 的患者的典型先兆症状是简单的幻听（响铃或嗡嗡声）、低沉或扭曲的听觉感知（如回声），以及头晕、不稳或眩晕的感觉。

颞叶癫痫发作的常见症状是意识丧失、伴目的

表 81.1 癫痫先兆的定位和定侧价值

先兆类型	症状产生区	定侧	常见的伴发局灶性癫痫综合征
感觉（发麻、蚁爬感）	初级感觉皮质	对侧	顶叶癫痫
	次级感觉皮质	身体同侧（如果为一侧的症状）	顶叶和颞叶癫痫
	辅助感觉运动区（supplementary sensorimotor area，SSMA）	对侧（大多数）	额叶和顶叶癫痫
简单视觉（闪光、火花等）	初级视觉皮质	对侧	枕叶癫痫
复杂视觉（有形视幻觉）	颞枕联合区、颞底、边缘系统	对侧（如果为一侧的症状）	枕叶和颞叶癫痫
简单听觉（简单的声音或听力下降）	初级听觉皮质	对侧（如果为一侧的症状）	颞叶癫痫
复杂听觉（噪声、说话声音、乐声）	听觉相关皮质和边缘系统	对侧（如果为一侧的症状）	颞叶癫痫
头晕	颞枕联合区	不能定侧	颞叶癫痫
嗅觉相关	眶额皮质、杏仁核、岛叶	不能定侧	颞叶内侧、额叶癫痫
味觉相关	顶盖、颞底	不能定侧	颞叶癫痫
腹部症状	前岛、额盖、SSMA	不能定侧	颞叶内侧癫痫
恐惧	杏仁核、海马、额叶内侧	不能定侧	颞叶和额叶癫痫
似曾相识感、复杂记忆再现	钩突、内嗅皮质、颞叶新皮质、边缘系统	不能定侧	颞叶癫痫
全身的感觉	杏仁核、内嗅皮质、次级感觉皮质、辅助感觉运动区	不能定侧	颞叶和额叶癫痫
自主神经症状（心悸、呼吸急促、感觉热或冷、性冲动）	杏仁核、岛叶、前扣带、前额叶内侧	不能定侧（无明显侧别性）	颞叶和额叶癫痫

Adapted from *Epilepsy & Behavior,* Volume 20, issue 2, Nancy Foldvary-Schaefer, Kanjana Unnwongse, Localizing and lateralizing features of auras and seizures, pp. 160–6, Copyright (2011), with permission from Elsevier.

表 81.2　癫痫客观症状的定位和定侧价值

发作症状	常见症状产生区或机制	定侧	常见的伴发局灶性癫痫综合征
肌阵挛、负性肌阵挛	初级运动皮质、运动前区	对侧（如果为一侧的症状）	额叶癫痫
阵挛	初级运动皮质、运动前区、SSMA	对侧（如果为一侧的症状）	额叶癫痫
强直性收缩或强直性姿势	初级运动皮质、SSMA、基底节区的激活	对侧（如果为一侧的症状）	额叶和颞叶癫痫
非对称性姿势	SSMA、中央前区	不能定侧	额叶和颞叶癫痫
肢体不动	负运动区的激活或初级、运动前皮质发作性功能障碍	对侧	额叶癫痫
自动症	眶额回、扣带回、岛盖或岛叶、SSMA 前的额叶内侧	不能定侧	颞叶、额叶、顶叶癫痫
保留意识的自动症	眶额回、扣带回、岛盖或岛叶、SSMA 前的额叶内侧	不能定侧	颞叶、额叶、顶叶癫痫
头眼偏转（偏向一侧，多于颈肌的过伸有关）	额眼区、纹状皮质、前运动区	对侧	额叶癫痫，也可见于颞叶、顶叶或枕叶癫痫的继发全面性发作过程中
发作或发作后失语[1]	语言区的前部或后部、弓形束	优势侧	颞叶和额叶癫痫
发作性言语[2]	非优势半球兴奋或优势半球抑制	非优势侧	颞叶和额叶癫痫
发笑	下丘脑、额前内侧、颞底	不能定侧	颞叶和额叶癫痫

SSMA，辅助感觉运动区

[1] 发作 / 发作后失语是指与部分意识损失一致的语言功能损害

[2] 发作性言语是指虽存在意识障碍，但仍可以说出有意义的言语

性口咽部和手部的自动症以及对侧肢体的肌张力障碍（Kuba et al.，2010）。一些患者表现出更复杂的行为，如游走、饮酒或接吻，后两者与非显性发作有关（Rashid et al.，2010）。自主神经症状，如瞳孔散大、多汗、呕吐、勃起和心率改变等。在 TLE 中，症状往往在几十秒钟内逐渐演变。癫痫发作后表现以神志不清和遗忘症为特征。演变的语言障碍，从全面性失语症到找词困难，是优势侧颞叶癫痫常见的发作后症状。

额叶癫痫（frontal lobe epilepsy，FLE）的典型发作特征反映了额叶内部以及与邻近颞区、岛区和顶区的复杂功能联系。FLE 的先兆通常不具有特异性。患者可能会主诉或表现出焦虑或恐惧的面部表情，上腹部先兆和似曾相识感（von Lehe et al.，2012），或者诉说头部有一种模糊的运动感（“头部先兆”；见 Canuet et al.，2008），有时与视力模糊有关（Beauvais et al.，2005）。涉及前额叶的癫痫发作症状多为不自然或怪异的表现，例如骑自行车或剪腿自动、颤抖、骨盆推动、跳跃、踢打、抽搐、爬行和喉间发声（Wehner et al.，2017）。涉及辅助感觉运动区（SSMA）的癫痫发作表现为面部、喉咙和肢体肌肉的对称或不对称强直性收缩（Unnwongse et al.，2012），而涉及初级运动皮质则表现为单侧阵挛性抽搐，通常为“杰克逊式扩布”（即依次涉及面部、上肢和下肢，反之亦然）。姿势张力的丧失（失张力发作）可能导致头部下垂或跌倒。在涉及初级运动系统的局灶性癫痫发作中，即使存在双侧的运动特征，意识也常常是可以保留的。FLE 的发作通常是突发突止的，发作常出现在睡眠期，发作持续时间较 TLE 短（约 30 秒 ±15 秒）。

顶叶癫痫的特征性先兆是对侧肢体的麻木、刺痛或蚁走的感觉，这在杰克逊扩布中尤为典型。其他主观的症状包括体像障碍、运动错觉、眩晕和复杂的视觉或听觉错觉。客观的行为表现是非特异性的，可能反映的是发作传播到初级运动区或 SSMA（癫痫发作侧对侧的局灶性阵挛活动、姿势性强直），或颞叶边缘系统（行为终止、自发症）（Wehner et al.，2017）。因此，顶叶癫痫常无明显的特征性（除外躯体感觉症状先兆），被称为局灶性癫痫综合征中的“伟大模仿者”（Ristic et al.，2012）。

枕叶癫痫（occipital lobe epilepsy，OLE）多存在视觉先兆，包括闪光、视物变形、视物颜色的改变、视幻觉等。癫痫视觉先兆（几秒到几分钟）比偏头痛患者的视觉先兆时间短（4~20 分钟）（Adcock and Panayiotopoulos，2012）。感觉异常、上腹部感觉

和经验性症状的出现，表明邻近的顶叶或颞叶边缘区受累（Bien et al.，2000；Jobst et al.，2010）。OLE的客观发作表现为快速眨眼或眼睑颤动（Kun Lee et al.，2005；Tandon et al.，2009）和眼球跟踪运动或眼球震颤（Adcock and Panayiotopoulos，2012）。根据癫痫发作的传播情况，进一步的症状类似于TLE（如失神、口腔和手部自动症）和FLE（如姿势性肌张力障碍和过度运动自动症；见Jobst et al.，2010）。

值得注意的是，癫痫发作的运动症状随年龄变化。虽然双侧强直性肌阵挛和婴儿痉挛是婴幼儿癫痫发作的主要症状（Nordli，2013），但随着大脑发育成熟，运动特征和偏侧体征就会凸显出来（Fogarasi et al.，2007）。在老年人，继发全面性癫痫发作的发作后症状，如神志不清、记忆障碍和Todd麻痹等症状的持续时间比年轻患者更长（Stefan et al.，2014）。

癫痫持续状态

大多数情况下，癫痫发作多在数分钟内自发停止。癫痫持续状态是指癫痫发作的极端状态，即不能自发停止。近年来，ILAE重新定义了癫痫持续状态，指出这是（在时间点之后）终止癫痫发作的机制失效或由导致异常长时间癫痫发作的机制启动的结果，这种情况下可以导致神经元死亡、神经元损伤和神经元网络的改变，这取决于癫痫发作的类型和持续时间（Trinka et al.，2015）。超过一半的癫痫持续状态患者在发病时有急性或远期的中枢神经系统损害或内科系统疾病。从临床角度看，全面性强直阵挛发作应在5分钟内终止，意识受损的局灶性发作应在10分钟内终止。如果有需要，应迅速升级治疗方案，将长期的不可逆损伤降至最低。

虽然癫痫持续状态的临床表现遵循前面讨论的癫痫发作的相同原则，但由于癫痫持续状态的高度动态性质，发作症状和体征可能会在短时间内发生变化。重要的是，在全面性痉挛状态时，癫痫发作的突出运动症状往往会随着时间的推移而减弱，这可能是由于导致这些症状产生的潜在神经网络耗尽所致。然而，大脑中的病理性发作活动可能会持续（非惊厥性癫痫持续状态）。因此，在伴有不可解释的昏迷或意识改变，或急性脑损伤后未恢复意识的患者中，非惊厥癫痫持续状态需要通过脑电图监测来评估。

部分性癫痫持续状态（epilepsia partialis continua，EPC）是指身体某一部位持续有规律或无规律地阵挛性抽搐，通常在身体的远端而不在近端。这一般都涉及初级运动皮质，偏瘫或其他皮质功能损伤通常亦与此相关（Bien and Elger，2008）。EPC一般有明确的病因，最常见的是血管或炎症性疾病、肿瘤和代谢毒性疾病。

癫痫的结构性病因

在神经外科的实际工作中，确定癫痫的结构性病因非常重要，因为切除癫痫灶可以最大程度上实现癫痫无发作（**专栏**81.2）。局灶性皮质发育不良（focal cortical dysplasias，FCD）是癫痫手术中最常见的皮质发育畸形（malformation of cortical development，MCD）。大脑皮质的功能分层发育是一个多阶段的过程，包括细胞增殖、分化、迁移、突触形成和细胞重组。皮质分层、神经元迁移、分化和生长过程中的任何一点的破坏都可能导致皮质发育异常，甚至可能影响一个脑区、多个脑叶或整个大脑半球。2011年，ILAE发布了一个结合组织学、临床表现和放射学的分类系统（Blümcke et al.，2011，见**表**81.3）。

FCDⅠ型和Ⅲ型是由于迁移后期皮质缺损或损伤所致。FCDⅠ型的可能原因有严重早产、缺氧缺血性损伤、头部创伤、颅内出血或产前/围产期卒中。通常认为，Ⅰ型FCD是一种单纯的畸形，表现为异常的皮质柱状结构紊乱，呈放射状（Ⅰa；**图**81.1）、切线状（Ⅰb）或混合状（Ⅰc）。FCDⅢ型伴有发育早期出现的其他结构病理改变，包括海马硬化（Ⅲa）、引起癫痫的肿瘤[如胚胎发育不良性神经上皮肿瘤（DNT，Ⅲb）]、邻近血管畸形（例如AVM、海绵状血管瘤）和其他致痫性病变（包括头部损伤、脑炎、缺氧缺血性损伤）。MRI可显示这些典型的病变，但可能无法确定其中的因果关系。

FCDⅡ型的原因是细胞发育和成熟异常，其特征是皮质分层异常和异形神经元（**图**81.2）。FCDⅡ型

专栏81.2 癫痫的结构性病因

局灶性皮质发育不良
皮质发育异常
海马硬化
神经皮肤综合征
血管畸形
下丘脑错构瘤
脑肿瘤
获得性损伤
  脑脓肿
  炎症和感染
  缺血性和出血性卒中

表 81.3　局灶性皮质发育不良分类

继发于皮质损伤或皮质发育迁徙过程中异常所致的局灶性皮质发育不良	Ⅰ型 皮质分层不良	Ⅰa 放射状皮质分层异常 Ⅰb 切线状皮质分层异常 Ⅰc 放射状和切线状皮质分层异常
	Ⅲ型 伴有病理性病变	Ⅲa 海马硬化 Ⅲb 肿瘤相关癫痫（比如胶质瘤、胚胎发育不良性神经上皮肿瘤） Ⅲc 血管畸形（如，海绵状血管瘤） Ⅲd 生命早期的其他病变（如，脑外伤、缺氧缺血性损伤、脑炎）
细胞发育和成熟异常所致的皮质发育不全	Ⅱ型 皮质分层异常伴异形神经元	Ⅱa 大量异形神经元 Ⅱb 大量异形神经元伴气球样细胞

患者表现为较小的患病年龄、难治性癫痫、较重的认知障碍。气球样细胞是 FCD Ⅱb 的主要细胞类型，该细胞可表达神经元核抗原（NeuN）、胶质纤维酸性蛋白（GFAP）、微管相关蛋白 1B（MAP1）、波形蛋白和巢蛋白，这说明这些细胞具有混合起源和未成熟特征。气球样细胞也可能表达包括 Sox2、c-Myc 和 Klf4 在内的干细胞标志物，这些标志物与增强的哺乳动物雷帕霉素（mTOR）靶信号通路有关。使用抑制剂抑制 mTOR 通路可能是一种很有前途的新疗法（Guerrini et al.，2015）。

癫痫 MRI 序列扫描包括 1.5 T 或 3.0 T 的 T1 和 T2 加权图像以及液体衰减反转恢复（FLAIR）图像（Duncan et al.，2016）。FCD 的特征包括皮质增厚、异常的脑回和脑沟，和最常见于 FCD Ⅱb 型的“transmantle 征”（图 81.3）。“transmantle 征”表现为延续至脑室的皮质下白质高信号，FLAIR 序列上最清楚，且与 FCD Ⅰ型患者相比，术后癫痫控制效果更好（Wang et al.，2013）。目前尚不清楚这是否与内在的低致痫性或解剖上更容易识别该类致痫组织有关。对气球样细胞的电生理学研究表明，气球样细胞是电“沉默”性的，并且有人假设气球样细胞的存在可以促进周围皮质的突触重组，从而导致组织中兴奋性的增加（Cepeda et al.，2003）。有相当一部分患者，仅通过影像学检查确定病灶并手术切除后仍处于药物难治状态，因此，癫痫发作是发生在发育不良的皮质内，还是来自周围的大脑，或者两者兼而有之，这仍是目前争论的焦点。

在治疗药物难治性癫痫的外科治疗中，海马硬化（hippocampal sclerosis，HS）是最常见的病理类型之一，占 33%~66%（综述见 Thom，2014）。海马硬化 ILAE 分类以海马不同亚区内神经元缺失和胶

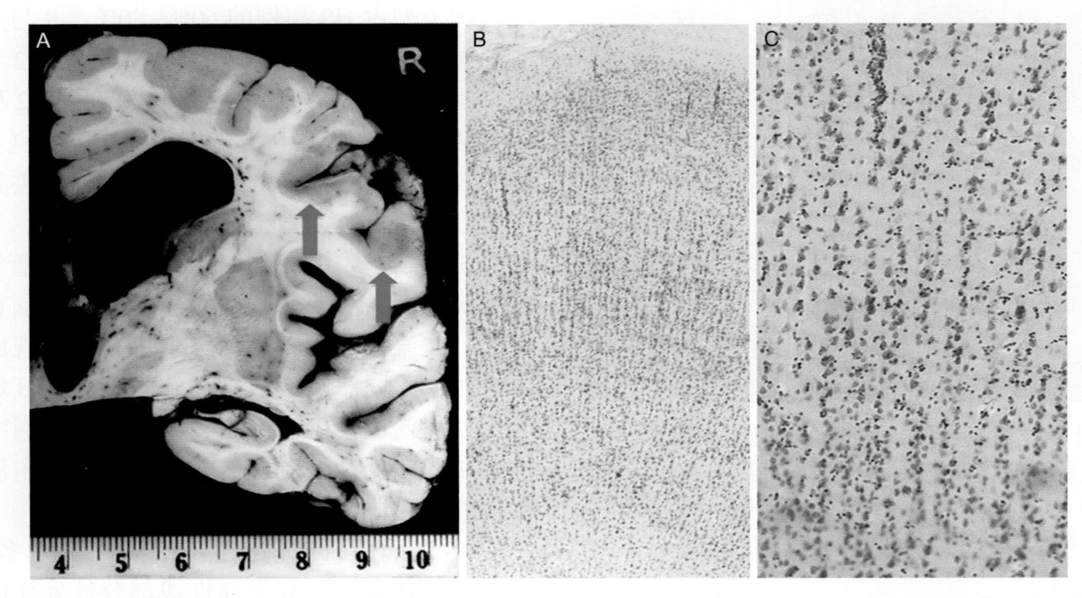

图 81.1　FCD Ⅰa 的病理组织学特征。（A）尸检标本，22 岁女性，患有癫痫（SUDEP），1 岁起病（全面性和部分性癫痫），20 世纪 70 年代 5 岁时行大脑半球切除术。右半球切片检查显示局灶性皮质发育不良累及额叶和颞叶，呈斑片状分布。（B、C）ILAE 2011 分类中的 FCD Ⅰa 型：异常组织的 Nissl 染色显示皮质柱状结构保留，典型的小尺寸神经元呈放射状排列（B：10×；C：20×）

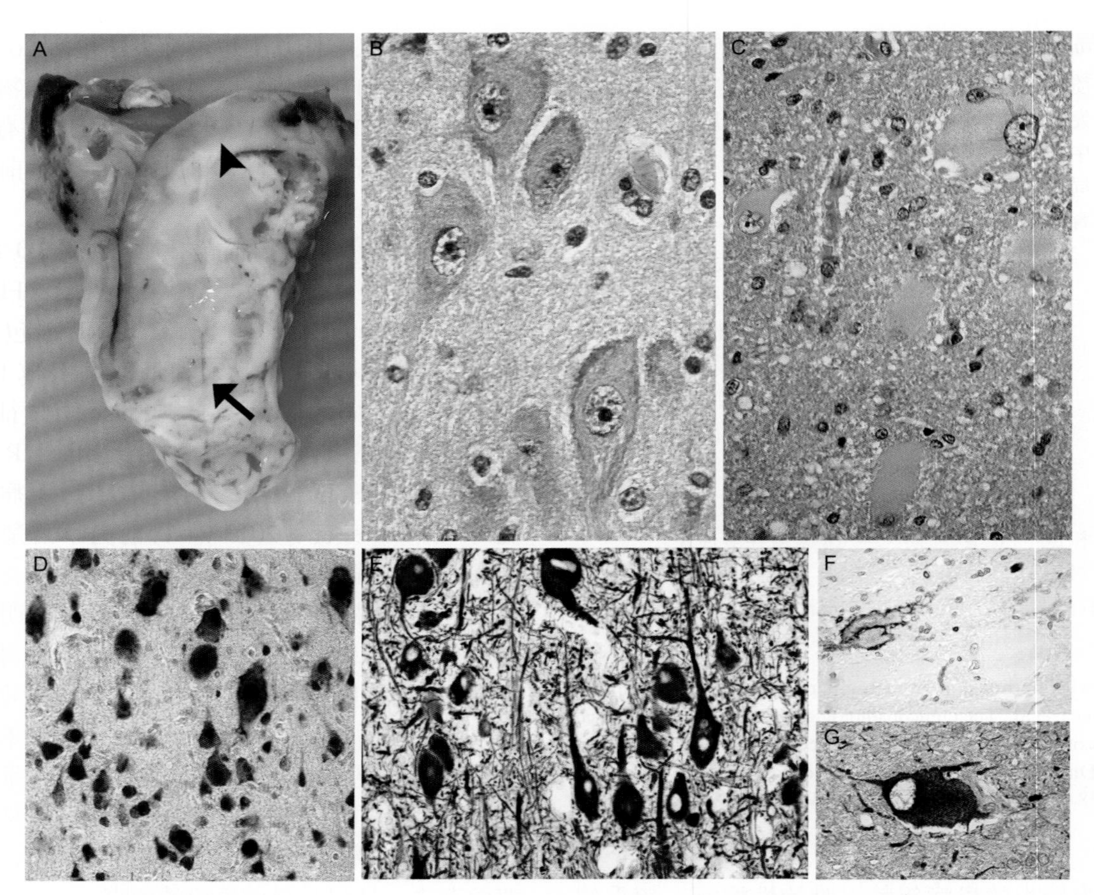

图 81.2 FCD Ⅱb 的病理组织学特征。（A）FCD Ⅱb 的大病理，与相邻的界限清楚的皮质（箭头）相比，FCD Ⅱb 灰白质交界不清（箭头）。（B）苏木精和伊红染色显示 FCD 皮质（50×）和（C）白质中含有气球样细胞（20×）。（D）异常神经元大于正常神经元，如 NeuN 染色示神经丝染色过度，如（E）所示。（F）气球细胞 CD34 和 nestin（G）的染色多样性

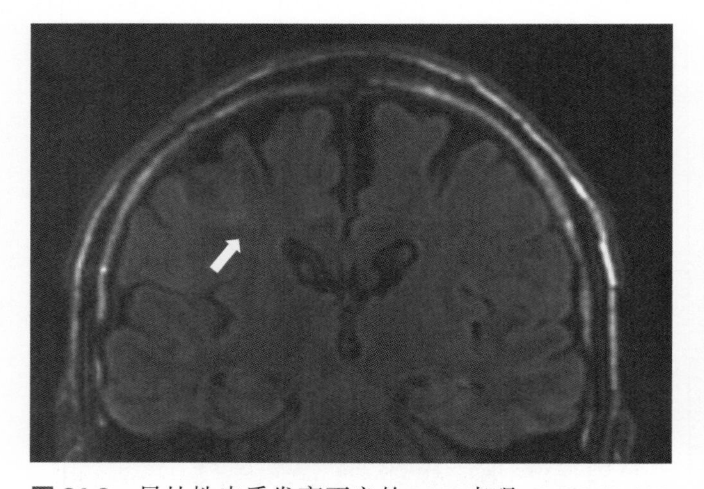

图 81.3 局灶性皮质发育不良的 MRI 表现。MRI FLAIR 序列显示局灶性皮质增厚，异常的脑回和脑沟，以及最常见于 FCD Ⅱb“transmantle 征”（箭头）。“transmantle 征”表现为延伸至脑室的皮质下白质高信号

质增生的模式为硬化的客观指标对 HS 进行了分类（Blümcke et al.，2013）（**图 81.4**）。在 HS 1 型（以前称为经典硬化症）中，CA1 亚区的神经元丢失和胶质增生程度更大，CA4 和 CA3 区也有，CA2 区较少。该病理类型占 HS 病例的 60%~80%，并与热性惊厥有共同的联系。术后癫痫无发作率更高，2 年的无发作率为 70%~85%，10 年为 50%。在 HS 2 型中，神经元丢失和胶质增生主要见于 CA1 亚区（占 HS 病例的 5%~10%）。在 HS 3 型中，神经元丢失和胶质增生仅出现在 CA4 亚区，伴有终板硬化（占 HS 病例的 3%~7%），并与如 DNT 或海绵状血管瘤这样的双重病理有关。HS 2 型和 3 型，通常癫痫首发年龄较大，在某些病例系列中，术后很难实现癫痫无发作。对于不同海马亚区锥体细胞丢失的区域选择性问题目前尚不清楚。但是，不同的调节网络、兴奋性通路的改变和抑制性传入以及有效的内源性神经保护机制可能都与此有关。

HS 的病因目前仍有争议，但可能是多因素的。癫痫持续状态、反复全面性或部分性发作以及长期热性惊厥发作并不是导致 HS 的必然因素。虽然 HS 被认为是一种散发性疾病，但也可能涉及其他易感因素。先天性免疫系统和获得性免疫系统的激活引

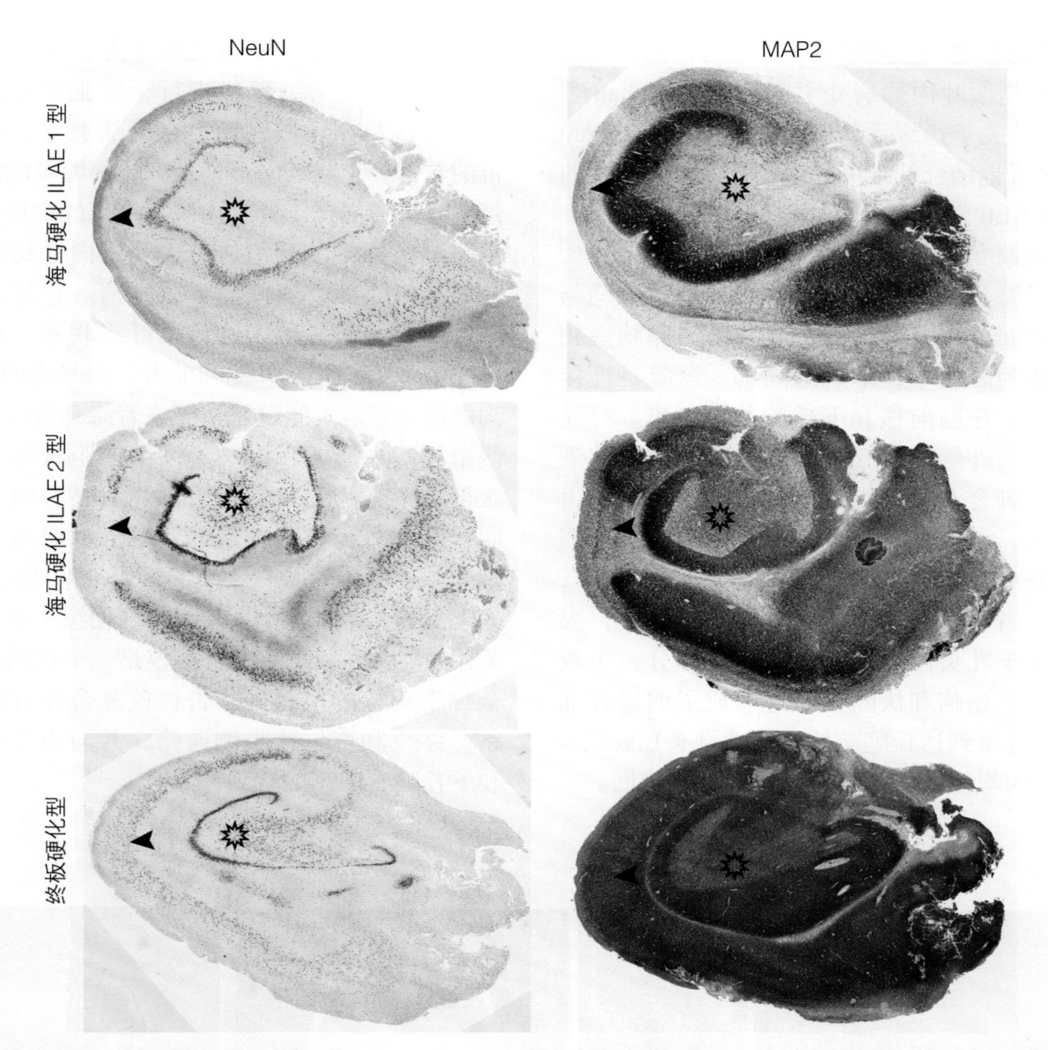

图 81.4　海马硬化（HS）亚型。左侧显示海马切片，NeuN（神经元细胞核）染色，右侧 MAP2（神经元胞体和树突）染色。星号表示 CA4，箭头表示 CA1。这些是决定 2013 年 ILAE 海马硬化分类中 HS 模式的主要区域。在 HS 1 型，CA4 和 CA1 有神经元丢失。在 2 型，主要神经元丢失仅限于 CA1。在最下面一行，CA4 神经元缺失最少。注：在 HS 3 型中，仅在 CA4 区可见神经元丢失和胶质增生，而在 CA1 区未见神经元丢失和胶质增生。
NeuN，神经元核抗原；MAP2，微管相关蛋白 -2

起的炎症反应在 HS 中已有报道，癫痫发作诱导的神经元缺失机制和发育过程中的异常可能是原因之一（Thom，2014）。HS 的影像学特征包括海马萎缩，T1 加权像体积减小，T2 加权像和 FLAIR 信号强度增加（图 81.5）。自动分割分析可以量化海马硬化，因此强烈推荐使用。

边缘系统的解剖

Papez 环路起自海马体，经穹隆至乳头体，然后通过乳头丘脑束传递到丘脑前核，并通过纤维投射至扣带回和海马回。边缘系统包括 Papez 环路及其相关的皮质下核团，包括杏仁核、下丘脑和隔核。它由白质和灰质组成，是大脑中涉及情感、记忆和学

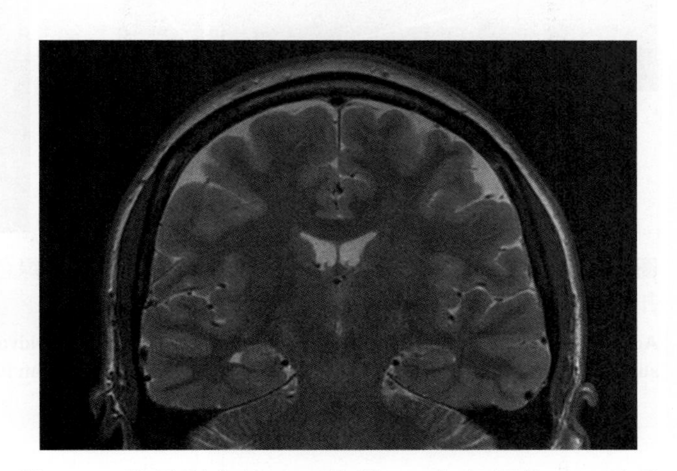

图 81.5　海马硬化的 MRI 特征：T2 加权冠状 MRI 显示右侧海马硬化，信号强度增加，海马萎缩，致脑室颞角更突出

习的最原始的部分之一。边缘系统是癫痫传播网络的一部分，尤其是颞叶内侧病变引起的癫痫。Shah 等（2012）发表了关于边缘系统的解剖学综述，Catani 等（2013）最近也结合纤维束成像修订了边缘系统的模型（另见**图** 81.6）。

海马构成颞角底壁的内侧部分，位于下托上，而下托构成了海马旁回的上表面。海马沟将海马与下托和海马旁回分离。海马的白质纤维与侧脑室相邻，向后延伸为海马伞，形成穹隆脚。穹隆是连接海马与乳头体、丘脑前核和下丘脑的投射束。穹隆脚向上弯曲并向外侧绕过丘脑枕。在胼胝体压部下方与对侧穹隆脚合并形成穹隆体。穹隆的两个脚由海马连合连接。穹隆体向前延伸至丘脑前端，两侧的纤维再次分离，并在 Monroe 脑室孔前向下拱起，形成穹隆柱。当穹隆的纤维接近前连合时分裂，大多数纤维终止于乳头体，形成了后连合部分，少数纤维与隔核、下丘脑和伏隔核相连形成了前连合部分。上升白质纤维到达丘脑前核，形成乳头丘脑束；从丘脑前核与内囊前肢的纤维汇合，到达扣带回。

扣带是一个位于胼胝体上方、平行于胼胝体的联合束。在前方，纤维走行于胼胝体嘴部下方的胼胝体下区。在后方，扣带在压部上方变窄，形成扣带的峡部。它继续向下延伸到毗邻海马的海马旁回前部。海马旁回位于颞叶内侧和下部的交界处。内嗅区由海马旁回的前部组成，内嗅区内含钩回，钩内含杏仁核。然而，后侧面界限不清。它与海马、皮质联系区包含较多传入和传出纤维联系，形成一个重要的中继中心。在外侧和前方，海马旁回受鼻沟（侧沟的前方延续）的限制，标志着海马旁回内嗅区的外侧范围。在后方，海马旁回由前距状沟分为扣带回峡部，上方为扣带回，下部为海马旁回，继续为舌回，下部分为扣带回峡部和下部的海马旁回，分别称为扣带回和舌回 [在后部，海马旁回由前距状沟分为上方的扣带回峡部（与扣带回相续）和下方的海马旁回（与舌回相续）]。杏仁核是一个核团复合体，完全位于钩核的范围内。杏仁核复合体有两条主要通路，终纹和杏仁核腹侧通路，并与边缘系统、丘脑和下丘脑有广泛的联系。

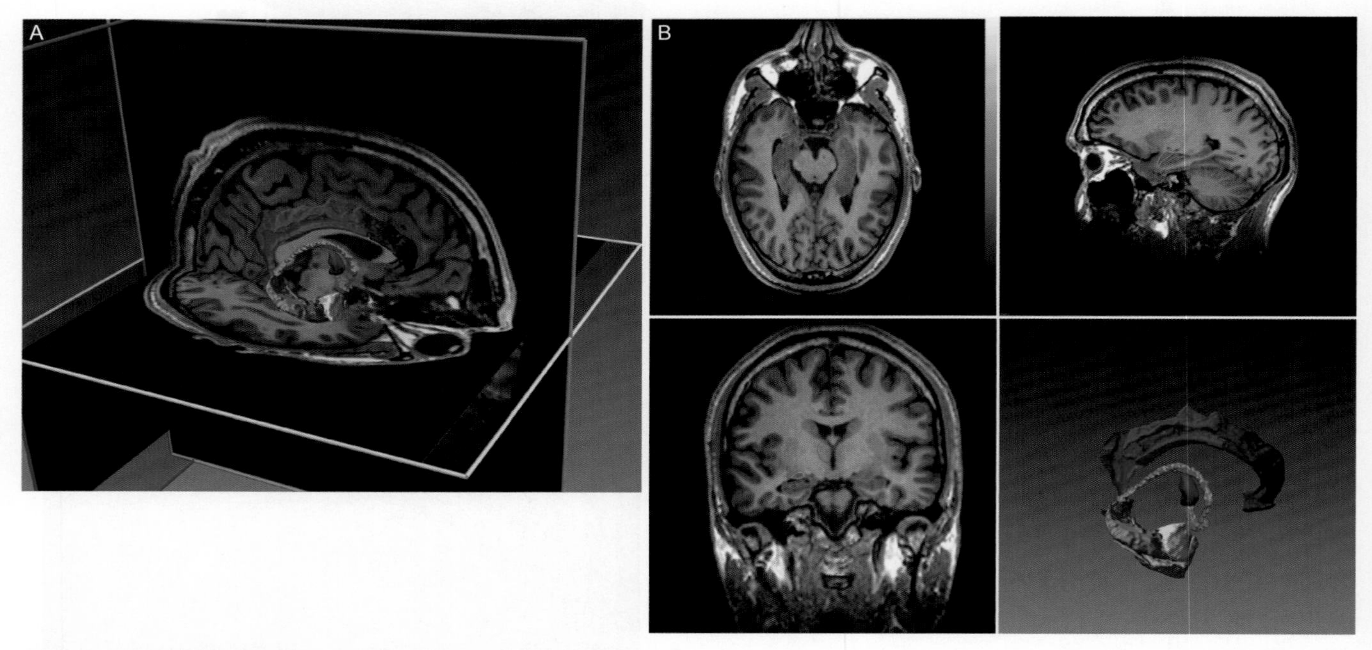

图 81.6　边缘系统 MRI T1 加权序列分割：海马穹隆 = 绿色，乳头体 = 红色，乳头丘脑束 = 粉红色，丘脑前部 = 紫色，扣带回 = 蓝色，海马旁回 = 橙色，杏仁核 = 黄色

Adapted from *Epilepsy & Behavior*, Volume 20, issue 2, Nancy Foldvary-Schaefer, Kanjana Unnwongse, Localizing and lateralizing features of auras and seizures, pp. 160–6, Copyright (2011), with permission from Elsevier.

延伸阅读、参考文献、EBRAIN 的相关链接

扫描书末二维码获取。

第 82 章　癫痫的诊断和评估

Richard Selway 著
韩春雷、解自行、张超男 译，孟凡刚、邵晓秋 审校

引言

关于癫痫的描述最早可追溯到公元前 2 世纪，苏美尔文及后来的巴比伦文称其为“跌倒性疾病（falling sickness）”。癫痫“epilepsy”一词源自希腊语“epilambanein”，意为“夺取（seize）”或“攻击（attack）”。发作（seizure）一词则来自于拉丁文的 sacire，意为 to claim。

因此，尽管希波克拉底在其 5 世纪著名的“神圣疾病（the sacred disease）”论文中已意识到癫痫起源于大脑，但在其大部分历史中，癫痫被认为是一个被邪灵附体的超自然发作性疾病。

19 世纪，随着神经病学发展成为一个独立的学科，大家对癫痫的理解也在进步。John Hughlings Jackson 将局灶性癫痫与脑局部病变联系起来，并开始了关于原发性癫痫（大脑在宏观上是正常的）和继发性癫痫（具有确切的基础病变）之间的区别以及哪一个才代表“真正的癫痫”的长期争论。

Jackson 和 Todd 提出了异常放电的概念，随着 Hans Berger 在 1929 年描记出脑电图之后，这种观点得到了进一步的证实。

如今，癫痫被认为是一种电磁方面的疾病，但其长期被曲解。在 19 世纪的大部分时间里，情绪、行为或人格障碍也认为是癫痫。

最近，人们认识到癫痫的社会经济负担，该病仍然带有重要的社会特征。此外，随着对神经网络的理解的提高，已经出现了新的神经调控技术，作为传统药物和切除性手术治疗的辅助手段。

什么是发作？

是由大脑内神经元异常、过度、同步化的电活动所引起的一过性体征和（或）症状。

什么是癫痫？

是以持久易感、易产生发作为特征的脑部疾病。临床上一般指间隔至少 24 小时以上，有 2 次突发的发作。

2014 年，国际抗癫痫联盟（International League Against Epilepsy，ILAE）工作组提出了更加实用的定义（Fisher et al.，2014）：

满足以下任何一条即可诊断为癫痫：

1. 至少两次非诱发性（或反射性）发作，两次发作间隔 24 小时以上；
2. 一次非诱发性发作，并且在未来 10 年中再次发作的可能性与两次非诱发性发作（非反射性）后再发风险（至少 60%）相当；
3. 诊断为癫痫综合征。

非诱发性是指没有潜在的急性病变，如戒酒、电抽搐治疗、脑炎、头部外伤或低血糖，这些病变可能会使健康人出现发作。

在小部分患者中，发作可由不会引起普通人群发作的特定刺激诱发（闪光灯、视觉模式、音乐、阅读、智力活动），称为反射性发作。有关发作分类和定义的完整讨论，请参见**第 82 章**。

流行病学

癫痫是最常见的严重神经系统疾病。全世界癫痫患者超过 6000 万人，无性别和种族差异，发达国家的年发病率为 45~50 例 /10 万人。在发达国家和发展中国家，癫痫的时点患病率（point prevalence）为 1%，终生发病率为 4% ~5%。

癫痫的发病率随年龄变化很大（见**图 82.1**）。

癫痫的发病在发达国家有两个高峰期：年轻人，尤其是出生的头几个月（一半的病例开始于儿童期或青春期）；65 岁以上的人群（由于脑血管疾病）。

总体而言，儿童的发病率正在降低，而老年人的发病率却急剧上升。的确，老年已经成为一生中最常见的癫痫发病阶段。在发展中国家，年轻人中有第三个发病高峰，这可能与脑外伤有关。

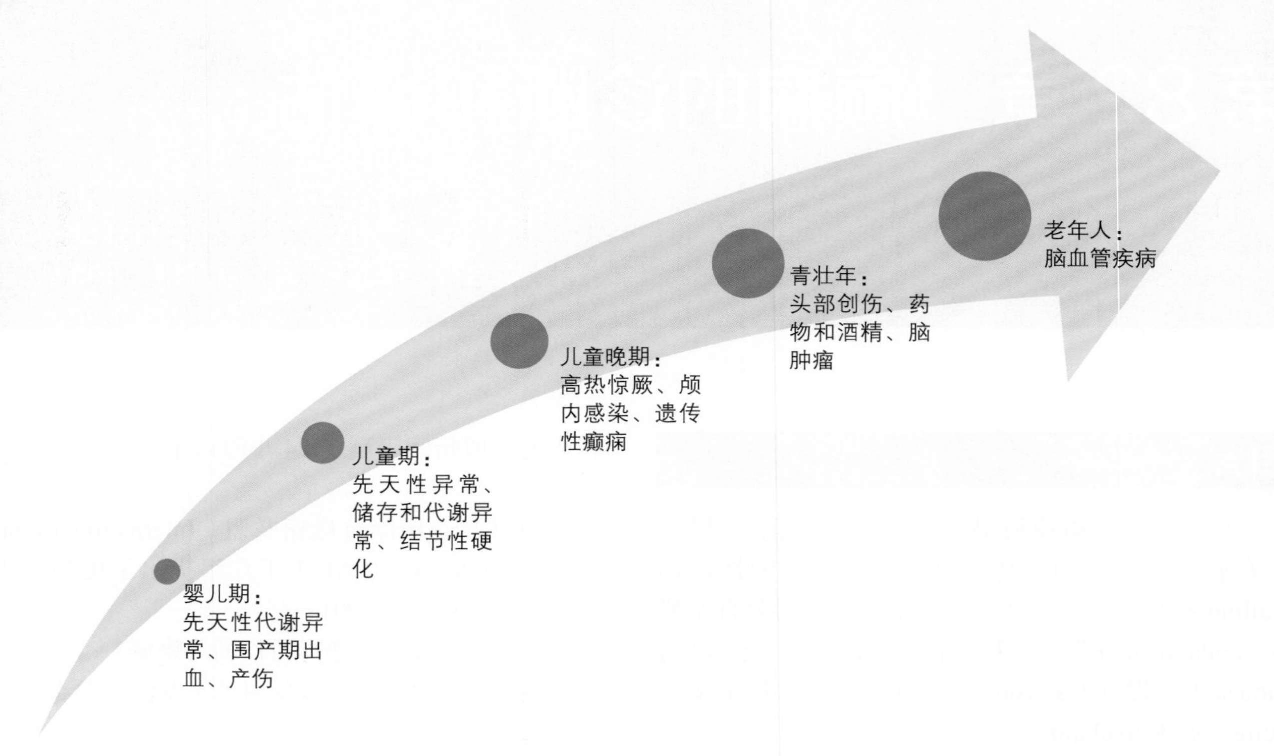

图 82.1 癫痫的病因按年龄进行划分。明尼苏达州罗切斯特市癫痫的发病率、患病率、累积发病率和死亡率，1935—1984 年

Reprinted from Mayo Clinic Proceedings, Volume 71, issue 6, W. Allen Hauser, John F. Annegers, Walter A. Rocca, *Descriptive Epidemiology of Epilepsy: Contributions of Population-Based Studies From Rochester, Minnesota*, pp. 576–86, Copyright (1996), with permission from Elsevier.

癫痫也是导致精神性疾病的第二大常见原因，尤其是在年轻人中。1/3 的患者会严重担忧自己的情绪问题。抑郁、焦虑和精神病常见，并且对患者的生活质量影响重大。抑郁症往往不能得到充分认识和治疗，伴有抑郁症的癫痫患者的总体自杀率是普通人群的 5 倍。焦虑会明显损害患者的社会心理功能，据报道，15%以上的颞叶癫痫患者中患有精神病。

癫痫会影响日常生活的方方面面，影响社交、就业和驾驶，并且经常需要对生活方式进行重大调整。因此，尽管发作的多少与患者的生活质量不成正比，但它在疾病本身之外又承担了巨大的负担（Gillam，1982）。

尽管如此，大多数癫痫患者预后良好，虽然这在很大程度上取决于具体病因。许多儿童癫痫综合征会在十几岁末期或成年早期消失。相反，很大一部分人癫痫会复发或患有终生无法治愈的发作。预后不良的标志包括症状性的病因、脑电图（EEG）上的广泛的癫痫样活动，对初始抗癫痫药（antiepileptic drug，AED）治疗的反应较差，并发的精神病史和癫痫家族史。

据估计，2/3 的癫痫患者可通过服用抗癫痫药物来控制发作。其余未控制发作的患者可选择外科治疗，因为一定比例患者（比例取决于选择标准，最高可达 60%）可从中受益，外科治疗可显著改善其发作，甚至在某些情况下可达到治愈（Brodie et al., 2012）。

癫痫的突然意外死亡

标准化死亡比（standardized mortality ratio，SMR），即观察到的死亡人数 / 预期死亡人数，用以比较特定疾病人群与年龄和性别相匹配的对照人群的死亡率。癫痫患者的标准化死亡比是普通人群的 2~3 倍。

当除去因潜在病因、事故和创伤及相关心理并发症导致的死亡，癫痫患者仍有不明原因突然死亡的风险。癫痫的意外死亡（sudden unexplained death in epilepsy，SUDEP）可能占所有癫痫死亡的 17%（年发生率为 0.35~10/1000）。

SUDEP 是指“癫痫患者突然的、难以预料的、有或没有目击者、非创伤性的、非溺水的死亡，并且尸检显示没有毒性或解剖性的死亡原因”。尽管其中一些死亡可能与未监测到的发作有关，但也有一些可能是心律不齐引起的。

遗传综合征

遗传易感性可能是综合征或非综合征的，其病因范围很广，包括形态、代谢和血管的异常。当有相关特征或家族史时，应考虑对有发作的儿童进行基因筛查。

发热惊厥

发热惊厥很常见，占所有发作的5%，与发热有关（通常在快速上升阶段），并且没有任何其他病因的证据。根据定义，发热惊厥发生在5个月 ~5岁，如果没有并发症，通常认为是良性的，尽管每3个儿童中就有1个会复发，而5%的儿童随后会发展为癫痫（50%以上的内侧颞叶硬化患者有发热惊厥史）。在指定年龄段以外出现的发作不应以上述相同的方式考虑，并且预后要差得多。

当发热惊厥具有局灶性癫痫、持续时间超过15分钟、24小时内复发、局灶性神经功能异常或癫痫家族史等不良特征时，发生癫痫的风险会增加3倍。

治疗通常采用对症和支持治疗，并加用解热药，如扑热息痛（对乙酰氨基酚）。在无并发症的情况下，不建议进行温水擦拭和长期的AED治疗。

诊断

从广义上讲，发作可分为部分性（局灶性）或全面性发作。前者起源于皮质结构，尽管可能继发为全面性发作，但通过其症状学可将发作定侧于特定的半球或定位于特定的脑叶或该脑叶内特定的区域（例如外侧颞叶新皮质与内侧颞叶结构）。相反，全面性发作则认为是起源于深部的中线结构，并同时扩散至双侧半球（“中心脑理论”）。

在发作的传统命名规则中，如果意识保留，则将其称为“简单性”发作；如果意识丧失，则称为“复杂性”发作。

一个发作可能特征性的表现为前驱症状、先兆、发作和发作后期，所有这些都可能有助于发作在中枢神经系统的定位。

前驱症状是指行为或情绪变化，可能出现在发作之前，有时甚至是发作前几个小时。不能将其视为癫痫电发作的一部分。

先兆即患者在发作之前的主观感受，例如颞叶发作时的胃部感觉。先兆属于癫痫电发作的一部分（简单部分性发作，其可扩散到更广的大脑范围从而产生客观发作）。发作后，患者可表现出定向不能或出现自动症状，即所谓的发作后期。

发作症状学

对发作的描述（“症状学”）是定位发作起源和扩散的第一步。虽然下表描述的症状是典型的发作传播，但实际情况常更复杂。例如，大多数枕叶部分性发作可能会扩散至颞叶内侧结构，从而产生具有两个部位特征的症状。仔细询问病史并观察视频中的典型发作，可以更好地了解起源部位和传播途径（**表82.1**）。

颞叶癫痫

颞叶癫痫是一组异质性疾病，在解剖学上大致分为起源于颞叶外侧新皮质和颞叶内侧区域（杏仁核和海马）的癫痫。

内侧颞叶癫痫的发病率是普通癫痫的2倍，最常继发于海马硬化，因此称为内侧颞叶硬化。其他原因包括肿瘤（特别是胚胎发育不良性神经上皮瘤，即DNET）、皮质发育不良、错构瘤和血管病变（如海绵状血管瘤）。

内侧颞叶硬化

内侧颞叶硬化是耐药性颞叶癫痫中最常见的病理类型，也是最明确的癫痫综合征之一，在MRI上具有明确的海马病变，海马CA1和CA3区神经元丢失是其典型的临床表现，而且至关重要的是手术切除后症状可缓解。

内侧颞叶硬化可能占癫痫患者的20%，接受颞叶切除术后65%患者的发作可得到控制。

发作通常在青春期之前出现，12岁左右，其中一半患者在儿童期都有热惊厥史。发作通常以自主神经性先兆开始，胃气上升感最常见，也可出现复杂的嗅觉或味觉感觉。随后是复杂部分性发作，伴意识障碍，最初为行为中止和凝视，随后是口咽和手部自动症（咀嚼、咂嘴、摸索或拽衣服），持续数分钟，患者不能回忆。对侧肢体通常伴有肌张力障碍性姿势异常。发作后意识模糊及情感症状如精神病或焦虑常见。继发全面性发作非常罕见。

影像学上特征性表现为MRI海马萎缩，T2或FLAIR序列为高信号，EEG上呈现前颞叶发作间期

表 82.1 发作的定侧和定位特征

定侧特征	
优势半球	发作期和发作后语言障碍
非优势半球	发作期言语 发作期自动症伴意识保留
同侧半球	单侧眨眼 手部自动症
对侧半球	单侧发作期阵挛（即有节奏的抽搐）或肌张力障碍性活动（持续的肌肉收缩） 上肢肌张力障碍
定位特征	
额叶	发作时间短（小于 2 分钟），特征刻板，意识保留 经常是夜间丛集性发作 运动症状突出（“过度运动发作”），有时剧烈但动作协调，可能误认为是夜惊、梦游或愤怒
初级感觉运动区	强直、阵挛、肌阵挛或失张力 Jackson 扩布 Todd 麻痹
眶额皮质	重复性手势自动症 认知障碍：意识或反应能力改变 幻嗅 自主神经症状
额极皮质	认知障碍 自主神经症状 轴向抽搐导致跌倒 最初的同侧头和眼偏转 强迫思维
额叶背外侧皮质	经常的强直运动 头眼对侧偏转（额眼区） 强迫思维和动作（即强迫地盯着某一物体） 优势侧可出现言语障碍
扣带回皮质	发作时伴随意识丧失的姿势自动症 情感先兆（如恐惧、抑郁、快乐、愤怒） 自主神经特征（如心悸、排尿或排便冲动） 痴笑自动症
中央区（辅助运动区、额顶岛盖、旁中央小叶）	不对侧强直姿势突然出现 / 中止，小于 60 秒，发作意识模糊轻 向癫痫起始半球对侧伸展上肢 同侧上肢屈曲（双上肢姿势似“4”字症） 头眼对侧偏转 发作时大叫或言语停止
岛盖 / 岛叶	面部阵挛动作 喉部症状 发音困难 多涎 味觉幻觉

（续表）

定位特征	
顶叶	对侧感觉先兆，同侧为感觉障碍 +/- 麻木、刺痛、蠕动感 可表现为 Jackson 扩布模式 疼痛，多为烧灼感 身体扭曲的幻觉 身体缩小 / 肿胀感（micro/macrosomatognosia） 身体延长 / 缩短（hyper/hyposchematica） 若中央旁小叶的生殖器感觉区受累可出现性冲动 以阅读、计算及书写为主的语言障碍
枕叶	发作起源对侧视野视觉先兆 多色形状（如圆形或闪光） 视觉受损（如：黑矇、暗斑、黑斑或白斑） 视觉幻觉（往往累及更前面的结构甚至延伸至颞叶） 静止或移动的人、动物或场景的图片 视错觉 非优势顶叶受累出现视空间知觉的改变 视物变大变小 物体显得小而远（teleopsia） 视像存留（视觉保留） 癫痫性眼震 快成分远离致痫灶，慢成分朝向致痫灶 眼球运动特征（如眼睑扑动、强迫闭眼）
颞叶	复杂先兆（如似曾相识感，常有胃气上升感，或听觉嗡嗡声） 行为中止——患者停止他们正在做的事情，凝视 意识丧失，表示颞叶癫痫的扩散同时累及对侧（复杂部分性癫痫） 自动症：口咽部 +/- 姿势性 自主神经特征：面色苍白、心悸 发作后意识模糊和头痛
内侧颞叶	一种独特的先兆，或孤立地出现，或随后伴有意识缓慢进行性障碍的行为中止，以及口咽部和手部的自动症 上腹胀感或腹部不适 似曾相识感（déjà-vu）、识旧如新（jamais-vu） 咀嚼、咂嘴、吞咽 自主神经特征 同侧瞳孔扩张 对侧上肢肌张力障碍，头眼偏转 持续时间长于外侧颞叶发作
外侧颞叶新皮质	伴有听觉、复杂视觉、幻觉或眩晕特征的起始先兆 嗡嗡声或鸣叫声，如仅在一只耳中听到，提示起源于对侧半球 先兆更短，意识改变更早和发作时间更短 更容易演变为双侧抽搐

棘波。参见**图** 82.2。

虽然大多数海马硬化患者以单侧病变为主，但大部分患者在脑电图上也会出现双颞叶棘波，至少30% 的患者在视频脑电监测上会出现明显的双侧发作期 EEG 改变。11% 患者的发作期 EEG 出现于真正起源侧的对侧。这既可能反映双侧致痫灶发作起源，也可能反映由单一起源迅速扩散至对侧引起的双侧功能紊乱。采用常规头皮电极记录时，致痫灶往往距离很远，且可迅速传播到对侧结构，然后首先传播至对侧半球的表面。在这种情况下，在行颞叶切除前，评估语言优势侧和对侧半球的记忆储备往往是有用的。

颞叶癫痫最初可能对 AED 反应良好，但从成年早期开始，发作逐渐耐药。手术切除（前颞叶整块

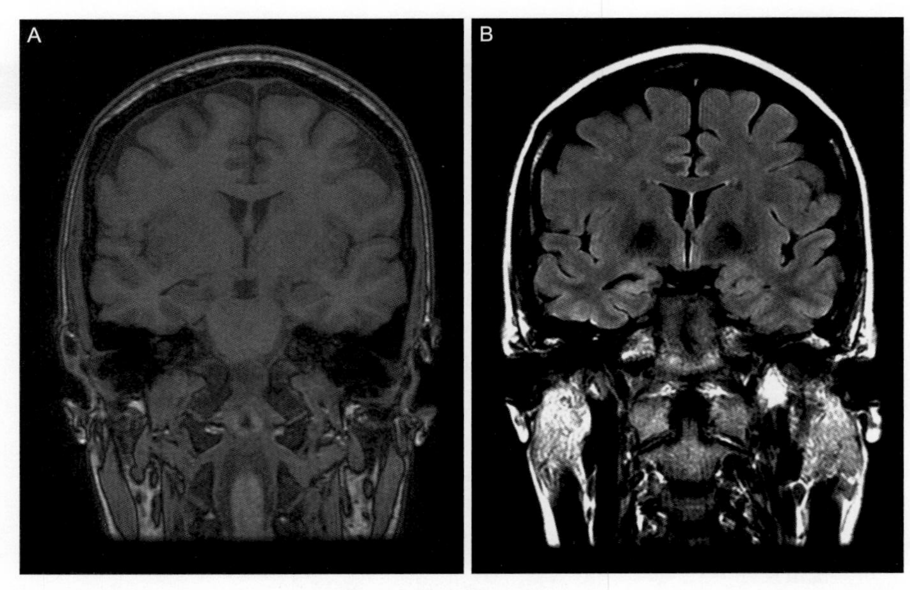

图 82.2 MRI 冠状位显示海马体积缩小、继发性颞角扩大及信号改变。冠状位 SPGR（A）和 FLAIR（B）MR 序列显示右侧海马低 T2 信号和体积缩小

切除术或选择性的海马杏仁核切除术）具有极好的效果，癫痫无发作率可达 80%。

检查

癫痫外科医生需要怎样的信息？一旦出现药物难治性，就需要进一步研究以定位致痫灶并确定潜在的病变。

这通常包括高分辨率的含有 FLAIR 序列的 MRI 扫描，以识别肿瘤性、血管性或发育性病理，以及头皮视频脑电监测。

脑电图

脑电图记录大脑不同区域的电活动，它记录的是神经元活动产生的复合电场（主要来自大脑皮质的突触后电位）。

脑电图记录通常通过头皮电极（头皮脑电监测）获得。视频脑电监测可同步记录电发作和临床发作，以促进致痫灶的定位。

表面电极为银质盘状，放置于患者头皮表面，以覆盖临床相关区域。电极放置最常用的惯例是“10-20”系统，其中电极的放置和识别采用字母和数字，例如 F（额部）、T（颞部）、Fp（额极），奇数覆盖左半球，数值越小代表位置越靠前和内侧（例如 F7 表示左侧额后外侧的位置）。

脑电图记录的是两个电极之间的电位差（以毫伏计）。若记录相邻电极的电位差，即为双极导联。另一种参考导联方法可以突出特定的脑电特征或尽量减少伪迹（即干扰），例如，参考单级导联法是将某个特点的电极触点与所有其他导联进行比较。

背景活动就是指持续的电活动。其中可见几种随年龄、时间、部位、临床活动相关的节律。需要重点关注阵发性活动，因为其本质上可能是发作。

图 82.3 是展示了闭眼时出现 α 活动爆发的脑电图。

侵入性 EEG

侵入性脑电图（invasive EEG，iEEG）需要在颅内放置记录电极，在一些患者中用于癫痫的术前评估或在手术中进行监测。而通过插入脑实质或病变内部的深部电极记录的脑电则称为立体定向脑电图技术（stereoencephalography，SEEG）。通过放置在暴露的脑表面硬膜下的网格或条状电极记录的脑电称为皮质脑电图（electrocorticography，ECoG），它可以在术中或术后进行记录。电极置入后，停用抗癫痫药，视发作频率记录 3~14 天，以确定致痫区的位置。

当头皮脑电图的信息不足以精确地定位致痫区或界定致痫区的边界时，就需使用侵入性脑电图。当无创性检查结果不一致、发作间期数据与发作症状学不一致或存在双重病理 / 发作部位不明确时，采用 iEEG 是有价值的，比如在头皮脑电图上看到双侧放电。两个进一步的例子是颞叶癫痫手术前头皮

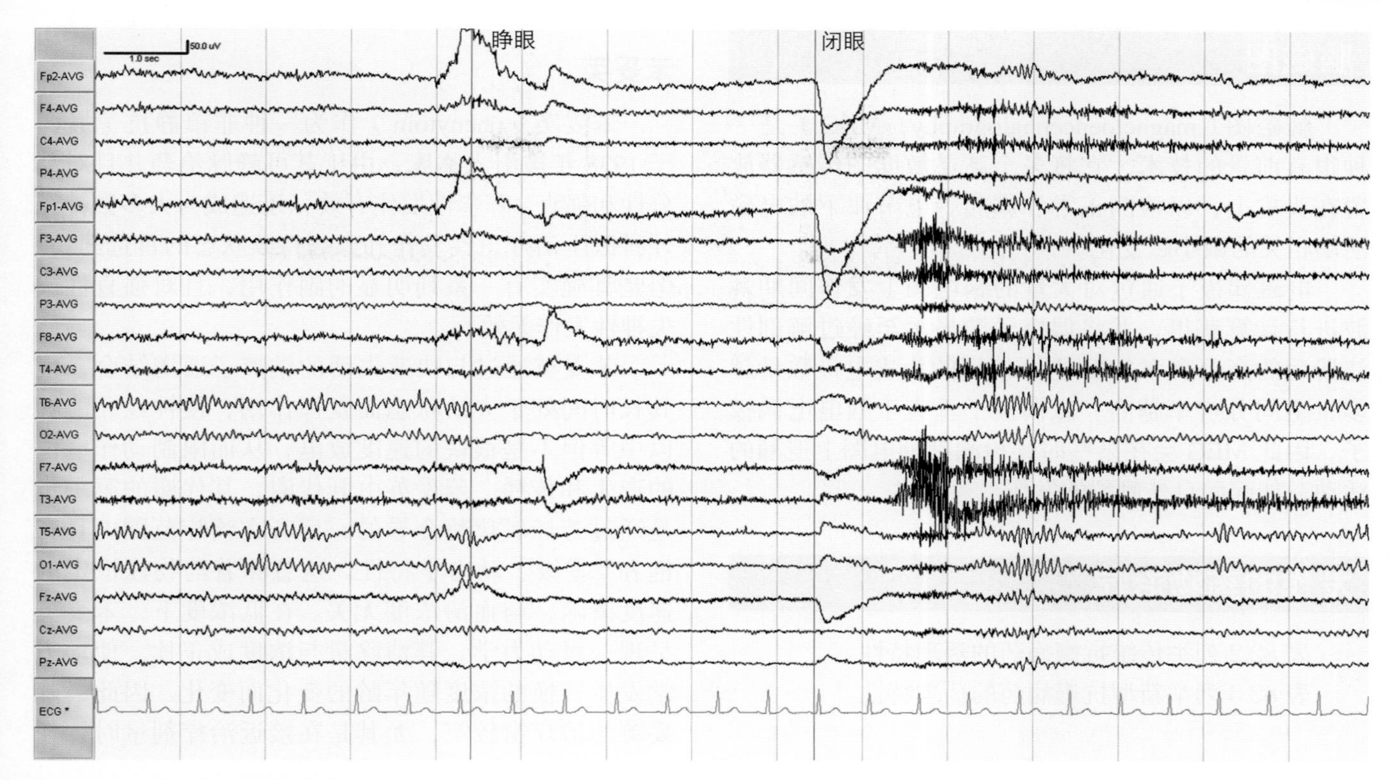

图 82.3　正常脑电图示闭眼时 α 活动爆发

Courtesy of Mr Robert Morris, Addenbrooke's Hospital, UK.

EEG 示双侧颞叶存在独立棘波和 MRI 上存在双侧海马硬化。颞叶外或非病变性颞叶癫痫手术前需进行侵入性脑电记录。此外，在功能区附近新皮质切除术前，可通过这些电极进行刺激和记录诱发的反应来鉴别和界定功能区。

硬膜下条状电极的触点呈单列排列，而硬膜下栅状电极在电极排列上则具有不同的设计构型和尺寸。这些电极通常是不锈钢的，但是铂电极是非磁性的，因此 MRI 兼容但价格昂贵。这些方法的采样脑区有限，因此术前计划对这些电极的放置至关重要。深部电极在神经导航或机器人辅助下通过颅骨钻孔放置的套管植入。一根电极通常有 4~10 个触点，但采样区域仍然有限，通常是针对深部的区域，如岛叶、海马或杏仁核。平行于海马旁回，从枕部入颅放置双侧电极，可以使多个记录触点覆盖到内侧颞叶起源的发作活动。

硬脑膜下栅状电极的放置需要开颅暴露皮质表面，特别注意在半球间及颞下放置时硬脑膜下桥静脉的阻挡。栅状电极可以覆盖更广泛的皮质，但无法达到深部结构。不建议放置双侧硬膜下栅状电极。尽管硬膜下条状电极可以通过钻孔放置，但是安全性要低于开颅放置，且易出现位置偏差。在一些复杂病例中，可以同时放置硬膜下电极和深部电极，从而结合使用 SEEG 和 ECoG 进行脑电图采集。

核医学成像

当 EEG、MRI 和发作模式在定侧或脑叶定位上不一致时，或确实存在 MRI 阴性但确凿的电生理异常时，发作间期 FDG-PET 扫描或（如可能）发作期单光子发射计算机断层扫描（SPECT）扫描的核成像或可提供有用的信息。

FDG-PET 检测的是发作间期区域性脑组织的糖代谢水平。包括致痫灶在内的皮质区域的低代谢是很典型的，而且左右对比代谢是否对称，可以区分真正的致痫灶和一些常表现低代谢的区域，如双侧丘脑。

相反，致痫灶在发作期 SPECT 上是高代谢的。SPECT 检查需要在发作开始后，发作尚未扩散之前，尽早注射示踪剂。示踪剂将稳定存在于在大脑内，其浓度与那一刻的血流成正比。可在接下来的几个小时内进行图像采集。在几秒内向发生自发性发作的患者注射放射标记的化合物，在技术方面极具挑战性，这使得这项检查成为一个困难和特殊的检查。

这两项检查获得的图像分辨率低，均需要与 MRI 融合以获得更好的分辨率和解剖学定位。

脑磁图

脑磁图（magnetoencephalography，MEG）是一种很有前景的技术，它将多个高灵敏度的传感器放置在头皮上，以检测正常和癫痫脑电节律下的电磁活动相关的微小磁变化。

电磁偶极子通过对大量的脑电图上发作间期棘波进行计算获得，并将偶极子源显示至经过解剖性注册后的高分辨率 MRI 上。使用的头皮电极数量越多，空间分辨率越高。磁偶极子垂直于脑电电偶极子，因此 MEG 会在某些时候检测到脑电图上遗漏的活动，如起源自外侧裂的发作。

发作的药物治疗

表 82.2 列举传统抗癫痫药的药理特性。

表 82.3 列举新型抗癫痫药的药理特性。

苯妥英

苯妥英（phenytoin）作为一种非镇静抗惊厥药于 1938 年被引入临床，由于其可静脉给药并且对部分性和强直 - 阵挛性发作有效，迅速成为大多数神经外科医生治疗急性发作和癫痫持续状态的首选药物。但是其确实有一系列明显的副作用，且对强直性或失神性发作无效。

苯妥英通过与快速失活的钠离子通道结合，使其长时间处于失活状态而发挥作用，使神经元能够以中等但不是很快的速度放电，从而限制动作电位的产生和传播。苯妥英由肝代谢，其代谢的第一步是通过芳烃氧化酶介导的，后者在治疗范围内具有饱和（零级）动力学特性。这意味着药物以恒定的速度清除，与血清浓度无关。在低浓度下，苯妥英呈现一级动力学，其清除量与浓度成正比。使动力学发生转换的浓度随年龄的变化而变化。因此，苯妥英的治疗窗较窄，尤其是在接近治疗剂量时，任

表 82.2　传统抗癫痫药的药理特性

药物	主要作用方式	适应证（发作类型）	吸收率（生物利用度%）	蛋白质结合率（结合%）	清除半衰期（小时）	清除途径	目标血清浓度
卡马西平	钠离子通道阻断	部分性、全面性	慢（75~80）	80	24~48	肝代谢	4~12 mg/L
氯巴占	GABA 能	部分性、全面性、部分性癫痫持续状态	快（90~100）	90	10~30	肝代谢	无
苯巴比妥	GABA 能	部分性、全面性、肌阵挛性、癫痫持续状态	慢（95~100）	50	72~144	肝，25% 排泄不变	10~40 mg/L
苯妥英	钠离子通道阻断	部分性、全面性、肌阵挛性、癫痫持续状态	慢（85~90）	90	24（9~40）	可饱和的肝代谢	10~20 mg/L
丙戊酸钠	多效应	部分性、全面性、肌阵挛性、失神性	快（100）	90	7~17	肝代谢	50~100 mg/L

表 82.3　新型抗癫痫药的药理特性

药物	主要作用方式	适应证	吸收率（生物利用度%）	蛋白质结合率（结合%）	清除半衰期（小时）	清除途径
加巴喷丁	结合钙离子通道	部分性	慢（60）	0	6~9	不代谢，肾排泄
拉莫三嗪	钠离子通道阻滞	部分性、全面性	快（95~100）	55	22~36	葡萄糖醛酸化代谢
左乙拉西坦	不确定	部分性、全面性	快（95~100）	<10	6~8	非肝水解，肾排泄
奥卡西平	钠离子通道阻滞	部分性、全面性	快（95~100）	40	8~10	肝转化为活性成分
普瑞巴林	结合钙离子通道	部分性	快（95~100）	0	6	不代谢，肾排泄
拉考沙胺	钠离子通道阻滞	部分性	快（95~100）	<15	13	肝，40% 排泄不变
唑尼沙胺	多效应	部分性、全面性	快（95~100）	50	**50~70**	肝代谢，肾排泄

何微小的剂量变化都可能导致血药浓度的不成比例变化。

苯妥英可诱导肝酶，因此可降低其他 AED（如丙戊酸钠）和脂溶性药物（如华法林）的血清水平。早期非剂量相关的不良反应包括 5% 的患者出现皮疹（很少进展为全面的 Stevens-Johnson 综合征）。剂量相关的神经毒性副作用在血清水平低于 30 mg/L 时少见，通常在口服剂量后 8~12 小时出现，包括扑翼样震颤、共济失调、构音障碍、眼球震颤等。

长期用药与可逆的畸形作用（痤疮、面部特征变粗、牙龈肥大和几个月后出现的多毛症）以及多年治疗后出现的骨质疏松症（拮抗维生素 D）、周围神经病变和小脑萎缩有关。苯妥英因具有类似利奈卡因的抗心律失常作用，在Ⅱ度心肌梗死患者中禁用。苯妥英也可能引起骨髓抑制和 SLE 样综合征。妊娠期间用药与胎儿海因综合征（fetal hydantoin syndrome）有关，表现为面部畸形、唇腭裂、心脏缺陷。

卡马西平

卡马西平合成于 1953 年。它通过阻断电压依赖的钠通道，抑制去极化神经元动作电位的重复放电。卡马西平能诱导自身代谢，并能加速几种脂溶性药物的肝代谢，最常见的是口服避孕药。可抑制卡马西平代谢导致毒性的药物包括苯妥英和红霉素。

卡马西平是治疗部分性和强直 - 阵挛发作的一线有效药物，应尽量避免用于失神发作，因为可能会加重失神发作。起始剂量要低，并且逐渐增加剂量，以利于耐受其中枢神经系统副作用，并允许肝自动诱导。尽管如此，许多患者即使在低于治疗剂量时也不能耐受药物的神经毒性作用。

复视、头晕、头痛、恶心、呕吐是中枢神经系统（central nervous system，CNS）毒性最常见的征象。也可出现各种特异性反应，最常见的是 5%~10% 的患者出现麻疹样皮疹。血液障碍和中毒性肝炎少见，轻度白细胞减少也不罕见。在较高浓度时，卡马西平具有抗利尿激素样作用，导致低钠血症，常无症状。与大多数抗惊厥药一样，卡马西平具有潜在致畸作用。

奥卡西平

在功能上，奥卡西平是一种前体，在肝中迅速被还原成其活性代谢产物。与卡马西平一样，它阻断钠离子通道，还调节钙、钾通道。奥卡西平具有与卡马西平相似的疗效谱，并具有更好的耐受性和较少的神经毒性副作用。皮疹不太常见，但与卡马西平相似，可能很少与 Stevens-Johnson 综合征有关。低钠血症更常见。奥卡西平似乎不会引起血液紊乱或肝毒性。此外，对其自身代谢无影响。

加巴喷丁

加巴喷丁是通过在 GABA（γ 氨基丁酸，主要的抑制性神经递质）中加入环己基而形成的，可使其能够跨越血脑屏障。然而，尽管具有这样的结构，加巴喷丁并不与 GABA 受体结合。相反它与神经元电压门控钙通道的 alpha-2-delta 亚基结合，抑制突触前末梢的钙离子流动和神经递质释放。

加巴喷丁是治疗部分性发作的有效辅助药物，无论继发或不继发全面性发作。它也广泛应用于治疗神经病理性疼痛。

不良反应轻微且短暂，以共济失调、嗜睡和眼震最为常见。胃肠道症状，如胀气和腹泻，偶有报道。5% 的患者可体重增加，特别是高剂量用药时。因加巴喷丁不经肝代谢，不诱导或抑制肝酶，因此它不与其他药物相互作用。它全部经肾排泄。

丙戊酸钠

丙戊酸钠通过对钠离子通道发挥一种使用和电压依赖性作用，限制持续重复放电而发挥其抗癫痫作用。它还可促进 GABA 的作用，可用于所有类型的发作，特别适用于特发性全面性癫痫。它由肝代谢，但不影响口服避孕药的激素成分。因为它没有明显的浓度效应 - 毒性关系，常规的治疗监测是无益的。

副作用包括剂量相关的震颤、食欲刺激引起的体重增加、一过性脱发和月经紊乱。较不常见的是血小板减少症和隐匿性帕金森病，二者都是可逆的。传统上，接受神经外科干预的患者在择期干预前会因出血性风险而停用丙戊酸钠，但这种做法现已落伍。3 岁以下的儿童有肝毒性的危险，特别是当他们有并发的代谢紊乱时；高氨血症引起的昏迷和脑病少见。

对于育龄妇女，应该避免服用，因为有 3% 的神经管缺陷的风险，特别是每天服用的剂量超过 1000 mg。

氯巴占

氯巴占是苯二氮䓬类药物，是治疗部分性和全面性发作的有效辅助药物。它对 Lennox-Gastaut 综合征的儿童也有效。与其他苯二氮䓬类药物一样，它能增强 GABA 介导的氯通道效应，与 γ 亚基上的

$GABA_A$ 受体结合，增加通道开放频率，从而增强突触后抑制。其镇静效应弱于安定。它在肝中转化为许多代谢物。

由于存在药物耐受性，并不是所有的有反应者都能在长期服用氯巴占时在发作上得到满意的控制。间歇性使用药物可以减少这种情况。副作用包括抑郁、烦躁和嗜睡。它可能加重先前存在的行为和情绪障碍。

苯巴比妥

合成于 1912 年，是临床上最古老的抗惊厥药，通过延长 $GABA_A$ 受体的氯离子通道开放来增强 GABA 的作用，导致神经元超极化。

尽管苯巴比妥成本低，以及治疗发作和难治性癫痫持续状态的有效性确保了它仍然是发展中国家最重要的 AED 之一，但由于其易于引起镇静和行为问题，这使得此药有些过时了。

苯巴比妥的半衰期长达 4 天，因此，调整给药剂量时可能需要 3 周才能达到稳定血药浓度。它由肝代谢，是肝代谢的强效诱导剂，加速许多脂溶性药物的清除。副作用包括躁动、抑郁、极端年龄多动、过敏性皮疹、骨质疏松、Dupuytren 挛缩等。具有致畸性。要缓慢减药，否则会因撤药导致癫痫复发。

拉莫三嗪

拉莫三嗪是最有效的新型 AED 之一，对所有类型的发作均有效。它对伴有多种发作类型的患者有效，尤其是伴学习困难的患者，可能是因为它能减少发作间期棘波，有助于提高觉醒。

拉莫三嗪选择性阻断钠通道缓慢失活状态，从而阻止兴奋性氨基酸递质的释放，特别是天冬氨酸和谷氨酸。它不影响华法林或其他 AED 等脂溶性药物的代谢。

拉莫三嗪单药治疗时，其半衰期为 24 小时。当它与苯妥英等酶诱导剂结合时，下降到 15 小时。丙戊酸抑制拉莫三嗪的葡萄糖醛酸化，使其半衰期延长至 60 小时。因此，停用苯妥英会导致拉莫三嗪循环浓度升高，而停用丙戊酸钠会导致血浆拉莫三嗪水平下降。与丙戊酸钠合用时，拉莫三嗪剂量常规减半。

拉莫三嗪单药致畸的风险较低，使其成为希望怀孕且无法或不愿停用 AED 的育龄妇女的首选药物。共济失调、复视、头痛、失眠和震颤时有报道。3% 的患者在单药治疗（如果联合丙戊酸钠治疗的话，发生率为 8%）时出现自限性丘疹。采用渐进的药物滴定方案，成人发生报道所称的 1/1000 的严重皮肤反应风险的可能性微乎其微。

左乙拉西坦

左乙拉西坦是吡乙酰胺乙基类似物的对映异构体，其确切作用机制尚不清楚。但是，已知它可与突触囊泡胞吐作用相关的突触囊泡蛋白 2A（SV2A）结合，介导神经递质的释放。

左乙拉西坦的问世标志着癫痫治疗的一项重大突破，并迅速确定了自己在所有新型 AED 中最重要的地位。它对所有发作类型均有效，不会被肝代谢，因此没有明显的药物相互作用，不需要治疗监测，通常以其起始剂量就可以治疗，并且通常具有良好的耐受性。罕见的副作用包括虚弱和精神病，尤其是在有精神病和嗜睡史的年轻男性中。

癫痫持续状态

癫痫持续状态是指患者持续性发作或反复发作而间期意识未恢复，并超过 30 分钟以上。强直 - 阵挛性或惊厥性癫痫持续状态最易识别，它是致命性的紧急医疗事件。然而，1/4 的病例是非惊厥性的，无论是失神性还是复杂部分发作都需要通过电生理来诊断。

癫痫持续状态最常发生在 1 岁以内的婴儿和 65 以上的成人。最常见的原因是不规律服药及停用现有的抗癫痫药物。酒精滥用、药物中毒和急性代谢紊乱是新出现癫痫持续状态患者的最可能诱发因素。

发病率和死亡率反映了长期惊厥活动的潜在病因和生理后遗症，如心律不齐、循环衰竭、体温过高和缺氧。惊厥性癫痫持续状态的死亡率约为 10%，在体质不佳老年人中，死亡率可上升至 50%。创伤越严重（例如急性脑血管发作或创伤），死亡率也越高，而酒精中毒或 AED 停药引起的癫痫持续状态预后较好。

癫痫持续状态的治疗目的是及时终止发作以阻止由系统性或代谢性紊乱及电活动直接导致的兴奋性毒性引起的神经损伤。如果惊厥性癫痫持续状态超过 30 分钟，尤其超过 1~2 小时，持续性脑损伤的风险将会持续增加。这是因为 30 分钟内，自身代偿机制尚足以预防脑损伤，但是如果持续状态持续存在，自身代偿机制破坏，脑损伤则会迅速加重。即使不致命，神经损伤也会导致一过性或永久的神经系统的、癫痫引起的以及认知方面的后遗症。

因此，实际工作中，如果发作持续 5~10 分钟以上，大多数机构建议紧急治疗。任何延误都会使预后恶化，降低不需要全身麻醉而中止发作的可能性。见表 82.4。

选择合适的癫痫患者进行手术

癫痫外科的工作旨在逐步确定手术相关适应证，使发作得到有效控制，并使神经功能损害最小化。

- **第 1 步：确定手术的临床适应证**

首先要确定癫痫和发作的类型，尤其要排除非痫性发作。必须先尝试充分的药物治疗，尤其要正规服药。是否行手术治疗取决于无法控制的发作对患者及其生活质量造成了多大的影响。发作绝对频率多少时需行手术治疗因患者的观点及其职业的不同而异。这要求在考虑手术之前，有充足的时间以确定发作是充分不受控制的。另一方面，由于可能发生其他致痫灶的“点燃”，长期的癫痫病史会影响癫痫手术的成功。

- **第 2 步 确定手术切除的致痫灶**

对于大多数病例，进行发作症状学、影像学和头皮 EEG 记录的电信号进行临床评估就足够了。对于内侧颞叶硬化者，通过冠位 MRI 体积测量或 FLAIR 序列上异常的信号改变，再辅以 EEG，足以进行致痫灶定位。对于后者，就是在住院期间，在临时停药甚至诱发发作后，使用头皮视频脑电设备监测足够的时间以捕捉足够的发作。

当影像学和电生理结果不一致时，比如发作间期或发作期棘波源自对侧，则需要进一步的检查。实际上，发作期的 SPECT（如前所述）价值最大，因为间期改变模式可能不太清楚，并且鉴于所用放射性核素的半衰期非常短，发作期 PET 检查也不切实际。

更复杂的病例需要侵袭性评估方法，例如放置硬膜下栅状和（或）深部电极。这常用于颞叶外半球性癫痫，放置硬膜下栅状电极可覆盖此处的致痫灶。对于海马硬化患者，放置双侧的深部电极也可以定位或定侧致痫灶起源。经皮放置双侧卵圆孔（蝶骨）电极现已很少使用。

- **第 3 步：预测并使癫痫病灶切除术后的神经功能障碍最小化**

具有长期癫痫病史的患者，其致痫灶的功能转移也不多见。功能性移位的程度存在差异，这将取决于对侧半球以及可以代偿切除后丧失的神经功能的其他区域的完整性。对于致痫灶位于优势半球的颞叶癫痫，行保留颞叶新皮质的海马杏仁核切除术将有助于保留语言功能。在海马杏仁核切除术之前，

表 82.4 成人癫痫持续状态（SE）的治疗方案

阶段（时间）	操作
第 1 阶段 0~5 分钟 （可疑的 / 即将发生的癫痫持续状态）	• 通过注意反复发作的惊厥发作活动而无明显意识恢复来诊断 SE 或怀疑 SE • 建立并维持气道 • 氧含量（10 L/min） • 监测生命体征 • 建立静脉通路并开始输液（例如生理盐水 / 葡萄糖生理盐水） • 病因检查：抽血进行代谢化验、AED 水平和毒性筛查 • 如果怀疑有感染，考虑尽早使用抗生素 • 酗酒或酒精戒断使用硫胺素，纠正低血糖症
第 2 阶段 5~10 分钟 （癫痫持续状态早期）	• 应用速效苯二氮䓬类药物： 1. 劳拉西泮 0.1 mg/kg，2 mg/min 静脉注射 或 2. 地西泮（作用时间较短），0.2 mg/kg，5 mg/min 静注 • 如果 5 分钟后发作继续，则重复一次 • 如果无法静注，则考虑地西泮 500 μg/kg 灌肠，最大剂量 30 mg • 考虑使用咪达唑仑 10 mg
第 3 阶段 10~30 分钟 （进入癫痫持续状态）	采用长效抗惊厥药： 1. 苯妥英钠静注，15~20 mg / kg，成人速度不超过 50 mg/min；儿童不超过 1 mg/（kg · min）； 需要心电图（ECG）和血压监测 或 2. 左乙拉西坦静注 30~70 mg / kg，速度 500 mg / min 或 3. 拉考沙胺 5~6 mg/kg，速度 40~80 mg/min
第 4 阶段 30~60 分钟 （难治性癫痫持续状态）	• 在重症监护室全麻并监测脑电图以实现“爆发抑制” • 寻找潜在的病因并予以纠正 • 考虑进行颅内成像 • 考虑 1. 苯巴比妥静注 20 mg/kg（100 mg/min） 或 2. 咪达唑仑 0.2 mg/kg 静脉推注，然后 0.1~0.4 mg/kg/ 小时输注 或 3. 异丙酚 3~5 mg/kg 静脉推注，然后 5~10 mg/kg / 小时输注 或 4. 硫喷妥钠 2~3 mg/kg 静脉推注，然后 3~5 mg /（kg · h）输注

Source data from Shorvon, S. , Baulac, M. , Cross, H., Trinka, E. , Walker, M. and, (2008), The drug treatment of status epilepticus in Europe: Consensus document from a workshop at the first London Colloquium on Status Epilepticus. Epilepsia, 49: 1277–1285

明确对侧半球是否可以代偿记忆和认知功能是必要的。术前可采用具有记忆算法的 fMRI 进行评估，现已逐步取代了 WADA 试验。

神经心理学评估可评估认知功能并有助于制订术前计划以减少神经功能损害。它还可以识别并帮助最大程度减少手术造成的心理影响。

延伸阅读、参考文献、EBRAIN 的相关链接

扫描书末二维码获取。

第 83 章　癫痫的外科治疗

Johannes Schramm 著
刘冲、解自行、杨鹏达 译，孟凡刚、张凯 审校

引言

癫痫的外科治疗适用于药物难治性癫痫患者。根据国际抗癫痫联盟（International League against Epilepsy，ILAE）所述，药物难治性癫痫是指两种正确选择、可耐受的抗癫痫药物（antiepileptic drug，AED）经足够的疗程及剂量药物治疗仍未能控制发作的癫痫（Kwan et al.，2010）。在严重颅脑畸形导致的儿童早期灾难性癫痫病例中，可以在不进行 1~2 年抗癫痫药物治疗的情况下实施早期手术治疗。手术目的是切除致痫区和可能的致痫病变。姑息性治疗旨在减少癫痫发作频率。

术前

病史

病史记录是为了描述癫痫发作类型（局灶性与全身性），发现意识丧失（单纯部分性与复杂部分性）、先兆的发生、癫痫发作频率和严重程度，以及癫痫持续时间。仔细研究癫痫发作的症状学特征可以获取有关致痫区的重要提示。既往病史中可能发生过诱发因素，如幼儿热性惊厥、颅脑损伤、围产期脑缺氧、已知可引起脑炎的病毒感染，这需要与患者或家长讨论。仔细记录病史是至关重要的，也是术前评估的第一步。

影像

影像学检查主要采用 MRI，但 PET 和 SPECT 也经常使用。“标准”头颅 MRI 检查通常不能显示致痫病变，因此对药物难治性病例，建议遵循特殊的 MRI 检查方案（Wellmer et al.，2013）。这些作者提出了六种基本的 MRI 序列（FLAIR、T2 加权、T1 加权、含铁血黄素 / 钙化敏感序列）。T2 和 FLAIR 的断层厚度不得超过 3 mm。T1 像应该采用 3D 扫描方式，各向同性的体素值 1 mm。对于 T2 和 FLAIR 图像，海马角度至少需要两个断层方向。如果发现海马硬化以外的病变，则应在注射造影剂前后进行 T1 加权序列扫描（Wellmer et al.，2013）。fMRI 和基于 3D-T1 的形态学测量分析技术可分别用于语言区的定侧和重要功能白质束的可视化，从而提高了 MRI 的应用价值（Urbach et al.，2015）。SPECT 尤其适用于发作期 SPECT（即在发作开始后和发作期间注入放射性示踪剂）。发作期 SPECT 可以显示发作期高灌注区，并被认为是致痫区。根据注射示踪剂的时间点不同，可以更多地显示癫痫放电传播的区域，而较少显示癫痫起源区域。^{18}F 标记的氟脱氧葡萄糖的 PET 可以显示葡萄糖低代谢区域，被认为与致痫区一致。对于 MRI 未显示病变，但颞叶有明确 PET 阳性区域的患者，该技术尤其有用（Carne et al.，2004）。WADA 试验是指在颈内动脉注射一定量的异戊巴比妥溶剂，使同侧大脑半球在 4~5 分钟内失去功能，来判定语言的优势侧。目前主要用于大脑半球离断术和胼胝体切开术。在后一种情况下，可以排除将运动或感觉语言区域向对侧半球转移的可能性，如果计划进行全胼胝体切开术，可能会产生负面后果。

脑电图

手术患者行术前脑电图（electroencephalography，EEG）记录是必不可少的，但不同于常规脑电图检查。通常使用最高可达 68 通道的专门脑电设备进行记录，并采用分屏技术进行连续视频监控，癫痫症状可以与同一屏幕上实时显示的脑电图直接联系起来。为了记录典型的癫痫发作，术前视频脑电图需在停用 AED 药物后进行，以期获得癫痫起源的定位提示。如果 MRI 成像和视频脑电图具有一致结果，可以计划进行手术切除。若结果不一致或发作性活动区域与重要功能区有重叠，视频脑电图可作为脑深部电极或硬膜下电极植入术的依据。如果致痫病变和（或）致痫区与重要功能区靠近或重叠，则可能需

要植入更大的栅格电极，因为这也可进行患者清醒状态下术前重要功能区定位。采用栅格电极进行术前定位的优势在于，不仅可以定位功能区皮质，还可以从中记录癫痫发作，而在唤醒手术中，癫痫发作的记录通常是不可靠的。脑深部电极采用立体定向技术植入，可以到达脑沟底部的微小病变或是硬膜下电极难以到达的皮质深部。脑深部电极、硬膜下条状电极和栅格电极也可联合使用。

癫痫外科

癫痫手术通常是由癫痫外科中心的癫痫外科团队进行，是多学科协作的典型案例。在大多数癫痫外科中心，术前评估是由癫痫病专家和儿科癫痫病专家负责，他们的主要任务是确定药物难治性病例并从中确定适合手术的患者。团队中一部分是神经心理科医生和神经放射科医生，他们的检查可能会指出与认知障碍有关的特定脑区。由神经放射科医生和神经病理科医生专门处理癫痫手术病例是理想的选择。最终，由临床癫痫专家、脑电图专家、神经放射科医生和神经外科医生组成癫痫外科会诊团队来负责讨论每个病例，目的是形成一个假设，即癫痫发作起源于何处，是否有病变以及病变对癫痫的影响，最终要做哪种类型的切除手术。团队合作是必不可少的前提，也是术后护理、副作用管理、随访以及如何处理持续性癫痫发作的潜在决策的关键。

癫痫的外科治疗

癫痫手术包含一系列干预措施，通常分为颞叶切除术和颞叶外切除术。详见**表 83.1**。因为完全离断致痫区与周围脑组织后癫痫不再发作，因此也有人分为切除术与离断术，典型的离断术有胼胝体离断术或半球离断术。另一类是姑息性手术，这种手术很少能完全解除癫痫发作，其目的是显著降低癫痫发作频率。当无法切除时，常采取姑息性手术，例如重要功能区多处软膜下横纤维切断术。还有一些姑息性手术使用调控技术（迷走神经刺激、脑深部刺激）。

病灶切除术

病灶切除术有三种形式：单纯病灶切除术、包含病灶边缘的病灶切除术和扩大病灶切除术。常见的病变有血管畸形、肿瘤和局灶性皮质发育不良。只要有可能，就尝试病灶全切除。

表 83.1 癫痫手术谱

Bonn University Epilepsy Surgery Group, Germany, 1989– 2011

手术类型	全部数量		相对数量
全部疗法	2590		100%
颞叶切除术	1485		57%
AHE	715		48%
经外侧裂		514	
经皮质		77	
经颞下		72	
ATL	348		24%
合并海马切除		321	
不合并海马切除		39	
病灶切除术	345		23%
合并海马切除		121	
不合并海马切除		224	
二次手术 / 扩大性切除	65		
颞叶外切除术	456		
额叶		289	
其他		167	
离断术：			
大脑半球离断术 / 胼胝体离断术	196		7.5%
单纯 MST	28		1.1%
（MST 附加）	108		
VNS	425		16.4%

AHE，杏仁核 - 海马切除术；ATL，前颞叶切除术；MST，多处软膜下横纤维切断术；VNS，迷走神经刺激器植入术

当癫痫活动仅起源于病灶且重要功能区不包含病灶边缘时，即进行单纯病灶切除术。在非功能区，首选包含病灶边缘的病灶切除术。一个公认的假设是，癫痫发作起源于病灶边缘的皮质。基于该假设，常用的病灶切除技术是切除原有病灶本身以及周围皮质边缘，当然这一边缘的范围判断存在一定的主观性（例如距病变边缘 1 cm 的范围或直到下一个软脑膜层）。在实际临床工作中，通常会对非重要功能区进行病灶切除，包括周围皮质的小边缘及脑沟周围较深的皮质。有时，由于病变附近的变色、皮质异常粘连或神经胶质改变，术中可能会扩大切除边缘。在海绵状血管瘤中，可以肯定的是，大多数情况下，癫痫发作起源于海绵状血管瘤周围的含铁血黄素皮质边缘。

当术前评估显示致痫区远远超出了最近的病灶

周围皮质时，情况更为复杂（图 83.1）。病灶周围或附近的致痫区如何精确界定？并因此行扩大病灶切除术时，应同时切除多少致痫皮质？病灶联合皮质切除术可包括部分颞叶切除术或颞外侧病灶切除联合内侧杏仁核 - 海马 - 海马旁回切除术。在颞叶外（extratemporal lobe，ETL）手术中，扩大病变切除术包含范围更广泛时，可转变为额叶切除术或多脑叶切除术。最近的一项海绵状血管瘤引起的药物难治性性癫痫患者的大型队列研究显示，76 例患者中有 87%需要进行扩大病灶切除术（von der Brelie et al., 2013）。在同一队列中，37 例外侧新皮质海绵状血管瘤，7 例与内侧颞叶结构一并切除。确定扩大病灶切除术的切除范围通常需要用条状电极或栅格电极进行有创性的术前评估，特别是与重要功能区邻近时。一些团队在手术中使用皮质脑电图来确定切除范围，但其作用值得怀疑，因为不能记录癫痫发作，只有发作间期棘波。最好是依据发作记录来做出决定（Rostomily and Silbergeld，2006）。

颞叶手术

颞叶癫痫（temporal lobe epilepsy，TLE）手术方式的选择取决于 TLE 的类型：内侧颞叶癫痫（mesial temporal lobe epilepsy，MTLE）、外侧新皮质 TLE 和颞叶癫痫。新皮质 TLE 是最罕见的类型（Walczak, 1995），通常需要进行病灶切除术或扩大病灶切除术，并保留内侧结构。MTLE 的特征是癫痫发作起源于海马或海马旁回区。颞叶癫痫没有进一步明确涉及颞叶内侧和皮质结构。颞叶切除术主要有三种类型：

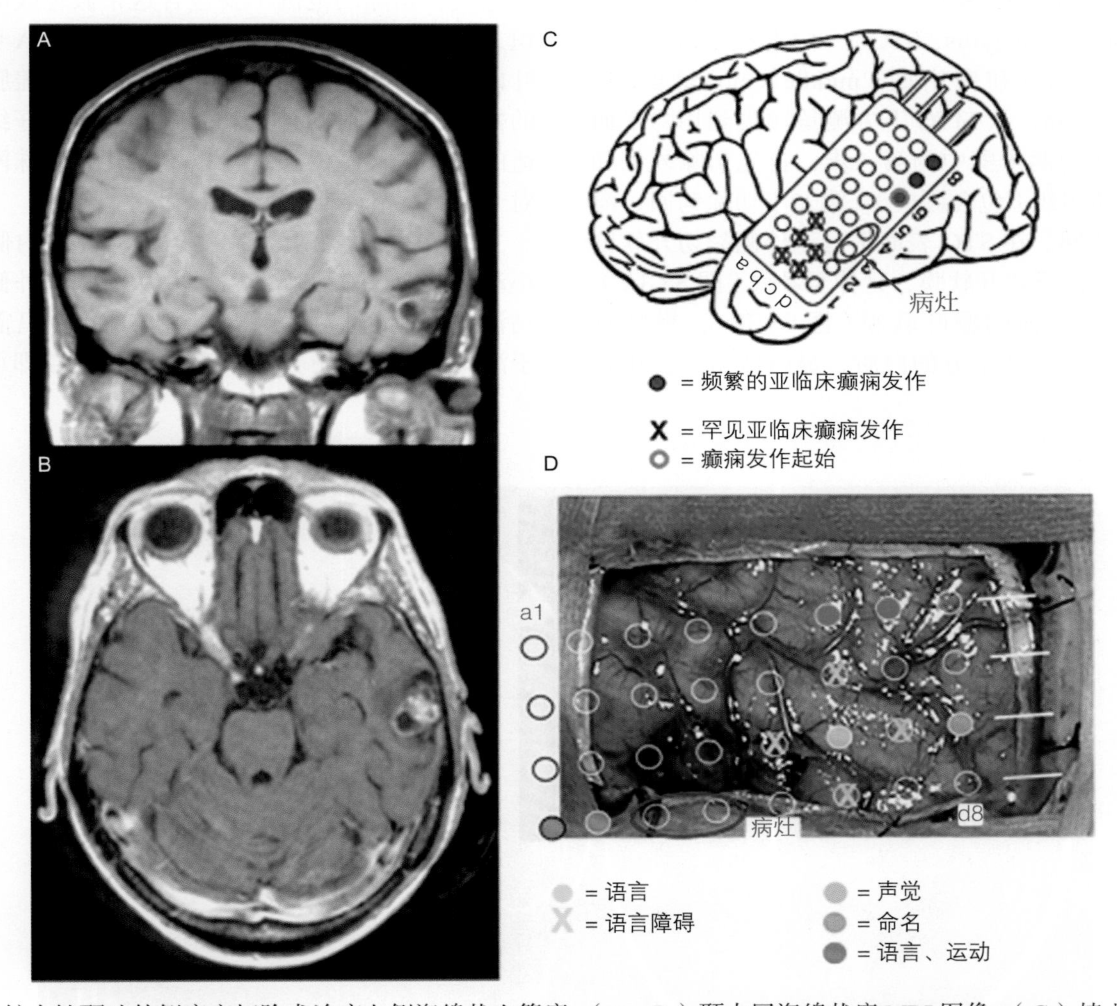

图 83.1　扩大性颞叶外侧病变切除术治疗左侧海绵状血管瘤。（A，B）颞中回海绵状瘤 MRI 图像。（C）植入式栅格电极示意图，显示栅状电极最下一行病灶后方临床下发作频繁的位置，b、c 两排位于病灶前方罕有临床下发作的位置，以及发作的起源位置。植入栅格电极是因为它与假定的语言区很近，发作活动也很广泛。这幅图是手术前定位的结果。（D）圆圈表示大脑表面电极触点的位置。功能定位的结果：蓝色椭圆表示病变部位，其上方的暗区是出血性皮质区。从图（C）的发作记录和（D）的功能定位结果可以清楚地看出，癫痫发作开始于出血皮质区的后方，临床下发作离之较远。扩大病灶切除术包括触点 b1~3、c1~5 和 d1~8。术后患者无言语障碍

前颞叶切除术（anterior temporal lobectomy，ATL）、外侧新皮质切除术、选择性杏仁核 - 海马切除术（selective amygdalohippocampectomy，SAH）。SAH 的单纯内侧切除术有三种入路：经皮质（Olivier，2000）、经外侧裂（Yasargil et al.，1985）和经颞下（Hori et al.，1993）。见**图 83.2**。许多团队使用 ATL（又称：前 2/3 颞叶切除术）或颞极联合扩大内侧切除术［又称：皮质 -（非皮质）杏仁核 - 海马切除术］治疗内侧颞叶癫痫。对颞叶切除术进行的唯一一项比较药物治疗和手术治疗的前瞻性随机研究证实了手术治疗优于药物治疗（Wiebe et al.，2001）。

ATL 是 TLE 的经典切除术式，被许多团队用作标准的 TLE 手术。切除范围包括在非优势半球从颞尖向后切除颞叶 5~5.5 cm，在优势半球切除颞叶 4.5 cm。内侧切除的范围比新皮质切除平面更靠后。作为一种改良术式，一些团队保留了颞上回（superior temporal gyrus，STG）。采用翼点入路开颅，显露额叶、STG 和颞中回（middle temporal gyrus，MTG）约 2 cm，从 MTG 上方测量颞尖到切除平面的距离。作为两步骤中的第一步，首先切除外侧和基底新皮质组织（包含颞极）；第二步切除钩回、海马和海马旁回。在 STG 表面平行于外侧裂切开软脑膜，并垂直向下切开软膜，延伸至颞底（**图 83.3A**）。保留外侧裂表面的颞叶软膜（**图 83.3B**），横断颞叶新皮质的皮质和下方的白质，显露颞角，使用超声外科吸引器（cavitron ultrasonic surgical aspirator，CUSA）从颞角向前分离至颞角的尖端。切除开放的颞角与外侧裂软脑膜之间的 STG，向前方直到颞极内侧的蛛网膜。在颞叶底面，此时新皮质组织仍然与内侧结构相连。使用 CUSA 沿后 - 前方向于海马旁回外侧、平行于海马 / 海马旁回（hippocampus/parahippocampal gyrus，HC-PHG）的方向，继续离断颞叶新皮质，直到与颞极前内侧的软脑膜切口相连。在下脉络点前方，杏仁核向基底外侧凸出，可以用超声吸引器吸除。脉络膜裂、脉络丛和穹隆伞部很容易识别。显微解剖沿着脉络膜裂将穹隆伞分离。切除钩回以及杏仁核（包括海马头和杏仁核之间的连接），杏仁核与内嗅皮质相对应。切除大部分海马头后，海马体部可被分离至前外方。使用 CUSA 切除杏仁核时，可在下脉络膜点到岛阈之间做一条假想线，切除的范围不要包含这条假想线的内侧组织，从而可以避免一些严重的问题。CUSA 可以在颞叶内侧薄层蛛网膜上直接操作，该层覆盖脑干周围的血管、第三对脑神经和大脑脚。通过仔细选择合适的 CUSA 设置，通常可以不打开内侧蛛网膜，但对于低龄儿童较难实现。

HC-PHG 仍然附着在几条小动脉的内侧，这些小动脉被双层软脑膜覆盖，并从内侧向外侧进入海马沟。从理论上讲，可以使用 CUSA，只需切除位于海马沟血管蒂下方的浅表 HC 和 PHG 即可。如果

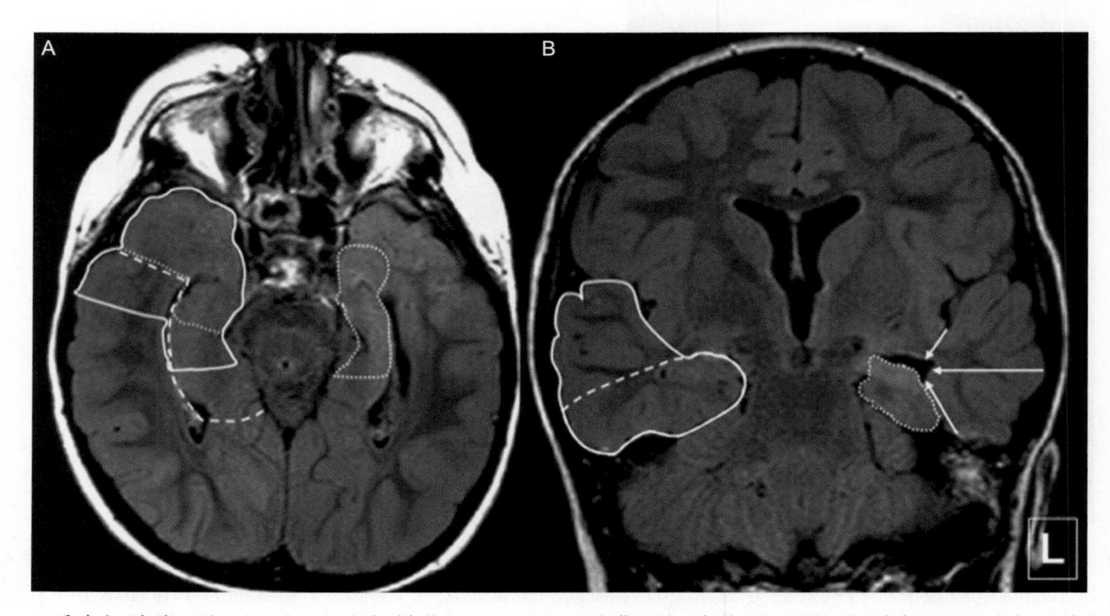

图 83.2 TLE 手术切除类型概述。（A）右侧轴位 MRI 显示三种典型切除范围：颞极切除加 SAH（点画线）、颞极切除联合广泛海马 / 海马旁回（HC-PHG）切除（虚线）、标准前颞叶切除包括内侧颞叶切除（实线）。左半球点画线显示标准 SAH 切除体积。（B）冠状位 MRI 显示标准 ATL 的轮廓（实线）和颞极后侧切除联合广泛杏仁核海马切除术（AHC）（虚线）。MRI 图像右侧，箭头标示三个 SAH 内侧切除入路。MRI 图像左侧，虚线标示切除范围

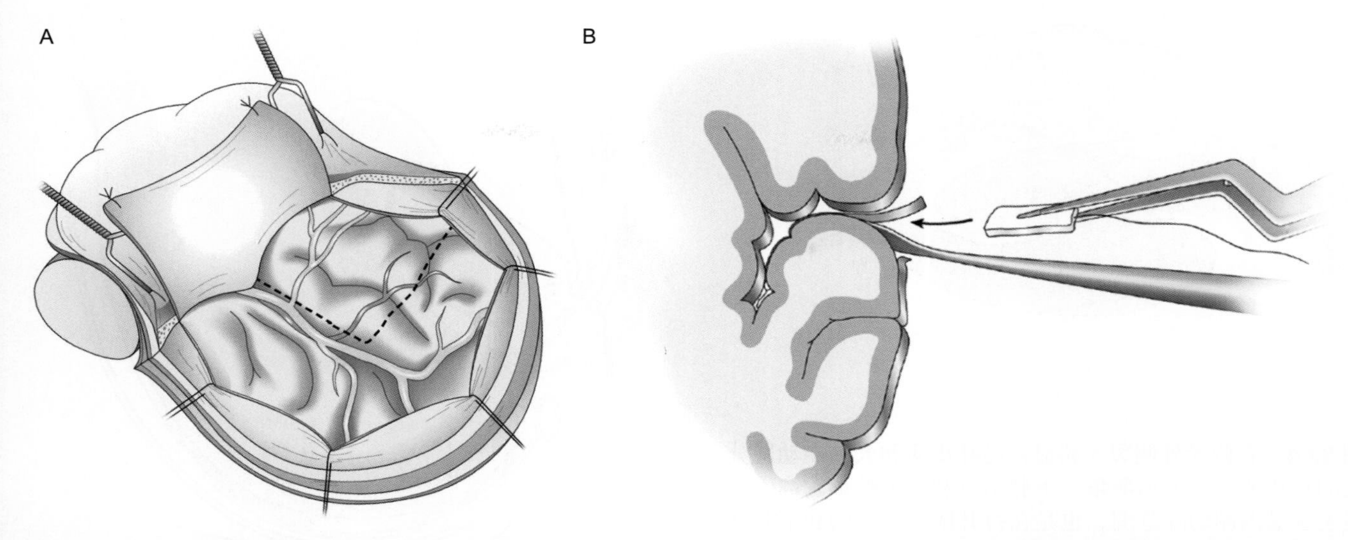

图 83.3 （A）标准右侧前 2/3 颞叶切除术开颅示意图。虚线表示软脑膜切口。（B）颞上回紧邻外侧裂的位置显示软脑膜平面的示意图，以保留侧裂动脉上的软脑膜层

Courtesy of Isabelle Christensen and Johannes Schramm.

想要得到一个良好的海马结构标本，就需要整块切除。通过抬高穹隆伞，可见覆盖在海马沟动脉上的双层软脑膜。然后使用 CUSA 从后方分离 HC-PHG，保留海马沟内的血管及双层软脑膜，作为残余的附着部分。最后一步是沿着脉络膜裂打开软脑膜，最好在海马沟内电凝血管并切断。然后切除下方的海马沟第二软脑膜层。在内侧和内侧基底部，保留完整的 PHG 上方的软脑膜层，将 PHG 向外侧分离，将其从软脑膜表面剥离。通常，可以获得长度 15~20 mm 的海马和海马旁回复合体。在大多数病例中，脑干上的内侧软脑膜和血管可以保留下来。双极电凝仅用于脑沟内的小动脉，这些小动脉需要在距离脑干周围大动脉不远处被切断。软脑膜层的微出血通常可以用氧化纤维素来止血。

颞极切除术与扩大颞叶内侧结构切除术相结合是颞叶癫痫标准切除术的常用替代方法［又称：Spencer 式切除术、皮质 -（非皮质）杏仁核 - 海马切除术］。这种术式在一些中心被用作治疗颞叶癫痫的标准方法，如果小病变（如海绵状血管瘤或良性肿瘤）位于颞极、杏仁核或海马头部，这种术式也非常有效。

采用类似标准 ATL 开颅术，切除颞极尖端后方 3 cm 的颞叶。软脑膜切口与外侧裂平行，并垂直向下延伸至颞叶底面。使用 CUSA 到达颞叶底面，穿过白质，打开颞角的尖端。完整保留大脑中动脉上方的蛛网膜，切除全部钩回，显露海马头部与对应的杏仁核。为了进一步暴露，以增加内侧结构的切除范围，应该在颞角开放水平的上方向后牵拉切开的颞叶。HC-PHG 复合体需从外侧、后方和内侧切除。前部切除包括大部分的杏仁核隆起部和海马头及其相连的内嗅皮质。外侧的分离最好使用 CUSA，或利用剥离子钝性分离，后方分离可使用 CUSA 或双极电凝加吸引器。内侧颞叶分离的方式与 ATL 的步骤类似。

SAH 被认为是一种治疗内侧颞叶癫痫合适的、理想的术式，其常见病因是阿蒙角硬化（又称：颞叶内侧硬化、海马硬化）。也可用于累及颞叶内侧结构、下脉络点后方的微小病变。共有三种入路：经外侧裂入路、经皮质入路和经颞下入路。

翼点开颅适用于经外侧裂 SAH（Yasargilet al., 1985），应显露额叶约 2 cm 和颞叶约 3 cm。分离外侧裂，仔细解剖大脑中动脉（middle cerebral artery, MCA），显露岛阀后方 15~20 mm 处的下环岛沟（图 83.4）。下一步是通过下环岛沟的切口打开颞角，切口距离岛阈后约 15 mm。用双极电凝穿过颞干以稍偏基底外侧的方式进行解剖，12~15 mm 后到达脑室（图 83.5）。脑室的开口向颞角的尖端扩大，首先绕过向内上侧突起的杏仁核。识别脑室内的脉络丛、脉络裂和下脉络点。可以看到 M1 升段外侧，接着切除钩回，完整保留内侧蛛网膜。然后分离穹隆伞，在下脉络点前方，用 CUSA 切除隆起的杏仁核，同时切除杏仁核与海马头之间的融合，这种分离直接到达钩回的空壳。同样，直接在内侧蛛网膜操作，需合理的 CUSA 设置。在这一阶段，需要分离 HC-PHG 内侧，然后用 CUSA 进行后方分离，然后用显微解剖或 CUSA 从外侧分离，保留完整的颅底软脑

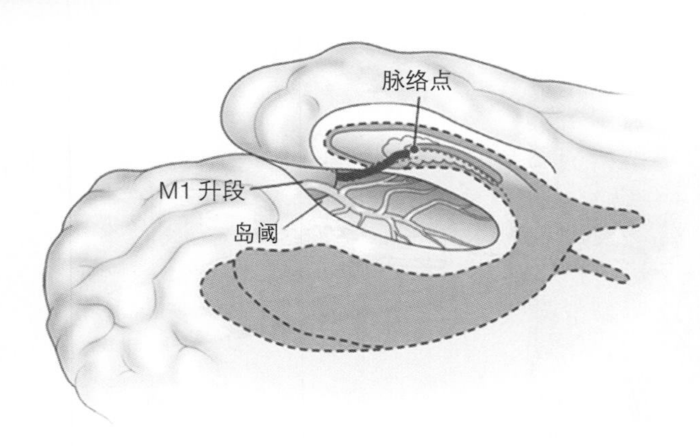

图 83.4 右侧经外侧裂入路显露岛叶皮质和大脑中动脉分支的示意图，并显示颞角、下脉络点和岛阈投影轮廓。红线表示最内侧切除范围，也是在打开脑室后岛阈和下脉络点之间的一条假想线。沿着这条线，从前外侧切除杏仁核和海马头部，无需担心会有不良反应。这是处理海马头部小肿瘤的一个重要标志

Courtesy of Isabelle Christensen and Johannes Schramm.

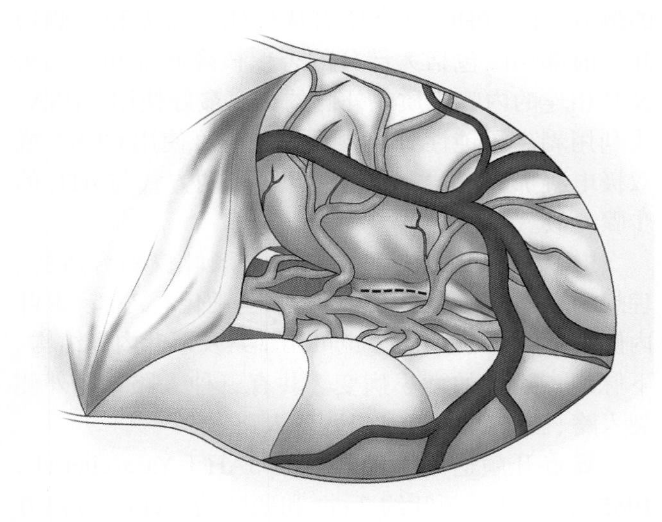

图 83.5 显露岛叶和岛阈以显示颞角入口区，为选择性海马杏仁核切除术入口区（虚线）。外侧裂的前部已打开，暴露下环岛沟和 M1 升段、M2~M3 分支

Courtesy of Isabelle Christensen and Johannes Schramm.

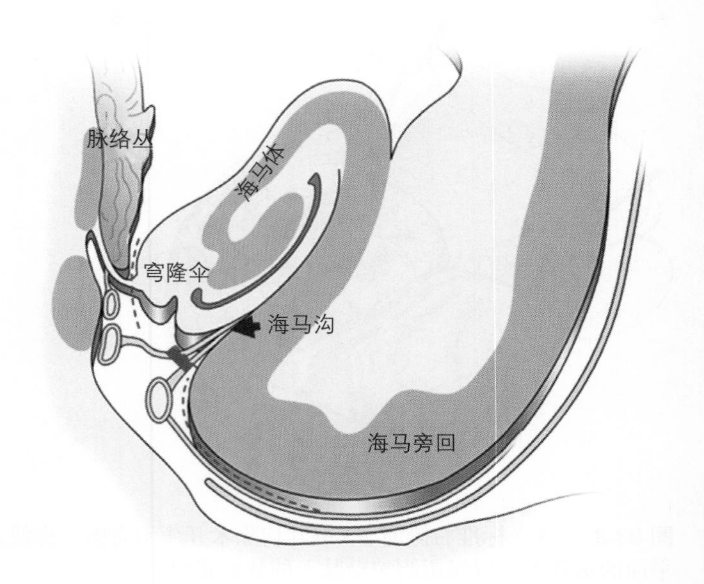

图 83.6 左侧颞叶内侧基底结构冠状位示意图。图示海马（HC）、海马旁回（PHG）和海马沟，实性红线表示横切海马沟内小血管的区域。短虚线表示可以用剥离子钝性抬起穹隆伞的区域，红色长虚线表示 PHG 和软脑膜基底内侧层之间的软膜下层面

Courtesy of Isabelle Christensen and Johannes Schramm.

膜。将包裹血管和海马沟的两层软脑膜剪开后，可以把附着于 PHG 的海马体中央部分从软脑膜盖上分离（图 83.6）。这样，可以获取 HC 和 PHG 的完整标本，在获得每位患者的许可下，从而允许以科学目的进行精确组织学诊断和分析。

外侧经皮质或经脑沟入路也可用于 SAH（Niemeyer，1958；Olivier，2000）。采用直切口和更小的颅骨开窗即可。要定位脑室并不容易，所以神经导航很有用。皮质在前后（anteroposterior，AP）方向的切口约为 15 mm。由于颞角顶壁有 Meyer 袢的存在，因此从低位进入脑室是有利的。HC-PHG 的分离和切除可从不同的角度进行操作，但需遵循与经外侧裂 SAH 相同的原则（即保留内侧蛛网膜完整并切断海马沟内血管）。在此入路中，还应全切钩回并切除杏仁核大部分。

SAH 的第三种途径是经颞下途径（Hori et al.，1993；Park et al.，1996）。常采用直切口和颅底的小骨瓣开窗术，内侧结构可以通过多种路径到达，例如梭状回、PHG 或侧副沟。为此，需要抬高颞叶，偶尔会受到颞底静脉的阻挡。在这种情况下，切开颞下回（inferior temporal gyrus，ITG）的软脑膜底面，抬起皮质，并使软脑膜留在颞底硬膜上。在极少数情况下，使用 CUSA 穿过 ITG 形成一个不高于 8~10 mm 小隧道，这明显改善了抬高颞叶其余部分的能力，且不会损伤基底静脉。可能很难定位脑室腔，冠状位 MRI 可清楚地显示术者在斜向上分离皮质到达脑室之前必须在颞叶底面的走行距离（22~25 mm）。进入脑室后，进一步延长经皮质的切口，可以更好地观察脑室内容物，并能识别标志物（穹隆伞、下脉络点、杏仁核隆起）。使用 CUSA 将 HC 头部、内嗅皮质和杏仁核一并切除，然后切除钩回，HC-PHG 以类似于经皮质和经外侧裂入路的方式被移除。

外侧新皮质颞叶切除术通常用于病变切除。它们可能是必要的，作为包含病变边缘的病变切除术或包括邻近皮质区病变的扩大切除术。在极少数病例中，可能会切除较大的外侧新皮质。开颅仅需要超过外侧裂以上数毫米。根据病灶位于后方的距离，采用弧形或问号切口。特别是在背侧的病变中，栅格电极已被用于绘制与语言相关的皮质。原则上要求切除指定脑区下的所有皮质组织，包括脑沟底部的皮质。并很容易使用常规吸引器或 CUSA 来完成。颞叶背外侧病灶切除术是唯一清醒开颅有助于定位语言相关皮质区的手术。较大的动脉分支或 Labbé 静脉需要保留，切除时不能延伸到颞叶的白质，以避免视辐射受损。

迷走神经刺激术

迷走神经刺激器植入术（vagal nerve stimulation，VNS）是一种姑息性手术，目的是减少药物难治性患者癫痫发作的频率。经过全面综合的术前评估后，没有显示可手术的致痫病变或区域，才可以进行该手术。对于药物难治性癫痫和可切除的病变，手术切除应始终优先于 VNS，因为它有治愈癫痫的潜力。VNS 目前用于全身性和部分性发作，在许多研究中，超过 50% 的患者癫痫发作频率可减少 50% 以上。在一些长期研究中，已经报道了癫痫发作频率降低 50% 至 70%~80%（Spanaki et al.，2004；Uthman et al.，2004）。VNS 适用于成人和儿童，但前提是身体可以容纳脉冲发生器，目前的型号为 45 mm × 32 mm × 7 mm。作为一种积极的作用，有文献表明 VNS 植入后患者的生活质量可得到改善（Cramer，2001；Spanaki et al.，2004）。

既往左侧颈部手术后的大面积瘢痕是 VNS 的排除标准。手术中不能使用单极热凝，只能使用双极电凝。

VNS 装置由脉冲发生器、迷走神经螺旋状电极和程控装置组成。手术过程中，用无菌袋覆盖手持程控装置，放置于脉冲发生器上，通过无线方式设置刺激参数。

将患者摆好体位，并用无菌单覆盖左侧两个手术切口，一个位于颈动脉分叉水平以下，另一个位于腋前线，用于制作锁骨下皮下囊袋。之所以选择左侧，是因为左侧迷走神经中通往心房的神经纤维比右侧的少。迷走神经与颈内动脉和颈内静脉伴行，应分离结缔组织鞘 3 cm。连接导线的颈端共有三个螺旋结构：两个电极和一个固定器。高柔韧性的螺旋电极缠绕于迷走神经上，并用两个塑料锚固定在更深的筋膜层，避免肌肉移动所致脱位。参见图 83.7。

三个锚中有一个将电极固定于更浅表的位置，但要在颈阔肌下面。从腋前线的短切口处在胸肌筋膜上制作一个皮下囊袋，大到足以放置脉冲发生器，因此缝合线应距离脉冲发生器约 2 cm。VNS 装置中提供的隧道器械用于将电极导线从颈部切口向下牵引至锁骨下囊袋。应将导线缠绕成袢，并将其放置在远离皮肤切口的发生器囊袋内，以避免更换发生器时造成损伤。发生器带有文字的一面朝上并将一根单线穿过缝合孔固定于囊袋深面。旧型号的脉冲发生器可能有不同的连接器插孔，详细信息应查阅制造商的使用手册。切口分两层缝合。在确定缝合切口之前，应进行术中导线测试、电极阻抗测试和刺激测试。

在极少数情况下，胸大肌下植入可能是首选（例如，对于皮下脂肪很少或没有的患者）。新式脉冲发生器的电池寿命为 5~8 年，具体取决于刺激参数的大小。术后可以立即开始刺激，但许多团队更倾向于在开始刺激前等待一段时间。向患者提供一个磁铁，当直接放在脉冲发生器上时，刺激会停止，直到移除磁铁。这对那些在刺激期出现嗓子嘶哑，抑或是想要唱歌或需要在公共场合说话的患者来说，这可能很有用。磁铁可以在脉冲发生器上滑动以触发按需刺激，在一些患者在可能出现癫痫发作之前

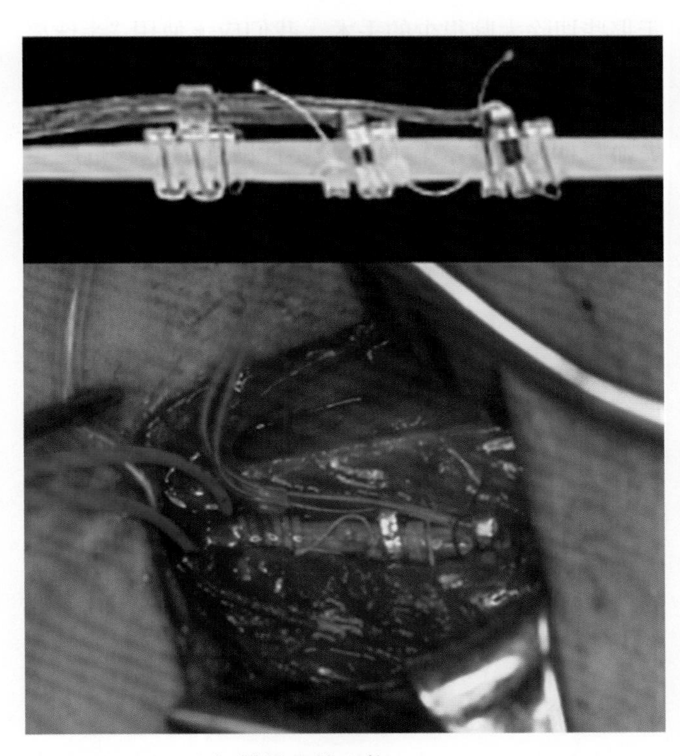

图 83.7　VNS 电极样品和植入物

感觉到先兆时使用这种刺激方式。扫描期间发生器输出编程为 0 mA 时，可以进行 MRI 头部扫描。患者刺激参数各不相同，但通常短时刺激之后是较长的静默期。详细信息可查阅 VNS 医师手册。

大脑半球切除术 / 大脑半球离断术

手术的适应证是针对导致难治性癫痫发作的单侧半球病变。这种半球损伤通常伴有一定程度的偏瘫、认知障碍和偏盲。在已知药物治疗无效的婴幼儿灾难性癫痫病例中，可能需要在出生后的前几个月进行早期手术。理想情况下，所有癫痫发作都应起源于受累半球。

传统的单侧大脑半球切除术在很大程度上被切除组织较少、离断组织较多的手术方式所取代，如 Rasmussen 功能性半脑切除术（Rasmussen，1983）。在过去的 25 年里，用大脑半球离断术和半球分离或传入神经阻滞等切开术来代替切除术的趋势已经发展起来。对于 Rasmussen 功能性半球切除术，在功能上相当于解剖切除，只做了一个大的颞叶切除和一个大的中央切除，其余部分是断开的，但仍保留在原位。切除的组织越少，大脑半球离断术这一术语就越合理，这包括背侧经皮质岛叶下半球离断术（Delalande et al.，2007）、经大脑皮质 - 脑室锁孔半球离断术（Schramm et al.，2001）和经外侧裂入路手术（Villemure and Mascott，1995）以及相关手术（Shimizu and Maehara，2000）。为了明确起见，对于那些切除大脑很少的手术，我们应该使用“半球离断术”这个术语。

现代半球离断术的优点是手术时间明显缩短，失血量明显减少，输血的必要性减少，显露范围更小和术中并发症的发生率低。这些优点在小婴儿和婴儿身上很明显，但在老年患者中也同样受益。

大脑半球常见的结构性病变有先天性发育缺陷（半侧巨脑症、多脑叶发育不良等）、Sturge-Weber 综合征和获得性病变（围产期梗死或出血、Rasmussen 脑炎或创伤后和脑炎后损伤）。

偶发的对侧癫痫发作或双侧致痫活动并不是必要禁忌证，因为可以达到令人满意的癫痫无发作率（Doring et al.，1999）。当优势半球受到影响时，明确进行大脑半球离断术和找到正确的时间点是困难的，有时甚至是有问题的，特别是在 Rasmussen 脑炎中。

手术技术

大脑半球离断术的技术要求很高，特别是在半侧巨脑症或广泛全半脑发育不良的病例中。现代半球离断术的共同之处在于，胼胝体切开术是从脑室内部进行的，通过打开外侧裂或岛盖开窗来到达脑室。额叶、颞叶和枕颞叶的分离也可以通过这个入路来实现。目前也已经做了多种方式的改良（Devlin et al.，2003）。参见图 83.8。背侧经皮质入路也可以经脑室途径将大脑半球与颞叶新皮质分离（更详细的描述，见 Schramm，2002）。其他技术，如偏侧大脑皮质切除术，应用较少。

Rasmussen 功能性大脑半球切除术需要一个大的开颅手术，显露大脑半球的中央部分，包括整个颞叶。手术切除包括颞叶和外侧裂上大部分中央区皮质（7~8 cm），显露大脑镰和胼胝体。然后进行胼胝体切开术，将额叶、顶枕叶与基底神经节组织离断。

经外侧裂锁孔技术（Schramm et al.，2001）是通过在外侧裂上方打开（4~5）cm×（4~6）cm 的颅骨，显露岛叶皮质周围的环岛沟来完成的。然后通过离断从基底神经节周围的颞角到额角尖端的皮质，打开整个脑室。接着沿着脉络裂进行颞叶内侧分离，从下脉络点延伸至钩回内侧的蛛网膜。为了获得组织学分析，可能需要切除部分 HC-PHG 组织。下一步采用经脑室入路分离额叶和顶枕叶的内侧，包括从脑室内部进行胼胝体切开。在开始进行额 - 基底离断前，从上升的 M1 到开放的额角尖端画一条假想线，电凝额叶基底的外侧面，并在显微镜下使用 CUSA 沿着 M1 及 A1 后方的轮廓分离额叶白质。这会自动通向大脑半球间的裂隙，离断线会沿着 A2 的轮廓定向然后绕过胼胝体的前部到达胼胝体的顶壁。然后

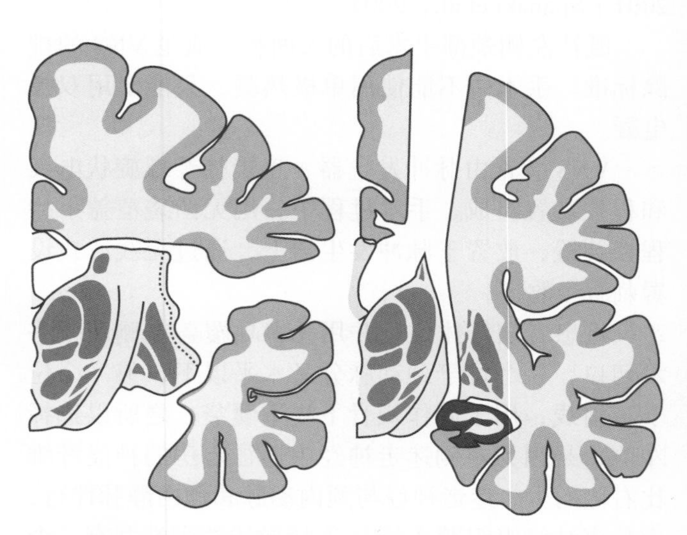

图 83.8 经外侧裂锁孔（左）和背侧经皮质半球切开术（右）的切开示意图
Courtesy of J. Schramm.

沿着胼周动脉横切胼胝体白质，并会自动终止于大脑镰的下缘，在此处大脑镰移行为颅底面的小脑幕。因此，在内侧离断的后半部分，它沿着镰幕边缘延伸。这将引导外科医生穿过三角区向下到达颞区，与最初的颞叶内侧离断面相交。在内侧离断的末端，孤立的基底节已被环状断开。建议在M2分支下方，用吸引器切除岛叶皮质，以消除持续癫痫发作的潜在来源。止血通常只需要用氧化纤维素和大量灌洗就能完成。切除M3~M4口径的小分支，但要保留所有M2、M3大分支及大脑后动脉。

外侧裂周区开窗手术（Villemure and Mascott，1995；Shimizu and Maehara，2000）在切除岛盖显露岛叶皮质后遵循同样的原则。

在背侧经皮质经脑室半球离断术（Delalande et al.，2007）中，采用约4 cm×5 cm的矢状窦旁骨窗，到达冠状缝后方约3 cm。经皮质进入侧脑室，显露室间孔和丘脑后部。通过此途径可进行旁正中胼胝体切开术。向外侧从丘脑和纹体之间进行离断，向深部直达侧脑室的颞角。从胼胝体前部切开术的额叶底面开始，切除直回的后部，横断线向外侧延伸穿过尾状体头，在此与外侧的纹状体下方横断面相交。用吸引器连通背侧纹状体下方离断面与胼胝体后部断面，从而将基底节与大脑半球分离。

经外侧和背侧经皮质半球切开术都具有失血少、显露小、输血率低的优点。背侧入路可保留所有浅表血管，并避免了对大脑中动脉的操作。对于有脑穿通畸形或明显萎缩的患者，经侧脑室锁孔技术是理想的，适用于接近正常大脑大小的患者，但对于半侧巨脑症的患者，建议不要与打开外侧裂相结合，而应该创建一个类似于外侧裂开窗技术的岛盖窗。

半球离断术有不可避免的副作用，如部分偏盲、患侧手精细运动的丧失，有时还会导致行走能力恶化。手术风险包括开颅手术的所有常规风险，发展为需要分流的脑积水，需要输血，以及极少情况下的死亡。现代手术中，手术死亡率约为1%，还存在一定的不完全离断和持续癫痫发作的风险。所有手术都有5%~30%的脑积水发生率（Schramm et al.，2012）。在其他连续队列中，目前大脑半球切除术的分流率分别为8%、16%、19%和23%，皮质切除术的分流率高达32%，在一项690名患者的半球切除术后脑积水的大型多中心研究中，平均分流率为23%。解剖性半球切除术是发展脑积水的重要危险因素（Lew et al.，2013）。每一种术式都有不完全离断率，即使是Rasmussen术式也是如此，不完全切除率也在2%~30%。分流率与病因和手术类型有关，半侧巨脑症患者中有着较高的分流率。分流手术时机可能非常晚，可在初次手术后6~8年。最近一项关于儿童大脑半球切除术的调查显示，153例患者的死亡率为0.7%（Koubeissi et al.，2009）。

癫痫的其他手术治疗

胼胝体切开术是一种成熟的术式，适用于跌倒发作、全身性强直阵挛性发作（generalized tonic-clonic seizures，GTCS）、失张力发作或Lennox-Gastaut综合征。通过阻断发作活动从一侧半球到另一侧半球的传播，对于减轻跌倒发作和（或）GTCS特别有效。通常仅限于胼胝体的前2/3或4/5，很少采用两阶段全胼胝体切开术（Spencer et al.，1988）。与其他癫痫切除术相比，具体的适应证（部分或完全胼胝体切开术）没有其他癫痫切除术明确。在许多悬而未决的问题中，有两个问题是：是否应该切断前连合，或者是否应该切断背侧的海马连合。适合胼胝体切开术的患者经常有多种癫痫发作类型，但主要是消除跌倒发作。需要注意的是，大约在25%的病例中，可以观察到局灶性发作的一过性增加。

在一项95例患者的研究队列中，77%的患者获得了令人满意的效果（即无癫痫发作和癫痫发作频率降低75%以上），这些患者中主要为跌倒发作和全身性强直-阵挛性发作。有研究发现前半段胼胝体切开术不如前2/3胼胝体切开术有效（Tanriverdi et al.，2009）。患者取仰卧位，单侧前额开颅，其中线内侧缘长6~7 cm，宽约4 cm，可绕过较大的桥静脉。可能需要离断一根较小的桥静脉。选择非优势半球进行半球间操作。在显微镜下仔细分离蛛网膜粘连，尤其是在两个半球粘连处。必须避免损伤扣带回，或至少限制在一侧。胼胝体很容易识别，这也得益于胼周的两条动脉。仔细分离动脉，并被垫棉覆盖。胼胝体的横切可以用双极和吸引器或CUSA低参数下完成。一些作者建议保留室管膜，但这通常是不可能的。取仰卧位时，通过单侧额部入路可以将横断面向后延伸到很远，但如果计划进行完全的胼胝体切开术，一些作者建议分别进行额部和顶骨开颅术。为了确定精确的离断范围，可以使用一小条毫米纸或术中导航。有些作者倾向于采取侧卧位，以使半脑向下塌陷，避免牵开器的牵拉。侧卧位时，仅通过一次开颅来进行完全的胼胝体切开术是比较困难的。

下丘脑错构瘤切断或切除术

错构瘤可有瘤蒂或具有广泛的基底，属于少数癫痫起源于病灶内的病变。切除具有一定困难，使用经脑室内镜时会更容易一些。广泛的病变首选内镜下切除。副作用包括记忆障碍和严重的内分泌功能障碍（多食、肥胖）。替代技术包括通过立体定向电极进行放射外科手术或电凝术。治疗效果好坏参半，通常癫痫无发作率远低于 50%。

多处软膜下横纤维切断术（multiple subpial transections，MST）属于姑息性手术，很少作为独立的干预手段。当病变区域与运动、语言或视觉皮质交界时，通常被用作病变切除或皮质切除的附加手段。因为没有较大规模的单纯 MST 病例报道，故很难评估该方法的有效性（Schramm et al.，2002）。很少可以达到 Engel Ⅰ级，但 45%~70% 的病例可以达到 Engel Ⅱ级和Ⅲ级，这在一定程度上取决于这种姑息性干预成功的定义标准（Spencer et al.，2002）。关于 MST 有效性具有不同的观点，有学者对支持和反对的观点进行了总结（Ojemann，2006；Wyler，2006）。MST 的原理是，通过阻断皮质内的短距离侧向连接纤维，而保留传出的长纤维，可以削弱皮质内通过双侧扩散的皮质神经元之间的同步性。将一钝钩插入软脑膜孔后，在脑回表面下方 5~6 mm 处，以间隔 5 mm 的距离进行平行切割。对脑回的侧壁做同样的动作比较困难，也比较危险。使用尖端朝下的钩状器械似乎是更安全的方法。小的出血点通常用氧化纤维素和填塞物处理，大出血很少见。术后运动皮质功能缺失是非常少见的，动作笨拙通常是暂时的。较大的皮质病变可以采取这种方式治疗。

脑深部电刺激是一种增强性姑息疗法。主要适应于药物难治性的部分发作，包括继发性全身发作。在一项前瞻性随机研究中（Fisher et al.，2010）发现 54% 的患者癫痫发作减少了至少 50%，14 名患者至少 6 个月没有发作。在刺激组中，14% 的受试者有抑郁症状，13% 有记忆障碍。这种手术在许多国家是免费的。最近的一篇综述比较了不同姑息手术的结果，包括 VNS、胼胝体切开术和 MST（Fauser and Zentner，2012）。

反应式皮质刺激器植入

最近的一项针对难治性部分性癫痫（191 例患者）的随机双盲研究（Morrell，2011）发现，12 周后癫痫发作频率显著降低 37.9%，而对照组为 19.3%。癫痫发作减少的中位数 1 年内增加到 44%，2 年内增加到 53%，3~6 年内增加到 48%~66% 不等（Bergey et al.，2015）。不同的医保系统将对植入这些昂贵的姑息设备做出不同的政策。

术后

预后

对癫痫预后的评估并不像看起来那么简单。理想的预后不仅应该考虑癫痫无发作率，还要考虑生活质量。理想的预后是癫痫完全无发作（包括发作先兆）、良好的生活质量和完全的社会重新融合。最常用的预后量表主要衡量癫痫发作的结果 :Engel 分级和 ILAE 分级（见**专栏 83.1**）。有些癫痫发作很严重，但有些在日常生活中很少注意到，所以癫痫发作的严重程度很难分类。

对于预后统计，至少随访 2 年。总的来说，TLE 手术效果好于非颞叶癫痫（Extratemporal lobe epilepsy，ETLE）手术效果（对于 TLE，Engel I 级在 65%~75%，ETLE 大约低 10%），但是在接下来的几年里，每年的癫痫无发作率约减少 1%。再次手术的成功率在 50%~69%（Grote et al.，2016），2006

专栏 83.1 癫痫发作预后分级

Engel 预后分级（Engel and Pedley，2008）

- Ⅰ级 - 无致残性癫痫发作
  - （完全无癫痫发作；非致残性，仅单纯部分性癫痫发作；一些致残性癫痫发作，但至少 2 年内无致残性癫痫发作；仅停用抗癫痫药物的全身性惊厥）
- Ⅱ级 - 罕见致残性癫痫发作
  - （最初无致残性癫痫发作，但现在罕见；手术后罕见致残性癫痫发作；多于罕见致残性癫痫发作，但至少 2 年内罕见癫痫发作；仅夜间癫痫发作）
- Ⅲ级 - 有意义的改善
  - （有意义的癫痫发作减少；长期无癫痫发作期相当于随访期的一半以上，但随访不少于 2 年）
- Ⅳ级 - 没有意义的改善
  - （癫痫发作显著减少；无明显变化；癫痫发作加重）

ILAE 预后分级

1 完全没有癫痫发作；没有先兆
2 只有先兆；无其他癫痫发作
3 每年发作 1~3 天；± 先兆
4 每年发作 4 天，相对于基线发作天数减少 50%；± 先兆
5 基线发作天数减少不到 50%；± 先兆
6 基线发作天数增加超过 100%；± 先兆

年 Ojemann 和 Jung 对 TLE 手术的预后评估问题和预后进行了充分的讨论（Ojemann and Jung，2006），Geller 和 Devinsky（Geller and Devinsky，2006）对 ETLE 手术做了相关讨论，同样 2005 年 Tellez-Zenteno 和他的同事也对这个问题进行了讨论（Tellez-Zenteno et al.，2005）。Schmidt 和 Stavem（Schmidt and Stavem，2009）比较了手术患者和非手术患者，得出的结论是“将手术与药物治疗相结合，患者癫痫无发作的可能性是单纯药物治疗的 4 倍”。

并发症

癫痫手术通常是在年轻且大多健康的患者中进行的，具有开颅手术的常规风险（感染、出血等），以及与不同癫痫手术类型相关的风险。发生率和文献参见 Tanriverdi 等（2009）。TLE 手术后的典型并发症包括视野缺损、短暂性言语障碍、腔隙性梗死和抑郁发作的发生率增加。左侧 TLE 手术后可观察到言语记忆减退等认知副作用，永久性发生率约为 2%。手术并发症（感染、血栓等）占 2%~5%，但很少引起永久性后遗症。死亡率远低于 1%，在大脑半球离断术中约为 1%。

争议：TLE 的小范围或大范围切除术

此讨论只与内侧 TLE 有关。希望的结果是有限的颞叶内侧结构切除术（SAH）引起的认知方面的副作用更少，但与大范围切除术相比，有相似的癫痫发作预后。

越来越多的证据表明，SAH 和颞叶切除术（temporal lobe resection，TLR）的癫痫预后非常相似（Schramm，2008）。在这篇综述中，大多数作者（6/8）发现 SAH 的癫痫预后与脑叶切除术相似。14 项研究中有 11 项表明 SAH 的神经心理预后会略好一些。然而，一项基于 11 项研究的 meta 分析（Josephson et al.，2013）发现，“与 SAH 相比，在 ATL 后，患者在统计学上更有可能达到 Engel Ⅰ级预后”。更有限的内侧切除术是否具有与 TLR 相当的癫痫发作预后，这个问题还没有明确的解决。已经广泛讨论了针对不同切除术类型进行对比研究的局限性（Schramm，2008）。

内侧切除术是否应最大限度地向背侧方向扩大的问题也是无定论的，因为在一篇综述中，12 项研究中有 7 项（58%）发现癫痫发作的预后与内侧切除的范围无关。重要的是要认识到，只有一项前瞻性随机研究测试了较大或较小的内侧切除范围的预后差异（Schramm et al.，2011）。意向治疗分析与 MRI 切除范围容积测定并没有显示后方达 3.5 cm 的切除组有不同的癫痫无发作率。与预期切除长度相比，由容积确定的真实切除长度的预后结果是相同的。

延伸阅读、参考文献、EBRAIN 的相关链接

扫描书末二维码获取。

第 84 章　大脑的发育性疾病

Colin Ferrie · Daniel Warren · Atul Tyagi 著
安旭 译，田永吉 审校

引言

大脑在出生前和出生后的发育是由复杂的遗传机制调控的。先天异常以及环境因素的影响可以引起一系列与脑畸形相关的发育性疾病。经典的胚胎发育理论依然是解释这些疾病的关键，了解原肠胚形成、腹侧和背侧的诱导发育、神经元的分化和增殖、组织发生和迁移以及神经元的髓鞘化，可以帮助神经外科医生了解临床实践中可能遇到的情况。在这一章中，对常见及罕见的大脑畸形进行综述，包括无脑畸形、全脑畸形、视间隔发育不良、裂脑畸形、灰质异位畸形、无脑回畸形/脑回肥厚畸形、多小脑回、脑穿通畸形、胼胝体发育异常、小头畸形、半脑畸形、后颅凹畸形和脑囊肿。本章重点是帮助读者理解概念和临床意义，而非关注细节。

大脑的发育：概述

经典的神经胚胎学对于理解大脑发育及发育不良仍然非常关键（Sarnat and Flores-Sarnat，2013）。大脑发育通常分为几个阶段，在这期间，病理过程（遗传和非遗传）会导致明显的畸形。然而，假设这些过程是必然出现的、互不关联的，有时间节点，而且其中一个节点在下一个开始之前结束，这种简化的方法非常有助于理解。

原肠胚形成

大约胚胎发育的第 3 周，被称为原肠胚发生（**图 84.1 和图 84.2**），形成由外胚层、中胚层和内胚层组成的三层结构。这一阶段发生问题，可能导致非神经系统（non-nervous system，CNS）和 CNS 结构的多种异常情况，包括脊髓异常、神经管囊肿、皮样和表皮样囊肿以及前脑膜囊肿。

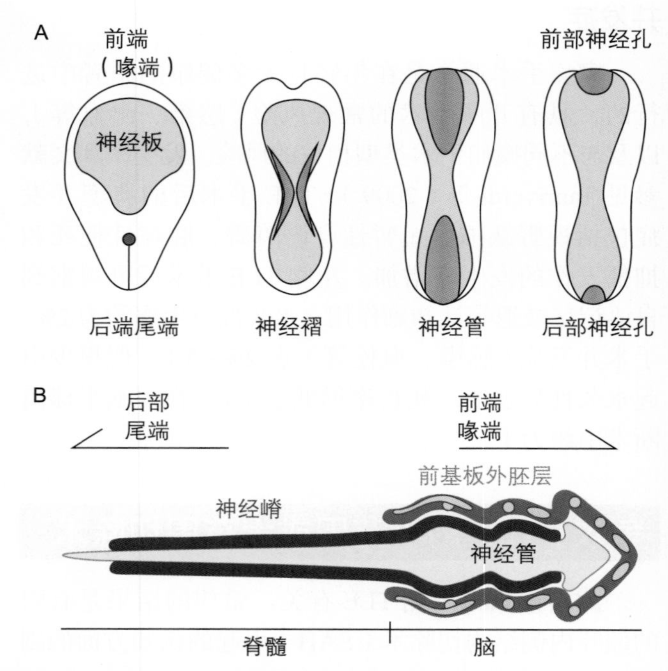

图 84.1　（A）在妊娠的第 3 周，背侧外胚层形成从前端到节点（黑色圆圈）的神经板。到第 3 周末期，神经板内翻形成一个神经折叠，然后闭合形成神经管。神经管的闭合从一个起点（接近将来颈部的位置）向喙端、尾端同时进行。两个开口（前部和后部神经孔）是神经管最后闭合的区域。（B）示意图显示三囊胚胎的背侧视图，喙端在右侧，尾端在左侧。直接包被神经管周边的是神经嵴，后者将来发育成周围神经系统的大部分。在发育中的胚胎的原始的头部区域内，神经上皮发育成前基板外胚层（蓝色区域），将来最终形成 7 对位于两侧的基板（黄色区域），其中的 5 对将发育成感觉神经元

背侧诱导分化

这一过程大约发生在妊娠 3~4 周，其关键结果是形成神经管。中胚层细胞向头端的原始节点（在原肠胚过程中形成）迁移，形成脊索，并诱导外胚层形成神经外胚层，包括神经板。然后分裂成两层，最

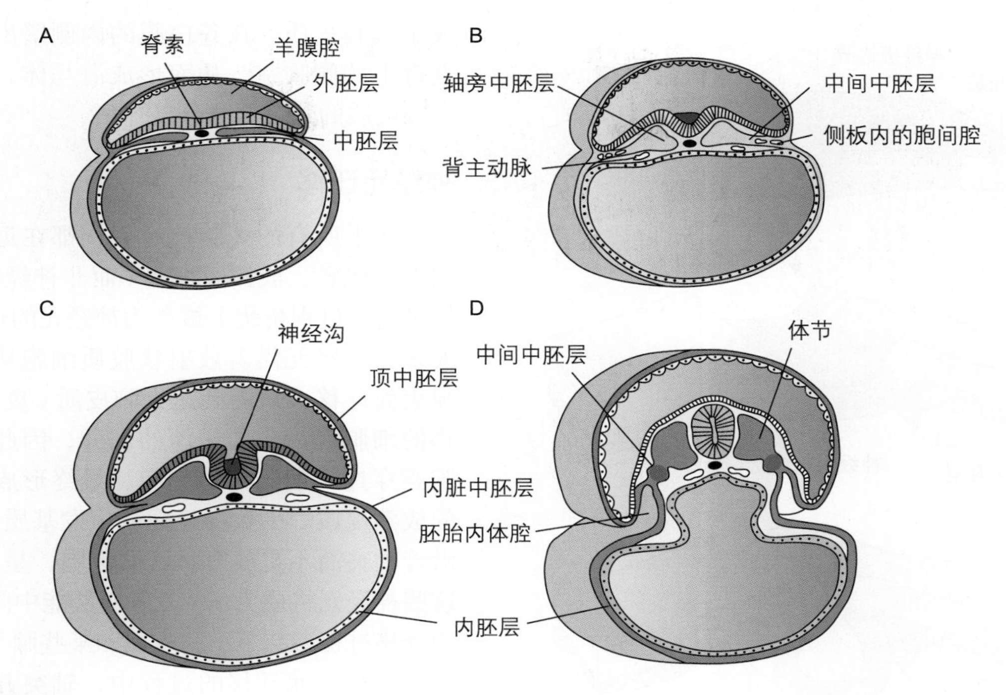

图 84.2 原肠胚形成

Reproduced from Thomas W. Sadler, *Langman's Medical Embryology*, 11th edition, Wolters Kluwer. Copyright 2009, with permission. http://www.lww.com.

终形成神经管和神经嵴。神经管形成的过程被称为神经胚形成，包括神经板的卷曲和融合。神经胚（**图84.3**）分为初级和次级神经胚，它们分别是神经管形成的关键阶段，神经管从脊索喙端到尾端（L1-L2 水平），也是分别形成下段腰椎、骶骨和尾骨等椎体的关键阶段。

神经嵴细胞的背向迁移与许多细胞群体和结构的形成相关，包括黑色素细胞、颅面软骨和骨、平滑肌、外周和肠道神经元以及胶质细胞。

腹侧诱导分化

腹侧诱导分化发生在妊娠的第 5~10 周，包括两个关键过程：从神经管的喙端形成数个原脑泡，这些原脑泡将形成大脑，其中的褶皱会把大脑分成不同的部分。

最初，三个原脑泡形成于神经孔关闭时期。前脑泡、中脑泡、后脑泡分别产生前部、中部、后部大脑。前脑的进一步分化形成端脑（前端）和间脑（尾端），后脑泡分化形成后脑和延髓。头部褶皱将前脑和中脑分开，而颈部皱褶将后脑和脊髓分开。

端脑憩室（端脑小泡）形成大脑半球，中心的腔隙形成侧脑室。间脑发育为丘脑、下丘脑、上丘脑、视杯和神经垂体，其中的中央腔隙形成第三脑室。端脑侧方外翻形成视网膜和视神经。生长迅速的端脑，尤其是外部区域覆盖间脑、中脑和后脑，最终形成“C”形特征的侧脑室，在发育中的大脑半球之间的间充质形成大脑镰。

中脑泡的发育远不如前脑泡的发育那么引人注目。中脑泡皱褶将其与后脑泡分离。缩小的中央腔隙形成导水管。神经管背面（翼板）的细胞向背部迁移，形成顶盖，包括上丘、下丘。另一些则向腹部迁移，形成红核和黑质。

后来，脑桥皱褶将后脑泡分为两部分。末脑形成延髓，后脑形成脑桥和小脑（部分由中脑泡形成）。后脑的扩张和顶板的拉伸形成了第四脑室。

神经的增殖、分化和组织发生

最初，一层神经上皮细胞排列在神经管上，以内、外限制性膜为界。神经上皮细胞的增殖产生假复层上皮，最外层的细胞向神经管腔中心移动。最内层（脑室区）与空腔毗邻，是有丝分裂的部位。未来的神经元（成神经细胞）随后向外迁移，形成外套层，后来成为灰质。外层是无细胞层，称为边缘区。它变成了白质。外套层中的神经元将轴突伸入边缘区，并以运动纤维的形式向外延伸到神经管之外。星形胶质细胞和少突胶质细胞也由脑室区的神经上皮细胞（成神经胶质细胞）有丝分裂形成，最后形成室管膜细胞，覆盖发育中的脑室系统。小胶质细胞

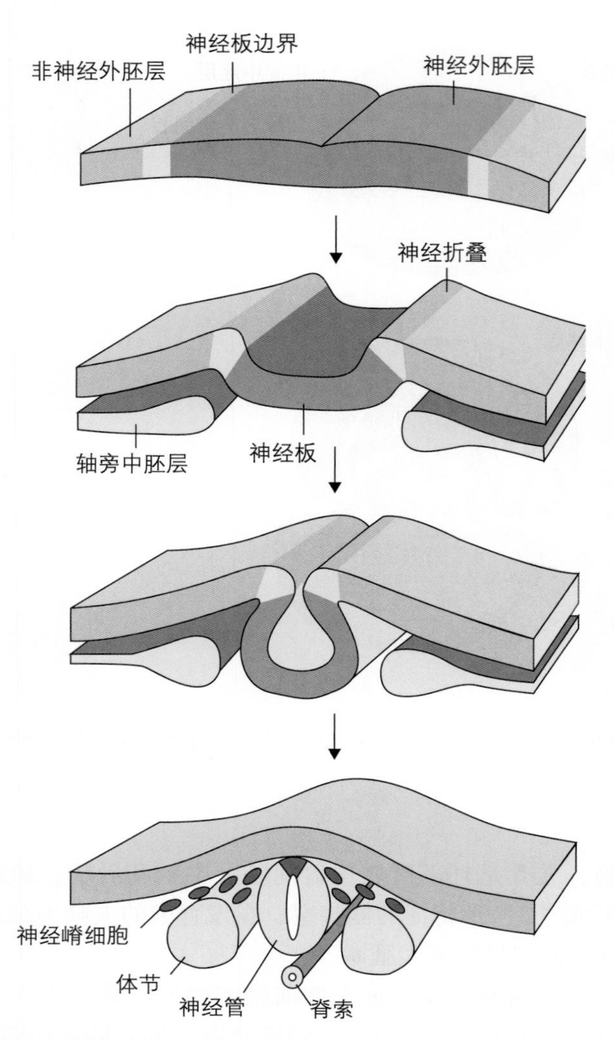

图 84.3　神经胚形成过程

Reproduced with permission from Laura S. Gammill, Marianne Bronner-Fraser, Neural crest specification: migrating into genomics, *Nature Reviews Neuroscience*, Volume 4, Issue 10, pp. 795–805, Copyright ©2003 *Nature Reviews Neuroscience*.

来自间叶细胞。

在胚胎的第四周，外套层增殖的成神经细胞在神经管的两侧（分别为基底板和翼板）使腹侧和背侧增厚，由脑室界沟隔开。随后，基板产生运动神经元，翼板产生感觉神经元。在脑干中，脑界沟分离运动性和感觉性颅神经核团。随后朝着不同方向的迁移从而最终使不同的脑干核团位于不同位置。翼板的边缘（菱唇）形成小脑。

发育中的端脑囊泡的外套层区域形成大脑半球的灰质、基底节和海马。纹状体来源于端脑囊泡基底部分外套层增厚的部分。后来下行的轴突纤维构成内囊，从而将纹状体分为内侧、外侧两部分。端脑囊泡的外套层其他部分较薄，称为苍白膜。它形成了大脑皮质。在苍白膜的内侧壁出现增厚并凸入发育中的侧脑室，从而形成海马体，海马沟将其与大脑皮质的其余部分分隔开来。

神经元迁移

几乎所有的大脑神经元，都在远离起源地的部位发育成熟。成神经细胞（而非神经元）也是如此，但是这个过程传统上被称为神经元的迁移（**图** 84.4）。大多数神经元沿着放射状胶质细胞从脑室下区向脑膜表面迁移，从而到达大脑皮质（皮质板）。最早迁移的细胞成为皮质最深的部分，因此之后迁移的细胞要穿过早期迁移的细胞，最终形成具有六层结构的成熟皮质。少数神经元从生发基质的神经节突起，沿着轴突而不是放射状胶质细胞，呈切线方向迁移，这些神经元将成为 γ-氨基丁酸能中间神经元。类似的迁移过程参与了小脑皮质和某些脑干核团的发育。

在神经元迁移的过程中，轴突开始发生。这个过程包括分别形成距离神经元胞体近处和远处的短轴突和长轴突。树突大多在迁移停止后形成，随后是突触形成。最初形成的神经元数量要多于最终组成成熟大脑的神经元，细胞凋亡是大脑发育的一个重要方面，它通常伴随突触的发生。

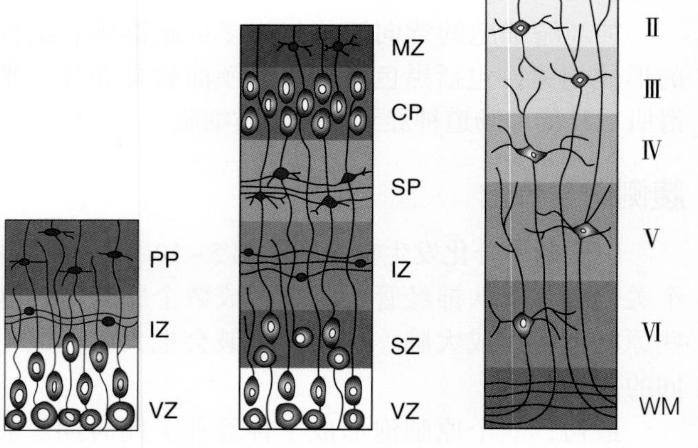

图 84.4　（左）最初的神经元迁移形成育板（preplate，PP）。（中间）第二批神经元分开 PP 进入边缘区（marginal zone，MZ）和板下区（subplate，SP），都是暂时的脑结构。（右）成熟的脑组织有 6 层发育好的皮质结构，但是没有胚胎性结构（MZ、SP、VZ）。中间的区域（intermediate zone，IZ）已经成为成熟的白质层

Source data from *The Fundamentals of Brain Development: Integrating Nature and Nurture* by Joan Stiles. Cambridge, MA: Harvard University Press Copyright © 2008 by the President and Fellows of Harvard College

髓鞘形成

髓鞘形成（在脊髓神经根、一些脑神经和脑干的一些长束纤维）从妊娠第 24 周时开始，大部分在两岁时完成。然而，直到第四十年，同侧前颞叶连接束才完全形成髓鞘。

大脑发育的控制

大脑发育处于精确的遗传机制控制之下，多种基因调控发育（Hu et al.，2014）。这些机制相互作用，许多只在特定的时间内表达。有一些仅控制神经系统内部的发育，另外一些在神经系统之外也发挥作用，有些则在发育不同的过程中发挥不同的功能。环境因素也很重要（Gressens et al.，2001）。例如，维甲酸（维生素 A）在控制 Hox 基因表达方面发挥重要作用，在控制大脑发育的局部调控中也很重要。

多种不同的机制已经被确认为是控制大脑发育的重要机制（Sarnat and Flores-Sarnat，2014）。诱导是指一个胚胎组织对另外一个胚胎组织的影响。因此，神经诱导是指非神经组织（例如脊索）对神经管发挥的影响作用。识别分子、黏附分子、细胞骨架成分和物理屏障（如背侧、腹侧正中间隔）都对神经元的迁移发挥着调节作用。

大脑发育异常（脑畸形）

分类

大脑畸形有许多种类型，一些相对常见，而另一些则非常罕见。分类与发现的顺序有关。传统上是基于形态学进行分类，以前是通过病理学检查确定，但近年来则是由神经影像学来确定。另外一种方法则是关注各种畸形在生命发育过程中发生的时间点。最近一些分类方法都是基于病因学尝试分类。这些分类方法中没有哪一个是完全成功的。纯粹的形态学分类没有考虑到遗传学的迅猛发展。然而，非遗传病因也很重要。

目前比较推崇将这些学说综合在一起的观点（de Wit et al.，2008）。

部分特定畸形的描述

无脑畸形

无脑畸形，连同脑膨出和脊柱裂，通常被归类为神经管缺陷，因为它们是神经胚发育障碍。在无脑畸形中，喙侧神经孔在 24 天内无法关闭，形成一个开放的缺陷（通常会非常大），涉及皮肤和颅骨；退化和出血的脑组织位于暴露的颅骨上。无脑畸形可能与其他神经管缺陷同时发生，也有可能合并各种中枢神经系统以外的问题。如果有遗传的因素参与，要注意明确这一点。

无脑胎儿在孕期易自然流产。在那些活着出生的胎儿最终结局无一例外的是死亡，常常发生在出生后数分钟内，也有存活了几个小时，偶尔可以存活几个星期。

尽管遗传和多种环境因素的相互作用很清楚，但导致无脑畸形的原因尚不清楚。家族内重复发生相对常见，与母亲年龄过小或高龄都有关。地理差异和生活习惯差异对发病率有显著的影响。营养不良，尤其是叶酸缺乏，似乎很重要。

无脑畸形可以在产前很容易诊断出来，并考虑终止妊娠。

前脑无裂畸形

前脑无裂畸形（图 84.5）是一组异质性疾病，其起源与妊娠前四周的致病过程有关。它主要影响前脑和面部，但颅后窝结构也有不同程度的影响。其病因多种多样，涉及遗传和获得性机制。它可以表现为孤立的畸形，或者以综合征的形式出现。已确定的致畸原因包括母体糖尿病、维甲酸和酒精。染色体组型异常，尤其是 13 号和 18 号染色体三倍体，是特别常见的，至少有 9 种不同的基因突变影响了背侧和腹侧发育模式（包括通常所说的 sonic hedgehog

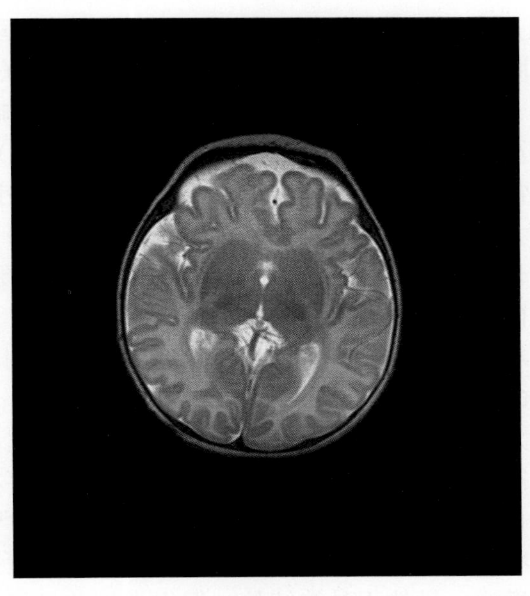

图 84.5　3 周龄儿童的轴位 T2 磁共振影像，半叶型前脑无裂畸形，表现为尿崩症。图像显示孤立的部分额叶融合

基因）。已知的突变似乎只导致一小部分散发性前脑无裂畸形病例。

习惯上，前脑无裂畸形分为未分叶、半分叶和已分叶。此外，它可以分为完整的和不完整的形式。所有这些都是由于解剖板的分离失败造成的。在未分叶前脑无裂畸形中，大脑半球没有分离，仅仅形成一个脑球和一个脑室。在已分叶前脑无裂畸形中，半球完全分离，但没有或仅有发育不全的嗅球和嗅束（无嗅脑畸形），深部灰质在不同程度上融合。

半分叶前脑无裂畸形表现为中线改变，通常有小的不同程度融合的额叶、分开的枕叶和后部一个大脑镰出现。最近新确认的一种形式是额叶、枕叶与深部灰质核团分离，但额叶后部和顶叶后凸融合，以及胼胝体的体部（但不是膝部或压部）的缺如。

前脑无裂畸形可能与许多其他脑畸形相关，包括：胼胝体的发育不全（没有 Probst 束），融合和（或）发育不良的脑干核团、小脑半球和（或）蚓部异常、Chiari 1 型畸形、菱脑融合、背侧囊肿、脑积水。背侧囊肿往往很大，位于矢状裂后部，或在未分叶前脑无裂畸形中位于脑球的后侧。这些表现有时反映了单个侧脑室的扩张或者第三脑室的极端扩张。

脑积水通常与背部囊肿有关，也可能是脑室内的生发基质挤压的结果。神经元迁移、皮质组织和髓鞘化的异常在前脑无裂畸形中很常见。这些问题一定程度上引起了相关的发育问题，如学习困难和癫痫。

有观点认为，在前脑无裂畸形中，面部情况反映大脑情况，因为面部异常越严重，大脑畸形一般越严重，但也有许多例外。面部可能是正常的，也可能是最极端的，表现为在中线只有一只眼眶（而没有眼球结构）的独眼畸形，无鼻畸形（或眼眶上长鼻），发育不全或缺失的下颌骨，无下颌并耳畸形。较不严重的面部异常包括低眼压（很少高眼压），鼻部异常（如后鼻孔闭锁和单鼻孔），裂腭或唇，小嘴。

大多数前脑无裂畸形的患儿在最初几个月内死亡，但越来越多的少数人存活到幼儿期甚至更久。死亡的原因可能是中枢神经系统畸形的影响，也可能是相关的非中枢神经系统问题。较轻的病例，预期寿命可接近正常人。

大多数前脑无裂畸形的婴儿肌张力低，这种症状可能持续存在，但痉挛通常会经常发生。存在学习障碍，在无分叶病例中，畸形的影响更加严重。在症状最轻的病例中，智力可能是正常或接近正常的。癫痫，虽然不是持续的，但很常见并且经常很严重、难以处理。

早期，详细的 MRI 成像来充分评估畸形是很重要的，有些病例，在与积水性无脑畸形和严重的脑积水相鉴别时有些困难。用血管成像来确定大脑前动脉和硬膜血管窦的位置和形态会很有帮助。除非致畸原因很明确，否则，非常有必要进行临床遗传评估，来确定是孤立的畸形还是综合征性畸形。内分泌和心脏的评估也很重要。当出现相关的背侧囊肿和（或）脑积水时，可能需要神经外科介入。

视中隔发育不良（视中隔 – 垂体发育不良复合体）

这种疾病是人们最为了解的大脑畸形之一（**图 84.6**）。它的三个主要特征——透明隔缺如、视神经发育不全和垂体功能障碍——可以作为孤立的表现或任意组合出现。可能与其他的脑畸形相关，这为可能的病因学提供了重要的线索。

单纯的透明隔缺如与人类已知的神经发育问题无关，尽管它可能会在大鼠产生导航问题。有一些病例描述了隔膜部分缺失的情况。穹隆和膈静脉的向前位移可能会使人误认为存在有部分透明膈。此外，还有一些透明隔间腔增宽的病例，与视神经发育不良和（或）垂体问题有关。视神经发育不全可为单侧或双侧（在这种情况下可对称或不对称），视力可能从正常到失明范围内的任何情况，也可能出现视野缺损和周围视野受限，这可能与视神经萎缩和发育不全相关，垂体功能减退可发生在新生儿期，同时伴有低血糖。然而，最常见的表现是由于生长激素的缺乏而导致的生长发育障碍。垂体其他激素可以因此而受到影响，少数患者出现全垂体功能减退。

最常见的相关的脑畸形是胼胝体发育不全、分叶的前脑无裂畸形、裂脑畸形和局灶性皮质发育不良。脑积水，前文已描述。

视中隔发育不良的核心特征提示是在腹侧诱导发育过程中发生了损伤。母亲年龄过小和初产妇都是重要的危险因素。大多数病例的病因可能是非遗传性的，尽管大量的基因突变可能导致这种疾病的各种特征。其他的致畸因素，包括医疗和非医疗的药物，以及先天性病毒感染，都可能有关。许多病例可能与血管性的致病因素有关，有一些与视中隔发育不良相关的中枢神经系统异常，可以用妊娠后期遭受到进一步的血管损伤来解释。

在产前和妊娠期可以通过测量与胎龄相关的视神经直径来发现视中隔发育不良。当然，只有在治疗性流产的可能性已经排除的情况下，才能诊断。

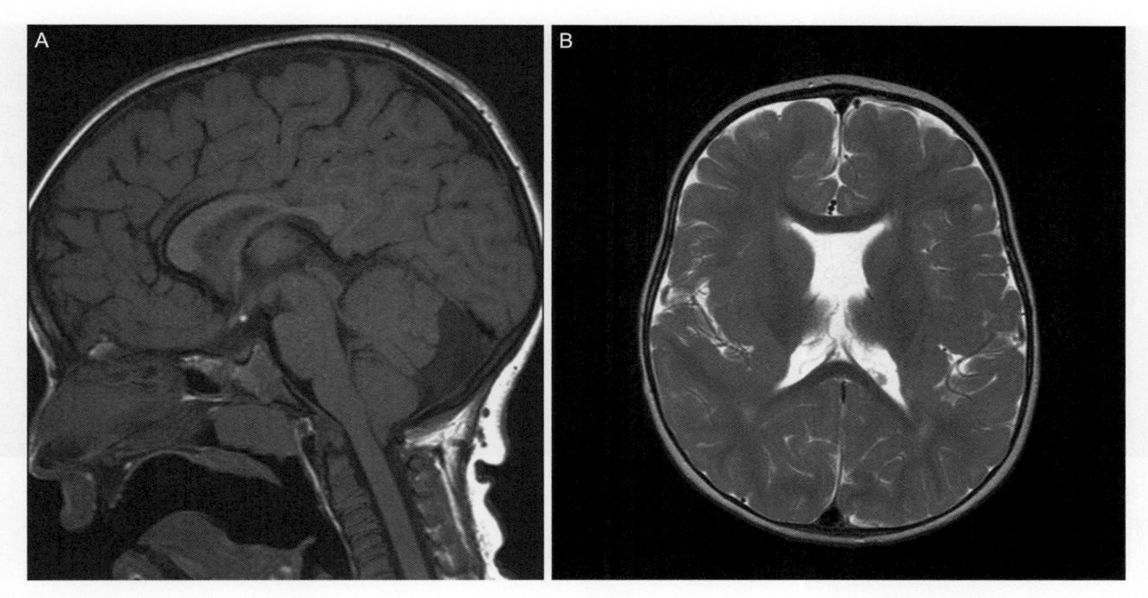

图 84.6　视中隔发育不良。T1 矢状位（**图** 84.6A）显示异位的垂体后叶，“亮点”位于视交叉后部，同时伴有一个偶然发现的 Chiari Ⅰ型畸形。T2 轴位（**图** 84.6B）确认透明隔缺失，伴随有外侧裂后部周围异常增厚的皮质，同时有外侧裂周围多小脑回

脑裂畸形

这类畸形的特征是从脑室的边缘到软脑膜表面的单侧或两侧裂隙（**图** 84.7）。这种裂隙通常伴随着异位的灰质，通常是多小脑回的。这种情况应该与脑穿通畸形相区别。裂口的两侧可分离或粘连（开放型、闭合型脑裂畸形），它通常位于大脑外侧裂区域，但可能更多地位于外侧裂前部或者后部。脑裂畸形可以单独发生，也可能与其他脑畸形相关，包括大脑半球其他部位的多小脑畸形、胼胝体不全、透明隔缺如、视隔发育不良等，也可以合并脑积水。

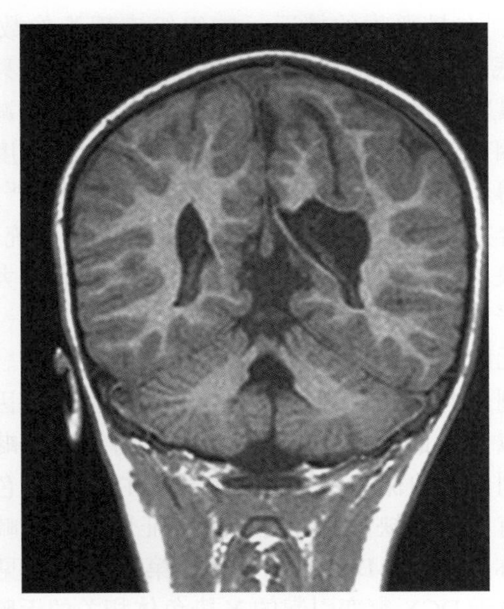

图 84.7　冠状位 T1 显示左侧半球闭合型唇脑裂畸形，可以看到垂直裂隙，从侧脑室边缘延续到软脑膜的表面，裂隙壁由异常增厚的皮质覆盖（多小脑回）。中线胼胝体缺如

这类畸形的临床表现复杂多样，同时也反映了裂隙的位置和严重程度以及裂隙合并的畸形。运动缺陷（半身或四肢）、学习困难（轻度至重度）和癫痫非常常见。癫痫发作，最常见的是局灶性发作，但也可以是全身性的，并且是药物控制无效的。

脑裂畸形是在神经元迁移和皮质组织过程中产生的畸形，很多病因假说认为是血管性的因素。通过对家族性病例的研究后发现，一些基因突变可以引起这类畸形。然而，大多数病例是散发性的，药物和感染性致畸剂在病因学方面也很重要。一些更严重的病例可以在产前被检测出来。

灰质异位

灰质异位的特征是神经元迁移到皮质外（**图** 84.8）。这里描述两种主要类型：结节型和条带型。

结节型异位是由正常神经元和胶质细胞组成的圆形肿块，没有条带状组织，可以位于脑室室管膜内侧和正常皮质之间的任何位置。异位的灰质具有正常灰质的信号特征，有助于将它们与结节性硬化的室管膜下结节相区分。最常见的形式是它们位于室管膜内侧附近，被称为室周结节异位。灰质异位可以是单发的或多发的，单侧的或双侧的，对称的或

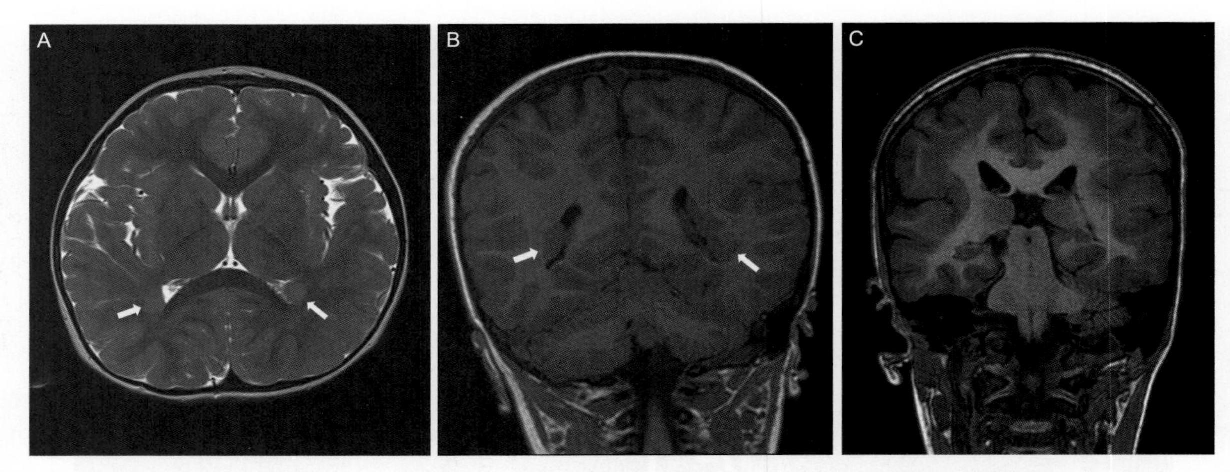

图 84.8 轴位 T2（A）和冠状位 T1（B）显示：一个 4 岁女孩，复杂癫痫，双侧脑室周围灰质异位（白色箭头），与脑组织的灰质相比，异位在 T1 和 T2 序列上均呈等信号。冠状位 T1（C）显示双侧条带型异位（双皮质综合征）

不对称的。结节型异位可能是无症状的，但它们经常引起局灶性或广泛性癫痫发作，后者提示畸形与丘脑皮质回路有功能联系。许多具有结节型异位的个体，智力在正常范围内，并且没有躯体障碍。然而另外一些患者，特别是那些在童年时即出现灰质异位的人，在学习和运动上有不同程度的障碍。结节型异位可阻塞导水管，引起脑积水。结节型异位通常孤立出现，但可与其他脑畸形合并发生，包括 Chiari Ⅱ型畸形。

结节型异位可与心脏、结缔组织和凝血功能异常有关。它似乎主要是 Filamin1（也称为 FilaminA）突变的结果，建议进行筛查。

双侧脑室周围结节型异位多见于女性。大多数病例是由 Filamin1 突变引起的，这是 X 染色体显性突变，通常在男性中是致命的。非遗传因素被认为是大多数单侧病例的原因。它们经常发生在三角区后部区域，后者是血管分水岭。常常合并海马异常。脑室周围结节型异位可以在产前检查检测到。

条带型异位的特征是大脑半球的两层皮质（因此也被称为双皮质综合征）。异位皮质位于真正的新大脑皮质下方的白质中，并且不分层。可以有不同的厚度，并且连接着正常的皮质，但是不会发生于扣带回和颞叶皮质。也有一些病例报道可以有两层非正常的皮质，覆盖的大脑皮质通常表现正常，也可能增厚。其他异常可能包括脑室增大、胼胝体变薄和小脑蚓部异常。异常条带的厚度与发育问题的严重程度相关。可能会发生癫痫，它通常始于儿童早期至中期，但发病可能更早或更晚。智力变化从轻度智力低下到严重的学习障碍都有可能发生。这类畸形也可能导致运动障碍。

条带型异位是一种神经元迁移的遗传性疾病。它主要是 X 染色体显性遗传，发病人群以女性为主，但在男性中是致命性疾病，是由于 doublecortin（DCX）基因的突变。一些 DCZ 突变在男性中是非致命的，但会导致无脑回，一种更严重的神经元迁移异常疾病。一小部分男性有带状异位，由体细胞 DCX 突变引起。

无脑回畸形（光滑脑）和巨脑回

经典的无脑回畸形（又称为 1 型无脑回畸形）

经典的无脑回畸形（通常简称为无脑回畸形），是一种大脑皮质缺乏（部分或完全）正常脑沟（脑回），而且皮质异常变厚（脑回肥厚）的脑畸形（**图 84.9**）。在最严重的情况，脑组织表现为像数字 8，和妊娠中晚期的形状相似。增厚的皮质通常只有四层。罹患畸形的患者通常在出生后因为肌张力减退和进食困难而明确诊断。可能发生重度到极重度的学习障碍和频率渐增的强直状态。癫痫通常是严重的。很少合并有其他相关的神经系统和非神经系统表现，这取决于遗传原因。畸形患儿的预期寿命会大大减少，严重的甚至在婴儿期死亡。

无脑回畸形是一种神经元迁移的遗传病。大多数病例是由于 LIS1 基因的突变所致。LIS1 基因的突变可以产生最严重的表型，表现为特征性的畸形从后部到前部的梯度变化。一些患者在 17 号染色体短臂上有明显的缺失，并有一种特征性的面部畸形外观，称为 Miller-Dieker 综合征。第二个最常见的原因是由于 DCX 突变引起的 X 染色体相关的无脑回畸形，具有从前部到后部的梯度。X 染色体相关的无脑回畸形也可能是由于 ARX 突变，这类型的患者有

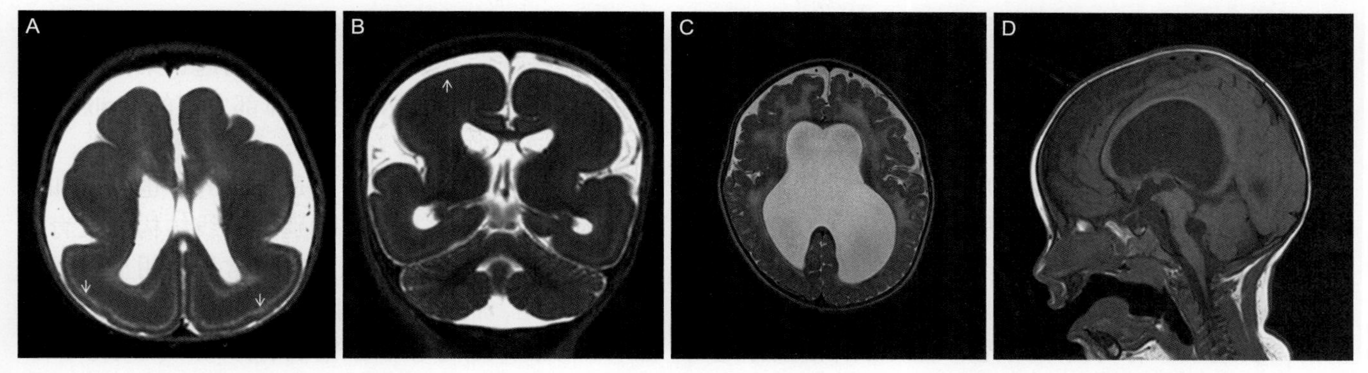

图 84.9　无脑回畸形（A、B）：6 月大婴儿，生长缓慢，全身性癫痫发作。轴位 T2 图像（A）和冠状位图像（B）显示典型的无脑回畸形，皮质的外形变薄，白质层细胞稀疏（白色箭头），与深部受限的神经元相分隔。很浅的大脑外侧裂形成"数字 8"的外形。（C、D）：14 月大的儿童诊断为 Dandy-Walker 综合征。轴位 T2（C）显示异常的双额浅沟和延迟的髓鞘形成，矢状位（D）显示额外的脑桥发育不良

模糊不清的生殖器。无脑回畸形也可作为肾小管病变的一种表现，特别是 TUBA1A 突变。这可能与胼胝体发育不良或发育不全和小脑发育不全有关。

在受影响的家庭中常可进行产前遗传诊断。神经影像学可以从孕晚期开始发现无脑回畸形。

鹅卵石样无脑回畸形（又称 2 型无脑回畸形）

鹅卵石样无脑畸形发生在三种相关疾病中，均有先天性肌肉营养不良和发育性眼部疾病（可能是轻微至严重）：Walker-Warburg 综合征、Fukuyama 综合征和肌肉眼脑病。它们由大量不同基因突变引起的 α- 肌营养不良蛋白聚糖的糖基化缺陷，从而引起 α- 抗肌萎缩相关糖蛋白病。在鹅卵石样无脑回畸形中，大脑表面胶质细胞界膜破裂，凹凸不平，导致软脑膜细胞、神经元和胶质细胞异位。鹅卵石样无脑回畸形几乎总是复杂畸形的一部分，特别是涉及小脑的畸形。脑积水在 Walker-Warburg 综合征中非常常见，偶尔出现肌肉眼脑疾病，但这不是 Fukuyama 综合征的特征。

多小脑回畸形

多小脑回畸形的特征是出现过度异常卷曲的小的融合脑回。在 MRI 上，它的外观是多变的。它表现为多个小脑回（可能与某些脑积水中看到的小脑回畸形混淆）。此外，它也可能表现为皮质增厚（与巨脑回畸形鉴别困难），有"凹凸不平"的灰白色交界处，或者是皮质的光滑区域（如果是广泛的光滑区域，可能与无脑回畸形混淆）。灰白质界线通常会"模糊"，其下的白质通常变薄。它可以是单侧的或双侧的（在这种情况下它可以是对称的或不对称的）、局部的或广泛的。已经发现，某些不同的分布区域，具有不同的病因学意义。这些分布区域包括双侧额叶、双侧额顶叶、双侧外侧裂周边、双侧顶枕叶矢状窦旁、双侧广泛的或单侧的外侧裂周边。经常有额外的脑畸形，反映了多小脑回畸形的广泛病因。

多小脑回畸形的临床表现反映了异常皮质的分布、范围、其他相关的畸形以及潜在的病因。有些病例在出生后不久，因为有严重的运动障碍（可以包括关节挛缩）、喂养困难和癫痫，就得以诊断。其他一些病例只是在偶然发作或家庭成员确诊后被发现。患有相对轻微的神经发育 / 神经精神疾病的人可能被发现有多小脑回畸形。局灶性或全身性癫痫发作很常见，在任何年龄都可能出现。然而，它绝不是持续性的，当它和其他脑部畸形合并出现时，发作时间可能是有限的和（或）对抗癫痫药物有反应。由于它倾向于外侧裂周边区域，假性延髓障碍在多小脑回畸形病例中很常见。

多小脑回畸形是由各种遗传性和获得性因素对发育中的大脑造成损伤引起的。组织学特征表明，很多病例出现在妊娠 20~24 周左右神经元迁移结束时。然而，其他一些组织学特征表明其起源可能更早。至少在某些情况下，可能发生在妊娠的第四个月之前，神经元正在迁移的阶段。血管损伤和子宫内感染（如风疹、巨细胞病毒和弓形虫感染）是多小脑回畸形重要的获得性因素。染色体异常在多小脑回畸形中很常见。特别重要的是涉及 22q11.2 的缺失，这种情况见于外侧裂周区的多小脑回畸形，常合并有先天性心脏缺陷和免疫系统缺陷。在多小脑回畸形的家族性病例中发现了几种特异性的基因突变，这些突变尤其出现在双侧畸形，但并不仅限于双侧畸形中。多小脑回畸形具有一些代谢疾病的特征，包括 Zellweger 综合征（一种过氧化物酶异常疾病）、有

机酸尿症、氨基酸尿症和线粒体疾病。因此，进行彻底的诊断检查是必要的。

脑穿通畸形

脑穿通畸形，这个术语仍然令人困惑。真正的脑穿通畸形囊肿是大脑半球内与脑室系统连通的局灶性囊腔。它似乎也与蛛网膜下腔空间连通，但总是有一个薄膜将两者分开。囊肿缺乏内部结构，囊壁由白质组成。有时会采用先天性或碎屑性脑穿通畸形来命名。脑穿通畸形也用来指被异常皮质覆盖的全厚囊肿（如多小脑回）。它可以被称为发育性脑穿通畸形，但术语裂脑畸形现在通常是首选，因为它的病因是不同的（见前文）

脑穿通畸形的临床特征反映了囊肿的大小、位置和潜在原因。常见的障碍包括脑瘫（痉挛类型、单侧或双侧）、学习障碍和癫痫。癫痫发生在大约 1/3 的患者中，可以从婴儿期开始直到成年。如果是前者，可能表现为癫痫性脑病，具有明显的广泛性发作表现；而后者，局灶性发作则是常见的。惊吓诱发的癫痫发作是被广泛认可的。少数脑穿通畸形囊肿因为脉络丛的搏动而增大并产生压力效应。

脑穿通畸形通常是由从妊娠中后期到产后早期大脑的获得性损伤引起的。从发病数量上看，缺血和出血是最重要的病因，但其他原因也包括创伤和感染。家族性常染色体显性的病例可能是由 COL4A1 基因突变引起的，该基因编码一种非常广泛表达的胶原蛋白。相关的白质异常和钙化可能有助于识别。COL4A1 表型是广泛的，因此进行遗传咨询是至关重要的。儿童和成年期间有发生出血性卒中的风险。

胼胝体发育不全以及胼胝体的其他发育异常

在胚胎发生过程中，联合体连接着大脑发育中的对侧区域。其中最重要的结构是从间脑延伸到视交叉的终板。其他结构包括前后联合和海马联合。胼胝体的形成包括终板的凋亡，从而使发育中的胼胝体纤维越过中线后投射。胼胝体发育不全是这一过程受到干扰而引起的，终板作为一个障碍而不是一个促进者。受阻的纤维束沿发育中的大脑半球内壁延伸变形，形成 Probst 束。这些组织的出现可以区别先天性胼胝体发育不全和后天胼胝体受损。胼胝体的形成是从喙端至尾端；在部分发育不全时，压部最有可能缺失，其次是嘴端，中间部分的缺陷最不常见。有一种胼胝体发育不全，各部位都存在，但胼胝体异常薄，这是由于各种原因造成的神经纤维缺陷引起的。Probst 束不会出现。

完全性胼胝体发育不全的神经影像学特征包括：较宽的侧脑室，缺乏正常的中线凸起；第三脑室向上移位；第三脑室上方侧脑室体部之间的 Probst 束，以及其他连合的显现。

胼胝体发育不全，可以是独立的，也可以和很多种脑的发育异常有关，特别是中线结构的发育异常。面部畸形，特别眼距过宽很常见。明显的发育问题很常见，包括学习缺陷（从轻度到重度）、运动障碍和癫痫。这些通常是相关发育异常的后果。孤立性的发育不全可能是无症状的，因为其他的半球间连接（正常和异常）接管了胼胝体的功能。然而，详细的神经心理评估通常会发现视觉处理、精细运动和特定的语言障碍。

胼胝体发育不全通常起源于遗传因素，是由某些染色体异常和单基因缺陷引起的后果。特别值得注意的是它经常与导水管狭窄引起的 X 染色体相关的脑积水有关，以及胼胝体发育不全而引起的精神发育迟缓和痉挛。两者都是由 L1CAM 的突变引起的，它编码一个细胞黏附分子。它也可能是由于各种代谢紊乱和致畸剂的影响，包括酒精。

小头畸形和大头畸形

小头畸形的定义是头围低于人群平均值的三个标准差以下。它几乎是，但不是完全与大头畸形（小脑）同义，因为脑组织可能很小，但头部大小正常。通常将其归类为先天性（或原发性）或后天性（或继发性），这取决于出生时头围大小是否正常。脑回的形状可能是正常的（真性小头畸形）、简化的、增厚的（微小无脑回畸形），或表现为多小脑回畸形。胼胝体可能缺失。显微镜检查可能显示神经元耗竭，特别是在皮质Ⅱ和Ⅲ层。

小头畸形的原因是多变的，包括可以影响脑组织的大多数病理过程。它的临床表现，可以从正常到严重残疾。显著的学习困难是常见的，但绝不是普遍的。

在出生前、婴儿期或儿童早期，任何导致脑组织破坏或干扰脑组织生长、活动的病理过程，都会导致小头畸形。先天性的小头畸形发生在常染色体隐性遗传、常染色体显性和 X 染色体相关遗传模式中。其中第一种模式最常见。目前至少已经识别 6 个基因，这些基因的突变会导致常染色体隐性小头畸形。许多导致小头畸形的基因在调节神经元增殖和细胞凋亡中具有重要作用。总体上来说，对先天性小脑畸形的研究非常有助于理解脑的发育（Gilmore and Walsh，2013）。

半巨脑畸形

这是一种复杂的大脑畸形，其特征是一侧大脑半球异常大。有时一个异常小的大脑半球（半小头畸形）会引起诊断混乱。虽然通常局限于前脑，但中脑、后脑也参与其中。病理上显示神经元和胶质细胞均有异常增殖。皮质的异常增厚和异位常见，通常有同侧侧脑室的扩大。

半巨脑畸形可能与同侧面部过度生长有关，有时与身体其他部位生长有关。此外，与神经皮肤疾病有很大的联系，包括结节性硬化症、Ⅰ型神经纤维瘤病、proteus 综合征、线性皮脂腺痣综合征和伊藤色素减少症。除了这些重要的关联，半巨脑的胚胎学仍有待确定。

临床表型是多样的。特殊的是，患者可能神经发育正常。更常见的是，它们有一系列的缺陷，可能包括偏瘫、视力缺陷、学习困难和癫痫。癫痫可能是小发作或明显大发作，经常非常严重，对抗癫痫药物耐药。半巨脑畸形是导致几种严重儿童癫痫综合征的重要原因，包括 Ohtahara 综合征、West 综合征和 Lennox–Gastaut 综合征。它是部分性癫痫持续状态的原因之一。

后颅凹畸形

小脑畸形并不少见。接下来将描述一些更具特征性的畸形种类。此外，完全性小脑缺如、广泛性小脑发育不全、小脑发育不良和巨大小脑，均已经被广泛认识。临床上，它们通常与大运动延迟、各种小脑体征和多变的整体发育延迟有关。经常会采用共济失调性脑瘫这一名称。后颅凹畸形的病因多样，包括孟德尔遗传疾病、染色体异常、单基因缺陷、神经代谢紊乱、致畸损伤和其他后天损伤。

Dandy-Walker 综合征包括小脑蚓部完全或部分缺失、抬高和向上旋转，第四脑室囊性扩张。脑积水很常见。在部分但并非所有的患者中，第四脑室出口被阻塞。Dandy-Walker 综合征可以是独立的疾病，也可以伴随其他畸形，特别是颅后窝和胼胝体发育不全，以及中枢神经系统以外的问题。常见颅内压升高的表现，小脑体征和智力损害也是常见的，但不是恒定的。

Dandy-Walker 综合征可以是几种少见常染色体异常、多种染色体异常的表现，也可以是单独的表现。在一些患病个体的家族里，发现一些可以导致其发生的特异性基因突变。

Joubert 综合征（图 84.10）是一种遗传性疾病，其最特征性的表现是小脑蚓发育不全或发育不良，突出的小脑上脚，深的脚间窝（放射学上表现为特征性磨牙征），以及形状异常并向喙侧移位的第四脑室，这可能涉及枕部脑膜膨出和神经系统之外的问题，尤其是视网膜营养不良和肾问题，包括肾结核。患病的婴儿身体十分脆弱，其特征是在早期异常的呼吸模式：间断呼吸急促——呼吸暂停，之后可能出现眼球运动障碍。

这类疾病是常染色体隐性遗传的，超过 20 个突变基因与之相关。这些突变会影响纤毛功能，常被归类为纤毛虫病。

菱脑融合是一种罕见的畸形，先天性小脑蚓部缺如，小脑半球内侧和齿状核融合。它通常是一种孤立的畸形，但可能伴有其他的中线缺陷。此外，

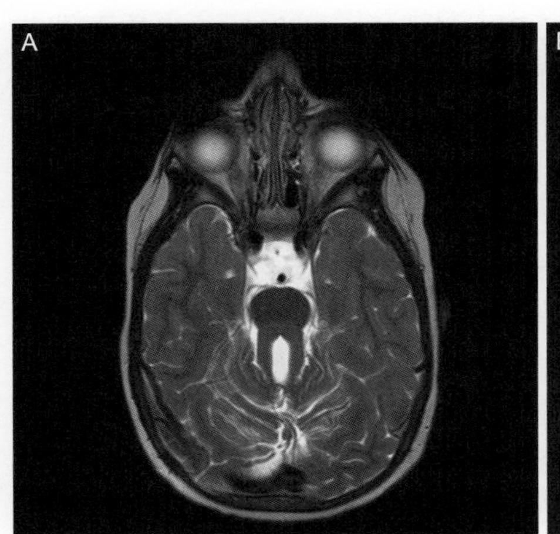

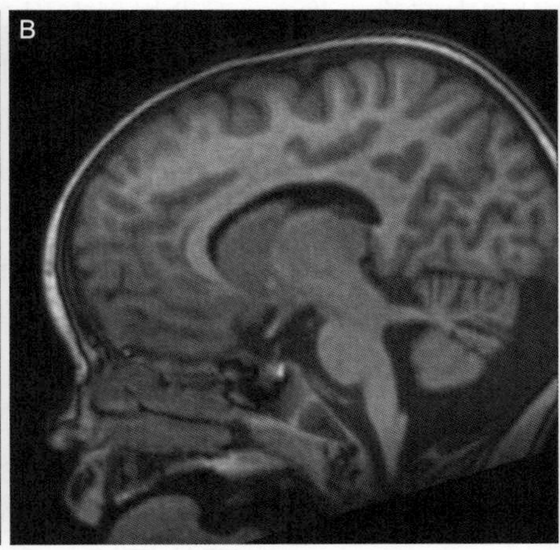

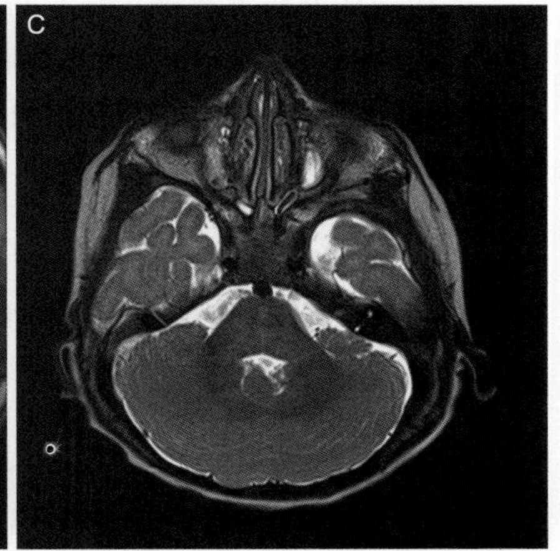

图 84.10　轴位 T2（A）和矢状位 T1（B）显示 Joubert 综合征，注意轴位 T2 图像上，特征性的“臼齿”征，是由于变厚的小脑上脚，在矢状位图像上可以看到第四脑室向喙端异位，此外还有小脑下蚓部发育不全。（C）轴位 T2 图像显示中线蚓部的缺如，以及与菱脑融合相同的小脑半球融合

还与 X 染色体相关性脑积水有关。其临床表现主要为小脑体征，不同程度的认知障碍。它被认为是由遗传起源的畸形，尽管文献中记录过孟德尔遗传模式，但经常是散在发生的。

巨大小脑延髓池，在大约 1% 的计算机断层扫描（computed tomography，CT）和 MRI 脑部扫描中可以发现这类畸形，目前认为是偶然发现的疾病，是指小脑后部脑脊液空间的非病理学扩大，不伴有相关的小脑异常。

脑膨出

脑膨出是硬膜囊内的神经组织通过颅骨缺陷突出。神经管未能完全闭合被认为是这种情况的胚胎学基础。脑膨出的发病机制是，神经管形成的最后阶段，神经和表面外胚层分离障碍（Hoving and Vermeij-Keers，2000）。高达 40% 的患者可能会有染色体异常。这类疾病发病率为 0.8~4/10 000 个活产婴儿（Simpson et al.，1984）。

典型的表现是从鼻 - 筛窦部到枕部区域的肿胀。可以分为基底、前顶部（额叶）、凸面和枕部。儿童可能表现为鼻梗阻、脑脊液漏或少见的反复性脑膜炎，特别是病变位于鼻筛骨部或者颅底区域。可能伴有脑积水、癫痫、神经功能缺陷或发育延迟。

产前超声波和胎儿磁共振成像可以帮助识别子宫内的病变。出生后，虽然超声可以提供有用的信息，但 MRI 扫描有助于展示囊内容和其他相关的颅内异常，如小头畸形、胼胝体发育不全、Chiari 畸形和蛛网膜囊肿（Da Silva et al.，2015）。鼻部脑膨出的辨别诊断包括皮样囊肿和罕见的鼻胶质瘤。CT 重建扫描有助于发现骨缺陷。

治疗方法取决于囊的大小、位置和内容物。关键的步骤是确定骨边缘和硬膜缺损，将疝出的神经组织复位至颅内，然后修复硬脑膜和颅骨。额筛骨的病变或者其他相关颅骨缺陷 / 畸形，因为疝出的组织复位距离较远，可以采用轨道推进技术（Mahapatra，2011）。颅底的病变损越来越多地通过内镜得以修复，且效果良好（Ma et al.，2015）。应注意缺损部位静脉窦的解剖结构，因为硬膜静脉窦通常与囊密切相关。如果有证据表明脑脊液漏，可能需要紧急进行手术。患者可能需要在矫正手术前或之后处理相关的脑积水。

与枕部相比，前部的（额筛骨部位）鼻脑膨出的生存率更高。幸存者的神经损伤率较高，只有 48% 发育正常（Lo et al.，2008）。一项对脑膨出的研究通过单变量分析，确定了几个预测发育迟缓的重要的独立预测因素（如：存在相关的颅内异常、脑积水、癫痫发作、小脑畸形和畸形内的脑组织）。在这些指标中，脑积水和颅内异常，对发育不良的累积预测效果最多。然而，病变的位置并不是一个重要因素（Lo et al.，2008）。在 Da Silva 等的另一项系统性回顾，在多维模型中脑积水与神经系统损伤有关。病变的位置再次被认为并不是影响脑积水或神经紊乱发生率的重要因素。脑积水的存在导致了更严重的神经系统结局。

神经外科手术的注意事项

患有脑畸形的儿童通常会有复杂的神经功能障碍，因此需要多学科协作。医疗照顾由一位神经疾病的顾问来协调完成最合适。此外，必须考虑是否存在神经系统以外的问题，并邀请相关专家加入团队。中线畸形常伴随内分泌异常，结节性异位患者可能会伴随心脏问题。神经外科医生参与治疗脑畸形儿童有三个主要原因：治疗颅内压升高；治疗癫痫；帮助治疗缓解痉挛（强直状态）。

正如已经提到的，许多畸形与脑积水有关，可以是几乎持续、频繁或偶尔伴随的。最常用脑室 - 腹腔分流术来缓解脑积水。然而，在一些畸形中（如 Dandy-Walker 畸形），囊肿腹腔（cyst-peritoneal）分流术或者联合手术被一些人提倡。

对于与癫痫相关的弥漫性和双侧畸形，切除手术永远不是一种选择，但功能性手术，包括胼胝体切开术、迷走神经刺激和多处软膜下切除可能会发挥作用。局灶性皮质发育异常是小叶和多叶切除的常见原因，癫痫学家对局灶性皮质发育异常进行了分类，对手术规划有用（Blümcke et al.，2011）。皮质下结节性异位也是癫痫手术的指征。半巨脑畸形，在非常年幼的儿童中经常表现为癫痫性脑病，也是半球切除术 / 切开术的重要指征。越来越多的证据表明，手术可能有利于认知发展，以及帮助控制癫痫发作。

脑畸形是导致脑瘫的一个重要原因。对于后颅凹畸形，这通常有肌张力减退或共济失调，不适合神经外科干预。痉挛和较小程度肌张力障碍在许多其他畸形中很常见，鞘内巴氯芬泵和选择性背根切断术可能在特定的病例中发挥作用。

延伸阅读、参考文献

扫描书末二维码获取。

第 85 章　脊髓发育与椎管闭合不全

Dominic Thompson 著
张衡、周文韬 译，田永吉 审校

引言

椎管闭合不全（脊柱裂）包括一组脊髓发育异常性疾病。在这组疾病中，它们由于胚胎学起源、临床表现和预后不同而被区分开来。椎管闭合不全的命名容易混淆，然而，根据胚胎发生的假定起始点，提出了一个简化分类。该简化分类不仅简化了术语，而且有助于指导正确的研究和管理。需要强调的是，虽然基于动物模型的胚胎发生的详细记录可用于解释一些开放性椎管缺陷，但对于闭合性椎管闭合不全，由于缺乏对椎管发育缺陷的客观证据，其机制不清。

脊髓的发生

虽然脊柱（中胚层）和脊髓（外胚层）的早期发育之间有密切的联系，但脊髓发生的不同阶段有助于理解椎管闭合不全。脊髓发生的全面描述详见 Pang 和 Thompson 的文献（Pang and Thompson，2010）。脊髓的发生可以分为三个阶段：原肠胚发育、初级神经胚发育和次级神经胚发育。

原肠胚发育

最原始的胚胎包括一个双层结构，即二胚层胚盘。在原始胚层的形成过程中，随着中轴线（原条）的形成，胚胎的极性得以确立。二胚层胚盘的外层细胞向原条迁移，然后在上、下胚层之间扩展，使之成为三层结构，这样就建立了三个生殖细胞层（内胚层、中胚层和外胚层）。随着胚胎的增大，原条从头向尾倒退，留下脊索。脊索是脊椎动物发育的基础，不仅维持着胚胎极性，而且还维持着背腹的同一性。在一个短暂的时期，通过脊索穿过胚胎有一个连接，它允许羊膜腔与卵黄囊（神经肠管）进行信号沟通。通过不同的信号传递过程，脊索将诱导覆盖的外胚层形成神经板，并开始将发育前的中胚层转化为体细胞中胚层。体细胞中胚层是脊柱形成的前驱。

初级神经胚发育

外胚层是早期胚胎的背侧部分，最终将形成中枢神经系统和体壁（皮肤及其附件）。在初级神经胚形成期间，在脊索的影响下，外胚层开始折叠，折叠边缘的褶将在中线相遇。不同物种的初始交汇点数量不同。然后，在这些“交汇点”之间拉链的过程就会发生，从而形成中枢神经系统的管状结构。褶皱外侧的外胚层将是未来的表面外胚层，这两个外胚层的衍生物（神经和皮肤）之后会在一个被称为分离的过程中分开。

由于初级神经胚分化而形成的神经管最终将形成大脑和脊髓，但仅限于第二个骶骨节段。终末脊髓、脊髓圆锥、终丝和马尾神经以不同的方式形成，称为次级神经胚形成。

次级神经胚发育

在胚胎的尾部有一组多能干细胞，称为尾状细胞团。这组细胞将有助于下泌尿生殖道、远端肛门直肠区和终末脊髓的发育。虽然对人类次级神经分化的细节了解不多，但目前多数认为，终将要分化成神经的细胞聚集在中央管腔周围，形成所谓的髓索，它将参与形成喙端脊髓，后者的形成，也是初级神经胚的结果。由次级神经胚形成的大部分脊髓会发生退化（退行性分化），导致圆锥明显上升，最终形成终丝。

椎管闭合不全分类

文献中有对椎管闭合不全的各种分类，但是基于假定的发育病理学的分类，其中大部分假设，可作为有用的临床指导（**图 85.1**）。基于此，我们可以依次研究那些由原肠胚发育、初级神经胚发育和次

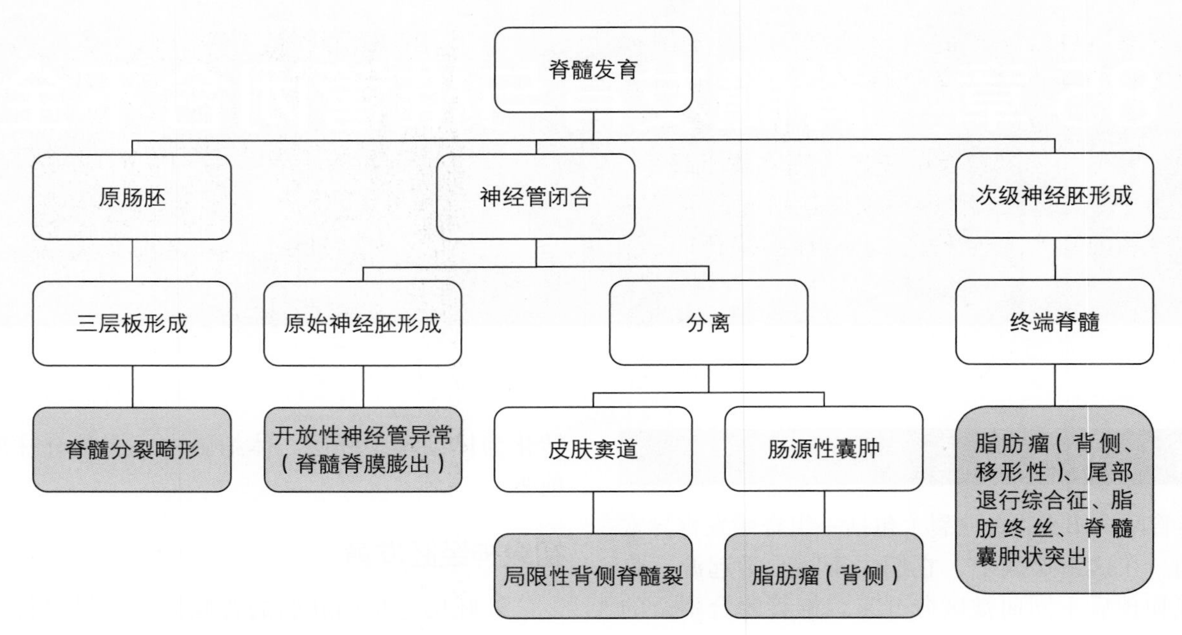

图 85.1 从胚胎学角度对椎管闭合不全的分类

级神经胚发育障碍引起的闭合不全。

原肠胚发育障碍

原肠胚的一个主要特征是三层生殖细胞层的建立，在这一阶段结束时，外胚层将形成面对羊膜腔的胚胎的背侧。因此，起源于早期发育阶段的闭合不全往往位于神经轴的腹侧，更可能与骨骼（中胚层）和内脏（内胚层）异常相关。在脊髓纵裂畸形中，可能存在重复的脊索导致两个神经管。由此产生的两个半侧脊髓可能分别位于不同的硬脊膜管内，中间有骨性中隔（Ⅰ型脊髓纵裂畸形），也可能包含在一个由纤维带分隔的单个硬脊膜管内（Ⅱ型脊髓纵裂畸形）（Pang，1992；Pang et al.，1992）。先天性椎体融合或椎体畸形通常与脊髓纵裂畸形并存，并可能导致脊柱畸形。

从背部到腹面横穿胚胎的神经肠管可能会持续存在，从而导致神经和肠道的衍生物之间以神经性或肠源性囊肿的形式异常连接。这些病变可能发生在从蝶骨枕骨联合到腰骶交界处的任何地方，但不会超过这些界限，因为神经管未沿着胚胎的全长延伸。同样，椎骨异常通常并存，这反映了三个生殖细胞层的受累。

初级神经胚发育异常

初级神经胚发育异常导致典型的开放性神经管缺损。外胚层没有形成管状结构，神经组织没有被皮肤覆盖，而是完全暴露，漏出脑脊液，或被未发育的脑膜覆盖。在脊髓，则导致脊髓膨出或脊髓脊膜膨出。这两个术语可以互换使用，但更准确来说，它们适用于神经基板与周围皮肤齐平的情况（脊髓膨出）或由于蛛网膜下腔积聚的脑脊液（cerebrospinal fluid，CSF）而导致神经基板高出皮肤的情况（脊髓脊膜膨出）。开放性神经管缺损是全中枢神经系统（central nervous system，CNS）畸形，除脊髓异常外，常见的几种脑部结构异常被称为 Chiari Ⅱ 型畸形；大约 80% 的病例也会出现脑积水。需要强调的是，Chiari Ⅱ 型畸形和脑积水与其他椎管（闭合性）闭合不全无关。

初级神经胚发育的一个重要特征是皮肤外胚层和神经外胚层的分离，这个过程被称为分离。根据这一过程是过早发生还是不完全发生，会导致两组不同的脊髓闭合不全。如果神经外胚层在管状突起形成之前过早分离，那么开放的神经管就会暴露于下层的中胚层；根据 McLone 的说法，这是基板表面脂肪形成导致脊髓脂肪瘤的第一步。因此，过早的分离被认为是背部脂肪瘤的潜在机制。重要的是，尽管这一假设符合背部脂肪瘤的解剖形态，但它与移行脂肪瘤或尾部（终丝）脂肪瘤不同，因为后者至少部分附着在圆锥上，因此与次级神经胚发育有关。

如果分离未能完全发生，那么皮肤和中枢神经系统的共同起源的一些残余会持续存在。这类疾病的命名复杂，诸如脑脊膜膨出、真假皮毛窦、长（短）拴系综合征以及局限性脊髓裂等术语（Martínez-Lage et al.，2010；Pang et al.，2013；Thompson，2013）。

可根据神经-皮肤连接的组织学性质区分不同类型的拴系综合征。在局限性脊髓裂（limited dorsal myeloschisis，LDM）中，主要是一系列的神经组织从脊髓的背面延伸到覆盖的皮肤，而在皮毛窦中，这种连接主要是上皮。区别不仅仅是用词，两者在临床表现和神经系统分化模式上也存在差异（见下文）。

次级神经胚发育异常

许多形式的神经管闭合不全涉及圆锥和马尾，因此被认为是由异常的次级神经胚发育或髓索退化受损引起的。如果髓索不能完全内卷成螺旋状，或仅部分内卷，结果是终丝增厚或脂肪增多，当脂肪瘤成分较大时，这被称为尾侧脂肪瘤或终丝脂肪瘤，在这两种情况下，圆锥在功能上趋于完整，但位置低于正常水平。移行性脂肪瘤也可起源于次级神经胚发育。之所以被称为移行性脂肪瘤，因为它们的位置居于背侧型和尾侧型之间，移行性脂肪瘤与圆锥和马尾结构的背根进入区密切相关，因此外科手术切除困难。

一些次级神经胚发育异常具有更广泛的局部关联，反映了尾部细胞群的多样性分化。一系列先天性生殖、泌尿系统异常的情况，都包含于部分尿道直肠瓣畸形（Partial UroRectal Spetal Malformations，PURSM），其中包括了泄殖腔异常、肛门闭锁、直肠阴道瘘和脊髓闭合不全等。有时，这些联系超出了尾部细胞群衍生的范围，包括前肠、心脏和脊椎疾病，并归类于各种缩写，包括 OEIS、VATER 和 VACTERL。

在尾部退化综合征中，似乎完全没有次级神经胚发育，脊髓的圆锥和末端骶节也发生缺失，这些导致了脊髓的高位终止（**图** 85.2）。骶骨发育不良，可能存在肛门直肠畸形。相比之下，在终端脊髓囊肿状突出的病例中，次级神经胚的发育是存在的，但导致了脊髓末端明显扩大。脊髓末端喇叭形扩展到皮下组织中，导致臀沟的中线处有一个大的肿胀（**图** 85.3）。

临床表现

广义上讲，椎管闭合不全有两种表现，第一种是皮肤异常覆盖脊柱，第二种是神经系统、泌尿系统或骨科的缺陷，即所谓的神经-骨科综合征。当然，这些方式间通常存在重叠。

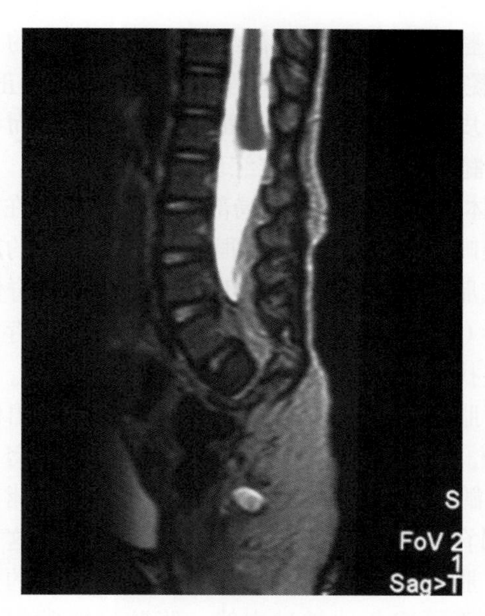

图 85.2 矢状位 T2 加权 MRI 扫描，一个有尾部退化综合征的儿童，脊髓圆锥缺如，脊髓末端有一个典型的被切断的表现，同时也有部分骶骨发育不全

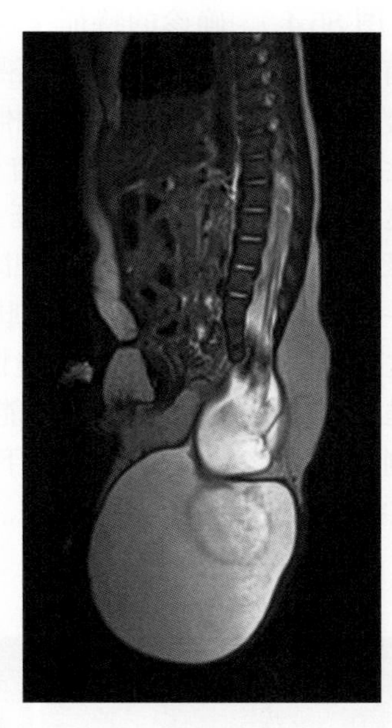

图 85.3 矢状位 T2 加权 MRI 扫描，一个婴儿有终端脊髓囊肿状突出。脊髓末端由于较大的囊性扩张，像是“被吹大”

椎管闭合不全的皮肤特征

开放性脊柱裂和闭合性脊柱裂这两个术语需要说明。“开放”一词是指神经组织暴露的情况，通常会漏出脑脊液，因此适用于脊髓脊膜膨出或脊柱裂，以及一些严重的脊膜膨出，其中神经组织仅被基本的脊膜覆盖。在所有其他形式的椎管闭合不全中，由于完整的覆盖皮肤，神经组织不是可见的，而是隐藏（隐匿）的。这并不是说上覆的皮肤是正常的，相反，皮肤通常在某些方面是异常的，从而导致所谓的脊髓闭合不全的皮肤红斑。

i. 局部体表多毛。中线的局部多毛皮肤是潜在的脊髓纵裂畸形的典型特征，很容易与新生儿的多毛体质或胎毛区分开来。由于骨骼异常常与脊髓纵裂畸形（split cord malformations，SCM）共存，因此应寻找脊柱畸形，如脊柱侧凸或后凸畸形。

ii. 皮下脂肪瘤。这代表了脂肪瘤性脊膜膨出的外部成分。上覆皮肤上偶尔会出现浅浅的酒窝，或出现“鹳”纹血管瘤。在脂肪瘤的深处，经常可以触诊到脊髓后部骨部分的缺损。正是通过这个骨缺损，脂肪瘤连接到脊髓的末端。脂肪瘤的全部或部分不可避免地越过中线。脂肪瘤通常很大，形状各异，有时呈尾状附属物。即使没有相关的神经体征，腰骶部中线脂肪瘤需进一步的评估。

iii. 皮肤窦道。中线的皮肤小点可能代表真皮窦道的皮肤末端（**图** 85.4）。确诊的特征是从缺陷处突出的毛发或有分泌物史，尤其是透明液体、间歇性肿胀或反复感染。这些病变易导致椎管内皮样形成和感染性并发症，如脊髓脓肿或脑（脊）膜炎。

iv. 上皮“瘢痕”，LDM 的典型皮肤特征是上皮变薄，有时被边缘隆起的区域包围，形成凹坑状的效果。LDM 的另一个典型病变是隆起的皮肤穹隆，通常有宽蒂。这些也分别称为非囊性和囊性 LDM。

重要的是，在某些时候，患者可能没有明显的外部迹象。例如，在终丝增厚的情况下，潜在的诊断可能只有在症状出现后才会显露出来。

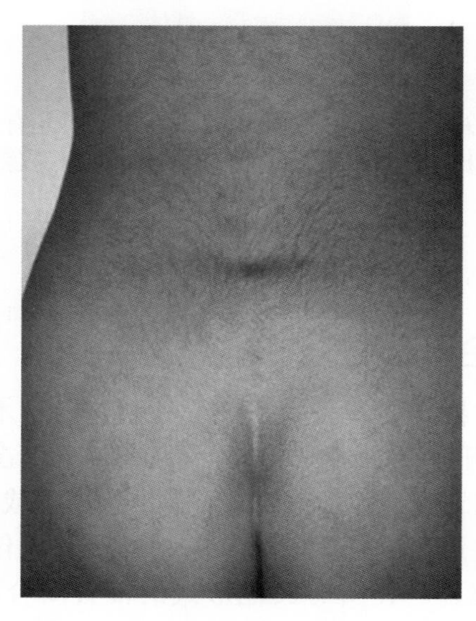

图 85.4 中线处皮肤凹陷，是典型的皮毛窦的痕迹

神经－骨科综合征

脊柱裂可能导致神经系统、泌尿系统和骨科症状和体征的不同组合，统称为神经 - 骨科综合征。

神经系统症状包括疼痛，这常是脊柱局部疼痛或运动引起的下肢疼痛，而不是典型的神经根性疼痛、麻木，通常是足部周围和下肢远端的无力，常常会影响脚踝和足部肌肉组织，且多不对称。

椎管闭合不全的骨科表现包括肌肉萎缩、关节畸形（例如马蹄内翻足）和步态异常。与神经系统症状一样，常表现为不对称性，这在脊髓纵裂畸形中尤其明显，与较小的半侧脊髓相对应的一侧，整个肢体或足都很小。包括先天性融合和半椎体在内的椎骨畸形会增加脊柱侧凸的风险。由于不对称的椎旁肌神经支配，神经肌肉脊柱侧凸也可能发生在高位脊髓脊膜膨出的患者。

由于骶神经根受累引起的泌尿系统异常，虽然可以发生在任何脊髓闭合不全，但是在脊髓脊膜膨出和脊髓脂肪瘤中特别普遍。复发性尿路感染、尿滴漏和尿失禁是典型的临床特征。在年龄较大的儿童中，先前的节制功能丧失、尿急或新发尿路感染可能是神经源性膀胱功能障碍的征兆。由于肠道控制受损导致的粪便感染，可能使一些更严重的椎管闭合不全的状态复杂化。当存在神经源性膀胱功能障碍时，这种情况基本都会发生。单纯的直肠失禁的症状很少起源于神经源性膀胱障碍。

脊髓拴系

“脊髓拴系”这一术语需要说明。在几乎所有的椎管闭合不全中，脊髓位于低于正常水平（L1/L2）的位置，因此从解剖学或影像学的角度来看，可能会被认为是被束缚的，但尾部退化综合征除外，因为在后者，其脊髓末端由于缺乏次级神经胚发育而处于高于正常水平的位置。然而，并非所有患有椎管闭合不全的儿童都具有皮肤异常以外的临床症状或体征，因此，脊髓拴系一词最好用于描述椎管闭合不全时发生的神经 - 骨科综合征的临床特征。与神经发育不良相反，脊髓拴系暗示其临床特征背后的机械病因；实际上，这两种机制都可能导致“脊髓拴系综合征”。

椎管闭合不全的检查方法

虽然检查、评估的时间和具体细节可能根据椎管闭合不全的类型有所不同，但一般原则包括疾病部位的准确影像学表现，建立神经和泌尿系统监测的基线，并放入治疗的计划方案中，将有助于改善长期的功能预后。

超声

在胚胎发生的前3个月里，在后椎体元素骨化之前，可以利用声学窗口的优势来观察脊髓末端。超声是一种十分实用的初始筛查试验，尽管通常需要MRI来确定诊断和制订手术计划，但超声已被证明对椎管闭合不全筛查十分敏感。

磁共振

MRI是可以明确识别椎管闭合不全的成像方式。脊髓圆锥的水平、瘘管的形成以及相关锥体的异常可以在磁共振影像上清晰地显示。在闭合型脊柱裂患者，通常只对脊髓进行影像学检查就足够了。但是在脊髓脊膜膨出患者，还需要行脑的影像学检查，以评估脑室形态和Chiari Ⅱ畸形的特征。

泌尿系统评估

在椎管闭合不全的病例中，泌尿系统功能需严格评估，应重点关注两方面：①肾和上泌尿道的安全；②控制能力。储存尿液的能力并能适时排空。确保肾的安全和健康是最首要的事项，特别是对于严重的椎管闭合不全（脊髓脊膜膨出、复杂型脂肪瘤和尾部发育不全综合征）。小容量、高压膀胱，特别是在泌尿系感染的情况下，可能易导致输尿管回流和肾损伤，需要紧急治疗，这可能包括膀胱造口术、持续或间歇性导管和预防性抗生素治疗。

获得“社交”上的控制，是随后的重要任务。许多患有椎管闭合不全的儿童在儿童早期，膀胱功能表面上会正常。除了识别“敌对的”膀胱外，婴儿期的早期膀胱功能测试还被用来试图识别神经源性膀胱功能障碍的早期迹象或预测这种情况发生的可能性。在婴幼儿童，膀胱功能和泌尿动力学研究的解读可能是非常困难的，需要泌尿系统专业知识。

康复评估

需要与年龄适当的肌肉力量记录，以作为运动缺陷的初步评估，并作为记录运动功能的一种手段，因为序贯的医学研究委员会（Medical Research Council，MRC）肌肉图表可以帮助识别恶化的早期迹象。物理治疗回顾也有助于识别肌力或步态中的缺陷，这些缺陷可能通过矫形辅助或整形外科的干预得到改善。

特定闭合不全的管理

脊髓脊膜膨出

脊髓脊膜膨出与其他椎管闭合不全性疾病不同，它是一种“泛中枢神经系统疾病”。因此，脊柱异常通常伴随着脑结构性改变和脑积水。典型的脑结构异常包括小脑、脑桥和第四脑室向下移位，顶盖弯曲，延髓变形和低位的发育不全的小脑幕。这些特征构成了Chiari Ⅱ型畸形（Geerdink et al.，2012）。Chiari Ⅱ型畸形可以导致脊髓球部功能不足（呼吸和吞咽障碍），特别是在婴儿期和年龄较大儿童的高位脊髓病。Chiari Ⅱ型畸形的症状可能提示脑积水或分流功能障碍。重要的是，Chiari Ⅱ型畸形可以是与开放性神经管缺陷独立的，并与Chiari Ⅰ型畸形无关。据报道，脑积水发生在高达80%的脊髓脊膜膨出病例中，可能在出生时出现或在脊椎缺陷闭合后出现。近年来，脊髓脊膜膨出相关脑积水的分流率有所下降，因为在许多病例中，脑室扩张程度可能稳定，没有明显的不良后果（Chakraborty et al，2008）。

虽然对于产前诊断出脊髓脊膜膨出患儿，剖宫产是其最常见的分娩方式，但没有证据表明正常的阴道分娩会造成额外的感染或神经系统风险。手术治疗脊髓脊膜膨出应在出生后48小时内进行，以降低感染的风险，减少对神经基板的持续损伤，同时满足外观的美容。分流管的放置可以在初始进行闭合手术时（如果有严重的脑积水），或者根据连续头围测量或超声检查，发现有明显的进行性脑积水的证据时再进行。

在闭合性椎管闭合不全的情况下，很少需要紧急手术。事实上，许多此类疾病的手术适应证和可能的预后尚不清楚。

脊髓脊膜膨出的手术要点

只要儿童的临床状况允许，而且没有绝对的手术禁忌证，如脓血症、凝血功能障碍或严重的呼吸障碍，脊髓脊膜膨出的产后修复最好应在出生后48小时内进行。

如果有严重的并发症，如危及生命的呼吸或心脏疾病，那么应该考虑非手术治疗。然而，即使在严重的脊髓脊膜膨出的病例中，远期功能可能很差，仍建议手术闭合。未经治疗患儿往往出现疼痛、慢性感染，并可出现明显的护理困难。

手术前外科评估

应评估脊柱缺损的大小和邻近皮肤的质量。直径大于 5 cm 的病变不易于初次闭合，可能会需要局部的皮瓣。在这种情况下，应该考虑做整形外科手术。运动功能评估是很重要的，记录下肢肌肉的力量将表明脊髓脊膜膨出的功能水平，并为持续的监测提供一个重要的基线。采用头围测量和颅骨超声来预测脑积水的进展，需要连续进行头围测量和脑室大小观测。生理盐水浸泡的纱布结合食品薄膜包裹可以保护病变免受干燥、创伤和污染。在手术治疗前可予以预防性抗生素。如没有感染迹象，在手术治疗后可停止上述治疗。

手术关键目标

手术主要目的是将脊髓放回到椎管内，重建硬膜囊，提供高质量的皮肤闭合，以保护修复并防止脑脊液漏。

手术关键步骤

手术时婴儿处于俯卧位，则需要对膝盖和面部等承受压力区域进行保护。手术是在全身麻醉下进行的。具体考虑的因素包括确保孩子保持温暖和灌注良好。大量失血通常少见，但可能在取大皮瓣或去除骨嵴时出现。

手术切口需要考虑病变的大小和形状，以及提高复杂皮瓣的潜在需要。除上述外，还需考虑：皮肤松弛、潜在的骨骼解剖结构以及接近肛门等。神经基板需要从周围异常的皮肤和黏膜上分离开来。在手术操作过程中，需要小心保护基板、脊髓和任何潜在的神经根，免受进一步的损伤。

手术的每一个层次都需要仔细缝合，以防止脑脊液漏、感染以及由于皮肤缝合时的过大张力导致的伤口裂开。

关键解剖

典型的病例，在病变中心可以见到神经基板，周围被脊髓脊膜膨出囊包绕，后者由发育异常的脊膜和皮肤组成。一旦基板被松解，囊肿壁被切除到正常的皮肤。重要的是要确保没有皮肤层的成分残留并附着在基板上，因为这可能会导致日后发生植入性的皮样囊肿。

椎体后部成分（棘突和椎板），在病变水平上往往是缺如的。确认最低的一个完整的椎板，有助于在病变的上极识别正常硬脊膜。这是将新的硬脊膜层从囊壁内层剥离下来的起点。

多层修复从基板的神经胚形成开始，将神经组织卷起以重建脊髓末端，可以采用 8/0 丝线间断缝合来实现。该步骤需保持缝合线张力适度，避免过度紧张，否则可能导致基板缺血损伤。偶尔会遇到异常的神经根进入囊内，这些神经根没有功能，可以清除。非常突出的骨嵴可予以切除，这样方便皮肤的闭合。此外，其他可能遇到的神经异常包括脊髓分裂、半脊髓脊膜膨出和终丝增厚。

注意修剪硬脊膜的边缘，然后用连续缝合线严密闭合，并保证水密性。如果担心硬脑膜闭合的完整性，可以通过采用相邻的骶棘肌筋膜的筋膜瓣来加强修复。

术后护理

术后患儿采用俯卧位或侧卧位，以避免手术伤口受压。应监测伤口是否有感染或脑脊液漏的迹象。

每天测量一次头围，并绘制在一个头围图表上。连续的颅内超声可以监测脑室的大小。如有进行性脑室增大或颅内压升高的迹象需进行脑室分流。

在出院前应进行泌尿系统检查以评估上、下尿路的结构和功能正常。下肢畸形，特别是踝关节和足部畸形，如足内翻，应进行评估，并由骨科医生和康复治疗师制订康复计划。

常见的并发症包括切口感染，靠近尿布区域，污染切口，增加感染风险。敷料污染后应及时更换。封闭敷料有助于保护切口，避免并发症。缝合线过度紧张，可发生局部坏死和切口裂开。

脑脊液漏可能是由局部因素（如伤口裂开）或进展性脑积水引起。脑脊液漏与高感染率相关，需要紧急治疗。脑脊液也可能聚集在皮肤下，引起局部肿胀。如发生皮肤的广泛破坏，可能会留下一个大的无效腔。在这种情况下，手术中放置引流管可以帮助降低这种风险。脑积水也可能导致假脑膜膨出。

至少 50% 的接受脊髓脊膜膨出治疗的患儿会出现脑积水。脑积水的体征包括头围增加、前囟张力增高、颅缝扩张、眼球“落日”征或超声示进行性脑室扩张。治疗需要放置一个脑室分流管。

其他少见的并发症包括脑干功能障碍。Chiari Ⅱ型畸形的影像学特点可以在大多数脊髓脑膜膨出的儿童中见到；然而，只有少数人会出现脑干功能障碍的症状。新生儿期的球部症状和体征包括呼吸暂停、误吸和喂养困难。这些缺陷可能由未处理或处理不当的脑积水造成。在考虑后脑部减压前，应充分治疗脑积水。

脊髓脊膜膨出修补术后下肢功能障碍的进行性恶化可能是由于脊髓空洞所致。这是一种罕见的早期并发症，它可发生在儿童后期，作为未治疗的脑积水或分流功能障碍的表现。

脂肪瘤

脊髓脂肪瘤是一种解剖学上复杂的椎管闭合不全的形式，在手术治疗方面可能是最具争议的。根据脊髓脂肪瘤的附着点，位于脊髓圆锥的上方、表面或者下方，可以分为背侧、过渡型和尾部型（末端）等三型脂肪瘤。第四型为复杂型脂肪瘤，最近被命名，脂肪瘤延伸到脊髓腹侧和神经根。背侧和尾部型脂肪瘤的手术治疗往往简单，因为圆锥和马尾的受累程度较少，从而降低了括约肌神经支配的风险。过渡型脂肪瘤则治疗困难，也是远期致残率最高的类型（**图 85.5**）。

在婴儿期出现的脂肪瘤病例中，多达 1/3 的病例没有临床症状，也没有神经骨科综合征的特征，仅表现为腰骶部皮下肿块。目前多数学者认为，脊椎脂肪瘤或许比当前认为的更加良性（Kulkarni et al.，2004；Pang et al.，2009；Pang et al.，2010；Wykes et al.，2012；Thompson et al. 2013）。这导致许多对传统松解手术有效性的质疑，特别是在没有症状的病例中，因为许多手术病例报道中远期效果令人失望。目前围绕脂肪瘤的外科争议在两个方面：首先，是否可以预防性脊髓栓系？其次，在电生理监测的指导下，根治性手术是否会带来更好的长期预后？在试图解决这些争议时，则需要考虑以下被接受的事实。

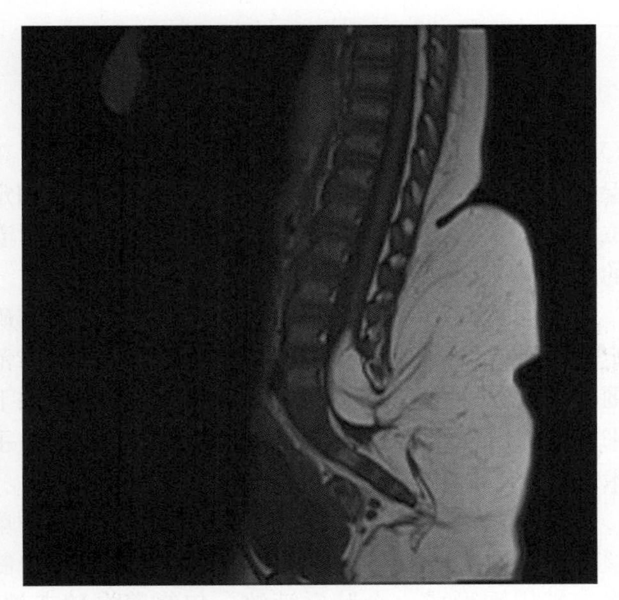

图 85.5　腰骶部脊柱的矢状位 T1 加权 MRI 像，显示一个复杂过渡型脊髓脂肪瘤。脊髓低位，椎管内脂肪瘤通过骶骨后部的缺陷与一个巨大的皮下脂肪瘤相连续

1. 多达一半未手术的脂肪瘤在随访过程中出现神经系统或泌尿系统恶化的证据。虽然移行脂肪瘤似乎有特别的风险，但所有的研究中都没有反映这一点，目前在诊断之初，还没有明确的可以预测病情恶化的特征。
2. 手术治疗脂肪瘤的风险并不小。这些风险包括至少 5% 病例出现新的神经系统或泌尿系统缺损，以及高达 20% 的病例中出现损伤并发症，如脑脊液漏。
3. 传统的松解手术技术具有较高的晚期恶化率。确切的比率因病例系列不同而异，但似乎与未手术病例的恶化率相当。
4. 虽然松解手术可明显缓解疼痛反应，但已形成的神经源性括约肌障碍很少能得到改善。
5. 恶化的确切机制尚不清楚，特别是机械栓系和潜在的神经发育不良的相对影响。

Pang 和同事的研究表明，用一种更激进的方法来进行最初的松解，其长期预后，要优于自然史或传统的松解术（Pang et al.，2009；Pang et al.，2010）。其基本原则是在术中电生理监测和定位引导下行脂肪瘤近全切除、神经基板的精细重建和硬脊膜扩大成形术。其优异的结果尚未被其他中心重复，但这很可能代表着这种疾病治疗方面的重大进步。不过将这项技术推荐为标准治疗方法可能还为时过早，尤其是在无症状的患儿中。考虑到刚刚提到的论点，我们目前的政策是仔细监测无症状儿童，定期进行神经学和泌尿学评估，当出现新的或进行性恶化的病例进行根治性手术。初始评估每 6 个月进行一次，直到达到排尿功能正常，此后每年进行一次评估。除非有恶化的证据，否则不需要磁共振成像扫描（**图 85.6**）。

脂肪瘤手术原则

手术关键目标

复杂脂肪瘤手术有三个主要目的，首先是将脊髓和脂肪瘤从周围组织上分离出来；其次将脂肪瘤从脊髓末端切除；最后重建脊髓末端和硬脊膜囊，以降低再次栓系的风险。

考虑到这些病变的解剖学复杂性，对现存的神经功能，特别是泌尿功能的风险，因此强烈建议使用术中神经电生理监测。监测包括运动诱发电位（motor evoked potentials，MEP）和神经根定位相结合，前者以评估运动通路的完整性，后者帮助识别和保存功能性神经根，特别是支配括约肌的神经根。监测和定位的肌群包括股四头肌（L4）、胫前肌（L5）、腓肠肌（S1）、拇展肌（S2）和肛门括约肌

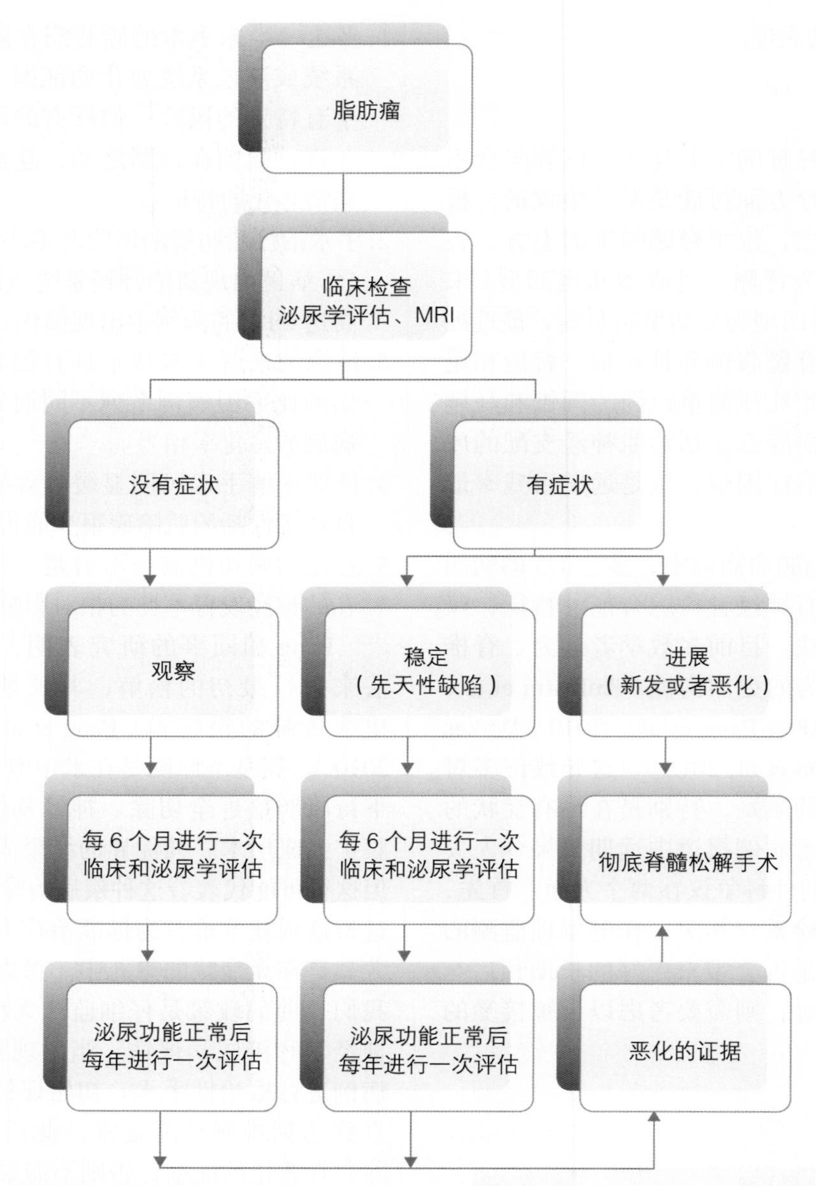

图 85.6 基于机构的脊髓脂肪瘤的治疗策略

（S3 和 S4）。这确保了每个腰骶水平都受到监测。

手术关键步骤

手术的第一步是定位脂肪瘤突出所通过的腰骶筋膜的缺损。然后进行椎旁肌反射，协助暴露筋膜缺损背侧的完整椎板。椎板切除是为了暴露硬脊膜，切除的范围应该足够高，以便能够直接进入并显示出脂肪瘤附着处上方的正常脊髓。脂肪瘤在附着到脊髓的过程中穿过硬脊膜的缺损，这种缺损可能相当古怪，通常需要行进一步的外侧骨切除，以便在脂肪瘤颈部的整个圆周上都能看到正常的硬脊膜。在手术显微镜下，硬脊膜打开范围，从正常的脊髓开始，一直持续到脂肪瘤对侧的颈部。在此步骤上识别和保护任何潜在的神经根都很重要，神经根刺激和定位有助于做到这一点。硬脊膜打开后，脊髓和附着的脂肪瘤应当没有任何周围的附着物。

手术的下一阶段是切除脂肪瘤。需要在两侧确定背根进入区，因为这将确定脂肪瘤切除的侧方范围。采用锐性分离，脂肪瘤从下面的脊髓上切除下来，显露出神经基板上的纤维性“白色平面”。在手术的这一步需要进行重复的 MEP 监测。

手术的最后阶段处理脊髓神经胚，这是用 8/0 单丝线缝合完成的。现在必须重建鞘囊，以便在脊髓终末端周围形成一个脑脊液池，包绕着脊髓末端。将人工补片修剪到适合硬脊膜缺损的确切尺寸，然后用连续的不可吸收缝合线固定到位，确保水密性。

覆盖的肌肉筋膜层和皮肤层随后应仔细缝合，以减少任何脑脊液漏或出现切口并发症的风险。

真皮窦道与 LDM

分离障碍与感染（脊髓脓肿或复发性脑膜炎）、包涵体囊肿形成（皮样或表皮样囊肿）和脊髓栓系有关（Thompson，2013）。风险因具体疾病诊断而异，如真皮窦道合并脑脊液漏感染并发症发生率高，而LDM 更易发生神经系统并发症。对于出现这种并发症的儿童，有明确的手术指征。在出现脊髓脓肿（通常是感染的皮样囊肿）的儿童中，最初的治疗应该仅限于脓液引流和积极的抗生素治疗，推迟手术治疗，直到感染得到充分治疗。即使没有并发症，出现典型的真皮窦道或 LDM 皮肤斑块的儿童也应该接受手术，因为手术风险低，远期预后良好。

真皮窦道或 LDM 的手术程序需要切除皮肤异物，找到潜在的根部，然后追踪到深层组织，进入硬膜内，最后切除与脊髓或圆锥的附着物。MRI 对病变的鞘内范围评估不准确，因此几乎所有病例都需要硬膜内探查（有时需要切开三个或四个椎板）。

终丝增厚

这是最轻微的异常，可能与正常变异有重叠。大多数学者认为：当终丝增厚（直径至少 2 mm）以及圆锥明显低于正常水平（L1/L2），随着儿童的成长，可能由于牵引力而发生损伤。在有神经骨科综合征特征的时候，手术治疗是明确的，即使在无症状或交界性的病例中也是如此，因为手术后发病率极低，且发生再次栓系的可能性很小，因此预防性干预是合理的。

在年幼儿童中，手术可以通过黄韧带开窗而不需要椎板切除术来进行。在手术显微镜下对终丝进行辨认和切开。几乎不变的是在终丝内有一根血管，需要在切开前进行明确的电凝止血，以避免将断端拉出术野之后，有持续出血的风险。

脊髓纵裂畸形（SCM）

在Ⅰ型 SCM（脊髓纵裂）中，在两个硬膜管之间存在骨刺，每个硬膜管包含一条半脊髓。症状可能包括由脊柱和脊髓的生长不同步引起的进行性疼痛、无力或肌肉萎缩，由于拴系或相关的脊椎畸形所致的进行性脊柱畸形也是危险因素（图 85.7）。这些畸形的儿童多数需要脊柱矫形手术，这可以降低在脊柱侧凸矫正过程中因牵张造成损伤的风险。

对于Ⅰ型 SCM，手术需要切除（通常是异常的）

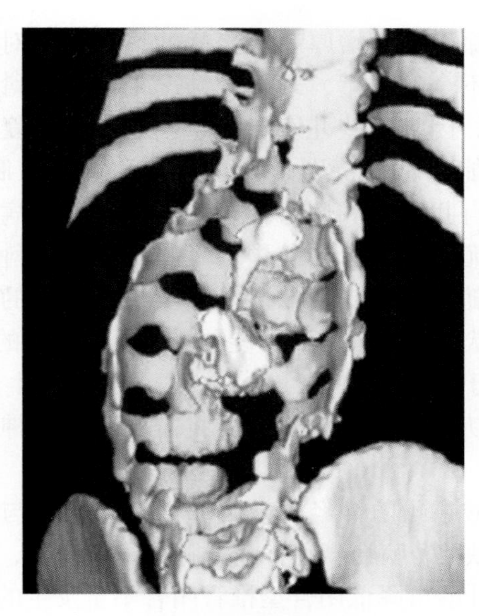

图 85.7　Ⅰ型脊髓纵裂畸形的腰骶部 3D CT 扫描，显示相关的骨性畸形。脊柱的后部成分发育缺陷，椎体有畸形，中线部位的骨嵴非常明显

椎板以暴露骨刺。用咬骨钳和磨除相结合的方法去除骨刺。骨刺的底部可能很宽，需要小心操作，以避免损伤邻近的神经组织。然后移除骨刺周围的硬脊膜鞘，重建硬脊膜，将两个半脊髓留在一个隔室内，腹侧硬脊膜不需要关闭。

Ⅱ型 SCM（双干脊髓）的外科解剖通常较简单。沿着裂开的脊髓长轴方向打开硬脊膜，辨认并移除任何夹杂的纤维带。从作者的经验看，Ⅱ型患者的病程可能非常缓慢，如果患者症状轻微或无症状，可选择观察随访。

末端脊髓囊肿状突出

这种情况罕见且复杂，是次级神经胚形成过程的疾病，但在严重的泌尿生殖系统和肛门直肠畸形的情况下，并不少见。这些被皮肤覆盖的末端脊髓囊性扩张位于臀沟的低位，囊肿可能巨大，护理困难，并且累及表面皮肤。在这种情况下，早期的运动功能恶化容易被观察发现，因此通常建议尽早治疗。术中电生理监测可以帮助确定功能性神经组织的最低水平，然后将其远端扩张的发育不良组织切除，继而进行鞘囊末端和覆盖皮肤的重建。

预后和预防

椎管闭合不全的预后因特定的闭合不全的个体而异，一般情况下，预后取决于诊断时候的神经、泌尿功能和骨科状况，以及是否存在并发的先天性畸形。除了终丝增厚等最轻微的情况外，对患有脊髓闭合不全的儿童，理想的情况是由多学科团队进行随访，因为这些儿童自童年期起通常有复杂和多变的功能需求，特别是自主活动和排便控制方面。他们的自我形象和性行为等相关的心理疾病常常很严重，尤其是在青少年中多发。从神经外科的角度来看，随访的主要目的之一是及早发现新的或进行性的症状和体征，它们可能预示着再次栓系的发生。

对于脊髓脊膜膨出的儿童，还有发生脑积水和延髓功能障碍的风险，这将需要终生的神经外科监护。

叶酸在预防神经管缺陷方面的作用只与开放型神经管缺陷（脑膨出和脊髓脊膜膨出）有关，没有证据表明叶酸可降低闭合型椎管闭合不全发生的风险。

争议

围绕椎管闭合不全仍有很多争议。许多情况罕见，局限于单中心的经验，缺乏大规模临床研究。在许多情况下，无症状时候的真实自然史记录很少，管理也是基于有限的证据。脊椎脂肪瘤尤其如此，预防性干预的作用还远未得到证实。根治性手术松解的效果在其他研究得到验证，将会非常重要。尝试识别或对那些可能从早期根治性手术获益的病例进行危险分层，也是非常重要。

一项随机临床对照试验表明，宫内手术治疗脊髓脊膜膨出的效果优于标准的产后修复。反对者对试验结论持怀疑态度，并对产妇风险以及对未来怀孕影响的伦理担忧。但这种手术可能会得到更广泛的应用，并利用微创技术改进手术。

结论

椎管闭合不全包括一组不同类型的先天性脊柱畸形。虽然目前很多病例的细节还不明确，但从胚胎学的角度可以很好地来理解这些疾病。早期、准确的解剖学诊断对判断预后、制订合适的治疗方案是非常必要的。

椎管闭合不全的手术非常复杂，应以优化远期功能结局为原则进行。术中神经生理监护和定位正在成为这些疾病手术中不可缺少的工具。

多学科团队护理在这些疾病的管理中也十分重要。

延伸阅读、参考文献、EBRAIN 的相关链接

扫描书末二维码获取。

第 86 章　颅缝早闭——症状性和无症状性颅面异常

Federico Di Rocco · Pierre-Aurelien Beuriat · Eric Arnaud 著
安旭 译，田永吉 审校

引言

颅缝早闭是指一个或者多个颅缝提前闭合，引起颅骨生长的改变，头颅外形的异常。头颅的形状和特定的颅缝相关，所以诊断是基于临床表现做出的。

该病的起因，很大程度上是未知的。基因研究人员已经确认了几个突变。

并发症可以导致颅骨的变形，还会导致面部形态异常。其中小脑扁桃体下垂、脑积水、颅内压增高、眼部保护不足、呼吸梗阻以及牙齿问题最为常见。

有一些因素会对手术指征产生影响。手术的目的是恢复功能和美观。手术技术几经演变，从简单的绑扎到头骨以及眶上的重新塑形、成骨性骨牵引以及内镜手术。对于所有的颅缝早闭症来说，长期的随访是必需的，因为有发生继发性骨缝（独立于最初受累的骨缝）早闭的风险。

定义

颅缝早闭症（craniosynostosis，CRS）这个术语源自 cranio（头骨）、syn（结合）以及 ostosis（骨形成）。它是指一个或者多个颅缝提前闭合，引起颅骨生长的改变，头颅外形的异常。正常来说，颅骨的生长是垂直于骨缝的。然而在 CRS 病例中，颅骨生长的方向是平行于骨缝，受累颅骨不能正常生长，为了补偿颅骨空间的不足，其余的颅骨也会异常生长。此外，由于颅骨生长直接关系到脑组织的生长，一个或者多个骨缝的闭合也会导致大脑的异常生长，因此，颅骨外形的改变，是代偿性生长和大脑变化的共同结果。

CRS 病例的头颅形状和受累的特定骨缝有关。颅骨拉长成船状是由于矢状缝的提前闭合（舟状头）（见**图** 86.1）。前额骨的生长受限形成三角形或者楔形是由于额缝的提前闭合（三角头）（见**图** 86.2）。由于单侧冠状缝或者人字缝提早闭合，会分别导致前斜头（见**图** 86.3）或者后斜头畸形。鉴别体位性后斜头畸形与真正的 CRS，非常重要的一点，前者骨缝依然是开放的，后者则是单侧人字缝提早闭合。在体位性斜头病例中，在受影响一侧的耳朵通常位置靠前但是和对侧在同一水平，而在真正颅缝早闭的患者中，患侧耳朵偏离向融合骨缝而且通常向下倾斜。当双侧冠状缝都闭合时（短头畸形），向前和向后的生长都会存在缺失，外观表现为短头。尖头畸形是指冠状缝和矢状骨缝都闭合。

CRS 也可以分为原发性（当颅缝闭合和骨质问题有关时）/ 继发性（当颅缝闭合和大脑发育的问题有关，这个问题妨碍了颅骨发育），综合征性的（当 CRS 和其他畸形相关，尤其是面部的畸形）/ 非综合征性的，简单型（仅有一个骨缝受影响）/ 复杂型（当多个骨缝受影响）。

流行病学

全球 CRS 发病率是 1∶2500 新生儿。这是人类最常见的颅面畸形。最常见的形式是非综合征性的 CRS（non-syndromic CRS，NSC）。它们占据了 80%~85% 的病例（Di Rocco et al.，2009）。NSC 中只影响一个骨缝的病例在 CRS 中占比超过了 70%。

舟状头畸形是最常见的类型。它大约占到了 NSC 50% 的比例（Lajeunie et al.，1996）。三角头畸形，过去是第三常见的 CRS，仅排在前斜头畸形之后，但是在过去 20 年，它的发病率上升了。现如今它是第二常见的 NSC 形式。后斜头畸形是最少见的，它大约占 NSC 的 3%。

对于舟状头畸形和三角头畸形，更倾向于发生于男孩，它们的男女比例分别是 2.5∶1 和 3.3∶1（Lajeunie et al.，1996），然而斜头畸形在女孩中更普遍（男女比例为 1∶2.3）（Lajeunie et al.，1996）。

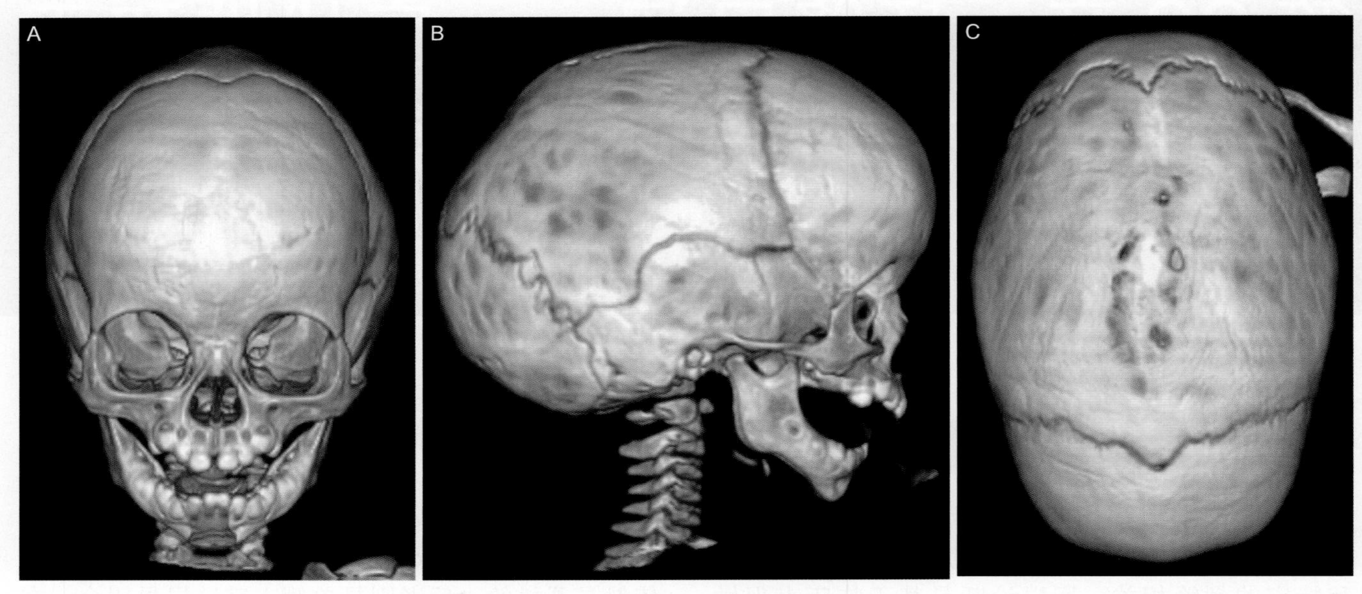

图 86.1 一个 6 月大男孩的颅骨 CT 的 3D 重建图片，典型的舟状头畸形，可以看到矢状缝闭合导致颅骨前后径延长

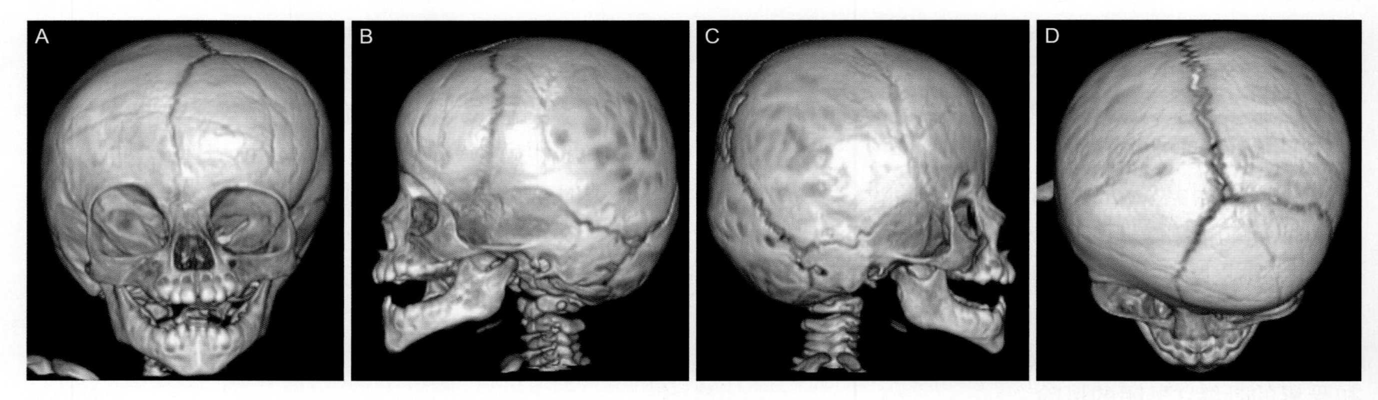

图 86.2 一个 8 月大女孩，颅骨 CT 的 3D 重建图片，右侧前斜头畸形。可以看到右侧冠状缝闭合，导致形成斜头形状

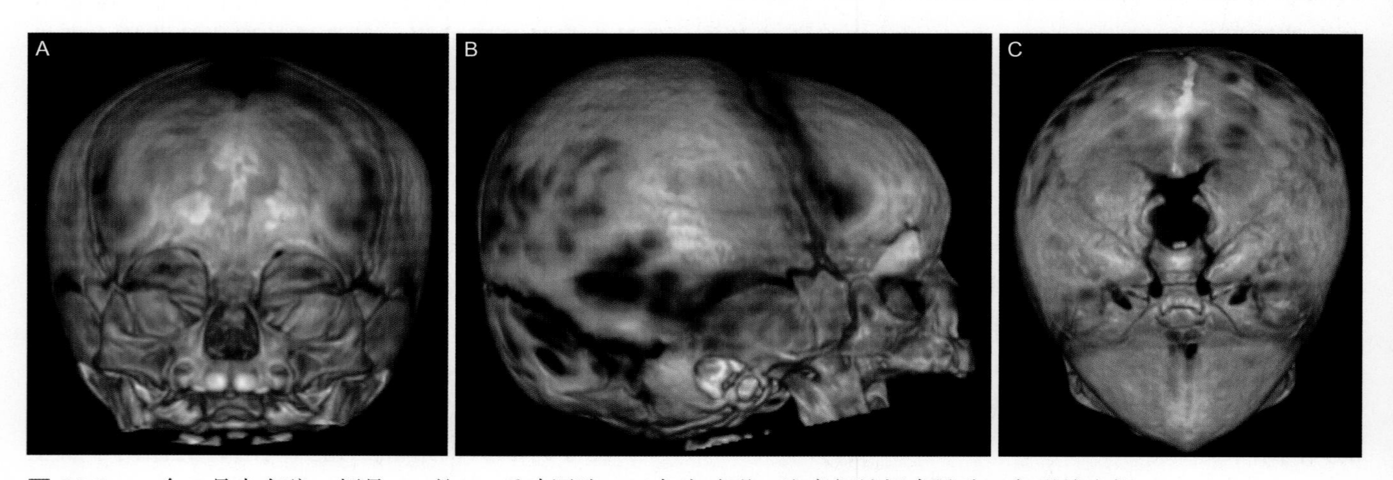

图 86.3 一个 7 月大女孩，颅骨 CT 的 3D 重建图片，三角头畸形，注意额缝闭合导致三角形前头部

大多数时候，NCS 是散发病例，但是任何一种颅缝早闭，都有可能有家族史。

综合征性 CRS（syndromic CRS，SCRS）占到全部 CRS 病例的 15%~20%。目前有超过一百种不同的综合征存在，但是最常见的包括 Crouzon 综合征（**图** 86.4 和**图** 86.5）、Pfeiffer 综合征、Apert 综合征、Saethre–Chotzen 综合征和 Muenke 综合征（**表** 86.1）。

病因和病理生理

遗传原因大部分还未知晓。分子层面的研究确认了一些在 CRS 中的突变，其中包括四种成纤维细胞生长因子受体（fibroblast growth factors，FGFR）中的三种，但是也确认了其他一些基因，例如 TWIST1、ERF、TCF12 以及 EFBN1，它们大多数存在于 SCRS 中。基因突变大多数是常染色体显性遗传，并且存在着很高的表型变异性。不同表型可以来自单一基因的突变。不同患者之间的表现存在着很大差异，从略低于正常到极端异常。与此相反，类似的表型可源于数个基因缺陷（Heuzé et al.，2014）。在 NSC 中，突变很少被发现（Wilkie et al.，2007）。其他因素，包括环境因素（子宫内胎儿受限、不健康的产前产妇生活习惯、围产期低氧血症）被认为促进 CRS 的发展。

从功能的角度来看，许多并发症可能源自 CRS。它们在数个骨缝受累的 SCRS 中更普遍。不只是颅骨的变形，面部异常变形也会导致多种并发症，因此，在处理这些复杂的病理情况时，整形外科、颅颌面外科以及神经外科医生进行协作非常必要。

从神经外科角度来看，大脑畸形中最常见的一种是小脑扁桃体下垂（cerebellar tonsillar prolapse，CTP）（有些时候被称为 Chiari Ⅰ型畸形）。CTP 被认为是颅后窝的容量变小和小脑容量之间不均衡导致的结果。这种不均衡是由提前闭合的人字骨缝和颅底骨缝以及与之相关的脑积水所造成的（Cinalli et al.，2005）。CTP 在 Crouzon 综合征和 Pfeiffer 综合征中非常常见（Cinalli et al.，2005）。尽管它通常是无症状的，但是有时也需要行后颅凹减压术。

颅内压（increased intracranial pressure，ICP）是另一个关注的要点。它继发于：颅缝早闭使得颅腔

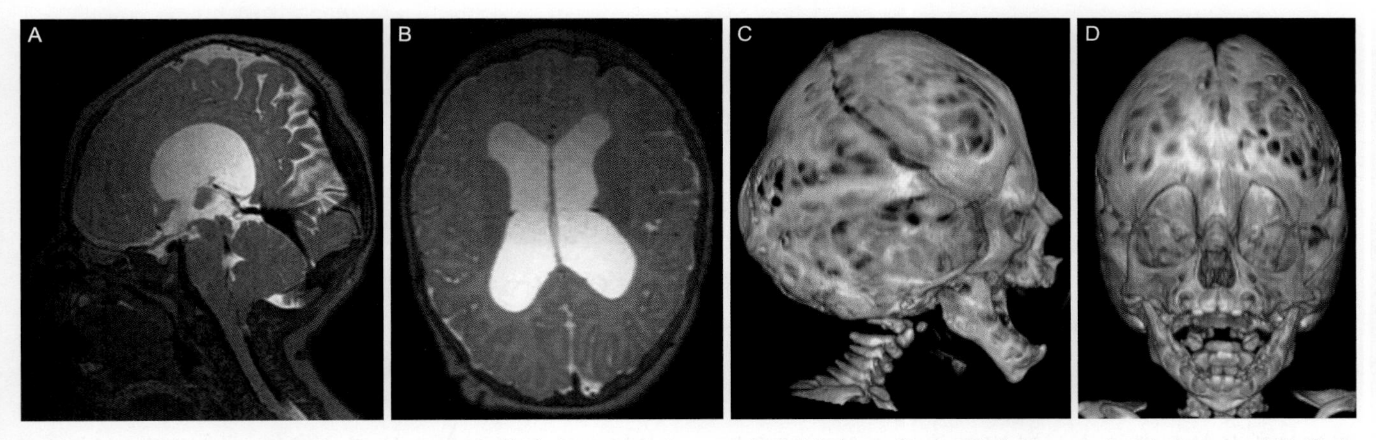

图 86.4　一个 19 月大男孩，患有 Crouzon 综合征，MRI（A、B）和颅骨 CT 的 3D 重建（C、D），注意 MRI 上小脑扁桃体下疝和侧脑室扩张。在颅骨 CT 上，可以看到"铜打碗征"

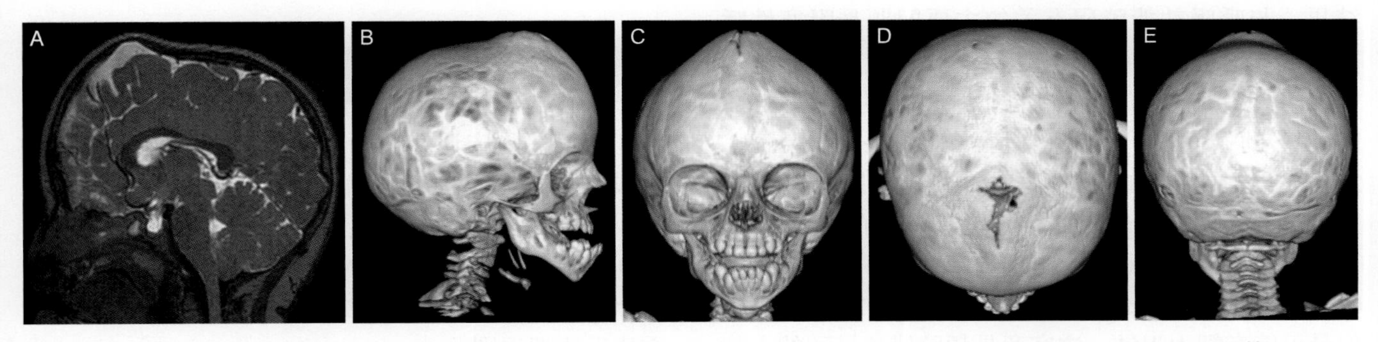

图 86.5　MRI（A）和颅骨 CT 3D 重建（B~E）：21 月大女孩，患有 Crouzon 综合征。注意 MRI 上没有小脑扁桃体的下疝，也没有脑室的扩张。在颅骨 CT 上，可以看到颅底骨缝早闭

表 86.1 最常见的颅面综合征特点

	临床特点	受累颅缝	基因发现
Crouzon 综合征	眼距过宽 喙状鼻子 眼球突出 神经发育不全	冠状缝 偶尔有颅底骨缝	FGFR2 新发或常染色体显性遗传的突变
Pfeiffer 综合征	眼距过宽 突眼 神经发育不全 宽、短、巨大脚趾 广泛偏离的拇指 手指过短	颅底骨缝早闭 三叶草头骨	FGFR2（95%）和 FGFR1（5%）突变新发或常染色体显性遗传
Apert 综合征	眼距过宽、眼下斜 薄上唇 面中部发育不全 并指、并趾	颅底骨缝早闭 冠状缝	FGFR2（S252W 和 P253R）突变大多都是新发的
Saethre-Chotzen 综合征	发际线低 鹰嘴鼻子 上睑下垂 耳朵异常（招风耳） 并指	冠状缝 额缝或者矢状缝已经被描述	TWIST1 新发或常染色体显性遗传的突变
Muenke 综合征	轻度的面中部发育不全 突眼	冠状缝	FGFR3（P250R）新发或常染色体显性遗传的突变

脑组织不匹配，从而导致颅腔容量下降；颈部静脉孔的狭窄导致的静脉流动异常；脑脊液动力学改变导致的脑室扩张。

脑积水在 Crouzon 综合征和 Pfeiffer 综合征中很常见（Cinalli et al.，2005；Di Rocco et al.，2010）。它的病理生理很复杂。它通常源自于静脉血流的异常以及 CTP 的结合（Cinalli et al.，2005；Di Rocco et al.，2010）。

从颅颌面手术的角度来说，面部形态和 CRS 中面部的生长的异常也会导致眼部保护不足、呼吸梗阻、齿颚矫正等问题。呼吸问题既是上呼吸道受阻导致的问题（Mathijssen et al.，2006），也是 CTP 的结果。与呼吸功能障碍有关的主要问题是阻塞性睡眠障碍，这也会加重颅内压增高。

另外有一个需要强调的非常重要的点是：CRS 的患儿的智力、行为以及情绪（Maliepaard et al.，2014）。结果是与畸形的类型、综合征以及相关脑部的畸形有关。Apert 综合征具有最差的精神预后（Renier et al.，1996）。Crouzon 综合征和 Saethre-Chotzen 综合征（Michael Cohen Jr.，2011）极少见，但是可能有智力迟钝。这究竟是颅脑错位导致的大脑白质病，还是由大脑本身基因变异导致的后果，要说明这一点，是非常困难的（Raybaud and Di Rocco，2007）。

诊断

CRS 有特异性表型，因此可以从临床进行诊断。

许多颅面畸形是可以进行产前诊断的，但是当前依然很罕见。当要确立诊断时，不仅要考虑头部变形，还要考虑大脑、面部以及四肢的异常情况。当超声检查发现异常体征的时候，建议做一个 MRI 以及羊膜腔穿刺手术，并进行标准核型分析和分子基因检测。

检查

当根据临床评估拟确立诊断以后，则需要做进一步的检查来评估相关联的异常。

X 线平片、计算机断层扫描（computed tomography，CT），以及最新的超声和 MR，可以用来发现具体哪一个骨缝受累。头骨和面部的形态改变可以在 CT 3D 重建后清晰识别。

在 SCRS 中其他检查非常必要：MRI 用于评估脑

积水、CTP以及其他可能的大脑畸形；眼科检查用于发现视盘水肿、突眼等颅内压升高的体征；耳鼻喉（ear，nose，and throat，ENT）检查来评估上气道梗阻；多导睡眠图检查，因为如果出现呼吸暂停的现象，可能需要改变手术方式。如果发现潜在的突变时，对患者及其家属进行基因检测，有利于正确的家长咨询。最后，建议进行神经心理学的随访。

手术原则

手术指征中有几个重要因素：患者的年龄、CRS的类型、颅内压增高、脑积水、CTP、呼吸道梗阻的严重程度、颅骨发育不全的程度、眼部问题，以及下颌骨/上颌骨、齿科、眼眶以及面部的形态。手术的目的是双重的：功能和美观。

在功能层面，手术的目的是为了治疗脑积水，预防颅内压增高、精神发育迟缓、眼部问题，以及改善呼吸道问题。在美观层面，手术的目的是矫正颅面畸形，预防形变从而预防心理学上的不良后果。

手术技术从简单的切除演进到整个头骨以及眶上的重建。当前，骨牵引术（Choi et al.，2010）和内镜手术（Jimenez and Barone，1998）成为受关注的备选方案（Sanger et al.，2014）。手术的范围、手术时机和手术指征至今仍是有争议的内容。但是人们应该记住NSC经常仅为了美观的原因进行手术（Di Rocco，2009）。由于不可能预测哪些患者将会出现神经认知障碍，因此，不论是否出于美观的考虑，手术都是有指征的（Barritt et al.，1981），接受手术越早，外观就会越好。而且，早期的手术可以获得一个更好的纠正，因为此时畸形更不明显，骨头更具延展性，以及它也允许了大脑自然的成长，从而实现被动术后重塑。因此这些患者应该在一岁之前实施手术。这些手术存在大量出血的风险（White et al.，2015），因此手术时机，依照手术方案，在很大程度上取决于CRS的类型和患者的体重。在我们的实践中，舟状头畸形患者通常在6个月龄之前进行手术；对于三角畸形和前斜头畸形患者，则是7~8月龄。

在SCRS中，手术的策略是更加复杂的。多次手术通常是必要的。实施第一次手术取决于出现颅内压增高的表现、脑积水、血小板减少症（thrombocytopenia，TCP）以及呼吸问题。如果视盘水肿存在，该手术应被视做紧急状况而立刻进行。

SCRS的经典手术是颅骨后部扩张、额-眶前移和面部矫正。颅骨后部扩张通常是Crouzon综合征或者Pfeiffer综合征的第一步。患有这些综合征的患者通常会有进展性脑积水，这是由于后颅凹发育不良，继发其中的神经血管结构拥挤所造成的。脑室内脑脊流引流会降低扩张力（这种扩张力可以促进颅骨生长），从而加重狭窄。因此，现在首推增加后颅凹容积的手术方式。它具有降低颅内压，重新稳定脑脊液动力学，以及为静脉结构减压的效果。有时候当CSF机械性梗阻导致脑积水，可以实施内镜脑室造瘘手术（Di Rocco et al，2010）。有多种技术可以采用，从单纯的后部开颅术到后部颅骨修复术，修复可以使用可吸收板或自由漂浮骨瓣。另一种非常有效的技术是进行后部开颅手术并使用扩张器以保证颅骨扩张。此外，当TCP出现时，可以实施枕骨大孔减压术，以降低颅颈交界处压力。为了纠正颅骨前部的畸形，则需要更多的手术。这些手术可以推迟，从而可以获得一个更好的以及更持久的美观结果。

当处理颅骨前部的时候，额-眶前移是手术的金标准，根据需要，可以随后进行面部前移。后者应当被尽可能推迟到患者11~12岁，以等到他们最后一次牙齿长出结束。如果面部后移严重，并且造成功能性（眼部、呼吸以及咀嚼）或者心理问题，也可以早一些进行手术。

额-眶前移手术的标准技术是水平舌槽矫正，将眶缘骨质切开并且向前推移。重建的部分采用生物吸收板材进行固定。

当讨论到面部矫正，由Tessier（Tessier，1967）描述的Lefort Ⅲ型是有手术指征的。可以采用骨质撑开技术，将骨质逐步扩张（Iannetti et al.，2006）。

在严重的眼球突出以及上呼吸道梗阻的病例中，Tessier建立了一种一期手术技术，将额-眶和面部矫正技术结合起来（Tessier，1971）。在大多数案例中，额面整体矫正手术，都需要联合骨质撑开术，因为已经有证据表明对于这种高风险的手术，可以显著降低并发症（Arnaud and Di Rocco，2012）。

最后，对于年龄较大的儿童和青少年，当面部生长已经几乎完成，患者的外表可以通过进一步的美容和正畸手术获得改善。

对所有的CRS患者，需要进行长期的随访，因为在原先受影响的骨缝之外，有继发第二个骨缝早闭的风险。

争议：对CRS行微创内镜手术

对于NSC患者，条状头骨切除手术和颅顶重塑手术之间仍存在争议。

支持：因为整个颅顶成形手术可能出现大量出血，因此，已经设计了多种技术以减少出血和输血。在这些技术中，微创内镜手术（minimally endoscopic procedures，MEP）（内镜下条状颅骨切除术，然后用颅骨头盔塑形数月）已经证明失血最少（Jimenez and Barone，2012），这样可以缩短住院时间，而且经济有效（Chan et al.，2013）。最后但是并非不重要，这种操作对几乎所有的单骨缝 CRS 都可能有效（Jimenez and Barone，2012）。

反对：手术结果依赖于术后保护头盔的应用。颅骨矫形术可能减少颅骨的生长，价格较贵而且费时费力。即使矫形手术，也存在不完全重塑的可能（Sauerhammer et al.，2014）。最后，近期研究表明，整个颅腔的塑形手术可以获得更好的长期智力结果（Hashim et al.，2014）。

延伸阅读、参考文献

扫描书末二维码获取。

第 87 章 儿童颅脑和脊柱损伤——特别注意事项

Andrew Kay · Desiderio Rodrigues · Melanie Sharp · Guirish Solanki 著
张衡 译，田永吉 审校

儿童创伤的发生率和流行病学

创伤性脑损伤（traumatic brain injury，TBI）是儿童死亡或残疾的最常见原因。

据估计，在英国每年约有 15 万名儿童发生颅脑损伤，但因创伤性脑损伤住院的儿童不到 1.4 万人。总死亡率为十万分之九，占所有儿童死亡的 1%（Royal College of Surgeons，1999）。

儿童 TBI 的主要发病机制与年龄有关。在 2 岁以下的儿童中，非意外性颅脑损伤（non-accidental head injuries，NAI）和地面摔倒是最常见的。从 2~4 岁，摔倒占主导地位。在 4 岁至青少年之间，摔倒或道路交通碰撞（road traffic collisions，RTC）是最常见的。在青少年中，RTC 是创伤性脑损伤的主要原因。

成人和儿童 TBI 的类型不同。颅骨骨折和硬膜外血肿在儿童患者中较为常见。

在所有儿童骨折中脊柱骨折仅占少数（1%~3%），约 60% 为颈椎损伤，其中只有 3% 会出现神经功能缺陷。儿童脊髓损伤（spinal cord injury，SCI）仍然是灾难性的事件，应尽一切努力减少损伤的程度和严重性以及损伤后的并发症（Eleraky，2000；Brown，2001）。

在 8 岁以下的儿童中，多达 87% 的损伤发生在 C3 或以上水平，C3 水平以下的损伤在年龄较大的儿童中更为常见，具有成人损伤模式。幼童中最常见的骨折类型是 C1 环和 C2（Hangman）骨折，而齿状突骨折在所有年龄段中分布平均，腰椎骨折发生在较大年龄组。

受伤的原因也取决于儿童的年龄，婴儿受伤是由于出生时的创伤或意外从父母的手臂、婴儿床、靠椅或沙发上坠落。2 至 8 岁的儿童会因从自行车上坠落或其他路面交通事故（road traffic accidents，RTA）而导致脊髓脊柱受伤。据报道，在这个年龄组中，多达 25%~60% 的人是由 RTA 导致的。年龄较大的儿童会因坠落或运动损伤而导致脊髓脊柱损伤。

儿童头部创伤的病理生理学

虽然儿童创伤性脑损伤的基本反应与成人相似，但儿童有独特的解剖和生理差异，新生儿和婴儿的头部比例较大、颈部肌肉力量较弱，这使他们在被旋转、加速 / 减速时受伤的风险增大。儿童的骨骼弹性更大、蛛网膜下腔间隙宽、大脑中水分含量高、脑组织的黏弹特性等都增加了弥漫性轴索损伤的可能性。

颅内压（intracranial pressure，ICP）随年龄而异，婴幼儿的正常颅内压低于 10 mmHg，年龄较大的儿童和成人的正常颅内压为 15 mmHg。

大脑血流量（cerebral blood flow，CBF）也显示出与年龄相关的变化：婴儿为 40 ml/（100 g · min），儿童为 75~110 ml/（100 g · min），青少年与成人一样为 50 ml/（100 g · min）。

颅脑损伤的治疗

所有 TBI 的早期治疗都应遵循 *Advanced Paediatric Life Support*（APLS）、*Advanced Trauma Life Support*（ATLS）、美国外科医生协会创伤委员会（1997）及英国国家临床规范研究院（National Institute of Clinical Excellence，NICE）指南。

所有因头部外伤入院的儿童都应在设有儿科重症监护室（paediatric intensive care unit，PICU）和小儿神外病房的专业创伤中心接受治疗。安全、及时的转运患者至关重要。

为测定儿童颅脑损伤的严重程度，可以应用格拉斯哥昏迷评分，对于尚不会说话的儿童和婴儿，可以使用其修改版本。

与成人类似，颅脑损伤早期的治疗重点是预防主要由缺氧和低通气量引起的继发性脑损伤，同时颈椎制动。对于重型 TBI（GCS 评分小于 8 分）或根据损伤机制和影像扫描结果预测神经功能恶化的患者，有必要尽早入住 PICU。

儿童气管插管的适应证与成人相同，对于需要行计算机断层扫描（computed tomography，CT）检查但不配合的儿童，也是行气管插管的指证。对儿童进行气管插管操作是困难的，8 岁以下的儿童应使用不带套囊的气管插管。

ICP 监测的适应证与成人颅脑外伤患者相似。婴儿颅内压可通过前囟进行定性评估。目前对积极降低儿童 ICP 阈值的共识是 20 mmHg（Adelson et al.，2003）。

儿童 ICP 的管理仍以成人患者的数据为基础，重点是维持氧饱和度和充足的通气量（包括避免过度通气）、使用镇痛镇静药物（包括阿片类药物、咪达唑仑加额外的骨骼肌松弛药），手术干预（如有必要），巴比妥类药物是二线治疗。异丙酚是一种广泛用于成人颅脑损伤的乳剂，在儿童中应用可能引起代谢性酸中毒和高血脂。

婴儿和儿童的正常脑灌注压（cerebral perfusion pressure，CPP）尚未确定，从婴儿的 40 mmHg 到青少年的 70 mmHg 的范围为被认为是合适的。

迄今为止，儿童去骨瓣减压术的临床试验规模很小。最大的随机对照试验有 27 例患者纳入，结果显示在 6 个月时功能预后改善（Taylor et al.，2001），远期预后尚未被回顾。与成人去骨瓣减压术临床试验的关注点一样，由关注死亡率到转化为关于增加功能性障碍的。有趣的是，考虑到远期生存结果尚不明确，小儿神经外科医生选择去骨瓣减压术的颅内压阈值仍然较低。

苯妥英钠在重型 TBI 的儿童患者中比在成人患者中更常用，以减少创伤后早期癫痫发生率。抗癫痫药物通常应用 1 周。早期癫痫在幼儿中更为常见，在年龄较大的儿童中则不那么常见。儿童早期癫痫发作对创伤后癫痫的预测作用不如成人。

低温虽然可降低 ICP，但其对儿童的有效性和安全性证据有限（参见“儿童创伤中的争议”部分）。

CT 头部平扫是 TBI 的首选检查。行颈椎 CT 检查，甲状腺会暴露于电离辐射，因此在轻微损伤时，X 射线可能就足够了。英国医院通常遵循 NICE 指南的 CT 扫描指征（**图** 87.1 和**图** 87.2）。

由于儿童韧带损伤和无明显影像学异常脊髓损伤（spinal cord injury without overt radiological abnormality，SCIWORA）发生率较高，又因此对于意识迟钝的儿童患者，“排除”颈椎比成人更困难。MRI 检查有助于识别脊髓信号的改变，如出血、韧带、肌肉及椎间盘的损伤等。急性骨损伤可以在短时反转恢复序列（short tau inversion recovery，STIR）的图像上很好地显示，这有助于区分急性和已经长期存在的变化。在儿童清醒之前，需要使用项圈对颈部制动（Lee et al.，2003）。

儿童颅脑损伤的预后

相当大比例的 TBI 患儿在到达医院前死亡。RTA 乘客的死亡率最高，坠落造成的死亡率最低（Parslow et al.，2005）。

当 CPP 小于 40 mmHg（高度提示死亡）、双侧躯体感觉诱发电位（somatosensory evoked potentials，SSEP）缺失（与严重残疾和死亡密切相关）或 ICP 长期高于 20 mmHg，都提示预后不良。

非意外性颅脑损伤

NAI 或虐待性头部外伤是导致 2 岁及以下的儿童严重或致命颅脑损伤的最常见原因，可能是由于撞击或摇晃头部，或两者兼有。与意外头部受伤的儿童相比，被诊断为 NAI 的儿童死亡的可能性高出 5 倍，然而，症状和体征并不总是明显的，因此诊断可能被忽视（Hinds et al.，2015）。

摇晃婴幼儿通常会导致近期内发生多灶性出血和（或）大面积慢性硬膜下出血，甚至会覆盖双侧大脑半球（**图** 87.3）。摇晃会导致桥静脉破裂，虽然出血量通常很小，但这是摇晃和撞击的区别。多发性、半球间、凸面及颅后窝出血与 NAI 之间有很强的相关性。

在意外创伤中确实会发生硬膜下血肿，在这个年龄组中也需要考虑到导致硬膜下血肿的其他原因，包括产伤（血肿通常在 4 周后消退）、凝血功能障碍，或罕见的代谢障碍（如戊二酸尿症 I 型）。

硬膜下出血、视网膜出血和先前状态良好的婴儿出现急性脑病，构成了所谓的三联征。在怀疑 NAI 时，需要进行完整的骨骼检查和血液学检查。神经影像学在确定 NAI 诊断中至关重要，因为 37% 的病例中可以检测到隐匿性损伤。有几个影像学特点被认为与 NAI 特别相关。出现硬膜下血肿，特别是在多个部位，如半球间、凸面及颅后窝，与 NAI 显著相关。对可疑的 NAI 患者，尽管 CT 是推荐的一线影像检查，但早期 MRI 越来越多地与 CT 一起应用，因为它能更好地评估剪切伤、缺氧缺血损伤以

NICE National Institute for Health and Care Excellence!

规则 2：需要进行 CT 扫描儿童的确定

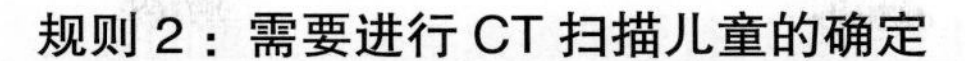

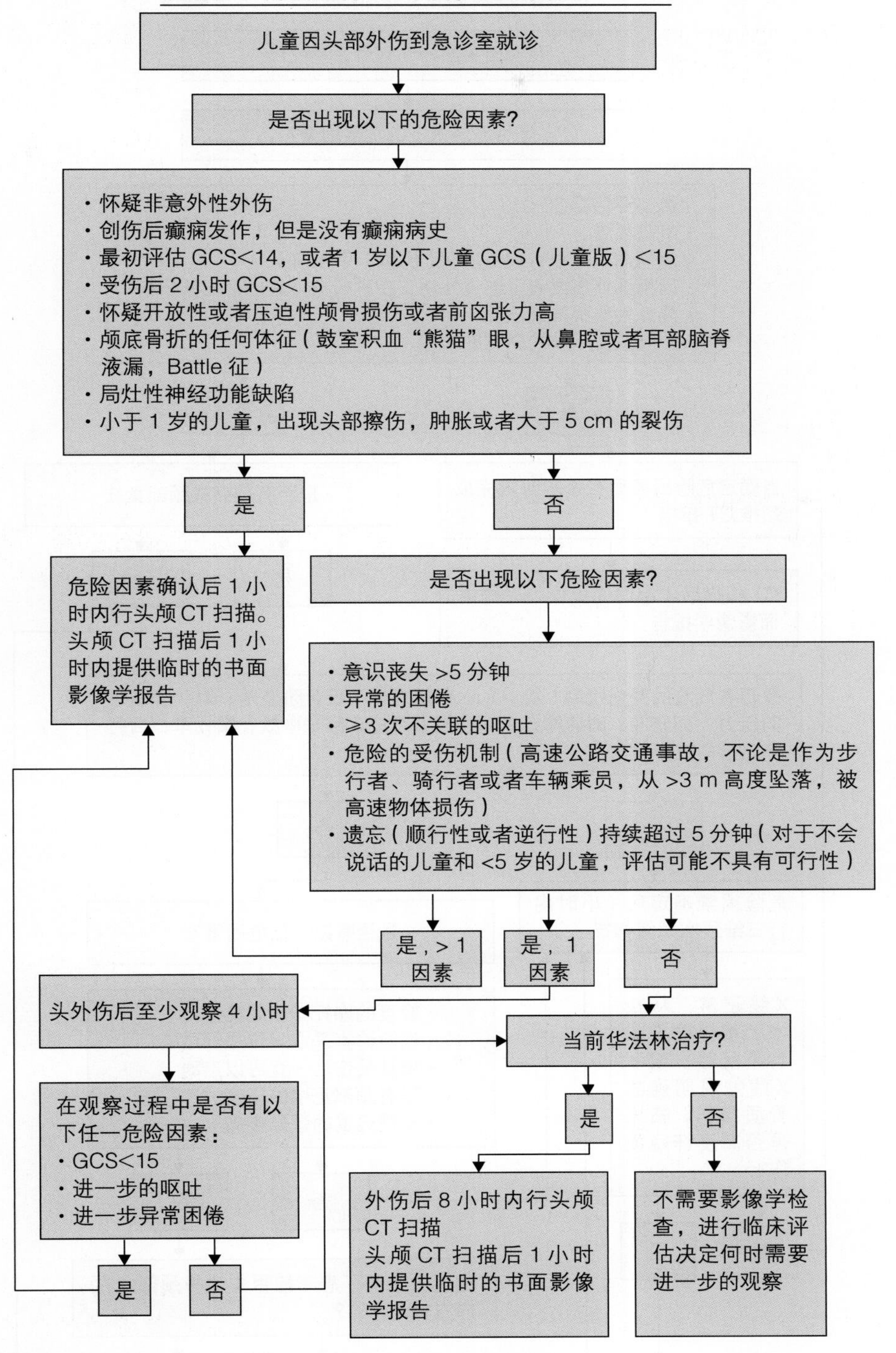

图 87.1　英国国家临床规范研究院制订的儿童需要进行头颅 CT 扫描的规范

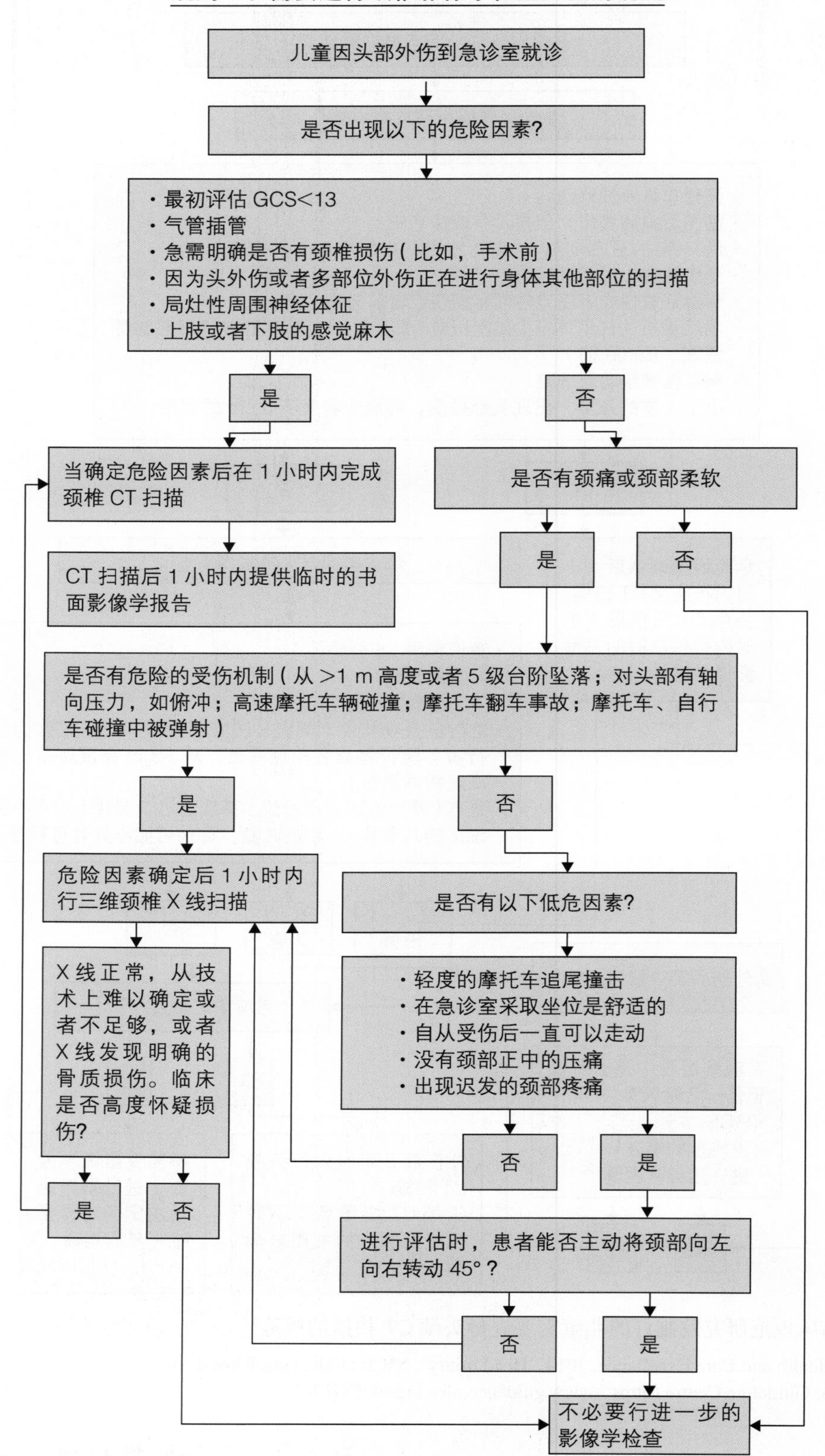

图 87.2 英国国家临床规范研究院制订的儿童需要进行颈椎影像学检查的规范

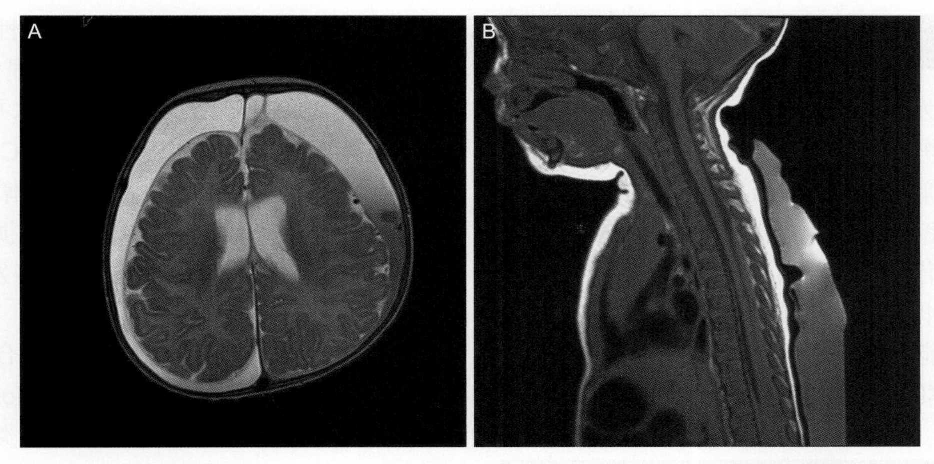

图 87.3　MRI 显示一个儿童复合非意外伤。(A) 显示双侧硬脑膜下血肿，注意交叉的前部静脉，缺少皮质血管，可以和脑外部积水相鉴别。(B) 脊髓硬脊膜下出血

及损伤发生的时间 (Vázquez et al., 2014)。

如果怀疑是 NAI，应立即请有关儿童保护部门作进一步调查。对怀疑 NAI 的患者急诊外科治疗应立即与该地区的小儿神经外科医生讨论。重症急性脑病的治疗需要儿科重症监护和儿童神经病学的专业知识。视网膜出血的处理需要眼科随访。

生长性骨折

生长性骨折是一种罕见的、出现于颅骨骨折后的病症 (**图 87.4**)。颅骨骨折后，由于大脑搏动和大脑生长，颅骨下面附着的硬脑膜和蛛网膜被撕裂，并随着时间的推移变宽，从而导致大脑通过硬脑膜和蛛网膜撕裂的缝隙疝出。

一种更罕见、严重的生长性骨折是“爆裂性骨折”，骨折后有较宽的哆开，其下方有显著的急性脑组织损伤。治疗包括创伤性脑损伤的 ICP 管理以及后续的手术修复覆盖缺损。

患病的儿童中半数在 1 岁以下，90% 在 3 岁以下。生长性骨折通常表现为无压痛性头皮肿胀，最常见的是在顶叶区。

一些因素预示较差的预后，包括年龄小于 8 岁，女性，缺陷小于 7 cm，缺陷越过中线，修复时间延迟超过 8 个月。

年龄小于 3 岁的线性骨折儿童应在损伤后 6 周进行临床评估，以排除有无生长性骨折。生长性骨折的治疗包括硬脑膜成形术或分开的颅盖骨硬膜颅骨成形术。

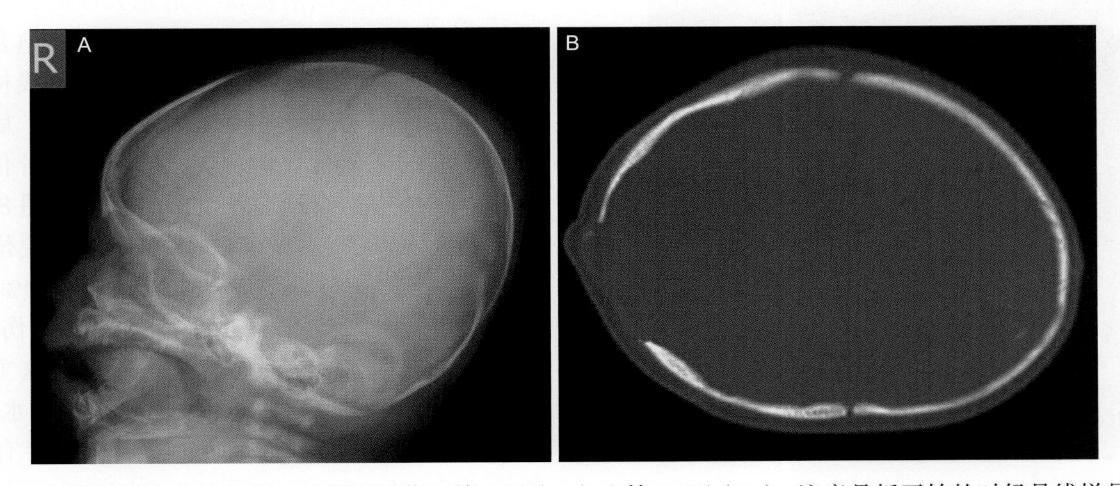

图 87.4　CT 扫描显示生长性骨折，分别于受伤后第 1 天 (A) 和第 50 天 (B)。注意骨折开始的时候是线样骨折，然后由于脑脊液 (CSF) 的搏动逐步变大

乒乓球骨折

乒乓球骨折发生在幼儿和新生儿中。发病机制包括产伤、意外伤害和非意外伤害。

它发生于有弹性的颅骨内板发生“弯折”后，但是颅骨外板（骨密质）连续性没有中断。颅骨骨膜保持完整，很少有潜在的脑损伤（见**图** 87.5）。

大多数在颅骨自然生长的重塑过程中恢复。对于那些有神经功能损伤或需要整形美容的患儿（经过大约 6 个月的观察），可以考虑进一步治疗。

儿童脊髓创伤

在创伤中，25%~50% 脊髓创伤儿童是合并有头部损伤。孩子越小，就越可能发生上颈椎损伤。这可能有几个原因：脊柱的完整性和椎体间的联合主要由强壮的韧带来维持，在颅颈交界处有一些重要的韧带，来维系部分骨化的上颈部和与之严重不成比例的沉重的头部之间的灵活运动。韧带也将 C1/C2 椎骨牢固联合在一起。年幼儿童的韧带更加灵活柔韧，头颈部大小比例更大。在年龄较大的儿童中，韧带没有那么灵活但更加坚韧，韧带和较重的颈部结构转移了颈椎中部的支点（C5/C6），使得损伤更容易发生在 C5/C6。

儿童 C1 软骨环后弓在 3 岁前发生骨化，而 C2 椎体在 6 岁时骨化，齿状突尖端骨化约在 12 岁。8 岁以下的儿童，C1 骨环的中线部分仍然较弱。C1

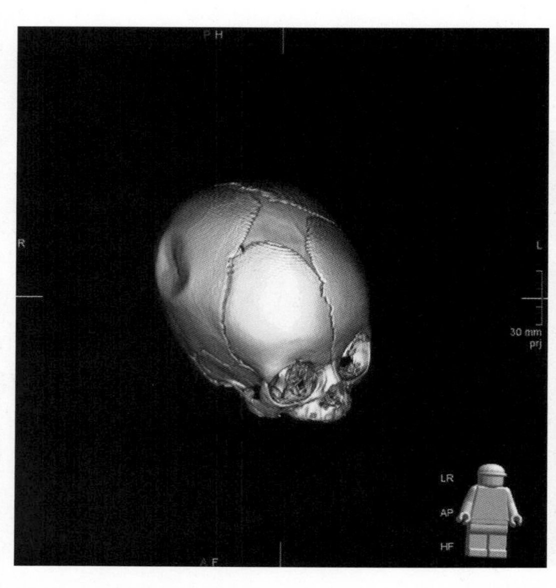

图 87.5 CT 扫描显示颅骨乒乓球骨折。这些骨折随着脑组织发育通常可以重新塑形

骨折通常发生在旋转性损伤和压缩性损伤中。同样，也可发生 C2 骨折。寰枢椎旋转性损伤很可能是由于韧带柔韧度不够，并且在 C1/C2 水平更容易发生创伤性破坏，骨折脱位也通常发生在 C1/C2 水平。

年幼儿童的关节面是水平的，增加了水平半脱位和移位的风险，从而导致脊髓继发损伤。SCIWORA 性损伤在年幼儿童中更常见，大多发生在 C3 以上，有很高的神经损伤风险。

一些隐匿性疾病，如唐氏综合征、黏多糖病（Hurler，Hurler-Scheie，Hunter，Morquio-Brailsford，Maroteaux-Lamy）、类风湿性关节炎和软骨发育不全，均与脊柱受累特异性相关。其病理学通常包括韧带松弛（唐氏综合征）和 GAG（糖胺聚糖）的沉积，可沉积在小关节和寰枢关节面。在 Maroteaux-Lamy 综合征，GAG 可沉积在硬脑膜、后纵向韧带和黄韧带。在类风湿性关节炎中，关节和骨骼会有炎性的变化。在软骨发育不全中，FGFR-3 异常会导致骨化加速，从而导致颅颈狭窄和脊髓受压。椎管狭窄可出现在某个节段或发生在多个节段，并伴有侧隐窝撞击。

在任何年龄，这些情况都会导致不同程度的椎管狭窄、寰枢椎不稳定，变形的表现主要是颈胸和胸腰椎后凸和脊柱侧凸，最终导致脊髓压迫，如果不治疗，将进展为脊髓病变。这些儿童因中度脊柱创伤，而面临着骨骼和神经损伤的巨大风险。

儿童脊柱发育解剖学和影像学

儿童脊柱只有到 10~12 岁时才能达到成人的比例。一些椎骨，包括 C1 环和 C2 的椎体及横突直到 3 岁才会骨化（Munk and Ryan，2007）。

游离齿状突以前被认为是先天性的，但现在认为是在 6 岁之前发生的齿状突骨折的不愈合。它是不稳定的，应该进行伸颈 / 曲颈的 X 射线检查。游离齿状突需要与持续性终末小骨相鉴别，后者是齿状骨中心的末端骨化融合失败导致的。骨化中心出现在 3~6 岁，融合通常发生在 12 岁时（**图** 87.6）。

在 8 岁以下，C2 和 C3 出现假性半脱位的概率分别是 46% 和 14%。上移 4 mm 或者 40% 的脱位可能是生理上的椎体假性半脱位。有多发伤的儿童，大约 1/5 的病例可能偶然有这种发现，这主要是由于不完全骨化、过度活动和幼儿关节面呈水平状态。假性半脱位在关节伸展时会减少，不伴有软组织肿胀。

在颈椎处于中立位或动态视图可评估寰枢椎间

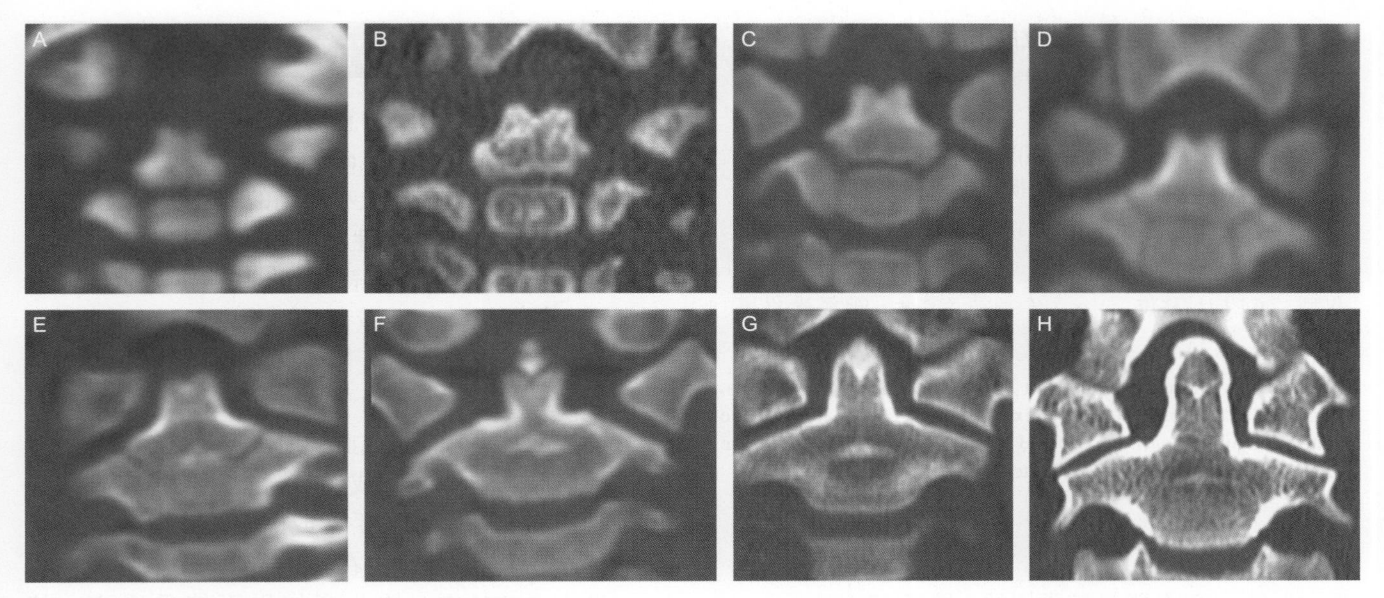

图 87.6 齿状突骨化发展过程的冠状位视图。（A）30 天。（B）5 月。（C）1.5 年。（D）2 年。（E）3 年。（F）5 年。（G）8.5 年。（H）14 年

隔（通常小于 5mm），可显示横突和翼状韧带损伤和水平方向的不稳定。梯状椎体、脊柱侧弯或偏置棘突，都会引起怀疑脊柱急性损伤。

产伤

这类损伤可能发生在胎儿胎位的机械复位或辅助分娩时。上颈和颈胸交界处发生损伤的可能性最大。这些损伤诊断往往不及时，主要是因为婴儿出生时缺乏影像检查，但出生相关脊髓损伤的死亡率很高，而且幸存者可能预后较差。不断改进产前监测和产科技术，有助于降低这些伤害的发生率。

婴儿臂丛神经损伤是由于在分娩过程中过度用力造成的。危险因素是生产困难、使用产钳、真空吸引、臀位分娩、胎儿巨大、婴儿肩难产和母亲糖尿病 / 肥胖。在臂丛神经损伤中，前三个月建议保守治疗的同时予以物理治疗，因为大多数损伤会自发愈合，后续可以进行神经转移或移植手术。

寰枢椎损伤

幼儿可能发生寰枕（C0/C1）和寰枢椎（C1/C2）脱位，因为头部体积相对较大，这些伤害往往是致命的。幸存者的治疗需要行颅颈或寰枢椎融合。在这类损伤中，寰枕关节增宽超过 5 mm，C1/C2 棘间距离扩宽超过 10~12 mm。这些损伤通常是严重 RTA 的结果，儿童的发生概率比成人大五倍。枕骨髁较小和寰枕关节表面呈水平方向，如果骨膜和翼状韧带撕裂，这使得发生脱位。

MRI 扫描有助于确认韧带损伤。韧带损伤经保守治疗通常愈合不好，严重的病例可能需要手术。

寰枢椎旋转半脱位

C1 在 C2 上的固定旋转可能会发生。这是儿童斜颈的常见原因，由半脱位或小关节脱位引起，表现为颈部疼痛，固定姿势的“歪曲”颈部，保持类似公鸡或知更鸟的姿势。另外可出现活动范围缩小，对侧胸锁乳突肌紧绷，儿童可能会头痛或咀嚼困难。症状平均出现在发病后 5 周左右，疾病诊断通常会延迟。

脱位可能是创伤后发生的，但是在儿童也可见于咽后感染性水肿，继发于上呼吸道感染导致的韧带松弛，被称为 Grisel 综合征。其他诱因包括唐氏症、类风湿性关节炎、颅后窝肿瘤和先天畸形。

如果横韧带完整，椎管狭窄只能在严重旋转和小关节脱位的情况下发生。然而，如果横韧带断裂，寰齿间隙（atlantodental interval，ADI）或前滑脱将超过 5 mm。只需旋转 45° 就可能发生椎管狭窄，椎动脉就有危险。

进行 CT 扫描时，先将头部处于中立位置，然后最大限度地向右和向左旋转。旋转半脱位时，C1 在 C2 上的半脱位不会发生变化。如果出现神经系统的症状或缺陷，应进行 MRI 检查，以排除脑干病变。

表 87.1 寰枢椎旋转半脱位的 Fielding 分类

Ⅰ型	单侧关节面半脱位，横韧带完整	常见，多数良性
Ⅱ型	单侧关节面半脱位，向前移位 3~5 mm，横韧带受损	
Ⅲ型	双侧关节面向前移位超过 5 mm，双侧侧块异位	罕见，神经受累风险较高
Ⅳ型	C1 向后移位	罕见，神经受累风险较高

Reproduced with permission from JW Fielding and RJ Hawkins, Atlanto-axial rotatory fixation. (Fixed rotatory subluxation of the atlanto-axial joint), *Journal of Bone & Joint Surgery*, Volume 59, Issue 1, pp. 37–44, Copyright © 1977 Wolters Kluwer Health, Inc.

Fielding 的分类是较常用的（见**表** 87.1）。

许多患者的症状在就医前可能会自发地减少。在半脱位出现时间不到 1 周的情况下，可以使用软领、抗炎药物和进行锻炼。如果半脱位持续时间较长，可以考虑在麻醉剂、肌肉松弛剂和硬领的情况下进行操作（对于年龄较大的儿童来说，头部吊带牵引和支撑是另一种选择）。有时可能需要圆环牵引或 C1-C2 融合。

儿童腰椎损伤

根据受伤脊柱的组合不同，骨折可分为压缩伤、爆裂伤、安全带伤或骨折脱位伤。

楔形压缩骨折是最常见的骨折，发生于屈曲时对椎体前部的轴向压缩负荷。这是一种稳定的损伤，没有椎管损害或脊髓损伤。后凸角度的发生是因为椎体前部高度的降低。

铰链骨折或安全带骨折是由突然加速减速引起极度弯曲造成的损伤。Chance 骨折常见于儿童。机制与安全带有关，因此经常与腹部损伤相关。

爆裂性骨折主要是因为轴向负荷，没有屈曲，影响前柱和中柱。15%~20% 的主要椎体骨折是这种类型。椎体后壁破裂，碎片进入椎管，则可能有脊髓损伤。

三柱损伤来自突然严重屈曲和旋转造成的剪切伤。这些本质上是不稳定的，因为三柱均失效是其特征。它们约占所有脊柱损伤的 20%，其 SCI 的可能性最高。大约 75% 的骨折脱位损伤患者有一定的神经功能缺损，其中 50% 有完全性 SCI。

无明显影像学异常的脊髓损伤

无明显影像学异常的脊髓损伤（spinal cord injury without overt radiographic abnormality，SCIWOR）发生在幼龄儿童中，临床上有明确的神经功能缺陷、X 光和 CT 扫描结果为阴性。然而，MRI 扫描可能显示脊髓、椎间盘或韧带异常。脊髓损伤可能从轻微到严重，原因可能是儿童脊柱弹性较强，韧带松弛，导致脊柱突然来回移位，造成脊髓损伤却没有明显脱位。神经功能缺损是由于过度伸展 / 过度屈曲或脊柱节段移位引起的脊髓或血管损伤。

当血肿压迫脊髓，或韧带断裂和不稳定导致继发性脊髓损伤，行减压手术或固定治疗时，应当行 MRI 扫描。这些损伤很少在平片或 CT 扫描中被发现。

患有 SCIWORA 的儿童如果不接受治疗，其复发和遭受更严重损伤的风险会增加。建议外固定 6~8 周，如果不稳定则可以考虑手术固定。

脊髓损伤的处理

创伤性 SCI 的治疗应该从受伤地点开始，立即给予复苏，脊柱固定后进行转运。PICU 的治疗包括通过强心药来维持足够的血压以改善脊髓灌注，必要时给予支持性通气。

儿童脊髓损伤的判断需要足够的成像，包括 CT 和 MRI，以便及时和清晰地识别所有通常在 X 光检查甚至 CT 扫描中看不到的损伤。需要认真识别韧带损伤、错乱排列骨折或变形、压迫性损伤、不稳定和脊髓损伤。可能需要动态屈曲 / 伸展位的图像。

清除压迫性血肿应作为急诊手术，以避免继发性脊髓损伤。伴有脊髓受压的畸形可能需要将儿童进行牵引治疗，在矫正后将其在环托支撑系统中进行外固定。随后，可能需要手术矫正和固定。无脊髓受压的颈椎骨折通常可以用环托装置治疗。在对骨折行固定治疗的病例，进行长期随访是至关重要的，因为随着时间的推移可能会出现渐进性畸形或不稳定。

脊髓损伤的康复

这通常和成人的治疗标准类似。ASIA 损伤评分被用来定义和描述脊髓损伤的范围和严重程度，并帮助确定未来的康复和恢复需求（American Spinal Injury Association，2002）。理想情况下，应该在受伤后 72 小时内完成评估。儿童的感觉和运动评估需要仔细测试和重复测试。SCI后的脊柱侧凸在儿童中很常见，尤其是当神经损伤发生在幼龄儿童时。

强化康复可以最大限度地恢复功能，或在现有缺陷的基础上发挥功能。脊髓康复是一项多学科的工作，脊柱单位应该受伤后尽快参与并在48小时内进行转诊。

儿童创伤中的争议

有研究关注低体温对儿童神经的保护作用。低温能有效降低颅内压和代谢需求，但也存在心律失常和凝血障碍的风险。早期研究显示没有增加不良事件，并进行一项更大规模的随机对照研究。2008年发表的试验显示，在受伤后8小时内开始并持续24小时的中等低温（32~33 ℃）治疗，并没有改善6个月时的功能结果，也没有改善3个月和12个月的功能和神经心理结果、在ICU或医院的住院时间，以及不良事件（Hutchison et al.，2008）。在儿童研究中还有另外四项研究显示没有任何益处。有14项针对成人的研究结果各不相同。低温治疗现在很少使用，但有时仍被认为是大型临床试验的潜在主题。

延伸阅读、参考文献、EBRAIN的相关链接

扫描书末二维码获取。

第 88 章 儿童脑肿瘤

Jonathan Roth · Shlomi Constantini 著
安旭 译，田永吉 审校

引言与流行病学

在儿童和所有脑肿瘤人群中，儿童脑肿瘤（paediatric brain tumours，PBT）是一个独特的部分。恶性儿童脑肿瘤（malignant paediatric brain tumours，MPBT）发病率仅次于急性淋巴白血病（acute lymphatic leukaemia，ALL），而且近年来发病率持续上升。大约 30% 的儿童癌症死亡是由 MPBT 引起的，是 ALL 的 3 倍。PBT 的发生率为 4.5/10 万（Ostrom et al.，2015），明显低于成人脑肿瘤的发病率，后者是 16.5/10 万。PBT 的发病率在男性患儿略高（男：女比值 4.5：4）。白人儿童的发病率约是黑人儿童的两倍。这种差异也存在于其他癌症中，其原因尚不清楚。大约 50% 的 PBT 是恶性的。年龄对 PBT 的发病率、组织学类型和预后有重要影响。年幼儿童（特别是 5 岁以下的儿童）的发病率为 3.5~4/10 万，5 年生存率约为 50%。年龄较大的儿童（10~20 岁）的发病率为 2~2.5/10 万，5 年生存率约为 75%。所有儿童患者的 5 年生存率约为 65%。随着年龄的增长，生存率不断下降，在 45~54 岁的患者中下降到 23% 左右。

对儿童患者的治疗有几个目标。首先，治愈或控制疾病，增加其长期生存的概率。其次，预防及减少各种诊断和治疗策略带来的远期并发症。最后，尽量减少诊断和治疗对儿童和家庭的心理社会影响。

常见儿童脑肿瘤

儿童脑肿瘤在几个方面与成人不同，包括组织学（和肿瘤的遗传特征）、位置、治疗方案和预后。

在成人中，约有 2/3 的原发性脑肿瘤位于大脑，在儿童，只有 1/4 的脑肿瘤位于大脑（**表** 88.1 和**表** 88.2）。近 30% 的 PBT 位于颅后窝（包括脑干和小脑），而在成人原发脑肿瘤的比例约为 7%。儿童中线肿瘤（包括下丘脑、视神经通路、松果体和垂体区域以及脑室系统）发病率较成人高（Ostrom et al.，2015）。

表 88.1　原发脑和中枢神经系统肿瘤的部位和年龄分布

<19 岁	成人
小脑 16%	3%
脑干 12%	4.3%
脑室 5.6%	1.8%
大脑 24%	65%
松果体 3%	—
垂体 8%	7%
脑神经 4.6%	1%
脊髓 5.6%	4.2%

Data from Ostrom, Q.T., De Blank, P.M., Kruchko, C., Petersen, C.M., Liao, P., Finlay, J.L., Stearns, D.S., Wolff, J.E., Wolinsky, Y., Letterio, J.J., & Barnholtz-Sloan, J.S., Alex's Lemonade Stand Foundation Infant and Childhood Primary Brain and Central Nervous System Tumors Diagnosed in the United States in 2007–2011, *Neuro-Oncology*, Volume 16, Issue s_10, pp. x1–x36, Copyright © 2014 Oxford University Press.

两个群体之间的组织学也不同，某些肿瘤被认为是“儿童”组织类型，如毛细胞星形细胞瘤、髓母细胞瘤和生殖细胞肿瘤。而其他亚型如胶质母细胞瘤和脑膜瘤，在儿童中则很少见（Ostrom et al.，2015）。

低级别胶质瘤

儿童低级别胶质瘤（low-grade gliomas，LGG）约占 PBT 的 40%，最常见的亚型是 WHO Ⅰ级毛细胞星形细胞瘤（pilocytic astrocytoma，PA），约占儿童 LGG 的一半。其他更常见于儿童的 LGG 亚型包括胚胎发育不良性神经上皮肿瘤（dysembryonal neuroectodermal tumour，DNET，WHO Ⅰ级）、神经节细胞胶质瘤（WHO Ⅰ级）、毛黏液样星形细胞瘤

表 88.2 依据年龄分组的原发性脑和中枢神经系统肿瘤组织学分布。最常见的病理类型用加粗字体

0~14 岁	15~19 岁	成人
毛细胞星形细胞瘤	**14%**	**脑膜瘤 30.1%**
20.9%	6.7%	**胶质母细胞瘤 20.3%**
胚胎性（包括髓母细	3.2%	神经鞘 8%
胞瘤）**16.8%**	**10.4%**	垂体 6.3%
胶质母细胞瘤 2.8%	4.6%	星形细胞瘤（2~3
其他星形细胞瘤	6.8%	级）9.8%
10.5%	2.7%	少突胶质细胞瘤
室管膜瘤 7%	**10.1%**	3.7%
生殖细胞肿瘤 3.9%	36%	淋巴瘤 3.1%
颅咽管瘤 3.1%		室管膜瘤 2.3%
垂体 0.8%		颅咽管瘤 0.7%
其他 32%		其他 14%

Data from Ostrom, Q.T., De Blank, P.M., Kruchko, C., Petersen, C.M., Liao, P., Finlay, J.L., Stearns, D.S., Wolff, J.E., Wolinsky, Y., Letterio, J.J., & Barnholtz-Sloan, J.S., Alex's Lemonade Stand Foundation Infant and Childhood Primary Brain and Central Nervous System Tumors Diagnosed in the United States in 2007–2011, *Neuro-Oncology*, Volume 16, Issue s10, pp. x1–x36, Copyright © 2014 Oxford University Press.

（WHO Ⅱ级）、多形性黄色星形细胞瘤（pleomorphic xanthoastrocytoma，PXA，WHO Ⅱ级）。弥漫性星形细胞瘤（Ⅱ级）和少突胶质细胞瘤（Ⅱ级）也可见于儿童，但与成人相比，发生率较低。在 2016 年版 WHO 中枢神经系统肿瘤分类中，这些肿瘤亚型被细分（Louis et al.，2016）。

LGG 可发生在任何位置，但下列位置的发生率较高，包括小脑、脑干、视神经通路、下丘脑和颞叶。

细胞遗传学研究揭示了大多数毛细胞星形细胞瘤的核型正常（Sanoudou et al.，2000）。在观察到异常的地方，并没有确认一致的核型异常。

神经纤维瘤病 1 型（NF1）的患者有较高的毛细胞星形细胞瘤的倾向，特别是在视神经 / 下丘脑区。由于散发性（非 NF1）毛细胞星形细胞瘤偶尔在 17q 染色体（NF1 抑癌基因的位置）上表现出杂合性丢失，人们预测 NF1 基因的突变会在散发性毛细胞星形细胞瘤中发现，从而导致表达丢失。事实上，情况似乎并非如此。NF1 抑癌基因在散发性毛细胞星形细胞瘤中的表达是明显上调的，可能是对细胞过度增殖的反应。这与 NF1 患者发生的毛细胞星形细胞瘤形成对比，后者 NF1 基因表达必然是缺失的。NF1 基因产物在 NF1 和非 NF1 毛细胞星形细胞瘤中不同贡献的确切根源，尚未阐明。

与成人的 LGG 相比，肿瘤抑制基因 TP53 与代谢基因 IDH1 和 IDH2 的突变，在儿童 LGG 中极其罕见（Chalil and Ramaswamy，2015）。

更进一步的基因分析表明，PA 中最常见的染色体异常是染色体区域 7q34 的扩增，包括 BRAF 的位点。这包括 BRAF 癌基因的复制，随后是几个融合基因的嵌入。这可以激活 MAPK 通路，从而导致了肿瘤的发生（Chalil and Ramaswamy，2015）。

在一小部分 LGG 中发现 BRAF V600E 突变，激活并导致 MAPK 通路下调。近年来，MAPK 通路已成为含有这种 BRAF 基因突变或复制的肿瘤化疗的靶点。

小脑毛细胞星形细胞瘤

颅后窝毛细胞星形细胞瘤被认为是最“经典”的 PBT 之一。通常表现为步态异常及脑积水继发的颅内压（intracranial pressure，ICP）增高症状，且这些肿瘤通常位于小脑半球；然而，中线 - 小脑蚓部或肿瘤突出到第四脑室部分也有描述。这些肿瘤通常含实性成分，很多也带有囊性成分。囊可能位于肿瘤内或邻近肿瘤的部位，囊壁在磁共振成像上可表现出增强。

小脑毛细胞星形细胞瘤需要与其他肿瘤进行鉴别诊断，包括血管母细胞瘤，后者可能有一个增强的结节并伴有囊肿。重要的是，PA 的实性成分可能没有任何增强，因此，磁共振其他序列，如液体衰减反转恢复序列（fluid attenuated inversion recovery，FLAIR）可能有助于显示肿瘤轮廓。有趣的是，儿童 PA 可能看起来像成人高级别胶质瘤，有多个实体 - 囊性成分，有非均质性强化。然而，高级别胶质瘤在儿童人群中是罕见的，发生在小脑部位更少。

对小脑 PA 的治疗包括最大限度安全的手术切除，这个通常是基于标准的显微外科技术。这些肿瘤经常会影响脑干或小脑脚的功能，因此，手术时需要仔细判断什么时候结束手术。

在儿童，尤其是婴儿，小脑半球外侧组织通常可以切除，其术后很少出现或没有长期的神经后遗症。可以通过这种方式建立一个安全、方便的手术通道，从而避免过度的小脑牵拉。

外科医生经常面临的问题之一是需要切除囊性成分的囊壁。囊壁在增强磁共振会有强化，因此被认为是肿瘤的一部分。然而，我们此前进行局部活检表明，如果在手术时检查囊壁并且囊壁看起来是透明的，没有肿瘤结节，则无需进行切除（Beni-Adani et al.，2000）。

一般认为肿瘤全切除（经 MRI 证实）后，远期复发率一般很低。然而，最近的一篇论文表明，即使在外科医生认为做到了全切，而且术后 MRI 显示切除干净，5 年无进展生存率（无复发）为 95%（大多数发生在术后前 3 年）（Dodgshun et al.，2016）。最近另一项研究发现，在 10 年的随访中，小脑 PA 在全切后的复发率为 19%（Kim et al.，2014）。因此，即使是全切后患者也必须进行长期随访。

脑干肿瘤

儿童的脑干胶质瘤（brainstem gliomas，BSG）包括一组肿瘤，表现出具有不同症状和肿瘤特性，从而导致了各种不同的生物学行为和不同的预后。BSG 占所有儿童脑肿瘤的 10%~20%，占幕下肿瘤 20%~30%。BSG 可以发生于所有年龄阶段。然而，它们很少在 5 岁之前被诊断出来，发病高峰年龄在 10 岁左右。男女患病概率大致相同。

与小脑和许多幕上肿瘤不同，BSG 累及非常重要的神经组织，以前曾经被认为是手术禁区。然而，Epstein 等表明，在特定的肿瘤亚组，在术中定位和监测下进行切除是可行的，并取得了可以接受的神经和肿瘤学结果（Constantini and Epstein，1996）。随着温和化疗和现代放射治疗技术的发展，综合治疗方案的决策变得更加复杂。目前，对于 BSG，还没有统一的治疗方法。治疗取决于肿瘤的位置、构造和生物学表现。

BSG 包括所有 WHO 的Ⅰ～Ⅳ级星形细胞瘤。Ⅰ级肿瘤（也称为毛细胞星形细胞瘤）通常表现为离散病变，常有囊性成分，然而，它们可能表现位于顶盖背外侧或延髓（和颈髓）肿瘤。注射钆造影剂后通常增强，可能有明显的水肿相关（例如，在颈椎），肿瘤也经常有非增强的成分。

WHO Ⅱ级肿瘤（弥漫性低级别星形细胞瘤）可能发生于脑干的任何部位。其生物学行为非常多样。顶盖和外生型肿瘤，通常进展缓慢。另一方面，弥漫性脑桥胶质瘤（diffuse pontine gliomas，DPG）也可能具有 WHO Ⅱ级肿瘤的组织学表现，但具有侵袭性行为。WHO Ⅱ级肿瘤通常不增强，在 T1 上呈低信号，T2 和 FLAIR 上呈高信号。

WHO Ⅲ级和Ⅳ级肿瘤（间变性星形细胞瘤和多形性胶质母细胞瘤）可以起源于任何位置，其通常更常见于脑桥（作为 DPG）。磁共振上可以表现为边界不清的强化（Ⅲ级）或坏死，环形强化的成分（Ⅳ级）。

其他胶质瘤病理类型很少发生在脑干中，包括神经节细胞胶质瘤、少突胶质细胞瘤和毛黏液样星形细胞瘤。

室管膜瘤

室管膜瘤是儿童第三常见的脑肿瘤，尤其常见于低龄儿童。室管膜瘤常位于第四脑室，有时通过 Luschka 或 Megandie 孔，可包绕脑干，当然也可以位于其他部位。

室管膜瘤的标准治疗包括手术全切除，当肿瘤侵袭低位脑干时，甚至可能需要进行气管切开或胃造口术。

对于后颅凹室管膜瘤，可以在切除术后对瘤床行放射治疗。然而，对于室管膜瘤全切术后放射治疗的必要性仍然存在争议，尤其是在幕下的病例（Ailon et al.，2015）。化疗在室管膜瘤中的疗效尚不明确，因此对于 3 岁以下的儿童也建议放射治疗（Purdy et al.，2014）。

非典型畸胎样横纹肌瘤

非典型畸胎样横纹肌瘤（atypical teratoid rhabdoid tumour，ATRT）是侵袭性中枢神经系统肿瘤，经常累及婴儿和幼儿，它通常位于颅后窝。预后一般较差，中位生存期低于 1 年。ATRT 类似髓母细胞瘤，直到 1980 年代才被认识。ATRT 显示 22q11.2. 染色体长臂的缺失。进一步的基因学研究发现 INI1/hSNF5 肿瘤抑制基因位于这个部位。该基因的体细胞突变，使儿童容易发生 ATRT。一些患有 ATRT 的儿童出生时就患有 HSNF5 基因的杂合子胚系突变，表明这些儿童很容易患上 ATRT（Taylor et al.，2000）。然而，在大多数情况下，这些胚系突变都是初次发生的。

髓母细胞瘤

髓母细胞瘤可能是 PBT 进行分子分型的标志，过去一些年之前，后颅凹髓母细胞瘤（posterior fossa medulloblastomas，PFMB）的患儿，根据年龄、肿瘤残留大小和有无播散，被分为两个亚组——一般风险组和高风险组。用于指导患者的治疗和预后。然而，近年来，髓母细胞瘤根据基因测序被分为四个亚组，每个亚组都在人口统计学、临床、分子和预后特征上不同（Taylor et al.，2012）。这些亚组包括

WNT 型、SHH 型、Group 3 型和 Group 4 型。不同亚组在手术细微差别（如脑干侵袭）、影像学（如磁共振波谱 MRS）和治疗选择上有所不同（Northcott et al.，2012）。这些 PFMB 亚组已被纳入 2016 年 WHO 中枢神经系统肿瘤分类中（Louis et al.，2016）。

可以期待，遗传性肿瘤标志物将会为患者的辅助治疗提供指导，因此，收集肿瘤组织样本进行基因学分析至关重要。此外，多中心合作也至关重要。目前也在建立肿瘤组织样本库以利于目前以及将来的基因学研究。

视路胶质瘤

视路胶质瘤（optic pathway gliomas，OPG）是低级别胶质肿瘤，起源于视觉通路的任何位置，如视神经、视交叉、视束或者视放射。OPG 属罕见病，约占 PBT 的 5%，其中大部分发生于儿童期的第一个 10 年。许多 OPG 与神经纤维瘤病 Ⅰ 型（NF1）相关，然而，约 40% 与 NF1 不相关（Shofty et al.，2015）。OPG 的病理学通常是毛细胞星形细胞瘤，但毛黏液样星形细胞瘤的诊出率不断提高，特别是在婴儿中。

关于 OPG 的许多问题仍然存在争议，包括分类、诊断、活检必要性、手术指征和手术目标，以及化疗和放疗的作用和时机。在下面的段落中，我们将对此进行简要概述，但是我们并没有试图尝试解决很多相关的争议。

OPG 分类通常以解剖学为指导，然而，目前各种分类系统与肿瘤进展的自然史或临床方面（特别是视觉预后）并没有很好的相关性。

出现的症状可能与肿瘤侵犯或视觉通路受压引起的视觉功能损伤有关，与脑脊液通道阻塞引起的脑积水有关；可继发于间脑畸形，压迫或侵犯导致间脑综合征（恶病质、头小畸形和视力下降）；由下丘脑 - 垂体轴紊乱引起的各种内分泌紊乱引起。特别是在婴儿期，视觉功能难以准确评估，给临床评估带来了很大困难。

诊断 OPG 经常是基于影像学表现，不需要行活检。视神经增粗，特别是出现强化时，伴有或者不伴有视交叉累及，都是诊断的依据。当与 NF1 相关时，视交叉 - 下丘脑肿瘤就可以诊断为 OPG。尽管 MRI 对 OPG 的诊断很重要，但不典型的病例，如大龄儿童的非 NF 相关病变，不能明确看到起源于视神经，或没有视交叉肿胀，这些患者应该进行活检。根据解剖的不同，肿瘤活检技术选择不同。可以经过额底入路暴露视交叉，对于病变累及第三脑室并导致脑积水的病例可以采用内镜下手术或立体定向活检。活检的作用是明确病理，同时确定分子改变，如 BRAF-KIAA1549 融合，既能指导预后，也能有治疗意义（Shofty et al.，2015）。

OPG 的自然病史无法预测。有些患者肿瘤可以保持稳定多年，有些患者肿瘤不断进展。经常见到有些患者视力下降但是肿瘤的形态没有明显变化。一般来说，与散发型病例相比，与 NF1 相关的 OPG 的病程更稳定。

OPG 的治疗需要多学科团队合作，涉及临床（尤其强调眼科评估）、放射治疗学、手术治疗以及神经肿瘤学方面。

一般情况下，肿瘤大小相对稳定，如果视力稳定，可以定期随访。然而，对于体积较大的肿瘤，如果具有明显的外生成分突入到额下区，或向上延伸到第三脑室导致脑积水或压迫脑干的肿瘤应考虑手术治疗。手术入路可选择额颞 / 额底入路或各种半球间 / 脑室入路。手术目标并非完全切除肿瘤，而是去除大部分外生肿瘤，并打通脑脊液通路。术中成像可用于协助确定切除范围（Millward et al.，2015）。

OPG 患者的腹水可能与脑室腹腔分流相关（Gil et al.，2001），其原因尚不清楚，但是必要时可以转流到心房。

化疗是大多数 OPG 的主要治疗方法，治疗方案多样，大多数从长春新碱 - 卡铂开始。尽管广泛使用化疗治疗 OPG，但长期的视力结局仍较差（Shofty et al.，2011）。放疗有不同的成功率，然而，可能会导致血管病（烟雾病）、内分泌异常和继发恶性肿瘤。

OPG 的预后一般较好，10 年生存率可以达到 85%~90%。因此治疗 OPG 的主要目标是保护视力。正如前述，尽管有争议，视力的远期预后仍然不容乐观。

环境中的危害因素

病原体，特别是某些病毒，可以增加某些癌症的风险。人类多瘤病毒可增加脑肿瘤风险。蛋白质从病毒向周围细胞转移，从而导致细胞增生调节异常。这可能是由于肿瘤抑制基因的灭活或细胞增殖上调。Weggen 等在髓母细胞瘤、脑膜瘤和室管膜瘤中也发现了人多瘤病毒序列的证据。目前，对于这些序列的临床意义尚不清楚。

辐射也增加患脑肿瘤的风险。头部照射治疗儿童头癣已被证明是未来发生良恶性肿瘤的主要危险因素。在患有神经纤维瘤病的儿童中，这种风险增加甚至更高。数据表明，即使是低剂量辐射（如计算机断层扫描，CT）也可能导致继发性恶性肿瘤，因此应该尽可能减少。肿瘤发生的机制可能是辐射可诱导基因改变，导致肿瘤抑制基因下调或致癌基因上调。

过去一些年，手机暴露一直是各种流行病学研究的重点。到目前为止，还没有明确的证据支持或反驳儿童使用手机带来的潜在风险，但不鼓励过度使用。在成人中，目前的文献表明，暴露于手机的低剂量辐射不会对发生脑肿瘤造成额外的风险。

有文献报道了儿童成髓母细胞瘤发病率具有季节倾向性。秋季（尤其是10月份）出生的儿童，患髓母细胞瘤的风险增加。造成这种季节性联系的潜在原因可能是怀孕和婴儿早期社区感染增加，或接触各种化学物质的季节性变化有关。然而，目前还没有建立出明确的病理生理学机制。

诊断、检查和手术前准备

病史和体检

许多儿科脑肿瘤位于中线位置，导致缺乏局灶神经系统体征，往往被延迟诊断，等明确诊断时，肿瘤可能已经很大。儿童脑肿瘤的表现包括颅内压升高（继发于肿瘤占位效应或者继发性脑积水）、局灶性神经体征、癫痫、认知和行为障碍，和（或）内分泌和生长障碍。一项meta分析回顾了儿童中枢神经系统肿瘤的临床表现（Wilne et al.，2007）。头痛、恶心和呕吐是最常见的症状，然而，只出现在30%~40%的患者（**表**88.3）。出现的症状与肿瘤位置密切相关（**专栏**88.1）。

表88.3 儿童脑肿瘤的症状和体征

在3702名<18岁儿童中	在232名<4岁儿童中
• 头痛（33%） • 恶心和呕吐（32%） • 步态异常或共济失调（27%） • 视盘水肿（13%） • 癫痫发作（13%） • 无特异症状的颅内压升高（10%） • 斜视（7%） • 行为或学业表现改变（7%） • 巨头畸形（7%） • 脑神经麻痹（7%） • 昏睡（6%） • 眼球运动异常（眼球震颤、Parinaud征）（6%） • 偏瘫（6%） • 体重减轻（5%） • 局灶性运动无力（5%） • 未明确的视力或眼睛异常（5%） • 意识水平改变（5%）	• 巨头畸形（41%） • 恶心呕吐（30%） • 情绪易怒（24%） • 昏睡（21%） • 步态异常或共济失调（19%） • 体重减轻（14%） • 临床上有明显症状的脑积水（囟门突出、颅缝扩张）（13%） • 癫痫（10%） • 头痛（10%） • 视盘水肿（10%） • 非特异的局灶性体征（10%） • 颅内压升高的非特异性症状（9%） • 局灶性运动无力（7%） • 头部倾斜（7%） • 意识水平下降（7%） • 斜视（6%） • 眼球运动异常（6%） • 发育迟缓（5%） • 偏瘫（5%）

Reprinted from *The Lancet Oncology*, Volume 8, issue 8, Sophie Wilne, Jacqueline Collier, Colin Kennedy, Karin Koller, Richard Grundy, David Walker, Presentation

儿童中常见的主诉是头痛。在瑞典学龄期儿童中，到7岁时，曾经有40%儿童经历过头痛，到15岁时，这个比例达到75%。在美国，大约20%的儿童患有慢性头痛。虽然大多数病例是良性原因，但有些可能是脑肿瘤表现出来的症状。认识到并非所有的脑瘤都伴有头痛，尤其是在年轻人群。在一项研究中，出现头痛的儿童中，18%的5岁以下儿童，52%的6~10岁，68%的11~20岁的儿童发生了脑肿瘤。在另一项研究中，62%的脑瘤儿童出现头痛，超过50%的儿童至少有三种相关症状，如恶心、呕吐、视觉影响、步态异常、力弱或性格改变、在学校内的改变、言语障碍。在我们的PBT病例中，40%的人出现头痛，只有3%的人以头痛作为唯一症状。

年幼儿童脑肿瘤的症状通常不具有特异性，很容易被首诊医生忽略。症状可能包括“小脑痉挛”，这可能被错误地认为是癫痫发作，但实际上是昏迷的急性期表现，代表早期症状和脑干受到压迫的危险水平，因为颅后窝空间狭窄。视觉模糊也可能表明颅内压增高。这些表现增加手术干预的迫切性。症状可能间断性地“出现或者消失”，患儿神经功能完整，给人一种“功能性”的印象，从而延误诊断。先前针对延迟诊断的研究发现，从第一次出现症状到明确诊断的中位时间［诊断前症状间隔（prediagnostic symptomatic interval，PSI）］约为2个月，与儿童年龄呈负相关（Kukal et al.，2009）。PSI也与肿瘤组织学相关。高级别肿瘤与短PSI相关，而低级别肿瘤与长PSI相关。Kukal等也表明，PSI与预后并不独立相关，而是与肿瘤组织学和患者年龄相关。

头围是体格检查的重要组成部分，特别是在婴儿中，应记录在头围表格上。视力下降在幼儿中多被忽略，直到视力丧失加重，因为儿童不会注意到并报告视力下降。如果可能的话，视力应该进行规范的检测。应记录视力和视野，特别是病变累及视

专栏 88.1 与肿瘤位置相关的症状和体征

- 幕上肿瘤：
  - 非特异性的颅内压升高（47%）
  - 癫痫发作（38%）
  - 视盘水肿（21%）
- 颅后窝肿瘤：
  - 恶心或呕吐（75%）
  - 头痛（67%）
  - 步态异常或共济失调（60%）
  - 视盘水肿（34%）
- 脑干肿瘤：
  - 步态异常或共济失调（78%）
  - 脑神经受损（52%）
  - 锥体束征（33%）
  - 头痛（23%）
  - 斜视（19%）
- 中心区域的肿瘤（第三脑室区域）：
  - 头痛（49%）
  - 眼球运动异常（20%）
  - 恶心和呕吐（20%）
  - 斜视（21%）

觉通路时。呆滞扩大的瞳孔是颅内压严重增高的征兆，也是神经系统功能即将恶化的征兆。只有大约20% 的 PBT 患儿会有视盘水肿，大约 50% 的患儿神经系统检查是正常的。因此，仔细的病史询问可能比临床检查更重要（Shay et al.，2012）。听力也应该进行正规检查，特别是有发育延迟或病变可能涉及听力通路时。

儿童神经病学家及儿科医师

在诊断阶段，特别是对于有复杂的神经系统情况或者合并癫痫的患者，请儿童神经病学家介入，将会非常有帮助。可能存在一般的医疗问题和（或）合发育、行为学、家族问题，需要儿科医生的专业知识。术前言语功能和物理治疗评估也是重要的。在许多西方国家，儿童神经病学家，是磁共振（magnetic resonance，MR）检查的守门人，他们接受培训以区别 PBT 的重要和不重要的体征。为了获得一个向上的学习曲线，儿童神经病学家及小儿神经外科医生之间必须建立良好的沟通。

神经心理和发育评估

对于 4 岁以上的儿童，术前应完成神经心理学的基线评估。一些有限的神经心理学测试甚至可以在一些 3 岁的孩子身上进行。使用 Vineland Adaptive Behavior Scale 量表进行正式的发育评估，也可以用于 3 岁以下的儿童。任何神经心理学评估的结果都可能因颅内压升高或情绪变化而产生干扰。然而，这将有助于预测术后认知功能恢复的程度，具有重要的法医学意义。

内分泌

任何术前有内分泌或生长障碍，以及术后可能发生内分泌并发症的儿童，应在术前由内分泌学家进行内分泌评估。应记录儿童的体重、身高和青春期发育状况，并评估其营养状况和体液平衡。

内分泌异常，在患有颅咽管瘤或视路 / 丘脑胶质瘤的患儿中常见。内分泌筛查在术前和术后都很重要，主要的内分泌异常需要后续治疗。

癫痫

应充分研究癫痫发作特点，最好用脑电图（electroencephalogram，EEG）。更频繁的发作可以采用视频 EEG 监测。所有局灶性癫痫发作的检查均应包括磁共振成像。手术前应尝试控制癫痫。对于小脑幕上病变，通常在术前开始预防性抗癫痫药物治疗；当然，这仍然是一个有争议的问题（Fattal-Valevski et al.，2013）。

神经影像

为了达到手术的目标，完整的中枢神经系统成像（包括脊柱成像）非常重要，手术目标可以是肿瘤全切除，或者是仅行活检。**图** 88.1~ **图** 88.4 展示了不同的儿童脑肿瘤的典型图像。

钆 -DTPA 强化的 MR 要优于 CT，可以明确病变的准确位置和范围，有助于制订肿瘤切除术的计划。

所有患者术前均应完善 MR 检查。对于中线部位的肿瘤，矢状位和冠状位图像特别有帮助，可以显示肿瘤与脑干、脑室系统和其他周围结构的关系，从而有助于制订手术计划。在处理有潜在播散可能的肿瘤（如生殖细胞肿瘤、室管膜瘤和髓母细胞瘤）时，应在完善头颅 MR 检查的同时进行脊柱的 MRI 筛查，

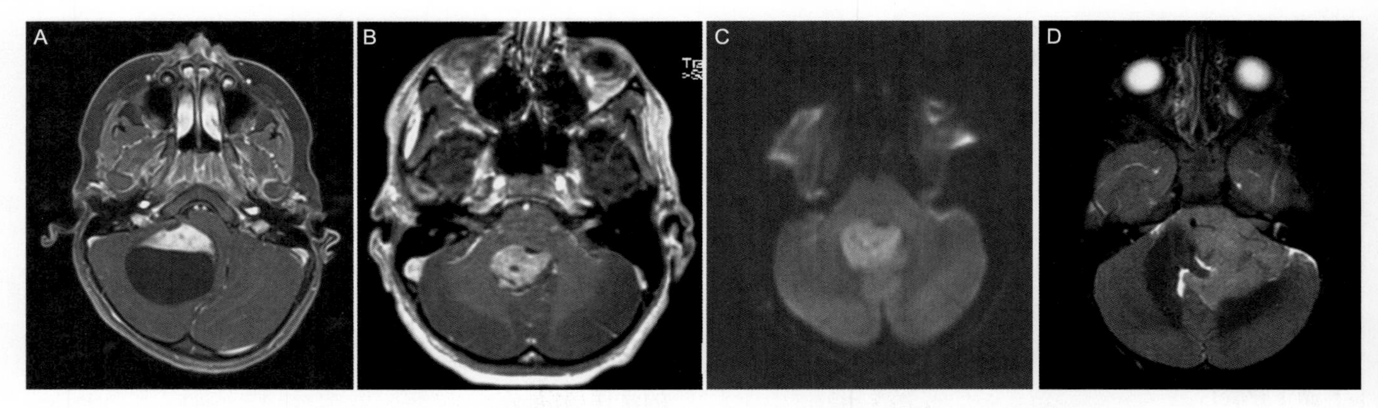

图 88.1 典型的儿童后颅凹肿瘤。（A）毛细胞星形细胞瘤；（B、C）髓母细胞瘤；（D）室管膜瘤

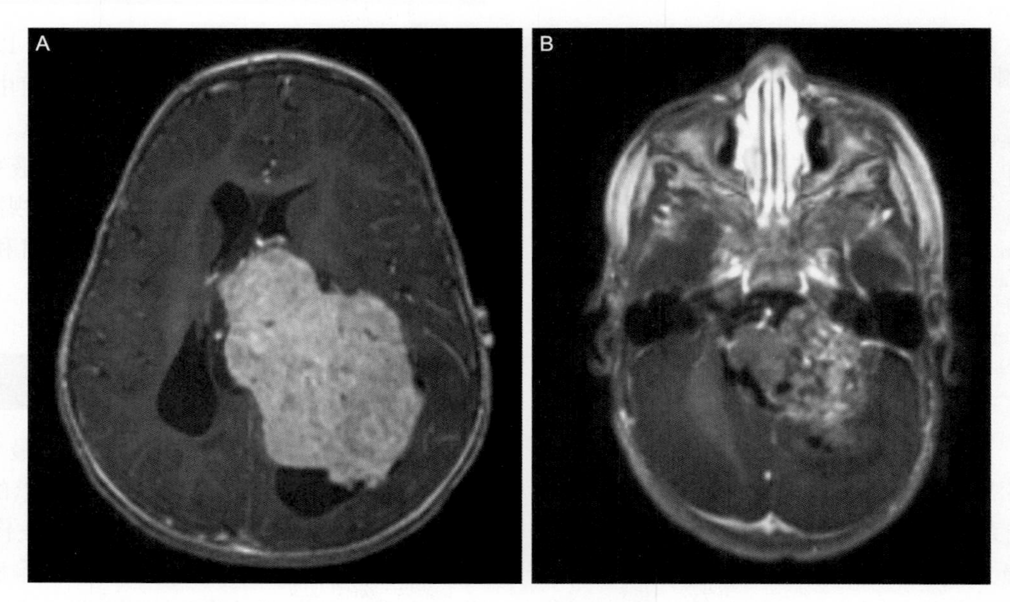

图 88.2 婴儿肿瘤。（A）脉络丛乳头状瘤；（B）颅后窝非典型畸胎样横纹肌瘤（ATRT）

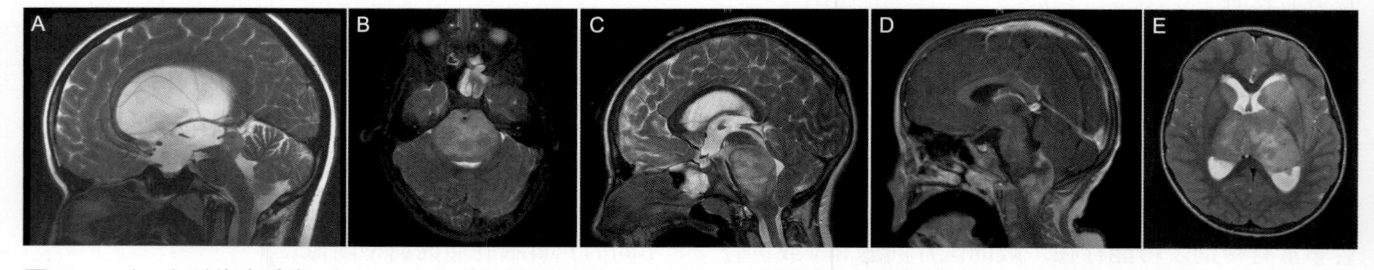

图 88.3 （A）顶盖胶质瘤；（B、C）弥漫脑桥胶质瘤（DPG）；（D）颈髓神经节胶质瘤；（E）双侧丘脑间变星形细胞瘤

以便发现脊柱和脑膜的播散，以免手术中血液流到椎管内，导致难以区分是血液还是播散的肿瘤。弥散加权和灌注磁共振成像有助于区别肿瘤，并评估治疗反应。

最近，白质的弥散张量成像（diffusion tensor imaging，DTI）非常有助于区别功能性神经通路和它们与肿瘤的位置关系。尤其是将DTI整合到导航工作站，可以增加手术的安全性。

值得注意的是，一些儿童是在急性事件后被诊断出来的。CT扫描，比MRI更迅速便捷，经常是

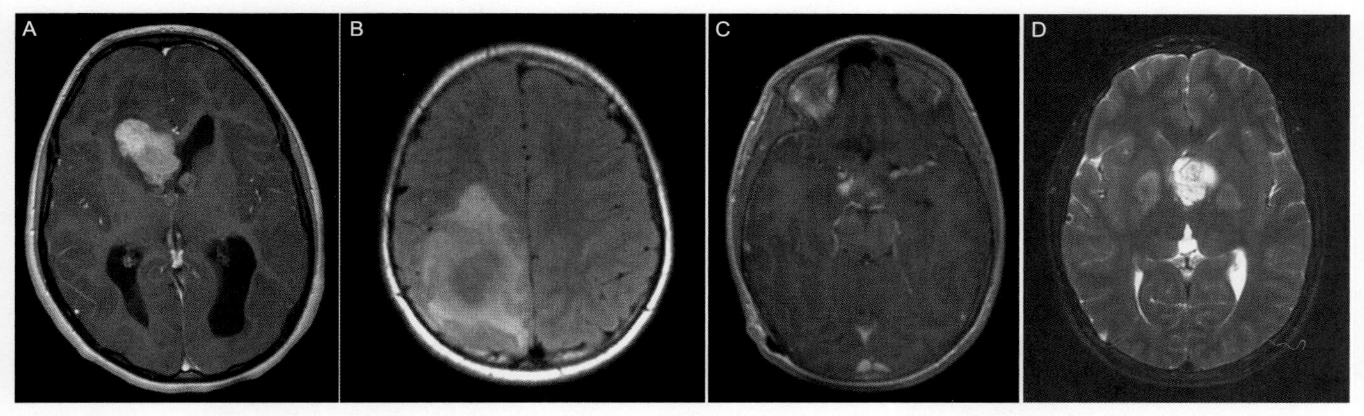

图 88.4　（A）结节硬化患者的室管膜下巨细胞星形细胞瘤（SEGA）;（B）错配修复综合征患者的胶质母细胞瘤；（C、D）神经纤维瘤病Ⅰ型患者的视交叉 - 下丘脑胶质瘤

主要的诊断工具。CT 成像在一些方面优于 MRI，可以明确颅骨受累情况，或显示出肿瘤相关的钙化（如颅咽管瘤），并且在评估可能侵袭颅骨的颅底肿瘤时非常重要。然而，这些肿瘤在儿童中并不常见。应该准备计划导航 / 立体定向技术，并在成像前在儿童头部指定部位放置标记。

还有各种其他的成像工具是可用的。并且在特定的场景下非常有用。头颅超声（ultrasound，US），特别是那些囟门未闭合的低龄儿童，可以作为一种筛查工具，但仍需 MR 的进一步评估。MRS 已广泛应用于肿瘤的诊断、复发与放射性坏死的鉴别以及随访和预后。MRS 的敏感性和特异性不高，因此 MRS 只能作为其他检查或组织学诊断的补充工具。核医学在脑肿瘤儿童的诊断和随访中起着重要作用。骨扫描可用于显示颅骨受累肿瘤的“热区”，如尤因肉瘤和骨肉瘤。FDG-PET 扫描显示与肿瘤相关的高代谢区，但该技术空间分辨率不高，也是一项补充工具。同样，SPECT 扫描可显示放射物摄取增加，特别是在星形细胞瘤，但这些也仅作为补充工具。

神经成像的时间

每当新的神经功能障碍发生时，比如运动功能、脑神经相关的或者眼科检查有异常发现，需要进行神经影像学检查。斜颈可能提示颅椎或后颅凹病变，因此，当没有其他原因解释新发的斜颈时，可行中枢神经系统成像以明确诊断。当头围增大超过正常的基础生长曲线时，需要进行神经系统成像，因为此时提示脑积水或颅内肿物。

新发的癫痫发作可能是脑肿瘤的表现。然而，大多数儿童癫痫发作不是继发于肿瘤，而是继发于皮质发育不全、创伤和代谢性疾病。文献中已经讨论了 MR 在儿童不明原因癫痫发作中的作用。只有不到 0.5% 的儿童患有脑肿瘤。目前，基于已有数据，推荐不明原因癫痫发作患者进行 MRI 随访复查。如果儿童持续有一个局灶性功能缺陷，在几个小时内不能缓解（例如在 Todd 瘫痪中），或者癫痫持续状态持续时间延长，数小时仍不能缓解，则应行急诊 MR 检查。在不明原因的局灶性发作（有或没有泛化发作）之后，当脑电图不提示儿童良性癫痫，任何其他原发性癫痫综合征或 1 岁以下儿童，建议行非急诊 MR 检查。

其他检查方法

其他诊断性检查包括生殖细胞肿瘤标志物，如血清和脑脊液中的甲胎蛋白（αFP）、人绒毛膜促性腺激素（β-HCG）以及胎盘碱性磷酸酶。在某些治疗方案中，这些标志物作为决策的主要指标，同时也是肿瘤随访的基线标志（Echevarria et al.，2008）。

地塞米松

在手术前几天开始应用类固醇，以减少瘤周水肿。这种药物可以明显改善儿童的身体状况。应避免长期大剂量使用，以免引起库欣样效应。

偶然发现的脑肿瘤

随着 MR 扫描在儿科疾病评估过程中使用的增加，导致偶然发现的脑肿瘤数量明显增加。目前，关于这些偶然发现脑肿瘤的自然病程和治疗的文献不多。在最近的一项研究中，Roth 等总结了在两个医学中心（美国、以色列）诊断的47例偶然发现的肿瘤。只有三例最终诊断为高级别肿瘤。他们认为，许多病变是良性的，可以密切观察随访（开始的时候每2~3个月复查一次）；然而，应根据影像学对肿瘤良恶性的判断、病变大小的变化或者强化程度、神经系统状态变化、手术风险以及父母的倾向性，制订个体化方案（Roth et al.，2012）。

不需要活检或者切除的肿瘤

有一些儿童脑肿瘤的诊断主要基于影像学和临床表现，不需要手术切除，甚至不需要活检。这些肿瘤可能会引起继发影响，如脑积水，后者需要治疗。但可以在没有肿瘤组织标本的情况下进行肿瘤学治疗。这些肿瘤包括：经典的弥漫内生型脑干胶质瘤（diffuse intrinsic brainstem glioma，DIPG）、经典的顶盖胶质瘤、双灶性肿瘤（总是与生殖细胞瘤有关）、视路胶质瘤（特别是与神经纤维瘤病1型相关）和室管膜下巨细胞星形细胞瘤（与结节性硬化症有关）。

手术原则

手术的目的是准确地辨认肿瘤的范围，包括是否存在软脑膜侵袭，在不引起进一步明显的神经功能缺损的前提下，尽可能多切除肿瘤，并治疗继发性脑积水同时重建脑脊液通路。最大限度的切除范围同时将致残率降到最低，为实现此目的，可利用手术辅助手段，如术中导航系统、实时成像、术前以及实时功能监测。在下一节中，我们将讨论用于实现这些目标的各个方面。针对特定类型肿瘤，最大范围切除肿瘤的目标是需要调整的，比如生殖细胞肿瘤，对辅助治疗非常敏感。收集脑脊液用于分析细胞学和肿瘤标志物检测，对那些有进入脑脊液循环通路倾向的肿瘤具有重要的预后意义。请注意，腰穿CSF比脑室CSF具有更好的预测价值和更高的阳性率（Gajjar et al.，1999）。

儿童生理学

儿童并不是一个小的成人，外科医生必须清楚，与成人相比，儿童所需的外科技术和麻醉技术存在差异。需要特别考虑气道，血容量，头皮和颅骨较薄，组织娇嫩，体表面积和体重比，静脉输液的要求和药物代谢的特点。儿童容易出现体温过低、低血容量和贫血，所有这些都应该预防。在一般的身体处理和手术过程中，幼龄儿童需要特别轻柔对待，外科医生必须细致止血来减少失血。

此外，还需注意，幼儿脑沟和大脑外侧裂发育尚不完全，还不能像成熟的脑组织那样，可以很容易地作为解剖界面或者手术通道。

手术时机

患有颅后窝肿瘤和梗阻性脑积水的儿童病情紧急，对于神经外科医生也是一个挑战，特别是手术的时机和顺序。脑积水通常在切除肿瘤后可以得到控制，但意识状态是手术时机的重要决定因素。意识模糊的患者属于外科的急诊，需要尽快手术。如果意识状态只受到轻微下降，类固醇类药物可以暂缓手术的紧急性。可以将患者放在后续择期手术的名单上，如果患者出现昏迷，则应立即行手术治疗。在存在巨大颅后窝肿瘤时，放置脑室外引流可能是有危险的，因为可能会出现上疝和继发脑干出血，而且可能会出现进一步的意识不清，并由于大脑后动脉被压迫在小脑幕缘而导致失明。据报道，上疝的风险为3%（Albright，1983），小脑蚓部巨大肿瘤患者的风险性更高。治疗方法是夹闭外引流并立即行肿瘤切除手术。第三脑室底造瘘术是脑室外引流的代替方案。

对于后颅凹肿瘤，目前倾向于立即行确切的肿瘤切除术，而不是先处理脑积水。即使患者出现反应迟钝，也建议立即放置外脑室引流和切除肿瘤，因为肿瘤本身可能会导致相当严重的脑干压迫并导致意识下降。这种情况下，脑室外引流和压力降低应该尽可能小，直到颅后窝减压，以防止发生上疝。如果患者长期呕吐，电解质紊乱脱水，营养不良，一般情况不佳，并且出现意识下降，非常有必要通过控制脑脊液引流来改善脑积水。这将改善患者的一般状况，准备迎接后续的肿瘤切除术，必须严密观察患者，警惕由于上疝或者脑干压迫加重导致的任何恶化。

由松果体区域肿瘤引起的梗阻性脑积水最好采用内镜下第三脑室底造瘘术。第三脑室底造瘘时可同时进行肿瘤活检（Roth and Constantini，2015）。如果有指证，可以行二次手术，切除肿瘤（Cultrera，2006）。导水管部位肿瘤最近被描述为一类独立的肿瘤。手术方式包括内镜下第三脑室底造瘘和活检（Roth et al.，2015）。

一个有争议的问题是颅内小肿瘤出现癫痫发作，没有占位效应或继发性脑积水。尽管缺乏文献资料，但低级别肿瘤转变为高级别肿瘤在儿童中似乎极其罕见。因此，只要影像学上保持稳定，癫痫可以通过药物控制，加以密切随访观察。

体位

儿童脑肿瘤手术的体位本质上取决于肿瘤的位置。外科医生必须能够直视肿瘤并且能舒适地到达肿瘤的边界。颅后窝肿瘤和枕部幕上病变通常采用俯卧体位。

外科医生在选择坐位时必须权衡风险和效益。在一些上蚓部、脑干或松果体病变，主要向小脑幕下延伸，坐位比俯卧位更适合，但每个病例都必须单独判断，并取决于外科医生的经验。4岁以下的儿童通常不选择坐位。坐位的优点是肿瘤暴露良好，有利于显微镜进入，出血和脑肿胀可以降到最低。缺点是外科医生必须坐在一个不方便的和不舒服的姿势，手臂长时间抬高并伸展进行手术，容易变得疲劳。此外，患者有心血管不稳定，容易出现体位性低血压、静脉空气栓塞（venous air embolism，VAE）和反常空气栓塞的风险增加。后者罕见，但是会出现灾难性后果。儿童发生空气栓塞的风险和处于坐位手术的成人一样，是30%~45%，而且儿童比成人更容易受到这种并发症的威胁。对VAE的检测方法、临床效果、治疗和预防方法的讨论不在本章范围，但在文献中有进一步的阐述（Jadik et al.，2009）。患者坐位手术时可能会发生颅内积气、颅内血肿、脑血流灌注不足。躺椅姿势，臀部倾斜，膝盖抬高至接近肩高，可以保持全坐姿手术的优势，同时可显著降低低血压、脑血流下降和空气栓塞的风险。

对于18个月至5岁之间儿童，使用3钉式固定必须非常小心。18个月以下儿童应禁止使用。如果施加过多的压力，可导致脑脊液漏和凹陷性颅骨骨折。对于6个月至14岁的儿童可使用马蹄环形和头钉系统固定（Gupta，2006）。

神经麻醉

在摆放手术体位之前，应行动脉穿刺、脉搏血氧监测并放置导尿管。当患者需要取俯卧位时，需要避免过度屈颈，下巴不要接触胸部。眼睛需要小心的保护，尤其是当患者取俯卧位的时候。虽然眼睛已经完全覆盖，但是仍应该在头部的两侧放置毛巾并固定，以防止消毒剂进入眼睛。当取俯卧位时，面部放在马蹄环上，小心衬垫，特别是眼睛。外科医生应该检查患者的眼睛，确保没有与马蹄环本身紧密接触。外科医生还应检查周围皮肤受压点用软垫充分保护。在儿童的臀部下方放置保护性胶带或者硅胶棒，以防止旋转手术台时儿童发生滑动。如果使用经鼻气管插管，不论采用坐位或者俯卧位，很少发生气管插管弯曲打折。一旦患者体位摆放完成，麻醉医师将需要检查气管内插管的位置，以确保其没有进入右主干肺支气管。

麻醉诱导时给予预防性广谱抗生素。我们目前使用万古霉素和头孢曲松，或头孢噻吩。麻醉时应该仔细注意保温措施，尤其患者是较年幼的孩子，体温过低往往是由于身体暴露的时间过长。后续的类固醇药物可在麻醉诱导时静脉注射。对颅后窝肿瘤患者无需使用抗癫痫药物，如果影像学上显示颅内结构紧密，可在切皮时静脉注射0.25~0.5 g/kg甘露醇，这可以降低颅内压，并有助于术区暴露，也可对脑组织起到保护作用。当患者处于坐位时，进行心前区多普勒和呼吸末CO_2监测。

手术入路

外科医生必须练习掌握灵活多样的手术入路，以求最安全最直接地达到肿瘤病灶。对位于颅底或基底池的肿瘤，儿童的手术原则与成人颅骨底手术相同，目的是最大限度地暴露肿瘤，同时最低限度对脑组织的牵拉，颅底手术入路越来越多地用于儿童来切除肿瘤，如脊索瘤、脑膜瘤和肉瘤。经蝶窦入路可以用于一些特定的蝶区和鞍旁病变（Kassam et al.，2007），这种入路适用于位于蝶鞍内颅咽管瘤和蝶鞍上球状肿物（鞍膈下）以及垂体瘤切除。采用内镜的经鼻经蝶入路非常适合那些小鼻腔的儿童（Kassam et al.，2007）。

神经外科手术的辅助策略

立体定向手术

肿瘤切除的各种辅助技术可以提高手术的精确度并降低致残率。术中超声是一种简单方法，可以识别皮质下较大的病变。无框立体定向正成为脑肿瘤手术中不可缺少的辅助技术，使外科医生能够准确规划手术路径，选择进入点（在许多情况下帮助设计更小的手术切口），并提供有效的术中导航（Roth et al.，2006）。无框立体定向可用于立体定向活检，而有框立体定向则适用于较小的深层病变活检。

神经内镜

经脑室内镜手术已经被广泛用于各种疾病。在脑脊液引流相关的手术，如内镜下第三脑室底造瘘（endoscopic third ventriculostomy，ETV）和透明隔切开术中被广泛使用（Oertel et al.，2009），此外，对于有脑积水或者无脑积水患者，可以采用内镜进行脑室内肿瘤切除术（Souweidane，2008）。对于因中线位置脑肿瘤（松果体、顶盖、丘脑）而继发梗阻性脑积水的患者，通常进行内镜活检，同时进行或者不进行ETV（Roth et al.，2015；Roth and Constantini，2015）。使用1~2 mm可伸缩内镜可以让外科医生从不同寻常的角度近距离观察肿瘤和肿瘤基底。该技术可以使外科医生能够尽量减少手术的并发症并提高病灶全切除率。可结合内镜和无框立体定向系统来改善内镜的定位和导航的准确度（Souweidane，2008）。

功能磁共振和弥散张量成像

基于血氧水平依赖性（blood-oxygen-level-dependent，BOLD）图像的术前功能MRI用于可配合的大于5岁的儿童，可以确定语言优势功能区，并有一定的可信度（Hertz-Pannier et al.，2014）。可以将定位感觉运动皮质区的功能磁共振（functional magnetic resonance，fMRI）图像，整合到无框立体定向图像，与电生理定位的感觉运动皮质准确相关联。也可以将功能MRI定位的语言皮质区注册到无框立体定向系统。这种技术对靠近或者位于语言或感觉运动皮质区域的肿瘤提供有效的帮助，更加自信地切除。

弥散张量成像（diffusion tensor imaging，DTI）已被用于主要白质纤维束的影像重建，比如锥体束（Hendler et al.，2003）。术前DTI与导航的结合可能还有助于术中识别出高功能性的白质纤维束，从而帮助外科医生切除位于锥体束附近的肿瘤，如脑干肿瘤或邻近丘脑或运动纤维束的大脑半球肿瘤。

静息态fMRI（rsfMRI）是通过测量连通性来研究大量神经网络的一种新方法。rsfMRI的基础是自发活动而不是任务诱导活化或者BOLD。目前，rsfMRI在识别具有潜在手术意义的特殊神经网络方面精度较低；然而，这是一种对儿童人群有潜在辅助意义的新工具（Hertz-Pannier et al.，2014）

电生理监测

电生理监测包括几种模式，如运动诱发电位（motor evoked potentials，MEP）、躯体感觉诱发电位（somatosensory evoked potentials，SSEP）、脑干听觉诱发反应、皮质刺激和脑神经核刺激（Sala et al.，2002）。MEP和SSEP在邻近椎体束和感觉束的病变切除过程中可提供持续的监测，这些病变最常见的解剖学区域是脑干。早期识别MEP或SSEP反应降低可提醒外科医生手术注意潜在的损伤，并有助于调整手术，在最大限度地保证患者安全的同时，最大限度地切除肿瘤。皮质刺激（无论清醒的患者或是借助EMG记录的处于麻醉中的患者，无需肌松药物）有助于识别运动带，并设计一个非功能区的手术通道。在低龄儿童中，虽然在全身麻醉下的运动阈值过高，无法获得准确的运动区域分布，但SSEP可以成功地用于识别感觉皮层。

SSEP或者位相反转，可以通过电极条带予以测量或确定。脑神经核刺激有助于脑干肿瘤的切除。刺激脑干表面（通常是第四脑室底部）绘制脑干的功能区，从而有助于在非功能区找到肿瘤入路（Morota et al.，1996）。

皮质定位与唤醒手术的对比

皮质定位对于切除靠近或者位于语言或感觉运动皮质的病变非常有帮助。对于8岁以上的清醒患者进行大脑皮质的电刺激定位是可行的，但这对孩子来说是一个非常不愉快的经历。在多伦多的研究小组中，610名患者中最小的也是12岁（Serletis and Bernstein，2007）。如果在儿童患者，语言或运动皮质功能定位的重要性大于肿瘤的完全切除，我们更倾向于先插入皮质电极，术前进行皮质功能定位，然后在二期手术中切除病变。这种分期手术的方法，通常在当孩子有癫痫发作和脑组织结构性病变时使用。标准电极网的电极间距为1 cm，不能使用额外刺激进行准确定位。特殊需求的电极网上的电极间距为0.5 cm。

术中成像

术中实时成像系统可基于术中获得的图像进行导航。这些成像系统包括术中MR（intraoperative MR，iMR）、CT扫描或超声（ultrasound，US）系统。通过获得术中图像，可以在手术中更新导航数据，从而实时校正诸如大脑、肿瘤或脑室等解剖位置的变化（Roth et al.，2006）。使用iMR系统进行导航成像和术后成像，可以缓解额外的术前和术后早期CT或MR扫描的需要。术中MR系统可以获取各种序列图像，如T1（有/无增强剂）、T2和FLAIR，从而有助于从正常脑组织中辨别病变组织并最大限度地切除肿瘤。增强的 FLAIR MR 提供明显的强化，可以清晰显示肿瘤边界，是检测肿瘤残留或复发的敏感方法（Essig et al.，1999）。需要注意的是，在儿童人群中，完全切除低级别胶质瘤已被证明是一个良好的预后因素（Black，2000；Cohen et al.，2001）。

术中超声（intraoperative ultrasound，IOUS）系统可获得高分辨率的 IOUS 图像。结合三维重建后可以作为导航的基础，新的、更新后的图像与术前图像重建在相同的空间方向同时呈现，以改善术中解剖定位。IOUS，如 Sono Wand 系统也显示了类似的结果：可以区分正常脑组织和胶质瘤组织（Tronnier et al.，2001）。在某些情况下，使用 IOUS 系统对脑组织和肿瘤组织的区分度更好，尤其是在对高端超声设备和低端 iMR 机器进行对比时（Roth et al.，2007）。IOUS 系统最大化提升了神经导航的准确性和有效性，使外科医生能够最有效地提高切除效果。

术后护理

根据手术等级，手术后可以在普通病房或神经重症病房进行加强护理。任何潜在的或明显的内分泌缺陷或下丘脑口渴中枢失调节都需要密切监测，并需要在儿童内分泌科医生的协助下管理，持续性癫痫则需要神经病学专家的持续参与。

在脑瘤儿童手术后的护理中，另外需要特别强调的是镇痛。这包括对较大龄儿童的患者自控镇痛或对幼龄儿童的阿片类药物注射。术后神经功能障碍，如颅后窝手术后的小脑症状和缄默症、由脑干相关手术引起的脑神经病变和（或）靠近延髓闩部手术后的恶心和呕吐，都会对儿童和家庭造成额外的不适与压力。因此，经常需要在由多学科儿童专家参与的环境中进行康复。此外，还需要为家庭提供咨询和支持。

长期来看，脑肿瘤儿童有获得正常生活质量的可能（Kulkarni et al.，2013）。在诊断和治疗后，应尽一切努力保留功能。

术后影像复查的时间

识别残余或复发性肿瘤对制订治疗计划、观察治疗反应和判断预后至关重要。手术导致的 MR 上的强化和细胞外甲基化血红蛋白的沉积，均发生在手术完成后的 24 小时内，这些强化，会影响检测少量的残留肿瘤。在这个时间窗内进行一次扫描，往往非常困难。因此在开颅术后 72 小时内进行 MR 检查以明确肿瘤是否完全切除。对于有转移倾向的肿瘤，如果术前不能进行脊柱磁共振扫描，那么术后也应该行全脊髓的磁共振扫描。外科医生应该意识到从颅后窝留到椎管内的血液在术后的几天里，可能会掩盖一些病变。

为了减小术后扫描次数，并且根据复发的频率，更加容易发现阳性结果，每类肿瘤都有相应的神经影像学检查方案。监测成像时间应根据肿瘤等级 / 恶性程度进行调整，这对低级别肿瘤和高级别肿瘤都很有效。

再次手术或者“二次探查”手术

对于残留病灶的二次手术，可以实现肿瘤的全切除。这尤其适用于室管膜瘤或脉络丛肿瘤，因为这些肿瘤，完全切除是影响长期生存的最重要因素，可能需要几次手术来完成全切（如果肿瘤可以切除的话）。术中成像可明确肿瘤是否全切除了，从而减少二次手术的可能。

病理的解读

儿童神经病理学是一门具有挑战性的学科，因为有很多罕见肿瘤类型，而且这些肿瘤具有细微而多变的组织学特征。基于儿科神经病理的预后判断，比成人患者更加难以预测，尤其是对于具有间变特性的神经胶质瘤。儿童罕见肿瘤类型，比如婴儿促结缔组织增生的胶质母细胞瘤（Al-Sarraj and Bridges，1996）、多形性黄色瘤性星形细胞瘤、非典型畸胎样 / 横纹肌样肿瘤，可被误认为是胶质母细胞瘤和 PNET 肿瘤（Parwani et al.，2005）。非典型畸胎样 / 横纹肌样瘤侵袭性强，对化疗反应不敏感，应与髓母细胞瘤相区分，否则任何对于治疗效果和化疗反应性的分析都是片面的（Squire et al.，2007）。非典型的脉络丛乳头状瘤需要与脉络丛乳头状瘤（choroid plexus papilloma，CPP）和脉络丛癌（choroid plexus carcinoma，CPC）相鉴别。现在越来越强调肿瘤标志物、免疫组化、增殖指数和细胞遗传学，以更准确地分类脑肿瘤和预测预后，这些在本书的其他章节讨论。

通过分流系统的肿瘤播散

脑室腹腔分流术或者脑室心房分流术后，发生神经轴外转移的病例并不常见（Pollack et al.，1994）。髓母细胞瘤有最高的风险，松果体肿瘤也可能以这种方式转移。与其他病理类型相比，经过分流的视路胶质瘤的儿童容易出现腹水。

辅助治疗

手术的作用根据肿瘤的不同类型而不同。对于部分肿瘤，主要依靠激进的手术治疗，如室管膜瘤、低级别神经胶质瘤（包括 1、2 级星形细胞瘤）、脉络丛乳头状瘤（包括非典型性）、垂体腺瘤和大多数脑膜瘤。

但是，某些肿瘤因侵袭到关键结构可能有较高的致残率而不适合全切，例如侵袭脑干，视束和下丘脑的肿瘤。有些肿瘤尽管"完全切除"，但复发率较高，这可能继发于局部侵袭（如高级别胶质瘤、CPC 和髓母细胞瘤）或并发转移（例如髓母细胞瘤、室管膜瘤、生殖细胞肿瘤）

多年来，各种辅助治疗方法不断发展，包括放射治疗和化学治疗。

某些肿瘤对辅助治疗非常敏感。当权衡各种治疗方法（包括手术、化疗和放疗）的风险和获益时，一些肿瘤的治疗方案主要通过化疗和（或）放疗，而手术（如果有的话）仅是用于诊断。这种治疗方法的一个典型例子是生殖细胞肿瘤。这类肿瘤位于中线部位，如鞍区或者松果体区，对化疗和放疗非常敏感。在过去的一些年中，它们的诊断和治疗已经从手术切除，转换为基于血清（或脑脊液）的肿瘤标志物——AFP、β-HCG 和胎盘碱性磷酸酶的诊断，只有所有标记为阴性，才有活检的指征（Echevarria et al.，2008）。然而，当导水管受压迫出现梗阻性脑积水时，这些患者可以进行 ETV 和内镜活检治疗（Shono et al.，2007）

治疗模式转变的另一个例子是在颅咽管瘤。它是一种良性肿瘤，通常位于蝶鞍上的区域，经常生长到第三脑室。直到几年前，最终的治疗方法仍是完全彻底切除。尽管复发率较低，但神经认知和激素分泌的预后不佳，主要是由于对下丘脑 - 垂体轴邻近结构的损伤。虽然手术仍然是主要治疗，以最大切除为目标，但是已经有一些有效的辅助治疗方案，使相对不激进的手术成为可能，从而降低手术相关致残率和良好的肿瘤控制效果。这些治疗方法包括放射治疗、内部化疗（如博莱霉素或干扰素）和肿瘤内放疗（Puget et al.，2006）。

本章的重点是儿童脑肿瘤的手术治疗，对于辅助治疗仅作简要回顾，重点关注它们的必要性和主要相关的肿瘤类型。

放射治疗

对于许多儿童中枢神经系统肿瘤，放射治疗对治疗起着至关重要的作用。对于大多数儿童脑肿瘤来说，化疗并不能清除所有的癌细胞，因此经常使用放射治疗。尽管放疗有益于溶解癌细胞，但也有潜在的、长期的并发症。婴幼儿的大脑容易受到辐射的影响，尤其是白质（Kitajima et al.，2007）。

神经认知功能下降、神经内分泌病、脑神经病，视网膜病、血管病（包括继发性烟雾病）、脊髓病和脊柱生长障碍都与辐射对大脑、脊柱和邻近区域的损伤有关。

微血管损伤后可能发生继发性海绵状血管瘤（Duhem et al.，2005）。继发性肿瘤（良性肿瘤如脑膜瘤，恶性肿瘤如高级别胶质瘤与甲状腺癌）由各种遗传损伤导致发生，并可能在放射治疗很多年后发生（Umansky et al.，2008）。对于继发性肿瘤的风险，在综合征性儿童中较高，如神经纤维瘤病和痣样基底细胞癌综合征（Kleinerman，2009）。

不建议对 3 岁以下儿童给予全脑放射治疗，因为会对认知及神经内分泌功能产生持久且深远的影响。

由于普通放射治疗存在的风险，因此精准度更高的适形放疗的技术已经越来越多地用于治疗小儿脑肿瘤。

立体定向放射手术已应用于治疗儿童肿瘤和动静脉畸形。该技术的优势是可以迅速消减对病变周边的辐射剂量。然而，关于儿童普通放射治疗的安全性，仍然存在争议，尤其是对于病变邻近关键部位，如脑干、脑神经和下丘脑。

质子治疗是一种用于脑和脊柱脊髓肿瘤的相对较新的放疗技术。虽然在 PBT 中只有初步的研究，但目前对质子技术的认识正在发生转变，特别是颅咽管瘤。质子处理对其他 PBT 的应用正在研究中。

化学治疗

辅助化疗已经成为大多数成人脑肿瘤和部分儿童肿瘤的治疗方案的一部分。事实上，由于在幼龄儿童中，放射治疗可能导致毁灭性的神经认知损伤和神经内分泌后遗症，因此越来越需要足疗程的化疗。

化疗可以在手术前用作新辅助治疗，特别是在高风险的手术患者，如有巨大肿瘤的婴儿以及患有脉络丛癌的儿童。

对于室管膜下巨细胞星形细胞瘤（subependymal giant cell astrocytomas，SEGA）相关的结节性硬化，化疗已成为手术的有效替代方案。这些肿瘤对mTOR抑制剂（如雷帕霉素和依维莫司）反应良好，约40%的患者在6个月内至少减少了肿瘤体积的50%。mTOR抑制剂对结节性硬化患者有其他改善作用，可改善癫痫发作、肾肿瘤、皮疹，甚至认知能力，从而成为一种改变疾病的药物。

延伸阅读、参考文献、EBRAIN的相关链接

扫描书末二维码获取。

第 89 章　儿童脑积水

Matt Bailey · Chris Parks · Conor L. Mallucci 著
刘智明 译，田永吉 审校

引言

儿童脑积水是小儿神经外科医生治疗的最常见的疾病。脑积水不是一个单一的疾病过程，而是由各种不同的病理过程或损害引起的，最终导致脑脊液产生和吸收的不失衡。如果不治疗，大多数病例是致命的（Laurence and Coates，1962），但在经过适当的手术治疗后，大多数患儿都存活了下来，有些甚至可以过着正常的生活，一直到成年。

治疗的主要方式是脑脊液分流术，但是随着影像和外科技术的进步，越来越多的患者被神经内镜手术成功治愈。这种疾病治疗非常复杂，许多患者需要多次手术和终生随访。

本章概述了小儿脑积水的病因和分类、分流手术和神经内镜治疗，阐述手术技术以及手术治疗的结果。

定义

"脑积水"一词来源于希腊语：hydro 意为水，cephalus 意为头，因此直译为头中的水（Oreskovic and Klarica，2011）。它通常指的是一种脑脊液生理的紊乱，导致脑室系统异常扩张，通常与颅内压升高有关（Kahle et al.，2015）。

尽管多年来已经提出了几个定义，但目前脑积水还没有普遍接受的定义。Rekate 在 2008 年提出的以下定义已经被外科学界的许多人接受："脑积水是脑室系统的主动扩张，是由于脑脊液在脑室内的产生和吸收到系统循环中之间的平衡失调而导致的"（Rekate，2008a）。

脑积水的病理生理学将在**第 92 章**讨论。

发生率及流行病学

脑积水的总发病率和患病率难以确定，因为它可以单独发生或并发于多种神经系统疾病。据报道，先天性脑积水的发病率为 0.6~0.8/1000 个活产新生儿（Blackburn and Fineman，1994；Persson et al.，2005；Persson et al.，2007；Jeng et al.，2011），但是，许多脑积水是继发于其他疾病（例如早产、肿瘤、感染、创伤）。脑积水的发生率在发展中国家被认为是最高的，这主要是由于新生儿感染率较高（Warf et al.，2011）。在发达国家，最常见的原因是早产儿出血后脑积水、先天性导水管狭窄、脊髓脊膜膨出和脑肿瘤（Kulkarni et al.，2013；Stone and Warf，2014）。某些因素已被确定与婴儿脑积水的风险增加相关，这些因素包括低出生体重、低社会经济地位、男性和种族，而亚裔的比例较低（Jeng et al.，2011；Tully et al.，2015）。

脑积水的分类

目前还没有普遍接受的脑积水分类系统，关于如何最准确地对这种疾病进行分类的争论仍在继续。由于脑积水不是单一病理性疾病，而是脑脊液动力学紊乱的一种情况，可伴随或不伴随潜在的疾病，其分类令人迷惑并且复杂（Oi，2011）。两种常用的分类是先天性和获得性脑积水，以及梗阻性和交通性脑积水。

根据 Dandy 在 20 世纪早期的研究成果，脑积水被分为梗阻性（或非交通性）脑积水和交通性脑积水（Dandy，1919）。Dandy 和他的合作者用脑室和腰椎穿刺来研究脑积水。他们将染料注入脑室系统，然后进行腰椎穿刺。如果在腰椎穿刺的脑脊液中发现了染料，那么脑积水就被归类为具有交通性。如果从腰椎穿刺中没有发现染料，则认为脑积水是梗阻性的。这种脑积水的分类法取决于检测的时间，并在美国传播使用（Kahle et al.，2015）。无论如何，对脑脊液生理学的理解已经进步，但仍然是一个有争议的问题。目前最广泛接受的观点是脑脊液是由脑室系统内脉络丛产生，呈整体流动，流入蛛网膜下腔，被蛛网膜颗粒吸收进入脑静脉系统，形成循环。还有其他的理论将在**第 92 章**讨论。

自从 1970 年代计算机断层扫描（computed tomography，CT）和 1980 年代磁共振成像（magnetic resonance imaging，MRI）等现代成像技术的引入，脑脊液通路中梗阻的确切位置现在常常可以确定。在外科学界，Rekate（Detwiler et al.，1999；Rekate，2001）提出的分类系统通常被使用，因为它提供了一种方法来定义任何特定患者脑积水的原因，并可提供潜在的治疗方案（**图** 89.1）。通过对梗阻部位的识别，临床医生可以针对特定的患者选择合适的手术方法（见**表** 89.1）。

儿童脑积水的病因

脑积水的原因可能是先天性的或获得性的。先天性原因包括 Chiari 畸形、脊柱裂、导水管狭窄、Dandy-Walker 畸形、蛛网膜囊肿和 Monro 孔闭锁。获得性的原因包括出血、感染、头部受伤以及肿瘤

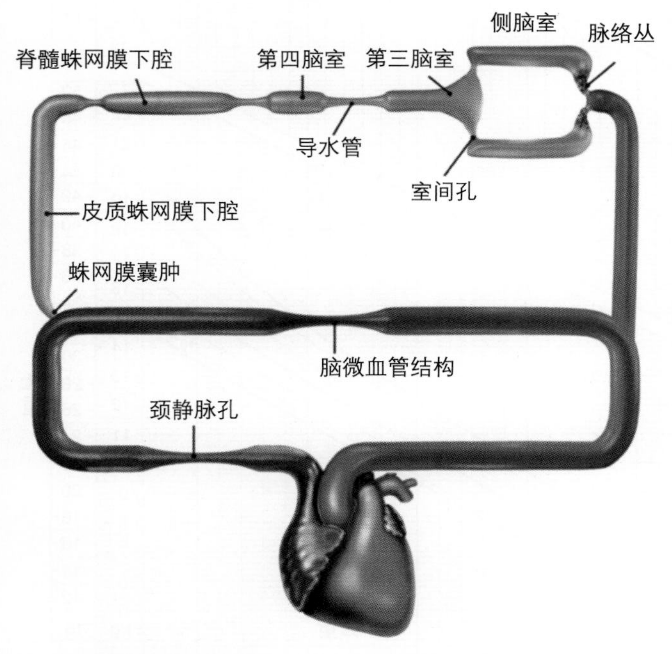

图 89.1 Rekate 分类法，描述脑脊液流动可能受限的六个位点：Monro 孔、中脑导水管、第四脑室出口、基底池、蛛网膜颗粒和静脉窦内的静脉血流出口（Rekate，2008；Rekate，2011）

Reproduced from Rekate, H. L., The definition and classification of hydrocephalus: a personal recommendation to stimulate debate, *Cerebrospinal Fluid Research*, Volume 5, Issue 2, Copyright © 2008 Rekate; licensee BioMed Central Ltd. With permission from Barrow Neurological Institute.

表 89.1 脑脊液通路上不同梗阻点导致脑积水的治疗选择

梗阻点	鉴别诊断	可以选用的治疗方案
Monro 孔	肿瘤	分流术（单侧或者双侧）
	先天性发育缺陷	脑室镜下透明隔开通
	脑室炎	
	功能性	
中脑导水管	肿瘤	分流术
	出生缺陷	ETV
	继发性	
第四脑室出口	感染	分流术
	肿瘤	ETV
	严重的 Chiari 畸形	手术打通
从脊髓到 CSAS	蛛网膜下腔	分流术
	出血	ETV
	LP 分流	
蛛网膜颗粒	出血或者感染	VP 或者 LP 分流
静脉高压	假瘤	VP 或者 LP 分流
	先天性脑积水	栓子溶解
	静脉窦血栓	肥胖相关的假瘤，行减肥手术

Reproduced from Rekate, H. L., A consensus on the classification of hydrocephalus: its utility in the assessment of abnormalities of cerebrospinal fluid dynamics, *Child's Nervous System*, Volume 27, pp. 1535–41 Copyright © 2011 Rekate.

等（Rekate，2008b；Kandasamy et al.，2011；Rekate，2011）。

来自分流设计试验（Drake et al.，1998）、脑积水研究网络（Kulkarni et al.，2013）和英国分流登记（Richards，2010）的数据给出了儿童脑积水最常见原因的分布，结果是大致相似。出血后脑积水占 25%，其他常见原因包括脊髓脊膜膨出、Chiari 畸形、肿瘤、导水管狭窄、感染、创伤和颅内囊肿。

不同年龄组的脑积水临床特征

尽管脑积水的病因多种多样，但各种病因导致的脑积水，其临床表现非常相似。发病时临床表现的不同与患儿发病时的年龄以及颅缝开放还是闭合有关。

颅骨骨缝通常在 12~18 个月大时闭合。由于在

此之前新生儿或婴儿的头骨发育有所不同，因此，脑积水的表现可能比较多变，包括发育不良、发育迟缓和头部控制不良。枕额头围（occipitofrontal circumference，OFC）可能会不成比例地增加，当绘制在百分位图表上时，可以看到它与百分位线相交（**图 89.2**）。易激惹、呕吐和喂养困难也很常见。随着脑积水的进展，颅骨骨缝裂开、前囟门膨隆、头皮静脉怒张。有些婴儿出现典型的"落日征"样表现，即由于第三脑室的压力传导到顶盖上，而导致上视不能。最终会出现心动过缓、低血氧饱和度和呼吸暂停。癫痫发作并不是单纯脑积水的常见表现特征，视盘水肿在这个年龄组也很少见（Abou-Hamden and Drake，2015）。在某些发展缓慢的脑积水病例中，体征可能很少，但总有头围不成比例地增长。

如果颅骨骨缝闭合后出现脑积水，大多数患者的头围正常。轻微的症状可能包括头痛、学习表现下降、记忆丧失或行为改变。一些急性的儿童病例，颅内压升高的症状和体征与成人相似，包括头痛、呕吐、视盘水肿、复视（第 6 脑神经麻痹）、嗜睡到最终昏迷。

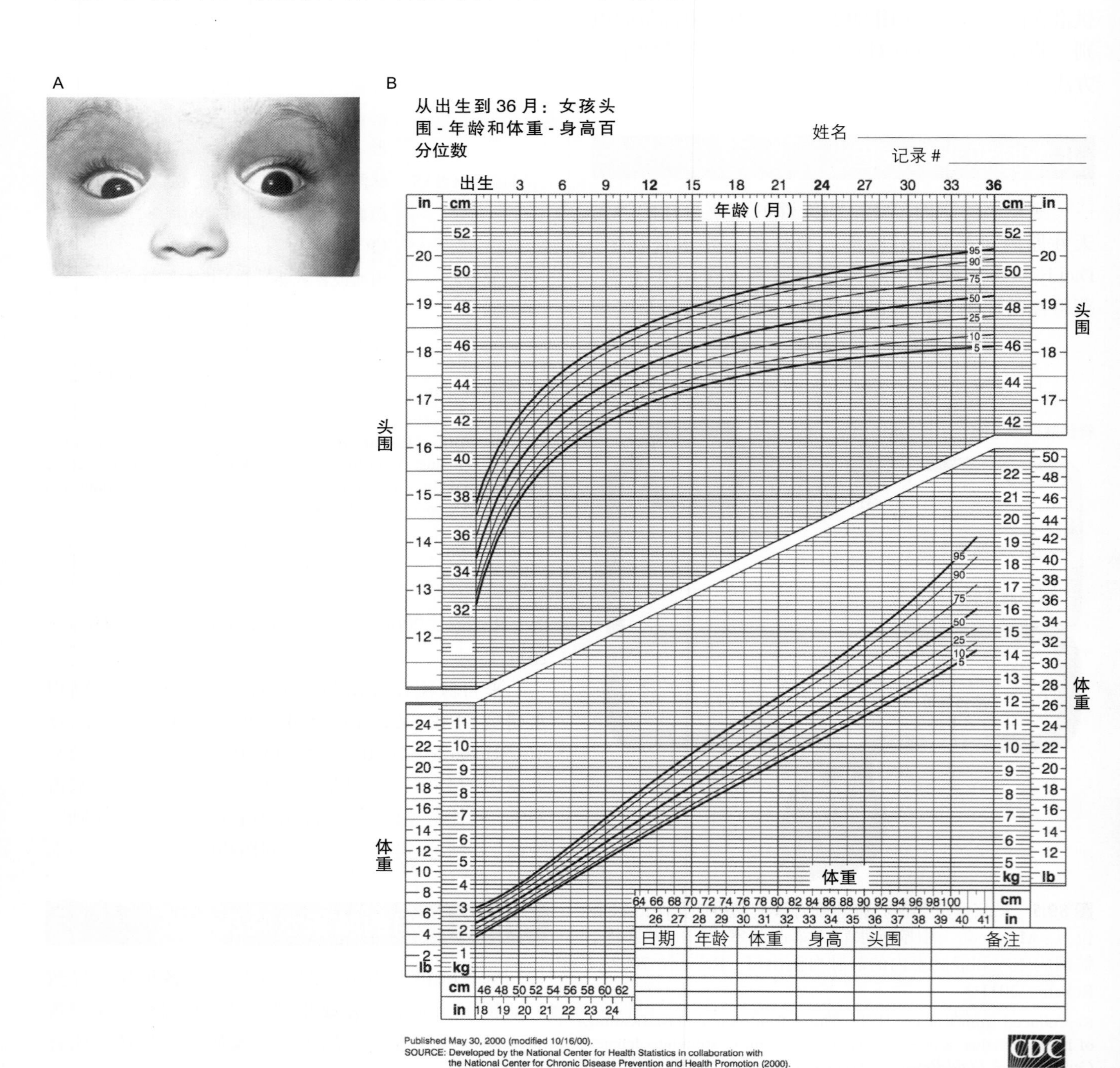

图 89.2 （A）儿童眼睛落日征。（B）女孩头围生长曲线，可以用来标记头部生长速度（Kandasamy et al.，2011）

婴幼儿脑积水的临床特征包括易怒、意识障碍、呕吐、发育不良、喂养困难、发育迟缓、头围过分增长、头部控制不良、前囟门张力增高、头皮静脉扩张、落日眼、心动过缓、呼吸暂停和癫痫。年龄较大的儿童，头痛、呕吐、困倦、复视、癫痫、上视障碍和视盘水肿是其主要特征。

脑积水影像学检查方法

头颅超声

出生后前12~18个月，前囟尚未闭合，头颅超声对大脑成像非常有帮助，许多医院新生儿病房常规使用超声对早产儿进行筛查。不需要镇静，而且这个过程可以根据需要反复进行，不会产生副作用。侧脑室的大小和形态在超声上很容易识别，但第三脑室和第四脑室、中脑导水管和颅后窝的内容物不能可靠评估（Dinçer and Özek，2011）。因此，脑积水的确切病因仅通过超声很难确定，如果需要对脑室扩大进行治疗，则需要进行其他的脑成像（Dinçer and Özek，2011）。

计算机断层扫描（CT）

CT方便、快速、可靠，并与生命急救支持系统兼容。由于图像采集时间短，在大多数情况下，儿童可不需要镇静进行CT检查。CT可显示脑室的大小和形态，并可揭示可能的病理，比如出血和肿瘤。脑室系统内梗阻的位置，可以通过梗阻近端脑室明显扩张，远端脑室大小正常（如导水管狭窄所见）来判断（Dinçer and Özek，2011）。CT对于脑脊液分流患者的复查随访也很有价值，因为CT上可以很好地显示分流管。然而，患有脑积水的儿童在其一生中往往需要进行许多影像学检查，而且人们担心暴露于电离辐射的长期影响（Koral et al.，2012；Krishnamurthy，2013）。鉴于此，一些中心现在使用快速序列磁共振成像对脑积水儿童进行急性评估和随访（Koral et al.，2012）。

磁共振成像（MRI）

MRI是对脑积水患儿的检查方法。

传统的T1和T2序列作为常规使用，可提供脑实质和病理特征（如导水管狭窄、肿瘤和Chiari畸形）的良好图像，并可评估脑室系统的大小和形状。现代序列如3D-CISS、快速自旋回归序列和脑脊液电影相位对比序列，可以对脑脊液从脑室到蛛网膜下腔循环通路的解剖和脑脊液在不同部位的流动进行良好的评估，并得到了广泛认可（Dinçer and Özek，2011）。脑脊液循环通路内膜的精细解剖细节，如Monro孔、脑导水管和第四脑室流出口都可以被显示出来。同样，颅内囊肿和脑室间分隔的解剖结构也可以进行显影，这对于决定每个患者最合适的手术策略非常具有参考价值。

MRI的局限性包括相对较长的图像采集时间，对较小的儿童通常需要全身麻醉或镇静。然而，在大多数病例中，在手术干预前均有足够的时间让儿童接受高质量的磁共振成像。MRI也广泛用于脑积水患者的随访，以评估脑室大小，并显示内镜手术的结果和分流管的位置。具有可调压分流泵的患者在成像后可能需要重新调整压力，因为有些分流泵会受到磁场干扰。

越来越多的MRI也被用于检查胎儿期的中枢神经系统（central nervous system，CNS）异常（包括脑积水），这些异常以前是通过母亲的超声波确定的。MRI可用于帮助临床医生进行预后判断。

不同年龄阶段患儿脑积水的管理

以下章节讨论不同年龄的儿童脑积水的评估和处理。首先我们将集中讨论早产儿脑积水的处理。接下来将介绍足月婴儿和儿童的管理。

早产儿脑积水

早产儿是指怀孕37周之前出生的婴儿。这些儿童的脑积水绝大多数是继发于与早产有关的脑室内出血（intraventricular haemorrhage，IVH）。**第90章**将讨论早产儿IVH的病理生理学。

15%~20%的出生体重低于1500 g的婴儿会发生IVH（du Plessis，2009；Robinson，2012）。出生体重越低，发生IVH的风险越高（Boop，2005）。IVH的表现可能是灾难性的，伴随快速的神经功能恶化，或进展为清醒状态降低、肌张力降低和呼吸损害，或可能是无临床症状（Robinson，2012）。因此，大多数新生儿单位常规用头颅超声（ultrasound，US）筛查早产儿来监测IVH，如果出现IVH，连续的头颅超声被用来记录出血的进展和监测脑室大小。影像学与临床特征相结合用于鉴别那些可能需要治疗的出血后脑积水（posthaemorrhagic hydrocephalus，PHH）的婴儿。

对 IVH 婴儿的病理研究表明，近一半的患儿出现脑室扩大，称为出血后脑室扩张（posthaemorrhagic ventricular dilatation，PHVD）。然而，PHVD 的存在并不总是会出现有症状的 PHH，可能是一种代偿现象，与静脉梗死或脑室周围白质缺血继发的脑实质减少有关（Boop，2005）。因此，临床医生必须结合影像学和临床表现来确定需要干预的潜在患者。

症状性 PHH 的临床特征包括头部生长速度（OFC）与公布的正常值相比增加，前囟门未闭合，颅缝延迟闭合和影像学上脑室进行性扩大。一些婴儿还表现出颅内压升高的特征，如嗜睡、呕吐、呼吸暂停和心动过缓。相比之下，代偿性 PHVD 的婴儿可能会有脑室指数的增加，但是 OFC 不会超过正常的百分位数（甚至低于百分位数），前囟柔软，颅缝可能是最重要的（Boop，2005）。

IVH 后婴儿出现症状性 PHH 的发生率，据报道，从 22%~29%，其中 9%~20% 的病例需要永久性脑脊液分流手术（Murphy，2002；Vassilyadi，2009；Limbrick，2010）。随着 IVH 的严重程度增加，婴儿发生 PHH 的可能性增加（Robinson，2012）。

早产儿出血后脑积水的管理

一旦诊断出有症状的 PHH，就应该实施治疗。这些婴儿比较虚弱，通常体重较轻。他们在临床上也可能不稳定，许多人还会有其他医学疾病。人们普遍认为脑室 - 腹腔分流术（ventriculoperitoneal，VP）不应作为有症状的早产儿 PHH 的初始治疗。这是因为这些患者的分流失败率很高，部分原因是脑脊液中大量的蛋白质和血液增加了 VP 分流阻塞的风险（Hislop，1988）。此外，这些婴儿的皮肤娇嫩，破裂风险或者感染率可能更高（Robinson，2012；Whitelaw and Aquilina，2012）。在大多数中心，只有当婴儿体重达到 2~2.5 kg 并达到足月年龄时才会行脑室 - 腹腔分流术（Whitelaw and Aquilina，2012；Leonard and Limbrick，2015）。鉴于此，有必要为有症状的 PHH 儿童提供临时性的治疗措施。

这些婴儿可能采取的临时治疗措施包括连续腰椎穿刺或脑室穿刺或者是通过神经外科手术放置脑室外引流管、脑室通路装置或脑室帽状腱膜下分流术（ventriculosubgaleal shunts，VSGS）。

腰椎穿刺与脑室穿刺

采用腰椎穿刺暂时缓解早产儿 PHH 已被广泛研究。大多数作者描述每次腰椎穿刺释放 10 ml/kg 的脑脊液（Kreusser et al.，1985；Robinson，2012；Leonard and Limbrick，2015），20 ml/kg 脑脊液被认为是可以释放的最大脑脊液量，因为释放更多的脑脊液可能会出现呼吸暂停、心动过缓和低血氧饱和度（Whitelaw and Aquilina，2012）。没有证据表明连续腰椎穿刺可以降低放置分流管的需要或避免脑积水的进展（Mazzola et al.，2014）。过去，连续多次经皮脑室穿刺被用于暂时性治疗 PHH，然而，由于相关的并发症，如穿刺性脑穿通畸形、感染和脑软化症，大多数中心已经放弃使用，除非是作为临床状态不好儿童等待进一步手术治疗期间的暂时性措施（Hudgins，2001；Shooman et al.，2009）。

脑室通路设备（VAD）、脑室帽状腱膜下分流装置（VSGS）和植入技术

放置临时分流管或者通路装置的目的是推迟永久性分流的植入，直到婴儿长大并有更好的营养和身体状况（Robinson，2012）。两个常用的选择是脑室通路设备（ventricular access devices，VAD）和脑室帽状腱膜下分流术（VSGS）。VAD 是由一段连接在低流量储液器上的脑室导管组成。一旦就位，就可以经头皮引流脑室脑脊液。穿刺抽吸 10ml/kg 的脑脊液，即可维持患儿病情稳定。脑室 - 帽状腱膜下分流类似于脑室通路装置，在头皮的帽状腱膜下内缠绕一小段远端导管。这在理论上的优点是允许持续的脑脊液引流，并通过帽状腱膜下的间隙进行吸收，从而持续降低颅内压（intracranial pressure，ICP），而不像通路装置仅能提供间歇性分流。尽管置入通路装置的原理是相似的，我们更倾向于用脑室 - 帽状腱膜下分流术来暂时缓解婴儿的病情进展（**图** 89.3）。

将婴儿全身麻醉后置于仰卧位。注意使用舒适的保暖床垫和毯子来保暖。术前给予单剂量抗生素。头部置于支撑头环上并处于中立位置（**图** 89.3A）。触诊头皮以确定前囟的边界，标记中线。设计一个弧形皮肤切口，这样可以使骨孔位于额骨后内侧，在冠状缝的前方。皮肤切口的曲线应指向中线，这样如果婴儿最终转换为 VP 分流手术，分流装置不会直接位于切口下方。可以采用右侧或左侧入路，并根据术前影像上患者的解剖结构进行调整。我们倾向于避免有血凝块的一侧，以减少导管阻塞的概率。在鼻根的中线处放置一个心电图贴，这样一旦铺好了手术无菌单，就可以触诊该点以帮助定位（**图** 89.3B）。

用洗必泰溶液氯己定对皮肤进行预处理。手术部位周围放置消毒敷料，然后将无菌纱布的反面贴附在上面，以尽可能减少纱布与皮肤的接触。然后再将手术无菌单贴附到上面，这样可以避免皮肤接触到手术无菌单上面的黏性部分。婴幼儿皮肤很娇嫩，当手术结束去掉手术无菌单时容易被撕裂。这样做的好处还有，在手术结束时去掉无菌单时，可以保护气管插管不被意外拔出（**图** 89.3C）。分流系统集中放置在一个单独的无菌推车上，并由助手护士负责递取。根据术前测量结果，将脑室端导管剪成一定长度，其目的是使导管位于侧脑室内，并指向 Monro 孔，长度通常为 3~4 cm。远端导管切成长度约为 15 cm，并在管壁上切开 4 或 5 个小孔，以便脑脊液流出。然后两者都连接到储存器，并用丝线固定。然后，我们将脑室导管导丝通过储液器置入脑室端导管，以便于放置，并在脑室导管放置到位后尽量减少操作（**图** 89.3D）。

用手术刀在皮肤表面浅浅切开，用皮肤钩拉开，然后用单极电刀逐层切开，以最大限度地减少出血（**图** 89.3E）。切口切开帽状腱膜，头皮瓣被反向拉起并用固定缝线固定。用单极电刀切开额骨的骨膜。然后用剪刀在帽状腱膜下层形成一个大囊袋。必须注意保持在正确的平面上，以确保前囟不裂开。将帽状腱膜和骨膜之间的纤维结缔组织分开，直到形成一个大口袋（**图** 89.3F~H），然后使用 15 号刀片的手术刀在额骨上旋转形成一个小的穿刺孔（**图** 89.3I）。使用动脉钳扩大该穿刺孔。穿刺孔大小需要能够容纳脑室端导管。用手术刀在硬脑膜上切开一个小口，用双极电凝硬脑膜边缘和皮质（**图** 89.3J）。然后垂直于颅骨插入脑室端导管（**图** 89.3K）。仅经过一小段距离即可正常进入脑室。脑脊液填充满储液囊即可证实进入侧脑室。然后保持导丝不动，将脑室端导管继续向前推进，直到储液囊达到并放置在颅骨上（**图** 89.3L）。然后从导管系统中取脑脊液样本并送去进行微生物检查（注意本例中的黄色脑脊液）。使用牵开器抬高帽状腱膜下腔隙，将远端导管盘绕放置在囊袋内（**图** 89.3M）。然后在关闭伤口前通过储液器向脑室内注入 5 mg 万古霉素（**图** 89.3N）。用可吸收缝合线（例如 4/0 vicryl）缝合帽状腱膜，用类似的可吸收线连续缝合皮肤（**图** 89.3O）。

脑室通路装置的置入是非常相似的，不同之处在于没有远端导管连接到储液器，也不需要帽状腱膜袋。我们更倾向于使用脑室帽状腱膜下分流术，而不是脑室通路装置，因为与脑室通路装置相比，它们需要的抽吸次数更少（Mazzola et al.，2014），我们认为这降低了感染的可能性。还有一些证据表明，与 VAD 治疗的婴儿相比，VSGS 治疗的婴儿需要永久性脑脊液分流手术的次数较少（Limbrick et al.，2010）。

术后前囟会立刻变软，帽状腱膜下分流管的轮廓常可透过头皮看到。帽状膜下囊袋会迅速充满脑脊液，家长和护理人员术前应注意这一点，因为婴儿经常有明显的帽状膜下脑脊液蓄积。每天都要监测 OFC，并检查和触诊皮下囊袋。工作正常的 VSGS 会导致帽状腱膜下囊袋饱满，但颅骨骨缝不能涨开，前囟（如果可触及）会变软，孩子的临床表现也会改善。

使用 VSG 分流术的婴儿状态会改善，囟门很软，颅缝不涨开，头围会符合生长曲线而不是偏离正常曲线。功能正常的分流会形成一个饱满的、甚至是紧绷的帽状腱膜下口袋；这是正常的，表明分流工作正常。

大多数植入了 VAD 或 VSGS 的婴儿会需要永久性脑脊液分流，通常一开始需要 VP 分流。在术后过程中，应监测 OFC 并绘制出正常值，并观察儿童有无症状性脑积水的迹象。如果需要额外的脑脊液引流，可以经皮穿刺帽状腱膜下囊袋。一旦儿童超过了矫正年龄，体重超过 2.5 kg，如果症状仍然存在，可以考虑进行 VP 分流。一小部分儿童不需要永久性脑脊液分流，可以在门诊定期随访。对于那些不需要进一步手术进行脑脊液分流的患者，我们在矫正年龄 2 个月左右，以择期手术去除他们的帽状腱膜下脑脊液分流。

足月婴儿和儿童期脑积水的评估和管理

决定何时需要治疗

如果儿童在影像学上表现出典型的颅内压增高的症状和体征，有脑室扩大的症状和体征，脑积水的诊断很容易确立。在这种情况下，决定是否进行治疗是很简单的。然而，在一些有“代偿性脑积水”的病例中，决定是否需要治疗是比较困难的。小儿神经外科医生经常会遇到临床表现相对良好的儿童，在影像学上发现有脑室扩大，这种情况并不罕见。有些患者可能有轻微的认知障碍、行为障碍或学习表现不佳，因此很难决定是否进行干预。有些患者就诊时非常年幼，认知障碍可能很难发现。一些学者认为，无症状的轻度或中度脑室扩大不需要治疗（Kalra and Kestle，2015），但另一些学者担心，如

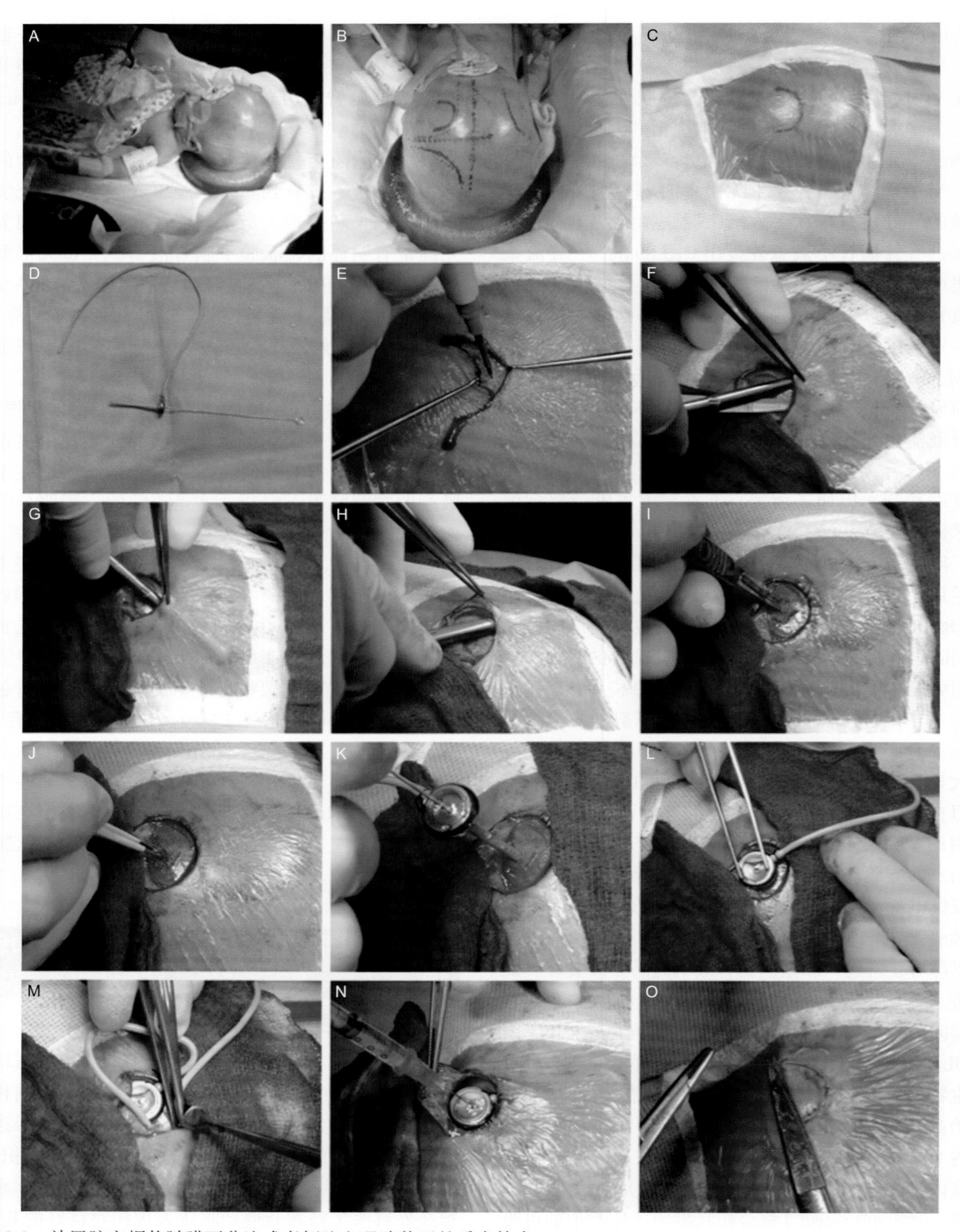

图 89.3 放置脑室帽状腱膜下分流或者侧脑室通路装置的手术技术

果儿童脑积水未得到治疗，可能无法实现其发育潜能。在这种情况下，处理策略包括连续成像来评估脑室大小是否增加，有时需要使用一段时间的颅内压监测来决定是否需要干预。

影像学上脑室扩大可由脑积水或周围脑组织萎缩引起。区分这些情况是很困难的。提示脑积水而不是脑萎缩的影像学特征包括第三脑室凹处扩大、颞角扩张、脑室周围间质水肿和脑沟萎缩（Dinçer and

Özek，2011)。

儿童脑积水的手术治疗方式

自 19 世纪 90 年代以来，脑积水的治疗一直采用外科手术。在 20 世纪早期，Dandy 等探索了脉络丛切除，并试图用开颅术打通梗阻的脑脊液通路。最初是通过额下入路和开放性第三脑室造口术进行。这些早期手术有很高的致残和致死率(10%~20%)(Warf，2014)。

脑脊液分流术

60 年前，硅胶导管和阀门被引入，外科治疗转向脑脊液分流。从那时起，大多数解剖腔被用作脑脊液引流的潜在储液器或导管，脑脊液分流术成为脑积水的标准治疗方法。目前最常见的分流术是脑室 - 腹腔分流术，但有时也在其他部位使用，如右心房(VA 分流)或胸膜腔。虽然分流术的引入对以前这种毁灭性的疾病产生巨大的影响，但是分流术相关的并发症也会给脑积水患儿带来灾难。

脑室外引流(external ventricular drains，EVD)通常用于临时脑脊液分流，例如在出现感染或出血时，直到可以建立永久性脑脊液分流。

内镜下第三脑室底造瘘术

20 世纪 90 年代，内镜设计的改进引发了神经内镜治疗脑积水的发展。内镜下第三脑室底造瘘术(endoscopic third ventriculostomy，ETV)包括将内镜置入侧脑室额角，经 Monro 孔进入第三脑室。然后在直视下在第三脑室的底部开一个口。这使得脑脊液绕过脑脊液通路的远端障碍进入桥前池(ETV 在**第 93 章**中描述)。这种技术现在在高收入国家的大多数小儿神经外科中心作为常规治疗手段，并使一些患者在不需要分流术的情况下接受治疗。ETV 也被用于那些曾经接受过分流手术但分流手术失败的患者(Chhun et al.，2015)。

内镜下第三脑室底造瘘术与脉络丛烧灼

最近，人们对脉络丛烧灼术(choroid plexus coagulation，CPC)重新产生了兴趣，并与 ETV 联合使用(Warf，2005)。该技术是使用柔性内镜通过单额钻孔进行。先进行 ETV，然后在同侧侧脑室内操作内镜，将脉络丛沿其整个长轴广泛烧灼到颞角。然后行透明隔切开，将内镜置入到对侧脑室，在另一侧脑室重复烧灼脉络丛(Warf，2005)。ETV 和 CPC 主要在撒哈拉以南的非洲进行，但是看到良好的结果以后，一些发达国家的团体也开始使用这项技术。

与单纯 ETV 相比，ETV 和 CPC 已被报道可以在婴儿获得更好的结果(Warf，2005)，并且在治疗由多种病因引起的脑积水(包括导水管狭窄和神经管缺陷)方面也有效果(Warf，2011；Warf et al.，2012)。目前认为这种手术的效果与脉络丛的烧灼量成正比(Warf et al.，2010)。由于它靠近重要解剖结构，一些外科医生担心脉络丛烧灼以后的潜在长期影响。对于许多脑积水的治疗，虽然有一些短期数据显示该技术与脑积水分流术有相似的认知结果，但其对神经认知结果的影响了解仍然有限(Warf et al.，2009)。

最优化治疗策略的选择

一旦诊断出脑积水，就需要计划治疗方案。通常患儿病情紧急，可能无法完善手术前的影像学检查，但在高收入国家的大多数病例中，可以在第一次手术治疗前完成 MRI 扫描。

仔细分析 MRI 扫描通常可以评估脑积水的病因，特别是脑脊液流动可能梗阻的位置。如果存在肿块病灶(肿瘤、脓肿、囊肿等)，在 MRI 扫描中很容易被发现，并且切除肿块病灶本身可能解决脑积水。

随着内镜技术使用的增加，对影像学的评估非常重要。如果发现梗阻点，可以使用内镜技术绕过梗阻点，从而避免分流。由于需要长期携带分流管和相关的并发症，许多小儿神经外科医生倾向于内镜手术。

至于选择 ETV 还是分流，仍有争议，目前还没有完全随机的对照试验来比较这两种治疗方案。当比较 ETV 和分流手术时，通常是比较每种手术方式的失败率，当失败时则需要进一步的手术来补救。在非特定的队列中，ETV2 年的失败率约为 35%(Kulkarni et al.，2010a; Kahle et al.，2015)。预后因素包括患者的年龄和脑积水的病因。这些都被纳入 ETV 是否能成功的评分中，这是一个有用的、经过验证的工具，可以对不同患者的 ETV 潜在成功率进行评估(**表 89.2**)(Kulkarni et al.，2010b)。我们对于有症状的脑积水的治疗路径，总结在**图 89.4**。

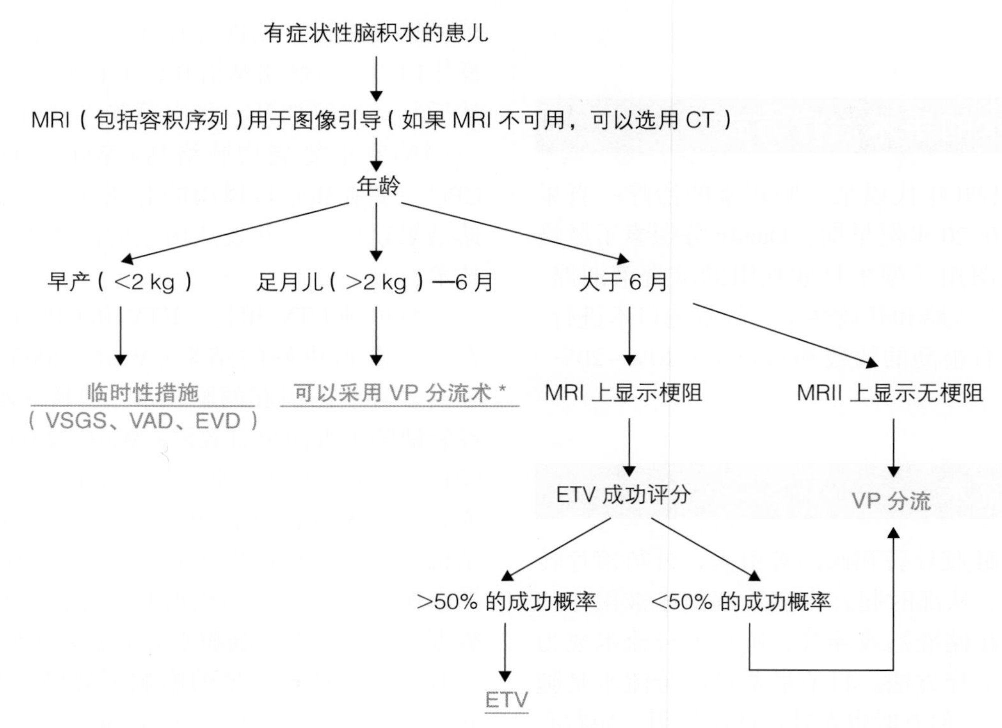

图 89.4 对于症状性脑积水的治疗策略

计算内镜下第三脑室底造瘘成功分数（endoscopic third ventriculostomy success score，ETVSS），将三部分的分数加在一起，就可以得到 ETV 成功概率的百分数。

所有患者术前都应行影像学检查，通常是 MRI，用于神经导航。2 kg 以下的早产儿采用脑室帽状腱膜下分流术。对于足月婴儿和儿童，术前影像上发现梗阻的，如果解剖上适合内镜手术，我们考虑采用 ETV。2 kg 以上但 6 个月以下的足月儿通常会接受 VP 分流术，因为这一年龄段的 ETV 成功率很低，但在某些情况下，例如当儿童患有腹腔内并发症或脑蛛网膜囊肿时，可以采用 ETV。

在 6 个月以上的患者中，如果 MR 上有梗阻的证据，我们进行 ETV 成功评分，如果成功的概率大于 50%，则将 ETV 作为初始治疗。在 MR 上无梗阻性特征或 ETV 成功率低于 50% 的情况下，多数情况下会进行分流。如果患者在未来出现分流失败，那么将重新考虑 ETV。

脑室腹腔分流术

VP 分流术是所有神经外科手术中失败率最高的手术之一，应该由训练有素且高效的团队进行。当仔细分析分流手术的生存曲线时，会发现在前 6 个

表 89.2 ETVSS 评分的计算方法

年龄	评分
<1 月	0
1~6 月	10
6~12 月	30
1~9 岁	40
10 岁或者更大	50
病因	**评分**
感染	0
脊髓脊膜膨出	20
IVH	20
非顶盖的脑肿瘤	20
导水管狭窄	30
顶盖肿瘤	30
其他	30
既往分流手术史	**评分**
既往曾经分流	0
既往无分流手术史	10

Source data from Kulkarni, A.V. et al. Predicting who will benefit from endoscopic third ventriculostomy compared with shunt insertion in childhood hydrocephalus using the ETV Success Score. *J. Neurosurg. Pediatr.* 6, 310–15 (2010).

月有高达 20% 的分流手术失败率 。早期分流失败的原因主要是感染、导管堵塞（分流管位置不佳）或分流元件移位（由于分流管断裂）。外科医生有可能减少这些早期分流失败的发生率，但是分流手术不能允许有技术上的错误。

图 89.5 以及后面的描述，是新生儿 VP 分流术的过程。手术步骤和各个年龄阶段患者基本是相似的。分流手术应该由经过适当训练的团队进行，分流手术最好是当天的第一台手术，为了将感染风险降到最低，人员在手术室周围、进出手术室的走动应该降到最低限度。我们在手术室的门上放置指示牌，除紧急出口外，保持手术室门紧锁（**图** 89.5C）。目前的国家临床卓越研究所（NICE）指南建议患者在手术前洗澡或用肥皂洗澡。许多研究都着眼于洗必泰沐浴液在减少手术部位感染方面的有效性，目前还不确定是否能减少手术部位感染（surgical site infection，SSI），尽管研究已经证明可以降低皮肤细菌水平（National Collaborating Centre for Women's and Children's Health，2008）。我们用洗必泰沐浴露和洗发水在手术前一天和手术的早上对所有患者进行清洗，发现自从采用这种方法以来，我们的手术部位感染率明显降低。

全麻气管插管成功后，将气管插管指向分流泵对侧，患者仰卧在手术台上，婴儿头部用头圈支撑，2 岁以上儿童头部用 Mayfield 马蹄枕支撑。将头部转向对侧，并在肩部下放置垫卷，使胸壁抬高，使头颅切口到腹部切口呈一条直线，以方便形成隧道（**图** 89.5A）。新生儿和婴儿，由于这个年龄段的头部相对于身体较大，经常需要使用大的胸部垫卷来抬高胸部。患者保温很重要，特别是在新生儿和婴儿中（National Collaborating Centre for Women's and Children's Health，2008），我们常规使用暖风床垫来帮助实现这一点（**图** 89.5A）。

在麻醉诱导时静脉注射抗生素，可以降低手术部位（National Collaborating Centre for Women's and Children's Health，2008）和 VP 分流感染（Klimo et al.，2014）。在切口处剪掉少量头发，以提高缝合质量，但脱毛并不能降低感染的风险（National Collaborating Centre for Women's and Children's Health，2008）。额部和顶枕部的钻孔是分流管脑室端最常用的进入部位。任何一种路径都是可以接受的，最近的一项系统回顾认为，没有证据可以显示其中一种路径优于另外一条路径（Kemp et al.，2014）。额部钻孔通常位于冠状缝前 1 cm，中线旁开 2~3 cm 处，顶枕部钻孔 位于耳郭上方及后方的 2~3 cm，但如果使用影像引导，这些穿刺点则可能会根据患者的术前影像而有所不同。由于部分儿童存在颅后窝囊肿或其他畸形，使得横窦位置比一般患者高，因此应该研究术前影像，必须相应地规划和调整顶枕入口点。头部和腹部皮肤切口均应标记（**图** 89.5B）。

皮肤采用恰当的皮肤制剂进行精心的术前准备。我们对所有年龄段的儿童都使用洗必泰溶液。术野边界用大的无菌棉签划定，并使用敷料包盖，同时将敷料妥善固定到位。然后将手术无菌单附着在棉签和敷料形成的固定结构上，因此黏合剂不会直接附着在患者的皮肤上。分流装置被集中在一个单独的小车上，由刷手护士取用（**图** 89.5D）。目前没有证据表明一种阀门设计优于另一种（Baird，2014）。我们使用低压定压阀作为标准阀（Miethke Paedigav），并针对复杂情况采用可调节阀门。**第 93 章**提供了更多有关阀门设计的内容。

我们用手术刀在皮肤上划开切口，然后用单极加深切口，以最大限度地减少失血。皮肤切口形状需要设计，使切口下面没有分流硬件，以最大限度地减少分流管处皮肤破裂从而使分流管暴露的风险。用高速磨钻形成一个骨孔（**图** 89.5E）。与此同时，腹部切口由助手打开。有多种腹部入口点。我们在脐部和肋缘之间的中线上做一个线形切口。向下分离直至打开腹直肌前鞘，将腹直肌纤维拉开，腹直肌后鞘和腹膜用镊子夹起（**图** 89.5F）。然后将这一层分开进入腹膜腔，可以通过置入钝器进入腹腔或直接看到网膜或肠道来确认进入腹腔。

然后用分流管通条经皮下脂肪层从一个切口穿刺到另一个切口（**图** 89.5G 和**图** 89.5H）。必须非常小心，以确保隧道不要太深，以免进入胸腔或者进入颅后窝。如果太浅表，就会造成皮肤撕裂。如果感觉到明显的阻力，有时需要在颈部做一个松解切口。如果颅骨钻孔在前额，则需要在耳后增加一个切口，那么皮下隧道穿刺需要分两步进行。然后将分流管的腹腔段通过通条隧道，同时将通条从一个切口中移除（**图** 89.5I）。拉动分流管，远端盘绕后用浸有碘伏溶液的纱布包裹。当放置脑室端导管时，用浸有碘伏的纱布包裹分流管阀门（需要使用的分流囊）。

有证据表明，如果导管脑室端远离脑室壁和脉络丛，那么发生堵塞的概率较低，大多数外科医生都有过导管脑室端位置不佳的经历。为了延长 VP 分流术的使用时间，本文介绍了各种改进脑室端导管放置位置的辅助技术，包括术中超声（Whitehead，

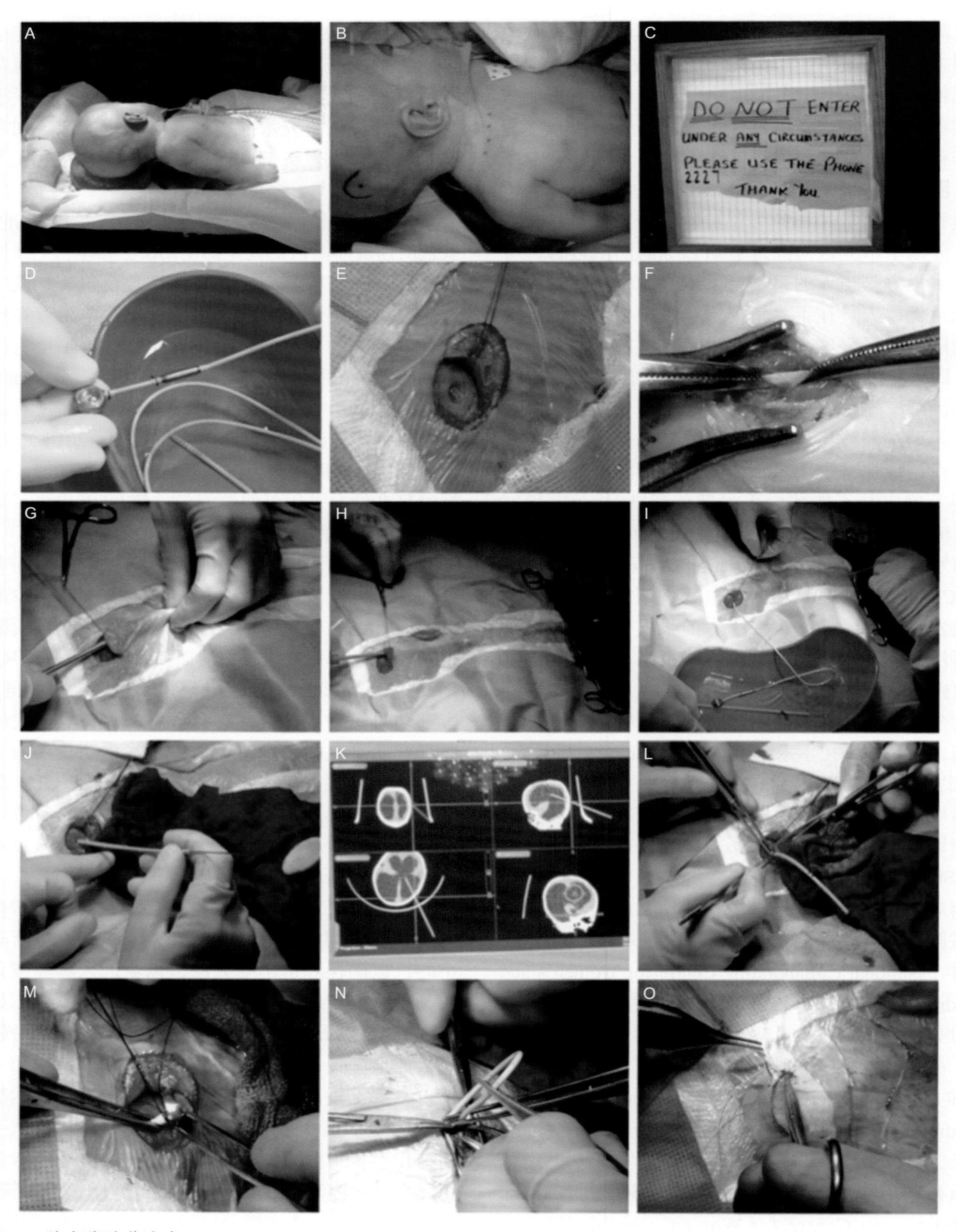

图 89.5 脑室腹腔分流术

2007）、电磁（electromagnetic，EM）或光学引导系统的无框立体定位。内镜下放置脑室端导管并未显示能延长分流管的寿命（Kestle et al.，2003；Kestle，2010）。我们对大多数脑室导管的放置使用EM导航引导，因为它改善了脑室导管的位置（Hayhurst et al.，2010；Levitt et al.，2012）并可能提高分流管的使用寿命（Hayhurst et al.，2010）。为此，从脑室导管中移除管芯，并用EM导航棒代替之。用手术刀在硬脑膜上切开小口，将皮质表面电凝处理。将分流管脑室端在导航系统引导下（**图89.5J**和**图89.5K**）对准脑室穿刺。当导管进入脑室时，通常会感觉到“突破感”，当脑脊液从导管中自由流出时，才能确认进入。常规采集脑脊液样本进行微生物学检查。然后，根据术前影像，将脑室导管剪短至预先确定的长度（**图89.5L**），导管连接到储液囊或阀门上。我们使用直角连接的储液囊，或者也可以将直角导轨与直通阀一起使用。轻微地弯曲导管也是可以接受的，但应该注意的是，在皮质层较薄的儿童中，导管可能会移动，从而几乎达到垂直方向。然后，轻柔地牵引远端导管，将阀门固定在帽状腱膜下的囊袋内，并将脑室导管用丝线固定在储液器上（**图89.5M**）。在将远端导管放入腹腔之前，确认脑脊液从远端管流出。

严密缝合皮肤是至关重要的，因为任何脑脊液漏都可能导致感染，并增加皮肤破裂的风险。帽状腱膜和皮肤要分层缝合。我们都用可吸收缝合线。同样，腹直肌前鞘和腹部皮肤切口也用可吸收缝合线缝合。然后无菌敷料包盖并保持48小时。

没有并发症的患者，留院观察2~3天后可以出院回家。术后我们不会常规使用抗生素。术后48小时内，如果伤口需要清洁，可以用无菌生理盐水清洗。48小时后，建议患者保持伤口清洁，如果愿意洗澡，可以根据目前关于手术部位感染的NICE指南进行（National Collaborating Centre for Women’s and Children’s Health，2008）。我们会让患者在两周内检查伤口的状况。门诊随访在2个月内进行，同时进行术后扫描，以评估脑室导管的位置和脑室的大小。我们还会在12~18个月进行一次扫描，作为将来参考的基线，因为分流设计试验的数据显示，脑室大小在术后3个月内继续缩小，但在术后大约14个月时稳定下来（Drake et al.，1998）。然而，术后早期扫描是有价值的，因为分流术在术后一年内失败率很高。然后在门诊对患者进行终身随访，最初每6个月随访一次，然后每年随访一次，在某些病例中，每两年随访一次。除非患者出现症状，否则我们不会增加额外的影像学检查。

脑室腹腔分流术的并发症

据报道，与脑室导管插入相关的脑实质出血发生在1%~4%的分流手术病例中（Savitz and Bobroff，1999；Kalra and Kestle，2015）。这些出血大多是无症状的（Savitz and Bobroff，1999），但根据出血部位的不同，它们有可能导致神经功能障碍。

在行VP分流术时，腹部或胸部器官可能会受到损伤。分流管有腐蚀内脏壁的报道，胃穿孔、小肠与大肠穿孔、膀胱穿孔和子宫穿孔均有报道（Wong et al.，2012）。

VP分流术有很高的失败率，约40%的儿童在他们第一次行分流术后的前2年内需要进一步干预（Kulkarni et al.，2013；Kahle et al.，2015）。大多数的失败原因是由于分流管阻塞。其他还包括感染、断开、移位、折断和过度引流等。2岁以下儿童的失败率更高，属于高危患者（Kalra and Kestle，2015）。

尽管分流管全长的任何地方都可能发生梗阻，但是阻塞最常见的部位是脑室端，在一项研究中脑室端梗阻占到梗阻病例的63%（Di Rocco et al.，1994）。近端导管梗阻最常见的原因是脑室导管腔内存在脉络丛。阀门堵塞往往在分流术或置换术后很早就发生，这可能是由于手术组织碎片或血液造成的（Kalra and Kestle，2015）。VP分流失败的患者通常表现为颅内压升高，影像学显示脑室增大。分流管梗阻的治疗是紧急手术，以替换阻塞的部分。在一些患者中，分流术失败的原因复杂，在分流翻修术前可能需要进行一段时间的ICP监测。

发生分流感染的患者死亡风险大约是未发生感染患者的2倍，接受分流相关手术的次数是未发生分流感染患者的3倍（Schoenbaum et al.，1975；Wong et al.，2012）。分流感染的死亡率在10%左右，从长远来看，出现这种并发症的患者在认知和学习成绩方面的表现较差（Vinchon and Dhellemmes，2006）。分流感染发病例占到所有分流手术3%~12%，大多数病例发生在手术后3个月内（Kulkarni et al.，2001）。症状包括发热、精神萎靡、易怒、分流装置的表面皮肤红肿和头痛。分流管穿刺取脑脊液分析显示白细胞计数升高，显微镜下可见微生物，脑脊液培养呈阳性。较少见的分流感染可表现为腹部假性囊肿，并伴有分流功能障碍和腹痛的症状。

分流感染中最常见的病原体是皮肤共生菌，如凝固酶阴性葡萄球菌和金黄色葡萄球菌（Thompson

and Hartley，2014；Kahle et al.，2015）。当分流管、脑脊液或伤口受到污染时可发生感染，这可能发生在手术时，术后段时间内通过手术伤口或通过邻近感染的扩散，如腹部感染（Thompson and Hartley，2014）。如果分流感染被证实，大多数神经外科医生会移除受影响的分流装置并植入EVD。患者给予静脉注射抗生素治疗，有时甚至鞘内注射抗生素，直到脑脊液无菌为止，此时可以考虑再置入分流管，也可以考虑内镜手术。

急性的分流过度可表现为轴外积液，慢性的则表现为裂缝脑室综合征。随着VP分流术后脑室的缩小，轴外液体或血液可能会积聚。这在脑室较大的大龄儿童中更为常见。可调压分流阀，可以设置为高阻力用于治疗这种情况或在高风险情况下，以防止发生这种情况。如果轴外积液确实发生，管理可能会很困难。处理策略包括减少过度引流，有时可以引流轴外积液。可以替换为具有较高压力的阀门或插入防虹吸装置。一旦过度引流减少，可以考虑通过适当位置的钻孔排出轴外积聚的液体。

裂隙脑室综合征

头痛在VP分流的儿童中很常见。一些儿童在VP分流术后脑室变得非常小，并伴有头痛，此时可被标记为裂隙脑室综合征。文献中对这种综合征没有一致、准确的定义，但通常这些儿童已经分流了几年，他们的脑室变得非常小（Kalra and Kestle，2015）。裂隙脑室综合征是由慢性引流过多引起的，颅腔相对于大脑显得太小。脑组织的顺应性降低，因此升高的脑脊液压力不会导致脑室扩张。

儿童可能表现为慢性低颅压性头痛或周期性头痛，提示颅内压力升高。这些患者的治疗选择是有争议的，包括颅内压监测，翻修分流管或改用可调压的或流量调节的阀门，以及使用颞下减压扩大颅腔容积（Kahle et al.，2015）。

儿童脑积水的远期预后

大多数接受分流术治疗的儿童在他们生命中的某个阶段需要进行分流翻修术。一项长期研究发现，32%的患者需要1~3次分流手术，另有52%的患者需要4次或4次以上的分流手术。约29%的患者报告有1或2次分流感染。高达70%的患者报告有抑郁症状，高达45%的患者需要治疗。大多数成年患者都是单身，只有1/4的女性患者有孩子。高达40%的成年患者在生活自理方面依赖父母（Gupta et al.，2007）。

脑积水患者的认知结果主要取决于脑积水的原因和任何相关的脑异常或原发性脑损伤。例如，患有单纯导水管狭窄的儿童具有接近正常的认知功能（Kahle et al.，2015）。而早产儿IVH患者的损伤率较高。智力、学习、记忆和执行功能可能会降低（Kahle et al.，2015）。癫痫很常见，对患者及其家人的生活质量有很大影响。

延伸阅读、参考文献、EBRAIN的相关链接

扫描书末二维码获取。

第 90 章　儿童神经血管性疾病

Helen G. McCullagh · Tufail Patankar · Tony Goddard · Atul Tyagi 著
刘智明 译，田永吉 审校

引言

小儿神经血管疾病包括几种常见的情况，如动静脉畸形、动脉瘤和发生在成人阶段的海绵状血管畸形。尽管儿童与成人的血管性疾病在病理上有相似之处，但在临床表现、部位和处理上存在差异。有一些疾病是儿科人群特有的，如 Galen 畸形或早产儿脑室内出血，还有一些主要发生在儿童，但也见于成人，如烟雾病。

最近在血管内治疗、放射外科和多种治疗方法的最新进展，增加了治疗儿童血管病变的选择。

对海绵状血管畸形和烟雾病潜在基因异常的鉴定有望进一步揭示这些疾病的发病机制。本章将讨论儿童人群中常见的神经血管疾病，重点放在那些主要见于儿童的疾病上。

早产儿脑室内出血

自发性脑室内出血（intraventricular hamorrhage，IVH）是早产的主要并发症之一，大量出血与致残和脑积水的高风险相关。

病因学

在早产儿中，出血的起源部位是室管膜下生发基质，位于 Monro 孔水平的尾状核和丘脑之间。该区域中的血管占据脑动脉和脑深部静脉收集区之间的边界区域，当受到缺氧和（或）静脉压升高时，其渗透性或生发基质脆性增加，这与脑血流（cerebral blood flow，CBF）的变化有关。早产儿 CBF 的波动与 IVH 有关，特别是与足月儿相比，早产儿 CBF 的自我调节功能受损。IVH 的危险因素包括导致血压变化的原因，例如快速输液时血压的变化，分娩时胎儿头部受压和气管抽吸导致的脑静脉压的增加。CBF 快速波动的原因包括高碳酸、窒息、酸中毒和低血糖。凝血功能异常常见于长时间的产时窒息和复苏，也是危险因素。

足月新生儿 IVH 多由脉络丛出血、深静脉窦血栓形成和丘脑梗死引起。最常见的临床症状是癫痫发作和喂养困难。

发病率

极低体重儿（＜1500 g）IVH 的发生率从 20 世纪 80 年代早期的 40%~50%，下降到 20 世纪 80 年代后期的 20%。然而，在过去的二十年中，IVH 的发生率保持平稳。在体重 500~750 g 的极早产儿中，大约 45% 的新生儿会发生 IVH（Ballabh，2010）。

临床表现

IVH 几乎总是发生在出生后的前五天，其中 50% 发生在出生的第一天。在一项研究中，出生体重小于 1750 g 的婴儿在出生后几分钟开始接受一系列的头颅超声检查，在出生后的第一个小时内检测到 20% 的婴儿发生 IVH。在同一研究中，阴道分娩和剖宫产分娩的 IVH 总发生率相似（Shaver et al.，1992）。

早产儿常规头颅超声检查发现的 IVH，其中有 25%~50% 的病例表现隐匿。然而，临床表现也可能是神经系统迅速恶化的灾难性综合征，在几分钟到几个小时内逐渐演变为昏迷、肌张力降低、紧张性姿势，或新生儿癫痫发作和缺乏自主活动。最常见的表现是警觉性和自发活动的亚急性恶化，时间从几小时到几天，通常伴有肌张力下降。呼吸可能会受到影响。

所有胎龄小于 32 周 +6 或出生体重在 1.5 kg 及以下的婴儿，均应进行常规头颅超声筛查。在英国，新生儿网络建议，对于在 23 周到 27 周 +6 之间出生的婴儿，在出生后 0~3 天进行筛查，在第 3~5 天、第 7~10 天重复筛查，在 28 天，在矫正孕期 36 周时再次筛查，或者出院前进行筛查。任何孕周出生的婴儿，如接受机械通气，都应该每周例行检查一次，出院时再检查一次（Periman and Rollins，2000）。

Ⅰ级IVH相当于轻度IVH，Ⅱ级中度IVH，Ⅲ级和Ⅳ级为重度IVH（**表90.1**）。每一级别的IVH可以是单侧或双侧的，也可以是对称性或不对称性的。

治疗

IVH和出血后脑室扩张的最佳治疗仍不明确。对这些患者的脑积水，一种常见的临时处理方法是进行脑室-帽状腱膜下分流术（ventriculosubgaleal shunt，VSGS）、脑室通路装置（ventricular access device，VAD）或脑室外引流术（external ventricular drain，EVD），直到患者明显需要并能够耐受永久性脑脊液分流。在对结果和并发症的系统回顾和meta分析中，VSGS、VAD和EVD的结果范围是相似的（Badhiwala et al.，2015）。出血后脑积水（posthaemorrhagic hydrocephalus，PHH）已在**第89章**详细讨论。

预后

脑室内出血的死亡率和短期致残率（Ⅰ级和Ⅱ级）。轻度IVH（Ⅰ级和Ⅱ级）的死亡率为5%，只有7%的幸存者出现PHH（Murphy et al.，2002）。在严重IVH Ⅲ级和室周出血性梗死（periventricular haemorrhagic infarction，PVHI）中，死亡率约为20%，75%的幸存者发展为PHH。严重的IVH也会增加脑室周围白质软化（periventricular leukomalacia，PVL）的风险（Kusters et al.，2009）。

IVH患儿存活的长期结局随着IVH严重程度的增加和胎龄的降低而恶化。在一项对1812名33周前出生的婴儿进行的前瞻性人群队列研究中，5岁时脑性瘫痪的患病率随着IVH的严重程度而增加。在5岁时被诊断为脑瘫的患儿中，8%为Ⅰ级IVH，11%为Ⅱ级，19%为Ⅲ级，50%为Ⅳ级（Beaino et al.，2010）。单纯性Ⅰ、Ⅱ级IVH的婴儿也有更高的感觉神经损伤风险（Bolisetty et al.，2014）。然而，在一项大型纵向观察性研究中，来自16个中心的1472名孕周不到27周的婴儿，随访18~22个月，患有Ⅰ级或Ⅱ级IVH的极低胎龄婴儿的神经发育结果与那些没有出血的婴儿没有显著差异（Payne et al.，2013）。

表90.1 IVH的严重程度和分级

Ⅰ级	仅位于生发基质
Ⅱ级	IVH填充10%~50%的脑室
Ⅲ级	IVH填充超过50%的脑室
Ⅳ级 脑室周围出血性梗死（PVHI）	除了单侧或者双侧IVH，还有脑实质内任何一个部位的出血。PVHI是一个更准确的病理生理学定义

Reproduced with permission from Lu-Ann Papile, Jerome Burstein, Rochelle Burstein, Herbert Koffler, Incidence and evolution of subependymal and intraventricular hemorrhage: A study of infants with birth weights less than 1,500 gm, *The Journal of Pediatrics*, Volume 92, Issue 4, pp. 529–34, Copyright © 1978 Elsevier.

争议

对于早产儿，常规使用连续腰椎穿刺术并不能降低分流手术的需要，也不能避免脑积水的进展。

脑室内溶栓药物包括组织型纤溶酶原激活剂（tissue plasminogen activator，tPA）、尿激酶或链激酶，并不推荐作为减少早产儿PHH行分流手术的方法。在一项使用DRIFT（引流、灌洗和纤溶疗法）的研究中，DRIFT与继发性IVH风险增加相关（Whitelaw，2007）。

有几项产后应用药物预防IVH的策略研究。没有证据表明使用苯巴比妥、吲哚美辛或维生素E对神经发育结果有整体益处。

Galen静脉畸形

概述

Galen静脉畸形（vein of Galen malformation，VGAM）是一种罕见的先天性中线血管异常，位于前髓帆间隙区域（大脑中央帆）。原发病理被认为是脉络膜动脉和大脑前正中静脉之间的异常连接，通过瘘管的血流阻止了大脑前正中静脉的正常消退。在儿童人群中，这些异常占动静脉畸形的1%，约占血管畸形的30%。

临床表现

VGAM可在产前、婴儿早期或儿童期出现，症状包括高输出性充血性心力衰竭（congestive heart failure，CHF）、脑积水、癫痫发作和颅内出血。

影像

影像显示新生儿或婴儿颅内中线部位大的静脉怒张，直径从几毫米到几厘米不等。大的静脉曲张常提示静脉狭窄，常与慢性缺血引起的脑室扩大和皮质下白质钙化有关。通过超声和胎儿MRI进行产前诊断，可以改善存活者的预后。

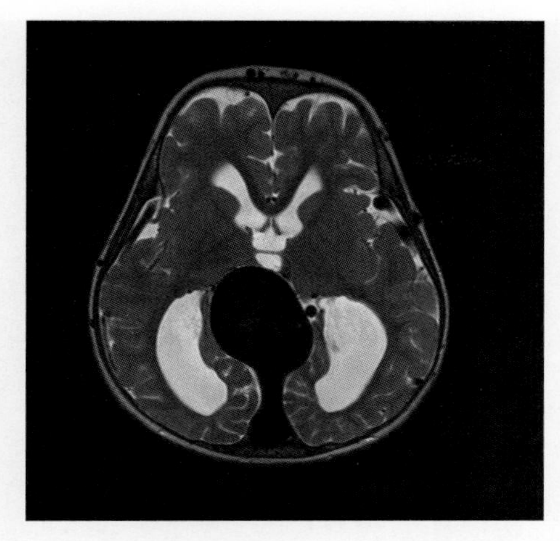

图 90.1 T2 轴位 MRI 图像，显示四叠体池的静脉怒张，伴有脑室扩大

鉴别诊断

VGAM 类似于永存的胚胎性矢状窦，引流单个或多个动静脉瘘。VGAM 根据其血管构筑分为壁型和脉络膜型。多条供血动脉，包括脉络膜动脉、丘脑穿支动脉和胼胝体周动脉，经常给脉络膜 Galen 动脉瘤畸形供血。相反，壁型 VGAM 通常由较少的供血动脉提供，包括胼胝体动脉和脉络膜后动脉。供血通常是单侧的。

VGAM 的鉴别诊断应包括引流到盖伦静脉的动静脉畸形或硬脑膜动静脉瘘。Galen 静脉动脉瘤样扩张引流至真正的 Galen 静脉。硬脑膜动静脉瘘是一种高流量的瘘管，通常由颈外动脉供血。软脑膜动静脉畸形有一个真正的病灶，在三岁以下的儿童中很少见。

与 VGAM 相关的静脉阻塞可发生在矢状窦水平或颅底。

治疗及预后

未经治疗的 Galen 静脉畸形预后很差。治疗可以通过动脉或静脉途径实现。线圈、Onyx 和黏合材料可以用来处理瘘管。静脉途径常用于动脉途径不能成功到达的患者。

初诊时年轻较小、CHF、癫痫发作和脉络膜血管结构是不良临床结果的预测因素。不良预后也可能与诊断时脑积水和栓塞不完全有关。

血管内治疗的目标因临床表现而异。对药物难治性 CHF 的新生儿需要进行紧急治疗，以建立血流动力学稳定性，并促进心脏和大脑发育。对于没有 CHF 的新生儿，治疗的目标是预防脑静脉高压、脑白质损伤和“融化脑综合征”。对于这些病例，治疗通常会推迟到孩子 5~6 个月大的时候，以便让大脑更成熟，动脉更扩大。脑脊液分流术在 VGAM 中是很有争议的，但在一些进行性脑室增大的患者中可能是必要的，特别是当患者有颅内压升高的特征时。

结果

一组病例中，26 例患者，19 年以上患者的总生存率为 76.9%。这包括 5 名因轻微症状或严重共病而未接受治疗的患者。超过 2/3 接受治疗的患者没有发育迟缓的证据（Li et al., 2011）

儿童烟雾病 / 烟雾综合征

烟雾病（moyamoya disease，MMD）是一种病因不明的脑血管疾病，最初的特征是双侧颈内动脉（internal carotid arteries，ICA）末端狭窄或闭塞，随后大脑前动脉或中动脉受累。多发性基底侧支血管通常随着脑血流量的减少而发展。Suzuki 和 Takaku 在 1969 年观察到侧支血管在脑血管造影上好像一股烟雾，并创造了“moya moya”一词。

烟雾综合征（moyamoya syndrome，MMS）是指与唐氏综合征、Ⅰ型神经纤维瘤病、颅骨辐射、自身免疫性疾病、脑膜炎和动脉粥样硬化等疾病相关的单侧或双侧血管改变的类似过程。

脑血流量的减少可能会导致儿童缺血性发作，通常是对过度换气的反应，比如哭泣时。

流行病学

烟雾病在所有种族群体中均可发现，但在东亚人群中的发病率是西方人群的 10 倍。在加利福尼亚州和华盛顿州进行的一项研究表明，MMD 和 MMS 的年发病率为 0.086/100 000，比日本的 MMD 发病率低 4~13 倍（Uchino et al., 2005）。

所有的研究都表明女性占优势，女性患病人数是男性的两倍。MMD 的发病年龄呈双峰分布，在 5~10 岁和第四个 10 岁之间出现两个高峰。在日本，10%~15% 的病例有家族史。

基因分析发现 RNF213 基因位于东亚人群的 17q25 区，是 MMD 的一个重要易感基因（Kamada et al., 2011）。95% 的家族性 MMD 患者和 79% 的散发性 MMD 患者中发现了 c.14576 G>A 在 RNF213 中的多态性。RNF213 与早发型和重型 MMD 相关

（Miyatake et al.，2012）。

病理学

ICA 狭窄的病理表现为纤维组织增厚的内膜和弹性纤维增生形成的板层。血管壁明显没有炎性改变。在不到 10% 的病例中，原发病变开始于单侧，但 75% 的病例在 3 年内变成双侧。

Suzuki 的血管造影分级（Suzuki and Takaku，1969）描述了 MMS/MMD 血管改变的进展，从Ⅰ级（颈内动脉末端狭窄）、Ⅱ级（脑底部侧支血管的出现）、Ⅲ级（烟雾样侧支血管明显增多）、Ⅳ级（从颈外动脉 ECA 形成跨越硬脑膜的侧支循环出现）、Ⅴ级（颅外侧支循环增多和烟雾样血管的减少）、到Ⅵ级（ICA 闭塞和烟雾样血管消失）。

临床特征

儿童最常见的表现是缺血性事件，不像成人既发生缺血性事件又发生脑出血（intracerebral haemorrhage，ICH）。

由于身体或智力活动、脱水、发热和哭泣而引起的换气过度可引发缺血性事件（Guzmann，2009）。在这些患者中，通常皮质血管在稳定状态下最大限度扩张，以代偿慢性脑缺血。过度通气导致二氧化碳减少，从而引起血管收缩，导致脑灌注减少和临床症状。

患者可能出现不典型症状，如头痛、晕厥和不自觉的舞蹈动作（Smith and Scott，2012）。

有报道，没有卒中病史的患者也可以有认知损害和下降，这表明慢性脑低氧血症对认知功能的有害影响，但有卒中病史的儿童这种影响更大（Kossorotoff，2012）。双侧疾病和症状持续时间是与认知缺陷相关的主要因素。

颅内出血在儿童中较为少见，主要表现为脆弱的深部侧支血管破裂伴深部脑实质内（基底神经节或脑室周围深部白质）或脑室内出血。蛛网膜下腔出血罕见的，有时是由位于 Willis 环的囊状动脉瘤破裂引起的，最常发生在椎基底系统。

辅助检查

数字减影血管造影（digital subtraction angiography，DSA）仍然是最好的检查，可以反映病情，并可以看到从 ECA 来的代偿情况（图 90.2）。MRI 和磁共振血管成像（magnetic resonance angiography，MRA）可以提供脑动脉、脑实质、脑灌注的信息，并越来越多地应用于患者的诊断评估和随访（图 90.3）。

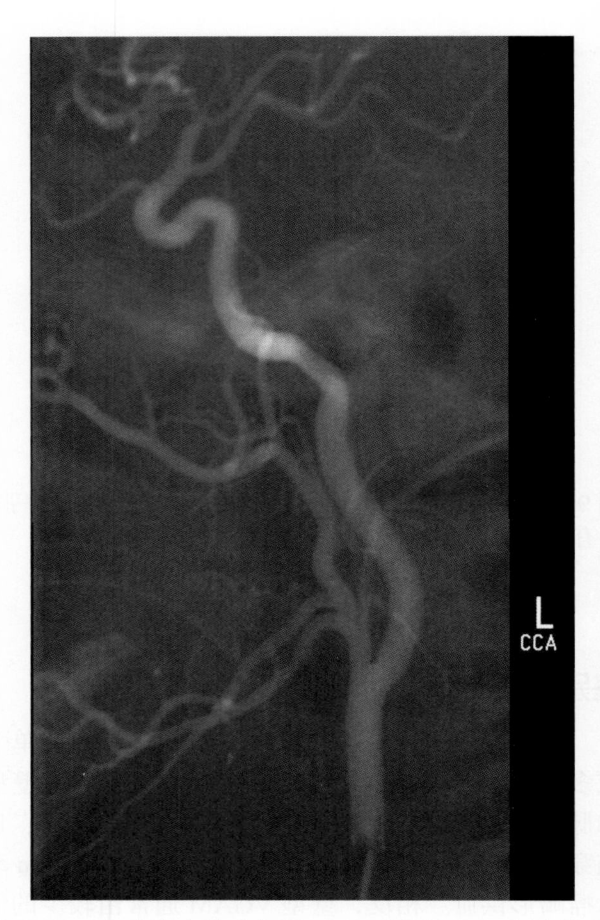

图 90.2 从颈总动脉进行的 DSA，先是 ICA 末端狭窄、ACA 近端和 MCA 出现脑底部的代偿血管。该图没有对颈外血管显影

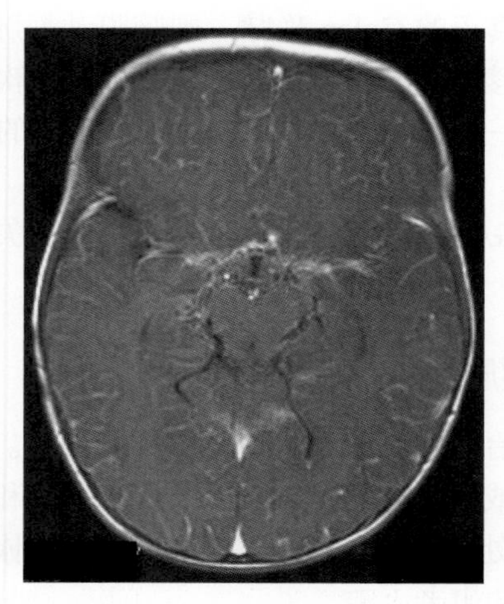

图 90.3 轴位 T1 强化后图像，显示在视交叉池和环池有大量的颅底侧支血管

MMD 的诊断标准最初是依据传统的血管成像制定的，当达到诊断标准时，MRI 和 MRA 就可以明确诊断。磁共振血管成像可以显示颈内动脉末端或大脑前动脉（anterior cerebral artery，ACA）和（或）

大脑中动脉（middle cerebral artery，MCA）狭窄或闭塞（图 90.3）。磁共振血管成像在闭塞或狭窄血管附近发现异常血管网络，或磁共振成像显示每个半球基底节区有两个或两个以上的血流空洞。

通过 SPECT、PET、氙气增强计算机断层扫描（computed tomography，CT）、动脉自旋标记 MR 和 CT 灌注等技术评估脑血流动力学，可能有助于识别有缺血性事件风险的患者并指导治疗。识别大脑半球和高危区域有助于有针对性的外科血管重建术。

治疗

治疗的目的是增加缺血大脑半球的脑血流量，降低缺血和出血事件的发生率。

建议采取避免低血压、脱水、过度换气等一般措施，以防止脑血流动力学障碍。开始长期口服抗血小板治疗，通常是阿司匹林，旨在减少血栓栓塞并发症的发生率。

手术选择包括直接或间接血运重建。直接血运重建术通过将 ECA 分支与皮质血管吻合，从而立即增加 CBF。最常见的是颞浅动脉到大脑中动脉分支（superfcial temporal artery to a middle cerebral arterial branch，STA—MCA）。间接血运重建是基于烟雾病的病理生理学，这可以避免使用颈外动脉及其分支。采用由颈外动脉分支供应的组织进行贴附，随着时间的推移增加颈内动脉循环的血流量。由 ECA 分支形成的脑血管新生，从而使脑血管再血管化。

一些间接血运重建的技术已经发展起来，所有这些都是基于血管贴敷的过程。在贴敷过程中，包含 ECA 分支的组织（硬脑膜、颞肌、帽状腱膜或颞浅动脉）直接与缺血脑表面接触。来自这些组织的新生血管被认为是通过从缺血性脑实质分泌血管生成因子来促进的。由于有效的新生血管生成至少需要 3 个月的时间，所以这个过程不会带来立竿见影的效果。

在外科血管重建手术之前，需要通过常规血管造影准确评估血管状态，以避免破坏由 ECA 自然发育而来的侧支血管。

间接增加血流的常见手术包括脑 - 硬脑膜 - 动脉贴敷术（encephaloduroarteriosynangiosis，EDAS），脑硬脑膜 - 动脉 - 肌肉贴敷术（encephaloduroarteriomyosynangiosis，EDAMS，图 90.4）和颅骨多点钻孔术（Oliveira et al.，2009）。在 EDAS 中，颞浅动脉与结缔组织一起分离，以保持其连续性。用软骨膜或硬脑膜缝合将颞浅动脉放置并固定在脑皮质表面。EDAMS 手术中，除 STA 外，还将颞肌置于脑皮质表面。

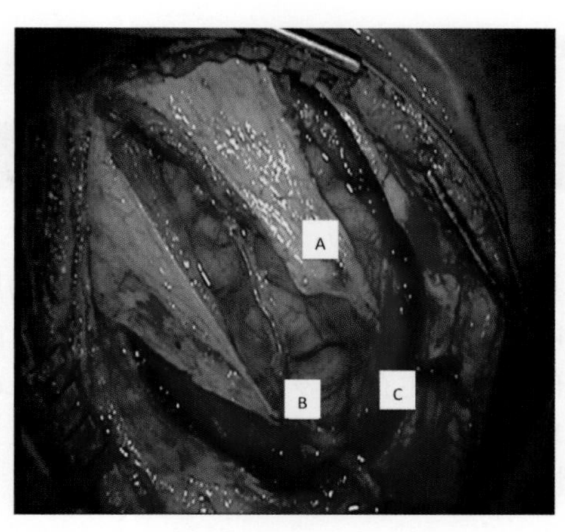

图 90.4 EDAMS 手术术中图片。（A）颞肌，（B）颞浅动脉，仍然保持连续性，（C）硬脑膜的边缘，在皮质处反折

如果行颅骨多点钻孔术，那么在受影响一侧的半球上钻 10~20 个孔，打开硬脑膜，使颈动脉外循环的血管可以进入颅内。

结果

对于有大脑半球症状的患者进行比较，结果显示 5 年内复发同侧卒中的风险，接受药物治疗的患者（65%）比接受手术治疗的患者（17%）明显更高。改善缺血大脑半球的血流量也有助于改善认知功能。

Guzman 等（2009）报道了一系列成人和儿童患者，主要采用直接手术搭桥治疗。他们报告的手术致残率和死亡率分别为每个治疗半球 3.5% 和 0.7%。

Scott 等（2004）分析了通过改良的 EDAS 技术进行间接血管重建术，在儿童中的结果。报告的手术致残率为每个治疗半球 4%。

根据专家共识，间接血管重建术更适合儿童，因为对于小直径血管，直接搭桥在技术上比较困难，更适合成人患者（Roach et al.，2008）。

麻醉问题

如果要避免围术期缺血性并发症，维持血流动力学稳定、正常血容量、避免低碳酸血症和低血压是重要的。

预后

儿童人群中未经治疗的症状性 MMD 的自然病史似乎是不佳的。该病的病程是多变的，可从迅速进展导致严重残疾到临床沉寂数年。在平均随访 7 年的情况下，有 TIA 型症状的儿童患者中有一半继续出现这些类型的发作（Fukuyama and Umezu，1985）。未经治疗的 MMD 与渐进性的神经和认知功能退化有关（Kurokawa et al.，1985）。

颅内动脉瘤

概述

儿童动脉瘤极为罕见，仅占所有颅内动脉瘤的0.5%~4%。在1966年对6368个破裂动脉瘤的研究中，只有41个发生在19岁以下的儿童身上（Locksley et al.，1966）。然而，在生命中的前20年里，它们占出血性卒中的10%~15%。

动脉瘤

患者的临床表现多种多样，可以表现为蛛网膜下腔出血（32%）、头痛不伴蛛网膜下腔出血（45%）、脑神经病变（16%）、恶心/呕吐（15%）、视觉症状（13%）、创伤（13%）、癫痫发作（4%）（Hetts et al.，2009）（**图 90.5**）。

这一人群中的动脉瘤不仅罕见，而且还表现出成人人群中未见的某些特征。

它们更多发生在不常见的位置，比如后颅凹（该部位的发生率是成人的两倍），并与远端血管相关。基底动脉干动脉瘤也比末端动脉瘤更常见。

它们更多的时候是纺锤形的和巨型的，并且以

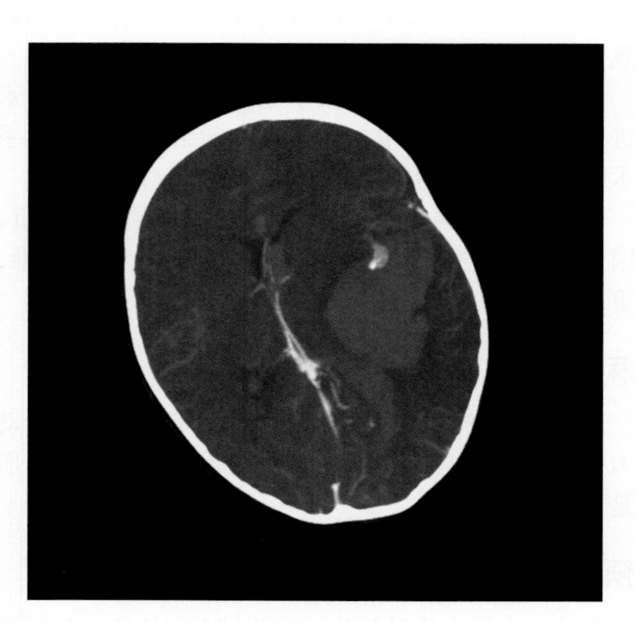

图 90.5 27岁女孩急诊入院，突发头痛，随后GCS下降到6分，左侧瞳孔固定并且散大。她转院时已经行气管插管并机械通气，行头颅CT及CT血管成像。结果显示左颞ICH，一个动脉瘤位于血肿前方。进一步的CT扫描显示血肿清除满意，但是MCA供血区域梗死。她然后接受了左侧去骨瓣减压术以稳定病情。随访2年后，她可以行走但是遗留轻度偏瘫（上肢＞下肢）。语言仅能说单词

轻微的男性占优势出现。它们具有多样性，特别是与血管病变和感染相关时（Jordan et al.，2009）。

据报道，儿童破裂动脉瘤中有5%~10%病例有自发性血栓形成，但在成人中非常罕见。已有自发性血管再通的报道，因此需要仔细的影像随访（Lasjaunias et al.，2005；Buis et al.，2006）。

青少年的动脉瘤更符合成人的表型。

Pierre Lasjaunias（2005）将儿科动脉瘤分为四种亚型（**表 90.2**）。在这个分型上，其他作者还增加了：肿瘤性动脉瘤、血流动力学动脉瘤和极罕见的家族性动脉瘤。

血流动力应激引起的动脉瘤可见于先天性血管缺失、动静脉畸形和高血压伴或不伴主动脉缩窄。

创伤性动脉瘤在儿童中更为常见，占所有病变的20%。这在颅底动脉固定的地方或者或硬脑膜的海绵窦段颈内动脉和胼胝体周动脉最常见。颈动脉海绵窦瘘可能是海绵窦段颈内动脉受累所致。大多数创伤性动脉瘤，即使在没有潜在动脉病变的患者中，也有增大的趋势。

从诊断的角度来看，已经逐渐转向非侵入性成像技术，如MRI和CT血管成像，脑导管血管造影可以用来治疗或制订治疗计划（**图 90.6A** 和**图 90.6B**）。

在超过35%的病例会出血，其中囊性动脉瘤出血是梭形动脉瘤（即使是感染病例）的两倍。在单纯性蛛网膜下腔出血的儿童患者中，高达57%的患者可能会发现动脉瘤（Jordan et al.，2009）。

梭形动脉瘤患者，其中较高比例的患者有潜在的诱发条件，如颅后窝畸形、血管瘤、动脉畸形、心脏缺损、主动脉缩窄、眼部异常和胸骨异常（PHACES）综合征、结节性硬化症、小头骨增生性原始侏儒症Ⅱ型、皮肤弹性过度综合征、成骨不全或神经纤维瘤病1型。

在生命的第一年，真菌性动脉瘤占颅内动脉瘤的10%（Buis et al.，2006），而且更有可能是多发性

表 90.2 Lasjaunias 儿童动脉瘤分型

1	梭形，没有感染或者创伤证据
2	囊状，没有感染或者创伤证据
3	感染性（真菌性）动脉瘤
4	创伤性动脉瘤

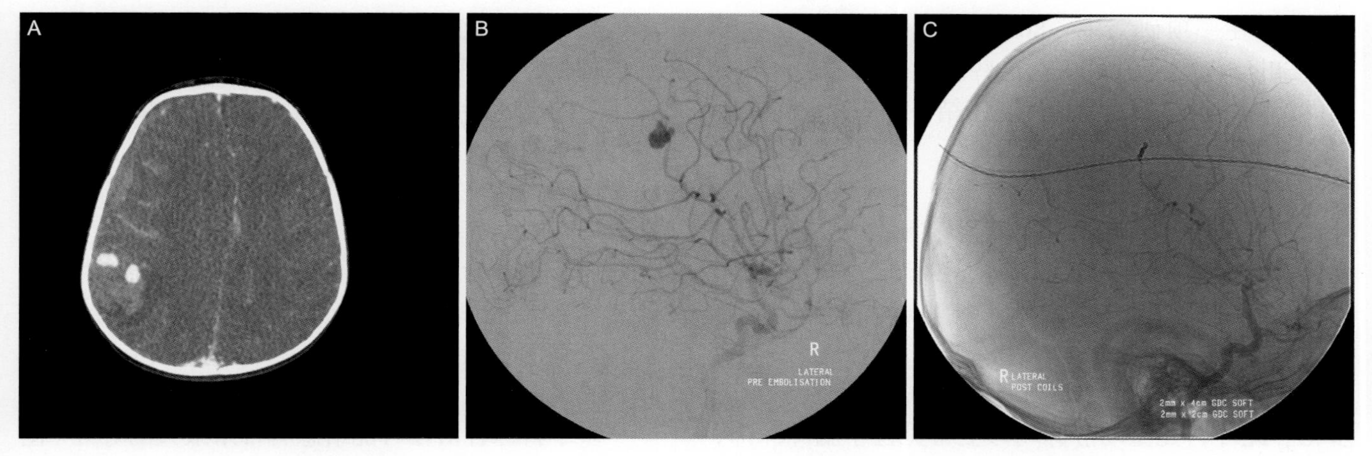

图 90.6 （A）一个6岁男孩的轴位头颅CT血管成像，主要表现为跌倒和癫痫发作，图像上显示一个双叶型病变，位于右顶叶，周围脑实质内有出血和硬脑膜下血肿；（B）脑血管造影侧面观，右侧颈内动脉末期，可见皮质动脉分支上的一个复杂动脉瘤；（C）将动脉瘤主体的近心端用线圈进行栓塞。微导管不能通过动脉瘤前端的狭窄，皮质支在狭窄处的远端有逆行显影，但是动脉瘤本身不再显影

的。相关的潜在疾病可能是心内膜炎、先天性与获得性免疫缺陷（包括 AIDS）和脑膜脑炎。在急性感染过程中可能会出现新的病变。与 HIV 感染相关的动脉瘤通常是多灶性的，形态学上通常是典型的长形接近端梭形病变。

我们遇到了一组与创伤相关的豆纹动脉远端动脉瘤患者。这些患者都经过仔细观察，而且有消退而不再出血的趋势。

儿童人群动脉瘤的治疗需要详细的病史和辅助调查，这些检查通常在成人中是不需要的，如败血症筛查或心脏结构检查。此外，所有病例都需要多学科治疗，包括心脏病学家、小儿神经学家、神经外科医生和介入神经放射学家。

在过去的几十年里，小儿颅内动脉瘤的治疗已逐渐从神经外科治疗转向非侵入性血管内治疗（图 90.6C）。

动脉瘤经血管内治疗后似乎有较高的再次治疗率，可以采用血管内治疗或外科治疗。真正的复发并不常见的，可能是对小的颈部残留有较低的接受性。

对于梭状动脉瘤，已经有报道显示采用复杂的神经外科搭桥手术具有良好的中期、长期的明显的临床结果。考虑到对患者成长的耐受性，这一点尤其令人鼓舞。

在儿童人群中，随着时间的推移，动脉瘤的增长率轻度增高（高达 10%）。部分原因是与血管病的相关性较高。不论是血管内治疗还是外科手术治疗，由于已经有多根血管受累，限制了对母动脉进行闭合的治疗选择。因为已经发育不良的血管承受血流动力学压力增加，形成新生动脉瘤的风险增加。

新的导流装置已被用于儿童人群中，治疗大型和梭状动脉瘤。这样的装置避免了对母动脉进行闭塞。需要更长期的随访来确认决定其持久性。有几个关于儿童动脉瘤患者的发人深省的病例系列，患儿出现晚期并发症，但成年后的全因死亡率也高于同龄人。晚期动脉瘤破裂似乎主要与最初手术或血管内治疗时动脉瘤闭合的程度有关（Koroknay-Pal et al., 2012）。因此，一些作者提倡终身随访。在一项研究中，59 名患者，中位随访时间为 34 年，其中 24 名（41%）患者有 25 个新生动脉瘤和 11 个复发动脉瘤，其中 25% 有症状（Koroknay-Pal et al., 2013）。7 例患者出现新的蛛网膜下腔出血。新发动脉瘤的年发生率为 1.9%。

吸烟是导致新的动脉瘤形成和蛛网膜下腔出血的重要危险因素。最初表现为多发性和梭状动脉瘤的患者特别容易发生新的病灶（Hetts et al., 2011）。

尽管需要更复杂的治疗策略，但在儿童人群中总体风险并未增加。然而，需要联合或序贯手术和血管内治疗的患者确实有额外的风险。

动静脉畸形

概述

尽管人们普遍认为动静脉畸形是发育中的病变，不像动脉瘤可能在出生后不久就出现，但它们非常罕见。然而，出血性表现比成人更常见（Hetts et al.,

2012），在一项研究中，86/135 例（63.7%）发生出血（Ellis et al.，2015）。在这些困难的情况下，多模式的评估和治疗是确保良好临床结果的先决条件。

动静脉畸形

虽然动静脉畸形的总体结构在病灶大小、硬脑膜供应或引流静脉数量方面与成人没有本质上的区别，但仍存在一些差异。这可能与成人人群的慢性高血流有关，因为静脉闭塞和狭窄、静脉扩张和动脉血流动脉瘤在成人中更常见。深静脉引流在儿童更多见。此外，儿童动静脉畸形更常见位于脑叶深部，在成人，皮质病变则更常见。与成人一样，儿童患者的深部动静脉畸形，以及有深部静脉引流和小脑幕下病，与出血表现有很强的关联。

如前所述，临床表现主要是出血（高达 80%）（**图 90.7A**），8.3% 表现为癫痫和偏头痛（6.3%）（Dinca et al.，2012）。由于确诊时年龄较小，计算出的终生破裂风险很高，通常倾向于更积极的治疗方法。

收治这类患者的中心应该有自己的处置流程，同时有小儿血管神经外科专家、神经介入医生和具备现代立体定向放射外科。

无论是否有术前靶向性的辅助栓塞，神经外科手术可以获得达到高达 90% 的闭塞率，致残率为 17%（主要是视野缺损）（Gross et al.，2015）。可以预见的是，Spetzler-Martin 评分较低的动静脉畸形患者的情况更好。初次就诊时候的 MRS 也强烈影响最终的临床结果。

立体定向放射手术对于小儿患者是一个很有吸引力的治疗选择，即使是那些有 AVM 破裂的患者。在特定的患者系列中，已报道了 71.3%~88% 的闭塞率，每年的出血率在 1%~2.2%（Dinca et al.，2012；Hanakita et al.，2015）。与成人患者一样，较小的病灶有较高的闭塞率。

血管内治疗的试验可能要少得多，单独使用血管内治疗的闭塞率低得令人无法接受，只有 20%，但并发症的发生率和动脉瘤一样，并不高（Zheng et al.，2014）。

多学科综合治疗可能给患者带来最大的好处（**图 90.7B**）。在大型神经科学中心，采用互补技术可以提高闭塞率，同时具有可接受的致残率。对于较大的病变，治疗可能持续数年，几乎总是需要联合治疗。出血的风险持续存在，直到完全闭塞。小病变临床结果可以很好，但是，较大病变治疗后的幸存者，仍然存在较高的长期依赖的风险。

海绵状血管畸形

海绵状血管畸形（cavernous malformations，CM）是儿童最常见的中枢神经系统（central nervous system，CNS）血管病变，虽然发病率比成人低 4 倍（Acciarri et al.，2009）。

发病年龄呈双峰分布，4 岁以下和 12 岁以上各有一个高峰。6 岁以下的患者被发现有明显更多的巨大海绵血管畸形（Bilginer et al.，2014）。

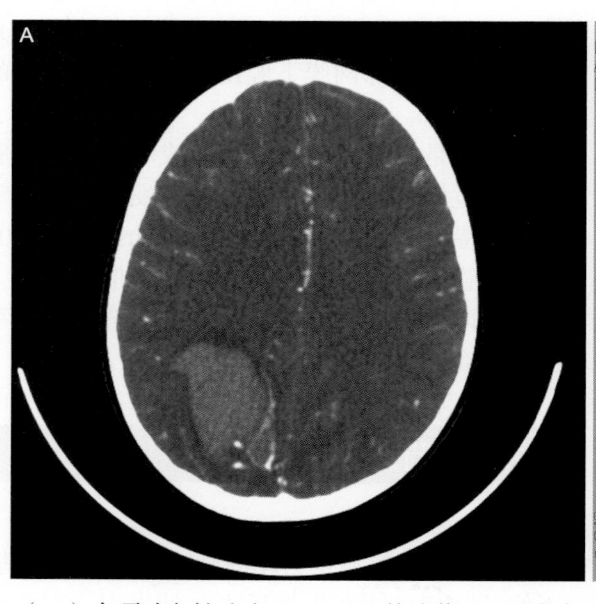

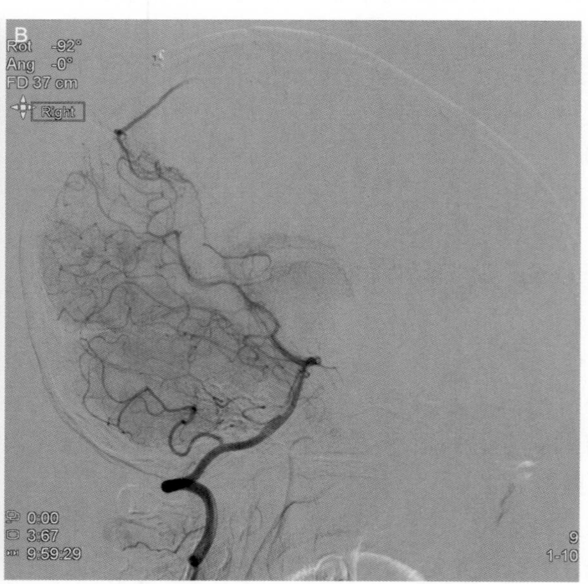

图 90.7 （A）右顶叶急性脑出血，CT 血管成像显示后部轻微血管密集，但是没有明显的病灶。（B）在脑血管造影上显示一个小的 AVM，位于右顶叶后部。通过手术切除联合立体定向放射外科，成功治愈

儿童整个神经轴的海绵状血管畸形的自然病史似乎比成人患者更具侵袭性，病变的生长率和出血率更高，体积更大，而且在诊断时往往影像学表现不典型。除了家族性疾病（通常与多发性病变和早期的临床表现有关），在儿童中发生海绵状血管畸形的主要危险因素似乎是头颅放射治疗（Acciarri et al.，2009）。这种风险是累积的，照射5年、10年、15年和20年的放射后海绵状血管畸形的发生率分别为2.24%、3.86%、4.95%和6.74%（Strenger et al.，2008）。治疗时越年轻，累积风险越高，病变形成的潜伏期越短。保守治疗是大多数无症状病变的常规治疗方法。

目前，对于这组患者进行影像学监测的益处或间隔时间尚无共识。

儿童脑内出血

结构性病变占儿童脑出血的50%。动静脉畸形仍然是最常见的病因，占到30%。海绵状血管畸形（15%）和动脉瘤（13%）是其他常见的结构性病变。其他原因包括镰状细胞病、烟雾病和极少的瘤内出血。10%~30%的脑出血继发于血液病，如血友病、血小板减少症和维生素K缺乏继发的凝血病。约25%的脑出血无法确定病因。

临床表现

高达45%的儿童可能表现出颅内压升高的特点，需要紧急处理。其表现包括严重头痛、呕吐、恶化的GCS评分和癫痫。多达50%的患者存在局灶性神经功能缺损（Beslow et al.，2010）。

辅助检查

CT扫描在早期发现出血是有用的。计算机断层血管造影（computed tomography angiography，CTA）或MRA可能有助于识别潜在的结构病变。DSA对于识别小的动静脉畸形可能是必要的，因为可能无法在非侵入性成像中看到。如果血肿消退后仍不能发现潜在病变，则需要重复DSA检查。

治疗

根据患儿出现症状时的GCS评分，可能需要对颅内压升高进行急性干预（如输入甘露醇、脑室引流，以及对高达50%的患者行急性血肿清除）。影像学检查有助于发现血肿的潜在原因和计划血肿的手术入路。手术的主要目的是清除血肿，在技术上可行的情况下，对潜在病变进行治疗或不进行治疗。在血肿清除过程中，清除潜在病变可能是必要的，因为血肿清除后，可能出现无法控制的出血。

预后

在确诊后3.5个月，71%的幸存者有神经功能缺陷，55%的患者有明显的临床残疾（Beslow et al.，2010）。脑出血5年后复发率为10%。

结论

儿童的神经外科疾病仍然造成一些独特的挑战。需要多学科的专家和多种治疗手段的密切协作。这些疾病需要长期的随访，因为患者可以长期生存，而且受到新发症状的威胁，以及出血和治疗可能造成残疾。

延伸阅读、参考文献、EBRAIN的相关链接

扫描书末二维码获取。

第91章 儿童癫痫

Sophia Varadkar・Martin Tisdall 著
解自行、李志保、周思宇 译，孟凡刚、王群 审校

引言

癫痫是一种以反复出现的自发性发作为特征的脑部疾病（Fisher et al.，2014）。癫痫较为常见，但准确估计发病率和患病率较困难；癫痫人群患病率为0.5%~1%，60%是从儿童期开始发病，其中20%~25%是药物难治性癫痫。

儿童癫痫的诊断

所有儿童、年轻人和成人，一旦出现疑似癫痫的新近发作，都应立即由具有癫痫专业知识的医生诊治，以避免误诊，确保癫痫的早期确诊，并排除严重的非神经系统诊断，特别是心脏疾病的诊断（Nunes et al.，2012）。

诊断是建立在临床病史基础之上的。需要儿童或年轻人以及任何目击者对事件的准确全面描述，视频非常有帮助。体格检查应寻找局部神经障碍的证据，以及神经皮肤综合征的皮肤症状，并考虑其他系统症状。还应该注意生长发育和受教育的情况。

脑电图（EEG）可为癫痫的诊断提供支持，但不能证实或排除癫痫的诊断。脑电图有助于确定癫痫类型和癫痫综合征，包括光刺激和过度通气诱发试验。在诊断不确定的情况下，长时程录像或动态脑电图可能是有帮助的。神经影像学可以识别引起癫痫的结构异常，磁共振成像（MRI）是标准检查。儿童时期第一次疑似癫痫发作后通常不需要进行常规检查，但是对于年龄小于两岁的儿童，所有病史、检查或脑电图提示局灶性发作的儿童，以及脑电图对一线用药无反应的儿童，应该进行影像学检查。

对于所有的病例，都应就再次发作时应采取的措施提出建议，必须讨论安全问题，在某些情况下还应交代紧急抢救（救援）措施。

儿童癫痫的症状

儿童癫痫的电-临床综合征是由一组特定临床表现、体征、症状构成的，这些综合征共同构成了一种独特的、可鉴别的临床疾病。综合征的重要因素包括发病年龄、癫痫类型、特定脑电图特征和结构代谢原因（Berg et al.，2010）。

广义上说，虽然新生儿癫痫发作常常是反应性/症状性的，但严重的早期婴儿癫痫性脑病（early infantile onset epileptic encephalopathies，EIEE）可能在出生到幼儿的任何时间出现。EIEE的特点是严重的癫痫发作，常常伴有婴儿痉挛、脑电图异常，以及在一岁以内出现发育迟缓、停滞或倒退。尽管MRI可能是阴性的，但也应寻找脑结构性改变。West综合征、Ohtahara综合征、早期肌阵挛性癫痫脑病、婴幼儿期癫痫伴迁移性局灶性发作和Dravet综合征（婴儿期严重肌阵挛性癫痫）在儿童癫痫中较为常见。该群体的遗传评估显示在阵列比较基因组中存在拷贝数变异。与EIEE相关的基因包括单基因SCN1A、STXBP1、ARX、CDKL5和女性PCDH19。在这个年龄段，还有可治疗的维生素反应性癫痫，包括维生素B6反应性癫痫，GLUT1功能丧失综合征和生物素酶缺乏综合征。

儿童中期（4~10岁）的癫痫以良性为主，患儿往往具有良好的发育和受到良好的教育，癫痫更可能自发缓解。最常见的是儿童失神癫痫和良性癫痫伴中央颞区棘波（benign epilepsy with centrotemporal spikes，BECTS）；较少见且容易被忽视的是早发型良性儿童枕叶癫痫（Panayiotopoulos综合征）。但是，更严重的癫痫也会出现。Lennox-Gastaut综合征（Lennox-Gastaut syndrome，LGS）的特征是全身性强直阵挛性发作、意识丧失、跌倒和强直性发作，并具有特殊的脑电图模式。肌阵挛性癫痫（Doose综合

征）预后不一。癫痫性脑病在睡眠中出现持续的棘慢波，并伴有 Landau-Kleffner 综合征（Landau-kleffner syndrome，LKS）出现。

在儿童后期（从 10 岁到青春期），常见的遗传性全面性（以前称为特发性）癫痫综合征表现为遗传性全面性癫痫、青少年肌阵挛性癫痫和青少年失神性癫痫。这些都是终身综合征。常染色体显性遗传性夜间额叶癫痫（autosomal-dominant nocturnal frontal lobe epilespy，ADNFLE）可能在儿童早期出现，但现在才被认识。

一些特定的病因在任何年龄都会引起癫痫，包括神经皮肤综合征，如结节性硬化症、Sturge-Weber 综合征、神经纤维瘤病以及其他结构病变，如肿瘤或多小脑回。如颞叶内侧硬化症、卒中、围产期损伤、感染和创伤等一些获得性病变（儿童较成人少见）也可以引起癫痫。另外一些特殊的病因也会看到，包括 Rasmussen 综合征、下丘脑错构瘤、偏瘫癫痫、痉挛性偏瘫、染色体异常（21 三体综合征和 20 号环状染色体综合征）。

药物治疗

在英国，儿童长时间癫痫发作和癫痫持续状态的治疗方案相对成熟（Advanced Life Support Group，2011）。

治疗上以服用抗癫痫药物（antileptic drugs，AED）为主。与成人相似，卡马西平、丙戊酸钠、拉莫三嗪和左乙拉西坦是最常用的药物。AED 通常缓慢增加，以达到最低有效剂量。药物副作用可能不同于成人。AED 是根据癫痫类型和癫痫综合征来选择的，这可能与成人的治疗不同。

癫痫共病的治疗在儿童中非常重要。应积极寻找和治疗运动障碍、认知和学习障碍、行为问题、自闭症、注意缺陷多动障碍或精神疾病等。

药物难治性是指“经两种耐受、适当选择和使用的抗癫痫药物（无论是单一疗法还是联合疗法）充分治疗仍无法达到癫痫无发作状态”（Kwan et al.，2010）。这一点很重要，因为在两种药物失效后，再服用一种药物控制癫痫无发作的概率小于 12%。如果第二次 AED 治疗失败，现在应及时转诊考虑其他治疗，包括癫痫手术、生酮饮食，对于不适合癫痫切除手术的儿童，应使用迷走神经刺激（vagus nerve stimulation，VNS）疗法进行神经刺激。

儿童癫痫外科的术前评估

癫痫手术切除、离断或热凝可能的致痫灶，其主要目的是在不损害功能的前提下实现癫痫无发作或显著改善癫痫发作。儿童癫痫应由专业的手术团队经仔细的术前评估（presurgical evaluation，PSE）后确定发作起始区，同时将手术损害风险降到最低（**图 91.1**）。2006 年国际抗癫痫联盟（International League against Epilepsy，ILAE）儿童癫痫外科小组委员会关于儿童转诊和评估的建议仍在被采用，并且正在更新（Cross et al.，2006）。术前评估技术的进步意味着 MRI 阴性的儿童也有可能接受手术治疗。

儿童的特殊考虑

术前评估没有最低年龄限制，应该尽早开始，以缩短病程，减少长期癫痫发作带来的不良影响。在儿童中，判断适合手术治疗的癫痫较为复杂。症状学带来的帮助较少，尤其是在低年龄组中，相比成人症状学具有更少的偏侧性。此外，儿童表现出明显的全身特征（如癫痫痉挛），但这可能是局灶性发作区发作活动迅速扩散的结果。儿童的影像学解释较为复杂，需要专业且精通儿童大脑外观时间变化规律的神经放射科医生来解释。在 2 岁以下的幼儿中，髓鞘形成完成之前，病变异常可能会被忽视，需要多年的重复影像检查来确定手术病例。儿童癫痫的心理社会影响在认知发展变化中产生的，因此手术时机会受到发展轨迹的影响。早期手术及药量减少将带来认知的改善（Boshuisen et al.，2015）。

术前评估的组成

PSE 的初始评估（现称为 1 期评估）内容与 2006 年的建议基本保持不变：发作间期头皮脑电图（包括睡眠）、专用 MRI 癫痫序列、可能的长期发作头皮视频脑电图、神经心理学评估和需要的功能磁共振成像（fMRI）（Ryvlin et al.，2014）。神经精神病学和神经 - 眼科学也应包括在内。扩展的 1 期评估还包括正电子发射断层扫描（PET）、脑磁图（MEG）、EEG-fMRI、脑电溯源分析和高分辨率脑电图。发作期和发作间期单光子发射 CT（SPECT）对发作期局灶性脑高灌注进行后处理分析，有助于结节性硬化症的结节定位和病变阴性病例的致痫灶定位。

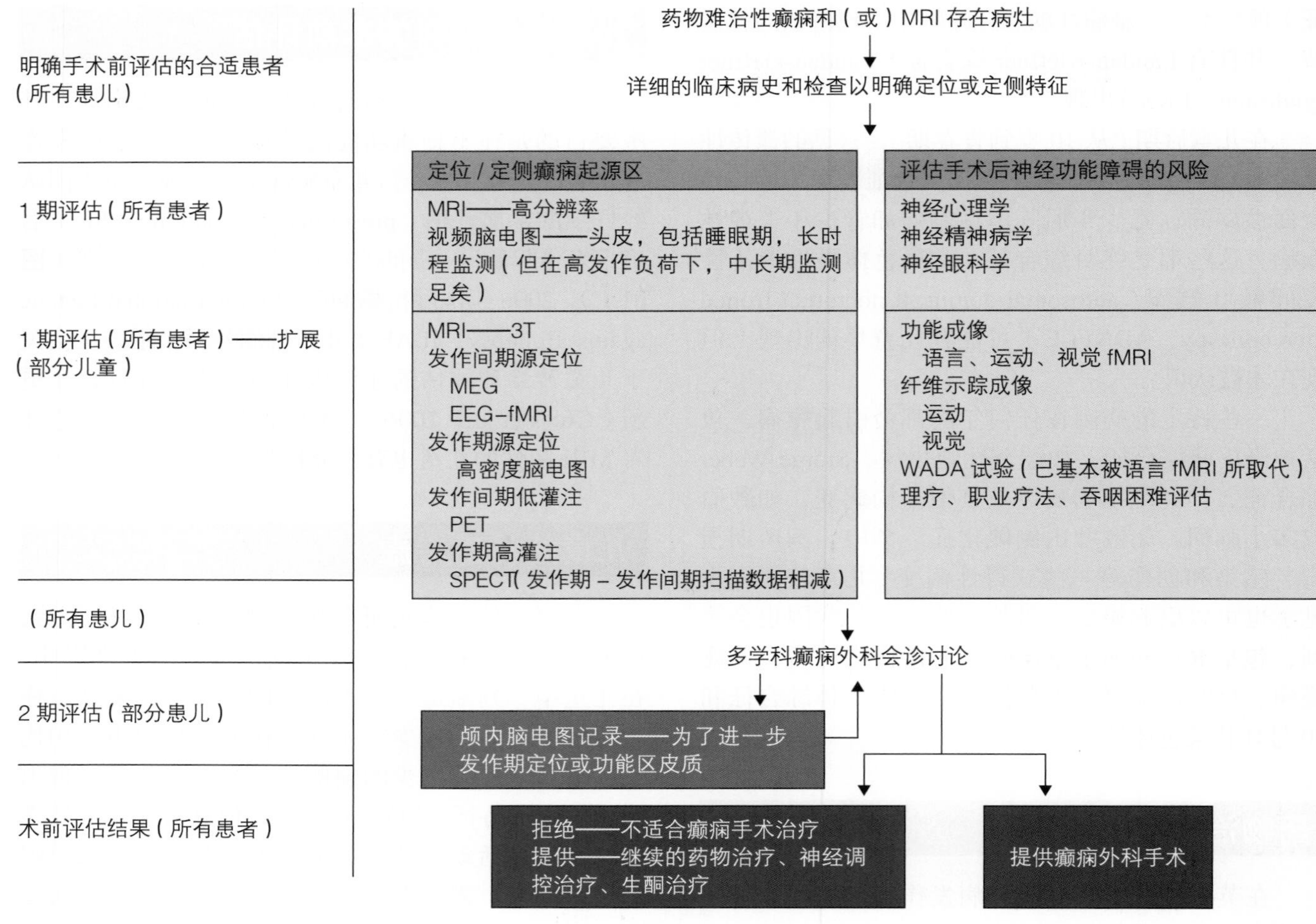

图 91.1 术前评估路径

表 91.1 小儿癫痫手术中潜在病因的发生率

病因	病例百分比
皮质发育不良	42%
肿瘤	19%
感染 / 卒中 / 创伤	10%
海马硬化	6%
结节性硬化症	5%
下丘脑错构瘤	4%
Sturge-Weber 综合征	3%
Rasmussen 综合征	3%
血管病变	1%
其他	7%

Source data from Pellock, J. et al., 2007. *Pediatric Epilepsy*, New York: Demos Medical.

潜在病因

2004 年，国际抗癫痫协会对世界上儿童癫痫中心进行了一次调查。在现代成人病例中占很大比例的海马硬化，在儿科病例中相对较少，而皮质发育不良是最大的一组（Pellock et al.，2008）。各种疾病的发病率如**表** 91.1 所示（Pellock et al.，2008）。

手术类型

在大多数儿科癫痫手术中心，脑叶切除和局部切除是外科手术的主要部分。然而，多脑叶和半球手术所占的比例要高于成人手术。2004 ILAE 调查显示了儿科中心外科手术的比例（**表** 91.2）（Pellock et al.，2008）。

手术注意事项

癫痫手术的原则在成人和儿科手术中相似，包括最大限度地切除病灶，同时尽量减少对有功能组织的损害。切除手术通常包括病变组织周围的下一个软脑膜边界。双重病理在儿科病例中更为普遍，尤其是颞叶切除。因此，与成人相比，在儿童海马硬化症的选择性切除策略方面的进展较少。癫痫

表 91.2　小儿癫痫手术的各手术类型所占百分比

外科手术类型	病例百分比
单脑叶 / 局灶性病变切除术	48%
半球切除术	16%
多脑叶切除术	13%
迷走神经刺激器植入术	16%
胼胝体切开术	3%
其他	4%

Source data from Pellock, J. et al., 2007. *Pediatric Epilepsy*, New York: Demos Medical.

的无发作率仍然是术后认知功能最重要的决定因素（Skirrow et al.，2015）。因此，一般认为包括新皮质和颞叶内侧结构更广泛的颞叶切除是有益的。因为尽管切除了潜在的功能性组织，但更大的切除量可能会改善癫痫发作结果。

在儿童，大脑重量与体重的比例高于成人。此外，年轻的患者通常需要更大的皮质切除，这可能导致明显的失血性缺血。外科医生和麻醉师必须高度重视，以确保充分止血和复苏，这表明儿童癫痫手术需要专业且经验丰富的外科和麻醉团队，以便能够预测和处理相关手术问题。

关于病灶切除术和杏仁核 - 海马切除术手术原则的详述请见**第 83 章**，此处不再赘述。

大脑半球离断或大脑半球切除

大脑半球切除术或大脑半球离断术的目的，是切除或断开一侧大脑半球的整个皮质。Dandy 和 L'Hermitte 于 1928 年首次提出用这种术式来治疗大脑半球胶质瘤。尽管没有改善胶质瘤患者的预后，但后来它成为了癫痫外科的一项重要技术。目前已经提出了多种改良手术，这些将在下一步进行讨论。为了方便起见，我们将使用术语大脑半球切除术来涵盖所有旨在大脑半球切除或离断的手术。

大脑半球切除术的适应证包括药物难治性的大脑半球性癫痫，或病理改变涉及多脑叶，或不合适小范围切除的癫痫，以及由一侧大脑半球引起的癫痫。患儿存在偏瘫且对侧大脑半球正常。随着时间的推移，大脑半球切除的适应证已经扩大了，以上适应证是相对的。所有可能病例都应该经过经验丰富的多学科癫痫外科团队会诊讨论。

手术决策的制订还将考虑癫痫负荷和生长发育轨迹，在某些情况下可能考虑“姑息性”大脑半球切除术。最近的研究表明，在选定的病例中，对侧半球 MRI 和 EEG 异常可能不会影响预后（Wyllie et al.，2007；Hallbook et al.，2010）。

大脑半球切除术的病理结果包括大脑半球性巨脑回、移行障碍、皮质发育不良、脑梗死、脑穿通畸形、Sturge-Weber 和 Rasmussen 综合征。

大脑半球切除术的功能结局

所有形式的大脑半球切除术都涉及同侧内囊和视神经辐射的中断。对侧偏瘫和同侧偏盲是无法避免的。手术后的效果取决于术前功能状态、患儿年龄和术前认知能力。相反，对于有围产期大脑半球梗死且术前伴有偏瘫和偏盲的儿童，大脑半球切除术后神经功能将不会改变或很少改变。另一方面，对于优势半球 Rasmussen 综合征患儿，手术后患儿的语言功能、运动功能和视力可能发生显著变化。后一种情况下的决策比较复杂，需要与患者和护理人员进行认真讨论。

技术演变

解剖性大脑半球切除术治疗癫痫在 1938 年首次报道。20 世纪 60 年代，这一手术被证明与术后皮质含铁血黄素沉积（继发于手术腔的出血）和脑积水导致的神经功能恶化有关（Beier and Rutka，2013）。随后解剖性大脑半球切除术就朝着脑皮质离断而不是切除的方向发展。Rasmussen 用功能性大脑半球切除术这一术语来描述大脑中央和颞部切除及额叶和枕叶离断。技术进一步发展产生了各种各样的半球离断术，包括很少或几乎不切除脑组织，目的是减少手术时间和失血（Villemure and Mascott，1995；Dorfer et al.，2013）。技术的选择将取决于团队的手术经验和潜在的大脑解剖结构。

技术

目前主要有两种方法，一种是大部分通过脑室系统完成以脑岛区为中心的大脑半球切除术，另一种是垂直矢状窦旁的大脑半球切除术。

无论采用哪种技术，都必须做到以下几点：离断同侧内囊，离断颞叶内侧结构，完成胼胝体切开术，离断额叶纤维。

并发症包括出血、感染、术后非感染性发热、无菌性脑膜炎、对侧偏瘫、脑梗死或水肿、脑积水（需要脑室分流术的占 10%~15%）和死亡（约占 1%~3%）。

大脑半球切除术的预后与其潜在的病理结果相关，总的癫痫无发作率为 70%~80%。获得性或进行

专栏 91.1 典型病例 1

一名5个月大的婴儿在2周时出现婴儿痉挛。在最初的检查中，她对药物有反应，除左手握拳外，她的智力发展良好。MRI显示右侧大脑半球皮质广泛发育畸形（**图91.2**），EEG显示右侧大脑半球出现多种形式癫痫放电。癫痫发作在12个月时复发，她接受了右半球切除术，无并发症。在1年的随访中，她没有癫痫发作，发育良好，只有左手有轻微的肌张力增加。

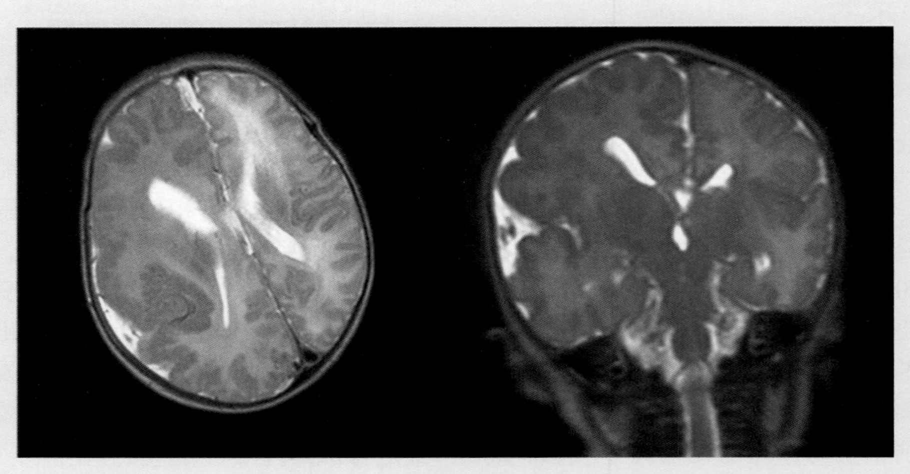

图 91.2 一名5个月大的儿童，轴位和冠状位T2 MRI表现为右侧大脑半球广泛的皮质畸形和多小脑回

性病变的预后优于发育性。所采用的手术技术不影响预后。见**专栏** 91.1。

有创监测（侵入性监测）监测

有创监测（侵入性监测）是一种将电极置于大脑表面或其内的技术，通过此技术记录到的发作期和发作间期活动，相比头皮脑电图，具有更高的空间分辨率。为了收集足够的数据，电极通常放置7 d左右。这项技术还允许通过电极对大脑进行电刺激，以描绘出皮质的功能区或识别致痫网络。这对于儿童可能是特别有用的，因为儿童开颅手术中是无法进行唤醒的。

两种技术占主导地位：通过开颅手术放置硬膜下栅状电极或经皮通过神经导航放置多个立体定向深部电极（stereoEEG）。这两种方法有不同的优势，但一般来说，硬膜下栅状电极具有更高分辨率的映射，而立体定向脑电图可更好覆盖深部和近中皮质区域，见**专栏** 91.2。

儿童癫痫的姑息性手术治疗

一部分患有严重和药物难治性癫痫的患者不适合做切除手术。在这组患者中，可以考虑采取姑息性手术，以减少癫痫发作的频率或严重程度，从而

专栏 91.2 典型病例 2

一名16岁男孩在8岁时出现了额叶症状的癫痫发作。他使用五种抗癫痫药物均治疗失败。除了一些特定的记忆障碍外，他的神经认知能力正常。磁共振成像最初被认为是没有病变。进一步的影像显示右额叶中回存在可疑病变，立体脑电电极植入（**图** 91.3）后，他接受了成功的病灶切除术。组织病理结果为局灶性皮质发育不良。术后1年随访，癫痫未再发作，也没有服用任何抗癫痫药物。

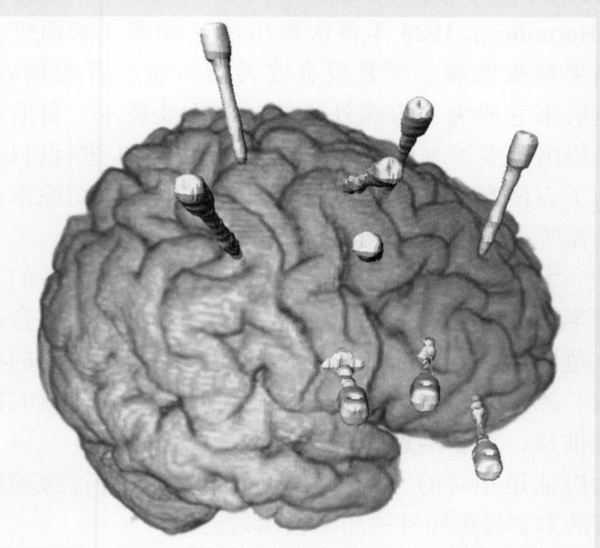

图 91.3 术后立体脑电图成像显示植入电极在皮质的位置

提高生活质量。

姑息性癫痫手术的适应证包括全身性或多灶性癫痫发作，其中无法定位发作源，或癫痫发作来自功能区，但功能区手术风险较大。

姑息性癫痫的手术技术包括胼胝体切开术、VNS和多软膜下横切术。

胼胝体切开术

胼胝体切开术对患有失张力（跌倒）发作癫痫的患者最有效，对强直性癫痫的疗效较低。在70%的患者中，完全胼胝体切开术可以减少大约70%的跌倒发作。与部分胼胝体切开术相比，完全胼胝体切开术减少癫痫发作的概率更高（Kasasbeh et al.，2014）。小儿术后离断综合征的发生率极低，这可能与大多数儿童有明显的发育迟缓和存在沟通障碍有关。与成人的做法相反，我们在绝大多数儿童中进行完全胼胝体切开术，但对于很少或没有认知障碍的儿童，我们进行部分或前2/3的胼胝体切开术。

经中线开颅，经大脑半球间入路进入胼胝体。蛛网膜瘢痕是经常遇到的，必须非常小心分开粘连。然后将胼胝体从喙部到压部分开。

迷走神经刺激（VNS）

1985年首次提出迷走神经刺激可减轻癫痫发作的假说。随后，动物研究和人类临床试验支持了该手术。VNS与胼胝体切开术疗效相似，但无颅内手术相应的风险。VNS是在左侧迷走神经上植入一个刺激电极（选择左侧是为了减少心脏不适的风险），并将其连接到一个胸部皮下刺激器上。刺激器设置一组背景基础刺激参数，并设定一组可通过刷刺激器磁铁触发的备用刺激参数。最新版本的设备可感知心率，并有一种算法，用于检测与癫痫发作相关的心动过速，然后自动触发备用设置，目的是终止癫痫发作（Schneider et al.，2015）。

多软膜下横切术（MST）

多软膜下横切术（multiple subpial transections，MST）是一种在假定的致痫区内垂直于脑回长轴，每间隔5 mm进行多处横断的手术技术。目的是毁损外侧皮质-皮质连接，使皮质区域没有维持癫痫发作所需的关键组织，同时保留功能所需的垂直的皮质-皮质下通路。

MST已用于起源于功能区皮质的癫痫，尤其是在Landau-Kleffner综合征的治疗中得到广泛应用。但该术式不太受欢迎，因为它会导致皮质损伤且有效性受到了质疑。

不同手术的选择

胼胝体切开术和VNS可能有协同作用。胼胝体切开术在失张力性癫痫患者中似乎更有效，但具有颅内手术的风险。对于失张力性癫痫占优势或被认为对生活质量有严重影响的癫痫患者，我们推荐胼胝体切开术作为初始手术方法。以前对接受VNS患者不能进行MRI扫描，但是现在MRI扫描仪设计已经解决了这一问题，VNS手术并不影响未来的癫痫手术评估。

儿童癫痫外科中的争议

优势半球Rasmussen综合征的手术时机

Rasmussen综合征以难治性癫痫发作、单侧皮质萎缩和相应的神经功能障碍为特征。大脑半球切除手术是唯一的治疗方法，可实现70%~80%的癫痫无发作（Bien and Schramm，2009）。然而，这种手术策略不可避免地会导致同侧偏盲、偏瘫，以及优势半球受累患者的语言功能障碍。这些缺陷可能在术前出现，但其严重程度和起病速度各不相同。认知能力下降较常见，但并非不可避免，对侧半球出现独立的发作间期癫痫样放电通常预示着认知能力下降（Longaretti et al.，2012）。通常情况下，癫痫手术前病程越短术后认知结果越好。因此，早期手术是有益的（Jonas et al.，2004）。大脑半球切除术后语言功能受损的程度主要与起病年龄有关，在合适的患者中术前可使用语言功能磁共振成像或Wada试验进行评估。在神经可塑性可能保留的情况下，通过早期手术使语言功能向对侧转移还是等待疾病进展使未受累大脑半球语言功能自然建立仍然存在争议（Hartman and Cross，2014）。即使手术侧位于大脑半球语言功能优势侧，也很少出现完全失语（Boatman et al.，1999）。尽管表达性语言功能可能显著减少，但感觉性语言功能一般仍保留。手术治疗时机的确定必须建立在癫痫发作严重程度和神经功能受损程度评估的基础上（Varadkar et al.，2014）。对于家庭成员和临床医生来说这是一种挑战，并需要评估手术和保守治疗可能导致的最终结果。

延伸阅读、参考文献

扫描书末二维码获取。

第十九篇　脑脊液循环障碍

第92章　脑积水和正常脑脊液动力学

Alexander Gamble・Harold Rekate 著
孙玉晨 译，张庆九 审校

引言

对脑脊液动力学的探索始于19世纪末。这些工作为20世纪20年代到60年代间脑脊液生理学研究铺平了道路。这些研究描述了脑脊液循环的基本原理，目前我们对脑脊液产生、循环和吸收的理解几乎都基于此。迄今为止，对脑脊液生理学和脑积水疾病的研究仍是神经外科界的热点领域。虽然脑脊液的流体力学在很早以前就已被详尽描述，但其潜在机制至今仍是神经科学界的一个争论热点。本章作为综述，或为有志于进一步探索脑脊液流体力学的读者提供入门知识。

脑积水

脑积水是指脑脊液形成（产生）和吸收之间的动态失衡，导致脑室体积增大的病理变化过程。脑脊液（cerebrospinal fluid，CSF）类似于水闸后面的水，CSF聚集在“水闸”之后，当到达足够的水位时，多余的CSF将通过水闸流出，排出的体积与其在水闸上方的高度成一定比例，从而自动保持循环体系中的CSF体积平衡。脑积水好比不适当地提高水闸高度，导致其后的液体量增加。对此，最初的解决方案是在水闸前后之间建立一个人工通道，以调节水闸前后的水量。如果在这个人工通道中存在一个合适的阀门来调控流量，便可使液体循环由被动的自我调节状态，转变为主动的虹吸状态。虽然这种比喻过于简单，但却说明了可以通过人工方案的介入，改变原有状态。神径外科医生处理复杂脑积水患者，就好比在自然界中通过人工干预原有生态系统，会产生意想不到的结果。

CSF分流术是脑积水的主要治疗方式，但其并发症多，治愈率低。20世纪中叶以前，脑积水基本上没有有效的治疗方法，直到CSF分流术的出现（Nulsen，1951），这些问题才得到解决。在发达国家，新生儿脑积水患病率为0.5‰～0.8‰（Garne et al.，2010；Jeng et al.，2011），他们中的大多数需要采用分流手术治疗。据估计在美国大约有70万人，在欧洲有200万人患有正常压力性脑积水（normal pressure hydrocephalus，NPH）（Jaraj et al.，2014）。对于采用分流术的患者，生活质量调整寿命年数一般为6年左右（Stein et al.，2006）。

脑脊液在中枢神经系统中的作用

脑组织是人体代谢最旺盛的器官。正常成人脑组织重量仅占体重的2%，流经脑组织的血液却占心输出量的15%，脑组织耗氧量占全身耗氧量的20%，脑葡萄糖消耗量约占体内葡萄糖消耗量的1/4。脑组织的复杂性和能量消耗量与CSF产生和吸收能力关系密切。CSF在维持脑稳态中发挥多种作用。首先，CSF可以提供一定浮力，起到缓冲保护神经组织的作用，同时，CSF可以减轻整个心动周期中血容量和血压的快速波动对脑组织的影响。另外，CSF循环可通过蛛网膜颗粒将几微米量级的颗粒转移到体循环中，不仅能够清除代谢废物，还能清除大分子量蛋白和细胞碎片。此外，越来越多的证据表明CSF中存在许多生长因子、激素、维生素和微量营养素，可通过CSF循环转运至远端靶细胞，并产生相应的作用。

神经元细胞生理功能的发挥需要稳定的细胞外环境。在脑组织细胞外液（extracellular fluid，ECF）和CSF中，离子和大分子浓度维持在相对稳定的范围。血脑屏障（blood-brain barrier，BBB）和血-脑脊液屏障（blood CSF barrier，BCSFB）的存在使得CSF的溶质浓度不同于血浆，如**表**92.1所示。BBB和BCSFB是脑组织特有的屏障结构，可选择性地允许分子和电解质通过。这些屏障对水的渗透性比其他大多数组织中有孔内皮细胞对水的渗透性低十倍，而对有机和无机溶质的渗透性至少低一千倍。溶质从

表 92.1　脑脊液与血浆成分的比较

浓度（mg/100ml）		
	CSF	血浆
蛋白质	16~38	6300~8500
葡萄糖	45~80	80~120
氨基酸	1.5~3	8~120
肌酐	0.5~22	0.7~2
尿素	5~39	22~42
乳酸	8~25	4.7
pH	7.3	7.4
电解质（mmol/kg）		
	CSF	血浆
钠	147	150
钾	2.86	4.63
钙	1.14	2.35
镁	1.1	0.8
氯	113	99
碳酸氢盐	23.3	26.8
磷酸盐	3.4	4.7
pH	7.3	7.4

Adapted with permission from Hladky, S.B. & Barrand, M.A., Mechanisms of fluid movement into, through and out of the brain: evaluation of the evidence, *Fluids and Barriers of the CNS*, Volume 11, Issue 1, p. 26. Copyright © 2014 Hladky and Barrand; licensee BioMed Central.

血浆转移到脑 ECF 和 CSF 是一个超选择性、主动的过程，而水可以被动、精准地随着溶质浓度变化在不同区域之间移动。组成 BBB 的内皮细胞和胶质细胞足突结构，使血脑屏障具有更强的抵抗静水压和渗透压增加的能力。当血压升高或血浆胶体渗透压降低导致滤过增加时，BBB 可以有效防止由此引发的脑组织水肿发生。因而中枢神经系统对由低蛋白血症引起的慢性高血压或水肿状态具有良好的耐受性。

年龄和疾病与脑脊液生理变化关系

随着神经元和胶质细胞的衰老，脑组织体积相应减少，加上脉络丛的纤维化，CSF 的产生会随着年龄的增长而减少。从中青年到老年，CSF 总体积大约会增加一倍（Courchesne et al.，2000）。即随着年龄的增长 CSF 的生成相对停滞，CSF 循环更新速率呈进行性减少。在儿童时期 CSF 更新速率高达 6 次 / 天，健康青年个体 CSF 更新速率为 4 次 / 天，而正常老年人的 CSF 更新速率下降到 3 次 / 天或更低（May et al.，1990；Serot et al.，2012）。

在 NPH 和阿尔茨海默病（Alzheimer's disease，AD）患者中，CSF 更新速率大大减少（**表** 92.2）。AD 和 NPH 的动物模型均证实由于 β 淀粉样肽（Aβ）和 τ 蛋白（tau protein）的特异性清除途径被破坏，导致两者在脑组织中蓄积（Shibata et al.，2000；Silverberg et al.，2010）。甲状腺素转运蛋白（transthyretin，TTR）由脉络丛上皮产生（Sousa et al.，2007），主要功能是转运甲状腺素（T4），与 Aβ 单体结合后，可抑制纤维蛋白原形成，并为淀粉样物质排泄出中枢神经系统提供途径（Redzic et al.，2005）。轻度认知损害的患者和 AD 患者的脑室容积与 CSF Aβ 水平呈明显负相关（Ott et al.，2010），这种相关性与原发病有关，但未必存在确切的因果关系。这可能与体液代谢紊乱参与衰老、AD 和 NPH 患者的病理生理过程有关。

AD 和 NPH 病理可能存在一定的重叠关系。CSF 标志物或组织活检无法明确区分这两种疾病是否可以同时存在（Golomb et al.，2000; Ott et al，2010）。Leinonen 等（2010）通过对 ICP 进行 24 小时监测，提高了疑似 NPH 的临床诊断率。Leinonen 等人收集了 219 例 NPH 患者在分流手术时获取的额叶脑组织标本。其中 168 例（77%）受益于分流术的患者中，52 例（31%）出现了 AD 相关病理表现，其中 13 例（25%）在随访结束时发展为临床 AD。69% 的患者脑组织标本未发现 AD 相关的病理表现，但其中仍有 6 例（5%）确诊为 AD。最近一项大型随机双盲对照试验对 215 例 AD 患者采用了低流量脑室 - 腹腔分流术治疗，未能显示任何 CSF τ 蛋白、Aβ 水平的下降或临床症状改善。这些阴性结果表明，虽然分流术可以引流 CSF，但它不能增加 CSF 的产量。因此，CSF 更新速率可能取决于脑室容积的变化程度。

表 92.2　脑脊液在正常压力性脑积水和阿尔茨海默病中的变化（Hladky and Barrand，2014）

	正常	NPH	AD
CSF 形成产生（ml/min）	0.4	0.25	0.2
体积（ml）	150	300	250
更新速率（次 / 天）	4	1.2	1.2

Adapted with permission from Johanson, C.E., Duncan, J.A., Klinge, P.M., Brinker, T., Stopa, E.G. & Silverberg, G.D., Multiplicity of cerebrospinal fluid functions: New challenges in health and disease, *Cerebrospinal Fluid Research*, Volume 5, Issue 10 Copyright © 2008 Johanson et al; licensee BioMed Central Ltd.

脑脊液的产生

脑组织

颅内 ECF 的总量约为 280 ml（Johanson et al., 2008），其中约 1/3 为脑脊液（目前的技术手段无法精确计算脑脊液占比）。并非所有离开血管腔进入细胞外的液体都可以被重吸收到静脉循环中，因此淋巴引流是一个必要的生理过程。输送到毛细血管的血浆中，约有 1% 会进入近端细胞外间隙。大约 90% 的滤液在最远端毛细血管后微静脉被重新吸收进入血液循环。因此，不同的组织器官，输送到终末器官的血浆中，约 0.1% 最终变成淋巴液。中枢神经系统不具有淋巴管结构，脑组织中 ECF 的功能类似于其他组织中的淋巴液，是神经系统清除细胞代谢废物（尤其是高分子量的代谢废物）的途径之一。除了代谢产生的水之外，细胞外液最终与脑脊液混合并流入脑室和蛛网膜下腔。与血脑屏障紧密连接的结构不同，室管膜细胞通过缝隙连接，使细胞外和脑室之间的溶质和水保持相对自由的平衡状态。来自脉络丛的脑脊液不同于 ECF，其中所含的代谢和细胞废物相对较少。这些生理特性形成了一个浓度梯度，驱使 ECF 溶质进入脑室 CSF，在本章后面将讨论其最终排泄到静脉循环的过程。

脉络丛

人脑脊液总量的 2/3 由脉络丛上皮细胞（CPe）产生。既往认为 CPe 在增强神经影像上呈明显强化，但其并不具有血脑屏障结构。这不代表 CPe 缺乏选择性，因为 CPe 在超微结构上存在高选择性血 - 脑脊液屏障（BCSFB）。立方上皮细胞之间的紧密连接限制了离子和水的转运。脉络丛富含血管，由前后脉络膜动脉以 3~4 ml/min 的血流速度供血，是脑灰质的 10 倍。与中枢神经系统内的其他内皮细胞不同，脉络丛中的血管内皮细胞结构间隙很大，可在基底外侧膜处获得大量血浆滤液。基底外侧膜包含许多皱褶，同时在脑室表面存在广泛的微绒毛结构，再加上分支状，叶状的结构，使得脑室脉络丛结构总质量接近 2 g，如图 92.1 所示。

脉络丛脑脊液形成机制

电解质的浓度具有高度可调节性。CPe 细胞从基底外侧吸收血浆超滤液。CPe 中的 Na^+-K^+-ATP 酶位于顶端膜，这与其在大多数其他组织中的位置不同。Na^+-K^+-ATP 酶建立了能量依赖性的电化学梯度，驱动离子的共同转运，并成为 CSF 中 Na^+ 的主要来源途径。Na^+-K^+-ATP 酶产生的细胞膜两侧 Na^+ 浓度差驱动基底侧的 H^+-Na^+ 交换体（NHE1）、Na^+ 依赖性 Cl^--HCO_3^- 交换体和 Na^+-HCO_3^- 共转运体进行离子转运。Na^+ 进入脑室可以驱动 Cl^- 转运，以保持中性电化学平衡。G 毒毛旋花苷是一种强效的强心苷，可使 Na^+-K^+-ATP 酶失活，并显著降低 CSF 生成量。利尿剂阿米洛利可以抑制 Na^+-HCO_3^- 共转运体进行离子转运，这也会导致 CSF 产生减少。除了细胞内的高 K+ 环境，循环利尿剂抑制顶端 Na^+-K^+-$2Cl^-$（NKCC1）协同转运体进行离子转运，也可抑制 CSF 的产生。

选择性水通道和水通道蛋白在脑脊液生理调控中具有重要作用，在中枢神经系统中，水通道蛋白 -1（AQP-1）几乎只在 CPe 的顶端膜高表达（Longatti et al., 2004; Praetorius and Nielsen, 2006）。AQP-4 在 CPe 低表达，其基本只在血脑屏障的星形细胞足突表达。敲除 AQP-1 的小鼠所产生的脑脊液比野生型小鼠少 20%~25%，平均 ICP 值比野生型小鼠低 50%（Oshio et al., 2003; Oshio et al., 2005）。有研究证实，在脑积水动物模型中 AQP-1 低表达（Paul et al., 2011）。在 CPe 顶端膜表达的 AQP-1 转运水的能力与 CPe 通过 BCSFB 转运水的能力相当。AQP-1 可以严格调控溶质运输，并使水分精准转运，这种特性与 BBB 相似，但较 BBB 调控能力更强。这些发现使 AQP-1 成为未来脑积水药物治疗的潜在的分子靶点。

碳酸酐酶（CA）存在几种亚型，其中部分亚型可与顶端膜和基底膜结合，另外几种亚型则以可溶的形式在胞质中发挥作用。尽管 CA 不直接参与离子转运，但在它催化下，H_2O 和 CO_2 发生反应，产生碳酸，后者再解离成 HCO_3^- 和 H^+。CA 抑制剂乙酰唑胺可减少用于共转运的 H^+ 和 HCO_3^-，增加细胞 pH 值，改变整体 CPe 生理特性，有效的抑制脑脊液生成。长期应用乙酰唑胺可减少顶端边缘的微绒毛，显著减少分泌所需的表面积（Azzam et al., 1978）。

脉络丛的营养和保护功能

CPe 中可以产生许多与神经元发育、维持和修复有关的蛋白质，并分泌到 CSF 中，例如：胰岛素样生长因子 2（IGF-2）、转化生长因子 β（TGF-β）家族成员、成骨蛋白（BMP）、成纤维细胞生长因子（FGFs）和视黄酸（RA）。它们对正常的中枢神经系统发育和损伤反应产生影响。在基底外侧膜上的 CPe GLUT1 转运体调节下，脑脊液葡萄糖含量约为血浆葡萄糖含量的 2/3。同样，CSF 中氨基酸的浓度通过它们各自的转运机制来维持稳定。CPe 中还包含特

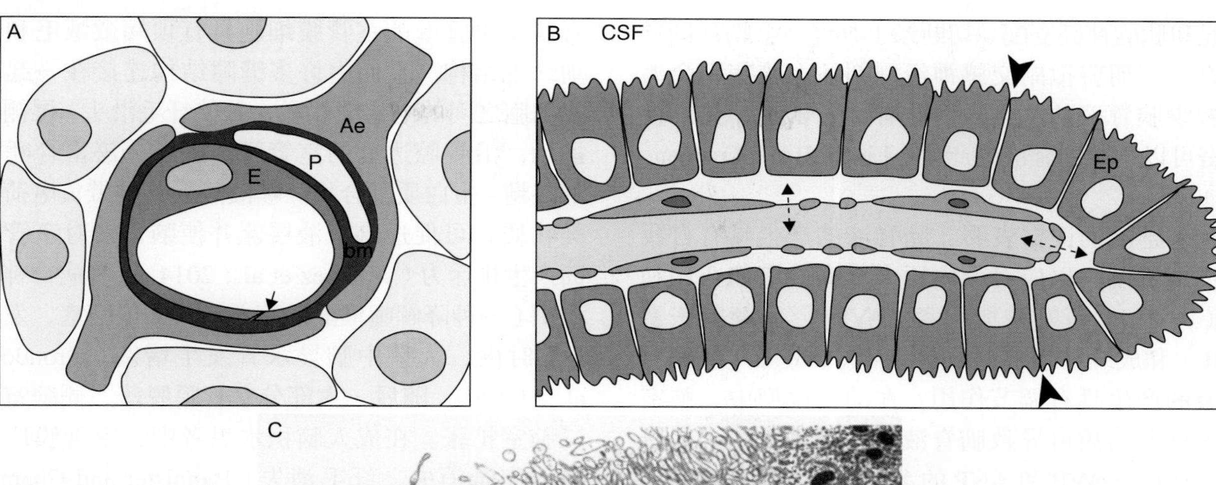

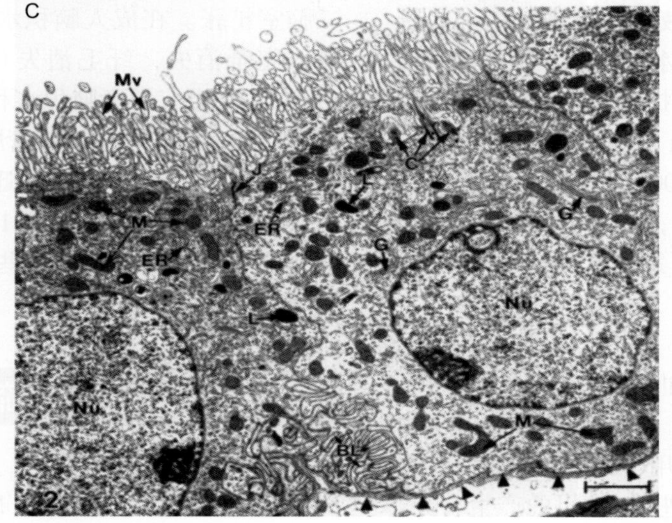

图 92.1 血脑脊液屏障和血脑屏障

颅内屏障示意图。颅内屏障界面用蓝色表示。血脑屏障（A）的原发部位是由周细胞（P）和星形细胞足突（Ae）支撑的脑血管内皮细胞（E）。脉络丛（B）上皮细胞（Ep）是血液 - 脑脊液屏障的屏障界面，内皮细胞在基质侧存在有孔结构（Stolp et al., 2012）。（C）脉络膜上皮超微结构。用 OsO4 固定成年 SD 大鼠侧脑室 CP，在电子显微镜下观察呈像。可见大量的顶膜（脑脊液面）微绒毛（Mv）和细胞内线粒体 (M)。J 是指在顶端两细胞间的紧密连接。C 代表中心粒。G 和 ER 分别代表高尔基体和内质网。细胞核（Nu）是椭圆形的，其中有核仁。箭头指的是上皮细胞靠近血浆的基底膜，底膜将上面的脉络膜细胞与下面的组织液分开。基底迷路（BL) 是由相邻细胞基底侧膜交织而成。比例尺 =2 μm

(A) Reproduced with permission from Stolp, H., Neuhaus, A., Sundramoorthi, R. & Molnár, Z., The Long and the Short of it: Gene and Environment Interactions During Early Cortical Development and Consequences for Long-Term Neurological Disease, *Frontiers in Psychiatry*, Volume 3, p. 50, Copyright © 2012 Stolp, Neuhaus, Sundramoorthi and Molnár.

(B) Reprinted from *Trends in Neurosciences*, Volume 31, issue 6, Norman R. Saunders, C. Joakim Ek, Mark D. Habgood, Katarzyna M. Dziegielewska, Barriers in the brain: a renaissance?, pp. 279–86, Copyright (2008), with permission from Elsevier.

定的核苷转运蛋白，可去除嘌呤和嘧啶代谢产物（如腺苷），明显改变神经元功能。在脉络膜丛中检测到非常高水平的解毒酶和结合酶，如环氧化物水解酶、谷胱甘肽过氧化物酶 UDP- 葡糖醛酸转移酶等，这表明 CPe 是脑内药物代谢的主要部位（Ghersi-Egea and Strazielle，2002）。此外，CPe 高表达溶质载体（SLC）和 ATP 结合蛋白，主要负责药物、毒素和其他有机蛋白从中枢神经系统中的主动排泄，这在神经肿瘤学中具有诸多意义。

脑脊液产生的调节

脑脊液的产生速率是可变的。有研究发现，许多先天性因素可以调节 CSF 产生。早期的有创性研究（Hayden et al.，1970）和最近的 MRI 研究都证实了脑脊液的每日产生量存在规律性周期变化。睡眠时脑脊液的分泌量可能是清醒时的两倍（Nilsson et al.，1992）。这种周期变化现象可能由 β- 肾上腺素的拮抗作用自主支配调节（Nilsson et al.，1994）。脉络丛含有血管活性肠多肽，可接受肾上腺素能神经、胆碱能神经和肽能神经支配。切断颈上神经节会增加脑脊液的产生，而将拟副交感神经制剂注入脑室则会大幅度减少脑脊液的产生，因此有学者认为，交感神经兴奋可以抑制脑脊液的产生（Lindvall and Owman，1981）。

越来越多的证据表明，脑脊液的产生具有自我调节反馈机制，以应对颅内压力增高，诸如心房利钠肽（ANP）、精氨酸加压素（AVP）、血管紧张素（AT-II）和成纤维细胞生长因子 -2（FGF-2）等都对脑脊液的产生具有调节作用。在动物模型中，脑室内注入这些物质可导致脑脊液产生减少。在人体研究中，脑脊液 AVP 和 ANP 的水平与 ICP 增加密切相关，而与无 ICP 升高时的脑室扩张不相关（Seckl and Lightman，1988；Tulassay et al.，1990；Yamasaki et al.，1997；Preston et al.，2003）。AVP 和 ANP 可诱导 CPe 暗细胞的比例增加，这种神经内分泌细胞与长期 CSF 产生量降低和氯离子传导降低有关（Johanson et al.，1999）。CPe 表达 AVP 受体，与 ANG 受体一样存在前馈机制。与其他外周组织不同，AT-Ⅱ降低了脑血管阻力，增加了脑血流量。AT-Ⅱ激活外周神经系统的交感神经，增加释放到血液中的 AVP。其降低脑脊液产生的作用与自主神经兴奋性无关，而与脑脊液中的 AVP 促进了 AT-Ⅱ的产生有关，它们相互之间存在正反馈关系（Chodobski et al.，1998）。由于 AT-Ⅱ不易透过 BBB 和 BCSF，其收缩血管的作用仅限于脉络膜小动脉，这是减少 CSF 产生的另一种辅助途径。

虽然 ANP 的合成和分泌至脑脊液的机制尚不明确，但已有证据表明，脑脊液中 ANP 含量可随脑脊液压力升高而增加，且 ANP 的含量可影响 CPe，产生对 ANP 的反馈。在脑积水动物模型中，脉络膜 ANP 受体表达高度上调（Mori et al.，1990），ANP 与受体的结合产生 cGMP，影响离子转运并减缓 CSF 的产生速率（Johanson et al.，2006）。与 AVP 相反，ANP 增加脉络膜血管的灌注（Schalk et al.，1992）。综合来看，ANP、AT-Ⅱ和 AVP 在维持 CP 灌注的同时，可以有效减少脑脊液的产生，并在由颅内压升高诱发脑缺血时，增加脑组织血流量。这些机制在急性颅内压升高和急性脑室扩张中起着重要作用，但与慢性脑积水或相对颅内压较低状态没有太大关系。

室管膜

室管膜不产生脑脊液，但为脑实质 ECF 和脑室 CSF 的连通提供了一个多孔屏障。排列在脑室壁和脊髓中央管壁的室管膜细胞具有顶端微绒毛和可运动纤毛结构。它们由许多缝隙结构连接在一起，调控细胞之间的电化学偶联，并使纤毛沿头 - 尾侧同步摆动。沿管腔边缘的室管膜细胞可分泌富含唾液酸的多糖 - 蛋白质复合物。唾液酸是一种带负电荷的糖类物质，可促进脑脊液层流并使脑脊液对室管膜表面产生排斥力（Jiménez et al.，2014）。将病毒神经氨酸酶（一种降解唾液酸的酶）注入大鼠脑室，发现在 4 小时内，大鼠中脑导水管发生堵塞（Grondona et al.，1996），随后，大部分室管膜脱落，侧脑室和第三脑室扩张。在成人脑积水患者中，室管膜广泛变薄或完全消失，纤毛消失（Bannister and Chapman，1980）。在患有中度脑积水和脊髓脊膜膨出的胎儿中可观察到室管膜剥脱、室管膜生发区（神经干细胞的位置）丢失和异常神经元迁移（Domínguez-Pinos et al.，2005；Sival et al.，2011）。室管膜对于大脑发育和功能不可或缺，其在这些病理生理过程中的作用机制有待进一步研究。

中枢神经系统中的流体动力学

一般流体动力学理论

苏格兰医生 Alexander Monro（Monro 孔就是以他命名的）和他的学生 George Kellie 于 19 世纪早期提出著名的 Monro-Kellie 假说。他们提出的压力 - 体积关系依然影响着现代医学教育。Monro-Kellie 假说认为，颅腔不可扩张，内容量固定，其内包含三种主要成分：脑组织、血液和脑脊液。脑组织是由神经细胞、胶质细胞和 ECF 组成。血管可分为动脉和静脉。颅内蛛网膜下腔（intracranial arachnoid space，SAS）可分为脑室和皮质 SAS，并可进一步细化为更多组成部分。

脑室系统包括两侧的侧脑室、第三脑室和第四脑室以及它们之间的连通通道。两侧侧脑室通过室间孔与第三脑室相连，第三脑室通过中脑导水管与第四脑室相连，第四脑室通过正中孔和两侧的侧孔分别与小脑延髓池和脑桥小脑角池连接。因此，在正常情况下，颅后窝的小脑延髓池与整个脑池、皮质和脊髓蛛网膜下腔相连通。脑组织在短期内可以承受一定压力，具有一定代偿空间。脑组织明显的体积变化，会影响到患者生命健康。在颅内占位性病变（如扩大的血肿），使脑脊液从脑室转移到脊髓蛛网膜下腔，硬脑膜静脉窦中的静脉血部分流入静脉系统汇入右心房。脑脊液通过脊髓蛛网膜下腔回流至静脉循环，脊髓蛛网膜下腔充当着类似于脑脊液体积和压力电容器的角色。脑脊液进入静脉循环的量与颅内压力呈直接线性关系。人的中枢神经系统具有很强的吸收能力。但当颅内蛛网膜下腔体积无法代偿时，诸如颅内血管或脑组织等部位就会受到影响。

虽然 Monro-Kellie 假说描述的是颅内占位性病变产生的影响，但其原理适用于涉及中枢神经系统内液体体积重新分布的所有病例。当中枢神经系统中任何一个部位体积发生变化时，其他部位对流体传导阻力会发生相应代偿性改变，其改变程度从高到低的顺序为：动脉、静脉和蛛网膜下腔。颅内空间是固定的，而脊髓 SAS 并不是。脊椎的硬膜外间隙主要包含脂肪和低压静脉丛，可压缩性很强。因此，脊髓 SAS 的主要功能之一是接受或者增加颅内蛛网膜下腔的脑脊液。

流体动力学障碍

在每个心动周期中，脑组织体积会随着动脉和静脉血容量的变化相应的增加或减少。因此，脑脊液的主要作用是充当缓冲液，保护大脑免受从收缩期到舒张期压力急剧波动的影响。正常的脑脊液流出要通过枕骨大孔，颅底和枕骨大孔周围的异常会干扰破坏正常的脑脊液生理循环。此外，脑脊液循环受到不同区域顺应性的影响。肥胖会降低脊髓顺应性，限制脑室静脉流出并降低脑室的顺应性。以上两种情况可见于特发性颅内高压（idiopathic intracranial hypertension，IIH）（以前称为假性脑瘤综合征）病例，并可发现 ICP 峰值升高和 ICP 平均值波动，以及 CSF 流速在枕骨大孔处增快。

Chiari Ⅰ型畸形患者有不同程度的小脑扁桃体下疝，并可能存在颅后窝发育不良。Chiari Ⅰ型畸形患者的小脑扁桃体位置很低，可能是脑脊液循环过程中的另一阻力因素。这个阻力来自枕骨大孔水平位置。当没有其他独立的病理因素存在时，只要脑室至脑皮质 SAS 的脑脊液循环保持畅通，脑积水就不会进展。然而通常可以在脊髓中央管水平观察到另一脑脊液间隙的扩张。Heiss 和他的同事们就这个问题撰写了大量的文章，揭示了 Chiari Ⅰ畸形中空洞形成的病理生理学过程（Heiss et al.，2012）。枕骨大孔处的高阻力提高了脑脊液在脊髓和脑室之间循环的流速和局部压力梯度。枕骨大孔和高位脊髓的局部蛛网膜下腔压力增大，脑脊液进入脊髓实质和中央管，并逐渐形成室管膜。当脊髓空洞形成后，随着每次心脏搏动，脊髓蛛网膜下腔和中央管之间产生的压力差梯度会进一步扩大。当脑和脊髓 SAS 之间脑脊液循环畅通时，脊髓空洞会逐渐消失。

脑池间的脑脊液流动

小脑延髓池（cisterna magna，CM）是脑脊循环的必经通道（见图 92.2），所有 CSF 都在此汇集。脑室系统的脑脊液经正中孔和成对的外侧孔流入 CM。很多学者认为，脑脊液自 CM 向下流至脊髓 SAS，然后返回向上进入基底池，进而与皮质 SAS 相沟通。这个观点与我们对解剖以及对脑脊液动力学的理解不一致。CM 是一个混合点、交叉点，其连接着各个空间的脑脊液，使它们之间的压力达到平衡。颅后窝减压术治疗 Chiari Ⅰ畸形及其多种变异，都为了重建畅通的小脑延髓池。CM 有多种流出途径：

- 从小脑后上方到四叠体池，然后通过环池与脚间池相连，包围中脑。
- 经桥小脑角池绕过桥脑 / 延髓到达脑桥池。脑脊液进一步的向上流动延伸并分散，最后到达大脑半球。
- 向下进入脊髓 SAS 和脊髓中央管。

脑池与脑脊液循环关系密切。在内镜下第三脑室底造瘘术（endoscopic third ventriculostomy，ETV）中，在第三脑室底部建立一个通道，将第三脑室与脚间池相连通。ETV 对于脑室和脚间池之间脑脊液

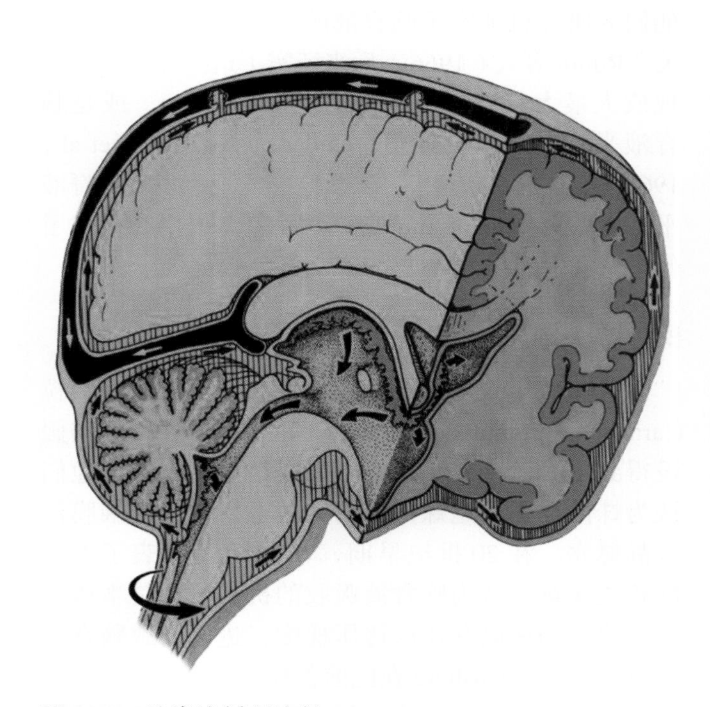

图 92.2 脑脊液循环途径

Reproduced from Rekate, H. L., The definition and classification of hydrocephalus: a personal recommendation to stimulate debate, *Cerebrospinal Fluid Research*, Volume 5, Issue 2, Copyright © 2008 Rekate; licensee BioMed Central Ltd.

流通受阻的患者是一个极好的选择。ETV 是继发性导水管狭窄或由第三室脑梗死引起的晚期脑积水的首选治疗方法。在部分蛛网膜下腔出血动脉瘤手术中，由于大脑前动脉及前交通动脉位于终板池内，第三脑室与基底池相连，通常可采用第三脑室前 - 下界终板造瘘。第三脑室前 - 下界终板造瘘的机制与 ETV 相同，所以这种术式在理论上是合乎逻辑。

脑脊液的吸收

我们目前对脑脊液吸收的认识源于：几十年前，科研人员将人工脑脊液输注到 SAS 进行的研究。在这些实验之前，人们就已发现，颅内压力高于静脉窦的压力，这种压力梯度促使 CSF 吸收。最初 Weed 和 Mortensen 在对狗的动物实验中发现，人工脑脊液输注量和脑脊液吸收量呈线性关系（Mortensen and Weed，1934；Weed，1935）。Pappenheimer 和他的同事以山羊作为实验动物，明确了脑脊液可随压力梯度汇入静脉系统（Pappenheimer et al.，1962）。他们研究表明，在某一压力阈值以下，脑脊液产生与吸收保持平衡，不发生脑脊液净吸收。一旦超过这个压力阈值，脑脊液压力和脑脊液吸收之间存在相应的线性关系，即脑脊液压力变化可导致 CSF 吸收程度发生改变，从而保持脑脊液总容量相对稳定。他们的研究也证实了脑脊液的产生与脑脊液压力无关。Rubin 等人（1966）后来证实了这些理论，并发现成人最大脑脊液吸收能力约 1.3 ml/min，或是脑脊液平均产生量的四倍。Cutler 等人（Cutler et al.，1968）进一步在儿童中证实了这些发现，发现脑脊液平均吸收阈值为 68 mm/H_2O。**图** 92.3 引用和描述了他们论文中的相关数据。

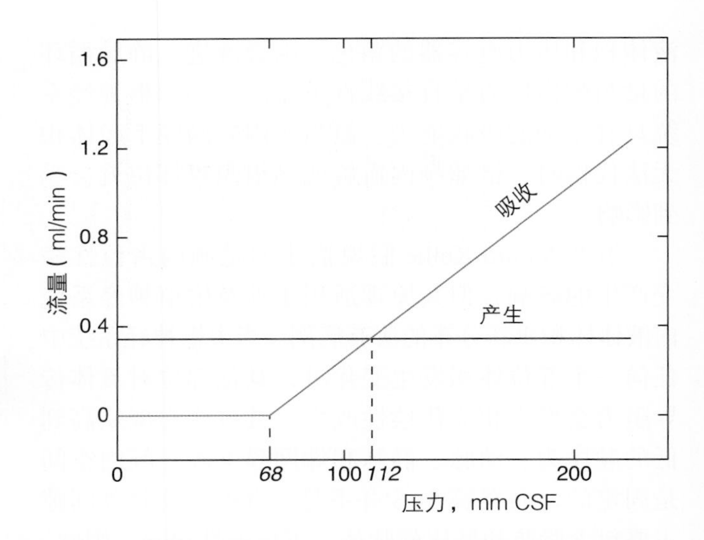

图 92.3 不同压力下的脑脊液吸收。脑脊液产生和吸收的叠加回归线作为吸收压力函数。横坐标为 112 mm 时，产生和吸收达到平衡。同时标注出了吸收为零时的压力值

蛛网膜颗粒

早在 18 世纪，就有解剖学家提出了蛛网膜颗粒（arachnoid granulations，AGs）的分泌作用。这些假设得到了 Luschka 和 Trolard 研究结果的支持，他们认为蛛网膜颗粒是蛛网膜的大绒毛，穿过硬脑膜汇入静脉窦。在 20 世纪早期，Weed 已经发表了大量的相关文章，认为脑脊液吸收的机制可能是半透性蛛网膜盲端两侧存在渗透压梯度，进而导致脑脊液的吸收。尽管 Cushing 在此前曾提出过这些增大的生物单向性通透结构理论，但直到半个世纪后他的观点才被证实是正确的。Welch 和他的同事们最先依靠光学显微镜在不同灌注压力下观察到灵长类动物的蛛网膜颗粒。他们观察到灵长类动物的蛛网膜绒毛在负压下变大，并形成复杂的迷宫状的细管状结构，这些细管结构可以允许微米级的颗粒通过（Welch and Friedman，1960；Welch and Pollay，1961）。随后，利用电子显微镜证实了细管结构是由内皮细胞形成的单向性液泡及孔道（Gómez et al.，1973；Tripathi，1974），同时，脑脊液压力与液泡 / 孔道形成的程度成正比（**图** 92.4）（Levine et al.，1982）。这些发现为多年前提出的脑脊液吸收行为理论提供了解剖学基础。这些吸收过程类似于瓣膜的功能。瓣膜开放需要一定压力，低于此压力时没有液体流动。一旦超过此压力，压力与液体流出量呈直接线性关系。随着时间的推移，机体自我调节使脑脊液的吸收与产生相匹配。诸如体位变化或脑血容量波动等因素，会以可代偿性的形式暂时使脑脊液的产生或吸收不平衡，但稳定的脑脊液循环容量可以长期维持。

脑脊液吸收的替代途径

传统观点认为，脑脊液仅由沿上矢状窦分布的蛛网膜颗粒吸收，然而这种观点并不完全正确。脑脊液吸收是一个综合的过程，除了蛛网颗粒外，脑脊液还可以通过淋巴、脊髓和神经根等途径被吸收。早在 1875 年，Key 和 Retzius 就发现了在尸体标本蛛网膜下腔注射台盼蓝示踪剂后，其在蛛网膜颗粒和颈部淋巴结中存在聚积。这些发现得到了 Weed 和他的同事们的证实，20 世纪许多研究也进一步印证了

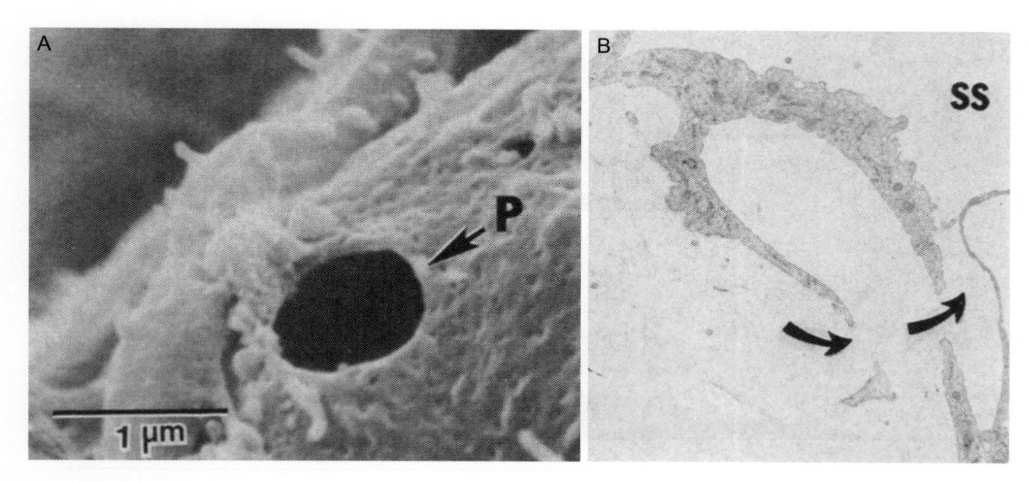

图 92.4　电镜下的蛛网膜颗粒

电子显微镜显示，在人工高压灌注脑脊液的情况下，蛛网膜绒毛突起形成到达静脉窦的小孔

这一观点。这些研究表明：脑脊液存在蛛网膜颗粒以外的其他吸收途径。在动物研究中发现，啮齿动物、兔子或猫中均不存在肉眼可见的 AGs。大型哺乳动物，如狗和反刍动物，AGs 的进化程度和数量都不如人类。我们只在灵长类动物中观察到接近人类大小和数量的蛛网膜颗粒，但相比于人类，在这些灵长类动物中观察到的 AGs 还是相对较少。从进化的角度来看，随着脑组织体积和复杂性的增加，脑脊液的产生比例也相应增加，同时这也相应需要更发达和高级的蛛网膜颗粒。除了这些解剖层面的观察了解，有实验表明，脑脊液传导性也随脑组织体积和复杂性的增加成比例增加（Mann et al.，1978）。

随着哺乳动物脑组织体积和复杂性的增加，脑脊液吸收从主要依赖神经周围和淋巴吸收途径，转变为更依赖于通过蛛网膜颗粒吸收入静脉循环的途径。人类脑脊液吸收主要通过蛛网膜颗粒，但蛛网膜颗粒以外的蛛网膜绒毛吸收途径同样起着很大的作用。这些因素共同构成了一个双重脑脊液吸收体系。蛛网膜绒毛在显微镜下才可观察到，一般在出生前后即可观察到蛛网膜绒毛，但到婴儿晚期或幼儿期才对脑脊液吸收产生作用（Gómez et al.，1982）。在胎儿发育期间以及婴儿早期，脑脊液吸收可能是通过更为原始的途径。这种原始途径主要依赖于蛛网膜颗粒以外的蛛网膜，而对蛛网膜颗粒的依赖相对较少（Oi and Di Rocco，2006）。随着神经系统的生长发育成熟，成人的脑脊液吸收主要以蛛网膜绒毛为主，如**图** 92.5 所示。因此，ETV 对新生儿及婴幼儿手术治愈率低可能与这一现象有关。

与正常受试者相比，脑积水患者随时间变化的压力 - 体积曲线也支持这种 CSF 双重吸收途径假说。有学者对正常人群进行人工脑脊液灌注研究，发现了一条平滑的半对数压力 - 容积曲线。研究表明，无论脑脊液灌注率高或低，吸收曲线均由明显的两种成分组成，这两种成分代表了不同的脑脊液吸收途径（Lorenzo et al.，1970；Nelson and Goodman，1971；Sokolowski，1976）。目前研究证实，在羊、狗和灵长类动物中，蛛网膜绒毛沿脊髓神经根分布（Welch and Pollay，1963；Gómez et al.，1974）。人类蛛网膜绒毛一般与神经根静脉并行或汇入其中（Tubbs et al.，2007）。Marmarou 等（1975）在对猫的脊髓和颅脑进行分离后发现脊髓蛛网膜绒毛吸收了脑脊液总产量的 15%。随后研究发现羊的脊髓蛛网膜绒毛可吸收 25% 左右的脑脊液（Bozanovic-Sosic et al.，2001）。据估计，在人类静息状态下，脊髓间隙可吸收约 40% 脑脊液，活动时，这一比例可增加到 75%（Edsbagge et al.，2004）。有证据表明，脑脊液在动物中还存在其他吸收途径，但其在人类尚缺乏相关证据，到目前为止，我们无法准确地量化人类脑脊液通过这些途径的吸收量。

脑脊液通过脑组织吸收途径存在争议。最近有许多关于脑脊液通过脑组织或淋巴重吸收的研究。此外，有些临床观察研究可以支持这一假设。在导水管梗阻患者中，由梗阻产生的脑室扩张速度远低于正常脑脊液的产生速度（Bering and Sato，1963），这种现象在不同动物模型中得到验证。在灵长类动物中，当导水管被堵塞时，首先表现为幕上脑室迅速扩张。一段时间后，这种扩张速率就会减缓，但这并不能代表脑室中脑脊液的产生减缓（Milhorat et al.，1970）。最近，通过磁共振电影成像（cine-MRI）观察脑脊液循环模型显示脑脊液在脑室内终末吸收

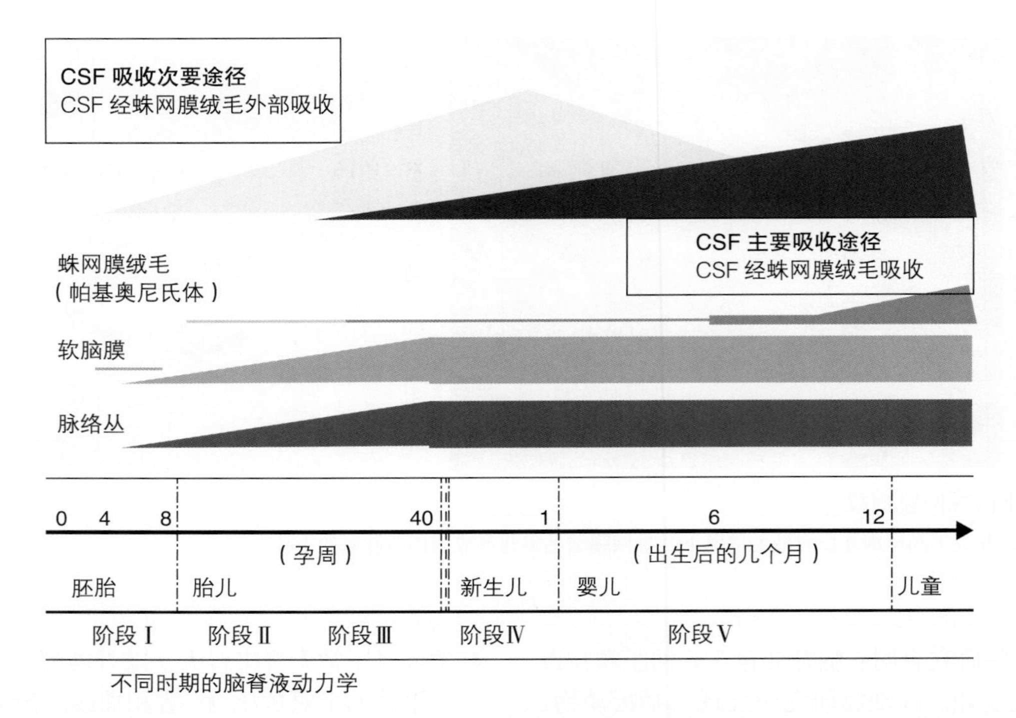

图 92.5 随着年龄的增长脑脊液吸收途径的发展变化。Oi 和同事提出的一岁以内脑脊液生产和吸收变化的理论

Reproduced with permission from Shizuo Oi, Concezio Di Rocco, Proposal of 'evolution theory in cerebrospinal fluid dynamics' and minor pathway hydrocephalus in developing immature brain, *Child's Nervous System*, Volume 22, Issue 7, Copyright © 2006 Springer Nature.

时出现回流逆转。这些发现是通过 MRI 对脑脊液流量进行评估，其依赖于专业软件、严格校准、数字减影、精确立体像素选择和高度衍生的数字模型。这些因素使这些结果的有效性受到质疑。此外，除了 MRI，尚缺乏其他脑脊液流量检查方法。

尽管目前没有直接精确量化方法，但我们可以认为脑脊液的很大一部分（大约 1/3）来自脑实质 ECF。近期，有许多文献介绍了脑脊液被脑组织吸收的特征。研究表明，各种示踪剂从颅内蛛网膜下腔通过组织间隙，汇入 Virchow-Robins 间隙内的小动脉或静脉微循环。这些示踪剂的转运是否能够真正代表脑脊液净流量或整体流量尚有待进一步考究。相对不通透的屏障严格调节着脑组织微环境中的溶质浓度。溶质是主动转运的，其严格地调节了水的流量。我们尚没明确除了从血浆进入脑脊液或细胞间隙以外的分子分泌的机制。虽然静水压力（ICP）可以增强细胞外液体在毛细血管重吸收，但如果没有从脑组织转运溶质的途径，就无法保持水分从脑组织向体循环转运。

在许多脑积水状态下，可以观察到的脑室周围水肿现象，称为脑室周围渗出。静水压力促使水通过室管膜进入脑室周围白质的细胞外间隙，降低其胶体渗透压。形成了一个渗透梯度，使细胞外水进入血管腔，并能转运大量的多余液体。水通道蛋白 4（AQP-4）在包绕着颅内血管的星形细胞足突上高表达，是血脑屏障不可分割的组成部分。大量研究表明：AQP-4 蛋白在脑积水动物模型的发生发展中起着一定作用，其对于室管膜的完整性是必要的（Li et al.，2009）。AQP-4 蛋白在脑积水模型和脑积水患者体内均表达上调（Castañeyra-Ruiz et al.，2013；Skjolding et al.，2013）。敲除 AQP-4 蛋白可诱发小鼠脑积水，脑积水程度远比正常小鼠严重。在细胞毒性水肿模型（如 TBI 和脑卒中）中，低表达 AQP-4 蛋白的小鼠比对照组水肿程度轻，恢复更好。在血管源性水肿（如肿瘤或脓肿）模型中，敲除 AQP-4 蛋白的小鼠水肿更明显，而且恢复明显比对照组差得多。这些发现表明 AQP-4 蛋白在水分调节中起着重要作用。

脑室扩张

我们可以很直观地观察脑室扩张的进展，但其潜在机制仍不明确。在不违反质量守恒定律前提下，如果脑组织和血容量保持稳定（我们假设它在短期内保持稳定），那如何解释脑室空间的大幅增加，如何解释脑室造瘘术或分流术后脑室大小迅速减小而头部并没有变小。

这些问题可以这样解释：通常 130~150 ml 脑脊

液中只有 50~60 ml 占据脑室空间，由此推测皮质 SAS 可以容纳大量脑脊液。脑室扩张初期，脑脊液体积不变，脑脊液重新分配到皮质蛛网膜下腔。脑室容量快速变化须伴随皮质蛛网膜下腔和脑池的相应变化，以保持脑组织和血管相对稳定。脑池和皮质蛛网膜下腔的体积变化很难用目前的成像技术来识别。**图** 92.6 示脑室和皮质 SAS 的理论模型。

皮层蛛网膜下腔厚度增加 2 mm，就可以代偿脑室容量减少 104 ml。皮质蛛网膜下腔容纳脑脊液的潜在能力，可能会通过脑沟、血管周围或 Virchow-Robins 间隙进一步增强。不适当的脑室过度引流会导致硬膜下积液，这其实是皮质蛛网膜下腔的大量扩张以代偿过度引流所致。如果脑脊液的产生和脊髓储备不能与引流相匹配，则可能发生桥静脉撕裂，导致血液流入硬膜下腔（转化为硬膜下血肿或 SDH）。

同样，对于未确诊的脑脊液漏患者，由于分流功能障碍而进行有创手术也同样存在弊端。由于脑室和皮质蛛网膜下腔之间的流动阻力大，任何位置的脑脊液漏都首先引流皮质 / 脑池蛛网膜下腔中的脑脊液。压力梯度、皮质 / 脑池的蛛网膜下腔容量和脑室 CSF 的持续产生将是脑室扩张的几个因素。还有一种情况是脑脊液压力低于瓣膜开启压力，放置脑室引流导管后只有在异常低位或负压引流时才能引流，进而导致脑室持续扩张。这种罕见的情况在神经外科文献中有诸多报道，这种情况下的脑室持续扩张，需识别和修复脑脊液漏。Rekate 等（2008）进一步强调了颅内脑脊液间隔之间的相互作用，他们在多个案例中证实，以弹性绷带对颈部稍加压力，可以迅速逆转脑室扩张，并可使患者恢复意识。压迫颈部静脉结构可增加脑血容量，增加脑肿胀或使脑顺应性降低。脑组织体积增加和脑顺应性的降低可使颅内压力增加，促进脑脊液吸收，这可以暂时减轻这类脑室扩张患者的症状，待明确脑脊液瘘的位置后，进一步采取有效的治疗。

脑积水按梗阻位置的分型

以往对于各种导致脑积水（梗阻性脑积水、交通性脑积水等）的病理生理学机制描述甚少（见**专栏** 92.1）。而事实上，所有形式的脑积水都具有梗阻性。在脑脊液循环中，梗阻的位置决定了脑室扩张的形式。于是，我们提出一种分类方法，即脑脊液从产生到终末吸收过程中，依据从近端到远端的梗阻位

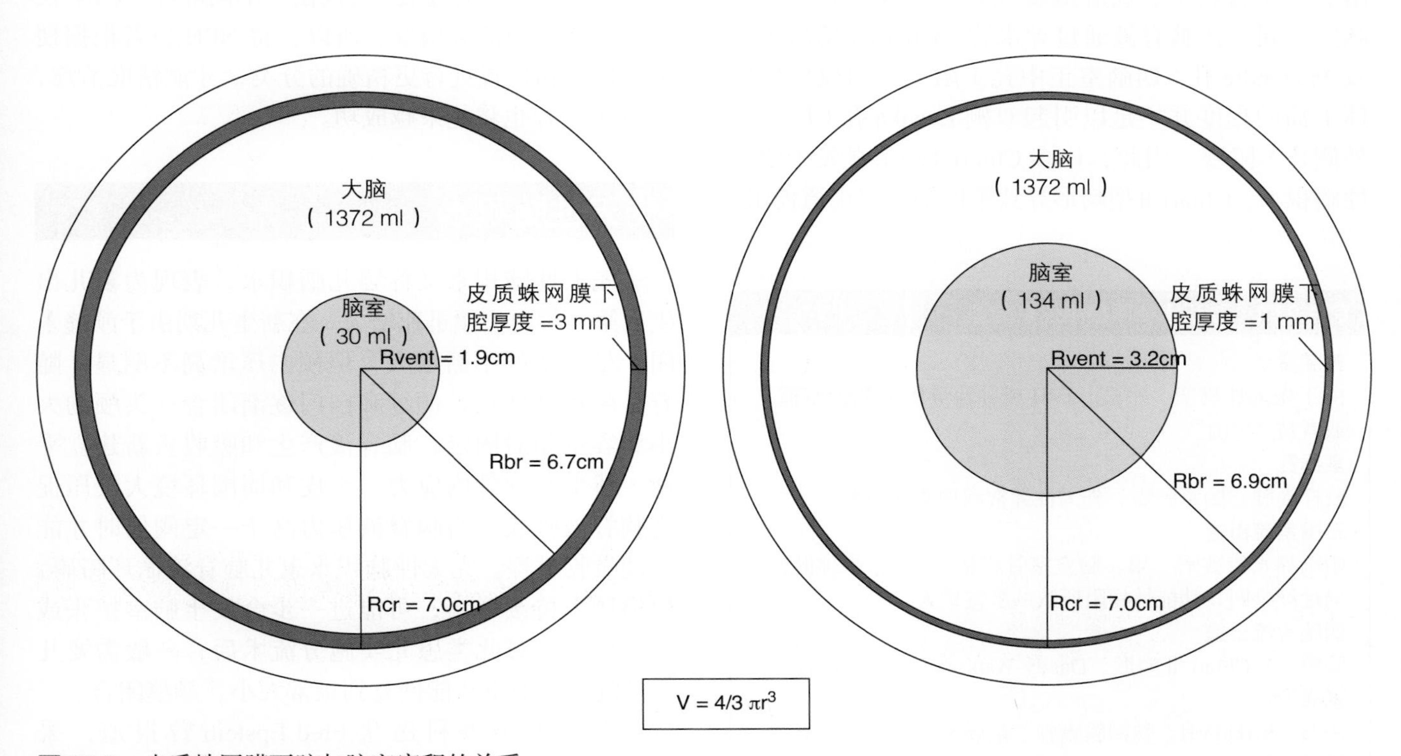

图 92.6 皮质蛛网膜下腔与脑室容积的关系

左图：显示正常或分流术后的正常脑室容积（V）。右图：当皮质蛛网膜下腔厚度从 3 mm 减少到 1 mm 时，脑室系统大小会发生可见性变化。在图示中，大脑的体积保持不变

点来分类。两个侧脑室脑脊液含量最多，且包含着四个脑室中绝大部分的脉络丛。因此，双侧侧脑室是脑脊液流向远端的驱动因素。从最近端开始，侧脑室本身可从内部发生阻塞。肿瘤、水肿或血肿对侧脑室的压迫可能会孤立脉络丛，导致“被孤立”的脑室进行性扩张，这常见于颞角，即“孤立颞角”，严重者可导致沟回疝，甚至危及生命。

一些病理因素可阻塞室间孔，导致一侧或两侧侧脑室进行性扩张。继发于单侧脑室过度引流的功能性梗阻已在前文描述。负压吸引使透明隔移位，在同侧尾状核头上方阻塞室间孔。分流产生的抽吸作用使相应的脑室处于隔离状态，如最初的病理因素持续存在，对侧脑室将进一步扩张。长期过度引流的另一个后果是室管膜内膜粘连或形成瘢痕。这种情况可能在第三脑室发生，导致侧脑室扩张，或发生在中脑导水管，导致三个幕上脑室全部扩张。虽然传统认为幕上三个脑室扩张是由导水管狭窄引起的，但是经分流术或ETV重建导水管后，发现存在功能性梗阻病例，如侧脑室后部扩张产生的压迫（Rekate，2007）。

第四脑室的Dandy-Walker囊肿（第四脑室中侧孔先天性闭锁）或其他病变导致第四脑室流出道梗阻、导水管狭窄。囊肿造瘘或切除病变可恢复第四脑室空间，使脑脊液通过导水管。Chiari Ⅰ畸形可导致Magendie孔（四脑室正中孔）阻塞，但仅凭扁桃体下疝的程度并不足以引起双侧Lushka孔（四脑室外侧孔）阻塞。因此，许多Chiari Ⅰ畸形继发于原发性脑积水。Chiari Ⅱ型畸形导致第四脑室流出道梗阻，

专栏 92.1 脑积水依照梗阻位点分型
侧脑室
由于先天性病变、瘢痕、IVH或肿块导致的侧脑室孤立或者被“包围”
室间孔
胶样囊肿、脑室肿瘤、先天性异常和功能性梗阻 *
三脑室流出道
中脑导水管狭窄、第三脑室室管膜粘连 *、松果体肿瘤、局灶纤维网、功能性梗阻所致的脑室扩大
四脑室流出道
脑膜炎、Chiari Ⅱ畸形、Dandy-Walker综合征、肿瘤
基底池
NPH、SAH/IVH、蛛网膜囊肿、脑膜炎
终端吸收
婴儿期静脉高压（Galen静脉畸形）、脉络膜丛乳头状瘤、维生素A不足
* 继发性过度引流

所有脑室扩张。羊水和脑脊液的混合液体通过发育存在缺陷的开放性神经管，导致在基底池产生密集瘢痕和粘连。再加上更大程度的下疝，脑室在功能上与脊髓和皮质蛛网膜下腔分离，这类患者由于ETV失败率高，更倾向于采用脑脊液分流术的治疗。

脑池内的脑脊液流动受阻将导致所有脑室扩张（大多数NPH病例的可能病因）。脑室外的脑脊液间隙梗阻可在神经影像学上有所表现，以推测其梗阻部位。这些资料有益于对患者选择最合适的手术方式。动脉瘤破裂导致的蛛网膜下腔出血（subarachnoid haemorrhage，SAH）引发的脑积水的原因与此相似，出血通过物理性阻碍脑脊液通过脑池，并可能在远期形成瘢痕。在极其罕见的情况下，个别患者可能产生脑脊液过多，比如自发性或脉络丛乳头状瘤等因素。如果脑脊液的产生量超过脑脊液的吸收能力，脑室就可能发生扩张。因此，脑脊液循环阻塞部位也可以发生在最远端点，如AGs。

研究显示，许多NPH病例是多病因的，ETV在治疗多病因导致的NPH的效果不明确。NPH的定义为脑室扩大与皮质萎缩不成比例，并具有一系列典型症状。NPH的病因包括从迟发性导水管狭窄、限制脑脊液从基底池近端到最远端皮质蛛网膜下腔，或婴幼儿脑积水的进展/失代偿等不同部位。ETV仅可以解决其中部分病变。所以，将NPH患者根据梗阻的性质和位置进行更精确的分类，才能精准治疗，NPH的治疗也将越来越成功。

先天性脑积水

先天性脑积水又称婴儿脑积水，表现为婴儿出生后第一年内头颅迅速增大。在新生儿期由于颅缝未闭，虽然头颅不断增大，但颅内压增高不明显。随着月龄逐渐增长，颅缝和囟门逐渐闭合，头颅的大小和容量相对固定，脑脊液产生和吸收重新建立平衡。新生儿颅骨内应力，头皮和周围环境大气压促进脑脊液吸收。当脑脊液压力高于一定阈值时才能启动吸收过程。先天性脑积水患儿脑脊液循环障碍，颅内压力持续增高，可能进一步会发生脑室扩张或头围变大。对此类患儿实施分流术后，一般需要几个月的时间脑室才能恢复到正常大小，颅缝闭合。

小儿神经外科医生Fred Epstein曾报道，采用加压包扎头部来治疗婴儿脑积水并取得了成功（Epstein et al.，1974）。其理论依据是：压迫头部使ICP超过脑脊液吸收压力阈值，促使脑脊液吸收。尽管神经外科界几乎从未有人采用这种治疗方

法，但 Epstein 表示已经成功治疗了 8/10 名婴儿，避免了采用分流术等有创治疗。ETV 治疗先天性脑积水的成功率与婴儿年龄成反比，小于 6 个月的患儿疗效较差。虽然在幕上脑室和基底池之间建立了有效的脑脊液循环通道，但在人工造瘘口远端存在较高的脑脊液吸收阻力。同时，新生儿颅骨无法产生足够吸收脑脊液所需的内应力。尽管 ETV 有效，但患儿脑室和头围仍持续增大。婴儿期颅内静脉高压引起的脑积水原理与以上相似。Galen 静脉畸形患儿的静脉流体静压力升高导致婴儿脑积水（因为皮质 SAS 的脑脊液压力必须超过静脉压力大约 5 cmH_2O，脑脊液才能发生净吸收）。

结论

脑积水不是一种单病因疾病，而是一系列诱发脑室扩张因素所致的复杂疾病。临床上经常存在没有仔细分析个体特有解剖学和生理学特征就进行脑脊液分流手术的情况。我们应根据不同患者制订个体化治疗方案。终身体内留置引流管严重影响患者生活质量。神经外科医生通常会让患者依赖于人工机械设备，而这些机械设备无法再现正常的生理机能。了解正常的脑脊液生理及病理状态，可使临床医生采用最佳方案治疗患者。脑积水虽然是常见的疾病，但治疗管理手段有限。我们需充分认识脑脊液动力学的复杂性。我们有责任创新 CSF 循环技术并开发能够调节 CSF 动力学的药物。

参考文献、EBRAIN 的相关链接

扫描书末二维码获取。

第 93 章　脑脊液分流术和神经内镜手术

Ian K. Pople・William Singleton 著
孙玉晨 译，张庆九 审校

引言

脑脊液（cerebrospinal fluid，CSF）的管理是一门复杂的“临床学科”，需要充分了解脑脊液生理和病理状态，全面了解现有分流类型的优缺点和各自特性。神经内镜技术快速发展成为神经外科的一项核心技能，为脑积水的治疗提供了新的选择。在本章中，我们将对脑脊液生理学、脑脊液分流原理以及分流类型进行详细描述。其中一节将专门介绍内镜下脑脊液分流技术，包括详细介绍第三脑室底造瘘术的应用。

脑脊液生理学

脑脊液主要有以下四种功能：

1. 浮力作用：维持脑组织“漂浮状态”，起到缓冲作用。
2. 排泄大分子量亲水性代谢废物。
3. 中枢神经系统（central nervous system，CNS）神经肽的循环和转运（在胎儿和婴儿早期发育过程中尤为重要）。
4. 维持中枢神经系统细胞内稳态。

脑脊液主要由脑室系统的脉络丛产生，其他约 1/3 的脑脊液由脑室壁的软脑膜 - 室管膜产生。脑脊液从侧脑室通过室间孔到达第三脑室，通过中脑导水管进入第四脑室，再通过第四脑室两个外侧孔和正中孔进入幕下池和脊髓蛛网膜下腔。

传统观点认为，大部分脑脊液主要由静脉窦旁的蛛网膜颗粒吸收。然而越来越多的证据表明，蛛网膜颗粒仅为脑脊液吸收途径之一。在正常生理条件下，大量 CSF 还可通过脑组织血管周围间隙被重吸收。脑脊液中的水分也可以通过水通道主动转运到颅内的毛细血管和星形胶质细胞终足（Brinker et al., 2014）。这些发现解释了急性脑积水在 CT 和 MR 上脑室周围水肿 / 高信号的影像学表现。

脑脊液动力学

成人脑脊液约占颅内容积的 9%。儿童脑室较小，颅内脑脊液相对于脑组织和血液较少。脑脊液循环的压力 / 动力学由以下三个因素控制：

1. 脑脊液产生
2. 脑室顺应性
3. 脑脊液吸收

正常情况下，不论颅内压（intracranial pressure，ICP）如何波动，脑脊液是以恒定速率产生的。脑脊液体积增大，脑室和脑组织的弹性就会降低。脑脊液吸收阻力定义为硬脑膜静脉窦的压力与脑脊液在蛛网膜颗粒的压力之差（假设大部分脑脊液在蛛网膜颗粒处被吸收）。在正常静息状态下，ICP 等于脑脊液压力。因此，ICP 可以定义为：

$$ICP=I_F \times R_O+R_D$$

其中 I_F= 脑脊液产生速率，R_o= 脑脊液吸收阻力，R_D= 硬脑膜静脉窦压力。

因此，从脑脊液动力学的角度来看，颅内压升高可能是由于脑脊液产生增加、脑脊液吸收阻力增加或硬脑膜静脉窦压力增加所致。这个公式解释了硬脑膜静脉窦闭塞如何直接影响脑脊液压力和 ICP。

脑脊液分流术和脑脊液分流原理

脑积水是一种因脑脊液体积增加而造成以脑组织损害为特征的疾病。脑积水通常合并颅内压升高，如果不及时治疗，严重者可导致死亡或严重功能障碍。脑积水的主要治疗方法是脑脊液分流术。

分流装置的流体动力学

在对患者进行治疗前，应熟知颅内压力和脑脊液流量之间的关系，从而选择个体化治疗方案（Chari

et al., 2014）。脑脊液分流的流量取决于诸多因素，包括脑室端压力（IVP）、流体静力压（p）、分流泵开启压力（OPV）和分流管远端压力（如腹腔内压力，IAP）。因此，标准脑室-腹腔分流术的压力梯度（ΔP）可以定义为：

$$\Delta P=IVP+p-OPV-IAP$$

流体静力压（p）是分流管直立时产生的压力、CSF 密度和重力的乘积。OPV 是一个常数，而 IVP 和 IAP 则会随着体位的改变而变化。影响流体静力压变化的主要因素是分流管直立时产生的压力（受分流管长度影响），因此临床上缩短远端分流管长度将影响脑脊液流量。

脑脊液通过分流管的流量（F）等于压力梯度（ΔP）除以管内阻力（R_T）和分流泵内阻力（R_V）。

$$F=\Delta P/(R_T+R_V)$$

分流管内阻力可以用泊肃叶（Poiseuille）定律计算（只要不缩短分流管长度，分流管内阻力就是一个恒定常数）。因此，脑脊液在分流管的流量受以下几种因素影响：

1. 患者基本条件和 IVP。
2. 患者的体位。
3. 分流系统的阻力。

虹吸作用

蛛网膜颗粒和静脉窦（脑脊液主要流出道）之间的压力差不受姿势体位的影响。然而，有些分流术后的患者坐起/站立时，分流管远端和脑室内压力差增加，分流流量会迅速增加，从而导致脑脊液的过度引流（Petrella et al., 2008; Farahmand et al., 2015）。临床上常表现为患者从平卧位转为站立位时出现相关症状（**表** 93.1）。长期过度引流是诱发裂隙脑室综合征的重要危险因素。

表 93.1　引流过度导致的症状/临床表现和影像学特征

症状	临床表现和影像学特征
站立位时头痛、恶心（平卧位时症状缓解）	脑神经麻痹（重症患者）
站立位时耳鸣、眩晕（平卧位时症状缓解）	Chiari 畸形
嗜睡、昏迷（重症患者）	硬膜下积液
	裂隙样脑室/脑室塌陷

脑脊液分流装置的类型

脑脊液分流术式的选择

脑脊液分流术指通过手术植入分流管，将脑脊液从脑室（或腰大池等）转移到体内其他部位。最常见的分流远端部位是腹腔、右心房或胸腔。**表** 93.2 汇总了近端和远端分流部位及各自优缺点。分流管的脑室端通常通过额部或顶枕部穿刺放置于脑室内，两种方法各有优缺点（**表** 93.2）。有医生提倡应用术中神经导航辅助，以确保分流管脑室端位于最佳位置。

分流泵

分流泵主要有两种类型：一种是流量调节分流泵（flow-regulated valve），另一种是压力控制分流泵（Czosnyka et al., 2002）。压力控制分流泵主要又分为固定压力分流泵、重力分流泵及可调压分流泵。大部分分流泵的治疗有效性数据是由厂家提供的，目前尚缺乏随机对照试验系统比较不同分流泵优劣。迄今为止只有一项随机对照研究对比了应用不同类型分流泵的临床预后，结果发现患者术后生存期没有任何临床差异（Drake et al., 1998）。因此，需要了解这些分流泵的特性，并根据患者个体情况选择最合适的分流系统。

流量调节分流泵

流量调节分流泵系统是通过调节 CSF 流出的阻力来维持 CSF 的稳定流量。例如 Integra OSV Ⅱ® 的分流泵系统中存在一个人工红宝石，嵌于一个可活动环内。它们以固定压力分流泵的形式工作，但当 ICP 超过一定阈值时，红宝石嵌入位置向下移动，流出孔变小，流动阻力增加。在一定的 ICP 范围内，脑脊液保持着恒定的流速。随着 ICP 进一步增加，可活动环向下位移，打开流出孔，减少流动阻力（**图** 93.1）。

有脑脊液过度引流风险或可能发展为裂隙脑室综合征的患者可考虑应用此类分流泵。目前的数据显示，与其他类型分流泵相比，其在改善低颅压症状方面存在优势（Drake et al., 1998; Hanlo et al., 2003）。但流量调节分流泵与固定压力分流泵对脑积水的治疗效果没有明显差异（Hanlo et al., 2003; Ziebell et al., 2013）。

表 93.2 分流管的近端位置、远端位置及其各自优缺点

分流装置位置	优点	缺点
近端		
侧脑室额角	• 没有神经导航系统辅助时，脑室的解剖位置相对明确，脑室穿刺置管较为简单（尤其在脑室较小的患者中） • 脉络丛较少	• 需要另行切口以置入分流管及分流泵（通常分流泵置于同侧耳郭后方） • 术后短期内脑室端分流管堵塞率较高 • 术中常需要调整头部位置
侧脑室枕角	• 手术过程中不需变换体位 • 导管脑室端部分较长，术后短期内脑室端分流管阻塞率较低 • 头部只需一个切口，调管更加方便	• 没有神经导航系统辅助时，脑室穿刺置管较为困难
腰大池	• 适合脑室较小（例如特发性颅高压患者）并需行分流手术的患者	• 存在体位性过度引流和诱发 Chiari Ⅰ型畸形的风险 • 需要添加更为复杂的重力分流泵
远端		
腹腔	• 腹腔容积较大，更容易吸收脑脊液 • 手术时腹腔易于探及 • 神经外科核心手术技能之一，目前广泛应用于临床	• 腹压高时可能影响分流效果 • 腹腔多处粘连的患者手术存在一定难度 • 脑脊液蛋白含量高时，可能影响腹腔对脑脊液的吸收效果（“CSF 腹水”）
右心房	• 远端分流阻塞发生率比脑室 - 腹腔分流和脑室 - 胸膜分流低 • 适用于脑脊液蛋白含量高的患者 • 腹腔或胸膜分流术后复发的脑积水患者，可优先选择右心房作为远端置管端	• 分流性肾炎 • 手术难度大，技术要求高（非常规手术）；如需二次手术（调整引流管位置等），手术难度与风险进一步增加 • 分流性感染可能会导致全身的症状表现，如心内膜炎 • 理论上存在诱发心律失常的风险
胸膜	• 手术相对简单	• 胸膜吸收脑脊液的能力低于腹膜 • 吸气时胸腔内负压可增加虹吸作用，导致过度引流 • 脑脊液蛋白含量高时，可能影响胸膜对脑脊液的吸收效果
CSF 脑池（小脑延髓池）“Torkildsen 分流”	• 绕过脑室梗阻部位，直接在中枢神经系统内进行脑脊液分流，目前很大程度已被脑室镜技术代替	• 手术难度大，技术要求高（非常规手术）
膀胱	• 目前尚未在临床中应用	• 感染 • 内脏受损 • 需二次手术时难度较大
胆囊	• 目前尚未在临床中应用	• 感染 • 内脏受损 • 需二次手术时难度较大

固定压力分流泵

固定压力分流泵的工作方式非常简单（开启压力和关闭压力）。当分流泵近端的 IVP 和分流泵远端的 CSF 压力差高于分流泵开启压力时，分流泵开始工作，允许 CSF 流动。但是，由于分流泵本身的工作机制，其关闭压力可能低于开启压力，在没有虹吸作用的情况下仍可能出现过度引流，进而引发相关症状。目前固定压力分流泵有多种类型，每种类型都会根据其压力范围（高、中、低）进行细分。按作用机制大致可分为四类：隔膜泵（diaphragm valve）、球锥形泵（ball-in-cone valve）、斜顶泵（mitre valve）和狭缝泵（slit valve）（**表** 93.3）。

重力分流泵

重力分流泵利用重力改变开启压力，减少患者体位变化带来的虹吸效应。它们属于球锥形泵，但带有额外的重力单元配件。当患者直立时，分流泵内的球体会移动到圆锥内，增加阻力，减少流出量

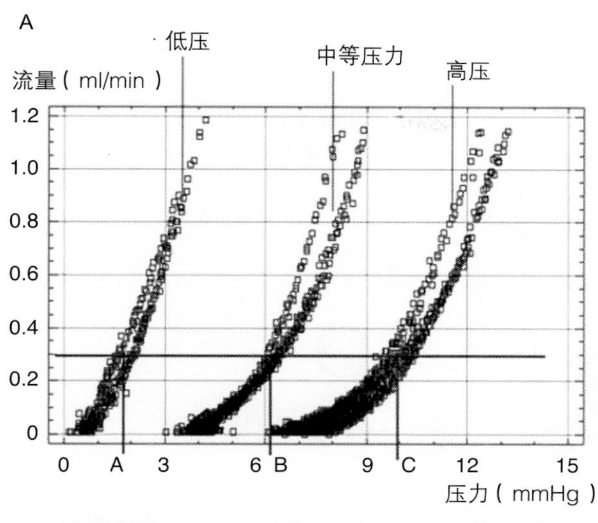

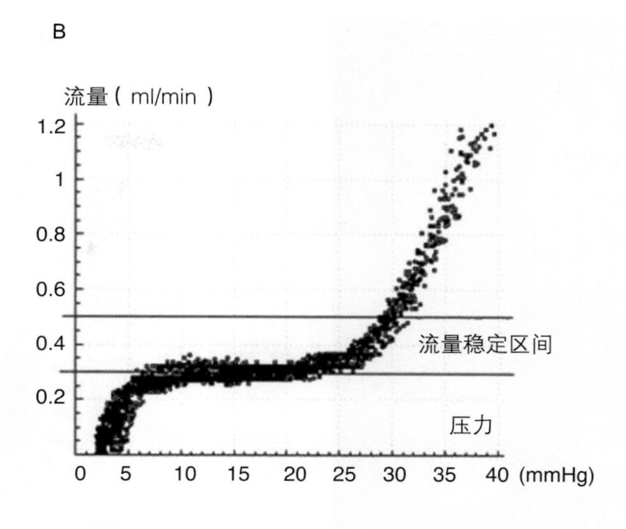

图 93.1　分流泵的压力/流量关系。(A)三种固定压力分流泵;(B)流量控制分流泵

表 93.3　固定压力分流泵示例与设计

固定压力分流泵	示例	优点	缺点
隔膜泵	• Sophysa Pulsar® • Medtronic Delta®	简易；储液囊靠近分流泵，CSF 采样相对容易	硅胶容易老化
球锥形泵	• Codman® Hakim	不容易老化	当 CSF 中存在絮状物或浑浊时，易发生阻塞
斜顶泵	• Integra™ Mischler Valve	具有直接流出道，即使 CSF 混浊，发生阻塞概率仍较低	硅胶容易老化
狭缝泵	• Sophysa Phoenix® • Holter-Hausner® • Codman® Unishunt	操作简单，性价比高。体积小(适用于新生儿)。可以放置在近端或远端	易发生虹吸。不能经分流泵采集 CSF

(例如 Integra™ H-V® 分流系统和 Mithke Pro-Gav® 分流系统)。与其他所有分流泵一样，此类分流泵也存在开启压力，其取决于分流管直立时产生的压力，因此应该根据患者的身高来选择。腰大池分流术应用重力分流泵，可以减少体位性过度引流。

可调压分流泵

可调压分流泵具有不同压力档位，可以通过外部磁场来调节。其优点是可以根据患者症状，无创性改变分流泵工作压力。缺点是强磁场(如 MRI)可能会干扰分流泵压力设置。因此需要充分告知患者避免接触强磁场。同时要注意患者在行 MRI 检查后，需检查分流泵参数设置(Lollis et al., 2010)(通常应用 X 线平片)(**图** 93.2)。

目前缺乏有关可调压分流泵与固定压力分流泵的疗效对比的数据资料。可调压分流泵主要用于先天性正压脑积水(idiopathic normal pressure hydrocephalus，iNPH)的治疗，根据患者临床表现逐步降低分流泵的开启压力，可有效降低 iNPH 患者术后脑脊液的过度引流和硬膜下积液的发生率。无创性调节分流泵工作压力，有助于降低脑室顺应性低的患者术后远期发生硬膜下积液的风险。对青少年或儿童脑积水患者，随着患儿身高的增长，逐步调整分流泵的开启压力，有助于降低术后远期发生硬膜下积液的风险。目前尚无数据表明，可调压分流泵是否可以降低部分儿童长期过度引流并发症的发生率或分流系统阻塞的发生概率。

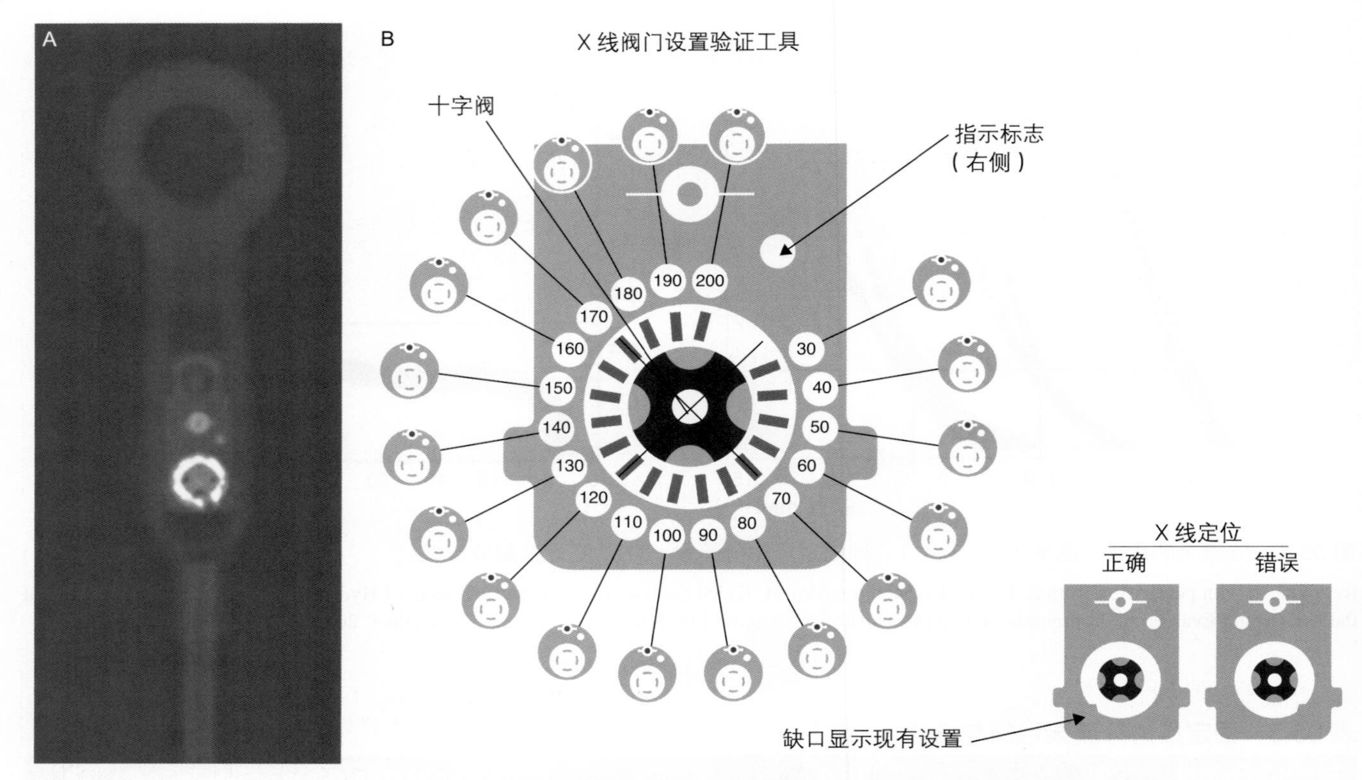

图 93.2 Codman Hakim®（Depuy-Synthes）可编程调节分流泵的平片影像和图解。可以用 X 线平片检查分流泵设置，并验证分流泵（A）与相对应的缺口位置设置（由英国 Codman Depuy-Synthes 提供）。其他分流泵设计也使用类似的方法来确定分流泵设置

手术治疗

脑室外引流术

脑室外引流术（external ventricular drain，EVD）是一种临时引流脑脊液的术式，是急性脑积水患者的抢救措施。适应证包括：脑室出血、颅内感染或者可逆性急性脑积水患者（不需行脑脊液分流术）。EVD 置管的手术步骤见**专栏** 93.1。

脑室 – 腹腔分流术

侧脑室枕角是最常用的分流管脑室端置入部位，也有医生为减少脉络膜丛阻塞分流管，倾向于穿刺额角。

目前临床广泛应用神经导航辅助（该技术逐渐普及且相关成本逐渐降低），以确保分流管置于脑室内的最佳位置。手术步骤见**专栏** 93.2。

脑脊液分流术失败的检查

对于怀疑有脑脊液循环功能障碍，存在分流手术指征的患者，应立即进行以下术前准备：

- 头颅 CT 平扫（包括脑室体积信息采集等，如需术中影像学引导，则需行颅脑 CT 三维重建）。
- 包括整个分流体系的 X 线平片：脑室 - 腹腔分流术患者需行颅骨、颈部、胸部、腹部平片（“分流系列平片”）。对于拟置入可调压泵分流系统的患者，还需行分流泵的切线位 X 线平片，以准确检查分流泵的参数设置。
- 实验室检查：包括血常规、凝血常规、血生化，脑脊液常规、脑脊液生化。当怀疑感染时，需检测 C 反应蛋白、血液和脑脊液培养。

记录拟植入的分流泵类型。对疑似分流失败的患者（尤其是复杂脑积水患儿）应尽快行 MRI 检查。

脑脊液分流术后感染

脑脊液分流术后感染后果严重（Di Rocco et al.，1994）。多种因素可导致脑脊液分流术后感染，遵循指南推荐方案可显著降低脑脊液分流术后感染率（Kestle et al.，2011）。目前已研制出一些预防术后感染的分流装置并已应用于临床。多项研究表明，应用抗生素浸泡分流装置（如 Bactiseal）或具有抑制细

专栏 93.1 脑室外引流术

- 垫高头部，保持头部微屈 30°（如使用神经影像导航系统，需钉子头架固定头部）。
- 如使用神经影像导航系统，需设置导航信息，将患者的信息准确录入。
- 若无明显禁忌（右侧脑室额角血肿，不对称脑室扩张），首选穿刺右侧脑室额角。
- 备皮，常规消毒，消毒备皮范围至少距手术切口 5 cm（术中形成皮下隧道置管引流）。
- 常规铺单，使双侧耳屏及同侧内眦可见或容易触及。
- 穿刺点位于冠状缝前 1~2 cm，中线旁开 3 cm，设计手术切口，使其不与计划内的其他手术（脑室镜手术或翼点开颅夹闭前循环动脉瘤手术等）切口冲突。
- 仔细止血，需特别注意骨缘（骨蜡止血）、硬脑膜和软脑膜出血（双极止血）。
- 朝向同侧内眦和耳屏连线汇合点（室间孔通常位于此），垂直于脑表面置入引流管，置入深度 5~6 cm（如果此时没有脑脊液流出，需拔出引流管调整穿刺方向重新穿刺）。
- 置管深度至少距皮缘 5 cm。
- 妥善固定引流管，避免引流管“脱出”，保持引流管通畅，妥善包扎。
- 连接外部引流装置（无菌条件下），固定引流瓶高度并记录。

** 外科医师可以根据具体情况决定是否应用神经影像导航系统（包括术中超声定位等）。神经影像导航系统尤其适用于解剖异常的患者（例如存在中线移位）。

菌黏附涂层的分流装置（如 Silverline®），可以降低术后感染发生。然而，这些具有抑菌涂层的分流装置仅对常见病原体存在一定的抑制作用，并不能完全消除术后感染发生风险，目前尚无证据支持其优于相对廉价的分流装置（Klimo et al.，2014）。一项英国的多中心前瞻性随机试验（https://www.basics.org.uk）刚刚完成，评估了不同类型分流管与标准分流管的对比疗效。我们饶有兴趣地等待结果公布。

神经内镜手术治疗脑积水

20 年前神经内镜技术就已经用于治疗脑积水，如第三脑室底造瘘术（ETV）。随着神经内镜技术的进步、光学设备的改进和图像显示的提升（包括高清晰度和最近的 3D 技术），使手术的准确性和安全性得到提高，神经内镜技术治疗脑积水又成为学界关注的焦点。越来越多的神经外科医生选择应用神经内镜治疗脑积水，避免了传统脑脊液分流术后较多的并发症，为脑积水患者提供了新的治疗手段。

专栏 93.2 脑室 - 腹腔分流术手术注意事项

- **术前注意事项**：术前备皮，预防性应用抗生素。
- **手术室准备**：尽可能减少手术室人员数量（确保手术安全为前提），减少人员往来。保持手术室门关闭，佩戴外科口罩。如条件允许，可应用层流手术室。
- **患者体位**：将气管插管置于远离术区一侧。确保患者体位可以顺利完成整个手术操作。
- **术区的准备**：标记手术切口。术区常规消毒铺单，手术切口注射局麻药物。
- **手术技术**：佩戴双层手套，尽量不要触碰手术切口边缘。消毒剂浸泡过的纱布覆盖手术切口边缘。
- **建立分流管隧道**，放置分流泵：应用通条建立皮下隧道（部分医生倾向于从远端建立皮下隧道，这样操作相对简便易行）。确保分流泵放置部位足够大，以容纳分流泵并避免分流管打折。
- **分流装置配件的处理**：在远离患者的区域更换新手套，打开分流装置，预装分流装置配件（术中应用无齿镊操作分流装置），向分流装置注入生理盐水并浸泡于生理盐水中。
- **止血和切口缝合**：缝合手术切口时，应充分止血，切口皮缘贴合对齐（这在婴儿手术中尤为重要）。
- **其他**：常规鞘内注射抗生素；使用特定的皮肤消毒剂或铺巾；使用抗生素液体浸泡分流装置。

神经内镜辅助第三脑室底造瘘术

历史

1923 年，Mixter 首次成功应用小型尿道镜对一位 9 月龄非交通性脑积水患儿实施了第三脑室底造瘘术（Mixter，1923）。早在 1935 年（Scarff，1936），Scarff 教授就主张应用 ETV 治疗梗阻性脑积水，但当时只有个例报道或小宗病例研究。直到 20 世纪八九十年代 ETV 才得以普及。ETV 的适应证见**专栏 93.3**。

专栏 93.3 神经内镜第三脑室底造瘘术适应证

绝对适应证：
- 导水管狭窄
- 梗阻性脑积水且脑室扩张明显
- 患有脊柱裂或分流管阻塞的老年患者
- 由松果体区或颅后窝肿瘤引起的梗阻性脑积水（治疗脑积水同时，可视具体情况应用神经内镜进行活检）

相对适应证：
- 导水管狭窄或有脊柱裂新生儿
- 交通性脑积水或分流管阻塞

解剖

ETV 的操作步骤见**专栏** 93.4。脑室镜进入侧脑室额角（通常为右侧）后，可沿丘纹静脉或透明隔静脉探及室间孔（两者通常于室间孔交汇），室间孔处的脉络丛在脉络膜裂中向前延伸或穿过（**图** 93.3）。将脑室镜穿过室间孔后（特别注意不要损伤或过度牵拉穹隆），可以识别出第三室底的典型特征。进而可探及乳头体、漏斗隐窝和终板（**图** 93.3）。透过变薄的第三脑室底可见桥前池中的基底动脉。

术前准备

所有患者术前均应完善颅脑 CT 平扫以明确梗阻性脑积水诊断，完善颅脑 MRI 检查明确梗阻位置。例如：矢状面 MRI 有助于显示第三脑室或导水管是否畅通（也可应用 Cine-MRI 辅助检查）。MRI 可辅助明确侧脑室、第三脑室和第四脑室的相对大小，以及基底动脉和桥前间隙的解剖结构，评估脑室镜进入桥前池在技术上是否可行。如果术中使用神经导航辅助，应进行 CT 三维立体成像检查。如条件允许，最好加做稳态干扰（constructive interference in steady state，CISS）序列或等效序列，提供正中矢状面的高分辨率 T2 MR 图像，从而清楚了解脑室内是否存在其他可以应用脑室镜治疗的梗阻性膜性结构（**图** 93.4）。

专栏 93.4 脑室镜下第三脑室底造瘘术基本步骤

- **仰卧位**：倾斜手术台或使患者颈部屈曲，使头部与水平面大约呈 30° 角。可以在一定程度上避免因脑脊液过度丢失而引发的颅内积气、硬膜下血肿及小脑上疝。
- **穿刺点位置的选择**：冠状缝前或冠状缝上，成人中线旁开 3 cm，儿童中线旁开 2 cm。
- **进入脑室的穿刺轨迹**：以双侧外耳道及内眦作为参考点，置管的头端应位于室间孔（成人约 6 cm，儿童约 4 cm）。
- **正中平面乳头体前三脑室底最薄弱处作为造瘘位置**：通常位于乳头体和漏斗隐窝之间前后轴的中间点。应用钝性手术器械（脑室镜探头、电极、球囊等）穿透三脑室底。
- **打开三脑室底后**，造瘘口通常可以通过球囊导管扩大，通过造瘘口可以清晰地显露基底动脉、脑干和斜坡。手术结束时，第三脑室底搏动振幅增加的患者远期预后较好。在保证安全的前提下，应尽可能的分离所有桥前池的 Lilliquist 膜。
- **术前影像学**：显示脑室解剖结构复杂的患者，建议应用神经导航辅助。

影像学诊断导水管狭窄通常基于矢状面 MRI 图像，但有时无法单纯通过影像学鉴别梗阻性脑积水和交通性脑积水。可以通过脑室置管或腰椎穿刺进行脑脊液循环检查，评估脑室相对顺应性，间接评估脑脊液循环梗阻程度。这类检查不作为常规检查，但对具体术式的选择有一定价值（Boon et al.，1997；Bech- Azeddine et al.，2007）。

禁忌证

桥前池或其他相关部位的解剖结构因肿瘤、严重脑膜炎或血管异常而发生严重病变患者，禁行第三脑室底造瘘术。早产儿脑出血后的脑积水治疗成功率低，第三脑室底造瘘术是否可行有待商榷。

手术技术

虽然具体手术细节因人而异，但是一些重要的手术步骤仍是手术成功的前提（**专栏** 93.4）。

由于生理盐水冲洗对脑组织和室管膜有明显的不利影响，在术中应尽可能使用人工脑脊液冲洗脑室。一些医生习惯在手术结束时临时留置脑室外引流管，而有医生不主张使用任何脑室外引流装置。作者通常于术中留置 Ommaya 储液囊并通过导管与脑室相通，在对患者术后随访中发现，留置 Ommaya 储液囊对患者的术后管理非常有利。比如，由于造瘘口阻塞导致的急性脑积水危及生命时，Ommaya 储液囊不仅可以立即引流脑脊液，还可以用于非手术时的颅内压监测。使用恒定速率输注方法分析研究患者术后脑脊液动力学，可用于预测这些患者的造瘘口功能，并可作为临床评估 ETV 术后效果的有效工具（Aquilina et al.，2012）。

预后

对于脑积水患者，ETV 因没有体内植入物，远期并发症较少，远期预后优于分流手术。2010 年 Kulkarni 等对 ETV 手术方案制订了量化评分表。（Kulkarni et al.，2010b）。临床医生可以根据患儿年龄、脑积水的病因以及是否有分流手术史对患儿进行评分，用于评估 ETV 远期成功率，评分越高，ETV 远期成功率就越高（这种评分方法尚未应用于成人）。脑积水发病 1 月内、感染后脑积水和既往曾行分流术的患者 ETV 评分较低。年龄>10 岁，导水管梗阻引起的脑积水，既往没有接受过分流术治疗的患者，ETV 远期成功率较高。

研究表明，术后短期内（小于 3 个月）ETV 疗效不如分流手术，但远期疗效较好（Kulkarni et al.，

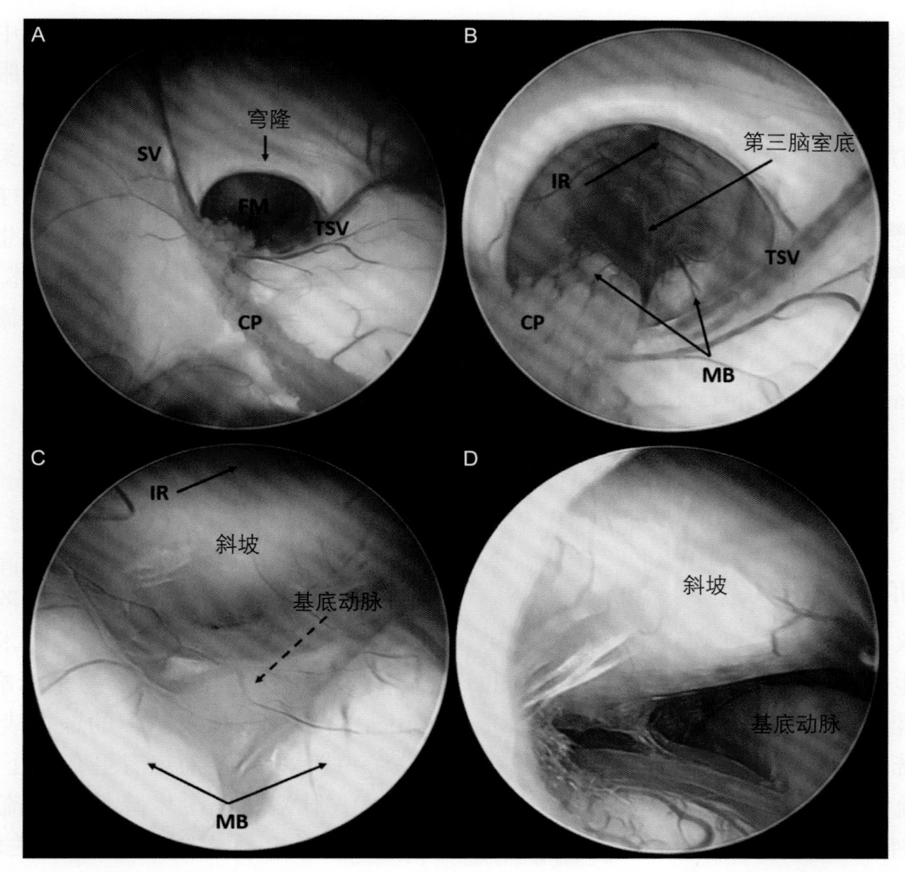

图 93.3　ETV 治疗导水管狭窄术中脑室镜图像。SV，透明隔静脉；TSV，丘纹静脉；CP，脉络丛；IR，漏斗隐窝；MB，乳头体；BA，基底动脉；FM，室间孔。

（A）标准右额入路进入到侧脑室室间孔。

（B）经由室间孔的第三脑室底视图。

（C）第三脑室底：本例由于慢性脑积水而使第三脑室底变薄，通过半透明的第三脑室底，可以观察到基底动脉。

（D）第三脑室底造瘘后桥前池基底动脉视图。应用内镜通过造瘘口以确保没有 Lilliquist 膜对脑脊液流动造成阻碍

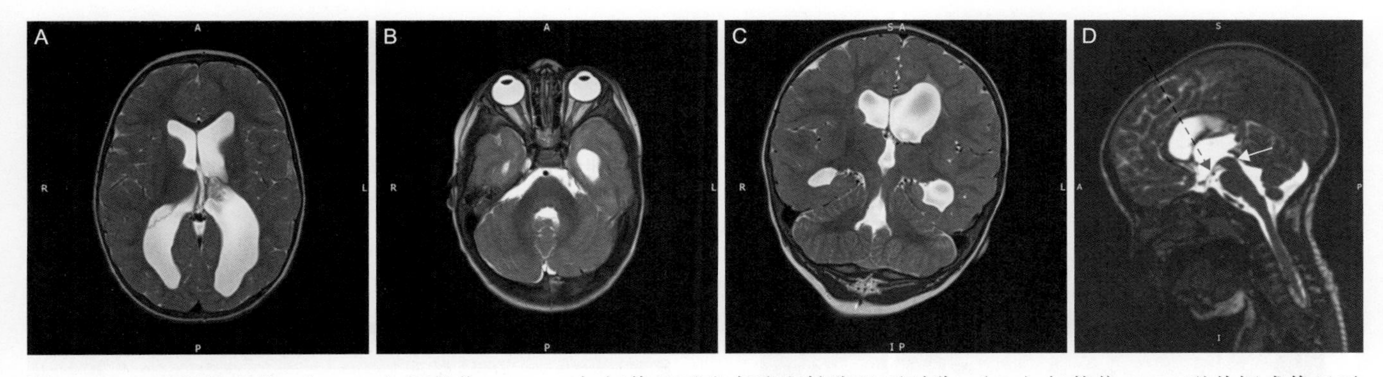

图 93.4　2 岁男性患儿，（A~C）冠状位 MRI T2 加权像显示患者脑室扩张且不对称。（D）矢状位 CISS 磁共振成像显示导水管阻塞（红色剪头）。红色虚线箭头表示脑室镜下第三脑室底造瘘术脑室镜通道轨迹

2010a)。这一观察结果还有待进一步的前瞻性研究验证，回顾性研究表明：ETV 对导水管狭窄所致的梗阻性脑积水患者的疗效优于对脑膜炎或脑出血所致的脑积水患儿的疗效。

其他神经内镜手术

透明隔造瘘术

通过内镜辅助的透明隔造瘘术治疗单室性脑积水 (monoventricular hydrocephalus，MH)，脑脊液可以绕过梗阻部位，将两侧侧脑室沟通。该手术作为脑脊液分流术和开放性手术的替代方案，降低了术后并发症，取得了良好的临床效果。

多房性脑积水的内镜治疗

多房性脑积水又称多间隔性脑积水，病理表现复杂，多见于新生儿，一般是由婴幼儿期脑室内出血和宫内脑室感染引发。可以通过多次分流手术，应用多个分流系统来进行治疗，这将产生一个复杂的分流系统。分流手术对多房性脑积水的治疗非常棘手 (**图** 93.5)。神经内镜对多房性脑积水的治疗具有明显优势，它可以分离脑室内的粘连，避免较多的穿刺损伤，通过将这些孤立区域沟通，恢复正常的脑脊液循环，并获得更令人满意的手术效果。

导水管成形术

神经内镜下导水管成形术 (aqueductoplasty，AP) 和导水管支架植入术治疗导水管狭窄引起的脑积水仍存在争议，目前尚未广泛应用于临床。这种手术易损伤导水管周围结构，如中脑损伤导致眼球运动障碍 (Parinaud 综合征)、动眼神经麻痹或滑车神经麻痹等，其诱发神经系统并发症的风险较高。此外，导水管的形状通常在正中矢状面呈 S 形，如果使用硬性脑室镜或导管，术中损伤中脑风险高。然而，该技术可以直接恢复 CSF 生理性通路，随着脑室镜技术的发展，实现这一技术指日可待。此外，脑室镜支架植入术可用于治疗分流术后产生的孤立性第四脑室。

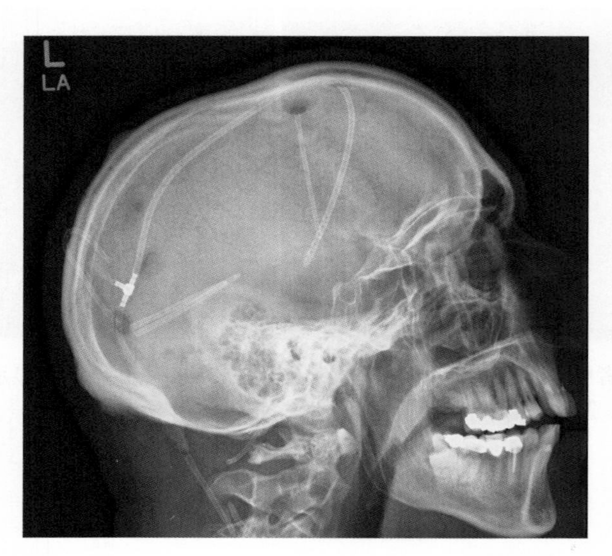

图 93.5 颅脑平片显示多个脑室端分流管。非常棘手的脑积水病例

脉络丛电凝术

在 20 世纪 50 年代脑脊液分流术应用之前，1918 年 Dandy 首次报道了切除脉络丛治疗婴儿脑积水的方法。这种手术死亡率极高，在脑脊液分流手术应用于临床之后，脉络丛切除术被淘汰。神经内镜技术的引入，使脉络丛电凝术的治疗效果有了显著改善，但还没有成为一种标准技术 (Pople and Ettles，1995)。越来越多的证据表明，其联合 ETV 作为一线治疗可能对患者更有益处 (Stone and Warf，2014)。脉络丛电凝术降低了分流术后脑积水复发率。脉络丛电凝术的适应证见**专栏** 93.5。

神经内镜下脉络丛电凝术的禁忌证：梗阻性脑积水和快速进展并伴有 ICP 升高的交通性脑积水。

进展性颅后窝囊肿的内镜治疗

神经内镜的快速发展 (导水管成形术，ETV 及分流术等使囊肿连通或引流等) 彻底改变了进展性颅后窝囊肿 (如 Dandy Walker 综合征和 Blake 袋囊肿) 引起的脑积水的治疗方法。

内镜下切除 / 吸除脑室内囊肿

蛛网膜囊肿

神经内镜下蛛网膜囊肿造瘘减压术对于脑室内、中线旁和鞍上池蛛网膜囊肿最有效。中颅窝蛛网膜囊肿的治疗方法仍存在争议，无论是内镜下手术还是

专栏 93.5 神经内镜下脉络丛电凝术适应证

婴儿缓慢进展的交通性脑积水：在十年的随访中，这类患者的手术成功率达到 64%。

脑脊液分泌过多导致的脑积水：如脉络丛乳头状瘤和脉络丛增生。神经内镜下直接处理诱发脑积水的病因。

无法进行分流手术的交通性脑积水：颅内反复出血后的脑积水且合并坏死性小肠结肠炎的患儿。

难治性脑积水患者：降低了分流管脑室端的阻塞。

开放手术，其远期失败率均较高（30%~50%）。四叠体池的蛛网膜囊肿可以在囊肿造瘘的同时，行第三脑室底造瘘术，手术成功率较高，预后较好。

第三脑室胶样囊肿

作者单位已于20世纪80年代初开展内镜治疗第三脑室胶样囊肿引起的梗阻性脑积水。神经内镜下微创切除胶样囊肿的优势大于开放性手术切除囊肿。然而这仍存在争议，有人仍然主张开颅经皮质或经胼胝体入路切除。也有其他学者报道，神经内镜在大多数此类病例的脑积水控制、症状改善和囊肿切除方面都取得了成功。这一般需要两个穿刺隧道，以大口径吸引器通过一个单独的通道，用于吸除部分黏稠性的囊肿内容物。当脑积水不严重时，内镜可以由立体定向引导进入脑室。与常规的ETV不同，术者可以借助神经导航规划最佳切除路径，力争顺利完整切除胶样囊肿。

总结

脑积水的外科治疗是一门复杂的“临床学科”。分流装置种类繁多，目前尚没有临床证据证明哪种装置更有优势。神经内镜技术和影像技术的发展为脑积水的治疗提供了更多的选择。现代的神经外科医生需要了解所有可用的术式，以便根据患者的个人情况做出最佳的决定。

延伸阅读、参考文献、EBRAIN的相关链接

扫描书末二维码获取。

第 94 章　正常压力性脑积水

Nicole C. Keong 著
张晓炜 译，张庆九 审校

引言

1965 年，Hakim 和 Adams 发表的一篇论文中首次提出正常压力性脑积水（normal pressure hydrocephalus，NPH）这一概念（Adams et al., 1965；Hakim and Adams，1965）。这篇具有里程碑意义的论文选取了三个病例为研究对象，其中两个是创伤后正常压力性脑积水，一个是特发性正常压力性脑积水（idiopathic normal pressure hydrocephalus, iNPH），由 Hakim 教授首先提出。目前的指南和研究主要集中于 iNPH，继发性正常压力性脑积水（secondary NPH）较少涉及。后者发生于蛛网膜下腔出血、脑部损伤、颅内手术或脑膜炎之后。

NPH 的说法有一定误导性，因为连续测量脑脊液压力所得的平均颅内压略高于正常值，且存在颅内压的波动性升高，特别是在快速眼动睡眠（rapid eye movement，REM）期间更明显。部分学者认为这种命名可能导致低估病情而延误诊断和治疗。因此，一些专家更倾向于使用成人特发性脑积水综合征或慢性交通性脑积水的专业术语。

病理生理学

病原学理论与研究证据

目前，已经有许多理论来解释 NPH 综合征发生的潜在机制。然而，其基本的病理生理过程仍然不清楚。目前大致分为结构、脑血流和脑脊液流动亚群三个方面，针对这些方面的具体观点在下文会有详细叙述，现在各个方面的系列研究还不能做到面面俱到（详见 Momjian et al.，2004；Keong et al., 2016）；**表** 94.1 为整体说明和补充参考。

结构

组织变形

Hakim 等提出假设，NPH 病理生理学的起始点是脑室内压力升高引起的组织变形（Hakim et al., 1976）。脑室压升高时压迫或拉伸软组织和血管，会导致其弹性丧失、萎缩和（或）缺血性损伤。这就产生了一种正常的脑脊液压力，导致了对大脑皮质的压力和压力梯度的逆向改变。

组织间压力增加

由于脑实质缺乏弹性，发生脑积水时，脑室和脑室周围组织和（或）凸性蛛网膜下腔与脑实质之间出现压力梯度，破坏静水压和渗透压平衡，使组织间液逆流导致水肿，而且血管活性代谢产物无法排出，局部脑血管反应性降低（Marmarou et al., 1980）。细胞和血管壁损伤又会导致体液进一步渗出到组织间隙。

生物力学

B 波出现可能导致颅内压间歇性升高，在快速眼动睡眠期间表现尤为明显。这种改变以及逐渐衰老的脑实质变性，使得老年人发生进行性脑室扩大的概率增加（Factora，2006）。在以慢性交通性脑积水为脑变形模型的研究中发现，组织间液向脑实质的逆流和组织弹性降低会发生联合作用（Pena et al., 2002），由此产生的流体压力从脑室到大脑半球面呈 U 形曲线（即最小值发生在脑组织中部），脑血流量（cerebral blood flow，CBF）曲线与其变化一致，这有助于解释进行性脑室扩大对白质产生不同程度的影响是如何实现的（Momjian et al.，2004）。也就是说，存在一个共同的生物力学过程使白质、脑室和脑血管内的结构完整性同时下降。

表 94.1 正常压力性脑积水的病因学说

	结构	脑血流	脑脊液流
主要概念	• 组织变形 • 弹性消失 • 间质液体流动反转 = 水肿 • 血管活性代谢物引流失败 • 脑组织变形 • U 形曲线	• 脑室扩张会扭曲基底神经节和额叶皮质之间的连线和(或)血管 • 深部腔隙性梗死 • 实质弹性消失	• 成人交通性脑积水 • 脑脊液生成与再吸收之间的不平衡 • 脑脊液生成减少 • 脑脊液流出阻力增加 • 无法清除有毒代谢产物
主要理论	• 组织变形 • 间质流体压力增加 • 生物力学	• 分水岭缺血 • 血管疾病	• 脑脊液流动障碍 • 脑脊液流体力学 • 血管活性代谢产物引流失败

Images Courtesy of Dr Nicole Keong©

脑血流量

分水岭缺血

正电子发射断层扫描（positron emission tomography, PET）、氙气增强计算机断层扫描（xenon-enhanced computed tomography）和单光子发射计算机断层扫描（single photon emission computed tomography，SPECT）的研究一致表明 NPH 患者存在广泛的大脑皮质和皮质下代谢水平下降以及脑血流循环障碍的现象（Tedeschi et al.，1995），这可能导致局部脑自动调节功能失调和放射冠分水岭缺血。然而各项研究中脑血流量的测定缺乏统一标准，只有少部分将脑血流量测定与结构成像匹配起来，为脑血流量的数据比较提供良好的解剖学基础（Owler et al.，2004）。

血管疾病

部分 NPH 患者的 MRI 图像表现为深部白质高信号（deep white matter hyperintensities，DWMH），引发了学者关于脑小血管病变和血管性脑病的争论。脑室扩张可能会使基底神经节和额叶皮质之间的连接和（或）血管扭曲，造成深部腔隙性梗死，或导致实质失去弹性。额叶下行纤维以及参与步态和排尿反射的白质缺血可能是 NPH 发病机制的根本。研究证实深部白质高信号（DWMH）与改善程度呈负相关（Krauss et al.，1996），与术后不良结果无相关性（Tullberg et al.，2001）。因此，这种病变的存在可能并不影响手术治疗效果。

脑脊液

脑脊液循环障碍

成人交通性脑积水被认为是脑脊液循环障碍的一种形式，涉及脑脊液产生和再吸收之间的不平衡（**专栏** 94.1）（Pickard，1982）。脑脊液的过量蓄积被认为是脑室扩大的原因。异常的脑部衰老（神经上皮、细胞外基质和实质的弹性丧失）对其也有影响。B 波压力表现为“水锤”的形式，对薄壁组织施加间歇性的压力。因此，除了脑脊液循环受到干扰之外，进行性脑室扩大的压力和脑实质内与之相反的结构压力之间也存在不平衡。

脑积水

上述不平衡现象存在是有生物学证据的。Czosnyka 等通过对一组有症状且颅内压（intracranial pressures，ICP）正常的脑积水患者进行脑脊液灌注研究，研究了脑脊液压力 - 容量补偿的年龄依赖性问题（Czosnyka et al.，2001）。研究证明，脑脊液流出阻力（定义为 Rout 或 Rcsf）随着年龄的增长以非线性方式增加，并与脑脊液产生率的下降相关，脑脊液产生率随着年龄的增长而下降；随着年龄的增长，ICP 波形图的振幅和振幅 -ICP 回归曲线的斜率均明显增大；弹性系数随年龄呈非线性增加，提示进行性脑实质僵硬。一些学者提出了“二次打击”假说，即婴儿期患有“良性外部性脑积水”的成人，在成年后期患血管疾病再次遭受深部白质缺血的打击时，启动导致 iNPH 综合征的一系列过程（Bradley et al.，2006）。

专栏 94.1 脑脊液调节障碍

蛛网膜下腔血流缺损和脑脊液循环障碍

软脑膜炎
感染
出血
脑膜炎癌症
异物
小脑扁桃体延伸 / 脱垂或扁平颅底
肿块（肿瘤性或非肿瘤性）
蛛网膜下腔阻滞（如由于上述原因，以及其他蛛网膜或导水管脉络丛、膜状物和非汇合的脑脊液室）

蛛网膜颗粒吸收脑脊液的障碍

先天性缺陷（即没有蛛网膜颗粒）
脑静脉窦压升高

脑脊液异常

脑脊液产生过多或脑脊液容量异常升高
脑室内脑脊液脉冲压升高，例如脉络丛乳头状瘤
蛋白质含量高导致脑脊液黏度增加，例如 Froin 综合征（脑脊液表现为蛋白质含量增高、呈黄褐色并且有高凝性）中描述的那样存在脊髓神经纤维瘤

Data from Pickard, J. D., Adult communicating hydrocephalus, *British Journal of Hospital Medicine*, pp. 27–40, Copyright © 1982.

血管活性代谢物清除障碍

脑脊液产生和循环的异常也可能导致清除有毒分子低效或失败。如果不能清除潜在的有毒代谢产物（如淀粉样肽 Aß 和 tau 蛋白），可能会导致它们在脑组织间液中的浓度增加，从而产生对神经元功能和生存不利的潜在环境。在衰老中发现的两个变化，减少脑脊液的产生，增加对脑脊液流出的抵抗力，可能与阿尔茨海默病和 NPH 的病理生理学机制有关。脑脊液产生和回流减少占主导可能表现为阿尔茨海

默病。相反，NPH可能是由于对脑脊液流出的阻力显著增加造成的。然而，Silverberg等进行的一项前瞻性、随机、双盲、安慰剂对照试验中，评估了215名可能患有阿尔茨海默病的受试者手术植入分流器的安全性和有效性（Silverberg et al.，2008），并没有证明低流量脑脊液分流对轻度至重度阿尔茨海默病受试者有任何益处。与分流改善相关的Rout阈值的争议目前仍无定论，或许只有脑脊液循环障碍达到一定程度后才能从分流术中获益。也可能导致该疾病发生的因素不止一个，还存在另一种因素的作用，两种因素可能同时发生，也可能一方起主导作用。

术前

典型正常压力性脑积水的临床表现

NPH容易诊断过度和诊断不足，因为支持NPH诊断的临床特征在老年人或患有其他神经退行性疾病的患者中也较为常见（Relkin et al.，2005）。这给诊断带来了挑战，比如许多潜在可治愈的NPH患者经常被误诊为患有阿尔茨海默病或血管性痴呆，相反的情况也有发生。因此，NPH的确切发病率和患病率仍存在争议，这取决于所使用的诊断标准和样本人群，其估计值的变化范围从罕见的0.0013%到频繁的0.4%。NPH的经典临床表现三联征是步态障碍、痴呆和尿失禁。患者常表现为三联征的症状不同时出现，尤其是在相对早期进行诊断时。

步态障碍

NPH患者的典型表现是站立不稳、倾向于跌倒和两脚分开的站立姿势。步态步幅会减少，患者可能会像脚粘在地板上一样拖着脚走路（即磁性步态）。Fisher进一步提出了“脑积水性共济失调”这一经典术语来描述这种表现，即身体前倾姿势、左右摇晃、不能保持平衡，闭眼时可能会加重这种不平衡（Fisher，1977）。常见的症状包括步幅、抬脚高度和行走时速度的降低以及整体转向。NPH所致的步态障碍可能与其他类型的额颞叶疾病有共同的特征。NPH也与帕金森病有很多相似之处。如果退行性疾病的典型特征如震颤、强直和面具样面容表现不明显，则很难与之进行鉴别诊断（Keong et al.，2011）。步态障碍的表现无局灶性缺损、肌张力高和反射亢进，这些都支持其他神经退行性疾病。标准化的步态检查方法也已进行了尝试（见**表**94.2）。

认知障碍

传统的认知障碍评估采用床旁简易精神状态量表（mini-mental state examination，MMSE），对出现局灶性皮质缺损如失认症或失语症者，再进行进一步检查。然而，这些方法有很大的局限性。多个操作员对测试分数的可还原性提出了质疑。神经心理学测试对于将正常颅压性脑积水中的痴呆模式与其他疾病（如与年龄相关的认知能力下降、萎缩和阿尔茨海默病）区分开来至关重要（见**表**94.2）。正式的神经心理学使用一系列集中测试，例如荷兰的研究中（Boon et al.，1998）将测试应用于相关性小的群体。现已证实，认知障碍的特征性表现为额叶-皮质下执行功能障碍（Iddon et al.，1999）。一篇关于iNPH指南的综述（Klinge et al.，2005）指出，虽然认知测试没有标准化，但其结果有助于对术后效果进行客观评估。

尿失禁

这是NPH的第三个典型临床表现，表现为发作性或持续性排尿功能障碍，少数可有尿失禁和便失禁同时出现。对症状较轻者尿失禁的诊断，iNPH指南要求至少具备以下症状中的两条：尿急、尿频、夜尿增多（Relkin et al.，2005）。尿动力学检查可能有助于区分NPH的尿功能障碍和其他一些常见的并发症（男性前列腺炎、女性反复出现的尿路症状或膀胱肌张力障碍/自主神经功能障碍），以及“神经源性膀胱综合征”系列中的其他疾病。

复杂的正常颅压性脑积水

并发症

NPH综合征的临床表现与其他神经退行性疾病有所交叉。Silverberg等提出假设，存在一个早期的诱因会导致阿尔茨海默病或正常颅压性脑积水（Silverberg et al.，2003），这可能有助于解释在这两种疾病均存在大脑淀粉样蛋白沉积。NPH需要与非典型性帕金森病进行鉴别诊断，后者属于“血管性帕金森症”的系列，还包括其他类型的严重的步态障碍和认知障碍。NPH独特的、已被广泛认可的认知表现（包括行为变化、情绪低落、偏执和幻觉）可能很难与抑郁症和精神分裂症等精神疾病区分开来。尿功能障碍也可能与步态和（或）认知状态有关，以早期为主，部分可有迟发性尿失禁的表现同样可能见于其他神经系统疾病。因此，对于合并有严重并发症

表 94.2 用于正常压力性脑积水评估的标准

评估	参考	分级	说明
步态	（Boon et al.，1997）	2~40	步态的 10 个特征进入行走评分（0~20），步数和 10 米步行的秒数（0~20）
	（Hellström et al.，2012b）	0~100	通过测量以自由步速行走 10 米所需的步数和秒数，以及步态的序数评估步态范围。结果得到两组连续数据（11 个步态类别）和两组有序数据（8 个等级类别）
	（Tinetti，1986）	16 个平衡	
	（Podsiadlo and Richardson，1991）	12 步态 以秒为单位计时	日常活动中的平衡和动作步态性能测试。平衡部分包括按顺序分级为正常、适应性或异常的 9 次演习。步态部分评定 7 项步态特征为正常或异常。测试体弱老年人的功能活动能力。从标准扶手椅站起来所需的时间，走 3 米，转身，走回扶手椅坐下
认知	（Boon et al.，1997）	组合测试	痴呆量表包括 10 字测验、数字跨度前后、步道制作、手指敲击
	（Iddon et al.，1999）	组合测试	Kendrick 物体学习测验（KOLT），选择性 CANTAB battery 评估（语言流畅性、记忆力和注意力）
	（Kubo et al.，2008）	组合测试	简易动作，正面评估系列，跟踪测试部分 A
	（Hellström et al.，2012a）	结合	钉板，雷伊听觉语言学习任务，瑞典斯特鲁普测试
结果	（Stein and Langfifitt，1974）	0~4 级	0 级（能够工作），1~2 级（回家可能需要帮助），3~4 级（可以独立运作但仍需要监护），4 级（无独立运作能力）
	（Black，1980）	6 级	优良 ~ 良好（无或无缺陷）、一般 ~ 短暂（改善）、差 ~ 死亡（不良结局）
	（Wilson et al.，2002）	7 级	改良 Rankin 量表（mRS）=0（无症状），1~2（无明显或轻微症状），3~4（中度至中度严重），5（严重），6（死亡）
	（Larsson et al.，1991）	结合	在行走时的步态 =0(正常)，1~2(无手杖或有手杖时不安全)，3~4(辅助器具)，5（轮椅） 生活条件 =0~1（独立生活或家庭辅助），2~3（辅助生活设施），4（医院）
	（Boon et al.，1997）	结合	荷兰 NPH 量表（4 个临床结果类别，但也提供了一个短神经心理学检查系列，用于提供痴呆症量表和 10 个步态特征进行行走评分），mRS 被用于残疾结果评估
	（Kubo et al.，2008）	结合	3 个 NPH 域（认知障碍、步态障碍、排尿障碍）。每个域名从 0 到 4 打分，得分越高，症状越严重。与 MMSE、步态状态量表（GSS）、TU> 及国际尿失禁咨询量表（ICIQ-SF）相关
	（Hellström et al.，2012b）	结合	欧洲 iNPH 多中心研究——使用步态、认知、平衡、自制四方面评估的综合量表

（如心脏病和血管病高风险）的患者来说，找到一个可靠的测试标准来确定脑脊液分流治疗 NPH 的适应证，权衡手术干预的相对风险和益处是至关重要的。

变异

NPH 患者也可以出现嗜睡、兴趣丧失、困倦和视觉空间障碍等表现，对不伴有上述典型三联征临床表现的患者，需要进一步观察。其他形式的脑积水也可能出现 NPH 综合征。成人长期显性脑室扩大（longstanding overt ventriculomegaly in adults，LOVA）是脑积水的一种形式，在儿童时期开始发展，但症状出现在相对较晚的成年。患者可以出现各种脑积水症状，可表现为亚急性症状和颅内压升高，也可表现为更危险的 NPH 三联征，即步态障碍、认知能力下降和（或）尿失禁（Keong et al.，2011）。在这种情况下，成人患者典型的表现为严重的脑室扩大，累及侧脑室和第三脑室，影像学上显示脑皮质沟回的消失。另外，患者可表现为长期巨颅，即头围测量值高于平均标准差的两倍，和（或）神经放射学证据表明蝶鞍明显扩大或破坏。LOVA 可通过分流治疗（需要使用压力可编程阀门进行仔细控制），而内镜下第三脑室造瘘术是最有效的治疗手段（Oi et al.，2000）。在其他表现为 NPH 综合征的脑积水亚群中可能存在不完全的中脑导水管狭窄，可能是由内源性（固有性）不完全梗阻（如导水管内部丛带）或外部压迫（如中颅窝蛛网膜囊肿扭曲）导致的。由于导水管的狭窄可能是继发性的，第三脑室造瘘术可作为一种选择，但在某些情况下脑室-腹腔分流可能更有效。精细的脑脊液室成像（如额外的三维T2加权和CISS磁共振序列）有助于评估脑脊液病灶信号的增强或减弱，从而为手术选择提供可靠的信息。

检查和鉴别诊断

常规的CT或磁共振成像（MRI）扫描是明确诊断NPH的基础。需要考虑的重要鉴别诊断包括肿瘤或类似病理引起的脑脊液通路阻塞（参见**专栏** 94.1）、明显的脑萎缩、缺血性脑血管疾病和（或）神经退行性病变。脑室增大不应完全归因于脑萎缩或先天性增大（Evans指数≥0.3或类似测量）（Relkin et al.，2005）。Evans指数的定义是额角的最大宽度除以颅骨的横向最大内径。另一种方法是双尾指数（脑室扩大的定义为BCI≥0.25），具体为尾状核头层面侧脑室宽度和该层面沿尾状核同一条线的大脑宽度的加值（见**图** 94.1）。

补充测试

相关指南指出，iNPH的预后评估缺乏一个单一的标准（Marmarou et al.，2005a）。"脑脊液放液试验"（使用腰椎穿刺抽出40~50 ml脑脊液）虽然特异性高至100%，但由于它的敏感性低至26%，所以不能作为排除试验。然而，腰椎穿刺常被用作确定脑脊液压力在正常范围内（5~18 mmHg/7~24 cmH_2O）

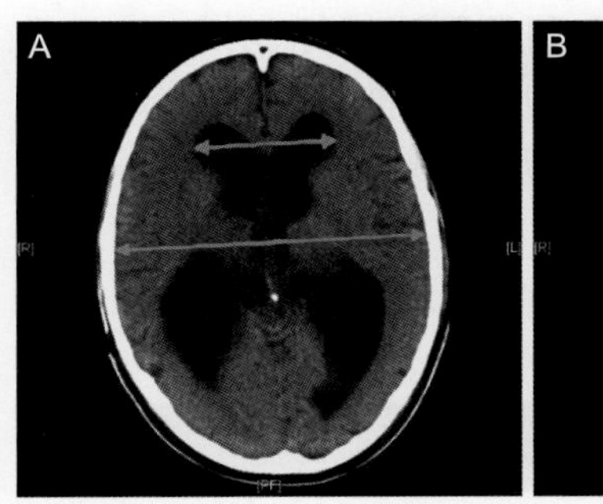

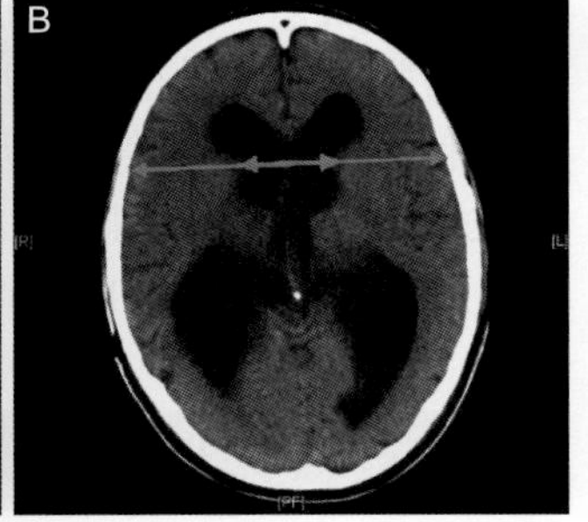

图 94.1 脑室扩大的测量

（A）Evans指数/比率：侧脑室额角的最大宽度除以在同一水平测量的颅骨最大内径；侧脑室额角宽度最大的轴性层；显著脑室扩大，Evans指数≥0.3

（B）双尾指数。沿着尾状核测量的同一条线，用脑宽度划分的两个尾状核尖之间的最小距离：轴状层，其中尾状核在侧脑室产生最大的凹陷；显著脑室扩大，双尾指数（bicaudate index，BCI）≥0.25

的第一线检查工具，而且未出现生化或微生物异常。现已证实，放置一个外置腰椎引流管，在5天内提取300 ml脑脊液，具有更高的灵敏度和特异性——分别为50%和80%（Walchenbach et al.，2002）。虽然这种方法被认为是金标准，但这种方法需要住院，并且存在一定的感染和神经根刺激的风险。

脑脊液流出阻力测量（Rout）是评估NPH患者水动力状态的另一种方法，就是将液体注入脑室或腰椎蛛网膜下腔（推注或输液）。脑脊液流出阻力是基于压力-容积模型计算的，在荷兰NPH研究中表明，当流出阻力大于18 mmHg/（ml·min）时，敏感性为46%，特异性为87%（Boon et al.，1998）。最近的meta分析显示，Rout阈值为12 mmHg/（ml·min）时可获得较高的准确性（72.95%）、高灵敏度（80.26%）和中等特异性（46.79%）（Kim et al.，2015）。这项技术的优点是，可以通过植入式脑室储液装置进行，检测迅速，只需要一天的时间（**图** 94.2B为输液研究数据示例）。

药物管理

药物治疗的选择（如连续腰椎穿刺和并注射乙酰唑胺）对临床症状的改善往往是有限的。因此，通常建议根据临床表现和补充试验得出的支持性证据进行手术干预。

手术治疗

NPH的自然病程是逐渐发展的，有些患者可能在一段时间内保持稳定，但大多数患者在最初评估后的3个月就表现出症状加重。

对手术干预的思考

手术包括放置分流器或内镜下第三脑室造瘘术。目前为止，脑室-腹腔分流术（VP）和腰大池腹腔分流术（LP）是比脑室-右心房分流术或脑室-胸腔分流术更好的选择。虽然压力控制阀和流量控制阀的使用可能取决于手术偏好，但在NPH的患者中，需要根据患者脑脊液的分流程度做出可调整的对策（请参阅**第** 92 **章**和**第** 93 **章**了解分流插入技术和分流技术）。

在阀门回路中增加的可穿刺储液囊可以为脑脊液检测提供便利，同时最大限度地降低碎片被直接吸入阀门装置的风险。在NPH范围内，一些患者在小脑幕上间隙和第四脑室之间存在一种相对不匹配的通道狭窄。尽管这是一个小的亚群，作者也报道了

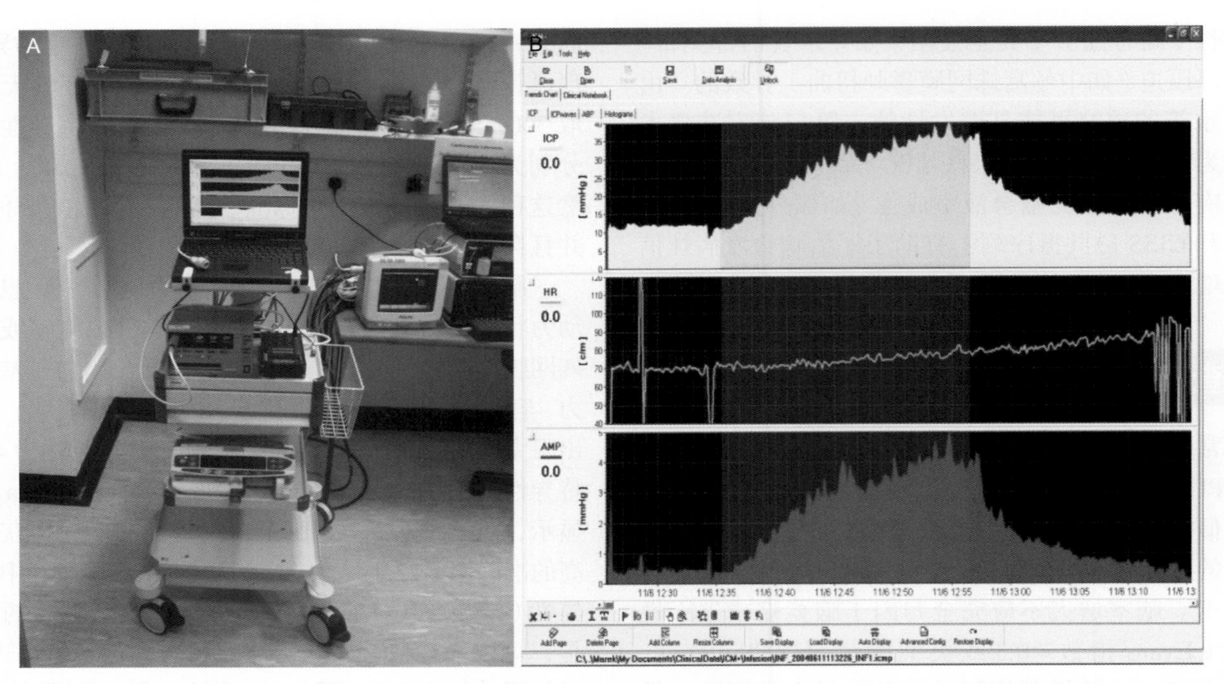

图 94.2 建立脑脊液注射研究。（A）用于计算机化测试的移动单元堆栈（可以进行计算机化的输液测试以查询 CSF 流体力学并提取各种参数）。（B）输液研究数据采集示例。脑脊液流出阻力（Rout）的计算方法为平衡末期脑脊液压力与基线脑脊液压力之差（即平衡期 - 基线 ICP）除以注射速度

Courtesy of Dr Zofia Czosnyka and Dr Marek Czosnyka.

使用神经内镜第三脑室造瘘术的良好效果。Gangemi 等的一项研究显示，72% 的患者病情好转，并发症（颅内出血）发生率为 4%（Gangemi et al.，2004）。仔细考虑亚组（包括前面讨论的成人长期显性脑室扩大），对于患者的个体化手术选择是非常重要的。

对于明显的脑室扩大的病例，导航并不比解剖标志有更多的优势，但对于适度的脑室扩大的病例，导航会是一个有用的工具，它可以优化尖端放置的最佳轨迹，避免穿过血管。在影像引导技术的帮助下，脑室导管的最佳放置也有助于减少因近端导管故障和（或）阻塞而引起的分流术翻修的长期并发症。在腹腔镜引导下放置远端导管可以降低由于腹腔外放置导管或远端导管移动引起的假脊膜膨出的发生率。如果已知有粘连或由于之前的手术造成了腹腔假分隔，在与普通外科同事协作的情况下，可优先选择脑室 - 胸腔 / 心房入路。

危险分层

一般来说，如果不积极解决老年 NPH 患者中出现的并发症以及相关的疾病，可能导致住院时间过长并且需要进行后期康复治疗。系统的术前多学科评估，通过识别高危患者进行手术并在必要时进行优化，可以有助于预防麻醉下发生意外、昏迷或心脏事件的风险。Kiefer 并发症指数（Kiefer et al.，2006）和其他心脏 / 整体风险评分在个体患者的风险评估中是有用的，因为它们为伴有并发症的患者提供了在血管、心脏和神经退行性疾病方面的客观评价（见 ISHCSF 回顾更全面地讨论 iNPH 并发症的影响；Malm et al.，2013）。

对于手术干预的讨论来说，对手术结果的期望值是至关重要的，因为许多患者症状出现较晚，腰椎引流术后有临床症状轻度改善，或者有明显的其他症状改善。对分流有利的预测指标包括：Rout 升高，对腰椎置管外引流或反复腰椎穿刺的有效反应，以及脑血流对乙酰唑胺的反应减弱（SPECT）。并发症被认为对预后影响较大，而年龄本身不作为判断预后的主要因素（Halperin et al.，2015）。

术后

并发症的管理

对 NPH 的外科干预有感染风险，包括脑膜炎、出血、癫痫、脑脊液漏和神经功能缺失（即卒中、分流道错位或功能障碍需要进行再手术）。在导管远端置管的穿隧道过程中，可能造成颈部组织结构损伤（如血管损伤）、胸部损伤（如气胸）。在试图进入

腹膜腔进行远端导管插入时，可能出现医源性肠浆膜或黏膜的开放，需要立即手术修复。腹腔污染是远端分流放置的禁忌证。严重风险为1%~2%，有3%~4%的颅内出血风险（Black et al.，1985）。明显的脑内出血比消化道出血更需要清除血肿，去除分流管并插入室外引流，但这是全部出血风险的一个罕见亚组。

硬膜下积液伴或不伴出血是更常见的，报道的发生率从2%到17%不等（Klinge et al.，2005）。这可能与分流引流过度或一些患者原有的皮质萎缩有关。并不是所有的积液都与临床相关。在少数病例中，需要以钻孔引流慢性硬膜下血肿的方式进行外科干预，可能还需要暂时性分流结扎术。通过一段时间的监测成像，调整阀门以减少引流通常是一种有效的策略。下引流的风险同样重要，需要一般的分流或阀门调整来优化症状。患者也可能经历分流管完全堵塞、断裂或故障。这可能会急性发作，甚至在以前只有隐伏症状的患者中发作。一些患者对安置分流阀表现出较高的敏感性，其中一组患者可能受益于选择性的瓣膜调整设置选项。Hashimoto等（SINPHONI）2010年发现，总体上严重事件发生率为3%，较轻事件发生率为20%（Hashimoto et al.，2010）。

然而，分流后未改善的患者仍有改善的潜在可能性。Klinge等报道，在欧洲iNPH的研究中，11%的未改善患者存在“寂静”分流功能障碍，但在瓣膜调整后可转变为分流适应者（Klinge et al.，2012）。虽然使用现代可变电阻阀可以实现这一点，但其他选择，如在分流回路中加入额外的反虹吸和反重力装置，则需要手术修改。正如Marmarou（Marmarou et al.，2005b）所报道的，并发症平均发生率为9.8%，为了追求手术结果的优化，再次手术率为33%（McGirt et al.，2005）。更引人注目的是，Pujari等发现53%的修正率仍然与74%的改进率相一致，进一步表明这种优化可以通过手术干预实现（Pujari et al.，2008）。

管理术中因素可能有助于减少分流相关感染。手术室因素，如在分流术中受限的流量、早些的手术时间、耗时短的步骤、高资历的手术团队和选择使用抗生素浸没导管，都可以用来改善手术效果。分流术后早期到晚期的一系列并发症强调了维持区域和国家分流登记的重要性，以支持出现分流后未改善患者的临床信息空白。

结果

2005年发表在iNPH指南上的一篇综述（Klinge et al.，2005）指出，由于NPH患者入选标准、临床改善定义、术后随访方案和时间、术后管理没有统一标准，使得NPH研究结论不一致。对此，Klinge等提出以下建议：在3、6和12个月时进行随访；对分流无改善者进行仔细评估和治疗；在改进的方法中使用客观量表。短期结果更有可能受到与分流相关的风险的影响，而长期结果则可能与伴随的脑血管和血管疾病有关。目前认为分流后第一年可能决定了分流的结局。此外，研究表明，在分流术的临床表现中，其死亡和发病与伴发的心脑血管疾病有关。

专家小组意识到缺乏iNPH分流治疗的结果评估标准。目前常用的几种量表通常是基于日常生活能力（activities of daily living，ADL）或残疾评估的功能分级，以及对三联征的单个组成部分的评级量表（Ishikawa，2014）。研究小组还开发了他们自己的综合评估量表，如“荷兰正常压力性脑积水量表”和欧洲多中心研究的iNPH量表（参见**表**94.2尾部）。作者在最近的实践指南报告中得出结论，分流可能对iNPH有效，在6个月时超过80%的步态得到了改善，严重不良事件风险为11%（Halperin et al.，2015）。

神经影像生物标志物的争议

目前iNPH的挑战主要在于优化分流手术适应证的确认。由于现有的症状分级方法和并发症的特异性，使得在NPH工作中很难再现更佳的手术结果。脑脊液和神经影像学生物标志物的进展可能有助于iNPH的鉴别诊断，并为亟待解决的预后及结果相关性研究提供参考。神经外科医师都会对两种特殊的神经成像感兴趣，因为MRI技术可以直接在各个中心开展——基于NPH和弥散张量成像的关键结构特征的定量评估。已有研究证实前者的可靠性；在一项针对100名iNPH患者的前瞻性研究中，SINPHONI作为一种基于MRI的诊断（异常增大的蛛网膜下腔积水的证据，即致密的高凸度、蛛网膜下腔和扩大的侧裂与脑室扩大有关），在69%~77%的患者中取得了良好的结果，结果差异多由于采用的结果分级量表的不同（Hashimoto et al.，2010）。

弥散张量成像（diffusion tensor imaging，DTI）已经被纳入一些病例的标准MR序列中，在iNPH与其他重叠疾病（如阿尔茨海默病）的鉴别诊断和描述急性脑积水的可逆性方面显示出了一些前景。利用DTI技术，可以证明NPH中共存的不同类型的白质损伤，并检测脑脊液对手术干预的相对反应性（Keong et al.，2017）。进一步阐明白质损伤模式的工作将支持早期预测和预测分流反应。多模态可能也有助于发展潜在分流反应的生物标志物，比如用其他成像技术了解脑血流、脑脊液动力学、血流、脑血管反应性和脑弹性。然而，在iNPH的多阶段、多学科评估中增加其复杂性是不可取的。虽然大多数成像方法都是非创伤性的，但没有一种成像方法能够达到腰椎外引流试验的敏感性和特异性的水平。由此得出，即使在iNPH的鉴别诊断中，资源也更倾向于尽可能广泛和持续的检查，而非仅限于应用在学术范围的分析比较手段。类似的问题也适用于脑脊液生化标志物这一新的研究方向，作为一种检查手段，其解释阈值和广泛的可用性还需进一步研究证实。

改变iNPH神经影像学的研究重点，在于最可能的正常压力性脑积水的病理生理学过程达成共识，即损伤的可逆性研究的突破，并找到相应的可重复和可量化的最佳检查方式。iNPH代表了一种独特的非永久性白质损伤模型，在此基础上有利于我们对其他类型的亚急性神经退行性疾病的认知。

延伸阅读、参考文献、EBRAIN的相关链接

扫描书末二维码获取。

第 95 章 假性脑瘤综合征

John Pickard・Nicholas Higgins 著
贾亮 译，张庆九 审校

引言与分类

1851 年 Helmholtz 发明了眼底镜，1891 年 Quincke 发明了腰椎穿刺术，1904 年 Nonne 提出了“假脑瘤”一词，用于治疗无颅内占位但存在视盘水肿和颅内压升高的病例。假性脑瘤综合征（pseudotumour cerebri syndrome，PTCS）指的是一组表现为颅内压增高而无局灶性神经功能障碍和结构异常的综合征。最常见的患者是围产期的肥胖女性。

文献中曾使用过的术语包括良性颅内压增高、特发性颅内压增高等，但这些词语直观上反映的是非恶性的、非凶险的疾病。而假性脑瘤综合征强调无颅内占位，之所以叫综合征与库欣综合征、库欣病有异曲同工之处（Johnston et al.，2007）。假性脑瘤综合征一词越来越多得到了大家的认可（Friedman，2013）。

假性脑瘤综合征虽然不是恶性的肿瘤性疾病，但许多患者往往因头痛和抑郁而痛苦不堪。

此类疾病在育龄期肥胖女性群体中较为常见，由于病因尚不明确，因此诊断为特发性颅内压增高（idiopathic intracranial hypertension，IIH）。严格意义上讲，IIH 应只包括那些病因不明的病例，由于许多被诊断为 IIH 病例的病因并未进行充分的探究，因此许多 IIH 病例其实包括许多继发性颅内压增高的病例。

诊断标准

假性脑瘤综合征的诊断标准由 Dandy 于 1937 年提出，并统计了 22 例该类患者临床资料，详细阐述了其临床特征。随后诊断标准被不断修正完善，目前主要依据：颅内压增高、无局灶性神经功能缺失（展神经麻痹除外）、脑脊液成分正常、影像学检查正常（包括 MRV）。有时会合并有侧脑室变小和空蝶鞍。

对于假性脑瘤综合征的患者，视盘水肿不一定出现。2013 年，Friedman 等将假性脑瘤综合征的诊断标准进一步完善（**专栏 95.1**）（Friedman et al.，2013）。

病理生理学

脑脊液的吸收是一个被动的过程，并符合由 Davson（Davson et al.，1970）提出并阐述的公式：

$P_{csf}-P_{sss}=I_f \times R_{out}$（+搏动成分）。

专栏 95.1 假性脑瘤综合征诊断标准

1. 假性脑瘤综合征的诊断[a]
   A. 视盘水肿
   B. 神经系统检查正常（颅神经异常除外）
   C. 神经影像学：需要排除脑积水、颅内占位、脑组织损伤及 MRI 表现脑膜异常增强的病例
   D. 脑脊液检查正常
   E. 腰椎穿刺脑脊液压力升高（成人 ≥250 mmH$_2$O，儿童 ≥280 mmH$_2$O，如果儿童没有镇静且不肥胖，则为 ≥250 mmH$_2$O）
2. 无视盘水肿的假性脑瘤综合征的诊断

   如果条件 BE 满足，无视盘水肿，但患者有单侧或双侧展神经麻痹，可以诊断假性脑瘤综合征

   如果条件 BE 满足，无视神盘水肿、展神经麻痹，假性脑瘤综合征可以初诊但是不能确诊。确诊需要至少满足以下三个神经影像条件：

1. 空蝶鞍
2. 蝶鞍后部扁平
3. 视神经周边蛛网膜下腔扩张，伴或不伴视神经移位
4. 横窦局限性狭窄

[a] 如果患者符合 A~E 诊断标准，则诊断为假性脑瘤综合征；如果患者符合 A~D 诊断标准，但脑脊液压力不达标，判定为可疑诊断。

其中 P_{csf} 是指脑脊液压力，P_{sss} 指上矢状窦的压力，I_f 指脑脊液生成率，R_{out} 指脑脊液流出阻力。通过计算机脑脊液输注研究，测量人工脑脊液注入蛛网膜下腔时脑脊液压力的变化，可以测量患者的流出阻力。

已提出多种机制作为 PTCS 的基础，并且不止一种机制发挥作用。

脑脊液分泌亢进

其他可能的发生机制还包括脑脊液分泌亢进，异常增多。在其他条件稳定不变前提下，单独多分泌一倍脑脊液，只会使颅内压增加 3 mmHg。脑脊液产生过多的原因主要有脉络丛组织增生和脉络丛乳头状瘤。在此类脑积水患者中，由于脑脊液产生异常增多，需要通过分流或脉络丛组织切除术去控制颅内压。在假性脑瘤综合征患者中并没有脉络丛组织的扩张，也就不需要上述方式降低颅内压。此外，颅内感染期也可以导致脑脊液产生异常增多。

脑水肿

脑水肿也可能是其发生的机制之一，主要依据明显缩小的脑室系统以及脑组织活检的组织学特征。但现代的弥散成像 MRI 技术证实，在假性脑瘤综合征患者中不存在细胞毒性或者血管源性脑水肿。

脑脊液吸收障碍

有许多试验和临床证据表明假性脑瘤综合征患者存在脑脊液的吸收障碍（Johnston et al.，2007）。脑脊液在蛛网膜颗粒水平吸收障碍时，脑室却不是扩张的。Foley 推测，在这种情形下，在脑皮质蛛网膜下腔空间和脑室之间没有阻碍，过多的脑脊液将潴留在皮质蛛网膜下腔空间。后来，脑池造影检查证实了这一推测。

脑脊液流出阻力（R_{out}）不是直接测量得出的。在脑脊液输注假设研究中，随着脑脊液压力的增加，上矢状窦压力 P_{sss} 仍能保持恒定。但近期许多研究结果推测这个假设是无效的。脑脊液的吸收可能不只有颅内蛛网膜颗粒单一途径。一些具有更高的基线颅内压力的患者，脊髓蛛网膜颗粒和其他脑脊液吸收通路可能被重新构建。

静脉回流障碍

长期以来，人们一直认为炎症时的耳旁静脉窦 ICP 升高和耳炎性脑积水有关。例如，Janny 通过关建孔开颅，用直接压力测定证实假性脑瘤综合征患者存在缩窄的上矢状窦。而横窦变窄的征象在早期的 MR 静脉期研究中经常被忽略。后来的研究证实这些静脉改变是真实的而非假象。逆行脑造影术证实，假性脑瘤综合征患者其缩窄的横窦之间经常有明显的压力梯度。继而通过静脉支架介入手术可以帮助此类视盘水肿的患者（Higgins et al.，2002；Higgins et al.，2004；Pickard et al.，2008）。

关键问题是在区分病理性的狭窄和腰穿导致的脑脊液减少所造成的狭窄。逆行静脉造影显示假性脑瘤综合征中肥胖年轻女性患者矢状窦压力与脑脊液压力是同步变化的。在假性脑瘤综合征患者中，脑脊液压力、脑脊液吸收和静脉引流之间存在一种正反馈回路，即当 ICP 增加时，静脉窦狭窄越明显，静脉流出减少，而 ICP 进一步增加。

尽管患者每天产生并更换 3 遍脑脊液，但腰椎穿刺放液却可以使症状缓解数周或数月。这一现象目前仍无法解释。如果通过脑脊液引流缓解了解静脉窦的狭窄，则静脉窦可能保持开放，直到再次达到临界脑脊液压力，这一过程可能需要数周或数月。

类固醇代谢机制

静脉阻塞不能解释 PTCS 与肥胖的关系，也不能解释 PTCS 脑脊液压力增加。而肥胖所产生的类固醇代谢和炎症反应可能与其相关。例如，肥胖可能与存在于脉络膜丛和蛛网膜颗粒内皮帽中的 11-β 羟类固醇脱氢酶Ⅰ型异常有关。高凝性和结缔组织疾病可能会改变这一内皮帽的特性。实验表明，使用类固醇后停用会增加 CSF 的流出阻力。Sinclair 等（Sinclair et al.，2010a，2010b）提出这一机制可能有双重作用，既增加产生脑脊液的脉络丛组织，也损害吸收受损的蛛网膜颗粒。

临床

表现

假性脑瘤综合征患者的头痛症状不同于脑瘤或者急性脑积水导致的头痛，后者是以晨起头痛、弯腰加重为特征。患者头痛可以不合并视盘水肿，也可以发生视盘水肿而无头痛。另外，有些患者存在过量使用止痛剂，以致其副反应引起头痛。通过腰椎穿刺释放脑脊液评估头痛的缓解程度是可行的。有些患者通过各种治疗后，视力问题得到了解决，但头痛往往持续存在。少部分患者有时自己会慢慢体会到过度换气可以帮助他们减轻头痛。但当他们以过度换气、手足痉挛就诊时，经常被误认为是癔症。

超过半数的PTCS患者会出现视觉症状，包括视力模糊和水平复视。当患者为男性时，通常与肥胖无关。但男性患者更有可能早期出现失明症状。

在首次就诊时恶心和呕吐是常见的症状（20%）。

耳鸣通常是搏动性的。压迫同侧颈内静脉可能会缓解症状，可能是由于它提高了横窦内的压力，扩大了可逆性狭窄的区域。释放脑脊液也可以缓解此类搏动性耳鸣。其他的耳部症状可能是由于脑脊液压力升高，并将此压力通过耳蜗导水管传入内耳所致。

四肢的神经根症状也偶有发生，可能是由于根袖扩张所致。而脑脊液引流可改善这些症状。

有些患者会有自发性脑脊液鼻漏。可能是脑脊液通过空蝶鞍、鼓膜盖裂开或前半规管漏至鼻腔。合并PTCS的患者实施颅底手术后并发的脑脊液漏，包括经蝶窦垂体手术或治疗Chiari畸形的枕骨大孔减压术，常规修补方法难以治愈脑脊液漏。

在儿童时期，PTCS比较少见，确诊前需要除外先天性视盘异常（如玻璃膜疣）。而且需要注意儿童的脑脊液压力应在平静条件下测量才比较准确。

另外要重视病史的采集，并对患者进行全身检查。测量血压以排除恶性高血压，并进行神经系统检查，以确定任何相关疾病（**专栏**95.2）。

例如，过多的口服维生素A是假性脑瘤综合征的原因之一，对于缺铁性贫血的治疗可能会逆转那些通过保守和手术处理后效果不佳的难治性假性脑瘤综合征。

尽管许多因素和假性脑瘤综合征有联系，但很少有研究能完全符合因果关系，即：撤出这些条件导致逆转假性脑瘤综合征，重新引入又会使得症状复发。

大多数患者会出现视力异常，包括视盘水肿、视野改变、视敏度减少、水平复视等。关于眼部的详细检查是必不可少的，可以排除先天性的眼部缺陷和视神经-脑-黄斑玻璃疣等。眼科检查可以评估病情是否进展。值得注意的是，视盘水肿并不总是随着PTCS的复发而复发。如果伴有视神经萎缩，即使没有视盘水肿，患者仍然有失明的危险。

专栏 95.2　继发性假性脑瘤综合征的病因

脑静脉畸形

脑静脉窦血栓形成
头部受伤伴随主要的鼻窦与颅底处的骨折
双侧颈静脉血栓形成或结扎
中耳乳突感染
右心房高压
上腔静脉阻塞
巨大的蛛网膜颗粒
鼻窦脑膜脑炎
动静脉瘘
脑脊液吸收障碍（颅内感染或出血所致）
高凝状态

药物和暴露

抗生素类：四环素、二甲胺四环素（米诺环素）、强力霉素（多西环素）、萘啶酸、磺胺类药物
维生素A：过多，异维甲酸，用于早幼粒细胞白血病的全反维甲酸，过量摄入肝
激素：人类生长激素，甲状腺素（儿童），醋酸左旋肾上腺素，左炔诺孕酮（Norplant系统），合成代谢类固醇
停用糖皮质激素
锂
十氯锂酮

医疗条件

内分泌：艾迪生病、甲状旁腺功能减退症
高碳酸血症：睡眠呼吸暂停、匹克威克综合征（Pickwichian syndrome）
感染：系统性红斑狼疮、白塞综合征
贫血
肾衰竭
特纳综合征
唐氏综合征
埃勒斯-当洛综合征

其他

家族性
太空飞行

Reproduced with permission from Deborah I. Friedman, Grant T. Liu, Kathleen B. Digre., Revised diagnostic criteria for the pseudotumor cerebri syndrome in adults and children, *Neurology*, Volume 81, Issue 13, pp. 1159–65, Copyright © 2013 Wolters Kluwer Health, Inc.

辅助检查

头颅CT扫描检查可以排除占位和脑积水。MR检查可以发现视神经鞘的扩张、伴眼球后部变平坦、皮质沟回扩张、空蝶鞍和横窦变窄（**图**95.1）。CT静脉成像（CTV）在判断颅内静脉窦异常与否方面优于MRV。通过脑脊液引流术可以在CTV上看到横窦

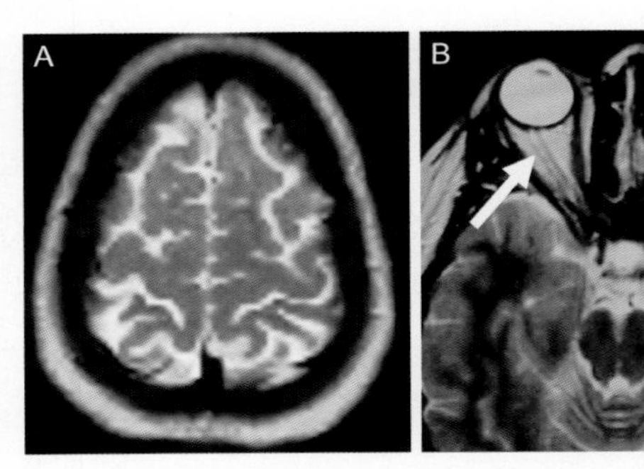

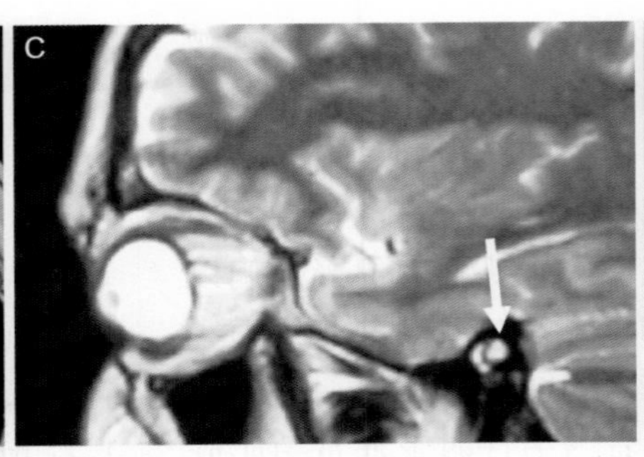

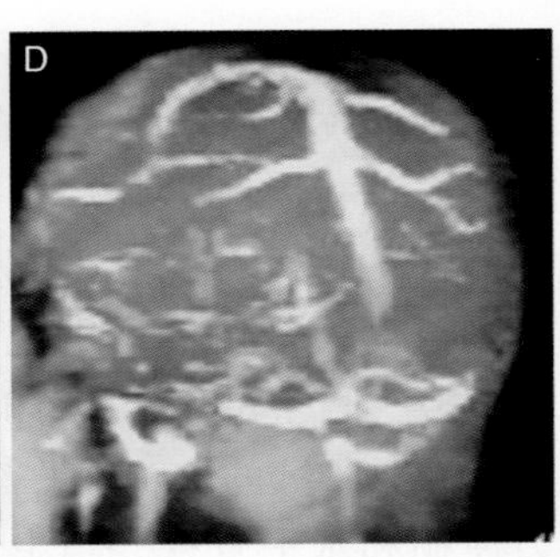

图 95.1 假性脑瘤综合征的头颅 MRI 特征，显示脑膜积液的各个方面。（A）凸面处有多余的脑沟下脑脊液。（B）视神经鞘内过多的脑脊液（箭头所指）。（C）部分空蝶鞍（箭头所指）。（D）MR 静脉造影显示右侧横窦严重狭窄

和其他颅内静脉窦狭窄的部分逆转。血管造影与逆行静脉造影不仅可以排除硬脑膜瘘管，而且可以量化静脉窦狭窄产生的压力梯度。

腰穿时需要除外占位病变和 Chiari 畸形。给肥胖的患者做腰穿是具有挑战性的。建议由有经验的高年资医师来操作，可以在 X 射线引导下穿刺，并且监测压力不短于 20 分钟。儿童做腰穿时可以酌情镇静，注意儿童哭闹时过度换气，从而降低动脉内二氧化碳水平，降低脑脊液压力，而影响结果的判断。有时候腰穿测压可能会低估真实的脑脊液压力。

关于假性脑瘤综合征患者脑脊液压力增加的原因目前仍有很多争论，特别是对于病态的肥胖者和阻塞性睡眠呼吸暂停者，其脑脊液压力有时波动较大，因此不应以单次腰椎穿刺作为最终结果，而应以多次或者持续性的压力测定为准。比如，有部分患者单次腰椎穿刺测量显示脑脊液压力为 10~20 mmHg，但持续的脑脊液压力监测时往往压力会超过 20 mmHg（图 95.2）。

因此，需要通过对颅内压力进行持续监测。电子记录过程中出现的脑脊液压力升高波也是脑脊液压力升高的重要指标。只有少数患者在脑脊液压力小于 10 mmHg 时出现 PTCS 的症状和体征。当合并 Chiari 畸形时，静脉造影术显示的横窦特征性狭窄不足以明确诊断。

PTCS 患者脑脊液的葡萄糖浓度通常正常，但蛋白质水平有时会正常或者略低于正常。而 PTCS 患者脑脊液中是否有特异性的生物标志物仍处于研究阶段。

治疗

PTCS 患者视力的恶化程度决定了其治疗策略。而在其治疗过程中，进行多学科团队管理至关重要。一些过度减肥或者过量使用止疼药物以及疾病诊断前需进行多次腰椎穿刺有创检查的患者会出现沮丧情绪，甚至出现心理问题，针对此种情况美国和英

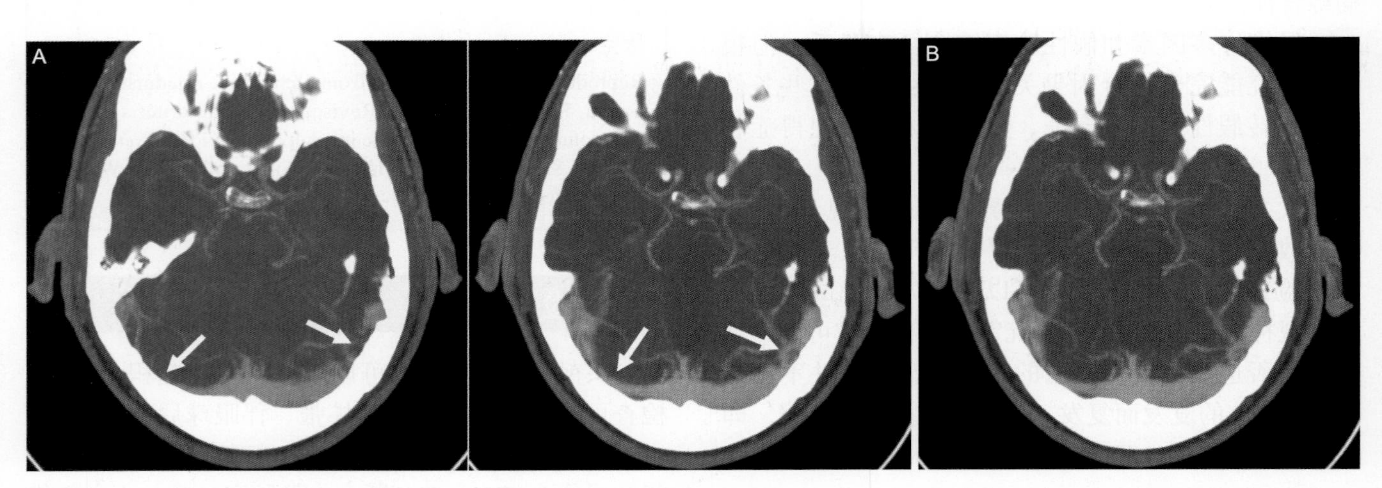

图 95.2 腰椎穿刺对静脉窦狭窄的影响。CT 静脉造影下可压缩性横窦的变化，腰椎穿刺释放脑脊液的即时影响。增加脑脊液压力和受到压迫的静脉窦会降低脑脊液吸收的能力并进一步增加脑脊液压力

国专门成立了PTCS慈善机构。对于视力迅速恶化的患者，要及时给予处理，否则可能面临诉讼。

医学治疗

应积极寻找致病因素。通过节食或减肥手术可以改善视力，减轻头痛的严重程度，但许多患者不能很好长期控制体重。一项关于减肥手术与PTCS关系的随机对照试验正在英国进行。

药物

碳酸酐酶阻断剂（乙酰唑胺、托吡酯）可以缓解假性脑瘤综合征患者的症状，但是许多患者不能耐受该药物的副作用。这些药物通过减少脑脊液分泌起作用，副作用可能导致肾衰竭，因此应该定期监测血液生化指标。托吡酯较温和，具有相对柔和的碳酸酐酶阻断作用，并且兼具抑制食欲和抗偏头痛的特点。

传统利尿剂呋塞米会使体重增加，因此应用很少。糖皮质激素仅限于视力急剧恶化的情况下使用，常与需要紧急脑脊液引流术联合使用。奥曲肽应用很少，而且应用前要谨慎。

多次腰椎穿刺

经历过多次腰椎穿刺且症状缓解欠佳的患者往往心理会受到一定的创伤。另外，多次腰椎穿刺可能增加蛛网膜下腔感染的风险，也给再次穿刺带来困难。此类患者的生活质量会明显降低。但经腰椎引流术释放大量脑脊液后可延长患者缓解期。

外科治疗

手术治疗适用于视力迅速恶化和药物治疗无效的患者。长期吸烟或者体型肥胖患者的伤口往往难以愈合。

颞肌下减压术

在分流手术被引入之前颞肌下减压术是首选的外科治疗方式。实施颞下减压术时应该避免颞叶癫痫的风险。

如果之前做过枕骨大孔减压手术，则不应实施此手术，以免引起小脑扁桃体疝、瘘管形成、中脑移位、脑萎缩等。

为了避免损伤面神经及其分支，应沿着肌纤维线方向分离颞肌，并保留颞肌在颞骨上的附着点。颅底的颞骨鳞部需广泛移除。避免减压窗太小。硬膜可以线样剪开，以使其部分扩张。值得注意的是静脉支架植入似乎可以避免颞肌下减压，并达到同样的效果。

脑脊液分流术

假性脑瘤综合征患者的脑室可能正常或者缩小，对其实施脑脊液分流操作是具有挑战性的（Tarnaris et al.，2011）。条件允许的话，建议在神经影像导航系统辅助下确定脑室端分流管位置。避免脑室端导管位置不佳出现阻塞、引流不通畅的情况。极度肥胖患者腹腔端导管的正确放置亦并非易事。有些术者推荐腹腔镜下放置腹腔端导管。脑室-腹腔分流的手术技巧在**第89章**有详细描述。

腰大池腹腔分流术也是一种术式选择，但是也有一些问题，比如导管扭曲或者过度引流导致小脑扁桃体移位下降。具有抗虹吸阀特点分流管可以避免此类并发症。腰大池胸腔引流也可作为一种术式选择。尽量选择具有可调压和抗虹吸的分流装置。此术式优点是连接两个较大的空间（腰部和胸腔），另一个优点是胸腔的负压可以随着呼吸将分流保持开启。少部分患者可能出现难治性的胸膜渗出、小脑扁桃体下疝等并发症。

手术时患者采取侧卧位。减少手术间的人员数量，阻止不相关人员的进出手术间，预防性应用抗生素，严格的无菌操作，可以降低感染的风险。

在腰椎中线处皮肤作1.5 cm的直线切口。皮肤切开后继续向棘突尖端分离。然后用Tuohy针进行腰椎穿刺，要注意确保斜面成一定角度，以便分流管能向上下方向滑行。避免通过穿刺针取出分流管，避免在导管就位后旋转穿刺针，否则会有分流管被穿刺针切断的危险。一旦分流器进入腰椎囊，就可以取出针，让分流器留在原位。

开腹手术或腹腔镜手术都可以使用，但是对于侧卧的肥胖患者，要找到腹膜是非常困难的。另一种选择是选择胸膜腔，在肋骨上表面进行穿刺并留置分流管，以避免损伤肋间束。术后X线检查确认分流管的位置，并为以后的复查随访提供一个基线标准。

对于症状复发的患者，首先要检测腹膜端分流管是否阻塞。双平面X线可以确定分流的位置，腰囊输注研究可用于评估流出阻力，但大多数最终仍需要探查并断开分流泵来确定分流管是否阻塞。

视神经减压术

视神经减压术对头痛症状缓解率低且有并发症，因而许多眼科医师弃用该术式。其相关手术并发症包括眼球运动障碍、视神经血肿、视盘梗死、视网膜中央分支动脉阻塞、术后突然失明、泪囊炎和纤维化（Alsuhaibani et al.，2011）。

静脉支架植入术

由于横窦狭窄引起常见症状的患者，静脉支架植入术是未来的发展趋势。第一例实施该术式的是2002年的一个患者。后来，越来越多的病例证明该术式对于假性脑瘤综合征患者是安全的（Higgins et al.，2003；Ahmed et al.，2011）。但也有一些严重的并发症发生，比如：支架移位、静脉窦穿孔、支架内血栓形成和硬膜下出血等。

在颈静脉孔水平静脉有狭窄的 PTCS 患者，或者此水平静脉被颅底骨质和茎突挤压，可以采取茎突切除联合静脉支架植入术式，参见**图** 95.3。

预后

PTCS 患者的预后是不确切的。有的患者单次腰椎穿刺后病情稳定，有的患者症状持续多年。患者的症状可能会改善，但几年后又会复发，尤其是在体重减轻后又反弹的情况下。

致谢和利益冲突

JDP 得到了剑桥 NIHR 生物医学研究中心神经科学主题的支持，NIHR 脑损伤医疗保健技术合作（名誉主任）和过去 NIHR 高级研究员奖。JDP 与 Ian Johnston 和 Brian Owler 合著的专著假性脑瘤综合征（The Pseudotumor Cerebri Syndrome）偶尔会获得版税（Johnston et al.，2007）。

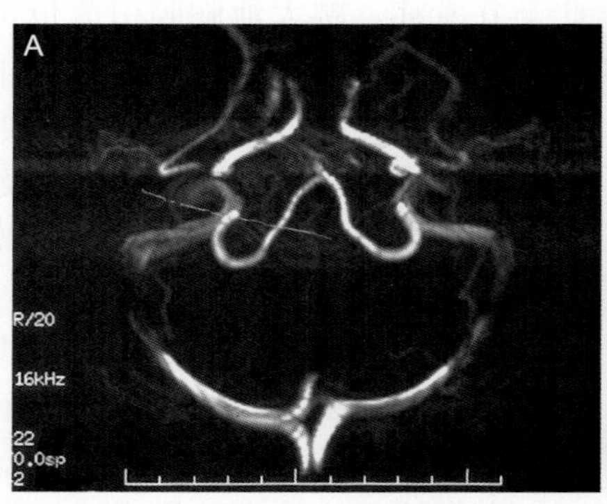

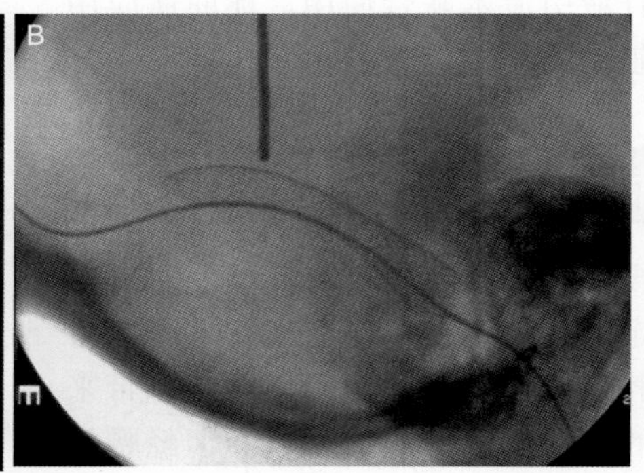

图 95.3 静脉窦支架植入术。在有固定静脉窦狭窄的病例中，血管内支架已经被证明可以缓解 PTCS 的症状。（A）三维相位对比磁共振静脉造影。轴向最大强度投影显示两个横窦远端信号较差，提示低血流。（B）右横窦静脉支架置换术后数字减影血管造影，患者症状得到改善

延伸阅读、参考文献、EBRAIN 的相关链接

扫描书末二维码获取。

第 96 章　蛛网膜囊肿

Ruichong Ma · Stana Bojanic 著
贾亮 译，张庆九 审校

引言

蛛网膜囊肿（arachnoid cysts，AC），首次报道于 1831 年，占颅内病变的 1%。椎管内蛛网膜囊肿比较少见。大多数蛛网膜囊肿位于中颅窝，男性稍多于女性，左侧大脑半球多于右侧。大多数的蛛网膜囊肿是无症状、偶然发现的。而症状性的蛛网膜囊肿主要见于儿童，典型症状包括头痛、头颅异常增大、发育迟缓以及癫痫发作等。无症状蛛网膜囊肿采取何种外科治疗方式（开颅、内镜下囊肿造瘘或分流）仍然是有争议的。

病理

蛛网膜囊肿的分类和构成

蛛网膜囊肿分为原发性和后天获得性。后天获得性的蛛网膜囊肿常继发于颅内出血或脑膜炎。Galassi 等根据中颅窝蛛网膜囊肿的发生部位与基底池的关系将其分为三类（**表** 96.1，**图** 96.1）。大体上看蛛网膜囊肿跟正常蛛网膜相似，但在显微镜下两者仍有一些不同之处。蛛网膜囊肿具有以下特点：①囊肿的边缘呈分裂状；②囊壁胶质层增厚；③没有横向交叉的小梁网；④囊壁出现高增生性蛛网膜细胞（Rengachary and Watanabe，1981）。颅内蛛网膜囊肿主要发生于额叶及中、颅后窝（**表** 96.2），但需与正常扩大的蛛网膜下腔相鉴别。蛛网膜囊肿形成于原始神经管和蛛网膜下腔脑池形成时期，是由于蛛网膜病理性撕裂导致。

发病机制

尽管有许多学者提出多种假说试图阐述蛛网膜囊肿的发病机制，但其具体形成、进展机制尚未明确。

表 96.1　颅中窝蛛网膜囊肿的 Galassi 分类

Galassi 分类	CT 脑池造影描述	与基底池是否沟通
Ⅰ	囊肿较小，局限于前颅窝	是
Ⅱ	向上沿外侧裂延伸并伴有颞叶移位	是
Ⅲ	囊肿较大，占据整个中颅窝并伴随额叶顶叶移位	否

Reprinted from *Surgical Neurology*, Volume 17, issue 5, Ercole Galassi, Francesco Tognetti, Giulio Gaist, Leo Fagioli, Franco Frank, Giorgio Frank, Ct scan and metrizamide CT cisternography in arachnoid cysts of the middle cranial fossa: Classification and pathophysiological aspects, pp. 363–69, Copyright (1982), with permission from Elsevier.

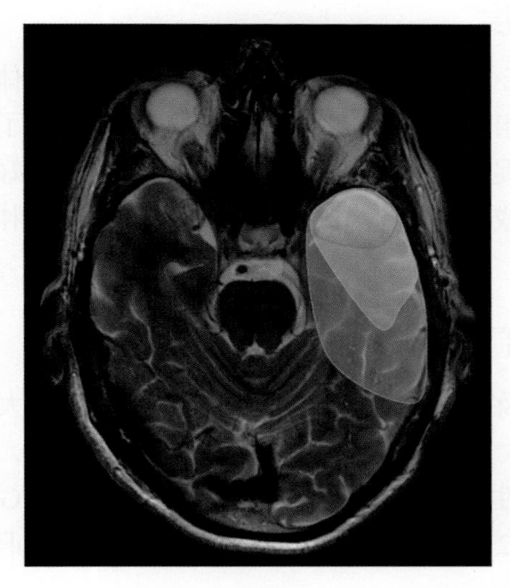

图 96.1　图示基于 Galassi 分类的中颅窝蛛网膜囊肿的相对大小和位置。蓝色所示的是Ⅰ型，囊肿较小，局限于中颅窝的前极。Ⅱ型，为黄色区域，向后上方延伸伴有颞叶移位，呈平行四边形。Ⅲ型，为红色区域，囊肿填满整个中颅窝，呈梯形状，伴有额叶和顶叶移位

脑脊液分泌异常

1964 年，Robinson 发现蛛网膜囊肿液体成分与

表 96.2 颅内蛛网膜囊肿的相对分布

位置	概率
外侧裂	49%
桥小脑角	11%
上丘	10%
小脑蚓部	9%
蝶鞍－蝶鞍上	9%
半球间	5%
大脑凸面	4%
脚间池	3%

正常脑脊液不同（Robinson，1964），包括磷酸盐、蛋白质、铁蛋白和乳酸脱氢酶（Berle et al.，2010）。一项关于囊壁的超微结构和细胞化学研究表明，蛛网膜囊肿壁和蛛网膜颗粒的神经上皮在结构上有相似性。最近的一些定量 PCR 研究发现，Na-K-2Cl 共转运体是液体转运导致囊肿扩张的潜在机制（Helland et al.，2010）。

渗透梯度

另一种理论认为，蛛网膜囊肿内的液体和 CSF 这两种组成成分存在差异，这种差异形成了渗透压梯度，促使脑脊液流入囊肿。这一理论很好解释了脑出血或炎症反应导致的继发性蛛网膜囊肿的形成特点。

单向阀门机制

小及中等蛛网膜囊肿一般较稳定，增大的趋势不明显。而较大或者进展性的蛛网膜囊肿，可能存在阀门性结构，导致单向的脑脊液流动（Galassi et al.，1982）。这种阀门结构在术中也得到了证实。

诊治策略

临床表现

大多数蛛网膜囊肿是偶然发现、无症状的。有无临床症状取决于患者的年龄和部位（表 96.3）。但在头部受到外伤时可能出现蛛网膜囊肿壁的破裂，继而导致急性出血，或者急、慢性硬膜下血肿、水囊瘤等。

表 96.3 蛛网膜囊肿在不同位置所表现出的症状和体征

位置	症状
中颅窝	头疼、癫痫、对侧肢体无力、精神错乱 儿童：发育迟缓、头围增长过快、发育停滞、颅面畸形
颅后窝	头疼、共济失调、三叉神经痛、听力缺失、眼肌麻痹、延髓功能障碍
额叶	垂体功能障碍、视力下降、脑积水、点头玩偶综合征
脊髓	脊髓神经根症状

中颅窝

大多数的蛛网膜囊肿位于中颅窝或外侧裂附近（占比 49%），男性多于女性、左侧大脑半球多于右侧大脑半球（图 96.2A）。主要症状是占位效应导致的颅压增高及颞叶、额叶皮质的刺激导致的头痛、癫痫、对侧肢体运动障碍。对于儿童，还会出现异常增大的头围、不对称的头颅形状，以及发育迟缓。颞叶蛛网膜囊肿与精神异常或者神经心理异常是否相关仍然有争议。

颅后窝

幕下蛛网膜囊肿占蛛网膜囊肿总数的 20%~30%。大多数位于桥小脑角区（图 96.2B）。当出现脑积水、压迫小脑半球及周边脑神经时会导致头痛、听力下降、三叉神经痛、复视、延髓性麻痹等。可以通过第四脑室的形状、小脑蚓部及神经结构的移位来鉴别颅后窝蛛网膜囊肿、扩大的脑池和 Dandy-Walker 畸形。

额部

鞍区或鞍旁蛛网膜囊肿起自于基底池蛛网膜下腔，与视神经、垂体、下丘脑和中脑比邻（图 96.2C）。因此会出现垂体功能减退、视力视野缺失。对于巨大的蛛网膜囊肿，可能会压迫第三脑室造成脑积水。在这些病例中，患者可能出现“点头玩偶综合征”（bobble head doll syndrome），即以 2~3 Hz 频率不自觉的前后头部摆动。

脑室内或脑室旁

比较少见，需要高分辨的磁共振才能鉴别出囊肿壁。鞍上囊肿压迫第三脑室前部可能会被误认为第三脑室型脑积水。起自四叠体池的蛛网膜囊肿可

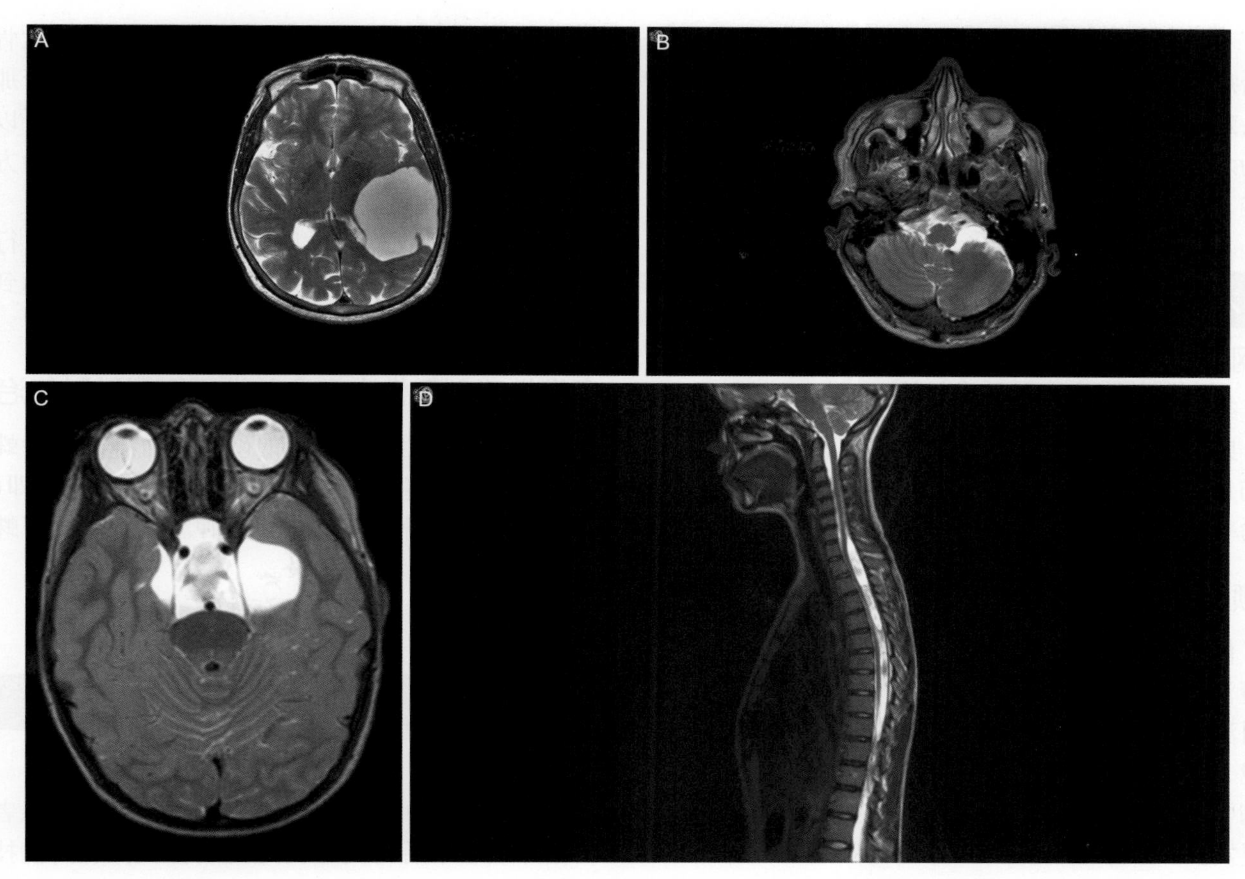

图 96.2　头颅 T2 加权像显示（A）左侧颅中窝蛛网膜囊肿，（B）左侧桥小脑角蛛网膜囊肿，（C）鞍上蛛网膜囊肿，（D）脊髓前移 T1~T3 期脊髓蛛网膜囊肿

能会压迫第三脑室后部和中脑导水管。

脊髓

脊髓蛛网膜囊肿（**图** 96.2D）由于压迫脊髓轴索或神经根从而产生典型的脊髓症状：共济失调、进展性的痉挛性瘫痪、部分患者会出现囊肿对应脊髓平面以下感觉异常等；神经根症状：神经痛、局部运动 - 感觉缺失。部分患者以后背疼痛为主要症状。

检查

当患者出现局部神经症状时，医生需要详细询问病史和查体。对于蛛网膜囊肿的诊断主要依靠影像学，尤其是磁共振。典型影像学表现为：T1 低信号，T2 高信号，类似于脑脊液。目前动态、功能磁技术不仅可以显示异常解剖，也可以描绘脑脊液流动形态和脑功能组织的改变。CT 脑池造影不推荐作为常规检查。蛛网膜囊肿的鉴别诊断详见**表** 96.4。

无症状的蛛网膜囊肿采取保守治疗，并进行影像学随访以了解囊肿有无增大。当患者出现急性梗阻性脑积水时，需要急症外科干预和处理。患者出现慢性硬膜下血肿时，需要治疗血肿，而不需要处理潜在的蛛网膜囊肿。相反，蛛网膜囊肿患者合并硬

表 96.4　蛛网膜囊肿的鉴别诊断及其影像学差异

鉴别诊断	影像学差异
蛛网膜下腔池生理性扩大	正常脑脊液间隙的生理性扩张
表皮样囊肿	MRI FLAIR 上的不均一性信号 DWI 序列可见弥散受限 呈分叶状
囊性肿瘤 • **毛细胞星形细胞瘤** • **血管母细胞瘤**	轴内经常可见异常强化的成分
非肿瘤性囊肿 • **神经肠源性囊肿** • **神经胶质囊肿** • **脑穿通性囊肿**	轴内与前肠衍生物（神经肠源性囊肿）沟通 通常被灰质（神经胶质囊肿）或胶质细胞（脑穿通性囊肿）组织包围
感染 • **包虫囊肿** • **脑囊尾蚴病**	身体其他部位的囊肿，如肝（包虫病） 病变较小而多发（神经囊虫病）

膜下积液并出现症状时，可以应用乙酰唑胺进行保守治疗。有症状的患者建议外科手术治疗。但对于仅有头痛症状的蛛网膜囊肿患者，手术治疗需要慎重。因为术后患者症状缓解与否仍不确定，且头痛原因众多，需要除外其他原因引起的头痛。

手术方式

蛛网膜囊肿分流术

类似于脑积水，可以将囊液分流到身体其他腔隙。典型的是将其分流至腹腔或者硬膜下。这种方式损伤最小，围术期风险最低。但在长期随访中，其成功率仅有 26%（Helland and Wester，2006）。

开颅囊壁切除 / 造瘘术

传统治疗方式为开颅囊壁切除或者造瘘术，以使囊液引流至硬膜下空间。大多数是囊壁造瘘将囊液引流至脑脊液自然腔隙中，使之循环起来（比如基底池、脑室系统）。一些外科医师会推荐造两个瘘口至脑脊液自然腔隙，以利于脑脊液的流动，避免囊肿复发。

内镜入路

近些年，内镜技术也越来越多用来处理颅内蛛网膜囊肿，通过内镜器械将囊肿壁造瘘，使囊液引流至基底池或脑室（图 96.3）。这样可以避免大骨瓣开颅，锁孔入路即可完成，更微创。有时对于那些囊壁较厚的、解剖部位难到达的蛛网膜囊肿可以在神经导航系统辅助下进行手术。对于选择哪种方式处理蛛网膜囊肿更合适目前仍有争议。

理想情况下，可采用“双重造瘘术”：进行囊肿－脑室、囊肿－脑池双重造瘘，以使 CSF 达到最佳流动状态（Kirollos et al.，2001）（图 96.3）。

自发性或创伤性出血合并蛛网膜囊肿时的治疗

对于自发性或创伤性的硬膜下血肿，合并蛛网膜囊肿时，大多数病例采用硬膜下血肿引流术即可，少部分采用小骨窗开颅清理血肿。一般情况下蛛网膜囊肿不需要外科处理。

脊髓的蛛网膜囊肿采用后椎板入路处理。

术后

结果

蛛网膜囊肿术后效果较好，76%~95% 的患者症状在开颅手术后得到了良好的改善，神经内镜技术的应用使开颅手术的改善率明显提高（Helland and Wester，2006；Johnson et al.，2011）。手术的失败与囊肿的位置没有明确的关系。额叶蛛网膜囊肿采用内镜技术治疗会有更高的症状改善率（74%）（Helland

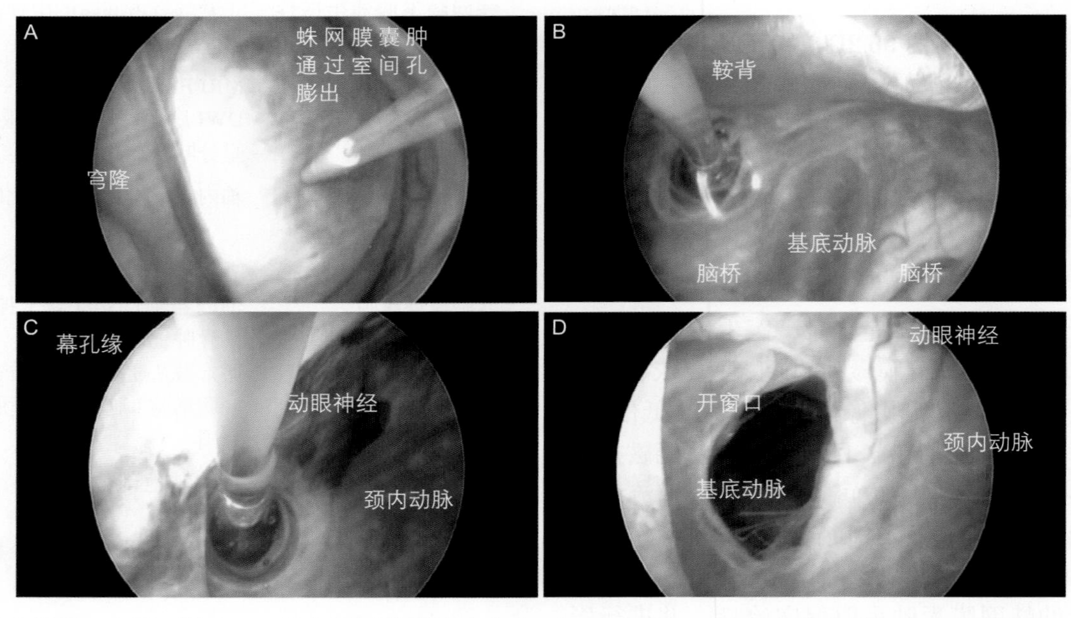

图 96.3 术中所见，内镜下鞍上 / 三脑室蛛网膜囊肿造瘘术。（A）在 Monro 孔处行囊室造口术进入侧脑室，（B）在囊肿基部行囊池造瘘术至基底动脉外侧的桥前池。术中中窝蛛网膜囊肿经内镜造瘘至枕间池和枕前池（C）在动眼神经后方使用 Fogarty 球囊扩大造瘘，（D）基底池基底动脉视图

and Wester，2006）。

并发症

总体手术并发症发生率为16.9%，需要二次手术的比率为7.2%（Helland and Wester，2006）。颞叶蛛网膜囊肿患者并发症发生率更低。颞叶蛛网膜囊肿术后，最常见的并发症是硬膜下积液的形成，其中开颅显微技术为4%~6%，内镜技术为9%（Cincu et al.，2007；Johnson et al.，2011），脑脊液漏发生率为6%，（Pradilla and Jallo，2007）。内镜操作有时会出现术区出血而不得不转为开颅手术。尽管分流手术的风险较小，但是术后近期并发症发生的比率却并不低（Helland and Wester，2006）

争议

大部分的蛛网膜囊肿是偶发的。手术的选择很重要，尤其是出现不相关的头痛症状和其他不明显的症状时。

对于具体实施哪种手术方式仍有争议（**表96.5**）。分流术式是一种微创技术，手术风险低，并且可以通过可调压分流装置控制囊肿体积。有数据显示囊肿切除或造瘘不增加近期手术并发症风险（Helland and wester，2006）。内镜技术使得传统开颅术后患者长期症状改善率提高到95%（Johnson et al.，2011），而分流手术的成功率仅为74%。大多数神经外科医生首选开颅或内镜手术治疗囊肿，分流作为第二治疗选择。

表96.5 治疗蛛网膜囊肿的手术技术及其优缺点

手术技术	优点	缺点
分流	微创，手术时间短	长期成功率较低，分流感染和其他并发症多
微创开颅	复发率低	需要开颅，时间长，感染风险高
内镜	复发率低，微创	术中出血风险高，术后硬膜下积液风险高，需要经验丰富的医师

运动与蛛网膜囊肿破裂风险研究

蛛网膜囊肿患者和正常人一样参加运动是否会造成囊肿破裂的风险增加仍有争议。一些神经外科医生认为蛛网膜囊肿的存在增加了创伤后出血和脑损伤的风险，因此应该避免竞技类运动。为证实这一点，也有一些个例报道。最常见的损伤是创伤后硬膜下积液的发生，可能是由于囊壁的撕裂形成了一个单向活瓣造成的。创伤导致颅内出血流入蛛网膜囊肿是一种罕见的情况。然而，重要的是要认识到，即使没有蛛网膜囊肿的情况下，所有竞技类运动本身都有发生创伤性脑损伤的风险。目前还不清楚有多少患者接受保守治疗且效果良好。最近一项关于185名患有蛛网膜囊肿的儿童队列研究显示，最终有112名患者参加了261项不同的运动，总时间为4410个月（strahle et al.，2016）。在这个队列中，只有两名患者出现症状性硬膜下积液，但没有神经损伤。两名硬膜下积液患者均经保守治疗，随后好转。然而，这些患者大多是参加低水平、低竞技性运动的儿童。预计参加高水平运动的年龄较大的儿童和成人将面临更大的风险，并增加创伤性脑损伤的发生率。

任何运动都不能保证绝对的“安全”。运动有可能增加蛛网膜囊肿患者脑损伤的风险，但这种情况较罕见。每个患者都应得到单独的咨询和建议，能否继续参加运动应由医生和患者共同决定。

延伸阅读、参考文献、EBRAIN的相关链接

扫描书末二维码获取。

第二十篇　感染性疾病

第 97 章　微生物学

Walter A. Hall 著
吴嘉铭 译，魏俊吉 审校

引言

中枢神经系统（central nervous system，CNS）的感染可由各种病原微生物引起，包括病毒、细菌、真菌和寄生虫。CNS 感染的发生是多因素作用的结果，如微生物毒性、宿主免疫系统的状态、感染接种体的大小，以及遗传或者或药物相关免疫抑制的暴露或者缺失（Hall，2008）。现代影像技术的发展，如计算机断层扫描（computed tomography，CT）和磁共振成像（magnetic resonance imaging，MRI）等可以显示颅内细微的形态结构，非常有助于 CNS 感染的检出，同样也能对治疗的结果和反应进行良好的监测。现代影像引导技术，如神经导航或术中 MRI 技术还可以让神经外科医生通过外科手段快速获取那些隐藏在大脑深在位置的感染灶，这些手段能加快对病原体的识别和确诊，从而更迅速地开始恰当的治疗。如有必要，快速分离病原微生物并进行外科手术减压，从而改善临床预后，降低神经疾病的发病率和死亡率。神经外科手术后的院内感染与社区性中枢神经系统感染的病原体有显著的不同。我们将重点讨论那些需要神经外科手术干预的 CNS 感染，包括需要外科手段去确诊病原体的感染，通过外科干预去缓解颅内压增高及其造成的神经症状，以及因神经外科手术导致的颅内感染。CNS 相关的主要感染有脑膜炎（图 97.1）、脑炎（图 97.4）、硬膜外脓肿（图 97.2）、硬膜下积脓（图 97.3 和图 97.4）和脑脓肿（图 97.5）等。

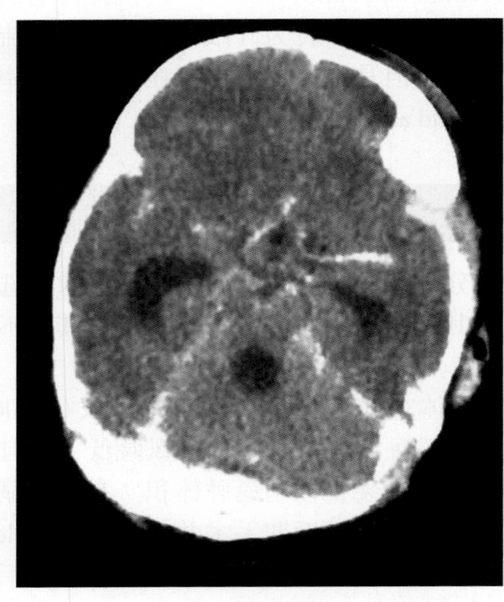

图 97.1　1 月新生儿，头部轴位 CT 扫描显示：脑积水以及脑干周围的弥漫性强化，此为大肠埃希菌引起的脑膜炎

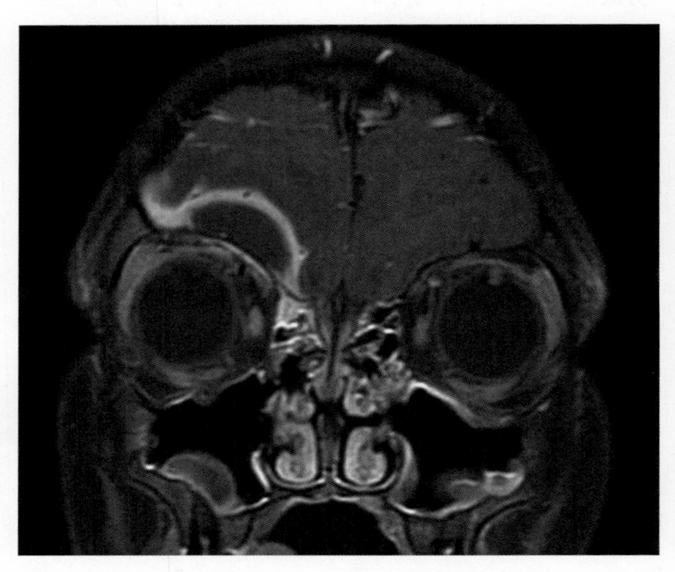

图 97.2　10 岁，男性儿童，冠状位 T1 增强 MRI 扫描显示：慢性鼻窦炎引起的硬脑膜外脓肿，因获得鼻窦内培养物前使用过抗菌药物，病原体一直未被确定

病原微生物分类

细菌

细菌应该是神经外科医生最为关注的中枢神经系统感染的病原体。患者皮肤定植的内源性菌群是导致神经外科术后感染的主要细菌，常见的细菌有金黄色葡萄球菌和表皮葡萄球菌；院内获得性病原

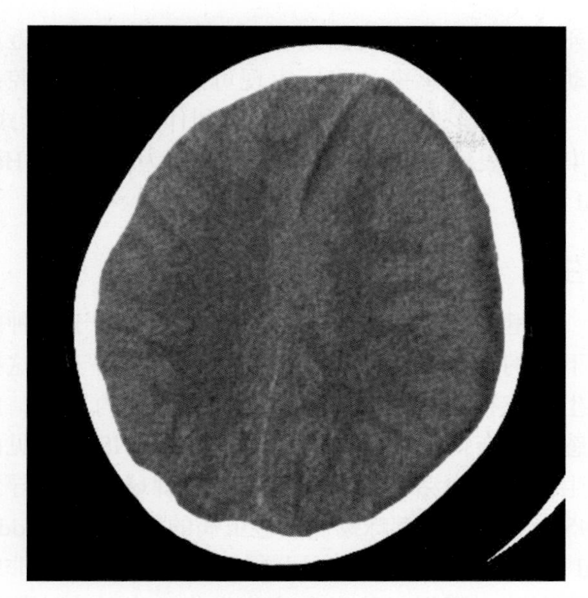

图 97.3　头部轴位CT平扫描显示：左侧硬膜下积脓蔓延至大脑纵裂并伴有占位效应，感染源为微小链球菌引起的双侧上颌窦炎

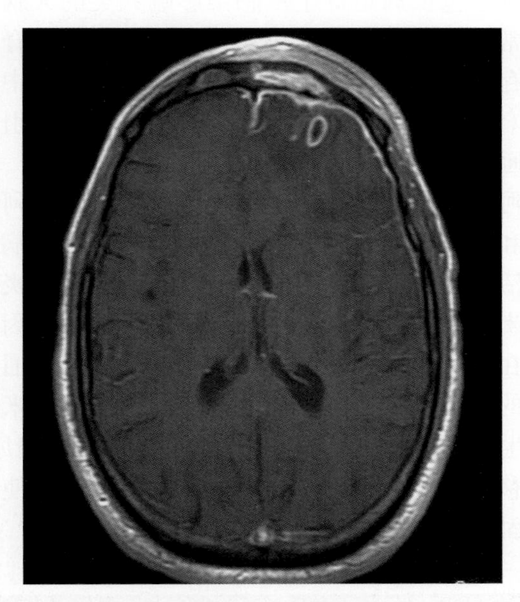

图 97.4　头部轴位T1增强MRI扫描显示：左额叶硬膜下积脓，同样可见伴有额窦炎引起的脑炎。引起感染的病原微生物是表皮葡萄球菌

体还包括革兰氏阴性菌和真菌，通常这些细菌对多种抗生素具有耐药性从而使临床治疗变得尤为困难。此外，导致自发性脑膜炎的细菌有b型流感嗜血杆菌、脑膜炎奈瑟菌、肺炎链球菌和李斯特菌。神经外科术后以及创伤性的脑脊液（cerebrospinal fluid，CSF）漏是脑膜炎的明确原因之一，其中一半的病原体是革兰阴性菌铜绿假单胞菌、克雷伯菌属和大肠埃希菌。结核分枝杆菌可引起软脑膜炎，也可演变

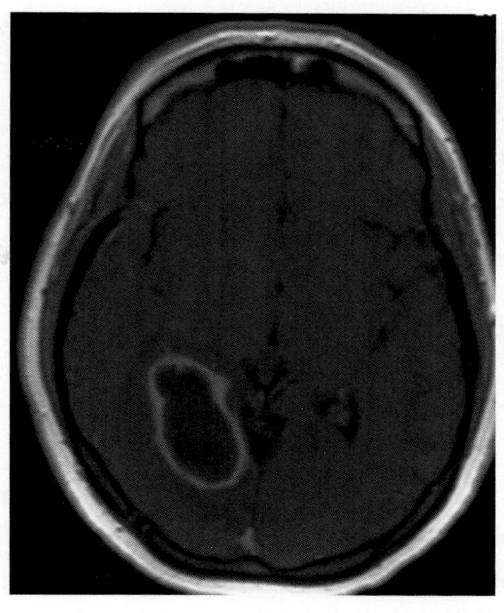

图 97.5　头部轴位T1增强MRI扫描显示：右侧枕部脑脓肿。从脓性标本中培养出脆弱拟杆菌，考虑是齿源性感染

为钙化的脑实质内病变，表现为微脓肿。

脑脊液分流感染最常见的病原菌是凝固酶阴性的表皮葡萄球菌（Naradzay et al.，1999），其他能引起分流感染的细菌有金黄色葡萄球菌、革兰氏阴性菌（包括鲍曼不动杆菌、大肠埃希菌、肺炎克雷伯菌和铜绿假单胞菌）、类白喉的痤疮丙酸杆菌，以及厌氧菌（Sacar et al.，2006）。免疫功能低下的患者也可能因念珠菌而发生脑脊液分流术后感染。11%~20%的分流术后感染是多种微生物感染（Grandhi et al.，2014）。

鼻旁窦和耳源性的需氧和厌氧微生物，尤其是微小链球菌，可引起硬膜外脓肿或硬膜下积脓。神经外科手术后，葡萄球菌和革兰氏阴性杆菌均可导致硬脑膜外脓肿和硬膜下积脓（Hall，2008）。来自耳源或齿源的厌氧微生物，如链球菌和拟杆菌属是脑脓肿发生的最主要原因。开放性颅脑创伤后脑脓肿常见的病原体包括金黄色葡萄球菌、链球菌和革兰氏阴性杆菌等需氧菌（Hall，2008）。静脉注射吸毒者和开颅手术后的脑脓肿最为常见的病原体为葡萄球菌，此与经污染的皮肤播种细菌密切相关（Kim and Hall，2014）。

病毒

中枢神经系统的病毒感染可引起脑膜炎、大脑脑炎和脊髓的横贯性脊髓炎。病毒性脑膜炎相对比较常见，且通常不需要神经外科手术干预，而病毒性脑炎并不常见，且严重得多，必要时需要手术干

预。虽然有许多病毒可以影响CNS，神经外科可能涉及的病毒有1型或2型单纯疱疹病毒（HSV-1或HSV-2）、1型或2型人类免疫缺陷病毒（human immunodeficiency virus，HIV），以及人类JC多瘤病毒。在美国，单纯疱疹病毒（herpes simplex virus，HSV）导致2%~5%的脑炎（Domachowske et al.，2014），这些病毒感染的病原体中超过90%是HSV-1（Whitley，2006），该病毒更倾向于感染颞叶和额叶下皮质，在MRI上最清晰可见，影像学现为弥散加权成像信号的高信号区域。病毒会跨越大脑侧裂这一特点可将这种感染与内在的脑肿瘤相区分。

在获得性免疫缺陷综合征（acquired immunodeficiency syndrome，AIDS）患者中，艾滋病毒可导致5%~10%的急性病毒性脑膜炎，在病毒获得时或血清转化阶段均会发生（Fukut and Byers，2014）。当艾滋病毒感染大脑时会引起脑炎，累及脊髓可导致急性横贯性脊髓炎。在免疫功能低下的患者和多达25%的艾滋病患者中，JC病毒导致进行性多灶性白质脑病（progressive multifocal leukoencephalopathy，PML）（Berger and Levy，1993）。

真菌

中枢神经系统的真菌感染通常表现为脑膜炎或脑脓肿。临床上重要的CNS真菌感染通常发生在免疫功能改变的患者，造成原因有艾滋病、糖尿病、药物诱导的免疫抑制（如糖皮质激素、化疗、抗器官移植排异反应的药物和广谱抗菌药物）、癌症、中性粒细胞减少、热损伤、胶原血管疾病、肝病、静脉注射毒品、慢性肺病、库欣综合征、脱水、酮症酸中毒、贫血、白细胞减少、营养不良、脾大、慢性肉芽肿病和既往开颅手术（Hall and Kim，2014）。脑膜炎最常由新型隐球菌和格特隐球菌引起，而脑脓肿最常由曲霉菌属引起。由于白色念珠菌多通过血液传播，其可导致微小和大型脓肿的形成。孢子菌引起的CNS受累最常见的形式是基底池软脑膜炎及其导致的脑脊液循环梗阻和脑积水。荚膜组织胞浆菌感染既可以表现为伴有脑积水的软脑膜炎，也可以表现为实质内小粟粒状肉芽肿或大的结节性组织胞浆病。慢性脑膜炎或大脑内芽生菌病是由皮炎芽生菌引起的。颅内血管的血管炎可以由白色念珠菌、粗球孢子菌、烟曲霉菌和毛霉菌属引起，并造成真菌性动脉瘤。毛霉菌属感染和毛霉菌病是进行性真菌感染，通常通过大脑中动脉和其他大动脉累及大脑，造成真菌性动脉瘤或表现为血管闭塞造成的颅内出血或缺血性脑梗死（Hall and Kim，2014）。梗死的脑组织成为真菌繁殖的理想介质。如果近端大动脉被真菌感染，临床表现可能为蛛网膜下腔出血。尖端赛多孢子菌是波氏假阿利什菌的无性形式，感染通常表现为脑脓肿，极少数表现为脑膜炎（Hall and Kim，2014）。

寄生虫

中枢神经系统的寄生虫感染主要是由于两种蠕虫下属的绦虫，造成囊虫病和包虫病。由于到这些寄生虫流行地区的国际旅行在世界范围内增加，此类感染正变得越来越普遍。囊虫病是CNS最常见的寄生虫病，由猪带绦虫引起。细粒棘球绦虫是导致CNS受累的囊性棘球蚴病或包虫病的原因（Akhaddar and Boucetta，2014）。囊尾蚴较多见于脑实质而非蛛网膜下腔，可引起脑炎和癫痫发作。当基底池软膜受累时会发生脑膜炎，而囊包阻塞中脑导水管或第四脑室时可导致梗阻性脑积水。

囊性包虫病是寄生虫感染影响人类的大脑和脊柱最常见的形式。棘球蚴囊包通常在大脑和脊柱中孤立存在，其中脊椎体在包虫病中比囊虫病中更常受累（Hall，2015）。在包虫病中，神经受压引起的症状通常与囊包在大脑或脊柱中的位置有关。

阿米巴病是一种由福氏阿米巴原虫、棘阿米巴原虫和巴拉姆西亚阿米巴原虫引起的寄生虫病。自由生活的阿米巴原虫容易引起脑炎或脑膜脑炎。大脑阿米巴病最近引起了医学界更大的关注，因为它可以在正常和免疫功能低下的个体中发展且通常是致命的。在免疫功能低下的个体中，与脑阿米巴病的发生发展相关的条件包括艾滋病、肝病、糖尿病、器官移植、肾衰竭、酗酒、静脉注射毒品、使用皮质类固醇或化疗（Hall，2012b）。

诊断技术

对于确定病原体和选择有效的抗菌治疗方法，获得适当的标本是十分重要的。对诊断神经外科植入物的感染术中获取标本进行细菌培养最关键，而皮肤或者伤口的表面培养可能并不可靠，因为最常见的致病微生物是正常皮肤菌群（Fukuta and Byers，2014）。理想情况下，抗菌药物治疗应该是收集足够多的标本后再启动，但是这种延迟启动对患者病情有潜在风险时则另当别论。

脑脊液

术后高度怀疑有脑膜炎可能时，如果影像学检查中没有脑疝等占位效应的证据，可以进行腰椎穿刺。脑膜炎时脑脊液（CSF）的开放压力可能升高，且液体的颜色可能变浑浊而非清澈。白细胞（white blood cell，WBC）计数可高于正常值 0~5 /mm³，以中性粒细胞为主。CSF 葡萄糖与血糖比值小于 0.5 为异常，CSF 蛋白水平可能升高。培养方面可留取 1~2 ml 脑脊液应用于细菌培养，5~10 ml 用于抗酸杆菌或真菌培养。脑脊液培养被认为是诊断的金标准，然而，如果留取标本之前已经开始了抗菌治疗，则识别出病原微生物的机会降低至不足 50%（Fukuta and Byers，2014）。对脑脊液标本采取聚合酶链反应（polymerase chain reaction，PCR）等核酸扩增检测对于排除细菌性脑膜炎或在已开始抗菌药物治疗且培养结果为阴性时可能有效。CSF 的革兰氏染色在 50% 的病例中会显示出单核增生杆菌或革兰氏阴性杆菌。90% 的肺炎链球菌病例中可以涂片阳性（Fukuta and Byers，2014）。在疑似脑室 - 腹腔分流感染的患者中，通过分流阀门的储液囊穿刺或从脑室导管获得的脑脊液标本比通过腰椎穿刺收集的脑脊液更容易培养到微生物。采用齐 - 内染色法和抗酸染色法可以检测到结核性脑膜炎中的抗酸分枝杆菌。

在单纯疱疹病毒性脑炎中，CSF 可显示单核细胞增多，血糖水平下降和蛋白质水平升高，存在红细胞提示出血性坏死（Domachowske et al.，2014）。PCR 检测脑脊液是明确诊断 HSV 和 HIV 的金标准。由于 HSV 很少从脑脊液中培养出来，通常需要进行脑活检来确诊。当单纯疱疹病毒性脑炎患者出现脑疝征象时，神经外科手术干预有助于进行紧急的颅内减压（Domachowske et al.，2014）。在 PML 中，CSF 通常是正常的，用 PCR 检测病毒 DNA 是首选的诊断测试（Domachowske et al.，2014）。CSF 中蛋白 14-3-3 的检测对典型克 - 雅病（Creutzfeldt-Jakob disease，CJD）的诊断具有高度特异性和敏感性（Defebvre et al.，1997）。

通过 PCR 检测和测定念珠菌特异性甘露聚糖抗原滴度，可在 CSF 中检测到白色念珠菌（Hall and Kim，2014）。针对隐球菌抗原、组织胞浆抗原、曲霉半乳甘露聚糖和球虫属的补体结合抗体可以识别脑脊液中的真菌感染。采用墨汁染色可以检测及诊断脑脊液中的新型隐球菌，通过手术方法获得感染的脑组织，可以使用 GMS（Gomori methenamine sliver stain）染色来诊断曲霉属或毛霉属（Hall and Kim，2014）。

囊虫病和包虫病的脑脊液不具备典型特点，当存在明确颅内占位效应或者颅内压增高的情况下腰椎穿刺取样，有发生脑疝的风险。阿米巴脑膜脑炎的脑脊液可能具有出血性并且白细胞计数升高。偶尔可在脑脊液的湿片检查中发现阿米巴原虫，检测脑脊液抗体和进行 PCR 检测有助于明确诊断（Hall，2012b）。在原发性阿米巴性脑膜炎中，应使用脑脊液的吉姆萨或瑞特染色来显示阿米巴滋养体（Fukuta and Byers，2014）。

血液

C 反应蛋白（C-reactive protein，CRP）在几乎所有颅内感染病例中均显著升高。红细胞沉降率（erythrocyte sedimentation rate，ESR）在 CNS 感染中也通常升高，但不像 CRP 那样敏感。ESR 和 CRP 水平同样可用于监测患者对抗菌治疗的治疗反应。血培养在诊断脑室 - 心房分流感染中很有效，然而在诊断脑室 - 腹腔分流感染时可能意义不大。

血清学检测可用于球孢子菌病的诊断，隐球菌属和荚膜组织胞浆菌的抗原检测可用于播散性疾病的诊断（Hall and Kim，2014）。尽管酶联免疫电转移印迹检测对单个脑病变的敏感性只有 30%，却是囊尾蚴病的血清学可靠诊断方法，具有 98% 的敏感性和 100% 的特异性（Akhaddar and Boucetta，2014）。CNS 包虫病的血清学诊断检测是基于酶联免疫吸附试验（enzyme-linked immunosorbent assay，ELISA）或免疫印迹试验来检测棘球蚴囊包内液来源的天然或重组抗原 B 亚单位的免疫球蛋白 G 抗体（Akhaddar and Boucetta，2014）。

其他测试

单纯疱疹性脑炎的脑电图显示可能为阵发性单侧癫痫样放电（Domachowske et al.，2014）。

TORCH 感染

围产期感染可能导致胎儿先天性异常。子宫内或分娩期间发生的感染可导致胎儿或新生儿死亡，以及儿童早期或晚期发病。五种常见疾病具有相似的症状特点，如皮疹和眼部症状的感染。它们被统称为 TORCH：弓形虫病、其他（梅毒、肠道病毒、水痘 - 带状疱疹病毒和细小病毒 B19）、风疹、巨细胞病毒（cytomegalovirus，CMV）、单纯疱疹病毒感染（Stegmann and Carey，2002）。在这组成首字母缩略词 TORCH 的五类病毒中，CMV 已成为最常见的先天性病毒感染。这些感染引起轻微的母体发病，但可能对胎儿产生严重的后果，即使母亲接受治疗，也不改变胎儿预后（Stegmann and Carey，2002）。

高度警惕围产期感染有助于及时诊断和启动相关治疗。提示先天性TORCH感染的临床表现包括头围增大、癫痫、听力丧失、白内障、皮疹、胎儿水肿、先天性心脏病、肝脾肿大、黄疸和血小板减少。但这些临床表现并不局限于TORCH感染，也可以在其他疾病和情形中看到。先天性弓形虫病的典型三联征是脉络膜视网膜炎、脑积水和颅内钙化，但大多数患有这种疾病的婴儿出生时没有明显的异常症状。新生儿单纯疱疹病毒感染有三种表现形式：发生于皮肤、眼睛和口腔，发生于CNS，或全身播散。

无症状的婴儿常常不会进行感染相关的常规筛查，但可以根据其临床表现对其进行特定的病原体检测（de Jong et al.，2013）。尽管IgM抗体的鉴定可以提示新生儿的感染，通过测量TORCH滴度不加选择地筛查先天性感染代价太大，且诊断率很低（Khan and Kazzi，2000）。实验室检测异常如血小板减少、贫血、转氨酶升高、血清直接和间接胆红素水平升高均可以在先天性巨细胞病毒感染中看到。对先天性巨细胞病毒感染的诊断是通过从尿液或唾液中分离病毒来确定的，通常是培养1~3天后呈阳性（Demmler，1991）。

不建议对无症状感染的新生儿进行直接的治疗，但是，慎重甄别后，可使用更昔洛韦治疗有症状的巨细胞病毒疾病。

抗菌药物使用原则

脑部对炎症损伤极其敏感，由抗原激发的有限免疫反应被称为免疫豁免（Nigam and Lesniak，2014）。CNS的脉管系统负责防止离子和溶质进入脑实质，并在需要时增强局部脑血流供应（Nigam and Lesniak，2014）。血脑屏障（blood-brain barrier，BBB）由包括微脉管系统的血管壁、周细胞和星形胶质细胞在内的内皮细胞组成。内皮细胞之间的紧密连接抑制了亲水分子扩散进入大脑。在有CNS感染的情况下，WBC会以血球渗出的方式通过内皮细胞穿过炎症状态的血脑屏障，而同时保持紧密连接的结构完整性（Engelhardt and Wolburg，2004）。

抗菌药物对CNS的渗透性是可变的，这取决于选择使用哪种抗菌药物治疗感染以及脑膜炎症的程度。亲脂性药物如万古霉素和氟喹诺酮类药物能很好地通过血脑屏障。氨基糖苷类和β-内酰胺类抗菌药物由于是亲水性化合物，不易穿过血脑屏障（Kim and Hall，2014）。在感染的情况下，BBB的损伤通常会使亲水抗菌药物进入CNS和CSF。从抗菌药物分类中的抑菌剂或杀菌剂分析，抑菌性的抗菌剂需要一个完整的免疫系统来杀死细菌。

脑室内或称鞘内抗菌药物的使用途径通常包括脑室外引流管或腰椎引流管，以确保充分进入脑脊液。脑室内抗菌药物已被推荐用于脑室炎的治疗和儿科分流手术时的预防（Gruber et al.，2009）。但是，部分血脑屏障通透性差却容易诱发癫痫高风险的抗菌药物，如β-内酰胺类药物，不应在脑室内使用。

抗菌药物的不规范使用导致对部分药物具有耐药性的微生物以惊人的速度出现，其中耐甲氧西林金黄色葡萄球菌（methicillin-resistant Staphylococcus aureus，MRSA）是最令人担忧的菌株之一。万古霉素的开发是为了防止细菌耐药性的发展，但目前出现了新的耐药菌株，如万古霉素耐药肠球菌（vancomycin-resistant enterococci，VRE）和万古霉素耐药金黄色葡萄球菌（vancomycin-resistant S. aureus，VRSA）。万古霉素耐药的菌株目前多使用利奈唑胺治疗，然而后续仍会再出现对该药物的耐药性。洗手液和酒精消毒液的使用降低了医院环境中如MRSA这样的耐抗菌药物细菌菌株的流行（Kim and Hall，2014）。在MRSA感染高风险的手术中，万古霉素可能是比头孢唑林更好的术前预防性抗菌药物。

围术期感染预防与控制

神经外科手术感染的预防可以通过直接干预两个方面来实现，包括术前抗菌药物的使用和无菌手术区域的维护。术前使用抗菌药物的时机对于预防手术部位感染（surgical site infections，SSI）很重要。一般而言，在手术切皮前应静脉使用抗菌药物，以确保皮肤切开时组织中抗菌药物具有杀菌浓度（Hall，2015），即必须保证在细菌接触到组织之前抗菌药物存在于该组织中（Kainth et al.，2014）。没有证据支持在手术结束后继续使用抗菌药物，且不推荐将治疗时间延长到24小时以上以防止耐药微生物的发展。此外，与单次抗菌药物相比，没有证据支持在神经外科手术预防性使用多次抗菌药物（Kainth et al.，2014）。北美脊柱外科协会为复杂脊柱手术的预防性抗菌药物使用组织了一个循证指南，建议单次使用能覆盖革兰氏阳性菌的广谱抗菌药物，且在皮肤切开之前，留有足够的时间使组织内药物达到足量浓度（Kainth et al.，2014；Hall，2015）。如果手术时间很长，或者发生大量失血，可以允许再次使用抗菌药物。手术结束后如果继续给药，会因正常宿主菌群受抑制而导致泌尿道和胃肠道的感染，如艰难梭菌结肠炎（Hall，2015）。用于治疗耐药微生物的抗菌药物不应用于外科手术预防用药，以防止耐药微生物的进一步传播。选择用于预防的抗菌药物应对那些最可能在机体组织内引起感染的微生物有效。

虽然肠外使用抗菌药物是神经外科预防感染的主要方式，局部抗菌药物给药也被认为是可以普遍接受的一种方法，尤其是当植入异物时。长期以来，像杆菌肽这样的抗菌药物溶液一直被用来在手术缝合前冲洗伤口，用于冲洗液的药物应对手术部位的菌群具有杀菌作用，且应有着最小的潜在毒副作用（Kainth et al.，2014）。实施神经外科洁净手术备皮时，必须综合考虑如下问题。关于是否有必要去除头皮毛发的问题一直有很大争议。在一项包含 11 个随机对照试验并涵盖超过 5000 名患者的大型回顾性研究中，对于术前去除毛发是否降低了 SSI 发病率的问题进行了分析（Tanner et al，2008）：三名独立的回顾分析人员得出结论，没有证据表明头发的存在或缺失会影响 SSI 的发病率。然而，研究发现，与电动剃须刀或脱毛膏相比，使用刮刀备皮的患者 SSI 发病率更高（Hall，2012a）。

当需要放置一个体内的永久植入物如脑室 - 腹腔分流管时，尽管文献未支持在儿童或成人患者中去除头发，但更多的神经外科医生会选择去除头发，希望这可以阻止可能的分流相关感染，因为一旦发生感染就需要移除分流设备（Hall，2012a）。保留患者的头发，特别是在切除像脑膜瘤这样的良性肿瘤时，可以提高患者的满意度而不会增加术后感染的风险。

但是必须要实施一些额外的措施，以确保进行皮肤切开前皮肤无菌。有研究发现，2111 例神经外科手术的术后感染率为 0.8%，其手术擦洗液包括三种成分。首先使用必妥碘手术擦洗液（普渡制药，斯坦福，加利福尼亚）处理皮肤，以保证位于毛囊深处的细菌暴露于消毒液下，其次用酒精溶液除去初步擦洗产生的泡沫。最后，使用 DuraPrep（3M，圣保罗，明尼苏达）或 ChloraPrep（康尔福盛，圣地亚哥，加利福尼亚）消毒液，待干后铺巾。如果未去除头发，则不应使用 DuraPrep 和 ChloraPrep，且头发和手术部位必须在手术开始前完全干燥，以防止术中使用电切时潜在的起火风险，这会显著推迟手术开始的时间。

手术器械的消毒和灭菌是防止感染性病原体感染神经外科手术患者的必要条件。不遵守消毒和灭菌的基本原则可导致感染暴发。根据使用这些手术器械相关的感染风险程度，用于手术和治疗的器械被分为高度危险性、中度危险性和低度危险性三类（Rutala and Weber，2004）。高度危险性器械，指用于神经外科手术的操作器械，如果被任何微生物污染，都有很高的感染风险。高度危险性器械的消毒是必须严格的，因为任何由病原微生物引起的污染都很可能首先导致局部感染，然后继发广泛严重感染。建议神经外科使用的操作器械应在购买时即进行过无菌消毒或蒸汽灭菌。如果危险器械是热敏性的，那么应该用环氧乙烷、过氧化氢气体等离子或液体化学灭菌剂处理（Rutala and Weber，2004）。用于手术的化学灭菌剂包括 2.4% 或更高浓度的戊二醛基制剂、1.12% 戊二醛与 1.93% 苯酚 / 苯酚盐、7.5% 稳态过氧化氢、7.35% 过氧化氢与 0.23% 过氧乙酸、0.2% 或更高浓度过氧乙酸，以及 1.0% 过氧化氢与 0.08% 过氧乙酸（Rutala and Weber，2004）。这些化学灭菌剂的暴露时间从 3~12 小时不等，但是如果使用 0.2% 或更高浓度过氧乙酸，在 50~56°C 下的杀孢子时间仅为 12 分钟（Rutala and Weber，2004）。在用蒸气或化学方法进行器械消毒之前，应先进行器械清洗以除去任何有机或无机物质。液体化学灭菌剂存在一些局限性，包括不能在手术器械处理后进行无菌包装，这意味着不可能在存储期间保持绝对无菌，或者接触了化学灭菌剂的器械应在使用后用水冲洗，而冲洗用水一般并非绝对无菌（Rutala and Weber，2004）。

朊病毒病

朊病毒病或传染性海绵状脑病（transmissible spongiform encephalopathy，TSE）是由一种不溶性细胞蛋白 PrP^c 在 CNS 的异常沉积引起的（Domachowske et al.，2014）。该病有三种形式：①散发性；②家族性；③暴露于蛋白质后的医源性（Belay，1999）。被认为具有家族性的 TSE 包括家族性克 - 雅病、Gersmann-Sträussler-Scheinker 病和致死性家族性失眠症（Belay，1999）。1996 年，英国的年轻人中出现了一种新发现的 CJD 变体（variant form of Creutzfeldt-Jakob disease，vCJD）（Belay，1999）。牛传染给人类的牛海绵状脑病现在被认为是 vCJD 的病因。当患者接触来源于人类遗体、硬脑膜移植物、角膜等制备的生长激素，或暴露于被污染的神经外科器械时，就会暴露于蛋白质抗原下（Domachowske et al.，2014）。该病的明确诊断通常需要脑组织活检并通过病理学检查、免疫细胞化学染色和蛋白免疫印迹检测来发现 PrP^c 蛋白质（Budka et al，1995）。

对疑似克 - 雅病（CJD）患者进行脑活检的神经外科器械要有严格的消毒去污程序，以防止传染源传播给使用相同手术器械的其他神经外科患者。在常规手术间进行脑部活检时，要用一次性材料覆盖工作面，这些一次性材料需要在手术后移除并焚烧。理想情况下，确保被污染的器械避免带来感染风险的最佳方法是丢弃并焚烧销毁（WHO，1999）。如果手术机构有能力在确诊之前隔离使用过的器械，那么这是一种可接受的替代办法，而且不需要在疑似病例中不必要地销毁昂贵的设备。如果销毁手术器械不现实，那么应按以下方法处理：①保持器械潮湿，直至去污完成；②器械使用后应尽快清洁；③不得将已污染的器械与未污染的器械混合；④采用推荐的方法去污及消毒（WHO，1999）。

手术过程中耐用器械的去污过程非常复杂。当对这些物品进行灭菌时，应结合两种或两种以上的去污方法。例如同时或先后进行加热和使用氢氧化钠（sodium hydroxide，NaOH）。热碱性水解既能清洁又能灭活大分子。用于清洗受污染设备的液体应在原地添加氢氧化钠或次氯酸钠，然后作为常规医疗垃圾处理。吸收溢出的被污染清洗液的材料应在使用后焚烧。对被污染的耐热器械进行清洗去污的推荐方法按照优先顺序见**专栏 97.1**。

专栏 97.1 用于克 - 雅病脑组织活检的耐热器械进行清洗去污的方法

1 浸泡在 1N（当量浓度）NaOH 中，在重力置换高压灭菌器内 121 ℃加热 30 分钟。清水冲洗干净后常规灭菌。
2 在 1N NaOH 或有效氯浓度为 20000 ppm 的次氯酸钠中浸泡 1 小时。在清洗和常规杀菌之前，转移到水中并在 121°C 的重力置换高压灭菌器内加热 1 小时。
3 在 1N NaOH 或次氯酸钠中浸泡 1 小时，然后取出并在水中冲洗。在清洗和常规杀菌之前，转移到一个开口的平底锅，并在重力置换（121 ℃）或多孔负载（134 ℃）高压灭菌器内加热 1 小时。
4 浸入 1N NaOH 中，并在大气压下煮 10 分钟。在常规消毒前用清水冲洗干净。
5 在室温下，在次氯酸钠（推荐）或氢氧化钠（备选）中浸泡 1 小时。在常规灭菌前用清水冲洗干净。
6 高压灭菌器内 134 ℃加热 18 分钟（WHO，1999）。

争议

神经外科手术中涉及一些与 CNS 感染预防和管理相关的争议性话题。近期的争议话题备受关注的是在复杂脊柱手术中局部应用万古霉素粉（vancomycin powder，VP）来预防 SSI。使用 VP 的基本原理是在感染最可能发生的部位聚集较高的局部药物浓度，而同时减少全身再分布。这种食品药品监督管理局规定适应证外的 VP 超说明书使用是经过了系统性回顾和 meta 分析的。最近一项关于在脊柱手术中局部使用 VP 预防感染的临床证据综述发现：接受 VP 的患者发生深部感染的概率是未接受 VP 的患者发生感染概率的 0.23 倍（Bakhsheshian et al.，2014）。根据估计，对每 100 名需要接受复杂脊柱手术的患者，使用 VP 可以节省高达 22 万 ~50 万美元的感染治疗费用。潜在的使用 VP 的缺点是患者对万古霉素耐药性的增加，万古霉素不能覆盖病原菌导致的硬件感染增加，万古霉素造成的系统性副作用如低血压、结肠炎、皮肤黏膜红斑（又被称为红人综合征）以及史斯 - 约综合征，还有药物可能对脊柱融合率产生影响。儿童和成人局部使用 VP 的合适剂量尚不清楚。

延伸阅读、参考文献、EBRAIN 的相关链接

扫描书末二维码获取。

第 98 章　颅内感染

Thangaraj Munusamy・Boon Hoe Tan・Eugene Yang 著
银锐 译，魏俊吉 审校

引言

颅内感染是全世界范围内致病及致死的重要原因之一。解剖学知识对理解颅内感染非常重要，因为它与致病机制、并发症和神经功能后遗症都有关系。由于微生物的固有属性和独特特征，颅内感染的临床症状相对特殊。最终的治疗取决于及时的微生物鉴定和抗菌治疗、减少微生物负荷、缓解颅内高压或占位效应，以及调节宿主的免疫反应，从而在尽可能控制炎症及水肿的情况下清除微生物。在本章中，我们将从神经外科的角度讨论常见颅内感染的处理及其相关的临床问题。

脑脓肿

脑脓肿是一种局灶性颅内感染，以局灶性脑炎起病，后逐渐发展形成囊性的脓液聚集。脑脓肿可由三个主要来源引起：

1. 邻近感染源的直接蔓延
2. 远处感染源的血行播散
3. 通过硬脑膜缺口直接进入颅内

邻近感染源直接蔓延的例子包括继发于化脓性中耳炎、乳突炎，或来自鼻旁窦前部的脑脓肿。这些直接蔓延通常影响到颞叶、小脑、额叶或鞍区和鞍旁区域。远处来源的血行播散包括感染性心内膜炎的菌栓，以及远处的感染源，如腹腔内积液或骨髓炎。身体的自然保护机制是通过肺部的毛细血管循环过滤这些病原体，但在存在房室分流的情况下，例如遗传性出血性毛细血管扩张症（Osler-Weber-Rendu 综合征）中的先天性发绀性心脏病或肺动静脉畸形，这些保护机制可能会失效（Helweg-Larsen et al.，2012；Chenran et al.，2014；Yakut et al.，2015）。

脑脓肿在免疫受损的患者中更常见，如 HIV 阳性、接受恶性肿瘤化疗、使用类固醇以及接受器官移植或炎症性疾病免疫抑制治疗的患者。

硬脑膜的直接破损可形成细菌入颅的直接入口，这通常是由于外伤（如颅骨凹陷性骨折和异物进入）或由神经外科手术导致。神经外科手术后的脓肿可能是由手术过程本身的性质造成的，如异物植入手术（电极、分流管）、脑室外引流、颅内压监测器，或在胶质瘤手术中使用的卡莫司汀植入剂（gliadel wafers）（McGovern et al.，2003）。

感染的阶段

一般认为，脑脓肿的形成可分为四个病理阶段：

1. 脑炎早期
2. 脑炎晚期
3. 脓肿形成早期
4. 脓肿形成晚期

脑炎早期（第 1~3 天）为脓肿形成的早期阶段，期间可出现组织坏死、中性粒细胞积聚、脑水肿。第 4~9 天起，早期的中性粒细胞积聚转变为以巨噬细胞和淋巴细胞为主的渗透。脓肿形成早期从第 10~13 天开始，此时脓肿囊的脑室面较薄。这可能导致脓肿破入脑室，引发脑室炎。脓肿形成晚期始于第 14 天后，其特征是形成了胶质细胞增生、胶原和肉芽层（Erdogan and Cansever，2008）。

病原体

引起脑脓肿的最常见微生物是链球菌，尤其是米勒链球菌，其次是厌氧菌、葡萄球菌和革兰氏阴性菌。肠道革兰氏阴性菌（如假单胞菌、变形杆菌和大肠杆菌）通常出现在有耳源性或鼻窦病灶、全身性菌血症或免疫功能低下的患者中。在脑脓肿患者中，链球菌约占 54%，葡萄球菌占 15%，革兰氏阴性菌占 8%，厌氧菌占 17%，诺卡菌占 2%（Helweg-Larsen et al.，2012；Chenran et al.，2014；Yakut et al.，2015）。

对免疫功能低下的患者（如 HIV、恶性肿瘤、移植受者、接受化疗或长期使用类固醇的患者），应考虑李斯特菌和诺卡菌等微生物感染。

诺卡菌脑脓肿的死亡率很高，为31%~77%，其治疗通常为长程（3~12个月）甲氧苄啶磺胺甲恶唑方案（Weerakkody et al.，2015）。

确诊结核性脑脓肿需要排除潜在的HIV暴露。Whitener在1978年提出的诊断标准是：①具有脑实质内形成脓肿的宏观证据（手术或活检）；②组织学证实脓肿中的炎症主要由血管肉芽组织组成，其中包含急性和慢性炎症细胞；③脓液培养阳性或有抗酸杆菌存在的证据。与男性相比，女性为易感患者，平均年龄为23.9岁。在没有HIV感染的情况下，结核性脑脓肿的发病率为中枢神经系统结核病的4%~8%（Mohindra et al.，2016）。

结核病对诊断提出了挑战，它在常规CT和MR影像上的表现与多种其他实体占位病变（包括转移性脑肿瘤、脑囊虫病、弓形体病和真菌性脑脓肿）都很相似（**图98.1**）。结核性脑脓肿是稳定的、无血管的球形占位，直径为2~10 cm，边界清楚，并含有结核杆菌的干酪样坏死区。孤立性结核的脑脊液评估通常不具有特异性。由于大多数结核性脑脓肿对足量的抗菌药物治疗和类固醇治疗反应良好，通常采取药物治疗，因此手术治疗的指征有限，仅在某些情况下需要手术干预以确诊或缓解明显占位效应或者潜在的对脑组织压迫（Chatterjee，2011；Monteiro et al.，2013）。

随着免疫抑制治疗（类固醇、免疫调节剂化疗）适应证的扩大、人类免疫缺陷病毒和艾滋病的流行以及器官移植受者的增多，真菌感染越来越常见。报道中常见的微生物感染包括中枢神经系统曲霉菌感染、赛多孢子菌感染、新型隐球菌感染和地方性霉菌病（Vergara et al.，2015）。真菌性脑脓肿的死亡率很高，尤其是在免疫功能低下的患者中。

临床表现

最常见的临床症状包括发热（60%）、颈部僵硬（25%）、恶心或呕吐（40%）、局灶性神经功能缺损（57%）、癫痫发作（21%）和意识障碍（45%）（Helweg-Larsen et al.，2012）。头痛、发热、恶心或呕吐的经典三联征仅在1/5的病例中出现。头痛、发热、局灶性神经功能缺损的三联征见于大约1/4的患者中。

头痛、意识模糊和嗜睡等精神状态改变，并伴有恶心和呕吐的症状可能提示颅内压升高，这可能是由大量脓肿聚集和病灶周围水肿引起的占位效应所致。

在脓肿破裂到脑室腔导致脑室炎和脑膜炎的情况下，可能会出现颈部僵硬或强直。

局灶性神经功能缺损取决于颅内脓肿的位置，导致大脑相应区域的功能丧失。可能表现为偏瘫、性格改变、视野缺损、失语、眼球震颤和共济失调。

影像学特征

磁共振成像具有准确、敏感的特点，被认为是脑脓肿首选的诊断性神经影像学检查。其经典表现为对比剂增强的T1加权图像上的环形增强病灶。MRI还可提供额外的信息，例如周围的增强边缘，以及脑脓肿病灶周围水肿的程度（**图98.2**）。

在脑炎阶段，化脓性脑脓肿呈T1低信号和T2高信号，较少有强化或非均匀的强化。结核性脑炎表现为脑回强化中一个不清晰的、低信号的区域。真菌性脑炎通常不强化，多位于基底节或深部脑白质。所有成熟的化脓性、结核性和真菌性脓肿都在T1像上呈低信号、在T2像上呈高信号，并且在对比增强序列上呈现显著的边缘增强。大多数化脓性和

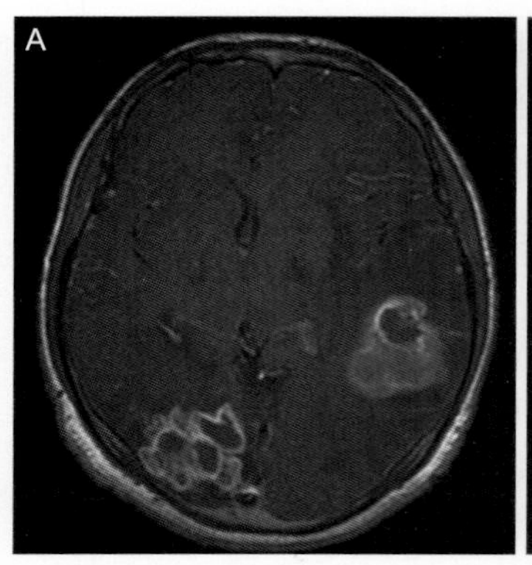

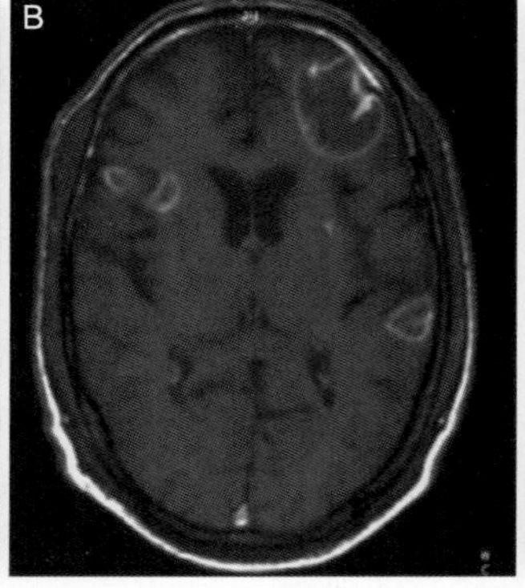

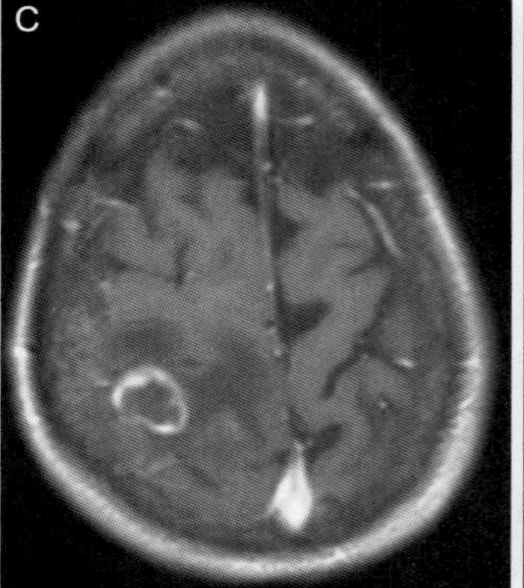

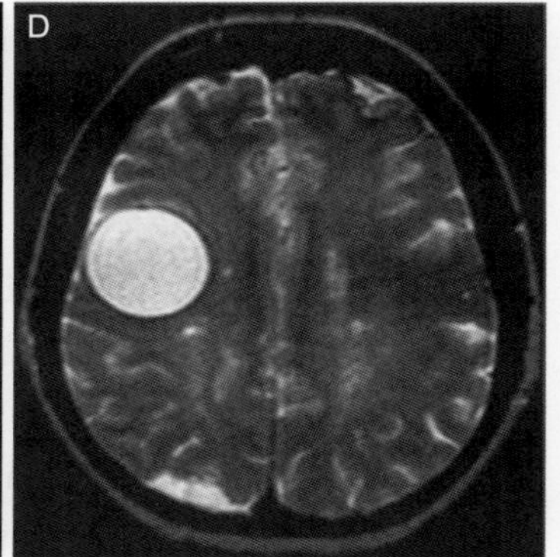

图98.1 中枢神经系统感染的MR影像。（A）脑结核（Helmy et al.，2011）；（B）脑弓形体病（Batra et al.，2004）；（C）真菌性脑脓肿（Bagla et al.，2016）；（D）脑棘球蚴囊（Seckin et al.，2008）

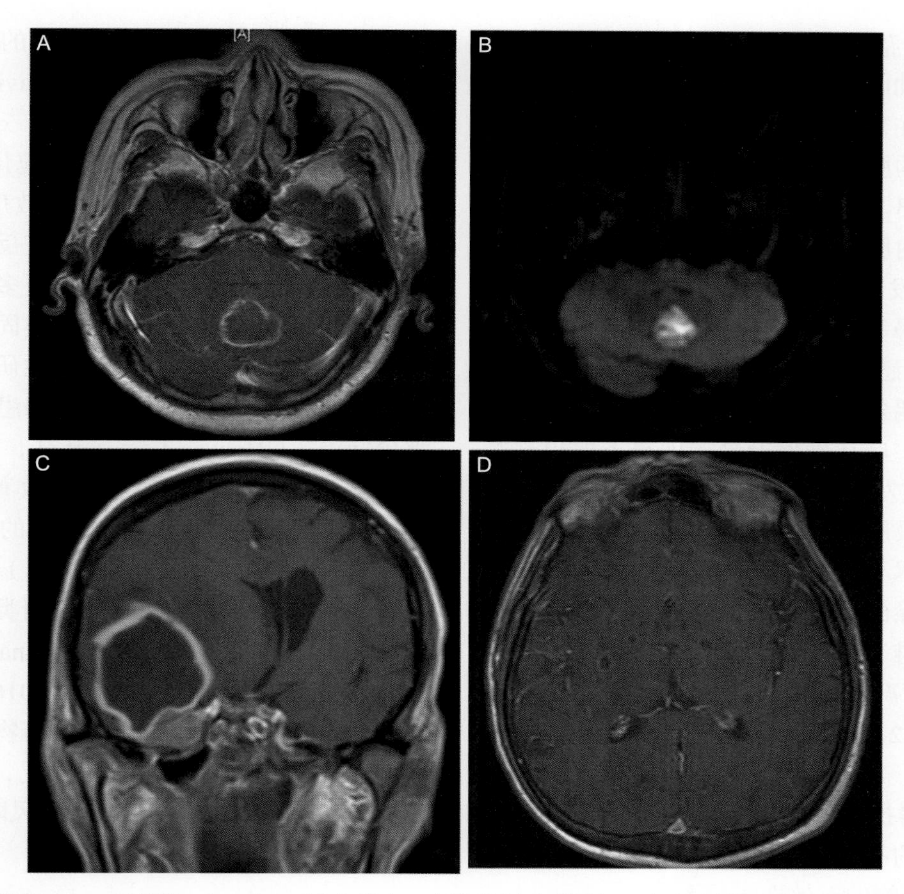

图 98.2　化脓性脑脓肿的 MR 影像。（A 和 B）（上排）：小脑脓肿在增强 T1 加权图像上表现为环形增强病变（A），在 DWI 上表现为高信号（B）。（C）晚期鼻咽癌患者的右颞部脓肿（放疗后）。（D）感染性心内膜炎患者的多个脓肿

结核性脓肿具有光滑或分叶状的外壁。大约一半的真菌性脓肿具有齿状外壁。真菌性脓肿也可表现出自外壁指向中央的腔内投影，而没有任何对比增强，这是其他类型脓肿的常规MRI影像不具备的（Cartes-Zumelzu et al.，2004；Luthra et al.，2007）。在免疫功能低下的患者中，对比剂增强可能相对较弱，可能会混淆诊断。2004 年有一例骨髓移植后免疫功能低下患者的病例报告，该例中发生了暴发性脑弓形体病，但影像上的增强很弱（Ionita et al.，2004）。

在化脓性脑脓肿的弥散加权成像序列上可以看到局限弥散区（**图** 98.2）。脓肿腔内可见坏死物质存在，其中含有炎症细胞、细菌和脓液，限制了水的流动。化脓性和结核性脓肿的 MRI 影像在弥散加权成像（diffusion-weighted imaging，DWI）呈高信号，脓腔内核心的表观扩散系数（apparent diffusion coefficient，ADC）值较低。相反，真菌性脓肿的 DWI 和 ADC 仅在脓肿边缘呈现局限弥散，而脓肿的核心部位却没有。

也有一些证据建议使用 DWI 来监测对药物治疗的反应性。DWI 信号从最初的高信号转变为低信号提示脓肿核心内的脓液消失，表明治疗反应性良好。

脑脓肿的 MR 波谱（MR spectroscopy，MRS）可见与缺氧和细胞分解有关的代谢物，如氨基酸、脂质、乳酸、醋酸和琥珀酸，不同脓肿中这些代谢物的量各异，可能有助于区分脓肿的亚型（Cartes-Zumelzu et al.，2004；Luthra et al.，2007）。

静脉对比剂增强的 CT 成像通常会显示中心低密度及周围边缘增强。

MRI 及 CT 还可协助进行立体定向引导下的脓肿抽吸，有助于微生物学诊断并减少细菌负荷。

管理

脑脓肿的管理和治疗需要神经外科医生、神经放射科医生和感染性疾病医生的多学科合作。应考虑的关键原则是从脓肿本身或潜在的感染源确定微生物学诊断。

虽然在手术干预的必要性方面没有绝对的脓肿大小的标准，但对于最大径超过 2.5 cm 的脓肿最好

通过开颅手术切除整个脓腔，或（通常）在立体定向引导下进行脓肿抽吸。完全切除脓肿可以改善影像学表现，但也存在额外的风险，尤其是术后癫痫发作的风险。较小的脓肿可以在影像引导下进行抽吸（Radoi et al.，2013）。

一旦发现颅内脓肿，都必须清除最初感染源和病原体以防止复发。应考虑将耳乳突炎病灶切除、化脓性中耳炎或鼻窦感染引流、远处感染源（如腹腔内积液）引流、感染伤口清创等与脓肿治疗同时进行。创伤后脓肿偶尔会含有异物，如骨片、枪弹颗粒、子弹或石头，应在确保安全的前提下取出这些异物以减少脓肿复发的风险。

立体定向抽吸脓肿的优点是操作简单、潜在的并发症比开颅手术少，但是它与更高的复发风险相关。开颅脓肿切除的复发率较低，尤其适合占位效应明显、诊断困难、创伤致异物进入引发脓肿或脓肿处于颅后窝等情况（Ratnaike et al.，2011；Helweg-Larsen et al.，2012；Radoi et al.，2013；Aras et al.，2016）。

脓肿壁是阻碍抗菌药物进入脓肿腔的物理屏障，降低了抗菌药物的有效性，此外，酸性的脓肿环境也可能抑制抗菌药物的有效性。

脓肿应送显微镜检和延长培养，以确定病原微生物。因此，抽吸脓肿将有助于基于药敏的针对性抗菌药物治疗。经验性抗感染治疗取决于几个因素，包括基于病史和检查判断的可疑细菌、革兰染色的初步结果，以及当地环境的微生物特点。

选择抗菌药物时应考虑到可疑的脓肿来源（鼻窦炎、耳源性或创伤性）、CSF渗透的药代动力学、持续时间和给药途径（即静脉或脑室内）。常见的经验性抗感染方案包括使用第三代头孢菌素和甲硝唑以覆盖更多的厌氧菌，特别是在有直接邻近感染源的情况下（即鼻窦炎、耳源性）。在有直接细菌播散情况下，如开放性外伤后或脑部手术后，可以联合使用抗菌药物，如覆盖革兰阳性菌的万古霉素联合第三代头孢菌素。一般来说抗感染治疗的持续时间为6~8周，通常建议使用大剂量静脉注射的途径，以克服药物血脑屏障通透性的问题。监测疗效需要根据影像学和相关的生化（如血浆C反应蛋白）标志物，从而调整抗感染疗程（Cartes-Zumelzu et al.，2004；Luthra et al.，2007）。

真菌性脑脓肿使用抗真菌药物治疗，例如伏立康唑治疗曲霉菌感染，两性霉素B治疗念珠菌和毛霉菌病。可以通过脑室引流管进行蛛网膜下腔给药，但并非普遍接受的做法。真菌性脑脓肿与较高的死亡率有关，特别是在免疫功能低下的患者中（Grannan et al.，2014；Ma et al.，2015；Gavito-Higuera et al.，2016；Patterson et al.，2016）。

皮质类固醇在脑脓肿中的应用也是有争议的，它可以减轻脑肿胀，缓解占位效应和脑疝。然而，它也可能导致宿主对感染的免疫反应降低，并可能减缓脓肿壁的形成，导致周围更多的正常脑组织被破坏，延迟遏制脓肿。手术前类固醇治疗似乎并没有明显改变预后：在一项回顾性研究中，21%接受治疗的患者与23%未接受治疗的患者出院时的GOS评分低于3（Helweg-Larsen et al.，2012）。术后接受类固醇治疗的患者的功能预后改善也不明显，25%使用类固醇的患者与20%未使用的患者GOS评分小于3（Helweg-Larsen et al.，2012）。在另一个病例系列中，与非类固醇组相比，使用类固醇与较高的死亡率相关（15.6% *vs.* 3.9%）（Ratnaike et al.，2011；Radoi et al.，2013；Aras et al.，2016）。

脑脓肿的治疗主张手术和药物治疗相结合。然而，也需要考虑患者的整体情况，即患者因素（围术期的麻醉、心血管和呼吸系统风险）以及病理因素（脓肿的大小、数量和位置）。

神经囊虫病和棘球蚴病

神经囊虫病是全球最常见的脑部寄生虫感染，第二位是棘球蚴病（包虫病）。神经囊虫病是由猪带绦虫的囊状幼虫引起的。可为实质型或实质外型。实质型最常见，通常累及灰/白质交界处，与实质外型相比，预后更佳。实质外型在整个中枢神经系统中累及的位置更广泛，与较高的寄生虫负荷和较差的预后相关。它可以导致蛛网膜炎、脑膜炎、颅神经卡压以及脑脊液流动受阻致脑积水。神经囊虫病的确诊往往较困难，因为大多数病例都没有手术指征，无法对寄生虫进行组织学鉴定。全面的神经影像学诊断标准可以提高诊断的准确性（**图 98.3**）。其治疗包括驱虫药（如阿苯达唑和吡喹酮）、抗癫痫药，以及抑制炎症的类固醇。手术可能包括囊肿切除或植入CSF分流装置以治疗脑积水（Baird et al.，2013；Del Brutto et al.，2017；Gripper and Welburn，2017）。

脑棘球蚴病是一种由棘球蚴幼虫引起的罕见的寄生虫病。它在中东、地中海、非洲、印度、澳大利亚和南美洲的部分地区流行。颅内棘球蚴病可表现为囊型（细粒棘球蚴）或泡型（多房棘球蚴）。最常发病在幕上区，以大脑中动脉的供血区域为主。症状与囊肿引起的局部占位效应或颅内压增高有关。诊

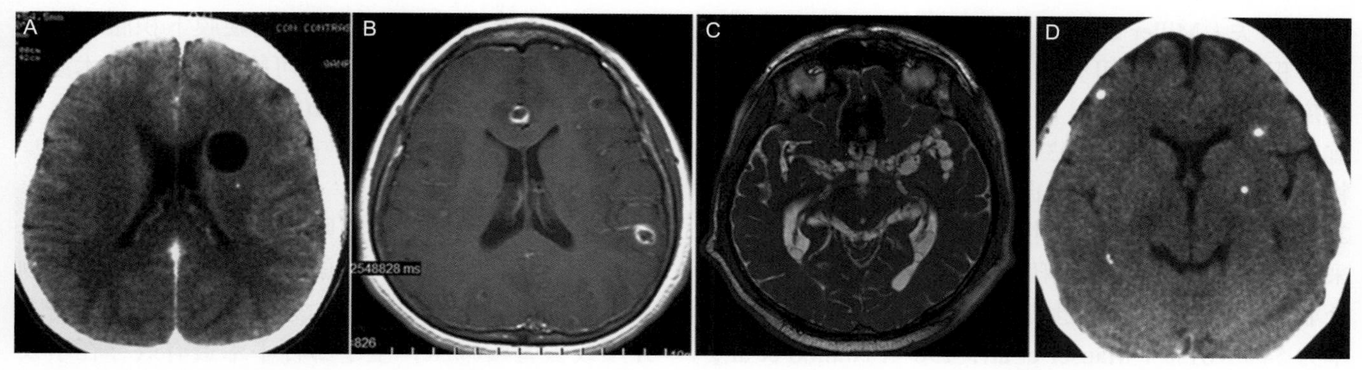

图 98.3　神经囊虫病的主要神经影像学诊断标准（Del Brutto et al.，2017）。没有可辨认头结的囊性病变（A），环形强化病变（B），基底蛛网膜下腔的多叶囊肿（C），以及典型的脑实质钙化（D）

断主要依靠计算机断层扫描和磁共振成像。从影像学角度看，囊肿呈球形，轮廓清晰，无强化、钙化或周围水肿（**图** 98.1）。泡型囊肿表现为清晰的多隔占位，由实体占位和囊性成分组成，其中实体部分存在钙化。囊液与 CSF 等密度。囊肿通常是单发的，但也有脑内多囊的报道。单发的脑囊肿常无颅外病变，但有必要对身体其他部位进行检查。鉴别诊断包括蛛网膜囊肿、表皮样囊肿、肠源性囊肿、囊性原发性脑肿瘤或转移瘤，以及脑脓肿。

Dowling 法是经典的囊肿手术切除方法：宽大的皮瓣，切除萎缩的皮质，降低手术台头端以利用重力，在囊肿和脑实质之间使用温盐水来剥离囊肿。操作过程中囊肿不慎破裂可能导致寄生虫扩散和过敏性休克（Bukte et al.，2004；Luo et al.，2013；Ulutas et al.，2015）。

硬膜外和硬膜下脓液聚集

积脓是指在正常解剖空间内的脓液聚集，因此硬膜下腔的聚集是积脓，而硬膜外只是一个潜在的空间，其脓液聚集被定义为脓肿。硬膜外脓肿通常位于额部，并受到骨缝的限制。硬膜外脓肿患者可能有轻微的临床症状，只有当脓液引起足够的占位效应时才会出现神经功能障碍。如果硬膜破损或通过硬膜静脉吻合口扩散，积脓可发展到硬膜下腔或引起血栓性静脉炎和脑炎。硬膜下积脓具有较高的发病率和死亡率，除了继发于硬膜外积脓，它还可以继发于血源性扩散或神经外科术后并发症。

硬膜下积脓

硬膜下积脓是一种神经外科急症，尽管有干预措施，其死亡率仍高达 20%，发病率为 50%（Le Beau et al.，1973；Nathoo et al.，1999）。在免疫功能正常的患者中，好发年龄为 11~20 岁，且男女性别比例为 3：1（Osborn and Steinberg，2007）。预后取决于年龄、并发症、原发微生物以及及时的诊断和治疗等因素。硬膜下积脓由于缺乏纤维蛋白囊和解剖屏障，更易迅速扩散。最常见的感染源是来自中耳炎和鼻旁或乳突气窦的感染。其他原因包括脑膜炎的直接蔓延、远处的血源性播散、手术部位感染以及发生颅骨骨折和硬膜撕裂的头部创伤（Munusamy and Dinesh，2015）。6%~22% 的病例可能同时发生实质内脓肿，9%~17% 发生硬膜外脓肿（Osborn and Steinberg，2007）。

临床表现

硬膜下积脓患者通常表现为发热、头痛和精神状态改变，随后神经系统状态迅速恶化。从症状出现到诊断的中位时间是 2 天（French et al.，2014）。癫痫发作也很常见，发生率高达 63%（Cowie and Williams，1983）。其他症状取决于潜在的病因，如鼻窦炎、乳突炎、中耳炎、脑膜炎、术后伤口感染、全身感染或头部外伤。病情进展为较大的占位病变后会出现颅内压升高相关的症状和体征。脑水肿和脑积水可能继发于脑血流或 CSF 流动的异常。皮质静脉或硬脑膜静脉窦血栓形成或化脓性栓子可导致静脉高压，并可能进展为脑梗死。

发病机制

硬膜下积脓的发病机制与脑脓肿的发病机制相似。致病的微生物因主要感染源而异。通常是单一菌种，但是多菌性的感染也不少见，尤其是来自于鼻旁窦的感染（Nathoo et al.，1999）。需氧和微需氧链球菌通常与继发于乳突炎或鼻窦炎的硬膜下积脓相关（Miller et al.，1987）。术后和创伤后硬膜下积脓中，通常可分离出金黄色葡萄球菌，而在免疫力低下的人群中，肺炎克雷伯菌往往是罪魁祸首（Greenlee et al.，2003）。其他已报道的致病微生物包括大肠杆菌和沙门菌（Munusamy and Dinesh，2015）。硬膜下积脓的微生物学诊断基于手术引流时采集的脓液或感染物的阳性培养，或从主要感染源处取样的结果。手术干预获取的硬膜下脓液培养成功率为 54%~81%（Mauser et al.，1987；Nathoo et al.，1999）。培养阳性率低的原因包括取样前经验性使用广谱抗菌药物进行抗感染治疗，以及厌氧菌培养方面的困难。

影像学特征

影像学诊断可利用增强 CT 或 MRI。硬膜下积脓表现为月牙形的聚集，在颅顶下或邻近大脑镰或大脑幕的脑表面跨越骨缝，通常在使用造影剂后呈边缘强化。然而，增强 CT 偶尔未见异常或仅有轻微的脑水肿，特别是在慢性病例中，硬膜下脓液可能无法产生周边强化（Moseley and Kendall，1984；Munusamy and Dinesh，2015）（**图 98.4**）。在这种情况下，MRI 更为敏感，尤其是在颅底、颅后窝或大脑镰处。硬膜下积脓在 DWI 上呈高信号，在 ADC 上呈低信号，与脑脓肿和脑室炎的表现相似。因此，弥散加权 MR 成像可以可靠鉴别硬膜下积脓与硬膜下血肿或反应性硬膜下积液（可能在创伤、手术或脑膜炎后出现）（Wong et al.，2004）。

治疗

硬膜下积脓的治疗原则包括手术干预以及尽早细菌学鉴定，清除原发感染病灶和充分的抗菌药物治疗（Miller et al.，1987）。手术干预方式有钻孔、开颅或去骨瓣减压，至于哪种手术最有效存在争议（Pathak et al.，1990）。只要能有效引流脓性物质和缓解占位效应，这三种方法的预后都是相当的（Bok and Peter，1993）。一般来说，如果积脓是非黏性并且没有固定的聚集，通过钻孔排脓便足够，并且可以避免手术时间过长或因复杂手术导致的相关手术并发症。然而，如果脓液较黏稠或组织紧密，则建议进行开颅手术，以便充分暴露和引流（Munusamy and Dinesh，2015）（**图 98.4**）。在某些情况下，脓肿周围脑组织可能明显肿胀，必要时需要进行去骨瓣减压术。如果术中怀疑骨瓣有骨髓炎，也应考虑在其后进行颅骨切除术，因为骨瓣可能作为持续感染的细菌来源。如果感染源来自耳或颅外病灶，必须对主要感染源进行探查和引流。如果患者因硬膜下积脓而出现败血症和相关临床症状，建议立即启动经验性抗菌药物治疗。后续抗菌治疗的调整应基于

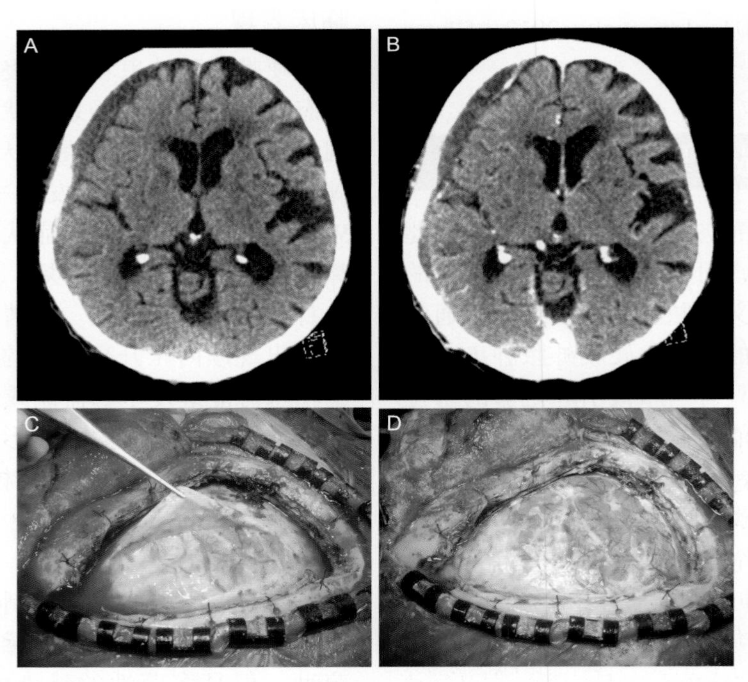

图 98.4　为一位硬膜下积脓患者进行开颅手术并排空硬膜下脓液。（A 和 B）（上排）：使用造影剂之前（A）和之后（B）的 CT 图像。此病例中造影剂增强不明显，硬膜下脓液组织紧密。（C 和 D）（下排）：脑表面揭起浓厚的硬膜下脓液（C），庆大霉素盐水冲洗硬膜下腔。其下脑组织充血但不肿胀（D），因此还纳了骨瓣，并继续进行抗菌药物治疗

革兰氏染色或特殊细菌染色、细菌培养的阳性结果，以及对原发感染部位的细菌情况的了解进行。根据临床和影像学上的反应，抗菌药物治疗通常要持续4~6周，并尽早征求传染病专家和微生物学家的专业意见（Leys et al.，1986）。

开颅术后可能出现硬膜下积脓，但极少与慢性硬膜下血肿的钻孔引流相关。据推测，这种相对简单和较小的手术可以最大限度地减少组织创伤，并降低细菌接种的程度。然而，它们的处理方式类似，手术的目标是实现充分减压和排空积脓。如有必要，可重新打开钻孔并排脓，但如果这还不够，则必须转为开颅手术。痤疮丙酸杆菌是一种无处不在的皮肤共生菌，很少直接诱发感染，其临床表现和进展过程并不典型（Gritchley and Strachan，1996）。

颅内硬膜外脓肿

颅内硬膜外脓肿是一种化脓性感染，由于邻近结构的连续蔓延而在颅骨内板和硬膜之间出现。传统上，它与鼻窦炎、乳突炎、中耳炎和颅骨骨髓炎相关（Calfee and Wispelwey，1999）。目前，常见的原因是继发于神经外科手术后的感染以及颅骨骨折和开放性伤口的头外伤。硬膜外脓肿的细菌学和发病机制与硬膜下积脓相似，但由于硬脑膜与颅骨的紧密粘连，它的边界很明显，进展速度较慢，病程也不长。因此，它起病隐匿，发热或头痛可能是唯一的临床表现。在某些情况下，症状可能需要数周时间才出现。然而，如果不加以治疗，感染可能会扩大和发展，导致颅骨骨髓炎、硬膜静脉窦血栓、化脓性脑膜炎、硬膜下积脓和脑脓肿等并发症（Pradilla et al.，2009）。增强CT和MRI显示出扁豆状的增强灶和增厚的硬膜表面，能够可靠地区分硬膜外脓肿和无菌性硬膜外积液。此外，CT还可显示患者潜在的颅骨骨髓炎或乳突炎以及骨质破坏和碎裂。有趣的是，DWI可成为区分硬膜下和硬膜外积脓的辅助手段。硬膜下积脓在DWI上呈高信号，而硬膜外积脓往往是低信号或混合信号强度（Tsuchiya et al.，2003）。颅内硬膜外脓肿的主要治疗和管理与硬膜下积脓相似。脓液可以通过钻孔或开颅手术进行充分引流。极少数情况下，如有严重的潜在骨髓炎，则需要切除颅骨（Tsai et al.，2003）。

颅骨骨髓炎

颅骨骨髓炎通常是由耳源性或牙源性感染的扩散、头部创伤的开放性伤口或涉及头皮或颅骨的手术引起的。患者表现为发热和与病因有关的症状。前额头皮肿胀见于额骨骨髓炎，是由于骨膜下脓肿的形成，1760年Percivall Pott爵士首次将其描述为Pott浮肿（Kombogiorgas and Solanki，2006）。Gradenigo-Lannois综合征是一种罕见的骨髓炎并发症，涉及颞骨岩部顶端，患者表现为三联征，包括因展神经麻痹导致的复视，与三叉神经受累有关的同侧口周或面部疼痛，以及与中耳炎有关的持续耳鸣（Heshin-Bekenstein et al.，2014）。面神经或后组脑神经麻痹可能见于假单胞菌感染引起的颅底骨髓炎所致的恶性外耳道炎。曲霉菌感染也被证明可以引起颅底骨髓炎而无任何外耳道炎的证据（Pincus et al.，2009）。颅骨骨髓炎的进展和扩展可能导致硬膜外脓肿、硬膜下积脓或脑脓肿（Johnson and Batra，2014）。由毛霉病引起的前颅底骨髓炎在世界许多地方都能见到，特别是在免疫力低下的患者身上。颅骨骨髓炎的细菌学取决于感染的部位和潜在原因。MRI是影像诊断的首选方式，可检测到板障或松质骨的变化，并可提供详细的颅底、脑神经和软组织情况。此外，白细胞增多和红细胞沉降率（erythrocyte sedimentation rate，ESR）升高也有助于诊断（Chang et al.，2003）。颅骨骨髓炎的治疗包括手术清创和活检或切除受感染的骨瓣，然后针对病原体进行长期抗菌药物治疗。根除主要感染源对确保治疗成功和减少复发风险同样重要（Pincus et al.，2009）。此外，高压氧治疗作为一种辅助治疗手段，在处理慢性难治性颅底骨髓炎方面可能有一定的作用。高压氧治疗被认为是这些病例的一种选择，因为它能增强吞噬细胞对需氧微生物的氧化杀伤，并促进血管生成和骨质生成（Prasad et al.，2014）。动态监测ESR或CRP是临床有意义的指标。使用镓-67骨扫描进行影像学随访也可用于确定颅底骨髓炎从活动至非活动的变化（Chang et al.，2003）。如果诊断和治疗得当，其预后通常良好。

脑膜炎、脑室炎和脑室腹腔分流感染

术后脑膜炎是神经外科手术的一种风险，在这类手术中硬膜会破损，报道中的比率在0.14%~9.2%。患者通常表现为头痛、发热、颈僵、精神状态改变，偶尔也有恶心和呕吐。如果患者的症状（如头痛）被归结为术后疼痛，而发热症状被退热药物掩盖，则可能延误诊断。然而，术后脑膜炎的临床过程不像社区获得性脑膜炎那样剧烈，死亡率也不高（Srinivas et al.，2011）。

脑膜炎的诊断通常需要CSF取样和分析，通常通过腰椎穿刺来实现。细菌性脑膜炎的CSF检查显示CSF总蛋白升高，CSF葡萄糖低或正常，CSF白细胞计数升高，并以中性粒细胞为主。术后脑膜炎中涉及革兰氏阴性菌的概率较高。在发达国家，最常见的致病菌是金黄色葡萄球菌。然而，也有地域差异，如在印度的一个病例系列中，最常见的微生物是革兰氏阴性杆菌、铜绿假单胞菌和克雷伯菌（Kourbeti et al.，2007；Dashti et al.，2008）。

术后脑膜炎需要适当的静脉或口服抗菌药物治疗。在第一种情况下，经验性抗菌药物通常包括万古霉素和第三代头孢类药物。如果CSF取样可对致病菌进行培养和药敏试验，则应相应地调整抗菌药物治疗。

脑室炎仍然是神经外科使用脑室外引流管进行临时CSF引流后常见的问题。还有一小部分患者是由于脑脓肿破裂进入脑室而发生脑室炎。在这种情况下，较大的细菌量会导致预后不良。

现代神经外科实践中推荐使用带有抗菌药物涂层或银离子的脑室导管以减少脑室炎的发生（Keong et al.，2012；Athanasios et al.，2015）。

降低EVD感染发生率相关的因素包括标准化的植入流程、较长的皮下隧道（>15 cm）、医疗和护理人员尽可能少的操作、CSF采样时的无菌技术以及较低的CSF采样频率（Lwin et al.，2012；Kubilay et al.，2013）。常规CSF采样已被证明不是早期发现CSF感染的必要条件（Hader and Steinbok，2000）。

脑室腹腔分流（VP分流）感染可被分为早期（6个月内）或晚期（超过6个月）感染。患者通常表现出非特异性症状，如发热、恶心和呕吐、烦躁以及精神状态改变。VP分流管感染也可能表现为分流管功能异常。VP分流感染最常见的病原体是皮肤菌群，如表皮葡萄球菌和金黄色葡萄球菌。

治疗的原则是取出被感染的分流管，同时使用全身抗菌药物和临时的CSF外引流，如脑室外引流、腰大池引流或腰椎穿刺。抗菌药物应持续使用至CSF指标恢复正常，以便随后植入新的脑室腹腔分流管。单纯使用抗菌药物的治疗效果较差（James et al.，1980；Tamber et al.，2014）。

脑膜炎和脑炎患者的颅内压监测和去骨瓣减压术

脑膜炎和脑炎患者的颅内压监测方面尚无明确的指南。然而，脑膜炎和脑炎可导致严重的脑水肿和皮质假性层状坏死，从而导致ICP升高以及脑疝（图98.5）。最近，瑞典的一项研究比较了急性细菌性脑膜炎患者的ICP干预组与对照组，显示干预组的死亡率明显下降（相对风险降低68%）；ICP干预组的神经系统恢复情况也更好（Sala et al.，2009；Glimåker et al.，2014）。另一例报道中，结核性脑膜炎导致了严重脑水肿，在ICP监测和采取ICP控制措施后反应良好，患者随后的神经系统恢复良好（Trendelenberg et al.，2011）。

脑炎患者中去骨瓣减压术并不常见，在药物治疗无效的情况下可以考虑抢救性应用。有研究表明，接受颅骨切除术的单纯疱疹性脑炎患者的长期神经系统预后与不需要颅骨切除术的患者没有明显区别（Youenn et al.，2015；Algahtani et al.，2016）。

神经外科的术后感染

CDC对术后手术部位感染（surgical site infection，SSI）进行了严格定义。SSI分为浅表切口SSI、深部切口SSI和器官/间隙SSI。

开颅手术后的SSI是神经外科术后患者发病和死亡的一个重要原因。神经外科术后SSI的发生率在3%~5%。开颅手术后的SSI范围很广，从单纯的伤口开裂和破裂，到头皮下感染的积聚，到颅骨瓣骨髓炎，再到硬膜下积脓或颅内脓肿。每种情况的处理都在相关部分中进行了阐述。

有几个危险因素与开颅术后SSI的风险增加有关。这些因素包括多次手术、脑脊液漏、手术时间延长、感觉改变、存在糖尿病等并发症以及同时使用皮质类固醇（Jiang et al.，2016）。马来西亚的一项研究显示，围术期ASA 2级的患者和清洁污染的伤口是发生SSI的重要危险因素（Buang and Haspani，2012）。在开颅手术后SSI中发现的主要细菌是金黄色葡萄球菌，其次是痤疮杆菌和肠杆菌（Buang and Haspani，2012）。

学界对预防SSI提出了许多建议，关于这些建议的详尽讨论可在WHO网站上查阅预防手术部位感染全球指南2016（http://www.who.int/gpsc/ssi-prevention-guidelines/en/）。预防性抗菌药物被广泛认作一种关键的预防措施。这需要选择合适的抗菌药物，在术前1小时内给药，并在术后24小时内停药。其他措施包括小心处理软组织、良好的止血以及伤口闭合。有人提出使用聚维酮碘冲洗可以降低开颅术后SSI的风险（Patel et al.，2014）。

头皮浅表感染是最常见的SSI形式。典型的表

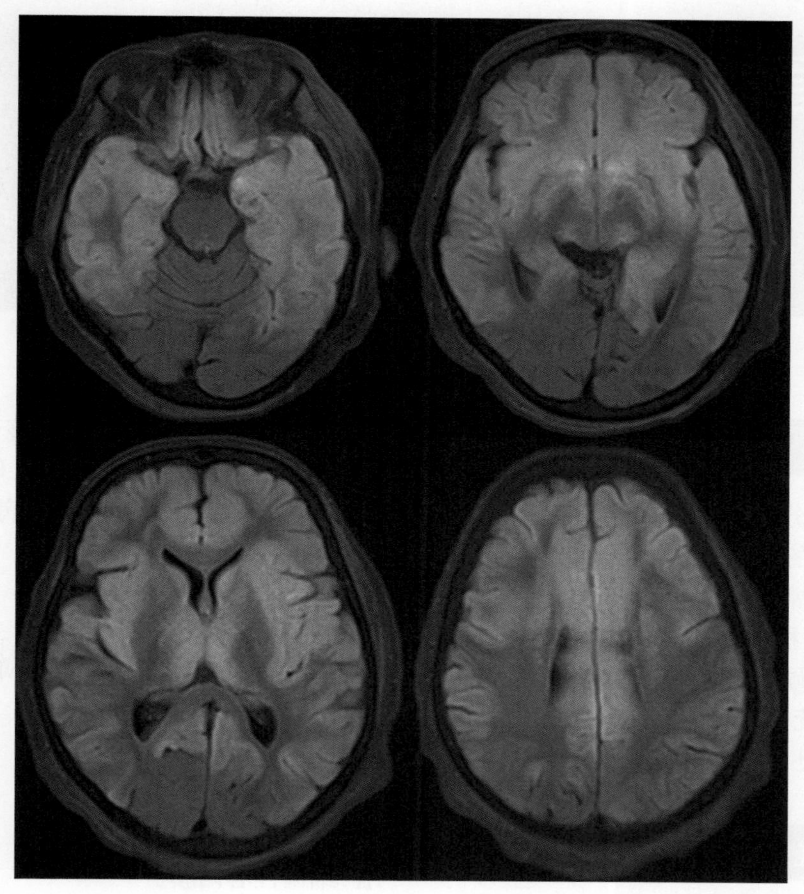

图 98.5　单纯疱疹病毒（herpes simplex virus，HSV）脑炎的 MR 图像显示额颞叶和基底神经节广泛受累，导致严重的脑水肿和假性层状坏死（Algahtani et al.，2016）

现包括局部红斑、肿胀和触痛，随着时间的推移，会发展成破溃伤口并形成脓液。一般来说全身症状，如发热、疲倦和嗜睡，属于晚期表现。颈僵、精神状态改变或出现新的局灶性功能缺失等症状则需要进行检查，以确保浅表感染没有扩展至深层结构，如硬膜下积脓或脑膜炎。在简单的病例中，其治疗主要是使用抗菌药物，尤其是能良好覆盖革兰氏阳性菌的抗菌药物。如果有广泛的感染或存在潜在的头皮下积液，可能需要对皮瓣进行手术清创。

延伸阅读、参考文献、EBRAIN 的相关链接

扫描书末二维码获取。

第 99 章　脊柱感染

Nicholas Haden・Edward White 著
文俊贤 译，魏俊吉 审校

引言

脊柱脊髓感染十分罕见，但其发病率正在逐步上升，并且具有很高的死亡率。由于其罕见和非特异性的临床表现，常常会导致诊断和开始治疗时间的延迟。高度警惕并积极治疗对脊柱感染患者的预后至关重要。本章对硬膜外脓肿、椎旁脓肿、椎间盘炎和椎体骨髓炎（统称为脊椎及椎间盘炎）以及术后脊柱感染进行了综述。

脊髓硬膜外及椎旁脓肿

脊髓硬膜外脓肿（spinal epidural abscess，SEA）是硬膜外间隙内的化脓性感染。鉴于 SEA 具有罕见、非特异性的临床表现以及其具有迅速进展为不可逆性瘫痪和严重脓毒症的可能性，临床很容易导致误诊。

流行病学

SEA 十分罕见，发病率约为 1.96 例 /10000 人。SEA 患者的平均年龄约为 57.5 岁，男性的发病率略高于女性（Reihsaus et al.，2000）。随着磁共振成像技术的进步、人口老龄化进展、HIV 发病率的上升以及静脉注射毒品的使用，这种疾病的发病率正在增加。

病理生理学

SEA 常出现在硬膜外间隙内脂肪较多的位置（如硬脊膜的背侧和外侧），此处血管分布少，这可能是其较容易受细菌侵染的原因之一。然而导致继发性脊髓功能障碍的病理生理机制目前尚不清楚。机械性压迫脊髓和血管损伤的综合作用可能是原因之一，长时间的脊髓压迫可能会导致不可逆转的脊髓缺血。

前位 SEA 十分罕见，其常继发于脊椎及椎间盘炎。SEA 最常见的发生部位是胸椎，其次是腰椎和颈椎，一般来说，SEA 只会蔓延至几个椎体的长度。细菌主要通过三种途径进入硬脊膜外腔，但仍有 30% 的病例我们无法确定其病原体来源（Darouiche et al.，1992）：

血源性

约 50% 的病例是血源性播散。潜在的原发灶包括：

ⅰ. 皮肤感染（最为常见）
ⅱ. 静脉注射毒品
ⅲ. 感染的血管通路
ⅳ. 细菌性心内膜炎
ⅴ. 尿路感染
ⅵ. 呼吸道感染
ⅶ. 咽部或口腔脓肿

直接蔓延

感染直接延伸至硬膜外腔的病例约占总体病例的 1/3。潜在的原发灶包括：

ⅰ. 脊椎及椎间盘炎
ⅱ. 腰大肌脓肿
ⅲ. 褥疮
ⅳ. 咽部感染导致颈椎 SEA
ⅴ. 纵隔炎导致胸椎 SEA
ⅵ. 穿透性损伤
ⅶ. 肾盂肾炎伴肾周脓肿

术中感染

ⅰ. 开放性手术

危险因素

与其他感染疾病一样，SEA 常见于患有糖尿病、免疫抑制、恶性肿瘤、HIV、酒精中毒和慢性肾衰竭的患者以及有静脉注射毒品的患者。少数患者有创伤史，后者成为细菌进入硬膜外腔的诱因。

临床表现

75% 的患者有明显的诊断延迟，只有少数患者（13%）在疾病早期表现为典型的背痛、发热和神经功能缺陷症状（Davis et al.，2004）。一项含有 915 名患者的 meta 分析中显示，背痛是与 SEA 相关的最常见症状（71%），其次是发热（66%）和神经功能缺陷（63%）。较不常见的临床症状和体征包括神经根病（20%）、局灶性压痛（17%）、头痛（3%）和颈部僵硬（3%）。而且术后 SEA 表现不明确，发热和神经功能障碍症状不常见（Reihsaus et al.，2000）。鉴于其可能迅速导致不可逆的瘫痪，需要对其高度警惕。

检验检查

实验室检查

患者的炎症指标，包括白细胞计数、血沉（erythrocyte sedimentation rate，ESR）和 C 反应蛋白（C-reactive protein，CRP）通常会升高。60%~80% 的患者会出现白细胞增多，而且一项纳入 25 例 SEA 患者的研究显示，患者的 CRP 平均值为 150 mg/L（Soehle and Wallenfang，2002）。

影像学检查

MRI 是首选的诊断性检查，因为它能将 SEA 与横贯性脊髓炎、脊髓缺血、脊柱脊髓肿瘤、椎间盘脱出、骨髓炎、椎间盘炎等疾病作出很好的鉴别（图 99.1）。对于合并 MRI 检查禁忌的患者，可以选择增强 CT 和 CT 脊髓造影。但它们的敏感性及特异性都较低。

微生物学检查

SEA 患者管理的关键在于对致病微生物的及时识别。对于无需手术的患者，我们可以通过引流及经 CT 引导下病灶穿刺获得脓肿样本。90% 的病例脓液微生物培养都呈阳性，而血培养阳性率只有大约 60%。最常见的病原菌是金黄色葡萄球菌（60%），其次是革兰氏阴性杆菌（包括大肠杆菌、铜绿假单胞菌和克雷伯菌）。10% 的病例会合并多重微生物感染（Sendi et al.，2008）。在取样前使用抗生素常常会导致微生物培养阳性率降低，所以在临床实践中，如果脓液标本获得较晚，则需要在识别致病微生物及防止患者病情恶化二者之间作出仔细权衡。

治疗

因为 SEA 的罕见性以及保守治疗会带来诸多潜在不良结果，使得随机对照试验变得不切实际，相关证据只能从几个病例队列研究中获得。治疗方法一般是手术引流加上针对性使用抗生素，或者根据药敏结果进行单纯抗生素治疗。保守治疗的主要困难在于即使接受了恰当的抗生素治疗也可能导致患者神经系统的快速恶化。

手术禁忌证包括：

ⅰ. 存在手术及麻醉禁忌

ⅱ. 存在广泛的脊髓受累

ⅲ. 完全瘫痪超过 48 小时

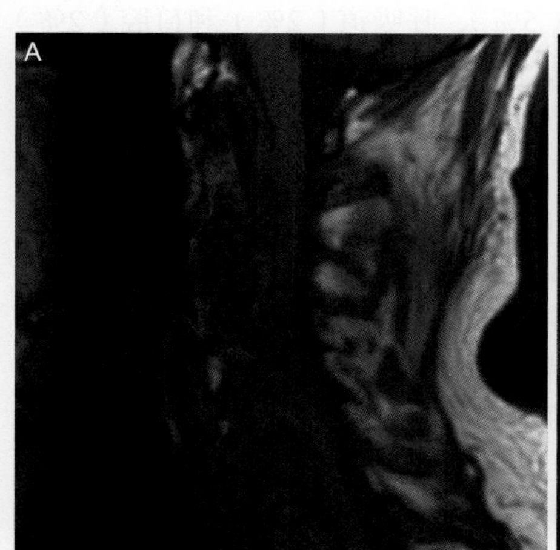

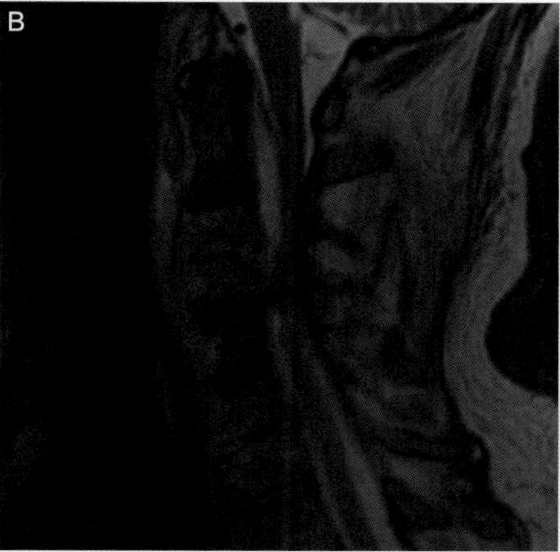

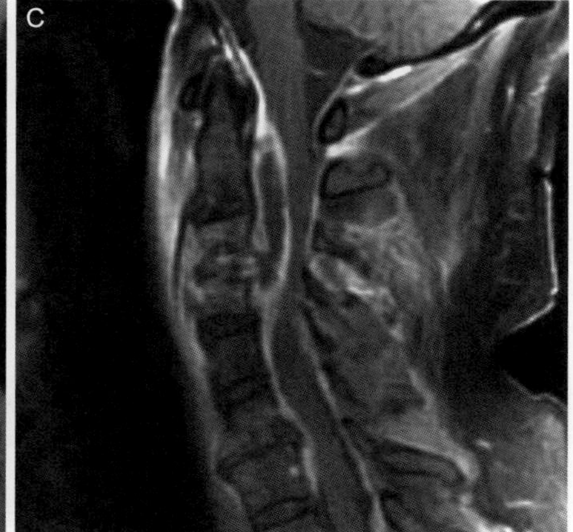

图 99.1　硬脊膜外脓肿的 MR 表现。颈椎 MRI 矢状面表现为 SEA 的特征性表现。在 T1 加权成像中（A），SEA 可表现为低或等信号，而在 T2 加权成像中（B），SEA 表现为高信号。常表现为均匀强化、不均匀强化、边缘强化三种强化形式（见图 C）。但是在急性期，聚集物常以脓为主，无肉芽组织，很少见到强化，预后不良的 MRI 预测表现为：椎管狭窄超过 50%；边缘增强；脊髓内信号改变；SEA 长度大于 3 cm（Tang et al.，2002）

ⅳ. 患者神经系统完好

如果不进行手术减压，应在 CT 引导下进行脓肿抽吸以确定致病微生物，并进行密切观察，以确保不会发生迅速的神经功能恶化，保守治疗失败的预测因素包括：

ⅰ. 年龄大于 65 岁

ⅱ. 糖尿病

ⅲ. 合并菌血症（特别是耐甲氧西林金黄色葡萄球菌，MRSA）

ⅳ. 神经损伤

ⅴ. 白细胞数量大于 12.5×10^9

ⅵ. CRP 超过 115（Kim et al.，2014）

手术干预的目的是清创肉芽组织和排出脓液，以减轻脊髓压迫和获得样本进行病原学分析。由于大多数 SEA 发生在后部，对于大多数病例，椎板切除术或使用椎板开孔术并用导管冲洗硬膜外间隙是适合的。如果 SEA 与脊髓植入物有关，则必须将植入物移除。对于范围广泛及位于前位的 SEA 来说，锥体内可能存在骨髓炎。在这些病例中，行椎板切除术后可能发生脊柱不稳定，应考虑使用经后路内固定融合术和（或）腔外入路，使用可扩张的笼式支架或植骨重建椎体。

经典的抗生素治疗方案包括使用三代头孢和万古霉素，直至除外 MRSA。一旦得到培养药敏结果，随后的抗生素治疗就因根据药敏结果进行修改。初次治疗时一般选择使用静脉注射，疗程通常至少需要 6~8 周。在脊椎及椎间盘炎或免疫抑制存在的情况下，可能需要长期治疗。

预后

自发性 SEA 的死亡率为 16%，瘫痪率为 15%，遗留神经功能缺损（不包括瘫痪）率为 26%，完全康复率为 43%（Reihsaus et al.，2000）。死亡通常是由于瘫痪的并发症或感染源所致。不良预后的标志包括手术前长时间、严重的神经功能缺损、MRSA 感染、类固醇使用、HIV 感染、血小板减少、颈椎 SEA、糖尿病、类风湿性关节炎和年龄超过 50 岁。

脊椎及椎间盘炎

椎间盘（椎间盘炎）和椎体骨髓炎之间有明显的重叠部分。这些疾病通常被称为脊椎及椎间盘炎。脊椎及椎间盘炎常与 SEA 共存。90% 的颈椎的脊椎及椎间盘炎伴有 SEA，而胸椎和腰椎部位合并 SEA 的比例分别为 33% 和 24%（Hadjipavlou et al.，2000）。

脊椎及椎间盘炎可分为化脓性、肉芽肿性（结核和真菌感染）或寄生虫性。化脓性椎间盘炎可进一步分为原发性和继发性（术后）。脊椎及椎间盘炎最常累及腰椎（58%），其次是胸椎（30%），然后是颈椎（11%）（Mylona et al.，2009）。

流行病学

据报道，脊椎及椎间盘炎的年发病率为 2.4/10 万，有证据表明发病率正在逐步上升，其原因可能是人口老龄化、脊柱内固定物的使用增加和静脉药物滥用。病例主要呈双峰分布，在 11~20 岁达到一个高峰，在 60 岁之后达到会更高的高峰。在年龄较大的病例群中，男性感染者大约是女性的两倍（Skaf et al.，2010）。

病理生理学

细菌可以通过血行途径、术中播种或从邻近感染部位直接蔓延来感染脊柱。在儿童时期，广泛的血管吻合网络通常会延伸到椎间盘。因此，感染性栓子通常局限于椎间盘，不太可能引起骨梗死。在 20~30 岁，血管吻合网络会逐步减少，并形成末端动脉，这使得感染性栓子可能引起骨梗死，感染累及椎间盘及临近骨质，并可能发展为病理性骨折和显著畸形。

鉴于脊柱后部血液供应相对较差，化脓性骨髓炎通常不会影响椎板、椎弓根、横突和棘突，累及这些结构大多是真菌性骨髓炎或结核性骨髓炎。

大约一半的脊椎及椎间盘炎病例可以发现远处的感染病灶。来源包括尿道（17%）、细菌性心内膜炎（12%）、皮肤和软组织（11%）、血管腔内装置（5%）、胃肠道（5%）、呼吸道（2%）和口腔（2%）（Gouliouris et al.，2010）。直接蔓延约占总体病例的 30%，最常发生在脊柱手术、腰椎穿刺和硬膜外麻醉后。

在世界范围内，结核是脊柱感染（Pott 病）最常见的病因，是因结核分枝杆菌从主要病灶血行播散引起的。除了结核，金黄色葡萄球菌是导致脊椎及椎间盘炎第二常见的病因，占 32%~67%。耐甲氧西林金黄色葡萄球菌（MRSA）脊椎及椎间盘炎目前仍然极为罕见。化脓性脊椎及椎间盘炎的第二大常见病原体是肠杆菌科（最常见的是大肠杆菌），占 7%~33%（Gouliouris et al.，2010）。链球菌和肠球菌占脊椎及椎间盘炎病例的 5%~20%，经常与细菌性心内膜炎相关（Mylona et al.，2009）。

危险因素

大多数脊椎及椎间盘炎患者至少有以下一种危险因素（Mylona et al.，2009）：

ⅰ. 糖尿病（24%）

ⅱ. 静脉药物滥用（11%）

ⅲ. 免疫抑制（7%）

ⅳ. 恶性肿瘤（6%）

ⅴ. 酒精中毒（5%）

ⅵ. 风湿病（5%）

ⅶ. 肝硬化（4%）

ⅷ. 肾功能衰竭（4%）

ⅸ. 既往放疗或脊椎骨折史

临床表现

疼痛是脊椎及椎间盘炎最常见的症状，90% 以上的患者都有这种症状。背痛通常是持续的，并在晚上及运动时加重。大约 50% 的患者会发热，但结核病患者不常发热。大约 1/3 的患者会出现神经功能缺损和神经根病（Mylona et al.，2009）。患者的临床表现通常是隐匿且非特异性的，特别是在非典型感染病例中，并且由于脊椎及椎间盘炎的罕见性和背痛频率不频繁，常常导致诊断延迟。在结核病病例中，这种诊断延迟时间通常较长，因为结核病起病隐匿，但在其晚期可导致硬膜外和椎旁积脓、神经功能缺损和严重畸形。

脊椎及椎间盘炎最常见的体征是脊柱压痛，并可能伴有椎旁肌肉痉挛和脊柱运动受限。罕见的表现包括伴疼痛的凸骨畸形、腰肌或咽后脓肿表现，窦道形成，甚至脊柱占位。儿童患者的临床表现包括易激惹、拒绝活动和腹痛（Gouliouris et al.，2010）。

检验检查

实验室检查

35% 的病例会合并白细胞计数升高，但老年人和合并免疫功能低下的患者通常正常。CRP 这项指标更为敏感，在超过 90% 的病例中升高。大约 70% 的患者合并贫血，50% 的患者血清碱性磷酸酶会升高（Gouliouris et al.，2010）。

微生物学检查

在疑似脊椎及椎间盘炎的病例中，除了从受累椎间盘或椎体采集标本外，还应进行血液和尿液培养。约 50% 的病例血培养呈阳性，85% 的培养结果与椎间盘或椎体病灶处取到的培养结果一致。具有较多毒性微生物以及发热的患者培养阳性率会更高。CT 引导下直接从感染椎间盘或者锥体处取得病灶，其诊断阳性率约 70%，24% 的病例能培养出一种以上的微生物（Hadjipavlou et al.，2000）。组织革兰氏染色，有氧和厌氧培养、真菌和结核培养以及结核病 PCR 检查都是必需的。组织学检查也有助于区分肉芽肿和化脓性脊椎及椎间盘炎，并排除潜在的肿瘤。

影像学检查

X 线平片常表现为终板不规则或终板侵蚀、椎间盘间隙狭窄、锥体高度减少并且逐渐畸形。这些变化在症状出现后 3~6 周开始出现。反应性骨硬化常在 8~12 周开始出现，并可能发展为大量骨赘形成和自发融合。然而，X 线平片的敏感性和特异性仍然很低，分别为 82% 和 57%（Modic et al.，1985）。CT 能更早地显示这些变化，在进行微生物学和组织学分析的活检时也十分有用。

MRI 是一项具有高灵敏度（96%）和高特异性（92%）的影像学检查，能够区分硬膜外和椎旁积脓（Dagirmanjian et al.，1999）（**图** 99.2 和**图** 99.3）。

锝 -99m 放射性核素骨扫描在感染的头几天高度敏感（90%），但特异性较低（78%），合并退行性病变时会导致假阳性。在鉴别困难的情况下，氟 -18 脱氧葡萄糖正电子发射断层扫描（FDG-PET）是一个非常有用的辅助手段，因为它能够区分感染和退行性变。

常规 MRI 在监测治疗反应方面的价值不太确定。好转的影像学标志包括骨质修复和不再增强。然而，这些改变往往出现较晚，并且在治疗开始后 4~8 周内的 MRI 扫描往往显示为增强信号和骨髓水肿的增加。

治疗

治疗的关键因素包括根除感染、减轻疼痛、保留脊柱结构和功能。在获得适当的组织样本后应立即开始抗生素治疗，即使在出现严重脓毒症或中性粒细胞减少症时，也应立即开始经验性抗生素治疗。一旦发现病原体，就应给予相应的静脉抗生素。

在一项开放标签、非劣效性、随机对照试验中，Bernard 等（2015）发现在 1 年随访结果中，6 周的抗生素治疗疗效（大约前 14 天静脉给药）不劣于 12 周的抗生素治疗。脊柱结核需要长期的抗结核治疗以及鉴定结核分枝杆菌耐药菌株。

脊柱固定的作用目前不太确定。如果有明显的椎

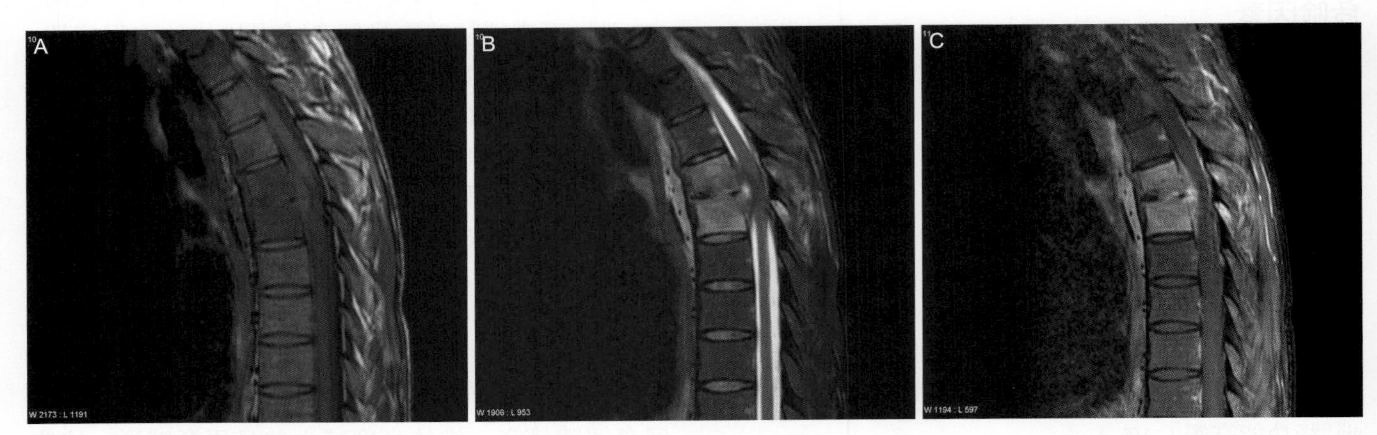

图 99.2 脊椎及椎间盘炎的 MR 成像。胸椎矢状面 MRI 能显示典型特征。最初的 MR 异常是由于椎体和椎间盘间隙的炎症和水肿。特征表现是 T1 加权序列上的骨髓低信号（A）。短 tau 反转恢复序列和 T2 加权序列上，可见骨髓和椎间盘间隙的高信号（B）。强化最初发生在终板 - 椎间盘界面，并随着骨质破坏的进展进入椎体（C）。这种增强提高了 MRI 的诊断价值，有助于区分感染和退行性病变

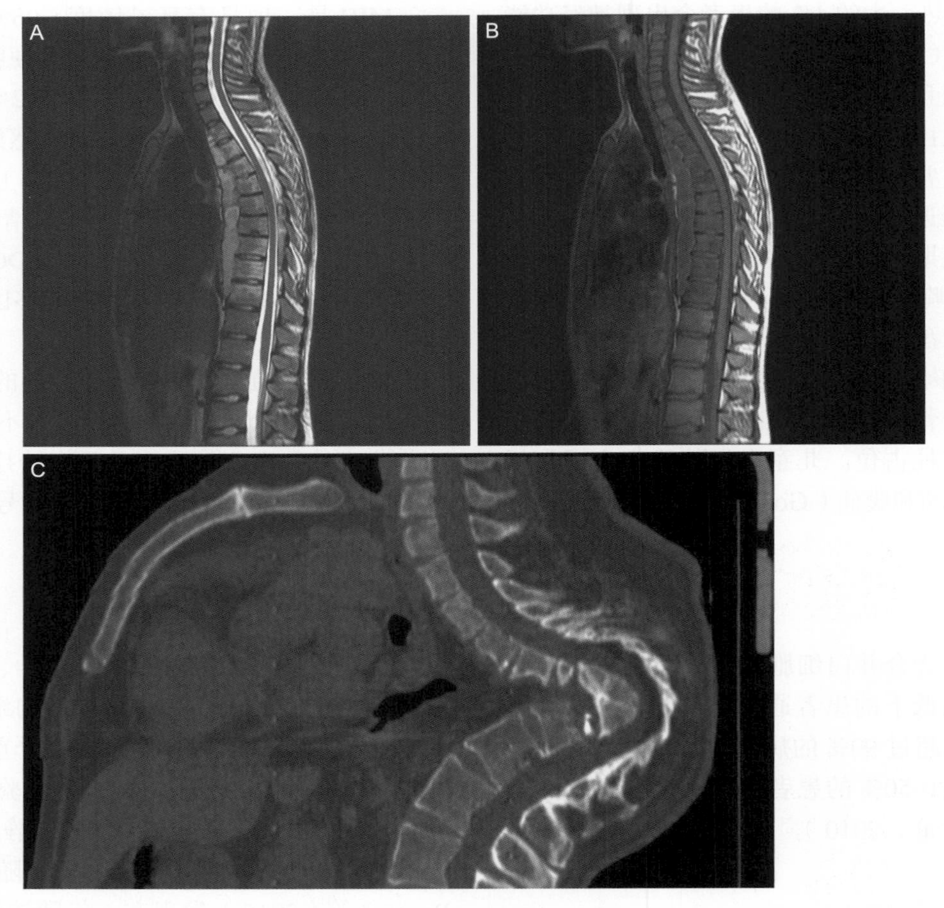

图 99.3 脊柱结核影像学表现。矢状位 T2 序列（A）和 T1 加权序列（B）MR 图像和矢状位 CT 扫描（C）能显示出脊柱结核的典型特征表现。通常情况下，脊柱结核累及椎体，而不影响后部，但涉及多个层面的感染会在韧带下传播，在前纵韧带下扩散，并且可能导致椎前脓肿（A，B）。因此，椎体前部不规则信号是早期影像学特征。并且可以进展为畸形（C）和椎旁大量积脓

体破坏，建议卧床休息。对于颈椎病灶，应当使用硬颈托。一旦疼痛缓解，胸椎或腰椎患者应使用胸腰骶矫形支具（thoracolumbar sacral orthosis，TLSO）或腰骶矫形支具（lumbar sacral orthosis，LSO）。

手术干预的指征包括：以进行性畸形或大量骨质丢失为特征的脊柱不稳定；由于神经压迫导致的严重神经功能障碍；保守治疗无效和顽固性疼痛。对于较大的椎旁脓肿，经皮引流通常优于手术引流。

多种外科技术可用于脊椎及椎间盘炎的治疗。在存在背侧 SEA 的情况下，可行椎板切除术，不过由于该病有累及椎体和椎间盘的倾向，可能会导致术后脊柱不稳定。对于颈椎病变，经前入路有利于清除感染骨质。多节段椎体切除术可辅以后路内固定。对于胸椎病变，胸廓可以起到保持稳定性的作用，因此使用适当的矫形器即可，可能不需要手术稳定。然而，如果需要减压和清创，则可能需要经胸或后外侧入路，并辅以经后路稳定手术。

结构完整性可以通过多种技术来维持，包括使用自体骨移植和钛网，自体移植，如肋骨和腓骨，以及同种异体移植。一部分学者担忧在感染病灶中植入内固定物的继发感染问题，但相关文献并未发现此类病例。

预后

脊椎及椎间盘炎的死亡率约为 5%，通常是由于继发严重的脓毒血症所致（Gouliouris et al.，2010）。大约 1/3 的患者会合并神经功能缺损。据报道，疾病复发率为 14%，而且多数在一年内复发。复发更常见于反复出现的菌血症、慢性鼻窦炎和椎旁脓肿。导致不良预后的危险因素包括延迟诊断 2 个月以上、运动无力以及院内感染（McHenry et al.，2002）。

术后伤口感染

据报道，脊柱手术后发生的术后手术部位感染（surgical site infection，SSI）在接受脊柱减压手术的患者中占 1.2%，在接受脊柱融合手术的患者中占 2.4%。在创伤性脊柱损伤的患者中，这一比例甚至更高，据报道，创伤性脊柱损伤的感染率高达 10%，这可能是由于长期卧床休息、暴露于院内感染环境和损伤后代谢状态改变综合所致（Hegde et al.，2012）。

危险因素

术后脊柱感染的危险因素见**专栏** 99.1。

病理生理学

导致 SSI 发生的原因可能是微生物，也可能与患者或手术过程有关。最常见的病原体是金黄色葡萄球菌，其他常见的病原体包括表皮葡萄球菌、粪肠球菌和铜绿假单胞菌（Weinstein et al.，2000）。尽管血行播散也可能发生，但最常见的是微生物在手术中进入伤口。预防 SSI 的关键因素是规范无菌操作和预防性使用抗生素。

许多患者的个人因素被证明与感染相关，增加 SSI 风险的术中因素包括手术时间，内固定物植入、翻修手术、手术室人员过多以及手术显微镜的使用（Hegde et al.，2012）。最大限度降低感染风险的方法包括避免过度使用电灼、定期松开牵开器、手术结束时清理伤口、使用抗生素冲洗伤口和封闭式负压引流管。

临床表现

感染的典型临床表现包括背部疼痛、伤口压痛、红斑和分泌物形成。严重的感染可能导致发热、低血压和精神错乱。来自如痤疮丙酸杆菌这样惰性的病原体感染，可引起较模糊的疼痛症状，比如假关节病和假体松动。临床表现也可以提示并发脊椎及

专栏 99.1 术后脊柱感染的危险因素

术前

1 高龄
2 肥胖
3 糖尿病
4 吸烟
5 既往化疗或放疗史
6 术前尿失禁
7 术前瘫痪
8 ASA 3 或 4 级
9 脊柱创伤

术中

1 颈椎后路手术
2 多节段手术
3 肿瘤切除
4 术中输血

术后

1 尿失禁
2 输血
3 使用类固醇

Source data from Olsen et al., 2003. http://thejns.org/doi/abs/10.3171/spi.2003. 98.2.0149

椎间盘炎或与 SEA 相关的神经功能障碍。

检验检查

实验室检查

CRP 测量是评估疑似 SSI 患者的关键。因为通常 CRP 在手术后两周内就会恢复正常。患者白细胞计数通常是正常的，而且由于皮肤可能有菌群污染，从浅表部位培养病原体不能明确诊断。因此，术中取组织培养对于诊断和指导抗生素治疗非常重要（Hegde et al.，2012）。如进行脊柱翻修手术，建议术中培养以排除低级别感染。

影像学检查

CT 可表现为植入物松动、器械周围透亮和椎间盘炎。对比增强 MRI 是诊断 SSI 和并发脊椎及椎间盘炎或 SEA 的首选成像方式。然而，由于金属伪影的存在和椎间盘切除术后正常改变（包括椎间盘间隙和椎间盘环内细微的强化，终板在 T1 加权序列上呈低信号，T2 加权序列上呈高信号），使得解读术后 MR 成像具有挑战性。脊椎及椎间盘炎往往会使椎间盘呈明亮的环状强化。骨扫描一般没有帮助，因为在术后一年内都会显示为反应性骨生成部位的摄取增加。

治疗

浅表脓肿可通过切开、引流、伤口清创和抗生素处理。先前讨论过外科引流 SEA 的指征。CT 引导下抽吸可治疗椎旁脓肿。感染毒性菌种或合并免疫缺陷的患者可能需要多次伤口冲洗。

对于合并感染的锥体融合手术患者，必须进行大量冲洗、并取下松动的植骨和金属植入物。使用椎间笼和经后路内固定一般可以控制感染（Weinstein et al.，2000）。当需要对多个伤口进行冲洗时，一些学者主张将抗生素珠植入伤口（Hegde et al.，2012）。对于已经融合合并晚期感染的患者，取出内固定物有利于控制感染。

单纯的术后椎间盘炎通过一个疗程的静脉抗生素便能得到有效的治疗。CT 引导下的椎间盘间隙活检获得的培养有很高的诊断效率。支具可以提高患者的舒适度。感染的消退通常与椎间盘间隙的自发融合有关。在少见的保守治疗失败的情况下，合并椎体破坏、进行性畸形、神经功能缺损或 SEA 时则需要进行腰椎间盘切除术和椎间融合术或椎体重建术。

争议：抗生素在椎间盘源性背痛中的作用

越来越多的证据表明椎间盘症状性退变、MRI 的轻度变化与低毒力厌氧病原体（如痤疮丙酸杆菌和丙棒状杆菌）导致的椎间盘间隙感染之间存在联系（Stirling et al.，2001）。但这些研究是有争议的，因为在这些研究中获得的阳性培养来源可能是围术期皮肤共生物污染。然而，一项双盲、随机、安慰剂对照试验（n=162）显示在通过阿莫西林根除这些病原体后，有腰椎间盘突出病史和 MRI1 型 Modic 改变的患者的腰痛和腿痛症状会得到显著的改善（Albert et al.，2013）。

关于该试验结果的有效性仍然存在很多争议。比如因腰椎间盘突出症而接受手术治疗的患者的数量和在各个治疗组之间的分布情况尚不清楚。有可能一部分患者在手术过程中发生了椎间盘间隙细菌污染，导致低度椎间盘炎，这可能导致随后患者对抗生素有反应。在 1 年的随访过程中，治疗组中有 2/3 的患者仍然有明显的疼痛感，使用安慰剂治疗的患者疼痛程度异常稳定，安慰剂疗效非常有限。最后，尚不清楚患者对其治疗方案是否知情。

总之，需要进一步研究来评估椎间盘低级别感染与影像学 Modic 改变和有症状的椎间盘退变之间是否存在联系。具体来说，需要一项设计合理的多中心、安慰剂对照、随机试验来确定抗生素治疗在这些患者中是否有作用。

延伸阅读、参考文献、EBRAIN 的相关链接

扫描书末二维码获取。

延伸阅读、参考文献、EBRAIN 的相关链接